This book is due for return on or before the last date shown below.

Fanaroff and Martin's Neonatal-Perinatal Medicine

Fanaroff and Martin's Neonatal-Perinatal Medicine

Diseases of the Fetus and Infant

9th EDITION

Richard J. Martin, MBBS, FRACP

Professor, Pediatrics, Reproductive Biology, and Physiology and Biophysics
Case Western Reserve University School of Medicine
Drusinsky/Fanaroff Chair in Neonatology
Director, Division of Neonatology
Rainbow Babies and Children's Hospital
Cleveland, Ohio

Avroy A. Fanaroff, MD, FRCP [E], FRCPCH

Professor, Pediatrics and Reproductive Biology
Case Western Reserve University School of Medicine
Eliza Henry Barnes Chair in Neonatology
Rainbow Babies and Children's Hospital
Cleveland, Ohio

Michele C. Walsh, MD, MSE

Professor, Pediatrics
Case Western Reserve University School of Medicine
Co-Director, Division of Neonatology
Medical Director, Neonatal Intensive Care Unit
Rainbow Babies and Children's Hospital
Cleveland, Ohio

ELSEVIER
MOSBY

ELSEVIER
MOSBY

3251 Riverport Lane
St. Louis, Missouri 63043

Library of Congress Cataloging-in-Publication Data

Fanaroff and Martin's neonatal-perinatal medicine : diseases of the fetus and infant / [edited by] Richard J. Martin, Avroy A. Fanaroff, Michele C. Walsh. — 9th ed.
   p. ; cm.
  Other title: Neonatal-perinatal medicine
  Includes bibliographical references and index.
  ISBN 978-0-323-06545-0
  1. Newborn infants—Diseases. 2. Fetus—Diseases. I. Martin, Richard J. II. Fanaroff, Avroy A. III. Walsh, Michele C. IV. Title: Neonatal-perinatal medicine.
  [DNLM: 1. Fetal Diseases. 2. Infant, Newborn, Diseases. 3. Perinatal Care. 4. Pregnancy Complications. WS 420 F1985 2010]
  RJ254.N456 2010
  618.92'01--dc22

Acquisitions Editor: Judy Fletcher
Developmental Editor: Arlene Chappelle
Publishing Services Manager: Julie Eddy
Senior Project Manager: Celeste Clingan
Design Direction: Lou Forgione

Printed in United States

Last digit is the print number: 9 8 7 6 5 4 3 2 1

To our spouses:
Patricia, Roslyn, and Larry

the Martin children and grandchild
Scott & Molly; Sonya, Peter, & Mateo,

the Fanaroff children and grandchildren
Jonathan & Kristy; Jodi, Peter, Austin, & Morgan;
and Amanda, Jason, & Jackson,

and the Walsh children
Sean and Ryan

with love, admiration, and deep appreciation
for their continued support and inspiration

Contributors

Jalal M. Abu-Shaweesh, MBBS

Associate Professor of Pediatrics, Case Western Reserve University; Attending Neonatologist, Rainbow Babies and Children's Hospital, Cleveland, Ohio
Respiratory Disorders in Preterm and Term Infants

Veronica H. Accornero, PhD

Assistant Professor of Clinical Pediatrics, University of Miami Miller School of Medicine, Miami, Florida
Infants of Substance-Abusing Mothers

Heidelise Als, PhD

Associate Professor of Psychiatry (Psychology), Harvard Medical School; Director of Neurobehavioral Infant and Child Studies, and Senior Associate in Psychiatry, Children's Hospital; Research Associate in Newborn Medicine, Brigham & Women's Hospital; Consulting Staff in Pediatric Psychology, Spaulding Rehabilitation Hospital, Boston, Massachusetts
Neurobehavioral Development of the Preterm Infant

Brenna L. Anderson, MD, MSCR

Assistant Professor of Obstetrics and Gynecology, Division of Maternal Fetal Medicine, Warren Alpert Medical School of Brown University, Providence, Rhode Island; Medical Staff, Women & Infant's Hospital, Pittsburgh, Pennsylvania; Consulting Physician, South County Hospital, South Kingstown, Rhode Island; Consulting Physician, Charlton Hospital, Fall River, Massachusetts
Perinatal Infections

Jacob V. Aranda, MD, PhD, FRCP(C)

Professor and Director, Neonatology, State University of New York Downstate Medical Center, Brooklyn, New York
Developmental Pharmacology

James E. Arnold, MS, FAAP

The Julius W. McCall Professor and Chair, Department of Otolaryngology, Head and Neck Surgery, Case Western Reserve University; Chairman, Department of Otolaryngology, University Hospitals Case Medical Center, Rainbow Babies and Children's Hospital, Cleveland, Ohio
Upper Airway Lesions

Sundeep Arora, MD

Attending Pediatric Gastroenterologist, Children's Hospitals and Clinics of Minnesota; Minnesota Gastroenterology, St. Paul, Minnesota
Disorders of Digestion

Komal Bajaj, MD

Reproductive Genetics Fellow, MonteFiore Medical Center, Albert Einstein College of Medicine, Bronx, New York; Research Associate, Human Genetics Laboratory at Jacobi Medical Center, Bronx, New York
Genetic Aspects of Perinatal Disease and Prenatal Diagnosis

Jill E. Baley, MD

Professor of Pediatrics, Case Western Reserve University School of Medicine; Medical Director, Neonatal Transitional Unit, Division of Neonatology, Rainbow Babies and Children's Hospital, Cleveland, Ohio
Perinatal Viral Infections; Schedule for Immunization of Preterm Infants

Eduardo H. Bancalari, MD

Professor of Pediatrics, University of Miami, Miller School of Medicine; Director, Division of Neonatology, University of Miami/Jackson Memorial Hospital, Miami, Florida
Bronchopulmonary Dysplasia

Emmalee S. Bandstra, MD

Professor of Pediatrics and Obstetrics and Gynecology, University of Miami Miller School of Medicine; Attending Neonatologist, Jackson Memorial Medical Center, Holtz Children's Hospital, Miami, Florida
Infants of Substance-Abusing Mothers

Edward M. Barksdale, Jr., MD

Professor of Surgery, Case Western Reserve University; Chief, Division of Pediatric Surgery, Rainbow Babies and Children's Hospital, Cleveland, Ohio
Selected Gastrointestinal Anomalies

Cynthia F. Bearer, MD, PhD

Mary Gray Cobey Professor of Neonatology, University of Maryland School of Medicine; Chief, Division of Neonatology, University of Maryland Medical System, Baltimore, Maryland
Occupational and Environmental Risks to the Fetus

Isaac Blickstein, MD

Professor, Hadassah-Hebrew University School of Medicine, Jerusalem, Israel; Senior Physician, Department of Obstetrics and Gynecology, Kaplan Medical Center, Rehovot, Israel
Fetal Effects of Autoimmune Disease; Obstetric Management of Multiple Gestation and Birth; Post-term Pregnancy

Jeffrey L. Blumer, MD, PhD

Professor of Pediatrics and Pharmacology, Case School of Medicine; Department of Pediatrics, Rainbow Babies and Children's Hospital, Cleveland, Ohio
Developmental Pharmacology

Samantha Butler, PhD

Instructor, Harvard Medical School; Staff Psychologist, Children's Hospital Boston, Boston, Massachusetts
Neurobehavioral Development of the Preterm Infant

Kara Calkins, MD

Clinical Instructor, David Geffen School of Medicine at UCLA, University of California; Attending Physician, Mattel Children's Hospital at UCLA, Department of Pediatrics, Division of Neonatology and Developmental Biology, Los Angeles, California
Developmental Origins of Adult Health and Disease

Michael S. Caplan, MD

Clinical Professor of Pediatrics, University of Chicago, Pritzker School of Medicine, Chicago, Illinois; Chairman, Department of Pediatrics, North Shore University Health System, Evanston, Illinois
Neonatal Necrotizing Enterocolitis: Clinical Observations, Pathophysiology, and Prevention

Waldemar A. Carlo, MD

Edwin M. Dixon Professor of Pediatrics; Director, Division of Neonatology, University of Alabama at Birmingham School of Medicine; Director, Newborn Nurseries, University of Alabama at Birmingham Medical Center, The Children's Hospital of Alabama, Birmingham, Alabama
Assessment of Pulmonary Function

Gisela Chelimsky, MD

Assistant Professor of Pediatrics, Case School of Medicine; Attending Physician, Rainbow Babies and Children's Hospital, Cleveland, Ohio
Disorders of Digestion

Valerie Y. Chock, MD

Instructor of Neonatology, Stanford University School of Medicine, Stanford, California
Biomedical Engineering Aspects of Neonatal Monitoring

Walter J. Chwals, MD

Professor of Surgery and Pediatrics, Tufts University School of Medicine, Boston, Massachusetts
Development and Basic Physiology of the Neonatal Gastrointestinal Tract; Selected Gastrointestinal Anomalies

Alan R. Cohen, MD, FACS, FAAP

Reinberger Chair in Pediatric Neurological Surgery; Professor of Neurological Surgery and Pediatrics, Case Western Reserve University School of Medicine; Surgeon-in-Chief and Chief of Pediatric Neurological Surgery, Rainbow Babies and Children's Hospital, Cleveland, Ohio
Disorders in Head Shape and Size; Myelomeningocele

Daniel R. Cooperman, MD

Professor of Orthopedic Surgery, Case Western Reserve University; Professor of Orthopedic Surgery, Rainbow Babies and Children's Hospital, Cleveland, Ohio
Musculoskeletal Disorders; Bone and Joint Infections; Congenital Abnormalities of the Upper and Lower Extremities and Spine

Timothy M. Crombleholme, MD

Richard G. and Geralyn Azizkhan Chair in Pediatric Surgery; Professor of Surgery, Pediatrics (Molecular and Developmental Biology), and Obstetrics and Gynecology, University of Cincinnati College of Medicine; Director, Fetal Care Center of Cincinnati, Division of Pediatric General, Thoracic, and Fetal Surgery, Cincinnati Children's Hospital, Cincinnati, Ohio
Surgical Treatment of the Fetus

Mario De Curtis, MD

Professor of Neonatology, Dipartimento di Scienze Ginecologiche, Perinatologia e Puericultura, University of Rome Faculty of Medicine; Director, Neonatology Unit, Patologia Neonatale e Terapia Intensiva Dipartimento di Scienze Ginecologiche, Perinatologia e Puericultura, Azienda Policlinico Umberto I, Rome, Italy
Disorders of Calcium, Phosphorus, and Magnesium Metabolism

Linda S. de Vries, MD, PhD

Professor in Neonatal Neurology, Department of Neonatology, Wilhelmina Children's Hospital, Utrecht, The Netherlands
Intracranial Hemorrhage and Vascular Lesions; Hypoxic-Ischemic Encephalopathy, Assessment Tools

Katherine MacRae Dell, MD

Associate Professor of Pediatrics, Case Western Reserve University; Chief, Division of Pediatric Nephrology, Rainbow Babies and Children's Hospital, Cleveland, Ohio
Fluid and Electrolyte Management; Acid-Base Management; The Kidney and Urinary Tract

Scott Denne, MD

Professor of Pediatrics, Indiana University School of Medicine, Riley Hospital for Children, Indianapolis, Indiana
Parenteral Nutrition; Enteral Nutrition

Sherin U. Devaskar, MD

Professor of Pediatrics, David Geffen School of Medicine at UCLA; Director, Neonatal Research Center, Division of Neonatology and Developmental Biology, Department of Pediatrics, David Geffen School of Medicine at UCLA, Los Angeles, California
Developmental Origins of Adult Health and Disease; Disorders of Carbohydrate Metabolism

Juliann Di Fiore, BSEE

Research Engineer, Department of Medicine, Case Western Reserve University, Division of Neonatology, Rainbow Babies and Children's Hospital, Cleveland, Ohio
Assessment of Pulmonary Function

Steven M. Donn, MD

Professor of Pediatrics, Division of Neonatal-Perinatal Medicine; Faculty Associate, Center for Global Health, School of Public Health, University of Michigan Health System; Staff Neonatologist, C.S. Mott Children's Hospital, Ann Arbor, Michigan
Assisted Ventilation and Its Complications

Morven S. Edwards, MD

Professor of Pediatrics, Baylor College of Medicine; Attending Physician, Texas Children's Hospital, Houston, Texas
Postnatal Bacterial Infections; Fungal and Protozoal Infections

William H. Edwards, MD

Professor of Pediatrics, Dartmouth Medical School, Hanover, New Hampshire; Vice Chairman, Department of Pediatrics, Neonatology Section Chief; Medical Director, Citad Nurseries, Dartmouth Hitchcock Medical Center, Lebanon, New Hampshire
Care of the Mother, Father, and Infant,

Francine Erenberg, MD

Assistant Professor, Cleveland Clinic Lerner College of Medicine of Case Western Reserve University; Staff, Pediatric Cardiologist, Cleveland Clinic Children's Hospital, Department of Pediatric Cardiology, Cleveland, Ohio
Fetal Cardiac Physiology and Fetal Cardiovascular Assessment; Congenital Defects

Avroy A. Fanaroff, MB, BCh, FRCP[E], FRCPCN

Professor, Pediatrics and Reproductive Biology, Case Western Reserve University School of Medicine; Eliza Henry Barnes Chair in Neonatology, Rainbow Babies and Children's Hospital, Cleveland, Ohio
Epidemiology; Perinatal Services; Obstetric Management of Prematurity

Jonathan M. Fanaroff, MD, JD

Assistant Professor of Pediatrics, Case Western Reserve University School of Medicine; Associate Medical Director, NICU; Director, Rainbow Center for Pediatric Ethics, Rainbow Babies and Children's Hospital, Cleveland, Ohio
Legal Issues in Neonatal-Perinatal Medicine

Ross Fasano, MD

Pediatric Hematology/Oncology Fellow, Children's National Medical Center, Washington, DC
Blood Component Therapy for the Neonate

Orna Flidel-Rimon, MD

Lecturer in Pediatrics, Hebrew University, Jerusalem; Attending Physician, Kaplan Medical Center, Rehovot, Israel
Post-term Pregnancy

Smadar Friedman, MD

Senior Lecturer, Hadassah University Hospital, Hadassah School of Medicine; Director, Neonatology Unit, Department of Neonatology, Hadassah Ein Kerem Hospital, University Hospital, Jerusalem, Israel
Fetal Effects of Autoimmune Disease

Susan E. Gerber, MD, MPH

Assistant Professor, Department of Obstetrics and Gynecology, Division of Maternal-Fetal Medicine, Northwestern University, Feinberg School of Medicine; Attending Physician, Department of Obstetrics and Gynecology, Division of Maternal-Fetal Medicine, Northwestern Memorial Hospital, Chicago, Illinois
Antepartum Fetal Surveillance; Evaluation of the Intrapartum Fetus

Jay P. Goldsmith, MD

Clinical Professor of Pediatrics, Tulane University School of Medicine, New Orleans, Lousiana; Neonatologist, Women's and Children's Hospital, Lafayette, Louisiana
Delivery Room Resuscitation of the Newborn, Overview and Initial Management; Chest Compression, Medications, and Special Problems

Bernard Gonik, MD

Professor and Fann Srere Chair of Perinatal Medicine, Department of Obstetrics and Gynecology, Wayne State University School of Medicine, Detroit, Michigan
Perinatal Infections

Jeffrey B. Gould, MD

Robert L. Hess Professor in Pediatrics and Director, Perinatal Epidemiology and Health Outcomes Research Unit, Department of Pediatrics, Division of Neonatal and Developmental Medicine, Stanford University School of Medicine, Stanford; Attending Neonatologist, Lucile Packard Children's Hospital at Stanford, Palo Alto, California
Evaluating and Improving the Quality and Safety of Neonatal Intensive Care

Pierre Gressens, MD, PhD

Chief, Inserm-Paris 7 University, Hopital Robert Debré, Paris, France; Professor of Perinatal Neurology, Imperial College London, Hammersmith Hospital, London, United Kingdom
Normal and Abnormal Brain Development; White Matter Damage and Encephalopathy of Prematurity

Susan J. Gross, MD

Professor, Department of Obstetrics and Gynecology, Women's Health and Department of Pediatrics, Albert Einstein College of Medicine; Chairperson, Department of Obstetrics and Gynecology, North Bronx Healthcare Network, Bronx, New York
Genetic Aspects of Perinatal Disease and Prenatal Diagnosis

Andrée M. Gruslin, MD, FRCS

Associate Professor, Division of Maternal Fetal Medicine, Department of Obstetrics & Gynecology and Newborn Care, Cellular and Molecular Medicine, University of Ottawa, Ottawa, Ontario, Canada
Erythroblastosis Fetalis

Balaji K. Gupta, MD

Clinical Assistant Professor, Department of Ophthalmology and Visual Sciences, University of Chicago Pritzker School of Medicine, Chicago, Illinois
The Eye, Examination and Common Problems

Maureen Hack, MB, ChB

Professor of Pediatrics, Case School of Medicine; Director, High Risk Follow-Up Program, Rainbow Babies and Children's Hospital, Cleveland, Ohio
Follow-up for High-Risk Neonates

Louis P. Halamek, MD

Associate Professor, Division of Neonatal and Developmental Medicine, Department of Pediatrics, Stanford University; Director, Center for Advanced Pediatric and Perinatal Education, Packard Children's Hospital, Palo Alto, California; Attending Neonatologist, Packard Children's Hospital, Palo Alto, California
Simulation in Neonatal-Perinatal Medicine

Aaron Hamvas, MD

The James P. Keating, MD, Professor of Pediatrics, Washington University School of Medicine, St. Louis Children's Hospital, St. Louis, Missouri
Pathophysiology and Management of Respiratory Distress Syndrome

Jonathan Hellmann, MBBCh, FCP(SA), FRCPC, MHSc

Professor of Pediatrics, University of Toronto; Clinical Director, Neonatal Intensive Care Unit, Hospital for Sick Children, Toronto, Ontario, Canada
Medical Ethics in Neonatal Care

Susan R. Hintz, MD

Associate Professor, Department of Pediatrics, Division of Neonatal and Perinatal Medicine, Stanford University School of Medicine; Attending Neonatologist, Lucile Packard Children's Hospital, Stanford, California
Biomedical Engineering Aspects of Neonatal Monitoring

Steven B. Hoath, MD

Professor of Pediatrics, University of Cincinnati College of Medicine, Division of Neonatology; Medical Director, Skin Sciences Program, Cincinnati Children's Hospital Medical Center, Cincinnati, Ohio
The Skin

Jeffrey D. Horbar, MD

Jerold F. Lucey Professor of Neonatal Medicine, University of Vermont College of Medicine; Chief Executive and Scientific Officer, Vermont Oxford Network, Burlington, Vermont
Evaluating and Improving the Quality and Safety of Neonatal Intensive Care

McCallum R. Hoyt, MD, MBA

Assistant Professor of Anesthesiology, Harvard Medical School, Boston, Massachusetts; Director of Gynecologic and Ambulatory Anesthesia; Staff, Obstetric Anesthesia, Brigham and Women's Hospital, Boston, Massachusetts
Anesthetic Options for Labor and Delivery

Petra S. Hüppi, MD

Professor of Pediatrics, University of Geneva Faculty of Medicine; Director, Child Development Unit, Department of Pediatrics, Children's Hospital, Geneva, Switzerland
White Matter Damage and Encephalopathy of Prematurity; Normal and Abnormal Brain Development

Lucky Jain, MD, MBA

Richard W. Blumberg Professor and Executive Vice Chairman, Department of Pediatrics, Emory University School of Medicine; Medical Director, Emory Children's Center, Children's Healthcare of Atlanta at Egleston in Atlanta, Georgia, Emory University Hospital Midtown, Atlanta, Georgia
The Late Preterm Infant

Alan H. Jobe, MD, PhD

Professor of Pediatrics, University of Cincinnati School of Medicine; Director of Perinatology Research, Cincinnati Children's Hospital, Cincinnati, Ohio
Lung Development and Maturation

Nancy E. Judge, MD, FACOG

Associate Professor of Reproductive Biology, Albert Einstein Medical School of Yeshiva University; Director of Obstetrics, Montefiore North Division, Montefiore Hospitals, Bronx, New York
Perinatal Imaging

Michael Kaplan, MD

Professor of Pediatrics, Faculty of Medicine of the Hebrew University; Director, Department of Neonatology, Shaare Zedek Medical Center, Jerusalem, Israel
Neonatal Jaundice and Liver Disease

Satish C. Kalhan, MBBS, FRCP, DCH

Professor, Department of Molecular Medicine; Staff, Department of Pathobiology, Gastroenterology and Hepatology, Cleveland Clinic Lerner College of Medicine of Case Western Reserve University Cleveland, Ohio
Disorders of Carbohydrate Metabolism

Reuben Kapur, PhD

Professor of Pediatrics, Molecular Biology and Biochemistry, Medical and Molecular Genetics, Microbiology and Immunology, Indiana University School of Medicine, Department of Pediatrics; Director, Program in Hematologic Malignancies and Stem Cell Biology, Herman B. Wells Center for Pediatric Research, Cancer Research Institute, Indiana University School of Medicine, Indianapolis, Indiana
Developmental Immunology

Ganga Karunamuni, MD

Graduate Research Assistant, Case Western Reserve University,Cleveland, Ohio
Cardiac Embryology

Lawrence M. Kaufman, MD

Clinical Associate Professor of Ophthalmology, University of Illinois at Chicago; Director of Pediatric Ophthalmology, Advocate Illinois Masonic Medical Center, Chicago, Illinois
Examination and Common Problems

Kathleen A. Kennedy, MD, MPH

Professor of Pediatrics, Department of Pediatrics, University of Texas Health Science Center at Houston; Director, Division of Neonatal-Perinatal Medicine; Director, M.S. in Clinical Research Degree Program, University of Texas Health Science Center at Houston, Texas
Practicing Evidence-Based Neonatal-Perinatal Medicine

John H. Kennell, MD

Professor of Pediatrics Emeritus, Department of Pediatrics, Case School of Medicine; Attending Physician, Division of Behavioral Pediatrics, Rainbow Babies and Children's Hospital, Cleveland, Ohio
Care of the Mother, Father, and Infant

Joseph A. Kitterman, MD

Professor of Pediatrics, University of California, San Francisco, School of Medicine, San Francisco, California
Fibrodysplasia Ossificans Progressiva

Marshall H. Klaus, MD

Professor of Pediatrics, Emeritus, University of California, San Francisco, School of Medicine, San Francisco, California
Care of the Mother, Father, and Infant,

Robert M. Kliegman, MD

Professor and Chair of Pediatrics, Medical College of Wisconsin; Pediatrician-in-Chief/Pamela and Leslie Muma Chair in Pediatrics, Children's Hospital of Wisconsin, Children's Corporate Center, Milwaukee, Wisconsin
Intrauterine Growth Restriction

Oded Langer, MD, PhD

Professor, Department of Obstetrics and Gynecology, Columbia University; Chairman, Department of Obstetrics and Gynecology, St. Luke's-Roosevelt Hospital Center, New York, New York
Pregnancy Complicated by Diabetes Mellitus

Noam Lazebnik, MD

Associate Professor of Reproductive Biology, Case Western University School of Medicine; Division of Maternal and Fetal Medicine, University MacDonald Women's Hospital, Cleveland, Ohio
Perinatal Imaging

Malcolm I. Levene, MD, FMedSe

Professor of Paediatrics and Child Health, University of Leeds School of Medicine Department of Pediatrics; Consultant Neonatologist, Leeds Teaching Hospitals NHS Trust, Leeds, West York, United Kingdom
Hypoxic-Ischemic Encephalopathy; Pathophysiology; Management

Foong-Yen Lim, MD

Assistant Professor of Surgery, Pediatrics and Obstetrics and Gynecology, University of Cincinnati College of Medicine; Pediatrics and Fetal Surgeon, Division of Pediatric General, Thoracic and Fetal Surgery, Cincinnati Children's Hospital, Cincinnati, Ohio
Surgical Treatment of the Fetus

Tom Lissauer, MB, Bchir, FRCPCH

Hon Consultant Neonatologist, Imperial College Healthcare Trust; Pediatric Program Director, Institute of Global Health, Imperial College, London, United Kingdom
Physical Examination of the Newborn

Suzanne M. Lopez, MD

Associate Professor of Pediatrics, Department of Pediatrics, University of Texas Health Science Center at Houston; Associate Professor of Pediatrics; Director, Neonatal Perinatal Medicine Fellowship, University of Texas Health Science Center at Houston, Houston, Texas
Practicing Evidence-Based Neonatal-Perinatal Medicine

Timothy E. Lotze, MD

Assistant Professor, Department of Pediatrics, Baylor College of Medicine; Section of Child Neurology, Texas Children's Hospital, Houston, Texas
Hypotonia and Neuromuscular Disease

Naomi L. C. Luban, MD

Division Chief, Children's National Medical Center, Department of Laboratory Medicine, Children's National Medical Center, Washington, DC
Blood Component Therapy for the Neonate

Lori Luchtman-Jones, MD

Associate Professor, George Washington University Medical School; Division Chief, Hematology, Children's National Medical Center, Washington, DC
Hematologic Problems in the Fetus and Neonate

David K. Magnuson, MD, FACS, FAAP

Department Chair, Pediatric Surgery, Cleveland Clinic Children's Hospital, Cleveland, Ohio
Development and Basic Physiology of the Neonatal Gastrointestinal Tract; Selected Gastrointestinal Anomalies

Henry H. Mangurten, MD

Professor of Pediatrics, Rosalind Franklin University of Medicine and Science/The Chicago Medical School, North Chicago, IL; Chairman Emeritus, Department of Pediatrics, Advocate Lutheran General Children's Hospital, Park Ridge, Illinois
Birth Injuries

Jacquelyn McClary, Pharm D

Clinical Pharmacist Specialist, Neonatal Intensive Care Unit, Rainbow Babies and Children's Hospital, Cleveland, Ohio
Developmental Pharmacology

Geoffrey Miller, MA, MB, BCh, MPhil, MD, FRCP, FRACP

Professor of Pediatrics and Neurology, Yale University School of Medicine; Clinical Director, Pediatric Neurology, Yale New Haven Hospital, New Haven, Connecticut
Hypotonia and Neuromuscular Disease

Marilyn T. Miller, MD

Professor of Ophthalmology, Department of Ophthalmology and Visual Sciences, University of Illinois at Chicago College of Medicine; University of Illinois Hospital, Chicago, Illinois
The Eye, Examination and Common Problems

Mohamed W. Mohamed, MD

Neonatology Fellow, The Hospital for Sick Children, Toronto, Ontario
Disorders of Calcium, Phosphorus, and Magnesium Metabolism

Thomas R. Moore, MD

Professor and Chairman, Department of Reproductive Medicine, University of California School of Medicine, San Diego, California
Erythroblastosis Fetalis; Amniotic Fluid and Nonimmune Hydrops Fetalis

Colin J. Morley MA, DCH, MD, FRCP, FRCPCH, FRACP

Professor of Neonatal Medicine, The Royal Women's Hospital, Melbourne, Australia, United Kingdom
Role of Positive Pressure Ventilation in Neonatal Resuscitation

Stuart C. Morrison, MD, ChB, FRCP

Clinical Faculty, Cleveland Clinic Medical School; Staff Radiologist, Cleveland Clinic Foundation, Cleveland, Ohio
Perinatal Imaging

Anil Narang, MD

Professor, Pediatrics (Neonatology), Department of Pediatrics, Postgraduate Institute of Medical Education and Research; Head, Department of Pediatrics, Advanced Pediatric Centre, Chandigarh, India
Perinatal and Neonatal Care in Developing Countries

Vivek Narendran, MD, MRCP, MBA

Associate Professor of Pediatrics, University of Cincinnati College of Medicine; Medical Director, University Hospital NICU, Cincinnati Children's Hospital Medical Center, Cincinnati, Ohio
The Skin

Mary L. Nock, MD

Assistant Professor, Department of Pediatrics, Case Western Reserve University School of Medicine; Attending Neonatologist, Rainbow Babies and Children's Hospital, Cleveland, Ohio
Tables of Normal Values

Mark R. Palmert, MD, PhD

Associate Professor of Paediatrics, University of Toronto Faculty of Medicine; Head, Division of Endocrinology, The Hospital for Sick Children, Toronto, Ontario, Canada
Disorders of Sex Development

Aditi S. Parikh, BA, MD

Clinical Instructor, Case Western Reserve University School of Medicine; Clinical Geneticist, University Hospital's Case Medical Center, Cleveland, Ohio
Congenital Anomalies

Robert L. Parry, MD

Associate Professor of Surgery and Pediatrics, Case Western Reserve School of Medicine; Pediatric Surgeon, Rainbow Babies and Children's Hospital, Cleveland, Ohio
Development and Basic Physiology of the Neonatal Gastrointestinal Tract; Selected Gastrointestinal Anomalies

Dale L. Phelps, MD

Professor of Pediatrics, University of Rochester School of Medicine, Rochester, New York
Retinopathy of Prematurity

Brenda Poindexter, MD, MS

Associate Professor of Pediatrics, Indiana University School of Medicine, Riley Hospital for Children, Indianapolis, Indiana
Parenteral Nutrition; Enteral Nutrition

Richard A. Polin, MD

Professor of Pediatrics, Department of Neonatology, Columbia University Medical Center; Director, Division of Neonatology, Morgan Stanley Children's Hospital of New York, Columbia University Medical Center, New York, New York
Developmental Immunology

Bhagya L. Puppala, MD

Assistant Professor of Pediatrics, Rosalind Franklin University of Medicine and Science, The Chicago Medical School, North Chicago, Illinois; Adjunct Professor of Pediatrics, Midwestern University, Downer's Grove, Illinois; Director, Neonatal Perinatal Medicine-Fellowship, Director, Neonatal Perinatal Medicine Research, Advocate Lutheran General Children's Hospital, Park Ridge, Illinois
Birth Injuries

Tonse N.K. Raju, MD, DCH

Adjunct Professor of Pediatrics, Georgetown University, Washington, DC; Program Scientist/Medical Officer, Pregnancy and Perinatalogy Branch, Eunice Kennedy Shriver National Institute of Child Health and Human Development, Bethesda, Maryland

From Infant Hatcheries to Intensive Care: Highlights of the Century of Neonatal Medicine

Ashwin Ramachandrappa, MD

Attending Neonatologist, Neonatology Associates, Ltd, Phoenix, Arizona

The Late Preterm Infant

Raymond W. Redline, MD

Professor of Pathology and Reproductive Biology, Case Western Reserve University School of Medicine; Pediatric Pathologist, University Hospital Case Medical Center, Cleveland, Ohio

Placental Pathology

Jacques Rigo, MD, PhD

Professor of Neonatology and Pediatrics Nutrition, University of Liège; Head, Department of Neonatology, CHR Citadelle, Liège, Belgium

Disorders of Calcium, Phosphorus, and Magnesium Metabolism

Barrett K. Robinson, MD, MPH

Clinical Fellow, Division of Maternal-Fetal Medicine, Department of Obstetrics and Gynecology, Northwestern University Feinberg School of Medicine, Chicago, Illinois

Evaluation of the Intrapartum Fetus

Susan R. Rose, MD

Professor of Pediatrics and Endocrinology, University of Cincinnati; Professor of Pediatric Endocrinology, Cincinnati Children's Hospital Medical Center, Cincinnati, Ohio

Thyroid Disorders

Florence Rothenberg, MS, MD, FACC

Assistance Professor, Department of Internal Medicine Staff; Cardiologist, VAMC Division of Cardiovascular Diseases, University of Cincinnati, Cincinnati, Ohio

Cardiac Embryology

Shaista Safder, MD

Assistant Professor, University of Central Florida and Florida State University, Arnold Palmer Hospital for Children, Orlando, Florida

Disorders of Digestion

Ola Didrik Saugstad, MD, PhD, FRCPE

Professor of Pediatrics, Department of Pediatric Research, Oslo University, Oslo, Norway

Oxygen Therapy

Katherine S. Schaefer, PhD

Associate Professor of Biology, Randolph College, Lynchburg, Virginia

Cardiac Embryology

Mark S. Scher, MD

Professor of Pediatrics and Neurology, Case Western University School of Medicine; Division Chief, Pediatric Neurology, Rainbow Babies and Children's Hospital, Cleveland, Ohio

Seizures in Neonates

Gunnar Sedin, MD, PhD

Professor, Perinatal-Neonatal Medicine, Uppsala University School of Medicine, Uppsala, Sweden

The Thermal Environment

Dinesh M. Shah, MD

Professor, Department of Obstetrics/Gynecology; Director of Maternal-Fetal Medicine and Maternal-Fetal Medicine Fellowship, University of Wisconsin School of Medicine and Public Health, Madison, Wisconsin

Hypertensive Disorders of Pregnancy

Eric S. Shinwell, MD

Clinical Associate Professor of Pediatrics, Hebrew University, Jerusalem, Israel; Director of Neonatology, Kaplan Medical Center, Rehovot, Israel

Obstetric Management of Multiple Gestation and Birth

Rayzel M. Shulman, MD, FRCPC

Research Fellow, University of Toronto, The Hospital for Sick Children, Toronto, Ontario, Canada

Disorders of Sex Development

Eric Sibley, MD, PhD

Associate Professor of Pediatrics, Division of Pediatric Gastroenterology, Stanford University School of Medicine, Stanford, California

Neonatal Jaundice and Liver Disease

Sunil K. Sinha, MD, PhD

Professor of Pediatrics, University of Durham, Durham, United Kingdom; Consultant Neonatologist, The James Cook University Hospital, Middlesbroug, United Kingdom

Assisted Ventilation and Its Complications

Carlos J. Sivit, MD

Professor of Radiology and Pediatrics, Case Western Reserve School of Medicine; Vice Chair, Clinical Operations, University Hospitals Case Medical Center, Cleveland, Ohio

Diagnostic Imaging

Ernest S. Siwik, MD

Associate Professor of Clinical Pediatrics, Louisiana State University Health Sciences Center; Director, Cardiac Catheterization Program, Children's Hospital of New Orleans, New Orleans, Louisiana

Principles of Medical and Surgical Management

Robert C. Sprecher, MD, FACS, FAAP

Chief, Pediatric Otolaryngology, Rainbow Babies and Children's Hospital, Case Western Reserve University, Cleveland, Ohio
Upper Airway Lesions

Robin H. Steinhorn, MD

Raymond and Hazel Speck Berry Professor of Pediatrics, Northwestern University Steinberg School of Medicine; Vice Chair of Pediatrics, Division Head of Neonatology, Children's Memorial Hospital, Chicago, Illinois
Pulmonary Vascular Development

David K. Stevenson, MD

Harold K. Faber Professor of Pediatrics; Vice Dean, Stanford University School of Medicine; Senior Associate Dean for Academic Affairs, Department of Pediatrics, Division of Neonatal and Developmental Medicine, Stanford University School of Medicine; Director, Charles B. and Ann L. Johnson Center for Pregnancy and Newborn Services, Lucile Packard Children's Hospital, Stanford, California
Biomedical Engineering Aspects of Neonatal Monitoring; Neonatal Jaundice and Liver Disease

Eileen K. Stork, MD

Professor of Pediatrics, Case Western Reserve University School of Medicine; Director, Neonatal ECMO Program, Rainbow Babies and Children's Hospital, Division of Neonatology, Cleveland, Ohio
Therapy for Cardiorespiratory Failure

John E. Stork, MD

Assistant Professor, Case Western Reserve University; Chief, Pediatric Cardiac Anesthesia, Rainbow Babies and Children's Hospital, University Hospitals Case Medical Center, Cleveland, Ohio
Anesthesia in the Neonate

Arjan B. te Pas, MD, PhD

Assistant Professor, Leiden University Medical Center; Paediatrician-Neonatologist, Department of Pediatrics, Division of Neonatology, Leiden University Medical Center, Leiden, The Netherlands
Role of Positive Pressure Ventilation in Neonatal Resuscitation

George H. Thompson, MD

Professor, Orthopedic Surgery and Pediatrics, Case Western Reserve University; Director, Pediatric Orthopedics, Rainbow Babies and Children's Hospital, Cleveland, Ohio
Musculoskeletal Disorders; Bone and Joint Infections; Congenital Abnormalities of the Upper and Lower Extremities and Spine

Philip Toltzis, MD

Professor of Pediatrics, Case Western Reserve University School of Medicine; Attending Pediatrician, Division of Pharmacology and Critical Care, Rainbow Babies and Children's Hospital, Cleveland, Ohio
Perinatal Viral Infections

Robert Turbow, MD, JD

Adjunct Professor, Department of Biology, California Polytechnic State University, San Luis Obispo, California; Attending Neonatologist, Phoenix Children's Hospital, Phoenix, Arizona
Legal Issues in Neonatal-Perinatal Medicine

Jon E. Tyson, MD, MPH

UT Medical School Master's Program—Co Director; Director, Center for Clinical Research and Evidence-Based Medicine; UT Medical School; Michelle Bain Distinguished Professor, Memorial Hermann Hospital, Lyndon Baines Johnson Hospital, Houston, Texas
Practicing Evidence-Based Neonatal-Perinatal Medicine

George F. Van Hare, MD

Louis Larnck Ward Chair in Cardiology; Professor of Pediatrics; Director, Division of Pediatric Cardiology, Washington University School of Medicine, St. Louis Children's Hospital, St. Louis, Missouri
Neonatal Arrhythmias

Maximo Vento, MD, PhD

Professor of Pediatrics; Director, Neonatal Research Unit, University Hospital La Fe, Valencia, Spain
Oxygen Therapy

Dharmapuri Vidyasagar, MD, MSs, FAAP, FCCM, DHC

Professor Emeritus, University of Illinois at Chicago, Department of Pediatrics, Chicago, Illinois
Perinatal and Neonatal Care in Developing Countries

Beth A. Vogt, MD

Associate Professor of Pediatrics, Case Western Reserve University; Attending Physician, Rainbow Babies and Children's Hospital, Cleveland, Ohio
The Kidney and Urinary Tract

Betty Vohr, MD

Professor of Pediatrics, Warren Alpert Medical School of Brown University; Director of Neonatal Follow-up Program; Medical Director, Rhode Island Hearing Assessment Program, Women and Infants Hospital, Providence, Rhode Island
Hearing Loss in the Newborn Infant

Michele C. Walsh, MD, MSE

Professor of Pediatrics, Case Western Reserve University School of Medicine; Co-Director, Division of Neonatology; Medical Director, Neonatal Intensive Care Unit, Rainbow Babies and Children's Hospital, Cleveland, Ohio
Epidemiology; Perinatal Services; Design Considerations; Myelomeningocele; Bronchopulmonary Dysplasia

Michiko Watanabe, PhD

Associate Professor, Departments of Pediatrics, Genetics, and Anatomy, Case School of Medicine; Staff, Division of Pediatric Cardiology, Rainbow Babies and Children's Hospital, Cleveland, Ohio
Cardiac Embryology

Diane K. Wherrett, MD, FRCPC

Associate Professor, Division of Endocrinology, Department of Pediatrics, University of Toronto, Toronto, Ontario, Canada
Disorders of Sex Development

Robert D. White, MD

Adjunct Professor of Psychology, University of Notre Dame, Notre Dame, Indiana; Clinical Assistant Professor of Pediatrics, Indiana University School of Medicine, Indianapolis, Indiana; Director, Regional Newborn Program; Memorial Hospital, South Bend, Indiana
The Sensory Environment of the Intensive Care Nursery; Design Considerations

Georgia L. Wiesner, MS, MD

Associate Professor of Genetics and Medicine, School of Medicine, Case Western Reserve University; Clinical Geneticist, Center for Human Genetics, University Hospitals Case Medical Center, Cleveland, Ohio
Congenital Anomalies

Jamie C. Wikenheiser, PhD

Assistant Professor, Department of Pathology and Laboratory Medicine, Division of Integrative Anatomy, University of California, Los Angeles
Cardiac Embryology

David B. Wilson, MD, PhD

Associate Professor, Department of Pediatrics, Washington University School of Medicine; Attending Physician, St Louis Children's Hospital, St Louis, Missouri
Hematologic Problems in the Fetus and Neonate

Deanne Wilson-Costello, MD

Professor of Pediatrics, Case Western Reserve University; Co-Director High Risk Follow-Up Program, Rainbow Babies and Children's Hospital, Case Western Reserve University, Cleveland, Ohio
Follow-up for High-Risk Neonates

Richard B. Wolf, DO, FACOG

Associate Clinical Professor, Department of Reproductive Medicine, University of California San Diego, School of Medicine, La Jolla, California; Attending Perinatologist, University of California San Diego Medical Center, San Diego, California
Amniotic Fluid and Nonimmune Hydrops Fetalis

Ronald J. Wong, MD

Senior Research Scientist, Department of Pediatrics, Division of Neonatal and Developmental Medicine, Stanford University School of Medicine, Stanford, California
Biomedical Engineering Aspects of Neonatal Monitoring; Neonatal Jaundice and Liver Disease

Mervin C. Yoder, MD

Richard and Pauline Klingler Professor of Pediatrics; Professor of Biochemistry and Molecular Biology; Professor of Cellular and Integrative Physiology, Indiana University School of Medicine, Department of Pediatrics; Director, Herman B. Wells Center for Pediatric Research; Associate Chair for Pediatrics Research, Herman B. Wells Center for Pediatric Research, Cancer Research Institute, Indiana University School of Medicine, Indianapolis, Indiana
Developmental Immunology

Thomas Young, MD

Professor of Pediatrics, School of Medicine, University of North Carolina Chapel Hill, Chapel Hill, North Carolina; Senior Neonatologist, WakeMed Faculty Physicians, Raleigh, North Carolina
Therapeutic Agents

Kenneth G. Zahka, MD

Professor of Pediatrics, Cleveland Clinic Lerner College Medicine, Case Western Reserve School of Medicine; Pediatric Cardiology, Cleveland Clinic Children's Hospital, Cleveland, Ohio
Genetic and Environmental Contributions to Congenital Heart Disease; Principles of Neonatal Cardiovascular Hemodynamics; Approach to the Neonate with Cardiovascular Disease; Congenital Defects; Cardiovascular Problems of the Neonate; Principles of Medical and Surgical Management

Arthur B. Zinn, MD, PhD

Attending Physician, University Hospitals Case Medical Center; Associate Professor, Case Western Reserve University, Cleveland, Ohio
Inborn Errors of Metabolism

Preface

The foundation for successful outcomes in neonatal-perinatal medicine has been the ability to apply knowledge of the fundamental pathophysiology of the various neonatal disorders to safe interventions. Molecular, biologic, and technologic advances have facilitated the diagnosis, monitoring, and therapy of these complex disorders. Advances at the bench have been transformed to the bedside, and survival statistics reveal steady improvements. Nonetheless, although the survival rates may give reason to rejoice, the high early morbidity and persistent neurodevelopmental problems remain cause for concern. Such problems include bronchopulmonary dysplasia, nosocomial infections, necrotizing enterocolitis, hypoxic-ischemic encephalopathy, cerebral palsy, and the inability to sustain the intrauterine rate of growth when the infants are born prematurely. These problems need to be addressed in addition to the complex birth defects and genetic disorders that now loom as major problems in the neonatal intensive care unit.

The field of Neonatal Perinatal Medicine has transformed from anecdotal medicine to evidence-based medicine. The problem is that evidence-based medicine predicts outcomes for groups but not individuals. The next frontier, individualized, or personalized medicine, requires application of the human genome project to the individual patient. That frontier is gaining momentum amidst a dizzying proliferation of newly acquired scientific knowledge. The translation of bench research to bedside innovation is proceeding smoothly as is the understanding of the underlying mechanisms of many disorders. Advances in genetics have helped solve the etiology of many disorders, and many previously mysterious diseases can now be attributed to mitochondrial disorders accompanied by cellular energy failure. We have also attempted to address these advances.

With the combination of print and electronic journals, the effort to stay current in a single subspecialty remains a daunting task. Indeed, presenting the current status of the field of neonatal-perinatal medicine, even in a two-volume textbook, has become extremely challenging. It is a tribute to the contributors to *Neonatal-Perinatal Medicine* that this text has reached its ninth edition. We are profoundly grateful to both our loyal and our new contributors who give so freely of their time and knowledge.

For this ninth edition, we have added several new sections ranging from problems of the late preterm infant to fetal origins of adult disease. We have, in addition, completely reorganized and rewritten a large number of chapters and significantly updated the rest. Our accomplished authors and careful editing continue to focus on the biologic basis of developmental disorders and evidence basis for their management. We have also increasingly sought to draw upon international leaders in the field of neonatal-perinatal medicine to provide a truly global perspective.

This book would not exist without the remarkable clinical and intellectual environment that constitutes Rainbow Babies and Children's Hospital in Cleveland. On a daily basis, we gain knowledge from our faculty colleagues and fellows, and wisdom from our nursing staff, who are so committed to their young patients. Once again, we have been blessed with an in-house editor, Bonnie Siner, to whom we cannot adequately express our thanks. She is the glue behind the binding in the book and has worked tirelessly with Elsevier staff members to bring this project to fruition. Elsevier has once again provided the resources to accomplish this mammoth task.

RICHARD J. MARTIN

AVROY A. FANAROFF

MICHELE C. WALSH

Contents

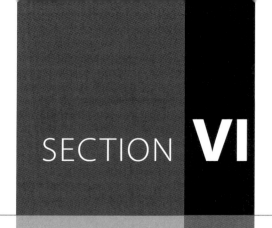

Development and Disorders of Organ Systems

CHAPTER 39

The Immune System

PART 1

Developmental Immunology
Reuben Kapur, Mervin C. Yoder, and Richard A. Polin

Developmental immunology can be defined as the study of how adaptive host defense blood cells in an individual sequentially respond to repetitive environmental challenges in a way that promotes the health and survival of the individual throughout maturation from fetal to adult life. According to classic principles, an individual becomes immune, or protected from reinfection, in response to an antigenic encounter during an initial infection. Mature immunologic competence is ultimately achieved through cumulative adaptive changes stimulated by exposure to a large repertoire of foreign antigenic material. Because the in utero fetal environment is sequestered from frequent encounters with microorganisms, the host defense system of the human newborn is inexperienced. This inexperience partially accounts for why newborns are so vulnerable to microbial attack during the first 6 weeks of life. Although many components of the immune system of the fetus are present early in gestation, some are immature and do not become fully functional (compared with the activity of immune defenses of adult subjects) until some time after birth. Despite these limitations, fetal host defense systems are capable of active engagement, and an immune response does occur when the fetus is infected in utero.

An understanding of the development of the immune system in a particular fetus or neonate must take into account the specific environment in which that individual is developing. Because more prematurely born neonates with very low birthweight are surviving, it is possible to ask how the immunologic development of these infants (in an extra-uterine environment) differs from in utero immunologic development of comparably aged fetuses. This chapter reviews the sequential appearance of the many components of the immune system in neonates and compares the functional activities of these components with those of immunologically competent adults.

The immunologic system may be divided into two systems of host defense mechanisms: innate, or nonspecific, immune mechanisms, and acquired, or specific, immune mechanisms.

By definition, *innate immunity* includes host defense mechanisms that operate effectively without prior exposure to a microorganism or its antigens. Some of these mechanisms include physical barriers, such as intact skin and mucous membranes, and chemical barriers, such as gastric acid and digestive enzymes. Beneath these important protective layers lie phagocytic cells, which constitute the first line of host defense against any microbes that breach the cutaneous and mucosal barriers. Soluble plasma and tissue proteins serve to amplify the function of the phagocytic cells as innate immune effectors. *Acquired,* or specific, *immunity* comprises primarily the cell-mediated (T lymphocyte) and humoral (B lymphocyte and immunoglobulin) systems.

Innate and acquired immune mechanisms are necessary for an individual to become fully immunocompetent. These systems are intimately interrelated and interdependent. Monocytes and macrophages are important components of natural immunity because these cells function to ingest and clear microbial pathogens from normal tissues. Monocytes and macrophages also play an important role in the processing and presentation of microbial antigenic material to T lymphocytes, a pivotal initiation step in the generation of a specific immune response. Monocytes and macrophages are important components of the innate and the acquired immune systems, and are necessary for an effective immune response.

OVERVIEW OF HEMATOPOIESIS

All the cellular components of the immunologic system have limited life spans; the cells must be constantly replenished from a pool of undifferentiated precursor cells derived from a pluripotent stem cell. Hematopoietic stem cells are capable of self-renewal, ensuring maintenance of a lifelong pool of available hematopoietic precursors. Through mechanisms that are not well understood, pluripotent stem cells are stimulated to divide and differentiate into multipotent stem and committed progenitor cells, which mature into circulating blood cells.[3] Fibroblasts, endothelial cells, and macrophages present in the microenvironment of the hematopoietic stem cells synthesize extracellular matrix molecules and growth factors that are crucial to the process of progenitor-derived blood cell production.

Evidence that mice could be protected from the lethal effects of total-body irradiation by exteriorizing and shielding of the spleen provided some of the first evidence that the hematopoietic system may be maintained through a population of precursor cells. Later, Till and McCulloch[50] showed that marrow withdrawn from a donor animal could repopulate the spleen of a lethally irradiated recipient animal with progenitor cells, giving rise to discrete colonies of red blood cells, megakaryocytes, granulocytes, and macrophages. The pluripotent hematopoietic stem cell was first isolated and characterized in mice. An equivalent cell in humans can be inferred from the successful long-term engraftment and proliferation of donor cells in recipient patients after bone marrow transplantation.

Development of other monoclonal antibodies that recognize cell surface molecules highly expressed by murine and human hematopoietic stem cells has permitted isolation and characterization of the growth and differentiation requirements of this rare hematopoietic cell population. In vitro colony-forming assays have been used to confirm that the proliferation and survival of hematopoietic progenitor cells are maintained by hematopoietic growth factors. Hematopoietic growth factors not only promote production of blood cells, but also enhance the maturation of cells; granulocyte ingestion and killing of invading microbes are stimulated by several hematopoietic growth factors. Hematopoietic growth factors play an important regulatory role in providing adequate numbers of functionally mature blood cells during systemic infections.

Fetal hematopoiesis begins in a primitive state early in gestation, before the development of a mature bone marrow hematopoietic microenvironment. The anatomic location of blood cell production changes several times during gestation as stem cells apparently home from one site to another.[61] Early hematopoietic activity is restricted to the yolk sac until 6 to 8 weeks of gestation, when the liver becomes the predominant site. As gestation proceeds to the 20th week, the bone marrow becomes the major site of hematopoiesis, and thereafter remains the primary reservoir for replenishing circulating populations of immune cells.

INNATE IMMUNITY
Cellular Components

The most primitive host defense mechanism involves the ingestion and killing of bacteria and other microorganisms by phagocytic cells. Polymorphonuclear neutrophils (PMNs), monocytes, and macrophages are the major cell types that accomplish this aspect of host defense. Natural killer (NK) cells are also important components of the innate immune system, but these cells kill invading pathogens by nonphagocytic mechanisms. All these cell types can eliminate pathogens from the host, but do so more efficiently when the pathogens are opsonized, or coated, by complement components and other soluble proteins of the innate immune system. Likewise, the nonphagocytic mechanisms of microbial cytolysis used by NK cells, PMNs, and monocytes are augmented in the presence of specific antibody to the target organism. This section provides an overview of the phagocyte and NK cell systems and highlights the areas in which phagocytes isolated from fetal and neonatal blood seem functionally immature.

POLYMORPHONUCLEAR NEUTROPHIL SYSTEM
Kinetics of Production and Circulation

The PMN system arises from a progenitor cell called the colony-forming unit granulocyte-macrophage (CFU-GM). As the name implies, this stem cell–derived progenitor cell may differentiate into PMNs or monocytes. The myeloblast is the first identifiable neutrophil precursor. Myeloblasts produce many daughter cells (myelocytes). These nonproliferating cells require 7 days to become fully differentiated PMNs. This postmitotic compartment of differentiating but immature PMNs (metamyelocyte and band forms) and mature bone marrow PMNs constitutes a reserve pool of cells that may be rapidly mobilized into the circulation in response to inflammation.

Positive and negative regulators of PMN production have been identified. Positive regulatory factors are interleukin (IL)-3, granulocyte-macrophage colony-stimulating factor (GM-CSF), and granulocyte CSF. Several negative regulators of PMN production have also been identified, including interferons (IFNs), transforming growth factor-α, macrophage inflammatory protein 1a, prostaglandins, and lactoferrin and other iron-binding proteins.

Although it is unclear what factors cause PMN release from the bone marrow under normal conditions, IL-1, tumor necrosis factor-α (TNFα), epinephrine, and complement component fragments are known to stimulate PMN release from the bone marrow during inflammatory states. When mature PMNs leave the marrow environment, they circulate for approximately 6 to 8 hours before migrating into tissues, where they live for an additional 24 hours. While in the bloodstream, half of the PMNs are found in a marginated pool (primarily in the pulmonary capillaries), and half are circulating in the peripheral blood. After PMNs emigrate from the blood vessels and enter a tissue, they do not reenter blood vessels, but age and die in the tissue. The actual site of PMN clearance is unknown, but macrophages ingest and degrade senescent apoptotic PMNs in vitro.

In the human fetus, PMN precursors are first identified in the yolk sac stage of primitive hematopoiesis.[61] Mature PMNs are not identifiable in the fetal liver or bone marrow until approximately 14 weeks of gestation. By 22 to 23 weeks of gestation, the circulating PMN count has increased, but still is only approximately 2% of the circulating PMN concentration measured in the cord blood of term gestation newborns. At the same time that circulating concentrations of PMNs are low, fetal blood contains high concentrations of circulating hematopoietic progenitors. This high concentration of circulating progenitors may not be indicative of a large total body pool of progenitors, however. The actual number of CFU-GMs in the human neonate is unknown. In comparative studies of fetal and neonatal rat hematopoiesis, the total-body CFU-GM pool was approximately 10% by weight of that of adult rats. One explanation for the high concentration of circulating progenitors is that these stem cells may be leaving one hematopoietic environment (the liver) for another (the bone marrow).

Circulating concentrations of PMNs increase dramatically at birth, peak at 12 to 24 hours, and then decline slowly by 72 hours to values that remain stable during the neonatal period. The PMN count rarely decreases to less than 3000/mm³ during the first 3 days and less than 1500/mm³ thereafter in term infants, although PMN counts in preterm infants may be 1100/mm³. When searching for the cause of neutropenia (<1500 PMNs/mm³) in infants, a strong suspicion of infection is warranted, although infants with preeclamptic mothers, premature birth, birth depression, intraventricular hemorrhage, and Rh hemolytic disease may have low peripheral PMN counts. Persistent neutropenia is one feature that is frequently seen in patients who succumb to overwhelming sepsis. Neutropenia in these infants may occur because of increased margination of activated circulating cells or may be related to rapid depletion of circulating and bone marrow storage pool PMNs. Whatever the mechanism, failure to provide adequate numbers of PMNs to areas of microbial invasion in tissues may be a factor that places the infant at increased risk for development of overwhelming sepsis.[25]

Overview of Polymorphonuclear Neutrophil Functions

The PMN is qualitatively and quantitatively the most effective killing phagocyte of host defense. Numerous coordinated steps are required to attract large numbers of PMNs from the circulating blood into a tissue at the site of microbial invasion (Fig. 39-1). When microorganisms penetrate cutaneous or mucosal barriers, macrophages and PMNs appear in the tissue, and along with the complement, kinin, and coagulation systems, initiate a series of events resulting in the release of complement fragments (particularly C5a) and other factors (IL-1, TNFα, and chemokines) that alter vascular endothelial cell morphology and function in the area of infection.

The initial recognition of invading microbes by the macrophages and PMNs is facilitated by the presence of pattern recognition receptors (Toll-like receptors [TLRs]) on the surface of the phagocytes that are specific for certain molecules distinctly expressed by bacteria, fungi, and viruses. Engagement of TLRs (see later) activates the phagocytes to release inflammatory mediators that affect endothelial cells in the immediate vicinity. These changes in the endothelial cell surface and the presence of numerous soluble inflammatory mediators cause circulating PMNs to withdraw from the circulation and adhere to the "inflamed" endothelium. After tightly adhering to the endothelium, the PMN begins a process of diapedesis through adjacent endothelial cells and the intact underlying basement membrane. When the PMN has penetrated the basement membrane, the cell emigrates from the blood vessel into the area of inflammation.

Initial random migration (chemokinesis) becomes highly directed (chemotaxis) by the increasing concentration of chemotactic factors secreted by activated monocytes and macrophages. Other chemotactic agents generated at the site of infection include products of complement activation and some byproducts of the microorganisms. On reaching the area of bacterial invasion, the PMN ingests encountered microbes and begins a process of biochemical activation resulting in generation of reactive oxygen intermediates and other metabolites, which are used to kill the pathogen. Selected aspects of this complex process are described further later on.

ADHESION

PMN adhesion to endothelial cells is a crucial step in the recruitment of these leukocytes to inflammatory sites. Although PMNs can adhere to normal or activated vascular endothelium, inflammation is associated with hemodynamic

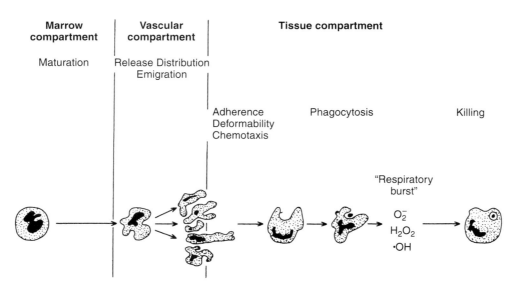

Figure 39-1. Overview of polymorphonuclear neutrophil (PMN) functions. PMNs are produced and mature in the bone marrow over a 2-week period. On release from the marrow, PMNs circulate for 6 to 8 hours before emigrating into tissues. At sites of infection, chemotactic factors enhance PMN adhesion to and emigration through vascular endothelium, and PMNs migrate in a directed fashion (chemotaxis) toward the pathogens. Phagocytosis of the offending organisms stimulates an increase in production of oxygen metabolites (respiratory burst), which facilitates PMN killing of the ingested microbes.

and biochemical changes in blood vessels that facilitate leukocyte adhesion to the vessel endothelial lining. It is now apparent that a series of changes in the expression of specific glycoproteins occurs on the leukocyte and the endothelial cell surface during inflammation.

One family of structurally and functionally related proteins found on the plasma membrane of all myeloid cells seems to mediate many adhesion-related neutrophil functions (i.e., chemotaxis, phagocytosis, degranulation, and aggregation). These cell surface glycoproteins belong to the integrin family of receptors and are designated CD11/CD18 leukocyte adhesion molecules. Each heterodimeric protein consists of one immunologically distinct α subunit (leukocyte functional antigen-1; CD11a, Mac-1; CD11b, P150, 95; CD11c), but all share a common β subunit (CD18). Monoclonal antibodies directed against CD11b/CD18 inhibit PMN aggregation, spread, chemotaxis, and adhesion to endothelial cells. CD11b/CD18 and CD11c/CD18 serve as complement receptors and mediate complement-coated (fragment iC3b) particle ingestion by PMNs. CD11a/CD18 has been shown to be important in PMN killing of target cells through antibody-dependent mechanisms. Patients with a heritable deficiency of these leukocyte cell surface glycoproteins have recurrent infections characterized by failure to accumulate granulocytes at sites of infection.

Neutrophil adhesion to vascular endothelium and to other phagocytes depends on several specific receptor-ligand interactions at the cell surface membrane (Fig. 39-2). Circulating neutrophils usually roll along vascular endothelial cells with transient interactions between neutrophil selectins on the cell surface and counter-receptors on the endothelium. When endothelial cells are activated during inflammation, more selectin counter-receptors (see Fig. 39-2) are expressed, and additional proteins (intercellular adhesion molecule [ICAM]-1 and ICAM-2 in Fig. 39-2) of the immunoglobulin supergene family, which serve as ligands for the neutrophil integrin family, are activated. The rolling neutrophil is slowed by the more concentrated interactions of the neutrophil cell surface selectins and the endothelial counter-receptors. Simultaneously, increased interactions of neutrophil cell surface integrins with endothelial ICAM-1 and ICAM-2 (see Fig. 39-2) occur, neutrophil cell surface selectins are shed, and a firm neutrophil-endothelial adhesive interaction is established. Neutrophils migrate between endothelial cells and emigrate into the tissue toward the nidus of microorganisms.

Adhesion of PMNs to artificial surfaces in vitro is comparable for unstimulated PMNs isolated from neonatal or adult blood. When PMNs from term neonates are stimulated with chemotactic factors, adhesion is greatly diminished, however, compared with cells isolated from adults. More profound deficits are displayed by PMNs from preterm infants. Less stimulated mobilization and overall expression of CD11b/CD18 glycoproteins on the plasma membrane is one important factor contributing to decreased stimulated adherence. Other causes of diminished stimulated adherence include impaired capacity to upregulate cell surface chemotactic receptors, lower granular content of lactoferrin, less fibronectin binding to the cell surface, and less shape change (failure to increase significantly overall cell surface area on chemotactic factor stimulation). Downregulation of L-selectin

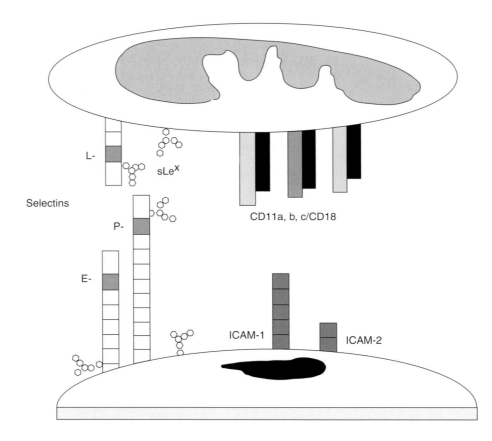

Figure 39–2. Adhesion of white blood cells to endothelial cells is mediated by several receptor-ligand pair interactions, including the selectin-carbohydrate (sialylated Lewis-x [sLe^x]) and integrin-immunoglobulin families. ICAM, intercellular adhesion molecule. (*From Bevilacqua MI: Endothelial-leukocyte adhesion molecules, Annu Rev Immunol 11:767, 1993, with permission.*)

expression on term newborn cord blood granulocytes and monocytes during acute inflammation has been shown, although the pattern and level of shedding vary from neutrophils isolated from adult subjects.[24]

Normal PMNs exhibit a biphasic pattern of aggregation, followed by disaggregation when exposed to chemotactic factors. Newborn cord blood PMNs readily aggregate, but do not disaggregate when stimulated. This irreversible aggregation of PMNs would represent an impairment to cellular emigration from inflamed blood vessels if this phenomenon occurred in vivo in newborns.

CHEMOTAXIS

Chemotaxis is defined as the directed migration of PMNs toward the origin of a chemoattracting substance (see Fig. 39-1). This movement involves a series of orchestrated events, including PMN binding of the chemoattractant (by cell surface receptors), generation of an intracellular second messenger that is coupled to the receptor-ligand binding, and remodeling of the plasma membrane and cytoskeleton to produce shape changes and proper orientation of the cellular contents toward the highest concentration of the chemoattractant. Morphologically, the PMN orients toward the chemoattractant, with the leading edge (lamellipodium) of the cell becoming more spread and possessing many ruffles. Most of the intracellular organelles remain at the posterior pole of the cell (uropod). As the cell moves, the leading edge adheres to available surfaces, and contraction of cytoskeletal microfilaments (actin and myosin) pulls along the rest of the cell. Many aspects of this process are poorly developed in PMNs isolated from neonatal blood. Some of the chemotactic defects of PMNs present during the neonatal period persist throughout early childhood.

PMNs must recognize a concentration gradient of the attracting substance to move in a directed fashion. Specific cell surface receptors at the leading edge of the cell bind the chemoattractant. The number of receptors for a commonly used in vitro chemoattractant, N-formyl-methionyl-leucyl-phenylalanine (f-MLP), seems to be equal on PMNs from neonates and adults. When stimulated with other chemoattractants, fewer receptors for f-MLP are redistributed, however, from intracellular granules to the plasma membrane in PMNs isolated from cord blood. These cells show an apparent defect in transduction of the signals of f-MLP binding. There are significant impairments in the generation of subcellular second messengers and associated alterations in intracellular and extracellular membrane potential that are normally associated with chemoattractant binding to PMNs from adult subjects.[60] In addition, chemotactic factor stimulation fails to mobilize sufficient CD11b/CD18 to the plasma membrane, and, as discussed earlier, this complement receptor is important in many adhesion-related processes. The in vivo functional relationship of these intracellular defects to impaired chemotaxis of PMNs from neonatal cord blood remains to be clarified.

PMN movement requires dynamic cytoskeletal involvement. Despite similar baseline concentrations of filamentous (F) actin, PMNs from newborns do not generate significant additional levels of F actin after chemotactic factor stimulation compared with PMNs from adults[18]; this may impair cell movement and orientation. PMNs from neonatal cord blood fail to orient as quickly and do not sustain the bipolar configuration of chemotactic factor–stimulated PMNs isolated from adult blood.

PMNs must be deformable to emigrate from the intravascular to the extravascular space and through the extracellular matrix of tissues. PMNs from neonatal cord blood are less deformable than cells from adults. Because the energy-dependent interaction of the contractile proteins actin and myosin influences cell deformability, differences in the extent or rate of microfilament polymerization between PMNs from neonates and PMNs from adults may be relevant. Decreased deformability may also be due to the failure to generate intracellular second messengers (cyclic adenosine monophosphate) after stimulation, to overall lower intracellular concentrations of adenosine triphosphate (necessary for microfilament contraction), or to differences in plasma membrane fluidity between PMNs isolated from neonates and PMNs from adults.[36]

PMNs from term neonates are deficient in in vitro chemotactic ability. PMNs from premature infants are even more impaired. Similar deficits in PMN mobility have been shown in human newborns in vivo. When the skin of newborns is inflamed by the skin window technique, leukocyte accumulation is delayed and less intense than in adults. Overall, impaired mobility is the most consistently observed defect in PMN function in human newborns, and it contributes in a large way to the increased infectious susceptibility of neonates.

PHAGOCYTOSIS

Phagocytosis is a process of particle ingestion. Most particulate matter must be opsonized (coated) with IgG, complement fragments C3b or iC3b, fibronectin, or other proteins before being recognized and engulfed by PMNs (Fig. 39-3). After binding of the opsonized microbe by an appropriate cell surface receptor, the PMN extends pseudopods to surround the particle and form a phagocytic vacuole.

PMNs of term and preterm infants have normal phagocytic activity under most normal in vitro test conditions. These cells express diminished amounts, however, and do not upregulate the complement receptor CR3 (CD11b/CD18) when stimulated with chemotactic factors to the same degree as PMNs from adults. When stressed by a high ratio of microbes to PMNs in vitro, phagocytosis of gram-negative organisms and yeast particles by PMNs of neonates is deficient. In addition, alterations in phagocytosis have been reported for PMNs isolated from clinically stressed premature newborns. PMNs of well newborns show normal phagocytic activity, but under stressful conditions, microbe ingestion may be altered.

MICROBICIDAL ACTIVITY

Oxygen-independent and oxygen-dependent mechanisms of microbial killing are used by the PMN. Microbe disruption occurs in the phagolysosome, which is formed when the phagosome fuses with primary and secondary neutrophil granules. Within the phagolysosome, cationic proteins, lysozyme, lactoferrin, and H^+ function as oxygen-independent microbicidal mechanisms. Oxygen-dependent killing begins with PMN membrane perturbation during receptor binding of the opsonized particle and phagocytosis. A respiratory burst (an increase in oxygen consumption) ensues as reactive

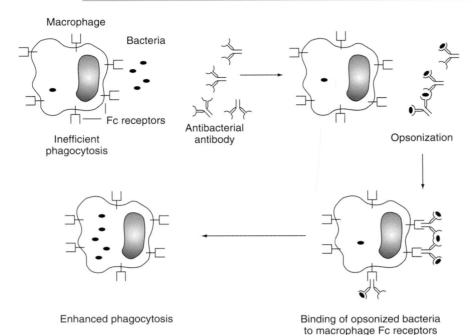

Figure 39–3. Antibody-dependent opsonization and phagocytosis of bacteria. Antibody binding to particles such as bacteria can markedly enhance the efficiency of phagocytosis. Enhancement of phagocytosis in macrophages involves increased attachment of the coated particle to the cell surface membrane and commensurate activation of the phagocyte, both of which are mediated through occupancy of Fc receptors. *(From Abbas AK et al, editors: Cellular and molecular immunology, 2nd ed, Philadelphia, 1994, Saunders, with permission.)*

oxygen intermediates are synthesized. First, a membrane oxidase is activated that ultimately leads to production of superoxide (O_2^-), which can lead to hydrogen peroxide (H_2O_2) synthesis. These intermediate products combine to form highly reactive hydroxyl radicals. In addition, myeloperoxidase present in PMN granules catalyzes the oxidation of halides (iodide, bromide, chloride) to hypohalous acids, which are powerful oxidants that cause bacterial cell wall dissolution.

PMNs isolated from well term neonates exhibit more rapid activation of the superoxide-generating system than PMNs from adults. These cells also produce more H_2O_2 than PMNs from adults; however, there are impairments in the later phases of oxidative metabolism. Decrements in hypochlorous acid production and in quantitative measures of reactive hydroxyl radical formation have been reported. Deficiencies in certain oxygen-detoxifying enzymes such as glutathione peroxidase and catalase may cause oxidative damage to the PMNs, may serve as a source of cell dysfunction, and may decrease neutrophil viability. Overall, microbicidal activity appears normal for PMNs of term and preterm infants, unless these infants are clinically ill. When stressed, defects in killing of group B streptococci, *Escherichia coli,* and other microorganisms become readily apparent and significant.

Summary

PMNs of term and preterm infants are as capable of ingesting and killing microbial pathogens as are PMNs of adults, unless the infants are clinically ill. Under conditions of stress, these PMNs do not function with normal phagocytic and microbicidal activities. PMNs isolated from the blood of neonates consistently display diminished chemotactic and adhesion capacities. It is unclear what role these disturbed PMN functions play in causing the neonate to be so highly susceptible to systemic infections.

A rationale for the use of hematopoietic growth factors to improve neutrophil function qualitatively and quantitatively has been well established.[49] In multiple studies involving neonatal animals and human infants, administration of granulocyte CSF or GM-CSF has been documented to increase the neutrophil storage pool, induce neutrophilia, and improve many neutrophil functions. A recommendation for the use of these growth factors to decrease the incidence of morbidity and mortality associated with sepsis in newborns cannot yet be made based on published work, however.

MONONUCLEAR PHAGOCYTE SYSTEM

Production and Differentiation

The mononuclear phagocyte system comprises bone marrow monocyte precursors, circulating monocytes, and mature macrophages.[8] As with the granulocyte lineage, mononuclear phagocytes are derived from CFU-GM progenitor cells. Several hematopoietic growth factors influence mononuclear phagocyte production. CSF-1 or macrophage CSF is the major hematopoietic growth factor influencing maturation and production of mononuclear phagocytes. Cells of this lineage seem to be unique in expressing cell surface receptors for CSF-1. On leaving the bone marrow, monocytes circulate for nearly 72 hours and then migrate into tissues, where the local extracellular milieu strongly influences monocyte-to-macrophage differentiation. Although the ultimate fate of macrophages is unclear, these cells have been observed to live for several months in many human tissues.

Monocyte-to-macrophage differentiation has been well characterized, but the control mechanisms involved remain elusive. As monocytes develop into macrophages, certain morphologic changes occur. The cells increase in diameter more than threefold and acquire more cytoplasmic granules and vacuoles. Differentiation is also associated with increased expression of cell surface receptors, biosynthesis of numerous biologically active molecules, and improved phagocytic activity.[40] Similar to PMNs, all mononuclear phagocytes have a well-developed cytoskeletal apparatus that is important in determining cell mobility and participation in many adhesion-related functions.

Macrophages may be first identified in the fetus in the hematopoietic foci of the yolk sac. Before the liver becomes the major site of hematopoiesis, macrophages constitute nearly 70% of the blood cells present in the liver. Over the next few weeks, erythroblasts increase in number and predominate, with hepatic macrophages declining to 1% to 2% of all differentiated blood cells. Few macrophages are present in the developing fetal lung, but at birth a rapid influx of macrophages is observed. Macrophage populations in the lung and other organs are maintained by local proliferation of macrophages and by influx of circulating bone marrow–derived monocytes. The stimulus for monocyte recruitment into tissues at homeostasis remains unclear.

Circulating monocytes do not appear in fetal blood before the fifth month of gestation; however, at 30 weeks' gestation, monocytes increase to 3% to 7% of the circulating formed blood cells. At birth and throughout the neonatal period, circulating monocyte concentrations exceed 500/mm^3, a value considered high for adults.

Mononuclear Phagocyte Functions
ADHESION
Mononuclear phagocytes adhere to various cells and tissues, and play central roles in wound healing, inflammation, and immune responses. Similar to neutrophils, mononuclear phagocytes must emigrate from blood vessels at inflammatory sites to eradicate invading microbes. Generally, mononuclear phagocyte recruitment and accumulation lag behind the brisk PMN influx by 6 to 12 hours, but the former process persists for several days. Mononuclear phagocytes are necessary not only for host defense at inflammatory sites, but also for tissue débridement and initiation of wound repair. Inability of PMNs and mononuclear phagocytes to accumulate at sites of inflammation or injury because of impaired adhesion-related functions results in recurring, poorly healing cutaneous abscesses.

Monocyte influx into inflammatory sites is impaired in neonates compared with adults. Whether this delay results from inadequate tissue release of monocyte attractants, impaired monocyte mobility, or impaired adhesion and emigration has not been clarified. Most evidence suggests that monocyte adhesion to artificial surfaces is unimpaired during the neonatal period. Deficits in other adhesion-related functions seem to explain the delayed accumulation of monocytes in injured tissues of neonates (see later).

CHEMOTAXIS
Monocyte chemotactic activity is decreased during the neonatal period, and this impaired mobility persists throughout early childhood. Although random migration of cord blood and peripheral blood monocytes seems unimpaired at birth, decreased migration in response to chemoattractants is noted soon after. Chemotaxis of cord blood monocytes is nearly normal, but monocytes isolated from the peripheral blood of newborns do not migrate normally. The chemotactic activity

of these cells sequentially declines over the first week of life before slowly improving and achieving (by age 6 years) the chemotactic activity of monocytes isolated from the blood of adults. Impaired migration in response to chemoattractants may be a primary factor in the delayed influx of monocytes at inflammatory sites during the neonatal period.

PHAGOCYTOSIS
The ability of mononuclear phagocytes to ingest a variety of soluble and particulate matter is vital to the role these cells play in the immune response. Endocytosis is important in microbial elimination, removal of senescent and transformed cells, and antigen processing for initiation of specific immune responses. Mononuclear phagocytes ingest microscopic fluid and soluble matter through a process of pinocytosis, whereas large particulate material is taken up through phagocytosis. Both processes involve cell surface membrane extension, particle enclosure, and translocation of the phagosome into the cell interior. As with neutrophils, macrophage phagocytosis is enhanced when particulate material is coated with IgG or complement fragments, and the opsonized particles engage cell surface Fc and C3b receptors.

Monocyte ingestion of *Staphylococcus aureus, E. coli, Streptococcus pyogenes, Toxoplasma gondii,* and herpes simplex virus type 2 seems quantitatively normal during the neonatal period, although the rate of ingestion may be slower. Similarly, alveolar macrophage ingestion of *Candida albicans* seems normal in newborns (who were intubated and receiving assisted ventilation) compared with the phagocytic capacity of alveolar macrophages isolated by bronchoalveolar lavage of adult volunteers.

Some evidence exists, however, of a selective impairment in phagocytosis of GBS. In these studies, monocytes isolated from neonatal cord blood ingested fewer organisms than monocytes isolated from adult peripheral blood. Phagocytosis of group B streptococci significantly increases when monocytes of newborns are incubated with organisms preopsonized with fibronectin and IgG.

MICROBICIDAL ACTIVITY
The generation of reactive oxygen intermediates is only one of several mechanisms used by mononuclear phagocytes to kill microbes. Similar to neutrophils, mononuclear phagocytes undergo a respiratory burst when particulate or soluble stimuli are engaged and ingested. The biosynthesis of O_2^-, H_2O_2, and hypohalous acids remains an important mechanism for killing of organisms by monocytes, but during the differentiation of these cells into macrophages, the magnitude of the respiratory burst diminishes, and myeloperoxidase-containing granules disappear from the cytoplasm. The reduced microbicidal function of macrophages is important because it permits these cells to remove small numbers of microorganisms from tissues without causing extensive tissue damage. Oxygen-independent microbicidal agents synthesized by macrophages include cationic proteins (defensins), lipid hydrolases, proteases, and nucleases. These agents, in combination with a highly acidified phagolysosome, seem to be cytolytically effective against many pathogenic microbes.

The microbicidal activity of mononuclear phagocytes can be regulated by cytokines. IFN-γ seems to be the most important activating agent; however, GM-CSF and TNFα also play important roles. Activated macrophages exhibit enhanced release of proinflammatory cytokines, upregulation of Fc receptors, and increased production of reactive oxygen intermediates. In contrast, IL-10 and transforming growth factor-α function as potent suppressors of some macrophage functions.

The ability of mononuclear phagocytes to generate reactive oxygen intermediates is normal during the neonatal period. Monocytes isolated from neonatal cord blood kill ingested bacteria and parasites as efficiently as cells from adult peripheral blood. Alveolar macrophages and monocyte-derived macrophages are also unimpaired in killing S. aureus and C. albicans during the neonatal period. IFN-γ production and the response of mononuclear phagocytes to exogenous IFN-γ are diminished, however, in newborns. How well fixed-tissue macrophages kill bacteria, parasites, and viruses and the response of these cells to cytokine stimulation remain untested.

Summary

The influx of mononuclear phagocytes to sites of inflammation is delayed and attenuated in newborns. This defect is most likely related to the impaired chemotactic activity displayed by the peripheral blood monocytes of these infants. Phagocytosis and microbicidal activity seem equivalent to the level displayed by mononuclear phagocytes of adults. In vivo studies of macrophage function at birth and during the neonatal period are limited, but pulmonary alveolar macrophages seem to function normally in the infants examined to date.

NATURAL KILLER CELL SYSTEM

Phenotypic and Functional Characteristics

Generally, NK cells are defined by their large granular morphology. These cells make up almost 15% of peripheral blood lymphocytes in adults and are found in several tissues, including liver, peritoneal cavity, placenta, and bone marrow. Human NK cells are defined by the expression of cell surface proteins CD56 and CD16 (low-affinity IgG receptor). NK cells lack the expression of T cell markers such as CD3. Murine NK cells are defined by the presence of the cell surface proteins NK1.1 and DX5. Similar to human NK cells, murine NK cells also lack the expression of CD3. In humans, NK cells have been subdivided further into two subsets on the basis of CD56 cell surface expression. These two NK cell subsets mediate distinct functions. CD56hi NK cells biosynthesize and secrete higher levels of cytokines such as TNFα, IFN-γ, GM-CSF, and IL-10 compared with CD56dim NK cells. CD56hi NK cells proliferate more efficiently in response to low doses of IL-2 compared with CD56dim NK cells. In contrast, CD56dim NK cells are more efficient at mediating NK cell cytotoxicity and antibody-dependent cell-mediated cytotoxicity compared with CD56hi NK cells; this is partly due to differences in the level of CD16 expression between these two subsets of NK cells.

NK cells play a crucial role in controlling viral infections and in eradicating tumor cells. NK cells recognize infected, transformed, and stressed cells in the body and eliminate them either by directly killing them or by synthesizing cytokines and chemokines, which activate several cellular components of adaptive immunity. NK cells not only play an important role in innate immunity, but also integrate various components of innate and adaptive immunity to mount an efficient immune response.

Mice that lack NK cells are susceptible to viral infections, including cytomegalovirus (CMV) infections. The gene that confers resistance to CMV infection has been mapped to an area on the chromosome that encodes several NK cell receptor genes.[62] NK cell receptors recognize virally infected cells and tumor cells and deliver a cytolytic response. Mice expressing defective NK cell cytolytic activity display impaired rejection of tumor cells in vivo. Restoration of NK cell function in NK cell–deficient mice suppresses tumor rejection and growth. Patients with mutations in the gene that encodes the transcription factor nuclear factor-κB (NF-κB) have defective NK cell activity despite normal numbers of NK cells, suggesting that NF-κB activity must regulate a crucial aspect of NK cell cytolytic function. Subsequent studies have shown that NF-κB plays an essential role in regulating the expression of perforin in NK cells. Perforin is known to play a crucial role in regulating NK cell cytolytic functions, and deficiency of perforin in NK cells impairs their cytolytic activity against virally infected host cells and tumor cells.

As discussed, NK cells recognize virally infected, stressed, and transformed cells through cell surface receptors. Generally, NK cells survey tissues and cells in the body for the expression of "self" major histocompatibility complex (MHC) class I molecules.[6,9] In the absence of adequate levels of MHC class I expression on autologous virally infected, transformed, or stressed cells, NK cells through their activating receptors deliver a "lethal hit," destroying them. In addition to expressing activating receptors, NK cells also express inhibitory receptors, however, that recognize normal levels of specific self MHC class I molecules on autologous cells and deliver an inhibitory rather than an activating signal, protecting normal cells from the cytotoxic effects of NK cells.

The mechanism by which an extracellular signal is converted into a series of intracellular events that eventually result in a cytotoxic response by NK cells is regulated partly by small signaling enzymes and adapter proteins in the cell. Activating NK cell receptors are associated with intracellular signaling molecules that contain a signature amino acid sequence known as the immunoreceptor tyrosine-based activation motif (ITAM).[6] ITAMs that activate NK cell receptors are essential for delivering the "lethal hit" to target cells, including virally infected and tumor cells. In contrast, inhibitory NK cell receptors are associated with intracellular signaling molecules that contain motifs crucial for inactivating NK cell cytotoxic functions. These motifs are known as the immunoreceptor tyrosine-based inhibitory motifs, and are closely associated with MHC class I molecules.

Together, immunoreceptor tyrosine-based inhibitory motifs and MHC class I molecules deliver a negative "off" signal to NK cells, protecting normal cells from the cytotoxic effects of NK cells. Under normal conditions, a fine balance between activating and inhibitory receptor function is maintained, which is essential for protecting normal autologous cells from the cytolytic activity of NK cells. In addition to using NK cell receptors, NK cells can mediate target cell killing by antibody-dependent cellular cytotoxicity on binding to IgG-coated cells through cell surface CD16 receptors. Collectively, these characteristics enable NK cells to act as a first line of defense, playing an important role in natural resistance against cancer and various infectious diseases.

Production and Differentiation of Natural Killer Cells

NK cells develop in human bone marrow from $CD34^+$ stem/progenitor cell precursors. The development of NK cells in the bone marrow requires the presence of the early-acting cytokines stem cell factor and Fms-like tyrosine kinase-3 (Flt3) ligand.[6] In addition to the requirement for stem cell factor and Flt3 ligand during the early phases of NK cell development, IL-15 is necessary for later stages of NK cell development and maturation. Mature NK cells express the IL-15 receptor α chain, the IL-2/15 receptor β chain, and the common cytokine receptor chain (γ-c), but do not express the IL-2 receptor α chain that is necessary for the formation of the high-affinity IL-2 receptor. Although high doses of IL-2 can stimulate NK cell proliferation, NK cell development is normal in mice that are deficient in the expression of IL-2 in vivo.

In contrast, NK cell development is impaired in vivo in mice that are deficient in the expression of either IL-2/IL-15 receptor β or γ-c genes.[6] These results suggest that IL-15 is indispensable for NK cell development, and that the α chain of the IL-15 receptor plays a unique role in the development of NK cells. Bone marrow stromal cells secrete IL-15, and exogenously added IL-15 supports NK cell development in vitro from human $CD34^+$ progenitor cells in the absence of bone marrow stromal cells. Likewise, in the murine system, IL-15 is necessary for the differentiation of functional NK cells in vitro.

Transcription Factors in the Development and Function of Natural Killer Cells

In addition to an essential role for cytokines in the development and maturation of NK cells, transcription factors play a crucial role in regulating the development of NK cells in vivo. Mice that lack the expression of the *ID2* gene show a significant reduction in NK cell numbers, although the generation of other lymphoid lineage cells is unaffected.[6] Genetic ablation of the Ets family of transcription factors also results in impaired NK cell lineage commitment. In mice, the production of IL-15 from bone marrow–derived stromal cells is partly regulated by the transcription factor, IFN regulatory factor-2. Deficiency of IFN regulatory factor-2 in mice results in impaired production of IL-15, and consequently these mice do not show terminal NK cell maturation. Genetic ablation of IFN regulatory factor-2 in mice also results in abnormal NK cell development and function. Taken together, the development of NK cells is complex and depends on several factors, including the regulation of cytokines by transcription factors.

Natural Killer Cell Function in Neonates

Most NK cells developing in human neonates express the CD16 and CD56 antigens. The percentage of NK cells in peripheral blood of newborns is similar to that of adult subjects. The absolute number of NK cells at birth is approximately twice that found in adult peripheral blood, presumably because of the higher total lymphocyte count. A small fraction of the neonatal NK cells fail to express CD56 and show poor cytolytic responses to target cells. In addition, compared with CD56-expressing NK cells, CD56-deficient NK cells do not respond well to exogenous IFN-γ stimulation. NK cell–mediated cytolysis in vitro generally is diminished during the neonatal period and early childhood. Defects in binding and lysis of target cells have been reported and are partly explained by impaired release of NK-derived IFNs and soluble cytotoxic factors. Baseline NK cell activity during the neonatal period is 30% to 80% of that of adult NK cells; however, treatment of NK cells with exogenous IL-2, IL-12, and IL-15 in vitro augments the cytolytic activity of NK cells derived from neonates. Nevertheless, the stimulated NK cell response in neonates remains suboptimal compared with adult NK cells. NK cells derived from neonates are functionally distinct from NK cells found in adults.

The functional defects in the development of NK cells in neonates have been proposed to be due partly to reduced expression of the γ-c chain on neonate-derived NK cells. The common γ-c chain is shared between cytokine receptors for IL-2, IL-4, IL-7, IL-9, and IL-15. Cord blood–derived NK cells express approximately one third of the level of γ-c chain expressed by NK cells. In vitro culture of the cord blood–derived NK cells induced a significant increase in the expression of γ-c chain, suggesting that reduced expression of γ-c chain in neonate NK cells may contribute significantly to infections in neonates.

Mutations in the γ-c chain in neonates have been linked to severe combined immunodeficiency (SCID) and profound reduction in NK cells. SCID is a rare, fatal syndrome characterized by profound deficiencies in lymphocyte function, including NK cells. Although most mutations resulting in SCID remain unknown, some studies have suggested a link between SCID and mutations in genes encoding adenosine deaminase, the γ-c chain of the IL-2 receptor and several other cytokine receptors, and Janus kinase 3, the intracellular signaling molecule that relays receptor-induced signals from the membrane to the nucleus.

Summary

NK cells are relatively normal in number in the neonatal period, but surface membrane expression of certain antigens is altered compared with adult NK cells. NK cell cytolytic activity against target cells in vitro is diminished during the neonatal period. The role of NK cell immaturity in contributing to the increased susceptibility of newborns to viral infection remains to be determined.

Humoral Components

OVERVIEW OF SERUM OPSONINS

The role of humoral factors in the enhancement of leukocyte phagocytosis of bacterial pathogens has been known since the turn of the 20th century. These heat-labile and heat-stable plasma proteins, called opsonins, consist mainly of serum antibodies and components of the complement system, although several other proteins seem to play important roles (see later). The opsonic activity of plasma or serum from newborn term infants is equivalent to activity measured in sera from adults until the test concentrations of plasma or serum are reduced to less than 10%. At low serum concentrations, opsonic activity against various bacteria and fungi is diminished during the neonatal period. Opsonic activity is reduced even more in premature infants and persists at test concentrations of plasma or serum greater than 10%. These deficiencies in opsonic activity may be related partly to lower complement and IgG and IgM concentrations in newborns. The complement system is described in the following section. The opsonic role and other functions of immunoglobulins are reviewed later, when antibodies are discussed as humoral components of specific immunity.

COMPLEMENT SYSTEM

Activation Pathways and Overview of Functional Products

The complement system plays an important role as one of the principal humoral effector pathways of immunity.[48] Its major function is to facilitate the neutralization of foreign substances either in the circulation or on mucous membranes. This function is accomplished by a series of plasma proteins that are involved in specific and nonspecific host defense mechanisms.

The classic pathway of complement activation requires the presence of specific antibodies against a particular antigen and the formation of immune complexes (Fig. 39-4). Two antibody molecules of the immune complex are bridged by the first component of complement, C1, which initiates a chain reaction in which one activated component serves as the enzyme that cleaves the next component in line. The order of component activation in the classic pathway is C1,

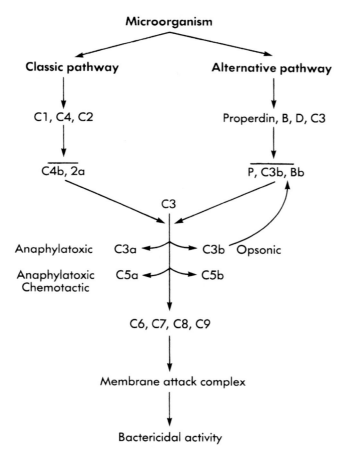

Figure 39–4. Complement system activation cascade. Activation of the classic pathway (*left*) and the alternative pathway (*right*) causes generation of soluble factors that amplify phagocyte functions and produces a membrane-bound attack complex that damages cell membranes. (*From McLean RH et al: Genetically determined variation in the complement system: relationship to disease,* J Pediatr *105:180, 1984, with permission.*)

C4, C2, and C3. Peptides with different biologic activities are created and either remain attached to the site of activation or diffuse into the milieu. The third component of complement, C3, is cleaved into membrane-bound C3b and the fluid phase C3a. With the generation of C3b, the classic pathway merges with the other mode of complement activation, the alternative pathway.

In contrast to the classic pathway, the alternative pathway may be activated by bacterial or mammalian cell surfaces in the absence of specific antibodies. This activation is possible because small amounts of C3 in the circulation are constantly being converted to C3b. This complement component can bind to cell surfaces, interact with the next alternative pathway components in sequence (factors B and D), and form a potent enzyme for further C3 activation (C3bBb). C3b originally generated by the classic pathway may involve this amplification loop of the alternative pathway and significantly enhance local C3 activation.

The central location of C3 in the complement pathway is important not only because the classic and alternative pathways converge at this point, but also because many biologic effects are determined by the interaction of this important molecule with various regulatory systems. The direction in which the complement pathway proceeds depends on the surface to which the C3b molecule is bound. Certain bacteria and other membranes offer a "protective surface" that favors the binding of C3b to factors B and D and the assembly of the enzyme that converts the next component in line, C5, into two biologically active fragments. The smaller product, C5a, acts as an anaphylatoxin to promote many aspects of acute inflammation, including chemoattraction of leukocytes and increasing vascular permeability. The larger fragment, C5b, remains attached to the C5 convertase on the membrane and assembles the components of the membrane attack complex: C5b, C6, C7, C8, and C9. Insertion of this complex into the cell membrane results in loss of membrane functions and cellular integrity.

In the absence of a protected site, C3b is exposed to factors I and H, which facilitate cleavage of C3b into iC3b and C3d. All these fragments of C3 can function as ligands for cellular receptors, which are located on erythrocytes and almost all immunocompetent cells. The C3b receptor (CR1) is known to mediate adherence of complement-coated complexes to erythrocytes, neutrophils, and mononuclear phagocytes and plays an important role in the clearance of immune complexes, bacteria, and cellular debris from the circulation. Other receptors also have been identified, such as the C3b-binding protein, CR2, which is found on B lymphocytes and eosinophils. Its function awaits clarification, but there is evidence that adherence of the Epstein-Barr virus is mediated by this receptor. Finally, the iC3b receptor (CR3, CD11b/CD18) seems to be important for the ability of the host to overcome bacterial invasion. As previously mentioned, patients with a genetic deficiency of leukocyte cell surface CR3 experience severe recurrent bacterial infections.

Ontogeny and Analysis of the Complement System in the Neonatal Period

Complement proteins are synthesized early in gestation. Synthesis of C2, C3, C4, and C5 can be confirmed between 8 and 14 weeks of gestation. Most evidence, derived through several methods, confirms that there is no transplacental passage of complement components.

The components of the classic complement system and their functional activity (measured by total hemolytic complement assay) in full-term neonates are nearly comparable with those of normal adults (Table 39-1). In some studies in which neonates were compared with their mothers, significant deficiencies in complement component concentrations were reported (approximately 50% of adult levels). These studies did not take into account that many complement components are acute-phase proteins, and their serum concentration during pregnancy is significantly elevated compared with other normal adults. Preterm neonates have significantly decreased concentrations, however, of C1q, C4, C3, and total hemolytic complement compared with term neonates. There is a statistically significant correlation between increasing birthweight or gestational age and serum concentrations of these components.

Alternative pathway activity and individual alternative pathway components are more deficient in concentration than classic pathway activity and components in term and preterm infants (see Table 39-1). Although the concentration of alternative pathway components in some newborn term infants is equivalent to the concentration in adults, most of these infants have lower measurable alternative pathway activity. In contrast to some classic pathway components, there is no correlation between factor B concentration and gestational age. Most serum alternative complement component values are equal to values measured in human adults by the first year of life (6 to 18 months of age).

TABLE 39-1   Summary of Published Complement Levels in Neonates

Complement Component	MEAN PERCENTAGE OF ADULT LEVELS	
	Term Neonate	Preterm Neonate
CH_{50}	56-90	45-71
AP_{50}	49-65	40-51
C1q	65-90	27-58
C4	60-100	42-91
C2	76-100	96
C3	60-100	39-78
C5	75	—
C6	47	—
C7	67	—
C9	14	—
B	35-59	36-50
P	33-71	13-65
H	61	—
iC3b	55	—

From Remington JS et al, editors: *Infectious diseases of the fetus and newborn infant,* 3rd ed, Philadelphia, 1990, Saunders, p 25.

Summary

Whether deficiencies in the complement system predispose a neonate to infection has not as yet been established.[48] Defects in the complement system and in the alternative pathway, in particular, are likely ultimately to be found to play a role in susceptibility to infection, especially in preterm infants. Newborns have a limited spectrum of antibody transmitted across the placenta; they receive IgG, no IgM, and little antibody to the entire range of gram-negative bacteria. The classic pathway has relatively little value at and shortly after birth. It follows that, in the absence of specific antibody, nonspecific activation of the biologically active fragments and complexes of the complement system through the alternative pathway becomes an extremely important defense mechanism for neonates during the first encounter with many bacteria. In most neonates, the functional deficiency of the alternative pathway, in conjunction with impaired functioning of PMNs, is likely to be clinically relevant.

FIBRONECTIN

Fibronectins are a class of multifunctional, high-molecular-weight glycoproteins that serve to facilitate cell-to-cell and cell-to-substratum adhesion. As adhesive ligands, fibronectins play an important role in directing cell migration, proliferation, and differentiation. Fibronectins seem essential for certain aspects of embryologic development of the fetus and for hemostasis, hematopoiesis, inflammation, and wound healing. In many pathophysiologic conditions (e.g., sepsis, thrombosis, cancer, organ fibrosis), the normal structure, physiology, and function of fibronectins are altered in a way that contributes to the underlying tissue or organ dysfunction.

Structure and Function

Fibronectins exist as soluble and insoluble dimeric molecules. Plasma fibronectin circulates at a mean concentration of 330 μg/mL in human adult peripheral blood. Soluble fibronectins have been identified in nearly every body fluid tested (synovial, ocular, pleural, amniotic, cerebrospinal, and others). Insoluble fibronectins are present in many connective tissues and extracellular matrices throughout the body. It is apparent that structural variants (isoforms) of fibronectin exist, and that expression of these isoforms is highly regulated in a cell-specific and tissue-specific fashion.

All fibronectins are capable of binding to multiple ligands simultaneously. The modular design of these glycoproteins translates into a linear array of active globular functional domains. Fibronectins display individual binding sites for some molecules and multiple sites for others. Fibronectins bind certain bacteria, heparin, fibrin, IgG, and DNA in several separate domains, but other bacteria, matrix molecules, actin, complement component C1q, and gangliosides are bound at unique sites in individual domains. In this way, fibronectin facilitates the interaction of cells with other cells, bacteria, tissues, particles, and soluble proteins.

Circulating plasma fibronectin concentrations are reduced in fetal cord blood (120 μg/mL) and in term infants (220 μg/mL). Premature infants of 30 to 31 weeks' gestation have significantly lower plasma concentrations (152 μg/mL) than term infants. Lower plasma concentrations in neonates are correlated with decreased synthetic rates, but plasma clearance of fibronectin also is measurably slower. Plasma fibronectin concentrations are reduced further in infants with respiratory distress syndrome, birth depression, sepsis, and intrauterine growth restriction.[13] Fibronectin biosynthesis by macrophages in vitro is decreased in the neonatal period.

Role in Immune Responses

Fibronectin improves leukocyte function in vitro. Plasma fibronectin and proteolytic fragments of fibronectins promote human adult peripheral blood neutrophil and monocyte chemotaxis, adhesion, and random migration. In addition, fibronectin enhances phagocyte ingestion, reactive oxygen intermediate production, and killing of opsonized (complement or IgG) yeast and bacterial organisms. Fibronectin seems to play an important role as an enhancer of phagocyte function.

Summary

Circulating concentrations of fibronectin are decreased in the neonatal period and are correlated with gestational age. Even lower plasma concentrations are measured in infants who are ill. Plasma fibronectin increases phagocyte function in vitro. The role of fibronectin in host immune defense in neonates remains uncertain, but in vitro data suggest a potential role as an enhancer of phagocyte function.

OTHER HUMORAL FACTORS

C-Reactive Protein

C-reactive protein (CRP) is an acute-phase reactant originally identified by its ability to bind to a pneumococcal polysaccharide antigen. This protein has strong functional similarity to the complement component C1q binding domain of IgG, and similar to IgG is able to activate the classic complement pathway by binding C1q. The polysaccharide antigen recognized by CRP is expressed by many bacteria and some fungi. When CRP binds to the antigen, and the complement system is activated, the organism is effectively opsonized, and rapid clearance occurs through neutrophil, monocyte, or macrophage phagocytosis.

CRP is synthesized by the fetus and the newborn. Serum concentrations seem equivalent in uninfected neonates and adults. CRP is one of the most rapidly responsive acute-phase proteins, with increases of 100-fold to 1000-fold (in adults) in the serum concentration detectable during an infection.[31] In surveys of infants with proven infections, an elevation of CRP serum concentration has been observed in 50% to 100% of patients. Normal values of CRP are less than 1.6 mg/dL on postnatal days 1 to 2 and less than 1 mg/dL thereafter. Diminished or absent increases in the CRP concentration have been observed during the first 12 to 24 hours of life in infected newborns, particularly in newborns infected with group B streptococci. CRP levels decrease rapidly in infants who clinically respond to antimicrobial therapy and return to normal in 5 to 6 days.

Lactoferrin

Lactoferrin is a positively charged iron-binding glycoprotein present in the specific granules of neutrophils. Lactoferrin is released into the phagosome after particle ingestion and is deposited on the cell surface membrane during stimulated degranulation. This glycoprotein seems to enhance neutrophil-endothelial adhesion interactions and neutrophil aggregation, reactive oxygen intermediate production, and chemotaxis. Deficient neutrophil adherence and directed migration have been reported in studies of patients with a heritable deficiency of lactoferrin-containing neutrophil-specific granules.

Neonatal cord blood neutrophils are profoundly deficient in lactoferrin. Stimulation of neutrophils with the synthetic chemoattractant f-MLP results in degranulation of lactoferrin that is quantitatively similar to the concentrations elicited from neutrophils of adults. In contrast, lactoferrin release is diminished when neutrophils are stimulated to spread and move on artificial surfaces. The role of lactoferrin deficiency in contributing to impaired neutrophil chemotaxis is uncertain.

Collectins

Collectins are soluble proteins that play a role in innate immunity.[53] These molecules include mannose-binding lectin (MBL) and surfactant proteins A (SP-A) and D (SP-D) in humans, and the bovine molecules conglutinin, CL-43, and CL-1. Collectins share several structural features, including a collagen domain, a neck region, and a globular carboxyl-terminal C-type (calcium-dependent) lectin-binding domain. Collectins specifically recognize the patterns of carbohydrates on the outer walls of microorganisms. In essence, collectins function by binding to microorganisms and enhancing uptake and clearance by phagocytes. MBL can also function to activate the classic complement pathway in much the same fashion as the complement component C1q. MBL, SP-A, and SP-D bind to one or more receptors on phagocytes and stimulate chemotaxis, the respiratory burst, and the opsonophagocytosis of a wide variety of microorganisms, including group B streptococci.

SP-A and SP-D are synthesized by type II alveolar cells and by nonciliated bronchiolar epithelial cells. As with other components of surfactant, the biosynthesis and secretion of these collectins increase dramatically during the third trimester of pregnancy. Acute injury or inflammation results in rapid increases in SP-A and SP-D biosynthesis. SP-D protein is also found in gastric mucosal cells, and SP-A is present in small intestinal cells.

MBL is synthesized in the liver and secreted into the circulation. MBL serum concentrations vary widely (1000-fold) in adult human subjects primarily related to inherited polymorphisms in the promoter region of the gene. A wide range in cord blood MBL concentrations has been reported. Neonatal serum MBL concentrations generally are lower than the levels measured in adult serum. Relative deficiency of MBL has been associated with increased susceptibility to infections in children and in some adults.

BIOLOGY AND ROLE OF CYTOKINES IN NEWBORNS

Overview

Newborn infants have an increased susceptibility to infection because of various host defense impairments that exist during the neonatal period. The generation and maintenance of acquired immune responses are controlled by a network of regulatory glycoproteins and phospholipids that mediate the interactions between cells. These cytokines and chemokines are responsible for the generation of the immune response and differentiation of a wide variety of immune and nonimmune cells. The infant's ability to generate the right balance of proinflammatory and anti-inflammatory cytokines when challenged with an infectious agent allows him or her to recover from the encounter with minimal residua. When the balance is not perfectly controlled, morbidity and mortality are increased.[23] Unregulated production of cytokines in neonates may contribute to the development of necrotizing enterocolitis, bronchopulmonary dysplasia, and hypoxic-ischemic brain injury. The number of newly discovered cytokines is increasing on a yearly basis. This section focuses on the major cytokines involved in the immune responses to infectious agents and noninfectious stimuli, their developmental patterns in fetuses and newborns, and their coordinated role in neonatal sepsis.

CYTOKINE AND CHEMOKINE BIOLOGY

Interleukin-1 Family
The IL-1 family comprises three polypeptides with similar tertiary structures (IL-1α, IL-1β, and IL-1 receptor antagonist [IL-1ra]). IL-1α and IL-1β are translated as precursor peptides. Pro-IL-1α is fully active and resides in the cytoplasm, but can be transported to the cell surface where it has a role in cell-cell communication. IL-1α appears in the circulation only during severe disease. IL-1α and IL-1β share little sequence homology, but bind to the same receptor and have the same tertiary structure. Pro-IL-1β (the main circulating member of this family) is inactive and must be cleaved by a cysteine protease (IL-1β-converting enzyme or caspase I) before it is secreted. IL-1ra is a competitive inhibitor of the other members of the family that has no agonist activity. There are two varieties of IL receptors: The type I receptor binds all members of the family; the type II receptor binds only IL-1β. Both receptors are members of the IL-1 receptor/TLR superfamily.

IL-1 is synthesized by a wide variety of immune and nonimmune cells, including monocytes, macrophages, neutrophils, endothelial cells, and epithelial cells. Synthesis of these ILs is triggered by microbial products of inflammation, and many of the features of the inflammatory response syndrome can be directly attributed to members of this family. IL-1 production by monocytes and macrophages from term and premature newborns is equivalent to that of adults. In preterm infants with sepsis, monocyte secretion may be diminished, however, during the acute phase of the disease.

Interleukin-6
IL-6 is secreted in a variety of different molecular forms as a result of post-translational modification. IL-6 synthesis is initiated by cytokines (including IL-1 and IL-6), platelet-derived growth factor, epidermal growth factor, viral and bacterial infections, double-stranded RNA, endotoxin, and cyclic adenosine monophosphate. The receptor for IL-6 consists of two subcomponents: (1) a ligand-binding molecule that is not responsible for signal transduction (IL-6R), and (2) a non–ligand-binding signal transducer (gp130). A soluble form of the IL-6 receptor (sIL6Ra) also exists. sIL6Ra can bind to IL-6 and then interact with gp130 on cells that do not express the IL-6 receptor. IL-6 injected intravenously into human patients is less toxic than IL-1β and TNFα, but does result in chills and fever. IL-6 is known to activate T and B cells, stimulate maturation of megakaryocytes, increase the production of acute-phase response proteins, and enhance NK cell activities. Monocytes from term infants produce adequate amounts of IL-6 after stimulation with lipopolysaccharide (LPS), but not IL-1. Cells derived from preterm infants exhibit decreased production no matter what the stimuli. Circulating levels of IL-6 in newborns are lower than corresponding maternal values; however, the percentage of IL-6-positive monocytes (after stimulation with LPS) is higher in preterm and term neonates.

Interleukin-10
IL-10 is a potent anti-inflammatory/immunosuppressive polypeptide synthesized by monocytes, macrophages, T cells, and B cells in response to bacteria, bacterial products, viruses, fungi, and parasites. IL-10 decreases the synthesis of a wide variety of proinflammatory cytokines, and increases the production of naturally occurring proinflammatory cytokine inhibitors (e.g., IL-1ra). The synthesis of IL-10 is enhanced by various other cytokines, including TNFα, IL-1, IL-6, and IL-12. In contrast, IL-10 enhances B cell function and promotes development of cytotoxic T cells. IL-10 receptors are members of the class II cytokine receptor family and consist of two subunits. IL-10 production in neonates is diminished.

Interleukin-12 and Interferon-γ
IL-12 is a heterodimer consisting of two subunits (p35 and p40) encoded by different genes. The p40 subunit mediates binding to the IL-12 receptor, whereas the p35 subunit is needed for signal transduction. The p40 subunit can also form homodimers with itself that bind to the IL-12 receptor with equal affinity, but without eliciting a cellular effect. The homodimers may help modulate the effects of IL-12. The synthesis of the p35 and p40 subunits is regulated independently. In response to a given stimulus, cells secrete 10 to 100 times more of the homodimer than the heterodimer. IL-12 is produced by phagocytic cells (e.g., monocytes and macrophages) in response to bacteria and bacterial products, intracellular pathogens, and viruses. The IL-12 receptor is a member of the gp130 cytokine receptor superfamily. The IL-12 receptor consists of two subunits, and both must be activated for signal transduction. The principal cellular targets of IL-12 are T cells and NK cells. IL-12 induces the production of interferon (IFN-γ), stimulates proliferation, and enhances cytotoxicity. The production of IL-12 by cord blood–derived mononuclear cells (in response to endotoxin) is diminished; however, normal IL-12 synthesis has been observed with heat-killed S. aureus as the stimulus.

IFN-γ is produced by NK cells, type 1 T-helper (Th) cells, and cytotoxic T cells in response to IL-12, TNFα, IL-1, IL-15, and IL-18. The receptor for IFN-γ has two subunits; one is responsible for binding, and the other is responsible for signaling. IFN-γ induces class II histocompatibility antigens and activates macrophages, and is important for host defenses against intracellular pathogens, among other functions (Box 39-1). Synthesis of IFN-γ is greatly diminished in neonates.

Tumor Necrosis Factor Family
The TNF family has two members: TNFα (cachectin) and TNFβ (lymphotoxin). TNFα exists as a transmembrane form (prohormone) and a smaller secreted form consisting of three

---

BOX 39-1   Functions of Interferon-γ

- Enhances macrophage microbicidal activity
- Promotes secretion of inflammatory mediators
- Enhances host cell resistance to nonviral intracellular pathogens
- Upregulates surface Fc receptors and class II major histocompatibility complex antigens on phagocytes
- Inhibits macrophage migration
- Promotes formation of giant cells
- Induces myelosuppression
- Augments functioning of mature neutrophils
- Enhances differentiation of cytolytic T cells, natural killer cells, and lymphocyte-activated killer cells
- Activates endothelial cells
- Suppresses host protein synthesis

monomers. The soluble form of TNFα is formed by the cleavage of the prohormone by a matrix metalloproteinase disintegrin. The transmembrane and the secreted forms of TNF can be biologically active. Similar to IL-1, synthesis of TNFα is triggered by microbial products of inflammation (and by IL-1 and TNFα themselves). A wide variety of cells are capable of producing TNFα; however, monocytes and macrophages represent the major sources of this circulating cytokine.

There are two varieties of TNF receptors—TNFR-1 and TNFR-2. Stimulation of TNFR-1 reproduces many TNFα functions, including cytotoxicity and upregulation of adhesion molecules. TNFR-1 contains a cytoplasmic sequence of 80 amino acids that regulates programmed cell death. TNFR-2 may facilitate binding of TNF to TNFR-1. TNFs share many of the proinflammatory effects of the ILs, but are more likely to result in leukopenia. The production of TNFα by neonatal monocytes and macrophages is less than that in adults. Endotoxin-stimulated cord blood cells from preterm infants secrete significantly less TNF than cells derived from term infants or adults. The expression of TNF receptors may also be diminished.

Platelet-Activating Factor

Platelet-activating factor (PAF) is a potent phospholipid inflammatory mediator that is rapidly degraded by acetylhydrolase. PAF is produced by many cell types; however, only macrophages and eosinophils exhibit regulated release. PAF primarily resides on the cell surface, where it acts as an intercellular messenger. Intravenous administration of PAF results in systemic hypotension, capillary leakage, pulmonary hypertension, neutropenia, thrombocytopenia, and ischemic intestinal necrosis in animals. At a cellular level, PAF is a potent activator of neutrophils. PAF production is increased by cellular exposure to lipopolysaccharide (LPS), hypoxia, hematopoietic growth factors, TNF, IL-1, thrombin, bradykinin, and leukotriene C₄. PAF stimulates the production of other mediators, including TNF, complement, oxygen radicals, prostaglandins, thromboxane, and leukotrienes. There is a strong association (but not a proven etiologic relationship) between neonatal necrotizing enterocolitis and increased concentrations of PAF.

Chemokines

Chemokines are the largest family of cytokines and are involved in the activation and recruitment of a wide variety of cell types. Chemokines are 8- to 12-kDa heparin-binding proteins ranging from 70 to 100 amino acids in length. All chemokines contain four cysteine motifs (forming double bonds) and are classified according to the arrangement of the cysteines at the amino-terminal end. Of the four subgroups (CXC, CC, C, and CX3C), the CC and CXC are the largest (Table 39-2). Chemokine receptors belong to the seven transmembrane–spanning family of G-protein–coupled

TABLE 39-2   Human CXC and CC Chemokines and Relative Receptors

Chemokines	Systematic Name	Chemokine Receptors
GRO α	CXCL1	CXCR2
GRO β	CXCL2	CXCR2
GRO γ	CXCL3	CXCR2
ENA-78	CXCL5	CXCR2
GCP-2	CXCL6	CXCR2, CXCR1
NAP-2	CXCL7	CXCR2
Interleukin-8	CXCL8	CXCR2, CXCR1
Mig	CXCL9	CXCR3
IP-10	CXCL10	CXCR3
I-TAC	CXCL11	CXCR3
SDF-1	CXCL12	CXCR4
BCA-1	CXCL13	CXCR5
MCP-1	CCL2	CCR2
MCP-2	CCL8	CCR3
MCP-3	CCL7	CCR1, CCR2, CCR3
MCP-4	CCL13	CCR2, CCR3
MIP-1α	CCL3	CCR1, CCR5
MIP-1β	CCL4	CCR5
RANTES	CCL5	CCR1, CCR3, CCR5
Eotaxin	CCL11	CCR3
Eotaxin-2	CCL24	CCR3
Eotaxin-3	CCL26	CCR3
LARC	CCL20	CCR6
TECK	CCL25	CCR9
CTACK	CCL27	CCR10
TARC	CCL17	CCR4
MDC	CCL22	CCR4
DC-CK1	CCL18	?
ELC	CCL19	CCR7
SLC	CCL21	CCR7

Adapted from Manzo A et al: Role of chemokines and chemokine receptors in regulating specific leukocyte trafficking in the immune/inflammatory response, *Clin Exp Rheumatol* 21:501, 2003.

receptors. Chemokines are constitutively produced in organs where cell attraction is required for maintenance of local homeostasis.[12] Most chemokines are inducible by inflammatory cytokines and endotoxin. In inflammatory states, chemokines are responsible for navigation and homing of effector leukocytes. In addition, chemokines induce a wide variety of leukocyte responses, including enzyme release from intracellular stores, oxygen radical formation, shape change through cytoskeletal rearrangement, generation of lipid mediators, and induction of adhesion to endothelium and extracellular matrix proteins. Chemokines are quite diverse in their target cell selectivity. CXC chemokines generally are more selective for neutrophils and T cells, whereas CC chemokines mainly attract monocytes and T lymphocytes. Considerable data suggest that chemotactic factor generation is deficient in newborn infants.

COORDINATED INFLAMMATORY RESPONSE IN NEONATAL SEPSIS

In human bacterial sepsis, cytokines are released in a sequential manner, resulting in a cytokine cascade. After a challenge with a low dose of endotoxin, TNFα peaks within 90 minutes. Other proinflammatory cytokines are released shortly afterward, and anti-inflammatory mediators follow in close sequence. The peak in IL-10 production may not occur for hours, however. In general, cytokines are not stored in intracellular compartments; they are synthesized and released in response to an inflammatory stimulus. Regulation of cytokine production occurs at the level of gene transcription. Specific transcription factors (e.g., NF-κB) bind to DNA response elements that either inhibit or promote gene transcription. Proinflammatory and anti-inflammatory cytokines or molecules are produced in response to an inflammatory stimulus. Counterinflammatory molecules include soluble cytokine receptors (resulting from proteolytic cleavage of the extracellular

binding domain), anti-inflammatory cytokines (e.g., IL-10), and cytokine receptor antagonists (e.g., IL-1ra).

Antigen-presenting cells (APCs) of the innate immune system (e.g., macrophages, NK cells, neutrophils, mucosal epithelial cells, endothelial cells, and dendritic cells [DCs]) play pivotal roles in the initiation of an inflammatory response to invading pathogens. As depicted in Figure 39-5, the macrophage is activated by endotoxin (LPS) binding to the CD14 receptor (the main LPS binding receptor) by an LPS-binding protein. CD14 also exists in a soluble form that is shed from the macrophage cell surface through the action of serine proteases. Circulating LPS-CD14 complexes can attach to endothelial cells or epithelial cells. Through this mechanism, endothelial cells are activated to produce other cytokines and mediators (e.g., PAF, nitric oxide, and IL-6) that contribute to the proinflammatory response. CD14 is also required for the recognition of other bacterial products, including peptidoglycans and lipoteichoic acid from grampositive bacteria. The formation of the CD14-LPS complex significantly reduces the concentration of LPS needed for activation.

CD14 lacks transmembrane and intracellular domains and cannot initiate a cellular response. Another pathway involving TLRs is responsible for cell activation and signal transduction.[1] CD14 seems to be able to discriminate between bacterial products and sort their signals to different TLRs. The TLRs are named from Toll, a plasma membrane receptor in *Drosophila*, which has a cytoplasmic domain homologous to the IL-1 receptor protein. Toll receptors induce signal transduction pathways that lead to the activation of the transcription factor NF-κB. In mammalian species, there are at least 10 TLRs (Table 39-3), which represent type I transmembrane proteins characterized by an extracellular domain, a transmembrane domain, and an intracellular domain. TLRs are pattern recognition receptors that recognize pathogen-associated molecular patterns. Pathogen-associated molecular patterns are shared by many pathogens, but are not

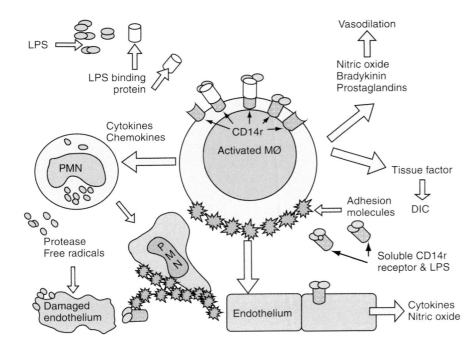

Figure 39–5. Role of macrophages in mediating the inflammatory response. Lipopolysaccharide (LPS) binding to the CD14 receptor (with or without LPS binding protein) activates the macrophage (MØ) to synthesize and secrete cytokines, chemokines, and other mediators. These soluble factors stimulate polymorphonuclear neutrophils (PMNs) to release proteases and oxygen free radicals that are important for microbial killing, but that also may injure endothelium and cause capillary leak. Binding of soluble LPS-CD14 complexes to endothelial cells promotes biosynthesis of other cytokines and small molecular mediators (e.g., nitric oxide, interleukin-6). Endothelial activation also results in upregulation of cell surface adhesive molecules that interact with neutrophil adhesive molecules and promote neutrophil extravasation. DIC, disseminated intravascular coagulation.

TABLE 39–3 Role of Toll-like Receptors (TLRs) in Pathogen Recognition and Pathophysiology of Human Disease

Toll-like Receptor	Ligands	Pathogens or Disease State
TLR1	Signals as a dimer only when combined with TLR2 for all its ligands; recognizes *Borrelia burgdorferi* OspA; required for adaptive immune response	Lyme disease
	Tri-acyl lipopeptides (bacteria, e.g., *Mycobacterium tuberculosis*)	
	Soluble factors (*Neisseria meningitidis*)	*N. meningitidis*
TLR2	Associates with CD11/CD18, CD14, MD-2, TLR1, TLR6, dectin 1; lipoprotein/lipopeptides (various microbial pathogens)	*M. tuberculosis*
	Peptidoglycan	Apoptosis of Schwann cells in leprosy
	Lipoteichoic acid	
	Lipoarabinomannan (mycobacteria)	
	Phenol-soluble modulin (*Staphylococcus epidermidis*)	
	Glycoinositolphospholipids (*Trypanosoma cruzi*)	Chagas disease
	Glycolipids (*Treponema maltophilum*)	Leptospirosis
	Porin (*Neisseria*)	
	Zymosan (fungi)	Fungal sepsis
	Atypical LPS (*Leptospira interrogans*)	
	Atypical LPS (*Porphyromonas gingivalis*)	Periodontal disease
	HSP70 (host)	
	CMV virions	CMV viremia
	Hemagglutinin protein of wild-type measles	Measles
	Bacterial fimbriae	
TLR3	Double-stranded RNA in viruses	Many
TLR4	Gram-negative enteric LPS (requires coreceptors MD-2 and CD14)	Gram-negative bacteria
	Additional ligands	Septic shock
	Chlamydial HSP60	*Chlamydia trachomatis, Chlamydia pneumoniae*
	RSV F protein	Certain viruses (e.g., RSV)
	Taxol (plant)	
	M. tuberculosis HSP65	*M. tuberculosis*
	Envelope proteins (MMTV)	Smallpox (vaccinia) blocks TIR domain of TLR4 and others
	HSP60 (host)	
	HSP70 (host)	
	Type III repeat extra domain A of fibronectin (host)	
	Oligosaccharides of hyaluronic acid (host)	
	Polysaccharide fragments of heparan sulfate (host)	
	Fibrinogen (host)	
	β-defensin$_2$	
TLR5	Flagellin (monomeric) from bacteria	Flagellated bacteria (e.g., *Salmonella*)

TABLE 39–3 Role of Toll-like Receptors (TLRs) in Pathogen Recognition and Pathophysiology of Human Disease—cont'd

Toll-like Receptor	Ligands	Pathogens or Disease State
TLR6	See TLR2 (as dimers with TLR2)	
	Phenol-soluble modulin	
	Di-acyl lipopeptides (mycoplasma)	
TLR7	Responds to imidazoquinoline antiviral agents (synthetic compounds)	May be useful as adjuvant for cancer therapy
	Loxoribine (synthetic compounds)	Viral infections
	Bropirimine (synthetic compounds)	
	Endogenous and exogenous ligands unknown	
	Single-stranded RNA	
TLR8	Imidazoquinoline (synthetic compounds)	Viral infections
	Single-stranded RNA	
TLR9	Bacterial DNA as "CpG" motifs	Viral infections
		Bacterial and viral infections (e.g., HSV)
		May be useful as adjuvant for vaccines and cancer therapy
		HSV type 2
TLR10	Unknown	Unknown

CMV, cytomegalovirus; HSP, heat-shock protein; HSV, herpes simplex virus; LPS, lipopolysaccharide; MMTV, mouse mammary tumor virus; RSV, respiratory syncytial virus; TIR, Toll/interleukin receptor.
From Abreu MT, Arditi M: Innate immunity and Toll-like receptors: clinical implications of basic science research, *J Pediatr* 144:421, 2004.

expressed in host cells. TLR4 is responsible for the recognition of bacterial endotoxin. It is essential for signaling, but requires a small protein (MD-2) to confer responsiveness. Other TLRs bind cell wall products from gram-positive bacteria and fungi.

When activated, TLRs initiate a signaling cascade that shares many of the same molecules used by the IL-1 receptor. Activated, macrophages synthesize and secrete the cascade of proinflammatory cytokines, chemokines, and mediators described earlier. Some of these cytokines activate neutrophils to release proteases and free radicals that have the capacity to damage endothelium and promote capillary leak. Upregulation of adhesion molecules on the neutrophils allows them to bind to counter-receptors on the endothelial cells and migrate to sites of inflammation. The proinflammatory cascade is interrupted by the initiation of counter-regulatory mechanisms. Because most patients with life-threatening infections (i.e., systemic inflammatory response syndrome) are not admitted early in the course of their sepsis episode, proinflammatory cytokines are detected in only a subset of patients. Anti-inflammatory cytokines (which appear later in the cascade) are found in most of these infected individuals.

The concentration of anti-inflammatory substances (e.g., IL-1ra and soluble receptors) increases substantially with time and has been termed the *compensatory anti-inflammatory response syndrome*. This is a response of the host to limit the toxicity of proinflammatory substances. Shortly after the onset of an infectious episode, the mononuclear cell becomes refractory and is unable to respond to proinflammatory cytokines. In contrast, the capacity to produce anti-inflammatory substances such as IL-1ra and IL-10 is preserved. This phenomenon has been referred to as monocyte deactivation or immunoparalysis. Although the mechanism responsible for monocyte deactivation is unclear, it probably involves increased production of IL-10. The risk of infection is greatly increased during this period of hyporeactivity.

ACQUIRED IMMUNITY
Cell-Mediated and Antibody-Mediated Responses
OVERVIEW

Lymphocytes constitute almost 20% of blood leukocytes and specialize in the recognition of invading foreign antigens in the context of major histocompatibility antigens. Lymphocytes are of two major types: (1) B lymphocytes that are produced in the bone marrow, mature in secondary lymphoid organs, and subsequently differentiate into antibody secreting plasma cells, and (2) T lymphocytes that mature and differentiate into CD4+

and CD8+ subsets in the thymus and subsequently seed the peripheral blood system, including the spleen and the lymph nodes.[21,57] T cell functions include helping B cells to make antibody; killing virally infected cells; regulating the level of the immune response; and stimulating the microbial and cytotoxic activity of the immune cells, including macrophages.

Each lymphocyte expresses a cell surface receptor that recognizes a particular antigen. In the case of T cells, it is called the T cell receptor (TCR), and in the case of B cells it is called the B cell receptor (BCR). Each lymphocyte is engineered to express a receptor that is specific for only one antigen. In this way, the lymphocyte population as a whole can recognize a wide range of antigens. The antigen receptors are generated during development by a process known as somatic mutation and recombination involving a few germline genes. The antigen receptors used by B cells and T cells are different. The BCR is a surface immunoglobulin, a membrane-bound form of the antibody that eventually gets secreted. The TCR is generated from a different set of genes that encode only the cell surface receptor.

T cells and B cells recognize antigens in different forms: B cells recognize an unmodified antigen molecule, either free in solution or on the surface of other cells. T cells recognize antigen only when it is presented to them in association with molecules encoded by the MHC. The functional consequence of these differences in antigen recognition is that T cells must be presented processed antigens in the form of short peptides by accessory cells such as macrophages or DCs, whereas B cells can directly recognize antigens in tissue fluids.

The acquired immune response arises through the process of clonal recognition. An antigen selects the clones of B and T cells that express the cell surface receptors that recognize the antigen. Because the number of different lymphocyte antigen specificities is large, the number of lymphocytes available to recognize each antigen is relatively small—only a few hundred lymphocytes in an adult. In addition, because so few cells are insufficient to eradicate an invading pathogen, the first step toward the generation of a specific immune response involves a rapid expansion of antigen-specific lymphocytes. This step is followed by further differentiation of antigen-specific cells into effector cells. These events underlie the difference between primary and secondary immune responses. During the primary response, the small number of specific cells increases, and the cells undergo differentiation. If the antigen is encountered again (or persists), there is a larger population of specific cells to react with the antigen, and these cells are able to respond more quickly because they have already undergone several steps along their differentiation pathway. These lymphocytes that have been stimulated by antigen (primed) and their progeny either may differentiate fully into effector cells or may form the expanded pool of cells (memory cells) that can respond more efficiently to a future (secondary) challenge with the same antigen.

T LYMPHOCYTES

Overview

T cells develop and differentiate in the thymus before seeding the secondary lymphoid tissues. T cells recognize antigen and MHC molecules through the TCR. This receptor consists of an antigen-binding portion formed by two different polymorphic chains in association with CD3, a complex of polypeptides involved in signaling cellular activation. The antigen-binding portion may consist of an $\alpha\beta$ chain heterodimer. In humans, the markers CD2 and CD5 are also present on all T cells (Table 39-4). Activated T cells also carry endogenously synthesized MHC class II molecules, although these are absent from resting T cells. Activated T cells may also be induced to express CD25, which forms part of the high-affinity IL-2 receptor and is important in clonal expansion.

There are two main subpopulations of T cells, which can be distinguished according to their expression of CD4+ or CD8+. These molecules act as receptors for class II (CD4+) and class I (CD8+) MHC molecules and contribute to T cell immune recognition and cellular activation. Most CD4+ T cells recognize antigen associated with MHC class II molecules, and these cells act predominantly as T-helper (Th) cells. CD8+ T cells recognize antigen-associated MHC class I molecules and are primarily responsible for cytotoxic destruction of virally infected cells.

Clones of mature CD4+ T cells fall into two major groups, which are functionally defined according to the cytokines they secrete: Th1 cells interact preferentially with mononuclear phagocytes, whereas Th2 cells tend to promote B cell division and differentiation. The balance of activity between these two subsets is related in part to how antigen is presented

TABLE 39–4 Cluster-Designated (CD) Molecules Found on Human T Cells

Antigen	Molecular Weight (kDa)	Comment
CD1a	49	Expressed on thymocytes
CD1b	45	Expressed on thymocytes
CD1c	43	Expressed on thymocytes
CD2	50	Sheep erythrocyte receptor
CD3	22	Part of T cell antigen receptor complex
CD4	55	MHC class II immune recognition
CD5	67	
CD6	120	
CD7	40	Possibly IgM Fc receptor
CD8	32	MHC class I immune recognition
CD25	55	Low-affinity interleukin-2 receptor
CD45	180	Expressed on memory T cells (also known as UCHLI)
CD45R	200	Expressed on virgin T cells (also known as Leu-18)

MHC, major histocompatibility complex.

to the cells, and it ultimately determines the type of immune response that develops.

The surface phenotypes of T cell populations change during T cell development. In humans, virgin T cells express the cell surface molecule CD45RA, whereas activated cells express the CD45RO isoform and higher levels of adhesion molecules, such as the β_1-integrins (CD29). The mechanism resulting in the generation of activated T cells from resting memory T cells is still unclear.

T Cell Development

Lymphocytes destined to become T cells must undergo several maturational steps in the thymus before they become mature effector T cells. In humans, the thymus develops embryologically as an outgrowth from the third and fourth pharyngeal pouches between weeks 6 and 7 of gestation. The cortex and medulla of the thymus begin to differentiate by the 10th week of gestation, and Hassall corpuscles appear the 12th week of gestation.

The undifferentiated cells that first enter the thymus (at approximately 7 weeks' gestation) do not express either the CD4+ or the CD8+ antigen, but do express the T cell markers CD7 and CD45 (CD7 may be the IgM Fc receptor, and CD45 is the common leukocyte antigen). In the thymus, T cell maturation is accompanied by the sequential appearance of surface phenotypic markers (see Table 39-4). CD1, CD2, and CD5 surface antigens appear soon after CD7

expression, whereas CD3 appears later. As gestation progresses, most cells leaving the thymus express either the CD4+ or the CD8+ surface antigen. Cells that lack both antigens (double-negative cells) retain stem cell function and possess a receptor (CD25, Tac antigen) for IL-2, which plays an essential role in T cell proliferation.

The first thymic cells to express CD4+ or CD8+ antigens express both antigens simultaneously and appear in the thymic cortex at approximately 10 weeks' gestation (Fig. 39-6). At this stage, transcribed TCR genes are first expressed on the cell surface. Production of the T cell α chain precedes production of the β chain. By the 12th week of gestation, occasional CD3$^+$ cells can be identified in human fetal peripheral blood. As gestation progresses, the percentage of CD3$^+$ cells in the peripheral blood increases, coming to represent more than 50% of T lymphocytes by 22 weeks' gestation. These CD3$^+$ cells also express either CD4+ or CD8+ antigen. By 13 weeks of gestation, CD3$^+$ T cells appear in the fetal liver and spleen, and these cells represent more than 50% of the T lymphocytes in those organs by the end of the second trimester.

Role of Cytokine Receptor Signaling in Lymphocyte Development

In humans, X-linked SCID (X-SCID) syndrome is characterized by defective T cell development and function. Affected patients lack T cells, but possess near-normal numbers of

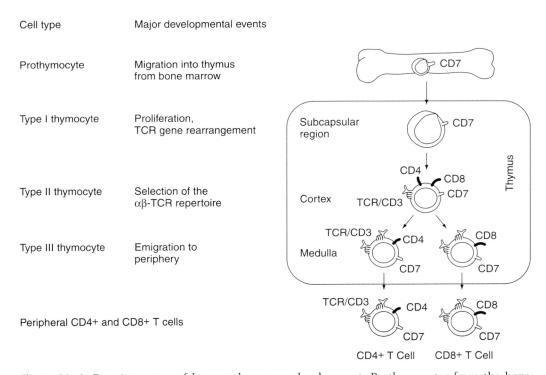

Cell type	Major developmental events
Prothymocyte	Migration into thymus from bone marrow
Type I thymocyte	Proliferation, TCR gene rearrangement
Type II thymocyte	Selection of the $\alpha\beta$-TCR repertoire
Type III thymocyte	Emigration to periphery
Peripheral CD4+ and CD8+ T cells	

Figure 39–6. Putative stages of human thymocyte development. Prothymocytes from the bone marrow enter the thymus and give rise to three major stages of $\alpha\beta$–T cell receptor ($\alpha\beta$-TCR) lineage thymocytes. TCR-α and TCR-β chain genes are rearranged during stage I; thymic selection occurs mainly during stage II; and emigration of mature CD4+ and CD8+ cells occurs in stage III. (*From Lewis DB et al: Developmental immunology and role of host defenses in neonatal susceptibility to infection. In Remington JS et al, editors: Infectious diseases of the fetus and newborn infant, 4th ed, Philadelphia, 1995, Saunders, with permission.*)

B cells. B cells from patients with X-SCID tend to secrete predominantly IgM antibody. Altered B cell–mediated antibody production in patients with X-SCID has been attributed to defective T cell help. The mapping of the gene that encodes the common subunit of cytokine receptors, including IL-2, has been linked to the X-SCID locus. Patients with X-SCID possess mutations in the common subunit, establishing a correlation between defects in this gene and the cause of X-SCID. Based on these observations, it was predicted that lymphocytes deficient in the expression of the IL-2 receptor would mimic some of the phenotypic abnormalities associated with patients with X-SCID. Deficiency of IL-2 or the IL-2 receptor does not result in any of the defects observed in patients with X-SCID, however. These observations have since been attributed to the presence of the common subunit of multiple cytokine receptors, including the IL-4, IL-7, IL-9, and IL-15 receptors. All these receptors are expressed on T cells, and mutations in the common subunit are likely to affect the function of all these receptors in patients with X-SCID and provide an explanation for the pathophysiologic process of this disease.

T Lymphocyte Activation and Maturation

The T cell receptor (TCR) is a multisubunit complex that consists of αβ chains noncovalently associated with the invariant CD3-γ, CD3-δ, CD3-ε, and TCR-ζ chains. T cell activation by APCs results in the activation of protein tyrosine kinases that associate with the CD3 and TCR-ζ subunits and the coreceptors CD4+ or CD8+. These activation events result in the transcriptional activation of many genes, resulting in T cell proliferation, differentiation, and acquisition of effector function.

Generally, interaction between the TCR and the antigen presenting cells (APC) results in the activation of intracellular enzymes and adapter molecules that consists of recognition sequences known as the Src homology (SH) 2 and SH3 domains containing signaling proteins that belong to the Src family of lymphocyte-specific kinase (LCK).[14] Activated LCK associates intracellularly with the TCR and with the CD8+ and CD4+ coreceptors. Activated LCK also activates the cytoplasmic domain of CD3-ζ, which contains a conserved amino acid motif, ITAM. ITAM allows the binding of additional signaling molecules such as SYK family kinase ZAP70. When recruited to ITAM, ZAP70 is activated, which subsequently activates a major adapter protein in T cell signaling termed *linker for activation of T cells* (LAT). Activation of LAT and several other signaling molecules in this cascade results in the activation of nuclear proteins, including transcription factors such as nuclear factor of activated T cells and mitogen-activated protein kinase.[14] Taken together, the successive activation of a series of intracellular signaling molecules on TCR engagement with MHC molecules on APCs results in the transcription of important T cell–specific genes that are crucial for development, differentiation, and function of T cells.

T cells require two signals for activation: a signal provided through the TCR, and a second, costimulatory signal. The CD28 molecule on T cells binds to B7-1 or B7-2 on APCs, providing the second of the two signals needed for initiation of naive T cell responses. A key feature of the costimulatory signal provided by CD28 is that, in conjunction with a TCR stimulus, it allows high-level IL-2 production and provides an essential survival signal for T cells. The combined costimulatory signal prevents T cell apoptosis or the induction of anergy (unresponsiveness) that may occur in response to activation of either signal alone.

Naive helper T cells can be divided into two subsets, based on the profile of cytokines they produce. Th1 cells produce IL-2, IFN, and TNF, and Th2 cells produce IL-4, IL-5, IL-6, IL-10, 1L-12, and IL-13. This differential pattern of cytokine expression contributes to differences in the function of these two subsets of T cells. Th1 cells are inflammatory cells responsible for mediating cell-mediated immunity. In contrast, Th2 cells act to help B cells produce antibodies. Naive T cells generally do not express mRNA for cytokines such as IFN, IL-4, TNF, or perforin. The decision of a naive T cell to mature into either Th1 or Th2 is partly regulated by the interaction between growth factors and growth factor receptors and transcription factors. For Th1 differentiation, interaction between naive Th cells and APCs results in the synthesis of IL-12. IL-12 in conjunction with transcription factors signals transducer and activator of transcription (STAT4), and T-bet drives the maturation of IFN-producing Th1 cells.[41] Likewise, IL-6, STAT6, and the transcription factor GATA-3 are essential for the generation of Th2 cells.[41] A balance between cytokines, signaling molecules, and transcription factors is essential for driving the differentiation of Th1 and Th2 cells from naive Th cells.

Role of Cytokines in T Cell Function

IL-2 was originally described as a T cell growth factor, but it is now known to have activity on various other cell types, including NK cells, B cells, macrophages, and monocytes. The synthesis and secretion of this cytokine are triggered by the activation of mature T cells. The binding of IL-2 initiates clonal expansion of activated T cells. High-affinity IL-2 receptor expression is induced on B cells by exposure to IL-4 and immunoglobulin receptor binding. The activity of IL-2 on other cell types (NK cells, macrophages, neutrophils, and lymphokine-activated killer cells) is mainly through the intermediate-affinity IL-2 receptor. A key role of the IL-2 receptor γ chain (which is also found in the receptors for IL-4, IL-7, IL-9, and IL-13) in the immune response is highlighted by the consequences of its genetic malfunction. Mutations in the IL-2 receptor γ chain are responsible for X-SCID in humans.

IL-4 is produced by a subpopulation of T cells and by mast cells. Its production follows T cell activation or cross-linkage of FcRI receptors on basophils or mast cells. IL-4 affects many cell types, promoting the growth of T cells, B cells, mast cells, myeloid cells, and erythroid cell progenitors. It promotes class switching in B cells to IgE and augments IgG1 production. Mice in which the IL-4 gene has been knocked out by targeted gene disruption are unable to make IgE. IL-4-overexpressing mice express very high IgE levels. The IL-4 effect on T cell development is to drive T cell differentiation toward a Th2 type at the expense of a Th1 response. The counterbalancing cytokine is IL-12, which cross-regulates IL-4. IL-4 has also been shown to initiate cytotoxic responses against tumor cells. The pleiotropic activity of IL-4 is reflected in the range of cell types that express IL-4 receptor. This high-affinity receptor is found on T cells, B cells, mast cells, myeloid cells, fibroblasts, muscle cells, neuroblasts, stromal cells, endothelial cells, and monocytes.

IL-7 signaling promotes cell-cycle entry and proliferation of developing T lymphocytes and B lymphocytes. In thymocytes, IL-7 signaling has been implicated in the induction and maintenance of the antiapoptotic protein Bcl-2 and has been shown to inhibit the expression of the proapoptotic factor Bax. These results suggest that one of the principal functions of IL-7 signaling in developing thymocytes is to promote cell survival.

IL-10 has important biologic effects on T cell function. Th0 and Th2 subsets of T cells synthesize IL-10, and production of IL-10 is inhibited by IFN-γ. IL-12 is made by B cells, monocytes, and macrophages, and acts synergistically with IL-2 to induce IFN production by T cells and NK cells. It is a key factor in the development of Th1 cells, stimulating their proliferation and differentiation. IL-12 enhances the cytotoxic activity of T cells. As noted earlier, IL-12 is a key cytokine for directing the T cell response to Th1.

T Cell Function in Neonates

In general, T cell responses in neonates are defective. Cord blood T cells have reduced ability to proliferate and synthesize cytokines such as IL-2, IFN-γ, IL-4, and GM-CSF. The defect in T cell functions in neonates has been attributed to qualitative and quantitative differences.[3,47] Studies showing reduced numbers of splenic T cells in neonates support the idea that lack of T cell responses in neonates is due to quantitative reduction in the overall numbers of T cells.[47] In addition to quantitative reduction, studies have also suggested that neonate T cells are primarily of the immature phenotype and lack the ability to mount a robust immune response. Additional studies have suggested a greater propensity of neonate naive Th cells to differentiate toward the Th2 phenotype rather than Th1 in the presence of endogenous neonatal APCs. The lack of Th1 differentiation from naive Th cells in neonates could result in impaired cell-mediated immunity. Taken together, studies so far point to multiple factors as contributors to neonatal tolerance (nonresponsiveness).

More recent studies have shown that neonatal T cells do not lack the ability to undergo proliferation and cytokine production when stimulated in a manner that does not require signaling through their TCR-CD3 complex. Studies comparing TCR-CD3–independent responses between adult and neonatal T cells have shown no differences in the ability of neonatal and adult T cells to synthesize IL-2 and undergo proliferation. Because efficient T cell responses in vivo require the presence of mature and functional APCs, studies using the ability of endogenous neonatal APCs to sustain proliferation in neonatal T cells showed that providing additional costimulatory signals to neonatal T cells in the context of endogenous APCs corrects the ability of these cells to induce proliferation and IL-2 production to adult levels. Neonatal T cells apparently do not possess intrinsic defects in T cell function; rather, the machinery necessary to provide costimulatory signals to neonatal T cells is defective.

Neonatal APCs such as dendritic cells (DCs) have been shown to express low levels of costimulatory molecules, including CD40, CD80, and CD86, compared with adult DCs.[10,28,44] The inability of neonatal DCs to deliver adequate levels of costimulatory signals to neonatal T cells is likely to be the cause of neonatal tolerance, in addition to lack of cytokine production, such as IL-12 by APCs and IFN-γ by naive Th cells, preventing the differentiation of these cells into Th1 cells. In addition to reduced CD40 signaling, the expression of MHC class II is also reduced on neonatal APCs, and may contribute to the reduced immune response of neonates.

As mentioned earlier, neonatal APCs show reduced expression of CD86 and CD40 costimulatory molecules. Treatment of these cells with a combination of IFN and CD40 ligand does not upregulate the expression of CD86 or CD40.[16] Neonatal APCs synthesize low levels of proinflammatory cytokines, including TNFα, IL-1β, or IL-12, in response to LPS stimulation (i.e., TLR4 ligand) and in response to other TLR ligands.[5,16,19,52] Upregulation of TLR4 and CD14 expression is not observed in neonatal APCs on LPS stimulation, and the expression of My88, a crucial adapter molecule in TLR signaling, is also reduced in neonatal APCs.[27,59] TLR4 expression is reduced on APCs derived from premature infants compared with full-term infants.[11] It is conceivable that premature infants are more susceptible to infections because of impaired TLR expression.

Examples of additional complexity in this process have also been documented. Studies have shown a differential response to TLR ligands on neonate APCs. TNFα synthesis is reduced in neonatal monocytes that are stimulated with LPS, whereas this response seems to be normal when these same cells are stimulated with R-848, a ligand for TLR7 and TLR8.[27] Neonatal APCs also show reduced IFN-γ responsiveness,[33,34] which is associated with defects in phagocytosis. The ability of neonatal monocytes to differentiate into DCs is significantly modulated, as reflected by differences in the morphologic characteristics of cord blood–derived DCs compared with adult DCs.[30] Taken together, studies so far implicate significant defects in TLR activation in neonatal monocyte/macrophage APCs.

Most studies related to neonatal DCs have been performed using in vitro generated monocyte-derived DCs (mDCs). These cells have several defects relative to adult mDCs. They tend to be immature based on low expression of MHC class II, CD80, and CD40. Even on LPS stimulation, the phenotype of these cells remains immature as reflected by continued lack of upregulation of MHC and costimulatory molecules.[26,58] The immaturity of neonatal DCs can be attributed to impaired TLR signaling, a phenomenon also observed in monocyte/macrophage–derived APCs discussed earlier. Additionally, neonatal DCs synthesize reduced levels of IL-12 in response to LPS.[15] This defect can be rescued, however, by providing exogenous IFN-γ to cultures.[15] Consistent with the above-described defects associated with neonatal DCs, these cells also show significant reduction in the priming of allogeneic cord blood–derived T cells relative to adult DCs.[15,29,30] Neonatal DCs apparently require additional mechanisms of activation to achieve the activation status of adult DCs.

When activated, they seem to be relatively competent, however.

In addition to monocyte-derived, cord blood–derived DCs, studies have suggested the presence of another group of DCs in cord blood that are characterized on the basis of lack of CD11c (a marker for myeloid DCs) expression and presence of CD123. CD123 is a marker used to identify plasmacytoid DCs (pDCs).[45] Cord blood contains a higher frequency of pDCs compared with peripheral blood. An enhanced ratio of pDC to mDC is also observed in cord blood compared with adults. Similar to mDCs, neonatal pDCs also show functional defects. They produce reduced levels of IFN-α/β.[7] Although cord blood pDCs respond to R-848 by upregulating the expression of CD40, CD80, CD86, and MHC antigens, the extent of upregulation is less in these cells compared with adult pDCs. Likewise, R-848-stimulated TNFα synthesis in cord blood pDCs is also reduced compared with adult pDCs. Neonatal mDCs and pDCs share similar functional characteristics. In adults, Flt3 ligand treatment of cells results in significant growth of cultured mDCs and pDCs derived from peripheral blood.[4] Treatment of hematopoietic progenitors from human fetal tissues and cord blood with Flt3 ligand induces differentiation of these cells into pDCs that synthesize significant amounts of IFN-α/β in response to viral stimulation.[39] Flt3 ligand could likely be used clinically to induce the expression of IFN in neonatal pDCs.

Neonatal DCs express reduced levels of MHC and costimulatory molecules such as CD80 and CD86. In addition, these cells express less IL-12 compared with adult DCs on activation of TLRs. IFN expression in cord blood pDCs is significantly reduced compared with adult pDCs. Recombinant Flt3 ligand given in vitro to cultures consisting of cord blood pDCs significantly enhances the number of pDCs, which are fully competent in secreting adult amounts of IFN subsequently.[54,56]

Compared with CD4+ neonatal Th cells, the status of CD8+ neonatal cytotoxic cells is poorly understood and remains controversial. Compared with neonatal CD4+ cells, neonatal CD8+ cells have a normal frequency of precursors; they are free of cytokine promoter modifications, such as the hypermethylation that is commonly associated with neonatal CD4+ Th cells.[55] Neonates show the presence of functional CD8+ cytotoxic T cells against congenital human CMV and Rous sarcoma virus. They also show the presence of functional memory CD8+ cells against congenital CMV.[20,32] These results suggest that under certain conditions of stimulation, despite the absence of adequate CD4+ T cell help, long-lived, functional memory CD8+ T cells can be generated by an in utero CMV infection. This type of antiviral immunity in neonates persists partly because of persistent and prolonged viral secretion associated with some viral infections, such as CMV infection. This type of infection is likely to result in sustained and continuous stimulation of CD4+ and CMV-specific, long-lived memory CD8+ T cells in utero. Whether in utero antigen stimulation could be used to develop infant vaccines for protecting neonates from viral infections is an area of active research.

In addition to defects in cell-mediated immunity, neonates manifest defects in humoral immunity. Generally, neonatal antibody responses to viral and bacterial infections are quantitatively and qualitatively different from adults. Although human neonates do mount an antibody response to pathogens, they predominantly produce IgM, and the magnitude of antibody response is significantly less than in adults.

B Cell Responses in Neonates

Several distinctions between neonatal and adult splenic B cells have been identified.[2] Neonatal B cells express reduced levels of costimulatory molecules CD40, CD80, and CD86, which results in defective T cell responses via CD40 ligand (CD40L) and IL-10. Marginal zone B cells derived from spleens of neonates tend to express reduced levels of CD21.[51] In addition, expression of a critical costimulatory receptor, TACI, is impaired in neonatal B cells, in particular in premature infants.[22]

Although these cell intrinsic factors contribute significantly to defects in antibody responses in neonates, B cell responses in neonates are also affected by external factors. Maternal derived antibodies can bind to vaccine antigens and inhibit neonatal B cells from recognizing them.[42] Additionally, serum complement levels, in particular, C3 levels, in neonates are reduced; this results in reduction in the formation of antigen-antibody complexes. The number of marginal zone macrophages in neonate spleens is also reduced compared with adults.[51] These cells play an essential role in trapping antigens. One also observes defects in the maturation of follicular DCs in neonates. Follicular DCs are crucial for attracting B cells and provide signals that result in somatic hypermutation and class switching of antibodies.

Additional defects include a lack of prolonged antibody response; this is due partly to impairment in the establishment and maintenance of antibody-secreting plasma cells in the bone marrow of neonates.[37] Although plasma cells in neonates do migrate to the bone marrow, they are impaired in their ability to thrive as long-lasting cells largely because of lack of survival and differentiation signals from bone marrow–derived stromal elements.[38] Finally, studies have also shown that in some instances administration of vaccines to neonates preferentially leads to the generation of memory B cells, rather than plasma cells. This situation has been largely attributed to reduced overall B cell receptor affinity of neonatal naive B cells for antigens resulting in an overall reduction in the strength of the intracellular signal, which may preferentially lead to the generation of memory B cells rather than plasma cells. In neonates, a significant number of B cell intrinsic factors and microenvironmental factors cooperate to regulate the development and maintenance of antibody-producing plasma cells and the preferential generation of memory B cells.[43]

Summary

Neonatal T cells are impaired in producing cytokines, notably IL-2 and Th1-type IFN-γ, under conditions of physiologic stimulation, including in response to TCR-CD3 stimulation. Neonatal T cells are not intrinsically incapable of mature function, however. Adult-level cytokine production can be elicited in human neonatal T cells by increasing the magnitude of Th1-promoting costimulatory signals. In contrast, neonatal cytotoxic T lymphocytes are capable of generating long-lasting memory effectors against several viral infections, including CMV and Rous sarcoma virus. These findings could be exploited in the future to generate vaccines for the treatment of viral infections.

Qualitative differences in neonatal T cells and APCs compared with adult cells might contribute to these deficient T cell–mediated responses of neonates. Compared with adult T cells, neonatal T cells seem to require more costimulation to achieve robust Th1 responses in vitro and in vivo. Neonatal APCs might be poorly functional in vivo and normally unable to promote vigorous Th1 responses. If APC function is augmented or supplemented, however, mature Th1 responses are promoted.

B LYMPHOCYTES AND ANTIBODY PRODUCTION

Overview of B Cell Function and Phenotypic Appearance
B lymphocytes represent 5% to 15% of circulating lymphocytes in the peripheral blood and are characterized by the presence of cell surface immunoglobulin.[21] Most B lymphocytes simultaneously express endogenously synthesized IgM and IgD and various other cell surface receptors (Table 39-5). Relatively few cells express cell surface IgG, IgA, or IgE. Cell surface immunoglobulin is similar in structure to secreted

TABLE 39–5 Cluster-Designated (CD) Molecules Found on Human B Cells*

Antigen	Molecular Weight (kDa)	Comment
CD5	67	B cell subset marker
CD10	100	Pre-B cell marker
CD19	95	
CD20	95	
CD21	35	Complement receptor CR2 (C3b receptor)
CD22	140	
CD23	45	IgE low-affinity receptor on activated B cells
CD25	55	Interleukin-2 receptor (low-affinity) chain
CDw32	40	Fc receptor (FcR11)
CD35	220	Complement receptor CR1 (C3d receptor)
CD45	180-220	Leukocyte common antigen
CD45R	220, 205	Restricted leukocyte common antigen

*All human B cells express surface immunoglobulin, and most B cells express class I and class II major histocompatibility antigens.

antibody and consists of four polypeptide chains (two identical heavy chains and two identical light chains) joined by disulfide bonds. Surface immunoglobulin is inserted into the lymphocyte membrane at the constant region of the immunoglobulin molecule.

Immune responses to foreign antigens can be classified as primary or secondary (Table 39-6). The primary immune response results in an increase in the titer of antibody, which plateaus and then is catabolized. In the secondary immune response, the antibody titer is usually greater, appears more quickly, and consists almost entirely of IgG antibody (versus IgM in the primary immune response). Most important, after the primary response, the host acquires an immunologic memory of that foreign antigen by expanding the population of antigen-specific T cells and B cells. Memory B cells are prone to making IgG earlier and exhibit higher affinity antigen receptors. Although a few foreign antigens are considered T cell independent (i.e., they do not require the help of T cells), the antibody response to most antigens requires the coordinated response of T cells, B cells, and APCs (B cells, macrophages, and DCs). Two kinds of signals are required to activate B cells: The first signal is provided by the interaction of the foreign antigen with surface immunoglobulin, and the second signal originates from Th cells, which are needed for amplification of the immune response.

B Cell Development
B cell maturation occurs in two stages. In the first stage, undifferentiated stem cells mature into cells identifiable as B lymphocytes; this is an antigen-independent phase that occurs in the fetal liver and bone marrow in humans. The second stage of lymphoid differentiation is antigen dependent; during this phase, B lymphocytes are transformed into plasma cells.

The first recognizable cell in the B cell lineage is the pre-B cell (Fig. 39-7). This cell can be detected in fetal liver by 7 to 8 weeks of gestation and is characterized by cytoplasmic staining for the heavy chain of IgM (μ chain). As gestation progresses, pre-B cells can be detected in the fetal bone marrow. Clonal diversity is generated at the pre-B cell stage of development. Intact immunoglobulin genes are formed by the rearrangement of gene segments composing each heavy-chain and light-chain family. Genes encoding the human heavy chain are located on chromosome 14; the κ light-chain genes are located on chromosome 2, and the λ light-chain genes are located on chromosome 22. The heavy-chain family consists of several hundred variable genes (*VH*), a smaller number of diversity genes (*DH*), and six joining genes (*JH*). The *JH* genes are linked to constant genes, which encode for the heavy-chain classes. The light-chain genes are similarly constructed. Antibody variable regions are generated from multiple smaller gene segments; the potential number of different antigen combining sites is the product of the number of *VH, DH,* and *JH* genes. Antibody diversity is additionally increased by the random addition of nucleotides at the splice site junctions of V, D, and J segments, and by point mutations in variable-region gene segments.

Pre-B cells give rise to immature B lymphocytes, which express surface IgM and complement receptors, but no other

TABLE 39–6   **Features of Primary and Secondary Antibody Responses**

Feature	Primary Response	Secondary Response
Lag after immunization	Usually 5-10 days	Usually 1-3 days
Peak response	Smaller	Larger
Antibody isotype	Usually IgM > IgG	Relative increase in IgG and, under certain circumstances, in IgA or IgE
Antibody affinity	Lower average affinity, more variable	Higher average affinity ("affinity maturation")
Induced by	All immunogens	Only protein antigens
Required immunization	Relatively high doses of antigens, optimally with adjuvants	Low doses of antigens, with adjuvants usually not necessary

From Abbas AK et al, editors: *Cellular and molecular immunology,* 2nd ed, Philadelphia, 1994, Saunders, p 188.

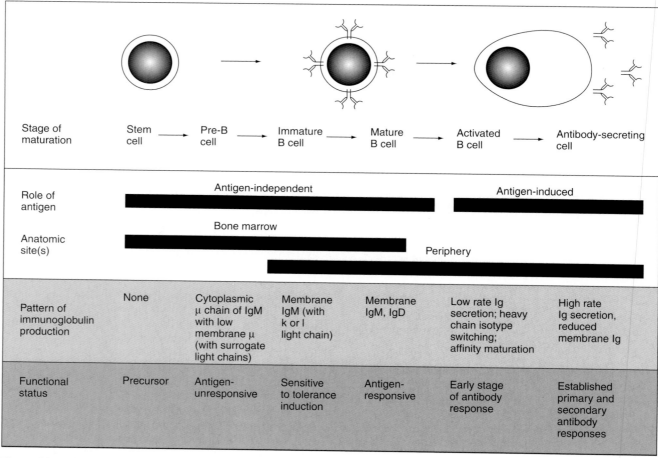

Figure 39–7. Sequence of B lymphocyte maturation and antigen-induced differentiation. Ig, immunoglobulin. (*From Abbas AK et al, editors:* Cellular and molecular immunology, *2nd ed. Philadelphia, 1994, Saunders, with permission.*)

immunoglobulin classes. These cells can be detected in the fetal liver at 8 to 9 weeks of gestation. Immature B lymphocytes have a unique functional property; when exposed to an antigen or ligand in the absence of activated T cells, they are rendered tolerant to additional stimulation with the same antigen; this process, called clonal anergy, accounts for the tolerance of B lymphocytes to self-antigens. Immunoglobulin class diversity occurs by a process of isotype switching, during which cells that express surface IgM with a particular specificity generate daughter cells that express another immunoglobulin class (Fig. 39-8). Cells that express other membrane immunoglobulin isotypes (IgG, IgA) can be shown by the 12th week of gestation. These other immunoglobulin classes almost always appear on cells that express membrane IgM concurrently.

At a later stage (the mature B cell stage), cells express membrane-bound IgG or IgA in association with membrane IgM and IgD. Cells that express surface IgD are incapable of being deactivated by antigen. In cells that express three heavy-chain classes, all three isotypes exhibit the same specificity and express the same variable-region genes. During the antigen-dependent phase of B lymphocyte differentiation, most B lymphocytes express only a single isotype, and plasma cells do not express surface immunoglobulin (see Fig. 39-7). By the 15th week of gestation, a normal fetus has levels of circulating B lymphocytes that are equal to or higher than the levels of adults. Fetal B lymphocytes can be shown in highest proportions in the spleen (30%), blood (35%), and lymph nodes (13%).

B Cell Activation by B Cell Antigen Receptors and Coreceptors

The BCR serves multiple functions on B cells that can differ substantially through various stages of their development. Proliferative expansion and differentiation are triggered through the pre-BCR and BCR complexes in pre-B cells and mature resting cells. At the opposite extreme, apoptosis is triggered in immature B cells on excessive clustering of newly expressed BCRs as a mechanism to eliminate autoreactive membrane IgM-expressing B cells. Strong BCR ligation in mature B cells has also been shown to inhibit V(D)J recombination at the membrane immunoglobulin locus, whereas weak ligation promotes recombination, presumably to generate higher affinity antibodies. Finally, the BCR serves as a specific receptor to internalize antigen efficiently for processing and peptide presentation to Th cells. The B cell has devised a complex network of BCR signaling cascades to perform such a diverse array of functions.

Role of Cytokines in B Cell Function

The cytokines IL-1, IL-2, and IL-4 affect B cell and T cell function. IL-2 stimulates the growth and differentiation of B cells. The ability of IL-4 to induce class switching in B cells has been documented earlier. This section deals in more detail with other cytokines having more specific effects on B cells.

IL-5 is produced by activated T cells. On B cells, IL-5 functions as a late-acting B cell differentiation factor, playing a major role in the production of IgA. IL-5 is perhaps better known, however, for its effect on eosinophil differentiation. It not only induces the generation of eosinophils from human bone marrow precursors, but also upregulates expression of CD11b on human eosinophils and activates IgA-induced eosinophil degranulation. T cell production of this cytokine is stimulated by parasitic infections.

IL-6 is a pleiotropic cytokine produced by many cell types, including T cells. Its effect on B cells is to promote growth and facilitate maturation of the B cells, causing immunoglobulin secretion. Resting B cells do not express the IL-6 receptor, but are induced to express the IL-6 receptor after activation.

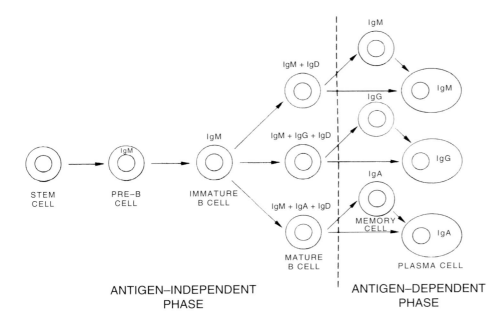

STEM CELL — PRE-B CELL — IMMATURE B CELL

IgM + IgD
IgM + IgG + IgD
IgM + IgA + IgD

MATURE B CELL

IgM
IgG
IgA

MEMORY CELL

IgM
IgG
IgA

PLASMA CELL

ANTIGEN–INDEPENDENT PHASE

ANTIGEN–DEPENDENT PHASE

Figure 39–8. Development of B cell surface immunoglobulin expression. Immunoglobulin class diversity occurs by a process of isotype switching. Immature B lymphocytes express surface IgM, but as cells mature, surface IgM and IgD in association with IgA or IgG are expressed. During the antigen-dependent phase of B cell maturation, B cells express a single immunoglobulin isotype, and mature plasma cells are devoid of surface immunoglobulin.

IL-7 has been described previously in the T cell section, but this cytokine, which is secreted by stromal cells, has a great effect on the development of progenitor B cells. IL-10 also affects T cells and B cells, acting synergistically with other cytokines on the growth of hematopoietic lineages, including those giving rise to B cells. Antibody depletion of IL-10 in vivo results in a reduced IgM and IgA response with an increase in IgG2 and a depletion of certain B cell subsets.

IL-13 is predominantly expressed in activated Th2 cells and regulates human B cell and monocyte activity. It acts as a costimulant with CD40 receptor engagement of human B cells. Interaction between CD40 and CD40 ligand in the presence of IL-13 induces isotype switching and IgE synthesis, as does IL-4.

IL-14 is believed to play a role in the development of B cell memory. IL-14 enhances the proliferation of activated B cells and inhibits the synthesis of immunoglobulin. It is produced by follicular DCs and activated T cells. IL-14 expression in reactive lymph nodes suggests that, during a secondary immune response, surface IgD B cells migrating through the lymph node encounter antigen, become activated, and express IL-14 receptor; after binding of IL-14, the increased Bcl-2 expression prevents apoptosis and permits B cell memory development.

Immunoglobulin Structure and Function

Specific antibody may be produced in response to direct microbial exposure or through immunization by an almost infinite spectrum of antigens (e.g., proteins, carbohydrates, bacteria, viruses, fungi, and drugs). Antibodies are synthesized and secreted by B lymphocyte–derived plasma cells that reside in the lymph nodes, spleen, mucosal linings of the gastrointestinal and respiratory tracts, and bone marrow.

Antibodies comprise a unique family of glycoproteins called immunoglobulin, which in humans consists of five major classes: IgG, IgA, IgM, IgD, and IgE. The basic structure of the IgG molecule is depicted in Figure 39-9. The IgG molecule is composed of four polypeptide chains—two heavy chains and two light chains—held together by covalent disulfide bonds and noncovalent forces. In a given IgG molecule, the two heavy chains and two light chains have identical amino acid sequences. The different immunoglobulin classes are distinguished by antigenic and amino acid sequence differences in their heavy chains. Some of the immunoglobulin classes are composed of subclasses; IgG has four subclasses—IgG1, IgG2, IgG3, and IgG4—that arise from antigenic differences in the heavy chains. In addition to these differences between the immunoglobulin classes and subclasses, there

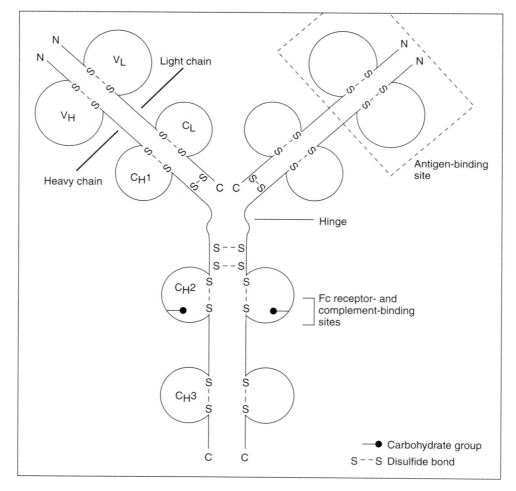

Figure 39–9. Schematic diagram of an immunoglobulin molecule. In this drawing of an IgG molecule, the antigen-binding sites are formed by the juxtaposition of light-chain (V_L) and heavy-chain (V_H) variable domains. The locations of complement-binding and Fc receptor-binding sites within the heavy-chain constant (C_H) regions are approximations. S-S refers to intrachain and interchain disulfide bonds; N and C refer to amino and carboxyl termini of the polypeptide chains. *(From Abbas AK et al, editors: Cellular and molecular immunology, 2nd ed. Philadelphia, 1994, Saunders, with permission.)*

are antigenic and amino acid sequence variations in the amino-terminal portions of the heavy chains and light chains in the so-called variable (Fab) regions. The structural variability in this region permits different antibody molecules to react specifically with different antigens. In contrast, the amino acid sequences of the carboxyl-terminal portions of the heavy (Fc region) and light chains do not vary between molecules of the same immunoglobulin class or subclass; these are called the constant regions. The variable regions of immunoglobulin molecules confer the antigen-binding specificity, and the constant regions differ among the various immunoglobulin classes; these regions' biologic properties and functions vary as well. Only IgM and IgG activate the complement system through the classic pathway, and only IgG can be actively transported across the placenta.

The chemical characteristics and biologic properties of the immunoglobulin classes are summarized in Table 39-7. IgG is the major immunoglobulin in the serum and interstitial fluid and has a long half-life of approximately 21 days. It is responsible for immunity to bacteria (particularly gram-positive bacteria), bacterial toxins, and viral agents. IgG antibodies can neutralize viruses and toxins, and facilitate the phagocytosis and destruction of bacteria and other particles to which they are bound. IgG can also activate the complement pathway and amplify the inflammatory response by increasing leukocyte chemotaxis and complement-mediated opsonization.

IgA is the second most abundant immunoglobulin in serum, but it is the predominant one in the gastrointestinal and respiratory tracts and in human colostrum and breast milk. In secretions, IgA occurs as a dimer joined by a J chain and bears an additional polypeptide chain, called the secretory component. This moiety endows the molecule with resistance against degradation by proteolytic enzymes. Secretory IgA is uniquely suited for functioning in the secretions of the respiratory and gastrointestinal tracts. IgA provides local mucosal immunity against viruses and limits bacterial overgrowth on mucosal surfaces. It also may limit absorption of antigenic dietary proteins. IgA does not activate the classic

complement pathway, but can activate the alternative pathway.

IgM antibodies exist in serum primarily as pentamers joined together by a J chain. IgM provides protection against blood-borne infection. It occurs only in small quantities in interstitial fluids and secretions. IgM antibodies are potent bacterial agglutinins and activate the classic complement pathway. Through activation of the complement system, IgM antibodies cause deposition of C3b on bacterial cell surfaces and facilitate phagocytosis. There are no phagocytosis-promoting receptors for IgM. Most serum antibodies to gram-negative bacteria are of the IgM type. Intrauterine and neonatal infections elicit the formation of predominantly IgM antibodies. Because IgM does not cross the placenta, the presence of specific IgM antibody in cord blood to spirochetes, rubella, CMV, or other microorganisms can be taken as reliable evidence of intrauterine infection with these agents. The absence of IgM does not exclude the possibility of congenital intrauterine infection, however.

IgE antibodies are present in extremely small quantities in serum and secretions. These antibodies play a major role in allergic reactions of the immediate hypersensitivity type. IgE antibodies bind to the cell membranes of basophils (mast cells) by a receptor for the carboxyl-terminal portion of the heavy chain. Binding of antigen (allergen) to the IgE fixed to the basophil results in the liberation of histamine, leukotrienes, and other pharmacologic mediators of immediate allergic reactions. IgD, which occurs in low concentration in serum, is present on the surface of B lymphocytes. The role of circulating IgD is unclear.

Antibody Production in Fetuses and Neonates
The fetus acquires the ability to produce serum immunoglobulins early in gestation. In vitro studies have shown the ability of fetal cells to produce antibody (IgM) by 8 weeks' gestation. IgG synthesis occur slightly later, and IgA synthesis begins at approximately 30 weeks' gestation. For numerous reasons (i.e., the sterile environment in utero, the inability of the fetus to respond to certain kinds

TABLE 39-7   Chemical and Biologic Properties of Human Immunoglobulin Classes

Variable	IgG	IgA	IgM	IgD	IgE
Heavy chains	γ	α	μ	δ	ε
Molecular weight (Da)	150,000	160,000 400,000*	900,000	180,000	190,000
Biologic half-life (days)	21	5	5	2	2
Adult serum concentration (mg/dL)	1000	250	100	2.3	0.01
Placental transfer	+	0	0	0	0
Binds complement (classic pathway)	+	0	+	0	0
Reaginic activity	0	0	0	0	+
Mucosal immunity	+	+++	+	0	++

*Secretory IgA.
0-+++ indicates increasing ability to protect mucosal surfaces from pathogen invasion.

of antibody, T cell suppression of B cell differentiation), the fetus makes little antibody before the time of birth. As discussed later, at the time of birth, most of the circulating antibodies are IgG antibodies that have been transported across the placenta from the maternal circulation. Low levels of "fetal" IgM (<10% of adult levels) are present at term gestation and reach adult levels by 1 to 2 years of age. The concentration of IgG decreases postnatally (because of the catabolism of maternal IgG) and reaches a nadir (physiologic hypogammaglobulinemia) at approximately 3 to 4 months of age. Adult concentrations of IgG are reached by 4 to 6 years of age, and adult levels of IgA are attained near puberty (Table 39-8).

Summary

The ability to mount cell-mediated or antibody-mediated immune responses to specific antigens is acquired sequentially during the course of embryonic development. Early in gestation, fetuses can respond to certain antigens, whereas other antigens elicit antibody production or cell-mediated immune reactions only after birth. The well-known inability of children younger than 18 months of age to induce antibodies to polysaccharides from *Pneumococcus* and *Haemophilus* organisms is a clinically important example of the sequential acquisition of antigen-specific immunocompetence in humans.

Antibody responses of fetuses and premature and full-term newborns differ from responses of children and adults. Fetuses and newborns do not respond to some antigens (e.g., pneumococcal polysaccharide), and the antibody responses to other antigens (e.g., rubella, CMV, *Toxoplasma*) are predominantly of the IgM type. T lymphocytes are less experienced in neonates and may tend to suppress rather than stimulate B cell differentiation. In addition, B cells of newborns differentiate predominantly into IgM-secreting plasma cells, whereas activated adult B cells produce IgG-secreting

TABLE 39-8 Normal Values for Immunoglobulins at Various Ages

Age	IgG (mg/dL)	IgA (mg/dL)	IgM (mg/dL)
Newborn	600-1670	0-5	5-15
1-3 mo	218-610	20-53	11-51
4-6 mo	228-636	27-72	25-60
7-9 mo	292-816	27-73	12-124
10-18 mo	383-1070	27-169	28-113
2 y	423-1184	35-222	32-131
3 y	477-1334	40-251	28-113
4-5 y	540-1500	48-336	20-106
6-8 y	571-1700	52-535	28-112
14 y	570-1570	86-544	33-135
Adult	635-1775	106-668	37-154

From Buckley RH et al: Serum immunoglobulins, I: levels in normal children and in uncomplicated childhood allergy, *Pediatrics* 41:600, 1968.

and IgA-secreting plasma cells as well. The adult pattern of B cell differentiation develops during the first year of life.

PASSIVE IMMUNITY

Passive immunity is the acquisition of specific antibody or sensitized lymphocytes from another individual, and it represents a means by which specific immunity can be acquired without previous exposure to antigen or the mounting of a specific immune response. Such immunity is transient, but nonetheless may provide sufficient antimicrobial protection during a vulnerable period of life. The development of an antibody response to an antigen seen for the first time requires 7 to 14 days. Active antibody-mediated immunity is of little value during the crucial first few days of an infection with a new microorganism. The presence of circulating specific antibody to that organism (i.e., passive immunity) permits the mobilization of multiple host defense mechanisms (e.g., complement system, neutrophils) to eliminate the invading microorganism and limit its colonization. In humans, the major avenues for the acquisition of passive immunity are the transfer of IgG across the placenta and the transfer of secretory IgA through colostrum and breast milk.

Placental Transport of Antibodies

Although B lymphocytes are present in a fetus by the end of the first trimester, there is little active fetal immunoglobulin production because this process depends on exposure to antigens. Serum immunoglobulin levels in fetuses are extremely low until 20 to 22 weeks of gestation, at which time an accelerated active transport of IgG across the placenta begins. Only maternal IgG is transported. The specificity of this transport process is due to the presence of specific placental receptors for the heavy chain (Fc region) of the IgG molecule. The transport of IgG is an active placental process, and the neonate's serum IgG concentration at birth is 5% to 10% higher than that of the mother. Prematurely delivered infants have lower IgG levels than infants delivered at term; infants who are very premature (24 to 26 weeks) may have acquired little maternal antibody before delivery. Infants who are small for gestational age have lower IgG levels than infants who are an appropriate size at any gestational age. The placental dysfunction that reduces the nutrient supply to these poorly growing infants may also limit transfer of IgG. This phenomenon is manifested further by the progressive decrease in IgG transport after 44 weeks of gestation, a period when the placenta is known to become increasingly dysfunctional.

Elevated levels of IgM or IgA in cord blood usually indicate that the infant has been exposed to antigen in utero and has synthesized antibody itself. Congenital infections with syphilis and rubella characteristically produce elevation of the cord blood IgM concentration, and specific fetal antibody of the IgM type directed against the infecting agent can be detected. Elevated levels of IgM and IgA also may be found if maternal-to-fetal transplacental bleeding has occurred.

Immunologic Properties of Human Breast Milk

Maternal transfer of immunity to the newborn infant is also possible through breast milk.[17] Table 39-9 lists specific and nonspecific protective factors that are transferred to the

TABLE 39–9   **Immunologically and Pharmacologically Active Components and Hormones Found in Human Colostrum and Milk**

Soluble	Cellular	Hormones and Hormone-like Substances
Immunologically specific	Immunologically specific	Epidermal growth factor
Immunoglobulin: secretory IgA (11S), 7S IgA, IgG, IgM	T lymphocytes	Prostaglandins
IgE, IgD, secretory component	B lymphocytes	Relaxin
T cell products	Accessory cells	Neurotensin
Histocompatibility antigens	Neutrophils	Somatostatin
Nonspecific factors	Macrophages	Bombesin
Complement	Epithelial cells	Gonadotropins
Chemotactic factors		Ovarian steroids
Properdin		Thyroid-releasing hormone
Interferon		Thyroid-stimulating hormone
α-fetoprotein		Thyroxine and triiodothyronine
Bifidus factor		Adrenocorticotropic hormone
Antistaphylococcal factors		Corticosteroids
Antiadherence substances		Prolactin
Epidermal growth factor		Erythropoietin
Folate uptake enhancer		Insulin
Antiviral factors		
Migration inhibition factor		
Carrier proteins		
Lactoferrin		
Transferrin		
Vitamin B_{12}-binding protein		
Corticoid-binding protein		
Enzymes		
Lysozyme		
Lipoprotein lipase		
Leukocyte enzymes		

From Ogra PL et al: Human breast milk. In Remington JS et al, editors: *Infectious diseases of the fetus and newborn infant,* 4th ed, Philadelphia, 1995, Saunders, p 114.

neonate by breast milk. Although all immunoglobulin classes can be detected in colostrum, secretory IgA constitutes most of the immunoglobulin in human breast milk. Secretory IgA consists of two "serum" IgA subunits, a J chain and a secretory component, which render it resistant to digestion by trypsin and pepsin and to hydrolysis by gastric acid. There is no evidence that immunoglobulins present in breast milk enter the systemic circulation of the human neonate.

The levels of IgA, IgM, and IgG have been studied serially in milk. The IgG concentration is relatively constant during the first 180 days of lactation, whereas IgM and IgA are highest in colostrum, decrease during the first 5 days of lactation, and remain relatively constant during the next 175 days. Breast milk contains antibodies to a broad spectrum of enteric bacteria and viruses (e.g., poliovirus, echovirus, coxsackievirus), and the antibody titers to these agents decrease in parallel to the decrease in concentrations of IgA in the milk.

Most immunoglobulins present in human breast milk are believed to be produced by plasma cells located in the breast itself, and very little milk immunoglobulin is derived from maternal serum immunoglobulins. Milk antibodies are directed predominantly against enteric bacterial and viral antigens; the concentration of such antibodies is much higher in colostrum than in maternal serum. The antibody composition of breast milk compensates partly for the deficiency of antibodies directed against enteric antigens in placentally transferred IgG. This unique spectrum of antibody specificity is achieved by the "homing" of B lymphocytes, sensitized in the mother's gastrointestinal tract, to her mammary glands. B cells stimulated by enteric bacterial or viral antigens in the Peyer patches of the small intestine migrate to the mucosal linings of the lactating mammary gland, where they differentiate into plasma cells and secrete their antibodies. Antigens introduced into the gastrointestinal tract stimulate the development of antibodies in breast milk; however, antibodies to these antigens do not develop in the serum. A mother transfers to her infant through breast milk antibodies specific for microbial agents present in her own gastrointestinal tract. As the neonate is being freshly colonized by primarily maternal flora, these antibodies limit bacterial growth in the gastrointestinal tract and protect against overgrowth.

The cellular components of human breast milk consist of macrophages, T and B lymphocytes, neutrophils, and epithelial cells. The cellular content of colostrum or early milk is higher than that of later milk and varies greatly among women. Neutrophils are present in significant numbers early in lactation, and their presence may be related to breast engorgement during the initial days of lactation. Although the function of the breast milk neutrophil is unclear, its presence does not imply infection. Epithelial cells occasionally present in milk may originate from the skin of the nipple.

Breast milk macrophages are mononuclear phagocytic cells that constitute approximately 80% of the leukocytes in milk. This is an active phagocytic cell that contains large amounts of intracytoplasmic lipid and IgA; bears cell surface receptors for IgG and C3b; and synthesizes several important host resistance factors, including lysozyme, C3 and C4 complement components, and lactoferrin. Milk macrophages are capable of phagocytizing and killing gram-positive and gram-negative bacteria and apparently interact with the lymphocytes present in breast milk.

The host defense factors that the breast milk macrophage synthesizes provide important nonspecific antimicrobial protection for neonates. Lysozyme is capable of lysing the cell walls of many bacteria. This enzyme is synthesized by the milk macrophage, and its concentration in human milk is 300 times that found in cow's milk. It is stable in an acid environment comparable with that of the gastric contents. Lactoferrin is synthesized by the milk macrophage, and its concentration in breast milk is higher than in any other body fluid. Lactoferrin antimicrobial activity derives from its ability to chelate iron, depriving bacteria of a cofactor important for their growth. The growth of *Staphylococcus* organisms and *E. coli* is limited by lactoferrin.

The C3 and C4 complement components are also actively synthesized by breast macrophages. The function of these proteins in milk is unclear because there is little IgG and IgM or the early complement components, C1 and C2, which are necessary for activation of C3 to its biologically active forms. IgA may activate C3 through the alternative pathway; however, it is found in highest concentrations in the breast macrophage itself. This macrophage-associated IgA is not synthesized, but rather is ingested by the macrophage. Viable in situ macrophages have been shown to release this IgA slowly, and this has led to the hypothesis that the breast milk macrophage may represent a vehicle for immunoglobulin transport down the neonate's gastrointestinal tract.

Viable T and B lymphocytes are present in human breast milk. T lymphocytes represent 50% of the milk lymphocytes early in lactation, declining to less than 20% as lactation progresses. The spectrum of responses of breast milk T cells differs from that of peripheral blood T cells from the same donor. Milk T cells are often unresponsive to *C. albicans* antigen, whereas peripheral blood T cells from the same donor are highly reactive. In contrast, milk T cells respond well to the K1 capsular antigen of *E. coli,* whereas peripheral blood lymphocytes exhibit minimal or no response to K1. This phenomenon may be related to the previously described homing of lymphocytes sensitized in the gastrointestinal tract to mammary glands.

The transfer of cell-mediated immunity from tuberculin-sensitive mothers to their breast-fed infants has been reported. If these reports are substantiated, this form of passive transfer of cellular immunity could be of major clinical significance. It is unlikely that intact T lymphocytes are passing from the mother's milk across the mucous membranes of the infant's gastrointestinal tract. A soluble T cell growth factor or lymphokine more likely is involved. The B lymphocytes present in milk have IgG, IgA, IgM, and IgD on their surfaces. These cells synthesize IgA almost exclusively, however. The contribution of B cells as passive immune effectors in breast milk is as yet unclear.

Summary

Maternal transfer of IgG antibodies across the placenta provides a newborn with a measure of immune protection. Antibodies to viral agents, diphtheria, and tetanus antitoxins, which are usually of the IgG class, are efficiently transported across the placenta and attain protective levels in the fetus. In contrast, antibodies to agents that evoke primarily IgA or IgM antibody responses are transported poorly or not at all, leaving the neonate unprotected against those organisms. An infant cannot be protected against agents to which the mother has not made significant amounts of antibody. Breast milk constituents may interact with the neonate's immune system in ways other than those already mentioned. A significant increase in the secretory IgA content of nasal and salivary secretions has been observed in breast-fed versus formula-fed newborns during the first few days of life. It is postulated that this increase may reflect the influence of a soluble factor in milk that acts to stimulate the mucosal immune system of breast-fed infants. Factors that enhance IgA synthesis by B cells and promote epithelial cell growth are also secreted by milk macrophages.

EVALUATION OF HOST DEFENSES IN NEONATES

Some disorders of immunologic function may become clinically apparent in the neonatal period or first year of life.[46] Because of differences in the developmental status of the newborn's host defense mechanisms and the lack of vast exposure to antigens, evaluation of the function of host defense mechanisms in the infant is different from the evaluation performed for older children and adults. Infants who have experienced two or more significant bacterial or fungal infections should be suspected of having a defect in host defense mechanisms. Patients with unusual infections (e.g., from *Pneumocystis jiroveci* [formerly *Pneumocystis carinii*]) or infections that respond incompletely to therapy and recur are also suspect. Growth failure, chronic diarrhea, chronic dermatitis, hepatosplenomegaly, and recurrent abscesses commonly occur in infants with immunologic deficiency. Primary immunodeficiency disorders are relatively uncommon, however, and numerous other predisposing conditions should be considered that may be predisposing an infant to multiple infectious episodes.

In evaluating a patient for a possible host defense mechanism defect, natural (cellular and humoral components) and acquired (cellular and humoral components) immune mechanisms should be considered and investigated. The evaluation should be divided into initial screening tests and definitive tests that allow one to establish a specific diagnosis (Box 39-2). Screening tests should be obtainable by physicians at all hospitals, but definitive tests may be available only at major medical centers.

BOX 39–2   Tests to Evaluate Neonatal Host Defense Mechanisms

NATURAL IMMUNITY

Cellular Components
- White blood cell count and differential*
- Nitroblue tetrazolium (NBT) dye reduction test*
- Random mobility and chemotaxis assay
- Phagocytosis assay
- Quantitative bactericidal assay
- Flow cytometric analysis of cell surface receptor expression
- Analysis of oxidative metabolism and enzyme activity

Humoral Components (Complement)
- Total hemolytic complement assay (CH_{50})*
- Determination of C3 and C4 concentrations*
- Assay of individual components of classic and alternative pathways
- Functional measurement of alternative pathway
- Functional assay for C3a and C5a

ACQUIRED IMMUNITY

B Lymphocytes and Antibody Production
- Quantitation of serum IgG, IgA, and IgM*
- Measurement of specific antibodies after immunization*
- Isoagglutinin titer (anti-A and anti-B)*
- Determination of IgE and IgD concentrations
- Flow cytometric enumeration and analysis of B cell phenotype
- Tests of B cell-to-plasma cell maturation and antibody production in vitro

T Lymphocytes
- Total lymphocyte count and morphology*
- Delayed hypersensitivity skin tests to common antigens*
- Chest radiograph for thymic size*
- Proliferative responses to mitogens, antigens, and allogeneic cells
- Flow cytometric enumeration and analysis of T cell subsets
- Cytotoxicity assays
- Lymphokine production assays

*Considered one of the initial screening tests.

REFERENCES

1. Abreau M, Arditi M: Innate immunity and Toll-like receptors: clinical implications of basic science research, *J Pediatr* 144:421, 2004.
2. Adkins B et al: Neonatal adaptive immunity comes of age, *Nat Rev Immunol* 4:553, 2004.
3. Adkins B: T-cell function in newborn mice and humans, *Immunol Today* 20:330, 1999.
4. Blom B et al: Generation of interferon alpha-producing predendritic cell (Pre-DC)2 from human CD34(+) hematopoietic stem cells, *J Exp Med* 192:1785, 2000.
5. Chelvarajan RL et al: Defective macrophage function in neonates and its impact on unresponsiveness of neonates to polysaccharide antigens, *J Leukoc Biol* 75:982, 2004.
6. Colucci F et al: Natural killer cell activation in mice and men: different triggers for similar weapons? *Nat Immunol* 3:807, 2002.
7. De Wit D et al: Blood plasmacytoid dendritic cell responses to CpG oligodeoxynucleotides are impaired in human newborns, *Blood* 103:1030, 2004.
8. Douglas S et al: The mononuclear phagocytic, dendritic cell, and natural killer cell systems. In Steihm E et al, editors: *Immunologic disorders of infants and children*, 5th ed., Philadelphia, Saunders, 2004, p 129.
9. Farag SS et al: Biology and clinical impact of human natural killer cells, *Int J Hematol* 78:7, 2003.
10. Flamand V et al: CD40 ligation prevents neonatal induction of transplantation tolerance, *J Immunol* 160:4666, 1998.
11. Forster-Waldl E et al: Monocyte toll-like receptor 4 expression and LPS-induced cytokine production increase during gestational aging, *Pediatr Res* 58:121, 2005.
12. Gale L, McColl S: Chemokines: extracellular messengers for all occasions? *Bioessays* 21:17, 1999.
13. Gerdes J et al: Tracheal lavage and plasma fibronectin: relationship to respiratory distress syndrome and development of bronchopulmonary dysplasia, *J Pediatr* 108:601, 1986.
14. Germain RN: T-cell development and the CD4-CD8 lineage decision, *Nat Rev Immunol* 2:309, 2002.
15. Goriely S et al: Deficient IL-12(p35) gene expression by dendritic cells derived from neonatal monocytes, *J Immunol* 166:2141, 2001.
16. Han P et al: Potential immaturity of the T-cell and antigen-presenting cell interaction in cord blood with particular emphasis on the CD40-CD40 ligand costimulatory pathway, *Immunology* 113:26, 2004.
17. Hanson L et al: The transfer of immunity from mother to child, *Ann N Y Acad Sci* 987:199, 2003.
18. Harris M et al: Diminished actin polymerization by neutrophils from newborn infants, *Pediatr Res* 33:27, 1993.
19. Hodge S et al: Cord blood leucocyte expression of functionally significant molecules involved in the regulation of cellular immunity, *Scand J Immunol* 53:72, 2001.
20. Holt PG: Functionally mature virus-specific CD8(+) T memory cells in congenitally infected newborns: proof of principle for neonatal vaccination? *J Clin Invest* 111:1645, 2003.
21. Insel R, Looney R: The B-lymphocyte system: fundamental immunology. In Steihm ER et al, editors: *Immunologic disorders in infants and children*, 5th ed., Philadelphia, 2004, Saunders, p 53.
22. Kaur K et al: Decreased expression of tumor necrosis factor family receptors involved in humoral immune responses in preterm neonates, *Blood* 110:2948, 2007.
23. Kobayashi K, Flavell R: Shielding the double-edged sword: negative regulation of the innate immune response, *J Leukoc Biol* 75:428, 2004.
24. Koenig J et al: Diminished soluble and total cellular L-selectin in cord blood is associated with its impaired shedding from activated neutrophils, *Pediatr Res* 39:616, 1996.
25. Koenig J, Yoder M: Neonatal neutrophils: the good, the bad, the ugly, *Clin Perinatol* 31:39, 2004.
26. Langrish CL et al: Neonatal dendritic cells are intrinsically biased against Th-1 immune responses, *Clin Exp Immunol* 128:118, 2002.
27. Levy O et al: Selective impairment of TLR-mediated innate immunity in human newborns: neonatal blood plasma reduces monocyte TNF-alpha induction by bacterial lipopeptides, lipopolysaccharide, and imiquimod, but preserves the response to R-848, *J Immunol* 173:4627, 2004.
28. Li L et al: Neonatal immunity develops in a transgenic TCR transfer model and reveals a requirement for elevated cell input to achieve organ-specific responses, *J Immunol* 167:2585, 2001.
29. Liu E et al: Tolerance associated with cord blood transplantation may depend on the state of host dendritic cells, *Br J Haematol* 126:517, 2004.
30. Liu E et al: Decreased yield, phenotypic expression and function of immature monocyte-derived dendritic cells in cord blood, *Br J Haematol* 113:240, 2001.
31. Malik A et al: Beyond the complete blood count and C-reactive protein, *Arch Pediatr Adolesc Med* 157:511, 2003.
32. Marchant A et al: Mature CD8(+) T lymphocyte response to viral infection during fetal life, *J Clin Invest* 111:1747, 2003.
33. Marodi L: Deficient interferon-gamma receptor-mediated signaling in neonatal macrophages, *Acta Paediatr Suppl* 91:117, 2002.
34. Marodi L et al: Cytokine receptor signalling in neonatal macrophages: defective STAT-1 phosphorylation in response to stimulation with IFN-gamma, *Clin Exp Immunol* 126:456, 2001.
35. Newton J et al: Effect of pentoxifylline on developmental changes in neutrophil cell surface mobility and membrane fluidity, *J Cell Physiol* 140:427, 1989.
36. Pihlgren M et al. Delayed and deficient establishment of the long-term bone marrow plasma cell pool during early life, *Eur J Immunol* 31:939, 2001.
37. Pihlgren M et al: Reduced ability of neonatal and early-life bone marrow stromal cells to support plasmablast survival, *J Immunol* 176:165, 2006.
38. Pulendran B et al: Flt3-ligand and granulocyte colony-stimulating factor mobilize distinct human dendritic cell subsets in vivo, *J Immunol* 165:566, 2000.
39. Schibler K: Mononuclear phagocyte system. In Polin R et al, editors: *Fetal and neonatal physiology*, 3rd ed., Philadelphia, 2004, Saunders, p 1523.
40. Seder RA, Ahmed R: Similarities and differences in CD4$^+$ and CD8$^+$ effector and memory T cell generation, *Nat Immunol* 4:835, 2003.
41. Siegrist CA: Mechanisms by which maternal antibodies influence infant vaccine responses: review of hypotheses and definition of main determinants, *Vaccine* 21:3406, 2003.

42. Siegrist CA, Aspinall R: B-cell responses to vaccination at the extremes of age, *Nat Rev Immunol* 9:185, 2009.

43. Simpson CC et al: Impaired CD40-signalling in Langerhans' cells from murine neonatal draining lymph nodes: implications for neonatally induced cutaneous tolerance, *Clin Exp Immunol* 132:201, 2003.

44. Sorg RV et al: Identification of cord blood dendritic cells as an immature CD11c– population, *Blood* 93:2302, 1999.

45. Steihm E et al: Immunodeficiency disorders: general considerations. In Steihm E et al, editors: *Immunologic disorders of infants and children*, 5th ed., Philadelphia, 2004, Saunders, p 289.

46. Stockinger B: Neonatal tolerance mysteries solved, *Immunol Today* 17:249, 1996.

47. Sullivan K, Winkelstein J: Deficiencies of the complement system. In Steihm ER et al, editors: *Immunologic disorders of infants and children*, 5th ed., Philadelphia, 2004, Saunders, p 652.

48. Suri M et al: Immunotherapy in the prophylaxis and treatment of neonatal sepsis, *Curr Opin Pediatr* 15:155, 2003.

49. Till J, McCulloch E: A direct measurement of the radiation sensitivity of normal mouse bone marrow cells, *Radiat Res* 14:213, 1961.

50. Timens W et al: Immaturity of the human splenic marginal zone in infancy: possible contribution to the deficient infant immune response, *J Immunol* 143:3200, 1989.

51. Upham JW et al: Development of interleukin-12-producing capacity throughout childhood, *Infect Immun* 70:6583, 2002.

52. van de Wetering J et al: Collectins: players of the innate immune system, *Eur J Biochem* 271:1229, 2004.

53. Velilla PA et al: Defective antigen-presenting cell function in human neonates, *Clin Immunol* 121:251, 2006.

54. White GP et al: Differential patterns of methylation of the IFN-gamma promoter at CpG and non-CpG sites underlie differences in IFN-gamma gene expression between human neonatal and adult CD45RO-T cells, *J Immunol* 168:2820, 2002.

55. Willems F et al: Phenotype and function of neonatal DC, *Eur J Immunol* 39:26, 2009.

56. Wilson C, Edelmann K: The T-lymphocyte system. In Steihm ER et al, editors: *Immunologic disorders in infants and children*, 5th ed., Philadelphia, 2004, Saunders, p 20.

57. Wong OH et al: Differential responses of cord and adult blood-derived dendritic cells to dying cells, *Immunology* 116:13, 2005.

58. Yan SR et al: Role of MyD88 in diminished tumor necrosis factor alpha production by newborn mononuclear cells in response to lipopolysaccharide, *Infect Immun* 72:1223, 2004.

59. Yang K, Hill H: Neutrophil function disorders: pathophysiology, prevention and therapy, *J Pediatr* 119:354, 1991.

60. Yoder MC: Embryonic hematopoiesis. In Christensen RD, editor: *Hematologic problems of the neonate*. Philadelphia, 2000, Saunders, p 3.

61. Yokoyama WM, Plougastel BF: Immune functions encoded by the natural killer gene complex, *Nat Rev Immunol* 3:304, 2003.

PART 2
Postnatal Bacterial Infections
Morven S. Edwards

NEONATAL SEPSIS

Despite the development of newer, more potent antimicrobial agents, infections are still an important cause of neonatal morbidity and mortality. Part 2 of this chapter focuses on bacterial infections; however, viral, fungal, and parasitic infections must be considered in the differential diagnosis of neonatal sepsis.

Incidence and Mortality

The term *sepsis neonatorum* is used to describe any systemic bacterial infection documented by a positive blood culture in the first month of life. Neonatal sepsis has distinct presentations based on the postnatal age at onset (Table 39-10): Early-onset sepsis occurs in the first 7 days of life and is acquired by vertical transmission from the mother. It usually has a fulminant onset with multisystem involvement, and has a higher case-fatality rate than late-onset sepsis (see Chapter 23). Late-onset sepsis usually is more insidious, but can have an acute onset. Late, late-onset sepsis occurs after 3 months of life and affects premature infants who are of very low birthweight (VLBW). Late, late-onset sepsis is often caused by *Candida* species or by commensal organisms such as coagulase-negative staphylococci (CONS), and often is associated with prolonged instrumentation, such as indwelling intravascular lines and endotracheal intubation. The incidence of neonatal sepsis ranges from 1 to 5 cases per 1000 live births. In the preantibiotic era, neonatal sepsis was almost uniformly fatal. Mortality rates decreased dramatically after the introduction of antimicrobial agents and with technological advances in neonatal care. Over the past two decades, the case-fatality rate has declined to approximately 5% to 10%.

Microbiology

The bacterial pathogens responsible for sepsis neonatorum tend to shift over time.[9] In the United States, gram-positive cocci, including group A *Streptococcus*, were common pathogens before the introduction of antibiotics, but this predominance shifted to gram-negative enteric bacilli after antimicrobial agents came into common use. In the 1950s and early 1960s, *Staphylococcus aureus* and *Escherichia coli* predominated as neonatal pathogens. In the late 1960s, group B *Streptococcus* (GBS) emerged as a perinatal pathogen, and it continues to be an important organism in newborn infections, as is *E. coli*. This predominance is reflected in the distribution of bacteria causing early-onset neonatal sepsis in active surveillance conducted over a multistate area during 1998-2000 (Table 39-11).[28] In neonates of VLBW with early-onset sepsis, GBS was the most frequent pathogen, followed by *E. coli* and *Haemophilus influenzae*.[65] An increase in the incidence of *E. coli* and a decrease in GBS has been noted over the last decade.[64]

TABLE 39-10   Characteristics of Neonatal Sepsis

	Early Onset (<7 Days)	Late Onset (≥7 Days to 3 Months)	Late, Late Onset (>3 Months)
Intrapartum complications	Often present	Usually absent	Varies
Transmission	Vertical; organism often acquired from mother's genital tract	Vertical or through postnatal environment	Usually postnatal environment
Clinical manifestations	Fulminant course, multisystem involvement, pneumonia common	Insidious or acute, focal infection, meningitis common	Insidious
Case-fatality rate	5%-20%	5%	Low

TABLE 39-11   Etiologic Agents in Neonatal Sepsis

Organism	No. (%)
Bacteria Causing Early-Onset Neonatal Sepsis*	
Group B *Streptococcus*	166 (41)
Escherichia coli	70 (17)
Viridans streptococci	67 (16)
Enterococcus species	16 (4)
Staphylococcus aureus	15 (4)
Group D *Streptococcus*	12 (3)
Pseudomonas species	9 (2)
Other gram-negative enteric bacilli	16 (4)
Other	37 (9)
Total	408 (100)
Etiologic Agents in Late-Onset Neonatal Sepsis†	
Coagulase-negative *Staphylococcus*	629 (48)
Staphylococcus aureus	103 (8)
Candida albicans	76 (6)
Escherichia coli	64 (5)
Klebsiella	52 (4)
Candida parapsilosis	54 (4)
Enterococcus species	43 (3)
Pseudomonas	35 (3)
Group B *Streptococcus*	30 (2)
Other bacteria	197 (15)
Other fungi	30 (2)
Total	1313 (100)

*Early onset, <7 days of age. Adapted from Hyde TB et al: Trends in incidence and antimicrobial resistance of early-onset sepsis: population-based surveillance in San Francisco and Atlanta, *Pediatrics* 110:690, 2002.
†Infants were all very low birthweight (<1500 g). Blood cultures were obtained after 72 hours of life. Adapted from Stoll BJ et al: Late-onset sepsis in very low birth weight neonates: the experience of the NICHD Neonatal Research Network, *Pediatrics* 110:285, 2002.

Other pathogens, including CONS, *Candida* species, and *S. aureus*, are more commonly etiologic agents in late-onset infection, as shown by data from a multicenter prospective registry in neonates with VLBW (see Table 39-11).[66] Community-acquired methicillin-resistant *S. aureus* (MRSA) strains have emerged as a significant cause of sepsis in neonates hospitalized in the neonatal intensive care unit since birth.[27] As history suggests, further changes in the etiologic agents of neonatal sepsis are likely and warrant continued observation.

Transmission

Infectious agents can be transmitted to a neonate in many ways. Transplacental transmission is well documented for congenital viral infections, but not for perinatal bacterial infections, with the exceptions of infections caused by *Treponema pallidum* and *Listeria monocytogenes*. Ascending intra-amniotic infection followed by aspiration of infected amniotic fluid can result in systemic neonatal infection, especially in the setting of prolonged rupture of membranes (ROM). Approximately 1% to 4% of neonates born to mothers with intra-amniotic infection develop systemic infection. Neonatal infection can also be acquired during vaginal delivery from bacteria colonizing the mother's lower genital tract. Inadequate hand washing by the nursery staff can promote the spread of microorganisms from an infected to an uninfected infant or from the hands of colonized caregivers to the newborn. The use of instrumentation, including endotracheal tubes, nasogastric feeding tubes, umbilical catheters, central venous catheters, and urinary catheters, also increases the risk of neonatal infection.

Early-onset infection is most often transmitted vertically by ascending amniotic fluid infection and by delivery through an infected or colonized birth canal. The pathogens that cause later onset disease can be acquired vertically in the peripartum period or horizontally from fomites in the environment or from colonized caregivers after delivery.

Risk Factors

MATERNAL RISK FACTORS

Maternal factors can influence the development of systemic bacterial infection in the neonate. (See also Chapter 23.) For reasons that remain unclear, the overall incidence of neonatal

GBS infections is higher among blacks than in other racial groups.[45] Maternal factors such as malnutrition and sexually transmitted diseases can also increase the risk of infection. The rates of prematurity and low birthweight, both of which predispose to neonatal infection, are inversely related to socioeconomic status. Maternal colonization with GBS is well documented as a risk factor for neonatal sepsis. Colonization during the third trimester in an uncomplicated pregnancy carries approximately a 1% risk of infection if acquisition by the neonate is not prevented by intrapartum antibiotic prophylaxis; this risk is increased if colonization is associated with prematurity, maternal fever, or prolonged ROM. Asymptomatic bacteriuria has been associated with premature birth. Colonization with genital mycoplasmas has been associated with low birthweight.

PERIPARTUM RISK FACTORS

Some peripartum factors associated with an increased risk of neonatal infection are untreated or incompletely treated focal infections of the mother (including urinary tract, vaginal, or cervical infections) and systemic infections, such as maternal septicemia or maternal fever without a focus. (See also Chapter 23.) Uncomplicated ROM lasting longer than 24 hours carries a 1% risk of neonatal sepsis above the baseline rate of 0.1% to 0.5%. The risk of infection increases fourfold if chorioamnionitis and prolonged ROM coexist. Prematurity and low birthweight are associated with an increased incidence of sepsis. In a population-based cohort study of neonatal GBS disease, attack rates of 5.99 per 1000, 2.51 per 1000, and 0.89 per 1000 live-born infants were noted for infants with birthweights of less than 1500 g, 1500 to 2500 g, and more than 2500 g.[56] Rates of first episode of late-onset infection per 1000 hospital days also decreased with increasing birthweight and gestational age, so that infants with a birthweight of 750 g or less had a fourfold higher rate than infants with a birthweight of 1000 g or more.[66]

Another peripartum risk factor is the use of fetal scalp electrodes. Deliveries using electronic fetal monitoring can be associated with subsequent development of neonatal scalp abscesses. Cephalhematomas rarely may be complicated by sepsis, meningitis, and osteomyelitis. Perinatal asphyxia, defined as a 5-minute Apgar score of less than 6, in the presence of prolonged ROM has been associated with an increased incidence of sepsis.

NEONATAL RISK FACTORS

Although no significant gender difference has been documented for infections acquired in utero, it was noted in the 1960s that male infants had a higher incidence of neonatal sepsis than female infants, possibly related to X-linked immunoregulatory genes. Immaturity of the immune system of the newborn host, as shown in Table 39-12, can also have a role in the predisposition to infection (see Part 1 of this chapter).[47] Metabolic disorders can predispose to infection. Among neonates of VLBW with late-onset sepsis, complications of prematurity associated with an increased rate of infection included mechanical ventilation, umbilical vessel catheterization, other vascular catheters, hyperalimentation, and duration of hospital stay.[66]

OTHER RISK FACTORS

It has been suggested that bottle feeding can predispose to infection. Prepared formulas lack several important biologic factors found in colostrum, such as bacterial agglutinins and iron-binding proteins, which have a local gastrointestinal protective effect against gram-negative enteric bacilli. Breast milk also contains immunoglobulins, macrophages, and lymphocytes, all of which play a role in immunologic defense.

TABLE 39–12	Host Responses to Bacterial Infection in Neonates		
Component	Function	Status in Neonate	Clinical Significance
Complement	Opsonization, chemoattraction	Decreased complement components, especially in preterm infants	Decreased production of chemotactic factors; decreased opsonization of bacteria
Antibody	Opsonization, complement activation	IgG concentration decreased in preterm infants; term infants have higher concentration than adults; IgA absent from secretions	Lack of antibody to specific pathogens results in increased risk of infection; increased risk of mucosal colonization with potential pathogens
Neutrophil	Chemotaxis	Impaired migration; impaired binding to chemotactic factors	Decreased inflammatory response; inability to localize infection
	Phagocytosis	Normal with sufficient quantities of opsonin	
	Bacterial killing	Normal in healthy neonates; diminished in stressed neonates	
Monocyte	Chemotaxis	Decreased	Decreased inflammatory response
	Phagocytosis	Controversial	Uncertain
	Bacterial killing	Controversial	Uncertain

Adapted from Polin RA et al: Neonatal sepsis, *Adv Pediatr Infect Dis* 7:25, 1992.

Factors that may affect late-onset neonatal infection include prior antimicrobial use, prematurity, a high infant-to-nurse ratio in the neonatal intensive care unit, and the presence of foreign materials such as endotracheal tubes and ventriculo-peritoneal shunts. Contaminated parenteral fluids, such as lipid emulsions, also have been associated with systemic infections.

Infants who acquire early-onset disease often have at least one major risk factor associated with pregnancy and delivery, such as prolonged ROM, preterm delivery, low birthweight, perinatal asphyxia, or maternal peripartum infection. By contrast, late-onset disease is seldom associated with obstetric complications.

Pathology

Histologic findings can be minimal in fulminant cases of neonatal sepsis.[58] When findings are present, they often reflect coexisting septic shock. Such findings may include renal medullary hemorrhage, renal cortical necrosis or acute tubular necrosis, adrenal cortical and medullary hemorrhage and necrosis, hepatic necrosis, intraventricular hemorrhage, and periventricular leukomalacia. Evidence of disseminated intravascular coagulation can be observed as well. In late-onset disease, pathologic changes consistent with the particular focal infection can be shown, including meningitis, pneumonia, hepatic abscesses, and arthritis or osteomyelitis. (Specific organ system infections are discussed later in the chapter.)

Diagnosis

SYMPTOMS AND SIGNS

The signs and symptoms of neonatal sepsis often are nonspecific. The temperature of an infant with sepsis may be elevated, depressed, or normal. Most, but not all, infants with sepsis have respiratory signs, including cyanosis or apnea. Other signs such as feeding difficulties or lethargy are nonspecific and may be subtle or insidious. A high index of suspicion is required to identify and evaluate at-risk infants.

CLINICAL MANIFESTATIONS

Bonadio and colleagues[10] evaluated prospectively a clinical observation scoring method for febrile infants younger than 2 months to determine its predictive value in distinguishing infectious from noninfectious illness. The variables examined were affect, feeding pattern, level of activity, level of alertness, respiratory status or effort, muscle tone, and peripheral perfusion. Inclusion criteria required that the infants had a rectal temperature of equal to or greater than 38°C ($\geq$100.4°F) and had received no antibiotics within the previous 72 hours. Infants underwent a complete sepsis evaluation, including lumbar puncture for blood cell count, glucose and protein determinations, and Gram stain and culture; blood and urine cultures; and urinalysis from a catheterized sample.

The mean score for infants with serious bacterial infection (meningitis, sepsis, or urinary tract infection) was significantly higher than the mean score for infants with aseptic meningitis or for infants with negative cultures and normal cerebrospinal fluid (CSF). Affect, peripheral perfusion, and respiratory status were the variables that best differentiated infected from noninfected febrile infants. Two of the 29 infants with serious bacterial infections had normal observation scores; however, both had abnormal clinical or laboratory findings suggestive of infection. The negative predictive value of this scoring system was 96%. Although observational findings alone cannot replace the physical examination and laboratory studies, they are an important aspect of the evaluation of a febrile neonate.

Although medical attention often is sought for young infants with fever, it is not a finding specific for infection. Many noninfectious processes can result in pyrexia, including dehydration, drug withdrawal, and extensive hematomas. Palazzi and associates[44] came to the following conclusions pertaining to the presentation of neonatal sepsis:

- Temperature elevation in full-term infants is uncommon.
- Temperature elevation is infrequently associated with systemic infection when only a single elevated temperature occurs.
- Temperature elevation that is sustained longer than 1 hour is frequently associated with infection.
- Temperature elevation without other signs of infection is infrequent.
- The infant's temperature can be helpful in suggesting an infectious or noninfectious process if the trend of temperatures and the newborn's clinical status is considered, but a single reading should not be taken alone as an indication of infection.

Septic infants can present with neurologic findings such as seizures and full fontanelle even in the absence of meningitis. Gastrointestinal symptoms include hepatomegaly, abdominal distention, vomiting, diarrhea, guaiac-positive stools, and jaundice. Cutaneous manifestations other than jaundice can be present, but are uncommon findings in neonatal sepsis.

Focal infections can precede or accompany neonatal sepsis; these can include cellulitis, impetigo, soft tissue abscesses, omphalitis, conjunctivitis, otitis media, meningitis, and osteomyelitis. The presence of certain focal infections can suggest the causative agent, such as streptococci with cellulitis, staphylococci with abscesses, and *Pseudomonas aeruginosa* with necrotic skin lesions.

Complications of neonatal sepsis include metastatic foci of infection, disseminated intravascular coagulation, congestive heart failure, and shock.

DIFFERENTIAL DIAGNOSIS

Because the signs and symptoms of neonatal sepsis are nonspecific, noninfectious etiologies should be considered in the differential diagnosis. Sepsis with or without pneumonia can manifest as respiratory distress, transient tachypnea of the newborn, and meconium aspiration. Central nervous system (CNS) symptoms can be caused by sepsis and meningitis, and by intracranial hemorrhage, drug withdrawal, and inborn errors of metabolism. Intestinal obstruction, gastric perforation, and necrotizing enterocolitis can manifest with some of the gastrointestinal signs and symptoms seen with sepsis. Some nonbacterial infections, such as disseminated herpes simplex virus (HSV) infection, can be indistinguishable from bacterial sepsis and must be considered in the differential diagnosis.

MICROBIOLOGIC TESTS

Cultures

A definitive diagnosis of neonatal sepsis can be made only with a positive blood culture. Blood, urine, and CSF should be obtained from all infants suspected to have sepsis. The optimal number of blood cultures and volume of blood per culture have not been established for neonates. Obtaining more than one blood culture can be helpful in distinguishing blood culture contaminants from true pathogens. A minimum of 0.5 mL of blood per bottle is recommended. To avoid contamination, blood should not be obtained from a capillary stick or from umbilical catheters except perhaps immediately after insertion. Several manual and automated methods are available for detecting growth in the blood culture medium. Many new automated radiometric techniques can detect growth 8 hours after collection, and almost always within 24 to 48 hours after collection.

The yield from a urine culture is low in early-onset sepsis and most often reflects spread to the bladder in the setting of bacteremia. Urine for culture should be obtained in a sterile manner, such as by catheterization or suprapubic bladder aspiration, and sent for chemical and microscopic analyses and culture before antimicrobial therapy is started for infants with suspected late onset of infection.

CSF should be obtained before antibiotic administration and sent for blood cell count, differential, and chemistry determinations, and for Gram stain and culture (see "Meningitis," later, and Appendix B for normal CSF indexes). Although controversial, some authorities believe that lumbar puncture may be postponed or excluded from the evaluation of an infant with suspected early-onset disease manifested by pneumonia. Meningitis accompanies sepsis, however, in approximately 10% of infants with early-onset disease and more often with late-onset disease. Meningitis cannot be diagnosed or excluded solely on the basis of symptoms, and blood cultures can be sterile in 10% to 15% of infants with early-onset meningitis and in one third of infants of VLBW with late-onset meningitis.[67]

Additional cultures should be obtained as indicated by clinical findings. Cultures of tracheal aspirates should be obtained in intubated neonates with a clinical picture suggestive of pneumonia, or when the quality and volume of the secretions change substantially and are consistent with a pneumonic process. Indiscriminate cultures of tracheal secretions can often be difficult to interpret, however. Aspirates or biopsy specimens of skin and soft tissue lesions can be sent for stains and cultures. If a bone or joint infection is suspected, evaluation of aspirated material is invaluable to establishing the diagnosis and determining susceptibility of the infecting pathogen. Stool cultures assist in the diagnosis of neonatal septicemia caused by enteric pathogens such as *Shigella, Salmonella,* and *Campylobacter,* but most often the bacteria recovered from stool cultures reflect gastrointestinal colonization, rather than infection. Cultures of gastric aspirates obtained on the first day of life reflect amniotic fluid infection and do not predict the development of neonatal infection.

Buffy Coat Examination

Leukocyte smears made from the buffy coat layer of centrifuged, anticoagulated blood can be stained with Gram stain and methylene blue or with acridine orange, then examined microscopically for intracellular bacteria. A positive buffy coat smear supports the diagnosis of sepsis and identifies the morphologic and Gram stain characteristics of the organism, but does not identify the infectious agent or include or exclude other foci of infection. Buffy coat examination is used infrequently since the advent of automated blood culture monitoring systems.

ANTIGEN DETECTION ASSAYS

Immunoassays that detect bacterial cell wall or capsule carbohydrate antigens in body fluids are an adjunct to diagnosis. Multiple studies have shown that antigen tests are an inappropriate substitute for properly performed bacterial cultures in the diagnosis of neonatal sepsis. With the available radiometric blood culture technology, rapid antigen testing is now infrequently required or indicated. In addition, these tests can provide results that are misleading. The only specimens recommended for testing with these devices are serum and CSF. A positive result should be taken to indicate the presence of antigen and not the presence of viable organisms.

OTHER LABORATORY TESTS

Leukocyte Counts

Many different aspects of the leukocyte count have been examined for their predictive value in diagnosing sepsis. Leukocytosis and leukopenia, defined as more than 20,000/mm^3 (leukocytosis) and less than 5000/mm^3 (leukopenia), have proven insensitive and nonspecific. A single leukocyte count obtained shortly after birth is not adequately sensitive for diagnosing sepsis.

Manroe and colleagues[37] established reference ranges for the absolute total neutrophil count, absolute total immature neutrophil count, and the ratio of immature to total neutrophils (I:T) for neonates during two time periods: the first 60 hours of life and from 60 hours to 28 days of life (Table 39-13). Mouzinho and associates,[40] from the same institution, observed that neonates with VLBW (weighing <1500 g and of ≤30 weeks' gestation) often had neutrophil indexes that did not fall within these ranges. Based on the results of combined retrospective and prospective study of infants with VLBW, the values for absolute total immature neutrophil count and I:T ratio were not significantly different from the ranges established by Manroe and colleagues,[37] but new absolute total neutrophil count ranges for infants with VLBW were proposed (Table 39-14). These ranges were based on small numbers of "normal, uninfected" neonates with VLBW. The latter reference range has higher specificity than the reference ranges of Manroe and colleagues,[37] suggesting that these ranges may be clinically useful in determining length of therapy in infants in whom cultures remain sterile.

The total neutrophil count has been examined for its value in predicting the presence of infection. Neutropenia, especially if it occurs in the first hours of life and is associated with respiratory distress, has a strong association with early-onset GBS sepsis. Many noninfectious processes are associated either with neutropenia or with neutrophilia

TABLE 39–13   Reference Ranges for Neutrophil (per mm³) Indexes in Neonates

Index	Birth	12 Hours	24 Hours	48 Hours	72 Hours	≥120 Hours
ANC	1800-5400	7800-14,400	7200-12,600	4200-9000	1800-7000	1800-5400
INC	≤1120	≤1440	≤1280	<800	<500	<500
I:T	<0.16	<0.16	<0.13	<0.13	<0.13	<0.12

ANC, absolute neutrophil count (mature and immature forms); INC, immature neutrophil count (all neutrophils except segmented ones); I:T, ratio of INC divided by ANC.
Adapted from Manroe BL et al: The neonatal blood count in health and disease, I: reference values for neutrophilic cells, *J Pediatr* 95:89, 1979.

TABLE 39–14   Proposed Reference Range for Absolute Total Neutrophil Count in Infants with Very Low Birthweight*

Age	ABSOLUTE TOTAL NEUTROPHIL COUNT†	
	Minimum	Maximum
Birth	500	6000
18 h	2200	14,000
60 h	1100	8800
120 h	1100	5600

*Defined as ≤1500 g.
†Neutrophils/mm³.
Adapted from Mouzinho A et al: Revised reference ranges for circulating neutrophils in very-low-birth-weight infants, *Pediatrics* 94:76, 1994.

(Table 39-15 and Box 39-3).[71] Many infants with documented sepsis have normal total neutrophil counts at the time of the initial evaluation.

The absolute total immature neutrophil count, defined as the absolute number of all neutrophils excluding the segmented neutrophils, has also been extensively studied. All newborns, but especially premature infants, have a relatively large number of immature neutrophils in the first few days of life. Infected neonates can have an increase above the upper limits of normal in immature cells released from the bone marrow in response to infection, but this response is inconsistent and sometimes delayed, and is an insensitive marker for the early diagnosis of infection. It is unusual, however, for uninfected infants to have an elevated absolute total immature neutrophil count above the reference ranges; if such a finding is present, further evaluation for occult infection should be considered.

The I:T ratio has been investigated as an early predictor of sepsis. The maximal I:T ratio in uninfected neonates is 0.16 in the first 24 hours, decreasing to 0.12 by 60 hours. The upper limit of normal for neonates of 32 weeks' gestation or less is slightly higher, at 0.2. The test has a good negative predictive value, that is, there is a high likelihood that infection is absent if the I:T ratio is normal. Most infected neonates have an elevated I:T ratio some time during the infection, so repeatedly normal I:T ratios can be reassuring. The usefulness of this test is limited because many noninfectious processes, including prolonged induction

with oxytocin, stressful labor, and even prolonged crying, are associated with increased I:T ratios.

Acute-Phase Reactants

The acute-phase response is a response of the body to infection or trauma clinically manifested by malaise, anorexia, fever, leukocytosis, negative nitrogen balance, and hepatic production of acute-phase proteins. Acute-phase reactants (APRs) are proteins produced by hepatocytes in response to inflammation. The inflammation can be secondary to infection, trauma, or other processes of cellular destruction. There are many different APRs, including CRP, fibrinogen, α_1-acid glycoprotein, α_1-antitrypsin, and elastase α_1-proteinase inhibitor. These APRs have different plasma half-lives and different incremental responses to inflammation. The method for the detection of APRs has improved with the development of rapid, automated, quantitative specific immunoassays. Numerous studies have evaluated APRs as early indicators of neonatal septicemia; an elevated APR does not distinguish between infectious and noninfectious causes of inflammation.

C-Reactive Protein

CRP is a globulin so named because it forms a precipitate in the presence of the C-polysaccharide of *Streptococcus pneumoniae*. It is believed to be a carrier protein involved in removing potentially toxic material. There is minimal transplacental passage of maternal CRP, and concentrations are unaffected by gestational age. Current methods are fully automated and provide a quantitative assessment of protein concentration. Normal concentrations in neonates are assay-dependent, but the upper limit of normal usually is 1 mg/dL. CRP is significantly elevated at the time of the initial evaluation in 50% to 90% of infants with systemic bacterial infections, but CRP has a low positive predictive value and should not be used alone to diagnose sepsis.

An increasing CRP value is usually detectable within 6 to 18 hours, and the peak CRP is seen at 8 to 60 hours after onset of an inflammatory process. The serum half-life is short, so the CRP usually declines to a normal concentration within 5 to 10 days in most infants with infection who have a favorable response to therapy. Serial determinations of CRP are valuable in excluding serious infections. The very high negative predictive value of several normal CRP values in sequence can allow for early discontinuation of empirical antibiotics in selected clinical settings. Nonbacterial infections can elicit a variable CRP response, with normal values in culture-positive viral meningitis and increased values in minor viral infections. Noninfectious processes, including

TABLE 39-15   Clinical Factors Affecting Neutrophil Counts

	TOTAL NEUTROPHILS		TOTAL IMMATURE NEUTROPHILS	I:T RATIO*	
	Decreased	Increased	Increased	Increased	Duration (Hours)
Maternal hypertension	++++	0	+	+	72
Maternal fever, healthy neonate	0	++	+++	++++	24
≥6 hours of intrapartum oxytocin	0	++	++	++++	120
Stressful labor†	0	+++	++++	++++	24
Asphyxia (5-min Apgar score <5)	+	++	++	+++	24-60
Meconium aspiration syndrome	0	++++	+++	++	72
Pneumothorax with uncomplicated respiratory distress syndrome	0	++++	++++	++++	24
Periventricular hemorrhage‡	+++	+	++	++++	120
Seizures§	0	+++	+++	++++	24
Prolonged crying (≥4 min)	0	++++	++++	++++	1
Asymptomatic hypoglycemia (≤30 mg/dL)	0	++	+++	+++	24
Hemolytic disease	++	++	+++	++	7-28 days
Surgery	0	++++	++++	+++	24
High altitude	0	++++	++++	0	6¶

*I:T, immature neutrophils/total neutrophils.
†Duration ≥18 hours, midforceps rotation, breech extraction, 10-minute second stage of labor.
‡No associated seizures.
§Seizures in the absence of hypoglycemia, asphyxia, or central nervous system hemorrhage.
¶Not tested after 6 hours.
+, 0%-25%; ++, 25%-50%; +++, 50%-75%; ++++, 75%-100%.
From Weinberg GA et al: Laboratory aids for diagnosis of neonatal sepsis. In Remington JS et al, editors: *Infectious diseases of the fetus and newborn infants*, 6th ed, Philadelphia, Saunders, 2006, p 1210.

BOX 39-3   Clinical Neonatal Factors Having No Effect on Neutrophil Counts

- Race
- Sex
- Maternal diabetes mellitus
- Route of delivery*
- Premature amniorrhexis, mother afebrile
- Meconium staining, no lung disease
- Uncomplicated respiratory distress syndrome
- Uncomplicated transient tachypnea of the newborn
- Hyperbilirubinemia, physiologic, unexplained
- Phototherapy
- Brief (≤3 minutes) crying
- Diurnal variation

*The total neutrophil count of the cord blood of infants delivered vaginally or by cesarean section after labor (2 to 14 hours) is twice that of infants delivered by cesarean section without labor.
From Weinberg GA, Powell KR: Laboratory aids for diagnosis of neonatal sepsis. In Remington JS et al, editors: *Infectious diseases of the fetus and newborn infant*, 6th ed, Philadelphia, 2006, Saunders, p 1210; data adapted from Manroe BL et al: The neonatal blood count in health and disease, I: reference values for neutrophilic cells, *J Pediatr* 95:89, 1979.

meconium aspiration pneumonitis, can have an elevated CRP 10 times the normal concentration.

Erythrocyte Sedimentation Rate

The erythrocyte sedimentation rate (ESR) is not a direct measure of an APR, but rather reflects changes in many serum protein APRs. A micro-ESR has been developed for use in infants. An approximation of the maximal normal rate in the first 2 weeks of life can be obtained by adding 3 to the age of the newborn in days. Beyond 2 weeks of life, the maximal rate varies between 10 and 20 mm/h. Owing to interlaboratory variation, each laboratory must develop its own reference range. The ESR is limited in that other factors unrelated to inflammation (e.g., anemia, hyperglobulinemia) can affect the rate. Micro-ESR values vary inversely with the hematocrit, but are affected little, if at all, by birthweight or gestational age. Slightly elevated micro-ESR values can occur with superficial infections and with noninfectious processes, including asphyxia, aspiration pneumonia, and respiratory distress syndrome. Markedly elevated values in the absence of infection are unusual, but have been observed with Coombs-positive hemolytic disease and physiologic hyperbilirubinemia. The long delay after onset of the inflammatory process before the peak ESR is reached and its long half-life render it of limited usefulness in monitoring the progress of bacterial infections in neonates.

Fibrinogen

Plasma fibrinogen concentrations are known to increase in association with infection, although some factors can result in a low fibrinogen level despite severe infection, including disseminated intravascular coagulation, exchange transfusion, and respiratory distress syndrome. Measurement of fibrinogen concentrations is not useful in the early diagnosis of infection because there is a large overlap in values between infected and healthy infants.

Fibronectin

Fibronectin is a multifunctional, high-molecular-weight glycoprotein produced primarily by the liver and endothelial cells, and widely distributed in the body, including in plasma and body fluids, on cell surfaces, and in the extracellular matrix. Fibronectin is involved in hemostasis, vascular integrity, and wound healing. It is important in embryogenesis, directing cell migration, proliferation, and differentiation. Fibronectin aids in the immune response by augmenting macrophage and neutrophil phagocytosis and acting as a nonspecific opsonin for the reticuloendothelial system. The plasma fibronectin concentration varies with age. In healthy neonates, it is approximately half that found in adults, whereas healthy premature infants have approximately one third of the amount in normal adults. After birth, the plasma concentration gradually increases, reaching adult values by 2 months of age. Fibronectin has been found to be decreased in neonates with infection and in neonates with asphyxia, respiratory distress syndrome, and bronchopulmonary dysplasia.

Cytokines

Cytokines such as IL-1β, IL-6, IL-8, TNFα, and others are endogenous mediators of the immune response to inflammation. There is evidence that measuring cytokine concentrations can be helpful in the early diagnosis of neonatal sepsis, but the study design employed and the method for each assay can affect the reported performance.[52] In some reports, such as that of Girardin and colleagues,[22] assay performance is excellent. These investigators found that 8 of 9 infants with systemic infection, but only 1 of 60 uninfected infants, had elevated serum TNFα. Confounding effects of maternal complications can affect findings, however. IL-6 and IL-8 can be elevated in infants with sepsis and in the setting of chorioamnionitis. Timing can have an impact on assay performance. Buck and coworkers[12] evaluated prospectively the use of IL-6 and CRP measurements in the diagnosis of early-onset sepsis in 222 neonates. Elevated IL-6 concentrations were observed in 73% of newborns with culture-positive infection and in 87% of infants with a clinical diagnosis of sepsis but negative cultures. Most newborns (78%) without evidence of infection had normal IL-6 concentrations. Of the infected newborns with normal IL-6 concentrations, 55% had elevated CRP measurements, suggesting that the peak IL-6 concentration was missed because of its short half-life.

Many investigators have evaluated colony-stimulating factors in the neonatal period. Data are conflicting, but suggest that concentrations of granulocyte colony-stimulating factors vary with gestational age and are influenced by mode of delivery, nutritional status, maternal hypertension, maternal glucocorticoid therapy, and infection.[4] A peak in granulocyte colony-stimulating factor concentration was observed approximately 7 hours after birth in healthy newborns, with a corresponding increase in the total neutrophil count 7 to 12 hours after birth. Infected newborns had a much higher peak concentration at 7 hours than uninfected infants.

Screening Panels

Excluding cultures, none of the previously mentioned tests, when used alone, is sensitive or specific enough to diagnose or exclude neonatal sepsis reliably. Numerous investigators have evaluated the predictive values of panels of tests for diagnosing sepsis. (Table 39-16 presents definitions of terms used in evaluating such tests.)

Krediet and colleagues[32] measured daily CRP values and I:T ratios in all newborns admitted to the nursery—185 patients during the first 4 days of life and 107 infants after the fourth day of life. A sepsis workup, including cultures, complete blood count, and radiologic studies, was performed as clinically indicated. For early-onset disease, the positive predictive value of either test alone was 18% to 23%, and the negative predictive value was 95% to 98%. When the tests were used together, the positive predictive value increased to 32%, and the negative predictive value decreased to 95%. For late-onset sepsis, the positive predictive value and negative predictive value for the tests, when used alone, ranged from 59% to 63% and 90% to 94%. When the tests were used together to screen for late-onset infection, the positive predictive value increased to 65%, and the negative predictive value decreased to 88%. These researchers concluded that a screening panel comprising CRP and the I:T ratio had limited value.

Tegtmeyer and coworkers[69] assessed a screening panel in 74 infected neonates. Their panel comprised CRP, I:T ratio, granulocyte count, and Eα1-PI. The sensitivity of each test alone ranged from 36% to 70% except for Eα1-PI, which

TABLE 39-16	Terms Used for Analyzing Accuracy and Reliability of Tests
Term	**Definition**
Sensitivity	Percentage of patients with infection who have an abnormal test result
Specificity	Percentage of patients without infection who have a normal test result
Positive predictive value	If test result is abnormal, percentage of patients with infection
Negative predictive value	If test result is normal, percentage of patients with no infection

From Weinberg GA et al: Laboratory aids for diagnosis of neonatal sepsis. In Remington JS et al, editors: *Infectious diseases of the fetus and newborn infant,* 6th ed. Philadelphia, Saunders, 2006, p 1208.

ranged from 87% (early-onset sepsis) to 100% (late-onset disease). When all the tests were used together, the sensitivity increased to 100%. Because the authors assessed only infected infants, they were unable to determine the specificity or predictive accuracy of their screening panel.

Philip and colleagues[46] evaluated the predictive accuracy of a three-part screen (Eα_1-PI, I:T ratio, and CRP) in more than 300 infected and uninfected infants admitted to the neonatal intensive care unit. When used alone, Eα_1-PI was more sensitive than the other two tests for diagnosing sepsis, but had a lower positive predictive value. When the three tests were used as a panel, the sensitivity was 23%, the specificity was 99.7%, the positive predictive value was 87.6%, and the negative predictive value was 99.7%. The use of screening panels does not significantly improve the positive predictive accuracy; however, the predictive accuracy of a negative panel often increases to 98% to 100%, and a panel with this accuracy of performance in excluding disease can provide useful information.

Treatment

EMPIRICAL ANTIMICROBIAL THERAPY

Although signs and symptoms of neonatal sepsis are often subtle and nonspecific, when the clinical diagnosis is obvious, the infant is often critically ill. Empirical antimicrobial therapy should be instituted immediately after obtaining samples for culture rather than waiting for the culture results. The choice of therapy should be based on several factors, including the timing and setting of the disease (e.g., early onset, late onset community acquired, health care associated late or very late onset), the microorganisms most frequently encountered, the susceptibility profiles for those organisms, the site of the suspected infection and the penetration of the specific antibiotic to that site, and the safety of the antibiotic. Caregivers should be aware of the susceptibility profiles for the most common neonatal pathogens isolated in their community and in their neonatal unit. Nonbacterial infectious etiologies must be considered in the differential diagnosis and, if deemed a significant possibility, appropriate antiviral or antifungal therapy must be started in addition to antibiotic therapy.

For early-onset disease in the United States, the antimicrobial regimen should provide coverage against GBS, E. coli and other gram-negative enteric bacilli, and L. monocytogenes. The combination of ampicillin and an aminoglycoside is frequently used. Listeria and GBS are uniformly susceptible to ampicillin, whereas the susceptibility of E. coli to ampicillin is less reliable. The aminoglycoside provides coverage against most gram-negative enteric bacilli and, with gentamicin specifically, has been found to act synergistically with ampicillin against GBS and Listeria organisms in vitro and in animal models. The choice of aminoglycoside should be based on susceptibility patterns for gram-negative enteric bacilli in the community. Gentamicin is used most frequently, with tobramycin and amikacin reserved for treatment of multidrug-resistant bacteria. If meningitis is suspected, especially gram-negative bacillary meningitis, many clinicians add or replace the aminoglycoside with the third-generation cephalosporin, cefotaxime, for better CNS penetration.

Empirical therapy for late-onset disease acquired in the community should provide coverage for the same neonatal pathogens discussed earlier and for potential community-acquired pathogens, such as S. pneumoniae and Neisseria meningitidis. Because meningitis frequently is a component of late-onset sepsis, antibiotics with good CNS penetration should be selected. Ampicillin and a third-generation cephalosporin (e.g., cefotaxime) are commonly recommended.

Health care–associated late-onset disease can be caused by the usual neonatal pathogens, but also by coagulase negative staphyloccus (CONS), enterococci, gram-negative enteric bacilli (including drug-resistant strains), and fungi. Therapy depends on the presence of risk factors for commensal organisms such as CONS (use of catheters or shunts) and the susceptibility profiles for common nosocomial pathogens isolated from the nursery. Virtually all staphylococci produce penicillinase and are resistant to ampicillin and penicillin. Vancomycin and gentamicin are commonly used for initial therapy. Vancomycin generally is active against all staphylococcal species, streptococci, and most enterococci, whereas the spectrum of activity of a penicillinase-resistant penicillin includes streptococci and only the methicillin-susceptible strains of CONS and S. aureus. Cefotaxime or ceftriaxone can be included when gram-negative meningitis is a concern. Cefotaxime does not have activity against L. monocytogenes, enterococci, or Pseudomonas species. Ceftazidime with an aminoglycoside should be used if Pseudomonas infection is suspected. Meropenem can be required when multidrug-resistant enteric gram-negative organisms are isolated. Many other combinations of antimicrobial agents can be effective therapy for nosocomial late-onset sepsis; however, it is prudent to use agents that have proven with experience to be safe.

The risks and benefits should be considered thoroughly if routine use of third-generation cephalosporins for late-onset disease is contemplated. One disadvantage is an increased risk for development of gastrointestinal colonization and perhaps subsequent infection with fungi and drug-resistant bacteria. With ceftriaxone, in particular, there is a theoretical risk of bilirubin displacement from albumin because of the drug's high protein-binding capacity. There are no clinical data to substantiate this effect in neonates. These cephalosporins are safe and effective against many of the common neonatal pathogens, and there is extensive experience with cefotaxime use during the neonatal period. Because third-generation cephalosporins do not cause the dose-related toxicities seen with agents such as aminoglycosides, monitoring of serum concentrations is unnecessary. Empirical therapy usually may be narrowed to one drug when final culture identification and susceptibility results are available.

The dosage and frequency of administration of antimicrobial agents vary with the newborn's gestational age, postnatal age, birthweight, and status of hepatic and renal function. Recommendations for antibiotic use in neonates are given in Tables 39-17 through 39-19 and in Appendix A.[41] These are guidelines only; specific doses and intervals may change frequently, especially in critically ill infants. Serum concentrations of aminoglycosides and, in some circumstances, vancomycin, should be monitored to ensure therapeutic efficacy while minimizing toxicity. The duration of therapy depends on the site of infection (see later).

TABLE 39–17   Recommended Dosage Schedule for Antimicrobial Agents Frequently Used to Treat Neonatal Sepsis

| | | DOSAGE (mg/kg/d) AND INTERVALS OF ADMINISTRATION | | | |
| | | BODY WEIGHT ≤2000 g | | BODY WEIGHT >2000 g | |
Antibiotic	Route	0-7 Days	>7 Days	0-7 Days	>7 Days
Ampicillin	IV, IM	100 div q12h	150 div q8h	150 div q8h	200 div q6h
Aztreonam	IV, IM	60 div q12h	90 div q8h	90 div q8h	120 div q6h
Cefotaxime	IV, IM	100 div q12h	150 div q8h	100 div q12h	150 div q8h
Ceftazidime	IV, IM	100 div q12h	150 div q8h	150 div q8h	150 div q8h
Ceftriaxone	IV, IM	50 once daily	50 once daily	50 once daily	75 once daily
Clindamycin	IV, IM, PO	10 div q12h	15 div q8h	15 div q8h	20 div q6h
Erythromycin	IV, PO	20 div q12h	30 div q8h	20 div q12h	30 div q8h
Metronidazole	IV, PO	15 div q12h	15 div q12h	15 div q12h	30 div q12h
Mezlocillin	IV, IM	150 div q12h	225 div q8h	150 div q12h	225 div q8h
Nafcillin	IV	50 div q12h	75 div q8h	75 div q8h	150 div q6h
Penicillin G	IV	100,000 U div q12h	200,000 U div q8h	150,000 U div q8h	200,000 U div q6h
Benzathine penicillin G	IM	50,000 U (one dose)	50,000 U (one dose)	50,000 U (one dose)	50,000 U (one dose)
Procaine penicillin G	IM	50,000 U q24h	50,000 U q24h	50,000 U q24h	50,000 U q24h
Ticarcillin	IV, IM	150 div q12h	225 div q8h	225 div q8h	300 div q6h

div, divided.
Adapted from Nelson JD: Antibiotic therapy for newborns. In: *Pocketbook of pediatric antimicrobial therapy,* Baltimore, 1998, Williams & Wilkins.

TABLE 39–18   Recommended Dosage Schedule for Aminoglycosides and Vancomycin in the Treatment of Neonatal Sepsis

| | | DOSAGE FOR WEEKS' GESTATION OR POSTCONCEPTIONAL AGE | | |
Antibiotic	Route	<30	30-37	>37
Amikacin*				
≤7 days	IV, IM	15 mg/kg 24h	15 mg/kg q18h	15 mg/kg q12h
>7 days		15 mg/kg q18h	15 mg/kg q12h	15 mg/kg q8h
Tobramycin[†‡]				
≤7 days	IV, IM	3 mg/kg q24h	3 mg/kg q18h	2.5 mg/kg q12h
>7 days		3 mg/kg q18h	2.5 mg/kg q12h	2.5 mg/kg q8h
Vancomycin[§]				
≤7 days	IV	20 mg/kg q24h	15 mg/kg q18h	15 mg/kg q12h
>7 days		20 mg/kg q18h	15 mg/kg q12h	15 mg/kg q8h

*Desired serum concentrations: peak 20-40 μg/mL, trough <10 μg/mL.
[†]Desired serum concentrations: peak 5-10 μg/mL, trough ≤2 μg/mL.
[‡]Gentamicin dosing: for <35 weeks' postmenstrual age, 3 mg/kg/dose q24h; for ≥35 weeks' postmenstrual age, 4 mg/kg/dose q24h.
[§]Desired serum concentrations: peak 20-40 μg/mL, trough <15 μg/mL.

TABLE 39-19   Indications, Pharmacology, and Toxicity of Antibiotics Commonly Used in Newborns

Antibiotic	Indications	Pharmacology	Toxicity	Comments
Amikacin	Aerobic gram-negative infections; use should be limited to treatment of gentamicin-resistant organisms	Renal excretion; activity in CSF low; not absorbed from GI tract	Possible ototoxicity, nephrotoxicity, and neuromuscular blockade	Toxicity rare if appropriate dosage is used, and blood concentration is monitored
Ampicillin	Initial treatment of sepsis and meningitis; gram-positive organisms except staphylococci; gram-negative organisms if susceptible (*Salmonella, Shigella, Haemophilus, Escherichia coli*)	Renal excretion	Seizures when high dosages are given	
Cefotaxime	Sepsis, meningitis caused by susceptible gram-negative organisms	Primarily renal excretion; good penetration into CSF		Active against streptococci; routine use can result in emergence of resistant gram-negative organisms
Ceftazidime	Can be used in combination with aminoglycoside for treatment of *Pseudomonas* infection	Renal excretion; penetrates blood-brain barrier		
Ceftriaxone	Sepsis, meningitis, soft tissue and bone/joint infections caused by susceptible organisms; not effective against staphylococci, *Listeria* species, enterococci, or *Pseudomonas* species	30%-65% excreted by kidneys, the remainder excreted in bile; penetrates blood-brain barrier	Potential gallbladder sludging	May displace bilirubin from albumin-binding sites in neonates
Clindamycin	Treatment of susceptible anaerobic infections		Pseudomembranous colitis in older children, but rare in neonates	
Chloramphenicol	Treatment of infections caused by bacteria resistant to all other antibiotics (e.g., *Salmonella* species)	Metabolized by liver, small amount excreted unchanged in urine; good penetration through blood-brain barrier	Gray baby syndrome (vasomotor collapse) related to immature hepatic function and associated with elevated concentrations of unconjugated chloramphenicol	Dose-related reversible bone marrow suppression; idiopathic irreversible aplastic anemia (rare); monitoring of blood concentration mandatory
Erythromycin	*Chlamydia, Pertussis* species, minor staphylococcal or streptococcal skin infections	Excreted in urine, stool, and biliary system; crosses blood-brain barrier poorly	No significant toxicity	

Continued

TABLE 39–19   Indications, Pharmacology, and Toxicity of Antibiotics Commonly Used in Newborns—cont'd

Antibiotic	Indications	Pharmacology	Toxicity	Comments
Gentamicin	Can be used for initial treatment of neonatal sepsis; not effective alone, but can be synergistic when used with ampicillin against group B streptococci, enterococci, and *Listeria* species	Renal excretion; activity low in CSF; not absorbed from GI tract in normal host	Possible ototoxicity, nephrotoxicity, and neuromuscular blockade	Toxicity rare if appropriate dosage is used, and blood concentrations are monitored
Nafcillin, oxacillin	Penicillin-resistant *Staphylococcus aureus* infections; active against streptococci, but not a first-line agent	Excretion is renal and hepatic for nafcillin and oxacillin; nafcillin and oxacillin are highly protein bound		
Neomycin	Bacterial diarrhea, enteropathogenic *E. coli*	Not absorbed by GI tract	Ototoxic, nephrotoxic if absorbed	Do not use parenterally
Penicillin G	Most streptococci, *Treponema pallidum*, *Bacteroides* species (except *Bacteroides fragilis*), *Neisseria meningitidis*	Renal excretion; fair penetration of inflamed meninges		Can be used to treat infections caused by susceptible organisms
Streptomycin	*Mycobacterium tuberculosis*	Renal excretion	Vestibular and auditory damage, nephrotoxicity	Must be given IM
Ticarcillin	Expanded gram-negative activity; can be used to treat susceptible *Pseudomonas* infections	Renal excretion	Platelet dysfunction	Can be associated with hypernatremia and hypokalemia; electrolytes are monitored
Tobramycin	Broad coverage of gram-negative organisms	Renal excretion; low activity in CSF	Possible ototoxicity and nephrotoxicity	Blood concentrations are monitored
Vancomycin	Effective against coagulase-negative staphylococci, methicillin-resistant *S. aureus*; most gram-positive aerobic organisms are susceptible	Renal excretion	Possible ototoxicity; previous preparations associated with nephrotoxicity	Flushing or hypotension may result from rapid infusion
Sulfonamides	Contraindicated in newborns		Displaces bilirubin from albumin-binding sites	
Tetracyclines	Contraindicated in newborns		Permanent discoloration of teeth, enamel hypoplasia; inhibits bone growth in premature infants	

CSF, cerebrospinal fluid; GI, gastrointestinal.

SUPPORTIVE THERAPY

Although appropriate antimicrobial therapy is crucial, supportive care is equally important. Ventilatory support may be necessary, particularly for infants with fulminant early-onset disease. Intravenous hydration and perhaps parenteral nutrition, with close monitoring of electrolytes and glucose, should be considered. Septic shock, if present, should be treated appropriately with fluids and inotropes as indicated by the clinical situation.

IMMUNOTHERAPY

The newborn's immune system is compromised in many aspects, including the neutrophil's chemotactic response to pathogens, T cell production of proinflammatory cytokines, and functional complement activity (see Part 1 of this chapter). Preterm infants are compromised further by hypogammaglobulinemia because significant transfer of maternal IgG does not begin until 32 to 34 weeks' gestation. Even term infants can lack specific antibodies to the most common pathogens in early-onset neonatal infections because most adults have low concentrations of antibody against GBS and *E. coli*. With the increased risk of overwhelming bacterial infection in preterm neonates, researchers have studied the effect of intravenous immune globulin (IVIG) in preventing and treating neonatal infections.

Intravenous Immune Globulin

There have been numerous studies evaluating IVIG for treatment of infected neonates. A beneficial effect from IVIG and appropriate antibiotics was observed in several studies compared with antibiotics used alone for the treatment of sepsis. These studies were limited, however, by small numbers of patients, nonblinded investigators, lack of a placebo control, or lack of bacteria-specific analysis of the IVIG preparation used. Meta-analysis of studies of IVIG for the treatment of neonates with sepsis showed a significant decrease in the mortality rate compared with standard therapies.[30] Further studies are warranted before IVIG use in infections can be recommended as routine therapy.

Other Agents in Development

Other agents that may be beneficial in the treatment of neonatal infections include human monoclonal IgM antibodies and pathogen-specific hyperimmune globulins. An intravenous *S. aureus* polyclonal immune globulin was well tolerated in VLBW infants, but further investigation is needed to assess efficacy.[5] Fibronectin administration may be useful in the prevention and treatment of neonatal sepsis because of its multifunctional roles, including nonspecific opsonization that aids in clearing debris in the reticuloendothelial system, augmentation of phagocytic activity, and hemostasis. Fibronectin has been used in adults as a topical agent to improve wound healing with persistent corneal ulcerations and intravenously in uncontrolled studies of patients with multiorgan system failure. Preliminary results seem encouraging, but large, prospective, controlled studies are required before any recommendations about its use can be made. Early postnatal prophylactic granulocyte-macrophage colony-stimulating factor corrected neutropenia in a single-blind, multicenter, randomized controlled trial in preterm infants, but it did not reduce sepsis or improve survival and short-term outcomes.[13]

PREVENTION

Intrapartum antibiotic prophylaxis (IAP) for prevention of early-onset GBS disease has been in widespread use since 1996. The guidelines issued in 1996 recommended screening of pregnant women for GBS colonization either by lower vaginal and rectal cultures obtained at 35 to 37 weeks' gestation or by assessing clinical risk factors to identify candidates for IAP. A comparison of the two prevention strategies showed that culture-based screening was 50% more effective than a risk-based strategy in preventing early-onset disease in neonates.[55] An 80% reduction in early-onset GBS disease, to approximately 0.3 to 0.4 per 1000 live births, has been achieved in the IAP era.[45] The 2002 revised guidelines from the Centers for Disease Control and Prevention (CDC) recommend that all pregnant women be screened during each pregnancy for GBS carriage. Lower vaginal and rectal cultures obtained at 35 to 37 weeks' gestation should be placed in a non-nutritive transport medium, incubated in selective broth medium, and subcultured into 5% sheep blood agar for isolation of GBS.

All pregnant women identified as GBS carriers should receive IAP at the time of labor or ROM. Penicillin (5 million U initially and then 2.5 million U every 4 hours until delivery) is recommended.[15] Ampicillin (2 g initially and then 1 g every 4 hours until delivery) is an acceptable alternative. Penicillin-allergic women who are not at high risk for anaphylaxis should receive cefazolin (2 g initially and 1 g every 8 hours until delivery). Vancomycin is recommended for women with a high risk for anaphylaxis. Because of increasing rates of resistance, clindamycin and erythromycin are less effective as alternative agents. These drugs should be reserved for women with risk of anaphylaxis in whom testing has indicated that the isolates are susceptible.

Delivery of a previous infant with invasive disease and GBS bacteriuria is always an indication for IAP. IAP is not indicated for planned cesarean section before ROM and onset of labor. Risk factors (labor onset or ROM before 37 weeks' gestation, ROM ≥18 hours before delivery, or intrapartum fever) should be used only when the results of cultures are unknown at the onset of labor. An algorithm for IAP for women with threatened preterm delivery is included in the current recommendations.[15]

The management of infants born to women receiving IAP depends on the infant's status at birth, the duration of prophylaxis, and the gestational age of the infant. If a woman receives IAP for suspected chorioamnionitis, her infant should have a full diagnostic evaluation and empirical therapy pending culture results based on the infant's exposure to established infection. Symptomatic infants should undergo full diagnostic evaluation and empirical therapy. A lumbar puncture, if feasible, should be performed. Limited evaluation consisting of complete blood count with differential and blood culture and observation for at least 48 hours is indicated for asymptomatic infants of less than 35 weeks' gestation and for infants whose mothers received chemoprophylaxis for less than 4 hours before delivery. Observation is appropriate for asymptomatic infants of at least 35 weeks' gestation whose mothers received chemoprophylaxis at least 4 hours before delivery.

Exposure to antibiotics during pregnancy has not changed the clinical spectrum of GBS disease or the onset of clinical signs of infection within 24 hours of birth for term infants with early-onset GBS infection.[11] In reports that document increases in non-GBS sepsis, the increase has occurred only in infants born prematurely or with low birthweight. Surveillance in two cities found stable rates of sepsis caused by other organisms, but an increase in ampicillin-resistant *E. coli* among preterm but not term infants.[28] Intrapartum ampicillin exposure has been shown to be an independent risk factor for ampicillin-resistant, early-onset sepsis.[8] These trends indicate the importance of ongoing surveillance. A comprehensive program for prevention of neonatal bacterial infections awaits the development and licensure of vaccines, some of which are now under testing, and of strategies to prevent premature delivery.

INFECTION OF ORGAN SYSTEMS

Meningitis

INCIDENCE

The contemporary incidence of bacterial meningitis in neonates is approximately 0.3 per 1000 live births. Bacterial meningitis can occur in 15% of neonates with bacteremia. For GBS, a higher proportion of late-onset cases than of early-onset cases identified from 2003-2005 manifested as meningitis (27% versus 7%; *P* <.001).[45] Low birthweight (<2500 g) and preterm birth (<37 weeks of gestation) are associated with an increased risk for neonatal meningitis. Meningitis has a predilection for young age; the incidence is higher in the first month of life than at any other age.

ETIOLOGY

The causative agents for neonatal meningitis generally mirror the causative agents associated with neonatal sepsis (see Table 39-11). One review of 101 infants with a gestational age of at least 35 weeks found that GBS accounted for 50%, *E. coli* accounted for 25%, other enteric gram-negative rods accounted for 8%, and *Listeria* accounted for 6% of cases. Among the remaining patients, *S. pneumoniae*, group A *Streptococcus*, and nontypable *H. influenzae* each accounted for less than 5% of cases.[31] Among premature infants, and especially VLBW infants, *Enterococcus*, CONS, and α-hemolytic streptococci also must be considered potential pathogens.

PATHOGENESIS

There are three mechanisms by which the meninges can become infected: (1) primary sepsis with hematogenous seeding; (2) focal infection outside the CNS, with either secondary bacteremia and resulting hematogenous dissemination or direct extension (e.g., from an infected sinus); and (3) direct inoculation after head trauma or neurosurgery, or from an open congenital defect, such as myelomeningocele or dermal sinus. The most common mechanism in neonates is hematogenous spread associated with a primary bacteremia, so the perinatal risk factors that predispose an infant to neonatal sepsis also influence the risk of acquiring meningitis. Certain microbial factors

are associated with increased risk of meningeal invasion. Despite the presence of more than 100 different capsular polysaccharide K antigens in *E. coli*, the K_1 capsular type is isolated in 70% of neonates with meningitis. Similarly, type III strains are responsible for 70% of all early-onset or late-onset GBS meningitis. The IVb serotype of *L. monocytogenes* is more frequently isolated in late-onset *Listeria* meningitis than are the other serotypes.

PATHOLOGY

Berman and Banker[7] reviewed clinical data from 29 neonates with bacterial meningitis, including 25 with postmortem examinations. All but two of the infections were caused by gram-negative enteric bacilli. The pathologic characteristics closely resembled characteristics found in older infants and children. In the acute stage, brain edema was prominent, but had not led to herniation in any of the infants. A subarachnoid exudate located at the base of the brain or evenly distributed over the cerebral hemispheres or, less commonly, isolated to the convexity was observed. In the acute stage of meningitis, a neutrophilic exudate predominated, which progressed to a mononuclear exudate by the chronic stage. Ventriculitis, resulting from destruction of the epithelial lining of the ventricles after inflammatory cell infiltration, was common. Vasculitis and radiculopathy caused by inflammatory cell infiltration were seen. Parenchymal changes included gliosis, encephalopathy, and infarction. Microglial proliferation was observed in the cerebral and cerebellar hemispheres, in the marginal white matter of the spinal cord and brainstem, and in the ependymal lining of the fourth ventricle and aqueduct. This proliferation sometimes resulted in narrowing or obliteration of the foramen of Luschka and aqueduct of Sylvius. A diffuse encephalopathy of uncertain etiology occasionally was present, believed to be metabolic in origin.

Many of the known pathologic sequelae of meningitis were shown at autopsy. Hydrocephalus was observed in 14 of the 25 infants. Communicating hydrocephalus, defined as normal flow of CSF from the lateral ventricles through the fourth ventricle, but obstruction of flow from impaired resorption in the arachnoid villi, was noted in nine infants. Five infants had noncommunicating hydrocephalus, defined as obstructed CSF flow at the level of the aqueduct of Sylvius or the foramina secondary to purulent exudate or gliosis. Hydrocephalus ex vacuo also can be observed when the ventricles are enlarged owing to loss of cerebral cortical tissue and secondary white matter degeneration as a result of encephalopathy; however, CSF flow is not impeded. Infants with ventriculitis can have prolonged symptoms with delayed sterilization of CSF. Thrombosis and cerebral infarcts can develop as a result of the vasculitis. Brain abscesses and subdural effusions were not observed in the series by Berman and Banker.[7] When brain abscess formation does occur, it tends to be associated with certain organisms, such as *Citrobacter koseri* (previously *Citrobacter diversus*) or *Enterobacter sakazakii*.

CLINICAL MANIFESTATIONS

The early signs and symptoms of neonatal meningitis are nonspecific. The signs most frequently observed include lethargy, reluctance to feed, emesis, respiratory distress, irritability, and temperature instability. Signs suggestive of a CNS process are less commonly observed in neonates with meningitis than in older children. A review of the clinical signs of bacterial meningitis in 255 newborns from six medical centers found that 40% had convulsions, 28% had a full or bulging fontanelle, and only 15% had nuchal rigidity.[44] In preterm infants, the signs and symptoms can be subtle. Because of the high mortality rate and risk of serious sequelae in survivors, and the nonspecificity of signs and symptoms in meningitis, the clinician must have a high index of suspicion when evaluating ill neonates.

DIAGNOSIS

The diagnosis of neonatal meningitis requires growth of the microorganism from the CSF. A presumptive diagnosis can be made when the CSF indexes suggest a bacterial process, and a pathogen is isolated from a blood culture. A thorough evaluation of CSF for the presence of infection includes bacterial culture and Gram-stained smear, cell count with leukocyte differential, and glucose and total protein determinations. Normal values for CSF indexes in the neonate are different from normal values in older infants or children and can be difficult to interpret if the age of the patient is not considered. As a guide to interpretation, a CSF leukocyte count exceeding 20 to 30/mm³ is a threshold for the presence of meningeal inflammation and should warrant consideration of meningitis as a possible diagnosis.

Sarff and colleagues[53] analyzed the CSF findings in 117 neonates with signs and symptoms suggestive of infection, but with sterile CSF cultures and no laboratory evidence consistent with a viral or bacterial process. These neonates had obstetric or neonatal factors that increased their risk for infection, including maternal toxemia, prolonged ROM, chorioamnionitis, maternal fever, unexplained jaundice, and prematurity. The CSF protein and glucose determinations and leukocyte counts in these neonates were elevated compared with older infants and children (Table 39-20). The CSF cell count was observed to decrease during the first week of life in term infants, but to increase in preterm infants. An alteration in blood-brain barrier permeability was cited as a potential mechanism for these findings.

Rodriguez and colleagues[50] evaluated CSF indexes during the first 12 weeks of life in high-risk infants with VLBW. These infants had sterile CSF bacterial cultures, weighed less than 1500 g at birth with weights appropriate for gestational age, and had no ultrasound evidence of intracranial hemorrhage. The CSF values were analyzed by chronologic age of the infant and by postconceptual age, defined by the authors as gestational age plus the chronologic postnatal age. The CSF glucose and protein determinations were higher in infants 26 to 28 weeks of age than in other age groups (Table 39-21; see also Appendix B).

CSF findings in 135 neonates with bacterial infections, including 98 with gram-negative bacillary meningitis, 21 with GBS meningitis, and 16 with septicemia without meningitis, were analyzed by Sarff and colleagues[53] using the reference ranges derived from 117 high-risk infants without documented infection. Only 4% of neonates with gram-negative bacillary meningitis had CSF leukocyte counts within the normal range, whereas 23% and 15% had normal protein and normal CSF and blood glucose determinations. E. coli was isolated from a CSF sample with normal cell

TABLE 39-20   Cerebrospinal Fluid Indexes in High-Risk Neonates without Meningitis

	Term	Preterm*
White Blood Cells (cells/mm³)		
Mean	8.2	9.0
Range	0-32	0-29
Percentage PMNs	61.3	57.2
Protein (mg/dL)		
Mean	90	115
Range	20-170	65-150
Glucose (mg/dL)		
Mean	52	50
Range	34-119	24-63
CSF-to-Blood Glucose Ratio (%)		
Mean	81	74
Range	44-248	55-105

*Preterm infant defined as 28 to 38 weeks' gestational age.
CSF, cerebrospinal fluid; PMNs, polymorphonuclear neutrophils.
Adapted from Sarff LD et al: Cerebrospinal fluid evaluation in neonates: comparison of high-risk infants with and without meningitis, *J Pediatr* 88:473, 1976.

count, glucose, and protein determinations in one infant. The indexes on repeat CSF evaluation from this patient were consistent with bacterial meningitis. Because CSF may be obtained early in the course of meningitis, before the inflammatory process is evident, normal CSF parameters do not exclude a diagnosis of meningitis. Despite overlap in CSF findings from uninfected neonates and neonates with meningitis, most neonates have at least one abnormal finding on the initial CSF examination.

Other tests can be helpful in supporting or establishing a diagnosis of neonatal meningitis. The Gram-stained smear is the most useful. Antigen detection should not be used as a substitute for bacteriologic culture in the diagnosis of GBS meningitis. Results of antigen detection assays should be confirmed by culture.

Indications for obtaining CSF in the evaluation of infection are controversial. Some investigators have questioned the usefulness of lumbar puncture in the evaluation of asymptomatic newborns with maternal risk factors. In a retrospective study of 284 asymptomatic infants younger than 7 days of age with a sepsis workup that included lumbar puncture performed in response to maternal risk factors, Fielkow and associates[19] found no episodes of meningitis. Many authorities maintain that CSF should be obtained in any neonate with suspected sepsis neonatorum before antibiotics are given. Relying on a positive blood culture to determine when to evaluate CSF can miss 10% to 15% of neonates with meningitis and sterile blood cultures. The diagnosis of meningitis would have been missed or delayed in 16 of the 43 infants

TABLE 39–21   Cerebrospinal Fluid Values in Infants with Very Low Birthweight* by Postconceptional Age†

Postconceptional Age in Weeks (No. Infants)	Leukocytes/mm³ ± SD (Range)	PMN (%) ± SD (Range)	Glucose (mg/dL) ± SD (Range)	Protein (mg/dL) ± SD (Range)
26-28 (17)	6 ± 10 (0-44)	6 ± 13 (0-50)	85 ± 39‡ (41-217)	177 ± 60‡ (108-370)
29-31 (23)	5 ± 4 (0-14)	10 ± 19 (0-66)	54 ± 18 (33-94)	144 ± 40 (84-227)
32-34 (18)	4 ± 3 (1-11)	4 ± 11 (0-36)	55 ± 21 (29-109)	142 ± 49 (54-260)
35-37 (8)	6 ± 7 (2-22)	5 ± 14 (0-40)	56 ± 21 (31-90)	109 ± 53 (45-187)
38-40 (5)	9 ± 9 (0-23)	16 ± 23 (0-48)	44 ± 10 (32-57)	117 ± 33 (67-148)

*<1500 g.
†Postconceptional age = gestational age + chronologic postnatal age.
‡Group at 26 to 28 weeks had significantly higher glucose and protein levels than the other groups ($P < .04$).
PMN, polymorphonuclear neutrophil; SD, standard deviation.
Data from Rodriguez AF et al: Cerebrospinal fluid values in the very low birth weight infant, *J Pediatr* 116:971, 1990.

reported by Wiswell and associates[73] if lumbar puncture had been omitted as part of the early neonatal sepsis evaluation. In a multicenter study of infants with VLBW, one third of 134 infants with late-onset meningitis had negative blood cultures.[66] Compared with noninfected infants, infants with meningitis had extended requirement for mechanical ventilation and hospitalization, and were more likely to have seizures and to die.

These data support the need to include a lumbar puncture in the diagnostic evaluation of infants with VLBW with suspected late-onset infection. Lumbar puncture can be delayed until a critically ill infant's status has stabilized or until correction of a coagulopathy, but omitting lumbar puncture as part of the evaluation would cause the diagnosis of meningitis to be delayed or missed completely in some infants.

TREATMENT

When initiating antimicrobial therapy for neonatal meningitis, potential pathogens and their susceptibility patterns and the achievable concentrations of the drugs in CSF should be considered. In the United States, empirical therapy should provide coverage for GBS, gram-negative bacillary enteric organisms, and *L. monocytogenes*. Ampicillin reliably provides coverage for GBS and *Listeria* organisms, but its activity against gram-negative enteric organisms is variable. When used for meningitis, ampicillin must be given in a higher dosage than that used for infections outside the nervous system to achieve adequate CSF concentrations. Although gentamicin is active against most gram-negative enteric organisms, aminoglycosides in general do not achieve satisfactory activity in CSF and are rarely used as monotherapy for treatment of meningitis.

When gram-negative bacillary meningitis is suspected, many clinicians favor using ampicillin, gentamicin, and cefotaxime pending final culture and susceptibility reports. Therapy for hospitalized neonates with late-onset meningitis should include coverage against nosocomial pathogens. Vancomycin and an aminoglycoside are frequently chosen to provide activity against CONS in addition to GBS and enterococci. If GBS is suspected, ampicillin should be included in the regimen. If enteric gram-negative organisms are suspected, cefotaxime should be added to the regimen. Antimicrobial therapy often can be simplified when the etiologic agent and its susceptibility profile have been determined.

The duration of therapy for culture-proven bacterial meningitis depends on the etiologic agent recovered and the infant's clinical response. The minimal duration in uncomplicated GBS or *Listeria* meningitis is 14 days. Gram-negative bacillary organisms are more difficult to eradicate from CSF. These infants often have persistently positive CSF cultures 3 to 4 days after the initiation of appropriate antimicrobial agents. In an uncomplicated case, the duration of therapy should be a minimum of 3 weeks, or 2 weeks after documented sterilization of CSF, whichever is longer. Examination of CSF, Gram-stained smears, and culture should be repeated routinely at 24 to 48 hours after initiation of therapy to document CSF sterilization and again near completion of therapy to document adequacy of treatment.

Supportive care of a newborn with meningitis is similar to that described for sepsis. In addition, treatment of seizures and inappropriate secretion of antidiuretic hormone may be necessary (see Chapter 40, Part 5). Neuroimaging is useful to assess ventricular size and to assist in delineating potential intracranial complications of meningitis.

PROGNOSIS AND OUTCOME

The mortality rate of neonatal meningitis has declined from almost 50% in the 1970s to contemporary rates of less than 10%. Survivors are at a high risk for neurologic sequelae.[26] A poor early outcome after GBS meningitis correlates with coma or semicoma, need for pressor support, total peripheral leukocyte count less than 5000/mm³, absolute neutrophil count less than 1000/mm³, and CSF protein greater than 300 mg/dL at the time of presentation.[33] Seizures at presentation, the burden of bacteria observed on Gram stain, and the severity of hypoglycorrhachia on the initial CSF sample are not predictive of sequelae at hospital discharge. Factors associated with poor outcome in gram-negative bacillary meningitis include CSF protein level greater than 500 mg/dL, CSF leukocyte count greater than 10,000/mm³, persistence of positive CSF cultures, and presence and persistence of elevated IL-1α and TNF.[39] For *E. coli* meningitis, the presence and persistence of K_1 capsular polysaccharide antigen and the concentration of endotoxin in the CSF correlated with poor outcome. One fourth to one third of the survivors of gram-negative and gram-positive neonatal meningitis experience permanent sequelae resulting in significant neurologic damage, including hearing loss, language disorders, mental retardation, motor impairment, seizures, and hydrocephalus.[63] Clinical follow-up and neurodevelopmental assessment are appropriate after this disease.

Meningoencephalitis

Infection of the brain and meninges caused by viruses, fungi, or protozoal parasites can occur in the neonatal period. Transplacental infection with CMV, rubella virus, and *Toxoplasma gondii* and perinatal infection with HSV are discussed in other parts of this chapter. Poliovirus, coxsackievirus, echoviruses, varicella-zoster virus, and Epstein-Barr virus can be acquired before, at, or after delivery. Disorders caused by these agents, tuberculosis, and syphilis are discussed in greater detail later. When conventional bacterial cultures of CSF are sterile in an infant with clinical evidence of CNS infection or evidence of inflammation on examination of CSF, or both, these agents and *Mycoplasma hominis* should be considered. In young infants, it is usually impossible to distinguish clinically between meningitis, meningoencephalitis, and encephalitis. Identification of the etiologic agent and specialized radiologic studies can be helpful in this regard.

Pneumonia

INCIDENCE

Pneumonia is the most common form of neonatal infection and one of the most important causes of perinatal death worldwide.[42] (See also Chapter 44.) In the 1920s and 1930s, pneumonia was found at autopsy in 20% to 30% of stillborn and newborn infants. More recently, intrauterine pneumonia has been reported in 5% to 35% of autopsies.

ETIOLOGY

Neonatal pneumonia is caused by many of the same pathogens associated with neonatal sepsis. When the disease is acquired in utero or at the time of delivery, GBS is a common bacterial pathogen, although infections with *E. coli,* other gram-negative enteric organisms, *Listeria* species, *H. influenzae, T. pallidum,* staphylococci, and *S. pneumoniae* have been described. Other causative agents include *Chlamydia trachomatis, Mycoplasma pneumoniae,* CMV, HSV, enterovirus, adenovirus, and rubella. When disease is acquired in the nursery or at home, the same organisms can be responsible, but infection with *S. aureus, Pseudomonas, Serratia, Bordetella pertussis,* and *Candida* species should be considered, especially in premature infants with VLBW who receive care in intensive care units. Viral pneumonia can be noted at or shortly after birth, and reports of epidemic disease in the nursery have occurred with respiratory syncytial virus, echovirus, and adenovirus. Epidemic bacterial pneumonia has occurred after contamination of respiratory equipment and from personnel with suppurative staphylococcal lesions.

PATHOGENESIS AND PATHOLOGY

Pneumonia can be acquired (1) transplacentally, (2) by aspiration of contaminated amniotic fluid before or at the time of delivery, (3) by aspiration of infected materials during or after delivery, (4) by inhalation of aerosols from infected personnel or contaminated equipment in the newborn nursery, or (5) hematogenously during the course of septicemia or from another focus of infection. Congenital (intrauterine) pneumonia frequently follows prolonged ROM. Gasping from asphyxia can result in the aspiration of infected amniotic fluid. Pathologic findings of congenital pneumonia reveal a diffuse inflammatory process with neutrophils present in the alveoli, but bacteria often absent. Amniotic debris and maternal leukocytes can be found, suggesting that disease has followed aspiration rather than hematogenous dissemination of microorganisms. Features commonly observed in bacterial pneumonia in older patients are not seen, such as infiltration of bronchopulmonary tissue, fibrinous alveolar exudate, and pleural reaction.

Aspiration during or after delivery can result in bronchopneumonia, which is sometimes associated with hemorrhage and with evidence of pleural inflammation. Pathologic studies reveal areas of densely cellular exudate with bacteria present. Vascular congestion, hemorrhage, and necrosis can be observed. Microabscesses and empyema can be found when the infection is caused by *S. aureus* or *Klebsiella pneumoniae.* Pneumatocele formation, commonly associated with infection by *S. aureus,* has been described in neonatal disease caused by *E. coli* and *Klebsiella* species. Fatal cases of GBS pneumonia have had evidence of hyaline membranes similar to those found in respiratory distress syndrome.

CLINICAL MANIFESTATIONS

Pneumonia should be suspected when respiratory distress develops in any infant, but suspicion should be heightened if antecedent problems referable to pregnancy and delivery have been noted. Infants with congenital pneumonia often die in utero or are critically ill at birth. Spontaneous respirations may not occur or may be established with difficulty. If respirations are established, tachypnea, moderate retractions, and grunting may be observed. Fever may or may not be noted, but is often a prominent sign of neonatal herpes simplex and enteroviral disease. In most cases, there is no cough. Cyanosis can be constant or intermittent, and respirations may be irregular and punctuated by periods of apnea. Congestive heart failure, manifested by cardiac enlargement, hepatomegaly, and tachycardia, can complicate the pneumonic process.

Infants who acquire pneumonia during delivery or postnatally can have systemic signs, including fever, reluctance to feed, and lethargy. Respiratory signs can occur early or late in the course and include cough, grunting, costal and sternal retractions, flaring of the alae nasi, tachypnea or irregular respirations, rales, decreased breath sounds, and cyanosis. Congestive heart failure can be present in severe disease.

Postnatally acquired pneumonia can develop at any age. Infants with chlamydial pneumonia typically present at 4 to 11 weeks of age with a prodrome of nasal congestion followed by tachypnea and a paroxysmal, staccato cough. Conjunctivitis is present or occurred earlier in approximately half of these infants. Inspiratory rales may be present, but expiratory wheezes are not commonly seen. These infants are afebrile and frequently gain weight slowly.

DIAGNOSIS

Chest radiographs are necessary to support the diagnosis of pneumonia and to exclude other causes of respiratory distress. In some patients, no abnormality is found if imaging is performed soon after the onset of symptoms, but by 24 to 74 hours, a diagnosis should be possible. Radiographic findings can reveal bilateral homogeneous consolidation when pneumonia is acquired in utero or diffuse bronchopneumonia with postnatally acquired disease. Pneumatoceles can be observed, usually later in the course of illness, and occasionally hemothorax or pleural effusions are seen. Pneumonia caused by GBS can be difficult to distinguish radiographically from respiratory distress syndrome. This can be a diagnostic dilemma, especially in premature infants. Bilateral, symmetric interstitial infiltrates with hyperexpansion of the lungs are the typical radiographic findings seen in *C. trachomatis* pneumonia (see Chapter 37).

The radiographic pattern of segmental or lobar atelectasis can be difficult to distinguish from that of massive meconium aspiration. In meconium aspiration, opacities may be distributed in the same manner as in bronchopneumonia, but the radiologic changes tend to be maximal early and disappear rapidly during the ensuing days. In contrast, the patchy opacifications noted with bronchopneumonia tend to be minimal early and become more impressive during the subsequent days.

Blood cultures should be obtained in infants with pneumonia; positive cultures establish an etiologic diagnosis. If obtained before 8 hours of age, Gram-stained smears of tracheal secretions showing neutrophils and bacteria can help identify neonates with pneumonia. Bacterial cultures of tracheal secretions may not be helpful in establishing an etiologic diagnosis because they often reflect the flora present in the vaginal canal. In newborns with prolonged ventilation, tracheal aspirate cultures frequently fail to identify the cause of respiratory deterioration.[70] A definitive microbiologic diagnosis can be made if organisms are isolated from cultures of pleural fluid, material aspirated from lung abscesses, or open lung biopsy tissue, but these interventions often are not performed. Tracheal secretions should be processed for viral isolates when nonbacterial pneumonia is suspected.

A diagnosis of *Chlamydia* pneumonia can be assumed if the organism is isolated from nasopharyngeal samples or from secretions obtained by deep tracheal suctioning, but special culturing techniques are required. Culture of *B. pertussis* requires inoculation of nasopharyngeal secretions onto appropriate media for isolation. Cultures tend to grow slowly. Polymerase chain reaction of nasopharyngeal or endotracheal secretions provides a rapid and preferable means for diagnosis of pertussis.

TREATMENT

When a diagnosis of pneumonia is suspected, antimicrobial therapy should be initiated promptly. If the diagnosis is supported by historical and clinical findings, but initial radiographs fail to confirm the clinical suspicion, treatment should not be delayed and is continued until results of a repeat chest radiograph, taken at 48 to 72 hours, are available. Empirical antimicrobial therapy is the same as that for neonatal sepsis. Ampicillin and either an aminoglycoside or cefotaxime are indicated for early-onset or late-onset, community-acquired pneumonia, and vancomycin and an aminoglycoside are indicated for late-onset nosocomial infection (see Tables 39-17 and 39-18).[41] Pneumonia caused by *Chlamydia* or *Pertussis* organisms responds best to treatment with azithromycin. Acyclovir therapy should be administered promptly if HSV pneumonia is suspected. Treatment for bacterial pneumonia is continued for 10 to 14 days or longer as dictated by the clinical course of the patient. Adequate fluids and oxygen, as required to treat hypoxemia, are useful adjunctive measures.

PROGNOSIS

The outcome of intrauterine pneumonia is variable, but more critically ill infants are likely to die in utero or within the first 2 days of life despite meticulous care and administration of appropriate antibiotics. The prognosis is worse for premature than for term infants. In the absence of other problems, the prognosis for term infants who acquire pneumonia postnatally seems to be good.

Otitis Media

INCIDENCE

Acute otitis media is the most common infection diagnosed in young children, and it can occur in neonates. In one prospective study, 9% of infants had an episode of otitis media by age 3 months.[68] The exact incidence is uncertain. It is estimated that otitis media develops in a minimum of 0.6% of all live births during the first month of life, and that the rate may reach 2% to 3% in premature infants. Otitis media occurs more often in male than in female infants, in infants with cleft palate, and in infants requiring prolonged intubation.

ETIOLOGY

The microbiology of acute otitis media in neonates differs from acute otitis media seen in older infants and children. Although organisms from the respiratory tract are also the most commonly isolated pathogens in neonatal disease, GBS, *E. coli*, and other gram-negative bacteria can be causative agents in the first 2 to 6 weeks of life. Studies of infants younger than 6 to 8 weeks have shown that *S. pneumoniae* was the pathogen isolated in 19% to 30% of cases, *H. influenzae* was recovered in 14% to 25% of cases, and β-hemolytic streptococci (groups A and B) were recovered in 5% of cases. Gram-negative bacilli (*E. coli* and *Enterobacter, Klebsiella,* and *Pseudomonas* species) were found in 7% to 18% of neonates or very young infants with otitis media.[6,57] Of cultures obtained by tympanocentesis in this age group, 40% to 50% have been sterile or judged nonpathogenic. Included among the nonpathogenic bacteria are organisms such as *S. aureus, Staphylococcus epidermidis,* and *Moraxella catarrhalis,* which likely are responsible for purulent otitis media in some newborns. Because strict anaerobic culture techniques were not used in most studies, many sterile isolates may have contained anaerobic microorganisms. Viral infection also has been associated with neonatal middle ear disease.

PATHOGENESIS AND PATHOLOGY

Otitis media is more common in premature than in term infants. This increased risk of infection may be related to the small size of the eustachian tube, with resultant obstruction and secondary infection. Aspiration of infected amniotic fluid is probably a leading cause of otitis media in newborns. The disease increases in frequency in bottle-fed infants, a finding that may be related to use of the supine position during feeding or to the lack of local immunity that may be conferred by ingredients in breast milk. Secretory IgA and other components in breast milk may exert protection by preventing the attachment of otitis media–causing bacterial strains to retropharyngeal or buccal epithelial cells.

CLINICAL MANIFESTATIONS

The most common presenting symptoms are respiratory complaints such as cough or rhinorrhea and fever.[6] Irritability, lethargy, vomiting, poor feeding, or diarrhea can also be present. Young infants with otitis media often are asymptomatic. The ear is difficult to examine adequately in newborn infants. Erythema, dullness, and bulging of the pars flaccida of the tympanic membranes can be noted, and pneumatic otoscopy can reveal decreased mobility of the tympanic membrane. Infants with typical facial or submandibular GBS cellulitis often have ipsilateral otitis media.

DIAGNOSIS

The nonspecificity of clinical signs and symptoms combined with difficulties in visualizing the tympanic membrane early in life probably account in part for the discrepancy between incidence data derived from prospective clinical studies and data from postmortem studies. In infants who appear ill or fail to respond to initial therapy, a specific diagnosis should be made by culture and Gram-stained smears of purulent middle ear fluid obtained by myringotomy or tympanocentesis. Cultures of the nasopharynx can yield the same organism in some cases, but cannot be routinely relied on to guide selection of antibiotics. Blood cultures can be helpful in patients with concomitant septicemia. Lumbar puncture should be performed to exclude meningitis in ill infants. Meningitis that was not suspected before examination of CSF has been noted in some newborns with otitis media, but the frequency with which the two occur simultaneously is unknown.

TREATMENT

The empirical antibiotics chosen and the route administered depend on the age and the appearance of the infant. For neonates with acute otitis media in the first 2 weeks of life, a combination of ampicillin and either an aminoglycoside or cefotaxime provides effective initial treatment. Hospitalized premature infants require parenteral therapy as well. A regimen such as vancomycin and gentamicin is one option for empirical therapy. Oral therapy with amoxicillin can be considered for well-appearing term infants older than 3 weeks who have had an uncomplicated intrapartum and neonatal course. If the infant is toxic-appearing or has evidence of infection elsewhere, cultures of middle ear fluid, blood, and CSF should be obtained, and the infant should be hospitalized for broad-spectrum parenteral antimicrobial therapy.

When culture results are known, antibiotic therapy can be altered appropriately. Treatment should be continued for 10 days or longer, depending on the etiologic agent, the associated condition (e.g., sepsis or meningitis), and the clinical response to therapy.

PROGNOSIS

Recurrent or persistent disease can occur. Infants with onset of otitis media before 2 months of age are at high risk for development of chronic otitis media with effusion. In addition to young age at the onset of the first episode, other risk factors for recurrent infections include low socioeconomic status and the presence of smokers in the household. Careful follow-up evaluation for infection and hearing loss is important. Insertion of tympanostomy tubes may be indicated to ensure adequate drainage of the middle ear and to reduce the likelihood of recurrent middle ear infections.

Conjunctivitis

INCIDENCE

Neonatal conjunctivitis, also referred to as ophthalmia neonatorum, is the most common ocular disease in neonates.[23] Previously, gonococcal conjunctivitis was the leading cause of infant blindness. The epidemiology of ophthalmia neonatorum in the United States has changed significantly, however, in the past century with the introduction of ocular prophylaxis by Credé in 1881 and the advent of prenatal screening and treatment of maternal gonococcal infections. Gonococcal conjunctivitis remains an important neonatal disease in less developed countries. In developed countries, ophthalmia neonatorum can be caused by chemical irritation after prophylactic instillation of silver nitrate into the conjunctival sac. Chemical conjunctivitis can occur in 10% to 90% of infants so treated. Chemical conjunctivitis caused by topical therapy with erythromycin or tetracycline occurs less frequently. The incidence of other forms of conjunctivitis is difficult to assess, but has been estimated at approximately 8 cases of chlamydial infection per 1000 live births and 0.3 cases of gonococcal disease per 1000 live births.

ETIOLOGY

The differential diagnosis of infectious conjunctivitis in a newborn includes bacterial, chlamydial, and viral agents. *C. trachomatis* and *Neisseria gonorrhoeae* are the most important causes of conjunctivitis in the newborn period with respect to frequency of the former and severity of complications in untreated cases for both. Other bacteria, including *S. aureus,* GBS, *Pseudomonas* species, *S. pneumoniae,* and *Haemophilus* species, can also be causative. Conjunctivitis is the most common ocular manifestation of neonatal herpes simplex infections.

PATHOGENESIS

Conjunctivitis caused by *N. gonorrhoeae, C. trachomatis,* GBS, or HSV usually is initiated by infection with microorganisms acquired during passage through the birth canal and reflects the prevalence of sexually transmitted diseases in the community. Premature ROM and prematurity increase the risk of disease by *N. gonorrhoeae*. Infection with *S. aureus* or other organisms more commonly reflects infection acquired postnatally. *Pseudomonas* conjunctivitis occurs most often in hospitalized premature infants and often is associated with systemic complications.

CLINICAL MANIFESTATIONS

The typical age at onset of conjunctivitis varies depending on the etiology, although there is much overlap. Chemical conjunctivitis usually is noted soon after birth and becomes less prominent within 48 hours. Bacterial conjunctivitis is most prominent during the first week of life, but can occur at any time during the neonatal period. Chlamydial conjunctivitis usually develops during the second week of life.

The signs of bacterial conjunctivitis in a newborn are similar to the signs observed in older patients. A purulent ocular discharge, erythema and edema of the lids, and injection or suffusion of the conjunctiva can be found. Gonococcal disease typically manifests with abrupt onset of profuse, purulent ocular discharge. Conjunctivitis caused by *Haemophilus* species and *S. pneumoniae* has been associated with dacryocystitis. When *C. trachomatis* is involved, minimal inflammatory changes may be detected, or there can be intense inflammation, swelling, and a yellow discharge associated with pseudomembrane formation. The cornea is affected rarely. Chlamydial infections usually are bilateral, whereas unilateral disease is common when staphylococcal disease is present.

Complications are rare, but can be devastating, with loss of vision. If bacterial conjunctivitis is left untreated, corneal involvement with punctate epithelial erosions can occur. In the case of disease with *N. gonorrhoeae,* large, punctate, superficial lesions can be seen that can coalesce and progress to corneal perforation. Gonococcal conjunctivitis should be considered a medical emergency. Untreated disease can progress rapidly from purulent conjunctivitis without corneal involvement to corneal ulceration and perforation. Meningitis or arthritis can complicate gonococcal ophthalmia neonatorum, but systemic spread of infection occurs rarely when appropriate therapy is given promptly before corneal involvement develops. When staphylococcal conjunctivitis is complicated by corneal involvement, the lower portion of the cornea is infected more frequently than the upper half, and marginal corneal infiltrates with peripheral vascularization can be seen. When chlamydial conjunctivitis is not treated, inflammation persists for 1 or 2 weeks. A subacute phase follows with slight injection of the conjunctiva and an accumulation of purulent material along the lid margins. Necrosis of the cornea has been observed, followed by fibrosis and scarring of the lid margin. Occasionally, chronic disease develops. Untreated chlamydial conjunctivitis, especially when associated with nasopharyngeal colonization, can progress to pneumonia in some infants. Even without invasive eye disease, systemic complications such as bacteremia and meningitis often develop in infants with *P. aeruginosa* conjunctivitis.

DIAGNOSIS

A presumptive diagnosis of chemical or infectious conjunctivitis can be made based on the history and physical examination. There is such overlap in clinical appearance and age at presentation that a definitive etiologic diagnosis cannot be determined reliably without the aid of laboratory testing. Purulent material must be sent for Gram stain and bacterial culture. Conjunctival scrapings should be sent when evaluating for *Chlamydia* infection because the organism resides in the epithelial conjunctival cells and not in neutrophils.

When gonococcal disease is suspected, the purulent material should be placed in special transport media and sent to the bacteriology laboratory. Other organisms are less fastidious, and a swab of purulent material, cultured promptly, is sufficient to establish a diagnosis. The presence of intracellular gram-negative diplococci on a Gram-stained smear suggests a diagnosis of gonococcal disease.

Characteristic intracytoplasmic inclusions can be identified by examining a Giemsa-stained smear from material obtained by gently but firmly scraping the lower portion of the palpebral conjunctiva with a blunt spatula or loop. Care must be taken not to injure the conjunctiva during the process. Leber cells (macrophages containing cellular debris) and inclusion-bearing epithelial cells (hence the name inclusion blennorrhea or conjunctivitis) are characteristic. The Giemsa stain is a specific, but not a sensitive, method for detection of *Chlamydia* conjunctivitis. Culture is the gold standard, but many laboratories do not have the capability of performing cell cultures. Numerous antigen detection assays, such as nucleic acid amplification and direct fluorescent antibody tests, are also options with a high degree of accuracy for detection of *Chlamydia* from conjunctival specimens.

TREATMENT

Therapy of gonococcal conjunctivitis involves frequent irrigation of the conjunctival sac with sterile isotonic saline until the discharge has resolved and parenteral antimicrobial therapy. The recommended antimicrobial therapy for ophthalmia neonatorum is ceftriaxone (25 to 50 mg/kg, not to exceed 125 mg) administered intravenously or intramuscularly one time. Evaluation for disseminated infection should include cultures of blood and CSF. For disseminated neonatal gonococcal infection, the recommended therapy is ceftriaxone (25 to 50 mg/kg) given once daily for 7 days or cefotaxime (50 to 100 mg/kg daily) given in two doses for 7 days. If meningitis is documented, treatment should be continued for 10 to 14 days. Persistence of conjunctivitis after treatment may indicate coinfection with *C. trachomatis* and requires additional therapy directed against this agent. Because there are reports of high rates of *C. trachomatis* and *N. gonorrhoeae* coinfection in adults, empirical treatment with erythromycin in addition to cephalosporin often is indicated.

Parenteral treatment with an aminoglycoside and an antipseudomonal penicillin in addition to topical treatment is indicated for conjunctivitis caused by *Pseudomonas* organisms. Antibiotics containing various combinations of bacitracin, neomycin, and polymyxin, administered topically as an ophthalmic ointment or solution several times a day for 7 to 10 days, have been recommended for other forms of bacterial conjunctivitis.

An association between orally administered erythromycin and infantile hypertrophic pyloric stenosis has been reported in infants younger than 6 weeks. The efficacy of a single erythromycin course for treatment of *Chlamydia* conjunctivitis was approximately 80%. Preliminary data indicate that a short course of azithromycin treatment is an effective alternative to erythromycin,[25] and azithromycin now is the treatment of choice for infants with chlamydial conjunctivitis. Topical treatment is ineffective and is not indicated.

PREVENTION

The CDC and the American Academy of Pediatrics Committee on Infectious Diseases recommend erythromycin (0.5%) ophthalmic ointment, tetracycline (1%) ophthalmic ointment, or a 1% silver nitrate solution for prophylaxis of ophthalmia neonatorum. The prophylactic agent should be dispensed in a single-dose tube or ampule and given within 1 hour of birth.

In a large study by Hammerschlag and colleagues[24] in which the efficacy of three topical prophylactic agents was studied in 230 infants born to women diagnosed with cervical chlamydial infection during pregnancy, 20% of infants given silver nitrate at birth, 14% of infants given erythromycin, and 11% of infants given tetracycline topical prophylaxis developed neonatal chlamydial conjunctivitis. This observation and findings from several other studies suggest that the most effective way to prevent chlamydial conjunctivitis (and other chlamydial disease) in neonates is to screen and treat pregnant women harboring the infection. Infants born to mothers known to have untreated chlamydial infection are at high risk for infection; however, prophylactic antimicrobial treatment is not indicated because the efficacy is unknown.

Ceftriaxone, 25 to 50 mg/kg (maximum 125 mg), should be administered intravenously or intramuscularly as a single dose to infants born to mothers with untreated gonococcal infection. Cefotaxime, 100 mg/kg, is an alternative. Administration of one of the topical agents used for prophylaxis does not eradicate established gonococcal infection that is not yet clinically apparent. Caution should be exercised in providing ceftriaxone to premature infants of low birthweight with hyperbilirubinemia.

Gastroenteritis

INCIDENCE

Most neonatal diarrheal disease is sporadic. It is usually self-limited and brief, but may cause significant morbidity in some infants. Failure to take appropriate steps to control the spread of infection to other infants can result in an epidemic outbreak of the disease in the nursery. The incidence varies from nursery to nursery and within the same nursery from year to year.

ETIOLOGY

Neonatal diarrheal disease is more likely to be associated with noninfectious processes. The organisms that have been associated with epidemic and sporadic infectious diarrheal disease include certain strains of *E. coli; Salmonella, Shigella, Yersinia,* and *Campylobacter* species[49]; and rarely *Pseudomonas, Klebsiella,* and *Enterobacter* species and *Candida albicans.* An epidemic of enterocolitis has been attributed to infection by group A streptococci. Enteric types of adenovirus, rotavirus, and calicivirus have been identified as causative agents

for gastroenteritis in neonates. In many cases, the etiologic agent is not identified, and viruses are assumed to be responsible despite negative viral and serologic studies.

There are at least five pathotypes of diarrhea-producing *E. coli.* Enteropathogenic *E. coli* (EPEC) was associated classically with severe outbreaks of infantile diarrhea in the developed world through the 1960s, and now is a common cause of diarrhea in infants in the developing world. There is a predilection for this infection in infants who are not breast-fed. Enterotoxigenic *E. coli* also has been associated with neonatal diarrheal disease, but infection usually is delayed until the introduction of foods to supplement human milk.

All *Salmonella* organisms are closely related and are now considered a single species, *Salmonella enterica.* There are more than 2000 *Salmonella* types that cause human disease. Three surface antigens determine reactions to antisera: O (somatic), H (flagellar), and Vi (capsular) antigens. Serogrouping is based on O antigens and designates groups A through E. *Salmonella* serotype *typhi* is in group D. Commonly reported isolates in the United States include *Salmonella* serotype *typhimurium* (group B) and *Salmonella* serotype *enteritidis* (group D).

Shigella comprises four serogroups with more than 40 serotypes. In the United States, *Shigella sonnei* (group D) followed by *Shigella flexneri* (group B) are the most common isolates from patients of any age with shigellosis. The central event in pathogenesis for *Shigella* is its ability to cross the colonic epithelium and invade the colonic mucosa. All virulent *Shigella* organisms have virulent plasmid-associated antigens that provide the means for intracellular and intercellular spread. Hemolytic uremic syndrome, associated with production of Shiga toxin, can complicate bacillary dysentery secondary to *Shigella dysenteriae,* serotype 1.

Campylobacter, a comma-shaped, gram-negative bacillus, is recognized increasingly as a common cause of gastroenteritis. *Campylobacter fetus* causes prenatal and neonatal infections that result in abortion, premature delivery, bacteremia, and meningitis. *Campylobacter jejuni* and *Campylobacter coli* usually cause neonatal gastroenteritis. Health care–associated outbreaks in nurseries, although uncommon, have been described.

Although it is likely that some diarrheal episodes in neonates can be caused by *Clostridium difficile,* the diagnostic criteria used in older children and adults are inadequate to establish a definitive etiologic diagnosis in this age group. *C. difficile* is rarely isolated from the stools of healthy children older than 1 year or healthy adults, but the organism and its cytotoxin can be shown in the stools of more than 50% of healthy neonates. The pathogenicity of this organism in neonates has not been well defined.

PATHOGENESIS

The gastrointestinal tract is colonized initially by organisms that enter the oropharynx at delivery. Maternal carriers of *Salmonella, Shigella, Campylobacter,* and EPEC can serve as the initial source of these pathogens in the nursery. Person-to-person transmission also has occurred in neonates of infected mothers and has resulted in health care–related outbreaks in nurseries. Asymptomatic health care workers who are carriers of these organisms have proved to be the source of spread.

Fomite transmission has been observed, and in rare instances infection has followed ingestion of contaminated milk, water, or materials used for radiographic evaluation of the gastrointestinal tract.

CLINICAL MANIFESTATIONS

Gastrointestinal tract bacterial infection can manifest without clinical symptoms; as a watery diarrhea without other findings; or as a severe diarrhea with fever, vomiting, and abdominal distention. It is difficult to predict the etiology on the basis of clinical findings. Bloody diarrhea containing mucus suggests *Shigella, Yersinia,* or *Campylobacter* gastroenteritis, but these findings have been observed occasionally in neonates with gastroenteritis caused by *Salmonella* or EPEC. Infection with *Salmonella* is frequently asymptomatic or mild. Neonates with diarrhea usually have a self-limited infection with loose, mucoid stools and, rarely, hematochezia. *Salmonella* gastroenteritis in the first month of life can be associated with bacteremia or extraintestinal manifestations, including meningitis. Neonatal shigellosis is rare. The classic picture is that of dysentery, but asymptomatic infection occurs as well. Complications include hemolysis, hemolytic uremic syndrome, colonic perforation, and pseudomembranous colitis. Seizures associated with *Shigella* bowel infection are uncommon in the first 6 months of life. Sepsis occurs uncommonly, but the case-fatality rate is significant for infants with systemic infection.

Infections caused by *C. fetus* are the most common type of *Campylobacter* infection in the first 3 weeks of life and are associated with a high incidence of fetal and neonatal mortality. Systemic *C. jejuni* or *C. coli* infection in neonates is rare. A blue-green discoloration of the stools or diaper can be found when *Pseudomonas* species predominate. The isolation of *Pseudomonas* organisms does not represent disease. Dehydration, acidosis, electrolyte disturbances, and hypotension can occur during the course of disease caused by any of these enteric pathogens.

DIAGNOSIS

Stool for bacterial culture should be obtained from infants with gastroenteritis. Recovery of *Shigella, Yersinia, Campylobacter,* or *Salmonella* from the stool of an infant with diarrhea is presumptive evidence that disease is caused by that organism. The diagnosis of EPEC is difficult because most clinical laboratories cannot differentiate diarrhea-associated strains of *E. coli* from normal stool flora *E. coli* strains. Isolates of *E. coli* suspected to cause a case or outbreak should be sent to a state health or other reference laboratory for serotyping.

A stool smear for polymorphonuclear leukocytes can be valuable. Fecal leukocytes can be observed in stool smears from patients with diarrhea caused by EPEC, *Yersinia, Campylobacter, Salmonella,* or *Shigella,* but usually are not seen in patients with nonspecific or viral gastroenteritis. Blood cultures should be obtained from any neonate with isolation of *Salmonella, Shigella, Campylobacter,* or *Yersinia enterocolitica* from the stool. Lumbar puncture for examination and culture of CSF should be considered if the neonate is febrile or otherwise "toxic" in appearance, or if *Salmonella* or other potential pathogens are isolated from the blood culture.

TREATMENT

Supportive care and correction of fluid and electrolyte abnormalities are the most important aspects of management. Because many infections are self-limited, antimicrobial therapy may not be indicated except in certain situations. It may be unnecessary to treat an infant with diarrhea caused by EPEC. During nursery outbreaks, infants with EPEC isolated from stool should be treated independent of the symptoms, however. When antimicrobial therapy is given, nonabsorbable orally administered antibiotics (neomycin, colistin sulfate) are appropriate options, and the duration of treatment is 5 days.

Infants with *Salmonella* isolated from stool should be treated with cefotaxime after obtaining blood and CSF cultures. When bacteremia or meningitis is present, therapy with cefotaxime or ampicillin for susceptible strains should be given for 10 days (bacteremia) to 4 to 6 weeks (meningitis). Antimicrobial therapy is effective in shortening the duration of diarrhea caused by *Shigella* and eliminating organisms from the feces, and is recommended for patients with bacillary dysentery. For cases in which susceptibility is unknown, ceftriaxone or cefotaxime should be administered. For susceptible strains, ampicillin or trimethoprim-sulfamethoxazole are effective. Treatment should be administered for 5 days. *Campylobacter enteritis* may be treated with azithromycin. Benefit from antimicrobial therapy for patients with *Yersinia enterocolitis* has not been established. Patients with septicemia and compromised hosts, including premature infants, with enterocolitis should receive treatment, however. Cefotaxime and aminoglycosides are appropriate antimicrobials.

PREVENTION AND PROGNOSIS

In addition to standard precautions, contact precautions are indicated for infants with diarrhea. Clusters of infections should be investigated appropriately. During outbreaks of disease caused by EPEC, contact precautions should be maintained until tests of stools collected after completion of antimicrobial therapy are negative for the infecting strain.

Osteomyelitis and Septic Arthritis

INCIDENCE

Osteomyelitis occurs rarely in newborns and can be difficult to diagnose. Septic arthritis is frequently concomitant, probably reflecting spread of infection through blood vessels that penetrate the epiphyseal plate (see Chapter 54).

ETIOLOGY

The most frequent causative agents for community-acquired osteomyelitis and septic arthritis are *S. aureus, E. coli,* and GBS. Community-associated MRSA strains and health care–associated MRSA are common pathogens. Uncommon etiologic agents include *N. gonorrhoeae, H. influenzae,* group A streptococci, and *T. pallidum.* Various staphylococcal and streptococcal species and anaerobic bacteria have been cultured from scalp electrode–related cases of osteomyelitis. *Candida* species and gram-negative enteric bacilli have assumed major roles for nosocomially acquired bone and joint infections, especially in preterm infants with low birthweight. These infections are most commonly isolated in nursery outbreaks.

PATHOLOGY

Osteomyelitis usually originates in the metaphysis of long bones. Involvement of the small bones of the hands and feet, the vertebrae, and the ribs has been noted, however. Multiple foci of osteomyelitis are seen more frequently in newborns than in older individuals; 10% to 40% of newborns have more than a single focus of infection. The cortical bone is thin, permitting infection to extend readily into soft tissues. Infection extends readily from an affected bone into the adjacent joint via transphyseal vessels. Destruction of cartilage, dislocations, and pathologic fractures can occur and permanently affect bone growth.

PATHOGENESIS

Osteomyelitis almost invariably follows hematogenous dissemination of microorganisms. Infection of the skin, omphalitis, umbilical catheterization, and occasionally improperly performed femoral venipunctures are predisposing factors in cases principally caused by S. aureus. Occasionally, osteomyelitis can follow direct extension of a soft tissue infection to bone, especially if the underlying bone is fractured, as illustrated in cases of osteomyelitis of the skull associated with infected cephalhematomas. Transplacental acquisition with dissemination to bone has been observed with T. pallidum.

CLINICAL MANIFESTATIONS

Destructive changes in bone caused by osteomyelitis can be advanced by the time a definitive diagnosis is made. In some patients, the disease is not accompanied by systemic signs or symptoms. Fever is absent or is a very late, intermittent finding. Findings of swelling, tenderness, and decreased motion of an extremity usually prompt initial appraisal. In a patient with osteomyelitis of the clavicle, an incomplete Moro reflex can be the only finding on physical examination. Localized tenderness and erythema can be seen, and heat and fluctuance can be noted. Focal findings overlying affected sites occur commonly when S. aureus is the pathogen. Less often, infants have an acute onset of systemic illness with fever, icterus, hemorrhagic manifestations, and hypotension. GBS osteomyelitis commonly manifests during the third and fourth weeks of life. In contrast to the fulminant onset and poor outcome that occur in some patients with late-onset meningitis, GBS bone and joint infection often has an indolent nature and an almost uniformly good outcome.

DIAGNOSIS

When the history and physical examination suggest the possibility of osteomyelitis, imaging studies should be obtained. Plain radiographic bony changes are delayed for 7 to 10 days after onset of infection, but a plain radiograph provides a helpful baseline. The earliest finding is deep soft tissue swelling. Later in the course of infection, periosteal thickening, cortical destruction, irregularities of the epiphysis, and periosteal new bone formation are seen. Additional findings include localized areas of cortical rarefaction, periosteal elevation, a widened joint space, and subluxation or dislocation of the bone from the joint (e.g., the hip) (Fig. 39-10).

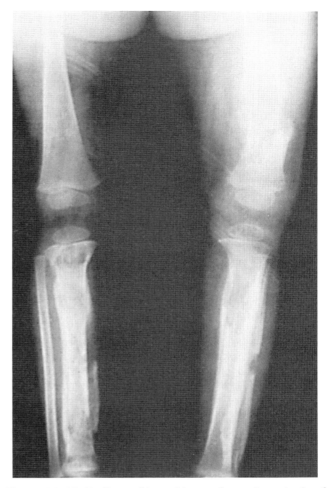

Figure 39-10. Radiographic evidence (posterior view) of multiple sites of osteomyelitis in an infant, the result of infection with *Staphylococcus aureus*. Clinical evidence of infection became apparent at 2 weeks of age. Osteolytic lesions can be seen in the right femur, right tibia and fibula, and left tibia. Periosteal new bone formation is visible in many areas.

Magnetic resonance imaging (MRI) is the diagnostic modality of choice for neonatal osteomyelitis. The diagnosis can be established within 24 to 48 hours after the onset of symptoms. The anatomic detail provided by MRI optimizes the definition of structural abnormalities and can guide surgical drainage. A technetium 99m phosphate scan can show areas of increased blood flow in the affected area, but this modality lacks the structural clarity of MRI and is rarely indicated.

Aspiration of soft tissues and bone is indicated, and samples should be sent for Gram stain and culture. Blood cultures are essential and have been reported to yield the causative agent in 60% of cases. Synovial fluid obtained from patients with joint involvement should be sent for Gram stain and culture. Because osteomyelitis frequently follows bacteremia, caregivers should consider obtaining CSF to exclude concomitant meningitis. Normal peripheral white blood cell counts are commonly seen in neonates with bone and joint infection, and ESR values less than 40 mm/h are reported in

25% of cases. Syphilis, tuberculosis, scurvy, rickets, and deep cellulitis must be considered in the differential diagnosis.

TREATMENT

Until the specific etiology has been clarified by culture, combination therapy should be initiated with vancomycin and either an aminoglycoside or an extended-spectrum cephalosporin for gram-negative coverage. When the infecting isolate and its susceptibility pattern have been identified, treatment should be continued with the most appropriate antibiotic. The dosages used should be the same as the dosages used for treatment of septicemia (see Tables 39-17 and 39-18). Parenteral therapy should be continued for 3 to 4 weeks or longer until clinical and radiographic findings indicate healing, and CRP and ESR are normal. Intra-articular administration of antibiotics is not indicated. Surgical drainage of purulent material is a key component of treatment, and consultation should be sought with a pediatric orthopedic surgeon in the management of this infection. When the hip or shoulder joints are involved, prompt surgical decompression and drainage are crucial.

PROGNOSIS

The degree of residual damage depends on the extent of disease before effective treatment. Permanent disability is more common when joint involvement has occurred. Growth disturbances can result from destruction of the epiphyseal plate. The number of foci of osteomyelitis in a patient who is effectively treated does not seem to correlate specifically with the extent or likelihood of permanent disability. Chronic osteomyelitis occurs infrequently. Overall, residual effects can be noted in 25% of neonates with infection of the bones and joints.

Urinary Tract Infection

The incidence of neonatal urinary tract infection varies from 0.1% to 1% of all infants, with a higher frequency in neonates with low birthweight. (See also Chapter 51.) In contrast to bacteriuria in all other age groups, neonatal disease is more commonly seen in male infants. This preponderance of male infants may reflect the increased risk of urinary tract infection in uncircumcised boys.[72] The presence of virulence factors in some bacteria also influences the development of urinary tract infections.

The organisms associated with neonatal urinary tract infection mirror those that cause neonatal sepsis. For community-acquired neonatal disease, infection with E. coli is most common. Although GBS can be isolated from the urine of infants with GBS sepsis, primary urinary tract infection is rare. The frequency of health care–associated urinary tract infection has increased with the survival of infants with VLBW. Pathogens causing health care–associated infections include E. coli, other gram-negative enteric bacilli, Enterococcus, Candida, and CONS.

Symptoms referable to the genitourinary system are rare. In most infants, the symptoms are nonspecific, similar to that of neonates with septicemia. Reluctance to feed, weight loss, and diarrhea can be the presenting features in some patients. An unexplained fever should prompt an investigation of the urinary tract in addition to an evaluation for sepsis and meningitis.

Urine culture need not be performed routinely in evaluation of infants with early-onset infection because isolation of a pathogen from the urine usually is a manifestation of sepsis, rather than an indicator of urinary tract infection. Definitive diagnosis of neonatal urinary tract infection for an infant evaluated beyond the first few days of life can be made only with culture of properly obtained urine. Samples collected by voiding into a bag are inappropriate. Catheterized specimens or samples obtained by suprapubic bladder aspiration are suitable. Isolation of any bacteria from a bladder aspirate is considered significant, whereas counts of 10^3 or higher colony-forming units per milliliter of catheterized urine are meaningful. Blood and CSF should be obtained as described in the evaluation for sepsis. Although the presence or absence of pyuria on examination of urine sediment is not conclusive evidence for diagnosing or excluding urinary tract infection, the presence of bacteria on Gram-stained smears of the sediment does support the diagnosis.

Empirical therapy for neonatal urinary tract infection should include ampicillin and an aminoglycoside in dosages used for sepsis. Administration should be parenteral because of the high incidence of sepsis in association with urinary tract infections in newborns, and because of the often erratic oral antibiotic absorption in infants. Vancomycin and an aminoglycoside should be considered for empirical therapy of health care–associated urinary tract infections.

Sterilization of the urine should be documented by repeat culture after 48 hours of therapy. Treatment duration is usually 10 days, but can be longer if there is persistent bacteriuria, anatomic obstruction, or a perinephric abscess. In uncomplicated cases of primary urinary tract infection, parenteral therapy can be given for 5 to 7 days, followed by oral antibiotic therapy to complete the course of treatment. Imaging studies, including renal ultrasound and voiding cystourethrogram or renal scan, should be performed to diagnose any anatomic or physiologic urinary tract anomalies.

Infections of the Skin

INCIDENCE

Infection of the skin is common and can be a result of bacterial, viral, or fungal disease. (See also Chapter 52.) The lesions may be localized or the cutaneous manifestation of systemic disease.

ETIOLOGY

Colonization of the skin begins at birth, and the organisms that initially are acquired reflect those present in the mother's birth canal. Subsequently, infants can acquire organisms from the environment or from the hands of family members or caregivers. S. aureus is the organism most often associated with neonatal skin infections. Application of triple dye, iodophor ointment, or chlorhexidine powder to the umbilical stump has been used to delay or prevent S. aureus colonization. Virtually any organism that causes disease in infancy can result in cutaneous infection, including group A streptococci and GBS, Listeria, P. aeruginosa, T. pallidum, HSV, and C. albicans.

PATHOLOGY

Histologic examination of the skin of patients with bullous impetigo can show intraepidermal bullae filled with polymorphonuclear leukocytes. Ritter disease, a severe generalized form of staphylococcal scalded skin syndrome, is caused by a toxin-elaborating strain of *S. aureus*. It is characterized by a severe bullous eruption with shedding of the epidermis. Histologic examination of the skin reveals an intraepidermal blister, cellular death and acantholysis, and a striking absence of inflammation. *Pseudomonas* or *Aeromonas hydrophila* infections cause ecthyma gangrenosum, which is characterized by the development of yellow-green pustules that progress rapidly to form hemorrhagic and necrotic ulcers. In most neonates with ecthyma gangrenosum, these lesions have developed as a consequence of bacteremia. Skin abscesses with minimal inflammation may be caused by *Candida* species; their occurrence should be considered diagnostic of invasive infection.[3]

PATHOGENESIS

Infection usually develops as a result of a small break in the skin and is caused by organisms that have colonized the skin and nares. Potential risk factors include abrasions after forceps use, scalp wounds associated with intrapartum fetal monitoring, the process of degeneration of the umbilical stump after cord clamping, intravascular catheter use, and circumcision. Infectious complications after severing the umbilical cord or circumcision were common before aseptic surgical techniques were introduced.

CLINICAL MANIFESTATIONS

Skin and soft tissue infections should be discovered promptly because clinical findings usually are apparent on casual observation. Lesions include pustules, vesicles, bullae, maculopapules, cellulitis, impetigo, abscesses, petechiae, purpura, and erythema multiforme.

The most frequently observed lesion is a maculopapular rash that is nonspecific and can be seen with bacterial infections (staphylococcal and streptococcal), fungal infections, and viral infections (measles, enteroviruses, rubella). Bullous lesions that appear after the second day of life usually suggest staphylococcal disease, in contrast to noninfectious blistering disease that is present at birth. Blisters can range in size from small vesicles to larger bullae filled with straw-colored fluid. When these lesions rupture, an erythematous, weeping, denuded area is present. In staphylococcal scalded skin syndrome, the epidermis can be shed in sheets, and intact bullae frequently are sterile. HSV, *T. pallidum*, *P. aeruginosa*, and GBS less frequently are associated with bullous lesions.

Pustules are a common manifestation of staphylococcal disease, but can be seen with listeriosis as well. Impetigo and erysipelas should suggest streptococcal infection. Less commonly, impetigo can be caused by *S. aureus* or *E. coli*. GBS has been associated with the triad of cellulitis, adenitis, and bacteremia. Cellulitis and soft tissue abscesses are the hallmark of infection with *S. aureus*, but occasionally can be caused by streptococci or *E. coli*. Erythema multiforme can occur during neonatal sepsis with *S. aureus*, streptococci, or *Pseudomonas*.

Congenital syphilis may be suggested by the presence of maculopapular lesions, and in some cases bullae have been noted at birth, particularly on the palms and soles. The blisters develop on an erythematous base and may consist of cloudy or hemorrhagic fluid that contains spirochetes. When the blisters rupture, a macerated area remains on which crusts form. A diagnosis of *Pseudomonas* or *Aeromonas* infection should be suspected in patients with ecthyma gangrenosum.

Candida infection may be localized to the oral cavity or the diaper area, or both. Early cutaneous lesions are vesicular with a surrounding area of erythema. Pustules may develop, and a confluent erythematous moist erosion is soon noted. Cutaneous manifestations of congenital candidiasis characteristically are present at birth or within hours of delivery. A diffuse, burnlike dermatitis has been described in several infants with low birthweight (<1500 g) as an early manifestation of systemic candidiasis.

In the early stages of infection with *S. aureus*, *Listeria*, GBS, or *Pseudomonas*, vesicles may be present. Herpes simplex and varicella zoster viruses produce vesicular lesions that are similar in appearance clinically and histologically.

DIFFERENTIAL DIAGNOSIS

Noninfectious processes that can be mistaken for the cutaneous manifestation of infection include milia, transient pustular melanosis, erythema toxicum, and sclerema neonatorum. (See Chapter 52.) Purpuric and bullous lesions can result from trauma, inherited skin disorders such as epidermolysis bullosa, acrodermatitis enteropathica, dermatitis herpetiformis, and mastocytosis. Coagulopathies and congenital leukemia can be associated with purpura.

DIAGNOSIS

A diagnosis should be based on stains and bacterial, fungal, and viral cultures of the lesion. In patients with staphylococcal scalded skin syndrome, microorganisms may not be present in the intact bullous lesions. *Candida* can be shown by use of a potassium hydroxide preparation that shows pseudohyphae. Skin biopsy may be required to document the depth of invasiveness. Dark-field examination of bullous lesions usually reveals *T. pallidum* in an infant with congenital syphilis. When this diagnosis is suspected, appropriate serologic studies must be performed, and contact precautions must be undertaken. Fluid obtained by aspiration of vesicles may permit identification of disease caused by various viral agents. Blood cultures should be obtained and may be positive in neonates with systemic infection or with staphylococcal or streptococcal disease.

TREATMENT

When lesions are localized and superficial, local therapy can suffice for neonatal staphylococcal pustulosis in an otherwise healthy term infant. Other manifestations of staphylococcal infections and most other bacterial infections of the skin should be treated by parenteral administration of antibiotics. Nafcillin is appropriate for methicillin-susceptible strains of staphylococci, and vancomycin should be used for MRSA. Streptococcal infections can be treated with penicillin G, ampicillin, or a third-generation cephalosporin. An aminoglycoside, an extended-spectrum penicillin, or ceftazidime should provide coverage for ecthyma gangrenosum caused by *P. aeruginosa*. Treatment of cutaneous fungal infections is discussed in Part 3 of this chapter.

Parenteral fluid therapy may be required to maintain hydration in patients with staphylococcal scalded skin syndrome. Specific attention should be paid to maintenance of adequate hemoglobin and serum albumin concentrations and of the body temperature. Incision and drainage are required if abscesses are found.

Full evaluation for disseminated disease should be carried out, and treatment should be initiated promptly with acyclovir for vesicular lesions presumed to be caused by HSV. Early initiation of treatment may prevent dissemination of localized infection and optimize outcome of generalized herpes infection heralded by cutaneous lesions. (See also Part 4.)

Omphalitis

INCIDENCE

Omphalitis was previously an important cause of neonatal disease and death worldwide. Since the introduction of simple umbilical cord hygienic measures, it is rarely seen in developed countries, but it remains an important cause of neonatal illness elsewhere. The incidence is unknown. Umbilical phlebitis and arteritis may develop spontaneously or may follow catheterization of umbilical vessels. Tetanus may follow contamination of the umbilical stump, but is rarely encountered in societies that practice routine immunization for tetanus and asepsis at the time of delivery. Necrotizing fasciitis is a life-threatening complication resulting from rapidly spreading destruction of the fascia and subcutaneous tissue around the umbilicus.

ETIOLOGY

Organisms that are found on the skin or that are introduced into the umbilical vessel by catheterization can produce omphalitis. *S. aureus* and *E. coli* are frequent pathogens, but group A streptococci, anaerobic bacteria, and polymicrobial infections may occur.[54]

PATHOGENESIS

Direct bacterial invasion of the umbilical cord and surrounding skin is common. Bacteria can invade the umbilical artery and spread across its lumen, causing necrosis of the loose connective tissue of the arterial wall. If the umbilical and iliac ends are occluded, a septic, loculated focus of infection may be found. When the umbilical end remains patent, purulent material may drain through the umbilicus. If the connective tissue of the artery is extensively involved, peritonitis can develop, or the infection can extend along its course and manifest as a scrotal or deep thigh abscess. If the iliac end of the artery is patent, but the umbilical end is sealed, septicemia can ensue.

CLINICAL MANIFESTATIONS

Purulent drainage can be noted from the umbilical stump at its base of attachment to the abdominal wall or from the navel after the cord has separated. The discharge can be foul smelling. Periumbilical erythema and induration may be noted. If extensive periumbilical edema or involvement of the abdominal wall is noted, the complication of necrotizing fasciitis should be considered.

DIAGNOSIS

Gram stain and culture for aerobic and anaerobic bacteria should be performed on the purulent material from the umbilical stump. Whenever septic umbilical arteritis is suspected, blood cultures should be obtained.

TREATMENT

Otherwise well-appearing infants who have moist or "smelly" cords, but no periumbilical erythema, edema, or exudate often respond to local measures. The exception is omphalitis caused by group A streptococci, which requires parenteral penicillin therapy. Parenteral administration of antibiotics is indicated if a neonate presents with periumbilical erythema, edema, and tenderness with or without purulent drainage. Combination therapy should be administered to provide broad-spectrum coverage. Vancomycin should be provided for gram-positive coverage. An aminoglycoside, or perhaps a third-generation cephalosporin for better tissue penetration, can be given for gram-negative coverage. The presence of crepitus or black discoloration of the periumbilical tissues suggests an anaerobic or mixed infection. In that case, consideration should be given to adding clindamycin or metronidazole for anaerobic coverage. Necrotizing fasciitis requires extensive surgical débridement and pathogen-directed antibiotic therapy and supportive care.

COMPLICATIONS

Omphalitis complicated by necrotizing fasciitis can be associated with bacteremia, coagulopathy, and shock, and frequently progresses to death despite heroic surgical and supportive measures. Septic embolization with metastasis to the lungs, kidneys, and skin can occur. Other infections complicating or occurring in the absence of cutaneous signs of omphalitis include pyelophlebitis (suppurative thrombophlebitis of portal or umbilical veins), liver abscess, septic umbilical arteritis, endocarditis, and subacute necrotizing funisitis.[20]

Mastitis (Breast Abscess)

Neonatal mastitis is most commonly caused by *S. aureus*. Infection with other organisms has been described, including *E. coli*, *Pseudomonas*, *Proteus*, *Salmonella*, GBS, and anaerobes. The incidence is low; in one center, only 21 cases of neonatal mastitis or breast abscess were seen in a 7-year period.[17]

Mastitis rarely develops during the first week of life, but is seen more frequently during the second and third weeks after birth. A preponderance of female infants has been observed when mastitis occurs beyond the second week of life. Breast abscesses are rare in premature neonates, presumably because of underdevelopment of the mammary glands. Infection probably results from invasion of the duct system of the breast by skin flora. The breast can be enlarged, erythematous, and tender, but is more likely to be firm than fluctuant. Systemic signs and symptoms are uncommon; only one fourth of infants have a low-grade fever. The disorder must be distinguished from enlargement that is physiologic or hormonally induced; hormonally induced cases more likely produce swelling bilaterally.

Aspiration of the abscess for Gram stain and culture and blood culture are indicated. If gram-positive cocci are seen on the Gram stain, vancomycin or clindamycin should be given until the results of susceptibility testing are available. An aminoglycoside or cefotaxime is indicated when gram-negative bacilli are present. If no organisms are noted on Gram stain, vancomycin or clindamycin and either an aminoglycoside or cefotaxime should be given pending culture results. Surgical incision and drainage may be necessary and should be performed by an experienced surgeon to minimize scarring of breast tissue.

Parotitis

Suppurative parotitis is a rare infection in newborns; only 32 cases have been described in English since 1970.[59] More than one third of the infants were born prematurely, and the causative organism in most cases was *S. aureus*. Infection is likely caused by the ascent of microorganisms from the oral cavity through the Stensen duct in the setting of salivary stasis or by invasion with blood-borne organisms. Dehydration has been noted before the onset of infection in some patients. Typically, infants present in the second week of life with parotid gland swelling and fever. The swollen parotid gland is accompanied by an area of erythema in the overlying skin. The gland may be tender, warm, firm, or fluctuant. Purulent material can drain spontaneously or be expressed from the Stensen duct. Septicemia may accompany localized infection.

The diagnosis is made by Gram-stained smear and culture of purulent material expressed from the duct or obtained by percutaneous aspiration of a fluctuant area of the parotid gland. A blood culture should obtained. Incision and drainage should be performed if the lesions are fluctuant. Empirical systemic antibiotic treatment should provide coverage for *S. aureus*, *E. coli*, and *Pseudomonas*. If the cultures are sterile, or the infant fails to respond to antimicrobial therapy, or both, addition of an antibiotic with anaerobic activity should be considered. Surgical drainage may be required if clinical improvement is not apparent within 48 hours. Complications include salivary fistulas, facial palsy, mediastinitis, and extension into the external auditory canal. Involvement of another salivary gland (most often the other parotid) or septicemia occasionally complicates cases of acute parotitis. The disease must be differentiated from infections of the maxilla and from lymphangiomas and hemangiomas.

MISCELLANEOUS BACTERIAL INFECTIONS
Anaerobic Infection
INCIDENCE

The true incidence of neonatal anaerobic bacteremia is difficult to ascertain. Surveys in the 1960s and 1970s suggested that anaerobic bacteria were the causative agents in one fourth of all neonatal bacteremias. A later retrospective review suggests that neonatal anaerobic bacteremia is less common even in the setting of significant gastrointestinal disease.[43] Anaerobes accounted for only 1% of isolates causing neonatal sepsis from 1989-2003 in another review.[9]

ETIOLOGY

With the exceptions of *Clostridium botulinum* and *Clostridium tetani,* most anaerobic bacteria are part of the normal flora of the gastrointestinal tract, the genital tract, or the skin, and can be potential neonatal pathogens. Gram-positive anaerobes associated with clinical disease in patients of any age include *Peptococcus, Peptostreptococcus,* microaerophilic streptococci, *Clostridium* species, *Propionibacterium,* and *Eubacterium.* Clinically significant gram-negative anaerobes include *Bacteroides fragilis,* other *Bacteroides* species, *Fusobacterium, Veillonella,* and *Prevotella melaninogenica.*

PATHOGENESIS

Anaerobic infections occur in association with aspiration, gastrointestinal ischemia or perforation, trauma, and tissue necrosis—events that have been associated with complicated deliveries or premature infants who are critically ill. Obstetric and neonatal factors associated with increased risk of sepsis neonatorum, including prolonged ROM, maternal chorioamnionitis, prematurity, and respiratory distress, are also risk factors for anaerobic sepsis.

CLINICAL MANIFESTATIONS

The signs and symptoms of anaerobic septicemia or peritonitis are indistinguishable from those described for other forms of neonatal septicemia or peritonitis. Neonatal anaerobic bacteremia occurs in two distinct settings. In the first 3 days of life, anaerobic bacteremia is associated with perinatal sepsis and chorioamnionitis, suggesting vertical transmission. In older neonates, anaerobic bacteremia is associated with a gastrointestinal process, including appendicitis, necrotizing enterocolitis, or other causes of ruptured viscus. The bacteria isolated vary, depending on the clinical setting. Gram-positive anaerobic bacteria susceptible to penicillin G were isolated from blood cultures from 8 of 12 neonates with sepsis in the first 48 hours of life, whereas 11 of 17 neonates older than 2 days of age with clinical evidence of necrotizing enterocolitis had penicillin-resistant, gram-negative anaerobes isolated from blood cultures.[43] This study suggests that gram-positive anaerobic bacteria are more frequently associated with early-onset sepsis and gram-negative anaerobes with gastrointestinal disease. The exception was observed in congenital pneumonia occurring in the absence of chorioamnionitis; *Bacteroides* was frequently isolated from blood cultures from these infants. Anaerobic infection caused by *Clostridium* can manifest as systemic illness or localized infection, such as cellulitis, omphalitis, or necrotizing fasciitis.

DIAGNOSIS

The diagnosis of anaerobic infection should be considered in neonates with clinical signs suggestive of sepsis associated with prolonged ROM, chorioamnionitis, intestinal perforation, or tissue necrosis. Anaerobic culture media are necessary to optimize recovery of these organisms. Use of an anaerobic transport tube or a sealed syringe is recommended for collection of clinical specimens.

TREATMENT

The choice of antibiotic therapy depends on the etiologic agent. Susceptibility testing for anaerobic bacteria is technically difficult and not readily available. Generally, penicillin is active against most gram-positive and some gram-negative anaerobic microorganisms. *Bacteroides* species of the gastrointestinal tract usually are penicillin-resistant. Because *B. fragilis* is commonly isolated from peritoneal fluid in newborns with intestinal perforation or necrotizing enterocolitis, anaerobic coverage is appropriate in those settings. *Bacteroides* species are predictably susceptible to metronidazole and sometimes to clindamycin. Metronidazole is favored over clindamycin for treatment of meningitis or when clindamycin resistance is a concern. A beta-lactam penicillin combined with a beta-lactamase inhibitor, such as piperacillin-tazobactam, can be useful for treatment in some infants.

PROGNOSIS

The reported case-fatality rate for neonatal anaerobic septicemia varies from 4% to 45%.

Infant Botulism

INCIDENCE

Infant botulism was first recognized in the United States in 1976, and more than 1500 cases have been confirmed since then. Cases have been reported from many countries and from most regions of the United States. The greatest proportion of cases have occurred in California and the eastern Pennsylvania–New Jersey–Delaware area.[34] The onset of illness peaks between 2 and 4 months of age, although disease occurring in the second week of life has been described. More than 90% of patients are younger than 6 months of age. The actual incidence is difficult to determine because most mildly ill infants go unrecognized, and many severely affected infants die suddenly and can be misdiagnosed as having sudden infant death syndrome.

ETIOLOGY

Infant botulism is caused by *C. botulinum,* a ubiquitous, gram-positive, spore-forming, toxin-elaborating obligate anaerobe. Seven serologically distinct types of toxin have been identified (types A to G), but disease in the United States has been caused almost exclusively by toxin A or B. *Clostridium barati* and *Clostridium butyricum,* other species of *Clostridium,* elaborate neurotoxins similar to botulinum toxin and have been associated with infant botulism in rare cases. *C. botulinum* spores have been found worldwide in soil, water, agricultural products, and honey. Although extensive epidemiologic studies have been performed, no single source has been identified.

PATHOGENESIS

Classic botulism follows ingestion of botulinal spores. Infant botulism occurs when ingested *C. botulinum* spores germinate in the intestine, releasing bacteria that colonize the colon and produce botulinum neurotoxin. Systemically absorbed toxin binds irreversibly to ganglionic and postganglionic cholinergic

synapses, preventing release of acetylcholine. Clinical manifestations include motor weakness in peripheral and cranial nerve distributions and autonomic instability.

Studies in a murine model suggest that infants at particular risk for development of botulism transiently lack competitive microbial intestinal flora, or that alterations in motility or pH permit overgrowth of vegetative forms of ingested spores. Infants who have been exclusively breast-fed and recently weaned are an at-risk group for botulism. Formula-fed infants with disease are hospitalized at a younger age than are breast-fed infants (7.6 weeks versus 13.7 weeks).

CLINICAL MANIFESTATIONS

The clinical features associated with infant botulism range from mild disease to sudden death. Most recognized cases require hospitalization. The onset can be insidious or fulminant. The symptoms for which most parents seek medical attention are lethargy, poor feeding, and progressive weakness. In retrospect, most parents acknowledge, however, that the infant has been constipated. Typically, the infant is afebrile unless a secondary infection has occurred. Other than hypotonia and weakness, the results of physical examination can be normal early in the course. Cranial nerve palsies soon develop and can manifest as poor head control, ptosis, expressionless facies, and weak cry. Airway protection becomes compromised if gag, swallow, and suck reflexes are impaired. Progressive descending symmetric flaccid paralysis can ensue. Deep tendon reflexes can be normal, but often become diminished or absent as the paralysis progresses. Paralysis of respiratory muscles can be complicated by aspiration pneumonia. Generalized weakness and hypotonia can persist for 1 to 3 weeks without evidence of improvement.

DIAGNOSIS

The diagnosis of infant botulism should be considered in any infant presenting with hypotonia, constipation, and poor feeding. Confirmation of the diagnosis requires isolation of *C. botulinum* or its toxin from the stool. The organism and occasionally the toxin can be isolated from stool for prolonged periods. Special culture techniques using enrichment and selective media are necessary to isolate *C. botulinum.* Toxin neutralization bioassay in mice performed on stool filtrate at a state laboratory or the CDC is the only reliable confirmatory test. A stool specimen for toxin assay is the test of choice for infant botulism.[34]

While awaiting the results of stool studies, a presumptive diagnosis can be made in infants with clinical features suggesting disease if typical findings are noted on electrodiagnostic studies. Nerve conduction study results are normal, but electromyography reveals abnormal spontaneous activity at the motor endplate with abundant brief, small-amplitude motor unit action potentials.

TREATMENT

A single dose of human-derived botulinum antitoxin, known as botulism immune globulin intravenous (BIG-IV) is efficacious in reducing hospitalization from 5.5 to 2.5 weeks and reducing by two thirds the rate of intubation required.[34] The U.S. Food and Drug Administration (FDA) licensed

BIG-IV for treatment of infant botulism in 2003. It now is under the proprietary name of BabyBIG and is available through the California Department of Health Services (510-540-2646) for treatment of botulism caused by types A or B *C. botulinum*.[35] BIG-IV should be administered as early as is feasible in the course of the disease to interrupt neuromuscular blockade.

Meticulous supportive care is also a mainstay of therapy. The goal is to provide nutritional and respiratory support, while avoiding potential complications. Patients should not be fed by mouth until adequate gag reflex and swallowing are observed. Gavage feeding can supply the necessary nutritional intake. Parenteral hyperalimentation may be necessary because normal bowel motility may not return for several weeks. Respiratory and cardiovascular status should be monitored closely. Intubation may be required for airway protection and respiratory failure. The average duration of hospitalization is approximately 1 month.

Antibiotics are not beneficial and can exacerbate the disease process by causing the release of neurotoxin into the gut when bacteria are killed. Antimicrobial therapy is indicated for treatment of pneumonia or urinary tract infection that may develop. The use of aminoglycoside antibiotics should be avoided because of the possibility of potentiation of neuromuscular blockade.

PROGNOSIS

Because the toxin binds irreversibly to the motor endplates, regeneration of nerve endings and their neuromuscular junctions is necessary for recovery. This often requires several weeks. Some centers have described relapse after initial improvement. A small percentage of infants have recurrence of symptoms after discharge home. No predictors of relapse are recognized. The case-fatality rate is estimated to be less than 2% for hospitalized patients.

Listeriosis

INCIDENCE

Listeria monocytogenes can produce disease in healthy individuals, but infection is more prevalent in pregnant women, neonates, and immunocompromised hosts. A population-based surveillance study by the CDC showed a geographic variation in the incidence of neonatal listeriosis. In the year after a large outbreak in California, the incidence was 24.3 per 100,000 live births in Los Angeles County, whereas in the rest of the United States, the incidence was 7.5 per 100,000 live births.

MICROBIOLOGY

Listeriosis is caused by *L. monocytogenes*, a nonsporulating, β-hemolytic, short, gram-positive bacillus. It is an intracellular pathogen and can be observed in polymorphonuclear leukocytes on Gram-stained smears of infected body fluids. *Listeria* is similar morphologically to diphtheroids and can be overlooked as a contaminant. *Listeria* organisms decolorize readily during the Gram-staining procedure and have been mistakenly identified as gram-negative organisms, including *Haemophilus*.

PATHOGENESIS

Listeria has been recovered from soil, sewage, and decayed vegetation. It is a well-known cause of sheep and cattle epizootics. Most non-neonatal human infections are acquired after ingestion of contaminated foods such as unpasteurized milk, soft cheeses, raw meat, and vegetables. Several epidemics of listeriosis in the general population have been reported in pregnant women and their offspring in association with consumption of Mexican-style soft cheese. Family contacts of patients with listeriosis can be colonized in their gastrointestinal tract.

Maternal disease is most frequently documented in the third trimester of pregnancy, probably in association with the decline in cell-mediated immunity that occurs at 26 to 30 weeks of gestation.[48] Infection acquired early in pregnancy can lead to abortion and, if acquired later, to stillbirth or premature labor and delivery. Transplacental transmission is believed to be the most significant mechanism for acquiring early-onset disease, although ingestion or aspiration of infected amniotic fluid before delivery and aspiration of infected secretions during delivery are possible.

The development of late-onset disease usually is not associated with symptomatic maternal infection. Transmission can be vertical from a colonized but asymptomatic mother or from other colonized or infected caregivers, or it can be nosocomial.

The distribution of *Listeria* serotypes from neonates with early-onset and late-onset disease differs. Early-onset disease is predominantly associated with serotypes Ia and Ib and occasionally IVb, whereas late-onset disease is associated most frequently with serotype IVb. Serotyping is useful in epidemiologic studies, but is not important clinically.

CLINICAL MANIFESTATIONS

The signs and symptoms of early-onset and late-onset disease are indistinguishable from signs and symptoms seen in other neonatal bacterial infections. In early-onset disease, the mother often has symptoms of a flulike illness before onset of labor. *Listeria* is frequently isolated from blood cultures obtained from febrile mothers. Evidence of neonatal infection is apparent in most infants at or soon after birth. Many appear meconium stained, even infants born before 32 weeks' gestation, and this is the result of a green-brown staining of the amniotic fluid. Sepsis and pneumonia are the most frequently observed clinical syndromes. Neonates can present with anorexia, lethargy, vomiting, respiratory distress, apnea, cyanosis, and a papular, pustular, or petechial rash.

Late-onset listeriosis most commonly manifests as meningitis. Fever and irritability can be present. The onset is often insidious.

DIAGNOSIS

A maternal history of stillbirth or repeated spontaneous abortions should prompt a high index of suspicion for listeriosis. Blood and CSF cultures should be obtained in all infants. *Listeria monocytogenes* isolated from cultures of the maternal amniotic fluid or placental tissue when infants have early-onset sepsis supports the diagnosis. Aspirates or biopsy specimens of the rash can reveal the organism.

CSF findings in cases of *Listeria* meningitis are characteristic of bacterial meningitides, with a predominance of polymorphonuclear leukocytes, an elevated protein concentration, and a depressed CSF glucose concentration. An increased number of mononuclear cells can be seen in CSF from some infants. On Gram stain, the organisms may be gram-variable and may look like diphtheroids, cocci, or diplococci. A peripheral leukocytosis with left shift, neutropenia, or thrombocytopenia can be observed. Anemia, possibly related to the production of hemolysin, is occasionally present.

TREATMENT

Cephalosporins have no activity against *Listeria*. Ampicillin is the first line of therapy. An aminoglycoside together with ampicillin is synergistic in vitro and in animal models of infection, and is suggested for initial treatment of neonatal infection. After clinical response occurs, ampicillin alone can be given for less severe infections. Treatment should be continued for approximately 14 days in uncomplicated infections. Repeat lumbar puncture should be performed at 24 to 48 hours after the start of treatment to document CSF sterilization.

PROGNOSIS

The case-fatality rate can approach 50% in early-onset infection with *Listeria*, but is less than 10% if disease occurs after the fifth day of life. In the absence of meningitis or other CNS complications, the prognosis is good even in premature infants. CNS sequelae can be observed in some infants after meningitis, but the prognosis has not been extensively studied.

Syphilis

INCIDENCE

The incidence of congenital syphilis parallels that of primary and secondary disease in women. The last national syphilis epidemic, which was followed by a congenital syphilis epidemic, occurred during the late 1980s and early 1990s. Congenital syphilis rates have declined yearly since 1991. During 2000-2002, the rate of congenital syphilis decreased 21% to 11.2 cases per 100,000 live births.[14] Lack of prenatal care and limited prenatal care are risk factors for congenital syphilis.

MICROBIOLOGY

Syphilis is caused by *T. pallidum*, a tightly coiled, motile spirochete. It is too narrow to be visualized by conventional light microscopy (0.09 to 0.18 μm wide × 5 to 15 μm long), but can be detected on dark-field microscopy. It can be propagated in animal models of infection, but has not been cultured in vitro.

PATHOGENESIS AND PATHOLOGY

Transmission of congenital syphilis is most frequently transplacental, although infection can be acquired by contact with genital lesions during delivery. Transplacental infection can occur at any stage of pregnancy and during any stage of maternal syphilis. Infants are more likely to become infected, however, if the mother had primary or secondary syphilis during pregnancy than if she acquired syphilis months or years before conception. The risk of fetal infection also increases with advancing gestational age. If early gestational infection is not recognized, potential outcomes include miscarriage, stillbirth, premature delivery, or neonatal death. Approximately 30% to 40% of fetuses with congenital syphilis are stillborn. Mothers of infants with congenital syphilis should have testing performed for other sexually transmissible infections, such as hepatitis B and hepatitis C, *Chlamydia*, human immunodeficiency virus (HIV), and gonococcal infection.

Previously, it was believed that fetal infection did not occur before 18 weeks' gestation. It is now known that early gestational infection can occur, but because of fetal immunoincompetence, the pathologic changes in fetal tissues are not observed until after the fifth month of gestation. The infection disseminates hematogenously from the placenta to the fetus, so diffuse involvement is common. The pathologic changes observed in congenital syphilis resemble the changes seen in acquired disease. Fibrosis and obliterative endarteritis with histiocytic, plasmacytic, and lymphocytic perivascular infiltrates are typical findings present in most affected organs. Examination of the placenta and the umbilical cord can assist in the diagnosis of congenital disease. Histologic examination reveals focal villositis with endovascular and perivascular proliferation in the placenta and necrotizing funisitis on umbilical cord sections. Spirochetes may be visible on silver-stained specimens of the placenta or umbilical cord.

CLINICAL MANIFESTATIONS

Congenital syphilis is classified into early and late stages based on age at onset. Early congenital syphilis occurs before 2 years of age and represents active infection and inflammation. Approximately two thirds of infected infants are asymptomatic at birth. A wide spectrum of clinical manifestations can be seen in symptomatic infants (Box 39-4). Most symptomatic infants have hepatosplenomegaly and bone changes on radiographs, and many are anemic. The enlarged liver is believed to be related to extramedullary hematopoiesis. A diffuse hepatitis with elevated aminotransferases and direct and indirect hyperbilirubinemia can be seen. Skeletal manifestations include metaphyseal osteochondritis, periostitis, and osteitis. Osseous destruction of the proximal medial tibial metaphysis (Wimberger sign) can be observed (Fig. 39-11). Symptomatic infants are more likely to have spirochetal invasion of the CNS, but laboratory evidence of CNS involvement is not always apparent.

Late manifestations reflect the body's response to early infection or to persistent inflammation. Cutaneous, dental, skeletal, ocular, auditory, and CNS involvement can occur (Box 39-5). The most frequently observed signs include frontal bossing, saddle nose deformity, short maxilla with high-arched palate, and Hutchinson triad.

DIAGNOSIS

As noted by Ingall and colleagues,[29] congenital syphilis should be considered in the differential diagnosis of any newborn with unexplained prematurity, hydrops fetalis of unknown etiology, or placental enlargement. An infant with persistent rhinitis; failure to thrive; or unexplained anemia, thrombocytopenia, jaundice, or hepatosplenomegaly should prompt consideration of congenital syphilis.

BOX 39-4 Clinical Findings of Early Congenital Syphilis*

- Nonimmune hydrops fetalis
- Intrauterine growth restriction
- Failure to thrive
- Generalized lymphadenopathy
- Bone abnormalities
  Periostitis
  Osteochondritis (Wimberger sign)
  Osteitis
- Hepatosplenomegaly (with or without elevated amino-transferases, jaundice)
- Mucocutaneous lesions
  Pemphigus syphiliticus (vesiculobullous eruption, contagious)
  Maculopapular eruption
  Mucous patches of palate, perineum, intertriginous areas
  Condyloma latum
- Persistent rhinitis (snuffles, contagious)
- Pneumonitis (pneumonia alba)
- Nephrotic syndrome
- Neurologic abnormalities
  Syphilitic leptomeningitis
- Hematologic abnormalities
  Leukocytosis
  Leukopenia
  Anemia, Coombs-negative hemolytic
  Thrombocytopenia
- Ocular abnormalities
  Chorioretinitis
  Uveitis

*Defined as age <2 years.

BOX 39-5 Clinical Manifestations of Late Congenital Syphilis*

DENTAL
Hutchinson teeth (notched, peg-shaped upper central incisors)[†]
Mulberry molars (multiple small cusps)

BONE
Frontal bossae of Parrot
Saddle nose deformity
Short maxillae
High-arched palate
Higouménakis sign (sternoclavicular thickening)
Flaring scapulae
Saber shins (anterior bowing of tibia)
Clutton joints (painless synovitis, hydrarthrosis)

CUTANEOUS
Rhagades (linear scars radiating from mouth, nares, and anus)

OCULAR
Interstitial keratitis[†]

NEUROLOGIC
Eighth cranial nerve deafness[†]
Mental retardation
Hydrocephalus
Cranial nerve palsies
Seizure disorder

*Defined as age >2 years.
[†]Features of Hutchinson triad.

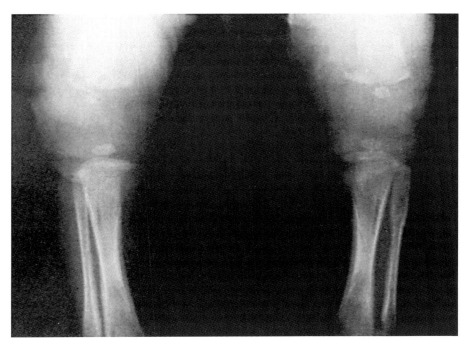

Figure 39-11. Osteochondritis and periostitis of the bones in both lower extremities of a patient with congenital syphilis. The radiolucent area seen at the medial aspect of the proximal tibial metaphyses is known as the Wimberger sign; the zone of translucency visible proximal to the epiphyseal ends of both tibias is called the Wegner sign.

T. pallidum cannot be cultured in vitro. Treponemes can be detected by dark-field examination or direct fluorescent antibody staining of material from mucocutaneous lesions, the umbilical cord or placenta, amniotic fluid, nasal discharge, or postmortem tissue.[51] More commonly, the diagnosis is suggested by the history or clinical and radiographic findings, or both, and confirmed by serologic testing. Serologic tests for syphilis (STS) include nontreponemal and treponemal antibody tests. Nontreponemal tests, such as the rapid plasma reagin test or the Venereal Disease Research Laboratory (VDRL) test, use a purified cardiolipin and lecithin antigen to detect reagin, a nonspecific antibody produced in response to *T. pallidum* infection. Biologic false-positive results can be seen with nontreponemal STS in patients with autoimmune disorders. Quantitative titers of nontreponemal tests can be followed to evaluate response to therapy.

Treponemal serologic tests include the fluorescent treponemal antibody absorption test and the *T. pallidum* particle agglutination test. Because both tests remain positive after initial infection, serial titers are not helpful for evaluating response to therapy. A fluorescent treponemal antibody absorption IgM test and a polymerase chain reaction technique for detection of *T. pallidum* in tissues and body fluids have been developed, but are not commercially available.

An infant should be evaluated for congenital syphilis when the maternal titer has increased fourfold, if the infant's titer is fourfold greater than the mother's, or if the infant is symptomatic. In addition, if born to a mother with positive nontreponemal and treponemal tests, the infant should be evaluated further if the mother had untreated, inadequately treated, or undocumented treatment for syphilis; if erythromycin was used for treatment during pregnancy; if treatment during pregnancy occurred less than 1 month before delivery; if the expected decrease in nontreponemal antibody has not been documented; or if there is insufficient serologic follow-up to document the response to treatment.

The evaluation of an infant with suspected congenital syphilis should include (1) physical examination; (2) quantitative nontreponemal test of serum (not cord blood) for syphilis;

(3) routine CSF evaluation and CSF VDRL; (4) long bone radiographs; (5) complete blood count and platelet count; and (6) other tests, such as chest radiography, as clinically indicated. Criteria for the diagnosis of proven or highly probable congenital syphilis include any of the following: (1) physical, laboratory, or radiographic evidence of active infection; (2) placenta or umbilical cord is positive for treponemes using specific direct fluorescent antibody staining or dark-field test; (3) active CSF VDRL result; or (4) an infant quantitative serum nontreponemal STS titer fourfold or more than that of the mother. A negative nontreponemal STS at delivery does not exclude recent maternal infection that has not yet elicited an antibody response, or has elicited only IgM antibodies that do not cross the placenta.

TREATMENT

Serologic tests on the infant and on the mother during pregnancy and at delivery, maternal antepartum antimicrobial therapy, and the infant's clinical status must be considered before treatment plans can be made. Treatment should be completed before nursery discharge for infants with proven or highly probable disease. It should be considered in infants who are asymptomatic with normal CSF and radiographic examination results under the conditions dictated by the maternal treatment history (Table 39-22).[1]

Jarisch-Herxheimer reactions, manifested by fever, tachypnea, tachycardia, hypotension, prominence of cutaneous lesions, and death, have been reported after initiation of treatment. The cause of this reaction is unknown, although release of endotoxin from the spirochetes has been suggested.

FOLLOW-UP

Infants with reactive nontreponemal STS must have serial quantitative tests after discharge home. Uninfected infants with reactive STS from transplacental transfer of maternal antibody should have a decrease in titer by 3 months of age and a nonreactive test at 6 months. To confirm therapeutic response, treated infants with suspected or proven disease

---

TABLE 39–22   Recommended Therapy for Neonates (<4 Weeks Old) with Congenital Syphilis*

Clinical Status	Treatment
Proven or highly probable disease	Aqueous crystalline penicillin G for 10 days[†]

Normal examination and nontreponemal test the same or less than four-fold the maternal result with maternal treatment history:
    None, inadequate penicillin treatment[‡]
	Aqueous crystalline penicillin G IV for 10-14 days[†]
	    or
	Clinical, serologic follow-up, and benzathine penicillin G IM, single dose[§]

Adequate therapy given >4 wk before delivery; mother has no evidence of reinfection or relapse	Clinical, serologic follow-up, and benzathine penicillin G IM, single dose[¶]

*If >1 day is missed, the course should be restarted.
[†]Aqueous crystalline penicillin G 50,000 U/kg IV given every 12 hours for the first 7 days of life and every 8 hours thereafter. Alternatively, procaine penicillin G 50,000 U/kg IM single daily dose for 10 days can be given.
[‡]Maternal treatment is termed inadequate when her penicillin dose is unknown, is undocumented, or was inadequate; if she received erythromycin or other non-penicillin regimen; if treatment was given <4 weeks before delivery; or the response to treatment was not documented by showing a fourfold decrease in titer of a nontreponemal test for syphilis.
[§]Benzathine penicillin G 50,000 U/kg IM. Some experts recommend aqueous crystalline penicillin G for proven or highly probable disease.
[¶]Some experts would not treat the infant, but would provide close serologic follow-up.
Adapted from American Academy of Pediatrics: Syphilis. In Pickering LK et al, editors: *Red Book: 2009 report of the Committee on Infectious Diseases,* 28th ed, Elk Grove Village, IL, American Academy of Pediatrics, p 645.

should have quantitative nontreponemal STS titers at 2 to 4 months, 6 months, and 12 months after completion of therapy, or until the test becomes nonreactive or the titer has decreased by fourfold. Retreatment should be considered for any child with persistent, unchanging nontreponemal STS titers.

CSF evaluations at 6-month intervals, in addition to serial serum quantitative nontreponemal titers, are recommended for infants with congenital neurosyphilis. Retreatment should be undertaken if the CSF VDRL is positive at 6 months of age.

Treatment of asymptomatic infected infants in the first 3 months of life usually prevents development of late stigmata. Late congenital syphilis can develop if congenital infection goes unrecognized and untreated. Stigmata of late congenital syphilis can develop in infants symptomatic at birth despite appropriate treatment in the neonatal period.

PREVENTION

Routine prenatal screening and penicillin therapy of infected women and their partners can prevent congenital syphilis. Prenatal screening consisting of nontreponemal STS in the first trimester and at delivery is recommended. Another test at the beginning of the third trimester should be considered in areas with a high prevalence of syphilis. Screening of the mother at delivery, in addition to the infant, is recommended to avoid potential false-negative infant serologic test results related to low antibody concentrations.

Tetanus Neonatorum

INCIDENCE

Tetanus neonatorum is rare in the United States, but remains a significant cause of neonatal morbidity and mortality in developing countries.

MICROBIOLOGY

Clostridium tetani is a slender, anaerobic, spore-forming, gram-positive bacillus. *C. tetani* is present in soil and can be found in human and animal feces. Risk factors associated with the higher incidence in developing countries include lack of maternal immunization against tetanus, childbirth under unhygienic conditions, use of contaminated umbilical stump dressings, and rituals involving the application of manure to the umbilicus.

PATHOLOGY

No specific pathologic lesions are attributed to this infectious agent, although changes in the brain and spinal cord have been described in patients dying of tetanus.

PATHOGENESIS

The signs and symptoms of tetanus are the result of toxin production, rather than invasive infection. The umbilical stump contaminated by soil or feces can serve as a portal of entry for the spores. When the spores germinate, the bacteria produce two toxins: tetanolysin, which hemolyzes red blood cells in vitro, but does not seem to be important in vivo, and tetanospasmin. Tetanospasmin is second only to botulinum toxin in potency. By inhibiting release of acetylcholine, it interferes with neuromuscular transmission, resulting in muscular contractions. Tetanospasmin affects the motor end-plates of skeletal muscle, the spinal cord and brain, and occasionally the sympathetic nervous system. When toxin becomes fixed to nervous tissue, it cannot be neutralized by antitoxin. The mechanism by which the toxin reaches the CNS is unclear. Transportation within the nerves is likely. The incubation period ranges from 2 to 21 days.

CLINICAL MANIFESTATIONS

The clinical syndrome differs from that seen in older children and adults. Most infants are irritable and show diminished suck and cessation of crying. Fever is often noted at presentation. The disease progresses to generalized rigidity with muscle spasms and seizures. Flexor spasms are exacerbated by stimulation. Some infants become cyanotic if the spasms are prolonged. Testing of deep tendon reflexes usually shows hyperreflexia. Extreme flexion of the toes is frequently observed. The hallmark of tetanus in older patients is lockjaw, also referred to as risus sardonicus. Lockjaw does not develop in most infants, but severe reflex spasms of the masseter muscles do occur if the jaw is moved for feeding.

Cardiorespiratory difficulties, including tachycardia, tachypnea, cyanosis, or apnea, can be observed. Laryngoglottal spasm can predispose to aspiration pneumonia. Pulmonary processes such as bronchopneumonia or hemorrhage are a frequent cause of death in neonatal tetanus.

DIFFERENTIAL DIAGNOSIS

Cultures of the blood and the wound (umbilical stump) are invariably sterile. Diagnosis is made by clinical presentation and exclusion of other possibilities. Infants can be misdiagnosed as having neonatal seizures.

TREATMENT

Supportive care is essential. Maintenance of a clear airway and provision of adequate ventilation are most important. Meticulous care must be exercised to decrease the likelihood of secondary bacterial pulmonary infections. The bladder may need to be catheterized if it does not empty spontaneously.

Because stimulation can precipitate spasms and seizures, timing of medical interventions should be coordinated, and exposure to nonessential external stimuli should be limited. Diazepam is an effective agent in controlling the tonic spasms of tetanus. Barbiturates may be helpful as an adjunct to therapy and may help sedate the patient.

Metronidazole should be given for a 10- to 14-day course to decrease the number of vegetative forms of *C. tetani* and is the treatment of choice. Penicillin G is an alternative antibiotic. Human tetanus immune globulin given intramuscularly in a single dose is recommended to neutralize circulating unbound toxin. Débridement of the entry site, an essential component of therapy in adult disease, is performed in some cases of neonatal tetanus, but wide excision is not indicated.

PREVENTION

A well-immunized mother offers the best protection against tetanus neonatorum. Because antitoxin crosses the placenta, infants born to mothers whose tetanus immunizations are current should have adequate antitoxin antibody concentrations. Aseptic obstetric and neonatal care minimizes the likelihood of introduction of *C. tetani* spores. Infants who recover from disease require routine tetanus immunizations because disease does not usually confer immunity.

Tuberculosis

INCIDENCE

Since the early 1990s, the incidence of tuberculosis in the United States has increased, especially among women of childbearing age. Perinatal tuberculosis is uncommon, but management of an infant born to a mother with tuberculous infection is common.

MICROBIOLOGY

Mycobacterium tuberculosis is the causative agent of tuberculosis. *M. tuberculosis* is a slow-growing, obligately aerobic, acid-fast bacillus (AFB). Neonatal infections with other strains of mycobacteria are uncommon. *Mycobacterium bovis* infections were occasionally seen before pasteurization of milk became standard. Neonatal infection with atypical or environmental mycobacteria is rare.

PATHOGENESIS AND PATHOLOGY

Infected mothers can transmit infection to their fetus transplacentally if primary tuberculous infection (asymptomatic or miliary) is acquired during pregnancy, or if the mother has tuberculous endometritis.[60,62] Postpartum transmission can occur if the mother has active pulmonary tuberculosis with cavitation. Neonatal tuberculosis can be acquired intrapartum from ingestion or aspiration of infected secretions and postnatally by inhalation of infected droplets. Before aseptic technique was routinely used, transmission from contamination of the skin or mucous membranes during circumcision was described.

The most common mode of transmission for perinatal disease is inhalation of infected droplets (Table 39-23). Coinfection with HIV increases the risk of extrapulmonary disease, and mothers with extrapulmonary tuberculosis, including pleural effusions, and endometrial, miliary, or meningeal disease are more likely to transmit infection to the fetus. Many infants born to infected mothers do not contract disease, however.

Primary complex formation in the porta hepatis of the liver occurs with congenital infection transmitted hematogenously. Miliary tubercles can be found in the spleen, bone marrow, lung, kidney, adrenal glands, and brain. Gross or microscopic placental lesions may be detected. Primary complex formation in the lung can reflect hematogenous spread, aspiration of infected amniotic fluid or vaginal secretions, or postnatal inhalation.

CLINICAL MANIFESTATIONS

Signs and symptoms of congenital tuberculosis are vague. Some infants may be symptomatic at birth, whereas others do not develop symptoms until late in the first month of life.[38] The appearance on chest radiographs frequently is abnormal. Many infected newborns are premature and have hepatosplenomegaly, respiratory distress, fever, reluctance to feed, and lethargy. Miliary tuberculosis, lymphadenopathy, and otitis media with tympanic membrane perforations, otorrhea, and facial nerve palsy can be seen as well. Meningitis, pleural effusions, and pulmonary cavitations are unusual.

Neonatal tuberculosis is manifested by fever, vomiting, cough, tachypnea, and weight loss. Hepatosplenomegaly occasionally occurs. Unless hepatic primary complex formation is present, it is often difficult to distinguish congenital from neonatal tuberculosis.

DIAGNOSIS

The diagnosis of tuberculosis can be established by demonstration of organisms on AFB smears and growth of *M. tuberculosis* in special culture media. The infant should have a tuberculin skin test (TST), a chest radiograph, and AFB stains and cultures of CSF and gastric and tracheal aspirates. The infant's TST is usually nonreactive even in the presence of active disease. Because treatment of an infected infant does not prevent the skin test from becoming reactive, repeat skin testing should be performed 3 months later if the initial skin test is negative. Other sites that can yield AFB growth include lung or liver tissue, lymph node, middle ear fluid, urine, and bone marrow aspirate.

TREATMENT

Because perinatal tuberculosis is uncommon, the safety and efficacy of antituberculous agents in neonates have not been determined. Standard therapy for older infants consists of

---

TABLE 39–23 Perinatal Transmission of Tuberculosis

Maternal Focus of Infection	Mode of Spread	Timing	Relative Frequency
Pneumonia with cavitary lesion*	Inhalation of infected droplets	Postnatal	Most common
Amniotic infection after rupture of placental caseous lesion	Aspiration or ingestion of infected fluid	Congenital or intrapartum	Less common
Placentitis after miliary or endometrial tuberculosis	Hematogenous through umbilical vein	Congenital	Rare
Cervicitis	Direct contact, aspiration, or ingestion	Intrapartum	Rare
Mastitis	Ingestion of infected milk	Postnatal	Extremely rare

*Any caregiver with cavitary pulmonary tuberculosis can transmit infection to the infant.

isoniazid, rifampin ethambutol, and pyrazinamide daily for 2 months followed by twice-weekly therapy with isoniazid and rifampin alone (Table 39-24).[61] An aminoglycoside is also initiated when treating potentially life-threatening disease, such as meningitis, until susceptibility testing is completed. The duration of therapy is 6 months in older children without meningitis. The optimal duration has not been determined for neonates, but prolonged treatment has been suggested because of potential neonatal immunoincompetence.

Corticosteroids have been used in tuberculous meningitis to reduce inflammation and decrease intracranial pressure and in endobronchial disease to reduce tracheal compression. Appropriate antituberculous agents must be administered concurrently with steroid therapy to avoid dissemination of infection.

The case-fatality rate for congenital tuberculosis is approximately 50%. Most deaths are related to undiagnosed and untreated disease. The prognosis is worse for premature infants than for term infants with congenital infection.

MANAGEMENT OF INFANTS BORN TO MOTHERS WITH POSITIVE PURIFIED PROTEIN DERIVATIVE SKIN TESTS

Regardless of the mother's clinical status, symptomatic newborns should have a thorough investigation for bacterial sepsis and tuberculous disease. Chest radiograph; CSF examination; blood and CSF bacterial cultures; and mycobacterial stains and cultures of CSF, gastric aspirates, and tracheal aspirates should be obtained. Decisions on antituberculous treatment of the infant should be based on the mother's status and on the results of the infant's evaluation.

For asymptomatic neonates, investigation and treatment are guided by the mother's clinical status. If a mother with a positive TST is clinically well, has a negative chest radiograph, and is not believed to have active disease, no intervention is necessary, provided that the household contacts have been investigated, and active disease has been excluded. Mothers with an abnormal appearance on chest radiograph must have an investigation for tuberculosis, including AFB stains and cultures of sputum and testing for HIV infection. Separation of the mother and the infant is recommended until the mother and infant have been evaluated; if tuberculosis disease is suspected, until the mother and infant are receiving appropriate antituberculous therapy, the mother wears a mask and understands and expresses her willingness to comply with infection control measures.

If there is no evidence of neonatal infection, the infant should be given isoniazid prophylaxis and reevaluated in 3 to 4 months with another TST. Isoniazid can be discontinued at 3 months if the second TST is negative, if the infant is well, and if there is no active infection in the household. Three- or four-drug antituberculous therapy should be started after cultures are obtained if there is evidence of disease in the infant. Bacille Calmette-Guérin immunization of the infant should be considered only in limited and select circumstances, such as if the mother or another household contact has possible multidrug-resistant tuberculosis or has poor adherence to treatment.

PREVENTION OF INFECTION IN THE NEONATAL INTENSIVE CARE UNIT
Barrier Nursing Technique

The use of masks and gowns by nursery personnel does not significantly alter staphylococcal colonization or infection rates in infants. Hand washing, if performed adequately, is

TABLE 39–24   Commonly Used Drugs for Treatment of Tuberculosis in Children

Drug*	Daily[†] (mg/kg/d)	Twice Weekly[†] (mg/kg per Dose)	Side Effects	Comments
Isoniazid	10-15; maximum 300 mg	20-40; maximum 900 mg	Mild hepatic enzyme elevation, hepatitis[‡], peripheral neuritis, hypersensitivity	Monitor liver function tests monthly
Rifampin	10-20; maximum 600 mg	10-20; maximum 600 mg	Hepatitis[‡], vomiting, thrombocytopenia, orange discoloration of secretions	Monitor liver function tests monthly
Pyrazinamide	20-40; maximum 2 g	50-70; maximum 2 g	Hepatotoxicity, hyperuricemia	Monthly uric acid and liver function tests
Streptomycin	20-40; maximum 1 g	20-40; maximum 1 g	Ototoxicity, nephrotoxicity	Monitor renal function, consider hearing test
Ethambutol	15-25; maximum 2.5 g	50; maximum 2.5 g	Optic neuritis, color blindness, decreased visual acuity	Monitor visual fields, visual acuity, and color discrimination frequently

*All drugs may be given PO except streptomycin, which must be given IM.
[†]See text for details and duration.
[‡]Incidence of hepatotoxicity increases when isoniazid and rifampin are used together, especially when the isoniazid dosage exceeds 10 mg/kg/d.
Adapted from Starke JR: Perinatal tuberculosis, *Semin Pediatr Infect Dis* 5:20, 1994.

effective in reducing the incidence of nosocomial nursery infections. A 3% solution of hexachlorophene soap is effective in reducing infection by gram-positive bacteria, and various iodinated preparations, including iodinated chlorhexidine (0.5%), are effective against gram-negative organisms. Studies suggest that alcoholic chlorhexidine hand washing agents are effective against drug-resistant strains of *Enterococcus faecium* and *Enterobacter cloacae*. Physicians should be aware that some organisms, including *P. aeruginosa*, can survive in many antiseptic solutions.

Bathing of Infants

Historically, infants were bathed with hexachlorophene to decrease the risk of gram-positive infections. In the 1970s, infants in France developed a toxic encephalopathy attributed to excessive amounts of hexachlorophene in talcum powder. Subsequent neuropathologic studies in the United States revealed an association between brainstem vacuolar lesions and hexachlorophene baths especially in premature infants. Routine bathing with hexachlorophene was discontinued in the early 1970s after this association was recognized.

The Committee on the Fetus and Newborn of the American Academy of Pediatrics recommends that the first bath be postponed until a newborn is thermally stable. Nonmedicated soap and water should be used. Sterile sponges soaked in warm water can be used. During nursery outbreaks of *S. aureus* infection, hexachlorophene bathing of the diaper area can be undertaken to prevent staphylococcal disease.[21] Surveillance of neonatal infections, prompt isolation and treatment of infected infants, and adequate hand washing should be used to prevent nosocomial infections. Crowding should be avoided, and cohort nursing techniques should be applied whenever possible. Hexachlorophene can still be used as an antibacterial agent by nursery personnel.

Cord Care

The umbilicus is a direct portal of entry to the bloodstream, and serves as a site from which other areas of the skin may become contaminated or colonized. No single method of cord care has proved superior in preventing colonization and the development of omphalitis. Options for cord care include application of alcohol, triple dye (brilliant green, proflavin hemisulfate, and crystal violet), or antimicrobial agents such as bacitracin ointment. Alcohol hastens drying of the cord, but probably is ineffective in preventing cord colonization or omphalitis.

Resuscitation and Ventilatory Equipment

Gram-negative microorganisms, particularly *Pseudomonas, Aeromonas,* and *Serratia,* have been associated with sporadic and epidemic infection in the nursery. Routine cultures of medications, nebulizers, and inhalation therapy equipment should be performed, and equipment should be changed frequently to prevent such infections. Use of umbilical, arterial, and venous catheters for parenteral alimentation also has been accompanied by an increased risk

of health care–associated infections. Meticulous care is required in the insertion and care of catheters and in the preparation of intravenous solutions for use in total parenteral alimentation. Administration of fluids should be discontinued if signs of inflammation, thrombosis, or purulence are observed. All apparatus used for intravenous administration should be replaced at intervals to decrease the hazard of extrinsic contamination.

Antibiotic Prophylaxis

The effectiveness of intravenous antimicrobial prophylaxis in newborns has not been proven. Indiscriminate use of antibiotics can result in colonization or infection with drug-resistant strains of bacteria or with fungi. The only role for antimicrobial prophylaxis in newborns is for the prevention of gonococcal ophthalmitis or tuberculous disease.

Immune Globulin

There have been numerous in vitro, animal model, and human studies evaluating the use of IVIG in the prevention of infections. Results of several well-designed human trials using IVIG to prevent nosocomial infections in preterm neonates have been published.[2,36] The results of the large, multicenter, randomized, controlled trial led by Fanaroff and associates[18] revealed no significant decrease in the incidence of nosocomial infections, in the number of days hospitalized, or in mortality rate in the premature infants given IVIG. One possible explanation for the lack of protection against health care–associated infections could be that pooled IVIG does not contain adequate amounts of specific antibody against the most common neonatal nosocomial pathogens—CONS and *Candida* species. Even specific antibody may not be protective against health care–associated infections, however, especially if they are associated with foreign bodies such as indwelling catheters. Administration of an IVIG derived from donors with high titers of antibody to surface adhesins of *S. aureus* and *S. epidermidis* failed to reduce the incidence of staphylococcal bacteremia in premature infants.[16] In the future, development of specific, high-titered immunoglobulin preparations against the specific pathogens may be beneficial in prevention of some neonatal infections.

REFERENCES

1. American Academy of Pediatrics: Syphilis. In Pickering LK et al, editors: *Red Book: 2006 report of the Committee on Infectious Diseases,* 27th ed, Elk Grove Village, IL, 2006, American Academy of Pediatrics, p 631.
2. Baker CJ et al: Intravenous immune globulin for the prevention of nosocomial infection in low-birth-weight neonates. The Multicenter Group for the Study of Immune Globulin in Neonates, *N Engl J Med* 327:213, 1992.
3. Baley JE, Silverman RA: Systemic candidiasis: cutaneous manifestations in low birth weight infants, *Pediatrics* 82:211, 1988.

4. Bedford Russell AR et al: Plasma granulocyte colony-stimulating factor concentrations (G-CSF) in the early neonatal period, *Br J Haematol* 86:642, 1994.

5. Benjamin DK et al: A blinded, randomized, multicenter study of an intravenous *Staphylococcus aureus* immune globulin, *J Perinatol* 26:290, 2006.

6. Berkun Y et al: Acute otitis media in the first two months of life: characteristics and diagnostic difficulties, *Arch Dis Child* 93:690, 2008.

7. Berman PH, Banker BQ: Neonatal meningitis: a clinical and pathological study of 29 cases, *Pediatrics* 38:6, 1966.

8. Bizzarro MJ et al: Changing patterns in neonatal *Escherichia coli* sepsis and ampicillin resistance in the era of intrapartum antibiotic prophylaxis, *Pediatrics* 121:689, 2008.

9. Bizzarro MJ et al: Seventy-five years of neonatal sepsis at Yale: 1928-2003, *Pediatrics* 116:595, 2005.

10. Bonadio WA et al: Reliability of observation variables in distinguishing infectious outcome of febrile young infants, *Pediatr Infect Dis J* 12:111, 1993.

11. Bromberger P et al: The influence of intrapartum antibiotics on the clinical spectrum of early-onset group B streptococcal infection in term infants, *Pediatrics* 106:244, 2000.

12. Buck C et al: Interleukin-6: a sensitive parameter for the early diagnosis of neonatal bacterial infection, *Pediatrics* 93:54, 1994.

13. Carr R et al: Granulocyte-macrophage colony stimulating factor administered as prophylaxis for reduction of sepsis in extremely preterm, small for gestational age neonates (the PROGRAMS trial): a single-blind, multicentre, randomized controlled trial, *Lancet* 373:226, 2009.

14. Centers for Disease Control and Prevention: Congenital syphilis—United States, 2002, *MMWR Morb Mortal Wkly Rep* 53:716, 2004.

15. Centers for Disease Control and Prevention: Prevention of perinatal group B streptococcal disease: revised guidelines from CDC, *MMWR Morb Mortal Wkly Rep* 51:1, 2002.

16. DeJonge M et al: Clinical trial of safety and efficacy of IHN-A21 for the prevention of nosocomial staphylococcal bloodstream infection in premature infants, *J Pediatr* 151:260, 2007.

17. Efrat M et al: Neonatal mastitis—diagnosis and treatment, *Isr J Med Sci* 31:558, 1995.

18. Fanaroff AA et al: A controlled trial of intravenous immune globulin to reduce nosocomial infections in very-low-birth-weight infants, *N Engl J Med* 330:1107, 1994.

19. Fielkow S et al: Cerebrospinal fluid examination in symptom-free infants with risk factors for infection, *J Pediatr* 119:971, 1991.

20. Fraser N et al: Neonatal omphalitis: a review of its serious complications, *Acta Paediatr* 95:519, 2006.

21. Freeman RK et al, editors: Infection control. In American Academy of Pediatrics Committee on the Fetus and Newborn: *Guidelines for perinatal care,* 3rd ed, Elk Grove Village, IL, 1992, American Academy of Pediatrics Press, p 3.

22. Girardin EP et al: Serum tumour necrosis factor in newborns at risk for infections, *Eur J Pediatr* 149:645, 1990.

23. Hammerschlag MR: Neonatal conjunctivitis. *Pediatr Ann* 22:346, 1993.

24. Hammerschlag MR et al: Efficacy of neonatal ocular prophylaxis for the prevention of chlamydial and gonococcal conjunctivitis, *N Engl J Med* 320:769, 1989.

25. Hammerschlag MR et al: Treatment of neonatal chlamydial conjunctivitis with azithromycin, *Pediatr Infect Dis J* 17:1049, 1998.

26. Harvey D et al: Bacterial meningitis in the newborn: a prospective study of mortality and morbidity, *Semin Perinatol* 23:218, 1999.

27. Healy CM et al: Emergence of new strains of methicillin-resistant *Staphylococcus aureus* in a neonatal intensive care unit, *Clin Infect Dis* 39:1460, 2004.

28. Hyde TB et al: Trends in incidence and antimicrobial resistance of early-onset sepsis: population-based surveillance in San Francisco and Atlanta, *Pediatrics* 110:690, 2002.

29. Ingall D et al: Syphilis. In Remington JS et al, editors: *Infectious diseases of the fetus and newborn infant,* 6th ed., Philadelphia, 2006, Saunders, p 545.

30. Jenson HB, Pollock BH: The role of intravenous immunoglobulin for the prevention and treatment of neonatal sepsis, *Semin Perinatol* 22:50, 1998.

31. Klinger G et al: Predicting the outcome of neonatal bacterial meningitis, *Pediatrics* 106:477, 2000.

32. Krediet T et al: The predictive value of C-reactive protein and I:T ratio in neonatal infection, *J Perinat Med* 20:479, 1992.

33. Levent F et al: Early outcomes from group B streptococcal (GBS) meningitis in the intrapartum antibiotic prophylaxis (IAP) era. Paper presented at Pediatric Academic Society Annual Meeting, 2009, Philadelphia, PA; Abstract 2848.470.

34. Long SS: Infant botulism, *Concise Rev Pediatr Infect Dis* 20:707, 2001.

35. Long SS: Infant botulism and treatment with BIG-IV (BabyBIG), *Pediatr Infect Dis J* 26:261, 2007.

36. Magny JF et al: Intravenous immunoglobulin therapy for prevention of infection in high-risk premature infants: report of a multicenter, double-blind study, *Pediatrics* 88:437, 1991.

37. Manroe BL et al: The neonatal blood count in health and disease, I: reference values for neutrophilic cells, *J Pediatr* 95:89, 1979.

38. Mazade MA et al: Congenital tuberculosis presenting as sepsis syndrome: case report and review of the literature, *Pediatr Infect Dis J* 20:439, 2001.

39. McCracken GH Jr et al: Cerebrospinal fluid interleukin-1β and tumor necrosis factor concentrations and outcome from neonatal gram-negative enteric bacillary meningitis, *Pediatr Infect Dis J* 8:155, 1989.

40. Mouzinho A et al: Revised reference ranges for circulating neutrophils in very-low-birth-weight neonates, *Pediatrics* 94:76, 1994.

41. Nelson JD: Antibiotic therapy for newborns. In Nelson JD, editor: *Pocketbook of pediatric antimicrobial therapy,* Baltimore, 1998, Williams & Wilkins, p 14.

42. Nissen MD et al: Congenital and neonatal pneumonia, *Paediatr Resp Rev* 8:195, 2007.

43. Noel GJ et al: Anaerobic bacteremia in a neonatal intensive care unit: an eighteen-year experience, *Pediatr Infect Dis J* 7:858, 1988.

44. Palazzi DL et al: Bacterial sepsis and meningitis. In Remington JS et al, editors: *Infectious diseases of the fetus and newborn infant*, 6th ed., Philadelphia, 2006, Saunders, p 247.

45. Phares CR et al: Epidemiology of invasive group B streptococcal disease in the United States, 1999-2005. *JAMA* 299:2056, 2008.

46. Philip AGS et al: Neutrophil elastase in the diagnosis of neonatal infection, *Pediatr Infect Dis J* 13:323, 1994.

47. Polin RA et al: Neonatal sepsis, *Adv Pediatr Infect Dis* 7:25, 1992.

48. Posfay-Barbe KM, Wald ER: Listeriosis, *Pediatr Rev* 25:151, 2004.

49. Rennels MB, Levine MM: Classical bacterial diarrhea: perspectives and update: *Salmonella, Shigella, Escherichia coli, Aeromonas,* and *Plesiomonas. Pediatr Infect Dis J* 5(suppl):S91, 1986.

50. Rodriguez AF et al: Cerebrospinal fluid values in the very low birth weight infant, *J Pediatr* 116:971, 1990.

51. Sánchez PJ: Congenital syphilis, *Adv Pediatr Infect Dis* 7:161, 1992.

52. Santana Reyes C et al: Role of cytokines (interleukin-1β, 6, 8, tumour necrosis factor-alpha, and soluble receptor of interleukin-2) and C-reactive protein in the diagnosis of neonatal sepsis, *Acta Paediatr* 92:221, 2003.

53. Sarff LD et al: Cerebrospinal fluid evaluation in neonates: comparison of high-risk infants with and without meningitis, *J Pediatr* 88:473, 1976.

54. Sawardekar KP: Changing spectrum of neonatal omphalitis, *Pediatr Infect Dis J* 23:22, 2004.

55. Schrag SJ et al: A population-based comparison of strategies to prevent early-onset group B streptococcal disease in neonates, *N Engl J Med* 347:233, 2002.

56. Schuchat A et al: Population-based risk factors for neonatal group B streptococcal disease: results of a cohort study in metropolitan Atlanta, *J Infect Dis* 162:672, 1990.

57. Shurin PA et al: Bacterial etiology of otitis media during the first six weeks of life, *J Pediatr* 92:893, 1978.

58. Singer DB: Infections of fetuses and neonates. In Wigglesworth JS et al, editors: *Textbook of fetal and perinatal pathology,* Boston, 1998, Blackwell Scientific, p 454.

59. Spiegel R et al: Acute neonatal suppurative parotitis: case reports and review, *Pediatr Infect Dis J* 23:76, 2004.

60. Starke JR: Tuberculosis. In Remington JS et al, editors: *Infectious diseases of the fetus and newborn infant,* 6th ed. Philadelphia, Saunders, 2006, p 581.

61. Starke JR: Perinatal tuberculosis, *Semin Pediatr Infect Dis* 5:20, 1994.

62. Starke JR: Tuberculosis: an old disease but a new threat to the mother, fetus, and neonate, *Clin Perinatol* 24:107, 1997.

63. Stevens JP et al: Long term outcome of neonatal meningitis, *Arch Dis Child Fetal Neonatal Ed* 88:F179, 2003.

64. Stoll BJ et al: Changes in pathogens causing early-onset sepsis in very-low-birth-weight infants, *N Engl J Med* 347:240, 2002.

65. Stoll BJ et al: Early-onset sepsis in very low birth weight neonates: a report from the National Institute of Child Health and Human Development Neonatal Research Network, *J Pediatr* 129:72, 1996.

66. Stoll BJ et al: Late-onset sepsis in very low birth weight neonates: the experience of the NICHD Neonatal Research Network, *Pediatrics* 110:285, 2002.

67. Stoll BJ et al: To tap or not to tap: high likelihood of meningitis without sepsis among very low birth weight infants, *Pediatrics* 113:1181, 2004.

68. Teele DW et al: Epidemiology of otitis media during the first seven years of life in children in greater Boston: a prospective cohort study, *J Infect Dis* 160:83, 1989.

69. Tegtmeyer FK et al: Elastase α1-proteinase inhibitor complex, granulocyte count, ratio of immature to total granulocyte count, and C-reactive protein in neonatal septicaemia, *Eur J Pediatr* 151:353, 1992.

70. Thureen PJ et al: Failure of tracheal aspirate cultures to define the cause of respiratory deteriorations in neonates, *Pediatr Infect Dis J* 12:560, 1993.

71. Weinberg GA et al: Laboratory aids for diagnosis of neonatal sepsis. In Remington JS et al, editors: *Infectious diseases of the fetus and newborn infant,* 6th ed. Philadelphia, 2006, Saunders, p 1207.

72. Wiswell TE et al: Declining frequency of circumcision: implications for changes in the absolute incidence and male to female sex ratio of urinary tract infections in early infancy, *Pediatrics* 79:338, 1987.

73. Wiswell TE et al: No lumbar puncture in the evaluation for early neonatal sepsis: will meningitis be missed? *Pediatrics* 95:803, 1995.

PART 3

Fungal and Protozoal Infections
Morven S. Edwards

FUNGAL INFECTIONS

Disseminated candidiasis is a frequent infection in infants with very low birthweight (VLBW). Other fungal infections are considerably less common in neonates. The increasing incidence of candidiasis is attributable in part to advances in the life-sustaining care provided by neonatal caregivers. Early recognition of infection is important because untreated infections, especially in infants with VLBW, are associated with considerable morbidity and mortality.

Candida

INCIDENCE

Mucocutaneous, cutaneous, and disseminated candidiasis have been reported in newborns. Systemic candidiasis occurs more frequently in premature infants with VLBW.

MICROBIOLOGY

Candida organisms are saprophytic yeasts that are ubiquitous and are constituents of the normal microbial flora of humans. The yeast, or blastospore form of the fungus, is round or egg-shaped and is important in tissue colonization. All *Candida* species form pseudohyphae that are important in invasion. *Candida albicans* is the predominant species associated with maternally acquired neonatal disease. *Candida parapsilosis* is a common species that can account for one quarter of all cases of invasive fungal infection in infants with VLBW.[8]

Other species, such as *Candida glabrata, Candida lusitaniae, Candida krusei,* and *Candida stellatoidea,* are reported less frequently. No special medium is required for growth of *Candida* in the laboratory.

PATHOGENESIS AND PATHOLOGY

C. albicans can be acquired from the vaginal flora of the mother at delivery or from person-to-person contact after birth. *Candida* usually has low pathogenicity for humans. Congenital cutaneous candidiasis seems to be more common if the pregnancy has been complicated by maternal vaginitis, the presence of an intrauterine device, or cervical cerclage.[42] Fungal colonization occurs on the skin and in the gastrointestinal tract before colonization of the respiratory tract.[22] A prospective study in intubated infants with VLBW suggested that there was an increased risk of systemic infection when infants became colonized in the respiratory tract in the first week of life.[40] Factors that alter host defense or that allow proliferation of the organism can increase the risk of invasion. Broad-spectrum antimicrobial use can expedite overgrowth of *Candida* in the gastrointestinal tract. Newborns in general, and infants with VLBW in particular, have qualitative and quantitative deficiencies in humoral and cellular immunity. The organism produces multiple virulence factors, such as adhesins, proteinases, and phospholipases, that promote attachment and invasion. After penetration of epithelial or endothelial barriers, in this setting, *Candida* can penetrate into lymphatics, blood vessels, and deep tissues, resulting in disseminated infection. Disseminated candidiasis can cause disease in any organ system. *Candida* microabscesses have been described in the liver, spleen, kidneys, heart, brain, eyes, bones, and joints.

CLINICAL MANIFESTATIONS

Clinical manifestations depend on the location and extent of the infection. Acute pseudomembranous candidiasis (thrush) manifests with white, curdlike patches that cover the buccal mucosa, gingiva, and tongue. These membranes can be adherent to underlying tissue and, when removed, reveal a denuded, erythematous, painful base. Severe thrush sometimes results in difficulty feeding, but usually no systemic symptoms are apparent. Thrush is frequently associated with cutaneous perineal infection. *Candida* diaper dermatitis begins with an erythematous vesiculopapular eruption that coalesces, producing large areas with satellite lesions that are surrounded by a fine, white, scaly collarette. These lesions usually are restricted to the intertriginous areas in the groin, but can be noted in any warm, moist area, including the neck, axilla, and antecubital and popliteal fossae. The peak incidence occurs at 3 to 4 months of age (see Chapter 52).

After an ascending in utero infection, generalized cutaneous lesions have been noted at birth in congenital cutaneous candidiasis. This condition typically manifests with intensely erythematous maculopapular lesions on the trunk and extremities that rapidly become pustular and rupture, leaving denuded skin with well-defined, raised, scaling borders.[42] Congenital cutaneous candidiasis is usually a benign, self-limited infection, unless it occurs in an infant weighing less than 1500 g, or is associated with respiratory symptoms, or both. In those circumstances, parenteral antifungal therapy is indicated.

Catheter-associated and systemic candidiasis occur later, at a mean of 30 days of age.[2] Infants with invasive neonatal candidiasis usually have one or more risk factors predisposing to infection (Box 39-6). These risk factors relate to immunologic immaturity, to bypassing of natural barriers, to the use of agents such as broad-spectrum antimicrobials that favor the growth of *Candida* species, and to the supportive care required by infants of VLBW. Prior fungal colonization is an important factor in the development of candidiasis. A blood culture obtained through an indwelling catheter, or peripherally while a catheter is in place, suggests the diagnosis. In catheter-associated fungemia, the blood culture becomes sterile concurrently with initiation of amphotericin B therapy and removal of the indwelling catheter. There is no involvement of distant organs, such as the liver, kidneys, or eye. A brief course of amphotericin B usually suffices for treatment. Catheter removal is mandatory. Failure to remove the colonized catheter promotes dissemination and increases the risk for an adverse outcome, including death.

The presentation of systemic candidiasis in an infant with VLBW is similar to that of bacterial sepsis. Infants also can have an insidious onset of symptoms with respiratory deterioration, enteral feeding intolerance, abdominal distention associated with guaiac-positive stools, temperature instability, hypotension, hyperglycemia, and glucosuria. In contrast to disseminated candidiasis in older children and adults, multiple foci of infection are common in infants with systemic disease. Meningitis occurs in approximately 40% of affected infants. Examination of cerebrospinal fluid (CSF) is mandatory. Renal involvement may manifest as candiduria, multiple renal abscesses, or fungus balls that can cause obstruction to the flow of urine. The latter complication may not become evident until later in the treatment course; renal ultrasonography should be performed at the initiation of treatment for all infants suspected to have disseminated candidiasis and repeated as clinically indicated. The ultrasound

---

BOX 39–6   Risk Factors for Invasive Candidiasis in Neonates

- Gestational age <32 weeks
- Birthweight ≤1500 g
- Male gender
- Apgar score <5 at 5 minutes
- Intubation/mechanical ventilation
- Placement of indwelling devices
  Umbilical catheters
  Peripheral or central venous catheters
  Urinary catheters
  Cerebrospinal fluid shunt devices
- Abdominal surgery
- Lack of enteral feeding
- Fungal colonization
- Use of intralipid
- Total parenteral nutrition use
- Corticosteroid use
- Use of histamine type 2 receptor blockers
- Administration of cephalosporins
- Prolonged administration of antibiotics

appearance of fungus balls may persist long after clinical resolution of infection. Surgical management can be required for decompression of obstructive candidiasis and drainage of abscesses.[19]

Endophthalmitis is more likely with prolonged candidemia; it most commonly manifests as retinitis, with fluffy or hard white infiltrates. A dilated retinal examination should be part of the diagnostic evaluation for all infants. Involvement of the liver or spleen with microabscesses; endocarditis among infants with indwelling catheters; and extension of infection to the lungs, bones, or joints occur less frequently. The presentation of bone or joint disease is usually indolent, and involvement may not be evident when amphotericin B is initiated, so a high index of suspicion is important. Percutaneous aspiration of an involved joint or bone at the bedside usually is sufficient to establish the diagnosis, and an open drainage procedure is rarely, if ever, required.

DIAGNOSIS

The diagnosis of systemic candidiasis is established by growth of *Candida* species in cultures from sites that are normally sterile. The isolation of *Candida* species from nonsterile sites, such as endotracheal tube secretions or the skin or mucous membranes, is an indication of colonization, and does not establish the diagnosis of disseminated infection. In contrast to adults, in whom the diagnosis of disseminated candidiasis is documented by blood culture in only one third of cases, 80% or more of neonates with invasive candidiasis have documented fungemia.[6] The use of special media for the isolation of fungi is not required. *Candida* species grow robustly in the routine blood culture media used in most clinical laboratories, and these media usually yield the organism within 48 to 72 hours of incubation.[44]

If catheter-associated candidemia is suspected, a blood culture obtained through the catheter and one obtained peripherally should be collected before catheter removal and the initiation of therapy. The peripheral culture should be repeated to document that fungemia has resolved with catheter removal.

If disseminated candidiasis is suspected, or if a positive peripheral blood culture is obtained, blood cultures should be repeated at intervals until sterility is documented. Urine culture should be obtained by suprapubic tap or catheter. The CSF should be evaluated. CSF evaluation usually reveals a modest pleocytosis, with several hundred cells or fewer, lymphocyte predominance, and mildly elevated protein. The inflammatory response in CSF can be minimal, and one half of infants with *Candida* meningitis can have normal CSF parameters.[9] Routine cultures yield yeast within 2 to 3 days.[34] Infants with disseminated candidiasis require a baseline abdominal ultrasound examination; ophthalmologic examination; and, if central venous access catheters have been in place, echocardiographic examination of the heart and the great vessels. Subsequent examinations can be conducted if there is evidence of focal infection of these organ systems, or if the clinical status indicates. Additional laboratory tests include a baseline complete blood count (CBC), blood urea nitrogen, creatinine, potassium, and liver enzymes. The CBC can reveal thrombocytopenia, and initial renal function abnormalities can be detected, particularly in infants with VLBW with disseminated candidiasis. These usually resolve as the infection is controlled.

TREATMENT

Treatment varies by the location and extent of infection and the age of the patient. Thrush usually responds to nystatin (Mycostatin) suspension (1 to 2 mL) given orally four times daily for 5 to 10 days. Nystatin cream or ointment three times daily for 7 to 10 days is usually effective for *Candida* diaper dermatitis, although secondary bacterial infection may require treatment with another topical or systemic antibiotic. Nystatin with a corticosteroid (Mycolog-II cream or ointment) can be useful in severe cases of *Candida* dermatitis. Congenital cutaneous candidiasis requires no therapy unless the infant has evidence of pneumonia, or weighs less than 1500 g at birth, or both, at which time parenteral antifungal therapy is indicated.[42]

Amphotericin B is the mainstay of treatment for systemic candidiasis in a newborn infant (Table 39-25). It is extremely well tolerated by infants with VLBW. Pharmacokinetic studies in neonates suggest that a single daily infusion administered over 4 hours is necessary to achieve detectable serum concentrations.[1] An initial dose of 0.5 mg/kg, administered over 1 to 2 hours, can be advanced to the 1 mg/kg per day dose after 12 to 24 hours. The duration of therapy varies, but a typical course for disseminated candidiasis is a 20 to 25 mg/kg cumulative dose. For catheter-associated candidiasis, the usual course of therapy is a cumulative dose of 10 to 15 mg/kg. This duration usually is required to ascertain that the sequential blood cultures obtained after catheter removal are sterile. Infants who have a delay in removal of central catheters are at higher risk of death and neurodevelopmental delay compared with infants whose catheters are removed promptly.[3]

Amphotericin B rarely causes nephrotoxicity in infants. Initially abnormal renal function usually improves as treatment is initiated, suggesting that renal dysfunction was caused by the fungemia, rather than precipitated by the treatment. Infants receiving the initial dose of amphotericin B should be monitored for cardiac arrhythmias, but this is a rare side effect. Because amphotericin B causes renal tubular wasting of potassium, the potassium should initially be monitored daily and supplemented as required to maintain the concentration at greater than 3 mEq/dL. If daily potassium, blood urea nitrogen, and creatinine levels are stable after the first week of therapy, these can be monitored twice weekly, and the CBC and liver enzymes can be determined weekly, for the duration of the treatment course.

The combination of flucytosine and amphotericin B has been used successfully to treat systemic candidiasis, especially when the meninges are involved. Flucytosine should not be used as monotherapy because resistance can develop. The dosage range is 50 to 150 mg/kg daily, given orally in divided doses every 6 hours. Bone marrow suppression, hepatotoxicity, and gastrointestinal symptoms associated with flucytosine administration are more common when serum concentrations exceed 70 to 100 μg/mL. The CBC and liver enzymes should be monitored, and serum concentrations of flucytosine should be measured.

Available data suggest that liposomal amphotericin B and amphotericin B lipid complex are safe and effective when used as initial therapy[18,27] or for therapy in neonates with systemic candidiasis who were intolerant of or refractory to conventional antifungal therapy.[49] Pharmacokinetic studies

TABLE 39–25   Antifungal Agents Used for Treatment of Systemic Infections in Neonates

Drug	Dosage* (mg/kg/d)	Interval/Route	Toxicity	Comments
Amphotericin B	1[†]	q24h IV	Anemia, hypokalemia	Monitor blood urea nitrogen, creatinine nephrotoxicity, and K⁺ daily initially and twice weekly if stable after 1 wk; hold dose until K⁺ <3 mEq/dL is corrected
Lipid formulations	3-7[‡]	q24h IV	Less nephrotoxic than amphotericin B	Monitor renal function and K⁺ as above for amphotericin B
Flucytosine	50-150	Divided q6h PO	Bone marrow suppression, hepatotoxicity, and gastrointestinal symptoms	Good penetration into CSF; must reduce dosage in patients with renal failure; monitor serum concentrations
Fluconazole	3-6	q24h PO, IV	Adjustment of dosage needed for renal impairment	Good penetration into CSF Limited experience
Itraconazole	5[‡]	q24h PO	Occasional hepatotoxicity	Limited experience
Caspofungin	1-2[‡]	q24h IV	Hepatotoxicity	Limited experience

*See text for details.

[†]Initial dose of 0.5 mg/kg should be followed 12-24 h later by 1 mg/kg dose administered daily. Dose should be increased to 1.5 mg/kg/d for neonates with invasive aspergillosis.

[‡]Optimal dose has not been established.

CSF, cerebrospinal fluid.

have not been performed in neonates, and randomized trials are lacking to establish the optimal and cumulative dosages, and whether these preparations should be used in combination with other antifungal agents.[43] Nephrotoxicity is less often observed with lipid formulations than with amphotericin deoxycholate. Lipid formulations have poor penetration of the kidney, however, and therapeutic failure has occurred in neonates with renal or systemic candidiasis. Until comparative data are available, the use of these products should be reserved for infants with dose-limiting toxicity attributable to conventional amphotericin B for whom renal fungal involvement has been excluded.

Among the echinocandin antifungal agents, limited clinical experience with caspofungin suggests that it is an effective, safe, and well-tolerated alternative agent to amphotericin B for neonates who have persistent fungemia, and are unresponsive to or are intolerant of amphotericin B deoxycholate. A dose of 1 mg/kg per day throughout the course of treatment and initial dosing with 1 mg/kg per day advanced to 2 mg/kg per day have been employed.[35,36] Potential toxicity in association with a daily dose of 6 mg/kg per day has been noted.[46] Early experience with micafungin revealed linear plasma pharmacokinetics over a broad dose range in experimental neonatal candidiasis, and indicated that a dose exceeding 2 mg/kg would be required to penetrate most compartments of the central nervous system.[15] Doses of 2 to 3 mg/kg have been well tolerated in premature infants.[14,37]

The efficacy and safety of fluconazole for the treatment of *Candida* fungemia have been studied in a few neonates. Treatment of infants with VLBW who had documented *C. albicans* infection has been carried out with fluconazole for 6 to 48 days.[16] An 80% cure rate was achieved, but four infants relapsed despite at least 14 days of therapy. Similarly, itraconazole has been used in a few cases, with a generally good

outcome. Until an efficacy trial is available that compares amphotericin B with fluconazole or itraconazole in a direct comparison, however, amphotericin B should remain the standard treatment for neonatal candidiasis.

PREVENTION

In 2001, administration of fluconazole during the first 6 weeks of life was shown to be an effective intervention to prevent fungal colonization and invasive candidiasis in infants with birthweights of less than 1000 g.[20] Fluconazole was administered intravenously at a dose of 3 mg/kg every third day for the first 2 weeks, every other day during weeks 3 and 4, and daily during weeks 5 and 6. The efficacy and safety of fluconazole prophylaxis in preventing invasive *Candida* infections in infants weighing less than 1000 g have subsequently been shown in additional multicenter, randomized trials, which, taken together, also show a significant decrease in invasive *Candida* infection-related mortality.[23,29] Longitudinal analysis during 4 years found continued benefit without the development of fluconazole-resistant *Candida* species.[13] This evidence base supports the use of fluconazole prophylaxis in high-risk infants weighing less than 1000 g at birth, and suggests that each neonatal intensive care unit should determine its incidence of infection and institute prevention in preterm infants at high risk for infection.[21]

Coccidioidomycosis

INCIDENCE

Coccidioidomycosis is endemic in the San Joaquin Valley in California and in other areas of the southwestern United States, Mexico, Argentina, Venezuela, and Paraguay. Most susceptible individuals living in endemic areas acquire asymptomatic infection within 5 years. Disease can occur in any geographic location after reactivation of infection. Despite the high incidence of infection in endemic areas, perinatal coccidioidomycosis rarely occurs.

MICROBIOLOGY

Coccidioides immitis, the causative agent of coccidioidomycosis, is a biphasic fungus. Highly contagious mycelia grow on culture media and soil, whereas the less infectious spherules grow in tissues. The spherule contains hundreds of endospores that, when released, can become spherules.

PATHOGENESIS

The infectious arthrospores can become airborne, or can be transferred from inanimate objects contaminated with dust. Infection is acquired from inhalation of arthrospores and less commonly from direct inoculation into cutaneous lacerations or abrasions. The incubation period is 7 to 21 days. Infection occurring in infants younger than 1 week of age has been described, suggesting vertical transmission.[4] Despite several reports of disseminated infection during pregnancy, placental and perinatal infections are rare.[7,26]

After arthrospore inhalation, mature spherules develop within several days. Granuloma formation with tracheobronchial lymph node involvement can follow. In extensive disease, polymorphonuclear leukocytes infiltrate the lung, similar to the process seen with bacterial pneumonia. Hematogenous dissemination occurs frequently in infants.

CLINICAL MANIFESTATIONS

In contrast to older children and adults, whose primary infection is often asymptomatic, pneumonia is usually present in most infants with recognized infection. Chest radiographs can show focal consolidation or diffuse nodular infiltrates, hilar adenopathy, and pleural effusions. Fever, anorexia, and respiratory distress often accompany neonatal coccidioidomycosis. If the disease becomes disseminated, lesions can develop in the skin, bone, lymph nodes, liver, spleen, and meninges.

DIAGNOSIS

Clinical and radiographic features of coccidioidomycosis can resemble features seen with histoplasmosis, pulmonary tuberculosis, and viral pneumonitis. If meningitis develops, an elevated protein concentration and hypoglycorrhachia can be seen on CSF examination. Early in the course, a neutrophilic pleocytosis can be seen, but this quickly progresses to a lymphocytic predominance.

The diagnosis is best established using serologic and histologic methods. An IgM response is usually detectable 1 to 3 weeks after the onset of symptoms. A high IgG titer indicates severe disease, and decreasing titers suggest improvement. Transplacental passage of complement-fixing antibody occurs, so an increase in the infant's titer must be shown to document neonatal infection. Antibodies are detectable in CSF in patients with meningitis. Spherules occasionally can be observed on silver-stained tissue samples. Culture of the organism is feasible, but is potentially hazardous to laboratory personnel. Coccidioidin skin tests are not helpful in the neonatal period, and these skin tests are not currently available in the United States.

TREATMENT

In older children and adults, primary infection is often self-limited and requires no therapy. The frequency of disseminated disease in young infants and the high case-fatality rate warrant treatment of all neonatal infections, however. Amphotericin B is the drug of choice for the initial treatment of infection (see Table 39-25). The duration of therapy is prolonged, and anecdotal therapy suggests that fluconazole administered orally can be given to complete the course of treatment.[7,26]

Cryptococcosis

INCIDENCE

Cryptococcosis occurs worldwide. Many infections are likely to be asymptomatic, and most symptomatic infections occur in individuals older than 30 years. Infection can occur in otherwise healthy individuals, but is more common in immunocompromised hosts, including patients with acquired immunodeficiency syndrome (AIDS), malignancies, and diabetes mellitus. Cryptococcal infection in the newborn period is an extremely rare disease.

MICROBIOLOGY

Cryptococcus neoformans is an encapsulated yeast that reproduces by budding. Its natural habitat is soil, and it has been commonly found in soil contaminated with pigeon excreta.

PATHOGENESIS AND PATHOLOGY

Cryptococcosis is acquired from inhalation of the yeast with resulting primary pulmonary infection. Ingestion or cutaneous inoculation is possible; a central venous catheter may have been the source of cryptococcemia in one neonate.[11] Case reports of disease with onset shortly after birth suggest that in utero or intrapartum transmission is possible. Otherwise, there has been no evidence of human-to-human transmission. Pulmonary infection can remain localized or can disseminate hematogenously to any organ, with the meninges most commonly affected. In adults, the infection is usually subacute or chronic, with large, solitary pulmonary nodules frequently observed. Diffuse pulmonary infiltration or miliary disease with dissemination is more common in infants.

Pathologic findings vary from minor inflammatory responses to abscess formation. Noncaseating granulomas, hepatitis, and cirrhosis of the liver are common findings. Meningitis frequently leads to obstructive hydrocephalus. Granulomas of the brain have been reported.

CLINICAL MANIFESTATIONS

Infantile cryptococcosis is a multisystemic infection. The signs and symptoms are similar to congenital infection caused by *T. pallidum, Toxoplasma,* cytomegalovirus, and rubella, and include failure to thrive, jaundice, hepatosplenomegaly, chorioretinitis, rash, and intracranial calcifications. Other symptoms suggestive of a central nervous system process, such as lethargy, irritability, vomiting, and seizures, can be observed. Respiratory symptoms are minimal, but occasionally interstitial pneumonitis can be present. Infants with meningeal involvement can show a pleocytosis ranging from

40 to 1000 leukocytes/mm^3 with a lymphocytic predominance, elevated protein, and slightly decreased glucose concentrations on CSF examination.

DIAGNOSIS

Definitive diagnosis of cryptococcosis requires isolation of the organism from body fluids or tissue specimens. Fungal cultures of CSF, blood, sputum or tracheal aspirates, material from abscess cavities, and bone marrow can yield growth of *Cryptococcus*. The presence of encapsulated, budding yeast on India ink-stained CSF or respiratory tract samples is usually indicative of cryptococcal disease. Serologic investigation includes antibody and antigen detection tests, but antigen detection is the preferred technique. Latex agglutination and enzyme immunoassay for detection of cryptococcal antigen in serum or CSF are excellent rapid diagnostic tests.

TREATMENT

In healthy adults, pulmonary cryptococcosis is usually self-limited and requires no therapy. Pulmonary disease frequently disseminates in immunocompromised patients if left untreated, however. Before the introduction of amphotericin B, cryptococcosis was almost uniformly fatal. The case-fatality rate has significantly decreased with amphotericin B therapy, but at least one third of adults fail to respond to therapy, and another one fourth have relapse after discontinuation of therapy. The combination of amphotericin B and flucytosine or fluconazole is indicated as initial therapy for patients with meningeal and other serious manifestations of cryptococcal infection. Because only six cases have been reported in neonates, only anecdotal data exist for treatment. One infant with VLBW survived cryptococcemia after receiving a 6-week course of therapy with amphotericin B.[11]

Histoplasmosis

INCIDENCE

Histoplasmosis is one of the most common pulmonary fungal infections in immunocompetent humans. It occurs worldwide in temperate climates and is endemic in the Ohio and Mississippi river valleys of the United States. In older children and adults, most infections are asymptomatic; however, in young infants, infections are often apparent and frequently disseminate. Despite the high incidence of infection in endemic areas, neonatal histoplasmosis is rare.

MICROBIOLOGY

Histoplasma capsulatum is the causative agent. It is not encapsulated, but artifacts resembling a capsule can be seen with some staining techniques. It is a thermally dimorphic fungus, growing as mycelia (mold) with microconidia and macroconidia (spores) in soil and converting to yeast form at human body temperatures. Soil is its natural habitat, and it thrives in moist soil contaminated with avian or bat excreta.

PATHOGENESIS

Inhalation of conidia is the most common mode of transmission. Other routes, such as ingestion or cutaneous inoculation, occur rarely. Human-to-human transmission, if possible, has not been well described. Several days after inhalation, the spores germinate in the alveoli, releasing yeast forms. An inflammatory response, initially neutrophilic, followed by an influx of lymphocytes and macrophages, ensues. The yeasts are phagocytosed, but not killed, and begin to proliferate within macrophages and can spread hematogenously to the liver, spleen, and other organs or to regional lymph nodes through the lymphatics. The inflammatory response can result in discrete granulomas resembling sarcoid, or caseating lesions that frequently calcify during resolution.

CLINICAL MANIFESTATIONS

The clinical spectrum of histoplasmosis in children includes asymptomatic infection, pulmonary disease that can be complicated by mediastinal lymphadenopathy and subsequent tracheobronchial obstruction, primary cutaneous infection, and disseminated infection. Asymptomatic infection occurs in most older children and adults, whereas acute disseminated infection with pulmonary disease is most common in young infants.[24] The most frequently observed signs and symptoms in disseminated disease are prolonged fever, hepatosplenomegaly, anemia, and thrombocytopenia. Because the infection can disseminate to the lymph nodes, adrenal glands, gastrointestinal tract, bone marrow, central nervous system, kidneys, heart, and bones, many other signs and symptoms can be present.

DIAGNOSIS

Fungal cultures from patients with acute, self-limited pulmonary infection rarely yield the organism, but frequently are positive from patients with disseminated disease. *Histoplasma* can be isolated from lower respiratory tract specimens, blood, bone marrow, hepatic and splenic biopsy specimens, and CSF, but growth may not be detected for 8 to 12 weeks. Lysis-centrifugation of blood samples submitted for fungal culture has increased the sensitivity and reduced the interval until cultures become positive. Demonstration of intracellular yeast forms supports the diagnosis when the clinical picture is compatible. Detection of *H. capsulatum* polysaccharide antigen in serum, urine, or bronchoalveolar lavage specimens is a rapid and specific diagnostic method. Complement fixation titers greater than 1:32 or a fourfold increase in yeast-phase or mycelial-phase titers suggests acute infection.

Chest radiographs in pulmonary histoplasmosis often are negative or reveal nodular infiltrates with mediastinal and hilar adenopathy. In disseminated disease, chest radiographs most frequently are negative, but hilar adenopathy, bronchopneumonia, or miliary nodules can be present. Pulmonary and splenic calcifications can be seen on subsequent radiographs after recovery from infection. Findings common in adult disease, including pleural effusions or cavitary formation associated with chronic pulmonary infection, are not seen in infantile disease.

TREATMENT

Primary pulmonary histoplasmosis in a healthy child usually does not require treatment. Therapy is recommended for disease in infancy because the risk of dissemination is higher, and untreated disseminated disease is almost uniformly fatal.[24] Amphotericin B is effective for initial treatment of disseminated disease and other serious infections. In patients older than neonates, itraconazole is effective, either as initial treatment or after clinical improvement has been observed.

Other Fungi

Malassezia yeasts are dimorphic, lipophilic fungi that are the causative agent of pityriasis versicolor (formerly tinea versicolor). Neonates acquire *Malassezia* through direct contact with their mothers or hospital personnel.[50] *Malassezia furfur* is the most commonly isolated of the several *Malassezia* species, and has been associated with fungemia and occasionally pneumonia in premature infants with low birthweight receiving lipid emulsion alimentation through central venous catheters.[38,48] Sporadic bloodstream infections have been described, with transmission probably by the hands of medical personnel. Because it requires high concentrations of medium-chain and long-chain fatty acids to grow, *Malassezia* cannot be cultivated on Sabouraud medium without the addition of sterile olive oil. Most infections respond to temporary cessation of lipid infusions and removal of the central venous catheter. Amphotericin B should be used for treatment until a clinical response and negative blood culture are documented.

Blastomyces dermatitidis is a dimorphic fungus endemic to the midwestern, southeastern, and Appalachian areas of the United States. Blastomycosis occurs more commonly in adults than in children and is rare in neonates. Infections can be asymptomatic, limited to the respiratory tract, or disseminated. Cutaneous and skeletal lesions are the most common extrapulmonary sites of infection. Cutaneous and genital disease have been documented during pregnancy and, if inadequately treated, can result in neonatal blastomycosis.[30] The diagnosis should be considered in infants with reticulonodular pneumonia born to mothers with chronic skin infections who live in endemic areas.

Candida diaper dermatitis is the most common superficial cutaneous fungal infection in young infants; however, tinea capitis and tinea corporis have been described.[12,47] Dermatophyte infections, caused by *Microsporum*, *Trichophyton*, or *Epidermophyton*, are acquired postnatally from contact with contaminated soil, infected animals, or household members. Because lesions associated with dermatophytosis can resemble the lesions seen with psoriasis, seborrhea, or impetigo, they can easily be misdiagnosed.

Invasive fungal dermatitis is an entity that is recognized increasingly with the survival of infants with VLBW. These infants have the same risk factors for invasive fungal infection as described for neonatal candidiasis. It is believed that the skin serves as the portal of entry for colonizing species. Diffuse involvement with a buff-colored crust suggests *Candida* species, but *Aspergillus* and *Trichosporon* have been seen.[41] Discrete erythematous lesions that become purple or black suggest *Curvularia* or one of the Zygomycetes.[39] The diagnosis is established by a full-thickness skin biopsy showing fungal invasion of the dermis. Treatment should be initiated with amphotericin B while awaiting the histopathologic and culture results from skin biopsy.

PROTOZOAL INFECTIONS

Malaria

INCIDENCE

Worldwide, there are 300 to 500 million cases of malaria annually and greater than 2 million deaths, most of which occur in children. Malaria remains an important cause of abortion, stillbirth, and neonatal death in many parts of the world. The 81 cases of congenital malaria reported in the United States from 1966-2005 occurred almost exclusively in infants of foreign-born women who were exposed within the year before the infant's delivery.[25]

MICROBIOLOGY

Malaria is caused by an obligate, intracellular protozoan of the genus *Plasmodium*. Congenital malaria has been recorded with each species, including *Plasmodium vivax*, *Plasmodium malariae*, *Plasmodium ovale*, and *Plasmodium falciparum*. Most congenital cases have been caused by *P. vivax* and *P. falciparum*.

PATHOLOGY AND PATHOGENESIS

Malaria is transmitted by the bite of infected female *Anopheles* mosquitoes or from transfusions (maternal-fetal, blood products, or contaminated needles) of infected blood. Anemia is the result of hemolysis. Parasites can be found in other organs of the body, including the intestinal tract, liver, spleen, lung, and brain. Because *P. falciparum* and *P. malariae* have no persistent exoerythrocytic phase, relapses do not occur. *P. vivax* and *P. ovale* are associated with relapses from dormant exoerythrocytic organisms. Transfusion-related malaria and congenital malaria have no exoerythrocytic phase.

The placenta is involved in most women who acquire malaria during pregnancy. It is unclear whether transmission to the infant is transplacental or from direct contact with maternal blood during labor or parturition. Most pregnancies resulting in congenital malaria are associated with a malaria attack during pregnancy; however, congenital infection has been described after uncomplicated asymptomatic pregnancies.

Host factors that can decrease the risk of malarial infections include abnormal hemoglobin and malaria-specific antibodies. Erythrocytes with fetal hemoglobin or hemoglobin S are less likely to become infected than erythrocytes with hemoglobin A. Women living in endemic areas are continuously exposed to malaria and develop antimalarial antibodies. Maternal antibody is believed to exhibit a protective effect for the fetus. One survey found that 7% of infants born to women evaluated at seven African sites had congenital malaria.[10]

CLINICAL MANIFESTATIONS

Most infants with congenital malaria have onset of symptoms by the eighth week of life, with an average age at onset of 10 to 28 days. Occasionally, onset has been documented at several months after birth. The most common clinical findings are fever, anemia, and splenomegaly. Approximately one third of infants have jaundice and direct or indirect hyperbilirubinemia. Hepatomegaly can be present. Nonspecific symptoms include irritability, failure to thrive, loose stools, and reluctance to feed. Congenital malaria often is complicated by bacterial illnesses in developing countries. In rare cases, malaria can be complicated by hypoglycemia; central nervous system infection; splenic rupture; renal failure; and, in *P. falciparum* infections, blackwater fever (severe hemolysis, hemoglobinuria, and renal failure). Untreated *P. falciparum* infection is associated with a high case-fatality rate.

DIAGNOSIS

Although a maternal history of a febrile illness during pregnancy can be elicited in most cases, congenital disease after an asymptomatic pregnancy in women has been reported. The diagnosis of congenital malaria should be considered in any infant presenting with fever, anemia, and hepatosplenomegaly born to a mother who at any time resided in an endemic area. The diagnosis depends on demonstration of parasites in the bloodstream. Thin and thick smears should be prepared and examined on several different occasions to maximize the possibility of parasite detection.

TREATMENT

Several types of antimalarial drugs act at different stages of the *Plasmodium* life cycle. Tissue schizonticides such as primaquine are effective against exoerythrocytic forms, whereas blood schizonticides such as chloroquine, quinine, and quinidine act only on parasites in the erythrocytic phase. Because transfusion-acquired disease, including congenital infection, does not have an exoerythrocytic phase, primaquine is not required. Chloroquine, given in an initial dose of 10 mg of chloroquine base per kilogram of body weight administered orally, followed by doses of 5 mg base/kg at 6, 24, and 48 hours after the initial dose, is frequently used. For treatment of congenital disease caused by chloroquine-resistant *P. falciparum,* quinidine gluconate or the combination of quinine administered orally and clindamycin has been suggested. Mefloquine is effective against most *P. falciparum* strains, but is not approved for use in infants. Experience with newer treatment options, such as artemisinin derivatives, in young infants is limited. Severe congenital malaria can require intensive care, and exchange transfusion can be necessary for high-grade parasitemia. Current recommendations regarding treatment of congenital malaria can be obtained from the malaria branch of the Centers for Disease Control and Prevention in Atlanta, Georgia.

Pneumocystis

INCIDENCE

Pneumocystis pneumonia occurs in patients with congenital immune defects or hematologic malignancies, or patients receiving immunosuppressive medications for organ transplantation. *Pneumocystis* is an unusual cause of pneumonia in the first year of life, but it can be observed as epidemic disease, first recognized during World War II and presumed to be related to malnutrition, and as sporadic disease associated with congenital immunodeficiency or AIDS. Some surveys suggest that rare cases can develop in healthy infants.

MICROBIOLOGY

Because of difficulties in laboratory cultivation, the taxonomy of *Pneumocystis jiroveci* (formerly *Pneumocystis carinii*) is inconclusive; it has features in common with protozoan parasites and fungi. *Pneumocystis* is a unicellular organism that can be found in three forms: a thick-walled cyst, a thin-walled trophozoite,

and an intracystic sporozoite. Each cyst can contain up to eight sporozoites. Organisms can be detected on tissue samples stained with Grocott-Gomori methenamine silver nitrate.

PATHOLOGY AND PATHOGENESIS

Serologic studies suggest that asymptomatic infection with *Pneumocystis* is widespread and commonly occurs in the first years of life. The organisms are believed to persist in a latent stage until impairment in host defense mechanisms permits their reactivation. Disease associated with *Pneumocystis* usually is limited to the lungs. There is now evidence that person-to-person transmission is the most likely mode of acquiring new infections. Airborne transmission from mother to infant has been proposed.[33]

Postmortem examination reveals a diffuse process, with the posterior and dependent regions of the lung most significantly affected. Microscopic examination reveals an eosinophilic, foamy, honeycombed intra-alveolar exudate composed of cysts. In epidemic infantile disease, a plasma cellular infiltrate is observed (hence the name interstitial plasma cell pneumonia), whereas in sporadic disease associated with immunodeficiency or immunosuppression, there is hyperplasia of the cells lining the alveoli and minimal cellular infiltrate with a paucity of lymphocytes.

CLINICAL MANIFESTATIONS

The clinical characteristics of sporadic *Pneumocystis* pneumonia are different from the characteristics observed in epidemic infantile disease. In sporadic cases associated with congenital or acquired immunodeficiency, there is an abrupt onset of high fever, coryza, nonproductive cough, and tachypnea. There is a quick progression to dyspnea and cyanosis. Radiographic findings most commonly reveal diffuse infiltrative disease. Concurrent infections, most commonly with cytomegalovirus, occur in more than 50% of immunocompromised infants with *Pneumocystis* pneumonia.

In epidemic infantile *Pneumocystis* pneumonia, a rare disease in developed countries, the onset is slow and insidious, with nonspecific symptoms such as anorexia, diarrhea, and restlessness.[28] Cough is not prominent initially, and fever is absent. In the subsequent weeks, infants become tachypneic, cyanotic, and dyspneic, with sternal retractions and flaring of the nasal alae. Auscultatory findings are minimal, consisting of fine, crepitant rales on deep inspiration. The chest radiograph can be negative early in the course, or can reveal a perihilar or diffuse haziness that progresses to a finely granular, interstitial pattern. Coalescent nodules can form in the periphery. Pneumothorax with interstitial and subcutaneous emphysema and pneumomediastinum can occur.

DIAGNOSIS

Typical findings on radiographic studies can suggest *P. jiroveci* pneumonia, but are not diagnostic. Demonstration of *Pneumocystis* cysts or extracystic trophozoite forms establishes the diagnosis. *P. jiroveci* can be detected in induced sputum or in tracheal or gastric aspirates, but the yield is low, and detection does not imply disease.[28] Bronchoalveolar lavage or open lung biopsy can yield the organism. Serologic tests are not useful.

TREATMENT

Trimethoprim-sulfamethoxazole is the drug of choice for treatment of *P. jiroveci* pneumonia in infants. It must be used with caution in young infants because of its potential for displacement of bilirubin from albumin-binding sites. The therapeutic dose is 15 to 20 mg/kg per day of the trimethoprim component in divided doses every 6 to 8 hours. The intravenous route of administration is preferable in infants with moderate or severe disease. Treatment is usually continued for 3 weeks. In infants who do not respond to trimethoprim-sulfamethoxazole or in whom adverse reactions develop, pentamidine isethionate, 4 mg/kg given parenterally as a single daily dose for 14 days, can be used.

Although radiographic improvement can take several weeks, clinical improvement is usually seen within 4 to 6 days after beginning therapy.[28] Local reactions at the injection site, tachycardia, hypotension, pruritus, hypoglycemia, and nephrotoxicity have been associated with pentamidine administration. Trimethoprim-sulfamethoxazole is the standard for prophylaxis against *Pneumocystis* pneumonia and has been used for that purpose in infants 2 months old and older with human immunodeficiency virus (HIV) infection.

Toxoplasmosis

INCIDENCE

Among 22,845 pregnant women analyzed by the Collaborative Perinatal Research Study in the United States, 38% had *Toxoplasma* IgG antibodies, reflecting past infection, and the incidence of acute maternal infection during pregnancy was estimated to be 1.1 per 1000 women.[45] A higher incidence is seen in women born in Cambodia or Laos.[17] In the United States, 1 to 3 infants per 1000 live births have *Toxoplasma*-specific IgM antibody. Worldwide, 3 to 8 infants per 1000 live births are infected in utero. An estimated 400 to 4000 cases of congenital toxoplasmosis occur in the United States each year.

MICROBIOLOGY

Toxoplasmosis is caused by *Toxoplasma gondii,* an obligate intracellular protozoan parasite. This ubiquitous organism exists in three forms: an oocyst excreted by infected cats that produces sporozoites, a proliferative form (trophozoite or tachyzoite), and a cyst (cystozoite) found in tissues of infected animals. *Toxoplasma* can be propagated in tissue cell cultures or by animal inoculation in research laboratories.

TRANSMISSION AND PATHOGENESIS

The cat is the only definitive host, but other mammals can be infected incidentally. Farm animals (cattle, pigs, sheep) can acquire infection after ingestion of food or water contaminated with infected cat feces that contain oocysts. Humans can acquire infection by ingestion of raw or poorly cooked meat containing the *Toxoplasma* cysts or by ingestion of food or water contaminated with oocysts. Risk factors include any exposure to cat feces, such as changing cat litter boxes, playing in sandboxes, or gardening in areas used by cats.

Congenital toxoplasmosis occurs almost exclusively as a result of primary maternal infection during pregnancy. Rarely, reactivation of infection in immunocompromised women during pregnancy can result in congenital toxoplasmosis. Most maternal infections are asymptomatic or result in mild illnesses. Fatigue and lymphadenopathy involving only a single posterior cervical node or generalized lymphadenopathy may be the only manifestation. Less commonly, acute maternal infection can manifest as an infectious mononucleosis-like syndrome with fever, nonsuppurative lymphadenopathy, headache, fatigue, sore throat, and myalgias. The general risk of transmission of acute infection from mother to fetus is estimated to be 40%; however, the actual risk and the severity of congenital infection vary with gestational age. The risk of transmission increases with increasing gestational age, but the earlier during pregnancy that fetal infection is acquired, the more severe the manifestations of congenital disease.

CLINICAL MANIFESTATIONS

The classic clinical presentation of congenital toxoplasmosis is the triad of hydrocephalus, chorioretinitis, and intracranial calcifications, but there is a wide spectrum of manifestations, and more than 75% of infected newborns are asymptomatic in early infancy. As described by McAuley and colleagues,[31] the four most common presentations include (1) a healthy-appearing term infant with subclinical infection in whom symptoms develop later in childhood, (2) a healthy-appearing term infant in whom clinical evidence of disease develops in the first few months of life, (3) an infant with generalized disease at birth, and (4) an infant with predominantly neurologic involvement at birth.

Many infants with subclinical infection who were believed to be normal at birth have evidence of infection on closer evaluation, including CSF abnormalities, such as lymphocytic pleocytosis, hypoglycorrhachia, and elevated protein concentrations. If the disease goes unrecognized and untreated, these infants can present with chorioretinitis, late-onset seizures, mental retardation, developmental delay, and hearing loss later in infancy or childhood. The second group of healthy-appearing, infected infants present with hydrocephalus and chorioretinitis in the first few months of life. Manifestations of generalized infection at birth include prematurity and intrauterine growth restriction, jaundice, hepatosplenomegaly, pneumonitis, temperature instability, lymphadenopathy, and cutaneous lesions (e.g., exfoliative dermatitis, petechiae, ecchymoses, and maculopapular lesions). Other signs of generalized infection include myocarditis; nephrotic syndrome; and gastrointestinal symptoms such as vomiting, diarrhea, or feeding difficulties. The fourth group of infected infants has predominantly neurologic disease, but can have systemic manifestations as well. Subtle neurologic deficits, obstructive hydrocephalus, or acute encephalopathy can be seen. Unilateral or bilateral macular chorioretinitis frequently occurs, and infants often have rash, hepatosplenomegaly, thrombocytopenia, granulocytopenia, and typical CSF findings. The most common manifestations of congenital toxoplasmosis during the first few months of life are compared with the manifestations of congenital rubella and cytomegalovirus infection in Figure 39-12.

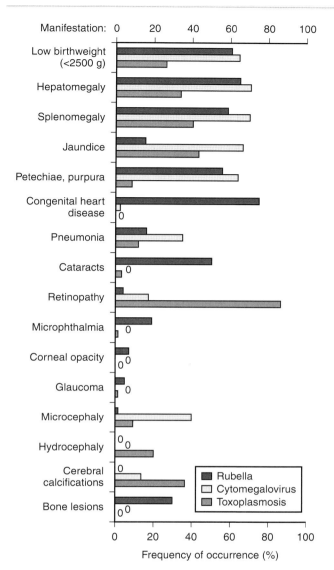

Figure 39–12. Manifestations of symptomatic congenital rubella, cytomegalovirus infection, and toxoplasmosis in neonates. *(From Overall JC Jr: Viral infections of the fetus and neonate. In Feigin FD et al, editors:* Textbook of pediatric infectious diseases, *4th ed, Philadelphia, 1998, Saunders, p 863.)*

DIAGNOSIS

Maternal infection occurring during gestation can lead to fetal infection. Most infants with congenital toxoplasmosis have normal results on physical examination at birth. Visual and neurologic impairment results when the infection is not diagnosed and adequately treated. Generally, all suspected maternal, fetal, and neonatal infections should have confirmatory diagnostic testing performed in an experienced reference laboratory, such as the Palo Alto Medical Foundation (550-853-4828).[5] Screening for IgG antibody in pregnancy is usually performed by indirect fluorescent antibody test or enzyme-linked immunosorbent assay and confirmed by the Sabin-Feldman dye test.

Several tests are available to determine the duration of maternal infection when IgG and IgM antibodies are positive. Fetal infection is best determined using amniotic fluid polymerase chain reaction amplification of the *Toxoplasma* gene *B1*.

Infection of an infant is best established definitively by intraperitoneal inoculation of placental tissue into laboratory mice, yielding cultivation of *Toxoplasma* organisms. When this is not feasible, strong evidence for the diagnosis is provided by the presence of *Toxoplasma*-specific IgM, IgA, or IgE antibody. Infants with suspected toxoplasmosis should undergo computed tomography (CT) scanning of the brain, evaluation of CSF, and indirect ophthalmologic examination.

TREATMENT

Pyrimethamine combined with sulfadiazine and supplemented with folinic acid is recommended for treatment of symptomatic and asymptomatic congenital infection. Therapy is continued for 1 year. Consultation with appropriate specialists should be sought when treating congenital toxoplasmosis.

PROGNOSIS

McLeod and colleagues[32] published the results of the national collaborative Chicago-based treatment trial for 120 infants with congenital toxoplasmosis. The duration of follow-up was a mean of 10.5 ± 4.8 years. A normal outcome was documented for 100% of infants treated with pyrimethamine and sulfadiazine for 1 year when there was not evidence of substantial neurologic disease at birth. Cognitive, neurologic, and auditory outcomes all were normal for these children. Normal neurologic or cognitive outcomes were also observed in greater than 72% of infants who did have moderate or severe neurologic disease at birth. None had sensorineural hearing loss, and most children in each group did not develop new eye lesions. These outcomes in patients treated for 1 year were markedly better than the outcomes in earlier years for infants who were untreated and infants who received only a 1-month course of therapy.

REFERENCES

1. Baley JE et al: Pharmacokinetics, outcome of treatment, and toxic effects of amphotericin B and 5-fluorocytosine in neonates, *J Pediatr* 116:791, 1990.
2. Bendel CM, Hostetter MK: Systemic candidiasis and other fungal infections in the newborn, *Semin Pediatr Infect Dis* 5:35, 1994.
3. Benjamin DK Jr et al: Neonatal candidiasis among extremely low birth weight infants: risk factors, mortality rates, and neurodevelopmental outcomes at 18 to 22 months, *Pediatrics* 117:84, 2006.
4. Bernstein DI et al: Coccidioidomycosis in a neonate: maternal-infant transmission, *J Pediatr* 99:752, 1981.
5. Boyer KM: Diagnostic testing for congenital toxoplasmosis, *Concise Rev Pediatr Infect Dis* 20:59, 2001.
6. Butler KM, Baker CJ: *Candida*: An increasingly important pathogen in the nursery, *Pediatr Clin North Am* 35:543, 1988.

7. Charlton V et al: Intrauterine transmission of coccidioidomycosis, *Pediatr Infect Dis J* 18:561, 1999.

8. Clerihew L et al: *Candida parapsilosis* infection in very low birthweight infants, *Arch Dis Child Fetal Neonatal Ed* 92:F127, 2007.

9. Cohen-Wolkowiez M et al: Neonatal *Candida* meningitis: significance of cerebrospinal fluid parameters and blood cultures, *J Perinatol* 27:97, 2007.

10. Fischer PR: Congenital malaria: an African survey, *Clin Pediatr* 36:411, 1997.

11. Gavai M et al: Successful treatment of cryptococcosis in a premature neonate, *Pediatr Infect Dis J* 14:1009, 1995.

12. Ghorpade A, Ramanan C: Tinea capitis and corporis due to *Trichophyton violaceum* in a six-day-old infant, *Int J Dermatol* 33:219, 1994.

13. Healy CM et al: Fluconazole prophylaxis in extremely low birth weight neonates reduces invasive candidiasis mortality rates without emergence of fluconazole-resistant *Candida* species, *Pediatrics* 121:703, 2008.

14. Heresi GP et al: The pharmacokinetics and safety of micafungin, a novel echinocandin, in premature infants, *Pediatr Infect Dis J* 25:1110, 2006.

15. Hope WW et al: The pharmacokinetics and pharmacodynamics of micafungin in experimental hematogenous *Candida* meningoencephalitis: implications for echinocandin therapy in neonates, *J Infect Dis* 197:163, 2008.

16. Huttova M et al: *Candida* fungemia in neonates treated with fluconazole: report of forty cases, including eight with meningitis, *Pediatr Infect Dis J* 17:1012, 1998.

17. Jara M et al: Epidemiology of congenital toxoplasmosis identified by population-based newborn screening in Massachusetts, *Pediatr Infect Dis J* 20:1132, 2001.

18. Juster-Reicher A et al: High-dose liposomal amphotericin B in the therapy of systemic candidiasis in neonates, *Eur J Clin Microbiol Infect Dis* 22:603, 2003.

19. Karlowicz MG: Candidal renal and urinary tract infection in neonates, *Semin Perinatol* 27:393, 2003.

20. Kaufman D et al: Fluconazole prophylaxis against fungal colonization and infection in preterm infants, *N Engl J Med* 345:1660, 2001.

21. Kaufman DA: Fluconazole prophylaxis decreases the combined outcome of invasive *Candida* infections or mortality in preterm infants, *Pediatrics* 122:1158, 2008.

22. Kaufman DA et al: Patterns of fungal colonization in preterm infants weighing less than 1000 grams at birth, *Pediatr Infect Dis J* 25:733, 2006.

23. Kicklighter SD et al: Fluconazole for prophylaxis against candidal rectal colonization in the very low birth weight infant, *Pediatrics* 107:293, 2001.

24. Leggiadro RJ et al: Disseminated histoplasmosis of infancy, *Pediatr Infect Dis J* 7:799, 1988.

25. Lesko CR et al. Congenital malaria in the United States: a review of cases from 1996 to 2005, *Arch Pediatr Adolesc Med* 161:1062, 2007.

26. Linsangan LC, Ross LA: *Coccidioides immitis* infection of the neonate: two routes of infection, *Pediatr Infect Dis J* 18:171, 1999.

27. López Sastre JB et al; Grupo de Hospitales Castrillo: Neonatal invasive candidiasis: a prospective multicenter study of 118 cases, *Am J Perinatol* 20:153, 2003.

28. Maldonado YA et al: *Pneumocystis* and other less common fungal diseases. In Remington JS et al, editors: *Infectious diseases of the fetus and newborn infant*, 6th ed. Philadelphia, 2006, Saunders, p 1129.

29. Manzoni P et al: A multicenter, randomized trial of prophylactic fluconazole in preterm infants, *N Engl J Med* 356:2483, 2007.

30. Maxson S et al: Perinatal blastomycosis: a review, *Pediatr Infect Dis J* 11:760, 1992.

31. McAuley J et al: Early and longitudinal evaluations of treated infants and children and untreated historical patients with congenital toxoplasmosis. The Chicago Collaborative Treatment Trial, *Clin Infect Dis* 18:38, 1994.

32. McLeod R et al: Outcome of treatment for congenital toxoplasmosis, 1981-2004: the national collaborative Chicago-based, congenital toxoplasmosis study, *Clin Infect Dis* 42:1383, 2006.

33. Miller RF et al: Probable mother-to-infant transmission of *Pneumocystis carinii* sp. *hominis* infection, *J Clin Microbiol* 40:1555, 2002.

34. Moylett EH: Neonatal *Candida* meningitis, *Semin Pediatr Infect Dis* 14:115, 2003.

35. Natarajan G et al: Experience with caspofungin in the treatment of persistent fungemia in neonates, *J Perinatol* 25:770, 2005.

36. Odio CM et al: Caspofungin therapy of neonates with invasive candidiasis, *Pediatr Infect Dis J* 23:1093, 2004.

37. Queiroz-Telles F et al: Micafungin versus liposomal amphotericin B for pediatric patients with invasive candidiasis: substudy of a randomized double-blind trial, *Pediatr Infect Dis J* 27:820, 2008.

38. Richet HM et al: Cluster of *Malassezia furfur* pulmonary infections in infants in a neonatal intensive care unit, *J Clin Microbiol* 27:1197, 1989.

39. Robertson AF et al: Zygomycosis in neonates, *Pediatr Infect Dis J* 16:812, 1997.

40. Rowen JL et al: Endotracheal colonization with *Candida* enhances risk of systemic candidiasis in very low birth weight neonates, *J Pediatr* 124:789, 1994.

41. Rowen JL et al: Invasive fungal dermatitis in the ≤1000-gram neonate, *Pediatrics* 95:682, 1995.

42. Santos LA et al: Congenital cutaneous candidiasis: report of four cases and review of the literature, *Eur J Pediatr* 150:336, 1991.

43. Scarcella A et al: Liposomal amphotericin B treatment for neonatal fungal infections, *Pediatr Infect Dis J* 17:146, 1998.

44. Schelonka RL, Moser SA: Time to positive culture results in neonatal *Candida* septicemia, *J Pediatr* 142:564, 2003.

45. Sever JL et al: Toxoplasmosis: maternal and pediatric findings in 23,000 pregnancies, *Pediatrics* 82:181, 1988.

46. Smith PB et al: Caspofungin for the treatment of azole resistant candidemia in a premature infant, *J Perinatol* 27:127, 2007.

47. Snider R et al: The ringworm riddle: an outbreak of *Microsporum* canis in the nursery, *Pediatr Infect Dis J* 12:145, 1993.

48. Stuart SM, Lane AT: *Candida* and *Malassezia* as nursery pathogens, *Semin Dermatol* 11:19, 1992.

49. Walsh TJ et al: Amphotericin B lipid complex in pediatric patients with invasive fungal infections, *Pediatr Infect Dis J* 18:702, 1999.

50. Zomorodain K et al: Molecular analysis of *Malassezia* species isolated from hospitalized neonates, *Pediatr Dermatol* 25:312, 2008.

Perinatal Viral Infections

Jill E. Baley and Philip Toltzis

Certain viruses seem to have a predilection for the fetus and may cause abortion, stillbirth, intrauterine infection, congenital malformations, acute disease during the neonatal period, or chronic infection with subtle manifestations that may be recognized only after a prolonged period. It is important to recognize the manifestations of viral infections in the neonatal period not only to diagnose the acute infection, but also to anticipate the potential abnormal growth and development of the infant.

HERPESVIRUS FAMILY

The herpesvirus family consists of numerous closely related viruses. They all have a DNA core and are enveloped in an icosahedral (20-sided) nucleocapsid. Eight viruses in the family infect infants: herpes simplex viruses (HSV) types 1 and 2; cytomegalovirus (CMV); varicella-zoster virus (VZV); Epstein-Barr virus (EBV); and human herpesviruses (HHV) 6, 7, and 8. These viruses are also characterized by the development of latent states after the primary infection.

Herpes Simplex

Neonatal herpes simplex infections are being diagnosed with increasing frequency, at a rate of 1 in every 3200 live births per year in the United States, resulting in an estimated 1500 new cases per year. The primary source of HSV infection for neonates is acquisition of the virus during delivery, yet far more women have infected genital tract secretions than there are neonatal infections. In addition, in numerous countries, neonatal infection is less common than in the United States, despite the high prevalence of genital infections, suggesting other, unknown means of protection to the neonate.

HSV are a group of large double-stranded DNA viruses within an icosahedral nucleocapsid and a lipid envelope. There is considerable cross-reactivity between the two serotypes, HSV-1 and HSV-2. Glycoprotein G is responsible for the antigenic specificity between them, as shown by the antibody response. The seroprevalence of HSV in the United States has continued to increase for HSV-1 and HSV-2. HSV-1 is now responsible for nearly 20% of neonatal infection, probably resulting from its increased seroprevalence and its increased maternal-to-neonatal transmission during reactivation of genital infection. The virus enters via breaks in the skin and mucous membranes, then attaches to the epithelial cells and begins to replicate. The virus is transported by retrograde axonal flow from the sensory nerve endings in the dermis to the sensory ganglia, where at least some portion of the viral DNA persists for the lifetime of the individual.

Fever, ultraviolet light, stress, and many undetermined reasons may cause the virus to reactivate, at which time the virus is transported antegrade down the sensory nerve axon to the skin or mucous membrane, where it again results in either symptomatic or asymptomatic disease. Either way, the virus is infectious. Analyses of viral DNA from individuals with recurrent lesions indicate that the identical virus is virtually always responsible. Superinfection with a differing viral strain is uncommon. Infection is not seasonal, and humans are the only known carriers of the infection.

HSV infections are labeled first episode, primary infections when the individual who has neither HSV-1 nor HSV-2 antibody (indicating prior infection) acquires either HSV-1 or HSV-2 in the genital tract. A first episode, nonprimary infection occurs when an individual who already has HSV-1 antibody acquires HSV-2 genital infection or vice versa. Recurrent infections occur with reactivation of latent infections.[68]

EPIDEMIOLOGY AND TRANSMISSION

Labial and oropharyngeal infections are predominantly caused by HSV-1 and may be transmitted by respiratory droplet spread or by direct contact with infected secretions or vesicular fluid. Most HSV-1 infections occur in childhood and are usually asymptomatic, sometimes causing a gingivostomatitis or mononucleosis-like syndrome. Girls have a higher seroprevalence than boys. Black children have a 35% seroprevalence by age 5 compared with 18% in white children, and the seroprevalence remains twice as high through the teen years, but is equivalent by 60 years of age.[68]

Because genital infections are usually transmitted by direct sexual contact with HSV-2, transmission most often occurs during or after adolescence. Symptomatic and asymptomatic individuals may transmit infection. Primary genital infection may cause localized pain and burning of the labia and vaginal mucosa 2 to 7 days after contact. After a period of paresthesia, vesicles full of seropurulent fluid develop. These vesicles break down easily, forming shallow ulcers and releasing numerous infectious virus particles. There is often copious watery vaginal discharge, edema, dysuria, and bilateral pelvic and inguinal lymphadenopathy, accompanied by systemic symptoms of fever, malaise, and headache. Healing may occur several weeks later. Many primary genital infections are asymptomatic, however.

Seroprevalence rates among pregnant women have indicated that at least 30% of women have serologic evidence of infection with HSV-2, but that most of these women lack a history or symptoms of infection. Not only was this seroprevalence largely unsuspected among these pregnant women, but asymptomatic viral shedding also occurred among them at a rate (roughly 1% viral shedding at any time in pregnancy) similar to that in women with symptomatic recurrences. Seroprevalence increases dramatically as the number of sexual partners increases. Recurrence is higher among women with genital HSV-2 infection than among women with HSV-1, probably because HSV-2 is more likely than HSV-1 to establish latency in the inguinal dorsal root ganglia. When viral replication is not medically suppressed, there are a median of four HSV-2 recurrences in the first year after a primary infection. HSV-1 recurs about once a year. Finally, for 70% of all women whose infants develop HSV infection, there is no history of infection or symptoms or of intercourse with a partner who has had the infection.

About 10% of HSV-2 seronegative women have HSV-2 seropositive partners. These women may remain uninfected with HSV-2 over prolonged periods despite continued, unprotected contact with a partner who is HSV-2 seropositive.

Because the seroconversion rate is 20% per year for these women, and most genital HSV-2 infections are asymptomatic, these women are at high risk of an unsuspected, primary HSV-2 genital infection during pregnancy.[68] Seroconversion rates are similar among pregnant and nonpregnant women. It is estimated that about one third of women who asymptomatically shed HSV in labor have been recently infected, and that their infants have a 10-fold or more greater risk of being infected than the infants of mothers with recurrent disease.

Women who are seronegative for HSV-1 and HSV-2 and have HSV-1–seropositive partners may acquire HSV-1 genital infection with oral sex. Oral sex has become more popular among teens because they believe it is safer sex. Overall, a woman who is seronegative for HSV-1 and HSV-2 with a discordant partner has a 3.7% chance of acquiring infection with either virus during pregnancy, and a woman who is seropositive for HSV-1 and seronegative for HSV-2 with an HSV-2–seropositive partner acquires HSV-2 infection in 1.7% of pregnancies.[68]

Transmission from mother to infant may occur via many different routes, including transplacental, intrapartum, and postnatal acquisition. Transplacental transmission (5%), responsible for in utero infection, is inferred by the documentation of HSV skin lesions and viremia at birth and by elevated specific cord IgM levels. Primary and recurrent maternal infections have been associated with congenital infection.

Intrapartum transmission is responsible for 85% of neonatal infections. The actual transmission is influenced by the type of maternal infection. A high titer of viral particles ($>10^6/0.2$ mL inoculum) is excreted for about 3 weeks with a primary maternal infection, which is more likely to involve cervical shedding than a recurrent maternal infection, in which 10^2 to 10^3 viral particles per 0.2 mL inoculum are shed for only 2 to 5 days. Maternal neutralizing antibodies may also be partially protective for a newborn in recurrent infections and may not yet be present (and available to cross the placenta) in a primary maternal infection. In a 20-year trial, 0.3% of women were found to be shedding either HSV-1 or HSV-2 asymptomatically at delivery. Neonatal disease resulted in 57% of first episode primary maternal infections (defined as having HSV-1 or HSV-2 isolated from genital secretions without having concurrent HSV antibodies), 25% of first episode nonprimary maternal infections (defined as HSV-2 isolated from genital secretions of a woman with only HSV-1 antibodies, or HSV-1 isolated from a woman with only HSV-2 antibodies), and 2% of recurrent maternal infections (present when the virus isolated from genital secretions was the same type as antibodies present in the serum at the time of labor).[20]

Because recurrent infections are so much more common, half of all neonatal HSV-2 infections occur secondary to recurrent maternal infection, even though transmission from mother to infant occurs in only 2% of the cases. The amount of neutralizing antibody also affects the severity of neonatal disease. Infants who do not receive much transplacental transfer of antibody are more likely to develop disseminated disease. Prolonged rupture of membranes (>4 to 6 hours) also increases the risk of viral transmission, presumably from ascending infection. Delivery via cesarean section, preferably before rupture of membranes, but at least before 4 to 6 hours of rupture, can reduce the risk sevenfold.[20]

Neonatal infection does still occur, however, even with cesarean delivery. Fetal scalp electrodes may accelerate transcervical infection and breach the infant's skin barrier, also increasing risk of infection. It was shown more recently that vacuum extraction may cause scalp lacerations resulting in HSV skin lesions at the site of application. The relative risk of vacuum extraction resulting in HSV infection was nearly 7.5 times that of spontaneous vaginal or cesarean delivery. Antenatal maternal viral culture screening for HSV shedding is of no predictive value in determining who will be shedding virus at delivery.

Finally, transmission may occur postnatally (10%). Restriction enzyme DNA analysis has been used to document postnatal acquisition of HSV and its spread within a nursery by identifying infection with the same herpes strain in infants born to different mothers. The father and the mother and maternal breast lesions have been implicated in neonatal infections. There is also concern regarding symptomatic and asymptomatic shedding among hospital personnel, one third of whom may have a history of HSV-1 lesions, and 1% of whom still have recurrent labial lesions. Individuals with a herpetic whitlow should be removed from the nursery. Removal of health care workers with other lesions would pose significant risk to neonates because it would cause significant disruption of care. Orolabial lesions should be covered with a mask, and skin lesions should be covered with clothing or a bandage. Workers should be counseled on good hand hygiene and not to touch a lesion.

CONGENITAL HERPES SIMPLEX VIRUS INFECTION

Congenital infection was found in 5% of the infants in the National Institute of Allergy and Infectious Disease (NIAID) Collaborative Antiviral Study Cohort.[159] These infants with growth restriction characteristically have skin lesions, vesicles and scarring, neurologic damage (intracranial calcifications, microcephaly, hypertonicity, and seizures), and eye involvement (microphthalmia, cataracts, chorioretinitis, blindness, and retinal dysplasia). Congenital infections are described throughout pregnancy and after primary and recurrent infections, but are most likely with a primary infection, or if the mother has disseminated infection and is in the first 20 weeks of pregnancy. Most cases are due to HSV-2. The manifestations probably result from destruction of normally formed organs, rather than defects in organogenesis, because the lesions are similar to lesions of neonatal herpes. A few children, usually in association with prolonged rupture of membranes, have isolated skin lesions that may be more amenable to antiviral therapy.

NEONATAL HERPES SIMPLEX VIRUS INFECTION

Although asymptomatic HSV infections are common in adults, they are exceedingly rare in neonates. Of all neonatal infections, 20% are caused by HSV-1 rather than HSV-2. Half of the infants are born prematurely, usually between 30 and 37 weeks of gestation, and many have complications of prematurity, particularly respiratory distress syndrome. Two thirds of the term newborns have a normal neonatal course and are discharged before the onset of disease. They may also have simultaneous bacterial infections. One fourth of the infants present on the first day of life, and two thirds present by the end of the first week.

Clinically, neonatal infections are classified as (1) disseminated, involving multiple organs, with or without central nervous system (CNS) involvement; (2) encephalitis, with or without skin, eye, or mouth involvement; and (3) localized to the skin, eyes, or mouth. Approximately 25% of cases are disseminated; 30% have CNS involvement; and 45% are localized to the skin, eyes, or mouth.

Among the 202 infants with HSV infections followed in the NIAID Collaborative Antiviral Study Group, mortality was significantly greater with disseminated infection (57%) than with encephalitis (15%), and did not occur with disease limited to the skin, eyes, or mouth.[159] The relative risk of death was 5.2 for infants in or near coma at onset of treatment, 3.8 for disseminated intravascular coagulopathy, and 3.7 for prematurity.[158] Among infants with disseminated disease, the infants with pneumonitis had a greater mortality. Sequelae among survivors were more common with encephalitis or disseminated infection, particularly with HSV-2 infection, or in the presence of seizures, but also were more likely in infants with skin, eye, or mouth infection who had three or more recurrences of vesicles within 6 months.[158] Sequelae were found in 75% of survivors with HSV-2, and only 27% of survivors with HSV-1 infection, which may be related to the in vitro susceptibility of HSV-1 to acyclovir.[160]

Disseminated Infection

Infants with disseminated infections have the worst prognosis. Disseminated infections may involve virtually every organ system, but predominantly involve the liver, adrenal glands, and lungs. Infants usually present by 10 to 12 days of life with signs of bacterial sepsis or shock, but often have unrecognized symptoms several days earlier. Although the presence of cutaneous vesicles is helpful in diagnosis, 20% of infants never develop vesicles. Disseminated intravascular coagulation with decreased platelets and with petechiae and purpura are common, and bleeding often occurs in the gastrointestinal tract. Pneumatosis intestinalis may also be present. Hepatomegaly or hepatitis, or both, is usually present, with or without jaundice. Respiratory distress, often with pneumonitis or pleural effusion on the chest x-ray, has a poorer prognosis.

Many infants die before manifesting symptoms of CNS involvement, which is common. These infants may present with irritability, apnea, a bulging fontanelle, focal or generalized seizures, opisthotonos, posturing, or coma. Cerebrospinal fluid (CSF) may be normal or may show evidence of hemorrhage. Virus can be isolated from CSF of only one third of infants with CNS symptoms. The routine use of polymerase chain reaction (PCR) on CSF has aided considerably in recognition of disease. Death usually occurs at about 2 weeks of age, roughly 1 week from the onset of symptoms, and often involves respiratory failure, liver failure, and disseminated intravascular coagulation with shock.

Encephalitis

Encephalitis may occur as a component of disseminated disease, via blood-borne seeding of the brain, resulting in multiple lesions of cortical hemorrhagic necrosis often in association with oral, eye, or skin lesions, at 16 to 19 days of life.

Brain involvement results from neuronal transmission of the virus. Regardless of the source of neurologic infection, only about 60% of infants have skin vesicles, and less than half have virus isolated from the CSF. Although the CSF is occasionally normal, it usually shows a mild pleocytosis, with a predominance of mononuclear cells, an elevated protein concentration, and a normal glucose concentration. Lethargy, poor feeding, irritability, and localized or generalized seizures may be the presenting manifestations. Nearly all electroencephalograms have nonspecific abnormalities.

In 12 infants with HSV-2 encephalitis, diffusion-weighted magnetic resonance imaging (MRI) showed extensive, often bilateral changes not visible on computed tomography (CT) or conventional MRI in 8 infants. Disease was found in the temporal lobes, cerebellum, brainstem, and deep gray nuclei. Hemorrhage and watershed distribution ischemic injury were also seen. These areas progressed to cystic changes on follow-up imaging.[152] Nearly half of untreated children die from neurologic deterioration 6 months after onset, and virtually all survivors have severe sequelae (microcephaly and blindness or cataracts).

Fever is a known symptom of HSV infection and is a common reason for an infant to be taken to the emergency department in the first month of life. The American Academy of Pediatrics (AAP) Committee on Infectious Diseases recommends considering HSV infection in neonates with fever, irritability, and abnormal CSF findings, especially in the presence of seizures. In a study of nearly 6000 infants with laboratory-confirmed viral or serious bacterial infections admitted from the emergency department, only 30% of the infants with HSV infections were febrile; 50% were fever free, and 20% were hypothermic. Of the febrile infants with CSF pleocytosis, bacterial meningitis (1.3%) was more common than HSV infection (0.3%), but not statistically so. Similarly, febrile infants with mononuclear CSF pleocytosis were not statistically more likely to have HSV infections (1.6%) than bacterial meningitis (0.8%), and 1.1% of hypothermic infants presenting with a sepsis-like syndrome had HSV infection.[22] All these infants should be considered for HSV infection when presenting in the first month of life, especially if they fail to improve on antibiotics and bacterial cultures remain negative for the first 24 to 48 hours.

Skin, Eye, and Mouth Infections

Infants with disease localized to the skin, eyes, or mouth usually present by 10 to 11 days of life. More than 90% of these infants have skin vesicles, usually over the presenting part at birth and appearing in clusters. Recurrences are common for at least 6 months. Infants at risk should be monitored for localized infections (vesicles) of the oropharynx. Either HSV-1 or HSV-2 can cause keratoconjunctivitis, chorioretinitis, microphthalmos, and retinal dysplasia, later possibly leading to cataracts. One third of these infants later develop neurologic sequelae indicative of undiagnosed neurologic involvement.

DIAGNOSIS

Isolation of virus is definitive diagnostically. Cultures of the newborn (scrapings of mucocutaneous lesions, CSF, stool, urine, nasopharynx, and conjunctivae) should be delayed to 24 to 48 hours after birth to differentiate viral replication in the newborn from transient colonization of the newborn at birth. The specimens for culture may be combined to save money because it is not important where the virus is located, but whether the virus is present, with the exception of CSF specimens, which are needed to determine CNS involvement.[68] If the culture shows cytopathic effects, typing should be done. Serologic testing is not useful in neonatal disease because transplacentally transferred maternal antibody confounds the interpretation. PCR testing has become invaluable, especially for the CSF, which has a very low recovery rate for HSV cultures. PCR can also be used to test blood, scrapings of lesions, the conjunctiva, or the nasopharynx.

THERAPY

Vidarabine was the first antiviral agent used to treat HSV that was efficacious despite the toxicity. When a low-dose acyclovir (30 mg/kg per day in three divided doses) was compared with vidarabine, the morbidity and mortality were equivalent, but the ease of acyclovir administration and decreased toxicity resulted in it readily supplanting vidarabine in use. High-dose intravenous acyclovir (60 mg/kg per day in three divided doses) was then compared with low-dose acyclovir for a longer treatment duration (21 days for disseminated or CNS disease and 14 days for disease localized to skin, eyes, or mouth). High-dose acyclovir resulted in a much improved survival rate: Infants with disseminated infection had an odds ratio of survival of 3.3, and infants with CNS disease had a similar survival. The likelihood of developmentally normal survival had an odds ratio of 6.6 compared with infants treated with the lower dose.[70,71]

Infants with an abnormal creatinine clearance need to have the acyclovir dose adjusted, and all infants need to be monitored for neutropenia. Infants with CNS disease need to have a repeat lumbar puncture at the end of the course of treatment. Treatment should be continued until the CSF is PCR negative. Infants who continue to have detectable HSV DNA in the CSF by PCR at the end of therapy are more likely to die or have moderate to severe impairment. Poor prognostic indicators are lethargy and severe hepatitis in disseminated disease, and prematurity and seizures in CNS disease.[70,71]

Mortality has been tremendously decreased with high-dose acyclovir and is now 29% for disseminated disease; 4% for CNS disease; and 0% for skin, eye, or mouth disease.[70,71] Although the percentage of survivors with normal development (31%) has not changed for CNS disease, normal development among survivors of disseminated disease is now 83%, and for skin, eye, or mouth disease is greater than 98% (Figs. 39-13 and 39-14).[70,71] Neonates with skin, eye, or mouth disease with neurodevelopmental abnormalities on follow-up may represent undetected CNS disease, adverse effects of inflammation secondary to disease, or seeding from recurrent skin lesions.

To improve outcome, earlier recognition and treatment of infection is needed. Initiation of therapy in the high-dose acyclovir trial usually began 4 to 5 days after onset of symptoms, which is no better than occurred in the low-dose trial.[70] Topical ophthalmic antiviral drugs should be given to infants with ocular involvement in addition to parenteral therapy. This may include 1% trifluridine, 0.1% iododeoxyuridine, or 3% vidarabine. All other therapy is supportive.

Oral prophylactic acyclovir therapy after completion of treatment has been used to suppress recurrence in infants

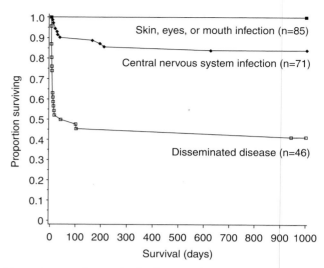

Figure 39–13. Survival of infants with neonatal herpes simplex virus infection, according to the extent of disease. (*From Whitley R et al; National Institute of Allergy and Infectious Diseases Collaborative Antiviral Study Group: Predictors of morbidity and mortality in neonates with herpes simplex virus infections,* N Engl J Med *324:450, 1991.*)

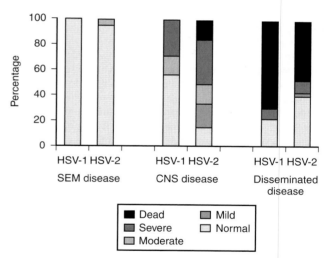

Figure 39–14. Morbidity and mortality among patients after 12 months of age by viral type, 1981-1997. CNS, central nervous system; HSV, herpes simplex virus; SEM, skin, eyes, or mouth. (*From Kimberlin DW et al: Safety and efficacy of high-dose intravenous acyclovir in the management of neonatal herpes simplex virus infections,* Pediatrics *108:223, 2001.*)

with skin, eye, and mouth disease.[67] There is a significant reduction in the recurrence of skin lesions, but it is unclear if this is safe, or if it would prevent neurologic disease. A trial is currently under way.[17,128]

In the United States, increased demand for parenteral acyclovir resulted in a national shortage. The U.S. Food and Drug Administration (FDA) and AAP allowed the Canadian affiliate of APP Pharmaceutical to supply its acyclovir product to the

United States during the shortage because the product differs only in labeling. Intravenous acyclovir remains the drug of choice for neonatal HSV disease and HSV encephalitis, whereas oral acyclovir is the first choice for skin recurrences after HSV disease. If parenteral acyclovir is unavailable, intravenous ganciclovir may be used as a second-line therapy and intravenous foscarnet as a third-line of therapy for neonatal HSV disease or HSV encephalitis. Skin recurrences may be treated with oral valacyclovir.

None of these drugs have been evaluated in controlled trials in neonates for these conditions. Ganciclovir and foscarnet toxicity is significantly greater than with acyclovir and include myelosuppression for ganciclovir and metabolic derangements (hypocalcemia and hypercalcemia, hypophosphatemia and hyperphosphatemia), and possibly irreversible nephrotoxicity for foscarnet.[66] Oral valacyclovir hydrochloride is a prodrug of acyclovir. It is rapidly absorbed via the gastrointestinal tract and converted to acyclovir, reaching higher plasma levels than acyclovir used alone.

PREVENTION

In 1999, the American College of Obstetrics and Gynecology recommended that cesarean delivery be performed if a mother had HSV genital lesions or prodromal symptoms at the time of delivery. Seventy percent of mothers of infants with neonatal disease do not have a history or symptoms of HSV infection, however, and their partners do not have a history of HSV infection, and neonatal infection may still occur even if a cesarean delivery is performed. Repetitive cervical cultures do not predict whether a mother will be shedding virus at delivery. Mothers should be counseled regarding the signs and symptoms of disease, and some may then recognize infection. If rupture of membranes has been present longer than 6 hours, some experts still recommend cesarean delivery in the face of genital lesions, but data are lacking, and controversy exists. Scalp electrodes should be avoided. There is also no consensus for treatment with ruptured membranes in a mother with lesions but a very immature fetus.

If an infant is delivered vaginally to a mother with recurrent genital lesions (5% risk of infection), most experts do not recommend treating the infant. Cultures and PCR of the neonate should be obtained at 24 hours of life, and the infant should be observed carefully. Circumcision should be delayed until cultures are known to be negative. Hand washing should be emphasized. Breast feeding may be allowed if there are no lesions on the breast. The mother needs to be taught the signs and symptoms of neonatal disease because the cultures do not always detect neonatal disease.

Whenever a mother has active genital lesions at the time of the birth of the baby, and she has no history of prior herpetic infection, both a herpes culture and PCR need to be sent, regardless of whether the birth is via Cesarean section or vaginal. Type-specific serology can be used to determine if this is a recurrent infection or if it is a first episode infection. Since the risk of infection to the newborn is greater than 50% in a primary, first-episode infection and 25% in a non-primary, first-episode infection in the mother, these infants should have surface cultures and blood and surface PCR for HSV, serum ALT and CSF cell count, chemistries, and PCR for HSV sent at 24 hours of life, earlier if the baby is ill or premature or had prolonged rupture of membranes. Acyclovir should be started after the evaluation. If it is a recurrent infection, the acyclovir may be discontinued after a negative evaluation. Empiric acyclovir treatment should be considered for 10 days for any first-episode infection, whether primary or non-primary, even if the baby's evaluation is negative. If a CSF infection is suspected, treatment should be continued for 21 days, after which a repeat CSF PCR needs to be sent. Another seven days of acyclovir should be given whenever the PCR is positive for HSV.

There is also considerable controversy concerning the prevention of a primary HSV genital infection in a seronegative pregnant woman. Although some authorities advocate for type-specific serologic screening for HSV in all pregnant women, arguing that many mothers want the information, that they may be counseled against oral or unprotected sex, and that strategies may be devised from the data that are collected, others argue against testing, stating that it is not cost-effective, there is no recommended intervention, and the unexpected positive test can cause significant psychological and social distress. Targeting women for testing who are at high risk for infection misses too many seronegative women. Some treatment strategies do exist, however. It has been shown that the use of condoms in at least 70% of sexual intercourse between a woman seronegative for HSV and a man seropositive for HSV reduced transmission by more than 60%.[68] Antiviral suppression with valacyclovir for 8 months in seropositive male partners reduced the transmission of HSV-2 infection to pregnant women by 48% and symptomatic infection by 75%.[28]

Many obstetricians now routinely recommend antiviral prophylaxis (valacyclovir or acyclovir usually) in the last trimester of pregnancy to suppress viral recurrences. Although no major malformations have been associated to date with the use of acyclovir in pregnancy, the safety to the fetus has not been determined. In a Cochrane Database meta-analysis of third-trimester antiviral prophylaxis, women were less likely to have a recurrence at delivery (relative risk 0.28), a cesarean delivery for genital lesions (relative risk 0.30), and HSV detected at delivery (relative risk 0.14).[55] Although there were no cases of neonatal disease among the infants, there were too few patients to draw a conclusion about neonatal risk. Neonatal infection may occur because viral shedding does still occur. There has been some success in vaccine development for women who are seronegative for HSV-1 and HSV-2, but the trials still need to be performed.

Cytomegalovirus

The cytomegaloviruses are the largest viruses in the herpesvirus family and are noted for their worldwide distribution among humans and animals. The virus is highly species specific, and humans are the only known reservoir for disease among humans. After primary infection, the virus enters a latent state, from which reactivation may frequently occur. Reinfection may also result from any of the thousands of human strains, which are homologous, but not identical. The differing antigenic makeup of the various strains may make it possible to identify the source of the viral infection.

The virus has a double-stranded DNA core surrounded by an icosahedral, or 20-sided, capsid. This capsid is surrounded by amorphous material, which is surrounded by a lipid envelope, probably acquired during budding through the nuclear membrane. The virus is named for the intranuclear and paranuclear inclusions seen with symptomatic disease—cytomegalic inclusion disease. These inclusion bodies often yield an "owl's eye" appearance to the cells. The virus does not code its own thymidine kinase or DNA polymerase, which is important when considering treatment. The virus is cultured in the laboratory only in human fibroblasts, although it replicates in vivo primarily in epithelial cells.

EPIDEMIOLOGY AND TRANSMISSION

CMV is currently the most common intrauterine infection. CMV is responsible for congenital infection in 0.15% to 2% of newborns, and it is a leading cause of deafness and learning disability. Infection is more prevalent in underdeveloped countries and among lower socioeconomic groups in developed countries, where crowding and poor hygiene are more common. Each year, 2% of middle to high socioeconomic class women of childbearing age seroconverts compared with 6% of women from lower socioeconomic groups. Seropositivity also increases with age, breast feeding for more than 6 months, nonwhite race, number of sexual contacts, and parity.

Transmission of CMV requires close contact with contaminated secretions because the virus is not very contagious. The virus can be cultured from urine, cervical secretions, saliva, semen, breast milk, blood, and transplanted organs, and all these sites intermittently excrete virus. Viral excretion is particularly prolonged after primary infection, but also occurs with reactivation of infection. Congenitally infected infants may shed virus for years and serve as a large reservoir for spreading infection to others. Toddlers also may shed the virus for prolonged periods compared with adults, in whom the humoral and cellular defense mechanisms lead to a latent state within a few months.

Transplacental transmission is responsible for congenital infection in 1% of newborns, and intrauterine fetal death may be more likely. Congenital infection may occur after either a primary or a reactivated infection in the mother. Overall, only 5% to 10% of congenital infections are symptomatic, and these are more likely after a primary maternal infection, although symptomatic infections have been reported in women with reactivation infections. Data implicate reinfection as the cause of some of these symptomatic infections. Symptomatic infants have a mortality of 20% to 30%, and two thirds of survivors may have sequelae. The 90% of infants with asymptomatic infection at birth also have a 5% to 15% risk of later sequelae, however.

Even with primary maternal CMV infection during pregnancy, transplacental infection occurs in only 30% to 40% of the fetuses, and only 10% to 15% of these infected fetuses develop symptomatic disease. With recurrent maternal CMV infection during gestation, only 1% to 3% of fetuses are infected. Although transmission seems to be increased in the third trimester, the risk of malformations (which occur during the period of organogenesis) lessens. The fetus may be infected throughout gestation. Infection seems to be more significant in the first half of pregnancy when the virus has considerable teratogenic potential. Neurons migrate from the periventricular germinal matrix to the cortex between 12 and 24 weeks of gestation. This process may be interrupted by infection, resulting in CNS malformations. In the second half of pregnancy, during the period of myelination, white matter lesions may develop, as seen on MRI.[87]

Perinatal infection is responsible currently for an additional 3% to 5% of infections among newborns, resulting from exposure to cervical secretions and blood during delivery or via breast milk. Transmission in early childhood may occur from child to child and from child to other family members. There is also an implication that infection may occur via fomites because virus may survive in urine for hours on plastic surfaces and has been cultured from toys in daycare centers. Nearly half of mothers of premature infants infected in the nursery seroconvert within 1 year and the same proportion of susceptible family members seroconvert when a single family member is infected.

Daycare compounds the problem. There is a 15% rate of infection among parents of children in daycare, particularly if the child is younger than 18 months. Mothers of children in daycare, particularly if they are of middle socioeconomic status and previously seronegative, are at significant risk of developing a primary CMV infection in a subsequent pregnancy; this may account for 25% of symptomatic congenital infections. Seronegative women who work at daycare centers have an 11% seroconversion rate per year, well above any predictable rate, and are at considerable occupational risk.

Similar concern has been expressed about women health care workers and their occupational risk. Although these women are exposed to virus, the data do not support an increased risk of transmission of the virus.

After early childhood, viral transmission seems to be minimal until puberty, when sexual activity begins. Infection rates are highest among adults with multiple sexual partners. An additional risk of infection occurs with blood transfusions and organ transplants to seronegative individuals. Transmission may be prevented by requiring all blood products to come from seronegative donors. Alternatively, the white blood cells carrying the virus may be removed by using frozen, deglycerolized red blood cell transfusions or by using filters to remove the leukocytes. Neither the transfusion method nor using filters completely protects against transmission of virus, however.

CMV transmission via human breast milk feeding has been reported to result in infection in premature infants (<32 weeks' gestation), resulting in a sepsis-like infection. Freeze-thawing of milk does not prevent transmission. Long-term outcome has not yet been determined, but in a report of 40 preterm infants who developed viruria in the nursery, most likely from breast milk feedings, neonatal outcome was not different from that of control infants. The infants exhibited cholestasis, elevation of C-reactive protein, mild neutropenia, and thrombocytopenia, but these symptoms resolved.[102]

MATERNAL CLINICAL MANIFESTATIONS

Most women are asymptomatic during either primary or recurrent infection, and pregnancy does not alter the clinical picture. A mononucleosis-like illness, which is heterophil negative, may develop in 5% to 10% of women. Other manifestations are rare.

ASYMPTOMATIC CONGENITAL INFECTION

Although 85% to 90% of all infants with congenital CMV are asymptomatic at birth, 15% may be at risk for later sequelae. The results of follow-up of 330 infants with asymptomatic infection who were mostly of low socioeconomic status are shown in Table 39-26. The most important sequela seems to be sensorineural hearing loss, which is often bilateral and may be moderate to profound. The presence of periventricular radiolucencies or calcifications on CT is highly correlated with hearing loss. The hearing loss may be present at birth or may appear only after the first year of life, and is frequently progressive, owing to continued growth of the virus in the inner ear. There is a very low risk of chorioretinitis; it may not be present at birth, but may develop later secondary to continued growth of the virus. A further finding may be a defect of tooth enamel in the primary dentition, leading to increased caries. Neurologic handicap may occur, but is uncommon. Premature infants are most at risk.

SYMPTOMATIC CONGENITAL INFECTION

Cytomegalic inclusion disease occurs in only 10% to 15% of infected infants and results in multiorgan involvement, particularly of the reticuloendothelial system and CNS. Death may occur at birth or months later, resulting in an overall mortality of 20% to 30%, usually from disseminated intravascular coagulation, bleeding, hepatic failure, or bacterial infection.

CNS involvement may be diffuse. Infants may be microcephalic, have poor feeding and lethargy, and have hypertonia or hypotonia. They may also exhibit intracranial calcifications of the basal ganglia and cortical and subcortical regions, ventricular enlargement, cortical atrophy, or periventricular leukomalacia. Most commonly, an infant who is small for gestational age or premature has hepatosplenomegaly and abnormal liver function tests. Hyperbilirubinemia, which occurs in more than half of infants, may be transient, but is more likely to be persistent, with a gradual increase in the direct component. Petechiae, purpura, and thrombocytopenia (direct suppression of megakaryocytes in the bone marrow) usually develop after birth and may persist for weeks. Approximately one third of infants with congenital infection are thrombocytopenic, and one third of those have severe thrombocytopenia, with platelet counts less than 10,000/dL. There may also be a Coombs-negative hemolytic anemia. Diffuse interstitial or peribronchial pneumonitis is possible, but less common than with perinatally acquired disease. Table 39-27 lists the clinical findings in 24 newborns with symptomatic CMV infection.

Prognosis

Fowler and colleagues[39] showed that although maternal antibody may not prevent congenital CMV infection, it lessens the severity (Table 39-28). Sequelae were found in 25% of infants after primary infection, but in only 8% after recurrent infection. Likewise, mental impairment (IQ <70), sensorineural hearing loss, and bilateral hearing loss were found in 13%, 15%, and 8% of infants after primary maternal infection, but only 15% of infants born after recurrent maternal infection had sensorineural hearing loss, and none had mental impairment or bilateral hearing loss. These infants also showed the progressive nature of sequelae after primary and recurrent infection (Fig. 39-14).

Ramsay and colleagues[121] looked at the 4-year outcome of 65 neonates with symptomatic congenital CMV in Britain and found a better prognosis than previously reported from

TABLE 39-26	Sequelae in Children after Congenital Cytomegalovirus Infection	
Sequelae	Symptomatic Infection (%)	Asymptomatic Infection (%)
Sensorineural hearing loss	58	7.4
Bilateral hearing loss	37	2.7
Speech threshold, moderate to profound	27	1.7
Chorioretinitis	20.4	2.5
IQ <70	55	3.7
Microcephaly, seizures, or paresis/paralysis	51.9	2.7
Microcephaly	37.5	1.8
Seizures	23.1	0.9
Paresis/paralysis	12.5	0
Death	5.8	0.3

From Stagno S: Cytomegalovirus. In Remington JS et al, editors: *Infectious diseases of the fetus and newborn infant,* 5th ed, Philadelphia, 2001, Saunders, p 408.

TABLE 39-27	Clinical Findings in the First Month of Life in 24 Newborns with Symptomatic Cytomegalovirus Infection after Primary Maternal Infection
Finding	No. (%)
Jaundice	15 (62)
Petechiae	14 (58)
Hepatosplenomegaly	12 (50)
Intrauterine growth retardation	8 (33)
Preterm birth	6 (25)
Microcephaly	5 (21)
Hydranencephaly	1 (4)
Death	1 (4)

From Fowler K et al: The outcome of congenital cytomegalovirus infection in relation to maternal antibody status, *N Engl J Med* 326:663, 1992. Copyright © 1992 Massachusetts Medical Society. All rights reserved.

TABLE 39–28	Sequelae in Children with Congenital Cytomegalovirus Infection According to Type of Maternal Infection		
Sequelae	Primary Infection*	Recurrent Infection*	P Value
Sensorineural hearing loss	15 (18/120)	5 (3/56)	.05
Bilateral hearing loss	8 (10/120)	0 (0/56)	.02
Speech threshold ≥60 dB	8 (9/120)	0 (0/56)	.03
IQ ≤70	13 (9/68)	0 (0/32)	.03
Chorioretinitis	6 (7/112)	2 (1/54)	.20
Other neurologic sequelae	6 (8/125)	2 (1/64)	.13
Microcephaly	5 (6/125)	2 (1/64)	.25
Seizures	5 (6/125)	0 (0/64)	.08
Paresis or paralysis	1 (1/125)	0 (0/64)	.66
Death	2 (3/125)	0 (0/64)	.29
Any sequelae	25 (31/125)	8 (5/64)	.003

*Percentage (number with sequelae/total number evaluated).
From Fowler K et al: The outcome of congenital cytomegalovirus infection in relation to maternal antibody status, N Engl J Med 326:663, 1992. Copyright © 1992 Massachusetts Medical Society. All rights reserved.

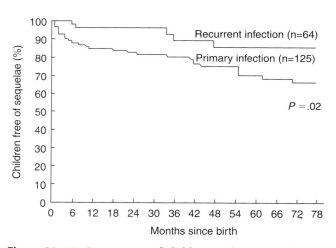

Figure 39–15. Percentages of children with congenital cytomegalovirus infection who remained free of sequelae, according to the type of maternal infection. P value was obtained by log-rank test. (*From Fowler K et al: The outcome of congenital cytomegalovirus infection in relation to maternal antibody status,* N Engl J Med 326:663, 1992.)

the United States (Table 39-29). Overall, the rate of neurologic abnormalities was 45%. Infants who presented with abnormal neurologic findings other than microcephaly had the worst prognosis, with a 73% rate of gross motor and psychomotor abnormalities compared with a 30% rate among children who did not present with neurologic findings. A Japanese study of 33 congenitally infected infants found that abnormal fetal ultrasound abdominal findings (ascites or hepatosplenomegaly) were associated with liver dysfunction and a 53-fold increase in mortality; infants who had no abdominal findings survived.[89] Data are also accumulating that neonatal viral blood load (>1000 copies per 10^5 PMN via quantitative PCR) may also predict infants who will develop sequelae, regardless of whether the infants were symptomatic or asymptomatic after birth.[76]

PERINATAL INFECTION

Mothers with recurrent CMV infection usually transfer significant antibody to the infant in utero. Even if this antibody transfer does not occur, a term infant who acquires infection after birth, denoted a perinatal infection, is usually asymptomatic. Transmission may occur in passage through the birth canal, via breast milk, or secondary to blood transfusion. Breast-feeding infants largely seroconvert. The incubation period is 4 to 12 weeks. Term infants may develop pneumonitis secondary to CMV, and present with cough, tachypnea, congestion, wheezing, and apnea. Although the mortality rate may be 3%, few infants require hospitalization. In contrast, premature infants, often infected through blood transfusion, have a high rate of serious or fatal illness. They also may develop pneumonitis, but with a picture of overwhelming sepsis, hepatosplenomegaly, thrombocytopenia, and neutropenia. There may be an increased risk in these infants of neuromuscular handicaps, although there does not seem to be a higher rate of sensorineural hearing loss, microcephaly, or chorioretinitis.

NEUROLOGIC IMPAIRMENT

Not all infants with symptomatic disease at birth have neurologic impairment. One third of these infants may have a normal neurologic outcome; however, 5% to 15% of asymptomatic infants may have sequelae. Increasing data are correlating abnormal findings on cerebral ultrasound, CT, or MRI with long-term neurodevelopmental or neurosensory sequelae. The numbers of infants per report are small, but collectively all show this correlation.* Of symptomatic infants with abnormal CT findings, 90% had neurodevelopmental or neurosensory sequelae,[13] whereas all infants with abnormal ultrasound findings had either one or more sequelae or death; however, none of 45 infants with normal ultrasound results had long-term sequelae (Table 39-30).[6] MRI may be particularly useful in detecting white matter or gyral abnormalities.[106,148] Finally, a β_2-microglobulin concentration in the CSF also seems to indicate the severity of brain involvement in congenital disease.

HEARING AND VISUAL IMPAIRMENT

Congenital CMV is the most significant cause of sensorineural hearing loss in childhood: 10% to 15% of all infants experience loss, but hearing loss may be detected in 30% to 65% of symptomatic infants.[87] The hearing loss tends to be more severe and to occur earlier in infants with symptomatic infection. The loss can be progressive or fluctuate and may not

---

*References 6, 12, 13, 46, 106, 148.

TABLE 39–29   Outcome of Symptomatic Congenital Cytomegalovirus Infection

| Neonatal Presentation | No. Infants | Normal* | DISABILITY | |
			Motor or Psychomotor*	Sensorineural Deafness*
Group 1	22	6 (27)	14 (64)	2 (9)
Group 2	35	22 (63)	8 (23)	5 (14)
Group 3	8	8 (100)	0	0
All groups	65	36 (55)	22 (34)	7 (11)

Group 1: Abnormal neurologic findings at presentation.
Group 2: Hepatomegaly, splenomegaly, or purpura at presentation without neurologic abnormality.
Group 3: Microcephaly or respiratory problems at presentation without neurologic abnormality.
*Number of infants (percentage).
From Ramsay MEB et al: Outcome of confirmed symptomatic congenital cytomegalovirus infection, *Arch Dis Child* 66:1068, 1991.

TABLE 39–30   Value of Cranial Ultrasound (US) Scanning in Predicting Outcome in 57 Patients with Congenital Cytomegalovirus Infection

| | NO. (%) NEWBORNS WITH POOR OUTCOME | | | | | |
	Normal US Results	Pathologic US Results*	Odds Ratio (95% CI)	P Value	PPV (%)	NPV (%)
DQ ≤85	0/45	8/11 (72.7%)	NE	< .001	72.7	100
Motor delay	0/45	6/11 (54.5%)	NE	< .001	54.5	100
SNHL	3/45 (6.7%)	6/11 (54.5%)	16.8 (3.2-89)	< .001	54.5	93.3
Death or any sequela	3/45 (6.7%)	11/12 (91.7%)	154 (17.3-1219.6)	< .001	91.7	93.3

*One newborn with pathologic US results died during the neonatal period. Follow-up data were available for 11 of the 12 patients who lived.
CI, confidence interval; DQ, developmental quotient; NPV, negative predictive value; NE, could not be estimated; PPV, positive predictive value; SNHL, sensorineural hearing loss.
From Ancora G et al: Cranial ultrasound scanning and prediction of outcome in newborns with congenital cytomegalovirus infection, *J Pediatr* 150:157, 2007.

occur until 6 years of age. Less than half of all neurosensory hearing loss secondary to CMV is detected by newborn screening. The viral burden of the newborn, as determined by PCR of the dried blood spots on Guthrie cards or in the urine or peripheral blood, seems to correlate well with the risk of developing hearing loss and deafness, and may provide a means of determining which infants should receive antiviral therapy.[12,14,154]

Chorioretinitis may be found in 15% to 30% of symptomatic newborns. Children often have impairment or strabismus secondary to chorioretinitis, optic atrophy, or central cortical lesions and macular scarring.

ANTENATAL DIAGNOSIS

Because most women remain asymptomatic with CMV infection, screening for primary infection is necessary to determine risk. CMV IgG, which has high sensitivity and specificity, reliably diagnoses primary infection. Few European or American countries routinely screen for seroconversion, however, because there is no consensus for treatment of either a newly infected pregnant woman or her infant. Detection of CMV IgM may indicate a recent infection, but IgM also increases with reactivation of latent infection. CMV IgG avidity testing may be helpful: the binding capacity or avidity of IgG is low just after an infection and

increases with time. CMV DNA may also be detected during acute infection from the peripheral blood.

If a primary maternal infection is suspected, or ultrasound shows abdominal or cerebral findings or intrauterine growth restriction, fetal diagnosis may be undertaken. Cordocentesis is unnecessary because the sensitivity is lower and the risks are greater than with amniocentesis. CMV may be detected in the amniotic fluid by viral culture or by PCR for CMV DNA with great sensitivity if the amniotic fluid is sampled at 21 to 23 weeks of gestation and at least 5 to 6 weeks after onset of maternal infection.[78] A high viral load seems to correlate with the development of a symptomatic infection and neurodevelopmental sequelae.

NEONATAL DIAGNOSIS

Virus isolation in tissue culture remains the most sensitive and specific test for diagnosis of congenital CMV in newborns. Isolation of virus from an infant within the first 2 to 3 weeks of life confirms the presence of a congenital infection. The virus is usually isolated from urine, but may be isolated from saliva, peripheral blood leukocytes, and other body fluids. Urine specimens should be refrigerated (4°C), but never frozen or stored at room temperature. The recovery rate remains at 93% in urine after 7 days of refrigeration and decreases to 50% after 1 month. Using hyperimmune sera or monoclonal antibodies, early antigens may be detected in tissue culture 24 hours after inoculation.

The diagnosis may also be made from urine, using DNA hybridization or PCR DNA amplification. A fourfold increase in IgG titers in paired sera or a strongly positive IgM anti-CMV may be used to make a presumptive diagnosis. The detection of serum IgM is complicated, however, by frequent false-positive and false-negative findings. As reported earlier, detection of CMV DNA by PCR in peripheral blood or on dried blood spots on Guthrie cards may be prognostic.

TREATMENT

In contrast to other herpesvirus infections, CMV does not induce its own thymidine kinase. Because acyclovir requires thymidine kinase, it has no efficacy in CMV. Ganciclovir has shown efficacy against acquired CMV in patients infected with human immunodeficiency virus (HIV), particularly for retinitis, but has significant toxicity (primarily reversible neutropenia and thrombocytopenia), and there is a high relapse rate after cessation of therapy. Very little is known about its safety and efficacy in neonates.

Kimberlin and coworkers[72] randomly assigned neonates with symptomatic disease to receive 6 weeks of therapy with ganciclovir versus no treatment and followed the hearing with brainstem auditory evoked response. When tested at 6 months, 84% of treated infants maintained normal hearing or improved their hearing, in contrast to 59% of control infants. None of the treated infants had worsening of hearing at 6 months compared with 41% of untreated infants. When tested at 1 year, 21% of treated infants and 68% of control infants had worsening of hearing. Neutropenia was three times more common (63%) in treated infants than in untreated infants. This study raises many questions. It is unknown whether improvement in hearing would be maintained long-term or what the impact of improved hearing is in infants with a high risk of developmental problems. Viral excretion in urine returns to pretreatment levels within 2 weeks after ganciclovir is discontinued, as does viral load. Treatment with ganciclovir can be considered for symptomatic infants, but cannot be routinely recommended.

PREVENTION

Several reports have looked at the pharmacokinetics of a commercial grade valganciclovir oral solution, but the results cannot be extrapolated to the use of currently available drug. The Collaborative Antiviral Study Group has begun a 6-week versus 6-month study of oral valganciclovir to determine if longer viral suppression is more efficacious.[2,69]

Prevention is the most important available means to avoid infection. Women childcare workers, especially when their children are younger than 2 years, need to be counseled about the risks of CMV in pregnancy and taught good hand washing procedures, as do women health care workers, particularly in nurseries. CMV is readily destroyed with soap, detergents, or antiseptics. Good hygiene, including hand washing and not kissing on the mouth, should be actively taught to all pregnant women. Transmission of CMV via blood transfusions may be largely eliminated by the use of blood from antibody-negative donors; by using leukocyte-depletion filters; or by using frozen, deglycerolized red blood cells. Vaccines are being studied for their safety and efficacy, but at present are years away from being clinically available.

When a pregnant woman has been infected with CMV, and her fetus has been diagnosed with infection, few options have existed, apart from abortion. The use of passive immunization with CMV-specific hyperimmune globulin, primarily given intravenously (a few had intra-amniotic injections), is promising. It seems to be safe. Only 1 of 31 infants whose mothers received CMV hyperimmune globulin developed symptomatic disease (37%) compared with 7 of 14 infants of untreated women (50%).[103] In a later study, three infants infected with CMV who had fetal cerebral abnormalities and whose mothers were treated with CMV hyperimmune globulin had regression of ultrasound findings and normal neurodevelopmental outcome at 4 to 7 years of age.[104]

Varicella-Zoster Virus

Varicella (chickenpox) is one of the most highly communicable human diseases. It is the result of a primary infection with VZV, which is one of the human DNA herpesviruses. After infection, latent virus persists in the dorsal root ganglia. The localized rash of herpes zoster results from a reactivation of infection, in which the virus begins to multiply within the ganglia and to propagate down the sensory nerves to its dermatomes.

EPIDEMIOLOGY AND TRANSMISSION

Humans are the only known reservoir of VZV. Immunity is lifelong and widespread. Of young adults, 70% to 80% have a history of chickenpox, and this has been found to be quite reliable. Conversely, only 10% to 20% of individuals lacking a history of chickenpox have been found to be seronegative, even though asymptomatic infection is believed to be unusual. Chickenpox may rarely occur in seropositive individuals, and this has been reported among pregnant women. Most reinfections are mild, however.

The initial protection against VZV depends on IgG. Neonates become ill because they are exposed to high titers of the virus from the mother, yet have an absence of antibody. In contrast, limitation of the severity of the infection and recovery from infection largely depend on cellular immunity, or T cells. Pregnant women are immunosuppressed with decreased T cell immunity, so disease can be very severe.

Chickenpox is seen year-round, with some increase in winter months, and is worldwide in distribution. In household contacts, 90% of susceptible individuals are infected. Transmission of the virus occurs via airborne respiratory droplet spread or via contact with the virus in the vesicular lesions of either varicella or, rarely, zoster. Although it is well documented that susceptible individuals may develop varicella after exposure to zoster lesions, varicella-zoster does not develop after exposure to chickenpox. Transmission may occur from 1 to 2 days before the onset of the rash until all vesicular lesions are dried and crusted, at least 6 days after onset of the rash. The incubation period is 10 to 21 days after exposure, unless the individual has been given varicella-zoster immune globulin, which may delay the onset of the infection for 28 days.

After replication of the virus within the nasopharynx and invasion of the local lymph nodes, there is a transient viremia, which seeds the viscera. Viral multiplication continues, causing a greater viremia and widespread cutaneous involvement. Subsequent viremias result in crops of vesicles, followed by the development of latency within the dorsal root ganglia.

CLINICAL MANIFESTATIONS

After a short prodrome of fever, headache, and malaise, there is a generalized exanthem, which begins on the face and trunk and proceeds centripetally. Recurrent crops of vesicles appear for 2 to 5 days, then crust and scab, usually healing without scarring. Secondary bacterial infection of the cutaneous lesions is the most common complication. Most other complications are rare, including encephalitis, myocarditis, arthritis, and glomerulonephritis.

Varicella pneumonia is the most common cause of mortality. The onset of fever and cough usually occurs within 2 to 4 days after the development of the rash, but may occur later. Radiographic changes consist of diffuse, nodular lesions with perihilar prominence. Dyspnea, cyanosis, rales, and chest pain may be severe, and there may be hemoptysis. Although only 15% of adults develop pneumonia, 90% of all cases of chickenpox pneumonia occur among adults. Immunocompromised individuals are also at increased risk.

VARICELLA IN PREGNANCY

There does not seem to be an increased risk of spontaneous abortion or prematurity as a result of maternal chickenpox, although prematurity and intrauterine growth restriction are common among infants with congenital varicella syndrome. Despite early reports of increased mortality, there is no evidence that chickenpox, in the absence of pneumonia, is more severe in pregnant women than among nonpregnant individuals. Mortality of 40% with chickenpox pneumonia has been reported among pregnant women who did not receive antiviral therapy. Reports of the use of intravenous acyclovir for varicella pneumonia suggest that it may improve the outcome. To date, there have been no congenital anomalies attributed to the use of acyclovir in pregnancy.

Because of the potential for increased mortality, varicella-zoster immune globulin (VZIG) may be useful for passive immunization of a susceptible pregnant woman after a significant exposure to varicella. Controlled trials are unavailable, however. VZIG needs to be administered within 96 hours of exposure and, preferably, after susceptibility has been confirmed serologically. VZIG is available only as an investigational new drug at the time of publication, and may be requested by calling 800-843-7477, a 24-hour number at FFF Enterprises. If VZIG is unavailable, immune globulin intravenous can be used. There are no controlled trials, but the VZV IgG titer can be significant, although the titers vary from preparation to preparation. If VZIG is unavailable, or more than 96 hours have passed since exposure, some infectious disease experts recommend the use of intravenous acyclovir for prophylaxis in a pregnant woman. Uncertainty continues regarding its effect on the fetus. VZIG may not protect the fetus from infection. Likewise, the absence of signs of maternal chickenpox after the use of VZIG does not indicate that the fetus is protected. Ultrasound evaluation revealing a wasted limb may assist in the diagnosis of an infected fetus, although this is, of necessity, a late diagnosis.

CONGENITAL VARICELLA SYNDROME

Maternal varicella has been shown to be teratogenic. Intrauterine infection occurs as a result of hematogenous dissemination across the placenta and can occur even with mild maternal infection.[33,111] The risk is highest (2%) in the first 13 to 20 weeks of gestation, but may occur after 20 weeks. A later maternal infection is more likely to result in less severe fetal manifestations. Before 13 weeks' gestation, the risk is only 0.4%.[48] Although portions of the congenital syndrome have been seen after maternal zoster, the full syndrome has not been seen, presumably because viremia is uncommon with zoster, and some preexisting immunity is present. Theoretically, the fetal lesions result from the development of zoster in utero. Infants born to mothers infected with varicella in pregnancy, yet who did not develop symptomatic congenital infection, have presented with zoster early in life without having been infected with varicella postnatally.

The typical features of the congenital syndrome include cicatricial cutaneous lesions with limb involvement, ocular abnormalities, and severe mental retardation. The condition usually progresses to an early death. The skin lesions usually are over an involved limb, sometimes over the contralateral limb, and are often depressed and pigmented in a dermatomal distribution. Cataracts, microphthalmia, chorioretinitis, cerebral atrophy, seizures, and mental retardation may occur; sometimes bowel and bladder dysfunction also may occur. Hypoplasia of the bone and muscle of a limb is prominent.

Maternal counseling is difficult because the incidence of the syndrome is so low as to preclude routinely recommending abortion. Maternal infection may have a 25% incidence of fetal varicella, but this does not indicate that the fetus will develop congenital varicella syndrome. Similarly, chorionic villus sampling with PCR to show virus and cordocentesis to show fetal VZV IgM indicate only fetal infection, not the development of the congenital syndrome.

The most helpful prenatal test is fetal ultrasound. Although the abnormalities do not develop immediately, most are present before 20 weeks' gestation. Limb abnormalities carry a 50% risk of mental retardation and early death. Hydrocephalus, liver calcifications, hydrops fetalis, and polyhydramnios may also be seen.

PERINATAL CHICKENPOX

Chickenpox is considered congenital when it occurs within the first 10 days of life, and it results from transplacental transmission of the virus from mother to fetus. Maternal varicella, particularly occurring from 5 days before delivery until 2 days after delivery, results in a higher neonatal mortality (20% to 30%) because there has not been enough time for maternal antibody to develop and transfer across the placenta to the fetus. The fetal attack rate is 24% to 50%. The incubation period is shorter—9 to 15 days from the onset of maternal rash to the development of fetal or neonatal disease. Infants may have a very mild infection with few lesions or may have severe disease, with widespread cutaneous and visceral involvement, including encephalitis and hepatitis. Death most often occurs secondary to pneumonia.

Zoster may also occur and represents an intrauterine infection. Dried blood spots from the Guthrie cards of more than 400 children with cerebral palsy were compared with case controls for the presence of neurotrophic viruses as determined by PCR.[42] Although seroprevalence was high even in control infants (nearly 40%), the presence of VZV DNA nearly doubled the risk of cerebral palsy.

Postnatally acquired chickenpox occurs between 10 and 28 days of life. The infection is usually mild and is unlikely to result in death. An outbreak may occur within the neonatal intensive care unit (NICU), but is much less common than in pediatric units.

LABORATORY DIAGNOSIS

Viral isolation from vesicular fluid or other tissues is definitive, but not easy to do. Demonstration of the VZV antigen can be accomplished with immunofluorescence, and PCR can be used to detect VZV DNA. Serologic testing can detect an increase in antibody titer and document infection. The presence of specific IgM usually indicates recent infection, but is an unreliable indicator.

THERAPY AND PREVENTION

The primary approach to varicella should be preventive. With the licensure of the live, attenuated varicella vaccine, it may be possible to immunize women of childbearing age actively before pregnancy. The vaccine seems to protect 85% of individuals vaccinated. Pregnancy should be avoided for at least 1 month after vaccination, but nursing mothers may be immunized. Infants should be vaccinated promptly, as per the immunization schedule, at 12 to 18 months.

VZIG should preferably be given within 96 hours of exposure. It modifies infection, but does not prevent it. Passive immunization should be administered to any infant born to a mother who develops varicella from 5 days before delivery until 2 days after delivery. Because a high dose would be needed, it is not recommended that the mother be given VZIG before the birth for passive immunization of the infant.

Acyclovir is the antiviral drug of choice for any infant with severe or potentially severe chickenpox, whether congenital or postnatal in origin. No acute toxicity has been shown after acyclovir use for neonatal HSV infections, although the dosage for neonatal chickenpox is much higher, and the long-term toxicity is unknown.

Although nosocomial cases of chickenpox are uncommon in the nursery, they may occur. Strict respiratory droplet isolation of any patients with active lesions or in the incubation period needs to be implemented, and only visitors and staff with prior immunity should be allowed in the room. Strict hand washing is a necessity. Postnatal exposure of a term infant 2 to 7 days old should carry little additional risk. Infants with low birthweight or preterm infants may be at considerable risk, however, because they were born before the transfer of maternal antibody across the placenta. All hospitalized exposed preterm infants with birthweight 1000 g or less or gestational age less than 28 weeks should receive VZIG or intravenous acyclovir, regardless of the maternal immune status. Hospitalized, exposed preterm infants who were 28 weeks' gestation or more should receive VZIG or intravenous acyclovir if the mother lacks a reliable history of chickenpox or serologic evidence of immunity. VZIG cannot be used to control the spread of varicella in a nursery because it only modifies, but does not prevent, the development of chickenpox.

Strict preventive measures are also necessary in the delivery and nursery services. If the mother has active lesions of chickenpox at delivery, she must be isolated from patients and staff. If the maternal lesions appear within 5 days before delivery and 2 days after delivery, the infant should be protected further with VZIG. If the mother had chickenpox before delivery, and her lesions have healed, she need not be isolated, but the infant should be, preferably in the mother's room, while in the incubation period. An infant with congenital chickenpox also needs isolation and treatment, but may remain with the mother. If a mother was exposed to chickenpox 6 to 20 days before delivery, and she has no history of chickenpox, she and her infant need to be isolated while it is confirmed by serology whether she is susceptible, and VZIG should be given to the infant if the mother develops lesions within 48 hours of delivery. The mother and infant may be discharged home together. If a mother develops the varicella rash postnatally, the infant has already been heavily exposed, and breast milk antibodies may decrease the severity of the infant's infection.

Epstein-Barr Virus

EBV, a B-lymphotropic herpesvirus, is among the most prevalent of human viruses. More than 95% of pregnant women are seropositive. When EBV infects adolescents, it may cause infectious mononucleosis, but most infections are asymptomatic. Humans are the only natural host for the virus; as is typical of herpesviruses, the virus is excreted intermittently during reactivations for the remainder of the individual's life. Transmission seems to require close, personal contact, via saliva. Infection is endemic year-round. Blood transfusion has also been documented to transmit virus occasionally.

Primary infection is rare during pregnancy because nearly all pregnant women are immune. The virus can be detected in cervical secretions by DNA hybridization. IgG and IgM to the viral capsid antigen can be detected in the acute infection, whereas IgG to the EBV nuclear antigen is detectable during latent infection.

Several studies have associated the occurrence of a primary infection in the first trimester of pregnancy with an adverse outcome, including prematurity, spontaneous abortion, and growth restriction. EBV can cross the placenta and has been shown to cause placental infection, but the pregnancy outcome seems to be normal, with rare cases of congenital anomalies reported.

A case-control study of more than 400 children with acute lymphoblastic leukemia showed an association of maternal infection with EBV at 12 to 14 weeks' gestation.[81] Further study indicated reactivation may also be associated with non–acute lymphoblastic leukemia childhood leukemia.[143] Finally, using quantitative real-time PCR to detect viruses in the tissue of infants who died of sudden infant death syndrome compared with controls, there was a statistical association with EBV and HHV-6[5] and sudden infant death syndrome.

Human Herpesvirus 6 and 7

The role of the T-lymphotropic viruses HHV-6 and HHV-7 in human infection is just emerging because HHV-6 was identified relatively recently in 1986, and HHV-7 was identified even later. They are double-stranded DNA members of the *Roseolovirus* genus of the herpesvirus family. There is only one variant of HHV-7, but two variants of HHV-6, A and B. Reflecting the high seroprevalence in adults, most infants have maternally acquired HHV-6 and HHV-7 IgG antibody, which wanes over the first 6 months of life, at which time these infants become seronegative and more susceptible to infection. HHV-6B infection is common in infants 6 to 12 months old, and most children are seropositive by 2 years of age. HHV-7 is acquired later than HHV-6, but is usually acquired by 5 to 6 years of age. After infection, the virus persists for life and is shed in the saliva, which is recognized as the major source of transmission.

About half of infants with primary HHV-6 infection are afebrile, although infants infected at younger than 6 months of age were more likely to be febrile than infants infected after 6 months.[164] Symptoms were present, however, in more than 90% of cases of primary infection, and one fourth of the infants were diagnosed with infantum subitum (roseola). Persistent and reactivated infection has not been shown to cause illness, but does persist in the brain, and HHV-6 has been implicated in a few cases of meningitis and encephalitis in infants and in children younger than 2 years. It is also associated with status epilepticus in these febrile infants. In a study of hospitalized children with encephalitis or severe febrile seizures, HHV-6B and HHV-7 were shown to be equally responsible for nearly one fifth of the cases in the first 2 years of life.[155]

HHV-6 is the only herpesvirus that can integrate its genome into the human chromosome, and many authorities hypothesized that HHV-6 congenital infection is inherited chromosomally and not transferred across the placenta.[142] There are no cases of congenital HHV-7, which also cannot integrate into the chromosome.[47] About one third of congenital HHV-6 infections are caused by HHV-6A. The remaining two thirds are caused by HHV-6B. All cases seem to be asymptomatic.[47] This is in contrast to later HHV-6 infections in infancy, all of which are due to HHV-6B. Congenital HHV-6 infections can be inherited from the chromosomes of either parent or both. Congenital infection was found in 1% of American infants, a rate similar to other Western European countries.[47]

Diagnosis remains difficult. Indirect immunofluorescence can be used to distinguish HHV-6 from HHV-7 IgG antibody and can be followed in serial titers. Also, antigen detection can be used to determine active HHV-6 and HHV-7 infections.

PARAMYXOVIRUSES

Paramyxoviruses are being increasingly noted as significant causes of human disease. Their spectrum has been greatly expanded with the discovery of human metapneumovirus (hMPV). They are single-stranded, RNA viruses with a lipid envelope. Among the human pathogens, there are two subfamilies. The Paramyxovirinae subfamily includes the parainfluenza viruses (PIV) and the mumps and measles viruses. HMPV belongs to the other subfamily, the Pneumovirinae, along with the related respiratory syncytial virus (RSV).

Parainfluenza Virus

PIV are enveloped RNA viruses in the Paramyxoviridae family. The four antigenic types (1 through 4) belong to the same subfamily as the mumps and measles (rubeola) viruses. Spread occurs through direct contact with infected respiratory secretions, via either respiratory droplets or contact with contaminated secretions on fomites. PIV 3 has been shown to survive for at least 10 hours on nonabsorptive surfaces (countertops) and 4 hours on absorptive surfaces, such as hospital coats, but die within minutes on finger pads.[7,16] Infection may occur year-round, but seasonal or nosocomial outbreaks also occur. PIV 1 and 2 outbreaks of croup or other respiratory illnesses tend to occur in the fall, whereas PIV 3 outbreaks are more likely in the spring and summer.

Nearly everyone is infected with all PIV types by 5 years of age. PIV 3, the most common cause of respiratory illnesses of all the serotypes, is also the most common type in infants younger than 12 months of age, infecting about half of them in that first year.[157] PIV 3 seems to spare infants in the first 4 months of life, owing to the presence of transplacentally acquired neutralizing antibodies, but it is the usual source of nosocomial nursery outbreaks, spread via health care workers.[43,92,99] Older, convalescing preterm infants seem to be at increased risk of severe disease in nursery outbreaks, consistent with waning levels of maternally acquired antibody.[99] The incubation period is 2 to 6 days, and virus may be shed for 3 weeks or more from infected infants. Immunity is incomplete, so reinfection may occur with all of the serotypes, but mostly only cause mild upper respiratory infections.

Parainfluenza infections have been regarded as second in frequency to RSV as a cause of respiratory infections. Rhinovirus seems to be more common in respiratory infections, however, and the more recently discovered hMPV is also probably more common than parainfluenza. As a group, PIV are responsible for upper respiratory infections, laryngotracheitis (croup), bronchiolitis, and pneumonia. PIV 1 and 2 are more likely to cause croup, whereas PIV 3 is highly associated with bronchiolitis and pneumonia, particularly in infants and young children. Respiratory infections from PIV may be difficult to differentiate clinically from infections caused by RSV. In young children and infants, they tend to be mild and have a very low mortality. Infected children may require supplemental oxygen, but rarely need ventilatory support. A few infants are asymptomatic. PIV have been identified as a cause of 13% of community-acquired pneumonia in infants.[80] Coinfection with other respiratory viruses may occur in 20% to 60% of infants and may worsen the severity of the infection.[26] In newborns, the infection is more similar to a severe RSV infection. Infants may have apnea, bradycardia, and pneumonia and there may be worsening of chronic lung disease.[43,92,99,157]

PIV may be diagnosed by isolating the virus from nasopharyngeal secretions; by rapid antigen detection techniques, such as immunofluorescent detection; and by PCR antigen detection. Serologic detection is not helpful. Prevention of nosocomial infections requires strict adherence to contact and respiratory precautions and strict hand washing. Severely ill infants must be monitored closely for oxygenation and need of ventilation. Severe laryngotracheobronchitis has been treated with epinephrine and corticosteroid aerosols, which decrease symptom severity and duration of hospitalization. Antibiotics may be used if there is bacterial superinfection.

Mumps

The mumps virus is another paramyxovirus, and humans are the only natural host. The virus is transmitted via respiratory droplets, saliva, and fomites. The incubation period ranges from 7 to 23 days, but is generally 14 to 18 days. The virus is readily isolated from saliva, urine, and CSF. Diagnosis is made by showing an increasing antibody titer. Respiratory isolation of any individual within the incubation period or with active mumps is recommended.

Clinically, the virus causes a prodrome of fever, malaise, and myalgia, usually followed by salivary gland swelling within 24 hours, then resolving within 1 week. The parotitis is usually bilateral and more often involves the parotid glands than the submaxillary glands; the sublingual glands are involved only rarely. Orchitis may rarely develop in infancy, but is usually found only in postpubertal boys, and rarely causes sterility. Likewise, aseptic meningitis and pancreatitis are uncommon complications usually found in older children. CSF pleocytosis is common, even without CNS symptoms. Finally, infection may be asymptomatic. Therapy is nonspecific and supportive.

There is no evidence that mumps is either more common or more severe among pregnant women compared with nonpregnant women. Deaths are exceedingly rare. Siegel and Fuerst[131] found no significant increase in risk of low birthweight among infants born to mothers with mumps when studied prospectively. In contrast, there is a considerable increase in the risk of a first-trimester (but not a second-trimester or third-trimester) abortion; the risk can be 27% among women with first-trimester mumps compared with a risk of 13% for uninfected, control women.

Although there have been multiple reports of birth anomalies after mumps in pregnancy, proof of association has been lacking, and studies using controls failed to find any increase in congenital malformations. There has been considerable discussion about a possible association of gestational mumps and infants with endocardial fibroelastosis. Statistical evidence is lacking, however, and the issue remains debatable.

Congenital and postnatal cases of mumps are exceedingly rare, and nearly always subclinical or very mild. Mumps as a cause of parotitis or aseptic meningitis is rare; even mothers with active mumps rarely infect their infants. There have been a few cases of mumps pneumonia in infants causing severe respiratory distress and death. There have been no reports of nosocomial epidemics of mumps in the nursery; transmission within the hospital is possible, although rare.

Rubeola (Measles)

The measles virus is also a paramyxovirus, has an RNA core and a lipid envelope. Humans are the only natural hosts.

TRANSMISSION

Rubeola is the most infectious of the childhood viral illnesses. It is most commonly found in late winter and in spring in temperate climates. The virus is usually transmitted via respiratory droplets, but may be airborne. Individuals are infectious from the onset of the prodrome (3 to 5 days before onset of the rash) until 4 days after the onset of the exanthem. The incubation period is usually 10 to 12 days, but it is difficult to recognize the time of exposure because patients are infectious during the prodrome. There is a 5% vaccine failure rate in individuals who receive only a single dose of the vaccine, and most endemic cases in the United States occur in these individuals with waning immunity or in infected individuals who have just entered the United States.

Transplacental, hematogenous transmission may also occur. In this instance, the fetus may have onset of disease virtually simultaneously with the mother, implying a large enough initial viral titer so as not to require further viral replication and viremia in the fetus.

LABORATORY DIAGNOSIS

Although the virus may be cultured from nasopharyngeal secretions, blood, urine, or other specimens, it is difficult to isolate, so most diagnoses are made by serology. A significant increase in IgG antibody concentration can be used if acute and convalescent sera are obtained, but, most commonly, serum IgM titers are used. IgM may stay elevated for at least 1 month after the onset of the rash.

CLINICAL MANIFESTATIONS

Clinically, the prodrome of measles begins with fever, cough, coryza, and conjunctivitis (with photophobia) and ends with the development of myriad Koplik spots, tiny, red-ringed white spots on the buccal mucosa. The maculopapular exanthem then begins over the head and neck, spreading to the trunk and upper extremities, then to the lower extremities, and finally fading in the same order over 7 to 10 days.

Measles pneumonia, often complicated by bacterial superinfection, is the most serious complication and is the usual cause of death in children younger than 1 year. The mortality in the United States is only 0.1%, however. Measles encephalitis, leading to drowsiness, seizures, and coma, is uncommon, but may occur in newborns and has a mortality of 11% and the potential for significant morbidity. Otitis, croup, purpura, myocarditis, and subacute sclerosing panencephalitis may also occur.

EFFECTS ON THE PREGNANT WOMAN

The clinical course of rubeola in either a pregnant or postpartum woman is the same as in a nonpregnant woman. The earliest reports of overwhelming pneumonia (often associated with congestive heart failure) caused by infection during pregnancy were tempered by many others in which maternal morbidity and mortality were not increased. In the measles epidemic in the United States from 1988-1991, infection during pregnancy was again associated, however, with the more serious complications of pneumonia and hepatitis. The mortality was 3% to 8%.

EFFECTS ON THE FETUS

Measles during pregnancy does not seem to be teratogenic because few to no malformations have been reported among infants born to mothers infected during epidemics. There are reports of fetal losses with infection during pregnancy. Measles also seems to be responsible for premature delivery, and these deliveries occur during or shortly after the acute illness. Some infants have experienced growth restriction.

PERINATAL MEASLES

Perinatal measles includes infections acquired transplacentally and infections acquired postnatally. Infection is assumed to be transplacental in origin if it occurs before 10 days of life. Most infants born to mothers with measles at or just before delivery remain uninfected, however, and are later susceptible to disease. The disease itself may be mild, but may also be fatal, and is often associated with pneumonia, particularly among infants born prematurely. Postnatally acquired rubeola is usually mild with minimal mortality. Of great concern are more recent reports of infants infected with measles before 2 years of age who have gone on to develop subacute sclerosing panencephalitis without the prolonged incubation period normally seen. They become ill with rapidly progressive disease before 5 years of age.[30]

THERAPY AND PREVENTION

The therapy for measles is usually symptomatic. No specific antiviral therapy is available. Ribavirin is not licensed for use in the treatment of measles. Vitamin A is recommended in regions where vitamin A deficiencies are recognized, or where the mortality of measles is greater than 1%. Some infants and children in the United States have vitamin A deficiencies. Infected patients should be isolated, and the isolation should include precautions against airborne transmission. Exposed, unimmunized individuals may be given measles vaccine, which sometimes affords protection.

Nonimmunized pregnant women and newborns who have no history of rubeola and who are exposed should be given immune globulin, 0.25 mL/kg preferably within 72 hours of exposure. The live attenuated measles vaccine should be administered to infants at 12 to 15 months of age, when maternally transferred antibodies are beginning to wane. The dose should be repeated at school entry to ensure that individuals with waning immunity are protected. The vaccine is contraindicated in pregnancy. Susceptible women who deliver in the incubation period or with rubeola need to be isolated from their infants if the infant is not born with a rash. Only immune staff and visitors may be allowed in the room. Immune globulin should be given to the mother and infant, preferably within 72 hours of exposure or immediately after delivery, if no rash is present. If siblings at home have measles when a susceptible mother and infant are discharged, the mother and infant should receive immune globulin.

True prevention of rubeola lies in maintaining a highly immune status in the population. This maintenance of immunity necessitates second vaccine doses to young adults, which is particularly important now that women are becoming pregnant at an older age, at which time their immunity may be waning, especially if they received only a single vaccination as a child. It has also been shown that preterm infants, born before 32 weeks' gestation, have very low levels of transplacentally transferred antibody, and are susceptible to infection by 6 months postnatally. Extremely preterm infants vaccinated at 15 months of age show an antibody response that is similar to that of term infants, however. It is particularly important that pediatricians continue to emphasize to their patients' families that MMR vaccination has *never* been shown to have a causal relationship with autism, despite the performance of numerous very large studies.

Respiratory Syncytial Virus

RSV is now recognized to be the most common respiratory pathogen in infants and children, infecting nearly all children by 2 years of age and reinfecting about 50% of children each year. In the United States, about 2% to 3% of infants younger than 1 year are admitted to the hospital with bronchiolitis, and most of them (60% to 70%) are infected with RSV. The mortality is roughly 2 per 100,000 infants. RSV usually causes a mild upper respiratory infection, but may be responsible for severe pneumonia and bronchiolitis, especially in high-risk populations. RSV usually occurs in the winter to early spring months in temperate climates, with a few relatively isolated infections during the rest of the year. This season overlaps that of other respiratory viral pathogens, so coinfections are common (about 20%). It is unclear how this affects disease severity. HMPV has roughly the same season as RSV and is increasingly being found to coinfect with RSV, now that it can be identified, but rhinovirus and adenovirus are also commonly found with RSV; influenza, parainfluenza, and newer coronaviruses are found less commonly. Infection is predominant in tropical climates during the rainy season.

RSV is a single-stranded, enveloped RNA paramyxovirus that can be divided into A and B types and divided further into subtypes. Both types may be present during epidemics, although one type is usually predominant. Although viral load seems to correlate with severity of infection, the subtype does not seem to correlate with severity, clinical course, or outcome. Because there is a 50% sequence divergence between type A and type B, infection with one type does not protect against infection with the other. Also, immunity is incomplete, and reinfection commonly occurs among infants, children, and adults. The viral genome encodes for 10 different proteins. Two surface proteins are particularly important. The fusion (F) protein is similar in all strains. It is responsible for the cell fusion, or syncytium, for which the virus is named. The G glycoprotein is an attachment protein, and it is responsible for the strain differences.

A few infants are infected with RSV during the first 3 weeks of life when levels of transferred maternal neutralizing antibody are at their highest. Infants with the highest antibody concentrations may have less severe infections. The effect of antibody in breast milk is inconsistent.

TRANSMISSION

Transmission of RSV most commonly occurs by direct contact with infected secretions from hand to nose or eye. Humans are the only source of the virus. Hospital staff play a major role in nosocomial spread of RSV via this mechanism, which can be addressed effectively with good hand washing. Transmission may also occur via aerosolized droplets or via fomites because live virus may be isolated for 1/2 hour from skin, 2 hours from gowns and gloves, and 1 day from glass or plastic. Viral shedding usually occurs over 3 to 8 days, but may last for weeks in high-risk or immunocompromised children. Incubation may be 2 to 8 days. Nursery epidemics have been described for RSV bronchiolitis and pneumonia, some simultaneously with parainfluenza and rhinovirus. In such epidemics, a third of the nursery staff may be infected, and this may be the cause of much of the spread within the nursery.

CLINICAL MANIFESTATIONS

Children in high-risk groups, particularly children who have pulmonary hypertension, heart disease, and lung disease, have a greater likelihood of severe disease, hospitalization, and mortality. Premature infants are particularly likely to require hospitalization if they have bronchopulmonary dysplasia, but are still 10 times more likely to be rehospitalized than term infants with RSV even if they do not have chronic lung disease. They are also more likely to be rehospitalized with RSV disease if they are discharged between September and December. Children with cyanotic or complex congenital heart disease are noted to have a higher mortality, and children who are immunocompromised or have cystic fibrosis are more likely to have severe disease, a higher mortality, and pneumonia. Long-term corticosteroid therapy seems to prolong the duration of viral shedding, and has not been shown to decrease the severity of disease. Finally, healthy infants younger than 6 weeks of age are more likely to develop lower respiratory tract infection, have a prolonged hospitalization, and require intensive care.

There have been numerous studies to determine risk factors for infection with a fair amount of variation in results. Because 3% to 5% of all infected infants are born at 33 to 35 weeks' gestation, the cost of administering palivizumab to all is prohibitive, and palivizumab is usually limited to infants at higher risk. High risk factors include preterm birth, chronic lung disease of prematurity, postnatal age of less than 6 to 10 weeks at the onset of the RSV season, congenital heart disease, neurologic disease, and immunodeficiency. Most studies report increased risk from other children, but this is variously documented as having two or more siblings, having school-age siblings or preschool-age siblings, or attending daycare.

Some reports find disease associated with the adverse effects of maternal prenatal smoking on lung growth and development in the fetus, whereas others indicate a worse effect secondary to smoking within the home. In the United States, Hispanic infants and Native American and Alaskan infants are more likely to be hospitalized than infants in the general population. Other reported risk factors include small for gestational age (<10% birthweight), male gender, multiple birth, cystic fibrosis, and family history of eczema. Reports vary concerning a family history of asthma or the effects of breast feeding.[15,37,119,125,126]

Young infants with infection may be asymptomatic. When symptoms occur, they are often nonspecific or are mild upper respiratory symptoms, such as a clear nasal discharge, cough, and coryza. Some infants have presented with respiratory arrest secondary to apnea. Others have simply developed bradycardia. Dyspnea, cyanosis, pulmonary infiltrates on chest radiograph, wheezing, respiratory decompensation, and fever all are well described. About two thirds of young children develop bronchiolitis, and one third develop pneumonia. Very premature infants may have minimal respiratory symptoms at first and may simply present with poor feeding, irritability or lethargy, and apnea. Fifty percent of infants may also have otitis media.

Although most febrile infants with bronchiolitis have a low risk of concurrent bacterial infection, the risk is significantly higher in preterm infants. Resch and colleagues[123] reported that 9.5% of infants born at less than 37 weeks' gestation had concurrent bacterial infections compared with 3.1% of term infants. Hospital stay was more than doubled. Infections tend to be in the urinary tract and tracheal aspirate, and some occur in the bloodstream.

The diagnosis is usually made rapidly from anterior nasopharyngeal or nasal swabs using immunofluorescent and enzyme immunoassay techniques that have a variable sensitivity, depending on the assay used. Culture of secretions or lung biopsy is possible, but results in a delayed diagnosis. Serologic testing is of limited value, particularly in young infants. PCR may also be used to detect antigen. Infections with parainfluenza, rhinovirus, adenovirus, and hMPV may mimic RSV infection in an infant.

SUBSEQUENT RESPIRATORY MORBIDITY

Infection with RSV, particularly in the first year of life, in term infants may result in chronic respiratory sequelae; this has been documented consistently in all clinical studies.[138] Term infants hospitalized for RSV bronchiolitis are three times as likely to have recurrent wheezing and 10 times more likely to need bronchodilators at 10 years of age.[105] Likewise, the prevalence of asthma at $7\frac{1}{2}$ years of age was 30% among infants hospitalized for RSV bronchiolitis, but only 3% in controls.[132] In contrast, the incidence of asthma as a diagnosis is significantly less (50%) among 7-year-olds who had two or more uncomplicated upper respiratory infections, or "colds," before 1 year of age.[57,73,138] RSV bronchiolitis in the first year of life increases the likelihood of recurrent wheezing, but may or may not increase atopy.[52] The incidence of recurrent wheezing seemed to decrease in the longer duration studies, but there may be some abnormalities in pulmonary function even in adults. It is unclear why these infants are more predisposed to recurrent wheezing. Severe infection may be a marker for a genetic predisposition, or RSV bronchiolitis may induce long-term changes in the lungs when infection occurs at a certain developmental stage.[73]

Preterm infants are more likely to be infected with RSV and to develop more severe lower respiratory tract disease than term infants. Preterm infants, particularly if they develop chronic lung disease of prematurity, have smaller airways and are more likely to become obstructed with mucus, necrotic tissue, and edema. They are also more likely to have immature immunity and to lack significant maternal transfer of antibodies. Likewise, term infants with abnormal pulmonary function resulting in a smaller size of the airways are predisposed to developing severe lower respiratory tract infection with RSV. Similarly, Broughton and colleagues[18] showed that preterm infants with increased respiratory resistance at discharge from the NICU at 36 weeks' corrected gestational age were more likely to develop symptomatic RSV infections. On follow-up at 1 year of age, preterm infants who had RSV infections have significantly higher airway resistance, but similar lung volume, as controls.[19] Finally, preterm infants treated with palivizumab who were not hospitalized for RSV were less likely to develop recurrent wheezing (13%) compared with all preterm infants who did not receive palivizumab (26%) and compared with untreated preterm infants who were also not hospitalized for RSV (23%).[134]

PROPHYLAXIS AND THERAPY

The primary treatment for RSV infection is supportive care and includes oxygen therapy to correct hypoxemia, mechanical ventilation as needed, and hydration. Care must be taken to prevent hyponatremia because infants with bronchiolitis have elevated levels of antidiuretic hormone. Bronchodilators are frequently used. A Cochrane review of eight randomized trials of bronchodilators showed a significant improvement in clinical scores, but no improvement in oxygenation or rates of hospitalization.[64] Likewise, nebulized epinephrine has not been shown to be beneficial. Corticosteroids are not recommended for bronchiolitis in infants. Palivizumab is also not recommended for treatment of infection because it has not shown any efficacy.

A Cochrane review of 12 trials lacked the power to provide firm conclusions regarding the use of ribavirin. Three small trials within the 12 studies may indicate reduced days of mechanical ventilation and hospitalization and, possibly, recurrent wheezing,[149] but this was unclear. Weighing against these findings are the cost of treatment and potential toxic risks to the patient and staff, so ribavirin use is extremely limited, or it is not used at all. Inhaled nitric oxide and extracorporeal membrane oxygenation have been used for respiratory failure. Most infants do not need antibiotic coverage; possible exceptions are infants needing intensive care and preterm infants.

Infected infants should be isolated with contact precautions. Use of gowns and gloves supplemented with mask and goggle use has decreased hospital spread. Staff members should not care for infected and uninfected infants simultaneously. The education of staff and family must include hand washing before and after patient care. In the event of an epidemic, there should be laboratory screening for RSV infection and segregation of infected and uninfected patients and staff. There are no data on the use of RSV immune globulin in an epidemic.

The primary defense against RSV infection should be avoidance of high-risk settings. The families of all high-risk infants should be instructed in avoidance behavior and careful hand washing.

RSV immune globulin intravenous was made from donors who have high serum titers of neutralizing antibody to RSV and was licensed in 1996 by the FDA for prophylaxis of severe lower respiratory tract disease in children younger than 2 years of age at high risk because of bronchopulmonary dysplasia or preterm birth at 35 weeks' gestation or less. It is no longer available, having been replaced by palivizumab.

Palivizumab, a humanized mouse monoclonal IgG$_1$ antibody, was licensed by the FDA in 1998. The product consists of 95% human amino acids and 5% mouse amino acids. The mouse sequence for antigen binding was grafted to gene segments coding for human IgG; this prevents an antimouse reaction on repeated use. This antibody binds to the F protein of the virus and is active against A and B viral strains. It is given intramuscularly every 30 days, beginning in early November, for a total of five doses, at a dose of 15 mg/kg. Efficacy is similar to that of RSV immune globulin intravenous (a 55% reduction in hospitalizations because of RSV in high-risk infants),[58] but it does not prevent otitis media or hospitalizations for other respiratory viruses. It is much

easier to administer.[45] There was no increase in adverse effects over controls. Also, palivizumab does not interfere with other vaccinations. It is not effective, and not approved, for treatment of RSV infections.

A trial of palivizumab for infants with acyanotic and cyanotic congenital heart disease showed a 45% reduction in RSV hospitalizations (9.7% versus 5.3%) with the larger decrease in infants with acyanotic lesions.[35] Adverse events and deaths were similar in treated infants compared with infants who received a placebo. Also, a 58% reduction in palivizumab serum concentrations was noted after cardiopulmonary bypass.

In Spain among infants less than 33 weeks' gestation, the rate of rehospitalization was at least 13.4% for lower respiratory disease because of RSV, when the infants did not receive any RSV prophylaxis. In addition, 11% of the infants were rehospitalized twice in 1 year for RSV. Prophylaxis for RSV should be continued for the entire season, even after the infant has been infected during the season. Cost-benefit analyses vary widely, but prophylaxis with palivizumab is very expensive, to the point that the cost is prohibitive for prophylaxis of all preterm and other at-risk infants. Recommendations for prophylaxis vary from country to country depending on population data.

The AAP recommends RSV prophylaxis for the following[94]:

1. Infants and children younger than 2 years old with chronic lung disease of prematurity who have required medical therapy (oxygen, bronchodilator therapy, diuretics, or steroids) within the 6 months before the onset of the season. These children may receive a maximum of five monthly doses. This may extend to two seasons, although the efficacy of treatment for a second season is not proven.
2. Infants born before 32 weeks' gestational age (31 weeks, 6 days, or less), even in the absence of chronic lung disease of prematurity.
   a. Infants born at or before 28 weeks, 0 days' gestational age, may benefit in their first season, whenever it occurs in the first 12 months of life.
   b. Infants 29 to 32 weeks' gestational age may benefit when they are 6 months of age or younger at the beginning of the season (a maximum of five monthly doses).
3. Infants who are 32 weeks and 0 days' gestational age to 34 weeks and 6 days at birth, and younger than 3 months of age at the start of the RSV season, and either attend daycare or have a sibling younger than 5 years of age.
   a. These infants may receive a maximum of three monthly doses, so that they are protected when they are at greatest risk for hospitalization.
   b. Table 39-31 provides a guideline for use of palivizumab.
4. Children who are 24 months or younger who have hemodynamically significant cyanotic and acyanotic congenital heart disease. Infants most likely to benefit include:
   a. Infants receiving medication for congestive heart disease.
   b. Infants with moderate to severe pulmonary hypertension.
   c. Infants with cyanotic heart disease.

TABLE 39–31 Maximal Number of Palivizumab Doses for Respiratory Syncytial Virus (RSV) Prophylaxis of Preterm Infants without Chronic Lung Disease, Based on Birth Date, Gestational Age, and Presence of Risk Factors*

Month Of Birth	MAXIMAL NUMBER OF DOSES		
	<28 Weeks, 6 Days' Gestation and <12 Months of Age at Start of Season	29 Weeks, 0 Days through 31 Weeks, 6 Days' Gestation and <6 Months of Age at Start of Season	32 Weeks, 0 Days through 34 Weeks, 6 Days' Gestation, and with Risk Factor[†]
Nov. 1–Mar. 31 of previous RSV season	5[‡]	0[§]	0[¶]
April	5	0[‡]	0[¶]
May	5	5	0[¶]
June	5	5	0[¶]
July	5	5	0[¶]
August	5	5	1[¶]
September	5	5	2[¶]
October	5	5	3[¶]
November	5	5	3[¶]
December	4	4	3[¶]
January	3	3	3[¶]
February	2	2	2[¶]
March	1	1	1[¶]

*Shown for areas beginning prophylaxis on November 1. If infant is discharged from the hospital during RSV season, fewer doses may be required.
[†]Risk factors: infant attends childcare or has a sibling <5 years old.
[‡]Some of these infants may have received one or more doses of palivizumab in the previous RSV season if discharged from the hospital during that season; if so, they still qualify for up to five doses during their second RSV season.
[§]Zero doses because infant will be >6 months old at beginning of RSV season.
[¶]Zero doses because infant will be >90 days of age at beginning of RSV season.
[¶]On the basis of the age of patients at the time of discharge from the hospital, fewer doses may be required because these infants will receive one dose every 30 days until 90 days of age.
American Academy of Pediatrics: Respiratory Syncytial Virus. In: Pickering LK, Baker CJ, Kimberlin DW, Lang SS, eds. Red Book: 2009 Report of the Committee on Infectious Diseases. 28th ed. Elk Grove Village, IL: American Academy of Pediatrics 566, 2009.

The AAP also recommends:

1. The RSV season usually begins in November or December, peaks in January or February, and ends in March or April. In the United States, the season tends to start the earliest in the South and the latest in the Midwest, but timing and severity may vary from year to year. When palivizumab is begun in early November and continued for five total doses, the infant has protective serum levels beyond the 20 weeks of treatment. The use of any additional dose is costly and not recommended.
2. The influenza vaccine should be given after 6 months of age before and during the influenza season.
3. Infants who have had cardiopulmonary bypass for surgical procedures experience a 58% decrease in serum levels and should be redosed as soon as they are medically stable.
4. There is no increased RSV risk in the following circumstances, and palivizumab is not indicated:
   a. Infants with hemodynamically insignificant heart disease, including:
      (1) Secundum atrial septal defect.
      (2) Small ventricular septal defect.
      (3) Pulmonic stenosis.
      (4) Uncomplicated aortic stenosis.
      (5) Mild coarctation of the aorta.
      (6) Patent ductus arteriosus.
   b. Infants with lesions adequately corrected surgically, unless still needing medication for congestive heart failure.
   c. Infants with mild cardiomyopathy, not receiving medical therapy.
5. Palivizumab has not been evaluated in randomized trials for immunocompromised children, so specific recommendations cannot be made. Prophylaxis may benefit a child with severe immunodeficiency, however.
6. Palivizumab is not effective in treating RSV disease or licensed for treatment of infection.
7. Prophylaxis should be continued even if a child experiences a breakthrough RSV infection during the season because some infants have been hospitalized more than once in a season for RSV lower respiratory tract infection. Also, multiple RSV strains may circulate during the same season.

8. The drug should be used within 6 hours of opening the vial because there is no preservative.
9. Patients with cystic fibrosis may be at increased risk of RSV infection, but the effectiveness of palivizumab is unknown.
10. If an RSV outbreak occurs in a high-risk unit, proper infection control measures should be used. Data do not support the use of palivizumab.
11. Palivizumab does not interfere with the responses to other vaccines.

Efforts toward development of a vaccine for active prevention of disease have been hampered by the results of the trial of the formalin-inactivated RSV vaccine, in which vaccinated infants had more severe disease and were more likely to die than nonvaccinated infants, possibly because the vaccine interfered with the secretory and neutralizing antibody response to the virus, allowing more active replication.

Human Metapneumovirus

Discovered in Holland in 2001, hMPV is an enveloped, negative-sense RNA virus of the Paramyxoviridae family, in the same subfamily with and sharing many clinical characteristics of RSV. There are four major genotypes: A1, A2, B1, and B2. All four genotypes circulate simultaneously throughout the season, but in varying proportions. It is unclear what effect this simultaneous circulation has on immunity, and whether certain genotypes are more virulent than others. hMPV is difficult to grow in the laboratory and has escaped detection, but can now be identified by PCR.

A large proportion of previously unidentifiable causes of respiratory tract disease in children and adults have been attributed to hMPV, and it is associated with upper and lower tract disease. Virtually all children are infected by 5 years of age,[8] and infection may be recurrent throughout life. hMPV seems to be second only to RSV as a cause of bronchiolitis in children younger than 1 to 2 years of age.[21] Although RSV is most common in infants younger than 6 months of age, hMPV is more common in infants 6 to 12 months old.[40,108] hMPV occurs in epidemics, mostly in the winter and spring months, and overlaps seasonally with RSV. It may cause a coinfection with other respiratory viruses.[86] During epidemics, bronchiolitis may be caused by RSV or hMPV alone or together, and various other respiratory viral pathogens have been reported as coinfections. Under these circumstances, disease severity has variably been reported as more severe or unchanged. hMPV is also present in smaller numbers year-round. The virus is worldwide in distribution. Humans are the only known source of infection.

In one study of nasal wash specimens obtained over a 25-year period from newborns to 5-year-olds, hMPV was responsible for 20% of previously virus-negative lower respiratory tract infections, indicating that 12% of lower respiratory tract infection in these children (newborns to 5-year-olds) was due to hMPV.[162] In this cohort, the mean age of infected children was 11.6 months. Three quarters of all infections occurred in the first year of life. Infection primarily occurred between December and April and resulted in a 2% hospitalization rate.

Infection seems to be slightly less severe than with RSV. The disease spectrum included upper respiratory tract infection (15%), bronchiolitis (59%), croup (18%), pneumonia (8%), and asthma exacerbation (14%). Asymptomatic infection may occur, particularly in healthy children or adults. Others present with rhinitis, mild fever, a wet cough, or wheezing. Otitis has also been reported.[122] It is unclear whether premature infants or infants with underlying chronic pulmonary disease or cardiovascular disease are at greater risk. Pulmonary function seems to be adversely affected in preterm infants, but recurrent wheezing is seen in term infants as well. Infection is believed to occur via contact with contaminated secretions, and the incubation period apparently is 3 to 5 days. The duration of viral shedding is unclear, but may be prolonged in the face of immunodeficiency.

Hospitalized patients should be isolated with contact precautions and an emphasis on careful hand washing. Treatment is supportive. Respiratory monitoring is important and may indicate a need for oxygen or mechanical ventilation. Bacterial superinfection seems to be unusual.

HUMAN IMMUNODEFICIENCY VIRUS
Epidemiology

HIV-1 is the principal cause of AIDS. (See also Chapter 23.) In the United States, homosexual men still constitute most domestic cases. Disease contracted through intravenous drug abuse or heterosexual activity also is prominent, however, and in some areas, nonhomosexual transmission outranks that seen in gay men. The U.S. Centers for Disease Control and Prevention (CDC) estimated in 2006 that approximately 27% of all Americans diagnosed with HIV infection were women, most of whom were of childbearing age. Approximately 80% of women newly diagnosed with HIV infection acquired it through heterosexual contact. Women from minority populations are disproportionately HIV-positive. In the 2006 CDC estimates, the incidence of new HIV infection in African-American women was 56 per 100,000 and in Latina women was 14 per 100,000 compared with less than 4 per 100,000 in white women.

In contrast to the United States, most adult HIV infection in the developing world is contracted through heterosexual means. The incidence is highest in east and central sub-Saharan Africa, Southeast Asia, and parts of South America. In these areas, most HIV-positive patients are middle-aged adults, with the prevalence among childbearing women in some urban centers exceeding 30%. The debilitation and fatality from AIDS lead to the depletion of the heart of the workforce in tenuous economies and the orphaning of numerous uninfected offspring.

Currently, virtually all HIV-infected infants acquire disease from an infected mother. Consequently, most mothers of infected infants in the United States fall into a high-risk category—intravenous drug use or sexual activity with a man at high risk (bisexuality or intravenous drug use). Infected children follow a socioeconomic pattern nearly identical to that seen in HIV-1-infected women, and greater than 85% are from minority populations. Reflecting a medical success story of remarkable proportions, the incidence of perinatal HIV in the United States decreased nearly 80% in the latter half of the 1990s. In the first decade of the 2000s, only 100 to 200 cases of perinatally acquired HIV infection per year were reported to the CDC. Much of this decline was the result of increased voluntary HIV testing during pregnancy and the widespread application of intragestational prophylaxis with antiretroviral drugs. By contrast, in the developing world, where such care is largely unavailable, hundreds of thousands of infants are infected through perinatal transmission each year.

Pathogenesis

HIV is an RNA-containing retrovirus with an approximately 9.7-kb genome. The virus infects cells containing the surface molecule CD4+, most notably helper T lymphocytes and macrophages. An infected adult initially exhibits a robust immune response to the virus, with the appearance of HIV-specific antibodies and CD8+ cytotoxic T lymphocytes. After an initial mononucleosis-like syndrome, adults experience a prolonged period of clinical latency, characterized by the establishment of stable, low-level plasma viral titers (referred to as the *set-point*) and near-normal CD4+ T lymphocyte counts. During this period, the number of target cells destroyed by HIV is balanced by CD4+ cell repletion. This state may last for years.

Despite the healthy appearance of latently infected patients, HIV actively replicates in lymph nodes and circulating CD4+ cells and ultimately overwhelms the host, leading to increasing concentration of virus in plasma and tissues, clinical deterioration, and CD4+ cell depletion. This last phenomenon results in profound disruption of the immune system because CD4+ T cells coordinate many aspects of immunity. The host thereafter is placed at risk for acquiring infections with organisms that normally possess low pathogenicity (opportunistic infections) and AIDS-related cancers. The strongest predictor of progression of disease in adults is the concentration of plasma-borne virus, commonly referred to as the *viral load*. The viral load is measured by a quantitative reverse transcriptase PCR test, which is widely commercially available. The number of CD4+ T cells also is an additional independent predictor of disease progression in adults.

Generally, untreated children with perinatal HIV-1 infection experience more rapidly progressive disease than adults. Similar to other intracellular pathogens, it is likely that HIV infection of the fetus early in gestation, when NK and T cells are low in number and immature in function, results in particularly severe disease. Even in a full-term newborn, however, T cells possess multiple functional deficiencies that render the host particularly susceptible to pathogens such as HIV. Early HIV-specific cytotoxic T cell lymphocyte responses, which are crucial for the initial control of HIV infection in adults, frequently are sluggish or absent in infected newborns. There is evidence that fetal and newborn immune cells may provide better substrates for HIV infection or replication than mature cells because neonatal macrophages and memory T cells support HIV replication better than cells derived from adults. Consequently, infected newborns typically show very high plasma viral loads early in life, frequently registering hundreds of thousands to millions of viral RNA copies per millimeter of plasma by 4 weeks of age. Infants usually are unable to establish a set-point, reflecting poor early control of viral replication, and, as a result, show unmoderated high viral loads throughout early childhood.[130]

As in adults, the strongest predictor of disease progression in perinatally acquired HIV-1 is the plasma-borne viral titer. High viral loads in infancy presage major manifestations of HIV and death early in life. Several factors other than viral load also have been associated with disease progression in perinatally acquired HIV-1. Thymic dysfunction, manifested by the early depletion of CD4+ and CD8+ T cell populations, occurs in a small percentage of HIV-1-infected infants and is strongly associated with early severe disease. Coinfections with other pathogens in early life may detrimentally affect disease progression further. CMV in particular, long suspected of enhancing HIV-1 replication in adults through transactivating transcription factors, results in higher mean titers of HIV-1 and the early appearance of HIV-1–associated signs and symptoms and death in infants infected with CMV and HIV-1.

Mother-to-child transmission occurs in approximately 25% to 30% of infants born to mothers who have not taken antiviral medications during gestation. Intrauterine transmission has been shown directly by detection of virus in aborted fetal tissue. Most infants are negative for HIV immediately after birth, however, and become positive within the first several weeks after delivery, supporting the contention that most perinatal transmission occurs near the time of delivery or as the child traverses the birth canal. Cervical secretions harbor HIV in concentrations proportionate to concentrations in the bloodstream. Infection at or near the time of delivery, when the mucous membranes of the infant are exposed to infected maternal secretions and blood, is assumed to be the principal mode of acquisition of HIV perinatally.

The primary factor that places an infant at risk for perinatal HIV transmission seems to be the degree of maternal viremia during pregnancy and its correlates—severity of maternal clinical illness and CD4+ cell depletion.[41] In several studies, the risk of transmission was proportionate to maternal viral load. No level of maternal viremia is absolutely safe for the fetus, and transmission occasionally has been reported even when maternal viral load has been undetectable. Nevertheless, vertical transmission rates approaching zero have been associated with viral loads smaller than 500 to 1000 HIV RNA copies per mm of plasma. Other risk factors for perinatal transmission are less well established. The presence of chorioamnionitis and the occurrence of premature rupture of membranes have been suggested as risks for perinatal HIV transmission. Instrumentation during delivery, with the associated exposure of the newborn to infected maternal blood and cervical secretions, also increases risk of transmission. There also has been speculation that some viral genotypes may be more likely to cross from mother to child than others.

HIV infection from mother to child also may occur though the ingestion of contaminated breast milk. Breast milk contains virus in macrophages and in the cell free fraction, and the viral concentration in breast milk correlates with the concentration measured in the bloodstream. In the United States, where alternative infant nutrition is available, the impact of breast milk-related HIV transmission is negligible. The effect in the developing world is substantial, however. The excess incidence of mother-to-child transmission of HIV attributable to breast feeding is estimated to be 4% to 22%.

Although the risk of breast milk–related late postnatal transmission is highest in the first 6 months postpartum, transmission occurs throughout the duration of breast milk exposure.

Breast milk–transmitted HIV is believed to enter the infant either through the gastrointestinal mucosa or possibly through tonsillar lymphoid tissue. Several factors have been identified that increase the risk of breast milk transmission, including the duration of breast feeding, severity of infection in the mother, presence of breast lesions, and inflammation of the infant's gastrointestinal mucosa (particularly by *Candida* infection). Several immunologic and chemical factors in breast milk have been found to inhibit HIV growth in vitro, and the relative concentrations of these factors in a particular specimen may influence the risk of transmission.

Care of the Mother and Prevention of Vertical Transmission

Advanced HIV infection in the mother can adversely affect the outcome of the pregnancy, even if the infant is not infected. Studies performed in Africa indicate that women ill with HIV infection bear infants who are smaller for gestational age and more premature compared with women without HIV infection. Perinatal mortality also is increased. Infants born to asymptomatically infected women have negligible effects. These data suggest that factors covariate with advanced HIV disease, particularly malnutrition, secondary and coexisting infections, and illicit drug and alcohol use, are the most important factors mediating the immediate health of the newborn, and must be addressed appropriately during the obstetric care of the mother. All women should be placed on multivitamin supplements, and these should be continued after gestation.

CARE OF THE MOTHER AND INFANT IN DEVELOPED COUNTRIES

Intragestational and postgestational administration of antiretroviral drugs is extremely effective in preventing vertical transmission of HIV-1 and has become the standard of care in the developed world.[97] In a landmark prospective, multicenter, randomized trial conducted in the early 1990s (PACTG 076), zidovudine prophylaxis resulted in a reduction in vertical transmission from 25.5% to 8.3%.[27] The regimen employed in this study included three phases: (1) a maternal oral dose of 100 mg five times a day beginning between 14 and 34 weeks of gestation; (2) intrapartum intravenous zidovudine at 2 mg/kg of body weight over the first hour, followed by 1 mg/kg hourly until birth; and (3) infant oral dosing of zidovudine at 2 mg/kg every 6 hours for 6 weeks. In response to the success of this study, the CDC recommended wide application of the PACTG 076 protocol to limit vertical transmission of HIV in the United States. Subsequent experience indicated that in some populations intrapartum and postpartum use of zidovudine could result in a 5% or less transmission rate.

Even as public health recommendations for this regimen were being established, significant changes in antiretroviral strategies in HIV-infected adults were evolving that produced dramatic reductions in plasma-borne viral loads and in AIDS-related deaths. These changes included the administration of multidrug regimens (rather than monotherapy) and the early institution of antiviral medication based primarily on viral load rather than CD4+ T cell depletion or the presence of symptoms. As a result, by the late 1990s, many HIV-infected women entering pregnancy already were taking multidrug regimens (termed *highly active antiretroviral therapy* [HAART]) comprising various combinations of nucleoside reverse transcriptase inhibitors (sometimes, but not always, including zidovudine), non-nucleoside reverse transcriptase inhibitors, and protease inhibitors, to maintain their own health.

Based on these realities, and the observation that low maternal viral loads strongly correlate with protection of the newborn, the CDC updated its recommendations in 2002 and again in 2008. The full text of these guidelines and updated information can be accessed at http://AIDSinfo.nih. gov. These recommendations, along with additional recommendations by the AAP,[51] can be summarized as follows:

1. Pregnant women found to be HIV-positive should be started on HAART using the same criteria as in nonpregnant patients, based on viral load, CD4+ count, and presence of HIV-related symptoms. Genotypic testing of the infecting isolate should be pursued before initiating therapy to determine preexisting resistance to antiretroviral drugs.

2. Therapy should be continued in women who are already on multidrug HAART at the time that pregnancy is identified, assuming that the woman has had a satisfactory response (reduction of viral load, improvement or stabilization in CD4+ T lymphocyte count, and improved or stable clinical condition). For women with persistently high or increasing viral loads during pregnancy, alterations of therapy should be considered based on genotypic testing of the woman's HIV isolate to detect drug resistance–conferring mutations in a manner identical to nonpregnant subjects.

3. The CDC recommends adding zidovudine if not initially included in the woman's HAART regimen, even if the drug had been discontinued because of the emergence of zidovudine-resistant HIV. This recommendation is based on the observation that trials have consistently shown a protective effect of zidovudine against vertical transmission of HIV even in the presence of zidovudine-resistant isolates in the mother. Zidovudine possesses pharmacologic qualities (high concentrations of active, intracellular drug in the placenta and efficient transplacental transfer of drug to the fetus) that render it particularly attractive in the prevention of mother-to-infant transmission. Intravenous zidovudine should be initiated during labor regardless of the mother's HAART regimen. The CDC recommendations allow that some women should continue non–zidovudine-containing regimens if they have resulted in sustained nondetectable viral loads before pregnancy, particularly women infected with documented zidovudine-resistant organisms or organisms intolerant of zidovudine. In such cases, it is preferable to use alternative drugs to zidovudine with good placental penetration; generally, nucleoside reverse transcriptase inhibitors cross the placenta well, and protease inhibitors do not.

4. In the unusual HIV-infected pregnant woman who has not received prior antiretroviral therapy and whose own

condition does not warrant initiating such therapy, zidovudine may be administered as monotherapy for prevention of vertical viral transmission using the schedule defined by PACTG 076. This schedule should be applied even in women with low or undetectable viral loads.

5. The CDC guidelines suggest discussing the relative risks of administering antiretroviral therapy during the first trimester with the mother, although in most instances initiation or continuation of HAART is recommended if such therapy would be standard in the nonpregnant patient.

6. Most antiretroviral drugs are available only for oral administration. During labor or before elective cesarean delivery, the woman should continue to receive HAART according to her scheduled dosing with small sips of water whenever possible. Additionally, she should receive continuous-infusion intravenous zidovudine using the regimen employed by PACT 076 (a loading dose of 2 mg/kg followed by 1 mg/kg per hour) until the cord is clamped. This infusion is recommended even when zidovudine is not part of the woman's long-term regimen because of the possibility that zidovudine-susceptible viral subpopulations exist even in the face of overall zidovudine resistance.

7. The CDC recommends further that zidovudine continue to be used as monotherapy (2 mg/kg per dose orally, or 1.5 mg/kg intravenously, every 6 hours for 6 weeks) in the infant regardless of the mother's regimen or the length of her past experience with zidovudine, out of concern that the early institution of antiretroviral drugs other than zidovudine for prophylaxis may foster resistance to a broad range of agents. Dosing should be started as soon after birth as possible, ideally within 6 hours of birth. Despite this recommendation, many AIDS therapists choose to institute prophylaxis for the infant with the same drug combination that was effective in the mother, conceding that the safety and pharmacokinetics of many antiretroviral drugs other than zidovudine have not been determined in newborns. Some authorities recommend multiple-drug regimens, usually including zidovudine, for an infant born to a mother who received only intrapartum therapy or no antiviral therapy at all because in these circumstances the resistance phenotype of the mother's HIV isolate is unknown. The decision to use nonzidovudine antiretroviral drugs and the dosing of such therapy in the infant should be established in consultation with a pediatrician expert in the care of HIV infection. Because in many instances there is a delay in registering the infant for insurance, and because liquid forms of antiviral agents may be difficult to procure from community pharmacies, every effort should be made to supply the family with the infant's medications (not just a prescription) at discharge.

8. For premature infants (<35 weeks' gestation), zidovudine should be administered at 2 mg/kg per dose orally every 12 hours, or 1.5 mg/kg per dose intravenously, increasing to 2 mg/kg per dose every 8 hours at 2 weeks if 30 weeks' gestation or greater at birth or at 4 weeks if less than 30 weeks' gestation at birth. The dosing of antiretroviral agents besides zidovudine in premature infants has not been determined.

9. The mother should be counseled against breast feeding, whether or not she is continuing antiretroviral therapy after pregnancy.

10. HIV-exposed newborns should be immunized against hepatitis B, using the dose and schedule recommended for infants not exposed to HIV.

Other issues surrounding care of HIV-complicated pregnancy are discussed subsequently.

Safety

The effectiveness of HAART therapy in the mother and intrapartum and postpartum prophylaxis in the infant in decreasing the incidence of vertical HIV transmission is incontrovertible. By the early 2000s, transmission rates after applying this strategy were less than 2%. Despite a broad experience, concerns remain, however, regarding the safety of deliberate exposure of the pregnant woman, fetus, and young infant to antiretroviral drugs. The adverse effects of zidovudine exposure as defined by the PACTG 076 trial have been investigated through follow-up studies of mothers and children enrolled in this and similar trials. Mild and reversible anemia in infants occurs during the 6-week period of postnatal administration, but no further untoward effects have been consistently documented after years of observation.[98] Anemia may be more severe in an infant born to a mother who was receiving multiple antiretroviral drugs during pregnancy.

Some concern has been raised by European investigators that a small percentage of children exposed in utero to zidovudine may have persistent defects in mitochondrial function, a subcellular target of zidovudine in vitro. Older children and adults receiving long-term nucleoside reverse transcriptase inhibitors such as zidovudine occasionally develop a high anion gap acidosis because of mitochondrial dysfunction. Studies of a large cohort of European children exposed as fetuses and infants to antiretroviral therapy suggest that mitochondriopathies may occur in 0.26%, an incidence that is greater than 20-fold that expected in the general population. A retrospective evaluation of more than 16,000 uninfected, exposed American children failed to reveal any subject with symptoms consistent with a mitochondrial disorder.[98]

The safety of nonzidovudine drugs when administered during and immediately after pregnancy is less well studied. To date, these drugs seem to be remarkably free of adverse effects to the mother and the infant. The one probable exception is the non-nucleoside reverse transcriptase inhibitor efavirenz, which is teratogenic in primates at serum concentrations routinely achieved after conventional dosing in humans.[98] Although initial studies from Europe suggested that multidrug HAART therapy during pregnancy predisposed to preterm delivery, this finding was not supported by data collected in an American cohort of 369 women receiving combination therapy without protease inhibitors and 137 additional women receiving combination therapy with protease inhibitors.[146] Studies examining the effectiveness of zidovudine/lamivudine and short courses of the non-nucleoside reverse transcriptase inhibitor nevirapine in preventing vertical transmission of HIV in developing countries (see later) likewise have not shown toxicity from these drugs either to the mother or to the infant.

The use of selected agents should prompt careful monitoring of the mother. Prolonged courses of nevirapine occasionally have been associated with significant hepatotoxicity in pregnant women, especially when the CD4+ counts exceed 250/mm³; such dosing requires frequent, serial liver function tests. Nucleoside reverse transcriptase inhibitors, especially the combination of stavudine and didanosine, rarely may be associated with the development of lactic acidosis in the mother during pregnancy. Data regarding potential toxic effects of a wide range of other antiretroviral drugs are being collected through long-term follow-up studies, and the clinician is encouraged to record all cases of antiretroviral drug exposure with the Antiviral Pregnancy Registry (see http://www.APRegistry.com).

Truncated Prophylaxis

Currently available information suggests that there is value to prophylactic antiviral administration even when the pregnant woman presents late in pregnancy. Observational data collected in New York indicate that, in nonresearch settings, the full three-phase course of prophylactic zidovudine (as prescribed by PACTG 076), started during pregnancy and extending into the intrapartum and postpartum periods, results in a relative risk of HIV vertical transmission of 0.23 (compared with no prophylaxis); that drug started only intrapartum, but including administration to the newborn, results in a relative risk of 0.38; and that drug given only to the infant, but started within 48 hours of birth, results in a relative risk of 0.35.[153] Prophylaxis initiated in the infant on the third day of life or later in the absence of maternal prophylaxis has no detectable effect. These data argue for the immediate initiation of antiretroviral prophylaxis regardless of when during pregnancy or delivery the mother is found to be HIV-positive.

For a woman in labor who has not received prior therapy, the ideal regimen is not established. The CDC recommends one of the following regimens, based on data generated in trials conducted in nonindustrialized settings (see later): (1) single dose of nevirapine during labor followed by a single dose to the infant within 48 hours of life, or (2) zidovudine and lamivudine during labor followed by 1 week of zidovudine and lamivudine to the infant, or (3) intravenous zidovudine to the mother during labor followed by 6 weeks of zidovudine to the infant, or (4) a combination of these schedules. Infants delivered to mothers who have received no therapy at all should be offered 6 weeks of zidovudine, with the addition of other antiretroviral drugs if zidovudine resistance is known or suspected in the mother's isolate; this prophylaxis should be initiated as soon after delivery as possible.

Prenatal Testing

The availability of effective prophylactic regimens against vertical transmission of HIV mandates routine prenatal HIV testing.[50] It currently is standard practice to add voluntary HIV testing to other prenatal screening tests. Most authorities recommend an "opt-out" strategy for prenatal HIV testing; that is, the test is performed routinely unless the woman specifically requests that it be excluded, assuming such a strategy is consistent with state statute. For women with negative test results exhibiting high-risk behaviors or residing in high-incidence areas, the assay should be repeated during the third trimester. Problems still exist in reaching selected populations of HIV-infected women, particularly

women using illicit drugs, in a sufficiently timely fashion to prevent transmission to their offspring.

Given the effectiveness of even incomplete prophylactic schedules, rapid HIV testing should be offered to laboring women who have had no prenatal care. If the rapid test is positive, intravenous zidovudine should be initiated immediately in the mother until delivery, and oral zidovudine should be administered to the infant, even in the absence of a confirmatory HIV test (Western blot or viral detection assay). Breast feeding should be postponed until confirmatory testing is completed. Confirmation of the rapid test should be pursued as soon as possible after delivery, and the decision to continue zidovudine in the infant and to recommend or restrict breast feeding can be made according to the result of the confirmatory test. All women found to be HIV-positive during pregnancy should be screened for other frequently encountered coinfections—specifically tuberculosis, syphilis, toxoplasmosis, hepatitis B and C, CMV, and HSV.

Cesarean Delivery

Multiple studies have documented the benefit of delivering infants born to HIV-infected mothers by cesarean section. A meta-analysis of 15 observational studies indicated consistent and significant reductions in vertical transmission when elective cesarean delivery is offered to HIV-infected women. Nevertheless, the additional benefit gained by cesarean delivery is minimal in an adherent mother receiving HAART with a very low or undetectable viral load late in gestation. Cesarean section may be most appropriate for the HIV-infected woman unable to administer antiretroviral therapy to herself or her newborn or in a mother who has a persistently high viral load (>1000 copies/mL) despite multidrug therapy. Operative delivery also should be considered in an infected woman when viral load is unknown.

Elective cesarean sections should be scheduled at 38 weeks of gestation, and if possible should be performed while the membranes are intact. Premature rupture of the membranes decreases the benefit from cesarean delivery, but the duration of ruptured membranes beyond which operative delivery adds no benefit is unknown. Intravenous zidovudine should be initiated at least 3 hours before surgery, and other antiretroviral medications should be continued before and after delivery. Postpartum complication rates after elective cesarean section approximate the rates seen in noninfected women, although they are higher after emergent cesarean delivery and in women with advanced disease.

CARE OF THE MOTHER AND INFANT IN DEVELOPING COUNTRIES

The expense of perigestational prophylaxis using HAART, or zidovudine monotherapy as defined by the PACTG 076 protocol, prohibits use in most of the developing world, where most of the HIV burden lies. It is unusual for pregnant women in many nonindustrialized countries to present for prenatal care during the early stages of gestation. To have any practical applicability in these settings, regimens must be effective when offered late in pregnancy. Several trials conducted in the late 1990s and the early 2000s in Africa and Asia have shown the efficacy of selected abbreviated schedules of antiretroviral agents to interrupt vertical transmission of HIV in environments with limited health care resources. These protocols were developed with the recognition that they do not address at least some intrauterine infection, and that they do not provide prophylaxis against most breast milk–related transmission. The principal antiviral agents used in these trials have been zidovudine, lamivudine, and nevirapine. The results of representative seminal trials are described next.

Short-Course Zidovudine

Trials in Thailand (among non–breast-feeding women) and Côte d'Ivoire (among breast-feeding mothers) initially evaluated a truncated zidovudine regimen consisting of 300 mg twice daily to the mother starting at 36 weeks and then 300 mg orally every 3 hours during labor. No prophylaxis was administered to the infant. Compared with placebo, HIV vertical transmission at 6 months was reduced by half (9.4% versus 18.9% among placebo recipients).[129] This study was followed by a four-arm protocol in which zidovudine was initiated at either 28 weeks' gestation or 36 weeks' gestation in the mother, and infant prophylaxis was given either for 3 days or for 6 weeks. The long-long arm produced significantly better protection than the short-short arm (4.1% versus 10.5% at 6 months). The longer antepartum arm was also associated with a significantly lower incidence of in utero infection compared with the short antepartum arm.

These studies document protection by zidovudine even when administered for a shorter duration than that prescribed in the PACTG 076 protocol, although generally inferior to the protection produced by strategies employing the full PACTG 076 regimen or HAART regimens. Despite the additional benefit of longer treatment of the mother, it is uncertain if such a schedule can be successfully applied in practice. Experience in Kenya with a protocol initiating zidovudine at the relatively late date of 36 weeks of gestation documented that less than one quarter of HIV-infected mothers took the fully prescribed regimen.

Zidovudine and Lamivudine

The effectiveness of the combination of the two nucleoside reverse transcriptase inhibitors zidovudine and lamivudine in preventing vertical transmission of HIV compared with placebo was tested in a trial conducted in several African countries in breast-feeding mothers (PETRA trial).[114] The combination (300 mg of zidovudine and 150 mg of lamivudine twice a day) was initiated at 36 weeks' gestation and continued through labor and 1 week after delivery. The same two drugs were administered to the infant (4 mg/kg of zidovudine and 2 mg/kg of lamivudine orally twice a day) for the first week of life. Although significant benefit was seen at 6 weeks postpartum, there was only a nonsignificant trend toward benefit at 18 months (14.9% offspring infection versus 22.2% in the placebo group). Dosing limited to the intrapartum period resulted in vertical transmission rates equal to that recorded in the placebo group. Lamivudine-resistant HIV was subsequently isolated from some of the mothers who had received this drug, but frequently did not persist; the implications of this finding are uncertain.

Nevirapine

Nevirapine is a non-nucleoside reverse transcriptase inhibitor that characteristically produces a rapid, profound decrease in HIV viral load. Its prolonged use as a single agent is limited by the rapid emergence of resistance, but this phenomenon is less problematic when the drug is used short-term exclusively to prevent perinatal transmission of virus. HIVNET 012, a trial conducted in breast-feeding mothers in Uganda, administered a single 200-mg dose of oral nevirapine to the mother at the onset of labor and a single 2 mg/kg dose of nevirapine to the infant at 48 to 72 hours of age. The comparison group was administered zidovudine orally during labor (600 mg, followed by 300 mg every 3 hours), and zidovudine was administered to the infant for 1 week (4 mg/kg twice daily). The incidence of infection at birth was equal in both groups (approximately 9%), but significant advantages in the nevirapine group were apparent by age 6 weeks and continued until 18 months: 25.8% infection in zidovudine recipients versus 15.7% infection in nevirapine recipients ($P < .003$).[61] The nevirapine strategy has the advantage that only two doses are required, and maternal and infant doses can be given under direct observation. Although nevirapine-resistant HIV isolates have been detected in women enrolled in these trials, typically resistance disappears after several months, suggesting that the strategy can be reapplied to subsequent pregnancies.

Subsequent studies have been designed to examine the nuances of short-term antiretroviral drug administration to interrupt mother-to-child transmission of HIV. These studies have employed zidovudine, nevirapine, or a combination of the two, and have applied them either to the mother and the infant or only to the infant. Virtually all studies document superior interruption of vertical HIV transmission if the laboring mother and newborn infant receive an antiretroviral agent compared with administration only to the infant. Most studies suggest that when the infant receives single-dose nevirapine plus 1 or 6 weeks of zidovudine, the incidence of HIV transmission is lower than when only one of these drugs is used alone.

Clinical Manifestations

Virtually all infants born to an HIV-infected mother are asymptomatic at birth. Most HIV-infected offspring begin to show signs and symptoms within the first 1 or 2 years of life. A smaller proportion, termed *rapid progressors*, become symptomatic within 1 or 2 months after delivery. Infants with rapidly progressive disease have plasma viral loads early in life that are two or three times higher than the plasma viral loads of infants with more indolent infection.

With the exception of *Pneumocystis jiroveci* (formerly *Pneumocystis carinii*) pneumonia, most opportunistic infections occur late in the course of the child's illness. *P. jiroveci* pneumonia commonly manifests in the first months of life. In contrast to *P. jiroveci* pneumonia in adults, virtually all of whom have preexisting immunity to *Pneumocystis* before acquisition of HIV, *P. jiroveci* pneumonia in infants is due to primary infection in the absence of preexisting immunity, and results in severe, frequently overwhelming, bilateral pneumonia. Other characteristics of untreated or poorly controlled perinatal HIV infection are nonspecific. Recurrent bacterial infections are frequent in infants with HIV infection. Most of these are minor (e.g., otitis media), but some are severe (bacteremia, pneumonia, or meningitis). Other commonly encountered early manifestations include persistent mucocutaneous candidiasis, abdominal organomegaly, diffuse lymphadenopathy, chronic diarrhea, failure to grow, and developmental delay. Children also acquire a diffuse, interstitial pneumonia of uncertain origin termed *lymphocytic interstitial pneumonia*. HIV-specific cancers, such as B cell lymphomas, Kaposi sarcoma, and leiomyosarcomas, are unusual in children and generally occur late in the course of the illness.

Diagnosis and Care of Infants Exposed to Human Immunodeficiency Virus

All infants born to a known HIV-infected mother or to a mother who falls into a high-risk category should be longitudinally evaluated for HIV infection. The routine diagnostic HIV tests employed in adults (enzyme-linked immunosorbent assay [ELISA] and Western blot) are based on the detection of anti-HIV antibodies, most of which are IgG. Because these routine HIV tests cannot distinguish infant-derived IgG from that transplacentally acquired from a seropositive mother, these tests virtually always are positive in the newborn period whether the offspring is infected or not and are of little usefulness.

The definitive diagnosis of HIV infection in a newborn requires the detection of virus or HIV-specific nucleic acid. Virtually all untreated newborns have HIV viral loads well above the level of detection, and this test is greater than 90% sensitive and virtually 100% specific by 4 weeks of age. Viral load assays further give an estimation of the severity of the infection and a baseline for judging the success of antiretroviral therapy. Some experts recommend testing the infant with a nucleic acid detection assay or by viral culture on three separate occasions up to 6 months of life. Infants who are repeatedly negative by that time no longer need to be followed for the possibility of HIV infection. Infants who test positive should have a second, confirmatory test performed before the diagnosis is established.

The CDC recommends initiating antiretroviral therapy for any infant diagnosed with HIV infection before age 12 months. Extrapolating from the experience with adults, such therapy should include at least three drugs derived from the nucleoside and non-nucleoside reverse transcriptase inhibitor families and the protease inhibitor family. Published experience with many of these agents in young infants is small relative to information available in adults, but preliminary results suggest that children have poorer virologic responses to multidrug regimens compared with adults. The treatment of infants with multidrug regimens poses difficulties not encountered in older patients, including devising dosing schedules that can be followed by frequently ill mothers and timing the administration of medication around feeds that may interfere with or increase the drug's bioavailability, depending on the agent. Proper use of these complex and potentially toxic agents requires the advice of an expert with substantial experience in perinatal HIV infection.

In addition to 6 weeks of prophylactic zidovudine, as outlined earlier, care of HIV-exposed infants requires few additional interventions. Because *P. jiroveci* pneumonia is the major life-threatening complication during the first year of the HIV-infected infant's life, many experts recommend that prophylaxis for *P. jiroveci* pneumonia should be administered beginning at 4 to 6 weeks and continuing for at least 1 year, or until HIV infection can be definitively excluded. The most effective prophylactic regimen is trimethoprim-sulfamethoxazole, 75 mg/m^2 per dose, twice a day, 3 days a week. The immunization schedule for HIV-infected infants is identical to immunocompetent infants, including recombinant hepatitis B vaccine at birth.

PROGNOSIS

Before the introduction of HAART, the median survival of HIV-infected children in the United States and Europe was 8 to 13 years. In the absence of antiretroviral therapy, rapid progressors usually have multiple, life-threatening complications and die early in life. A few perinatally infected children have reached adolescence and remain symptom-free with their immune systems intact even without antiviral chemotherapy. The ultimate outcome of these unusual cases is unknown. As in adults, the survival of children in industrialized countries has markedly improved since the introduction of HAART, reflecting the benefits of HAART regimens seen in adults. Longitudinal studies conducted in the late 1990s, the period during which HAART became standard in adults and children, documented a dramatic decline in yearly mortality among HIV-infected children. The reduction in mortality was experienced by all subgroups defined by age, sex, CD4+ T lymphocyte counts, and ethnicity.

ENTEROVIRUSES AND PARECHOVIRUSES

Enteroviruses belong to the family Picornaviridae. The four traditional groups of enteroviruses are the polioviruses, echoviruses, coxsackieviruses, and enteroviruses. Among these four groups, presently 67 serotypes are recognized. Although these groupings are still widely employed, more recent molecular analyses have categorized enteroviruses into five genetically defined species, and have indicated that some of the original members belong to nonenterovirus genera altogether. In particular, hepatitis A, initially designated an enterovirus, has been reclassified as a distinct and unique genus. Two additional former enteroviruses, echovirus 22 and 23, are sufficiently genetically and structurally different from the other enteroviruses to be assigned to a new genus name, *Parechovirus*. Several new parechoviruses have been identified.

Epidemiology and Transmission

Humans are the true hosts for the enteroviruses, but these viruses have been described in various animals, probably secondary to contamination from humans. They are transmitted primarily by the fecal-oral route, but they have also been transmitted by the oral-oral route and have been isolated in swimming pools, from contaminated hands, and from flies. Typically, within a given geographically defined population, a narrow range of serotypes is responsible for most endemic disease. The community incidence of enteroviral disease peaks in temperate areas in summer and fall, but occurs throughout the year in tropical areas. In addition to geographically confined organisms, occasional strains cause epidemics that can reach worldwide proportions. In all four enterovirus groups, there are far more subclinical, undiagnosed infections than recognized disease, but when disease occurs, it is particularly severe in the neonatal period.

Perinatal infection can occur before, during, or after parturition. Enteroviruses may be transmitted transplacentally, presumably during maternal viremia, and congenital infections have been most often described after a maternal infection in the third trimester; such infections can result in fetal death. Most infection in the neonatal period is the result, however, of exposure of the oral or respiratory tract mucosa to organisms harbored by the mother at the time of birth or from secretions from the mother or other humans shortly thereafter.

Epidemics of enteroviral disease have been described in the nursery. The virus may be introduced by personnel, but more commonly the infant index case has acquired the virus from his or her mother at the time of delivery. Risk factors for infection in the nursery include low birthweight, administration of antibiotics or blood, proximity to the index patient, care by the nurse of the index patient in the same nursing shift, and nasogastric feeding or intubation.

Infection during Pregnancy

Enterovirus infection during pregnancy is common, especially during peak periods of enteroviral disease in the community, with some surveys documenting an intragestational incidence of 9% or more. Few data indicate any risk from either the polioviruses or the echoviruses for the development of congenital anomalies, but the situation is less clear for coxsackieviruses. Early investigations found an association of coxsackieviruses A9 and B2 to B4 with a higher rate of anomalies, particularly urogenital and cardiovascular, but others have found no such association. Reports of prematurity and stillbirth exist for all the enteroviral groups after infection late in pregnancy, but these effects seem to be uncommon. In most pregnant women, the infection is either asymptomatic or associated with mild, nonspecific illness. By contrast, mothers infected with echoviruses or coxsackie B viruses, the enteroviral groups most commonly associated with significant illness in newborns, frequently complain of fever and abdominal pain near the time of delivery.

Neonatal Infection

The nonpolio enteroviruses cause a wide spectrum of illnesses, and substantial data have been collected regarding specific types and strains. The severity of disease in a newborn is a function of the infecting strain, the titer of passively transferred specific antibody in the infant, and the timing of infection. Maternal infection just before delivery, before the mother can mount an antibody response, with high-titer viral transmission immediately before or during birth is associated with the most severe symptoms in the newborn.

Most neonatal enteroviral disease manifests as a nonspecific mild febrile illness. These infections probably are acquired postnatally. Signs and symptoms occur between the first and second week of life, usually after the infant has been discharged from the nursery, and consist of fever of 38°C to 39°C, irritability, vomiting or diarrhea, and poor feeding. These infants frequently are admitted to the hospital for a bacterial

sepsis evaluation and discharged 3 days later when the bacterial cultures have proved negative, and the infant's symptoms have spontaneously improved. Occasional infants exhibit respiratory distress, rash, or aseptic meningitis. The course is self-limiting, and recovery without residual is the rule.[84] A history of an intercurrent viral-like illness in a family member can usually be elicited. Nosocomial infection, acquired horizontally after birth, also frequently has this relatively mild course.

A more fulminant, life-threatening illness occurs as a consequence of vertical transmission at the time of birth but before the development of significant serotype-specific antibodies in the mother. The mortality is highest for echovirus-11, but other serotypes, particularly some coxsackie B viruses and several parechoviruses, also have been implicated.[65,151] Approximately one third to one half of infants with severe enteroviral disease are born prematurely.[1] In fulminant cases, onset of illness typically occurs within the first 2 to 5 days of life. Severe neonatal disease shares many characteristics of overwhelming bacterial infection, with extreme lethargy and hypoperfusion. Infants also present with fever, which may be greater than 39°C, poor feeding, and rash. The rash is usually macular or maculopapular, sometimes with petechiae. The most fulminant cases are complicated by hepatitis, first manifested by hepatomegaly and jaundice. Such cases can progress to necrosis of the liver and fulminant hepatic failure with intractable coagulopathy and hemorrhage, and profound hepatocellular dysfunction. Mortality from enteroviral hepatitis and coagulopathy ranges from 30% to 80%.[1]

Despite the life-threatening nature of the acute hepatic failure, recovery of hepatic function among survivors is the rule. Coincident with hepatitis, or sometimes separate from it, a newborn may have myocarditis, characterized by respiratory distress, tachycardia, and arrhythmias, with mortality approaching 50%. As with hepatitis, if the infant survives acutely, full recovery over a long course is usual. Both of these severe manifestations may occur coincidentally with meningoencephalitis. In these infants, the CSF examination often is typical for viral CNS disease, but some serotypes produce CSF changes typical of bacterial meningitis, including marked hypoglycorrhachia, and still others result in no CSF pleocytosis at all. Although there are a few reports of neurologic sequelae among survivors of aseptic meningitis, nearly all children develop normally. In contrast, neonatal encephalitis resulting from parechovirus may be severe, causing white matter injury and long-term sequelae in a significant proportion of affected infants.[150]

Enteroviral infection shortly after birth also has been implicated in a few cases of sudden infant death. Some infants have died within the first week of life. Mild prodromal symptoms usually precede the infant's death. Evidence of enterovirus has been found in the heart and respiratory tract at postmortem examination.

Laboratory Diagnosis

Traditionally, the diagnosis of enteroviral infection has been established by isolation of the virus in culture. Some serotypes of enterovirus are very difficult to grow in vitro, however. More recently, commercially available PCR technology has become available for enterovirus diagnosis, using primers that flank a highly conserved region in the 5′ noncoding region of the genome present in nearly all serotypes. When applied to infection in newborns and young infants, PCR diagnosis is more sensitive and much more rapid than viral culture. The widely used enteroviral PCR tests do not detect parechoviruses, however. Enterovirus can be identified by culture and PCR in serum, urine, CSF, nasopharynx, and stool. The usefulness of serology and antigen detection for diagnosis of enteroviral disease is precluded by the large number of non–cross-reacting serotypes.

Therapy and Prevention

The most important measure in limiting the spread of enteroviral disease is strict hand washing. Access to the nursery should be limited to healthy personnel. Cohort nursing care during nursery epidemics may be effective in limiting spread. There is some evidence that passive immunization with immune globulin during a nursery outbreak may be beneficial in limiting new cases and decreasing the severity of illness in affected infants.

High-dose intravenous immune globulin has been used in established neonatal disease, although there have been no controlled trials testing its effectiveness. Passive immunization has been shown to have a virologic effect in the infant only if the lot of immune globulin possesses very high titers against the offending serotype. The antiviral drug pleconaril is promising in neonatal enteroviral infection, but remains in development. This compound binds to sites on the enteroviral surface, prohibiting attachment to the target cell and subsequent uncoating. It has activity against numerous enteroviruses in vitro at concentrations that are readily achieved in the serum with human dosing. Preliminary experience, including data collected in neonates, indicates that the drug is highly bioavailable, has a large volume of distribution (including the CNS) and long half-life, and possesses few side effects. There have been numerous reports of pleconaril administration in infants with severe enteroviral disease, with recovery frequently occurring soon after drug initiation. Randomized trials in neonatal infection have not been published, however, and in the absence of controlled studies, the effectiveness of pleconaril in severe newborn enteroviral disease remains uncertain.

HEPATITIS VIRUSES

Hepatitis may result from various viral infections, including CMV, herpesvirus, rubella virus, EBV, VZV, and coxsackievirus. The disease usually occurs as part of a systemic infection. A primary infection of the liver, resulting in acute or chronic hepatitis, or both, may also be caused by specific hepatotropic viruses, as discussed in the following sections. (See also Chapter 48.)

Hepatitis A Virus

Hepatitis A virus (HAV) is a spherical, single-stranded, positive-sense RNA particle in the picornavirus group. HAV is distributed worldwide. The infection is highly contagious and is spread most commonly by the fecal-oral route. Common source outbreaks resulting from contaminated food,

particularly raw shellfish culled from tainted waters, also occur. Rarely, HAV is transmitted by blood transfusion or from mother to child. Fecal excretion of HAV begins 2 to 3 weeks before onset of the disease and may continue for 4 to 6 weeks. The average incubation period is 25 to 30 days.

HAV is a common infection in children, and children in daycare are at particular risk. Most pediatric infections are asymptomatic and anicteric. Children who do exhibit symptoms usually have a gastroenteritis-like syndrome and experience only mild hepatitis with virtually complete resolution. Adults are more likely to develop the typical signs and symptoms of hepatitis, with jaundice, abdominal pain, malaise, fever, acholic stools, dark urine, and vomiting. Fulminant disease is uncommon, and the mortality is less than 1%. The carrier state does not occur. The diagnosis is made by detecting anti-HAV IgM antibodies in the serum, which appear with the onset of disease and persist for several months. Detection of anti-HAV IgG, which persists throughout life, may indicate either recent or distant infection.

Acute HAV in pregnancy does not seem to increase the risk of congenital malformations, stillbirths, intrauterine growth restriction, or spontaneous abortion. The risk of perinatal transmission is minimal, even when the mother develops acute disease within the last weeks of pregnancy.[144] Perinatal transmission can rarely occur, however, and spread in special care nurseries has been reported. In most instances, neonatal disease is asymptomatic or mild and is self-limiting. Occasional reports suggest that maternal disease with HAV during pregnancy can result in meconium peritonitis in the fetus.

Although vertical transmission of HAV is unusual, some authorities recommend treating the infant with 0.02 mL/kg of immune serum globulin intramuscularly if maternal symptoms develop 2 weeks before to 1 week after delivery. The unusual nursery outbreak of HAV should be managed with the administration of prophylactic immune globulin to susceptible staff and infants and with emphasis on good hand washing. Two formalin-inactivated HAV vaccines are available in the United States and are highly protective, but are not yet licensed for children younger than 12 months of age.

Hepatitis B Virus

Hepatitis B virus (HBV) is the prototype of the family of viruses known as *hepadnaviruses* (hepatotropic DNA viruses). The complete infectious virion is a 42-nm sphere. Hepatitis B surface antigen (HBsAg) is found in the viral envelope and is produced in excess during infection, resulting in circulating, free spherical and tubular particles. It is detected (usually by radioimmunoassay [RIA] or ELISA) in acute and chronic infection. Subdeterminants of the surface antigen define four major serotypes. All four share an epitope designated "a"; antibody to HBsAg (anti-HBsAg) is directed against this common epitope and confers some protection against all four serotypes.

The viral inner core nucleocapsid contains hepatitis B core antigen (HBcAg), DNA polymerase, and partially double-stranded DNA. HBcAg is expressed on the surface of the infected hepatocyte, but does not circulate and cannot be detected by routine assays. Anti-HBcAg, total and IgM specific, can be detected by RIA or ELISA. HBeAg, a soluble polypeptide encoded within the same open reading frame as the core antigen, is detectable when HBV replication is rapid. Its appearance usually indicates a high concentration of HBV. HBeAg-negative individuals are infectious, but transmission of disease occurs at a lower rate. HBeAg and anti-HBe also can be detected by either RIA or ELISA. Several genotypes of HBV have been defined and designated types A through H. HBV DNA initially is transcribed into RNA intermediates, which serve as messages for viral proteins or as a template for progeny viral genomic DNA through reverse transcription by the viral polymerase.

CLINICAL MANIFESTATIONS AND HEPATITIS B VIRUS BLOOD TESTS

HBV infection is most often contracted by injection drug use, but may be transmitted through intimate physical contact or vertically from mother to infant. Blood products are routinely screened for HBV, and transfusion, previously the most common source of HBV infection, is now only rarely implicated. The incubation period is 50 to 180 days. HBsAg usually is present 1 to 3 months after exposure and appears before the onset of symptoms. Elevation of hepatocellular enzymes in the serum may be found 2 weeks to 2 months after HBsAg is detected. This period in adults frequently is characterized by a prodrome of nausea, vomiting, headache, and malaise, which progresses to jaundice.

Within 1 to 2 weeks of the onset of jaundice, HBsAg usually is cleared from the serum. With self-limited disease, there is often a window period between the disappearance of HBsAg and the development of anti-HBsAg so that both tests are negative. The appearance of anti-HBsAg is a marker of recovery and immunity against future reinfection. The IgM antibody response to HBcAg begins before the disappearance of HBsAg and persists through the window period. Testing for HBsAg and IgM anti-HBcAg is the most reliable strategy to document recent HBV infection. IgM anti-HBcAg disappears by 6 months, but the later appearing IgG anti-HBcAg may persist for life. HBeAg is variably expressed in HBV disease and denotes actively replicating, high-titer infection. The development of anti-HBeAg signals improved control of viral replication, but not eradication. HBV vaccines are composed of recombinant HBsAg; recipients of vaccine are positive for anti-HBsAg. Vaccine recipients can be distinguished from hosts who have recovered from wild-type infection by the absence of antibody to other viral components, particularly anti-HBcAg.

Most HBV-infected adults have a self-limited disease and become noncontagious. Less than 1% develop fulminant hepatic failure, but many of these patients die. The virus is not cytopathic for the infected hepatocyte, and hepatic damage and subsequent viral clearance are the results of the host's immune response. Chronic active or persistent hepatitis, which may develop in 30% of chronic carriers, is characterized by persistent serum HBeAg in the absence of anti-HBsAg and is particularly common in patients superinfected with the hepatitis D virus.

Infants born to antigen-positive mothers or mothers with acute hepatitis have a 35% incidence of prematurity and are more likely to be of low birthweight. The risk of preterm birth seems to be related to degree of maternal illness. Fulminant fatal cases of neonatal hepatitis secondary to vertically transmitted HBV are uncommon, but do occur (1% to 2% of all cases) and may be recurrent in successive pregnancies. More typically, infants infected with HBV develop a less robust immune response to the HBV-infected hepatocyte compared with adults and establish asymptomatic chronic infection ("chronic carriage"). The development of chronic carriage is strongly correlated to age: 95% of infants become chronic carriers compared with 30% of toddlers and 5% of adults.[56]

The consequences of chronic HBV carriage established in the newborn are not encountered until early adulthood, at which time the patient has a gradual onset of hepatic fibrosis and insufficiency. Carriers also may develop hepatocellular carcinoma after the initial infection. Hepatocellular carcinoma is most common in populations affected by a high incidence of vertically transmitted HBV and in populations with high cross-sectional prevalence of HBV surface and HBe antigenemia.[140] HBV itself is not oncogenic; the formation of tumor is probably the result of years of low-grade inflammation and repeated hepatocellular regeneration.

PERINATAL TRANSMISSION

Multiple studies have shown that vertical transmission of HBV is strongly associated with high-grade maternal HBe antigenemia, and that almost all infants born to HBeAg-positive mothers are infected in the first year of life, with 85% to 90% developing chronic viral infection. The risk of vertical transmission of HBV from an asymptomatic carrier mother to her infant increases from 10% to 85% when the mother is HBeAg-positive. Mothers may transmit HBV vertically in sequential pregnancies. The risk of vertical transmission of HBsAg from mother to infant at birth is higher in Asia than in Western industrialized countries.

Transmission occurs significantly more often at birth or in the postpartum period than transplacentally. Cord blood samples frequently are HBsAg-negative in infants who subsequently become infected. Peripartum transmission is implied further by observations made in mothers who acquire acute hepatitis B infection during pregnancy. The risk is very low with infection during the first two trimesters, but increases to 50% to 75% with hepatitis late in pregnancy or in the early postpartum period. Entry of virus through the infant's gastrointestinal tract is suggested by the finding that 95% of the gastric contents of infants born to carrier mothers are HBsAg positive after birth.

Although HBsAg can be found in the breast milk of 70% of carrier mothers, studies have not shown an increased risk with breast feeding, indicating that mothers who desire to breastfeed may do so with little risk. American studies indicate further that breast feeding carries no detectable risk of vertical HBV transmission in an infant who has received appropriate immunoprophylaxis at birth.[53]

There is also risk of transmission of HBV to family contacts of HBsAg carriers from close contact over long periods. The risk is higher from sibling carriers than from either parent, and is increased when the family member has evidence of liver disease. In the developing world, a significant proportion of infant infection is the result of horizontal transmission from the mother or other family member during the child's early life, rather than infection at the time of birth.

PREVENTION

Approximately 0.8% of women in the United States are HBsAg-positive in pregnancy. Active and passive immunization can prevent vertical transmission of HBV in 85% to 95% of cases, even in high-risk situations. The institution of immunoprophylaxis has had a profound impact on the incidence of newborn-acquired acute and chronic HBV infection and the associated hepatocellular carcinoma, particularly among high-prevalence populations in the United States (e.g., Alaskan Natives) and in areas of high endemicity in the developing world.[24,79]

Less than 50% of HBV-infected women in the United States have risk factors for HBV infection. Consequently, present recommendations mandate routine, universal screening of all pregnant women for HBV and universal vaccination of all infants. Current guidelines recommend that all pregnant women be tested for the presence of HBsAg early in gestation. Women at high risk for acquiring HBV, such as intravenous drug users or women with clinical hepatitis, should be tested again shortly before parturition. Hospitals are advised to develop systems that ensure the results of HBV screening tests are available to the pediatrician at the time of delivery. In everyday practice, some women without identified risk may acquire infection after the initial screening test, and others fail to be rescreened, and it may be impossible to transmit every woman's HBV status to the pediatrician in a timely fashion. In large centers that can perform HBV testing daily, screening at the time of delivery may overcome both of these potential problems.

Treatment of the infant varies, depending on whether the mother is HBsAg-positive, HBsAg-negative, or of unknown status at delivery. Infants of HBsAg-negative mothers do not need treatment with hepatitis B immune globulin (HBIG). They should be vaccinated before leaving the hospital with either Recombivax HB (5 μg in 0.5 mL) or Engerix-B (10 μg in 0.5 mL). Both must be given intramuscularly. Subsequent doses should be given at 1 and 6 months of age, although the last dose may be given up to 18 months of age. Combination vaccines currently are available that include HBV antigen and other childhood vaccines in the same vial. Only the monovalent preparation of hepatitis B vaccine should be used for the first dose, however, assuming it is administered at less than 6 weeks of age.

Infants of HBsAg-positive mothers should be passively immunized with HBIG (0.5 mL given intramuscularly) and hepatitis B vaccine at a different anatomic site within 12 hours of birth, although some benefit can be realized even if given 48 hours after birth. The vaccination schedule should be completed by 6 months to ensure rapid protection of the infant. In contrast to infants born to HBsAg-negative mothers, infants born to HBV-infected mothers should be tested for HBsAg and anti-HBsAg after the vaccine schedule has been completed (at age 9 to 15 months, to allow clearance of HBIG from the infant's bloodstream), to detect failure of seroconversion or vertical transmission despite vaccination.

If the mother's serologic status is unknown, maternal HBsAg should be tested at delivery, and the first dose of the vaccine should be given to the infant within 12 hours of birth. If the mother proves to be positive for HBsAg, HBIG

should be administered to the infant as soon as possible, but certainly within the first 7 days of life.

Early studies examining hepatitis B vaccine response in preterm infants indicated a lower seroconversion rate among infants with very low birthweight born to HBsAg-negative mothers compared with infants weighing more than 2000 g. Subsequent studies have determined that medically stable preterm infants immunized at 30 days of age have an antibody response similar to full-term infants regardless of gestational age or birthweight. In a preterm infant born to a mother who is HBsAg-negative, the first dose of HBV vaccine should be given at 30 days of life or when the infant reaches 2000 g, before hospital discharge. In preterm infants born to HBsAg-positive mothers, HBV vaccine should be given within 12 hours of birth (along with HBIG), but the full three-dose vaccine schedule should be initiated at 30 days of age (i.e., the infant should receive a total of four vaccine doses).

If a preterm infant is born to a mother with uncertain HBV status, and her status cannot be determined within 12 hours after delivery, HBIG should be administered to the infant immediately because the suboptimal immune response to vaccine alone precludes its use as a single intervention in the event that the mother proves to be HBV-positive. If the mother's HBV tests ultimately show she is negative for virus, the vaccine schedule can proceed using the same schedule for mothers known to be HBsAg-negative at delivery.

After nearly 20 years of widespread newborn vaccination, the hepatitis B vaccine seems to be exceedingly safe when given during infancy.[82] The original hepatitis B vaccine preparations contained the preservative thimerosal, a derivative of mercury. Concerns regarding the potential, albeit unproven, toxicity of thimerosal prompted a brief suspension of perinatal hepatitis B vaccination in the late 1990s and a mandate to develop vaccine formulations that did not contain this preservative. By 2001, all vaccines included in the childhood schedules were either thimerosal-free (including hepatitis B) or contained only trace amounts.

Hepatitis C Virus

Hepatitis C virus (HCV) is a single-stranded RNA virus of the family Flaviviridae. HCV is composed of six genotypes and multiple subtypes. The severity of the infection corresponds to the HCV strain, with genotype 1 producing the most aggressive course. HCV is the most common chronic blood-borne infection in the United States, and the most frequent condition requiring liver transplantation. The seroprevalence among volunteer blood donors in the United States is approximately 1% to 2%. At present, intravenous drug use is the most prominent risk factor for acquisition of HCV. Health care workers experiencing a needle-stick injury or mucous membrane exposure to blood products also are at risk. Sexual transmission of HCV is uncommon, and household contact results in viral transmission only rarely, if at all.

Historically, transmission occurred most frequently after exposure to blood or blood products, including sporadic lots of intravenous immune globulin. The practice of administering multiple small-volume transfusions to ill neonates during the 1960s and 1970s resulted in inadvertent HCV infection in a substantial proportion of the recipients. The screening of potential blood donors with newer generation antibody tests for HCV has greatly reduced the incidence, however, of transfusion-acquired infection in adults and children. Since the implementation of these screening programs, vertical transmission has become the most common mechanism of HCV infection in children.

HCV infection has a 30- to 60-day incubation period. In unusual circumstances, infection results in acute hepatitis with symptoms similar to those caused by other hepatotropic viruses—abdominal pain, jaundice, nausea, vomiting, fever, and malaise. Most acute infections in adults are asymptomatic, however. More than half of all HCV-infected adults develop chronic hepatitis, which may resolve or may progress in one fourth of patients to cirrhosis and eventually to hepatic failure.[124] As with chronic HBV infection, chronic HCV infection is a significant risk factor for hepatocellular carcinoma. Interferon-α therapy has been successful in generating long-term remission in some patients with chronic HCV infection, but the relapse rate is high. Concomitant ribavirin improves the response. Therapy is otherwise supportive.

Although HCV infection is relatively prevalent among young adults, almost every expert recommends against screening for HCV during pregnancy, unless the woman possesses known risk factors for infection, such as transfusion or organ transplantation before 1992 or infusion of clotting factor concentrates before 1987; intravenous drug abuse; presence of a tattoo or body piercing that was placed unprofessionally; or HIV infection. Pregnancy does not seem to worsen the severity of HCV infection, and HCV infection does not seem to increase maternal or fetal morbidity and mortality beyond that conferred by concomitant maternal drug use. As in nonpregnant adults, most pregnant women infected with HCV are asymptomatic with only mildly abnormal liver function tests. Interferon and ribavirin are contraindicated in pregnancy, and if therapy is indicated, it should be deferred until after delivery.

The incidence of mother-to-child transmission in women not coinfected with HIV is approximately 5%.[90] HIV coinfection in the mother increases the risk of vertical transmission of HCV twofold to fivefold. More recent data suggest, however, that effective multidrug therapies for HIV during pregnancy may reduce the risk of transmission of HCV as well. Maternal illicit drug use also increases the risk of vertical transmission of HCV to the newborn. Transmission seems to be a function of the degree of maternal viremia. If the mother's serum is HCV-negative by PCR, the rate of transmission to the newborn approaches zero.[36] Conversely, studies have indicated that transmission rates are roughly proportionate to maternal HCV plasma load.[59] No minimal level of viremia has been established below which the infant is safe, however.

Most infants probably are infected at or near delivery, and several investigators have documented that the risk of vertical transmission is increased by prolonged rupture of the membranes and invasive fetal monitoring, both of which heighten the exposure of the newborn to maternal blood.[90] Most series have been unable to document protection from HCV vertical transmission by cesarean section.[59] Some samples of colostrum and breast milk contain detectable HCV RNA, but studies indicate no increased risk of mother-to-child transmission attributable to breast feeding as long as the nipples are not damaged or bleeding.[141] Administration of immune globulin to a newborn has no role in preventing vertical transmission because donors for commercial immune globulin preparations are screened and rejected for the presence of HCV antibodies.

Infants born to mothers infected with HCV are virtually all asymptomatic at birth and remain so for years.[145] There are few long-term longitudinal studies of these infants. Progression of disease seems to be slower in children than in adults, and most children experience only mild to moderate intermittent elevations of serum liver transaminase levels through at least the first two decades of life. Liver histologic changes tend to be mild as well. It is uncertain how many of these children progress to cirrhosis or hepatocellular carcinoma later in life. A small proportion of children with vertically transmitted HCV clear the infection spontaneously over their first few years. Maternal HCV antibodies may be detectable in the infant for 18 months and cannot be used for diagnosis unless they persist beyond this time. HCV-specific RNA can be detected in the serum by PCR. Most infants born to a mother infected with HCV have negative HCV PCR at birth, but, if infected, PCR becomes positive after the first 1 or 2 months. Thereafter, the test is variably positive throughout life, reflecting intermittent episodes of viremia.

Hepatitis D Virus

Hepatitis D virus (HDV), formerly known as the δ agent, is a defective RNA virus that uses HBsAg as its surface coat and requires coinfection with HBV. Its epidemiology is the same as HBV. HDV is transmitted parenterally, and in the United States is most commonly found in drug addicts and hemophiliacs. HDV is worldwide in distribution. Perinatal transmission, which is rare, occurs only with HBV transmission and can be interrupted by interrupting HBV perinatal transmission.

Hepatitis E Virus

Hepatitis E virus (HEV) is a single-stranded, positive-sensed, nonenveloped RNA virus unrelated to the other hepatitis agents. HEV disease has been identified in Asia, Africa, the Middle East, and Central America.[136] Occasionally, a case is diagnosed in an immigrant in the United States or Europe. In endemic areas, HEV occurs sporadically, but several instances of large outbreaks have been reported, typically affecting thousands of people. Infection is transmitted through contaminated water supplies sullied by sewage; person-to-person spread is uncommon. The diagnosis can be made by identification of viral particles in the stool, by Western blot assays for anti-HEV IgM and IgG, and by detection of circulating viral RNA using PCR, but these tests are not routinely available in most hospitals in the United States. In nonpregnant adults, infection with HEV is similar to that caused by HAV. Most cases are characterized by self-limiting icteric hepatitis with full recovery. Subclinical and anicteric infections also occur. Fulminant hepatitis results from a small fraction of infections. HEV infection does not lead to chronic hepatitis.

There is a striking association between pregnancy and the development of overwhelming HEV-related hepatitis, particularly in women from the Asian subcontinent. In some endemic areas, HEV is the most common identifiable cause of clinically apparent hepatitis in pregnant women, even when the prevalence of HEV in the general population is lower than other hepatotropic pathogens. Massive hepatic necrosis is particularly prominent during the third trimester of pregnancy, when the mortality rate can exceed 20%.[3] The reasons for this predilection are unknown, but some data suggest that hormonal elevations during pregnancy promote viral replication.[63]

Mild HEV disease during pregnancy can result in abortion, intrauterine death, stillbirth, or preterm delivery.[112] Reports studying a few subjects have documented vertical transmission of HEV in more than half of infants born to mothers who were viremic during pregnancy. Blood-borne virus can be detected soon after birth, suggesting intrauterine transmission. All the affected infants had abnormalities of liver function tests, and approximately 20% to 25% died; one of these had hepatic necrosis at autopsy. Liver function returned to normal in survivors after 2 to 3 months.

Hepatitis G Virus and GB Virus Type C

Hepatitis G virus (HGV) and GB virus type C (GBV-C) were isolated independently, but subsequently proved to be nearly identical flaviviruses based on genetic sequence. HGV/GBV-C has a genomic organization similar to HCV. In adults, infection by HGV/GBV-C results in viremia that lasts for months to years, but the virus eventually is cleared by the appearance of antibody against the viral protein E2. Although initial studies suggested that HGV/GBV-C was a cause of hepatitis, subsequent surveys have failed to establish that HGV/GBV-C infection produces liver disease or any disease at all. This observation, along with data that suggest HGV/GBV-C primarily infects lymphocytes rather than hepatocytes, has prompted some experts to recommend that the name "hepatitis G virus" be discontinued.

HGV/GBV-C is transmitted through the same routes as HIV and HCV—transfusion, injection drug use, sexual activity, and vertical transmission from mother to infant. Occasional patients with HGV/GBV-C infection have none of these risk factors, suggesting that other modes of acquisition occur as well. Prevalence studies have documented that active infection, defined by the detection of circulating HGV/GBV-C RNA, and past infection, defined by the presence of antibody to HGV/GBV-C, are extraordinarily common in healthy individuals and patients with underlying conditions. Approximately 2% of blood donors have evidence of active HGV/GBV-C infection, and an additional 15% to 18% have evidence of past infection. Coinfection with HGV/GBV-C occurs in more than 20% of subjects with HCV infection. Ongoing or past infection by HGV/GBV-C is detected in two thirds or more of intravenous drug users and patients with HIV. Although no clinically apparent disease has been identified in individuals infected with HGV/GBV-C, interest in this virus has been rejuvenated by studies suggesting that active HGV/GBV-C replication in HIV-infected patients may slow the progression of HIV disease. The mechanism of this putative protective effect in HIV-infected hosts is uncertain.

HGV/GBV-C is efficiently transmitted from mother to child. Studies that have included healthy women and mothers coinfected with HCV or HIV have documented HGV/GBV-C transmission to more than half of their offspring. Typically, an infant becomes positive for HGV/GBV-C RNA by

3 months of age, and, similar to adults, active infection lasts for months. Most studies have failed to detect an independent association between HGV/GBV-C infection in vertically infected newborns and subclinical or clinically apparent liver disease. To date, no other clinical consequences have been identified in infected infants.[156]

ROTAVIRUS

Rotavirus is the predominant cause of acute viral gastroenteritis in infants and young children. It is a double-stranded RNA virus containing 11 genomic segments. The virus is composed of three concentric capsid shells. Strains are characterized by the electrophoresis migration patterns of the RNA segments and by structural differences of the capsid proteins VP6, VP7, and VP4. VP6 serotype A accounts for most of the rotaviruses that are pathogenic in humans. The virus replicates primarily in enterocytes in the proximal small intestine, where infection leads to denuding of the villus tips and mononuclear cell infiltration of the underlying lamina propria. The virus seems to remain localized to the intestine. It has not been identified in breast milk.

Epidemiology and Transmission

The distribution of rotavirus is widespread throughout the industrialized and developing world. The virus causes an estimated 150 million diarrheal episodes in infants and young children each year, and approximately 0.5 million deaths. Rotavirus infections are usually prevalent in temperate climates during the winter months, whereas in tropical areas, infection is endemic year-round. In some nurseries, endemic infection rates reflect the incidence in the community, but in others the incidence of disease is relatively constant. Rotavirus infection in neonatal units may also occur in the context of a clinically apparent outbreak. The distinction between endemic and epidemic rotavirus disease is blurred, however, in the nursery. Longitudinal prevalence surveys conducted in geographically diverse nurseries during periods without outbreaks indicate that 10% to 70% of infants admitted for more than 1 week excrete rotavirus at some time before discharge, often asymptomatically, and that typically only one or two strains account for all the infections over many months.

Epidemiologic aspects of rotavirus potentiate its spread in a confined environment, such as a nursery. The stool of infected individuals contains high titers of virus, and infection can be transmitted by very small inocula. Additionally, the virus survives on inanimate surfaces and is resistant to many commercial disinfectants. Rotavirus likely is introduced into the unit by a newborn who acquires infection during delivery after exposure to maternal stool, or by an infant or a staff member who imports the virus from the community. Thereafter, most infection is nosocomial, transmitted via the hands of personnel. Viral excretion in the stool begins 1 to 2 days before the onset of diarrhea, is highest after 3 to 4 days of diarrhea, then wanes 1 to 2 weeks later. Outbreaks may spread rapidly through the nursery, where the most important factors determining spread seem to be the frequency of handling the infants and the closeness of the bed spaces.

Clinical Manifestations

Nearly all reports indicate that rotavirus infection frequently is asymptomatic or mildly symptomatic in newborns. Some data suggest that maternally derived serum and intestinal antibodies and possibly breast milk antibodies may be responsible for preventing or ameliorating infection early in life. Additionally, a high proportion of nursery infections are caused by the VP4-serotype designated *P[6]*.[85] This serotype is not usually isolated from older children with community-acquired symptomatic infection. The reasons underlying the predilection of newborns for P[6] strains are unknown, but this observation suggests that the relatively mild disease in infants may partially be the result of intrinsic properties of the infecting virus.

Symptomatic infants develop irritability and poor feeding, followed by watery or mucous stools that are sometimes bloody and frequently contain increased reducing substances.[120] Occasionally, infants develop severe diarrhea and dehydration, but fatalities are rare. There has been speculation that rotaviral infection may predispose to necrotizing enterocolitis, but such an association has not been clearly established.

The diagnosis is usually made by detection of viral antigen in stools using ELISA. False-positive results may be 1% to 4%. Hand washing remains the most effective prophylactic measure. Hard surfaces should be washed with alcohol-containing disinfectants because quaternary ammonia-containing compounds are not active against the virus. Therapy consists of rehydration and maintenance of fluids and electrolytes. Some investigators have found that breast feeding prevents infection or lessens the severity of the illness.

A tetravalent vaccine approved by the FDA in 1998 was removed from the market in 1999 because postmarketing surveillance indicated a rare association with intussusception. Two additional oral rotavirus vaccines were introduced in the mid-2000s: a pentavalent product composed of five reassorted strains derived from human and bovine rotaviruses, and a monovalent vaccine composed of an attenuated human strain. Both vaccines seem to be protective and free of significant side effects, including intussusception. The first dose of each vaccine is preferentially administered at 2 months, although both may be given at 6 weeks. Immunization of preterm neonates is recommended at the same postnatal age if the infant is otherwise stable, and he or she has been discharged from the hospital.

PARVOVIRUS B19

Parvoviruses are small (23 to 25 nm), single-stranded DNA viruses of the family Parvoviridae (genus *Erythrovirus*) that lack an envelope, but form capsids. (*Parvum* is the Latin word meaning "small.") The viral genome consists of approximately 5600 nucleotides and encodes for only three proteins—a nonstructural protein, NS1, which functions in replication and is responsible for the destruction of the erythroid progenitors, and two structural proteins, viral protein 1 (VP1) and viral protein 2 (VP2).[163] VP1 differs from VP2 only in that it has 226 additional amino acids at its amino terminal. Although most of the capsid consists of VP2, which may assist in the entry of the virus into the cell, the additional 226 amino acids

of VP1 form loops that are external to the capsid and contain the epitopes recognized by neutralizing antibodies. Immunity to parvovirus occurs primarily through the antibody response, and IgG confers lasting immunity.

Parvoviruses are animal viruses, which seem to be species-specific. Parvovirus B19 replicates only in human erythroid precursors and is the only virus in the family definitely known to be pathogenic in humans. Parvovirus B19 was identified in 1975 in the sera of blood being screened for hepatitis B, and its name signifies the well in which it was identified. Parvovirus B19 is distributed worldwide, and infection occurs sporadically throughout the year, although there are seasonal increases in temperate zones, particularly in the spring, and epidemics occur every 4 years.

Transmission of infection occurs mainly through contact with respiratory secretions or droplets, but also occurs vertically from mother to fetus and via blood or blood products. IgG antibodies to parvovirus B19 are believed to confer lifelong immunity, and vertical transmission has not been documented in women with immunity before pregnancy. Secondary infection rates among nonimmune household contacts approach 50%, and childcare personnel and teachers have an occupational risk of approximately 20%. Although seroprevalence is found in only 5% to 10% of young children, it increases to approximately 50% in young adults and is nearly 90% in elderly adults. The annual seroconversion rate of women of childbearing age is estimated to be 1.5%. The risk seems to be greatest in homes with multiple children, especially between ages 3 and 10 years. The incubation period usually is 4 to 14 days, but can be 21 days. Rash and joint symptoms appear 2 to 3 weeks after infection. Individuals are most infectious before the onset of the rash, but are no longer so after the appearance of the rash, so school attendance with rash is not of concern. Hospitalized patients with aplastic crisis may remain contagious for a week after the onset of symptoms.

Clinical Manifestations

In most instances, infection with parvovirus B19 is asymptomatic and remains unrecognized. The most common illness is erythema infectiosum, or fifth disease. These individuals usually have a syndrome of malaise and low-grade fever, followed by the development of an erythematous, "slapped cheek" rash, sparing the nasal bridge and circumoral region, and a blotchy, maculopapular rash of the trunk and extremities. These areas develop central clearing, resulting in a reticular pattern. This rash may recur with heat or cold exposure. Individuals shed virus during the prodrome and are unlikely to be infectious by the time the rash aspect of the illness occurs. Another manifestation that is less common in children is a symmetric arthralgia or arthritis, particularly of the hands, wrists, and knees, which is usually self-limited. Both manifestations, rash and arthropathy, seem to be immune mediated.

Because the virus causes lysis of red blood cell precursors, it may cause a transient red blood cell aplasia, which is rarely significant in healthy individuals. Aplastic crises may result, however, in the presence of hematopoietic disease, such as sickle cell disease or thalassemia. Chronic infection and anemia may result in patients with immunodeficiency disorders. Other reports suggest an association of the virus with myocarditis,[110] peripheral nerve abnormalities, or vasculitis.

Fetal Infection

Fifty percent of pregnant women are susceptible to parvovirus. When infection occurs, transplacental transmission of parvovirus is estimated to be 30% to 50%; fetal loss occurs in 5% to 9% of the fetuses.[118] Most pregnancies result in apparently normal newborns despite proven fetal infection,[74] although there may be an increase in infants who are small for gestational age and spontaneous abortion. Although there have been a few reports of congenital anomalies, the relationship to parvovirus infection is not yet proven. In studies of viral causes of intrauterine fetal deaths, parvovirus was found in 13% of fetuses and was highly associated with chronic villitis and hydrops fetalis.[139] Parvovirus B19 attaches to the globoside glycolipid cellular receptor found on erythroid precursor cells (erythroblasts and megakaryocytes), erythrocytes, placental syncytiotrophoblast, fetal myocardium, and endothelial cells, but replication occurs only in the erythroid progenitor cells.[163]

The most common adverse fetal outcome reported in infected fetuses is hydrops fetalis; parvovirus B19 may be responsible for 20% to 30% of the cases of nonimmune hydrops, particularly during epidemics. The virus infects the erythroid progenitor cells in the fetal liver, causing a maturation arrest at a time that the fetus is expanding its red blood cell volume and has a shortened red blood cell life span, resulting in severe fetal anemia in most, but not all, instances. Fetal anemia results in congestive heart failure, a known cause of hydropic changes, such as generalized edema, ascites, and pleural effusions.

The virus may also cause myocarditis, after attachment to the globoside receptors in the myocardial cell, which also results in hydrops. Some fetuses develop thrombocytopenia and hepatic damage. Meconium peritonitis has resulted from small bowel obstruction and perforation. Placental damage, resulting in leakage of α-fetoprotein, is often linked to poor outcome. The risk of hydrops is greatest between 17 and 24 weeks of gestation, when fetal red blood cell precursors are developing, but hydrops may occur in the third trimester as well. Of fetuses with hydrops who received no treatment, half resolved spontaneously, and one third resulted in fetal death. Fetal death usually occurs 3 to 5 weeks after the maternal illness, but may occur 11 weeks later. The mother may also become ill with "mirror syndrome," which consists of a preeclampsia-like state, with anemia, hypertension, proteinuria, and swollen legs, mirroring the fetal infection.[31]

There are too few cases of hydrops secondary to parvovirus B19 to conduct a controlled trial, so most clinicians advocate intrauterine transfusion. Measurement of the middle cerebral artery peak systolic velocity on fetal ultrasound may be useful as an indicator of the need for fetal transfusion. When transfusion has been used, survival of the fetus has been 85%. One fetus with hydrops was also successfully treated with intrauterine fetal peritoneal injection of parvovirus B19 hyperimmune gammaglobulin.[91] Fetuses who survived intrauterine transfusion had a good neurodevelopmental outcome on follow-up.[32] Serial ultrasound studies and serum α-fetoprotein screening may be beneficial, but are unproven. Digitalization has also been used for fetuses with myocarditis. Surviving fetuses do not seem to have heart disease. A few cases have also been reported of encephalitis, meningitis, perivascular calcifications, and intrauterine stroke. In these cases, virus seems to infect the immature endothelial cells.

Diagnosis

Because parvovirus B19 is too fastidious to grow in the laboratory, serology remains the best means of diagnosis, with the measurement of specific IgM or an increase in titer of specific IgG. IgM antibodies appear 7 to 14 days after infection and are often present for at least 6 months. IgG antibodies appear within days and persist for the life of the patient. Not all fetuses make parvovirus B19 IgM, so viral DNA needs to be detected. Parvovirus B19 DNA may be detected in maternal serum, amniotic fluid, or fetal blood using PCR, but the presence of the antigen does not always indicate recent infection because a tiny percentage of healthy individuals can also have parvovirus B19 antigen isolated from their blood. Placental infection has been documented at 14 to 16 weeks' gestation, but it is rare for the amniotic fluid to be infected before 21 weeks of gestation, and detection of amniotic fluid infection usually requires a delay of at least several weeks after the maternal infection. Placental infection does not invariably result in fetal infection.

Isolation

Contact isolation with gown, gloves, and mask is indicated for hospitalized patients with aplastic crisis. Pregnant health care personnel should be aware of their risks, although the magnitude of this risk is uncertain. Serologic testing and the option not to care for a patient with an aplastic crisis may be offered. Patients with only the rash of erythema infectiosum are not contagious. A vaccine has been developed, but is unavailable, and the cost-effectiveness is questionable.

INFLUENZA A AND B

The influenza viruses are RNA viruses of the Orthomyxoviridae family. Although there are three antigenic types (A through C), type C has not played a significant role in neonatal infections and is associated primarily with coryza. Type B is responsible for about 10% of infections in humans, but is not usually associated with epidemics. Type A virus is also classified by the presence of two distinct glycoprotein surface antigens, the hemagglutinin and neuraminidase antigens. Hemagglutinin is responsible for viral binding to cell receptors, and neuraminidase is responsible for the release of virus after replication from the cell.[161] The H1, H2, and H3 hemagglutinin subtypes, and the N1 and N2 neuraminidase subtypes are particularly important in epidemics because immunity is largely due to the production of antibody to these antigens, and "drifts," or minor changes in the antigens, occur over time, requiring changes in the immune response to the virus.

An antigenic "shift," with the development of a new hemagglutinin or neuraminidase antigen, results in pandemic infection at infrequent intervals. In one 10-year study among

209 infants in the first year of life, influenza A (H3N2) occurred most commonly, followed by influenza B and influenza A (H1N1), with infections in 178, 96, and 26 infants.[44] More recent epidemics of avian H5N1 influenza A in humans have resulted from direct contact with birds. Disease has been particularly severe in infants and young children. There has been increasing concern that the genome of avian H5N1 influenza A could mix with human influenza A and be able to be transmitted directly from human to human and be able to cause widespread disease.

Influenza is rapidly and easily spread person to person by aerosol droplet or by contact with contaminated secretions. Viral shedding and infectiousness are greatest in the 24 hours before onset of symptoms and at the peak of symptoms. The virus may survive in the environment, although the role of fomites in transmitting infection is unclear. The incubation period is 1 to 3 days. Winter outbreaks are more common in temperate climates. School-age children have the highest attack rate and serve as a source of spread to adults and younger children. Hand washing and cohorting are the most effective means to interrupt epidemics within the NICU. Cohorting requires rapid diagnosis. PCR detection of influenza RNA is the most rapid and sensitive means of diagnosis. In addition, staff members should not work when ill, and family members should be carefully screened, particularly in season, for viral illness before admission to the NICU.

All women who may be pregnant during an influenza season should receive inactivated vaccine. The vaccine is safe throughout pregnancy and breast feeding.[161] Staff members in the NICU should also be encouraged to be vaccinated; compliance has traditionally been low. Also, inactivated vaccine should be given to family members of high-risk infants. Little is known about the safety and efficacy of using antiviral prophylaxis for staff members and parents in epidemics in the NICU, although they have been used.[49]

Most influenza infections in neonates are asymptomatic. Infection is less common in the first 6 months of life and usually less symptomatic, probably reflecting the transplacental transference of maternal antibody during pregnancy, which may protect the infant for the first 6 months, and antibody transferred via breast milk. Infants may present with high fever and an upper respiratory tract infection, however, and infection may be indistinguishable from bacterial sepsis. Infants younger than 6 months have also been reported to have the highest mortality. In the 2003-2004 influenza season, the mortality of infants younger than 6 months was 0.88 per 100,000 children. One third of the infants died at home, and one fourth had coinfections with bacteria. Only one third had conditions recognized as putting the infant at high risk, such as pulmonary or cardiovascular disease or immunosuppression. Chronic neurologic and neuromuscular conditions, not previously recognized as at-risk conditions, were present in one third of the children.[9]

Bronchiolitis, pneumonia or croup, fever, rhinorrhea, apnea, irritability, and feeding difficulties all may be primary symptoms. In a prospective study of the first year of life, one third of the infants were infected, but only 40% of the infants were infected in the first 6 months of life, and most lower respiratory tract disease and otitis media occurred in the latter 6 months, when the transferred maternal antibody would be expected to

have waned.[44] There was also a very significant increase in risk of infection with increasing numbers of siblings, ranging from a 20% infection rate with no siblings to a 59% rate with three or more siblings. Lower respiratory tract disease was, however, far less common than with RSV or PIV. One third of infants presenting to the emergency department during influenza epidemics had influenza infection, although they frequently had no respiratory symptoms. In contrast, one third of the infants presenting with a community-acquired pneumonia were also infected with influenza.[77,117]

Several influenza A and a few influenza B epidemics have been reported in NICUs. Low rates of immunization among staff members played a significant role in these epidemics. Prematurity and pulmonary disease, particularly bronchopulmonary dysplasia, seem to be risk factors.

There is no antiviral treatment licensed for use in infants younger than 1 year of age. Amantadine has been used in NICU outbreaks, but did not seem to decrease the length of illness, and in one instance resistance was quickly noted.[29,100] The safety of any of the antiviral drugs has not been determined in infants. Likewise, inactivated influenza vaccine is not licensed for infants 6 months or younger because it has not been shown to be immunogenic, even though infants, especially infants with bronchopulmonary dysplasia, may be at greater risk than older children. Instead, the risk of exposure to these infants should be minimized by immunizing health care workers and family members and other close contacts. Vaccination of preterm infants after 6 months of age, even in the presence of prolonged hypogammaglobulinemia, does result in a good antibody response.[127]

NOVEL H1N1 INFLUENZA A

Novel H1N1 influenza A was first recognized in Mexico and the United States in March and April 2009. It was initially called "swine flu" because it seemed to be genetically related to the influenza viruses that occurred in pigs in North America. It has now been shown, however, that novel H1N1 influenza A is a reassortment virus of two genes that circulate in swine in Europe and Asia and bird (avian) genes and human genes. In April 2009, the United States declared a public health emergency and began working on pandemic alert level; this was based on the spread of the virus rather than its severity. The virus continued to spread, and outbreaks occurred in the United States throughout the summer in 2009. The United States has the highest number of cases in the world, although most patients recovered and did not experience severe illness. In the Southern Hemisphere, when it entered its influenza season in 2009, cases of novel H1N1 virus spread in addition to the regular seasonal influenza virus.

At the present time, limited data are available regarding the spread, infection, prevention, and treatment of novel H1N1 influenza. The following data and recommendations are current as of the writing of this chapter, but will undoubtedly be changing as more data are accrued. These recommendations were obtained from the website of the CDC (www.cdc.gov/h1n1flu); this site should be consulted regularly for changes in recommendations.

The novel H1N1 virus seems to spread via the same mechanisms as the regular influenza virus, by large particle respiratory droplet transmission, which occurs when a person coughs or sneezes. The particles travel only a short distance (<6 feet) because of their size. Influenza virus may also survive and remain infectious on environmental surfaces for 2 to 8 hours. Small droplet or airborne transmission is also possible. It is not spread by eating food, including pork or pork products. The virus can be destroyed by heat (75°C to 100°C) or by numerous chemical germicides or household disinfectants, including chlorine, detergents, hydrogen peroxide, and alcohols. Most importantly, hand washing with soap and water and with alcohol-based hand cleaners is very effective. Individuals should cover their nose and mouth with a tissue when coughing or sneezing; wash their hands frequently; and avoid touching their eyes, nose, and mouth. Individuals with a flulike illness should remain at home.

Infection may be mild or severe. The symptoms are the same as for seasonal influenza: fever, cough, sore throat, aches, chills and fatigue, headache, running or stuffy nose, and vomiting and diarrhea. Young children may not develop fever, but are more likely to have diarrhea. Complications may be mild (otitis, febrile seizures) or severe (bacterial co-infeciton, pneumonia or worsened baseline conditions) and may progress very rapidly. Pneumonia was seen in nearly half of children who were less than five years of age.[61a] Hospitalization was required in 35% of one month old infants and 21% of two month old infants.[85a]

- Children younger than 5 years (highest risk is for children <2 years old)
- Pregnant women
- Adults 65 years old and older
- People with chronic conditions
  - Chronic pulmonary (asthma), cardiovascular, renal, hepatic, hematologic (sickle cell disease), neurologic, neuromuscular, or metabolic disorders (diabetes)
  - Immunosuppression, either by medication or HIV infection or cancer or chronic steroids
  - Individuals younger than 19 years old on long-term aspirin therapy

There are four influenza antiviral drugs available for use. The novel H1N1 influenza virus is sensitive to date to the neuraminidase inhibitors, zanamivir and oseltamivir, but resistant to the adamantine medications, amantadine and rimantadine. Treatment should be started as soon as possible after onset of symptoms in all hospitalized patients with suspected, probable, or confirmed novel H1N1 infection, and in patients who are in a high-risk group for seasonal influenza complications. Treatment benefit seems to be greatest when treatment is started within 48 hours of symptom onset, but data from patients with seasonal influenza indicate that there may be some decrease in mortality and hospital stay even when started after 48 hours. Treatment should continue for 5 days.

There are limited safety data for oseltamivir in children younger than 1 year of age, which indicate that serious adverse effects are probably rare, and this group has had significant morbidity and mortality from seasonal influenza. Infants less than three months should not receive chemoprophylaxis unless the situation is felt to be critical. Oseltamivir may be considered for treatment (3 mg/kg/dose twice daily for 5 days). Premature infants have immature renal function and may have slower clearance of oseltamivir. There are insufficient data to recommend a dose and drug concentrations that have been measured are highly variable.

Pregnant women infected with H1N1 influenza virus in 2009 had higher rates of hospitalization and represented about 6% of all the deaths in the United States. They should be vaccinated during prenatal visits and may receive both seasonal flu vaccine and H1N1 flu vaccine at the same time in different sites (one in each arm). Vaccination of the pregnant woman may offer some protection to her newborn infant, which is particularly important, as the vaccine is not licensed for infants less than six months of age. Certainly, all caregivers of infants less than six months should also be vaccinated in an effort to prevent them from bringing influenza to the infant. Pregnant women should receive the monovalent injectable, inactivated vaccine with or without themerosol preservative. Breast feeding is likewise compatible with vaccination and may offer some antibody protection to the infant. Both the nasal spray or injectable vaccine may be given to the breast feeding mother.

The virus has not been shown to cross the placenta to date, but the newborn may be exposed to contaminated secretions at birth. Thus, the newborn should be considered exposed rather than infected, and should be carefully observed. The baby may be separated from the mother in an incubator in the same room, or in a separate room until the mother has been treated with antivirals for at least 48 hours and has been free of fever while off antipyretics for at least 24 hours, and can control her cough and respiratory secretions. Breast feeding should be fully supported and the breast milk should be used to feed the newborn. When able to see her infant, the mother should wear a face mask, wash her hands with soap and water, and follow respiratory hygiene and cough etiquette guidelines for at least seven days after symptom onset or 24 hours after resolution of symptoms, whichever is longer.

In past pandemics, secondary bacterial infections, particularly caused by *Streptococcus pneumoniae* (pneumococcus), have also been the cause of increased morbidity and mortality. Continued pneumococcal vaccination is important.

RUBELLA VIRUS

Rubella virus is an RNA virus in the Togaviridae family. It is surrounded by a lipid-containing envelope, which is responsible for its infectivity. Only one immunologic strain has been identified; the epidemics that have occurred seem to be secondary to changes in the susceptibility of the population, rather than changes in the virulence of a strain.

Rubella produces a very mild but extremely contagious disease, sometimes referred to as German measles. The incubation period is 14 to 23 days. It primarily manifests in adults with a maculopapular rash that can last 3 days and spreads from the face to the trunk and extremities, and with postauricular, suboccipital, and posterior cervical lymph node enlargement. There may be conjunctivitis, headache, sore throat, and cough. Although arthralgias may occur, recovery is nearly always rapid and complete. Fever is slight. Thrombocytopenia and encephalitis are rare. Half of all infections may be asymptomatic.

Epidemiology and Transmission

Rubella virus exclusively infects humans and is spread via respiratory droplet contact. Infections are worldwide in distribution, but tend to peak in late winter and early spring. Presumably, the viral reservoir is maintained by mild or asymptomatic infections that occur constantly throughout the year and by prolonged viral shedding (possibly ≥1 year) from congenitally infected infants. Most individuals shed virus from 7 days before the onset of the rash until 14 days afterward. In the prevaccine era (before 1969), epidemics occurred every 6 to 9 years. The last major epidemic in the United States was in 1965. The goal of routine rubella vaccination in the United States, begun in 1969, was to eliminate congenital rubella syndrome. From 2001-2006, there were only four cases of congenital rubella syndrome in the United States. Three of the mothers were born outside of the United States.[93] In 2004, the CDC declared that rubella was no longer endemic in the United States. Rubella continues to occur among immigrants, however, and it is important that pediatricians continue to administer the vaccine. The current goal is global elimination.

Most cases of congenital rubella syndrome occur after a primary maternal infection that causes viremia and intrauterine transmission. A few cases have occurred after maternal reinfection with rubella, but these are very rare. Accidental vaccination with RA27/3 vaccine in pregnancy may result in fetal infection (2%), but congenital defects or congenital rubella syndromes have not been seen.

After a primary maternal infection in the first trimester, there may be fetal loss, stillbirth, placental infection, or congenital rubella syndrome, or the fetus may remain totally uninfected. Not all infected fetuses develop congenital rubella syndrome. The virus may cause persistent placental infection with or without persistent fetal infection. The placenta is a relatively effective barrier to fetal infection from 12 to 28 weeks' gestation, but is not so effective in the first and third trimesters, particularly in the last month of pregnancy.

Gestational age at the time of maternal infection is the most important determinant of fetal infection and of the development of congenital defects, although fetal infection may occur at any point in gestation. Among 273 infants delivered after maternal rubella infection, Miller and colleagues[95] reported that fetal infection occurred in 90% of infants after maternal infection before 11 weeks' gestation, in 67% of infants at 13 to 14 weeks' gestation, and in 25% of infants at 23 to 26 weeks' gestation. Infection increased to 53% of infants after maternal infection in the third trimester, however, and reached 100% in the last month of pregnancy.

In addition, the risk of fetal damage with fetal infection decreases with increasing gestational age. Peckham[113] followed 218 congenitally infected infants for 2 years and found that fetal damage occurred in 52% of infants infected before 8 weeks' gestation, in 36% of infants infected at 9 to 12 weeks' gestation, and in 10% of infants infected at 13 to 20 weeks' gestation. No fetal damage was shown after infection beyond 20 weeks' gestation. Rubella results in chronic infection of the fetal tissues, however, causing an inhibition of fetal cell multiplication. Many infants who show no apparent involvement at birth develop consequences years later. In concordance with the chronicity of the disease, Peckham[113] later noted that at 6 to 8 years of age, these same infants had an 82% risk of sequelae after infection in the first trimester. The risk of fetal damage reported by Miller and colleagues[95] was even higher, with sequelae shown in 90% of infants infected before 11 weeks' gestation, 33% infected from 11 to 12 weeks' gestation, 11% infected at 13 to 14 weeks' gestation, and 24% infected at 15 to 16 weeks' gestation.

Congenital Rubella Syndrome

Congenital rubella is not a static disease. Nearly three fourths of infected infants show no apparent involvement at birth, but develop consequences years later. More than half of infants with expanded congenital rubella syndrome have intrauterine growth restriction (birthweight is often <1500 g) and continue to fail to thrive postnatally. These infants often have myriad transient symptoms, including thrombocytopenia, petechiae and purpura, hemolytic anemia, hepatitis, jaundice, and hepatosplenomegaly. Nearly half of infants show "blueberry muffin" spots on the head, neck, and trunk, which represent dermal extramedullary hematopoiesis. Infants may also show myocarditis, cloudy cornea, long bone radiolucencies, interstitial pneumonia, and meningoencephalitis, manifested by an elevated CSF protein level and pleocytosis. Although most of these symptoms are transient, they may also indicate severity of infection. Fulminant hepatitis or pneumonia, myocarditis with congestive heart failure, meningoencephalitis, thrombocytopenia, and bony lesions all are associated with a higher mortality.

Congenital rubella is best known for causing deafness and defects of the eye, CNS, and heart. Three fourths of infants develop sensorineural deafness, usually bilateral. Deafness may be the only sequela of congenital infection and may occur with maternal infection up to 20 weeks' gestation.

Congenital heart disease occurs only when the fetus is infected during the first 8 weeks of gestation, the period during which organogenesis occurs, but is quite common with infection during that period. Patent ductus arteriosus, the most common lesion, may occur alone or in conjunction with pulmonary artery or valvular stenosis, or there may be stenoses of other vessels.

Microcephaly and neuropsychiatric problems are also common. Studies of long-term outcome show that 26% of children with congenital rubella syndrome were severely mentally retarded, 12% had neurologic problems, 18% had behavioral abnormalities, and 6% had autism. Most rubella survivors without mental retardation had learning disorders, behavioral problems, difficulties with balance, and muscle weakness.

Ophthalmologic abnormalities may include cataracts in one third of children, often bilateral and occasionally accompanied by glaucoma. Other children may have microphthalmos or characteristic salt-and-pepper chorioretinitis. Rubella RNA can be detected and quantified in the lens of affected infants.

Attention has focused more recently on the effects of HLA haplotypes, immune complexes, and autoantibodies in predisposing congenital rubella survivors to autoimmune conditions. In a 60-year follow-up of congenital rubella survivors, Forrest and colleagues[38] showed that 20% had died (mostly of cardiovascular disease and malignancy); 68% had mild aortic valve stenosis, 22% had diabetes mellitus, 19% had thyroid disease, 73% had early menopause, and 13% had osteoporosis. HLA-A1 and HLA-B8 antigens were increased in frequency.

Diagnosis

Diagnosis of maternal rubella on the basis of clinical findings is unreliable, and serologic testing must be used. If the maternal immune status is unknown at the time of rash illness, acute-phase titers should be obtained within 7 days of the illness; seropositivity usually indicates prior immunity with very little risk of current infection. Women with very low titers may be reinfected, which can result in a small risk of fetal infection. Latex agglutination, enzyme immunoassay tests, and immunofluorescence are now more commonly used than passive hemagglutination techniques.

Rubella-specific IgM may be determined 7 to 14 days after the illness. A high or moderate IgM titer is very helpful, but false-positive results may occur, and low IgM titers may be found in patients with subclinical reinfection. Testing IgG avidity can be very helpful in differentiating acute infection from reinfection, postvaccination, and false-positive IgM values.

Traditionally, an increase in serum antibody titers obtained initially in the acute phase, preferably within 7 days of illness, and repeated in the convalescent phase, 10 to 14 days later, is used to diagnose acute infection. The titers need to be run simultaneously in the same laboratory. If antibody is still not present 4 weeks after exposure, another serum sample should be tested at 6 weeks for certainty. Acute-phase titers may be obtained, with less accuracy, 28 days after illness, but are not interpretable thereafter.

The antenatal diagnosis of fetal rubella infection has been made with rubella cultures or detection of rubella-specific IgM or rubella-specific antigen or RNA by reverse transcriptase PCR from amniotic fluid or percutaneous umbilical blood sampling. Chorionic villus sampling has also been used, but less is known of its reliability.

Any infant born to a mother suspected of having had a rubella infection in pregnancy or born with clinical signs and symptoms consistent with congenital rubella syndrome should have a complete evaluation and diagnostic workup. Isolation of rubella virus from a newborn provides an absolute diagnosis. The virus is most often isolated from the nasopharynx, but has been grown in the blood, CSF, and urine, or even from the lens of the eye or CSF years later. The diagnosis may also be made by detecting rubella-specific IgM in cord or infant blood or by detecting stable or increasing concentrations of rubella-specific IgG in the infant's serum over several months, although hypogammaglobulinemic infants may fail to produce antibody. More recently, oral fluid testing for rubella-specific IgM or reverse transcriptase PCR for rubella antigen has been very helpful.

Prevention and Therapy

All children with postnatally acquired rubella should be isolated for 7 days after the rash appears. In contrast, children with congenitally acquired rubella should be considered contagious for at least 1 year, unless repeated urine and blood cultures are negative. In addition, the families of these infants should be counseled regarding the risks to pregnant women.

Susceptible pregnant women exposed to rash illnesses should have a laboratory workup performed for diagnosis, as should the individual who is the origin of the illness. Immune globulin is not recommended for prophylaxis in an exposed pregnant woman unless abortion is absolutely not a consideration because congenital rubella has occurred despite the lack of symptoms in women given immune globulin. Also, vaccination after exposure does not prevent infection from the current exposure, but might prevent exposure and infection in the future.

The goal in the United States is to eliminate rubella with vaccination. The RA 27/3 rubella virus vaccine is exclusively used in the United States and is highly effective. Infants should be vaccinated at 12 to 15 months of age and again at school entry. Preterm infants seem to lose maternal antibody to rubella at a much earlier age than term infants because the antibody is transferred primarily during the third trimester. The antibody response to vaccination is similar, however, to that of term infants. Postpartum and postpubertal women should be vaccinated unless contraindication exists. Breast feeding is not a contraindication. Women should not be vaccinated during pregnancy because 3% of fetuses may be infected, but birth defects have not been reported after vaccination of pregnant women, even if the fetus is infected. It is acceptable to vaccinate children of pregnant women because there is no evidence of transmission of virus after vaccination. Some parents continue to believe that vaccination with MMR may cause autism, despite numerous data and studies failing to show any association. The Immunization Safety Review Committee of the Institute of Medicine rejects any causal association.

RHINOVIRUS

Rhinoviruses are the most prevalent of human pathogens and are well known to cause the "common cold." They are small, nonenveloped RNA viruses classified as picornaviruses. There are three large groups of human pathogens among the Picornaviridae family: the enteroviruses (enteroviruses, polioviruses, coxsackieviruses, and echoviruses), the hepatoviruses (hepatovirus A), and the rhinoviruses. There are more than 100 rhinovirus serotypes, and even more serotypes are being described with improved methodology. Immunity to one serotype offers little immunity to another and is only of variable and brief duration to that serotype. The rhinoviruses are usually spread from person to person via contaminated hands and self-inoculation of the nasopharynx, but may also be spread by aerosol droplets. Infection may occur year-round, but may be epidemic in fall and spring, in temperate climates; the incubation period lasts 2 to 7 days. Shedding has been documented for up to 3 weeks. Cell culture of the nasopharynx has a low sensitivity of diagnosis. PCR shows the prevalence and importance of this virus, particularly in infancy and early childhood.

A series of reports on 285 infants at high risk of developing asthma, who were followed to 6 years of age, emphasized the importance that rhinovirus infections play in the first year of life.[60] Human rhinovirus was the most common etiology of upper respiratory tract infection (48%) and occurred early and repetitively in these high-risk infants. Coinfection with other viruses generally resulted in more severe upper respiratory tract infections.[62] Higher rates of infection were found in children enrolled in daycare or with siblings in the home. A wheezing illness caused by rhinovirus at any point in the first 3 years of life in these high-risk infants resulted in a 10-fold increase in risk of asthma at 6 years of age—much more of a risk than found with RSV wheezing illness in early childhood (Fig. 39-16).[60]

Because rhinovirus is now known to cause lower respiratory tract disease, it is likely that it enhances susceptibility to asthma in predisposed children. It is known that low interferon-γ responses in infancy increase the risk of viral illness and of wheezing during infancy.[60] Many other reports have now verified rhinovirus as the most important cause of upper and lower respiratory infections; it is responsible for five hospitalizations per 1000 children younger than 5 years of age each year, which is far more significant than found for RSV.[75,96]

There is no effective treatment, and the only prophylaxis is use of infection control measures, such as contact precautions and hand washing. Rhinoviruses have also now been shown to be the etiology of sporadic, individual infections, or outbreaks, in the NICU. Infants may present with apnea, feeding difficulties, cough or rhinitis, and fever. Signs and symptoms may be indistinguishable from RSV. Young infants seem to be particularly susceptible to rhinovirus. Infants with bronchopulmonary dysplasia may develop a lower respiratory tract disease that is as likely to require intensive care admission as RSV. Preterm infants with bronchopulmonary dysplasia who were readmitted with rhinovirus had significant worsening of their pulmonary status, necessitating prolonged increases in care.

SEVERE ACUTE RESPIRATORY SYNDROME

In 2003, an epidemic of severe acute respiratory syndrome (SARS) occurred in China, Hong Kong, Vietnam, and Canada, and was eventually reported in 16 countries, including the United States. A novel coronavirus, unrelated to the other known human and animal coronaviruses, has been shown to be the cause of the outbreak. The horseshoe bats of southern China were found to be the natural reservoir of this enveloped RNA virus, and it can spread to a wide variety of other animals. It is feared that the virus will again spread from animal to human and cause future outbreaks. Exposure and travel histories need to be obtained in all severe respiratory outbreaks.[10]

Virtually all cases of SARS in children have occurred via contact with infected adults, either in the home or in a health care setting. Coinfection may occur with other viral pathogens, but it is unknown what role coinfection plays. Less than 10% of infections have occurred in children. The virus causes a mild, nonspecific respiratory illness in younger children, in contrast to the very serious, life-threatening infection in adults and teenagers older than 12 years. Most children present with fever, but may have cough, coryza, myalgia, malaise, chills, or diarrhea.[83]

In young children, the physical examination is normal, and the course is shorter and milder. As a group, young children apparently do not develop significant respiratory distress or require oxygen, and they make a complete recovery. Chest auscultation is unimpressive. The chest radiograph shows mild focal alveolar infiltrates. (In some cases, high-resolution CT showed airspace disease even though the chest film was negative.) Less than 1% of children require mechanical ventilation.[83] Similar to adults, children have multiple laboratory findings, including lymphopenia from destruction of the CD4+ and CD8+ lymphocytes, thrombocytopenia, and mild disseminated intravascular coagulation. Lactic dehydrogenase is also elevated in most cases. No deaths have occurred in young children, and they are asymptomatic within 6 months. Most reports of infections in children begin with infants a few months old. One premature infant presented at 56 days of life, at a corrected age of 38 weeks. His illness was comparable to that of adults, requiring oxygen, continuous positive airway pressure, and NICU admission, although he made a complete recovery.[135]

No infants born to mothers infected with SARS-COV (coronavirus) have shown any evidence of transplacental or congenital infection. Pregnant women may be more severely affected, with mortality of 25%. Only one infant survived of seven pregnancies in women infected in the first trimester in Hong Kong, but two less severely affected women in the United States had infants with normal outcomes. Infants born to mothers infected in the second or third trimester seem to survive, whether born via cesarean section prematurely because of the mother's deteriorating condition or vaginally at term to a convalescent mother. None of the infants had evidence of infection. Infants born soon after the mother is infected tend to be appropriately grown, whereas infants born later have intrauterine growth restriction and oligohydramnios[83]; this could be secondary to the use of ribavirin or steroids for the mother's illness or because of the mother's illness itself. Infants born prematurely had a high incidence of necrotizing enterocolitis and jejunal perforation. Extensive fetal thrombotic vasculopathy with zones of avascular villi was noted in the placentae of two infants who survived a maternal SARS infection.[102]

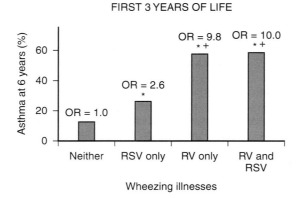

FIRST 3 YEARS OF LIFE

Figure 39–16. Risk of asthma at age 6 years in children who wheezed during the first 3 years of life with rhinovirus (RV), respiratory syncytial virus (RSV), or both (*P, .05 versus neither; +P, .05 versus RSV only). OR, odds ratio. (*From Jackson DJ et al: Wheezing rhinovirus illnesses in early life predict asthma development in high-risk children,* Am J Resp Crit Care Med *178:667, 2008.*)

Diagnosis of disease in children may be based on the World Health Organization definition of probable SARS (radiographic evidence and epidemiologic linkage) or the CDC definition of suspect SARS (radiographic evidence is unnecessary). Children seem more likely to have negative reverse transcriptase PCR tests and viral cultures, possibly because of a lower viral titer in the upper airway.

Infected individuals should be quarantined, preferably in a negative pressure room, and there should be strict adherence to infection control principles to prevent spread via aerosol, droplet, or fomites. There have been no documented cases of transmission of infection from children to adults, but there have been cases of not yet symptomatic parents infecting health care workers. This situation may represent lower viral titers in the children. Closed circuit scavenger systems should be built into ventilator systems, and continuous positive airway pressure, oxygen flow, or nebulizers should be used only within an isolette.

At this time, ribavirin does not seem to be useful in the treatment of most routine cases of SARS. The use of aerosols, such as albuterol, and continuous positive airway pressure may potentiate spread to other individuals. High-dose steroids, ribavirin, and oxygen and ventilation, as needed, have been the mainstays of treatment offered to date.

WEST NILE VIRUS

West Nile virus (WNV) is a single-stranded RNA flavivirus, transmitted to humans by the bites of infected mosquitoes. This arbovirus (arthropod-borne) survives in nature in a cycle that goes from mosquito to bird to mosquito, and primarily involves the *Culex* species of mosquitoes. It is a neuropathogen of humans, equines, and birds (especially crows). Infection has also been associated with transfusions or organ transplants from infected donors. Indigenous to Africa, Asia, Europe, and Australia, WNV was first reported in the Western Hemisphere in 1999 in an epizootic in New York City. Since then, it has rapidly spread throughout eastern and midwestern parts of the United States. Human infection may be asymptomatic (80%) or result in simple West Nile fever (20%) or invasive meningoencephalitis (<1%). Diagnosis is made by testing serum and CSF for WNV-specific IgG and IgM. The specificity, sensitivity, and predictive value of IgM and IgG in breast milk and neonatal or cord blood are unknown. There is no specific treatment for infection or vaccine to prevent infection. Preventive measures are the only defense and involve mosquito control and the education of the public to wear protective clothing, to use insect repellant on skin and clothing when outdoors, and to avoid the outdoors during peak mosquito hours (dusk to dawn).

There have been few reports of WNV infections in children younger than 1 year of age. Breast feeding was implicated in a report that came from Michigan, in 2002, when an infant was found to have WNV-specific serum IgM after breast feeding for 17 days. The mother developed WNV meningoencephalitis 9 days after receiving an infected transfusion, given after the birth of the infant. WNV genetic material was detected transiently in the breast milk. The infant remained well. No other cases of breast milk transmission have been proven, and transmission via human breast milk seems to be rare.[54] The benefits of breast feeding are well established, so there are no changes in the recommendations for breast feeding.

Intrauterine infection was probably documented in 2002 in the fetus of a mother who developed paraplegia secondary to WNV during the second trimester of her pregnancy.[4] The infant appeared well at term and had a normal physical examination, including head circumference. Ophthalmologic examination revealed marked chorioretinal scarring, however, and MRI of the brain showed generalized lissencephaly and marked white matter loss. In a survey in Colorado during an epidemic, 549 cord blood samples were screened for WNV-specific IgG and IgM. Of the cord samples, 4% were positive for IgG, indicating maternal infection, but none were positive for IgM, and all infants had normal growth and outcome.[109] Likewise, the CDC followed the outcome of 77 pregnancies in which the mothers were infected with WNV. There were four miscarriages and two elective abortions. Of the 72 live-born infants, none had conclusive evidence of congenital infection, although three infants developed infections that might have been congenitally acquired. Seven infants had major malformations, but only 3 of these could have been related to infection, and none of these infants had evidence of infection.[107]

The CDC has developed guidelines for the evaluation of infants born to mothers infected with WNV during pregnancy and a registry for pregnancy outcome.[147] Screening for WNV in asymptomatic, pregnant women is not recommended because there is no therapeutic intervention, and the outcome is currently unknown. A detailed ultrasound examination of the fetus should be obtained no earlier than 2 to 4 weeks after the onset of symptoms in an infected pregnant woman. Amniotic fluid, chorionic villi, and fetal serum may be tested for infection; in the event of a miscarriage or abortion, all products of conception should also be tested. Infants born to women known to be infected during the pregnancy should have a thorough physical examination, including measurements of head circumference, length and weight; a neurologic examination; and evaluation for dysmorphic features, any dermatologic lesions, or hepatosplenomegaly. The infant's serum should be tested for IgG and IgM specific for WNV, and the infant should have evoked otoacoustic emissions testing or auditory brainstem response testing. The placenta should also be examined by a pathologist.

An infant suspected to have WNV infection should undergo an extensive workup, including a CT scan of the head and an ophthalmologic examination. The infant should have a complete blood count and liver function tests. Examination of the CSF should be considered and should include an IgM for WNV. The infant should be examined by a dysmorphologist, and developmental milestones and growth measurements should be followed for the first year of life. At 6 months of life, the infant should have an additional hearing screen and determination of WNV IgG and IgM.

ADENOVIRUS

Adenoviruses are double-stranded, nonenveloped DNA viruses. The six groups (A through F) have multiple distinct serotypes, and the different serotypes cause different kinds of illness. The virus is most commonly found in the upper respiratory tract, and infection usually spreads via respiratory tract secretions. The virus is viable in the secretions for long periods, so fomites contaminated with secretions may transmit infection, in addition to aerosolized droplets and person-to-person contact. Viral shedding may occur intermittently for months after infection. Individuals may be reinfected and have asymptomatic infection. Health care workers and equipment, particularly ophthalmologic, have been implicated as sources of infection, so control requires careful hand washing and contact and droplet precautions. Infected health care workers should not participate in direct patient care for 2 weeks after onset, and should use gloves in addition to strict hand washing. Ophthalmologic medications should be single-dose in nature, and equipment needs careful sterilization. Daycare of young infants and children is another frequent source of infection, for which there are few effective control measures other than careful hygiene because the virus is also shed in the stool.

Adenovirus is most often associated with the "common cold," pharyngitis, otitis media, or pharyngoconjunctival fever. Respiratory infections are most common in late winter to early summer. Enteric strains cause gastroenteritis, more often in young infants and children, and occur year-round. Epidemic keratoconjunctivitis can be spread from contaminated water in inadequately chlorinated swimming pools in summer or from ophthalmologic equipment.

Although older children and healthy adults usually have self-limited, acute infections, infants and neonates, especially premature infants, may develop disseminated disease with a high mortality. The serotypes most commonly found (85%) in children are not as commonly found in infants younger than 6 months, suggesting that transplacental maternal antibody may be protective.[115]

Young infants, similar to immunocompromised individuals, may develop disseminated infections, pneumonia, bronchiolitis, or meningoencephalitis. In this instance, infection may be confused with invasive bacterial disease. The degree of inflammation is indicated by the considerable elevation of C-reactive protein. These infants are usually infected with subgroup B viruses (serotypes 3, 7, 21, and 35) and, less commonly, with subgroup D viruses (serotypes 2 and 32). Mortality, which may be 80%, is at its highest in the first 2 weeks of life. These infants may develop pancytopenia, disseminated intravascular coagulation, pleural effusion, wheezing, and hepatitis. Pneumonia may be fatal, and, if survived, may result in significant lung damage, necessitating increased respiratory support for months.

Several reports have documented outbreaks of epidemic keratoconjunctivitis secondary to serotype 8 in NICUs.[23,116] Affected infants have lid edema, erythema, fever, and, less commonly, conjunctivitis. They also develop acute and chronic respiratory manifestations.

Adenovirus type 30 was identified more recently as the source of an outbreak in the NICU affecting 21 infants.[34,115] Type 30 is a D group adenovirus not previously identified in NICU outbreaks, although D group adenoviruses have been known to cause gastrointestinal infections and keratoconjunctivitis. Eight infants developed pneumonia (of whom seven died), and eight infants developed conjunctivitis. Five asymptomatic infants were detected only by surveillance cultures. Several items of importance were noted in this report. The ophthalmologists, who had upper respiratory infections but continued to work, and who did not completely follow the American Academy of Ophthalmology infection control best practices, seemed to have a major role in this outbreak. Infection control measures were successful, but were discontinued too soon, before all infants had stopped shedding virus, and the outbreak began again. Finally, steroid use in the infants with pneumonia was highly associated with mortality.[34,115]

Reports of intrauterine or postnatal myocarditis owing to adenovirus have been increasing. Finally, evidence is accumulating for the rare case of congenital infection.[25] These infants die of disseminated disease and are small for gestational age. They may have necrotizing pneumonia, hepatitis, meningitis, myocarditis, and nephritis.

Diagnosis of adenoviral infection can be made by tissue culture, shell vial technique, or antigen detection via immunofluorescence in the pharynx, eye, body fluids, or stool. PCR is the most sensitive and specific test, although the most expensive. There is no effective, specific antiviral therapy that is not too toxic. Treatment is supportive.

HUMAN PAPILLOMAVIRUS

Human papillomavirus (HPV) is a double-stranded, nonenveloped DNA virus. The organism cannot be propagated in cell culture, and its presence is detected by the identification of viral DNA from tissue samples. Infection by HPV usually is asymptomatic. A few infected adults develop mucocutaneous lesions, most commonly cutaneous and genital warts and neoplasms of epithelial surfaces, especially the uterine cervix. HPV can be typed according to DNA sequence, and more than 100 genotypes have been identified. The different types can be distinguished by their propensity to cause low-grade warts (particularly types 6 and 11) versus high-grade, carcinomatous lesions (particularly types 16 and 18). Genital HPV infection in adults is usually transmitted by sexual contact. Nonsexual modes of acquisition, such as autoinoculation and heteroinoculation, are suspected, however.

Genital HPV is increasingly easier to detect in infected women during pregnancy, presumably reflecting increased viral activity. Virus can be transmitted to the newborn, but the timing, frequency, and consequences of vertical transmission of HPV are matters of debate. Although some studies suggest vertical transmission occurs in more than half of pregnancies involving women with known HPV-related genital lesions, more recent investigations indicate a far lower rate.[137] HPV isolated from the pharynx or genital tract of the infant soon after birth frequently is discordant from HPV found in the mother, suggesting at least some neonatal acquisition by horizontal routes. HPV detected soon after delivery usually causes no clinically detectable disease, and evidence of infection disappears within a few months[88]; seroconversion to the initially detected virus is unusual.

The childhood disease most strongly associated with vertically transmitted HPV is juvenile-onset recurrent respiratory papillomatosis (JORRP). This illness, which usually becomes clinically apparent by 2 to 3 years of age, is characterized by the development of multiple benign laryngeal papillomas. These lesions require repeated surgical excision to avoid airway obstruction. Occasionally, papillomas spread to the lower respiratory tract. JORRP is most strongly associated with HPV types 6 and 11, and often there is a history of condylomatous lesions in the mother caused by HPV of the same type.[133] The prevalence of JORRP is approximately 2 per 100,000 persons younger than 18 years, far lower than the prevalence of genital warts in pregnant women, suggesting that most infants exposed to HPV types 6 and 11 during birth remain unaffected.

Some, but not all, studies suggest a lower risk of JORRP if the infant is delivered by cesarean section, but operative delivery is not always protective, and it is not routinely recommended in a pregnant woman with genital warts. It is suspected that vertically transmitted HPV also can result in the development of anogenital warts in the child within the first several years of his or her life, presenting a dilemma to the child's caregivers because identical lesions can be associated with sexual abuse.

In the mid-2000s, a tetravalent recombinant HPV vaccine was introduced containing the major capsid proteins of HPV types 6, 11, 16, and 18. In the United States, this vaccine is recommended for females age 9 through 26 years, administered, it is hoped, before the natural acquisition of HPV through sexual activity. Because laryngeal and anogenital disease in newborns are caused primarily by HPV types 6 and 11, the broad application of this vaccine has the potential to reduce significantly mother-to-child transmission of HPV infection, although it is presumed to require many years of immunization before this potential is fully realized.

LYMPHOCYTIC CHORIOMENINGITIS VIRUS

Lymphocytic choriomeningitis virus (LCMV) is a member of the Arenaviridae family. Rodents, particularly the house mouse and pet hamsters, serve as the principal reservoirs for LCMV. Humans acquire the virus by inhaling aerosolized droppings or by coming into direct contact with an infected animal. Human infection is probably more common than appreciated. Serosurveys among healthy adults from various parts of the world have detected LCMV antibodies in 3% to 5%. Most cases in adults are mildly symptomatic or manifest with nonspecific, self-limited flulike symptoms. Uncommonly, these progress to aseptic meningitis or encephalitis.

LCMV crosses the placenta to cause intrauterine infection. Few cases of congenital disease have been published, but these reports describe a striking and common phenotype. Most manifestations in the newborn are confined to the CNS and the eyes.[11] Infants typically are born with either microcephaly or macrocephaly, the latter the consequence of aqueductal stenosis and hydrocephalus. Neuroimaging studies frequently reveal periventricular calcifications and patchy abnormalities of white matter. Most infants are left with severe visual and neurologic impairment. More than 90% of reported cases have chorioretinitis with scarring and visual impairment. Hearing usually is preserved. Manifestations outside the CNS (liver and heart dysfunction and thrombocytopenia) have occasionally been described, but are uncommon.

In many cases, the mother recalls an influenza-like illness early in pregnancy, but only a few remember exposure to rodents. The diagnosis is supported by measuring anti-LCMV IgM and IgG. Antibodies to LCMV are sufficiently uncommon in the general population that their presence in an infant with typical CNS findings is sufficient to establish the diagnosis, especially in the absence of alternative possibilities, such as toxoplasmosis and CMV.

REFERENCES

1. Abzug MJ: Prognosis for neonates with enterovirus hepatitis and coagulopathy, *Pediatr Infect Dis J* 20:758, 2001.
2. Acosta EP et al: Ganciclovir population pharmacokinetics in neonates following intravenous administration of ganciclovir and oral administration of a liquid valganciclovir formulation, *Clin Pharmacol Ther* 81:867, 2007.
3. Aggarwal R, Krawczynski K: Hepatitis E: an overview and recent advances in clinical and laboratory research, *J Gastroenterol Hepatol* 15:9, 2000.
4. Alpert SG et al: Intrauterine West Nile virus: ocular and systemic findings, *Am J Ophthalmol* 136:733, 2003.
5. Alvarez-Lafuente R et al: Detection of human herpesvirus-6, Epstein-Barr virus and cytomegalovirus in formalin-fixed tissues from sudden infant death: a study with quantitative real-time PCR, *Forensic Sci Int* 178:106, 2008.
6. Ancora G et al: Cranial ultrasound scanning and prediction of outcome in newborns with congenital cytomegalovirus infection, *J Pediatr* 150:157, 2007.
7. Ansari SA et al: Potential role of hands in the spread of respiratory viral infections: studies with human parainfluenza virus 3 and rhinovirus 14, *J Clin Microbiol* 29:2115, 1991.
8. Barenfanger J et al: Prevalence of human metapneumovirus in central Illinois in patients thought to have respiratory viral infection, *J Clin Microbiol* 46:1489, 2008.
9. Bhat N et al: Influenza-associated deaths among children in the United States, 2003-2004, *N Engl J Med* 353:2559, 2005.
10. Bitnun A et al: Severe acute respiratory syndrome-associated coronavirus infection in Toronto children: a second look, *Pediatrics* 123:97, 2009.
11. Bonthius DJ et al: Congenital lymphocytic choriomeningitis virus infection: spectrum of disease, *Ann Neurol* 62:347, 2007.
12. Boppana SB et al: Congenital cytomegalovirus infection: association between virus burden in infancy and hearing loss, *J Pediatr* 146:817, 2005.
13. Boppana SB et al: Neuroradiographic findings in the newborn period and long-term outcome in children with symptomatic congenital cytomegalovirus infection, *Pediatrics* 99:409, 1997.
14. Bradford RD et al: Detection of cytomegalovirus (CMV) DNA by polymerase chain reaction is associated with hearing loss in newborns with symptomatic congenital CMV infection involving the central nervous system, *J Infect Dis* 191:227, 2005.
15. Bradley JP et al: Severity of respiratory syncytial virus bronchiolitis is affected by cigarette smoke exposure and atopy, *Pediatrics* 115:e7, 2005.
16. Brady MT et al: Survival and disinfection of parainfluenza viruses on environmental surfaces, *Am J Infect Control* 18:18, 1990.
17. Braig S et al: Acyclovir prophylaxis in late pregnancy prevents recurrent genital herpes and viral shedding, *Eur J Obstet Gynecol Reprod Biol* 96:55, 2001.
18. Broughton S et al: Diminished lung function, RSV infection, and respiratory morbidity in prematurely born infants, *Arch Dis Child* 91:26, 2006.
19. Broughton S et al: Lung function in prematurely born infants after viral lower respiratory tract infections, *Pediatr Infect Dis J* 26:1019, 2007.

20. Brown ZA et al: Effect of serologic status and cesarean delivery on transmission rates of herpes simplex virus from mother to infant, *JAMA* 289:203, 2003.

21. Camps M et al: Prevalence of human metapneumovirus among hospitalized children younger than 1 year in Catalonia, Spain, *J Med Virol* 80:1452, 2008.

22. Caviness AC et al: The prevalence of neonatal herpes simplex virus infection compared with serious bacterial illness in hospitalized neonates, *J Pediatr* 153:164, 2008.

23. Chaberny IE et al: An outbreak of epidemic keratoconjunctivitis in a pediatric unit due to adenovirus type 8, *Infect Control Hosp Epidemiol* 24:514, 2003.

24. Chang MH et al: Hepatitis B vaccination and hepatocellular carcinoma rates in boys and girls, *JAMA* 284:3040, 2000.

25. Chiou CC et al: Congenital adenoviral infection, *Pediatr Infect Dis J* 13:664, 1994.

26. Cilla G et al: Viruses in community-acquired pneumonia in children aged less than 3 years old: high rate of viral coinfection, *J Med Virol* 80:1843, 2008.

27. Connor EM et al: Reduction of maternal-infant transmission of human immunodeficiency virus type 1 with zidovudine treatment. Pediatric AIDS Clinical Trials Group Protocol 076 Study Group, *N Engl J Med* 331:1173, 1994.

28. Corey L, Wald A, Patel R et al: Once-daily valacyclovir to reduce the risk of transmission of genital herpes, *N Engl J Med* 350:11, 2004.

29. Cunney RJ et al: An outbreak of influenza A in a neonatal intensive care unit, *Infect Control Hosp Epidemiol* 21:449, 2000.

30. Dasopoulou M, Covanis A: Subacute sclerosing panencephalitis after intrauterine infection, *Acta Paediatr* 93:1251, 2004.

31. de Jong EP et al: Parvovirus B19 infection in pregnancy, *J Clin Virol* 36:1, 2006.

32. Dembinski J et al: Long term follow-up of serostatus after maternofetal parvovirus B19 infection, *Arch Dis Child* 88:219, 2003.

33. Enders G et al: Consequences of varicella and herpes zoster in pregnancy: prospective study of 1739 cases, *Lancet* 343:1548, 1994.

34. Faden H et al: Outbreak of adenovirus type 30 in a neonatal intensive care unit, *J Pediatr* 146:523, 2005.

35. Feltes TF et al: Palivizumab prophylaxis reduces hospitalization due to respiratory syncytial virus in young children with hemodynamically significant congenital heart disease, *J Pediatr* 143:532, 2003.

36. Ferrero S et al: Prospective study of mother-to-infant transmission of hepatitis C virus: a 10-year survey (1990-2000), *Acta Obstet Gynecol Scand* 82:229, 2003.

37. Figueras-Aloy J et al: FLIP-2 Study: risk factors linked to respiratory syncytial virus infection requiring hospitalization in premature infants born in Spain at a gestational age of 32 to 35 weeks, *Pediatr Infect Dis J* 27:788, 2008.

38. Forrest JM et al: Gregg's congenital rubella patients 60 years later, *Med J Aust* 177:664, 2002.

39. Fowler KB et al: The outcome of congenital cytomegalovirus infection in relation to maternal antibody status, *N Engl J Med* 326:663, 1992.

40. Garcia-Garcia ML et al: Human metapneumovirus infections in hospitalised infants in Spain, *Arch Dis Child* 91:290, 2006.

41. Garcia PM et al: Maternal levels of plasma human immunodeficiency virus type 1 RNA and the risk of perinatal transmission. Women and Infants Transmission Study Group, *N Engl J Med* 341:394, 1999.

42. Gibson CS et al: Neurotropic viruses and cerebral palsy: population based case-control study, *BMJ* 332:76, 2006.

43. Glezen WP et al: Parainfluenza virus type 3: seasonality and risk of infection and reinfection in young children, *J Infect Dis* 150:851, 1984.

44. Glezen WP et al: Influenza virus infections in infants, *Pediatr Infect Dis J* 16:1065, 1997.

45. Groothuis JR et al: Prophylactic administration of respiratory syncytial virus immune globulin to high-risk infants and young children. The Respiratory Syncytial Virus Immune Globulin Study Group, *N Engl J Med* 329:1524, 1993.

46. Haginoya K et al: Abnormal white matter lesions with sensorineural hearing loss caused by congenital cytomegalovirus infection: retrospective diagnosis by PCR using Guthrie cards, *Brain Dev* 24:710, 2002.

47. Hall CB et al: Congenital infections with human herpesvirus 6 (HHV6) and human herpesvirus 7 (HHV7), *J Pediatr* 145:472, 2004.

48. Harger JH et al: Frequency of congenital varicella syndrome in a prospective cohort of 347 pregnant women, *Obstet Gynecol* 100:260, 2002.

49. Harper SA et al: Prevention and control of influenza. Recommendations of the Advisory Committee on Immunization Practices (ACIP), *MMWR Recomm Rep* 54:1, 2005.

50. Havens PL et al: HIV testing and prophylaxis to prevent mother-to-child transmission in the United States, *Pediatrics* 122:1127, 2008.

51. Havens PL, Mofenson LM: Evaluation and management of the infant exposed to HIV-1 in the United States, *Pediatrics* 123:175, 2009.

52. Henderson J et al: Hospitalization for RSV bronchiolitis before 12 months of age and subsequent asthma, atopy and wheeze: a longitudinal birth cohort study, *Pediatr Allergy Immunol* 16:386, 2005.

53. Hill JB et al: Risk of hepatitis B transmission in breast-fed infants of chronic hepatitis B carriers, *Obstet Gynecol* 99:1049, 2002.

54. Hinckley AF et al: Transmission of West Nile virus through human breast milk seems to be rare, *Pediatrics* 119:e666, 2007.

55. Hollier LM, Wendel GD: Third trimester antiviral prophylaxis for preventing maternal genital herpes simplex virus (HSV) recurrences and neonatal infection, *Cochrane Database Syst Rev* (1):CD004946, 2008.

56. Hyams KC: Risks of chronicity following acute hepatitis B virus infection: a review, *Clin Infect Dis* 20:992, 1995.

57. Illi S et al: Early childhood infectious diseases and the development of asthma up to school age: a birth cohort study, *BMJ* 322:390, 2001.

58. IMPACT-RSV Study Group: Palivizumab, a humanized respiratory syncytial virus monoclonal antibody, reduces hospitalization from respiratory syncytial virus infection in high-risk infants, *Pediatrics* 102:531, 1998.

59. Indolfi G, Resti M: Perinatal transmission of hepatitis C virus infection, *J Med Virol* 81:836, 2009.

60. Jackson DJ et al: Wheezing rhinovirus illnesses in early life predict asthma development in high-risk children, *Am J Respir Crit Care Med* 178:667, 2008.

61. Jackson JB et al: Intrapartum and neonatal single-dose nevirapine compared with zidovudine for prevention of mother-to-child transmission of HIV-1 in Kampala, Uganda: 18-month follow-up of the HIVNET 012 randomised trial, *Lancet* 362:859, 2003.

61a. Jain S, Kamimoto L, Bramley AM, et al and the 2009 Pandemic Influenza A (H1N1) Virus Hospitalizations Investigation Team: Hospitalized patients with 2009 H1N1 influenza in the United States, April-June 2009, *N Engl J Med* 2000, Epub Oct 8.

62. Jartti T et al: Serial viral infections in infants with recurrent respiratory illnesses, *Eur Respir J* 32:314, 2008.

63. Kar P et al: Does hepatitis E viral load and genotypes influence the final outcome of acute liver failure during pregnancy? *Am J Gastroenterol* 103:2495, 2008.

64. Kellner JD et al: Bronchodilators for bronchiolitis, *Cochrane Database Syst Rev* (2):CD001266, 2000.

65. Khetsuriani N et al: Neonatal enterovirus infections reported to the national enterovirus surveillance system in the United States, 1983-2003, *Pediatr Infect Dis J* 25:889, 2006.

66. Kimberlin D: Ganciclovir may be used during intravenous acyclovir shortage, *AAP News March* 2009.

67. Kimberlin D et al: Administration of oral acyclovir suppressive therapy after neonatal herpes simplex virus disease limited to the skin, eyes and mouth: results of a phase I/II trial, *Pediatr Infect Dis J* 15:247, 1996.

68. Kimberlin DW: Herpes simplex virus infections in neonates and early childhood, *Semin Pediatr Infect Dis* 16:271, 2005.

69. Kimberlin DW et al: Pharmacokinetic and pharmacodynamic assessment of oral valganciclovir in the treatment of symptomatic congenital cytomegalovirus disease, *J Infect Dis* 197:836, 2008.

70. Kimberlin DW et al: Safety and efficacy of high-dose intravenous acyclovir in the management of neonatal herpes simplex virus infections, *Pediatrics* 108:230, 2001.

71. Kimberlin DW et al: Natural history of neonatal herpes simplex virus infections in the acyclovir era, *Pediatrics* 108:223, 2001.

72. Kimberlin DW et al: Effect of ganciclovir therapy on hearing in symptomatic congenital cytomegalovirus disease involving the central nervous system: a randomized, controlled trial, *J Pediatr* 143:16, 2003.

73. Kneyber MCJ et al: Long-term effects of respiratory syncytial virus (RSV) bronchiolitis in infants and young children: a quantitative review, *Acta Paediatr* 89:654, 2000.

74. Koch WC et al: Serologic and virologic evidence for frequent intrauterine transmission of human parvovirus B19 with a primary maternal infection during pregnancy, *Pediatr Infect Dis J* 17:489, 1998.

75. Kusel MM et al: Role of respiratory viruses in acute upper and lower respiratory tract illness in the first year of life: a birth cohort study, *Pediatr Infect Dis J* 25:680, 2006.

76. Lanari M et al: Neonatal cytomegalovirus blood load and risk of sequelae in symptomatic and asymptomatic congenitally infected newborns, *Pediatrics* 117:e76, 2006.

77. Laundy M et al: Influenza A community-acquired pneumonia in East London infants and young children, *Pediatr Infect Dis J* 22(10 suppl):S223, 2003.

78. Lazzarotto T et al: New advances in the diagnosis of congenital cytomegalovirus infection, *J Clin Virol* 41:192, 2008.

79. Lee C et al: Effect of hepatitis B immunisation in newborn infants of mothers positive for hepatitis B surface antigen: systematic review and meta-analysis, *BMJ* 332:328, 2006.

80. Legg JP et al: Frequency of detection of picornaviruses and seven other respiratory pathogens in infants, *Pediatr Infect Dis J* 24:611, 2005.

81. Lehtinen M et al: Maternal herpesvirus infections and risk of acute lymphoblastic leukemia in the offspring, *Am J Epidemiol* 158:207, 2003.

82. Lewis E et al: Safety of neonatal hepatitis B vaccine administration, *Pediatr Infect Dis J* 20:1049, 2001.

83. Li AM, Ng PC: Severe acute respiratory syndrome (SARS) in neonates and children, *Arch Dis Child Fetal Neonatal Ed* 90:F461, 2005.

84. Lin TY et al: Neonatal enterovirus infections: emphasis on risk factors of severe and fatal infections, *Pediatr Infect Dis J* 22:889, 2003.

85. Linhares AC et al: Neonatal rotavirus infection in Belem, northern Brazil: nosocomial transmission of a P[6] G2 strain, *J Med Virol* 67:418, 2002.

85a. Louie JK, Acosta M, Winter K et al; for the California Pandemic (H1N1) Working Group: Factors associated with death or hospitalization due to pandemic 2009 influenza A (H1N1) infection in California, *JAMA* 302:1896, 2009.

86. Maggi F et al: Human metapneumovirus associated with respiratory tract infections in a 3-year study of nasal swabs from infants in Italy, *J Clin Microbiol* 41:2987, 2003.

87. Malm G, Engman ML: Congenital cytomegalovirus infections, *Semin Fetal Neonatal Med* 12:154, 2007.

88. Mammas IN et al: Human papilloma virus (HPV) infection in children and adolescents, *Eur J Pediatr* 168:267, 2009.

89. Maruyama Y et al: Fetal manifestations and poor outcomes of congenital cytomegalovirus infections: possible candidates for intrauterine antiviral treatments, *J Obstet Gynaecol Res* 33:619, 2007.

90. Mast EE et al: Risk factors for perinatal transmission of hepatitis C virus (HCV) and the natural history of HCV infection acquired in infancy, *J Infect Dis* 192:1880, 2005.

91. Matsuda H et al: Intrauterine therapy for parvovirus B19 infected symptomatic fetus using B19 IgG-rich high titer gammaglobulin, *J Perinat Med* 33:561, 2005.

92. Meissner HC et al: A simultaneous outbreak of respiratory syncytial virus and parainfluenza virus type 3 in a newborn nursery, *J Pediatr* 104:680, 1984.

93. Meissner HC et al: Elimination of rubella from the United States: a milestone on the road to global elimination, *Pediatrics* 117:933, 2006.

94. Meissner HC, Bocchini JA: Reducing RSV hospitalizations: AAP modifies recommendations for use of palivizumab in high-risk infants, young children. *AAP News*, August 2009.

95. Miller E et al: Consequences of confirmed maternal rubella at successive stages of pregnancy, *Lancet* 2:781, 1982.

96. Miller EK et al: Rhinovirus-associated hospitalizations in young children, *J Infect Dis* 195:773, 2007.

97. Mofenson LM: U.S. Public Health Service Task Force recommendations for use of antiretroviral drugs in pregnant HIV-1-infected women for maternal health and interventions to reduce perinatal HIV-1 transmission in the United States, *MMWR Recomm Rep* 51:1, 2002.

98. Mofenson LM, Munderi P: Safety of antiretroviral prophylaxis of perinatal transmission for HIV-infected pregnant women and their infants, *J Acquir Immune Defic Syndr* 30:200, 2002.

99. Moisiuk SE et al: Outbreak of parainfluenza virus type 3 in an intermediate care neonatal nursery, *Pediatr Infect Dis J* 17:49, 1998.

100. Munoz FM et al: Influenza A virus outbreak in a neonatal intensive care unit, *Pediatr Infect Dis J* 18:811, 1999.

101. Neuberger P et al: Case-control study of symptoms and neonatal outcome of human milk-transmitted cytomegalovirus infection in premature infants, *J Pediatr* 148:326, 2006.

102. Ng WF et al: The placentas of patients with severe acute respiratory syndrome: a pathophysiological evaluation, *Pathology* 38:210, 2006.

103. Nigro G et al: Passive immunization during pregnancy for congenital cytomegalovirus infection, *N Engl J Med* 353:1350, 2005.

104. Nigro G et al: Regression of fetal cerebral abnormalities by primary cytomegalovirus infection following hyperimmunoglobulin therapy, *Prenat Diagn* 28:512, 2008.

105. Noble V et al: Respiratory status and allergy nine to 10 years after acute bronchiolitis, *Arch Dis Child* 76:315, 1997.

106. Noyola DE et al: Early predictors of neurodevelopmental outcome in symptomatic congenital cytomegalovirus infection, *J Pediatr* 138:325, 2001.

107. O'Leary DR et al: Birth outcomes following West Nile Virus infection of pregnant women in the United States: 2003-2004, *Pediatrics* 117:e537, 2006.

108. Ordas J et al: Role of metapneumovirus in viral respiratory infections in young children, *J Clin Microbiol* 44:2739, 2006.

109. Paisley JE et al: West Nile virus infection among pregnant women in a northern Colorado community, 2003 to 2004, *Pediatrics* 117:814, 2006.

110. Papadogiannakis N et al: Active, fulminant, lethal myocarditis associated with parvovirus B19 infection in an infant, *Clin Infect Dis* 35:1027, 2002.

111. Pastuszak AL et al: Outcome after maternal varicella infection in the first 20 weeks of pregnancy, *N Engl J Med* 330:901, 1994.

112. Patra S et al: Maternal and fetal outcomes in pregnant women with acute hepatitis E virus infection, *Ann Intern Med* 147:28, 2007.

113. Peckham CS: Clinical and laboratory study of children exposed in utero to maternal rubella, *Arch Dis Child* 47:571, 1972.

114. Petra Study Team: Efficacy of three short-course regimens of zidovudine and lamivudine in preventing early and late transmission of HIV-1 from mother to child in Tanzania, South Africa, and Uganda (Petra study): a randomised, double-blind, placebo-controlled trial, *Lancet* 359:1178, 2002.

115. Piedra PA: Adenovirus in the neonatal intensive care unit: formidable, forgotten foe. *J Pediatr* 146:447, 2005.

116. Piedra PA et al: Description of an adenovirus type 8 outbreak in hospitalized neonates born prematurely, *Pediatr Infect Dis J* 11:460, 1992.

117. Ploin D et al: Influenza burden in children newborn to eleven months of age in a pediatric emergency department during the peak of an influenza epidemic, *Pediatr Infect Dis J* 22(10 suppl): S218, 2003.

118. Public Health Laboratory Service Working Party on Fifth Disease: prospective study of human parvovirus (B19) infection in pregnancy, *BMJ* 300:1166, 1990.

119. Purcell K, Fergie J: Driscoll Children's Hospital respiratory syncytial virus database: risk factors, treatment and hospital course in 3308 infants and young children, 1991 to 2002, *Pediatr Infect Dis J* 23:418, 2004.

120. Ramani S et al: Rotavirus infection in the neonatal nurseries of a tertiary care hospital in India, *Pediatr Infect Dis J* 27:719, 2008.

121. Ramsay ME et al: Outcome of confirmed symptomatic congenital cytomegalovirus infection, *Arch Dis Child* 66:1068, 1991.

122. Regamey N et al: Viral etiology of acute respiratory infections with cough in infancy: a community-based birth cohort study, *Pediatr Infect Dis J* 27:100, 2008.

123. Resch B et al: Risk of concurrent bacterial infection in preterm infants hospitalized due to respiratory syncytial virus infection, *Acta Paediatr* 96:495, 2007.

124. Resti M et al: Maternal drug use is a preeminent risk factor for mother-to-child hepatitis C virus transmission: results from a multicenter study of 1372 mother-infant pairs, *J Infect Dis* 185:567, 2002.

125. Rossi GA et al: Risk factors for severe RSV-induced lower respiratory tract infection over four consecutive epidemics, *Eur J Pediatr* 166:1267, 2007.

126. Sampalis JS et al: Development and validation of a risk scoring tool to predict respiratory syncytial virus hospitalization in premature infants born at 33 through 35 completed weeks of gestation, *Med Decis Making* 28:471, 2008.

127. Sasaki Y et al: Serum immunoglobulin levels do not affect antibody responses to influenza HA vaccine in preterm infants, *Vaccine* 24:2208, 2006.

128. Scott LL et al: Acyclovir suppression to prevent clinical recurrences at delivery after first episode genital herpes in pregnancy: an open-label trial, *Infect Dis Obstet Gynecol* 9:75, 2001.

129. Shaffer N et al: Short-course zidovudine for perinatal HIV-1 transmission in Bangkok, Thailand: a randomised controlled trial. Bangkok Collaborative Perinatal HIV Transmission Study Group, *Lancet* 353:773, 1999.

130. Shearer WT et al: Viral load and disease progression in infants infected with human immunodeficiency virus type 1. Women and Infants Transmission Study Group, *N Engl J Med* 336:1337, 1997.

131. Siegel M, Fuerst HT: Low birth weight and maternal virus diseases: a prospective study of rubella, measles, mumps, chickenpox, and hepatitis, *JAMA* 197:680, 1966.

132. Sigurs N et al: Respiratory syncytial virus bronchiolitis in infancy is an important risk factor for asthma and allergy at age 7, *Am J Respir Crit Care Med* 161:1501, 2000.

133. Silverberg MJ et al: Condyloma in pregnancy is strongly predictive of juvenile-onset recurrent respiratory papillomatosis, *Obstet Gynecol* 101:645, 2003.

134. Simoes EA et al: Palivizumab prophylaxis, respiratory syncytial virus, and subsequent recurrent wheezing, *J Pediatr* 151:34, 42 e1, 2007.

135. Sit SC et al: A young infant with severe acute respiratory syndrome, *Pediatrics* 112:e257, 2003.

136. Skidmore SJ: Tropical aspects of viral hepatitis: hepatitis E, *Trans R Soc Trop Med Hyg* 91:125, 1997.

137. Smith EM et al: Human papillomavirus prevalence and types in newborns and parents: concordance and modes of transmission, *Sex Transm Dis* 31:57, 2004.

138. Stein RT et al: Respiratory syncytial virus in early life and risk of wheeze and allergy by age 13 years, *Lancet* 354:541, 1999.

139. Syridou G et al: Detection of cytomegalovirus, parvovirus B19 and herpes simplex viruses in cases of intrauterine fetal death: association with pathological findings, *J Med Virol* 80:1776, 2008.

140. Szmuness W et al: Prevalence of hepatitis B virus infection and hepatocellular carcinoma in Chinese-Americans, *J Infect Dis* 137:822, 1978.

141. Tajiri H et al: Prospective study of mother-to-infant transmission of hepatitis C virus, *Pediatr Infect Dis J* 20:10, 2001.

142. Tanaka-Taya K et al: Human herpesvirus 6 (HHV-6) is transmitted from parent to child in an integrated form and characterization of cases with chromosomally integrated HHV-6 DNA, *J Med Virol* 73:465, 2004.

143. Tedeschi R et al: Activation of maternal Epstein-Barr virus infection and risk of acute leukemia in the offspring, *Am J Epidemiol* 165:134, 2007.

144. Tong MJ et al: Studies on the maternal-infant transmission of the viruses which cause acute hepatitis, *Gastroenterology* 80(5 pt1):999, 1981.

145. Tovo PA et al: Persistence rate and progression of vertically acquired hepatitis C infection. European Paediatric Hepatitis C Virus Infection, *J Infect Dis* 181:419, 2000.

146. Tuomala RE et al: Antiretroviral therapy during pregnancy and the risk of an adverse outcome, *N Engl J Med* 346:1863, 2002.

147. U.S. Public Health Service: Interim guidelines for the evaluation of infants born to mothers infected with West Nile virus during pregnancy, *MMWR Morb Mortal Wkly Rep* 53:15, 2004.

148. van der Knaap MS, et al: Pattern of white matter abnormalities at MR imaging: use of polymerase chain reaction testing of Guthrie cards to link pattern with congenital cytomegalovirus infection, *Radiology* 230:529, 2004.

149. Ventre K, Randolph AG: Ribavirin for respiratory syncytial virus infection of the lower respiratory tract in infants and young children, *Cochrane Database Syst Rev* (1):CD000181, 2007.

150. Verboon-Maciolek MA et al: Human parechovirus causes encephalitis with white matter injury in neonates, *Ann Neurol* 64:266, 2008.

151. Verboon-Maciolek MA et al: Severe neonatal parechovirus infection and similarity with enterovirus infection, *Pediatr Infect Dis J* 27:241, 2008.

152. Vossough A et al: Imaging findings of neonatal herpes simplex virus type 2 encephalitis, *Neuroradiology* 50:355, 2008.

153. Wade NA et al: Abbreviated regimens of zidovudine prophylaxis and perinatal transmission of the human immunodeficiency virus, *N Engl J Med* 339:1409, 1998.

154. Walter S et al: Congenital cytomegalovirus: association between dried blood spot viral load and hearing loss, *Arch Dis Child Fetal Neonatal Ed* 93:F280, 2008.

155. Ward K et al: Human herpesvirus-6 and -7 each cause significant neurological morbidity in Britain and Ireland, *Arch Dis Child* 90:619, 2005.

156. Wejstal R et al: Perinatal transmission of hepatitis G virus (GB virus type C) and hepatitis C virus infections—a comparison, *Clin Infect Dis* 28:816, 1999.

157. Welliver R et al: Natural history of parainfluenza virus infection in childhood, *J Pediatr* 101:180, 1982.

158. Whitley R et al: Predictors of morbidity and mortality in neonates with herpes simplex virus infections. The National Institute of Allergy and Infectious Diseases Collaborative Antiviral Study Group, *N Engl J Med* 324:450, 1991.

159. Whitley RJ et al: Changing presentation of herpes simplex virus infection in neonates, *J Infect Dis* 158:109, 1988.

160. Whitley RJ, Gnann JW Jr: Acyclovir: a decade later, *N Engl J Med* 327:782, 1992.

161. Wilkinson DJ et al: Influenza in the neonatal intensive care unit, *J Perinatol* 26:772, 2006.

162. Williams JV et al: Human metapneumovirus and lower respiratory tract disease in otherwise healthy infants and children, *N Engl J Med* 350:443, 2004.

163. Young NS, Brown KE: Parvovirus B19, *N Engl J Med* 350:586, 2004.

164. Zerr DM et al: A population-based study of primary human herpesvirus 6 infection, *N Engl J Med* 352:768, 2005.

CHAPTER 40

The Central Nervous System

PART 1

Normal and Abnormal Brain Development

Pierre Gressens and Petra S. Hüppi

MECHANISMS OF BRAIN DEVELOPMENT

Normal development of the human central nervous system (CNS) encompasses several steps, including neuroectoderm induction, neurulation, cell proliferation and migration, programmed cell death, neurogenesis and elimination of excess neurons, synaptogenesis, stabilization and elimination of synapses, gliogenesis, and myelination (Table 40-1).

These different steps of brain development and maturation are controlled by the interaction between genes and environment. Numerous genes involved in brain development have been identified: genes controlling neurulation, neuronal proliferation, neuronal size and shape, programmed cell death, neuronal-glial interactions, and synaptic stabilization.[105] However, it seems unlikely that the 30,000 genes in humans can totally control the organization of 100 billion neurons and trillions of synapses. A normal pattern of expression of these genes requires an adequate environment. Interactions with the intrauterine milieu (factors coming from the mother, placenta, or amniotic fluid) and with the postnatal environment critically modulate gene expression through reciprocal action with neurotransmitters, trophic factors, and hormones and their machinery. Accordingly, brain malformations can be due to environmental factors, genetic factors, or an interaction of both (Boxes 40-1 through 40-4).

This part of the chapter focuses primarily on the development of the neocortex. Detailed descriptions of the development of other CNS structures such as cerebellum can be found in texts by ten Donkelaar and colleagues[111] and Wang and Zoghbi.[121]

Neural Induction and Neurulation

During early stages of gastrulation, organizing centers produce inductive molecules that initiate genetic programs leading to the differentiation of the neural tissues from surrounding tissues.[108] Grafting experiments in amphibians have shown that the appearance of neural tissue depends on signals coming from mesodermic cells of the dorsal marginal zone (the Speeman organizing center) and that other signals deriving from this zone also allow the regionalization of the neuroectoderm along the rostrocaudal axis. Studies have identified some of the factors implicated in neural induction, including follistatin, noggin, Notch, dorsalin1, Wnt1, and Hedgehog.

Neurulation is the process by which neuroectodermal cells transform into a neural tube, which will differentiate into the brain and the spinal cord. Neurulation can be divided into four steps that overlap both in time and space: (1) neural plate formation, (2) neural plate modeling, (3) neural groove formation, and (4) closure of the neural groove to form the neural tube. In humans, the neural plate appears at the beginning of the third gestational week in the mediodorsal zone of the embryo, just ahead (in the rostrocaudal axis) of the Hensen node. The neural groove appears during the third gestational week. Neural tube closure starts at the beginning of the fourth gestational week, with the formation of the neural crests (which will give rise to dorsal root ganglia, Schwann cells, and cells of the pia and arachnoid). Neural tube closure begins in the region of the lower medulla and proceeds both rostrally and caudally.

The anterior neuropore closes at approximately 24 gestational days and the posterior neuropore closes at approximately 26 gestational days. This posterior site of closure is located around the lumbosacral level, and more caudal spinal cord is formed secondarily by a separate process involving canalization (4 to 7 gestational weeks) and retrogressive differentiation (seventh gestational week to after birth; giving rise to the ventriculus terminalis and the filum terminale). The neural tube is initially a straight structure. Before the closure of the posterior neuropore, the anterior part of the neural tube is shaped into three primary vesicles: the prosencephalon, the mesencephalon, and the rhombencephalon.

TABLE 40–1	Schematic Chronology of the Major Events During Human Neocortical Development
Neuroectoderm induction	3rd GW
Neurulation	3rd to end of 4th GW
Prosencephalic and hemispheric formation	5th-10th GW
Neuronal proliferation	10th-20th GW
Neuronal migration	12th-24th GW
Programmed neuronal cell death	28th-41st GW
Neurogenesis	15th-20th GW to ? postnatal months or years
Synaptogenesis	20th GW to puberty
Gliogenesis	20th-24th GW to ? postnatal years
Myelination	36th-38th GW to 2-3 postnatal years
Angiogenesis	5th-10th GW to ? postnatal years

GW, gestational week.

The prosencephalic phase and the formation of the hemisphere take place between 5 and 10 gestational weeks in humans.

CNS regionalization results from the combination of two mechanisms. Rostrocaudal regionalization creates transverse domains with distinct competences in the neural plate and tube,[57,106,123] whereas dorsoventral regionalization creates longitudinally aligned domains.[103] The combination of these two axes yields a grid-shaped pattern or regionalization.[101] Different genes involved in this regionalization have been identified. These include *BMP* (bone morphogenetic proteins), *PAX* (paired box genes), and *SHH* (sonic hedgehog) genes for the dorsoventral axis, and *HOX* (clustered homeobox-containing genes), *KROX20*, *FGF8* (fibroblast growth factor-8), *EN* (engrailed genes), *WNT*, *OTX* (homeobox genes homologous of the *Drosophila* orthodenticle gene), *EMX* (related to the "empty spiracles" gene expressed in the developing *Drosophila* head), and *DLX* (homeobox genes homologous to the distal-less genes of *Drosophila*) genes for the rostrocaudal axis (Fig. 40-1).

Neuronal Proliferation

There are no precise data concerning the number of neurons present in the brains of different mammalian species. In the human adult brain, estimates range from 3 billion to 100 billion neurons. Similarly, the precise proportion of glial cells is unknown, with a neuron-to-glia ratio estimated at between 1:1 and 1:10.

BOX 40–1   Environmental Factors and Maternal Conditions with Potential Impact on the Developing Brain

THERAPEUTIC DRUGS
Retinoic acid
Antithyroid drugs
Estroprogestative hormones, testosterone, and derivatives
Antimitotic drugs
Lithium and psychotropic drugs
Benzodiazepines and antiepileptic drugs

ADDICTION DRUGS
Tobacco
Caffeine
Ethanol
Cocaine
Opiates
Cannabis

PHYSICAL AND CHEMICAL AGENTS
Dioxins and heavy metals
Organic solvents
Ionizing radiation
Head trauma
Repeated shaking

MATERNAL FACTORS AND STATUS
Sex hormones
Catecholamines
Thyroid hormones
Diabetes mellitus
Peptides (vasoactive intestinal peptide)
Placenta and decidual hormones
Oxygen and hypoxia-ischemia
Hyperthermia

INFECTIOUS AGENTS
Herpes simplex I and II
Herpes zoster
Cytomegalovirus
Rubella virus
Parvovirus B19
Coxsackie virus, B group
Human immunodeficiency virus
Influenza virus
Benign lymphocytic meningitis virus
Toxoplasma gondii
Listeria monocytogenes
Syphilis

In some regions of the CNS, neuron production continues for the entire life span. This late neuronogenesis is clearly apparent in the olfactory bulb and the dentate gyrus. Its importance at the level of the neocortex, especially in physiologic conditions, remains to be demonstrated. In this context, production of neurons for the human neocortex is generally considered to be a phenomenon occurring during the first half of gestation.

The neocortex is composed of vertical units (neuronal columns): the number of neurons in a given unit seems stable

---

BOX 40–2   Major Etiologies of Human Holoprosencephaly

CHROMOSOMAL HOLOPROSENCEPHALY
Chromosome 13: trisomy, deletion or duplication of 13q, ring
Deletion 2p, duplication 3p, deletion 7q, deletion 21q
Triploidy

SYNDROMAL HOLOPROSENCEPHALY
Meckel syndrome
Varadi-Papp syndrome
Pallister-Hall syndrome
Smith-Lemli-Opitz syndrome
Velocardiofacial syndrome

NONSYNDROMAL GENETIC HOLOPROSENCEPHALY (SPORADIC OR MENDELIAN INHERITANCE)
SIX3: HPE2 locus on chromosome 2p21
SHH: HPE3 locus on chromosome 7q36
TGIF: HPE4 locus on chromosome 18p11.3
ZIC2: HPE5 locus on chromosome 13q32

ENVIRONMENTAL HOLOPROSENCEPHALY
Hypocholesterolemia
Retinoic acid
Ethanol

BOX 40–3   Classification of Human Congenital Microcephaly

PRIMARY GENETIC MICROCEPHALY
Micrencephaly vera and radial microbrain (autosomal recessive or X-linked for one locus):
■ *MCPH1* (microcephalin)
■ *MCPH5* (ASPM gene)
■ *SLC25A19* (deoxynucleotide carrier)
Microcephaly with simplified gyral pattern (autosomal recessive):
■ Normal or thin corpus callosum
■ Agenesis of the corpus callosum
Microlissencephaly (MLIS) (autosomal recessive):
■ With thick cortex (MLIS1 or Norman-Roberts syndrome)
■ With thick cortex, brainstem and cerebellar hypoplasia (MLIS2 or Barth syndrome)
■ With intermediate cortex (MLIS3)
■ With mildly to moderately thick cortex (MLIS4)

MICROCEPHALY ASSOCIATED WITH OTHER BRAIN MALFORMATIONS
MICROCEPHALY AS PART OF A SYNDROME
Neu-Laxova syndrome
Seckel syndrome
Rubinstein-Taybi syndrome
Cornelia de Lange syndrome
Microcephalic osteodysplastic dwarfism

MICROCEPHALY ASSOCIATED WITH BIOCHEMICAL DISORDERS
MICROCEPHALY SECONDARY TO ENVIRONMENTAL FACTORS
Hypoxia-ischemia
Severe malnutrition
Maternal hyperphenylalaninemia and phenylketonuria
Ionizing radiation
Ethanol
Infections (cytomegalovirus, benign lymphocytic meningitis virus, *Toxoplasma gondii*)

---

throughout studied mammals and is constant throughout the different cortical areas (with the exception of the visual cortex). In contrast, the time necessary to produce the neocortical neurons of a given column progressively increases with increasing mammalian evolutionary complexity. Indeed, the period of neuronogenesis takes 6 days in mice whereas it takes 10 weeks in humans (gestational weeks 10 to 20, approximately). This period of neuronogenesis corresponds to the production of neurons from precursors present in the germinative neuroepithelium.

Administration of bromodeoxyuridine or tritiated thymidine, which are incorporated into DNA during the S phase of the mitotic cycle, has allowed the different parameters of the mitotic cycle and their evolution during the progression of neuronogenesis to be studied both in rodents and monkeys. In the pioneering model described by Caviness and collaborators,[23] which is based on the existence of a homogeneous population of precursors in the periventricular germinative neuroepithelium, the length of the total mitotic cycle progressively increases during the neuronogenetic interval (Fig. 40-2). This progressive increase in length is due to the progressive increase in length of G_1 phase, while G_2, M, and S phases remain constant. However, interference with the γ-aminobutyric acid (GABA)-ergic or glutamatergic systems in monkeys has been shown to modulate the length of S phase during this period. The second major contribution of these studies is to show that the proportion of daughter cells that reenters the mitotic cycle (G_1 phase) or leaves the cycle (postmitotic G_0 cells that are going to migrate to the cortex) is variable and depends on the stage of progression in the neuronogenetic interval. Therefore, in this model, at each step of the neuronogenetic interval, the periventricular neuroepithelium can be characterized by two variables: the length of G_1 phase and the fraction of

daughter cells that will continue to divide. Although this model is based on the assumption that cell death is negligible in the germinative neuroepithelium, a report[15] suggests that a large part of the precursor cells die in the germinative neuroepithelium during the neuronogenetic interval. Also, the existence of a regionalized germinative neuroepithelium has been proposed,[93] where cell cycle parameters would depend on the location of the dividing cell. This regionalization would allow an early specification of the characteristics for the future cortical areas.

During the neuronogenetic interval, after the M phase of the mitotic cycle, daughter cells face a dual choice: to reenter the mitotic cycle (G_1) or to leave the cycle (G_0) and, by doing so, to become postmitotic for the rest of their lives. Some factors, like insulin-like growth factor type 1, fibroblast growth factor, or vasoactive intestinal peptide, stimulate mitoses of neuronal precursors, whereas factors like glutamate or GABA reduce the proliferation of these cells but do not push

BOX 40–4 Genes and Environmental Factors Identified in Human Neuronal Migration Disorders

GENES

FLN1 (filamin): X-linked periventricular heterotopia

LIS1: type I lissencephaly (generally sporadic) and Miller-Dieker syndrome (microdeletion 17p13.3)

DCX (doublecortin) or *XLIS*: X-linked double cortex syndrome (usually girls) and type I lissencephaly (usually boys)

RELN: autosomal recessive lissencephaly + cerebellar hypoplasia

PEX genes: Zellweger syndrome (autosomal recessive)

ENVIRONMENTAL FACTORS

Ethanol

Cocaine

Cytomegalovirus

Toxoplasma gondii

Ionizing radiation

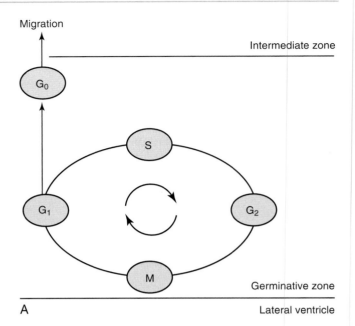

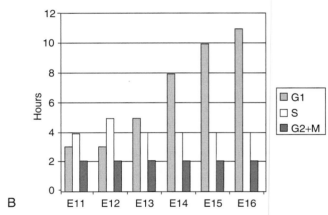

Figure 40–2. A, Schematic representation of the different phases of the mitotic cycle in the germinative neuroepithelium. Note the interkinetic movement of nuclei during the mitotic cycle: the relative position of the nucleus in the germinative zone is determined by the phase of the cycle. G_1, phase of protein synthesis; S, phase of DNA duplication; G_2, phase of protein synthesis; M, mitosis; G_0, postmitotic phase. B, Evolution of the length of the different phases of the mitotic cycle in the mouse germinative zone during the period of neuronogenesis (between embryonic days 11 and 16). During this interval, duration of the mitotic cycle increases from 8 hours up to 18 hours. This increased duration is secondary to a progressive increase in duration of G_1 phase.

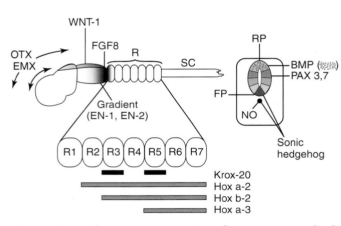

Figure 40–1. Schematic representation of some genes involved in the patterning of the rostrocaudal and dorsoventral axis of the central nervous system. FP, floor plate; NO, notochord; R, rhombomeres; RF, roof plate; SC, spinal cord. (*From Lagercrantz H, Ringstedt T: Organization of the neuronal circuits in the central nervous system during development,* Acta Paediatr *90:707, 2001, with permission.*)

these cells to become postmitotic. Very few factors have been described as capable of withdrawing precursor cells from the mitotic cycle. Pituitary adenylate cyclase-activating polypeptide seems to be one of these factors because it is able to prevent daughter cells from reentering the mitotic cycle and to initiate their migration to become cortical neurons.[73]

Neuronal Migration and Cortical Lamination

Neocortical neurons derive from the primitive neuroepithelium and migrate to their appropriate position in the cerebral mantle. In humans, migration of neocortical neurons occurs

mostly between the 12th and the 24th weeks of gestation.[104] The first postmitotic neurons produced in the periventricular germinative neuroepithelium (ventricular zone) migrate to form a subpial preplate or primitive plexiform zone (Fig. 40-3). Subsequently produced neurons, which will form the cortical plate, migrate into the preplate and split it into the superficial molecular layer (layer I or marginal zone containing Cajal-Retzius neurons) and the deep subplate. Schematically, the

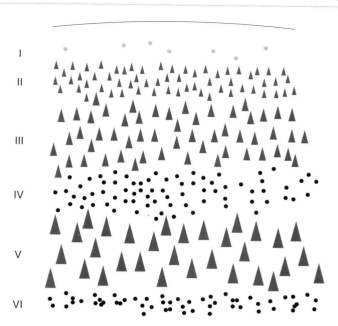

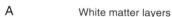

A

White matter layers

Figure 40–3. A, Schematic representation of the six layers of the mature mammalian neocortex. B, Schematic illustration of mammalian neocortical formation and neuronal migration. GZ, germinative zone; IZ, intermediate zone (prospective white matter); PPZ, primitive plexiform zone; SP, subplate; I, cortical layer I or molecular layer; II to VI, cortical layers II to VI. *Arrows* and *light gray circles* indicate migrating neurons; *black circles and triangles* represent postmigratory neurons.

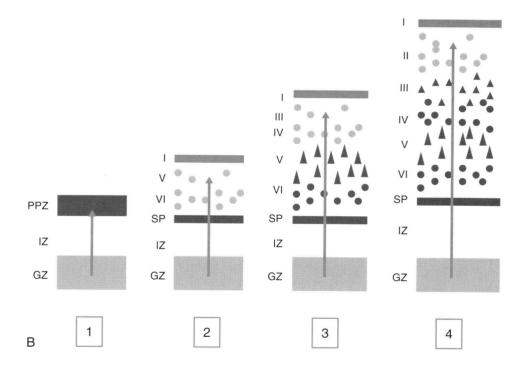

B

successive waves of migratory neurons pass the subplate neurons and end their migratory pathway below layer I, forming successively (but with substantial overlap) cortical layers VI, V, IV, III, and II (an inside-out pattern).

Neocortical migrating neurons can adopt different types of trajectories (Fig. 40-4)[43,95]:

1. A large proportion of neurons migrate radially, along radial glial guides, from the germinative zone to the cortical plate. Radial glia are specialized glial cells present in the neocortex during neuronal migration; these cells

display a radial shape with a nucleus located in the germinative zone, a basal process attached on the ventricular surface, and a radial apical process reaching the pial surface (Fig. 40-5). Rakic[96] postulated that these radially arranged glial guides keep a topographic correspondence between a hypothesized protomap present in the germinative zone (ventricular and subventricular zones) and the cortical areas.

2. An important group of neuronal precursors initially adopt a tangential trajectory at the level of the ventricular or subventricular germinative zones before adopting a classic

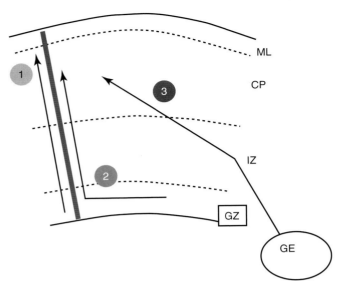

Figure 40–4. Schematic representation of the different migratory pathways adopted by neurons. **1,** Radial migration along radial glial cells of neurons originating from the periventricular germinative zone (GZ). **2,** Tangential migration in the germinative zone (GZ) followed by a radial migration along glial guides. **3,** Tangential migration in the intermediate zone (IZ) of neurons originating from the ganglionic eminence (GE). CP, cortical plate; IZ, intermediate zone (prospective white matter); ML, molecular layer.

radial migrating pathway along radial glia. This tangential migration could permit some dispersion at the level of the cortical plate of neurons originating from a single clone in the germinative neuroepithelium, increasing the clonal heterogeneity within a given cortical area.

3. Tangentially migrating neurons have also been described at the level of the intermediate zone (prospective white matter). Most of these neuronal cells displaying a migrating pathway orthogonal to radial glia originate in the ganglia eminence. Most GABA-expressing interneurons seem to be produced by this mechanism.

Using time-lapse imaging of clonal cells in rat cortex over several generations, it was shown that neurons are generated in two proliferative zones by distinct patterns of division.[83] Neurons arise directly from radial glial cells in the ventricular zone and indirectly from intermediate progenitor cells in the subventricular zone. Furthermore, newborn neurons do not migrate directly to the cortex; instead, most exhibit distinct phases of migration, including a phase of retrograde movement toward the ventricle before migration to the cortical plate.

The phenotype of radial glia seems to be determined both by migrating neurons and by intrinsic factors expressed by glial cells. Among the latter, the transcription factor Pax6, which is specifically localized in radial glia during cortical development, is critical for the morphology, number, function, and cell cycle of radial glia. From the appearance of the cortical plate, the radial glial fibers are grouped in fascicles of five to eight fibers in the intermediate zone.[61] The final

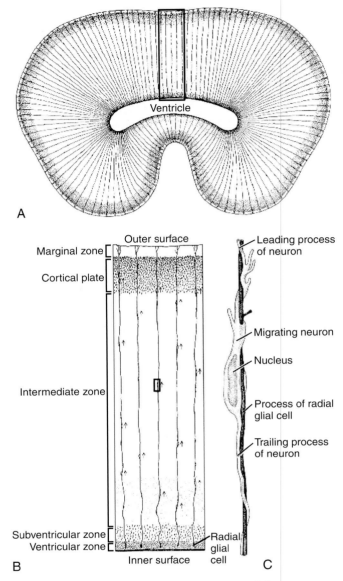

Figure 40–5. A, Schematic representation of the immature primate brain. **B,** Illustration of section (box in **A**) through the primate brain with the laminar organization of the immature brain, with ventricular, subventricular, intermediate zone, cortical plate, and marginal zone, and the arrangement of radial glial fibers illustrated in magnification. **C,** Three-dimensional reconstruction of a migrating neuron (magnified box in **B**) with radial fiber from radial glial cell having their origin in the ventricular zone and their relations to the migrating neuron. (*Modified from Rakic P: Mode of cell imigration to the superficial layers of fetal monkey neocortex.* J Comp Neurol 145:66, 1972.)

cortical location of the neurons, which could be determined by the guiding glial fascicle, partly determines the connections the neuron will be able to establish. The fascicles of glial fibers, filled with glycogen, could also provide the energy supply for migrating neurons, which are distant from developing blood vessels.

The ontogenic unit comprising the radial glial fascicle is very similar in the mouse, rat, hamster, cat, and human.[45] Because this glial unit is constant throughout the mammalian species studied, it could represent the basic developmental module of the developing cortex: the unit remains stable while the number of adjacent units gradually increases to permit brain expansion in the evolution of mammalian species. Knowledge of the genetic and environmental factors that control the organization, number, and function of these glial fascicles could, therefore, improve understanding of cortical development and evolution of the brain.

Studies over the last decade have identified several molecules involved in the control of neuronal migration and in targeting neurons to specific brain regions.[14,26] These molecules can be divided into four categories (Fig. 40-6):

1. Molecules of the cytoskeleton that play an important role in the initiation and progression (extension of the leading process and nucleokinesis) of neuronal movement. Initiation controlling molecules include Filamin-A (an actin-binding protein involved in periventricular nodular heterotopia) and Arfgef2 (ADP-rybosylation factor GEF2, which plays a role in vesicle trafficking and is involved in periventricular heterotopia combined with microcephaly). Progression controlling molecules include doublecortin (Dcx, a microtubule-associated protein [MAP] involved in double cortex and lissencephaly), Lis1 (a MAP and dynein

regulator involved in isolated type 1 lissencephaly and Miller-Dieker syndrome), and other molecules that are associated with migration defects in transgenic mice but that have not yet been associated with human disorders (phosphatase inhibitor 14-3-3epsilon, MAP1B, MAP2, and Tau).

2. Signaling molecules, which play a role in lamination. These molecules include the glycoprotein Reelin (involved in lissencephaly and cerebellar hypoplasia in humans and in the Reeler mouse mutant characterized by an inverted cortex) and other proteins generally associated with inverted cortex in transgenic or mutant mice, but which have not yet been associated with human disorders such as adaptor protein Disabled-1 (Dab1), ApoE receptor 2 (Apoer2), very low density lipoprotein receptor (Vldlr), two Reelin receptors, serine-threonine kinase Cdk5 (cyclin-dependent kinase 5), activator of Cdk5 p35, Brn1/Brn2, and transcriptional activators of Cdk5 and Dab-1.

3. Molecules modulating glycosylation which seem to provide stop signals for migrating neurons. These molecules include POMT1 (protein O-mannosyltransferase associated with Walker-Warburg syndrome), POMGnT1 (protein O-mannose beta-1,2-N-acetylglucosaminyltransferase involved in muscle-eye-brain disease), Fukutin (a putative glycosytransferase involved in Fukuyama muscular dystrophy), and focal-adhesion kinase (Fak involved in migration disorder in transgenic mice). These three human

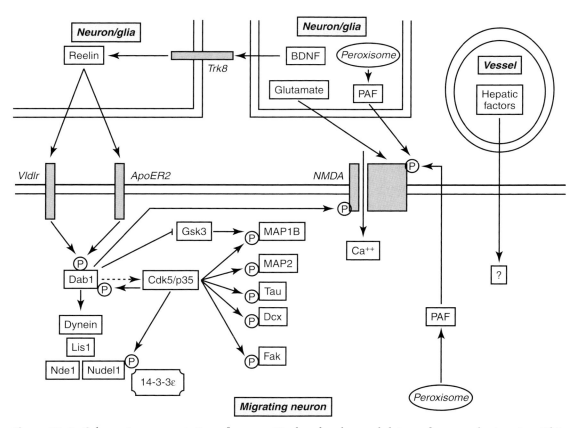

Figure 40–6. Schematic representation of some critical molecular modulators of neuronal migration. This scheme illustrates the cross-talk between different groups of molecules including cytoskeletal proteins, signaling molecules of the Reelin pathway, NMDA receptor-mediated pathway, and peroxisome-derived factors.

diseases comprise type 2 lissencephaly (cobblestone lissencephaly).

4. In addition to these three major groups of molecules, other factors have been shown to modulate neuronal migration, including neurotransmitters (glutamate and GABA),[10,12,75] trophic factors (brain-derived neurotrophic factor BDNF and thyroid hormones),[20] molecules deriving from peroxisomal metabolism, and environmental factors (ethanol and cocaine).

The application of diffusion-weighted magnetic resonance imaging (MRI) or diffusion tensor MRI to the evaluation of developing brain has opened up the possibility to study some of these developmental events in vivo. Quantitative indices derived from the diffusion tensor allow measurement of apparent diffusion and diffusion anisotropy, which ultimately depend on microstructural tissue development. Several different diffusion tensor imaging (DTI) parameters are available in this assessment. These include the three diffusion tensor eigen values ($\lambda 1$, $\lambda 2$, $\lambda 3$, which represent diffusion along the three tensor principal axes), the mean diffusivity (D_{av}) or apparent diffusion constant (ADC), and a mathematical measure of anisotropy, which describes the degree to which water diffusion is restricted in one direction relative to all others. Diffusion tensor MRI was used to study cortical development in human infants ranging from 26 to 41 weeks' gestational age; apparent diffusion of water in cortex was maximally anisotropic at 26 weeks' gestational age and declined to zero by 36 weeks' gestational age.[76] During this period, the major eigenvector of the diffusion tensor in cerebral cortex is oriented radially across the cortical plate. Vector maps illustrate diffusion anisotropy and direction of the major diffusion eigenvector. In the case of cortical gray matter, the vectors are oriented radially, consistent with the orientation of the radial glial fibers (Fig. 40-7).[76] Anisotropy changes are different in early intracortical maturation, where changes in fraction anisotrophy (FA)

are mainly due to changes in $\lambda 1$[28] confirmed also by studies in the developing rat brain.[51,107] One study on human fetal brain has shown that cortical anisotropy increases from 15 weeks' gestation to approximately 26 weeks' gestation and then shows a gradual decline to 32 weeks' gestation.[47] The increase of anisotropy in this time period coincides with active neuronal migration along the radial glial scaffolding, whereas the decrease coincides with the phase of neocortical maturation with transformation of the radial glia into the more complex astrocytic neuropil.

The use of new, ultrafast MRI sequences such as multiplanar, single-shot, fast spin-echo T2-weighted images provides high-resolution images of the fetus in utero with imaging times of less than 1 minute.[2] The normal MRI pattern of fetal brain maturation from 13 weeks' gestation has been described, documenting the presence of the primary sulci and the insula by 15 weeks' gestation. Operculization of the insula begins by 20 weeks' gestation and all the main sulci, except the occipital sulci, are present by 28 weeks' gestation.[2] From 28 weeks' gestation there is mainly an increase in secondary and tertiary sulcal formation. From 23 to 28 weeks in vivo[41] and from 15 weeks in vitro,[19,27] the typical multilayer pattern of the cerebral parenchyma can be observed with the innermost hyperintense signal (T1-weighted MRI) of the germinal matrix (Fig. 40-8). The five-layer pattern of the fetal forebrain, including the layers of neuroblast formation and migration, could be identified at 16 to 18 weeks' gestation in postmortem fetal brains.[27] During the last trimester, the gyri and sulci already formed become more prominent and more deeply infolded, with subsequent development of secondary and tertiary gyri at 40 to 44 weeks of gestational age (Fig. 40-9).

Komuro and Rakic[64] first reported that specific inhibitors of the N-methyl-D-aspartate (NMDA) glutamate receptor subtype slowed down the rate of in vitro neuronal migration. GABA is also involved in neuronal migration modulation

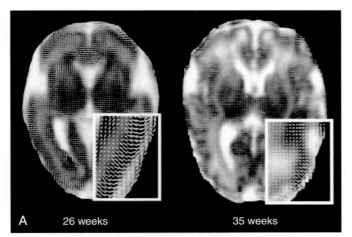

RADIAL ORGANIZATION OF CORTICAL LAYERS

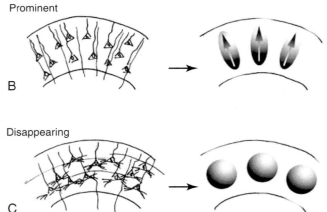

Figure 40–7. **A,** Diffusion tensor images of preterm infants at 26 weeks' and 35 weeks' gestation illustrating the direction of major eigenvectors in the immature cortex. **B,** Predominantly radially oriented diffusion in immature cortex at 26 weeks (high anisotropy) represented schematically by the diffusion ellipsoid with the *arrow* pointing in the direction of maximal diffusion. **C,** Absence of radial organization and isotropic diffusion after 35 weeks' gestational age with diffusion equal in all direction represented schematically by a sphere. (*From McKinstry RC, Mathur A, Miller JH, et al: Radial organization of developing preterm human cerebral cortex revealed by non-invasive water diffusion anisotropy MRI, Cereb Cortex 12:1237, 2002, with permission.*)

(layer I), mimicking some aspects observed in human status verrucosus deformans.

Central Nervous System Organization

SUBPLATE NEURONS

As mentioned previously, subplate neurons constitute a distinct structure during neocortical development.[66] Neurons of the subplate are generated at approximately the seventh week of gestation, and the subplate is generated from the preplate at approximately 10 gestational weeks. This structure localized beneath the neocortical plate reaches its maximal thickness between 22 and 36 gestational weeks. The subplate is present in preterm neonates but has disappeared in full-term neonates. Some authors have suggested that these neurons disappear by apoptosis, whereas others have suggested that they are incorporated into layer VI of the mature neocortex.

Subplate neurons express different neurotransmitters, neuropeptides, and growth factors, receive synapses, and make connections with cortical and subcortical structures. These neurons play several important roles during brain development: (1) they produce axons for the internal capsule that will serve as guiding axons for axons originating from neurons in layers V and VI; (2) between 25 and 32 gestational weeks, they produce axons for the corpus callosum; (3) they act as a waiting zone for thalamocortical axons (with which they establish synapses) before they invade the cortical plate and reach layer IV. This waiting zone is necessary for appropriate target selection by thalamocortical afferents.

The subplate neurons can be lesioned or destroyed in preterm neonates with periventricular white matter lesions.[102] These data have been recently substantiated in animal models of periventricular white matter damage (see Part 2 of this chapter).[77]

MRI has been used to visualize the developmental evolution of the subplate zone and other laminar compartments of the fetal cerebral wall between 15 and 36 weeks' gestation.

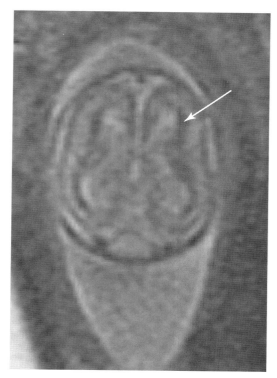

Figure 40–8. Germinal matrix illustrated by in vivo fetal T2-weighted MRI at 20 weeks' gestation. *Arrow* points to low signal intensity periventricular germinal matrix.

because it stimulates, in tissue culture, neuronal migration through calcium-dependent mechanisms.[11] Growth factors also have been implicated in the control of neuronal migration. Intraventricular injection of neurotrophin-4 or overexpression of brain-derived neurotrophic factor produces heterotopic accumulation of neurons in the molecular layer

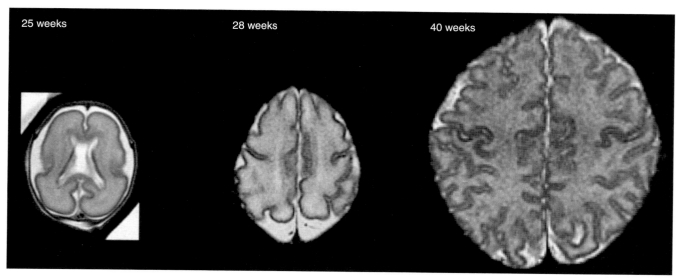

Figure 40–9. Cortical folding illustrated from 25 weeks' to 40 weeks' gestation by in vivo MRI. T2-weighted images at 25, 28, and 40 weeks' gestational age.

The combination of MRI and histochemical staining of the extracellular matrix enabled selective visualization of the subplate zone in the developing human brain. The tissue elements of the subplate zone are embedded in an abundant, very hydrophilic, and transient extracellular matrix that is most likely responsible for the low signal intensity on T1-weighted MRI in Figure 40-10 and the slightly higher signal intensity on T2-weighted MRI as seen in vivo at 26 weeks (Fig. 40-11).

AXONAL AND DENDRITIC GROWTH

When neurons near their final destination, they start to produce axons and dendrites, allowing connection with distant cerebral structures. This ontogenic step occurs largely, but

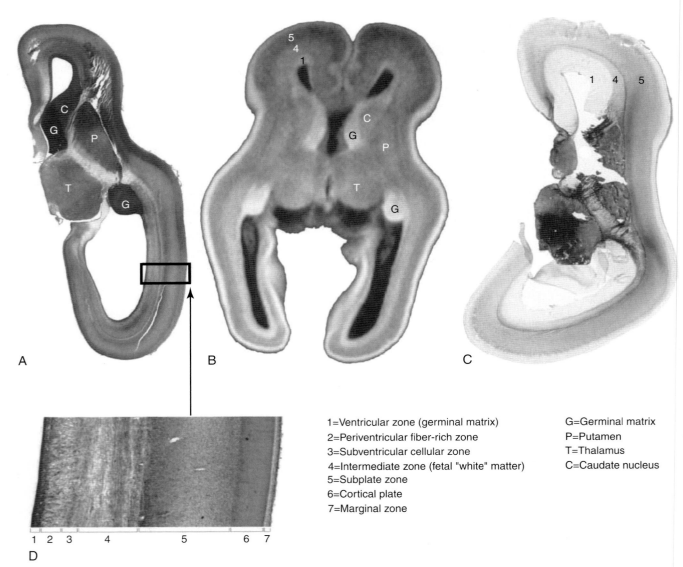

1=Ventricular zone (germinal matrix)
2=Periventricular fiber-rich zone
3=Subventricular cellular zone
4=Intermediate zone (fetal "white" matter)
5=Subplate zone
6=Cortical plate
7=Marginal zone

G=Germinal matrix
P=Putamen
T=Thalamus
C=Caudate nucleus

Figure 40–10. See color insert. The cerebral wall displays five laminar compartments of varying MRI signal intensity (**B**), which partly correspond to laminar compartments delineated on Nissl-stained (**A**) and histochemical (**C**) sections. Starting from the ventricular surface, these laminar compartments are as follows: The ventricular zone (germinal matrix) of high MRI signal intensity, which corresponds to the highly cellular ventricular zone in Nissl-stained sections and, therefore, is marked with number 1 (1 in **D**). The periventricular zone of low MRI signal intensity, which largely corresponds to the periventricular fiber-rich zone (2 in **D**). The intermediate zone of moderate MRI signal intensity, which encompasses both the subventricular cellular zone and the fetal white matter (3 and 4 in **D**). The subplate zone of low MRI signal intensity, which closely corresponds to the compartment marked with 5 in Nissl-stained section (5 in **D**) and acetylcholinesterase-stained section (5 in **C**); therefore it is marked with 5 on MR images (5 in **B**). The cortical plate of high MRI signal intensity, which closely corresponds to the compartment marked with 6 on Nissl-stained sections (6 in **D**) but on MR images cannot be separated from the marginal zone (7 in **D**); therefore, it is always described on MR images as a band of high signal intensity situated above the subplate zone. (*From Kostovic I, et al: Laminar organization of the human fetal cerebrum revealed by histochemical markers and magnetic resonance imaging,* Cereb Cortex 12:536, 2002, with permission.)

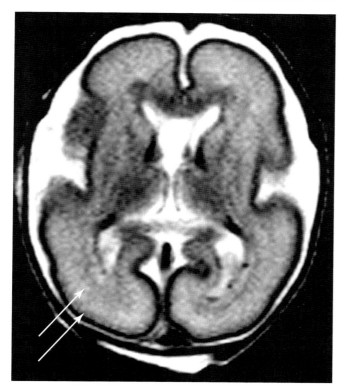

Figure 40–11. T2-weighted MRI (axial plane) of a preterm infant at 26 weeks' gestation with *arrows* indicating subcortical zone of higher signal intensity corresponding to the autopsy description of highly hydrophilic extracellular matrix in the subplate zone.

4. Growth cones can interact with various glycoproteins of the extracellular matrix that act as guiding cues.
5. At early stages of brain development, distances separating structures are rather small, facilitating the navigation of growth cones. These first-produced axons, called *pioneer axons*, serve as guides for later-produced axons, when distances between structures are significantly larger.

As for neuronal production, some axonal projections are produced in excess, connecting too many structures or neurons. This initial phase is followed by a regressive phase where redundant or misconnected axons are eliminated or retracted, allowing the emergence of adequate and functional connections. This balance between the maintenance or the elimination of axons is regulated by different mechanisms. Obviously, the survival of the neuron is determinant in this decision. Furthermore, competition for available trophic factors interacts with the genome to modulate this balance.[21] Also, electrical activity is a key determinant for the maintenance of axons. Accordingly, in utero and especially postnatal stimuli and experiences significantly shape the developing brain by modulating the maintenance or elimination of some axons.[24]

Some callosal connections, some "feedback" intracortical connections, and some corticofugal projections (such as the motor pathway) seem to be examples of connections largely under the control of this "overproduction-elimination" principle and therefore are highly dependent on the environment.[56] In contrast, some "feedforward" intracortical connections seem to be more genetically predetermined and therefore less susceptible to environmental cues.[92]

Studying white matter development with in vivo imaging was largely impossible before the advent of advanced MR techniques, with diffusion imaging being of particular interest in the assessment of the white matter microstructure. Diffusion characteristics differ between pediatric and adult human brain in two primary ways. First, apparent diffusion coefficient (ADC) values are higher for pediatric brain than adult. Second, ADC maps of pediatric brain show contrast between white and gray matter, with the ADC values for white matter being higher than those for gray. The precise cause of the decrease in ADC with increasing age is not known, although it has been postulated that the rapid decrease observed between early gestation and term is due to the concomitant decrease in overall water content. Brain water content decreases dramatically with increasing gestational age. As it does, structures that hinder water motion (e.g., cell and axonal membranes) become more densely packed, which further restricts the motion of the remaining water. The use of diffusion tensor MRI has allowed visualization of early white matter connectivity (Fig. 40-12) with demonstration of interhemispheric callosal fibers in the nonmyelinated stage at 28 weeks of gestation. During white matter development, decreases in diffusion are observed principally in $\lambda 2$ and $\lambda 3$ (and much less in $\lambda 1$), which reflect changes in water diffusion perpendicular to white matter fibers and may indicate changes due to premyelination (change of axonal width) and myelination.[40,80,87]

Relative anisotropy values for white matter areas are relatively low in newborns and increase steadily with increasing age.[81] They are particularly low for preterm infants.[54] This

not exclusively, during the second half of gestation and extends into the postnatal period. For example, evoked visual potentials can be produced as early as 24 to 27 gestational weeks in human neonates, confirming the existence of an established wiring at this early developmental stage.

Growing axons have to find their path through developing structures to reach their target. In this process, growing axons, and in particular their distal tip, called the *growth cone*, are helped by several mechanisms:

1. The transcriptome of each neuron contains information determining the types of connections this neuron can establish.
2. Target neurons or neurons on the pathway of growing axons secrete or express on their membranes chemoattraction or chemorepulsion factors that interact with receptors present on growth cones, resulting in attraction or repulsion of these axonal growth cones. Several ligand-receptor families have been described, including netrin, slit, comm, robo, semaphorin, cadherin, and ephrin receptors.[71] The interaction between these different ligands and receptors leads to changes in calcium levels in the growth cones, which seem to play a key role in the resulting behavior of the growth cone.
3. Neurotransmitters and trophic factors are liberated that will favor or inhibit the extension of the growing axons expressing the corresponding receptor.

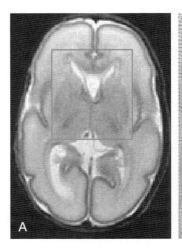
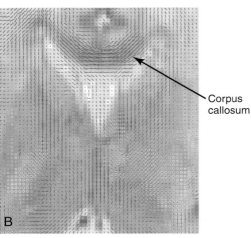

Figure 40–12. See color insert. **A,** Anatomic axial T2-weighted MRI. **B,** Diffusion tensor vector maps for the regions indicated by the box in **A,** showing nonmyelinated interhemispheric fiber connections in the corpus callosum at 28 weeks' gestational age. The blue lines represent the in-plane fibers, the out-of plane fibers are shown in colored dots ranging from green to red. (*Hüppi PS, et al: Microstructural development of human newborn cerebral white matter assessed in vivo by diffusion tensor magnetic resonance imaging,* Pediatr Res *44:584, 1998, with permission.*)

increase has been attributed to changes in white matter microstructure that accompany the "premyelinating state."[122] This state is characterized by a number of histologic changes, including an increase in the number of microtubule-associated proteins in axons, an axon caliber change, and a significant increase in the number of oligodendrocytes. It is also associated with changes in the axonal membrane, such as an increase in conduction velocity and changes in Na^+/K^+-adenosine triphosphatase activity. Myelination then further increases relative anisotropy values. Although myelin accounts for much of the change in relative anisotropy, diffusion anisotropy is present under any circumstance in which the cytoarchitecture of the tissue is arranged in such a way as to lead to greater hindrance of water motion in one direction compared with others.

Making proper connections through white matter structures is probably one of the determining factors for further cortical organization. One major hypothesis for the morphogenetic mechanism of cortical folding is based on mechanical tension along axons in the white matter.[114] A striking increase in cerebral cortical volume accompanies the axonal and dendritic growth described previously. That this growth is particularly rapid between approximately 28 and 40 weeks' gestational age has been shown by quantitative three-dimensional MRI techniques with use of postacquisition image analysis. Volumetric analysis of MRI data sets is achieved by segmentation of the imaged volume into tissue types depending on their difference in signal intensity, followed by three-dimensional renderings. Overall brain volume more than doubles between 28 and 40 weeks' gestation, and cortical gray matter volume increases fourfold in the same period.[55] This increase is thought to relate primarily to neuronal differentiation rather than to an increase in the total number of neurons. Cortical surface, changing from smooth, lissencephalic to highly convoluted, increases fivefold between 28 and 40 weeks' gestation (Fig. 40-13).

So far, several hypotheses have been put forward on the mechanisms that underlie the folding process during development, but the potential influence of genetic, epigenetic, and environmental factors is still poorly understood. According to postmortem observations of fetal brains,[36] the primary folds would form in a relatively stable spatiotemporal way during intrauterine life depending on physical constraints

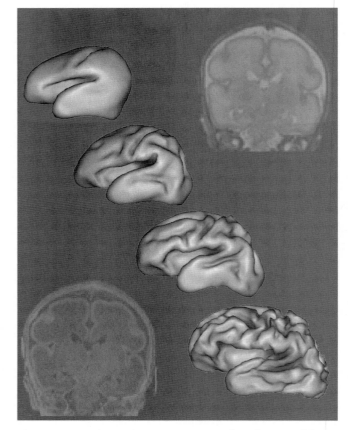

Figure 40–13. See color insert. External and internal brain surface at from 26 to 36 weeks' gestation illustrated by three-dimensional models generated from magnetic resonance imaging, which illustrates timing of regional cortical folding and permits quantitative measures of surface and sulcation index. (*Images reconstructed by specialized image analysis software, courtesy of Dubois J, Benders M, Cachia A, et al: Mapping the early cortical folding process in the preterm newborn brain,* Cereb Cortex *18:1444, 2008.*)

and mechanical factors.[97] An attractive theory suggests that the specific location and shape of sulci are determined by the global minimization over the brain of the viscoelastic tensions from white matter fibers connecting cortical areas.[48,49] This may explain why specific abnormalities in the sulcal pattern are observed in certain brain developmental disorders that are the result of subtle impairments in the neuronal migration and the set-up of corticocortical connections.[94,115] The emergence of the cortical foldings in the preterm newborn brain was recently studied by applying dedicated postprocessing tools to high-quality MR images acquired shortly after birth over a developmental period critical for the human cortex development.[33] Through the three-dimensional reconstruction of the developing inner cortical surface, a sulcation index was derived and allowed measurement of variations with age, gender, and presence of brain lesions and mapped the individual sulci appearance, highlighting early interhemispherical structural asymmetries that may be related to the cortical functional specialization of the brain. Females have lower cortical surface and smaller volumes of cortex and white matter than males, but equivalent sulcation. The highest sulcal index is found in the central region, followed by the temporoparieto-occipital region, with the lowest sulcation index in the frontal region, which confirms that the medial surface folds before the lateral surface and that the morphologic differentiation of sulci begins in the central region and progresses in an occipitorostral direction. Such spatiotemporal differences in brain maturation have been described in detail in older children through the analysis of cortical volume and thickness changes.[38] In particular, occipital regions grow much faster than prefrontal regions in newborns born at term,[39] and higher-order association cortices mature only after lower-order somatosensory and heterotopia visual cortices.[109]

The right hemisphere presents gyral complexity earlier than the left, which is particularly evident at the level of the superior temporal sulcus, which parallels early functional competence in response to auditive stimuli in newborns. Preterm birth may be responsible for the delay that we observed in sulci appearance in comparison with postmortem and fetal studies, in that both cortical volume[58] and surface area[1] of extremely preterm infants imaged at term equivalent age are decreased and less complex than in normal infants, and this impairment seems to increase with decreasing gestational age at birth.[62] Furthermore, preterm infants with intrauterine growth restriction had more pronounced reduction of volume in relation to surface area and increased sulcation with resultant changes in cortical thickness, which correlated with impaired behavioral functions.[32]

SYNAPTOGENESIS

The concept of synaptic stabilization (with the elimination of nonstabilized synapses) has been proposed.[25,34] During brain development, there are successive waves of overproduction of labile synapses, inducing redundant connections produced in a relatively random manner (Fig. 40-14). This step is under tight genetic control. Each wave of overproduction is followed by a period of stabilization of synapses that have a functional meaning and elimination of redundant or meaningless synapses. This period of stabilization and elimination is highly influenced by environmental stimuli and experi-

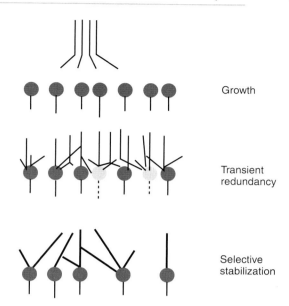

Figure 40–14. Schematic representation of the epigenetic hypothesis based on selective stabilization of synapses. Spontaneous or evoked activity of developing neuronal networks controls the selective elimination of redundant synapses formed during the transient phase of synaptic redundancy. *(Adapted from Changeux JP, Danchin A: Selective stabilisation of developing synapses as a mechanism for the specification of neuronal networks,* Nature 264:705, 1976.)

ence. In this model, a moderate increase in the number of genes would induce a richer substrate on which the environment could produce a more complex network. Neuronal activity-mediated glutamate release induces a postsynaptic calcium influx at the level of NMDA receptors. Calcium changes lead to production of trophic factors such as brain-derived neurotrophic factor, which stabilize labile synapses, protecting them against elimination. Nitric oxide, which is rapidly produced after glutamate binding to its NMDA receptor, is another key player in synaptic stabilization and plasticity. This model of synaptic stabilization and elimination does not exclude the existence of an instructive process where synaptic connections are adequately established right away.

In monkey occipital neocortex, five successive waves of synaptogenesis have been described.[18] Based on data obtained in human occipital cortex,[71] the following timetable for humans is proposed (Fig. 40-15): (1) a first phase starting approximately 6 to 8 weeks of gestation and limited to lower structures like the subplate; (2) a second phase starting after 12 to 17 weeks with relatively few synapses produced in the cortex (contacts on the dendritic shafts); (3) a third phase starting around midgestation and ending approximately 8 months after birth; this phase is characterized by an estimated rate of 40,000 new synapses per second in the monkey; (4) a fourth phase lasting until puberty and also characterized by a high rate of synapse production; and (5) a last phase extending until late adulthood but somewhat hidden by the intense loss of synapses characterizing these ages. Experimentally, the first two phases are not affected by lack of sensory stimuli. The third phase partially depends on this sensory input, whereas the fourth phase is highly dependent on sensory input and experience.

DENSITY OF SYNAPSES

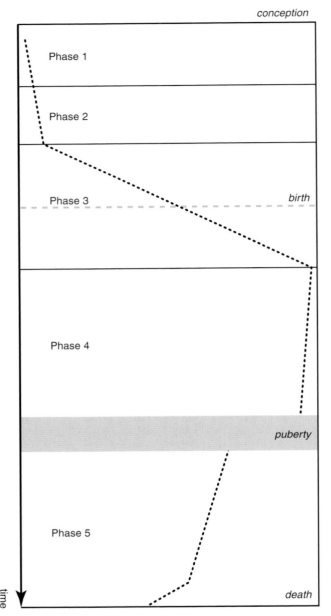

Figure 40–15. Schematic representation of the synaptic density in the visual cortex of the macaque monkey. *(From Bourgeois JP: Synaptogenesis, heterochrony and epigenesis in the mammalian neocortex, Acta Paediatr Suppl 422:27, 1997.)*

Current understanding of the mechanisms of synaptogenesis and of synaptic stabilization raises numerous questions in neonatal medicine and pediatric neurology. Very preterm infants are a typical example of such an issue:

1. What are the effects of environmental modifications of preterm birth on synaptic stabilization?
2. What are the influences (positive or negative) of too early sensory stimuli for synaptogenesis?
3. What are the effects on the synaptic equipment of drugs that interfere with the glutamatergic or the nitric oxide system?

PROGRAMMED CELL DEATH

Depending on brain area, between 15% and 50% of the initially formed neurons will be eliminated by a physiologic process called *programmed cell death,* or *apoptosis.* Approximately 70% of these neurons that are destined to disappear seem to die between 28 and 41 gestational weeks.[13]

Programmed cell death is a complex mechanism that involves a balance between death and trophic signals, death and survival genetic programs, and effectors and inhibitors of cell death (Fig. 40-16).[78,116] Under the influence of a combination of exogenous and endogenous factors, genetic programs are activated (hence the name, "programmed cell death") that are able to overcome the natural defenses of the neuron. The cell eventually dies and is rapidly removed by phagocytosis performed by neighboring glial cells. In this process, activation of the cascade of caspases (proteolytic enzymes) is a key step leading to DNA fragmentation and neuronal cell death. The caspase pathway can be activated by intrinsic and extrinsic mechanisms. The intrinsic mechanism or mitochondrial-dependent pathway is triggered by cytochrome C release by mitochondria and is controlled by members of the Bcl-2 family, whereas the extrinsic pathway is triggered by activation of death receptors, a subgroup of the tumor necrosis factor receptor superfamily. Neuronal apoptosis can be also triggered by a caspase-independent pathway involving AIF (apoptosis-inducing factor) release from mitochondria.

Electrical activity seems to be a critical factor for neuronal survival. During the period of brain growth spurt in rodents, administration of drugs that block electrical activity leads to a dramatic exacerbation of neuronal cell death in different brain areas. These drugs include NMDA receptor blockers (MK-801 or ketamine), GABA-A receptor agonists such as classic antiepileptic drugs (phenytoin, phenobarbital, diazepam, clonazepam,

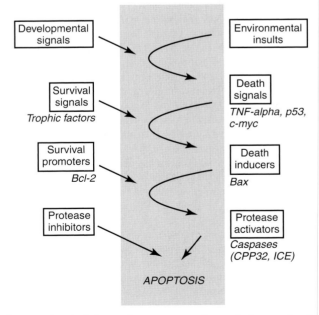

Figure 40–16. Schematic representation of the molecular cascade leading to neuronal apoptosis and showing the balance between pro-survival (left side) and pro-death (right side) factors.

vigabatrin, or valproic acid), and anesthetics (combination of midazolam, nitrous oxide, and isoflurane).[86] These effects on neuronal cell death are mimicked by acute administration of ethanol, which blocks NMDA receptors and activates GABA-A receptors. Although the mechanism is unknown, the systemic injection of a combination of sulfites (which are present in the excipient of some commercially available preparations of injectable glucocorticoids and vasoactive amines) and dexamethasone to newborn mouse pups led to an exacerbation of programmed neural cell death both in the neocortex and basal ganglia.[9,103]

Postnatal systemic steroid therapy had been widely used for chronic lung disease in the preterm infant until follow-up studies indicated higher rates of cerebral palsy and of subnormal (less than 70) cognitive function in steroid-treated infants (see Chapter 44, Part 7). Quantitative MRI studies have indicated a possible origin of these functional deficits by showing marked reduction of cortical gray matter volume after repetitive antenatal and postnatal steroid treatment.[79,82] Different roles have been attributed to programmed cell death, although final proofs are still lacking. These comprise elimination of "sick" neurons; increase of neuronal diversity by eliminating redundant neurons; and competition for trophic factors with elimination of neurons that have lower access to these trophic factors.

GLIAL PROLIFERATION AND DIFFERENTIATION, AND MYELINATION

Glia is composed of three types of cells: astrocytes, oligodendrocytes, and microglia (brain macrophages).

Astrocytes

Neocortical astrocytes have a dual origin (Fig. 40-17).[46] After the end of neuronal migration, radial glial cells (which are glial cells specialized in the guidance of migrating neurons)

transform into astrocytes, which are found mainly in the deep cortical layers and underlying white matter. In addition, the periventricular germinative zone produces, after the end of neuronal production, astrocytic precursors that will migrate mostly into the superficial neocortical layers.

The presence of low-intensity periventricular bands in the white matter on T2-weighted MRI has been recorded in studies of premature infants, predominantly less than 30 weeks' gestational age. These bands are thought to represent populations of migrating radial glial cells based on their position and on correlative neuropathologic data.[8,26] The presence of these bands on T2-weighted MRI is therefore thought to be a marker of normal brain development.

Transformation of radial glia into astrocytes involves an autophagic digestion of apical processes and a nuclear translocation from the germinative neuroepithelium toward the white matter. Molecular mechanisms controlling this transformation remain unknown. In vitro, it was shown that neurons are necessary to maintain the radial phenotype of these glial cells.

In human neocortex, this astrocytic proliferation probably starts at approximately 24 weeks of gestation, with a peak at approximately 26 to 28 weeks. The final stage of astrocyte production is not known, but one might assume that the bulk of astrocyte production is completed by the end of normal gestation. However, it is important to remember that astrocytes retain the capability to divide throughout their life span. This peak of astrocyte production at approximately 26 to 28 weeks might be particularly important for preterm neonates. Indeed, astrocytes play several important roles during brain development, including axonal guidance, stimulation of neuron growth, synaptic formation, transfer of metabolites between blood vessels and neurons (magnetic resonance spectroscopy [MRS] results), establishment of

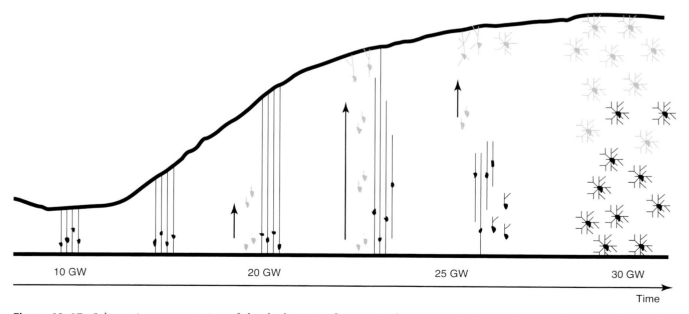

Figure 40–17. Schematic representation of the dual origin of neocortical astrocytes in human fetuses. Astrocytes destined to the white matter and deep cortical layers derive from the progressive transformation of radial glial cells (black cells), whereas most astrocytes destined to the more superficial cortical layers derive from precursors that migrate from the germinative neuroepithelium (gray cells). GW, gestational weeks. Arrows indicate migrating astrocytes.

scaffolding structures, production of extracellular matrix components, production of trophic factors, neuronal survival, myelination, and participation in the blood-brain barrier. For example, experimental transient blockade of astrocyte production in the rodent neocortex leads to increased neuronal programmed cell death and long-term changes in neocortical synaptic equipment.[125]

One of the essential contributors to progress in the noninvasive detection of tissue metabolism and in vivo biochemistry in recent years has been ^{1}H-MRS, which gives specific chemical information on the biochemistry of numerous intracellular metabolites (Fig. 40-18). Neurochemistry has particularly benefited from this technique, in that there is the possibility of detecting cerebral metabolites in vivo in otherwise inaccessible tissue. Astrocytes play a variety of complex nutritive and supportive roles in relation to neuronal metabolic homeostasis. For example, astrocytes take up glutamate and convert it to glutamine; removal of glutamate from the extracellular space protects surrounding cells from glutamate-induced excitotoxicity. Glutamate and glutamine are amino acids that are measured in ^{1}H-MRS when using short echo times. Alternatively, glutamate in the astrocyte can stimulate glycolysis with lactate production. Lactate is then released into the extracellular space and can also be taken up by neurons and used for energy generation.[88] In the immature brain, especially in the immature white matter, lactate is present in higher concentrations.[22,52]

Osmoregulation is another major metabolic task fulfilled by astroglia. Osmolytes synthesized by astrocytes or present in astroglia include taurine, hypotaurine, and myoinositol. Developmental changes in myoinositol have been described by Kreis and colleagues,[67,87] with a decrease of myoinositol during the first year of life and a marked reduction of myoinositol in the first weeks after birth regardless of the gestational age at birth. Studies indicate that astroglial cells are also able to synthesize creatine from glycine, which will need to be considered in interpreting

creatine concentrations in brain[12,31] and its role as a neuroprotective agent.

Oligodendrocytes and Myelination

Oligodendrocytes, which produce myelin, can be divided into four cell types according to their stage of maturation: oligodendrocyte progenitor (NG2+), preoligodendrocyte (O4+, O1−), immature oligodendrocyte (O4+, O1+), and mature myelinating oligodendrocyte (O4+, O1+, MBP+, PLP+).

The progenitors originate from the proliferative subventricular zone and are bipolar and mitotically active. They are produced during the last months of gestation and in the early postnatal period. During migration in the white matter, differentiation into preoligodendrocytes occurs, which are multipolar cells retaining a proliferative capacity. This second cell type is the dominant one in the second half of gestation in the periventricular white matter. The immature oligodendrocyte is a multipolar cell that starts in the third trimester to ensheathe the axons in preparation for myelination. The last stage is differentiation into the mature, myelinating, highly multipolar cell. Each stage of differentiation can be marked by specific monoclonal antibodies (Fig. 40-19).[3]

Growth factors, hormones, and cytokines (basic fibroblast growth factor, neurotrophin-3, platelet-derived-growth factor, insulin-like growth factor type 1, interleukin-6, thyroid hormone) are implicated in oligodendrocyte maturation, but up to 50% of oligodendrocytes undergo programmed cell death (apoptosis) during development.[118] Preoligodendrocyte progenitors are highly vulnerable to oxidative stress, excitotoxic cascade (through α-3-amino-hydroxy-5-methyl-4-isoxazole propionic acid [AMPA]-kainate and NMDA receptors), and hypoxic-ischemic insults.[118]

^{1}H-MRS as an in vivo technique to assess metabolic composition of brain tissue can help in characterizing integrity of developing white matter. N-acetylaspartate (NAA), an amino acid specific to the CNS, has been shown to be uniquely localized in neuronal tissue of the adult brain, whereas during

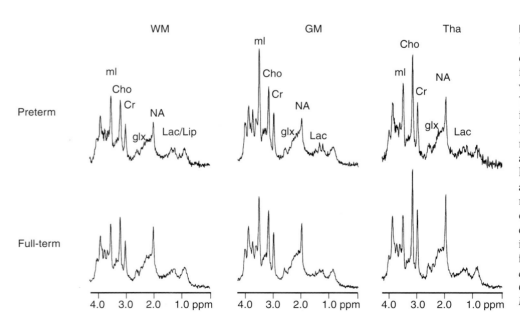

Figure 40–18. Averaged in vivo [1]H-MR spectra during human development in function of different regions of the brain: WM, white matter; GM, gray matter; Tha, thalamus. Metabolites identified are Lac, lactate; NA, N-acetyl-aspartate; glx, glutamine and glutamate; Cr, creatine and phosphocreatine; Cho, choline; mI, myoinositol. Spectra are scaled identically. Developmental changes in metabolite concentrations are illustrated by different peak heights comparing spectra from preterm and full-term newborns. (*Spectra analyzed by Roland Kreis, MR Center, Inselspital, University of Berne, Switzerland.*)

OLIGODENDROCYTE LINEAGE

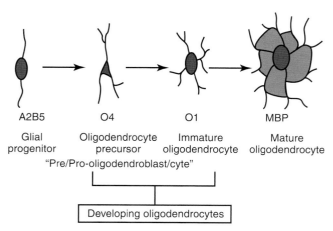

Figure 40–19. Schematic representation of the oligodendrocyte development showing their morphology and some major immunohistochemical markers (A2B5, O4, O1, and MBP [myelin basic protein]). (*Adapted from Back SA, et al: Immunocytochemical characterization of oligodendrocyte development in human cerebral white matter,* Soc Neurosci Abst 20:1722, 1996.)

development it is also found in oligodendrocyte type 2 astrocyte progenitor cells and immature oligodendrocytes.[112] NAA has been shown to be an acetyl group source in the nervous system.[78] The major requirement for acetyl groups is lipid synthesis, which takes place immediately before myelin deposition in the developing brain. A marked increase of NAA shown in several studies (Hüppi and Lazeyras[53] for review) in the period from 32 to 40 weeks of gestation, just before the initiation of myelination, supports the importance of NAA in lipid synthesis (see Fig. 40-18). Regional differences in age-dependent changes of NAA concentrations during early brain development show stable concentrations in perithalamic voxels,[22] where myelination is already initiated at 32 weeks, and a marked increase in central cerebral white matter[68] between 32 and 40 weeks of gestation (see Fig. 40-18).

Myelination occurs over a protracted period, ending long after birth (Table 40-2). The chronology and rate of myelination vary with the brain structure. Structures that function first tend to be myelinated first. However, although myelination leads to a marked acceleration in nerve conduction, human and experimental studies have reported several examples of dissociation between the degree of myelination and the maturation of a given function. Myelination starts in the cerebral hemispheres around birth and is largely complete by the age of 2 to 3 years. There is no detectable myelination in the forebrain before the seventh gestational month, and this process continues in some parts until the years of maturity. Myelination is most intense in the telencephalon during the third trimester and postnatally.

TABLE 40-2   Sequence of Myelination Based on Histologic Analysis and Magnetic Resonance Imaging

Anatomic Region	MEDIAN AGE FOR DETECTION OF MYELIN: HISTOLOGY[124]	AGE FOR DETECTION OF MYELIN: MAGNETIC RESONANCE IMAGING[41]	
		T1-Weighted Images	T2-Weighted Images
Ventrolateral thalamus		28-30 wk	32 to 34 wk
Posterior limb of internal capsule	38/44 wk*	38-40 wk	Posterior portion 40-48 wk Anterior portion 56-70 wk
Anterior limb of internal capsule	50/87 wk	48-53 wk	70-90 wk
Central corona radiata	37/52 wk	38-56 wk	52-65 wk
Genu corpus callosum	50/53 wk	56-64 wk	64-72 wk
Splenium corpus callosum	54/65 wk	52-56 wk	56-64 wk
Occipital white matter			
Central	47/87 wk	52-60 wk	76-96 wk
Peripheral	56/122 wk	56-70 wk	90-102 wk
Frontal white matter			
Central	50/119 wk	52-64 wk	90-106 wk
Peripheral	72/119 wk	70-90 wk	96-114 wk

*The first number corresponds to earliest identification of some myelin tubules by microscopic examination of hematoxylin and eosin stained sections. The second number corresponds to mature myelin stained with blue dye by eye observation.

Pathways of the olfactory, optic, acoustic, and sensorimotor cortex are the first to be myelinated, whereas projection and association pathways are the last. Projection fibers begin myelination before association fibers. The myelination of association fibers lasts until adulthood.

Imaging Characteristics of Myelination

On histologic examination, mature myelin is present at 37 to 40 postconceptional weeks in the posterior limb of the internal capsule and in the lateral cerebellar white matter (see Table 40-2). Myelination advances at differing rates in different regions of the brain. Myelination occurs in an orderly and predictable fashion, proceeding cephalad from the brainstem at 29 weeks to reach the centrum semiovale by 42 weeks. Myelination advances at differing rates in different regions of the brain and is visible at different times on T1-weighted (lipid: high signal) and T2-weighted (water: high signal) MRI, the classic imaging sequences on conventional MRI.[5,8] The exact reasons for these differences are not clear. However, it is known that the T1 shortening correlates temporally with the increase in cholesterol and glycolipids that accompany the formation of myelin from oligodendrocytes.[90] Furthermore, the T2 shortening correlates temporally with the tightening of the spiral of myelin around the axon, the conformational changes in the myelin proteins, and saturation of polyunsaturated fatty acids in the myelin membranes. Portions of the proteins, cholesterol, and glycolipids that compose myelin are hydrophilic and form hydrogen bonds more strongly with water molecules. With an increase in bound water to the myelin building blocks, there is a consequent decrease in free water and an increase in T1 shortening times. This reduction in free water accompanying the preparation for myelination may explain the pattern of T1-weighted MRI changes preceding anatomic myelination by histologic analysis (see Table 40-2). Sensory pathways are the first to myelinate: vestibular, acoustic, tactile, and proprioceptive senses are myelinated at term birth. A shortened T2 relaxation time and therefore a T2 hypointense signal is observed in the ventroposterolateral nuclei of the thalamus as early as 28 weeks' gestation, in the posterior limb of the internal capsule as early as 36 weeks' gestation, and in the corona radiatae and the sensorimotor cortex at term. The signal alteration in the sensory motor cortex might also be due to a more advanced organization of cortical neurons, oligodendroglial cells, synaptic density, and dendrite formation, which would cause decreased interstitial water and a shortening of the T2 relaxation time (Fig. 40-20).[65] Phylogenetically older structures such as the inferior and superior cerebellar pedunculi and vermis are myelinated before term, whereas the cerebellar hemispheres are myelinated much later.[110] Similarly, the amygdala and hippocampus are partly myelinated at term.

Changes in the volume of myelinated white matter have also been determined by volumetric MRI studies, with myelin comprising less than 5% of total brain volume at 34 weeks' gestation and showing a rapid increase thereafter.[55] The dramatic fivefold increase in myelinated white matter after 34 weeks is of major interest for the understanding of brain injury during this period. This increase in myelin is presumed to be the result of the maturation of oligodendrocytes that have been actively differentiating during the immediately preceding period.

Microglia and Brain Macrophages

Microglia constitutes 5% to 15% of the total cerebral cellular population. The prevailing view is that microglial cells are derived from circulating precursor in the blood that originates from bone marrow.[72] During the first trimester of human gestation, penetrating cells have an ameboid morphology, with large ovoid cell bodies and no or few short processes, and express macrophage antigenic characteristics depending on their location and activation state. This macrophage-like morphology evolves into an intermediate and a mature phenotype with a smaller cell body and longer processes. At midgestation, macrophage-microglia populations are mostly detected in white matter pathways,

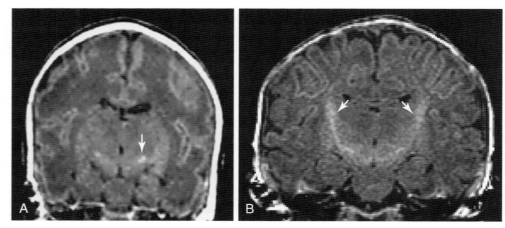

Figure 40–20. T1-weighted MR images illustrating progress of myelination. **A,** A 28 weeks' gestation distinct T1 shortening (high signal) is seen only in a small perithalamic region (*arrow*). **B,** At 40 weeks, distinct T1 shortening (high signal) is seen throughout the internal capsule reaching the central cortex (*arrows*).

such as the external and internal capsules and corpus callosum. As suggested from rodent studies, these cells could contribute to physiologic developmental remodeling through phagocytosis of cellular fragments produced by neurodevelopmental apoptosis and elimination of exuberant axons and dendrites.[74] However, the correlation between regressive events and the distribution of macrophages is not clear, suggesting other possible functions for these cells during development.

In the case of a cerebral lesion, experimental data support a neurotoxic role for the cerebral macrophage through the production of free radicals and nitric oxide. Under pathologic conditions, microglial cells can be transformed into functional brain macrophages with the reappearance of specific cell surface markers.

After development, mature microglia constitute a quiescent cellular population with small cell bodies, numerous long, thin processes, and a possible role in the regulation of the extracellular environment and immune protection of the brain.

Brain Vascular Development

Despite its major role in brain development and functioning, the ontogeny of the brain vasculature has not been the focus of numerous studies. Precise description of the successive steps of brain vessel development and its chronology is still lacking, and little information is available on the molecular mechanisms controlling the development and patterning of brain vessels. Accordingly, the exact timing of the switch from a neuronal anaerobic metabolism to an aerobic one is unknown, although this information might be critically important in understanding the potential consequences of hypoxia or ischemia at successive stages of brain development.

As soon as the neural tube is formed, blood vessels penetrate the primitive neuroepithelium. During migration of neocortical neurons, the density of blood vessels is rather low, with significant distances separating migrating cells from blood vessels. Penetration of vessels in the cerebral mantle is radial and ventriculopetal, starting from the leptomeningeal plexus and directed toward the ventricle.[69,84] No transventricular, paraventricular, or recurrent arteries ending in deep white matter have been identified. Horizontal collaterals progressively appear with a ventriculofugal gradient that reaches white matter at approximately 20 gestational weeks in the human fetus. The chronology of the horizontal ramification of vessels starts at approximately 20 weeks of gestation in the subplate and deep cortical layers, reaches layer III approximately at birth, and is completed (layers II and I) in the postnatal period.

Most neopallial vessels remain devoid of apparent muscularis until the final weeks of gestation.[70] Muscularis development follows a ventriculopetal gradient. The lack of muscular layers around neopallial arteries and the gradient of muscularization of these vessels could explain the high susceptibility of immature arteries to deep white matter and germinal matrix hemorrhages and the lack of vasomotor autoregulation in periventricular areas during a large part of the second half of gestation or the corresponding period in the preterm infant.

ABNORMAL BRAIN DEVELOPMENT AND DISORDERS

As a rule, the different categories of congenital malformations of the CNS reflect the time at which a noxious event disrupted the normal sequence of CNS development rather than the nature of the noxious event itself. Therefore in this section the congenital CNS disorders are arranged according to time of onset of the morphologic alteration. (See also Parts 7 and 8 of this chapter.)

Disorders of Neural Tube Formation and Prosencephalic Development

CRANIORACHISCHISIS TOTALIS, ANENCEPHALY, MYELOSCHISIS, ENCEPHALOCELE, MYELOMENINGOCELE, AND OCCULT DYSRAPHIC STATES

Craniorachischisis totalis is secondary to total failure of neurulation with the formation of a neural platelike structure without overlying tissue. The onset of this malformation is no later than 20 to 22 days of gestation and most cases are aborted spontaneously during embryonic life.

Anencephaly results from failure of anterior neural tube closure and occurs before 24 days of gestation. It is often associated with polyhydramnios. Approximately three fourths of these infants are stillborn, and the remainder die in the neonatal period.

Myeloschisis results from failure of posterior neural tube closure and occurs before 24 days of gestation. A neural platelike structure without overlying tissue replaces large parts of the spinal cord. Most of these infants are stillborn.

Encephalocele is usually considered to be a restricted disorder of anterior neural tube closure, although its precise mechanisms remain unknown. It occurs before 26 days of gestation. Encephalocele is occipital in three fourths of cases, sometimes frontal (where it may protrude into the nasal cavities), and rarely temporal or parietal. Neural tissue (most often from the occipital lobe) in the encephalocele usually displays a normal gyration and underlying white matter and is connected to the brain through a narrow neck (Fig. 40-21). Hydrocephalus is present in approximately half of the cases. In cases in which the encephalocele is located in the lower occipital region or upper cervical area, cerebellum is usually present in the encephalocele, occipital tissue is present in approximately half of the cases, and Chiari II malformation is associated (producing Chiari III malformation). Corpus callosum agenesis and anomalies of venous drainage are frequently associated. Encephaloceles are observed in a variety of chromosomal disorders (e.g., trisomies 13 and 18) and syndromes (e.g., Walker-Warburg, Meckel-Gruber, Dandy-Walker, Joubert, Goldenhar-Gorlin, Knobloch, and Robert syndromes).

Myelomeningocele is a restricted disorder of posterior neural tube closure that occurs before 26 days of gestation. (See also Chapters 8 and 11 for in utero diagnosis and treatment.) It involves all layers, including spinal cord, nerve roots, meninges, vertebral bodies, and skin. Approximately three fourths of myelomeningoceles have a lumbar localization

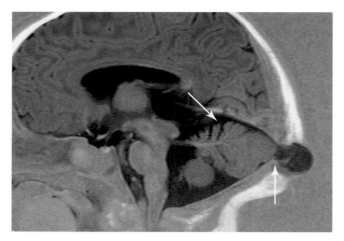

Figure 40–21. Occipital encephalocele *(right arrow)* with moderate displacement of the cerebellum *(left arrow)* and dilation of ventricular system, particularly the fourth ventricle. *(Image courtesy of J. Delavelle, Department of Radiology, University Hospitals of Geneva, Geneva, Switzerland.)*

be observed in chromosomal abnormalities and in single-gene disorders, the vast majority of isolated nonsyndromal cases are thought to be due to an interaction of genetic susceptibility (e.g., specific mutations in the methylenetetrahydrofolate reductase gene) with environmental factors (such as valproate exposure or maternal type 1 diabetes mellitus).

A newborn with a meningomyelocele presents the clinician with difficult decisions about what to tell the parents and whether to close the spinal defect surgically. Surgery should be undertaken within the first 24 hours after birth to prevent further deterioration of the spinal cord and nerve roots and to prevent infection (meningitis). Fetal and neonatal therapy of meningomyelocele is discussed in Chapter 11 and Part 8 of this chapter.

Factors that influence the decision for surgical closure include size and location of the lesion, the technical feasibility of closure, the prognosis for ambulation, the presence or absence of associated abnormalities (hydrocephalus, kyphosis, or other major structural abnormalities), the availability of personnel and a facility to provide adequate care for the infant, and the infant's family structure and the attitudes of the family toward the defect and its consequences. The usual decision is to proceed with early surgical closure of the spinal defect, followed by placement of a ventriculoperitoneal shunt if hydrocephalus is present (see Part 8 of this chapter). Thereafter, the infant requires long-term neurosurgical, orthopedic, and urologic follow-up to maintain shunt stability, promote ambulation if possible, and minimize the untoward effects of multiple urinary tract infections.

Occult spinal dysraphisms are considered to be disorders of caudal neural tube formation (secondary neurulation) and include distortion of the spinal cord or roots by fibrous

(thoracolumbar, lumbar, or lumbosacral). Hydrocephalus is present in 70% of cases, especially when the lumbar region is involved. Chiari II malformation is almost always present in lumbar myelomeningoceles (Fig. 40-22). Location and extent of the lesion determine the clinical symptoms. Thoracic myelomeningoceles have a generally poor prognosis. Varying degrees of paresis (often severe) of the legs and sphincter dysfunction are the major clinical signs. Although myelomeningocele can

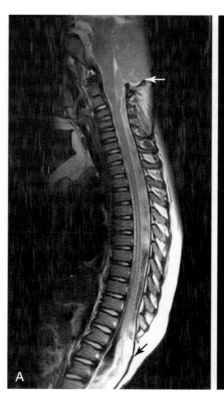

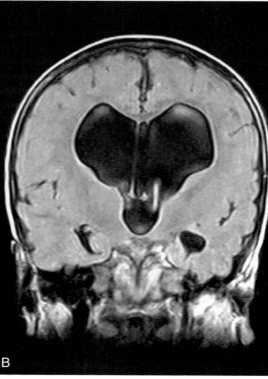

Figure 40–22. A, Lumbar myelomeningocele *(black arrow)* with distal displacement of medulla and cerebellum *(white arrow)* (Chiari malformation) with associated hydrocephalus **(B)**. *(Image courtesy of J. Delavelle, Department of Radiology, University Hospitals of Geneva, Geneva, Switzerland.)*

bands and adhesions, intraspinal lipomas, epidermoid cysts, fibrolipomas, subcutaneous lipomas, tethered cord (the most common condition), and diastematomyelia. Clinical symptoms are variable (absent, minimal, moderate, or severe) according to the degree of neural tissue involvement. Clinical signs include motor and sensory deficits in the lower and sometimes upper (when posterior fossa or cervical cord malformations are associated) limbs, bowel and bladder dysfunction, and ophthalmologic complications (when hydrocephalus is present).

HOLOPROSENCEPHALY AND AGENESIS OF THE CORPUS CALLOSUM

(See also Part 7 of this chapter.)

Holoprosencephaly refers to a large spectrum of brain malformations sharing a common embryologic origin. The frequency of holoprosencephaly is approximately 1 per 10,000 births, including miscarriages and terminations beyond 20 weeks of gestation, although it reaches approximately 40 per 10,000 if embryos are included, suggesting that holoprosencephaly is often accompanied by early embryonic loss.

Holoprosencephaly results from a defect in the cleavage of the prosencephalon in the rostrocaudal axis (between the diencephalon and the telencephalon) and in the transversal axis (division into two hemispheres). Holoprosencephaly can be divided into alobar variants (absence of interhemispheric fissure, corpus callosum, and third ventricle; unique ventricle; fusion of thalami), semilobar variants (presence of the interhemispheric fissure in the caudal part), and lobar (presence of a third ventricle; frontal horns partially formed; presence of the corpus callosum; hypoplastic frontal lobes) according to the severity of the malformation (Fig. 40-23). There seems to be a continuum between lobar holoprosencephaly and septo-optic dysplasia (Fig. 40-24). In all forms of holoprosencephaly, the septum pellucidum and the trigone are missing, whereas the olfactory bulbs and tracts are usually hypoplastic or absent (arhinencephalia).

The most severe forms of dysmorphic facies are usually found in alobar holoprosencephalies, but this is not a general rule and facial anomalies do not always reflect the severity of the brain malformations. Malformations affecting mainly cardiac, skeletal, genitourinary, and gastrointestinal organs

are frequent. In the most severe cases, neurologic signs are already present in the neonatal period and include apneas, seizures, tonic spasms, lack of neurologic development, and death.

Causes of holoprosencephaly are variable, with genetic, chromosomal, syndromic, and environmental etiologies (see Box 40-2). Most cases are sporadic, although some familial cases have been reported. Several maternal factors have been associated with holoprosencephaly, such as maternal diabetes or ethanol consumption. Holoprosencephaly is also observed in several syndromes, including the Smith-Lemli-Opitz syndrome characterized by abnormalities in cholesterol metabolism.

Approximately 12 loci, located on 11 chromosomes, have been identified for holoprosencephaly (HPE1 through HPE12). Genes *SIX3* (coding for a homeoprotein), *SHH* (transduction factor; see earlier), *ZIC2* (zinc finger transcription factor), and *TGIF* (TG-interacting factor, interacting with Smad2) have been identified as corresponding to loci HPE2, HPE3, HPE5, and HPE4, respectively. Among these genes, *SHH* is considered to be the most important one. Interestingly, abnormalities affecting genes located downstream to *SHH* in the *SHH* pathway also induce holoprosencephaly.

Agenesis of the corpus callosum is a relatively frequent malformation. Its prevalence in the general population is unknown because it might occur in a totally asymptomatic manner. Its prevalence in a population with mental retardation reaches 2% to 3%. Agenesis of the corpus callosum represents approximately 50% of the malformations of the midline.

Agenesis of the corpus callosum can be partial (affecting in most cases the posterior portion, except when it is associated with holoprosencephaly) or complete. The lateral ventricles are deformed by the fibers of the cerebral hemispheres that were destined to form the corpus callosum and that form the Probst bundles running longitudinally along the lateral ventricles. The Probst bundles are inconsistently present, and their presence has been considered a sign of better prognosis.

Corpus callosum agenesis can be associated with other brain malformations (such as neuronal migration disorders) or with extracerebral malformations. In the presence of associated malformations, the prognosis of agenesis of the corpus callosum is considered poor in most cases. In contrast, the prognosis of isolated agenesis of the corpus callosum (partial or complete) is much more variable, with some

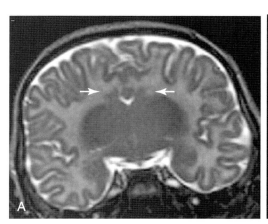
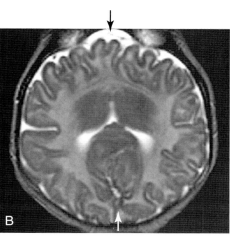

Figure 40-23. Semilobar holoprosencephaly (**A**) with absence of corpus callosum, anterior interhemispheric fissure (*black arrow* in **B**), and frontal horns of lateral ventricle (*white arrows*), but with presence of interhemispheric fissure (*white arrow*) in the posterior caudal part (**B**). (*Image courtesy of J. Delavelle, Department of Radiology, University Hospitals of Geneva, Geneva, Switzerland.*)

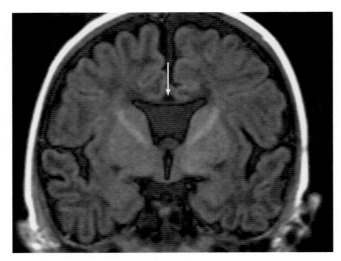

Figure 40–24. Septo-optic dysplasia with agenesis of the corpus callosum and septum pellucidum *(arrow)*. *(Image courtesy of J. Delavelle, Department of Radiology, University Hospitals of Geneva, Geneva, Switzerland.)*

cases having a totally normal or near-normal neurologic outcome, some cases with moderate or severe neurologic handicap, and some cases evolving toward death within the first days or months after birth. Because of the relatively low number of reported cases and the relatively short follow-up in many of these cases, providing reliable figures for the neurologic outcome of the isolated malformation remains difficult.

DANDY-WALKER MALFORMATION

Although it does not primarily affect the cerebral hemispheres, we include the Dandy-Walker malformation in this chapter because it is frequently associated with malformations of the cerebral hemispheres (important for differential diagnosis and for determination of the outcome), it often has neonatal signs, and it is the prototype of cerebellar malformations observed in the neonatal period.

Dandy-Walker malformation results from abnormal development of the rhombencephalon, probably occurring between the 7th and the 10th gestational weeks. Dandy-Walker

malformation is observed in approximately 1 per 25,000 to 30,000 births. This malformation is usually sporadic, with a few reported familial cases. Its etiology is unknown, and environmental factors (e.g., ethanol, warfarin sodium, viral infection) have been reported in a few cases.

Dandy-Walker malformation classically consists of three major abnormalities: (1) enlargement of the posterior fossa and elevation of the tentorium, (2) cystic dilation of the fourth ventricle, and (3) partial or complete agenesis of the corpus callosum. Hydrocephalus is often present but may appear late during pregnancy or even after birth. Other brain malformations (in particular, abnormalities of the midline and neuronal migration disorders) are observed in up to 70% of cases (Fig. 40-25). Extraneurologic malformations involving the heart, kidneys, limbs, and face are also frequent. The associated neurologic and extraneurologic abnormalities have a major impact on the prognosis of the Dandy-Walker malformation, with better prognosis often (but not always) associated with cases of isolated Dandy-Walker malformation.

As reviewed by Volpe,[119] a prominent posterior fossa cerebrospinal fluid collection can be divided into three categories: (1) enlargement of the fourth ventricle (including Dandy-Walker malformation, other disorders with agenesis of the cerebellar vermis such as Joubert syndrome and other familial vermian ageneses, and trapped fourth ventricle); (2) enlarged cisterna magna; and (3) arachnoid cyst.

Abnormalities of Neuronal Proliferation

MICROCEPHALY

(See also Part 7 of this chapter.)
Microcephaly is defined by an occipitofrontal circumference below −2 standard deviations (SD) for age and sex. Severe microcephaly refers to a circumference below −3 SD. Skull growth is determined by brain expansion, which takes place during the normal growth of the brain during pregnancy and infancy. Microcephaly most often occurs because of failure of the brain to grow at a normal rate. Any condition that affects brain growth can cause microcephaly. Primary microcephaly is distinguished from secondarily acquired microcephaly, in which the brain attains the expected size during pregnancy

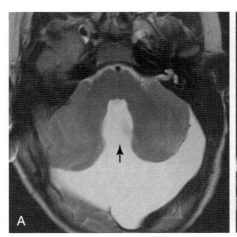

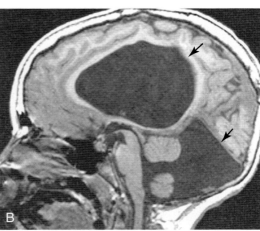

Figure 40–25. Dandy-Walker malformation with enlargement of posterior fossa. **A,** Axial T2-weighted MRI with absence of cerebellar vermis *(arrow)*. **B,** Sagittal T1-weighted MRI with elevation of the tentorium *(bottom arrow)* and hydrocephalus *(top arrow)*. *(Image courtesy of J. Delavelle, Department of Radiology, University Hospitals of Geneva, Geneva, Switzerland.)*

but subsequently fails to grow normally. Microcephaly can be divided into acquired etiologies (e.g., anoxic/ischemic brain damage, severe malnutrition, fetal alcohol syndrome, intra-uterine infection, maternal hyper-phenylalaninemia and phenylketonuria, anticonvulsant drugs, irradiation) and primary developmental microcephaly (see Box 40-3). The latter can be divided into (1) isolated microcephaly (primary microcephaly); (2) microcephaly associated with other brain malformations; (3) microcephaly associated with chromosome disorders; (4) microcephaly as part of a syndrome with multiple congenital anomalies (e.g., Neu-Laxova, Seckel, Rubinstein-Taybi, and Cornelia de Lange syndromes, microcephalic osteodysplastic dwarfism); and (5) microcephaly associated with biochemical disorders.

Primary Genetic Congenital Microcephaly

A standard classification of malformations of abnormal cortical development[6] divides lesions into those due to neuronal and glial proliferation in the germinal zones versus those due to cellular migration. Abnormal neuronal and glial proliferation leads to micrencephaly vera, microcephaly with simplified gyral pattern and, when combined with migration defect (see later), microlissencephaly.[121] The head circumference is very small in all those disorders, often in the range of 24 to 28 cm at birth. Brain weights have been among the smallest ever reported (below 100 gm). Precise classification of this group remains fluctuant and consensus has not been reached. The incidence of congenital microcephaly below –2 SD is approximately 3 to 4 per 100 births. Congenital microcephaly below –3 SD occurs in approximately 1 to 2 per 1000 births.

Micrencephaly Vera

Micrencephaly vera (or true micrencephaly or radial microbrain) (Fig. 40-26) is a genetic condition in which the brain is abnormally small because of a reduced number of neurons, but in which a normal or subnormal gyral pattern is present and no other gross pathologic abnormality is present. Brain weight is typically less than 500 g (one third of normal values and comparable with that of early hominids). Mental retardation is usually moderate. Eight different loci have been mapped, and 5 genes are currently cloned: *MCPH1* (microcephalin), *CDK5RAP2* (MCPH3), *ASPM* (MCPH5), *CENPJ* (MCPH6), and deoxynucleotide carrier (DNC). Inheritance is autosomal recessive or X-linked recessive (XLR) for one locus.

The *MCPH1* locus located in 8p22-pter encodes microcephalin, which could play a role in the initiation of chromosome condensation during mitosis, in DNA repair following ionizing radiation damage, or in cell cycle timing in neural progenitors. Microcephalin is mainly expressed in brain, liver, and kidney. In mouse, it is expressed in fetal brain during neurogenesis (forebrain, germinative area) and, in human cells, it is localized at the centrosome level. The gene is poorly conserved in vertebrates: 57% sequence identity between mouse and human orthologs (mean human-mouse protein sequence identity: 85%). So far, mutation has been exclusively reported in inbred Pakistani families.[40]

The MCPH3 locus located in 9q33.3 encodes the cyclin-dependent kinase 5 regulatory associated protein 2 gene (*CDK5RAP2*). Nonsense mutations were identified as a cause for MCPH3 in two Northern Pakistani families.[13,15] CDK5 is a protein kinase, active in the central nervous system, with numerous neuron-specific roles in processes including neurogenesis, neuronal migration, and neurodegeneration. *CDK5RAP2* is an inhibitor of CDKR1 and thus also an inhibitor of CDK5. Human *CDK5RAP2* shows centrosomal localization in HeLa cells at various stages of mitosis.[15,17,24,85] In murine embryos at E15.5, CDK5RAP2 was widely distributed, but was most prominent in the brain and the spinal cord.[13,117] In *Drosophila*, the *CDK5RAP2*-homolog centrosomin (cnn) is required to recruit various proteins to the centrosome.[18,113] In cnn mutant embryos, centrosomes fail to function during mitosis as major microtubule organizing centers, leading to dramatic mitotic defects in embryos.

The MCPH5 locus in 1q31 corresponds to the *ASPM* gene, a human ortholog of the *Drosophila* melanogaster "abnormal spindle" gene (asp), identified by homozygosity mapping and found responsible for approximately one half of the micrencephaly vera (MV) cases in all ethnic backgrounds. The gene contains multiple repeats of 20-amino-acid sequence beginning with isoleucine (I) and glutamine (Q), called *IQ repeat*. All published mutations lead to loss of function.[17] In *Drosophila*, asp is essential for normal mitotic spindle function in embryonic neuroblasts.[120] The protein encoded shows consistent increase in size through evolution. The predominant difference between Asp and ASPM is a single large insertion coding for « IQ domains ». The number of IQ domains seems related to CNS complexity: roundworm: 2 IQ; *Drosophila*: 24 IQ; mouse: 61; human: 72-80.

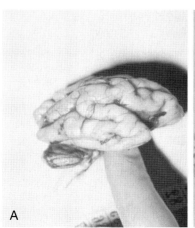
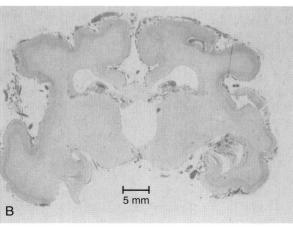

5 mm

Figure 40–26. Radial microbrain. A, Gross specimen. B, Microscopic section. (*From Barkovich AJ, et al. Formation, maturation, and disorders of brain neocortex, AJNR Am J Neuroradiol 13:423, 1992, with permission.*)

The MCPH6 locus in 13q22.2 encodes the centrosome associated protein J (CENPJ, also known as CPAP for centrosome protein 4.1 associated protein). CENPJ is located in the centrosome through the cell cycle and interacts with the non-erythrocyte 4.1 protein 135 variant (4.1R-135). The E1235V mutation found in an affected patient occurs in a Tcp10 domain of CENPJ, which interacts with 4.1R-135. During cell division, this protein plays a structural role in the maintenance of centrosome integrity and normal spindle morphology, and it is involved in microtubule disassembly at the centrosome.[7] CENPJ is widely distributed in the developing embryo. It is expressed at E15 in the neuroepithelium lining the lateral ventricles of the mouse forebrain and has a higher expression in the newly forming layers of the cortical plate. CENPJ may have a role in the control of centrosome microtubule production during neurogenic mitosis.[16]

The DNC-SLC25A19 gene (17q25) is responsible for the Amish type of micrencephaly vera (MV), a unique autosomal recessive disorder observed in Amish, characterized by extreme microcephaly (−6 to −12 SD), death within the first year, and associated with alpha-ketoglutarate aciduria. SLC25A19 encodes for a nuclear mitochondrial DNC.[100] The gene is composed of 9 exons coding for a protein of 16,5 kb. Slc25a19 knockout mice do not survive after E12. Affected embryos at E10 have neural tube closure defect and increased alpha-ketoglutarate in the amniotic fluid.

Other loci have been mapped for micrencephal vera/microcephaly with simplified gyral pattern (MV/MSG). These include MCPH2 (19q13.1-q13.2),[99] MCPH4 (15q15-q21),[59] and MRXS9 (Xq12-q21.31). About 20% of families are still unlinked.

Microcephaly with Simplified Gyral Pattern

Microcephaly with simplified gyral pattern are disorders defined by congenital severe microcephaly, reduced number and shallow appearance of gyri, and normal to thin cortex. Two clinical variants are delineated, one with a normal or thin corpus callosum and one with agenesis of the corpus callosum. Inheritance is autosomal recessive. Micrencephaly vera and microcephaly with simplified gyral pattern are likely part of a continuous phenotype, with mild microcephaly with simplified gyral pattern being seen in some patients from families with typical micrencephaly vera.[98]

Beyond the three genes described previously, several other loci have been mapped for micrencephaly vera or microcephaly with simplified gyral pattern. Approximately 20% of families are still unlinked.

MICROLISSENCEPHALY

The microlissencephaly disorders have simplified gyri but are distinguished from microcephaly with simplified gyral pattern by a cortex that is thicker than in normal brains. At least four different types have been identified on imaging and clinical grounds: microlissencephaly with thick cortex (MLIS1, or Norman-Roberts syndrome), microlissencephaly with thick cortex, severe brainstem, and cerebellar hypoplasia (MLIS2, or Barth syndrome), microlissencephaly with intermediate cortex and abrupt anteroposterior gradient, and microlissencephaly with mildly to moderately thick (6 to 8 mm) cortex. Inheritance is autosomal recessive. No gene has been mapped.

MEGALENCEPHALY

(See also Part 7 of this chapter.)
Megalencephaly (or macrocephaly) corresponds to an excess increase of the brain volume. It can affect one (hemimegalencephaly) or both hemispheres (symmetric megalencephaly).

Symmetric megalencephaly can be associated with other brain malformations, including hydrocephaly, tumors, or gyration abnormalities (e.g., pachygyria). Some cases of symmetric megalencephaly have a familial transmission with different modes of inheritance. Some of these transmissible forms are accompanied by familial mental retardation. Megalencephaly can also be part of a syndrome, such as Weaver and Proteus syndromes. In the absence of associated malformation or familial history, the prognosis of isolated symmetric megalencephaly is difficult to determine because some cases have a normal evolution, whereas mental retardation can be observed in other cases. Symmetric megalencephaly must be differentiated from congenital macrocrany with normal brain volume but increased pericerebral spaces. This entity, sometimes called external hydrocephaly, can have a familial transmission (usually autosomal dominant) and often has an excellent neurologic prognosis.

Hemimegalencephaly is characterized by increased growth of one hemisphere or a part of it. This hemisphere is abnormal, with foci of pachygyria, polymicrogyria, heterotopias, and white matter gliosis. Brainstem and cerebellum can also be affected. Hemimegalencephaly can be isolated or associated with hemihypertrophy (as part of a syndrome such as Protée syndrome, Klippel-Trenaunay-Weber syndrome, or Ito hypomelanosis) or, in some cases, with other malformations as part of Bourneville sclerosis. Hemimegalencephaly is usually sporadic. Its pathophysiologic process remains unclear but could involve genes implicated in brain symmetry such as LEFTY1, LEFTY2, or ZIC3. Patients with hemimegalencephaly usually display a macrocrania, hemiplegia, severe or intractable epilepsy, and developmental delay that can be severe and exacerbated by the epilepsy.

Disorders of Neuronal Migration

Abnormalities of neuronal migration have been described in a large variety of syndromic, genetic, and environmental conditions (see Box 40-4).

CLASSIC LISSENCEPHALIES (TYPE I LISSENCEPHALIES)

Classic lissencephalies form a genetically heterogenous group with highly variable neuroradiologic signs. Complete agyria (lack of gyration) has to be distinguished from pachygyria (incomplete gyration with a reduced number of flat and broad gyri separated by shallow sulci).[4] The shallow sylvian fissures result in a figure-eight appearance of the axial brain sections. Aspect and severity can vary according to the cortical area and generally follow a rostrocaudal gradient. Hippocampus and temporal cortex are often less affected. Dobyns and Truwit have proposed a radiologic score of severity based on the presence and location of agyria, pachygyria, and subcortical band heterotopias.[30] On MRI, the cortex appears thickened: 5 to 20 mm, whereas the normal thickness is between 2.5 and 4 mm. The microscopic cytoarchitecture is abnormal (reduction of the number of cortical layers and abnormal neuronal densities), yielding a neuropathologic pattern that is specific for each molecular abnormality described thus far. Lateral ventricles can be enlarged in their posterior portion (colpocephaly). Lissencephaly variants are characterized by major abnormalities of the corpus callosum and of the cerebellum. By definition, head circumference is greater than −3 SD in classic lissencephalies and is less than −3 SD in microlissencephalies (see earlier). The incidence of classic lissencephaly is estimated to be 1.2 cases per 100,000 live births.

LIS1 Mutations (Isolated Lissencephaly and Miller-Dieker Syndrome)

Abnormalities of the *LIS1* gene (platelet-activating factor acetyl-hydrolase isoform 1B alpha subunit gene, PAFAH1B1), which encodes the *LIS1* (PAFAH1B1) protein, account for the pathology seen in 40% of patients with lissencephaly. Deletions and nonsense mutations of *LIS1* induce an agyri-pachygyric phenotype with a posterior-anterior gradient (posterior being more severe; grade 2-3, according to Dobyns and Truwit[30]). Missense mutations can induce less severe phenotypes (grade 4, according to Dobyns and Truwit[30]). The cortex is thickened (10 to 20 mm), disorganized, and generally composed of four layers: a large molecular layer, a layer of superficial neurons, a paucicellular layer containing myelinated fibers, and a deep layer containing neurons that failed to reach their final target. The 17p13 deletion, which contains the *LIS1* gene, is responsible for the Miller-Dieker syndrome, which combines a grade 1 lissencephaly and dysmorphic features (prominent forehead, bitemporal hollowing, micrognathia, malpositioned and/ or malformed ears, short nose with upturned nares and low nasal bridge, long and thin upper lip, and late tooth eruption) (Fig. 40-27). Septum calcifications are sometimes observed.

DCX Mutations

The *DCX* or *XLIS* gene, encoding doublecortin or DCX and located on the X chromosome, is responsible for the disease in about 40% of patients with lissencephaly and in 85% of patients with subcortical laminar heterotopia.[29,42,89] In boys, mutations induce a classic lissencephaly (grade 1 to grade 4) with a thickened cortex (10 to 20 mm) and a rostrocaudal gradient (i.e., a gradient reverse to that observed in patients with *LIS1* mutations). Heterozygous girls display a subcortical laminar heterotopia, which consists of a gray matter layer of variable thickness located between the normally located superficial cortical gray matter and the lateral ventricle ("double cortex"). This double cortex can be limited to the anterior part of the hemispheres. The clinical phenotype in females is variable and ranges from a complete lack of neurologic signs to mental retardation and epilepsy. Female carriers do not have a preferential X chromosome inactivation and, therefore, a normal MRI finding does not exclude the presence of a carrier status. Results of neuropathologic studies have shown that brains from patients with *LIS1* mutations exhibited the classic inverted four-layer lissencephalic architecture and unique cytoarchitectural findings, including a roughly ordered 6-layer lamination in male patients with *DCX* mutations and lissencephaly.

TUBA3 Mutations

Alpha 3 tubulin gene *TUBA3* mutations have been described recently[63] in one male patient and in one female patient. The first patient presented with a classic lissencephaly with a thick disorganized cortex and, clinically, with severe epilepsy, mental retardation, and motor deficits. The second patient exhibited less severe cortical abnormalities with temporal and rolandic pachygyria and abnormal organization of the hippocampus. Both patients had corpus callosum agenesis, inferior vermis abnormalities, and brainstem hypoplasia. The *TUBA3* gene is the human homolog of the murine *Tuba1*, which is expressed during early embryonic development. *Tuba1* mutations impair the ability of the protein to bind GTP (guanosine triphosphate) and to form native heterodimers with β-tubulin, which is very important for microtubule function. Mutation in murine *Tuba1* induces abnormal neuronal migration with disturbances in layers II/III and IV of the visual, auditory, and somatosensory cortices.

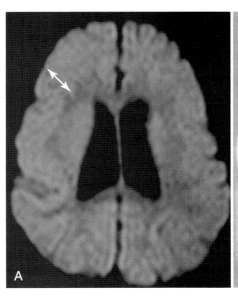
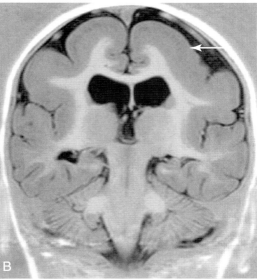

Figure 40–27. Type 1 lissencephaly, or Miller-Dieker syndrome, with (**A**) pachygyric "four-layered" thickened cortex (*arrow*). **B**, Axial diffusion weighted image also characterizes thickened cortex compared with underlying white matter (*arrow*). (*Image courtesy of J. Delavelle, Department of Radiology, University Hospitals of Geneva, Geneva, Switzerland.*)

ARX Mutations

ARX (Aristales-related homeobox) gene mutations cause a particular classic X-linked lissencephaly with or without corpus callosum agenesis. The cortex in three layers of ARX lissencephalies is less thick (5 to 10 mm) than in the other classic lissencephalies and the cortical abnormality displays a rostrocaudal gradient (frontal regions being more affected). Female carriers can have isolated or combined corpus callosum agenesis, epilepsy, and/or mental retardation.

XLAG syndrome is also associated with mutations of the ARX gene. Affected boys have lissencephaly, corpus callosum agenesis, facial dysmorphic features, ambiguous genitalia, thermoregulation troubles, and severe epilepsy, which can begin prenatally. ARX gene mutations are implicated in a wide spectrum of X-linked disorders extending from mild forms of X-linked mental retardation without apparent brain abnormalities to severe lissencephaly. Phenotypes include corpus callosum agenesis with mental retardation, X-linked West syndrome, and Partington syndrome (hand dystony). A phenotype-genotype correlation has not been established.

The ARX gene is expressed mainly in telencephalic structures. In adults, ARX gene expression becomes restricted to a population of GABAergic neurons.[91] ARX seems to be implicated in interneuron migration from the ganglionic eminence (future thalamus); however, its role in cell differentiation and neuronal migration needs to be further clarified.

Lissencephaly with Cerebellar Hypoplasia

Lissencephaly with cerebellar hypoplasia (LCH) is a heterogeneous group of lissencephalies associated with a cerebellar hypoplasia preferentially of the vermis and hemispheres that display sulci. A temporary classification comprising eight subtypes has been proposed. While the phenotype of type A LCH is caused by LIS1 or DCX gene mutations, patients with type B LCH have/display RELN gene mutations.[50] The latter lissencephaly is more severe than type A LCH but has a rostrocaudal gradient similar to that seen in patients with DCX gene mutations. The cortex is quite thick (5 to 10 mm), while the cerebellum is hypoplastic and smooth.

Further genes responsible for other forms of LCH are unknown. Type C LCH patients usually have a cleft palate. Type D LCH patients (patients with Barth syndrome) display a neuropathology that includes massive brain, cerebellum, and corticospinal tract hypoplasia; their cortex is thick (10 to 20 mm). Type E is close to type A LCH, but with a marked gradient from frontal agyrya to occipital pachygyrya. Type F LCH includes a corpus callosum agenesis. Moreover, two new types of LHC have been reported: LCH with corpus callosum agenesis and cerebellar dysplasia and a subtype with cerebellar hypoplasia, Dandy Walker malformation, and myoclonic epilepsy.

Syndromic Lissencephaly

Two types of lissencephalies are included in the group of syndromic lissencephalies: lissencephalies associated with other neurologic abnormalities (e.g., lissencephaly/pachygyria associated with peripheral demyelinating axonopathy) and lissencephalies observed in syndromes of multiple malformations (in which lissencephaly is generally inconstant and not necessary for diagnosis). Among these syndromes, craniotelencephalic dysplasia (extensive craniosynostosis, microphthalmy, encephalocele), Warburg micro syndrome (corpus callosum agenesis, microphthalmy, microcephaly, cataract, dysmorphic features), Goldenhar syndrome (hemifacial microsomia, branchial arch development abnormalities, hemifacial microsomia, microtia) or Baraitser-Winter syndrome (hyperthelorism, ptosis, coloboma, pachygyria/lissencephaly with a frontal predominance) have been reported.

COBBLESTONE LISSENCEPHALIES (TYPE II LISSENCEPHALIES)

Cobblestone lissencephalies are characterized by a pachygyric or granular brain appearance with shallow sulci and hypomyelination with subcortical cystic cavitations. Lateral and third ventricle dilation, which can be severe, vermis hypoplasia, or general cerebellar and brainstem hypoplasia with small pyramids can be observed. Additional brain anomalies such as hypoplasia/agenesis of corpus callosum, occipital encephalocele, and Dandy-Walker malformation have been described. Hemispheres can be merged on the median line by gliosis. The cortex is thickened (7 to 10 mm), disorganized, and invaded by gliovascular fascicles. White matter contains many heterotopic neurons. Typically, the brain is surrounded by a neurofribroglial envelope, which is not observed in classic lissencephalies and which induces a bumpy (hence "cobblestone") rather than smooth aspect to the cortical surface. The cortical development defect occurs most likely between 6 and 24 weeks of gestation. Many neurons migrate too far through a defective glial-limiting membrane into the subpial space, that is, beyond the cortical plate. Cobblestone lissencephalies are linked to abnormal O-glycosylation of alpha dextroglycan. POMT1 (9q34 locus) and POMT2 genes encode the two O-mannosyltransferases proteins 1 and 2 (POMT1, POMT2). POMGnT1 encodes an O-mannosyl-beta-1,2-N-acetylglucosaminyltransferase. The FCMD gene on chromosome 9q31 (FKTN) encodes the fukutin protein.

Clinically, cobblestone lissencephalies are observed in three autosomal recessive syndromes, which have been shown to display a significant overlap on the basis of recent molecular genetic discoveries. The incidence of cobblestone lissencephalies is not known, but is most likely around 1 case in 100,000 live births.

Walker Warburg syndrome (WWS) is the most common and the most severe form of cobblestone lissencephaly. It is characterized by the combination of brain malformations such as hydrocephalus, agyria, retinal dysplasia, and sometimes occipital encephalocele (HARD+/-E syndrome) with structural eye abnormalities and muscular dystrophy. Newborns die within the first postnatal months. Eye abnormalities include cataracts, microcornea and microphthalmia, retinal dysplasia, hypoplasia or atrophy of the optic nerve, and glaucoma. In 30% of the patients, this phenotype is linked to POMT1 or POMT2 mutations.

The severity of the brain involvement in Fukuyama syndrome is milder than that in WWS and MEB (muscle-eye-brain) syndrome, and the eyes are only occasionally affected severely. MEB syndrome is characterized by eye involvement (congenital myopia and glaucoma, retinal hypoplasia), mental retardation, and structural brain involvement (pachygyria, flat brainstem, and cerebellar hypoplasia).

Fukuyama disease is linked to mutations of the FCDM gene. MEB syndrome is linked to POMGnT1 gene mutations.

TYPE III LISSENCEPHALY

Type III lissencephaly is characterized by severe microcephaly, agyrya, corpus callosum agenesis, cerebellar, basal ganglia hypoplasia, a thin six-layered cortex, and blurred white matter borders. This lissencephaly has been reported in three autosomal recessive syndromes: Neu-Laxova syndrome, Enchara-Razavi-Larroche lissencephaly (microcephaly, corpus callosum agenesis, cystic cerebellum brain stem hypoplasia and fetal akinesia[35]), and a syndrome reported with lissencephaly, severe microcephaly, corpus callosum agenesis, cerebellar hypoplasia, dysmorphic features and punctuate epiphysis. Neuropathologic findings are similar in these three entities and thereby suggest that they are either allelic diseases or linked to genes implicated in the same function or pathway.

X-LINKED PERIVENTRICULAR HETEROTOPIA

The human X-linked dominant periventricular heterotopia is characterized by neuronal nodules lining the ventricular surface (Fig. 40-28). Hemizygously affected males die within the embryonic period, and affected females have epilepsy, which can be accompanied by other manifestations such as patent ductus arteriosus and coagulopathy. The gene responsible for this disease, Filamin A gene *FLNA*,[37] encodes an actin-cross-linking phosphoprotein,

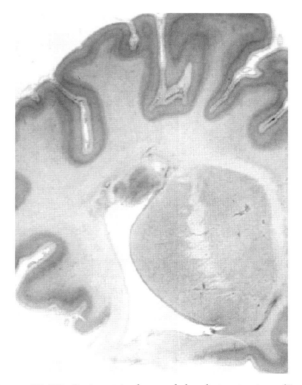

Figure 40–28. Periventricular nodular heterotopias. (*From Barkovich AJ, et al: Formation, maturation, and disorders of brain neocortex,* AJNR Am J Neuroradiol *13:423, 1992, with permission.*)

which transduces ligand-receptor binding into actin reorganization. Filamin A is necessary for locomotion of several cell types and is present at high levels in the developing neocortex.

Null mutations in the *FLNA* gene induce, through a loss-of-function mechanism, X-linked periventricular heterotopias and extraneural abnormalities (cardiac valvular anomalies, propensity to premature stroke, small joint hyperextensibility, gut dismobility, and persistent ductus arteriosus).

ZELLWEGER SYNDROME

The Zellweger cerebrohepatorenal syndrome is a fatal autosomal recessive disease caused by an absence of functional peroxisomes. One hallmark of this human disease is the presence of heterotopic neurons in the neocortex, the cerebellum, and the inferior olivary complex. Patients display severely retarded and/or rapid regression of psychomotor development, facial dysmorphisms, and severe muscular hypotonia; they usually die within the first postnatal months.

Animal models of this human disease have been produced by inactivation of a gene critically involved in peroxisomal assembly.[44] The analysis of these models showed (1) that the migration defect was partially caused by altered NMDA glutamate receptor-mediated calcium mobilization, (2) that this NMDA receptor dysfunction was linked to a deficit in PAF synthesis, and (3) that normal neocortex development requires a normal peroxisomal metabolism in brain and in liver.

EFFECTS OF ENVIRONMENTAL FACTORS ON NEURONAL MIGRATION

Neuronal migration disorders have been described in humans or in animal models after in utero exposure to several environmental factors, including infection with cytomegalovirus or toxoplasmosis (Fig. 40-29), ethanol (Fig. 40-30), cocaine, or ionizing radiation.[43] In most cases, the mechanisms by which these factors disturb neuronal migration remain unclear. Cocaine exposure during gestation has been shown to disturb neuronal migration and cortical addressing both in mice and monkeys. Cocaine exposure in mice was also shown to specifically decrease GABA neuron migration from the ganglionic eminence to the cerebral cortex but not to the olfactory bulbs, suggesting a degree of specificity in the effects of cocaine on neuronal migration. In the human fetal alcohol syndrome, neuronal molecular ectopias have been described in several cases although this sign is not restricted to this syndrome. (See also Chapter 12.) Animal studies have identified abnormalities of radial glia and disturbances of transformation of radial glia into astrocytes.

Disorders of Central Nervous System Organization and Maturation

Disorders involving subplate neurons, axonal and dendritic growth, synaptogenesis and synaptic stabilization, programmed cell death, and glial proliferation and differentiation are likely to have a major impact on brain functions. Unfortunately, little is known about these disorders, largely because the tools to investigate these steps adequately are usually not available even with postmortem tissues. The clinical consequences are rarely obvious in the neonatal

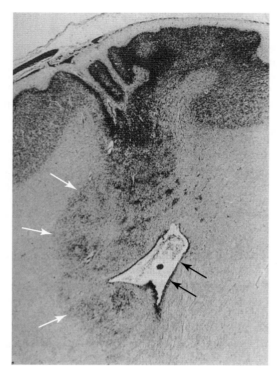

Figure 40–29. Combined polymicrogyria, white matter cystic lesion (*black arrows*) and white matter heterotopic neurons (*white arrows*) in a case of congenital toxoplasmosis. (*From Barkovich AJ, et al: Formation, maturation, and disorders of brain neocortex,* AJNR Am J Neuroradiol *13:423, 1992, with permission.*)

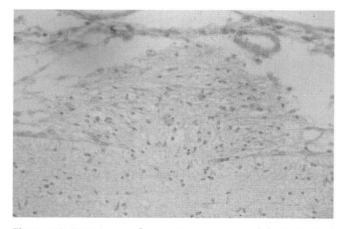

Figure 40–30. Neuronal ectopia in a case of fetal alcohol syndrome. (*From Barkovich AJ, et al: Formation, maturation, and disorders of brain neocortex,* AJNR Am J Neuroradiol *13:423, 1992, with permission.*)

period and usually occur later in life. These disorders can be schematically classified into primary (e.g., idiopathic mental retardation, Down syndrome, fragile X syndrome, Angelman syndrome, Rett syndrome, neurofibromatosis type I, tuberous sclerosis [Bourneville disease], Coffin-Lowry syndrome, Rubinstein-Taybi syndrome, Duchenne muscular dystrophy,

thyroid deficiency, and autism) or potentially acquired (e.g., malnutrition deficiencies or effects of prematurity and related environmental factors, including therapeutic and illicit drugs, such as cocaine, acting on the CNS and inducing organizational disorders).[60,119] In most of these disorders, several steps of brain development are affected, such as cortical lamination, dendritic branching and arborization, synaptic contacts, axonal development, and myelination. For example, in tuberous sclerosis, neuronal proliferation and later glial differentiation and proliferation are disturbed.

REFERENCES

1. Ajayi-Obe M, Saeed N, Cowan FM, et al: Reduced development of cerebral cortex in extremely preterm infants, *Lancet* 356:1162, 2000.
2. Andreasen NC, Harris G, Cizadlo T, et al: Techniques for measuring sulcal/gyral patterns in the brain as visualized through magnetic resonance scanning: BRAINPLOT and BRAINMAP, *Proc Natl Acad Sci U S A* 91:93, 1994.
3. Back SA, Luo NL, Borenstein NS, et al: Late oligodendrocyte progenitors coincide with the developmental window of vulnerability for human perinatal white matter injury, *J Neuro Sci* 21:1302, 2001.
4. Barkovich AJ, Gressens P, Evrard P. Formation, maturation, and disorders of brain neocortex, *AJNR Am J Neuroradiol* 13:423, 1992.
5. Barkovich AJ, Kjos BO, Jackson DE Jr, Norman D: Normal maturation of the neonatal and infant brain: MR imaging at 1.5 T, *Radiology* 166:173, 1988.
6. Barkovich AJ, Kuzniecky RI, Jackson GD, et al: Classification system for malformations of cortical development: update 2001, *Neurology* 57:2168, 2001.
7. Basto R, Lau J, Vinogradova T, et al. Flies without centrioles, *Cell* 125:1375, 2006.
8. Battin MR, Maalouf EF, Counsell SJ, et al: Magnetic resonance imaging of the brain in very preterm infants: visualization of the germinal matrix, early myelination, and cortical folding, *Pediatrics* 101:957, 1998.
9. Baud O, Laudenbach V, Evrard P, Gressens P: Neurotoxic effects of fluorinated glucocorticoid preparations on the developing mouse brain: role of preservatives, *Pediatr Res* 50:706, 2001.
10. Behar TN, Smith SV, Kennedy RT, et al: GABA(B) receptors mediate motility signals for migrating embryonic cortical cells, *Cereb Cortex* 11:744, 2001.
11. Behar TN, Schaffner AE, Scott CA, et al: GABA receptor antagonists modulate postmitotic cell migration in slice cultures of embryonic rat cortex, *Cereb Cortex* 10:899, 2000.
12. Behar TN, Scott CA, Greene CL, et al: Glutamate acting at NMDA receptors stimulates embryonic cortical neuronal migration, *J Neurosci* 19:4449, 1999.
13. Bhutta AT, Anand KJ. Abnormal cognition and behavior in preterm neonates linked to smaller brain volumes, *Trends Neurosci* 24:129, 2001; discussion 131-122.
14. Bielas S, Higginbotham H, Koizumi H, et al: Cortical neuronal migration mutants suggest separate but intersecting pathways, *Annu Rev Cell Dev Biol* 20:593, 2004.
15. Blaschke AJ, Staley K, Chun J: Widespread programmed cell death in proliferative and postmitotic regions of the fetal cerebral cortex, *Development* 122:1165, 1996.

16. Bond J, Roberts E, Springell K, et al: A centrosomal mechanism involving CDK5RAP2 and CENPJ controls brain size, *Nat Genet* 37:353, 2005.
17. Bond J, Roberts E, Mochida GH, et al: ASPM is a major determinant of cerebral cortical size, *Nat Genet* 32:316, 2002.
18. Bourgeois JP: Synaptogenesis, heterochrony and epigenesis in the mammalian neocortex, *Acta Paediatr Suppl* 422:27, 1997.
19. Brisse H, Fallet C, Sebag G, et al: Supratentorial parenchyma in the developing fetal brain: in vitro MR study with histologic comparison, *AJNR Am J Neuroradiol* 18:1491, 1997.
20. Brunstrom JE, Pearlman AL: Growth factor influences on the production and migration of cortical neurons, *Results Probl Cell Differ* 30:189, 2000.
21. Cabelli RJ, Shelton DL, Segal RA, Shatz CJ: Blockade of endogenous ligands of trkB inhibits formation of ocular dominance columns, *Neuron* 19:63, 1997.
22. Cady EB, Penrice J, Amess PN, et al: Lactate, N-acetylaspartate, choline and creatine concentrations, and spin-spin relaxation in thalamic and occipito-parietal regions of developing human brain, *Magn Reson Med* 36:878, 1996.
23. Caviness VS Jr, Goto T, Tarui T, et al: Cell output, cell cycle duration and neuronal specification: a model of integrated mechanisms of the neocortical proliferative process, *Cereb Cortex* 13:592, 2003.
24. Chae T, Kwon YT, Bronson R, et al: Mice lacking p35, a neuronal specific activator of Cdk5, display cortical lamination defects, seizures, and adult lethality, *Neuron* 18:29, 1997.
25. Changeux JP, Danchin A: Selective stabilisation of developing synapses as a mechanism for the specification of neuronal networks, *Nature* 264:705, 1976.
26. Childs AM, Ramenghi LA, Evans DJ, et al: MR features of developing periventricular white matter in preterm infants: evidence of glial cell migration, *AJNR Am J Neuroradiol* 19:971, 1998.
27. Chong BW, Babcook CJ, Salamat MS, et al: A magnetic resonance template for normal neuronal migration in the fetus, *Neurosurgery* 39:110, 1996.
28. Deipolyi AR, Mukherjee P, Gill K, et al: Comparing microstructural and macrostructural development of the cerebral cortex in premature newborns: diffusion tensor imaging versus cortical gyration, *Neuroimage* 27:579, 2005.
29. des Portes V, Pinard JM, Billuart P, et al: A novel CNS gene required for neuronal migration and involved in X-linked subcortical laminar heterotopia and lissencephaly syndrome, *Cell* 92:51, 1998.
30. Dobyns WB, Truwit CL: Lissencephaly and other malformations of cortical development: 1995 update, *Neuropediatrics* 26:132, 1995.
31. Dringen R, Verleysdonk S, Hamprecht B, et al: Metabolism of glycine in primary astroglial cells: synthesis of creatine, serine, and glutathione, *J Neurochem* 70:835, 998.
32. Dubois J, Benders M, Borradori-Tolsa C, et al: Primary cortical folding in the human newborn: an early marker of later functional development, *Brain* 131:2028, 2008.
33. Dubois J, Benders M, Cachia A, et al: Mapping the early cortical folding process in the preterm newborn brain, *Cereb Cortex* 18:1444, 2008.
34. Edelman GM: *Group selection as the basis for higher brain function.* Cambridge, Mass, 1981, MIT Press.
35. Encha Razavi F, Larroche JC, Roume J, et al: Lethal familial fetal akinesia sequence (FAS) with distinct neuropathological pattern: type III lissencephaly syndrome, *Am J Med Genet* 62:16, 1996.
36. Feess-Higgins ALJ: *Development of the human fetal brain anatomical atlas.* 1987 Paris, France, Institut Natl de la Sante.
37. Fox JW, Lamperti ED, Eksioglu YZ, et al: Mutations in filamin 1 prevent migration of cerebral cortical neurons in human periventricular heterotopia, *Neuron* 21:1315, 1998.
38. Giedd JN, Blumenthal J, Jeffries NO, et al: Brain development during childhood and adolescence: a longitudinal MRI study, *Nat Neurosci* 2:861, 1999.
39. Gilmore JH, Lin W, Prastawa MW, et al: Regional gray matter growth, sexual dimorphism, and cerebral asymmetry in the neonatal brain, *J Neurosci* 27:1255, 2007.
40. Giorgio A, Watkins KE, Douaud G, et al: Changes in white matter microstructure during adolescence, *Neuroimage* 39:52, 2008.
41. Girard N, Raybaud C, Gambarelli D, Figarella-Branger D: Fetal brain MR imaging, *Magn Reson Imaging Clin N Am* 9:19, vii, 2001.
42. Gleeson JG: Neuronal migration disorders, *Ment Retard Dev Disabil Res Rev* 7:167, 2001.
43. Gressens P: Mechanisms and disturbances of neuronal migration, *Pediatr Res* 48:725, 2000.
44. Gressens P, Baes M, Leroux P, et al: Neuronal migration disorder in Zellweger mice is secondary to glutamate receptor dysfunction, *Ann Neurol* 48:336, 2000.
45. Gressens P, Evrard P: The glial fascicle: an ontogenic and phylogenic unit guiding, supplying and distributing mammalian cortical neurons, *Brain Res Dev Brain Res* 76:272, 1993.
46. Gressens P, Richelme C, Kadhim HJ, et al: The germinative zone produces the most cortical astrocytes after neuronal migration in the developing mammalian brain, *Biol Neonate* 61:4, 1992.
47. Gupta RK, Hasan KM, Trivedi R, et al: Diffusion tensor imaging of the developing human cerebrum, *J Neurosci Res* 81:172, 2005.
48. Hilgetag CC, Barbas H: Role of mechanical factors in the morphology of the primate cerebral cortex, *PLoS Comput Biol* 2:e22, 2006.
49. Hilgetag CC, Barbas H: Developmental mechanics of the primate cerebral cortex, *Anat Embryol (Berl)* 210:411, 2005.
50. Hong SE, Shugart YY, Huang DT, et al: Autosomal recessive lissencephaly with cerebellar hypoplasia is associated with human RELN mutations, *Nat Genet* 26:93, 2000.
51. Huang H, Yamamoto A, Hossain MA, et al: Quantitative cortical mapping of fractional anisotropy in developing rat brains, *J Neurosci* 28:1427, 2008.
52. Huppi PS, Fusch C, Boesch C, et al: Regional metabolic assessment of human brain during development by proton magnetic resonance spectroscopy in vivo and by high-performance liquid chromatography/gas chromatography in autopsy tissue, *Pediatr Res* 37:145, 1995.
53. Hüppi PS, Lazeyras F: Proton magnetic resonance spectroscopy ((1)H-MRS) in neonatal brain injury, *Pediatr Res* 49:317, 2001.
54. Huppi PS, Maier SE, Peled S, et al: Microstructural development of human newborn cerebral white matter assessed in vivo by diffusion tensor magnetic resonance imaging, *Pediatr Res* 44:584, 1998.
55. Huppi PS, Warfield S, Kikinis R, et al: Quantitative magnetic resonance imaging of brain development in premature and mature newborns, *Ann Neurol* 43:224, 1998.

56. Huttenlocher PR, Bonnier C: Effects of changes in the periphery on development of the corticospinal motor system in the rat, *Brain Res Dev Brain Res* 60:253, 1991.

57. Hynes M, Porter JA, Chiang C, et al: Induction of midbrain dopaminergic neurons by Sonic hedgehog, *Neuron* 15:35, 1995.

58. Inder TE, Warfield SK, Wang H, et al: Abnormal cerebral structure is present at term in premature infants, *Pediatrics* 115:286, 2005.

59. Jamieson CR, Govaerts C, Abramowicz MJ: Primary autosomal recessive microcephaly: homozygosity mapping of MCPH4 to chromosome 15, *Am J Hum Genet* 65:1465, 1999.

60. Johnston MV, Alemi L, Harum KH: Learning, memory, and transcription factors, *Pediatr Res* 53:369, 2003.

61. Kadhim HJ, Gadisseux JF, Evrard P: Topographical and cytological evolution of the glial phase during prenatal development of the human brain: histochemical and electron microscopic study, *J Neuropathol Exp Neurol* 47:166, 1988.

62. Kapellou O, Counsell SJ, Kennea N, et al: Abnormal cortical development after premature birth shown by altered allometric scaling of brain growth, *PLoS Med* 3:e265, 2006.

63. Keays DA, Tian G, Poirier K, et al: Mutations in alpha-tubulin cause abnormal neuronal migration in mice and lissencephaly in humans, *Cell* 128:45, 2007.

64. Komuro H, Rakic P: Modulation of neuronal migration by NMDA receptors, *Science* 260:95, 1993.

65. Korogi Y, Takahashi M, Sumi M, et al: MR signal intensity of the perirolandic cortex in the neonate and infant, *Neuroradiology* 38:578, 1996.

66. Kostovic I, Judas M: Correlation between the sequential ingrowth of afferents and transient patterns of cortical lamination in preterm infants, *Anat Rec* 267:1, 2002.

67. Kreis R, Ernst T, Ross BD: Development of the human brain: in vivo quantification of metabolite and water content with proton magnetic resonance spectroscopy, *Magn Reson Med* 30:424, 1993.

68. Kreis R, Hofmann L, Kuhlmann B, et al: Brain metabolite composition during early human brain development as measured by quantitative in vivo 1H magnetic resonance spectroscopy, *Magn Reson Med* 48:949, 2002.

69. Kuban KC, Gilles FH: Human telencephalic angiogenesis, *Ann Neurol* 17:539, 1985.

70. Kuban K, Teele RL: Rationale for grading intracranial hemorrhage in premature infants, *Pediatrics* 74:358, 1984.

71. Lagercrantz H, Ringstedt T: Organization of the neuronal circuits in the central nervous system during development, *Acta Paediatr* 90:707, 2001.

72. Ling EA, Wong WC: The origin and nature of ramified and amoeboid microglia: a historical review and current concepts, *Glia* 7:9, 1993.

73. Lu N, DiCicco-Bloom E: Pituitary adenylate cyclase-activating polypeptide is an autocrine inhibitor of mitosis in cultured cortical precursor cells, *Proc Natl Acad Sci U S A* 94:3357, 1997.

74. Mallat M, Chamak B: Brain macrophages: neurotoxic or neurotrophic effector cells? *J Leukoc Biol* 56:416, 1994.

75. Marret S, Gressens P, Evrard P: Arrest of neuronal migration by excitatory amino acids in hamster developing brain, *Proc Natl Acad Sci USA* 93:15463, 1996.

76. McKinstry RC, Mathur A, Miller JH, et al: Radial organization of developing preterm human cerebral cortex revealed by noninvasive water diffusion anisotropy MRI, *Cereb Cortex* 12:1237, 2002.

77. McQuillen PS, Sheldon RA, Shatz CJ, Ferriero DM: Selective vulnerability of subplate neurons after early neonatal hypoxia-ischemia, *J Neurosci* 23:3308, 2003.

78. Mehta V, Namboodiri MA: N-acetylaspartate as an acetyl source in the nervous system, *Brain Res Mol Brain Res* 31:151, 1995.

79. Modi N, Lewis H, Al-Naqeeb N, et al: The effects of repeated antenatal glucocorticoid therapy on the developing brain, *Pediatr Res* 50:581, 2001.

80. Mukherjee P, Miller JH, Shimony JS, et al: Diffusion-tensor MR imaging of gray and white matter development during normal human brain maturation, *AJNR Am J Neuroradiol* 23:1445, 2002.

81. Mukherjee P, Miller JH, Shimony JS, et al: Normal brain maturation during childhood: developmental trends characterized with diffusion-tensor MR imaging, *Radiology* 221:349, 2001.

82. Murphy BP, Inder TE, Huppi PS, et al: Impaired cerebral cortical gray matter growth after treatment with dexamethasone for neonatal chronic lung disease, *Pediatrics* 107:217, 2001.

83. Noctor SC, Martinez-Cerdeno V, Ivic L, Kriegstein AR: Cortical neurons arise in symmetric and asymmetric division zones and migrate through specific phases, *Nat Neurosci* 7:136, 2004.

84. Norman MG, O'Kusky JR: The growth and development of microvasculature in human cerebral cortex, *J Neuropathol Exp Neurol* 45:222, 1986.

85. Ohshima T, Ward JM, Huh CG, et al: Targeted disruption of the cyclin-dependent kinase 5 gene results in abnormal corticogenesis, neuronal pathology and perinatal death, *Proc Natl Acad Sci USA* 93:11173, 1996.

86. Olney JW, Wozniak DF, Jevtovic-Todorovic V, et al: Drug-induced apoptotic neurodegeneration in the developing brain, *Brain Pathol* 12:488, 2002.

87. Partridge SC, Mukherjee P, Henry RG, et al: Diffusion tensor imaging: serial quantitation of white matter tract maturity in premature newborns, *Neuroimage* 22: 1302, 2004.

88. Pellerin L, Pellegri G, Martin JL, Magistretti PJ: Expression of monocarboxylate transporter mRNAs in mouse brain: support for a distinct role of lactate as an energy substrate for the neonatal vs. adult brain, *Proc Natl Acad Sci USA* 95:3990, 1998.

89. Pilz DT, Matsumoto N, Minnerath S, et al: LIS1 and XLIS (DCX) mutations cause most classical lissencephaly, but different patterns of malformation, *Hum Mol Genet* 7:2029, 1998.

90. Poduslo SE, Jang Y. Myelin development in infant brain, *Neurochem Res* 9:1615, 1984.

91. Poirier K, Van Esch H, Friocourt G, et al: Neuroanatomical distribution of ARX in brain and its localisation in GABAergic neurons, *Brain Res Mol Brain Res* 122:35, 2004.

92. Polleux F, Dehay C, Goffinet A, Kennedy H: Pre- and postmitotic events contribute to the progressive acquisition of area-specific connectional fate in the neocortex, *Cereb Cortex* 11:1027, 2001.

93. Polleux F, Dehay C, Moraillon B, Kennedy H: Regulation of neuroblast cell-cycle kinetics plays a crucial role in the generation of unique features of neocortical areas, *J Neurosci* 17:7763, 1997.

94. Provost AC, Pequignot MO, Sainton KM, et al: Expression of SR-BI receptor and StAR protein in rat ocular tissues, *C R Biol* 326:841, 2003.

95. Rakic P: Developmental and evolutionary adaptations of cortical radial glia, *Cereb Cortex* 13:541, 2003.

96. Rakic P: Specification of cerebral cortical areas, *Science* 241:170, 1988.

97. Regis J, Mangin JF, Ochiai T, et al: "Sulcal root" generic model: a hypothesis to overcome the variability of the human cortex folding patterns, *Neurol Med Chir (Tokyo)* 45:1, 2005.

98. Roberts E, Hampshire DJ, Pattison L, et al: Autosomal recessive primary microcephaly: an analysis of locus heterogeneity and phenotypic variation, *J Med Genet* 39:718, 2002.

99. Roberts E, Jackson AP, Carradice AC, et al : The second locus for autosomal recessive primary microcephaly (MCPH2) maps to chromosome 19q13.1-13.2, *Eur J Hum Genet* 7:815, 1999.

100. Rosenberg MJ, Agarwala R, Bouffard G, et al: Mutant deoxynucleotide carrier is associated with congenital microcephaly, *Nat Genet* 32:175, 2002.

101. Rubenstein JL, Shimamura K, Martinez S, Puelles L: Regionalization of the prosencephalic neural plate, *Annu Rev Neurosci* 21:445, 1998.

102. Sarnat HB, Flores-Sarnat L: A new classification of malformations of the nervous system: an integration of morphological and molecular genetic criteria as patterns of genetic expression, *Eur J Paediatr Neurol* 5:57, 2001.

103. Shimamura K, Hartigan DJ, Martinez S, et al: Longitudinal organization of the anterior neural plate and neural tube, *Development* 121:3923, 1995.

104. Sidman RL, Rakic P: Neuronal migration, with special reference to developing human brain: a review, *Brain Res* 62:1, 1973.

105. Simeone A: Towards the comprehension of genetic mechanisms controlling brain morphogenesis, *Trends Neurosci* 25:119, 2002.

106. Simon H, Hornbruch A, Lumsden A: Independent assignment of antero-posterior and dorso-ventral positional values in the developing chick hindbrain, *Curr Biol* 5:205, 1995.

107. Sizonenko SV, Camm EJ, Garbow JR, et al: Developmental changes and injury induced disruption of the radial organization of the cortex in the immature rat brain revealed by in vivo diffusion tensor MRI, *Cereb Cortex* 17:2609, 2007.

108. Smith JL, Schoenwolf GC. Notochordal induction of cell wedging in the chick neural plate and its role in neural tube formation, *J Exp Zool* 1989;250:49-62.

109. Sowell ER, Peterson BS, Thompson PM, et al: Mapping cortical change across the human life span, *Nat Neurosci* 6:309, 2003.

110. Stricker T, Martin E, Boesch C: Development of the human cerebellum observed with high-field-strength MR imaging, *Radiology* 177:431, 1990.

111. ten Donkelaar HJ, Lammens M, Wesseling P, et al: Development and developmental disorders of the human cerebellum, *J Neurol* 250:1025, 2003.

112. Urenjak J, Williams SR, Gadian DG, Noble M: Specific expression of N-acetylaspartate in neurons, oligodendrocyte-type-2 astrocyte progenitors, and immature oligodendrocytes in vitro, *J Neurochem* 59:55, 1992.

113. Vaizel-Ohayon D, Schejter ED: Mutations in centrosomin reveal requirements for centrosomal function during early *Drosophila* embryogenesis, *Curr Biol* 9:889, 1999.

114. Van Essen DC: A tension-based theory of morphogenesis and compact wiring in the central nervous system, *Nature* 385:313, 1997.

115. Van Essen DC, Dierker DL. Surface-based and probabilistic atlases of primate cerebral cortex, *Neuron* 56:209, 2007.

116. Vaudry D, Falluel-Morel A, Leuillet S, et al: Regulators of cerebellar granule cell development act through specific signaling pathways, *Science* 300:1532, 2003.

117. Venturin M, Moncini S, Villa V, et al: Mutations and novel polymorphisms in coding regions and UTRs of CDK5R1 and OMG genes in patients with non-syndromic mental retardation, *Neurogenetics* 7:59, 2006.

118. Volpe JJ: Neurobiology of periventricular leukomalacia in the premature infant, *Pediatr Res* 50:553, 2001.

119. Volpe JJ: *Neurology of the newborn*. Philadelphia, 2001,WB Saunders.

120. Wakefield JG, Bonaccorsi S, Gatti M: The *Drosophila* protein asp is involved in microtubule organization during spindle formation and cytokinesis, *J Cell Biol* 153:637, 2001.

121. Wang VY, Zoghbi HY: Genetic regulation of cerebellar development, *Nat Rev Neurosci* 2:484, 2001.

122. Wimberger DM, Roberts TP, Barkovich AJ, et al: Identification of "premyelination" by diffusion-weighted MRI, *J Comput Assist Tomogr* 19:28, 1995.

123. Yamada T, Pfaff SL, Edlund T, Jessell TM: Control of cell pattern in the neural tube: motor neuron induction by diffusible factors from notochord and floor plate, *Cell* 73:673, 1993.

124. Zheng D, Purves D: Effects of increased neural activity on brain growth, *Proc Natl Acad Sci USA* 92:1802, 1995.

125. Zupan V, Nehlig A, Evrard P, Gressens P: Prenatal blockade of vasoactive intestinal peptide alters cell death and synaptic equipment in the murine neocortex, *Pediatr Res* 47:53, 2000.

PART 2

White Matter Damage and Encephalopathy of Prematurity

Petra S. Hüppi and Pierre Gressens

Brain injury in the premature infant is composed of multiple lesions, principally described as germinal matrix intraventricular hemorrhage (IVH), posthemorrhagic hydrocephalus (PHH), and periventricular leukomalacia (PVL). With the reduction of the incidence of IVH and PHH, the third entity now appears to be the most important brain lesion[88,107] determining the neurodevelopmental outcome of premature infants. Periventricular leukomalacia has classically been described as a disorder characterized by multifocal areas of necrosis, forming cysts in the deep periventricular cerebral white matter, which are often symmetric and occur adjacent to the lateral ventricles. These focal necrotic lesions correlate well with the development of spastic cerebral palsy in infants with very low birthweight (VLBW). With the advances in neonatal care and survival at increasingly low gestational ages, a large number of infants with VLBW is now seen with mild motor impairment and often considerable cognitive and behavioral deficits,[103] which may relate to a more diffuse injury to the developing brain.

This chapter presents the current concepts of brain injury to the immature brain, which has recently been termed *encephalopathy of prematurity*,[108] summarizing the old and new neuropathologic findings, mechanisms of pathogenesis through animal models, and the characteristics of this type of lesion in modern neuroimaging.

NEUROPATHOLOGY OF WHITE MATTER INJURY

Historical View

Congenital encephalomyelitis was the term first used by Virchow in 1867 to describe a disease in newborns who demonstrated pale, softened zones of degeneration within the periventricular white matter at autopsy. Microscopically, these lesions were characterized by glial hyperplasia with the presence of foamy macrophages and signs of tissue destruction with necrosis. Interestingly, Virchow related the disease to acute infection, in that many of the cases were seen in infected mothers.[106] Clinically he suggested that these lesions might be related to a disease described earlier by Little,[60] in which the patients suffered from spasmodic limb contractures, diplegia, and mental retardation, occasionally with an additional epileptic condition. Parrot, in 1873, first linked the pathologic entity to premature birth and proposed that the lesions were due to a particular vulnerability of the immature white matter as a result of nutritional and circulatory disturbances resulting in infarction.[82] Much later, Rydberg again proposed a hemodynamic etiology with a reduction of cerebral blood flow to the vulnerable regions of the immature white matter.[94] Banker and Larroche in 1962 first introduced the term *periventricular leukomalacia* to define this characteristic lesion they found in 20% of autopsies of infants who died before 1 month of age. They described the macroscopic and microscopic neuropathology in more detail.[9]

Periventricular Leukomalacia

MACROSCOPIC NEUROPATHOLOGY

The topography of the lesions as described was uniform, primarily affecting the white matter in a zone within the subcallosal, superior fronto-occipital and superior longitudinal fasciculi, the external and internal border zone of the temporal and occipital horn of the lateral ventricles, and some parts of the corona radiata.[31] These areas appeared pale, usually bilateral, but without definite symmetry (Fig. 40-31). Although not unanimously accepted, it has been noted that the anatomic distribution of PVL correlates with the development of perforating medullary arteries and areas that represent arterial border or end zones that arise between ventriculopetal and ventriculofugal arteries within the deep white matter (Fig. 40-32).[47] Immunohistochemical studies further confirm a low vessel density in the deep white matter between 28 and 36 weeks' gestation, whereas in the subcortical white matter, the vessel density is low, between 16 and 24 weeks, and thereafter increases (Fig. 40-33).

MICROSCOPIC NEUROPATHOLOGY

The earliest recorded changes were of coagulation necrosis of all cellular elements with loss of cytoarchitecture and tissue vacuolation. Axonal swelling and intense activated microglial reactivity and proliferation were observed as early as 3 hours after insult. In addition, in the periphery of these focal lesions, a marked astrocytic and vascular endothelial hyperplasia characterized the brain tissue reaction at the end of the first week. After 1 to 2 weeks, macrophage activity with characteristic

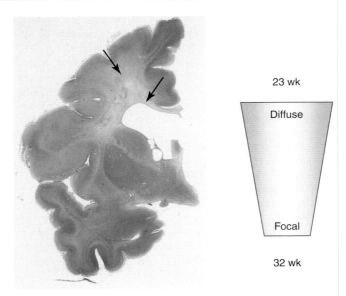

Figure 40–31. See color insert. Neuropathology showing periventricular lesions primarily affecting the white matter and characterized by pale softened zones of degeneration (hematoxylin preparation) (*left arrow*) and thinning of the corpus callosum with ventriculomegaly (*right arrow*). Lesions detected in infants with very low gestational age at birth tend to be diffuse with more focal cystic lesions in infants with higher gestational age at birth.

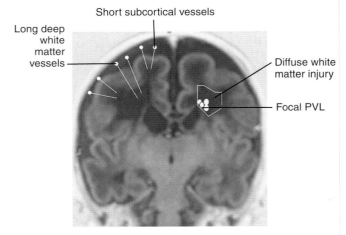

Figure 40–32. Schematic representation of vascular supply characterized by short subcortical end-arteries and long deep end-arteries and their relation to the diffuse and focal component of immature white matter injury (according to Rorke LB: Anatomical features of the developing brain implicated in pathogenesis of hypoxic-ischemic injury, *Brain Pathol* 2:211, 1992). PVL, periventricular leukomalacia.

lipid-laden macrophages was predominant over the astrocytic reactivity, with progressive cavitation of the tissue and cyst formation thereafter. During subacute and chronic stages of PVL, swollen axons calcify, accumulate iron, and degenerate, particularly at the periphery of the injured zone. Additional minor changes were also found within the gray matter with

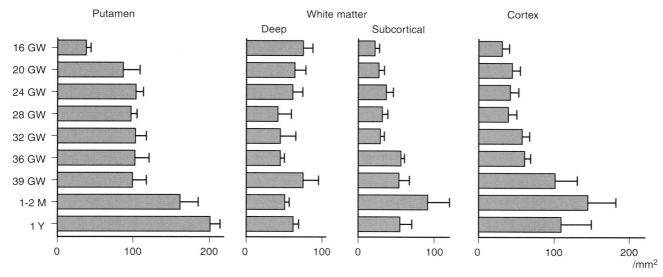

Figure 40–33. Developmental changes in vessel density in the human brain illustrate decrease in vessel density in long deep white matter arteries between 28 and 36 weeks. Note the low density of subcortical end-arteries before 32 weeks of gestation (GW). (*From Miyawako T, et al:* Early Human Dev *53:2025, 1998, reprinted with permission.*)

some diffuse neuronal loss, especially in lower cortical layers, the hippocampus in the cerebellar Purkinje cell layer. Since these early studies, many conventional neuropathology studies have noted a widespread diffuse central cerebral white matter astrocytosis, often with abnormal glial cells, which were called *perinatal telencephalic leukoencephalopathy.* From these studies, Leviton and Gilles introduced for the first time a differentiation between focal and diffuse white matter damage.[56]

NEW NEUROPATHOLOGIC INSIGHTS

This diffuse white matter damage is macroscopically characterized by a paucity of white matter, thinning of the corpus callosum, and in later stages, ventriculomegaly and delayed myelination.[33,56] With the use of immunocytochemical techniques, the assessment of autopsy tissue has allowed further localization of cell-specific injury in white matter damage. Deep periventricular white matter is prone to focal necrosis regionally consistent with the presumed vascular end zones/border zones, whereas in the peripheral white matter, diffuse injury could be characterized by preferential death or injury of late oligodendrocyte progenitors and immature oligodendrocytes, or pre-OLs (see Part 1).[8]

Vulnerability of Oligodendroglia Cell Line

Several lines of evidence implicate damage to immature oligodendrocytes during a specific window of vulnerability as a significant underlying factor in the pathogenesis of PVL (see Models of Encephalopathy, later). Oligodendrocyte progenitor cells proliferate and die by programmed cell death (see Part 1) regulated by trophic factors such as platelet-derived growth factor (PDGF) and insulin-like growth factor (IGF). The activation of cytokine receptors on the surface of oligodendrocytes can lead to the death of these cells. Studies in vitro have shown that the inflammatory cytokines TNF-α and interferon-gamma are toxic to cultured oligodendrocyte

progenitor cells.[4] Selective injury to oligodendrocytes is mediated by induction of "death" receptors such as Fas on the surface of oligodendrocytes. Direct axonal contact appears to be another important factor for the survival of oligodendrocytes.[16] Oligodendrocytes are further susceptible to oxidative damage mediated by free radicals such as reactive oxygen and nitrogen species and as a consequence of the depletion of the main antioxidant glutathione.[6] Injury-induced swelling and disruption to axons within the white matter leads to locally elevated glutamate, which also induces oligodendrocyte cell death and/or injury. Glutamate toxicity depends on the maturational stage of the oligodendrocyte and is mediated via the alpha-3-amino-hydroxy-5-methyl-4-isoxazole propionic acid (AMPA) receptor and potentially through N-methyl-D-aspartate (NMDA) receptors.[23,52,54]

Recent experimental data show, on the other hand, an important increase in NG2 (high molecular weight, integral membrane chondroitin sulphate proteoglycan)-positive oligodendrocyte progenitor cells within the area of the injury.[97] The role of this increase in NG2 cells is currently unknown, but this population is distinct from neurons, oligodendrocytes, astrocytes, and microglia. This cell population could comprise multipotent cells capable of differentiating into any other type of cell and playing a role in axonal growth and myelination, and in regeneration after injury with functional integration in neural circuitry.

Microglial Activity

Specific immunocytochemical markers (e.g., CD68) have identified a marked increase of activated microglia in diffuse white matter injury.[38] Microglia are already widely dispersed throughout the immature white matter by 22 weeks' gestation. These cells are fully capable of producing potentially toxic inflammatory mediators, free radicals, and reactive oxygen intermediates.[90] The phagocytic activity of microglia and their capacity for oxidative-mediated injury are potently enhanced by inflammatory mediators (IFN-γ, TNF-α, IL-β, and bacterial lipopolysaccharide, or LPS).[101] Studies of preoligodendrocytes of the same maturational stage as those populated in the immature white matter of the human premature infant show that cells are exquisitely vulnerable to attack by reactive oxygen species (ROS) and reactive nitrogen species (RNS) produced by activated microglia.[71] Presence of activated microglia inducing cell death in immature white matter, both in preoligodendrocytes as well as in astrocytes, has been widely confirmed.[28,102] So far, it also seems that microglia and resident mononuclear phagocytes are the primary sources for the proinflammatory cytokines in PVL brains.[53]

Neuronal/Axonal Damage

Indirect assessment of axonal damage in classic PVL was done by immunostaining for beta amyloid precursor protein, a neuronoaxonal protein. Immunostaining of damaged axons was predominant in the acute phase of PVL and was no longer detectable in the chronic stage. Swollen axons calcify (probably due to glutamatergic overactivation), accumulate iron, and degenerate; this has been shown to occur without overt coagulation necrosis of all tissue components.[39] Axons from the corticospinal tract, thalamocortical fibers, optic radiation, superior occipitofrontal fasciculus, and the superior longitudinal fasciculus may be affected and result in motor, sensory, visual, and higher cortical function deficits. Thalamocortical projections that course through the white matter develop before the functional development of cortical neurons. Therefore, the ensuing disruption to these circuits and to the subcortical plate may not only affect the function, but also the density, survival, and organization of cortical neurons and the cortex itself (see later).[46]

In addition, there is evidence for death of progenitor cells, not neural stem cells, in the subventricular zone after hypoxia-ischemia.[93] These destructive effects are paralleled with potential trophic reactions such as the proliferation of potentially pluripotent progenitor cells, also called *polydendrocytes*, in the area of injury.[97] These cells are known to differentiate into oligodendrocytes, to a lesser extent into gray matter astrocytes, and potentially even into neurons.[78]

Subplate Damage

Damage to the early developing subplate neurons with their critical role for the organization of the cortical plate (see Part 1 of this chapter) has long been postulated as a possible mechanism by which injury to the immature brain results in long-lasting motor and cognitive deficits.[109] McQuillen and colleagues[70] were able to show specific cell death in subplate neurons after hypoxia-ischemia in very immature animals. Lack of guidance for the thalamocortical connections as a result of a loss of subplate neurons may represent one of the major developmental disturbances after injury to the immature brain.[55]

The current concept of pathogenesis of encephalopathy of prematurity is based on the combination of destructive and developmental disturbances, which are schematically summarized in Figure 40-34.

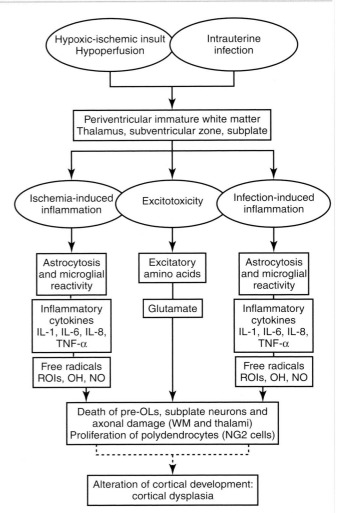

Figure 40–34. Schematic representation of the current main pathogenetic factors involved in immature white matter injury. IL, interleukin; NO, nitric oxide; OH, hydroxyl ion (reactive oxygen species); OL, oligodendrocyte; ROI, reactive oxygen intermediate species (like Fe superoxide anion); TNF, tumor necrosis factor; WM, white matter. (*Adapted from Rezaie P, Dean A: Periventricular leukomalacia, inflammation and white matter lesions within the developing nervous system* Neuropathology 22:106, 2002.)

MODELS OF ENCEPHALOPATHY OF PREMATURITY: IMPLICATIONS FOR PATHOGENESIS

The etiology of white matter injury and encephalopathy of prematurity in human neonates has been widely described as multifactorial rather than linked solely to cardiovascular instability and hypoxia-ischemia. The many preconceptional, prenatal, perinatal, and postnatal factors potentially implicated in the pathophysiology of these lesions include hypoxia-ischemia, endocrine imbalances, genetic factors, growth factor deficiency, abnormal competition for growth factors, overproduction of free oxygen radicals, maternal infection with overproduction of cytokines and other proinflammatory agents, exposure to toxins, maternal stress, and malnutrition. Although some of these potentially noxious factors may suffice to permanently injure the developing brain, some researchers have developed a "two-hit" hypothesis in which early exposures increase the susceptibility of the brain to subsequent insults (Fig. 40-35).

The development and characterization of distinct yet complementary animal models should help unravel the complex cellular and molecular pathophysiologic mechanisms underlying perinatal white matter lesions and encephalopathy of prematurity. In animal models or in vitro paradigms, the insults most often used to induce white matter damage or oligodendrocyte cell death, respectively, are generally hypoxia, hypoxia-ischemia, infection, inflammatory factors, oxidative stress, or excitotoxic agents. The relevance of white matter damage produced in these animal models to human white matter injury is largely based on neuropathologic data, although some studies are also based on MRI parameters or on neurologic and behavioral deficits.[24]

This section focuses on the most studied models of perinatal white matter damage, highlighting their major contributions to the understanding of the pathophysiology of these lesions. The reader interested in a deeper insight will find more information and a more comprehensive bibliography in published reviews on this topic.[37,72]

Hyoperfusion and Hypoxia-Ischemia

Hypoxic-ischemic or hypoperfusion insults have been used in a large variety of neonatal species including rats, mice, rabbits, pigs, and dogs. In most cases, these insults produce specific gray matter damage (mimicking lesions observed in human full-term infants), which have been the focus of most of these studies, whereas observed white matter damage is generally considered to be an extension of gray matter damage in the most severe cases. However, notable "exceptions" highlight some potentially important features of perinatal white matter damage.

In dog pups, hypoxic-ischemic insult by bilateral carotid ligation selectively induces white matter damage mimicking human PVL.[115] This selective vulnerability of white matter could underlie a genetic predisposition of the dog to white matter hypoxic-ischemic damage. Modern tools of genomics could unravel important genes involved in the pathophysiology of perinatal white matter damage.

In rats, the classic Rice-Vannucci model performed on postnatal day 7 or 9, predominantly leads to gray matter lesions. However, analyses have shown the involvement of the periventricular white matter with the involvement of immature oligodendroglial and progenitor cells.[7,99] More importantly, adaptation of this paradigm to more immature newborn rats (postnatal days 1 or 3) has allowed production of important lesions in the periventricular white matter with relative sparing of the classic intracortical injuries (Fig. 40-36).[70,98] These studies have also highlighted the specific involvement of subplate neurons in brain damage. Altogether, these data obtained in newborn rats further support the notion of an ontogenic window of white matter sensitivity and subplate vulnerability to insults such as hypoxia-ischemia.

Asphyxia of sheep fetuses (around 65% of gestation) has been shown to induce periventricular (focal and diffuse) and subcortical (diffuse) white matter disease, accompanied by acute astrocyte and oligodendrocyte loss, and marked reactive microgliosis.[65] These studies support the concept of the association of focal (e.g., cystic lesions) and diffuse (e.g., diffuse microglial activation) white matter lesions, the pathophysiology of which being potentially distinct. Furthermore, it was shown by microdialysis that white matter glutamate levels were significantly increased following asphyxia, supporting a role of excitotoxicity in the pathogenesis of such white matter lesions (see later).[62]

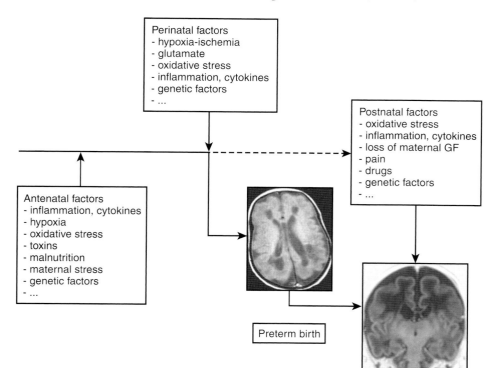

Figure 40–35. Schematic representation of the "multiple-hit" hypothesis in which a combination of two or more environmental or genetic factors occurring during the prenatal, perinatal, or postnatal period induces or modulates brain lesions. GF, growth factors.

Perinatal factors
- hypoxia-ischemia
- glutamate
- oxidative stress
- inflammation, cytokines
- genetic factors
- ...

Postnatal factors
- oxidative stress
- inflammation, cytokines
- loss of maternal GF
- pain
- drugs
- genetic factors
- ...

Antenatal factors
- inflammation, cytokines
- hypoxia
- oxidative stress
- toxins
- malnutrition
- maternal stress
- genetic factors
- ...

Preterm birth

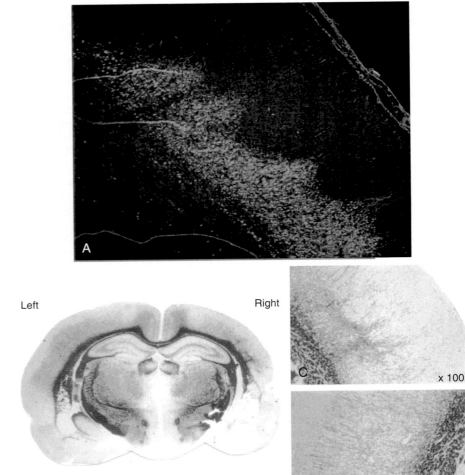

Figure 40–36. Pattern of injury after hypoxic-ischemic injury in the P3 rat brain **A,** Degenerating neurons 24 hours after hypoxic-ischemic insult at P3 stained with Fluoro-Jade. Ipsilateral brain with severe damage: a columnar aspect of positive cells is present with confluence of positive cells in the deep layers IV-VI (100×). The outer layers I-III remained unaffected. **B,** Myelin basic protein immunostaining of the brain at P21 after hypoxic-ischemic injury at P3. Coronal section of brain at the level of the dorsal hippocampus (10×). A reduction of the cortical and myelinated areas in the ipsilateral right hemisphere extending from the cingulum to the rhinal sulcus. At 100×, the alteration of the myelin pattern in the deep cortical layers is shown in the ispsilateral right cortex (**C**) when compared with the left normal cortex (**D**).

Exposure of pregnant rats[11] or postnatal rat pups[104] to hypoxia induces pathologic changes in the periventricular white matter which are reminiscent of human periventricular leukomalacia, with inflammation, astrogliosis, and myelination delay in the prenatal model, and white matter atrophy, ventriculomegaly, and alteration of synaptic maturation in the postnatal paradigm. Although the initial insult is a pure hypoxia, the observed effects are likely the result of the combination of different mechanisms, such as hypoperfusion, ischemia, inflammation, and/or oxidative stress induced by the protracted hypoxia and the subsequent reoxygenation phase.

Infection and Inflammation

Systemic administration of LPS to immature cats, dogs, or rabbits induces white matter lesions. Systemic administration of LPS can induce a marked systemic inflammation and immune changes in the central nervous system such as an increased expression of CD14. Furthermore, high doses of LPS can induce hypotension, hypoglycemia, hyperthermia, and lactic acidosis, all potential factors predisposing to brain damage. However, low doses of LPS, which do not induce significant hypotension, have also been shown to induce white matter damage in fetal sheep.[37,64] In fetal sheep, the comparison of white matter damage induced by cord occlusion and by LPS injection, revealed distinct patterns of microglia-macrophage activation, suggesting separate or partly separate underlying mechanisms.[64] On the other hand, systemic administration of LPS to newborn rats failed to induce detectable white matter lesions, although increased cytokine production and microglial activation were observed in the white matter.[15,30,113] These data suggest species differences that might be linked to species-related genetic susceptibility of the developing white matter to infectious-inflammatory factors. Interestingly, in vitro studies have shown that macrophages are necessary for LPS to induce preoligodendrocyte cell death.

Live infectious agents have also been used by a few research groups to produce models of white matter lesions. In pregnant rabbits, ascending intrauterine infection with *Escherichia coli* caused focal white matter damage in 6% of live fetuses,[114] whereas direct inoculation of *E. coli* in the uterine cavity combined with early antibiotics produced focal white matter cysts in about 20% of live fetuses and diffuse white matter cell death in almost all live fetuses (Fig. 40-37).[22] Cystic lesions are accompanied by macrophage-microglia activation and reactive astrogliosis, while diffuse white matter cell death does not induce such glial responses. These results suggest that these two types of brain damage have distinct pathophysiologic mechanisms.

In addition, a recent study has shown that infection of pregnant mice with *Ureaplasma parvum*, an organism frequently isolated in chorioamnionitis, induces central microgliosis and disrupted brain development as detected by decreased number of calbindin-positive and calretinin-positive neurons in the neocortex as well as myelination defect in the periventricular white matter.[79]

Finally, intrauterine inoculation of Border disease virus to pregnant sheep induces decreased expression of white matter molecules, including myelin basic protein in the fetuses.[3] However, the virus also infects the thyroid and the pituitary gland, raising the question of the precise etiology of the white matter damage (low thyroid hormones versus infectious-inflammatory insult).

Excitotoxicity and Oxidative Stress

Glutamate can act on several types of receptors including NMDA, AMPA, kainite, and metabotropic receptors. Excess release of glutamate has been suggested to represent a molecular mechanism common to some of the risk factors for brain lesions associated with cerebral palsy. In keeping with this possibility, injection of glutamate agonists into the striatum, neocortex, or periventricular white matter of newborn rodents (rats, mice, or hamsters), rabbits, or kittens produces, according to the stage of brain maturation, histologic lesions that mimic those seen in humans with cerebral palsy, such as neuronal migration disorders, polymicrogyria, cystic periventricular leukomalacia, and hypoxic-ischemic or ischemic-like cortical and striatal lesions.[1,67,69]

Studies exploring the pathophysiology of these excitotoxic white matter lesions in newborn rodents and rabbits have permitted the following contributions (Fig. 40-38)[89]:

1. Both NMDA and AMPA-kainate agonists can induce periventricular cystic white matter lesions.

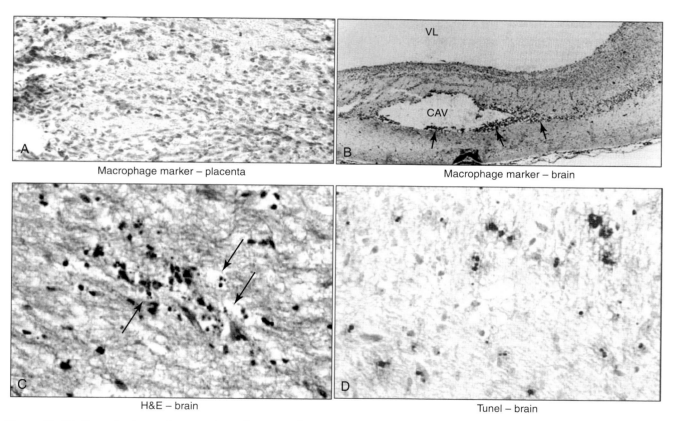

Macrophage marker – placenta

Macrophage marker – brain

H&E – brain

Tunel – brain

Figure 40–37. See color insert. Intrauterine infection with *Escherichia coli* in pregnant rabbits induces a combination of placental and brain abnormalities. **A,** Macrophage activation is observed in all placentas. The numerous red cells correspond to activated macrophages labeled with a specific antigen. **B,** Focal cystic periventricular white matter lesions with macrophage activation are detected in some fetuses. Brown cells identified by *arrows* correspond to activated macrophages/microglia labeled with a specific antigen. CAV, cystic lesion; VL, lateral ventricle. **C** and **D,** Diffuse white matter cell death without detectable inflammatory response is observed in all fetuses on hematoxylin-eosin stained sections (**C,** *Arrows* point to examples of apoptotic nuclei in the periventricular white matter) and on Tunel (a marker of fragmented DNA and of accompanying cell death)-stained sections (**D,** Purple-blue nuclei correspond to diffusely distributed dying white matter cells). (*From Debillon T, et al: Intrauterine infection induces programmed cell death in periventricular white matter,* Pediatr Res 47:736, 2000, *and Patterns of cerebral inflammatory response in a rabbit model of intrauterine infection-mediated brain lesion,* Brain Res Dev Brain Res 145:39, 2003, *with permission.*)

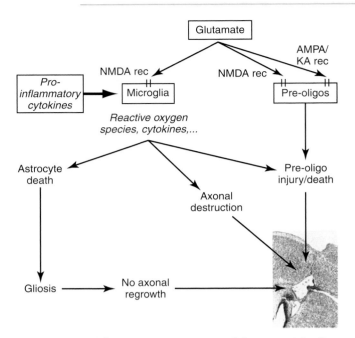

Figure 40–38. Schematic representation of the potential cellular and molecular pathways by which excess release of glutamate and proinflammatory cytokines may lead to white matter lesions. AMPA, alpha-3-amino-hydroxy-5-methyl-4-isoxazole propionic acid; KA, kainate; NMDA, N-methyl-D-aspartate; oligo(s), oligodendrocyte(s); rec, receptors.

2. NMDA receptor–mediated white matter lesions involve an early microglia-macrophage activation and astrocyte cell death, whereas AMPA-kainate receptor–mediated lesions involve preoligodendrocyte cell death. In addition, NMDA receptors expressed by preoligodendrocytes could participate in the injury of these preoligodendrocytes.

3. The periventricular white matter of newborn rodents and rabbits exhibits a window of susceptibility to excitotoxic insults.

4. Transient expression of NMDA receptors on white matter microglia-macrophages and transient expression of high levels of AMPA-kainate receptors on preoligodendrocytes are likely important factors to explain the window of sensitivity of the white matter to neonatal excitotoxic insults.

5. The study of NMDA receptor-mediated white matter lesions in newborn rabbits revealed that the excitotoxic white matter lesion extended into the subplate but not in the overlying neocortical layers. Based on the use of antioxidant molecules, excitotoxic white matter lesions involve excess production of reactive oxygen species, which play an important role in the pathophysiology of the lesions.

Extensive in vitro studies have confirmed the exquisite susceptibility of preoligodendrocytes to AMPA-kainate agonists and to oxidative stress.[52]

Combined Insults

In order to further support the hypothesis of a multifactorial cause of perinatal brain damage (see Fig. 40-35), different groups have combined insults in newborn rodents.

Pretreatment of newborn mice with systemic proinflammatory cytokines (e.g., IL-1β, IL-6, or TNFα) before an excitotoxic insult significantly exacerbates excitotoxic white matter lesions, demonstrating a causative link between circulating proinflammatory cytokines and white matter damage.[27] Preliminary results suggest that this effect of proinflammatory cytokines is more pronounced with NMDA receptor agonists when compared with AMPA-kainate receptor agonists (see Fig. 40-38). The precise mechanism by which these systemic cytokines act on white matter excitotoxicity remains to be determined but could potentially involve activation of brain cyclooxygenase (COX) or activation of microglia with increased white matter production of reactive oxygen species and cytokines.

Similarly, systemic pretreatment with IL-9, a Th2 cytokine, was shown to exacerbate NMDA receptor-mediated white matter lesions.[27,84] The mechanism of IL-9 toxicity involves brain mast cell degranulation and excess release of histamine. Interestingly, increased circulating levels of IL-9 around birth had been demonstrated in a subgroup of human infants who later developed cerebral palsy.[77] Recently, chronic mild stress of pregnant mice was shown to induce a significant exacerbation of excitotoxic white matter lesions in pups.[89a]

LPS was also used to sensitize the newborn brain to hypoxia-ischemia. A low dose of this endotoxin, given 4 hours before a mild hypoxic-ischemic insult in the P7 rat, induced extensive brain damage, while each insult given separately did not induce any detectable brain lesion.[30]

Recent years have seen the emergence of several experimental paradigms to study white matter diseases of the preterm infant. These animal models have permitted identification of some of the potentially key cellular players (e.g., preoligodendrocytes, microglia-macrophages) and molecular players (e.g., glutamate, cytokines and other inflammatory mediators, reactive oxygen species) involved in the pathophysiology of perinatal brain damage. These studies have also delineated potential targets for neuroprotection. Future studies should incorporate imaging and behavioral studies to facilitate comparison with the human situation. Although it is clear that studies with rodents, due to their cost and availability, are absolutely necessary to generate and test multiple hypotheses, the use of larger models such as sheep, pigs, and monkeys will remain a key for testing in a more reliable fashion the relevance of the obtained data for the human situation.

NEUROIMAGING OF WHITE MATTER INJURY
Neonatal Sonography

Neonatal sonography is the one major bedside technique to image the neonatal brain. Leviton and colleagues postulated in 1990 that ultrasonographic white matter echodensities and echolucencies in infants with low birthweight predicted later handicap more accurately than any other antecedent.[57]

Unlike intraventricular hemorrhage, damage to the white matter can have different appearances and depending on the timing of the injury, the imaging characteristics can be non-specific with generally an increase in echogenicity in the acute phase of the injury (Fig. 40-39). In clinical practice, at least in the older preterm infant, the condition of white matter is judged by its echogenic potential as compared with that of the choroid plexus. Generally, the echogenicity found in early periventricular leukomalacia is similar in intensity to that of the choroid plexus. The echogenicity is bilateral, but slightly asymmetric in appearance, can be sharply delineated, and may have nodular components. This has to be differentiated from normal peritrigonal flaring, which is perfectly symmetric and has a radial appearance. Evolution of such hyperechogenicity can be twofold, either complete disappearance or evolution into cysts and/or ventricular dilation. Cyst formation is typical during the second week (10 to 40 days) after the insult. de Vries and associates[26] postulated an ultrasound-based classification for PVL of four grades. Increasing grades are associated with increasing neurodevelopmental handicap.

Grade I is defined as transient (persisting less than 7 days) periventricular densities without cyst formation. If cysts develop and are few in number, localized primarily in the frontal and frontoparietal white matter, this is classified as grade II. When they are widespread and extend into the parieto-occipital region, they are referred to as grade III; these may grow and gradually disappear, leaving an irregularly dilated lateral ventricle. Grade IV cysts are present all the way into the subcortical area and resemble porencephaly (Table 40-3). In a pooled analysis based on data from 15 published studies, 11% of infants with small, 35% of those with medium, and 60% of those with large ultrasound-defined white matter echolucencies had an intelligence or developmental index less than 70,[40] which outlines the importance of potentially associated microstructural alterations in cortical development after white matter injury. Ultrasound can be viewed as the ideal mode of imaging to detect cystic PVL, but has very limited value for detecting diffuse white matter injury and the processes leading to encephalopathy of prematurity as shown in studies comparing neonatal sonography with MRI.[18,25,49,91]

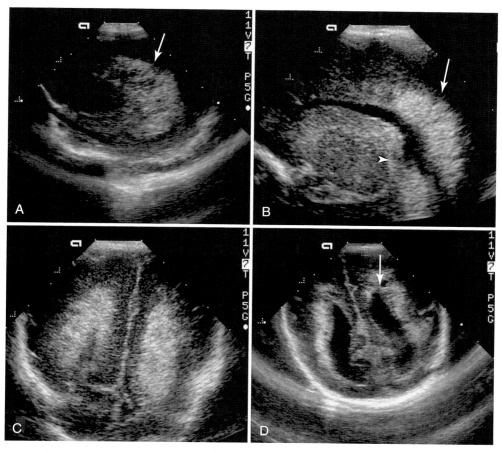

Figure 40–39. Ultrasound scans of periventricular echodensity in a preterm infant born at 27 weeks' gestational age with premature rupture of membranes and neonatal sepsis. Note: bilateral echodensities in sagittal view at 5 days of age (**A, B;** *arrows*) with echogenicity of similar intensity to echogenicity of choroid plexus (**B;** *arrowhead*). **C,** Bilateral echodensities in coronal view. **D,** Cystic transformation noted by echolucency developing at 12 days in sagittal view (*arrow*).

TABLE 40-3	Ultrasound Classification of Periventricular Leukomalacia[26]
Grade I	Transient periventricular echodensities (PVE) (<7 days)
Grade II	PVE evolving into localized frontoparietal cystic lesions
Grade III	PVE evolving into extensive periventricular cystic lesions
Grade IV	Echodensities evolving into extensive periventricular and subcortical cysts

Classification needs longitudinal assessment with daily to weekly ultrasound evaluations.

Conventional Magnetic Resonance Imaging

Conventional T1- and T2-weighted imaging can show signal abnormalities in the periventricular white matter that are different from the cystic lesions detected by ultrasound. The typical conventional MRI pattern in the subacute phase consists of punctate periventricular areas of T1 signal hyperintensities and T2 signal hypointensities (Fig. 40-40). The precise neuropathologic correlate of these signal abnormalities is not completely known, but may be due to some hemorrhagic component of the lesions. The abnormal signal most likely represents the cellular reaction of glial cells and macrophages, which are known to contain lipid droplets (see microglia activation), accounting for the high signal intensity in T1-weighted MR images.[95] These abnormalities have been associated with the presence of markers of oxidative stress in the cerebrospinal fluid (CSF).[48] Most of these lesions disappear by term age and their significance for later neurodevelopmental problems is still unclear.[29]

Conventional MRI features of chronic white matter injury in the immature brain are characterized either by cysts comparable to ultrasound, but also and more importantly, by a persistent high signal intensity of the white matter in T2-weighted images representing diffuse white matter injury

(Fig. 40-41).[43] This imaging characteristic is later associated with thinning of the corpus callosum and loss of white matter volume, resulting in deep prominent sulci (see later). In several studies on the preterm infant brain, diffuse excessive high signal intensity (DEHSI) in the cerebral white matter on T2-weighted imaging was reported to be present in up to 40% to 75% of preterm infants with low birthweight imaged at term (Fig. 40-42).[63] MRI is further ideally equipped to assess delayed myelination. The absence of myelination in the posterior limb of the internal capsule (missing T1 high signal intensity, T2 low signal intensity) at term age is a good indicator of later neuromotor impairment (Fig. 40-43).[2,10,21]

Woodward and associates[112] in a population-based study showed that 21% of preterm infants at term age had MR-defined moderate to severe white matter abnormalities, but an even larger proportion of 49% had gray matter abnormalities characterized by poor cortical development. Furthermore, about half of the preterm infants showed mild white matter abnormalities, and these infants had only marginal mental developmental indices at age 2 years (Table 40-4).

Diffusion Magnetic Resonance Imaging

Diffusion-weighted MR imaging (DWI) or diffusion tensor imaging (DTI) measures the self-diffusion of water. The two primary pieces of information available from DWI studies—water apparent diffusion coefficient (ADC) and diffusion anisotropy measures—change dramatically during development, reflecting underlying changes in tissue water content and cytoarchitecture (see Part 1 of this chapter).

DWI parameters also change in response to brain injury. ADC decreases in acute injury and possible mechanisms leading to this decrease are: decrease in extracellular fluid due to cellular swelling (cytotoxic edema), swelling of mitochondria and reduction of cytoplasmic diffusion, axonal swelling, and other mechanisms such as membrane changes due to fatty acid peroxidation.

Early assessment of periventricular white matter in preterm infants with DWI can reveal bilateral periventricular diffusion restriction similar to the typical distribution of PVL

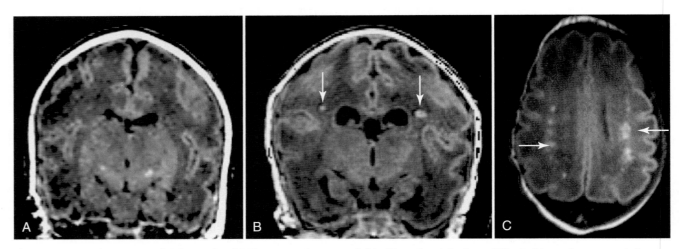

Figure 40–40. Conventional T1-weighted MR images in coronal (**A, B**) and axial plane (**C**). **A,** Normal preterm infant at 31 weeks' gestational age. **B, C,** Bilateral periventricular lesions with high signal intensities in a preterm infant of 31 weeks' gestational age (*arrows*).

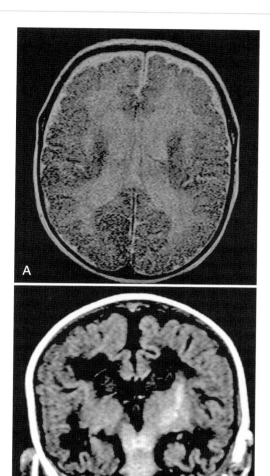

Figure 40–41. Conventional T2-weighted MRI (**A**) and inversion recovery MRI with T1-weighted signal characteristics (**B**) in an ex-preterm infant of 25 weeks' gestational age imaged at 40 weeks' gestational age, with severe bronchopulmonary dysplasia and repetitive episodes of severe hypoxia. **A,** Widespread markedly increased T2 signal intensity in the central white matter. **B,** Low signal intensity on the inversion recovery image in the central white matter, representative of diffuse white matter injury.

when ultrasound and conventional MRI show no or nonspecific abnormalities (Fig. 40-44).[14] A reduced ADC in an otherwise normal preterm brain is considered an early indicator of white matter damage (just as a reduced ADC is seen shortly after the onset of an acute cerebral ischemic lesion in adults). The typical histologic changes in the acute phase of PVL outlined earlier are characterized by some of the same mechanisms leading to restriction of water diffusivity. These changes are responsible for the diffusion changes described earlier in that they considerably change the microstructure of white matter and therefore change water diffusivity.

The chronic phase of white matter injury again is characterized by cyst formation (Figs. 40-45 and 40-46) and by T2-weighted hyperintensities of the white matter or DEHSI for which studies demonstrate higher ADC values in the area of T2 hyperintensities, which confirms the locally higher

tissue water content in those areas (see Fig. 40-42).[20,74] These high ADC values are similar to those seen in the very immature healthy white matter; therefore a potential explanation for the failure of ADC to decline from high levels in the extremely premature infant to lower levels in the term infant in the presence of DEHSI might be related to prior injury with destruction of normal cellular elements (i.e., preoligodendrocytes) as discussed in the models of white matter injury.[107] Further quantitative measures of diffusion at term among premature infants with perinatal white matter lesions, when compared with preterm infants without white matter injury, showed lower anisotropy values in the area of the previous injury (i.e., central periventricular white matter), but also in the underlying posterior limb of internal capsule (Fig. 40-47).[44,76] The lower anisotropy in the injured cerebral white matter suggests that white matter fiber tracts were destroyed or their subsequent development was impaired. Whether this effect involves axon bundles per se, their packing density, or their encasement by premyelinating oligodendroglia is unknown. The lower anisotropy in the internal capsule further suggests a disturbance in the development of the descending corticospinal tracts.[42] Fiber tracking is another technique applied to the developing brain to study quantitative assessment of specific pathway maturation in white matter.[110] Berman and coworkers[12] showed significant differences in the maturational changes in fractional anisotropy and transverse diffusion between the motor and the somatosensory pathway in premature infants between 30 and 40 weeks' gestational age. This approach further allowed the measurement of diffusion changes across multiple levels of the functional tract and, therefore, the assessment of myelination progress over a given white matter fiber tract.[12,83]

The subsequent neurologic deficits after cerebral white matter injury are grouped together under the term of cerebral palsy. Structural correlates of cerebral palsy have been assessed using DTI.[41] Tract-specific evaluation of children with cerebral palsy after PVL identified most frequent alterations in white matter fiber tract development in the retrolenticular part of the internal capsule, posterior thalamic radiation, and superior corona radiata, and in commissural fibers of the corpus callosum.[75]

The clinical relevance of injury and related modification of white matter architecture detected in this fashion is not yet known, and long-term follow-up studies of prematurely born children are currently underway linking functional outcome to structural white matter development assessed by DTI.[5,10,19,32,100]

DWI with diffusion tensor analysis has provided new insights into microstructural white matter development and seems to be an ideal tool to assess alteration of white matter pathways in neurologic disease.

Magnetic Resonance Spectroscopy

One of the essential contributors to the progress in noninvasive detection of tissue metabolism and in vivo biochemistry in recent years has been magnetic resonance spectroscopy (MRS), which gives specific chemical information on the biochemistry of numerous intracellular metabolites. The biochemical characteristics of white matter damage in preterm

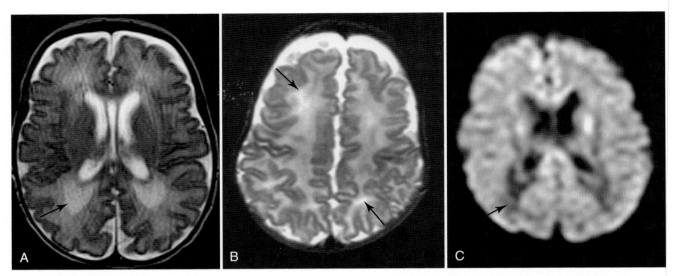

Figure 40–42. A, B, Conventional T2-weighted MRI illustrating the typical diffuse excessive high signal intensity (DEHSI) *(arrows)* associated with chronic phase white matter injury. C, T2-weighted hypersignal *(arrow)* is associated with low intensity on diffusion-weighted images.

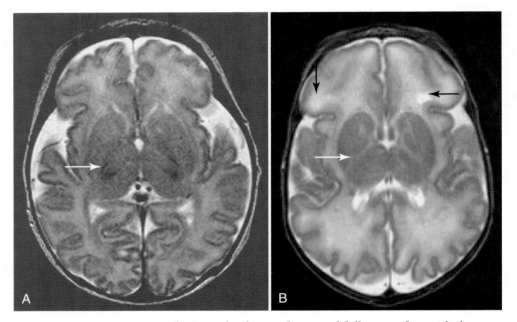

Figure 40–43. A, Conventional T2-weighted MRI of a normal full-term infant with thin area of low signal in the T2-weighted MRI corresponding to myelin deposition in the posterior limb of the internal capsule *(arrow)*. B, Corresponding T2-weighted MRI with diffuse white matter lesions *(black arrows)* and missing signal change in the posterior limb *(white arrow)* of the internal capsule, indicating delay in myelination.

infants have been studied in vivo using MRS.[35,92] Similar to the high diagnostic value of MRS in term asphyxia, MRS in acute phase immature white matter injury can detect indicators of anaerobic glycolysis with increased intracerebral lactate.[86] Data suggest that white matter damage in the preterm infant studied around term gestational age resulted in high lactate-to-creatinine and high myoinositol-to-creatinine ratios.[92] The increased presence of lactate at this chronic stage was not associated with changes in pH,[92] whereas N-acetylaspartate as a marker of neuroaxonal integrity was reduced in the damaged periventricular white matter.[35] As outlined in part 1 of this chapter on brain development, astrocytes further play a variety of complex nutritive and supportive roles in relation to neuronal metabolic homeostasis. For example, astrocytes take up glutamate and convert it to glutamine. This removal of glutamate from the

TABLE 40–4   **Neurodevelopmental Outcomes at Two Years' Corrected Age**

Outcome Measure	WHITE-MATTER ABNORMALITY, n = 167				P Value
	None n = 47 (28%)	Mild n = 85 (50%)	Moderate n = 29 (17%)	Severe n = 6 (3.5%)	
MDI score (mean ± SD)	92.50 ± 15.63	85.32 ± 15.46	77.93 ± 19.16	69.67 ± 25.30	<0.001
Severe cognitive delay (%)	7	15	30	50	0.008
PDI score (mean ± SD)	94.63 ± 13.45	90.73 ± 12.75	80.11 ± 18.18	56.17 ± 23.50	<0.001
Severe motor delay (%)	4	5	26	67	<0.001
Cerebral palsy (%)	2	6	24	67	<0.001
Neurosensory impairment (%)	4	9	21	50	0.003
Any neurodevelopmental impairment (%)*	15	26	48	67	<0.001
Number of impairments	0.22 ± 0.47	0.40 ± 0.71	1.15 ± 1.20	2.33 ± 1.97	<0.001

*Presence of severe impairment defined as MDI or PDI score less than 70, cerebral palsy, or hearing or visual impairment.
MDI, mental development index; PDI, psychomotor development index.
Adapted from Woodward LJ, Anderson PJ, Austin NC, et al: Neonatal MRI to predict neurodevelopmental outcomes in preterm infants, *N Engl J Med* 355:685, 2006.

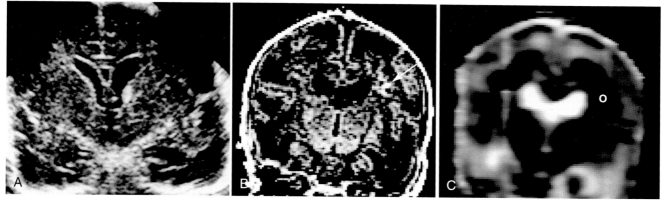

Figure 40–44. Ultrasound scan (**A**) and T1-weighted MR image (**B**) in coronal plane in an infant of 30 weeks' gestational age at 5 days' postpartum age. **A,** Negative ultrasonographic scan. **B,** Small, possibly hemorrhagic lesion (*arrow*) in the left periventricular white matter. Apparent diffusion coefficient maps in coronal plane (**C**) and axial plane (**D**) from diffusion-weighted image illustrate bilateral periventricular lesions with low D_{av} (0.8 $\mu m^2/ms$; *circle*) indicating acute periventricular leukomalacia.   (*In part from Inder T, et al: Early detection of periventricular leukomalacia by diffusion-weighted magnetic resonance imaging techniques,* J Pediatr *134:631 1999.*)

extracellular space protects surrounding cells from glutamate excitotoxicity. Glutamate uptake into astrocytes further stimulates glycolysis within the astrocyte with production of lactate that can be used by neurons as energy substrate.[85] Given that chronic phase white matter injury is characterized by widespread cerebral white matter astrocytosis, this change in metabolite composition might be an expression of altered cellular composition and substrate use.

Other metabolites become visible with short echo-time spectroscopy such as the macromolecules/lipids at 0.9 ppm and 1.3 ppm (see Fig. 40-18). These resonances show important changes in adult hypoxia-ischemia[34] and in experimental data on in vitro apoptosis.[13] Preliminary data suggest that these metabolites are also present in acute periventricular white matter injury of the immature brain and might represent metabolites

from membrane peroxidation. Consistent with the observation of these resonances, one study found elevated neonatal levels of lipid peroxidation and oxidative protein products in cerebrospinal fluid of infants with PVL documented by MRI.[48]

IMPAIRMENT OF BRAIN GROWTH AND LONG-TERM DEVELOPMENT

Periventricular white matter injury has been strongly associated with long-term neurodevelopmental deficits in preterm infants.[81,87,88] The significance of abnormalities in myelination in relation to functional (neurologic) development has been extensively studied. Correlation was found between neurodevelopmental delay and delay in myelination.[25,36,96,111]

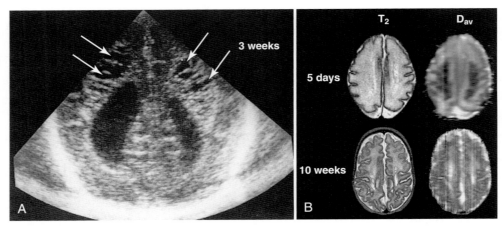

Figure 40–45. Ultrasound scan (**A**) of bilateral cystic periventricular leukomalacia (*arrows*). **B**, The evolution of the lesions identified on DWI (D_{av}) at 5 days of age with the development of cystic lesions on T2-weighted MRI and apparent diffusion coefficient map (D_{av}) at 10 weeks of age. (*In part from Inder T, et al: Early detection of periventricular leukomalacia by diffusion-weighted magnetic resonance imaging techniques,* J Pediatr *134:631 1999.*)

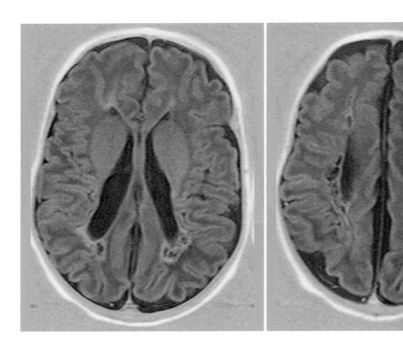

Figure 40–46. Axial inversion recovery MR images with T1-weighted contrast illustrating chronic phase of periventricular leukomalacia with multiple bilateral cystic lesions with high signal gliotic scars and calcifications in the periphery of the cystic lesions. Note the loss of white matter volume with cerebral atrophy.

The major long-term morbidity of the focal component of periventricular leukomalacia is spastic diplegia. This motor disturbance has as its central feature a spastic paresis of the extremities with greater effect on lower than upper limbs. More severe lesions with lateral and posterior extension into the centrum semiovale and corona radiata are associated with effects on the upper extremities or visual and cognitive deficits.

The development of three-dimensional MRI methods combined with image postprocessing techniques has allowed volumetric assessment of brain development and an absolute quantitation of myelination.[17,45] These techniques allow exact definition of brain volume and can, therefore,

accurately monitor brain growth and measure cerebrospinal fluid volume and changes in cortical gray matter volume. Three-dimensional MRI volumetric techniques were used to evaluate the effect on subsequent brain development of early white matter injury in premature infants. Three groups of infants were studied at 40 weeks' postconceptional age: premature infants with preceding evidence for periventricular white matter injury by cranial ultrasound and MRI; premature infants who had no prior evidence of white matter injury; and control term infants (Fig. 40-48).

In premature infants with preceding white matter injury, the volume of myelinated white matter at term was significantly lower than in premature infants without prior white

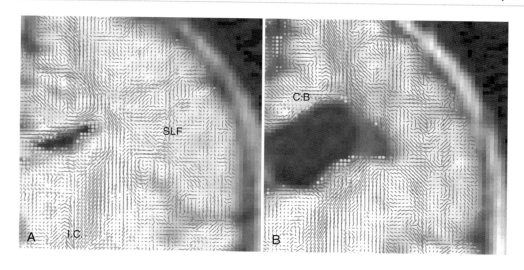

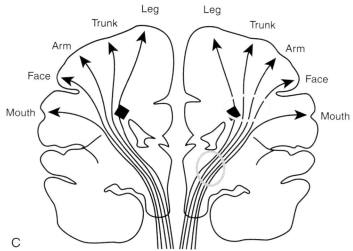

Figure 40–47. See color insert. Diffusion vector maps overlaid on coronal diffusion-weighted images for a premature infant at term with no white matter injury (**A**) and a premature infant at term with perinatal white matter injury (**B**). The posterior limb of the internal capsule (I.C.) in **A** shows more homologous directed vectors that are longer and more densely packed than in the internal capsule of **B**. Anteroposterior-oriented white matter fibers in the area of the superior longitudinal fasciculus (SLF; yellow and green dots with yellow representing higher anisotropy than green) in **A** indicate the presence of fiber bundles that are missing or are less prominent in **B**. The only discrete anteroposterior fiber bundles that definitely are present in **B** are the cingulate bundles (C.B.). Fibers of the corona radiata appear less well organized in **B** than **A**. Loss of axons in the central white matter (*yellow area*) and the posterior limb (*red area*) will result in neuromotor disturbances illustrated schematically in **C**. (**A**, **B**, *From Hüppi P, Murphy B, Maier S, et al: Microstructural brain development after perinatal cerebral white matter injury assessed by diffusion tensor magnetic resonance imaging,* Pediatrics *107:455, 2001.*) **C**, *Schema reproduced from Volpe JJ:* Neurology of the newborn, *4th ed, Philadelphia, 2001, Saunders, p 362.*)

matter injury and infants born at term, providing a measure of the degree of delay of myelination. Furthermore, this study showed a marked decrease in cortical gray matter volume in preterm infants with prior periventricular white matter injury indicating impaired cerebral cortical development after early white matter injury. This finding may explain the intellectual deficits associated with periventricular leukomalacia in preterm infants.[51] Assessing moderately preterm

infants without signs of white matter injury revealed cortical development similar to that of full-term infants.[116] Regional assessment of white matter myelination in preterm infants further revealed particular delay in myelination in the central and posterior part of the brain.[73] When assessing cerebellar volume at term there was a significant reduction of cerebellar volume of preterm infants when compared to term infants.[58] Unilateral cerebral white matter lesions resulted in contralateral

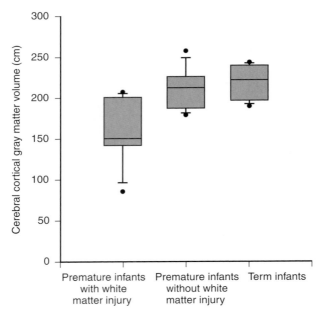

Figure 40–48. Figure illustrating the effects of perinatal white matter injury on subsequent cortical gray matter development at term with a significantly lower cortical gray matter volume determined by three-dimensional MRI with postacquisition image analysis in a group of preterm infants with perinatal white matter injury compared with control preterm and full-term infants. (*From Inder T, et al: The postmigrational development of polymicrogyria documented by magnetic resonance imaging from 31 weeks' postconceptional age,* Ann Neurol *46:755, 1999, with permission.*)

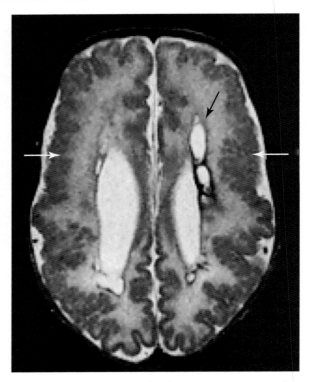

Figure 40–49. Axial T2-weighted MRI in a preterm infant of 25 weeks' gestational age at birth imaged at 31 weeks' gestational age showing cystic lesions in the periventricular white matter (*black arrow*) associated with bilateral polymicrogyria (*white arrows*). (*From Inder T, et al: The postmigrational development of polymicrogyria documented by magnetic resonance imaging from 31 weeks' postconceptional age,* Ann Neurol *45:798, 1999, with permission.*)

reduction of cerebellar volume indicating a trophic interplay from cerebrocerebellar connectivity.[59]

Long-term follow-up studies of preterm infants have confirmed the permanent character of these disruptive/adaptive changes in brain development. Evaluations of 8-year-old preterm infants with volumetric brain assessment showed persistence of cortical gray matter reduction in preterm infants accompanied by a reduction in the volume of hippocampus, which correlated with cognitive scores indicating long-term functional consequences. Both cortical volume and cortical thickness were shown to be reduced in 15-year-old adolescents born prematurely.[68] Studying a larger cohort of preterm subjects at the same age, Nosarti and colleagues[80] noted widespread alterations in both gray and white matter volumes throughout the brain. Of note, volumes of several gray matter regions, including the middle temporal gyrus, superior temporal gyrus and sensorimotor region, and precentral and postcentral gyri were linearly related to gestational age for the preterm group. Furthermore, decreases in both gray and white matter volumes in the middle temporal gyrus were associated with cognitive impairment in the preterm group.

Human brain development is characterized by several interrelated steps. Neuronal and radial glial proliferation and migration are early events in brain development that are followed by a series of organizational events that result in the complex circuitry of axons and dendrites characteristic of the human brain. Elaboration of dendritic and axonal ramifications and attainment of proper alignment and orientation is most likely one of the driving forces for the folding of the cerebral cortex during development.[105] Such primary cortical folding may be influenced by preterm birth and intrauterine growth restriction. Infants with early white matter lesions have shown a trend toward increased sulcation in the overlying cortex. Early alteration of white matter connectivity, ensuing disruption to the white matter circuits and to the subcortical plate may, therefore, alter subsequent density, survival, and organization of cortical neurons. In severe cases, secondary polymicrogyria after primarily early white matter injury has been described (Fig. 40-49).[50] Neuropathologic study of cerebral cortex in preterm infants has revealed cortical dysplasia in areas overlying destroyed white matter.[66] These abnormalities of cortical development may be found secondary to disturbances of afferent input to and efferent output from areas of the cortex, as caused by disruption of the respective white matter axons.[66] Cortical volume changes in three-dimensional MRI[51] as described earlier are probably representative of these cortical alterations and may explain the increased risk of cognitive impairment and epilepsy in infants with classic motor deficits (spastic diplegia) after injury to the immature white matter.

REFERENCES

1. Acarin L, Gonzalez B, Castro AJ, Castellano B: Primary cortical glial reaction versus secondary thalamic glial response in the excitotoxically injured young brain: microglial/macrophage response and major histocompatibility complex class I and II expression, *Neuroscience* 89:549, 1999.

2. Aida N, Nishimura G, Hachiya Y, et al: MR imaging of perinatal brain damage: comparison of clinical outcome with initial and follow-up MR findings [see comments], *AJNR Am J Neuroradiol* 19:1909, 1998.

3. Anderson CA, Higgins RJ, Waldvogel AS, Osburn BI: Tropism of border disease virus for oligodendrocytes in ovine fetal brain cell cultures, *Am J Vet Res* 48:822, 1987.

4. Andrews T, Zhang P, Bhat NR: TNF alpha potentiates IFN-gamma-induced cell death in oligodendrocyte progenitors, *J Neurosci Res* 54:574, 1998.

5. Anjari M, Srinivasan L, Allsop JM, et al: Diffusion tensor imaging with tract-based spatial statistics reveals local white matter abnormalities in preterm infants, *Neuroimage* 35:1021, 2007.

6. Back SA, Gan X, Li Y, et al: Maturation-dependent vulnerability of oligodendrocytes to oxidative stress-induced death caused by glutathione depletion, *J Neurosci* 18:6241, 1998.

7. Back SA, Han BH, Luo NL, et al: Selective vulnerability of late oligodendrocyte progenitors to hypoxia- ischemia, *J Neurosci* 22:455, 2002.

8. Back SA, Luo NL, Borenstein NS, et al: Late oligodendrocyte progenitors coincide with the developmental window of vulnerability for human perinatal white matter injury, *J Neurosci* 21:1302, 2001.

9. Banker B, Larroche J: Periventricular leukomalacia of infancy, *Arch Neurol* 7:386, 1962.

10. Bassi L, Ricci D, Volzone A, et al: Probabilistic diffusion tractography of the optic radiations and visual function in preterm infants at term equivalent age, *Brain* 131:573, 2008.

11. Baud O, Daire JL, Dalmaz Y, et al: Gestational hypoxia induces white matter damage in neonatal rats: a new model of periventricular leukomalacia, *Brain Pathol* 14:1, 2004.

12. Berman JI, Mukherjee P, Partridge SC, et al: Quantitative diffusion tensor MRI fiber tractography of sensorimotor white matter development in premature infants, *Neuroimage* 27:862, 2005.

13. Blankenberg FG, Storrs RW, Naumovski L, et al: Detection of apoptotic cell death by proton nuclear magnetic resonance spectroscopy, *Blood* 87:1951, 1996.

14. Bozzao A, Di Paolo A, Mazzoleni C, et al: Diffusion-weighted MR imaging in the early diagnosis of periventricular leukomalacia, *Eur Radiol* 13:1571, 2003.

15. Cai Z, Pan ZL, Pang Y, et al: Cytokine induction in fetal rat brains and brain injury in neonatal rats after maternal lipopolysaccharide administration, *Pediatr Res* 47:64, 2000.

16. Casaccia-Bonnefil P: Cell death in the oligodendrocyte lineage: a molecular perspective of life/death decisions in development and disease, *Glia* 29:124, 2000.

17. Caviness VS, Kennedy DN, Richelme C, et al: The human brain age 7–11 years: a volumetric analysis based upon magnetic resonance images, *Cereb Cortex* 6:726, 1996.

18. Childs AM, Cornette L, Ramenghi LA, et al: Magnetic resonance and cranial ultrasound characteristics of periventricular white matter abnormalities in newborn infants, *Clin Radiol* 56:647, 2001.

19. Constable RT, Ment LR, Vohr BR, et al: Prematurely born children demonstrate white matter microstructural differences at 12 years of age, relative to term control subjects: an investigation of group and gender effects, *Pediatrics* 121:306, 2008.

20. Counsell SJ, Allsop JM, Harrison MC, et al: Diffusion-weighted imaging of the brain in preterm infants with focal and diffuse white matter abnormality, *Pediatrics* 112:1, 2003.

21. de Vries LS, Groenendaal F, van Haastert IC, et al: Asymmetrical myelination of the posterior limb of the internal capsule in infants with periventricular haemorrhagic infarction: an early predictor of hemiplegia, *Neuropediatrics* 30:314, 1999.

22. Debillon T, Gras-Leguen C, Leroy S, et al: Patterns of cerebral inflammatory response in a rabbit model of intrauterine infection-mediated brain lesion: intrauterine infection induces programmed cell death in rabbit periventricular white matter, *Brain Res Dev Brain Res* 145:39, 2003.

23. Deng W, Rosenberg PA, Volpe JJ, Jensen FE: Calcium-permeable AMPA/kainate receptors mediate toxicity and preconditioning by oxygen-glucose deprivation in oligodendrocyte precursors, *Proc Natl Acad Sci U S A* 100:6801, 2003.

24. Derrick M, Luo NL, Bregman JC, et al: Preterm fetal hypoxia-ischemia causes hypertonia and motor deficits in the neonatal rabbit: a model for human cerebral palsy? *J Neurosci* 24:24, 2004.

25. de Vries L, Eken P, Groenendaal F, et al: Correlation between the degree of periventricular leukomalacia diagnosed using cranial ultrasound and MRI later in infancy in children with cerebral palsy, *Neuropediatrics* 24:263, 1993.

26. de Vries L, Eken P, Dubowitz L: The spectrum of leukomalacia using cranial ultrasound, *Behav Brain Res* 49:1, 1992.

27. Dommergues MA, Patkai J, Renauld JC, et al: Proinflammatory cytokines and interleukin-9 exacerbate excitotoxic lesions of the newborn murine neopallium, *Ann Neurol* 47:54, 2000.

28. Dommergues MA, Plaisant F, Verney C, Gressens P: Early microglial activation following neonatal excitotoxic brain damage in mice: a potential target for neuroprotection, *Neuroscience* 121:619, 2003.

29. Dyet LE, Kennea N, Counsell SJ, et al: Natural history of brain lesions in extremely preterm infants studied with serial magnetic resonance imaging from birth and neurodevelopmental assessment, *Pediatrics* 118:536, 2006.

30. Eklind S, Mallard C, Leverin AL, et al: Bacterial endotoxin sensitizes the immature brain to hypoxic—ischaemic injury, *Eur J Neurosci* 13:1101, 2001.

31. Gilles FH, Murphy SF: Perinatal telencephalic leucoencephalopathy, *J Neurol Neurosurg Psychiatry* 32:404, 1969.

32. Gimenez M, Miranda MJ, Born AP, et al: Accelerated cerebral white matter development in preterm infants: a voxel-based morphometry study with diffusion tensor MR imaging, *Neuroimage* 41:728, 2008.

33. Golden J, Gilles F, Rudewilli R, Leviton A: Frequency of neuropathological abnormalities in very low birth weight infants, *J Neuropathol Exper Neurol* 56:472, 1997.

34. Graham GD, Hwang JH, Rothman DL, Prichard JW: Spectroscopic assessment of alterations in macromolecule and small-molecule metabolites in human brain after stroke, *Stroke* 32:2797, 2001.

35. Groenendaal F, van de Grond J, Eken P, et al: Early cerebral proton MRS and neurodevelopmental outcome in infants with cystic leukomalacia, *Dev Med Child Neurol* 39:373, 1997.

36. Guit G, Van der Bor M, Den Ouden L, Wondergrem J: Prediction of neurodevelopmental outcome in the preterm infant: MR-staged myelination compared with cranial US, *Radiology* 175:107, 1990.

37. Hagberg H, Peebles D, Mallard C: Models of white matter injury: comparison of infectious, hypoxic-ischemic, and excitotoxic insults, *Ment Retard Dev Disabil Res Rev* 8:30, 2002.

38. Haynes RL, Folkerth RD, Keefe RJ, et al: Nitrosative and oxidative injury to premyelinating oligodendrocytes in periventricular leukomalacia, *J Neuropathol Exp Neurol* 62:441, 2003.

39. Hirayama A, Okoshi Y, Hachiya Y, et al: Early immunohistochemical detection of axonal damage and glial activation in extremely immature brains with periventricular leukomalacia, *Clin Neuropathol* 20:87, 2001.

40. Holling EE, Leviton A: Characteristics of cranial ultrasound white-matter echolucencies that predict disability: a review, *Dev Med Child Neurol* 41:136, 1999.

41. Hoon AH Jr, Belsito KM, Nagae-Poetscher LM: Neuroimaging in spasticity and movement disorders, *J Child Neurol* 18 Suppl 1:S25, 2003.

42. Hoon AH Jr, Lawrie WT Jr, Melhem ER, et al: Diffusion tensor imaging of periventricular leukomalacia shows affected sensory cortex white matter pathways, *Neurology* 59:752, 2002.

43. Hüppi PS: Advances in postnatal neuroimaging: relevance to pathogenesis and treatment of brain injury, *Clin Perinatol* 29:827, 2002.

44. Hüppi P, Murphy B, Maier S, et al: Microstructural brain development after perinatal cerebral white matter injury assessed by diffusion tensor magnetic resonance imaging, *Pediatrics* 107:455, 2001.

45. Hüppi P, Warfield S, Kikinis R,, et al: Quantitative magnetic resonance imaging of brain development in premature and mature newborns, *Ann Neurol* 43(2):224, 1998.

46. Iai M, Takashima S: Thalamocortical development of parvalbumin neurons in normal and periventricular leukomalacia brains, *Neuropediatrics* 30:14, 1999.

47. Inage YW, Itoh M, Takashima S: Correlation between cerebrovascular maturity and periventricular leukomalacia, *Pediatr Neurol* 22:204, 2000.

48. Inder T, Mocatta T, Darlow B, et al: Elevated free radical products in the cerebrospinal fluid of VLBW infants with cerebral white matter injury, *Pediatr Res* 52:213, 2002.

49. Inder TE, Anderson NJ, Spencer C, et al: White matter injury in the premature infant: a comparison between serial cranial sonographic and MR findings at term, *AJNR Am J Neuroradiol* 24:805, 2003.

50. Inder TE, Huppi PS, Zientara GP, et al: The postmigrational development of polymicrogyria documented by magnetic resonance imaging from 31 weeks' postconceptional age, *Ann Neurol* 45:798, 1999.

51. Inder T, Hüppi P, Warfield S, et al: Periventricular white matter injury in the premature infant is associated with a reduction in cerebral cortical gray matter volume at term, *Ann Neurol* 46:755, 1999.

52. Jensen FE: The role of glutamate receptor maturation in perinatal seizures and brain injury, *Int J Dev Neurosci* 20:339, 2002.

53. Kadhim H, Tabarki B, Verellen G, et al: Inflammatory cytokines in the pathogenesis of periventricular leukomalacia, *Neurology* 56:1278, 2001.

54. Karadottir R, Cavelier P, Bergersen LH, Attwell D: NMDA receptors are expressed in oligodendrocytes and activated in ischaemia, *Nature* 438:1162, 2005.

55. Kostovic I, Judas M: Prolonged coexistence of transient and permanent circuitry elements in the developing cerebral cortex of fetuses and preterm infants, *Dev Med Child Neurol* 48:388, 2006.

56. Leviton A, Gilles F: Ventriculomegaly, delayed myelination, white matter hypoplasia, and periventricular leukomalacia. How are they related? *Pediatr Neurol* 15:127, 1996.

57. Leviton A, Paneth N: White matter damage in preterm newborns—an epidemiologic perspective, *Early Hum Dev* 24:1, 1990.

58. Limperopoulos C, Soul JS, Gauvreau K, et al: Late gestation cerebellar growth is rapid and impeded by premature birth, *Pediatrics* 115:688, 2005.

59. Limperopoulos C, Soul JS, Haidar H, et al: Impaired trophic interactions between the cerebellum and the cerebrum among preterm infants, *Pediatrics* 116:844, 2005.

60. Little WJ: The influence of abnormal parturition, difficult labours, premature birth, and asphyxia neonatorum on the mental and physical condition of the child, especially in relation to deformities, *Trans Obstet Soc London* 3, 293–344, 1861.

61. Lodygensky GA, Rademaker K, Zimine S, et al: Structural and functional brain development after hydrocortisone treatment for neonatal chronic lung disease, *Pediatrics* 116:1, 2005.

62. Loeliger M, Watson CS, Reynolds JD, et al: Extracellular glutamate levels and neuropathology in cerebral white matter following repeated umbilical cord occlusion in the near term fetal sheep, *Neuroscience* 116:705, 2003.

63. Maalouf EF, Duggan PJ, Counsell SJ, et al: Comparison of findings on cranial ultrasound and magnetic resonance imaging in preterm infants, *Pediatrics* 107:719, 2001.

64. Mallard C, Welin AK, Peebles D, et al: White matter injury following systemic endotoxemia or asphyxia in the fetal sheep, *Neurochem Res* 28:215, 2003.

65. Mallard E, Rees S, Stringer M, et al: Effects of chronic placental insufficiency on brain development in fetal sheep, *Pediatr Res* 43:262, 1998.

66. Marin-Padilla M: Developmental neuropathology and impact of perinatal brain damage. II: White matter lesions of the neocortex, *J Neuropathol Exp Neurol* 56:219, 1997.

67. Marret S, Gressens P, Evrard P: Arrest of neuronal migration by excitatory amino acids in hamster developing brain, *Proc Natl Acad Sci U S A* 93:15463, 1996.

68. Martinussen M, Fischl B, Larsson HB, et al: Cerebral cortex thickness in 15-year-old adolescents with low birth weight measured by an automated MRI-based method, *Brain* 128:2588, 2005.

69. McDonald JW, Silverstein FS, Johnston MV: Neurotoxicity of N-methyl-D-aspartate is markedly enhanced in developing rat central nervous system, *Brain Res* 459:200, 1988.

70. McQuillen PS, Sheldon RA, Shatz CJ, Ferriero DM: Selective vulnerability of subplate neurons after early neonatal hypoxia-ischemia, *J Neurosci* 23:3308, 2003.

71. Merrill JE, Ignarro LJ, Sherman MP, et al: Microglial cell cytotoxicity of oligodendrocytes is mediated through nitric oxide, *J Immunol* 151:2132, 1993.

72. Mesples BM, Plaisant F, Fontaine RH, Gressens P: Pathophysiology of neonatal brain lesions: lessons from animal models of excitotoxicity, *Acta Paediatr* 94(2):185, 2005.

73. Mewes AU, Huppi PS, Als H, et al: Regional brain development in serial magnetic resonance imaging of low-risk preterm infants, *Pediatrics* 118:23, 2006.

74. Miller SP, Vigneron DB, Henry RG, et al: Serial quantitative diffusion tensor MRI of the premature brain: development in newborns with and without injury, *J Magn Reson Imaging* 16:621, 2002.

75. Nagae LM, Hoon AH Jr, Stashinko E, et al: Diffusion tensor imaging in children with periventricular leukomalacia: variability of injuries to white matter tracts, *AJNR Am J Neuroradiol* 28:1213, 2007.

76. Neil J, Miller J, Mukherjee P, Huppi PS: Diffusion tensor imaging of normal and injured developing human brain—a technical review, *NMR Biomed* 15:543, 2002.

77. Nelson KB, Dambrosia JM, Grether JK, Phillips TM: Neonatal cytokines and coagulation factors in children with cerebral palsy, *Ann Neurol* 44:665, 1998.

78. Nishiyama A, Komitova M, Suzuki R, Zhu X: Polydendrocytes (NG2 cells): multifunctional cells with lineage plasticity, *Nat Rev Neurosci* 10:9, 2009.

79. Normann E, Lacaze-Masmonteil T, Eaton F, et al: A novel mouse model of *Ureaplasma*-induced perinatal inflammation: effects on lung and brain injury, *Pediatr Res* 65:430, 2009.

80. Nosarti C, Giouroukou E, Healy E, et al: Grey and white matter distribution in very preterm adolescents mediates neurodevelopmental outcome, *Brain* 131:205, 2008.

81. Okumura A, Hayakawa F, Kato T, et al: Developmental outcome and types of chronic-stage EEG abnormalities in preterm infants, *Dev Med Child Neurol* 44:729, 2002.

82. Parrot J: Etude sur le ramollissement de l'éncephale chez le nouveau-né, *Arch Physiol Norm Pat* 5, 59–73, 1873.

83. Partridge SC, Mukherjee P, Berman JI, et al: Tractography-based quantitation of diffusion tensor imaging parameters in white matter tracts of preterm newborns, *J Magn Reson Imaging* 22:467, 2005.

84. Patkai J, Mesples B, Dommergues MA, et al: Deleterious effects of IL-9-activated mast cells and neuroprotection by antihistamine drugs in the developing mouse brain, *Pediatr Res* 50:222, 2001.

85. Pellerin L, Pellegri G, Martin J, Magistretti P: Expression of monocarboxylate transporter mRNAs in mouse brain: support for a distinct role of lactate as an energy substrate for the neonatal vs. the adult brain, *Proc Natl Acad Sci USA* 95:3990, 1998.

86. Penrice J, Cady E, Lorek A, et al: Proton magnetic resonance spectroscopy of the brain in normal preterm and term infants, and early changes after perinatal hypoxia-ischemia, *Pediatr Res* 40:6, 1996.

87. Perlman JM: Neurobehavioral deficits in premature graduates of intensive care— potential medical and neonatal environmental risk factors, *Pediatrics* 108:1339, 2001.

88. Perlman J: White matter injury in the preterm infant: an important determination of abnormal neurodevelopment outcome, *Early Hum Dev* 53:99, 1998.

89. Plaisant F, Clippe A, Vander Stricht D, et al: Recombinant peroxiredoxin 5 protects against excitotoxic brain lesions in newborn mice, *Free Radic Biol Med* 34:862, 2003.

89a. Rangon CM, Fortes S, Lelièvre V, et al: Chronic mild stress during gestation worsens neonatal brain lesions in mice, *J Neurosci* 27:7532, 2007.

90. Rezaie P, Male D: Colonisation of the developing human brain and spinal cord by microglia: a review, *Microsc Res Tech* 45:359, 1999.

91. Rijn AM, Groenendaal F, Beek FJ, et al: Parenchymal brain injury in the preterm infant: comparison of cranial ultrasound, MRI and neurodevelopmental outcome, *Neuropediatrics* 32:80, 2001.

92. Robertson N, Kuint J, Counsell T, et al: Characterization of cerebral white matter damage in the preterm infant using 1H and 31P magnetic resonance spectroscopy, *J Cereb Blood Flow Metab* 20:1446, 2000.

93. Romanko MJ, Zhu C, Bahr BA, et al: Death effector activation in the subventricular zone subsequent to perinatal hypoxia/ischemia, *J Neurochem* 103:1121, 2007.

94. Rydberg, E: Cerebral injury in newborn children consequent on birth trauma: with an inquiry into the normal and pathological anatomy of the neuroglia, *Acta Pathol Microbiol Scand* S7-10, 1–247, 1932.

95. Schouman-Claeys E, Henry-Feugeas MC, Roset F, et al: Periventricular leukomalacia: correlation between MR imaging and autopsy findings during the first 2 months of life, *Radiology* 189:59, 1993.

96. Sie L, Van der Knaap M, van Wezel-Meijler G, Valk J: MRI assessment of myelination of motor and sensory pathways in the brain of preterm and term-born infants, *Neuropediatrics* 28:97, 1997.

97. Sizonenko SV, Camm EJ, Dayer A, Kiss JZ: Glial responses to neonatal hypoxic-ischemic injury in the rat cerebral cortex, *Int J Dev Neurosci* 26:37, 2008.

98. Sizonenko SV, Sirimanne E, Mayall Y, et al: Selective cortical alteration after hypoxic-ischemic injury in the very immature rat brain, *Pediatr Res* 54:263, 2003.

99. Skoff RP, Bessert DA, Barks JD, et al: Hypoxic-ischemic injury results in acute disruption of myelin gene expression and death of oligodendroglial precursors in neonatal mice, *Int J Dev Neurosci* 19:197, 2001.

100. Skranes J, Vangberg TR, Kulseng S, et al: Clinical findings and white matter abnormalities seen on diffusion tensor imaging in adolescents with very low birth weight, *Brain* 130:654, 2007.

101. Smith ME, van der MK, Somera FP: Macrophage and microglial responses to cytokines in vitro: phagocytic activity, proteolytic enzyme release, and free radical production, *J Neurosci Res* 54:68, 1998.

102. Tahraoui SL, Marret S, Bodenant C, et al: Central role of microglia in neonatal excitotoxic lesions of the murine periventricular white matter, *Brain Pathol* 11:56, 2001.

103. Taylor HG, Burant CJ, Holding PA, et al: Sources of variability in sequelae of very low birth weight, *Neuropsychol Dev Cogn Sect C Child Neuropsychol* 8:163, 2002.

104. Turner CP, Seli M, Ment L, et al: A1 adenosine receptors mediate hypoxia-induced ventriculomegaly, *Proc Natl Acad Sci U S A* 100:11718, 2003.

105. Van Essen D: A tension-based theory of morphogenesis and compact wiring in the central nervous system, *Nature* 385:313, 1997.

106. Virchow R: Zur pathologischen Anatomie des Gehirns I Congenitale Encephalitis und Myelitis, *Virchows Arch Pathol Anat* 38, 129–142, 1867.

107. Volpe JJ: Cerebral white matter injury of the premature infant-more common than you think, *Pediatrics* 112:176, 2003.

108. Volpe JJ: Brain injury in premature infants: a complex amalgam of destructive and developmental disturbances, *Lancet Neurol* 8:110, 2009.

109. Volpe J: Subplate neurons-missing link in brain injury of the premature infant? *Pediatrics* 97(1):112, 1996.

110. Watts R, Liston C, Niogi S, Ulug AM: Fiber tracking using magnetic resonance diffusion tensor imaging and its applications to human brain development, *Ment Retard Dev Disabil Res Rev* 9:168, 2003.

111. Welch R, Byrne P: Periventricular leukomalacia (PVL) and myelination, *Pediatr* 86:1002, 1990.

112. Woodward LJ, Anderson PJ, Austin NC, et al: Neonatal MRI to predict neurodevelopmental outcomes in preterm infants, *N Engl J Med* 355:685, 2006.

113. Xu J, Ling EA: Induction of major histocompatibility complex class II antigen on amoeboid microglial cells in early postnatal rats following intraperitoneal injections of lipopolysaccharide or interferon-gamma, *Neurosci Lett* 189:97, 1995.

114. Yoon BH, Kim CJ, Romero R, et al: Experimentally induced intrauterine infection causes fetal brain white matter lesions in rabbits, *Am J Obstet Gynecol* 177:797, 1997.

115. Yoshioka H, Goma H, Sawada T: [Cerebral hypoperfusion and leukomalacia], *No To Hattatsu* 28:128, 1996.

116. Zacharia A, Zimine S, Lovblad KO, et al: Early assessment of brain maturation by MR imaging segmentation in neonates and premature infants, *AJNR Am J Neuroradiol* 27:972, 2006.

PART 3

Intracranial Hemorrhage and Vascular Lesions

Linda S. de Vries

Intracranial Hemorrhage

Even though white matter damage is now considered to be the main determinant of cerebral palsy later in infancy, germinal matrix hemorrhage-intraventricular hemorrhage (GMH-IVH) is still a serious condition in premature infants, associated with a high mortality rate. Large IVHs, complicated by posthemorrhagic ventricular dilation or associated with a unilateral parenchymal hemorrhage, are associated with an increased risk of adverse neurologic sequelae. The widespread use of cranial ultrasonography since the early 1980s has shown a gradual decrease in incidence of IVH and has helped with the identification of risk factors. The increased use of magnetic resonance imaging (MRI) has helped to better define the site and extent of the lesion and to visualize associated white matter damage.

INCIDENCE

GMH-IVH mainly occurs in premature infants, and the risk is higher with decreasing maturity.[143] A 2003 study, however, also showed that an IVH, sometimes associated with a thalamic hemorrhage, can be seen in full-term infants, and this can be associated with a sinovenous thrombosis.[162]

The first studies, using computed tomography (CT) and ultrasonography, were performed between 1978 and 1983 and showed an incidence of 40% to 50% in infants with a birthweight of less than 1500 g.[15] In the 1990s, many groups noted a decline in the incidence to approximately 20% of infants with very low birthweight,[8,65] but this decline has not

been confirmed by others,[6] and no further decline was noted in a cohort of the Vermont Oxford Network.[67] Since the early 1980s, the incidence of intraparenchymal hemorrhage has also shown a decline, although this decline was not found in all studies.[76] The average incidence for intraparenchymal hemorrhage is now 5% to 11%.[8,30,32,76] An even lower incidence of 3% was reported in a French population-based cohort.[74] The decrease in the incidence of GMH-IVH is mainly attributed to the increased use of antenatal corticosteroids and the postnatal use of surfactant.[44,65,124,130]

Timing of the Hemorrhage

Accurate timing of GMH-IVH is possible only when sequential ultrasonographic studies are performed. A diagnosis of a hemorrhage of antenatal onset can be made only when the first ultrasonogram is performed on admission, within a few hours after delivery.[79] Many studies have shown that almost all hemorrhages develop within the first week after birth, and many of them within the first 48 hours after birth. Progression of a GMH-IVH over 1 to 2 days is not uncommon, and this applies especially to an IVH progressing to an intraparenchymal hemorrhage.[30] Venous infarction is the most likely underlying mechanism for this progression (see Neuropathology later). Only approximately 10% of cases of GMH-IVH occur beyond the end of the first week, in contrast to periventricular leukomalacia, where late onset is not uncommon.[2] Lesions seen in the caudothalamic groove after several weeks are probably not hemorrhagic in origin and are better referred to as *germinolytic necrosis*.[127] They are more common in infants with chronic lung disease and can also be seen in infants with postnatally acquired cytomegalovirus infection.

NEUROPATHOLOGY

Ruckensteiner and Zollner[126] were the first to point out that GMH-IVH developed after hemorrhage in the subependymal germinal matrix, a structure that is most prominent between 24 and 34 weeks of gestation and has almost completely regressed by term. Germinal matrix tissue is abundant over the head and body of the caudate nucleus, but can also be found in the periventricular zone. More recently, MRI has confirmed just how extensive this tissue is in preterm infants. The germinal matrix contains neuroblasts and glioblasts that undergo mitotic activity before migrating to other parts of the cerebrum. Bleeding into the caudothalamic part of the germinal matrix was predominant in the large autopsy series from New Jersey, but more than a third of cases also had bleeding into the temporal or occipital germinal matrix outer zones.[110] The germinal matrix receives its blood supply from a branch of the anterior cerebral artery known as the Heubner artery. The rest of the blood supply is derived from the anterior choroidal artery and the terminal branches of the lateral striate arteries.[58] Vessels in the germinal matrix are primitive and cannot be classified as arterioles, venules, or capillaries and are often referred as the *immature vascular rete*. Venous drainage of the deep white matter occurs through a fan-shaped leash of short and long medullary veins through which blood flows into the germinal matrix and subsequently into the terminal vein, which is positioned below the germinal matrix.[140] The anatomic distribution of parenchymal lesions associated with GMH-IVH suggest venous infarction due to obstruction of this vein.[54]

Germinal Matrix Hemorrhage

Most GMHs arise in the region of the caudate nucleus. Although GMHs at the level of the caudate nucleus are identified with ultrasonography, MRI has shown that GMH also occurs in the germinal matrix in the roof of the temporal horn. The size of the GMH changes with the maturity of the infant: the less mature the infant, the larger the GMH. The site also varies with maturity, with occurrence over the body of the caudate nucleus in the less mature infant and over the head of the caudate nucleus in the more mature infant.[58] When the GMH is followed longitudinally with ultrasonography, a subependymal cyst is seen as a sequel after several weeks, and this cyst is often still present at term equivalent age.

Intraventricular Hemorrhage

Hemorrhages occurring in the germinal matrix often rupture through the ependyma into the lateral ventricle and are then referred to as an *IVH*. These hemorrhages can vary considerably in size and, if large, can lead to acute distention of the lateral ventricle. Large clots can be present, seen as casts at postmortem examination or with cranial ultrasonography, and these can sometimes change position with repositioning of the infant. The blood can fill part of or the entire ventricular system, spreading through the foramen of Monro, the third ventricle, the aqueduct of Sylvius, the fourth ventricle, and the foramina of Luschka and Magendie to collect eventually around the brainstem in the posterior fossa. Clot formation can lead to outflow obstruction at any level, but most commonly at the level of the aqueduct of Sylvius, or more diffusely at the level of the arachnoid villi. More gradual progressive ventricular dilation occurs especially in those with a large GMH-IVH; this is known as *posthemorrhagic ventricular dilation*. This can be transient or persistent. In a small group, it can be rapidly progressive and noncommunicating, usually because of obstruction at the level of the aqueduct of Sylvius or the outlet foramina of Luschka and Magendie. Unilateral outflow obstruction at the level of the foramen of Monro can lead to unilateral hydrocephalus (Fig. 40-50). In cases of communicating progressive posthemorrhagic ventricular dilation, the increase in ventricular size is more gradual and is considered to be caused by an obliterative arachnoiditis due to blood collecting in the subarachnoid spaces of the posterior fossa, leading to an imbalance between cerebrospinal fluid (CSF) production and reabsorption.

Parenchymal Hemorrhage

The most severe type of hemorrhage involves the parenchyma. This type of lesion occurs in approximately 3% to 15% of all hemorrhages.[74,76] A recent study made us aware of the different veins involved in this type of lesion.[35] Direct extension into the parenchyma from pressure of blood in the ventricle is now considered unlikely. Some still take the view that all parenchymal hemorrhages are originally ischemic in origin, with any bleeding being a secondary complication. However, most agree that a unilateral parenchymal lesion accompanying GMH-IVH is most often caused by the presence of the GMH leading to impaired venous drainage and venous infarction. Gould and colleagues[54] showed that the ependyma remained intact, indicating that there had not been an extension of the preceding IVH. These lesions almost invariably show a moderate to large IVH on the ipsilateral side. The parenchymal hemorrhage is mostly unilateral but can occur in both hemispheres. A score was recently introduced, taking into account whether the lesion is unilateral or bilateral, the presence of a midline shift, and the number of regions that are involved.[6] The appearance of the intraparenchymal hemorrhage has changed since the early 1990s. Instead of a unilateral globular hemorrhagic lesion, in continuity with the lateral ventricle and evolving into a single

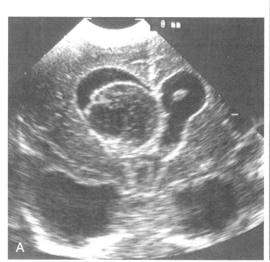

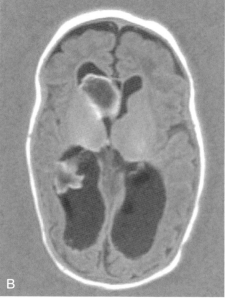

Figure 40–50. Cranial ultrasonography, coronal view, shows large right-sided intraventricular hemorrhage of antenatal onset in an infant born at term (**A**). The clot has started to resolve and has become less echogenic. The foramen of Monro appears to be (partially) occluded, leading to severe posthemorrhagic ventricular dilation, especially of the right ventricle. Magnetic resonance image, T1-weighted sequence, of this infant at 6 weeks after birth still shows the resolving intraventricular clot, irregular outline of the ventricular system, and bilateral absence of myelination of the posterior limb of the internal capsule (**B**).

porencephalic cyst, a smaller, triangular parenchymal lesion can be seen, with the tip of the triangle toward the lateral ventricle. There may be partial or even no communication of the parenchymal hemorrhage with the lateral ventricle, and an evolution into a few cystic lesions, separate from or partially in communication with the lateral ventricle, can be seen after several weeks (Figs. 40-51 and 40-52).[30] This type of lesion is sometimes classified as *unilateral periventricular leukomalacia* (PVL), but in view of the later MRI appearance, with very focal instead of diffuse gliosis, this appears to be incorrect. It is possible that improvement in neonatal care is associated with the change in appearance seen over time.

Intracerebellar Hemorrhage

Cerebellar hemorrhage was always considered uncommon, but the increased use of routine MRI in preterm infants has shown that this condition is not as rare as previously thought.[97] Some suggest that this problem is especially common in very immature infants. The condition has been reported in 2.5% of high-risk preterm infants.[81,97] Ultrasonography performed through the posterolateral fontanelle is more successful in making the diagnosis, but is still inferior to MRI. Cerebellar atrophy without an apparent cerebellar hemorrhage has also been reported as a common sequel of severe immaturity.[12,98] Reduced cerebellar volumes were only shown on three-dimensional MRI in preterm infants at term equivalent age, in association with supratentorial pathology, such as hemorrhagic parenchymal infarction, IVH with dilation, and periventricular white matter damage.[136]

PATHOGENESIS

The precise nature and origin of GMH-IVH remain uncertain. Although some groups have suggested that the capillaries in the germinal matrix do not rupture easily, others have suggested that they can rupture because the vessels are immature in structure with little evidence of basement membrane protein and they are of relatively large diameter. Early neuropathologists considered subependymal bleeding to be entirely venous in origin. This theory was rebutted by the work of Hambleton and Wigglesworth[58] and Pape and Wigglesworth,[111] who suggested from their injection studies that capillary bleeding was more prominent than terminal vein rupture. There has been a return to the concept that most parenchymal hemorrhages are due to venous infarction[54,140] or to a reperfusion injury after an ischemic insult.[152] An anatomic analysis of the developing cerebral vasculature did not show precapillary arteriole-to-venous shunts.[3]

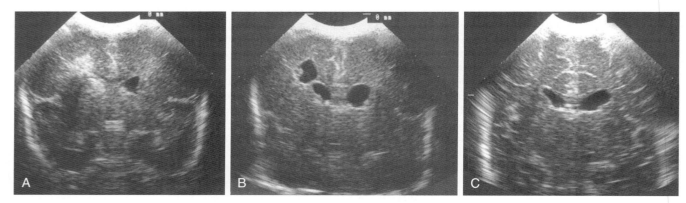

Figure 40–51. A, Cranial ultrasonography, coronal view, shows intraventricular hemorrhage and parenchymal hemorrhage not in communication with the lateral ventricle. B, Three weeks later, a single cystic lesion is present after resolution of the hemorrhage. C, At term, the cyst is no longer seen.

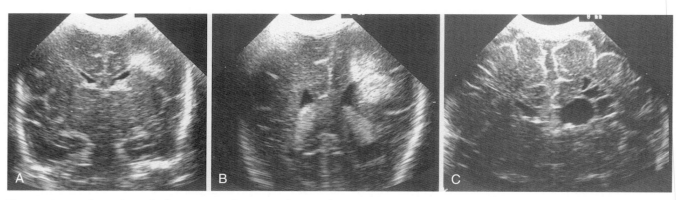

Figure 40–52. A, B, Cranial ultrasonography, coronal view, shows intraventricular hemorrhage and parenchymal hemorrhage not in communication with the lateral ventricle. C, At term age, multiple cysts are seen adjacent to the lateral ventricle.

Prenatal Factors

Histologic signs of amniotic infection have been shown to increase the risk of GMH-IVH.[141] This fits in well with acute inflammatory placental lesions[149] and increased serum levels of interleukin (IL)-1β, IL-6, and IL-8, noted to be associated with severe IVH in extremely premature infants.[62,141,164] In one of these studies, a correlation was shown between blood cytokine concentrations and altered hemodynamic function.[164] Cord blood IL-6 concentration correlated inversely with newborn systolic, mean, and diastolic blood pressures. The number of infants with an IVH was limited, but in the five infants with an IVH, the placenta significantly more often showed evidence of fetal inflammation.[164] An increase in total leukocytes during the first 72 hours after birth,[114] as well as an increased ratio of immature to total white blood cells, was also recognized as independent risk factors for GMH-IVH.[164]

Maternal preeclampsia has been associated with a reduced risk of GMH-IVH.[27,130] The protective effect appears to be due to enhanced in utero maturation of the fetus. Administration of antenatal corticosteroids is, according to several studies, the most important protective factor against development of GMH-IVH.[130] The effect may be due to a direct maturational effect on the brain, but other factors may also be involved, like the reduction of the severity of lung disease and the decreased need for inotropes. One study did not find a protective effect of antenatal corticosteroid administration.[114]

Intrapartum Factors

Whether the mode of delivery plays a role is still uncertain.[59,90] A reduced mortality but not a reduced risk of a GMH-IVH was recently reported in a Swedish population-based study for preterm infants with a gestation of 25 to 36 weeks.[64] In a cohort study, a protective effect of a cesarean section was seen only for the most immature infants (less than 27 weeks' gestation).[143] A vaginal breech delivery is in some studies associated with a higher risk of large GMH-IVH, but this effect was lost in a multivariate analysis.[130] Neonatal transport for infants born outside a tertiary center has also been shown to be a risk factor.[143] A decrease in the number of infants who need transportation will reduce the number of infants with GMH-IVH.

Delayed cord clamping was recently associated with a reduction in GMH-IVH as demonstrated by five infants (14%) in the delayed clamping group compared with 13 infants (36%) in the nondelayed group ($P = .03$).[94] The impact of delayed cord clamping on IVH was evaluated, adjusting for gestational age and cesarean section. The final model indicated that the IVH rate was more than three times higher in the immediate cord clamping group (OR 3.5, 95% confidence interval [CI] CI 1.1–11.1). In a systematic review, there were no significant differences for infant deaths, but a significant difference in the incidence of IVH was reported in 7 of the 10 published studies ($P = .002$).[119]

Neonatal Factors

Respiratory problems, particularly respiratory distress syndrome (RDS), have been recognized as important risk factors in the development of GMH-IVH. This association is most likely not causal but due to the associated complications occurring during mechanical ventilation for RDS, such as hypercarbia, pneumothorax, and acidosis. Because of improvement in ventilatory techniques, including an increased use of nasal continuous positive airway pressure, hypercarbia and severe acidosis have become less common. Hypercarbia, a potent cerebral vasodilator, was noted in the past to be associated with GMH-IVH, and Levene and colleagues showed a very high risk for an IVH when a combination of hypercarbia and severe acidosis was present.[78]

Cardiovascular Factors

The immature brain is considered vulnerable to fluctuations in blood pressure owing to limitations in autoregulation of cerebral bloodflow.[84] Impaired autoregulation renders the cerebral circulation "pressure-passive" and hence unprotected from any wide swings or changes in blood pressure. This applies especially to sick preterm infants. Data initially obtained using a radioactive xenon tracer[84] showed a direct linear relationship between blood pressure and cerebral bloodflow in a small number of infants. Similar findings were obtained using near-infrared spectroscopy.[145] Using these techniques, it was recently shown that routine caregiving procedures in critically ill preterm infants were associated with major circulatory fluctuations and that these cerebral hemodynamic changes were associated with early parenchymal ultrasound abnormalities.[83] Muscle paralysis was noted to stabilize the fluctuating bloodflow pattern and was followed by a reduction in GMH-IVH.[115] Looking at a selected population of ventilated infants with evidence of asynchronous respiratory efforts, a significant reduction in intraventricular hemorrhage (any grade and severe IVH) was found, using muscle paralysis.[15a] The fluctuating pattern may be exaggerated in hypovolemia.[118] Hypotension is common in infants with severe RDS, and in the presence of a pressure-passive cerebral circulation, may lead to hypoxia-ischemia of the germinal matrix. Several groups have shown that arterial hypotension precedes the development of GMH-IVH,[153] with the hemorrhage occurring during a period of reperfusion. This finding is supported by a continuous ultrasonography study, which showed occurrence of the hemorrhage during an increase in blood pressure after a period of lower blood pressure.[43,108] The researchers showed a low flow in the superior vena cava, detected during the first few hours of life preceding an IVH. The antenatal administration of steroids is associated with a reduction in the need for blood pressure support. Following a reduction in the severity of RDS, this effect on the blood pressure may be most protective for the development of a GMH-IVH.[101] Early administration of fresh frozen plasma does not reduce the incidence of GMH-IVH.[107] A reduction in GMH-IVH has been seen during an era of closer attention to blood pressure, gentle handling, synchronous ventilation, and less severe RDS because of antenatal steroid and postnatal surfactant therapy, rather than because of any specific drug used as prophylaxis.[155] Measurement of cardiac troponin (cTnT) and N-terminal-pro-B type natriuretic peptide (NTpBNP), both markers of cardiac function at 48 hours after birth, has shown that infants with a patent ductus arteriosus and IVH grades III or IV and/or death had significantly higher median cTnT/NTpBNP levels compared with infants with a patent ductus arteriosus without IVH grades III or IV and/or death and those with spontaneous patent ductus arteriosus closure.[36]

Genetic Factors

Thrombophilic disorders, including the factor V Leiden mutation, which renders factor V resistant to cleavage by activated protein C, and the prothrombin G20210A mutation, which was found to be associated with raised plasma concentrations of prothrombin, were suggested to play a role in the development of GMH-IVH. However, a large prospective study was unable to confirm previously reported associations of hemostasis gene variants and development of IVH in infants with very low birthweight.[61] Interleukin-6 CC genotype increased the risk of the development of severe hemorrhagic lesions (OR 3.5; 95% CI 1.0-12.2; P = .038).[60] This observation could, however, not be confirmed in a considerably larger sample size.[53] Antenatal porencephaly was recently reported to be associated with a mutation in the collagen 4A1 gene (COL4A1) encoding procollagen type 4α1, a basement membrane protein in two preterm siblings and preterm twins.[11a,34]

DIAGNOSIS

With ultrasonography largely available in neonatal units, most high-risk preterm infants have routine ultrasonographic examinations soon after admission or within the first few days after birth. Three clinical syndromes, however, can be recognized in preterm infants not paralyzed or heavily sedated on the ventilator.[152] The first is known as *catastrophic deterioration*, noted by a sudden deterioration in the infant's clinical state, such as an increase in oxygen or ventilatory requirement, a fall in blood pressure, or acidosis. More often, however, a drop in hematocrit is seen without a clear change in the infant's condition. The *saltatory syndrome* is more common and gradual in onset, presenting with a change in spontaneous general movements. The third and most frequent presentation is *asymptomatic*; 25% to 50% of infants with GMH-IVH have no obvious clinical signs.

A classification system suitable for describing early and late ultrasonographic appearances and based on that suggested by Volpe[152] is given in Table 40-5.

Ultrasonography is a noninvasive bedside technique, using the anterior fontanelle as an acoustic window. Good correlations of ultrasonographic GMH-IVH signs with autopsy findings have been reported. With the increased use of MRI, it has

become apparent that GMHs at sites other than at the level of the caudate nucleus, like the roof of the temporal horn, are not always identified using ultrasonography. With ultrasonography, it also is not always possible to be certain about the presence or absence of a small associated IVH. Immediate access to ultrasonography in contrast to MRI, and the fact that the examination can be repeated as often as indicated, still makes this technique the first method of choice.[87]

Timing of the examination depends on the questions raised. An examination within hours after delivery helps in timing the lesion as antenatal or postnatal. When trying to determine risk factors, sequential scans until the GMH-IVH is diagnosed are also important. A single scan at the end of the first week shows 90% of all hemorrhages as well as their maximum extent. Further ultrasonographic examinations (up to two to three times weekly) are required in infants with any degree of hemorrhage to detect the occurrence of posthemorrhagic ventricular dilation, which occurs in approximately 30%, and the occurrence of associated PVL[77,103]; the more severe the hemorrhage, the higher the risk for development of post-hemorrhagic ventricular dilation. Posthemorrhagic ventricular dilation tends to develop 10 to 20 days after the onset of GMH-IVH.

Experts from the American Academy of Neurology, the Child Neurology Society, and the American Academy of Pediatrics have published recommendations on the use of ultrasonography to evaluate premature neonates.[92] It is recommended that all neonates younger than 30 weeks' postmenstrual age be screened with cranial ultrasonography because 23% of this group have significant abnormalities detected. Optimal timing of the ultrasonography allows detection of clinically unsuspected IVH and evidence for PVL or ventriculomegaly. At a minimum, it is recommended that scans be performed at 7 to 14 days of age and at 36 to 40 weeks' postmenstrual age. Data do not support routine MRI for all neonates with abnormal results on screening ultrasonography.

Unilateral intraparenchymal hemorrhage associated with a bilateral or ipsilateral GMH-IVH is now considered to be due to impaired drainage of the veins in the periventricular white matter, resulting in venous infarction.[30,140] This type of lesion is classically triangular or fan-shaped, with the apex at the outer border of the lateral ventricle. In some cases the lesion is globular with the apex of the triangle at the midline and a smooth outer border. The globular type of lesion (usually unilateral) evolves over 2 to 3 weeks into a porencephalic cyst (Fig. 40-53), whereas those intraparenchymal hemorrhages that are clearly separate from the ventricle at the start often form multiple small cysts (see Fig. 40-53).[30]

TABLE 40–5   Grading System for Neonatal Intraventricular Hemorrhage*

Description	Generic Term
Grade I: Germinal matrix hemorrhage	GMH
Grade II: Intraventricular hemorrhage without ventricular dilation	GMH-IVH
Grade III: Intraventricular hemorrhage and with acute ventricular dilation (clot fills >50% of the ventricle)	GMH-IVH ventriculomegaly
Intraparenchymal lesion—describe size, location	Intraparenchymal hemorrhage

*This represents an evolution of the system described in Papile LA, et al: Incidence and evolution of the subependymal intraventricular hemorrhage: a study of infants with birth weights less than 1500 grams, *J Pediatr* 92:529, 1978.
GMH, germinal matrix hemorrhage; IVH, intraventricular hemorrhage.

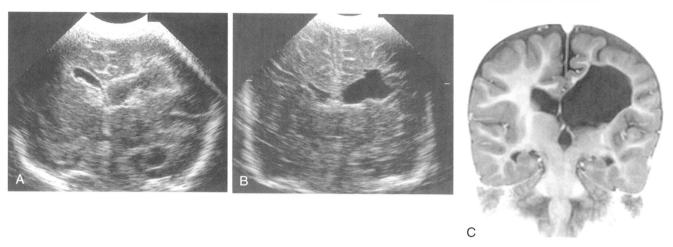

Figure 40–53. Cranial ultrasonography, coronal view, shows large intraventricular hemorrhage and parenchymal hemorrhage in communication with the lateral ventricle. A, The clot has started to resolve. B, At term age, a porencephalic cyst is present after resolution of the hemorrhage. C, Magnetic resonance image, T1-weighted sequence, of this infant at 18 months of age shows a large porencephalic cyst, loss of white matter, and reduced myelination on the affected side.

MANAGEMENT

Clinical management of children who have a GMH-IVH is not different from that of other at-risk preterm infants. Minimal handling, prevention of fluctuations in blood pressure or CO_2 levels, prevention of breathing against the ventilator, and optimization of any coagulopathy may be warranted in an attempt to prevent extension of the initial hemorrhage.[21] A blood transfusion may be needed in case of a large IVH associated with a drop in hemoglobin. Continuous electroencephalographic monitoring may be helpful in the detection of subclinical seizures (see Part 5 of this chapter). The use of fibrinolytic therapy in an attempt to resolve the initial clot has been disappointing and can even result in rebleeding.[157] Repeat ultrasonographic scans are indicated to diagnose posthemorrhagic ventricular dilation. Ventricular dilation seen on cranial ultrasonography usually precedes the development of clinical symptoms by several weeks. The clinical signs are a full fontanelle, diastasis of the sutures, and a rapid increase in head size. Sunsetting of the eyes is a late sign. Posthemorrhagic ventricular dilation is transient in approximately half of the infants and is persistent or rapidly progressive in the remaining cases.[103] Once it is recognized that the ventricles have begun to enlarge, the baseline size should be measured using ultrasonography. The most widely adopted measurement system is that of Levene and Starte.[77] This "ventricular index" is the distance between the midline and the lateral border of the ventricle measured in a coronal view in the plane of the third ventricle. Another useful measurement is the depth of the frontal horn taken just in front of the thalamic notch, with a height of more than 3 mm being used to define ventriculomegaly and one greater than 6 mm to suggest posthemorrhagic ventricular dilation.[22] Measuring the occipital horn in a sagittal plane can also be useful because there can be a discrepancy between the anterior and posterior horn width. Any measurement greater than 24 mm also suggests severe posthemorrhagic ventricular dilation (Fig. 40-54). Accurate measurement of the CSF pressure is

required to make a distinction between infants with progressive hydrocephalus (i.e., those with raised intracranial pressure) and those in whom the dilation is due to cerebral atrophy (low pressure).[70] Raised CSF pressure can cause symptoms, including visual disturbance, seizures, feed intolerance, and apneas. In the long term, pressure-induced destruction of neuronal tissue can lead to motor handicap and mental retardation. Short-term adverse effects on the nervous system have been confirmed using somatosensory and visual evoked potentials, Doppler estimates of cerebral bloodflow velocity, and near-infrared spectroscopy. Soul and colleagues[133] showed a pronounced effect of CSF removal on cerebral perfusion, regardless of the opening pressure and the amount of fluid removed. The impact of removal of CSF on cerebral tissue was also assessed using advanced volumetric three-dimensional MRI, showing an increase in both cortical gray and myelinated white matter volume.[68] CSF hypoxanthine levels IL-8, IFN-γ and sFas (soluble Fas) were noted to be raised in infants with posthemorrhagic ventricular dilation and especially so in those with associated PVL.[10,39,132]

Even so, there is no direct evidence that early drainage of CSF alters the natural history or outcome of posthemorrhagic ventricular dilation. In two large, retrospective, observational studies, a significant reduction in the need for shunt placement was noted when intervention was started before the 97th percentile +4 mm line of the graph of Levene and Starte was crossed and when the threshold for inserting a subcutaneous reservoir was low.[14,31] The initial data of the drainage, irrigation, and fibrinolytic therapy (DRIFT) study showed a reduced need for shunt insertion, 22% compared with approximately 60% in other multicenter studies.[69,148,158] A subsequent randomized controlled trial was discontinued due to a high risk (33%) of rebleeding in the group allocated to DRIFT without an apparent positive effect on the need for a ventriculoperitoneal shunt.[159] A prospective international randomized study, randomizing for early or later placement of a subcutaneous reservoir, is now in progress.[14]

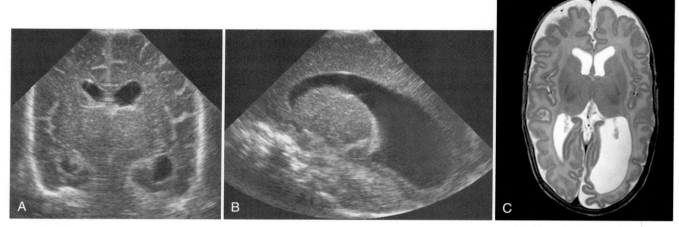

Figure 40–54. **A,** Cranial ultrasonography, coronal view, shows mild ventricular dilation. **B,** Parasagittal view obtained during the same examination shows severe dilation of the left occipital horn. **C,** The magnetic resonance image, T2-weighted, spin echo sequence still shows marked occipital dilation at term-equivalent age.

NEURODEVELOPMENTAL OUTCOME

Data about long-term neurologic and developmental outcome mainly deal with children who had a large IVH with or without parenchymal involvement. These follow-up data are still mainly based on neonatal ultrasonographic data. Associated PVL may have been missed using this technique, especially in children with posthemorrhagic ventricular dilation, in whom the periventricular white matter is more difficult to visualize. Children with small hemorrhages were until recently not considered to be at increased risk for development of a major handicap, even though they score lower on tests assessing visual-motor integration.[85,150] Recent three-dimensional volumetric imaging studies, however, have shown reduced gray matter volumes at term-equivalent age[113,146,147] associated with a reduced mental development index (MDI) on the Bayley Scale of Infant Motor Development (BSID)-II, but this was only significant in the most immature infants with gestation less than 30 weeks. The risk of poor outcome increases significantly with the presence of posthemorrhagic ventricular dilation (50%) and even further in those who require shunt insertion (75%).[117,148]

Children with ventriculomegaly present at term are at higher risk of a poor outcome.[91] In this study, ventriculomegaly was significantly more common after high-grade GMH-IVH and bronchopulmonary dysplasia. Outcome data for children with a unilateral parenchymal hemorrhage show a major neurodevelopmental disability in approximately 80%. The most common handicap is a hemiplegia contralateral to the side of the parenchymal hemorrhage. Ten infants with a porencephalic cyst following a parenchymal hemorrhage were followed into adolescence.[131] At all ages assessed, rates of motor, cognitive, and overall impairment were significantly higher compared with those in preterm control subjects ($P \leq .002$ for all tests). Six of the ten children were ambulatory when seen at 16-19 years required learning assistance in school, and had social challenges. In a retrospective hospital-based population study, outcome was considerably better than reported previously, with cerebral palsy occurring in only 7.4% of the infants with a large IVH (grade III) compared with 37 (48.7%) of the 76 infants with a parenchymal hemorrhage ($P < .001$).[14] Whether this better neurodevelopmental outcome was related to earlier treatment of posthemorrhagic ventricular dilation or due to a cohort with more localized lesions and of more mature preterm infants needs to be established, and a prospective randomized controlled trial is now underway.[14]

The data[14] are very much in contrast to those of a recent study looking at a large group of infants with a grade III-IV hemorrhage with and without a shunt.[1] Of the 562 infants with a grade III hemorrhage, 103 (18%) needed a ventriculoperitoneal (VP) shunt, compared with 125 of the 436 (29%) with a grade IV hemorrhage. Children with severe IVH and shunts had significantly lower scores on the BSID II compared with children with no IVH and children with IVH of the same grade and no shunt. An MDI less than 70 was found in 183 of 424 (43%) infants with a grade III hemorrhage without a shunt compared with 59 of 99 (60%) in those with a shunt. In those with a grade IV hemorrhage without a shunt, 143 of 295 (48%) had an MDI less than 70, compared with 87 of 115 (76%) of those requiring a shunt. Infants with shunts were at increased risk for cerebral palsy and head circumference at the less than 10th percentile at 18 months' adjusted age. Infants with a grade III hemorrhage without apparent associated white matter involvement are more likely to do well or may develop a diplegia, whereas those with a venous infarction are more at risk of developing a hemiplegia, depending on the site and extent of the lesion. A score introduced recently was helpful in predicting outcome.[7] Early prediction of development of a hemiplegia is now possible using MRI at 40 to 42 weeks. At term, myelination of the posterior limb of the internal capsule should be present (Fig. 40-55). In infants in whom hemiplegia subsequently developed, asymmetry and even lack of myelination of the posterior limb of the internal capsule were noted (Fig. 40-56).[29] Using diffusion tensor MRI, visualization of

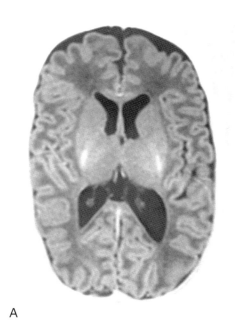

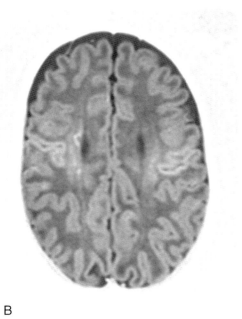

A   B

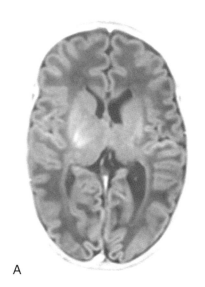

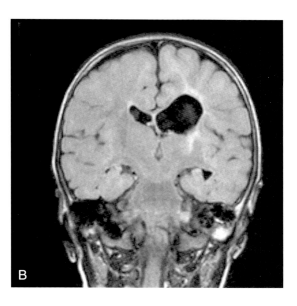

A   B

Figure 40–55. A, Magnetic resonance image, T1-weighted sequence, at term age, in same infant as in Figure 40-51. A symmetric high signal at the level of the posterior limb of the internal capsule is seen. **B,** At a higher level, a small triangular area of high signal intensity is still seen as a sequel of the parenchymal hemorrhage.

Figure 40–56. Magnetic resonance image, T1-weighted sequence, at term age, in same infant as in Figure 40-52. **A,** There is no symmetric high signal at the level of the posterior limb of the internal capsule **B,** A FLAIR sequence at 18 months of age shows high signal intensity suggestive of gliosis adjacent to the porencephalic cyst and across the internal capsule.

the tracts is possible at an earlier stage, but data are only available in preterm infants with a unilateral intraparenchymal hemorrhage examined later in infancy.[15b]

Outcome data of preterm infants with a cerebellar hemorrhage were recently reported and are reason for concern.[82] Neurologic abnormalities were present in 66% of infants with an isolated cerebellar hemorrhage compared with 5% of the control group. Infants with isolated cerebellar hemorrhagic injury versus controls had significantly lower mean scores on all tested measures performed at a median age of 32 months, including severe motor disabilities (48% versus 0%), expressive language (42% versus 0%), delayed receptive language (37% versus 0%), and cognitive deficits (40% versus 0%). The researchers concluded that cerebellar hemorrhagic injury in preterm infants is associated with a high prevalence of long-term pervasive neurodevelopmental disabilities. In a few other smaller studies of prematurely born children with cerebral palsy, involvement of the cerebellum was not uncommonly seen on MRI and these children showed a distinct clinical type of cerebral palsy with clinical features, including striking motor impairment and variable degrees of ataxia and athetosis or dystonia. Most were severely damaged, with cognitive, language, and motor delays, and all but one were microcephalic.[12,98]

PREVENTION

Both prenatal and postnatal pharmacologic prophylaxis have been used to reduce the incidence of GMH-IVH. With improvement in general neonatal care, a reduction has also been reported in many large neonatal units without the use of any drugs. Neonatal intensive care unit (NICU) characteristics were shown to affect the incidence of severe GMH-IVH, with NICUs with high patient volume and high neonatologist-to-staff ratio having a lower rate of severe GMH-IVH.[139]

The most promising specific prophylactic drugs are antenatal steroids.[44,130] A systematic review published in 2007 involving more than 4000 babies showed a significant reduction in the risk for GMH-IVH diagnosed by ultrasonography (OR 0.54; 95% CI 0.43-0.69). There was also a strong trend toward improved long-term neurologic outcome (OR 0.64; 95% CI 0.14-2.98).[124] It is not certain whether the effect is mainly due to increased lung maturation and therefore less severe RDS, stabilization of postnatal blood pressure, or perhaps a direct protective effect on the brain. It is not recommended that courses of antenatal corticosteroids be repeated because there may be a negative effect on brain growth.[18,100] Betamethasone instead of dexamethasone is recommended because dexamethasone has been associated with an increased incidence of PVL.[9]

Antenatal phenobarbital was shown to be protective in some but not all studies. The quality of some of these studies was not good because of lack of randomization or a placebo group. When these studies were excluded from a systematic review, no protective effect could be shown.[20]

Studies of antenatal administration of magnesium sulfate yield different results. No reduction in the incidence of either a small or a large GMH-IVH was found in a large, randomized, multicenter study.[17] Long-term follow-up, however, did show an improvement in gross motor function, but no significant reduction in development of cerebral palsy. In a recent multicenter randomized controlled trial, no significant reduction was found for the incidence of a large GMH-IVH (2.1% versus 3.2%; relative risk [RR] 0.64; 95% CI 0.38-1.06). Moderate or severe cerebral palsy occurred significantly less frequently in the magnesium sulfate group compared to the control group (1.9% vs. 3.5%; RR 0.55; 95% CI 0.32-0.95).[125] Other tocolytic drugs have also been studied in relation to occurrence of GMH-IVH. Ritodrine was noted to be associated with a significantly reduced risk for development of a grade III or IV GMH-IVH, in contrast to administration of indomethacin and magnesium sulfate.[154]

Maternal vitamin K administration was associated with a trend toward reduction in the overall rate of GMH-IVH (RR 0.82; 95% CI 0.67-1.00).[19]

Phenobarbital was the first drug used postnatally in the prevention of GMH-IVH. Although the first studies were promising, a meta-analysis of 10 trials was unable to show a reduction in the incidence or severity of GMH-IVH (RR 1.04; 95% CI 0.87-1.25).[160]

The most promising prophylactic drug administered postnatally is indomethacin. The results of a meta-analysis involving 19 trials and a total of 2872 infants showed a significant reduction in the incidence of grades III and IV hemorrhage (pooled RR 0.66 [0.53-0.82]).[41] The children of the original cohort, studied by Ment and colleagues,[89] were assessed at 8 years of age and no effect of indomethacin was seen on long-term outcome.[151] Analysis of the original cohort by gender, however, showed that indomethacin halved the incidence of IVH, eliminated parenchymal hemorrhage, and was associated with higher verbal scores at 3 to 8 years in boys.[93] Another large trial was also unable to show an improvement in survival without sensory impairment at 18 months, despite a reduction in incidence of severe GMH-IVH.[128] A meta-analysis of ibuprofen involving 15 studies did not show a reduction in the incidence of IVH.[104]

OTHER HEMORRHAGES

See also Chapter 28.

Subdural and subarachnoid hemorrhages are probably underdiagnosed because they are difficult to recognize using cranial ultrasonography. Clinical signs may be mild or absent. A significant subdural hemorrhage is most often related to birth trauma, but a small subdural was noted to be a common occurrence in an MRI study looking at 111 consecutive full-term infants.[156] Nine infants had a subdural hemorrhage, three following a normal vaginal delivery (6.1%), five following forceps assisted delivery after an attempted ventouse delivery (27.8%), and only one following traumatic ventouse delivery (7.7%). Underlying mechanisms can be a tear of the dura, occipital diastasis, or rupture of bridging veins. A tear of the dura can occur after a precipitous delivery or from use of instrumentation, both of which are not very common with preterm delivery. A dural tear results in extensive bleeding from the adjacent sinus. Occipital diastasis can occur during a vaginal breech delivery with excessive extension of the neck of the infant, although vaginal breech deliveries are not commonly performed as a consequence of results of multicenter, randomized studies.[66] Rupture of the bridging veins is the most common etiology of a subdural hemorrhage and may be seen in association with a subarachnoid hemorrhage. These children are usually born at term and present with a full fontanelle, lethargy, apneas, or seizures. In case of a severe hemorrhage, a midline shift may be seen and surgery needs to be considered. The diagnosis usually is made using CT or MRI (Fig. 40-57). Hydrocephalus can develop from outflow obstruction and temporary external drainage, sometimes followed by permanent drainage, may be needed. Secondary cerebral infarction has also been reported and has been related to prolonged arterial compression.[55]

A small subarachnoid hemorrhage is sometimes (7%) seen in preterm infants at postmortem examination and does not usually cause any symptoms.[110] Blood can leak into the subarachnoid space after an IVH, by flowing through the aqueduct into the fourth ventricle and subsequently through the foramina of Luschka and Magendie into the subarachnoid space. Once again, the diagnosis is hard to make using ultrasonography unless the lesion is large and causes compression of brain tissue. Hydrocephalus is less commonly seen than in children with a subdural hemorrhage.

Vascular Lesions

CEREBRAL ARTERY INFARCTION

Because of increased access to neonatal MRI, infarction of a major artery, or a branch arising from it, is better recognized. This condition is often referred to as *neonatal stroke* or *perinatal arterial stroke*.[120] Information about incidence is becoming available with the introduction of neonatal registries.[25,86] Newborn infants are susceptible to neonatal stroke because of

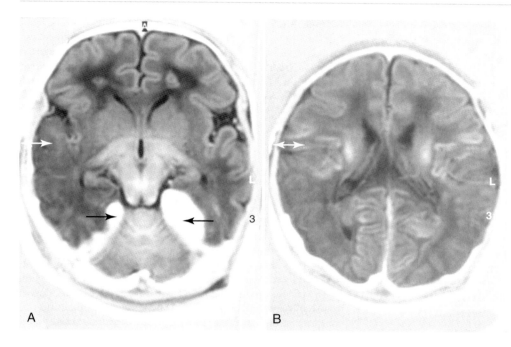

Figure 40–57. A, Magnetic resonance image, T1-weighted sequence, shows a large collection of blood in the posterior fossa with blood along the tentorium bilaterally (*black arrows*). B, At a higher level, extensive cortical highlighting is seen posteriorly and in the region of the sylvian fissure (*white arrows*). A posterior trunk middle cerebral artery infarct is also seen on the right.

a number of factors present around the time of delivery, such as the hypercoagulable state of the mother, mechanical stress during delivery, the transient right-to-left intracardiac shunt, and the risk of dehydration during the first few days after delivery often associated with a high hematocrit and blood viscosity.[105] Neonatal stroke can be divided into sinovenous thrombosis and arterial ischemic stroke.[25] Both conditions still are not always detected because presenting symptoms may not always be clear and appropriate imaging is not always performed. Arteriovenous malformations are discussed in Chapter 45.

Sinovenous Thrombosis

An incidence of 41 per 100,000 newborn infants with sinovenous thrombosis was found in the Canadian Pediatric Ischemic Stroke Registry.[25] Most (66%) come to medical attention within 48 hours of birth, although infants can also develop symptoms 10 to 14 days after delivery, sometimes associated with dehydration or infection.[106] Almost half of the children (43%) with sinovenous thrombosis in this registry were newborns. Seizures are the most common presenting symptom and were reported in 70% of the infants from the Canadian Registry. Lethargy is also commonly present.[40,123] The fontanelle can be full and scalp veins may be prominent.

During the birth process, molding of the skull and overriding of the sutures of the different parts of the skull may occur and affect the underlying sinus, resulting in the occurrence of sinovenous thrombosis. Perinatal asphyxia is a commonly associated risk factor, seen in 24% of the newborns in the Canadian Registry. The superior sagittal sinus and the lateral sinuses are most commonly involved. Involvement of the straight sinus, the vein of Galen, and the internal cerebral vein has also been reported.[40] An associated IVH and especially a unilateral thalamic hemorrhage or periventricular congestion may help in clarifying the diagnosis.[70b,162] Wu and coworkers[162] noted that sinovenous thrombosis was significantly more

common in full-term infants with an IVH and a unilateral thalamic hemorrhage (4 of 5) compared with newborns with an IVH only (5 of 21). They strongly recommend the diagnosis of sinovenous thrombosis be considered in any full-term neonate presenting with an IVH.

In another study by the same group, risk factors were analyzed in 30 full-term infants with a sinovenous thrombosis.[161] They reported that 29% of these newborn infants had been on extracorporeal membrane oxygenation and 23% had congenital heart disease. Only seven infants were tested for a genetic thrombophilia, and four of these seven were found to be positive.

A diagnosis can be made using Doppler flow ultrasonography, which may demonstrate absent or decreased flow in the affected sinus. Contrast-enhanced CT can also be used, showing the so-called empty delta sign, the lack of contrast filling. The best method is MRI and especially the use of magnetic resonance venography, which helps make a definitive diagnosis by showing a reduction or absence of venous flow in the affected venous sinus (Fig. 40-58).

There is no agreement about the use of antithrombotic therapy in this age group, but recommendations were recently made.[102] Different treatment policies were noted with physicians in the U.S. being less likely to treat neonates with CSVT with antithrombotic medications compared to physicians at non-U.S. centers, 25% versus 69% of neonates.[69a] The number of infants is limited, requiring many centers for performance of a randomized study.

More than 90% of newborns with sinovenous thrombosis survive, and 77% of survivors were considered to be normal at a mean follow-up of 2.1 years.[26,40] Data from the Canadian Registry are not so encouraging, with 61% of survivors having a neurologic deficit and 9% experiencing a recurrence of cerebral or systemic thrombosis.[25]

In the retrospective chart study by Fitzgerald and associates assessing 42 newborn infants, 57% presented with seizures and 60% had associated parenchymal infarcts, which

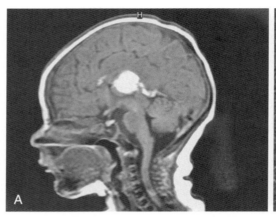
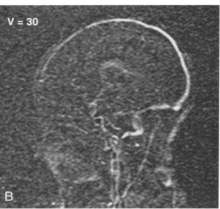

Figure 40–58. Magnetic resonance images obtained at 10 days' of age. T1-weighted sequence showed an area of high signal intensity compatible with hemorrhage in the thalamus. **A,** There is high signal at the level of the straight sinus. **B,** Magnetic resonance venography shows presence of flow in the superior sagittal sinus, but absence of signal at the level of the straight sinus.

were mainly hemorrhagic.[40] Seventy-nine percent had any form of impairment with 59% having cognitive impairment, 67% cerebral palsy, and 41% epilepsy. Infarction was associated with the presence of later impairment ($P = .03$).

Perinatal Arterial Ischemic Stroke

Cerebral infarction in the neonate has been defined as a severe disorganization or even complete disruption of both gray and white matter caused by embolic, thrombotic, or ischemic events.[5] In infants dying in the acute stage of the condition, the hemisphere is swollen and deeply congested. There is involvement of both white matter and cortex, with secondary hemorrhagic infarction in some cases. In infants who survive for longer, contraction of the affected area is seen with softening and multiple cystic degeneration, giving a honeycomb appearance on sectioning. A distinction between a unilateral parenchymal hemorrhage, which usually occurs in the preterm infant and evolves into a porencephalic cyst, and an infarct in the region of the middle cerebral artery, which usually occurs in a term newborn and evolves into an area of parenchymal cavitation, is recommended. A porencephalic cyst following a parenchymal hemorrhage of antenatal onset has, however, been referred to as *fetal stroke* and small porencephalic cysts following antenatal venous infarction have also been included within the spectrum of presumed perinatal stroke.[72,109]

Lesions involving the left hemisphere are three to four times more common than those of the right hemisphere. This may be due to hemodynamic differences early after birth related to the patent ductus arteriosus or a preferential flow across the left common carotid artery. Middle cerebral artery infarction occurs twice as often as involvement of any other artery.

Both de Vries and colleagues[28] and Mercuri and coworkers[95] used a classification system based on the main artery involved. Infarcts in the territory of the middle cerebral artery were further subdivided into main branch, cortical branch, and lenticulostriate branch infarction.

INCIDENCE

In the Canadian Registry, the incidence of perinatal arterial ischemic stroke was as high as 93 per 100,000 newborn infants, which is much higher than reported previously. Estan

and Hope[37]studied a 7-year cohort and reported a prevalence of 0.025%, which is similar to the finding of Perlman and colleagues,[116] who found a prevalence of 0.02%. Several groups found neonatal stroke to be the second most common cause of neonatal seizures.[37,80] Data about focal infarction in preterm infants are scarce. In a recent hospital-based study we found an incidence of 7 per 1000 preterm infants with a gestational age less than 35 weeks.[11]

Convulsions are the most common presenting symptom.[71,135] They are usually of the focal clonic variety, but multifocal tonic or subtle seizures also may be seen (see also Part 5 of this chapter). Many of the infants show no major clinical neurologic abnormality between seizures. The largest population reported to date showed that 77% of the 215 infants presented with seizures, which were focal in almost all. Thirteen percent were admitted because of apneas, and 10% showed only hypotonia as a presenting symptom.[73] Symptoms can also be very subtle, especially in the preterm infant,[11,28] and the diagnosis can be easily missed. Presentation with a hand preference later in infancy may lead to a diagnosis, with an area of cavitation on CT or MRI, suggestive of a perinatal or in utero arterial ischemic stroke, which is now referred to as *presumed perinatal stroke*.[72,75]

DIAGNOSIS

After presentation with focal seizures in a child without an obvious history of perinatal asphyxia, care should be taken not to miss the diagnosis of arterial ischemic stroke. The middle cerebral artery is most commonly involved, and the infarct occurs more often on the left than the right side. Arterial infarcts of the anterior and posterior cerebral artery are less often diagnosed, possibly because of the lack of clinical symptoms in the neonatal period (Fig. 40-59). Involvement of the smaller branches of the middle cerebral artery is more often seen in preterm infants, whereas obstruction of the main branch is less common in this age group.[11,28] Infarcts can be hemorrhagic in 20%, and bilateral infarcts can be seen in 10% to 15% (Fig. 40-60).

In the absence of abnormalities on ultrasonography, MRI is recommended to confirm or exclude the diagnosis. Ultrasonography has not been considered reliable in making a diagnosis; this applies especially when the examination is made soon after the clinical presentation.[47] By the end of the first week, a wedge-shaped area of echogenicity, often with a linear demarcation line, restricted to the territory of

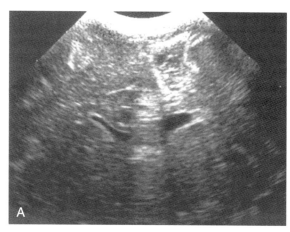
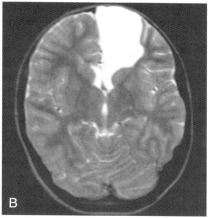

Figure 40-59. Preterm infant, gestational age 32 weeks. **A,** Routine ultrasonographic scan at 2 weeks showed an area of cystic evolution in the region of the left anterior cerebral artery. Mild ex vacuo dilation of the left ventricle is also present. **B,** T2-weighted magnetic resonance image, spin-echo sequence, at 7 years of age shows the parenchymal cavity in the same distribution.

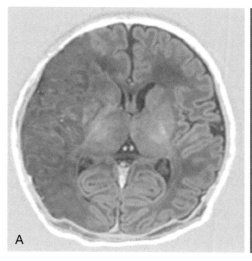
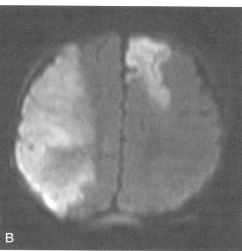

Figure 40-60. Full-term infant, magnetic resonance images obtained at 4 days of age. **A,** T1-weighted sequence shows low signal intensity in the distribution of the right middle cerebral artery suggestive of main branch involvement. **B,** Diffusion-weighted image shows high signal intensity in the same area, as well as a smaller area of high signal intensity in the distribution of the left anterior cerebral artery.

one of the main arteries, usually becomes apparent.[16] Cystic evolution can take place over the next 4 to 6 weeks, often associated with ex vacuo dilation of the ipsilateral lateral ventricle. Doppler ultrasonography can show asymmetry of arterial pulsations. Perlman and associates[116] noted decreased pulsations on the affected side, whereas Taylor[142] noted an increase in size and number of visible vessels in the periphery of the infarct and increased mean bloodflow velocity in vessels supplying or draining the infarcted areas in four of eight infants.

The threshold for performing MRI should be low in infants presenting with neonatal seizures. MRI plays an important role in making the diagnosis. If performed early after clinical presentation, diffusion-weighted MRI is very helpful. This technique shows abnormalities, indicating cytotoxic edema, at a very early stage, preceding abnormalities seen on conventional MRI. This technique also enables visualization of acute damage to the corticospinal tracts at the level of the midbrain.[33,71] Preliminary data suggest that these findings predict wallerian degeneration and development of subsequent hemiplegia.[33,71] A repeat scan can show asymmetry at the level of the mesencephalon, which can be seen as early as 6 weeks after onset of the infarction.[13] Magnetic resonance angiography, which allows investigation of the main vascular bed, can be used and can sometimes show dissection or occlusion of one of the main

vessels. This may be rare, however, and this technique may also fail to show small vessel occlusion. Early assessment of structure-function relationship is possible using functional MRI. This technique was shown to provide additional information in a child with a posterior cerebral artery infarct.[129]

Reorganization of the somatosensory cortex can be followed using a combination of transcranial magnetic stimulation (TMS) and functional MRI.[38,129,137,138] Staudt and colleagues[138] showed that when a lesion abolishes the normal contralateral corticospinal control over the paretic hand, the contralesional hemisphere develops (or maintains) fast-conducting ipsilateral corticospinal pathways to the paretic hand. This reorganization with ipsilateral corticospinal tracts can mediate a useful hand function. Normal hand function, however, seemed only possible with preserved crossed corticospinal projections from the contralateral hemisphere. Guzzetta and colleagues also recently suggested that ipsilesional reorganization is more effective in the restoration of a good motor function as opposed to the contralesional reorganization.[57]

RISK FACTORS

Perinatal complications have been reported in more than 50% of newborn infants with a perinatal stroke.[46,75] Stroke among infants admitted with neonatal encephalopathy is an uncommon observation.[121] Cardiac disease, extracorporeal membrane oxygenation, and portal vein thrombosis have all been reported as associated risk factors.[112] Stroke was especially common (31%) among infants with transposition of the great arteries and this was associated with balloon septostomy.[88,99] Maternal cocaine abuse has also been considered to cause stroke. In a study of 43 women who abused crack cocaine during pregnancy, 17% of their infants had evidence of cortical infarction, compared with only 2% of the matched control group.[63] Studies conducted since the late 1990s have illustrated the importance of extensive investigations for an underlying genetic prothrombotic disorder.[23,46,73] In particular, activated protein C resistance caused by factor V Leiden mutation is an increasingly common associated finding.[23,70a] Factor V Leiden mutation, prothrombin mutation, increased lipoprotein-α, methylenetetrahydrofolate reductase C677T (MTHFR), and congenital protein C and protein S deficiency have also been reported as associated findings.[73] Population-based studies using case-matched controls found diverse etiologic factors responsible for perinatal arterial stroke in term infants. Infertility, preeclampsia, prolonged rupture of membranes, and chorioamnionitis have been identified as independent maternal risk factors.[26,75] A recurrence risk of 3% to 5% was given by both the Canadian and the German population-based studies.[73] A lower recurrence risk of 1.2 % was recently reported among 84 newborn infants with perinatal stroke.[42] Association with elevated maternal antiphospholipid antibodies (anticardiolipin antibodies, lupus anticoagulants) has also been reported (see also Chapter 18).[24] Data on risk factors in preterm infants are scarce.[11,51] Using case-matched controls (three controls per case, matched for gestational age), etiologic factors responsible for perinatal arterial stroke in preterm infants were recently studied and it was noted that these were different from those born at term. Twin-twin transfusion syndrome (19% versus 3%; OR 31.2; CI 2,9-340,0; P = .005), fetal heart rate abnormality (58% versus 26%; OR 5.2; CI 1.5-17.6; P = .008), and hypoglycemia (42% versus 18%; OR 3.9; CI 1.2-12.6; P = .02) were identified as independent risk factors for preterm stroke.[11]

PROGNOSIS

The outlook in most cases is relatively good. Published follow-up data from case reports suggest that the majority of the infants achieve independent walking before 13 months and more than half of all infants surviving neonatal stroke are entirely normal at 12 to 18 months of age.[48] Spastic hemiplegia is the most important sequela, particularly after infarction of the main branch of the middle cerebral artery. An increased incidence has been shown for male infants.[155] Two thirds of children with hemiplegia are of normal intelligence.[4,122] In a cohort studied by Mercuri and colleagues,[95] a hemiplegia developed in only 5 of 24 infants (20%). An additional two had mild asymmetry, and two had mild global delay. Hemiplegia or asymmetric tone tended to develop only in those cases with involvement of the hemisphere, basal ganglia, and internal capsule on first scan. When 22 of these 24 children were seen again at school age, 30% showed a hemiplegia and another 30% showed some neuromotor abnormality. Involvement of the internal capsule was always associated with some motor disturbance.[96] Deficits in higher-level cognitive skills may, however, become apparent during school, and this is more common in males.[155a] Homonymous hemianopia may follow posterior cerebral artery infarction.

Outcome data depend very much on the threshold for performing MRI, on the artery involved, and on whether the main branch is involved or only a cortical branch or one of the lenticulostriate branches. Mercuri and colleagues[95] found an abnormal background pattern, even when recorded on a two-channel electroencephalogram, to be the best early predictor of adverse neurologic outcome. Involvement of the internal capsule was also shown by this group to be a predictor of motor outcome.[96]

de Vries and coworkers[11,28] noted that involvement of the lenticulostriate branches was more common in preterm infants. Only 3 of 16 infants with involvement of a cortical branch or one or more lenticulostriate branches had cerebral palsy, in contrast to all five survivors with main branch involvement. Govaert and associates[56] suggested that cranial ultrasonography was important in the prediction of hemiplegia. In the parasagittal view, attention should be paid to involvement of the central groove, which is usually present in those with involvement of the main branch or the anterior trunk of the middle cerebral artery.

Seizures are a common complication and occur beyond the neonatal period in 25% to 67% of affected infants.[49] An infarct on prenatal ultrasonography (P = .0065) and a family history of epilepsy (P = .0093) were significantly associated with postneonatal epilepsy in the univariate analysis. As epilepsy may first develop later in childhood, the rate of epilepsy will be higher when follow-up is longer. Hippocampal tissue was examined in children in whom intractable epilepsy developed after a middle cerebral artery infarct. Hippocampal sclerosis was noted to be less common in those with early-onset stroke (before 28 weeks' gestation).[134]

Goodman[52] noted that half of all children with hemiplegia have psychiatric disorders (i.e., problems with behavior, emotions, or relationships interfering with the child's everyday life). They usually present with irritability, anxiety, and hyperactivity/inattention. This finding was not supported by another long-term follow-up study.[144]

The overall prevalence of cerebral palsy is approximately 1 in 2000 children. On the basis of the estimated incidence of perinatal cerebral vascular infarction, it might be expected that this condition is the cause of the neurologic deficit in up to 20% of children with cerebral palsy. This is supported by recent data showing that 22% of 377 infants with cerebral palsy showed focal arterial infarction on head imaging.[163]

REFERENCES

1. Adams-Chapman I, et al for the NICHD Research Network: Neurodevelopmental outcome of extremely low birth weight infants with post-hemorrhagic hydrocephalus requiring shunt insertion, *Pediatrics* 121:e1167, 2008.
2. Andre P, et al: Late-onset cystic periventricular leukomalacia in premature infants: a threat until term, *Am J Perinatol* 18:79, 2001.
3. Anstrom JA, et al: Anatomical analysis of the developing cerebral vasculature in premature neonates: absence of precapillary arteriole-to-venous shunts, *Pediatr Res* 52:554, 2002.
4. Ballantyne AO, et al: Plasticity in the developing brain: intellectual, language and academic functions in children with ischaemic perinatal stroke, *Brain* 131:2975, 2008.

5. Barmada MA, et al: Cerebral infarcts with arterial occlusion in neonates, *Ann Neurol* 6:495, 1979.
6. Bassan H, et al: Ultrasonographic features and severity scoring of periventricular hemorrhagic infarction in relation to risk factors and outcome, *Pediatrics* 117:2111, 2006.
7. Bassan H, et al: Neurodevelopmental outcome in survivors of periventricular hemorrhagic infarction, *Pediatrics* 120:785, 2007.
8. Batton DG, et al: Current gestational age-related incidence of major intraventricular hemorrhage, *J Pediatr* 125:623, 1994.
9. Baud O, et al: Antenatal glucocorticoid treatment and cystic periventricular leukomalacia in very preterm infants, *N Engl J Med* 341:1190, 1999.
10. Bejar R, et al: Increased hypoxanthine concentrations in cerebrospinal fluid of infants with hydrocephalus, *J Pediatr* 103:44, 1983.
11. Benders MC, et al: Maternal and infant characteristics associated with perinatal arterial stroke in the preterm infant, *Stroke* 38:1759, 2007.
11a. Bilguvar K, et al: Pacifier and Breastfeeding Trial Group: COL4A1 mutation in preterm intraventricular hemorrhage, *J Pediatr* 155:743, 2009.
12. Bodensteiner JB, Johnsen SD: Magnetic resonance imaging (MRI) findings in children surviving extremely premature delivery and extremely low birthweight with cerebral palsy, *J Child Neurol* 21:743, 2006.
13. Bouza H, et al: Prediction of outcome in children with congenital hemiplegia: a magnetic resonance imaging study, *Neuropediatrics* 25:60, 1994.
14. Brouwer AJ, et al: Neurodevelopmental outcome of preterm infants with severe intraventricular hemorrhage and therapy for post-hemorrhagic ventricular dilatation, *J Pediatr* 152:648, 2008.
15. Burstein J, et al: Intraventricular hemorrhage in premature newborns: a prospective study with CT, *Am J Radiol* 132:631, 1997.
15a. Cools F, Offringa M: Neuromuscular paralysis for newborn infants receiving mechanical ventilation, *Cochrane Database Syst Rev.* 2:CD002773, 2005.
15b. Counsell SJ, et al: Thalamo-cortical connectivity in children born preterm mapped using probabilistic magnetic resonance tractography, *Neuroimage* 34:896, 2007.
16. Cowan F, et al: Does cranial ultrasound imaging identify arterial cerebral infarction in term neonates? *Arch Dis Child Fetal Neonatal Ed* 90:F252, 2005.
17. Crowther CA, et al: The Australasian Collaborative Trial of Magnesium Sulphate: effect of magnesium sulfate given for neuroprotection before preterm birth, *JAMA* 290:2669, 2003.
18. Crowther CA, et al, ACTORDS study group: outcomes at 2 years of age after repeat doses of antenatal corticosteroids, *N Engl J Med* 357:1179, 2007.
19. Crowther CA, Henderson-Smart DJ: Maternal vitamin K prior to birth for preventing neonatal periventricular hemorrhage, *Cochrane Database Syst Rev* 1:CD 001691, 2001.
20. Crowther CA, Henderson-Smart DJ: Phenobarbital prior to preterm birth for the prevention of neonatal periventricular hemorrhage (PVH), *Cochrane Database Syst Rev* 3:CD 000164, 2003.
21. Dasgupta SJ, Gill AB: Hypotension in the very low birth weight infant: the old, the new and the uncertain, *Arch Dis Child Fetal Neonatal Ed* 88:F450, 2003.
22. Davies MW, et al: Reference ranges for the linear dimensions of the intracranial ventricles in preterm neonates, *Arch Dis Child Fetal Neonatol Ed* 82:F219, 2000.
23. Debus O, et al: Factor V Leiden and genetic defects of thrombophilia in childhood porencephaly, *Arch Dis Child* 78:F121, 1998.
24. deKlerk OL, et al: An unusual cause of neonatal seizures in a newborn infant, *Pediatrics* 100:E8, 1997.
25. deVeber G, Andrew M: Canadian Pediatric Ischemic Stroke Study Group: cerebral sinovenous thrombosis in children, *N Engl J Med* 345:417, 2001.
26. deVeber GA, et al: Neurologic outcome in survivors of childhood arterial ischemic stroke and sinovenous thrombosis, *J Child Neurol* 15:316, 2000.
27. Developmental Epidemiology Network Investigators: The correlation between placental pathology and intraventricular hemorrhage in the preterm infant, *Pediatr Res* 43:15, 1998.
28. de Vries LS, et al: Infarcts in the distribution of the middle cerebral artery in preterm and full-term infants, *Neuropediatrics* 28:88, 1997.
29. de Vries LS, et al: Asymmetrical myelination of the posterior limb of the internal capsule: an early predictor of hemiplegia, *Neuropediatrics* 30:314, 1999.
30. de Vries LS, et al: Unilateral haemorrhagic parenchymal infarction in the preterm infant, *Eur J Pediatr Neurol* 5:139, 2001.
31. de Vries LS, et al: Early versus late treatment of posthaemorrhagic ventricular dilatation: results of a retrospective study from five neonatal intensive care units in the Netherlands, *Acta Paediatr* 91:212, 2002.
32. de Vries LS, et al: Ultrasound abnormalities preceding cerebral palsy in high-risk preterm infants, *J Pediatr* 144:815, 2004.
33. de Vries LS, et al: Prediction of outcome in newborn infants with arterial ischemic stroke using magnetic resonance diffusion-weighted imaging, *Neuropediatrics* 36:12, 2005.
34. de Vries LS, et al: COL4A1 mutation in two preterm siblings with antenatal onset of parenchymal hemorrhage, *Ann Neurol 65:12*, 2009.
35. Dudink J, et al: Venous subtypes of preterm periventricular haemorrhagic infarction, *Arch Dis Child Fetal Neonatal Ed* 93:F201, 2008.
36. El-Khuffash AF, Molloy EJ: Influence of a patent ductus arteriosus on cardiac troponin T levels in preterm infants, *J Pediatr* 153:350, 2008.
37. Estan J, Hope P: Unilateral neonatal cerebral infarction in full-term infants, *Arch Dis Child Fetal Neonatal Ed* 76:F88, 1997.
38. Eyre JA, et al: Is hemiplegic cerebral palsy equivalent to amblyopia of the corticospinal system? *Ann Neurol* 62:493, 2007.
39. Felderhoff-Mueser U, et al: Soluble Fas (CD95/Apo-1), soluble Fas ligand and activated caspase 3 in the cerebrospinal fluid of infants with posthemorrhagic and nonhemorrhagic hydrocephalus, *Pediatr Res* 54:659, 2003.
40. Fitzgerald KC, et al: Cerebral sinovenous thrombosis in the neonate, *Arch Neurol* 63:405, 2006.
41. Fowlie PW, Davis PG: Prophylactic intravenous indomethacin for preventing mortality and morbidity in preterm infants, *Cochrane Database Syst Rev* 3:CD000174, 2002.
42. Fullerton HJ, et al: Risk of recurrent childhood arterial ischemic stroke in a population-based cohort: the importance of cerebrovascular imaging, *Pediatrics* 119:495, 2007.
43. Funato M, et al: Clinical events in association with timing of intraventricular hemorrhage in preterm infants, *J Pediatr* 121:614, 1992.
44. Garland JS, et al: Effect of maternal glucocorticoid exposure on risk of severe intraventricular hemorrhage in surfactant-treated preterm infants, *J Pediatr* 126:272, 1995.

45. Gleissner M, et al: Risk factors for intraventricular hemorrhage in a birth cohort of 3721 premature infants, *J Perinat Med* 28:104, 2000.

46. Golomb MR, et al: Presumed pre- or perinatal arterial ischemic stroke: risk factors and outcomes, *Ann Neurol* 50:163, 2001.

47. Golomb MR, et al: Cranial ultrasonography has a low sensitivity for detecting arterial ischemic stroke in term neonates, *J Child Neurol* 18:98, 2003.

48. Golomb MR, et al: Independent walking after neonatal arterial ischemic stroke and sinovenous thrombosis, *J Child Neurol* 18:530, 2003.

49. Golomb MR, et al: Perinatal stroke and the risk of developing childhood epilepsy, *J Pediatr* 151:409, 2007.

50. Golomb MR, et al: Cerebral palsy after perinatal arterial ischemic stroke, *J Child Neurol* 23:279, 2008.

51. Golomb MR, et al: Very early arterial ischemic stroke in premature infants, *Pediatr Neurol* 38:329, 2008.

52. Goodman R: Psychological aspects of hemiplegia, *Arch Dis Child* 76:177, 1997.

53. Göpel W, et al: Interleukin-6-174-genotype, sepsis and cerebral injury in very low birth weight infants, *Genes Immun* 7:65, 2006.

54. Gould SJ, et al: Periventricular intraparenchymal cerebral haemorrhage in preterm infants: the role of venous infarction, *J Pathol* 151:197, 1987.

55. Govaert P, et al: Traumatic neonatal intracranial bleeding and stroke, *Arch Dis Child* 67:840, 1992.

56. Govaert P, et al: Perinatal cortical infarction within middle cerebral artery trunks, *Arch Dis Child* 82:F59, 2000.

57. Guzzetta A, et al: Reorganisation of the somatosensory system after early brain damage, *Clin Neurophysiol* 118:1110, 2007.

58. Hambleton G, Wigglesworth JS: Origin of intraventricular haemorrhage in the preterm infant, *Arch Dis Child* 51:651, 1976.

59. Haque KN, et al: Caesarean or vaginal delivery for preterm very-low-birth weight (≤1,250 g) infant: experience from a district general hospital in UK, *Arch Gynecol Obstet* 277:207, 2008.

60. Harding DR, et al: Does interleukin-6 genotype influence cerebral injury or developmental progress after preterm birth? *Pediatrics* 114:941, 2004.

61. Härtel C, et al: Genetic polymorphisms of hemostasis genes and primary outcome of very low birth weight infants, *Pediatrics* 118:683, 2006.

62. Heep A, et al: Increased serum levels of interleukin 6 are associated with severe intraventricular hemorrhage in extremely premature infants, *Arch Dis Child Fetal Neonatal Ed* 88:F501, 2003.

63. Heier LA, et al: Maternal cocaine abuse: the spectrum of radiologic abnormalities in the neonatal CNS, *AJNR Am J Neuroradiol* 12:951, 1991.

64. Herbst A, et al: Influence of mode of delivery on neonatal mortality and morbidity in spontaneous preterm breech delivery, *Eur J Obstet Gynecol Reprod Biol* 133:25, 2007.

65. Heuchan AM, et al: Perinatal risk factors for major intraventricular haemorrhage in the Australian and New Zealand Neonatal Network, 1995–97, *Arch Dis Child Fetal Neonatal Ed* 86:F86, 2002.

66. Hofmeyr GJ, Hannah ME: Planned caesarean section for term breech delivery, *Cochrane Database Syst Rev* 3:CD000166, 2003.

67. Horbar JD, et al: Trends in mortality and morbidity for very low birth weight infants, 1991–1999, *Pediatrics* 110:143, 2002.

68. Hunt RW, et al: Assessment of the impact of the removal of cerebrospinal fluid on cerebral tissue volumes by advanced volumetric 3D-MRI in posthaemorrhagic hydrocephalus in a premature infant, *J Neurol Neurosurg Psychiatry* 74:658, 2003.

69. International PHVD Drug Trial Group: International randomised trial of acetazolamide and furosemide in posthaemorrhagic ventricular dilatation, *Lancet* 352:133, 1998.

69a. Jordan LC, et al: Antithrombotic treatment in neonatal cerebral sinovenous thrombosis: results of the International Pediatric Stroke Study, *J Pediatr* 156:704, 2010.

70. Kaiser A, Whitelaw A: Cerebrospinal fluid pressure during posthaemorrhagic ventricular dilatation in newborn, *Arch Dis Child* 60:920, 1986.

70a. Ken G, et al: Impact of thrombophilia on risk of arterial ischemic stroke or cerebral sinovenous thrombosis in neonates and children: a systematic review and meta-analysis of observational studies, *Circulation* 121:1838, 2010.

70b. Kersbergen KJ, et al: Anticoagulation therapy and imaging in neonates with a unilateral thalamic hemorrhage due to cerebral sinovenous thrombosis, *Stroke* 40:2754, 2009.

71. Kirton A, et al: Quantified corticospinal tract diffusion restriction predicts neonatal stroke outcome, *Stroke* 38:974, 2007.

72. Kirton A, et al: Presumed perinatal ischemic stroke: vascular classification predicts outcomes, *Ann Neurol* 63:436, 2008.

73. Kurnik K, et al: Recurrent thromboembolism in infants and children suffering from symptomatic neonatal arterial stroke: a prospective follow-up study, *Stroke* 34:2887, 2003.

74. Larroque B, et al: White matter damage and intraventricular hemorrhage in very preterm infants: The EPIPAGE study, *J Pediatr* 143:477, 2003.

75. Lee J, et al: Maternal and infant characteristics associated with perinatal arterial stroke in the infant, *JAMA* 293:723, 2005.

76. Lemons JA, et al: Very low birthweight outcomes of the National Institute of Child Health and Human Development Neonatal Research Network, January 1995 through December 1996. NICHD Neonatal Research Network, *Pediatrics* 107:E1, 2001.

77. Levene MI, Starte DR: A longitudinal study of posthaemorrhagic ventricular dilatation in the newborn, *Arch Dis Child* 56:905, 1981.

78. Levene MI, et al: Risk factors in the development of intraventricular haemorrhage in the preterm neonate, *Arch Dis Child* 57:410, 1982.

79. Leviton A, et al: The epidemiology of germinal matrix haemorrhage during the first half day of life, *Dev Med Child Neurol* 33:138, 1991.

80. Lien JM, et al: Term early-onset neonatal seizures: obstetric characteristics, etiologic classifications and perinatal care, *Obstet Gynecol* 85:163, 1995.

81. Limperopoulos C, et al: Cerebellar hemorrhage in the preterm infant: ultrasonographic findings and risk factors, *Pediatrics* 116:717, 2005.

82. Limperopoulos C, et al: Cerebral hemodynamic changes during intensive care of preterm infants, *Pediatrics* 122:e1006, 2008.

83. Limperopoulos C, et al: Cerebral hemodynamic changes during Intensive care of preterm infants, *Pediatrics* 122:e1006, 2008.

84. Lou HC, et al: Impaired autoregulation of cerebral blood flow in the distressed newborn infant, *J Pediatr* 94:118, 1979.

85. Lowe J, Papile LA: Neurodevelopmental performance of very low birth weight infants with mild periventricular, intraventricular hemorrhage, *Am J Dis Child* 144:1242, 1990.

86. Lynch JK, et al: Report of the National Institute of Neurological Disorders and Stroke workshop on perinatal and childhood stroke, *Pediatrics* 109:116, 2002.

87. Maalouf EF, et al: Comparison of findings on cranial ultrasound and magnetic resonance imaging in preterm infants, *Pediatrics* 107:719, 2001.

88. McQuillen PS, et al: Balloon atrial septostomy is associated with preoperative stroke in neonates with transposition of the great arteries, *Circulation* 113:280, 2006.

89. Ment LR, et al: Low-dose indomethacin and prevention of intraventricular hemorrhage: a multicenter randomized trial, *Pediatrics* 93:543, 1994.

90. Ment LR, et al: Antenatal steroids, delivery mode and intraventricular hemorrhage in preterm infants, *Am J Obstet Gynecol* 172:795, 1995.

91. Ment LR, et al: The etiology and outcome of ventriculomegaly at term in very low birth weight infants, *Pediatrics* 104:243, 1999.

92. Ment LR, et al: Practice parameter: neuroimaging of the neonate, *Neurology* 58:1726, 2002.

93. Ment LR, et al: Prevention of intraventricular hemorrhage by indomethacin in male preterm infants, *J Pediatr* 145: 832, 2004.

94. Mercer JS, et al : Delayed cord clamping in very preterm infants reduces the incidence of intraventricular hemorrhage and late-onset sepsis: a randomized, controlled trial, *Pediatrics* 117:1235, 2006.

95. Mercuri E, et al: Early prognostic indicators of outcome in infants with neonatal cerebral infarction: a clinical, electroencephalogram, and magnetic resonance imaging study, *Pediatrics* 103:39, 1999.

96. Mercuri E, et al: Neonatal cerebral infarction and neuromotor outcome at school age, *Pediatrics* 113:95, 2004.

97. Merrill JD, et al: A new pattern of cerebellar hemorrhages in preterm infants, *Pediatrics* 102:e62, 1998.

98. Messerschmidt A, et al: Preterm birth and disruptive cerebellar development: assessment of perinatal risk factors, *Eur J Paediatr Neurol* 12:455, 2008.

99. Miller SP, et al: Abnormal brain development in newborns with congenital heart disease, *N Engl J Med* 357:1928, 2007.

100. Modi N, et al: The effects of repeated antenatal glucocorticoid therapy on the brain, *Pediatr Res* 50:581, 2001.

101. Moise AA, et al: Antenatal steroids are associated with less need for blood pressure support in extremely premature infants, *Pediatrics* 95:845, 1995.

102. Monagle P, et al: Antithrombotic therapy in neonates and children: American College of Chest Physicians Evidence-Based Clinical Practice Guidelines (8th Edition), *Chest* 133 (6 suppl):887S, 2008.

103. Murphy BP, et al: Posthaemorrhagic ventricular dilatation in the premature infant: natural history and predictors of outcome, *Arch Dis Child Fetal Neonatal Ed* 88:F257, 2003.

104. *Cochrane Database Syst Rev* 23(1):CD003481, 2008.

105. Nelson KB, Lynch JK: Stroke in newborn infants, *Lancet Neurol* 3:150, 2004.

106. Nwosu ME, et al: Neonatal sinovenous thrombosis: presentation and association with imaging, *Pediatr Neurol* 39:155, 2008.

107. Osborn D, Evans N: Early volume expansion for prevention of morbidity and mortality in very preterm infants, *Cochrane Database Syst Rev* 2:CD002055, 2004.

108. Osborn DA, et al: Hemodynamic and antecedent risk factors of early and late periventricular/intraventricular hemorrhage in premature infants, *Pediatrics* 112:33, 2003.

109. Ozduman K, et al: Fetal stroke, *Pediatr Neurol* 30:151, 2004.

110. Paneth N, et al: Brain damage in the preterm infant, *Clin Dev Med* 131:1, 1994.

111. Pape KE, Wigglesworth JS: Haemorrhage, ischaemia and perinatal brain, *Clin Dev Med* 69/70:133, 1979.

112. Parker MJ, et al: Portal vein thrombosis causing neonatal cerebral infarction, *Arch Dis Child Fetal Neonatal Ed* 87:F125, 2002.

113. Patra K, et al: Grades I-II intraventricular hemorrhage in extremely low birth weight infants: effects on neurodevelopment, *J Pediatr* 149:169, 2006.

114. Paul DA, et al: Increased leukocytes in infants with intraventricular hemorrhage, *Pediatr Neurol* 22:194, 2000.

115. Perlman JM, et al: Reduction in intraventricular hemorrhage by elimination of fluctuating cerebral blood flow velocity in preterm infants with respiratory distress syndrome, *N Engl J Med* 312:1353, 1985.

116. Perlman JM, et al: Neonatal stroke: clinical characteristics and cerebral blood flow velocity measurements, *Pediatr Neurol* 11:281, 1994.

117. Persson EK, et al: Disabilities in children with hydrocephalus—a population-based study of children aged between four and twelve years, *Neuropediatrics* 37:330, 2006.

118. Pryds O: Control of cerebral circulation in the high-risk neonate, *Ann Neurol* 30:321, 1991.

119. Rabe H, et al: a systematic review and meta-analysis of a brief delay in clamping the umbilical cord of preterm infants, *Neonatology* 93:138, 2008.

120. Raju TN, et al, and NICHD-NINDS Perinatal Stroke Workshop Participants: Ischemic perinatal stroke: summary of a workshop sponsored by the National Institute of Child Health and Human Development and the National Institute of Neurological Disorders and Stroke, *Pediatrics* 120:609, 2007.

121. Ramaswamy V, Miller SP, Barkovich AJ, et al: Perinatal stroke in term infants with neonatal encephalopathy, *Neurology* 62:2088, 2004.

122. Ricci D, et al: Cognitive outcome at early school age in term-born children with perinatally acquired middle cerebral artery territory infarction, *Stroke* 39:403, 2008.

123. Rivkin MJ, et al: Neonatal idiopathic cerebral venous thrombosis: an unrecognised cause of transient seizures or lethargy, *Ann Neurol* 32:51, 1992.

124. Roberts D, Dalziel S: Antenatal corticosteroids for accelerating fetal lung maturation for women at risk of preterm birth, *Cochrane Database Syst Rev* 3:CD004454, 2006.

125. Rouse DJ, et al, Eunice Kennedy Shriver NICHD Maternal-Fetal Medicine Units Network: a randomized, controlled trial of magnesium sulfate for the prevention of cerebral palsy, *N Engl J Med* 359:895, 2008.

126. Ruckensteiner E, Zollner F: Uber die Blutungen im Gebiete der Vena Terminalis bei Neugeborenen, *Frank Z Pathol* 37:568, 1929.

127. Schlesinger AE, et al: Hyperechoic caudate nuclei: a potential mimic of germinal matrix hemorrhage, *Pediatr Radiol* 28:297, 1998.

128. Schmidt B, et al: Trial of indomethacin prophylaxis in preterm investigators: long-term effects of indomethacin prophylaxis in extremely-low-birth-weight infants, *N Engl J Med* 344:1966, 2001.

129. Seghier ML, et al: Combination of event-related fMRI and diffusion tensor imaging in an infant with perinatal stroke, *Neuroimage* 21:463, 2004.

130. Shankaran S, et al: Prenatal and perinatal risk and protective factors for neonatal intracranial hemorrhage, *Arch Pediatr Adolesc Med* 150:491, 1996.

131. Sherlock RL, et al: Long-term outcome after neonatal intraparenchymal echodensities with porencephaly, *Arch Dis Child Fetal Neonatal Ed* 93:F127, 2008.

132. Sival DA, et al: Neonatal high pressure hydrocephalus is associated with elevation of pro-inflammatory cytokines IL-18 and IFNgamma in cerebrospinal fluid, *Cerebrospinal Fluid Res* 31;5:21, 2008.

133. Soul JS, et al: CSF removal in infantile posthemorrhagic hydrocephalus results in significant improvement in cerebral hemodynamics, *Pediatr Res* 55:872, 2004.

134. Squier W: Stroke in the developing brain and intractable epilepsy: effect of timing on hippocampal sclerosis, *Dev Med Child Neurol* 45:580, 2003.

135. Sreenan C, et al: Cerebral infarction in the term newborn: clinical presentation and long-term outcome, *J Pediatr* 137:351, 2000.

136. Srinivasan L, et al: Smaller cerebellar volumes in very preterm infants at term-equivalent age are associated with the presence of supratentorial lesions, *AJNR Am J Neuroradiol* 27:573, 2006.

137. Staudt M, et al: Two types of ipsilateral reorganisation in congenital hemiparesis: a TMS and fMRI study, *Brain* 125:2222, 2002.

138. Staudt M, et al: Reorganization in congenital hemiparesis acquired at different gestational ages, *Ann Neurol* 56:854, 2004.

139. Synnes AR, et al: Neonatal intensive care unit characteristics affect the incidence of severe intraventricular hemorrhage, *Medical Care* 44:754, 2006.

140. Takashima S, et al: Pathogenesis of periventricular white matter haemorrhage in preterm infants, *Brain Dev* 8:25, 1986.

141. Tauscher MK, et al: Association of histologic chorioamnionitis, increased levels of cord blood cytokines, and intracerebral hemorrhage in preterm neonates, *Biol Neonate* 83:166, 2003.

142. Taylor GA: Alterations in regional cerebral blood flow in neonatal stroke: preliminary findings with color Doppler sonography, *Pediatr Radiol* 24:111, 1994.

143. Thorp JA, et al: Perinatal factors associated with severe intracranial hemorrhage, *Am J Obstet Gynecol* 185:859, 2001.

144. Trauner DA, et al: Behavioural profiles of children and adolescents after pre- or perinatal unilateral brain damage, *Brain* 124:995, 2001.

145. Tsuji M, et al : Cerebral intravascular oxygenation correlates with mean arterial pressure in critically ill premature infants, *Pediatrics* 106:625, 2000.

146. Vasileiadis GT, et al: Uncomplicated intraventricular hemorrhage is followed by reduced cortical volume at near-term age, *Pediatrics* 114:e367, 2004.

147. Vavasseur C, et al: Effect of low grade intraventricular hemorrhage on developmental outcome of preterm infants, *J Pediatr* 151:e6, 2007.

148. Ventriculomegaly Trial Group: Randomised trial of early tapping in neonatal posthaemorrhagic ventricular dilatation: Results at 30 months, *Arch Dis Child* 70:F129, 1994.

149. Vergani P, et al: Risk factors for neonatal intraventricular hemorrhage in spontaneous prematurity at 32 weeks gestation or less, *Placenta* 21:402, 2000.

150. Vohr BR, et al: Effects of intraventricular hemorrhage and socioeconomic status on perceptual, cognitive, and neurologic status of low birth weight infants at 5 years of age, *J Pediatr* 121:280, 1992.

151. Vohr BR, et al: School-age outcomes of very low birth weight infants in the indomethacin intraventricular hemorrhage prevention trial, *Pediatrics* 111:e340, 2003.

152. Volpe JJ: *Neonatal Neurology*, 4th ed, Philadelphia, 2008, WB Saunders.

153. Watkins AMC, et al: Blood pressure and cerebral haemorrhage and ischaemia in very low birthweight infants, *Early Hum Dev* 19:103, 1989.

154. Weintraub Z, et al, in collaboration with the Israel Neonatal Network: Effect of maternal tocolysis on the incidence of severe periventricular/intraventricular haemorrhage in very low birthweight infants, *Arch Dis Child Fetal Neonatal Ed* 85: F13, 2001.

155. Wells JT, Ment LR: Prevention of intraventricular haemorrhage in preterm infants, *Early Hum Dev* 42:209, 1995.

155a. Westmacott R, et al: Late emergence of cognitive deficits after unilateral neonatal stroke, *Stroke* 40:2012, 2009.

156. Whitby EH, et al: Frequency and natural history of subdural haemorrhages in babies and relation to obstetric factors, *Lancet* 363:846, 2004.

157. Whitelaw A, et al: Low dose intraventricular fibrinolytic treatment to prevent posthaemorrhagic hydrocephalus, *Arch Dis Child* 67:12, 1992.

158. Whitelaw A, et al: Phase 1 trial of prevention of hydrocephalus after intraventricular hemorrhage in newborn infants by drainage, irrigation and fibrinolytic therapy, *Pediatrics* 111:759, 2003.

159. Whitelaw A, et al: Randomized clinical trial of prevention of hydrocephalus after intraventricular hemorrhage in preterm infants: brain-washing versus tapping fluid, *Pediatrics* 119:e1071, 2007.

160. Whitelaw A, Odd D: Postnatal phenobarbital for the prevention of intraventricular hemorrhage in preterm infants, *Cochrane Database Syst Rev Oct* 17;(4):CD001691, 2007.

161. Wu YW, et al: Multiple risk factors in neonatal sinovenous thrombosis, *Neurology* 59:438, 2002.

162. Wu YW, et al: Intraventricular hemorrhage in term neonates caused by sinovenous thrombosis, *Ann Neurol* 54:123, 2003.

163. Wu YW, et al: Cerebral palsy in a term population: risk factors and neuroimaging findings, *Pediatrics* 118:690, 2006.

164. Yanowitz TD, et al: Hemodynamic disturbances in premature infants born after chorioamnionitis: association with cord blood cytokine concentrations, *Pediatr Res* 51:310, 2002.

PART 4

Hypoxic-Ischemic Encephalopathy
Malcolm I. Levene and Linda S. de Vries

Hypoxic-ischemic encephalopathy, severe enough to cause irreversible damage in the mature fetal brain, has an incidence of 1 to 2 per 1000 live births, but is 2 to 3 times more common in developing countries. Up to 25% of surviving infants may be irreversibly damaged by this condition. Neuroprotective therapy with hypothermia[11,29] has been shown to be effective in reducing the risk for disability and death in affected term babies and as such will offer an important therapeutic strategy to reduce brain damage in surviving babies. (See Management, later) Additional studies are needed to more clearly identify optimal candidates for therapeutic hypothermia.

I. Pathophysiology

Malcolm I. Levene

The immature brain is in some ways more resistant to hypoxic-ischemic (asphyxial) events than the central nervous system of the adult or older child. The reasons for this include a lower cerebral metabolic rate, particularly of glucose; immaturity in the development of the balance in functional neurotransmitters with potential neurotoxicity; and the plasticity of the immature central nervous system. Nevertheless, cerebral hypoxia-ischemia occurring in the fetus and newborn is a major cause of acute mortality and chronic neurologic disability in survivors. This is an even greater problem in the developing world than in Western nations. (See also Chapter 7.)

DEFINITIONS

Much confusion exists concerning the terminology of hypoxic-ischemic insults during fetal and neonatal life. The following discussion helps define the various widely used terms.

Hypoxic-Ischemic Encephalopathy

This term describes abnormal neurologic behavior in the neonatal period arising as a result of a hypoxic-ischemic event. The severity of hypoxic-ischemic encephalopathy (HIE) can be defined as mild, moderate, or severe depending on symptoms and signs; these are summarized in Table 40-6.[28]

Hypoxia or Anoxia

This denotes a partial (hypoxia) or complete (anoxia) lack of oxygen in the brain or blood.

Asphyxia

This is the state in which placental or pulmonary gas exchange is compromised or ceases altogether, typically producing a combination of progressive hypoxemia and hypercapnia. If the hypoxemia is severe enough, initially peripheral tissues (muscle and heart) and ultimately brain tissue develop an oxygen debt, leading to anaerobic glycolysis and production of a lactic acidosis. The lactic acid diffuses into the bloodstream, causing metabolic acidemia. This can be measured by blood gas analysis.

Ischemia

This is reduction (partial) or cessation (total) of bloodflow to an organ (e.g., the brain), which compromises both oxygen and substrate delivery to the tissue. Ischemia may occur as a result of perfusion failure alone (e.g., cardiac arrest or arterial infarction) or in the fetus in combination with hypoxia after a period of increasing compromise, as may happen during an abnormal labor. This usually results in increasing hypoxic acidosis with its consequent depressant effect on cardiovascular function.

SELECTIVE VULNERABILITY

It is impossible to generalize the diverse patterns of pathologic lesions seen after hypoxic-ischemic events. A number of factors influence the distribution of brain injury, summarized as follows:

- Cellular susceptibility
- Maturity
- Vascular territories
- Regional susceptibility
- Type of hypoxic-ischemic insult
- Others

There has been much debate as to the role of preexisting antenatal factors in exacerbating intrapartum HIE. An MRI study of term infants with neonatal encephalopathy has shown that the majority of the brain damage present in these babies occurred in the immediate perinatal period and was not the result of long-standing damage.[4]

Cellular Susceptibility

The neuron is the most sensitive cellular element to hypoxic-ischemic insult, followed by glia and cells comprising cerebral vasculature.

Maturity

Gestational age plays an important role in the changing susceptibility of cerebral structures to hypoxic-ischemic insult for a number of reasons, including rapid changes in neuronal development, changing vascular watersheds, and biochemical variables within cells, such as relative proportions of excitotoxic and inhibitory expression. Hypoxic-ischemic insult before 20 weeks' gestational age, such as may occur as the result of severe maternal illness, may lead to neuronal heterotopia or polymicrogyria[30] because the insult has hit the fetal brain during the stage of neuronal migration, which is not complete until 21 weeks of gestation (see also Part 1 of this chapter). Insults affecting the brain during midgestation (26 to 36 weeks) predominantly damage white matter, leading to periventricular leukomalacia (see also Part 2 of this chapter). Insults at term (35 weeks and beyond) result predominantly in damage to gray matter, particularly deep gray matter (posterior putamen and ventrolateral nucleus of the thalamus).

Vascular Territories

Watershed injury refers to tissue damage that occurs in regions that are most vulnerable to reduction in cerebral perfusion as the result of having the most tenuous blood supply. These tissues are at the furthest points of arterial anastomoses and are exposed to damage when perfusion pressure falls, usually as the result of impaired cardiac output and low blood pressure. Watershed areas change with advancing development. From 26 to 34 weeks' gestation, the periventricular white matter may be vulnerable because of its position between ventriculopetal and ventriculofugal arteriole distributions.

Periventricular leukomalacia has been described as being a watershed lesion, but more recently this has been challenged as the major factor in its pathogenesis.

TABLE 40–6   Clinical Staging of Hypoxic-Ischemic Encephalopathy

Variable	Stage I	Stage II	Stage III
Level of consciousness	Alert	Lethargy	Coma
Muscle tone	Normal or hypertonia	Hypotonia	Flaccidity
Tendon reflexes	Increased	Increased	Depressed or absent
Myoclonus	Present	Present	Absent
Seizures	Absent	Frequent	Frequent
Complex reflexes			
Suck	Active	Weak	Absent
Moro	Exaggerated	Incomplete	Absent
Grasp	Normal or exaggerated	Exaggerated	Absent
Doll's eye	Normal	Overactive	Reduced or absent
Autonomic function			
Pupils	Dilated, reactive	Constrictive, reactive	Variable or fixed
Respirations	Regular	Variations in rate and depth, periodic	Ataxic, apneic
Heart rate	Normal or tachycardia	Bradycardia	Bradycardia
Electroencephalogram	Normal	Low voltage, periodic paroxysmal	Periodic or isoelectric

Modified from Sarnat HB, et al: Neonatal encephalopathy following fetal distress: a clinical and electroencephalographic study, *Arch Neurol* 33:695, 1976.

In the term brain, a cortical watershed area (the parasagittal region) is present between the three main arteries supplying each hemisphere. The paracentral gyrus appears to be most vulnerable, with less sensitivity in the posterior parietal-preoccipital watershed area. The motor cortex is particularly liable to watershed injury, accounting for the observation that spastic cerebral palsy is the most common major sequela to hypoxic-ischemic insult at term. By corollary, the hippocampus, temporal lobe, and occipital lobes are most resistant to this type of insult. Volpe and colleagues,[32] using positron emission tomography to measure regional cerebral bloodflow in 17 full-term asphyxiated newborns, found a consistent decrease in bloodflow to the parasagittal region of both cerebral hemispheres in most of the infants.

The depths of the sulci are also sensitive to hypoxic-ischemic insult as the result of being watershed areas at term. Reduction in perfusion in small vessels at the base of sulci during hypoxia-ischemia leads to columnar necrosis and may lead to ulegyria in the older child's brain.

Arterial infarction (stroke) causes a characteristic pattern of damage on histologic examination wherein all cell elements die rather than just neurons, which bear the major burden of hypoxic-ischemic insult. Adverse perinatal events are reported to have been present in 46% of cases of arterial infarction,[19] but the relationship is probably not causal in most cases. In a group of 124 infants with neonatal encephalopathy, only 5% had a stroke lesion identified.[25] Infarction of a major cerebral artery should not necessarily be considered to be due to a hypoxic-ischemic insult because thrombosis and embolus are more common etiologic factors. The lesions typically involve the cerebral cortex and subcortical white matter, primarily in the territory of the middle cerebral artery and rarely in the distribution of the basilar artery.

Regional Susceptibility

Some regions of the brain are particularly sensitive to hypoxic-ischemic insult owing to the vascular factors discussed previously, but high metabolic rates of individual nuclei may predispose them to damage during cerebral hypoperfusion. This may account for the susceptibility of the posterior and lateral thalamic nuclei to damage after acute total asphyxia. Another factor accounting for regional variability to hypoxia-ischemia is the distribution of glutamate excitotoxic receptors. Regional cerebral glucose use also has been investigated with positron emission tomography after perinatal cerebral hypoxia-ischemia. Doyle and colleagues[6] investigated five newborns with positron emission tomography, using [18F]fluoro-2-deoxyglucose as the positron-emitting isotope. Localized decreases in cerebral glucose use were seen, corresponding to areas of hypodensity in cerebral gray and white matter structures noted on computed tomography (CT) scans. As with the cerebral bloodflow data, the alterations in regional cerebral glucose use presumably represented corresponding regions of tissue necrosis in which oxidative metabolism had declined below the rate of normal tissue.

Types of Hypoxic-Ischemic Insult

Animal studies on primates have modeled two different patterns of hypoxic-ischemic insult and have shown different patterns of neuronal injury depending on the type of insult.[3,20] Acute total asphyxia was produced in fetal monkeys by clamping the umbilical cord and preventing the animal from breathing. This produced injury to the thalamus, brainstem, and spinal cord structures. The longer the duration of the acute insult, the more extensive was the damage in these regions. Little damage was reported in higher structures.[20]

The second model attempted to mimic a partial asphyxial insult lasting 1 to 5 hours.[3] This produced damage predominantly in the cerebral hemispheres and particularly in the watershed distribution (see Vascular Territories earlier), often with sparing of brainstem, hippocampus, and temporal and occipital lobes. Damage was also seen not uncommonly in the basal ganglia and the cerebellum. In half the animals studied, significant asymmetry was seen between damage to the two hemispheres.

Others

Other types of hypoxic-ischemic insults include maternal fever during labor, which may accelerate fetal brain injury, fetal starvation with reduction in intracerebral glucose availability, sepsis, and twinning. The effects of these factors may act through one or a number of the variables discussed previously.

NEUROPATHOLOGY

For the reasons given previously, there are no consistent neuropathologic features of hypoxic-ischemic injury; rather, these vary depending on the type and duration of the insult and the gestational age of the child at the time of the insult. The pathologic features evident on examination also depend on the interval between the insult and death. If death occurs in close proximity to the hypoxic-ischemic insult, few if any changes may be seen, but if survival is prolonged for hours or days, then the neuropathologic features become more apparent as they develop in a temporal sequence. The following represent some of the more consistent features of hypoxic-ischemic injury.

Cerebral Edema

Brain edema is thought to occur frequently in infants who have sustained a severe cerebral hypoxic-ischemic insult, and is widely reported in autopsy studies. Cellular edema develops within an hour of the insult and resolves by 7 days after its onset.[30] In primate studies of intrapartum asphyxia, partial intermittent hypoxia-ischemia with marked and prolonged hypoxemia was associated with severe edema in all cases, whereas brain swelling was not a feature of severe, acute, total hypoxic-ischemic insults.[21] Edema particularly affects white matter and probably accounts for the abnormal signal on magnetic resonance imaging (MRI) seen in the region of the posterior limb of the internal capsule (see Neuroimaging later). Because of the higher water content in the neonatal brain cerebral edema cannot be reliably detected by magnetic resonance imaging until 24 hours after the event. The edema typically resolves by 7 days after onset. If the brain damage has been widespread and severe, on gross examination the brain appears swollen, with slitlike lateral ventricles, widening and flattening of the cerebral gyri with associated obliteration of the sulci, and herniation of hippocampal structures. In the most severe cases, herniation of the cerebellar tonsils and vermis through the foramen magnum has been described, but this is seen rarely in clinical practice.

Cellular Responses

Different cell lines in the brain react in varying ways to an acute hypoxic-ischemic insult. Neurons may undergo either necrosis or apoptosis (see Pathophysiology of Perinatal Hypoxic-Ischemic Brain Damage later). The nature of these two mutually exclusive processes can be distinguished to some extent by histologic staining. In necrosis, sections stained with hematoxylin and eosin show changes from 5 to 6 hours after the injury. Nuclear membranes degenerate, with release of nuclear chromatin and a secondary inflammatory reaction.[30]

Microglial cells (brain macrophages) respond rapidly within 2 to 3 hours after a hypoxic-ischemic insult and undertake the function of ingesting and lysing dead tissue. Activated microglia express a number of cytoxic cytokines. Hemoglobin released from damaged red cells is mobilized in this way, leaving residual hemosiderin present in the macrophage. Microglial cells present in the dentate gyrus are a reliable indication of previous hypoxic-ischemic insult in infants younger than 9 months of age.[5]

Glial cells respond to hypoxic-ischemic insult by enlarging, proliferating, and later developing fibrillary processes with the expression of glial fibrillary acidic protein, which can be recognized by specific staining. A glial response occurs from 17 weeks of gestational age.[30]

Calcification

Deposition of calcium in damaged neurons is commonly seen after hypoxic-ischemic insult and, if extensive enough, may be apparent on brain imaging. Insults other than those due to hypoxia-ischemia may also cause extensive calcification, including viral infection and certain metabolic disorders.

Chronic Lesions

Cerebral atrophy is the end stage of cellular loss in the brain. Atrophy affects particularly vulnerable areas of the brain (described earlier under Selective Vulnerability). Various specific forms of end-stage pathologic lesions have been recognized in the brain for many years.

Status marmoratus describes a patchy, marble-like appearance of the basal ganglia and thalamus that may develop approximately 6 months after a severe perinatal hypoxic-ischemic insult. Histologic study shows abnormal myelination of glial bundles rather than neurons.

Ulegyria refers to a particular form of pathology seen in the depths of the cortical sulci and is probably due to a particular watershed vulnerability (see Vascular Territories earlier). The chronic phase of this process produces the appearance of mushroom-like gyri because of loss of deep gray matter in the sulci.

SYSTEMIC ADAPTATION TO HYPOXIC-ISCHEMIC INSULT

Severe fetal hypoxic-ischemic injury affects the entire organism, and these effects have been well studied in animal models. Compromise resulting in hypoxic-ischemic injury may occur at any time during pregnancy, the birth process, or the neonatal period. The pattern of brain damage is reflected by the gestational age of the fetus at the time that the injury occurs. Fetal hypoxic-ischemic injury may result from maternal, uteroplacental, or fetal problems (Box 40-5). The

BOX 40–5 Causes of Fetal Hypoxic-Ischemic Insult

MATERNAL
Cardiac arrest
Asphyxiation
Severe anaphylactoid reaction
Status epilepticus
Hypovolemic shock

UTEROPLACENTAL
Placental abruption
Cord prolapse
Uterine rupture
Hyperstimulation with oxytocic agents

FETAL
Fetomaternal hemorrhage
Twin-to-twin transfusion syndrome
Severe isoimmune hemolytic disease
Cardiac arrhythmia

fetus may survive maternal hypoxia-ischemia such as transient hypoxia or hypotension. Correctable placental factors include hyperstimulation with oxytocic agents or intermittent cord compression, but these may cause irreversible brain damage before recovery occurs.

Brain damage as the result of in utero hypoxic-ischemic insult has been described.[30] Occasionally, there is a history of a catastrophic maternal illness, such as suffocation, anaphylaxis, or major physical trauma. In other situations, the antecedent pathogenic event is confined to the fetus, with or without an associated abnormality of the uteroplacental unit. Whatever the cause of the cerebral hypoxia-ischemia, the neuropathologic consequence is often devastating.

In the mature fetus, a period of mild to moderate hypoxemia produces a consistent pattern of responses (Fig. 40-61A).[1] Initially, there is fetal bradycardia with compensatory increase in stroke volume leading to an immediate rise in blood pressure, and in particular an increase in perfusion to the brain and other vital organs at the expense of the rest of the body. With ongoing hypoxemia, the fetal heart rate gradually increases to prehypoxic levels, but the blood pressure and carotid bloodflow remain elevated above prehypoxemic levels. The fetus is very resistant to mild or moderate hypoxemia and normal cardiovascular function will be maintained for up to an hour even with a PaO_2 of 15 mm Hg. If only moderate hypoxia is maintained, cerebral perfusion will remain normal, but if the situation persists for weeks then fetal growth restriction will occur. If moderate hypoxia is unrelieved, metabolic acidosis eventually develops with further adverse effects on physiologic and cellular integrity.

As the hypoxic insult becomes more severe, changes in regional cerebral bloodflow occur. The brainstem is able to extract sufficient oxygen to maintain metabolism despite very low PaO_2 at the expense of the cerebrum. Failing myocardial function may cause a fall in cardiac output, and the watershed areas of the cerebral hemispheres are most exposed to damage (see Vascular Territories earlier).

In some cases, the fetus sustains a much more acute hypoxic-ischemic insult, as may occur during cord prolapse or uterine rupture. The physiologic effects are shown in Figure 40-61B.

Under these circumstances, severe fetal bradycardia develops within a minute of the total asphyxial event, with an initially marked rise in blood pressure and carotid vascular resistance. In contrast to the more chronic situation, there is a reduction in cerebral bloodflow that is further exacerbated as blood pressure starts to fall owing to myocardial failure with unrelieved acute insult. This type of insult is likely to damage the basal ganglia and brainstem, in contrast to the more chronic insult, which leads to damage in the cerebrum.

Preconditioning

Preconditioning describes reduced sensitivity of the immature brain to injury depending on whether it has been exposed to previous nondamaging hypoxic events some hours before the main hypoxic-ischemic insult. Preconditioning of immature rat pups by exposure to moderate hypoxia before hypoxia-ischemia appears to be neuroprotective. Preconditioning may work through a number of pathways including induction of antiapoptotic genes, stimulation of growth factors (e.g., IGF), nitric oxide (NO), and free radical scavengers.

PATHOPHYSIOLOGY OF PERINATAL HYPOXIC-ISCHEMIC BRAIN DAMAGE

The most important advance in the neurobiology of hypoxic-ischemic brain damage in recent years has been the gradual (and as yet incomplete) unraveling of the processes leading to neuronal death. Our increasing understanding of these molecular and cellular changes is leading to strategies aimed at neuroprotection once a potentially damaging insult has occurred.

Acute hypoxic-ischemic insult leads to events that can be broadly categorized as early (primary) and delayed (secondary) neuronal death. The term *secondary* recognizes that many processes are involved and may extend up to 72 hours or even longer after the acute insult. Early neuronal death is predominantly due to necrosis, and delayed cell death is predominantly apoptotic.

Early or primary neuronal damage occurs as a result of cytotoxic changes due to failure of the microcirculation, inhibition of energy-producing molecular processes, increasing extracellular acidosis, and failure of Na^+/K^+-adenosine triphosphatase (ATPase) membrane pumps, which results in excessive leakage of Na^+ and Cl^- into the cell with consequent accumulation of intracellular water (cytotoxic edema). Free radical production is also initiated, which further compromises neuronal integrity. If not reversed, these processes lead to neuronal death within a short time of the acute insult, but recovery and reperfusion as occur with resuscitation fuel the pathways to late (secondary) neuronal damage through a relatively large number of known pathophysiologic mechanisms.

Secondary Neuronal Death

A complicated cascade of intracellular events is triggered by the initial hypoxic-ischemic insult, which results in either cell necrosis or apoptosis (Fig. 40-62).[1]

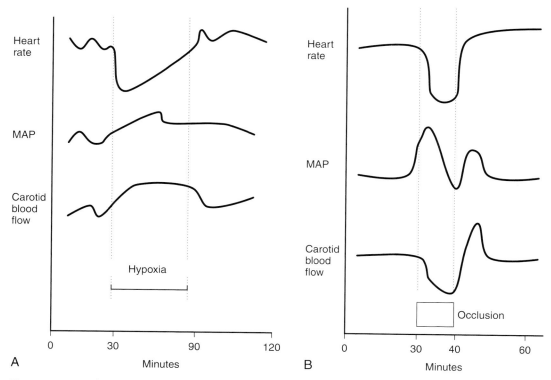

Figure 40–61. Physiologic responses to two models of asphyxia in the near-term fetal sheep. **A,** Moderate hypoxia lasting for 60 minutes. **B,** Complete umbilical artery occlusion for 10 minutes. MAP, mean arterial pressure. (*Data from Bennet L, et al: The cerebral hemodynamic response to asphyxia and hypoxia in the near term fetal sheep as measured by near-infrared spectroscopy, Pediatr Res 44:951, 1998.*)

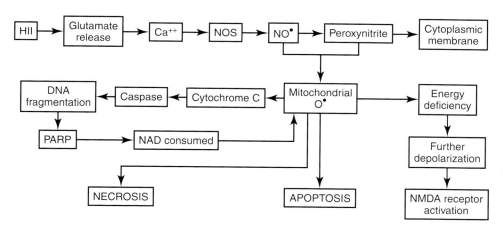

Figure 40–62. A summary of the intracellular cascade initiated by a hypoxic-ischemic insult. NAD, Nicotinamide adenine dinucleotide; NMDA, N-methyl D-aspartate; NO·, nitric oxide free radical; NOS, nitric oxide synthase; O·, oxygen free radical; PARP, poly(ADP-ribose)polymerase. (*Adapted from Johnston MV, et al: Neurobiology of hypoxic-ischemic injury in the developing brain, Pediatr Res 49:735, 2001.*)

Glutamate Injury (Excitotoxicity)

Excessive neuroexcitatory activity occurs as a result of the asphyxial event and this is mediated through glutamate toxicity. Glutamate activates N-methyl-D-aspartate (NMDA) receptors, which in turn cause calcium channels to open in an unregulated manner with excess entry of intracellular Ca^{2+}. In high concentration, this ion activates lipases, proteases, endonucleases, and phospholipase C, which in turn break down organelle membranes. This sets up a variety of abnormal processes with release of free radicals, including NO• and superoxide ions. This has further adverse effects on

cell membranes and leads to mitochondrial failure with the release of caspase-3 and eventual DNA fragmentation, poly (ADP-ribose) polymerase (PARP) which causes further energy failure of intracellular membrane function. This process also triggers an apoptotic response in the cell.

Free Radical Formation

Unstable free radicals cause peroxidation of unsaturated fatty acids, and because the brain is especially rich in polyunsaturated phospholipids, it is especially susceptible to free radical attack. Mechanisms for quenching and inhibiting free radical production exist within the brain, but in the immature organ these mechanisms may be underdeveloped. Consequently, the human neonatal brain is at particular risk for free radical formation. Brain arteriole endothelium is the main source of free radical production by the action of xanthine oxidase, but free radicals are also produced by activated neutrophils, microglia, and intraneuronal structures. During reperfusion, free radical production from the arteriolar endothelium results in blood-brain barrier leakage and release of platelet-activating factor, platelet adhesion, and neutrophil accumulation.[14] This has the effect of reducing cerebral reperfusion bloodflow with secondary failure to provide substrate to the brain.

Two particularly important mechanisms that expose the newborn brain to free radical attack are the presence of free iron and the presence of NO. Free iron that is not bound to protein is found in higher concentration in the immature animal because of low transferrin levels. Free iron catalyzes mildly reactive oxygen species to more toxic free radicals. There is evidence that after a hypoxic-ischemic insult there is an increased presence of intraneuronal free iron within the first 24 hours[22] that persists for several weeks.

NITRIC OXIDE

NO is produced by three isoforms of the enzyme nitric oxide synthase (NOS), designated neuronal (nNOS), endothelial (eNOS), and inducible (iNOS). NO production is accelerated by intracellular Ca^{2+} influx and in excessive concentrations is neurotoxic. It is thought that up to 80% of N-methyl-D-aspartate toxicity is mediated through NO. NO also combines rapidly with superoxide to produce peroxynitrous acid, which gives rise to the free radical peroxynitrate. Excessive NO can cause DNA strand breaks and induce neuronal apoptosis mediated through caspase-3 activation. Studies on immature animals rendered nNOS-depleted, reduced injury in brain regions usually rich in nNOS activity.[9,10] This beneficial effect has been shown to be due to caspase-3 inhibition.[8] iNOS has also been reported to aggravate injury in the immature brain.[15]

Apoptosis

See also Part 1 of this chapter.
Apoptosis or programmed cell death is now recognized to be the major cause of neuronal death. It can be distinguished histologically from necrosis by shrinkage of affected cells with retention of the cell membrane. By contrast, necrosis is associated with cell rupture, which induces secondary inflammatory processes. DNA degradation develops in the apoptotic cell, giving a characteristic ladder appearance on gel electrophoresis.

Apoptosis is a gene-regulated process,[7] and both proapoptotic and antiapoptotic genes influence the process, *including BCL2, Bax, APAF1,* and the caspase gene family. In particular, the antiapoptotic gene *cJUN* is thought to trigger the process.[7] A major role in the apoptotic mechanism is played by the caspase family of proteins, with caspase-3 identified as the "execution protein." Inhibitors of caspase can block apoptosis and attenuate injury.[33] Other factors that may initiate or accelerate apoptosis include intracellular alkalosis[26] and caspase-independent apoptosis-inducing factor.[35]

Cytokines

There is evidence that some proinflammatory cytokines (tumor necrosis factor-α, interleukin [IL]-1β, and IL-18) are activated after a hypoxic-ischemic insult in immature experimental animal models, and they may have neurotoxic properties.[13] All of these cytokines rely on caspase-1 as a converting enzyme for full activation. Caspase-1 has also been shown to be an important mediator of neonatal brain injury.[17] After hypoxic-ischemic insult, widespread expression of caspase-1 and IL-18 protein in microglia was found.[13] IL-18-deficient mice had significantly less brain injury than wild-type mice, suggesting that IL-18 may have an essential function in the pathway of events leading to posthypoxic ischemic brain injury.[13] These data suggest that hypoxic-ischemic insult may initiate an inflammatory response in the absence of infection, leading to neuronal injury.

Studies in animals and humans have shown that exposure to infection (gram-negative bacteria in animal models) and chorioamnionitis in pregnant women significantly exacerbate clinical and neuronal injury.[2,8]

Human Studies

New technologies have given considerable insight into the time scale of these events in human infants who have been subject to a presumed severe clinical asphyxial event before delivery. In the early 1980s, magnetic resonance spectroscopy showed a consistent pattern of metabolic disturbance in the brain.[27,34] The ^{31}P magnetic resonance spectroscopy spectra in affected term infants were usually normal within the first 6 hours after birth, suggesting that mitochondrial phosphorylation had initially recovered with resuscitation. By 12 to 24 hours, there was a significant decline in the energy ratio of phosphocreatine to inorganic phosphate (PCr/Pi), with a further decline in the most severely affected infants at 48 to 72 hours. In some infants, recovery occurred to normal values within 7 days. The delayed fall in PCr/Pi ratio represents secondary energy failure. [1]H magnetic resonance spectroscopy in other groups of asphyxiated infants showed a rise in intracerebral lactate peak simultaneous with the fall in PCr/Pi ratio.[12,23] Studies sampling specific voxels in the affected brain show regional differences, with increased lactate concentrations particularly in the thalamus compared with the occipitoparietal white matter.[12]

Near-infrared spectroscopy has also been used in the term newborn to study cerebral blood volume and bloodflow after severe presumed hypoxic-ischemic insult. These studies have shown a marked increase in blood volume and bloodflow in the brain with loss of normal CO_2 reactivity,[18,24] which suggests that secondary energy failure compromises cerebral arteriolar function with failure of small vessel reactivity that results in vasodilation and maximum bloodflow.[32]

II. Assessment Tools

Linda S. de Vries

Many different tools have become available to aid in the more precise prediction of neurodevelopmental outcome in the full-term infant with HIE. Both neurophysiology and neuroimaging play an important role and are discussed separately.

NEUROPHYSIOLOGY

See also Part 5.

Neonatal electroencephalography (EEG) is a well-recognized method to assess brain integrity after hypoxia-ischemia that results in neonatal encephalopathy. In newborn infants, the EEG commonly uses 16 channels and is in most centers only performed during the day; it requires skilled technicians and highly trained and experienced neurophysiologists to interpret the recordings. The 16-channel EEG provides detailed information and when performed with simultaneous video recording, helps to make a distinction between clinical and subclinical seizures.[45,79] A recent study showed that less than 10% of neonatal seizures were correctly identified by the neonatal staff, compared with simultaneous video-EEG recordings.[81] Normal and severely abnormal results on EEG have important predictive value. Normal traces almost invariably predict a normal outcome, whereas persistent, severely abnormal traces predict an adverse outcome (Fig. 40-63).[62,106] Prediction in children with mild to moderate EEG abnormalities is less reliable and requires sequential recordings. EEG activity is fully differentiated in full-term infants. During quiet sleep, a discontinuous pattern (tracé alternant)

alternates with a high-voltage continuous delta pattern. In wakefulness, the EEG is characterized by low-voltage mixed theta-delta activity. In active sleep, a mixed medium-voltage delta-theta activity is seen. Abnormalities on the EEG can be classified as background abnormalities, ictal abnormalities, and abnormalities in the organization of states and maturation.[62,74,75,103] Background pattern abnormalities are highly predictive of outcome (Fig. 40-64).[41,80] It should be taken into account that antiepileptic drugs can (transiently) affect sleep states and the background pattern, especially in children with severe encephalopathy.[103] The following background patterns can be recognized: isoelectric and extremely low voltage (less than 5 μV); burst suppression pattern, with long periods of inactivity (usually longer than 10 seconds) mixed with bursts of abnormal activity. Outcome is especially poor with long periods of inactivity[40,77] and brief periods of bursts (less than 6 seconds) with small-amplitude bursts and interhemispheric asymmetry and asynchrony.

To overcome the problem of difficult access and lack of continuity, a continuous monitoring device is now increasingly being used, the amplitude-integrated EEG (aEEG). This simple device was initially used as a single-channel EEG from a pair of parietal electrodes. The EEG signal is first amplified and passed through an asymmetric band-pass filter that strongly attenuates activity below 2 Hz and above 15 Hz to minimize artifacts from electrical interference. The EEG processing

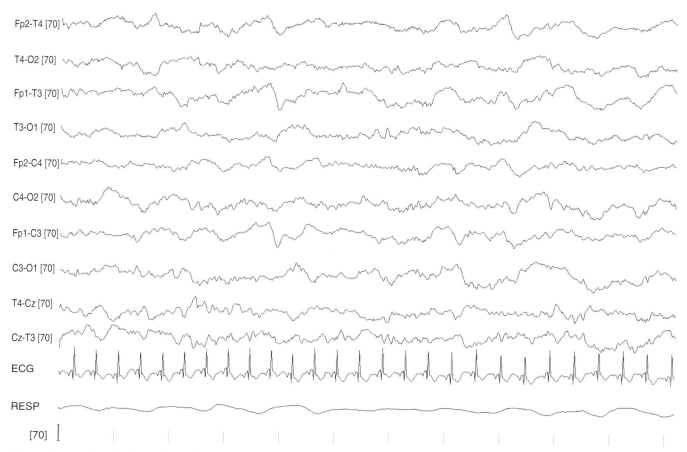

Figure 40–63. Standard 16-channel electroencephalogram showing a normal continuous-voltage background pattern. (*Courtesy AC van Huffelen, PhD, Department of Neurophysiology, University Medical Center, Utrecht, The Netherlands.*)

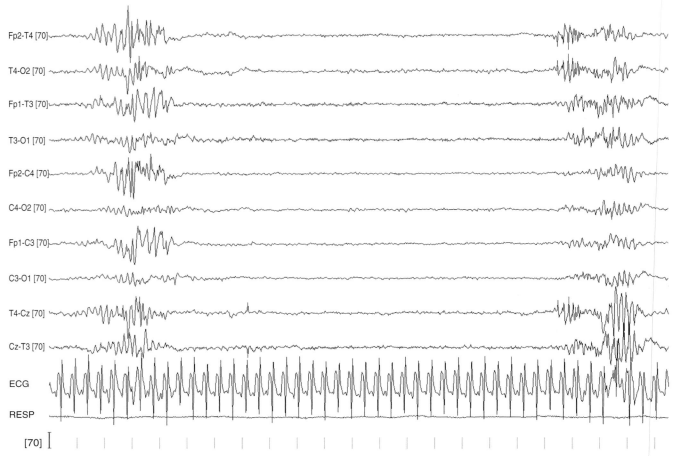

Figure 40–64. Standard 16-channel electroencephalogram showing a typically abnormal burst suppression background pattern. (*Courtesy AC van Huffelen, PhD, Department of Neurophysiology, University Medical Center, Utrecht, The Netherlands.*)

involves semilogarithmic amplitude compression, rectification, smoothing, and time compression.[85] The digital devices also provide the raw EEG and can use more than a single channel. Easy around-the-clock access and easy interpretation based on pattern recognition have led to an increase in continuous monitoring of brain activity in the neonatal intensive care unit. Several groups have compared simultaneous aEEG with a 16-channel EEG recording.[104] A good correlation was noted for the background pattern (Fig. 40-65). In a later study comparing a standard EEG with a single-channel aEEG from the C3-C4 position and without display of the raw-EEG, only 12% to 38% (mean 26%) of individual seizures were detected.[97] Seizures that will not be detected with aEEG are short seizures, low-amplitude seizures, and focal discharges (Fig. 40-66). Sensitivity of seizure recognition can be considerably improved when using a two-channel bilateral centroparietal aEEG recording with access to the corresponding raw EEG.[96] While the sensitivity for detecting seizures in one or two-channel aEEG recordings without access to the raw EEG was 27% to 56%, 76% of the seizures were detected when using two aEEG channels with the corresponding raw EEG. Performing at least one 16-channel EEG during the aEEG recording is therefore strongly recommended. Use of continuous aEEG recording provided information about the improvement that can occur in infants with very poor background patterns immediately after delivery. Recovery of a burst suppression pattern within the first 24 hours was sometimes noted to be associated with a normal outcome.[88] On the other hand, children with a continuous voltage pattern could deteriorate after 24 hours during a period of secondary energy failure, showing deterioration of their background pattern and late onset of seizures. In most infants, however, a good prediction of later neurodevelopmental outcome could be made on the basis of the aEEG background pattern obtained at 6 or even 3 hours after birth.[55,103] The early predictive value of the background pattern assessed with this technique has led to its use for selection of newborn infants in intervention studies, such as the hypothermia study.[58] A longer recording will also allow assessment of the presence, quality, and time of onset of sleep-wake cycling (SWC). The presence, time of onset, and quality of SWC reflects the severity of the hypoxic-ischemic insult to which newborns have been exposed.[83] The time of onset of SWC helps predict neurodevelopmental outcome based on whether SWC returns before 36 hours (good outcome) or after 36 hours (bad outcome). It was recently shown that recovery of background activity tends to be slower during hypothermia, and care should be taken when predicting outcome. The positive predictive value for predicting a poor outcome during the first 3 to 6 hours was only 59% in the infants receiving hypothermia compared to 84% in those with normothermia. Infants

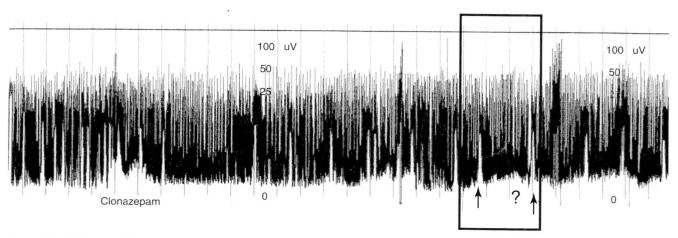

Figure 40–65. Same child as in Figure 40-64 showing burst suppression pattern on the amplitude-integrated electroencephalogram (aEEG). The box indicates a period of simultaneous EEG recording. The two arrows indicate an electrical discharge recognized by aEEG, and the question mark indicates a period when a focal discharge was seen only on the standard EEG (see Fig. 40-66).

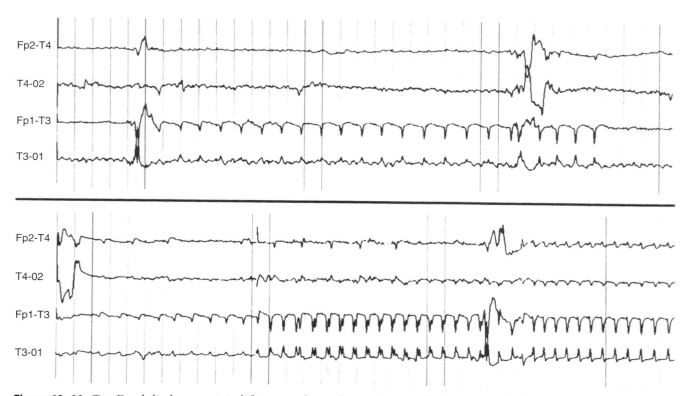

Figure 40–66. *Top,* Focal discharge, origin left temporal, not detected on amplitude-integrated electroencephalogram; *bottom,* focal discharge with spread. (*From Toet MC, et al: Comparison between simultaneously recorded amplitude integrated EEG [Cerebral Function Monitor] and standard EEG in neonates,* Pediatrics 109:772, 2002, with permission.)

with a good outcome normalized their background pattern by 24 hours, but by 48 hours if treated with hypothermia. Similar observations were made by Hallberg and colleagues.[58a,101b]

The presence of subclinical seizures can be better evaluated using aEEG, and it was noted that newborns very often show electroclinical dissociation, especially after administration of the first drug given for clinical seizures.[45,95] Scher and colleagues[95] found that 58% of infants with seizures persisting after treatment with phenobarbitone or phenytoin showed uncoupling of electrical and clinical seizures (see also Part 5 of this chapter). Status epilepticus (ongoing seizure activity for at least 30 minutes) is not uncommon and was noted in 18% in a cohort monitored with continuous aEEG.[89] In this study, there was a significant difference in background pattern, as well as in duration of the status epilepticus between infants with a poor outcome, compared with those with a good outcome.

Efficacy of treatment of seizures was noted to be poor, as already reported by others using intermittent 16-channel EEGs.[45,84] The most commonly used drugs (phenobarbital and phenytoin) were shown to treat seizures effectively in less than half of patients when given as a single drug.[84] Other drugs, like lidocaine, were noted to be more effective, but are not yet widely used.[47,61,76] Off-label use of antiepileptic drugs like levetiracetam and topiramate is not uncommon.[98]

Long-term outcomes in children who had neonatal seizures vary considerably in reports.[46,60,75] This is probably due to differences in inclusion criteria and methods of diagnosing neonatal seizures. Postneonatal epilepsy is not uncommon (20% to 50%) and was noted to be especially common after subtle seizures.[48,71] In two studies using aEEG and treating clinical as well as subclinical seizures, postnatal epilepsy developed in only 8% to 9% of the survivors.[60,105] There is no agreement in the literature over whether neonatal seizures themselves can lead to damage of the immature neonatal brain. Electroclinical and electrographic neonatal seizures produce an increase in cerebral bloodflow velocity. It is suggested that electrographic seizures are associated with disturbed cerebral metabolism and that treatment of neonatal seizures until electrographic seizure activity is abolished may improve outcome.[44,88a]

Animal studies have shown that neonatal seizures can permanently disrupt neuronal development.[63,64,74] Seizures superimposed on hypoxic ischemia in rat pups were noted significantly to exacerbate brain injury.[108] On the other hand, antiepileptic drugs are not without side effects, and data from a study published in 2002 have shown apoptotic neurodegeneration in the developing rat brain at plasma concentrations relevant for seizure control in humans.[42]

EVOKED POTENTIALS

Evoked potentials can further aid in the prediction of neurodevelopmental outcome of full-term infants with HIE. Brainstem auditory evoked potentials (BAEPs) or brainstem evoked response and visual evoked potentials (VEPs) are technically easier to perform than somatosensory evoked potentials (SEPs).

BAEPs are responses generated in the auditory brainstem pathway after an acoustic stimulus (see also Chapter 42). They are used to assess both the peripheral sensitivity and the neurologic integrity of the auditory pathway. Seven positive waves can be recognized; these are indicated with Roman numerals. BAEPs are regarded as the most objective and reliable method of evaluating peripheral auditory function in neonates. Because perinatal asphyxia is a well-known risk factor for sensorineural hearing loss, BAEPs should always be performed in at-risk infants. Initial studies using BAEPs to predict neurodevelopmental outcome were not as consistent as those using SEPs and VEPs. An increase in the I through V peak latency, considered to represent brainstem conduction time, was noted to be of predictive value. When children were assessed again at 4 to 12 years, the sensitivity, specificity, positive predictive value, and false-negative rate of neonatal BAEPs for subsequent neurodevelopmental outcomes were 40.5%, 87.8%, 75.0%, and 59.5%, respectively.[68] More recent

studies by the same group have used maximum-length sequence BAEPs with an increased repetition rate of clicks (90 to 910 per second) and have shown that this may be a better way to demonstrate the effect of HIE, which was most marked on day 3 (Fig. 40-67).[67]

The VEP is a gross electrical signal generated by the occipital area of the cortex in response to a visual stimulus. The stimulus can be either a diffuse flashing light or a patterned visual stimulus. In the neonatal unit, light-emitting diode goggles or small light-emitting diode screens are most widely used. The P200 and the N300 are the major components that can be recognized in the neonatal period. FVEPs (flash VEPs) are good predictors of cerebral visual impairment after perinatal asphyxia.[107] A high correlation between FVEPs and neurodevelopmental outcome was found by the same group.[101,107] Absent FVEPs carried a poor prognosis, whereas persistently abnormal FVEPs also predicted an abnormal outcome. Normal FVEPs, however, were not always associated with a good outcome, and FVEPs appeared to be more resistant than SEPs. When FVEP recording was performed within 6 hours after birth, a positive predictive value of 77% was found, slightly lower than for SEPs (82%) or aEEG (84%).[55] VEPs were recently shown to be predictive of cerebral visual impairment in full-term infants with symptomatic hypoglycemia and injury to the occipital visual cortex.[99]

SEPs are technically the most difficult to perform and by far the most time consuming. The median nerve is usually

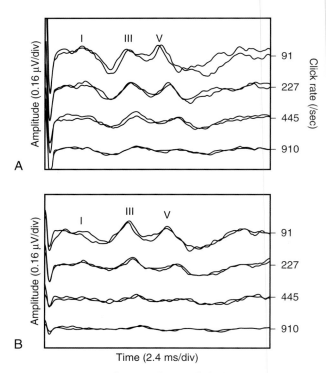

Figure 40–67. Sample recordings of the brainstem auditory evoked potential at 91, 227, 455, and 910 clicks per second. **A,** Normal term neonate. **B,** Asphyxiated term neonate; the amplitude of wave V is significantly reduced at 910 clicks per second. (*From Jiang ZD, et al: Maximum length sequence brainstem auditory evoked responses in term neonates who have perinatal hypoxia-ischemia,* Pediatr Res 48:639, 2000.)

stimulated because this is better tolerated than stimulation of the tibial nerve. At the scalp, contralateral to the site of stimulation and overlying the primary somatosensory cortex, wave N19 is recorded, which is considered to be cortically generated. In the newborn, this component is usually referred to as N1. The predictive value of SEPs in full-term infants with HIE was first shown by Hrbek and colleagues[65] and has been confirmed since by several groups.[52,57,94,101] When comparing FVEPs and VEPs, some studies showed SEPs to be superior in the prediction of neurodevelopmental outcome. Because the predictive value within the first 6 hours after birth was noted to be similar for aEEG and evoked potentials, aEEG is preferred because of easy access, application, and interpretation.[55]

NEUROIMAGING

See also Parts 1 through 3 of this chapter.
As discussed earlier, certain regions of the brain are preferentially affected under different circumstances. Different imaging modalities can be used, but recent data have shown MRI to be superior compared with ultrasonography and CT.

Cranial ultrasonography has a poor reputation when it comes to assessment of abnormalities of the brain of the full-term infant with HIE. Ultrasonography can be helpful, however, especially when performed sequentially during the first week of life.[54,90] Changes in the thalami and basal ganglia may be subtle, but usually become more clear by the end of the first week of life.[54] Alterations of the signal in the white matter can sometimes be seen on admission, suggesting that the insult is of antenatal onset. More often, echogenicity develops gradually over a period of days. In severe cases, the ventricles are difficult to visualize owing to edema and are referred to as *slitlike*. A Doppler signal can be obtained during the ultrasonographic examination, at the level of the anterior or preferably the middle cerebral artery. Several studies have shown that an increase in diastolic flow, resulting in a reduced resistance index (less than 0.55) and an increase in cerebral bloodflow velocity (greater than 3 standard deviations), is associated with a poor neurodevelopmental outcome.[66,72] Changes usually developed after the first 24 hours after birth. Color Doppler flow across the sagittal sinus can be used to diagnose or exclude a sinovenous thrombosis.

CT is less sensitive than MRI for detecting changes in the central gray nuclei, which is the most common problem in full-term infants with HIE.[50] A decrease in attenuation of white matter may be difficult to differentiate from normal unmyelinated white matter. CT is still useful in experienced hands and especially in a child admitted after a traumatic delivery and suspected of having an extra-axial hemorrhage. In such cases, ultrasonography may miss these collections unless they are large with an associated midline shift. CT may be more accessible than MRI, and in the likelihood of possible surgical intervention, a CT can be done soon after admission.

MRI is the most appropriate technique to use and is able to show different patterns of injury.[78] The basal ganglia and thalami are involved in the first pattern, which is especially common after an acute sentinel.[37,82] An altered, sometimes reversed signal at the level of the posterior limb of the internal capsule can be seen during the second half of the first week, and this has been noted to be of very high predictive value for

neurodevelopmental outcome (Fig. 40-68).[92] With the use of diffusion-weighted MRI, abnormalities in the thalami and basal ganglia can often be seen within days after birth, but the alterations in signal intensity may be more pronounced later during the first week (Fig. 40-69).[39] Calculation of apparent diffusion coefficients can be of further use to assess the severity of the insult.[93] Changes in the basal ganglia are often seen together with changes at the level of the central gyrus, and this combination carries a poor prognosis.[70] The second most common pattern of injury is injury to the watershed regions, which is especially well recognized with diffusion weighted MRI.[78] Signal intensity changes in the white matter can also be well recognized with MRI, as well as cortical highlighting. The severity of white matter abnormalities can vary from focal lesions, often with punctate white matter lesions, and these were recently noted to be especially common in infants with milder encephalopathy and of slightly lower gestational age.[73] White matter lesions can also be very diffuse with loss of gray-white matter differentiation, preceding cystic evolution. These more severe white matter abnormalities are often seen in association with abnormalities of the basal ganglia, and early changes on MRI correlate well with neonatal EEG, later MRI findings, and neurodevelopmental outcome.[41,51,91] Tanner and colleagues[100] used dynamic susceptibility contrast-enhanced MRI to calculate qualitative values of relative cerebral bloodflow. Values of regional cerebral bloodflow were generally larger in gray than white matter. Movement artifacts were common and only a small number of infants were studied during the first week of life.

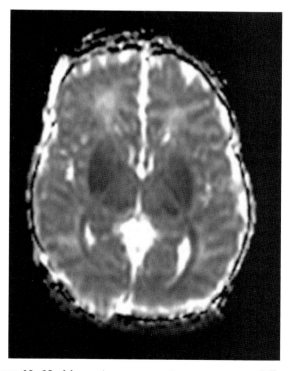

Figure 40–68. Magnetic resonance image, apparent diffusion coefficient map, performed on day 3 in a full-term infant with hypoxic-ischemic encephalopathy grade II. A decreased signal is seen in the lentiform nuclei, the ventrolateral thalami, and optic radiation.

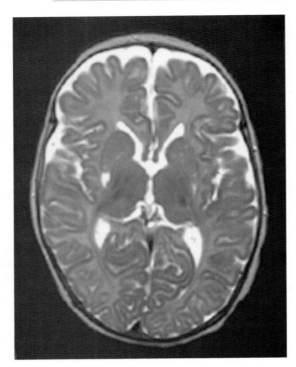

Figure 40–69. T2-weighted spin echo sequence at 3 months of age in the same child as in Figure 40-68. Cortical atrophy is noted anteriorly. Small areas with a signal intensity compatible with cerebrospinal fluid are seen at the level of the lentiform nuclei, more marked on the right side.

Focal ischemic lesions are also well detected using this technique. The middle cerebral artery, most often the left branch, is most commonly affected. Diffusion-weighted MRI allows detection of the area involved at a time when conventional MRI may not yet be very reliable. Involvement of the descending corticospinal tracts can be well visualized with diffusion-weighted MRI and is referred to as *pre-wallerian degeneration*, which is highly predictive of subsequent wallerian degeneration and development of a hemiplegia.[53,69] Magnetic resonance angiography can further aid in the visualization of abnormal flow across the artery involved in case of an embolism or dissection. The area of cavitation noted on a repeat scan performed a few months later usually is smaller than expected on the basis of the area of abnormal signal intensity seen on the initial scan, but the tissue surrounding the cavity is altered and shows gliotic scarring later in infancy. Sinovenous thrombosis was considered to be a rare condition, but with the introduction of MRI and MR venography, it is more often diagnosed.[108] Conventional MRI shows an increased signal in the sinus on a T1-weighted image, and magnetic resonance venography shows lack of flow across the sinus. The sagittal sinus, straight sinus, or the deep veins of the basal ganglia can be affected.[56] An associated unilateral thalamic hemorrhage can be present.[109] In such cases, prothrombotic factors should be checked (see also Part 3 of this chapter and Fig 40-58).

Metabolic assessment using proton or phosphorus spectroscopy can be performed during the MRI examination. This technique uses the intrinsic magnetic properties of some atomic nuclei (^{1}H, ^{31}P). The most commonly used nucleus for clinical applications is the proton (^{1}H) because it is the most abundant and strongest nucleus. N-acetylaspartate, creatine/phosphocreatine, choline-containing compounds, myoinositol, glutamine and glutamate, and lactate can all be recognized within the proton spectrum. The peaks described for the ^{31}P spectrum are β-ATP, α-ATP, and γ-ATP, PCr, phosphodiesters, inorganic phosphate (Pi), and phosphomonoesters. Depletion of ATP and an increase in Pi, associated with a change in the PCr/Pi ratio, have been reported using phosphorus spectroscopy.[49] A decrease in N-acetylaspartate and a high lactate peak have been reported for ^{1}H proton spectroscopy.[59,87] An increased lactate-to-creatine ratio (greater than 1) obtained within 18 hours after birth predicted neurodevelopmental impairment at 1 year of age with a sensitivity of 66% and a specificity of 95%.[59] In another study, the ratio of lactate to N-acetylaspartate was used, showing a sensitivity of 78% and a specificity of 90%.[36] Cerebral intracellular alkalosis was noted to persist for months after neonatal encephalopathy.[86] A comparison of proton spectroscopy and diffusion-weighted MRI on the first day after birth showed that proton magnetic resonance spectroscopy was better in accurately depicting the severity of injury at this early stage.[38] A recent meta-analysis comparing conventional MRI diffusion-weighted imaging and MRS as potential early biomarkers found deep gray matter Lac/NAA to be the most accurate quantitative MR biomarker within the neonatal period for prediction of neurodevelopmental outcome after neonatal encephalopathy.[101a]

Positron emission tomography has been infrequently used.[43,102] A study of regional cerebral metabolic rates of glucose (CMRgl) in six infants by Blennow and colleagues[43] showed localized increases in five, which were in good agreement with changes seen with other neuroimaging techniques. In another study of 20 infants, the deep subcortical areas, thalamus, basal ganglia, and sensorimotor cortex were identified as the most metabolically active brain areas. Total CMRgl were inversely related to the severity of HIE ($P < .01$).[102]

III. Management
Malcolm I. Levene

PRIMARY PREVENTION

Prevention of fetal asphyxia is far preferable to the prospect of managing the newborn who has suffered a hypoxic-ischemic insult in labor. The aim of modern obstetrics is to recognize the compromised fetus before irreversible organ damage occurs and rescue it from the hostile environment.

Electronic fetal monitoring (EFM) is widely used to identify hypoxic babies (see also Chapter 10). A Cochrane Review[110] of 12 randomized controlled trials showed a statistically significant decrease in the number of neonatal seizures in the infants born in the EFM group (RR 0.50; 95% CI 0.31-0.80). This effect was noted in only two of the larger studies, where the option of pH estimation was available for unfavorable traces. There was no significant difference in overall perinatal death rate (RR 0.85; 95% CI 0.59-1.23). These studies also showed a significantly increased risk of delivery by cesarean section in the EFM group (RR 1.66; 95% CI 1.30-2.13).

Follow-up of surviving infants was available in two studies and both failed to show any reduction in long-term neurologic adverse effects.

Fetal electrocardiogram (ECG) waveforms have been evaluated as a more sensitive method for detecting fetal hypoxia than EFM. Two different methods have been studied: the PR to R-R ratio and the ST waveform. In the PR to R-R ratio, there is normally a positive correlation between the PR interval and the R-R interval, so that when the heart rate increases, both the PR and R-R intervals shorten. The hypoxemic heart behaves differently, with shortening of the PR interval and lengthening of the R-R interval so that change in the PR to R-R ratio is a predictor of fetal heart hypoxic compromise. An alternative method assesses changes in the ST waveform in much the same way as exercise ECG assessment in adults with myocardial disease.

A Cochrane analysis of four randomized controlled trials of fetal ECG use in labor has been reported by Neilson.[155] All trials assessed fetal ECG as an adjunct to EFM alone in labor. The studies of ST waveform resulted in fewer babies born with severe metabolic acidosis (pH < 7.05) (RR 0.64; 95% CI 0.41-1.00), and fewer babies with neonatal encephalopathy (RR 0.33; 95% CI 0.11-0.95), although the numbers of babies with encephalopathy was very low when compared with standard EFM alone. There was no significant increase in numbers of cesarean section delivery or admissions to the neonatal unit. By contrast, analysis of PR interval showed no benefit in pregnancies monitored with this technique.

More recently a Cochrane review compared fetal pulse oximetry with EFM monitoring.[124] In the five trials published to date there was no overall reduction in cesarean section rate or neonatal outcome when EFM and oximetry were compared with EFM alone. One study reported a significant reduction in cesarean section rate in the group assessed by pulse oximetry following the detection of a nonreassuring EFM trace.

In summary, intrapartum assessment of severe hypoxia may result in improved condition at birth and reduce the risk of neonatal encephalopathy, but there is little evidence to support the notion that hypoxic-ischemic brain damage can be prevented.

RESUSCITATION

See also Chapter 26.

The key to resuscitation is to restore adequate oxygenation and perfusion of vital organs, particularly the brain. Systemic acidosis developing as a result of intrapartum asphyxia impairs cardiac contractility, but its effect on cerebral function is less clearly understood and there is some evidence that a degree of intracerebral acidosis may have a neuroprotective effect.[115]

Infants are born in unexpectedly poor condition and require immediate resuscitation. Most infants born in suboptimal condition can be anticipated (Box 40-6), and staff trained in neonatal resuscitation should be available at the birth. It is estimated, however, that approximately 20% of infants who require resuscitation do not fall into this group. The importance of expert resuscitation has been recognized and studied only comparatively recently, and every infant, wherever born, must have available to it personnel with expert resuscitation skills and all the appropriate equipment in good working order.

BOX 40-6 Conditions in Which the Need for Resuscitation at Birth May Be Anticipated

PRELABOR FACTORS

MATERNAL
Toxemia (eclampsia)
Diabetes mellitus
Drug addiction
Cardiovascular disease
Infectious disease
Collagen vascular disease

UTEROPLACENTAL
Placental abruption
Umbilical cord prolapse
Placenta previa
Polyhydramnios
Premature rupture of the membranes

INTRAPARTUM FACTORS
Isoimmunization
Multiple birth
Preterm birth
Cardiopulmonary abnormalities
Abnormal presentation
Precipitous delivery
Fetal distress
Thick meconium staining
Prolonged labor
Difficult forceps delivery
Intrauterine growth restriction
Prolonged pregnancy

SYSTEMIC MANAGEMENT

The diving reflex occurs during experimental asphyxia to maintain blood flow to vital organs such as the brain at the expense of less-vital organs. This is the basis of systemic complications after a clinically significant hypoxic-ischemic insult, and the heart, kidneys, and liver are the most vulnerable organs. Almost all babies with hypoxic-ischemic encephalopathy (HIE) show compromise in at least one organ system outside the brain.[166] The clinical course after a hypoxic-ischemic event in labor is unpredictable, so problems should be anticipated and the infant appropriately observed by trained staff in a clinical environment. Hypoxic-ischemic insult affects the whole organism and any organ system may be compromised. Brain-oriented management is discussed later; this section discusses management of systemic complications.

The Renal System

Renal impairment is reported to occur in 23% to 70% of asphyxiated infants.[166] Acute renal failure (plasma creatinine greater than 130 μmol/L [1.2 mg/dL] for at least 2 consecutive days) is reported in 19% of asphyxiated infants of greater than 33 weeks' gestation. In a study using a more sensitive measure of renal tubular function (N-acetylglucosaminidase), there was a relationship between elevated N-acetylglucosaminidase levels and degree of HIE in the infant.[166]

Because of the fear of renal failure and fluid overload, many clinicians have adopted a policy of fluid restriction in asphyxiated newborn infants, but there is no evidence that normal fluid volumes contribute to cerebral edema in the newborn. Fluid restriction is necessary in infants who have inappropriate antidiuretic hormone secretion or those with known renal tubular impairment. Fluid intake in these infants should be titrated against measurements of the infant's serum and urinary electrolytes.

Oliguria is managed by careful maintenance of fluid balance with daily measurement of plasma and urinary creatinine levels, and serum and urinary electrolytes, as well as daily assessment of the infant's weight. Acute renal failure and anuria lasting more than a day should be initially managed conservatively (see Chapter 36). Chronic renal failure and the need for dialysis is extremely rare in severely asphyxiated full-term infants.

Cardiovascular System

Myocardial contractility is impaired after hypoxic-ischemic insult, causing a significant reduction in cardiac output, hypotension, and further impairment of cerebral blood flow and perfusion of other organs. Myocardial dysfunction detected by Doppler ultrasonography has been shown to occur in 28% to 50% of asphyxiated newborn infants.[114,160] Other cardiac pathologic processes recognized to occur after a severe hypoxic-ischemic insult include acute cardiac dilation with functional tricuspid valve regurgitation, myocardial ischemia present on ECG assessment, and ischemic necrosis of papillary muscle. Tropinin has been suggested as a marker for perinatal myocardial damage but little objective data are available.

Hypotension is a common complication after severe hypoxic-ischemic insult,[166] and volume support is often ineffective in restoring normotension. The inotrope dopamine (5 to 15 μg/kg per minute) has been shown to be more effective in restoring blood pressure in asphyxiated infants.

Hepatic and Gastrointestinal Systems

Elevated liver enzymes occur in 80% to 85% of asphyxiated full-term newborn infants during the first week of life.[138,166] Irreversible liver damage appears to occur very rarely after birth asphyxia. Necrotizing enterocolitis is a well-recognized complication in asphyxiated infants, but is seen relatively rarely due to this cause.

Hematologic Complications

Coagulation impairment is relatively common after a severe asphyxial insult. The bone marrow may be transiently damaged, leading to thrombocytopenia. Disseminated intravascular coagulation is also well recognized to occur after birth asphyxia, with low levels of factor XIII and elevated thrombin-antithrombin complexes; D-dimer, fibrin, and fibrinogen degradation products; and soluble fibrin monomer complexes.[170]

Coagulation impairment should be anticipated and screening for hematologic abnormalities undertaken in all severely asphyxiated newborn infants. Supportive treatment with platelets, vitamin K, or clotting factors may be indicated by specific abnormalities on the coagulation screen. The management of disseminated intravascular coagulation is controversial, but there is no indication for systemic heparinization (see also Chapter 46).

BRAIN-ORIENTED MANAGEMENT

Hypothermia has become a standard of care for babies with moderate to mild HIE and four large studies have now confirmed the effectiveness and safety of this technique in preserving cerebral function.[111,126,132,167] This technique is discussed in detail below. In addition to hypothermia, careful attention must be paid to maintain cerebral homeostasis by anticipation of complications that may have a direct or indirect effect on brain function and recovery after a severe hypoxic-ischemic insult. More standard brain-specific complications affecting the infant after a severe hypoxic-ischemic insult are discussed here.

Glucose

Hypoglycemia has been shown to be an additional adverse factor for the immature brain in conjunction with a hypoxic-ischemic insult. Immature hypoglycemic animal models subjected to anoxia have a considerably increased mortality rate compared with anoxic, normoglycemic animals.[180] The presence of ketone bodies as an alternative brain fuel ameliorates this effect despite low levels of circulating glucose.[180] The facilitative glucose transporter proteins (GLUT1) transports glucose across the blood-brain barrier, and related proteins (GLUT3 and 45-kd GLUT3) mediate transport into the neuron and glial cells, but these proteins are in low concentration in the immature brain. Hypoxic-ischemic insult initially enhances both GLUT1 and GLUT3 expression in the brain, but GLUT3 decreases after 72 hours, associated with extensive cellular necrosis.[178] Asphyxia initially increases cerebral metabolic rates of glucose (CMRgl), and consumption of glucose during the hypoxic-ischemic insult causes depletion of intracerebral glucose. Very limited numbers of infants have been studied after asphyxial insults by positron emission tomography, with conflicting results. In five term infants, CMRgl was increased 2 to 3 days after the insult,[117] whereas another study of CMRgl in 20 human asphyxiated infants showed a high correlation between the more severe degree of HIE and lowest values of CMRgl.[173] These low levels were obtained at a median age of 11 days, which was later than the first study and may account for the differences in values.

Studies have shown that there are major differences in behavior of the mature and immature brain to glucose infusion.[176] The infusion of glucose in the immature organism, unlike in adults, before a hypoxic-ischemic event appears to have protective effects compared with subjects not given sugar supplementation. The pretreated hyperglycemic group had better preservation of PCr and ATP than the normoglycemic group.[177] Preconditioning the animal before a major hypoxic-ischemic insult may afford protection, which appears to be due to enhanced intracerebral glycogen levels,[119] increased expression of GLUT1,[141] and increased availability of alternative brain fuels.[122] The clinical question of whether glucose infusion after hypoxic-ischemic insult is of value remains controversial. Hattori and Wasterlain[139] have shown that glucose treatment after hypoxic-ischemic insult in 7-day-old rat pups protects against neuropathologic damage, but another study has shown in the same animal model a worsening in neuronal injury when glucose was given immediately after the insult.[168]

Although routine use of high-concentration glucose is not advised after a hypoxic-ischemic event in the neonate, it is clear that hypoglycemia must be avoided.

Seizures

See also Part 5 of this chapter.

Seizures occur in most infants who have sustained a significant hypoxic-ischemic insult; indeed, seizure is a feature of moderate and severe HIE. In general, the more severe or prolonged the hypoxia-ischemia, the more seizure activity the infant will have. There has been considerable debate as to whether seizure activity after a hypoxic-ischemic event confers an additional risk factor on the infant in terms of adverse neurodevelopmental outcome. If this is established, then there is an increased onus on the effective management of seizure activity. A hypoxic-ischemic insult sets in train a cascade of intraneuronal events that may result in cell death. Seizures may simply be a paraphenomenon indicating the process of neuronal demise.

Studies have shown that immature neurons are more susceptible to the development of seizures than the mature brain, but also less vulnerable to neuropathologic consequences. In animal studies, the induction of multiple short seizures over the first days of life does not result in neuronal loss, but does result in morphologic changes involving cortical activation and cell density evident when the brain was examined in adult life.[140] Furthermore, these animals exhibited impaired learning in the preweaning period[169] and lower seizure threshold in later life. Seizure activity in neonates after a hypoxic-ischemic insult usually shows a pattern of short but frequent convulsive episodes, although status epilepticus is well recognized.[118,175] There is often dissociation between clinically evident seizures and seizures recognized on EEG monitoring, so that the frequency of seizure activity after a hypoxic-ischemic insult may be underestimated by clinical observation. Therefore, asphyxiated infants are likely to have a significant seizure burden that may be underestimated by clinicians. There is evidence that although the majority of irreversible neuronal injury after recovery from hypoxic-ischemic insult is due to the underlying cause of the condition, additional functional injury may ensue secondary to the seizure burden. This strengthens the case for effective management of seizure activity following a hypoxic-ischemic event.

Fully effective anticonvulsant therapy in the neonatal period is not available at present for controlling either clinical or electrographic seizures. Phenobarbital is the mainstay of therapy, but it has been shown that although clinically evident seizures were reduced or abolished by this drug in most cases, electrographic seizures were reduced in only 4 of 14 infants after a loading dose.[118] In some infants, phenobarbital caused an increase in the duration of electrographic seizures despite a second loading dose. A study comparing the efficacy of phenobarbital against phenytoin in the management of EEG-diagnosed seizures found that in

a randomized, single-blind, controlled trial there was complete seizure control in less than 50% of infants with either drug. When both drugs were given, only 50% of infants had complete seizure abolition.[159]

In a study of term asphyxiated infants, high-dose phenobarbitone (40 mg/kg) was associated with a significant reduction in severe neurodevelopmental disability. In many cases, the phenobarbital was given before the first evidence of seizure activity.[135] A meta-analysis of five studies comparing barbiturates with conventional therapy following hypoxic-ischemic encephalopathy found no difference in risk of death, or severe neurodevelopmental disability in survivors.[128] Phenobarbital has also been shown to have toxic effects on brain growth, neuronal toxicity, and adverse cognitive and behavioral effects when given to immature animals.[143] Other anticonvulsants used to treat seizures occurring after a hypoxic-ischemic insult include phenytoin (no greater efficacy than phenobarbital),[159] benzodiazepines (clonazepam, midazolam, lorazepam), lidocaine, thiopentone, sodium valproate, and lamotrigine.[143] These drugs have been evaluated in an uncontrolled manner and the information on effect is largely anecdotal.

In Europe, lidocaine is more commonly used as a second or third-line anticonvulsant, but should not be used if phenytoin has been administered because cardiotoxicity may occur. Lidocaine was effective in abolishing electroconvulsive seizures in 76% of babies who continued to seize after both phenobarbitone and midazolam treatment.[150] Midazolam infusion has also been evaluated in a group of babies who were refractory to phenobarbitone treatment for status epilepticus. Midazolam infusion abolished electroconvulsive seizures in 10 of 13 such babies.[121] It is essential that new randomized, controlled trials be started to evaluate the efficacy of the newer anticonvulsant drugs in the management of seizures due to hypoxic-ischemic insult.

There has been accumulating evidence that antiepileptic drugs have adverse effects including apoptosis, inhibition of brain growth, adverse behavioral and cognitive effects in adult life when the drugs were administered to young animals.[116]

Therapeutic management of seizures following a hypoxic-ischemic event must be pragmatic, with attempts made to stop seizure activity, either clinical or electrographic. Phenobarbital remains the first-line drug. Phenytoin is often used as a second-line anticonvulsant. Realistically, the use of both these drugs will abolish seizure activity only in a little over 50% of cases. The duration of anticonvulsant administration should be minimized to avoid the potential adverse effects of prolonged exposure. The optimal duration of anticonvulsants is unknown. Some clinicians withdraw treatment as soon as the neurologic examination normalizes.

Cerebral Edema

Cerebral edema occurs commonly after a severe hypoxic-ischemic insult and has been shown to develop at the cellular level within 1 to 2 hours of insult in a monkey model. Studies of intracranial pressure monitoring in human infants who have suffered a severe hypoxic-ischemic insult have shown that severely raised intracranial pressure (greater than 15 cm H_2O) was found in a minority of infants monitored by a median time of 26 hours.[146] In this group of asphyxiated infants with raised intracranial pressure, successful treatment of the intracranial hypertension as judged by a significant benefit on outcome, was estimated to have occurred in less than 10% of cases. There is no evidence that routine monitoring of intracranial pressure is of benefit to the infant. Raised intracranial pressure is most probably an end result of the abnormal pathophysiologic processes that occur after hypoxic-ischemic insult and in itself is a marker of damage rather than a cause of it. Consequently, the management of raised intracranial pressure becomes relatively less important.

Corticosteroids

There are few data to suggest that corticosteroids are effective in the management of hypoxia-ischemia. Animal studies on immature rat pups have shown that pretreatment with dexamethasone before a hypoxic-ischemic insult resulted in less severe injury than in untreated control animals, but treatment with dexamethasone after the insult was ineffective in ameliorating cerebral edema. Steroids are routinely used in older children and adults with focal edema, as occurs in tumor or traumatic brain injury, but appear to be much less effective after a global hypoxic-ischemic insult.

There is concern about the long-term effects of large doses of dexamethasone given shortly after birth, particularly in preterm infants, in whom it is estimated that there is a significant increase in the risk of cerebral palsy.[136] There is no scientific justification for the use of steroids after an intrapartum hypoxic-ischemic insult to treat cerebral edema.

Hypothermia

In recent years, interest in neuroprotection by brain cooling has shown benefit in both animals and humans. Studies in animal models have shown that in a variety of immature species, varying degrees of mild hypothermia (2° to 5°C) for 3 to 72 hours was effective in maintaining brain function.[172] Hypothermia has been suggested to have an effect by reducing cerebral metabolism and ATP consumption and downregulating many intracerebral metabolic processes associated with rapid expression of early gene activation. These effects may account for the suggestion that hypothermia has a primary effect by inhibiting apoptosis.

Three major randomized controlled trials have now been published evaluating the neuroprotective role of hypothermia in the combined outcome of death and neurodevelopmental disability in mature babies.[111,132,167] All three studies shared similarities in design in that they aimed to produce hypothermia (rectal temperature of 34° to 35°C in one study[132] and 33.5°C in the other two)[111,167] for a total of 72 hours. The primary outcome in each study was death or disability at 18 months. Various differences in design of these three studies are shown in Table 40-7. The first neonatal study to be published[132] evaluated the role of selective head cooling in infants with both moderate to severe neonatal encephalopathy and abnormalities on aEEG, sufficiently severe to put the baby into a high risk of adverse outcome. The European TOBY study also used both neonatal encephalopathy and aEEG as entry criteria, but the NICHHD study[167] used only clinical criteria for entry. In regional brain cooling,

a cooling cap perfused with a coolant solution at 10°C was used to reduce brain temperature and maintain a rectal temperature of 34.5°C. In total body cooling, the infant is placed on a cooling mattress or under a cooling blanket and the infant's rectal temperature reduced to 33.5°C. All babies were cooled within 6 hours of birth and maintained at a temperature of 33.5°C for 72 hours. Outcome was assessed as death or neurodevelopmental outcome at 18 months.

Despite the relative minor differences between these studies, the outcome at 18 months is remarkably consistent. All three studies showed a strong trend toward reducing death or severe disability in cooled infants, and was statistically significant in one.[167] In the selective head cooling study, a subgroup analysis showed that in babies with moderate aEEG abnormalities, there was a statistically reduced outcome for death or disability.[132] The TOBY study (Azzopardi)[111] analyzed the number of babies surviving to 18 months without neurologic abnormality and showed a statistically significant improvement in the hypothermic group (RR 1.57; 95% CI 1.16-2.12). Meta-analyses of these three studies show significantly improved survival without neurologic abnormality and significantly reduced cumulative outcome of death and severe disability (Fig. 40-70). Babies classified as moderate, rather than those with severe asphyxia, are more likely to benefit, of interest, is the apparent observation that control infants who become hyperthermic have worse outcomes.

Hypothermia appears to be a remarkably safe therapeutic maneuver within the context of randomized controlled trials. There is no reported excess of complications in the hypothermic group. Although the safety of controlled hypothermia has been shown, it is important to note that the temperature control of the hypothermic babies has been very carefully maintained within preset limits. It is clear that more severe hypothermia (<33°C) may have a detrimental effect on the baby with short-term and potentially long-term complications. Therapeutic hypothermia has been confined to studies in mature infants of no lower than 35 weeks' gestation. Historical studies have shown a vast excess of deaths in very immature babies who have become cold, and this form of treatment is not recommended in premature infants.

In regional brain cooling, it has been shown that temperature gradients through the head may affect efficacy of mild hypothermia as a neuroprotective therapy.[142] A subgroup analysis of infants enrolled into the TOBY study[111] evaluated MR brain scans in 151 infants at a median age of 8 days.[164] Infants in the hypothermia group showed a significant reduction in both basal ganglia/thalamic ($P = .03$) and white matter ($P = .016$) abnormalities, but no significant differences in cortical lesions.

OTHER NEUROPROTECTIVE STRATEGIES

The pathophysiologic process of irreversible brain injury has been reviewed earlier in this section. The processes that lead to neuronal death are complicated and incompletely understood. A number of studies have attempted to make preliminary investigations into the role of different strategies in neonatal brain protection after a hypoxic-ischemic insult, but few useful clinical data are currently available.

The calcium channel blocker nicardipine was given to four infants who had sustained severe intrapartum hypoxic-ischemic insult. In three of the four, the mean arterial blood

TABLE 40–7   Hypothermia Studies in the Mature Newborn Infant

Methods	Patient Details	Entry Criteria	Outcome
Gluckman, et al[132] Head cooling 34°C-35°C for 72 hours	N = 234 GA ≥ 36 weeks	Apgar ≤ 5 at 10 min Or continued resuscitation at 10 min Or pH < 7.00 Or BD ≥ 16 mmol/L HIE grade 2 or 3 aEEG abnormalities	FU at 18 mo; 156 survived; 16 lost to FU
Eicher, et al[126] 33°C + 0.5°C for 48 hours Ice filled bags to head and body	N = 65 GA ≥ 35 weeks	1 of the following: Cord pH ≤ 7.0 or BD ≥ 13 Infant pH < 7.1 Apgar ≤ 5 at 10 min Continued resuscitation > 5 min Fetal HR < 80 bpm > 15 min Sao$_2$ < 70% or Pao$_2$ < 35 for 20 min 2 features of HIE No aEEG requirement	FU at 12 mo; 41 survivors; 13 lost to FU
Shankaran, et al[167] Cooling blanket 33.5°C for 72 hours	N = 208 GA ≥ 36 weeks	Acute perinatal event pH ≤ 7.0 or BD ≥ 16 mmol/L Apgar ≤ 5 at 10 min IPPV ≥ 10 min Encephalopathy or seizures	FU 18-22 mo; 146 survivors; 3 lost to FU
Azzopardi, et al[111] Cooling mattress, 33.5°C + 0.5°C for 72 hours	N = 325 GA ≥ 36 weeks	1 of: Apgar ≤ 5 at 10 min Resuscitation for ≥ 10 min pH < 7.0 or BD ≥ 16 mmol/L at 60 min and HIE grade 2 or 3 and aEEG abnormalities	FU at 18 mo; 237 survivors; 2 lost to FU

aEEG, amplitude integrated EEG; BD, base deficit; FU, follow-up; GA, gestational age; HIE, hypoxic ischemic encephalopathy; HR, heart rate; IPPV, intermittent positive pressure ventilation.

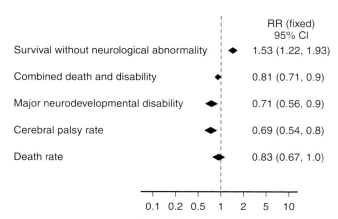

	RR (fixed) 95% CI
Survival without neurological abnormality	1.53 (1.22, 1.93)
Combined death and disability	0.81 (0.71, 0.9)
Major neurodevelopmental disability	0.71 (0.56, 0.9)
Cerebral palsy rate	0.69 (0.54, 0.8)
Death rate	0.83 (0.67, 1.0)

0.1 0.2 0.5 1 2 5 10

Figure 40–70. Meta-analysis of three randomized controlled trials with follow-up to 18 months or more. CI, confidence interval; RR, relative risk. *(Adapted from Azzopardi D, et al: Moderate hypothermia to treat neonatal encephalopathy: the TOBY randomized controlled trial and synthesis of data, N Engl J Med 361(14):1349, 2009.)*

pressure dropped precipitously with a fall in cerebral blood-flow. The systemic effects of the relatively nonspecific calcium channel blockers significantly limit their value for brain protection.

Magnesium sulfate ($MgSO_4$) is an N-methyl-D-aspartate receptor antagonist and has been proposed to be an effective agent for brain protection. A retrospective assessment of risk factors for cerebral palsy showed that maternal exposure to $MgSO_4$ reduced the risk of this condition in their offspring,[157] but there is little evidence that the mechanism for this effect is by way of reducing the incidence of intraventricular hemorrhage in premature infants. The Collaborative Eclampsia Trial[125] reported that infants of women who had been assigned to $MgSO_4$ before delivery were significantly less likely to be intubated or admitted to a neonatal unit. A recent large multicenter study has shown no improvement in the cumulative outcome of death or cerebral palsy at 2 years, but a subgroup analysis showed a significant reduction in moderate or severe cerebral palsy in surviving infants.[163] Although studies have evaluated the role of $MgSO_4$ in term asphyxiated infants, no reports of outcome exist. $MgSO_4$ in high dose is associated with neonatal hypotension,[144] which may override any potential beneficial effect.

Allopurinol is an inhibitor of xanthine oxidase and has free radical scavenging action, but in a study involving 32 severely asphyxiated infants given allopurinol (40 mg/kg) in a randomized, double blind, placebo controlled trial there was no reduction in mortality or morbidity in infants treated with this drug.[113]

PROGNOSTIC FACTORS

Cerebral hypoxia-ischemia due to perinatal asphyxia is an important cause of neonatal mortality and morbidity. The outcome of infants sustaining cerebral hypoxia-ischemia is influenced by several factors, including the duration and severity of the insult to the brain; gestational age; presence of seizures; and associated infectious, metabolic, and traumatic derangements. Although the prognosis for any single newborn often is difficult to formulate, certain clinical and laboratory abnormalities, along with perinatal cerebral hypoxia-ischemia, are associated with a high risk of neurologic morbidity (Box 40-7).

The degree of maturity at birth is an important predictor of mortality in infants asphyxiated at birth. In a group of infants who were either stillborn or without spontaneous respirations for a minimum of 20 minutes, 32% of preterm infants survived. Of the full-term infants, 70% survived. The long-term morbidity of the survivors was 11% in the premature infants, 36% in the term infants. Nelson and Ellenberg[156] also reported an appreciably higher death rate in premature infants, but an increased risk for cerebral palsy in the full-term survivors. The lower morbidity among the premature infants was related in part to the small number of survivors in this group.

Acidosis

Obstetricians have long used blood acid-base status to ascertain the presence or absence of asphyxia in the fetus during the intrapartum period. Obstetricians concentrate on more severe degrees of acidosis and on the extent to which the altered pH reflects an underlying metabolic (lactic) acidosis. In the study of Goldaber and associates,[133] 2.5% of 3506 full-term newborns exhibited an umbilical artery pH of less than 7.00, 66.7% of whom had a metabolic component to their acidosis. Significantly more of the severely acidotic newborns exhibited low (less than 3) 1- and 5-minute Apgar scores, compared with infants with higher umbilical artery pH values. In addition, neonatal death was significantly more frequent in the severely acidotic group. Low and colleagues[148] compared

---

| BOX 40–7 | Predictors of Mortality and Neurologic Morbidity after Perinatal Hypoxic-Ischemic Insult |

- Extended very low Apgar scores
- Time to establish spontaneous respiration
- Neonatal neurologic examination
- Brain imaging (ultrasonography, magnetic resonance imaging)
- Other investigations:
  EEG or amplitude-integrated EEG
  Evoked potentials (visual, brainstem auditory, and somatosensory)

---

59 full-term fetuses exhibiting metabolic acidosis with 59 fetuses with normal umbilical blood acid-base status and 51 fetuses exhibiting only a respiratory acidosis at birth. Various complications, including encephalopathy, were apparent in the majority of newborns experiencing a metabolic acidosis, compared with very low complication rates in those infants with either respiratory acidosis or no acidosis at all. In addition, Low and colleagues[147] had previously demonstrated a positive correlation between the severity and duration of intrapartum metabolic acidosis and neurodevelopmental outcome at 1 year, and the same positive correlation exists for premature infants, including those weighing less than 1000 g.[131]

Apgar Scores and Condition at Birth

Several studies have demonstrated the low sensitivity of the 1- and 5-minute Apgar scores in predicting long-term neurologic outcome. However, Nelson and associates[158] evaluated 39 full-term infants whose 20-minute Apgar scores were 3 or less. Six died in the early postnatal period, and of the 14 survivors, 8 exhibited cerebral palsy when examined at 7 years of age. Thus, the extended Apgar score is a reliable predictor of ultimate neurologic morbidity, especially when very low scores are obtained at 20 minutes. In term infants, low Apgar scores of 0 to 3 at 5 minutes was 8 times more accurate in predicting death than umbilical artery pH ≤7.[120]

The time from birth until onset of spontaneous, sustained respirations also has been correlated with long-term neurologic function. Mulligan and colleagues[154] reported a 19% immediate mortality rate and an 18% morbidity rate among 39 surviving full-term infants in whom spontaneous respirations did not appear for more than 1 minute after birth. D'Souza and associates[123] followed for up to 5 years 15 full-term infants who had survived apnea for 10 or more minutes at birth. Of the group, two exhibited severe neurologic deficit and five had delayed language development. Full-term infants who were apneic for 30 or more minutes were universally and severely damaged.[129] The data suggest that a prolonged delay in the initiation of spontaneous respirations is a reasonable indicator of irreversible brain damage.

Hypoxic-Ischemic Encephalopathy

Neurologic examination of the infant in the immediate newborn period provides a useful index for predicting later developmental outcome, especially in the full-term infant. Follow-up studies have shown that those infants assessed as having only mild HIE had virtually no risk of subsequent major neurodevelopmental disability, and in infants with moderate HIE approximately 75% survived without major neurologic deficit. There were very few deaths in the moderate HIE group. Infants with severe HIE had a very poor outcome, with 50% to 100% mortality rate and severe disability incidence in survivors of 65% to 75% (Table 40-8).

A numeric scoring system based on features of hypoxic-ischemic encephalopathy has been shown to be able to predict, with a high degree of accuracy, outcome at 12 months of age.[171] The maximum (worst) score was 22 and a score of 15 or more showed a positive predictive value of 92% and

TABLE 40–8   Adverse Outcome (Death or Disability) According to Degree of Hypoxic-Ischemic Encephalopathy

Study	N	PROPORTION SEVERELY ABNORMAL OR DEAD (%)			Duration of Follow-up (Yr)
		Mild	Moderate	Severe	
Sarnat and Sarnat[165]	21	–	25	100	1
Finer, et al[130]	89	0	15	92	3.5
Robertson and Finer[161]	200	0	27	100	3.5
Low, et al[149]	42	–*	27	50	1
Levene, et al[145]	122	1†	25	75	2.5

*Mild and moderate considered together.
†Disability due to congenital myopathy.

negative predictive value of 82% for abnormal outcome, with a sensitivity of 71% and specificity of 96%. Using a slightly different encephalopathy score, maximal abnormal features with seizures on day 1 predicted outcome at 30 months of age correctly in 87% of cases.[152]

Very few follow-up studies are available relating to the outcome of term babies born with HIE in developing countries. Ellis and associates[127] published the 1-year outcome in 131 infants born in Kathmandu, Nepal, in 1995. Only 36% of babies born with any grade of HIE were normal at 1 year of age compared with 94% of controls and, unsurprisingly, the outcome was worse by increasing severity of HIE (74% normal for grade 1, 26% for grade 2, and 3% for grade 3). The authors calculated the total prevalence for major neurodevelopmental impairment at 1 year in this Nepalese population to be 1.1 per 1000 live births.

Hypoxic-Ischemic Encephalopathy and Less Severe Neurodisability

In recent years it has become apparent that the outcome of HIE may be more heterogeneous than was previously thought. It has been suggested that if HIE caused an infant to be damaged, then the outcome involved severe cerebral palsy with or without intellectual impairment. More recently, data have been published on less severe forms of disability in older children who have survived a perinatal hypoxic-ischemic insult at term.[134,174]

A Canadian cohort born between 1974 and 1979 was carefully assessed at the age of 8 years and compared with a control group of similar-aged children.[162] The major disability rate was comparable with that in children assessed at a younger age, but important differences at 8 years were seen in the children with HIE, but without major neurologic deficit, compared with the control subjects. The mean full-scale IQ in the control group was 112 and that of the unimpaired children who had mild HIE was 106 (not significant). For the apparently unimpaired children who had moderate HIE, the mean IQ was 102 ($P < .001$) compared with both mild HIE and control subjects. The good prognosis for cognitive and motor outcome for the infants described as having "mild fetal intrapartum asphyxia" was confirmed by another Canadian study of 43 affected children compared with a similar number of control subjects and assessed at 8 years of age.[137] There were no differences between the two groups for tests of motor and cognitive development (Bayley and McCarthy scales).

A report on the later outcome of 68 term babies with depression at birth and neonatal encephalopathy found 36% had cerebral palsy. The surviving 34 who were apparently normal were assessed at 8 years, 8 (15%) had minor neurologic dysfunction and/or perceptual motor difficulties, only 2% had only cognitive impairment, and the rest were normal. Eighty percent of the infants with minor neurologic dysfunction had an abnormality on the MR brain scan usually involving basal ganglia or white matter.[112] Similar results were reported from Norway of surviving term infants with HIE who escaped cerebral palsy but who were found to be more likely to have minor motor impairments and attention deficit hyperactivity disorder requiring additional educational support.[153]

In another cohort of term infants born between 1992 and 1994 with neonatal encephalopathy lasting more than 24 hours, 50 survivors were examined who had escaped cerebral palsy and neuropsychological testing showed lower cognitive scores mainly in the group with severe neonatal encephalopathy. This group had a mean IQ that was 11.3 points below that of the controls.[151] In particular, infants with severe neonatal encephalopathy had memory and attention/executive functions impaired compared with controls. Infants who had suffered moderate neonatal encephalopathy in the neonatal period were not significantly different from their controls in neuropsychological testing but they were identified as having a greater need for special educational in school.

In summary, the prognosis for children with HIE depends on the severity and duration of the neurologic abnormality. Major neurodevelopmental problems occur only after moderate and severe HIE, and death is a significant risk in severe HIE. Emerging data strongly support the observations that a significant number of children with perinatal hypoxic-ischemic insult, previously considered to be without major problems, have significant perceptual-motor difficulties or a reduction in cognitive abilities. The predictive values of neuroimaging procedures and other investigative techniques are described earlier. MRI and EEG assessment provides the basis for the most accurate prediction of disability in later childhood.

REFERENCES

SECTION I—PATHOPHYSIOLOGY

1. Bennet L, et al: The cerebral hemodynamic response to asphyxia and hypoxia in the near term fetal sheep as measured by near-infrared spectroscopy, *Pediatr Res* 44:951, 1998.
2. Blume HK, et al: Intrapartum fever and chorioamnionitis as risks for encephalopathy in term newborns: a case-control study, *Develop Med Child Neurol* 50:19, 2008.
3. Brann AW, Myers RE: Central nervous system findings in the newborn monkey following severe in utero partial asphyxia, *Neurology* 25:327, 1975.
4. Cowan F, et al: Origin and timing of brain lesions in term infants with neonatal encephalopathy, *Lancet* 361:736, 2003.
5. Del-Bigio MR, Becker LE: Microglial aggregation in the dentate gyrus: a marker of mild hypoxic-ischaemic brain insult in human infants, *Neuropathol Appl Neurobiol* 20:144, 1994.
6. Doyle LW, et al: Regional cerebral glucose metabolism of newborn infants measured by positron emission tomography, *Dev Med Child Neurol* 25:143, 1983.
7. Dragunow M, Preston K: The role of inducible transcription factors in apoptotic nerve cell death, *Brain Res Rev* 21:1, 1995.
8. Eklind S, et al: Bacterial endotoxin sensitizes the immature brain to hypoxic-ischaemic injury, *Eur J Neurosci* 13:1101, 2001.
9. Ferriero DM, et al: Neonatal mice lacking neuronal nitric oxide synthase are less vulnerable to hypoxic-ischemic injury, *Neurobiol Dis* 3:64, 1996.
10. Ferriero DM, et al: Selective destruction of nitric oxide synthase neurons with quisqualate reduces damage after hypoxia-ischemia in the neonatal rat, *Pediatr Res* 38:912, 1995.
11. Gluckman PD, et al: Selective head cooling with mild systemic hypothermia after neonatal encephalopathy: multicentre randomised trial, *The Lancet* 365:663, 2005.
12. Groenendaal F, et al: Cerebral lactate and N-acetyl-aspartate/choline ratios in asphyxiated full-term neonates demonstrated in vivo using proton magnetic resonance spectroscopy, *Pediatr Res* 35:148, 1994.
13. Hedtjärn M, et al: Interleukin-18 involvement in hypoxic-ischemic brain injury, *J Neurosci* 22:5910, 2002.
14. Hudome S, et al: The role of neutrophils in the production of hypoxic-ischemic brain injury in the neonatal rat, *Pediatr Res* 41:607, 1997.
15. Ikeno S, et al: Immature brain injury via peroxynitrite production induced by inducible nitric oxide synthase after hypoxia-ischemia in rats, *J Obstet Gynaecol Res* 26:227, 2000.
16. Johnston MV, et al: Neurobiology of hypoxic-ischemic injury in the developing brain, *Pediatr Res* 49:735, 2001.
17. Liu XH, et al: Mice deficient in interleukin-1 converting enzyme are resistant to neonatal hypoxic-ischemic brain damage, *J Cereb Blood Flow Metab* 19:1099, 1999.
18. Meek JH, et al: Abnormal cerebral hemodynamics in perinatally asphyxiated neonates related to outcome, *Arch Dis Child Fetal Neonatal Ed* 81:110, 1999.
19. Mercuri E, Cowan F: Cerebral infarction in the newborn infant: review of the literature and personal experience, *Eur J Paediatr Neurol* 3:255, 1999.
20. Myers RE: Two patterns of perinatal brain damage and their conditions of occurrence, *Am J Obstet Gynecol* 12:246, 1972.
21. Myers RE, et al: Brain swelling in the newborn rhesus monkey following prolonged partial asphyxia, *Neurology* 19:1012, 1975.
22. Palmer C, et al: Changes in iron histochemistry after hypoxic-ischemic brain injury in the neonatal rat, *J Neurosci Res* 56:60, 1999.
23. Peden CJ, et al: Proton spectroscopy of the brain following hypoxic-ischaemic injury, *Dev Med Child Neurol* 35:502, 1993.
24. Penrice J, et al: Proton magnetic resonance spectroscopy of the brain in normal preterm and term infants and early changes following perinatal hypoxia-ischemia, *Pediatr Res* 40:6, 1996.
25. Ramaswamy V, et al: Perinatal stroke in term infants with neonatal encephalopathy, *Neurology* 62:2088, 2004.
26. Robertson NJ, et al: Brain alkaline intracellular pH after neonatal encephalopathy, *Ann Neurol* 52:732, 2002.
27. Roth SC, et al: Relation between cerebral oxidative metabolism following birth asphyxia and neurodevelopmental outcome at one year, *Dev Med Child Neurol* 34:285, 1992.
28. Sarnat HB, et al: Neonatal encephalopathy following fetal distress: a clinical and electroencephalographic study, *Arch Neurol* 33:695, 1976.
29. Shankaran S, Laptook, Ehrenkranz RA, et al: Whole-body hypothermia for neonates with hypoxic-ischemic encephalopathy, *N Engl J Med* 353(15):1574, 2005.
30. Squier W: Pathology of fetal and neonatal brain damage: identifying the timing. In Squier W, editor: *Acquired Damage to the Developing Brain: Timing and Causation*, London, 2002, Arnold, p 110.
31. Toet MC, et al: Cerebral oxygenation and electrical activity after birth asphyxia: their relation to outcome, *Pediatrics* 117:333, 2006.
32. Volpe JJ, et al: Positron emission tomography in the asphyxiated term newborn: parasagittal impairment of cerebral blood flow, *Ann Neurol* 17:287, 1985.
33. Wang X, et al: Caspase-3 activation after neonatal rat cerebral hypoxia-ischemia, *Biol Neonate* 79:172, 2001.
34. Wyatt JS, et al: Magnetic resonance and near infrared spectroscopy for the investigation of perinatal hypoxic-ischaemic brain injury, *Arch Dis Child* 64:953, 1989.
35. Zhu C, et al: Involvement of apoptosis-inducing factor in neuronal death after hypoxia-ischemia in the neonatal rat brain, *J Neurochem* 86:306, 2003.

SECTION II—ASSESSMENT TOOLS

36. Amess PN, et al: Early brain proton magnetic resonance spectroscopy and neonatal neurology related to neurodevelopmental outcome at 1 year in term infants after presumed hypoxic-ischaemic brain injury, *Dev Med Child Neurol* 41:436, 1999.
37. Barkovich AJ, et al: Perinatal asphyxia: MR findings in the first 10 days, *AJNR Am J Neuroradiol* 16:427, 1995.
38. Barkovich AJ, et al: Proton spectroscopy and diffusion imaging on the first day of life after perinatal asphyxia: preliminary report, *AJNR Am J Neuroradiol* 22:1786, 2001.
39. Barkovich AJ, et al: MR imaging, MR spectroscopy, and diffusion tensor imaging of sequential studies in neonates with encephalopathy, *AJNR Am J Neuroradiol* 27:533, 2006.
40. Biagioni E, et al: Constantly discontinuous EEG patterns in full-term neonates with hypoxic-ischemic encephalopathy, *Clin Neurophysiol* 110:1510, 1999.
41. Biagioni E, et al: Combined use of electroencephalogram and magnetic resonance imaging in full-term neonates with acute encephalopathy, *Pediatrics* 107:461, 2001.
42. Bittigau P, et al: Antiepileptic drugs and apoptosis in the developing brain, *Proc Natl Acad Sci U S A* 99:15089, 2002.

43. Blennow M, et al: Early (18F) FDG positron emission tomography in infants with hypoxic-ischaemic encephalopathy shows hypermetabolism during the postasphyctic period, *Acta Paediatr* 84:1289, 1995.

44. Boylan GB, et al: Cerebral blood flow velocity during neonatal seizures, *Arch Dis Child* 80:F105, 1999.

45. Boylan GB, et al: Phenobarbitone, neonatal seizures, and video-EEG, *Arch Dis Child Fetal Neonatal Ed* 86:F165, 2002.

46. Boylan GB, et al: Outcome of electroclinical, electrographic, and clinical seizures in the newborn infant, *Dev Med Child Neurol* 41:819, 1999.

47. Boylan GB, et al: Second-line anticonvulsant treatment of neonatal seizures, *Neurology* 62:486, 2004.

48. Brunquell PJ, et al: Prediction of outcome based on clinical seizure type newborn infants, *J Pediatr* 140:707, 2002.

49. Cady EB, et al: Non-invasive investigation of cerebral metabolism in newborn infants by phosphorus nuclear magnetic resonance spectroscopy, *Lancet* 1:1059, 1983.

50. Chau V, et al: Comparison of computer tomography and magnetic resonance imaging scans on the third day of life in term newborns with neonatal encephalopathy, *Pediatrics* 123:319, 2009.

51. Cowan F: Outcome after intrapartum asphyxia in term infants, *Semin Neonatol* 5:127, 2000.

52. de Vries LS, et al: Predictive value of early somatosensory evoked potentials in full term infants with birth asphyxia, *Brain Dev* 13:320, 1991.

53. de Vries LS, et al: Prediction of outcome in newborn infants with arterial ischemic stroke using magnetic resonance diffusion-weighted imaging, *Neuropediatrics* 36:12, 2005.

54. Eken P, et al: Intracranial lesions in the full term infant with hypoxic ischaemic encephalopathy: ultrasound and autopsy correlation, *Neuropediatrics* 25:301, 1994.

55. Eken P, et al: Predictive value of early neuroimaging, pulsed Doppler and neurophysiology in full term infants with hypoxic-ischemic encephalopathy, *Arch Dis Child* 73:F75, 1995.

56. Fitzgerald KC, et al: Cerebral sinovenous thrombosis in the neonate, *Arch Neurol* 63:405, 2006.

57. Gibson NA, et al: Somatosensory evoked potentials and outcome in perinatal asphyxia, *Arch Dis Child* 67:393, 1992.

58. Gluckman PD, et al: Selective head cooling with mild systemic hypothermia after neonatal encephalopathy: multicentre randomised trial, *Lancet* 365:663, 2005.

59. Hanrahan JD, et al: Relation between proton magnetic resonance spectroscopy within 18 hours of birth asphyxia and neurodevelopment at 1 year of age, *Dev Med Child Neurol* 41:76, 1999.

60. Hellström-Westas L, et al: Low risk of seizure recurrence after early withdrawal of antiepileptic treatment in the neonatal period, *Arch Dis Child* 72:F97, 1995.

61. Hellstrom-Westas L, et al: Lidocaine treatment of severe seizures in newborn infants: I. Clinical effects and cerebral electrical activity monitoring, *Acta Paediatr Scand* 77:79, 1988.

62. Holmes GL, Lombroso CT: Prognostic value of background pattern in the neonatal EEG, *J Clin Neurophysiol* 10:323, 1993.

63. Holmes GL, et al: Consequences of neonatal seizures in the rat: morphological behavioral effects, *Ann Neurol* 44:845, 1998.

64. Holmes GL: Seizure-induced neuronal injury, *Neurology* 59:S3, 2002.

65. Hrbek A, et al: Clinical application of evoked electroencephalographic responses in newborn infants, *Dev Med Child Neurol* 19:34, 1977.

66. Ilves P, et al: Changes in Doppler ultrasonography in asphyxiated term infants with hypoxic-ischaemic encephalopathy, *Acta Paediatr* 87:680, 1998.

67. Jiang ZD, et al: Time course of brainstem pathophysiology during first month in term infants after perinatal asphyxia, revealed by MLS BAER latencies and intervals, *Pediatr Res* 54:680, 2003.

68. Jiang ZD, et al: Brainstem auditory outcomes and correlation with neurodevelopment after perinatal asphyxia, *Pediatr Neurol* 39:189, 2008.

69. Kirton A, et al: Quantified corticospinal tract diffusion restriction predicts neonatal stroke outcome, *Stroke* 38:974, 2007.

70. Kägeloh-Mann I, et al: Bilateral lesions of thalamus and basal ganglia: origin and outcome, *Dev Med Child Neurol* 44:477, 2002.

71. Legido A, et al: Neurologic outcome after electroencephalographic proven seizures, *Pediatrics* 88:583, 1991.

72. Levene MI, et al: Severe birth asphyxia and abnormal cerebral blood-flow velocity, *Dev Med Child Neurol* 31:427, 1989.

73. Li AM, et al: White matter injury in term newborns with neonatal encephalopathy, *Pediatr Res* 2008.

74. Liu Z, et al: Consequences of recurrent seizures during early brain development, *Neuroscience* 92:1443, 1999.

75. Lombroso CT, Holmes GL: Value of the EEG in neonatal seizures, *J Epilepsy* 6:39, 1993.

76. Malingré MM, et al: Development of an optimal lidocaine infusion strategy in neonatal seizures, *Eur J Pediatr* 165:598, 2006.

77. Menache CC, et al: Prognostic value of neonatal discontinuous EEG, *Pediatr Neurol* 27:93, 2002.

78. Miller SP, et al: Patterns of brain injury in term neonatal encephalopathy, *J Pediatr* 146:453, 2005.

79. Mizrahi EM, Kellaway P: Characterisation and classification of neonatal seizures, *Neurology* 37:1837, 1987.

80. Monod N, et al: The neonatal EEG: statistical studies and prognostic values in full-term and pre-term babies, *Electroencephalogr Clin Neurophysiol* 32:529, 1972.

81. Murray DM, et al: Defining the gap between electrographic seizure burden, clinical expression, and staff recognition of neonatal seizures, *Arch Dis Child Fetal Neonatal Ed* 93:F187, 2008.

82. Okereafor A, et al: Patterns of brain injury in neonates exposed to perinatal sentinel events, *Pediatrics* 121:906, 2008.

83. Osredkar D, et al: Sleep-wake cycling on amplitude-integrated electroencephalography in term newborns with hypoxic-ischemic encephalopathy, *Pediatrics* 115:327, 2005.

84. Painter MJ, et al: Phenobarbital compared with phenytoin for the treatment of neonatal seizures, *N Engl J Med* 341:485, 1999.

85. Prior P, Maynard DE: Monitoring Cerebral Function: Long Term Recordings of Cerebral Electrical Activity and Evoked Potentials, *Amsterdam, Elsevier,* 1986.

86. Robertson NJ, et al: Cerebral intracellular alkalosis persisting months after neonatal encephalopathy measured by magnetic resonance spectroscopy, *Pediatr Res* 46:287, 1999.

87. Roelants-van RA, et al: Value of 1H-MRS using different echo times in neonates with cerebral hypoxia-ischemia, *Pediatr Res* 49:356, 2001.

88. van Rooij LG, et al: Recovery of amplitude integrated electroencephalographic background patterns within 24 hours of perinatal asphyxia, *Arch Dis Child Fetal Neonatal Ed* 90:F245, 2005.

88a. van Rooij LGM, et al: Effect of treatment of subclinical neonatal seizures detected with continuous amplitude-integrated electroencephalographic monitoring: a randomized controlled trial, *Pediatrics* 124:e358, 2010.

89. van Rooij LGM, et al: Neurodevelopmental outcome in full term infants with status epilepticus detected with amplitude-integrated electroencephalography, *Pediatrics* 120:e354, 2007.

90. Rutherford MA, et al: Cranial ultrasound and magnetic resonance imaging in hypoxic-ischaemic encephalopathy: a comparison with outcome, *Dev Med Child Neurol* 35:813, 1994.

91. Rutherford MA, et al: Hypoxic-ischaemic encephalopathy: early and late magnetic resonance imaging findings in relation to outcome, *Arch Dis Child Fetal Neonatal Ed* 3:F145, 1996.

92. Rutherford MA, et al: Abnormal magnetic resonance signal in the internal capsule predicts poor neurodevelopmental outcome in infants with hypoxic-ischemic encephalopathy, *Pediatrics* 102:323, 1998.

93. Rutherford M, et al: Diffusion-weighted magnetic resonance imaging in term perinatal brain injury: a comparison with site of lesion and time from birth, *Pediatrics* 114:1004, 2004.

94. Scalais E, et al: Multimodality evoked potentials as a prognostic tool in term asphyxiated newborns, *Electroencephalogr Clin Neurophysiol* 108:199, 1998.

95. Scher MS, et al: Uncoupling of EEG-clinical neonatal seizures after antiepileptic drug use, *Pediatr Neurol* 28:277, 2003.

96. Shah DK, et al: Accuracy of bedside electroencephalographic monitoring in comparison with simultaneous continuous conventional electroencephalography for seizure detection in term infants, *Pediatrics* 121:1146, 2008.

97. Shellhaas RA, et al: Sensitivity of amplitude-integrated electroencephalography for neonatal seizure detection, *Pediatrics* 120:770, 2007.

98. Silverstein FS, Ferriero DM: Off-label use of antiepileptic drugs for the treatment of neonatal seizures, *Pediatr Neurol* 39:77, 2008.

99. Tam EW, et al: Occipital lobe injury and cortical visual outcomes after neonatal hypoglycemia, *Pediatrics* 122:507, 2008.

100. Tanner SF, et al: Cerebral perfusion in infants and neonates: preliminary results obtained using dynamic susceptibility contrast enhanced magnetic resonance imaging, *Arch Dis Child Fetal Neonatal Ed* 88:F525, 2003.

101. Taylor MJ, et al: Prognostic reliability of somatosensory and visual evoked potentials of asphyxiated term infants, *Dev Med Child Neurol* 34:507, 1992.

101a. Thayyil S, et al: Cerebral magnetic resonance biomarkers in neonatal encephalopathy: a meta analysis, *Pediatrics* 125:e 382, 2010.

101b. Thoresen M, et al: Effect of hypothermia on amplitude-integrated electroencephalogram in perinatal asphyxia, *Pediatrics*, in press.

102. Thorngren-Jerneck K, et al: Cerebral glucose metabolism measured by positron emission tomography in term newborn infants with hypoxic-ischemic encephalopathy, *Pediatr Res* 49:495, 2001.

103. Toet MC, et al: Amplitude integrated EEG at 3 and 6 hours after birth in full term neonates with hypoxic ischemic encephalopathy, *Arch Dis Child* 81:F19, 1999.

104. Toet MC, et al: Comparison between simultaneously recorded amplitude integrated EEG (cerebral function monitor) and standard EEG in neonates, *Pediatrics* 109:772, 2002.

105. Toet MC, et al: Postneonatal epilepsy following amplitude-integrated EEG-detected neonatal seizures, *Pediatr Neurol* 32:241, 2005.

106. Watanabe K, et al: Behavioral state cycles, background EEGs and prognosis of newborns with perinatal hypoxia, *Electroencephalogr Clin Neurophysiol* 49:618, 1980.

107. Whyte HE, et al: Prognostic utility of visual evoked potentials in term asphyxiated neonates, *Pediatr Neurol* 2:220, 1986.

108. Wirrell EC, et al: Prolonged seizures exacerbate perinatal hypoxic-ischemic brain damage, *Pediatr Res* 50:445, 2001.

109. Wu YW, et al: Intraventricular hemorrhage in term neonates caused by sinovenous thrombosis, *Ann Neurol* 54:123, 2003.

SECTION III—MANAGMENT

110. Alfirevic Z, et al: Continuous cardiotocography (CTG) as a form of electronic fetal monitoring (EFM) for fetal assessment during labour, *Cochrane Database of Systematic Reviews* 2006, Issue 3. CD 006066.

111. Azzopardi D, et al: Moderate hypothermia to treat neonatal encephalopathy: the TOBY randomized controlled trial and synthesis of data, *N Engl J Med (submitted)* 2009.

112. Barnett A, et al: Neurological and perceptual-motor outcome at 5-6 years of age in children with neonatal encephalopathy: relationship with neonatal brain MRI, *Neuropediatrics* 33:242, 2002.

113. Benders MJNL, et al: Early postnatal allopurinol does not improve short term outcome after severe birth asphyxia, *Arch Dis Child Fetal Neonatal Ed* 91:F163, 2006.

114. Bennhagen RG, et al: Hypoxic-ischaemic encephalopathy is associated with regional changes in cerebral blood flow velocity and alterations in cardiovascular function, *Biol Neonate* 73:275, 1998.

115. Bennet L, et al: Pathophysiology of asphyxia. In Levene M, Chervenak F, editors: *Fetal and Neonatal Neurology and Neurosurgery*, Edinburgh, 2009, .

116. Bittigau P, et al: Antiepileptic drugs and apoptotic neurodegeneration in the developing brain, *Proc Natl Acad Sci* 99:15089, 2002.

117. Blennow M, et al: Early (18F) FDG positron emission tomography in infants with hypoxic-ischaemic encephalopathy shows hypermetabolism during the postasphyctic period, *Acta Paediatr* 84:1289, 1995.

118. Boylan GB, et al: Phenobarbitone, neonatal seizures and video-EEG, *Arch Dis Child Fetal Neonatal Ed* 86:F165, 2002.

119. Brucklacher RM, et al: Hypoxic preconditioning increases brain glycogen and delays energy depletion from hypoxia-ischemia in the immature rat, *Dev Neurosci* 24:411, 2002.

120. Casey BM, et al: The continuing value of the Apgar score for the assessment of newborn infants, *N Engl J Med* 344;467, 2001.

121. Castro Conde JR, et al: Midazolam in neonatal seizures with no response to phenobarbital, *Neurology* 64:876, 2005.

122. Dardzinski BJ, et al: Increased plasma beta-hydroxybutyrate, preserved cerebral energy metabolism and amelioration of brain damage during neonatal hypoxia ischemia with dexamethasone pre-treatment, *Pediatr Res* 48:248, 2000.

123. D' Souza SW, et al: Hearing, speech and language in survivors of severe perinatal asphyxia, *Arch Dis Child* 56:245, 1981.

124. East CE, et al: Fetal pulse oximetry for fetal assessment in labour, *Cochrane Database of Systematic Reviews* 2007, Issue 2. CD 004075.

125. Eclampsia Trial Collaborative Group: Which anti-convulsant for women with eclampsia? Evidence from the collaborative eclampsia trial, *Lancet* 345:1455, 1995.

126. Eicher DJ, et al: Moderate hypothermia in neonatal encephalopathy: efficacy outcomes, *Pediatr Neurol* 32:11, 2005.

127. Ellis M, et al: Outcome at 1 year of neonatal encephalopathy in Kathmandu, Nepal, *Dev Med Child Neurol* 41:689, 1999.

128. Evans DJ, et al: Anticonvulsants for preventing mortality and morbidity in full term newborns with perinatal asphyxia, *Cochrane Database Syst Rev* 3, 2007. CD001240.

129. Finer NN, et al: Hypoxic-ischemic encephalopathy in term neonates: perinatal factors and outcome, *J Pediatr* 98:112, 1981.

130. Finer NN, et al: Hypoxic-ischemic encephalopathy in term neonates: perinatal factors and outcome, *J Pediatr* 98:112, 1981.

131. Gaudier FL, et al: Acid-base status at birth and subsequent neurosensory impairment in surviving 500 to 1000 gm infants, *Am J Obstet Gynecol* 170:48, 1994.

132. Gluckman P, et al: Selective head cooling with mild systemic hypothermia after neonatal encephalopathy: multicentre randomised trial, *Lancet* 365:663, 2005.

133. Goldaber KG, et al: Pathologic fetal acidemia, *Obstet Gynecol* 78:1103, 1991.

134. Gonzalez FF, Miller SP: Does perinatal asphyxia impair cognitive function without cerebral palsy? *Arch Dis Child Fetal Neonatal Ed* 91:F454, 2006.

135. Hall T, et al: High-dose phenobarbital therapy in term newborn infants with severe perinatal asphyxia: a randomised, prospective study with three year follow-up, *J Pediatr* 132:345, 1998.

136. Halliday HL, et al: Early postnatal (<96 hours) corticosteroids for preventing chronic lung disease in preterm infants (review), *Cochrane Database Syst Rev* 1, 2003. CD001146.

137. Handley-Derry M, et al: Intrapartum fetal asphyxia and the occurrence of minor deficits in 4-8 year old children, *Dev Med Child Neurol* 39:508, 1997.

138. Hankins GD, et al: Neonatal organ system injury in acute birth asphyxia sufficient to result in neonatal encephalopathy, *Obstet Gynecol* 99:688, 2002.

139. Hattori H, Wasterlain G: Posthypoxic glucose supplement reduces hypoxic-ischaemic brain damage in the neonatal rat, *Ann Neurol* 28:122, 1990.

140. Holmes GL: Effects of seizures on brain development: lessons from the laboratory, *Pediatr Neurol* 33:1, 2005.

141. Jones NM, Bergeron M: Hypoxic preconditioning induces changes in HIF-1 target genes in neonatal rat brain, *J Cereb Blood Flow Metab* 21:1105, 2001.

142. Laptook AR, et al: Differences in brain temperature and cerebral blood flow during selective head versus whole-body cooling, *Pediatrics* 108:1103, 2001.

143. Levene M: The clinical conundrum of neonatal seizures, *Arch Dis Child Fetal Neonatal Ed* 86:F75, 2002.

144. Levene MI, et al: Acute effects of two different doses of magnesium sulphate in infants with birth asphyxia, *Arch Dis Child* 73:F174, 1995.

145. Levene MI, et al: Comparison of two methods of predicting outcome in perinatal asphyxia, *Lancet* 1:67, 1986.

146. Levene MI: The asphyxiated newborn infant. In Levene MI, et al, editors: *Fetal and Neonatal Neurology and Neurosurgery*, 3rd ed, London, 2001, Churchill Livingstone, p 471.

147. Low JA, et al: Factors associated with motor and cognitive deficits in children after intrapartum fetal hypoxia, *Am J Obstet Gynecol* 148:533, 1984.

148. Low JA, et al: Newborn complications after intrapartum asphyxia with metabolic acidosis in the term fetus, *Am J Obstet Gynecol* 170:1081, 1994.

149. Low JA, et al: The relationship between perinatal hypoxia and newborn encephalopathy, *Am J Obstet Gynecol* 152:256, 1985.

150. Malingre MM, et al: Development of an optimal lidocaine infusion strategy for neonatal seizures, *Eur J Pediatr* 165:598, 2006.

151. Marlow N, et al: Neuropsychological and educational problems at school age associated with neonatal encephalopathy, *Arch Dis Child Fetal Neonatal Ed* 90:F380, 2005.

152. Miller SP, et al: Clinical signs predict 30-month neurodevelopmental outcome after neonatal encephalopathy, *Am J Obstet Gynecol* 190:93, 2004.

153. Moster D, et al: Joint association of Apgar scores and early neonatal symptoms with minor disabilities at school age, *Arch Dis Child Fetal Neonatal Ed* 86:F16, 2002.

154. Mulligan JC, et al: Neonatal asphyxia: II. Neonatal mortality and long-term sequelae, *J Pediatr* 96:903, 1980.

155. Neilson JP: Fetal electrocardiogram (ECG) for fetal monitoring during labour, *Cochrane Database Syst Rev* 3, 2006. CD00116.

156. Nelson KB, Ellenberg JH: Neonatal signs as predictors of cerebral palsy, *Pediatrics* 64:225, 1979.

157. Nelson KB, Grether JK: Can magnesium sulfate reduce the risk of cerebral palsy in very low birth weight infants? *Pediatrics* 95:263, 1995.

158. Nelson KB, et al: Apgar scores as predictors of chronic neurologic disability, *Pediatrics* 68:36, 1981.

159. Painter MJ, et al: Phenobarbital compared with phenytoin for the treatment of neonatal seizures, *N Engl J Med* 341:485, 1999.

160. Perlman JM, et al: Acute systemic organ injury in term infants after asphyxia, *Am J Dis Child* 143:617, 1989.

161. Robertson C, Finer N: Term infants with hypoxic-ischaemic encephalopathy: outcome at 3.5 years, *Dev Med Child Neurol* 27:473, 1985.

162. Robertson CMT, et al: School performance of survivors of neonatal encephalopathy associated with birth asphyxia at term, *J Pediatr* 114:753, 1989.

163. Rouse DJ, et al: A randomized controlled trial of magnesium sulfate for the prevention of cerebral palsy, *N Eng J Med* 359:895, 2008.

164. Rutherford MA, et al: Neonatal MR imaging findings in a multicentre trial of moderate total body hypothermia (TOBY) in neonatal encephalopathy, *PAS abstract* 2009.

165. Sarnat HB, Sarnat MS: Neonatal encephalopathy following fetal distress, *Arch Neurol* 33:696, 1976.

166. Shah P, et al: Multiorgan dysfunction in infants with post-asphyxial hypoxic-ischaemic encephalopathy, *Arch Dis Child Fetal Neonatal Ed* 89:F152, 2004.

167. Shankaran S, et al: Whole-body hypothermia for neonates with hypoxic-ischemic encephalopathy, *N Engl J Med* 353:15, 2005.

168. Sheldon RA, et al: Post ischemic hyperglycemia is not protective to the neonatal rat, *Pediatr Res* 32:489, 1992.

169. Sogawa Y, et al: Timing of cognitive deficits following neonatal seizures: relationship to histological changes in the hippocampus, *Brain Res* 131:73, 2001.

170. Suzuki S, Morishita S: Hypercoagulability and DIC in high-risk infants, *Semin Thromb Hemost* 24:463, 1998.

171. Thompson CM, et al: The value of a scoring system for hypoxic encephalopathy in predicting neurodevelopmental outcome, *Acta Paediatr* 86;757, 1997.

172. Thoresen M: Thermal influence on the asphyxiated newborn. In Donn SM, et al, editors: *Birth Asphyxia and the Brain: Basic Science and Clinical Implications*, Armonk, NY, 2002, Futura, p 355.

173. Thorngren-Jerneck K, et al: Cerebral glucose metabolism measured by positron emission tomography in term newborn infants with hypoxic ischemic encephalopathy, *Pediatr Res* 9:495, 2001.

174. van Handel M, et al. Long-term cognitive and behavioural consequences of neonatal encephalopathy following perinatal asphyxia: a review, *Eur J Pediatr* 166:645, 2007.

175. van Rooij LG, et al. Neurodevelopmental outcome in term infants with status epilepticus detected with amplitude-integrated electroencephalography, *Pediatrics* 120:e354, 2007.

176. Vannucci RC, Mujsce DJ: Effect of glucose on perinatal hypoxic-ischaemic brain damage, *Biol Neonate* 62:215, 1992.

177. Vannucci RC, et al: The effect of hyperglycemia on cerebral metabolism during hypoxia-ischemia in the immature rat, *J Cereb Blood Flow Metab* 16:1026, 1996.

178. Vannucci RC, Vannucci SJ: Hypoglycemic brain injury, *Semin Neonatol* 6:147, 2001.

179. Willis F, et al: Indices of renal tubular function in perinatal asphyxia, *Arch Dis Child* 77:F57, 1997.

180. Yager JY, et al: Effect of insulin-induced and fasting hypoglycemia on perinatal hypoxic-ischemic brain damage, *Pediatr Res* 31:138, 1992.

PART 5

Seizures in Neonates

Mark S. Scher

Neonatal seizures are one of the few neonatal neurologic conditions that require immediate medical attention. Although prompt diagnostic and therapeutic plans are needed, multiple challenges impede the physician's evaluation of the newborn with suspected seizures (Box 40-8). Clinical and electroencephalographic (EEG) manifestations of neonatal seizures vary dramatically from those in older children, and recognition of the seizure state remains the foremost challenge. This dilemma is underscored by the brevity and subtlety of the clinical repertoire of the neonatal neurologic examination. Environmental restrictions of the sick infant in an intensive care setting, who may be confined to an incubator, intubated, and attached to multiple catheters, limit accessibility. Medications alter arousal and muscle tone and limit the clinician's ability to distinguish clinical neurologic signs

---

BOX 40–8   **Dilemmas Regarding Neonatal Seizures**

Diagnostic choices
- Reliance on clinical versus electroencephalographic criteria

Etiologic explanations
- Multiple prenatal/neonatal conditions as a function of time

Treatment decisions
- Who, when, how, and for how long?

Prognostic questions
- Mechanisms of injury based on etiologies versus intrinsic vulnerability of the immature brain to prolonged seizures

---

reflective of the underlying disease state. Brain injury from antepartum factors may precipitate neonatal seizures as part of an encephalopathic clinical picture during the intrapartum and neonatal periods, well beyond when brain injury occurred. Overlapping medical conditions from fetal through neonatal periods must be factored into the most appropriate etiologic algorithm to explain seizure expression before applying the most accurate prognosis. Medication options to treat seizures effectively remain elusive and may need to be applied on a specific etiologic basis. Potential neuroresuscitative strategies proposed for the encephalopathic neonate with seizures must consider maternal, placental/cord, and fetal disease conditions that cause or contribute to neonatal seizure expression and potential brain injury as part of both fetal and neonatal brain disorders of varying etiologies.

DIAGNOSIS: CLINICAL VERSUS ELECTROENCEPHALOGRAPHIC

Neonatal seizures are usually brief and subtle in clinical appearance, sometimes comprising unusual behaviors that are difficult to recognize and classify. Medical personnel vary significantly in their ability to recognize suspect behaviors, contributing to both overdiagnosis and underdiagnosis. The most common practice has been to classify clinical behaviors as seizures without EEG confirmation. However, abnormal motor or autonomic behaviors may represent age- and state-specific behaviors in healthy infants, or nonepileptic paroxysmal conditions in symptomatic infants. For these reasons, confirmation of suspect clinical events with coincident EEG recordings is now more widely recommended. Although in patients with few seizures, these may be missed as brief random events on routine EEG studies, synchronized video/EEG/polygraphic recordings potentially establish more reliable start points and endpoints for electrically confirmed seizures that require consideration for treatment intervention.[10] Rigorous physiologic monitoring also better integrates the diagnosis of the seizure state with etiologic, treatment, and prognostic considerations.

Clinical Seizure Criteria

Neonatal seizures are listed separately from the traditional classification of seizures and epilepsy during childhood. The International League Against Epilepsy's Classification adopted by the World Health Organization still places neonatal seizures in an unclassified category. Another classification scheme suggests a strict distinction of clinical seizure (nonepileptic) events from electrographically confirmed (epileptic) seizures with respect to possible treatment interventions.[55] Continued refinement of such novel classifications is needed to reconcile the variable agreement between clinical and EEG criteria for establishing a seizure diagnosis[7,96] in the context of nonepileptic movement disorders caused by acquired diseases, malformations, or medications.

Several caveats (Box 40-9) may be useful in the identification of suspected neonatal seizures, yet continue to raise questions regarding our diagnostic acumen.

The clinical criteria for neonatal seizure diagnosis were historically subdivided into five clinical categories: focal clonic, multifocal or migratory clonic, tonic, myoclonic, and

BOX 40–9   Caveats Concerning Recognition of Neonatal Seizures

- Specific stereotypic behaviors occur in association with normal neonatal sleep or waking states, medication effects, and gestational maturity.
- Any abnormal repetitive activity may be a clinical seizure if out of context for expected neonatal behavior.
- Attempt to document coincident electrographic seizures with the suspected clinical event.
- Abnormal behavioral phenomena may have inconsistent relationships with coincident electroencephalographic seizures, suggesting a subcortical seizure focus.
- Nonepileptic pathologic movement disorders are events that are independent of the seizure state and may also be expressed by neonates.

BOX 40–10   Classification of Neonatal Seizures Based on Electroclinical Findings

CLINICAL SEIZURES WITH A CONSISTENT ELECTROCORTICAL SIGNATURE (PATHOPHYSIOLOGY: EPILEPTIC)
Focal clonic

- Unifocal
- Multifocal
- Hemiconvulsive
- Axial

Focal tonic

- Asymmetric truncal posturing
- Limb posturing
- Sustained eye deviation

Myoclonic

- Generalized
- Focal
- Spasms

Flexor

- Extensor
- Mixed extensor/flexor

CLINICAL SEIZURES WITHOUT A CONSISTENT ELECTROCORTICAL SIGNATURE (PATHOPHYSIOLOGY: PRESUMED NONEPILEPTIC)
Myoclonic

- Generalized
- Focal
- Fragmentary

Generalized tonic

- Flexor
- Extensor
- Mixed extensor/flexor

Motor automatisms

- Oral-buccal-lingual movements
- Ocular signs
- Progression movements
- Complex purposeless movements

ELECTRICAL SEIZURES WITHOUT CLINICAL SEIZURE ACTIVITY

From Mizrahi EM, Kellaway P: *Diagnosis and management of neonatal seizures*, Philadelphia, 1998, Lippincott-Raven.

subtle seizures.[93] A subsequent classification expands the clinical subtypes, adopting a strict temporal occurrence of specific clinical events with coincident electrographic seizures to distinguish neonatal clinical "nonepileptic" seizures from "epileptic" seizures (Box 40-10).[55]

SUBTLE SEIZURE ACTIVITY

Subtle seizure activity is the most frequently observed category of neonatal seizures and includes repetitive buccolingual movements, orbital-ocular movements, unusual bicycling or peddling, and autonomic findings (Fig. 40-71A). Any subtle paroxysmal event that interrupts the expected behavioral repertoire of the newborn infant and appears stereotypical or repetitive should heighten the clinician's level of suspicion for seizures. However, alterations in cardiorespiratory regularity, body movements, and other behaviors during active (rapid eye movement [REM]) sleep, quiet (non-REM) sleep, or waking segments must be recognized before proceeding to a seizure evaluation.[74] Within the subtle category of neonatal seizures are stereotypical changes in heart rate, blood pressure, oxygenation, or other autonomic signs, particularly during pharmacologic paralysis for ventilatory care. Other unusual autonomic events include penile erections, skin changes, salivation, and tearing. Autonomic expressions may be intermixed with motor findings. Isolated autonomic signs such as apnea, unless accompanied by other clinical findings, are rarely associated with coincident electrographic seizures[16] (see Fig. 40-71B). Because subtle seizures are both clinically difficult to detect and only variably coincident with EEG seizures, synchronized video/EEG/polygraphic recordings are recommended to document temporal relationships between clinical behaviors and coincident electrographic events.[8,10,55] Despite the "subtle" expression of this seizure category, these children may have suffered significant brain injury.

CLONIC SEIZURES

Rhythmic movements of muscle groups in a focal distribution that consist of a rapid phase followed by a slow return movement are clonic seizures, to be distinguished from the symmetric "to-and-fro" movements of tremulousness or jitteriness. Gentle flexion of the affected body part easily suppresses the tremor, whereas clonic seizures persist. Clonic movements can involve any body part such as the face, arm, leg, and even diaphragmatic or pharyngeal muscles. Generalized clonic activities can occur in the newborn but rarely consist of a classic tonic followed by clonic phase, which is characteristic of the generalized motor seizure noted in older children and adults. Focal clonic and hemiclonic seizures have been described with localized brain injury, usually from cerebrovascular lesions,[10] but can also be seen with generalized brain abnormalities. As in older patients, focal seizures in the

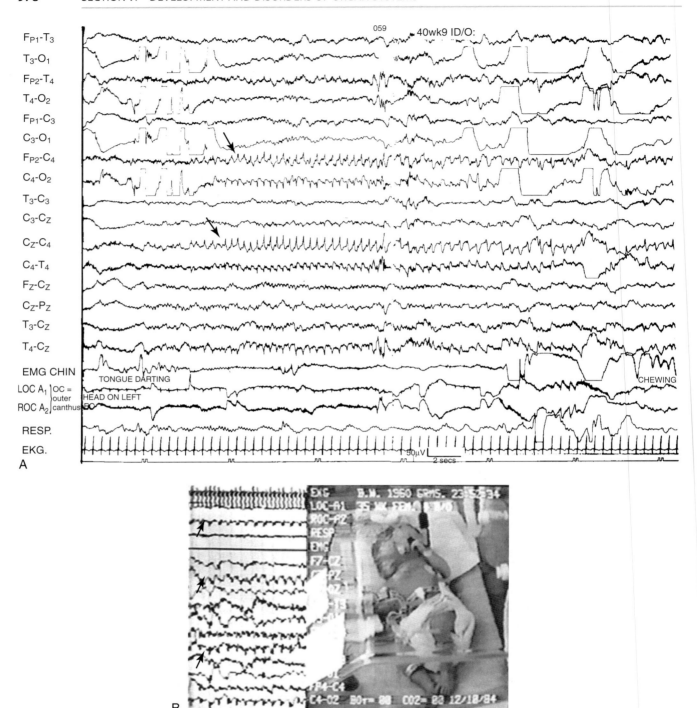

Figure 40–71. A, Electroencephalogram (EEG) segment of a 40-week gestation, 1-day-old girl after severe asphyxia resulting from rupture of velamentous insertion of the umbilical cord during delivery. An electrical seizure in the right central/midline region is recorded *(arrows)*, coincident with buccolingual and eye movements (see comments and eye channels on record). B, Synchronized video/EEG record of a 35-week gestation, 1-day-old girl with *Escherichia coli* meningitis and cerebral abscesses. The *top arrow* notes apnea coincident with prominent right hemispheric and midline electrographic seizures *(middle and bottom arrows)*. In addition to apnea, other motor signs coincident to EEG seizures were noted at other times during the record. (*A, From Scher MS, Painter MJ: Electrographic diagnosis of neonatal seizures: issues of diagnostic accuracy, clinical correlation and survival. In Wasterlain CG, Vert P, editors: Neonatal seizures, New York, 1990, Raven Press, p. 17, with permission; B, From Scher MS, Painter MJ: Controversies concerning neonatal seizures, Pediatr Clin North Am 36:288, 1989, with permission.*)

neonate may be followed by transient motor weakness, historically referred to as a *transient Todd paresis* or *paralysis*, to be distinguished from a more persistent hemiparesis over days to weeks. Clonic movements without EEG-confirmed seizures have been described in neonates with normal EEG backgrounds, and their neurodevelopmental outcome can be normal.[8]

MULTIFOCAL (FRAGMENTARY) CLONIC SEIZURES

Multifocal or migratory clonic activities spread over body parts either in a random or anatomically appropriate fashion. Such seizure movements may alternate from side to side and appear asynchronously between the two halves of the child's body. The word *fragmentary* was historically applied to distinguish this event from the more classic, generalized tonic-clonic seizure seen in the older child. Multifocal clonic seizures may also resemble myoclonic seizures, consisting of brief, shocklike muscle twitching of the midline or extremity musculature. Neonates with this seizure description either die or suffer significant neurologic morbidity.[70]

TONIC SEIZURES

Tonic seizures refer to a sustained flexion or extension of axial or appendicular muscle groups. Tonic movements of a limb or sustained head or eye turning may also be noted. Tonic activity with coincident EEG needs to be carefully documented because 30% of such movements lack a temporal correlation with electrographic seizures (Fig. 40-72). "Brainstem release" resulting from functional decortication after severe neocortical dysfunction or damage is one physiologic explanation for this nonepileptic activity (discussed later). Extensive neocortical damage or dysfunction permits the emergence of uninhibited subcortical expressions of extensor movements.[72] Tonic seizures may also be misidentified when the nonepileptic movement disorder of dystonia is the more appropriate behavioral description. Both tonic

movements and dystonic posturing may also simultaneously occur.

MYOCLONIC SEIZURES

Myoclonic movements are rapid, isolated jerks that can be generalized, multifocal, or focal in an axial or appendicular distribution. Myoclonus lacks the slow return phase of the clonic movement complex described previously. Healthy preterm infants commonly exhibit myoclonic movements without seizures or a brain disorder. EEG therefore is recommended to confirm the coincident appearance of electrographic discharges with these movements (Fig. 40-73). Pathologic myoclonus in the absence of EEG seizures also can occur in severely ill preterm or full-term infants after severe brain dysfunction or damage.[78] As with older children and adults, myoclonus may reflect injury at multiple levels of the neuraxis from the spine, brainstem, and to cortical regions. Stimulus-evoked myoclonus with either coincident single spike discharges or sustained electrographic seizures have been reported.[79] An extensive evaluation must be initiated to exclude metabolic, structural, and genetic causes. Rarely, healthy sleeping neonates exhibit abundant myoclonus that subsides with arousal to the waking state,[15] termed *benign sleep myoclonus of the newborn*.

Nonepileptic Behaviors of Neonates

Specific nonepileptic neonatal movement repertoires continually challenge the physician's attempt to reach an accurate diagnosis of seizures and avoid the unnecessary use of antiepileptic medications. Coincident paper or synchronized video/EEG/polygraphic recordings are now the suggested diagnostic tool to confirm the temporal relationship between the suspect clinical phenomena and electrographic expression of seizures. The following three examples of nonepileptic movement disorders incorporate a classification scheme,[55] based on the absence of coincident EEG seizures.

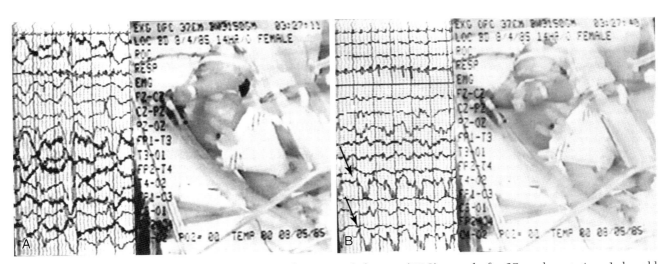

Figure 40-72. A, Segment of a synchronized video/electroencephalogram (EEG) record of a 37-week gestation, 1-day-old girl who suffered asphyxia, demonstrating prominent opisthotonos with left arm extension in the absence of coincident electrographic seizure activity. B, Synchronized video/EEG record of the same patient as in A, documenting electrographic seizure in the right posterior quadrant *(arrows)*, after cessation of left arm tonic movements and persistent opisthotonos. *(From Scher MS, Painter MJ: Controversies concerning neonatal seizures, Pediatr Clin North Am 36:292, 1989, with permission.)*

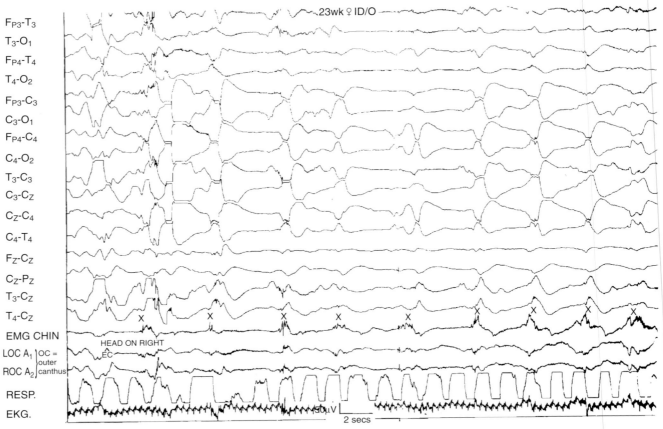

Figure 40-73. Electroencephalogram segment of a 23-week gestation, 1-day-old girl with grade III intraventricular hemorrhage and progressive ventriculomegaly. An electroclinical seizure is noted with coincident myoclonic movements of the diaphragm ("x" marks). *(From Scher MS: Pathological myoclonus of the newborn: electrographic and clinical correlations,* Pediatr Neurol 1:342, 1985, with permission.)

TREMULOUSNESS OR JITTERINESS WITHOUT ELECTROGRAPHIC CORRELATES

Tremors are frequently misidentified as clonic activity. Unlike the unequal phases of clonic movements described earlier, the flexion and extension phases of tremor are equal in amplitude. Children are usually alert or hyperalert but may also appear somnolent. Passive flexion and repositioning of the affected tremulous body part diminishes or eliminates the movement. Such movements are usually spontaneous but can be provoked by tactile stimulation. Metabolic or toxin-induced encephalopathies, including mild asphyxia, drug withdrawal, hypoglycemia, hypocalcemia, intracranial hemorrhage, hypothermia, and growth restriction, are common clinical scenarios when such movements occur. Neonatal tremors usually decrease with age; for example, in 38 full-term infants, excessive tremulousness resolved spontaneously over a 6-week period, with 92% being neurologically normal at 3 years of age.[88] Medications are rarely considered to treat this particular movement disorder.[63]

NEONATAL MYOCLONUS WITHOUT ELECTROGRAPHIC SEIZURES

Myoclonic movements are either (1) bilateral and synchronous or (2) asymmetric and asynchronous. Clusters of myoclonic activity occur predominantly during active (REM) sleep, more so in the preterm infant,[24] but also in healthy term infants. These benign movements are not stimulus sensitive and have no coincident electrographic seizure activity or changes in EEG background rhythms. When this movement occurs in the healthy term neonate, it is usually suppressed during wakefulness. This clinical entity of benign neonatal sleep myoclonus is a diagnosis of exclusion after an extensive consideration of pathologic diagnoses.[15]

Some infants with severe central nervous system dysfunction present with nonepileptic spontaneous or stimulus-evoked myoclonus. Metabolic encephalopathies (e.g., glycine encephalopathy), cerebrovascular lesions, brain infections, or congenital malformations may present with nonepileptic myoclonus.[78] Encephalopathic neonates may respond to tactile or painful stimulation by either isolated focal, segmental, or generalized myoclonic movements. Rarely, cortically generated spike or sharp-wave discharges as well as seizures may also be noted on the EEG coincident with these myoclonic movements[78] (Fig. 40-74). Medication-induced myoclonus as well as stereotypic movements have also been described.[85]

A rare familial disorder has been described in the neonatal and early infancy periods, termed *hyperekplexia*. These movements usually are misinterpreted as a hyperactive startle reflex. These infants are stiff with severe hypertonia, which may lead to apnea and bradycardia. Forced flexion of the

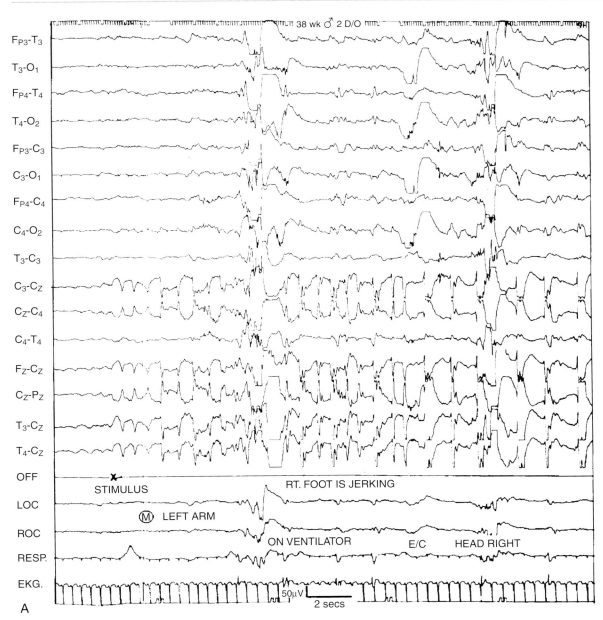

38 wk ♂ 2 D/O

Fp3-T3	
T3-O1	
Fp4-T4	
T4-O2	
Fp3-C3	
C3-O1	
Fp4-C4	
C4-O2	
T3-C3	
C3-Cz	
Cz-C4	
C4-T4	
Fz-Cz	
Cz-Pz	
T3-Cz	
T4-Cz	
OFF	
STIMULUS	RT. FOOT IS JERKING
LOC	ⓜ LEFT ARM
ROC	
RESP.	ON VENTILATOR E/C HEAD RIGHT
EKG.	50μV 2 secs

A

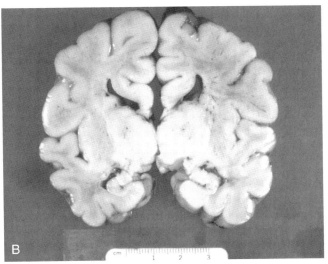

B

Figure 40–74. **A,** Segment of an electroencephalographic recording of a 38-week gestation, 2-day-old boy with glycine encephalopathy who has stimulus-sensitive generalized and multifocal myoclonus. Note the onset of a midline (C_z onset) electrographic seizure with a painful stimulus, followed by right foot myoclonus. **B,** Coronal section of the brain for the patient described in **A,** with agenesis of the corpus callosum and bat-wing shape of lateral ventricles. Spongy myelinosis was noted on microscopic examination. (*From Scher MS: Pathological myoclonus of the newborn: electrographic and clinical correlations, Pediatr Neurol 1:342, 1985, with permission.*)

neck or hips sometimes alleviates these events. EEG background is generally age appropriate. The postulated defect of these individuals pertains to regulation of brainstem centers facilitating myoclonic movements. Occasionally, benzodiazepines or valproic acid lessen the startling, stiffening, or falling events. Neurologic prognosis is variable.

NEONATAL DYSTONIA/DYSKINESIA WITHOUT ELECTROGRAPHIC SEIZURES

Dystonia or dyskinesia is a third commonly misdiagnosed movement disorder that is often misrepresented as tonic or subtle seizures, or may be expressed with nonepileptic tonic movements. These movements can be associated with either acute or chronic disease states involving basal ganglia structures or extrapyramidal pathways, commonly injured after antepartum or intrapartum severe asphyxia (termed *status marmoratus*),[93] or rarely with specific inherited metabolic diseases[46] or drug toxicity from neuropsychiatric medications given to the mother. Alternatively, posturing reflects subcortical motor pathways that remain functionally unopposed because of a diseased or malformed neocortex.[72]

Electrographic Seizure Criteria

Electrographic/polysomnographic studies have become invaluable tools for the assessment of suspected seizures.[10,12,55,67,95] Technical and interpretative skills of normal and abnormal neonatal EEG sleep patterns must be mastered before the clinician develops a confident visual analysis style for seizure recognition.[66,74]

Corroboration with the EEG technologist is always an essential part of the diagnostic process because physiologic and nonphysiologic artifacts can masquerade as EEG seizures. The physician must always anticipate expected behaviors for the child for a specific gestational maturity, medication use, and state of arousal in the context of potential artifacts.

For the epileptic older child and adult, it is generally accepted that the epileptic seizure is a clinical paroxysm of altered brain function with the simultaneous presence of an electrographic event on an EEG recording. Some advocate the use of single-channel computerized devices for prolonged monitoring given the multiple logistical problems using conventional multichannel recording devices. This device, however, may not detect focal or regional seizures because recording from a single channel will not detect localized disease processes distant from the channel.[67]

Epilepsy monitoring services for older children and adults readily use intracerebral or surface electrocorticography to detect seizures. Such recording strategies, however, are not ethically appropriate or practical for the neonatal patient. Subcortical foci therefore are difficult to eliminate definitively from consideration (see later).

ICTAL ELECTROENCEPHALOGRAPHIC PATTERNS— A MORE RELIABLE MARKER FOR SEIZURE ONSET, DURATION, AND SEVERITY

Neonatal EEG seizure patterns commonly consist of a repetitive sequence of waveforms that evolve in frequency, amplitude, electrical field, and morphology. Four types of ictal patterns have been described: focal ictal patterns with normal background, focal patterns with abnormal background, multifocal ictal patterns, and focal monorhythmic periodic patterns of various frequencies. It is generally suggested that a minimal duration of 10 seconds with the evolution of discharges is required to distinguish electrographic seizures from repetitive but nonictal epileptiform discharges.[10,13] Clinical neurophysiologists usually classify brief or prolonged repetitive discharges with a lack of evolution as nonictal patterns, but some argue that simply the presence of epileptiform discharges is confirmatory of seizures.[86] The specific features of electrographic seizure duration and topography are unique to the neonatal period.

SEIZURE DURATION AND TOPOGRAPHY

Few studies have quantified minimal or maximal seizure durations in neonates.[9,13,81] Most notably, the definition of the most severe expression of seizures that potentially promotes brain injury, status epilepticus, can be problematic. For the older patient, status epilepticus is defined as at least 30 minutes of continuous seizures or two consecutive seizures with an interictal period during which the patient fails to return to full consciousness. This definition is not easily applied to the neonate for whom the level of arousal may be difficult to assess, particularly if sedatives are given. One study arbitrarily defined neonatal status epilepticus as continuous seizure activity for at least 30 minutes, or 50% of the recording time[81]; 33% (11 of 34 term infants) had status epilepticus with a mean duration of 29.6 minutes before antiepileptic drug use, and another 9% (3 of 34 preterm infants) also had status epilepticus with an average duration of 5.2 minutes per seizure (i.e., 50% of the recording time). The mean seizure duration was longer in the full-term infant (i.e., 5 minutes) compared with the preterm infant (i.e., 2.7 minutes). Given that more than 20% of this study group fit the criteria for status epilepticus based on EEG documentation, concerns must be raised regarding the underdiagnosis of the more severe form of seizures that potentially contribute to brain injury.

Uncoupling of the clinical and electrographic expressions of neonatal seizures after antiepileptic medication administration also contributes to an underestimation of the true seizure duration, including status epilepticus (Fig. 40-75). One study estimated that 25% of neonates expressed persistent electrographic seizures despite resolution of their clinical seizure behaviors after receiving antiepileptic medications,[80] termed *electroclinical uncoupling*. Other pathophysiologic mechanisms besides medication effect also might explain uncoupling.[7]

Most neonatal electrographic seizures arise focally from one brain region. Generalized synchronous and symmetric repetitive discharges can also occur. In one study, 56% of seizures were seen in a single location at onset; specific sites included temporal-occipital (15%), temporal-central (15%), central (10%), frontotemporal-central (6%), frontotemporal (5%), and vertex (5%). Multiple locations at the onset of the electrographic seizures were noted in 44%.[10] Electrographic discharges may be expressed as specific EEG frequency ranges from fast to slow, including beta, alpha, theta, or delta activities. Multiple electrographic seizures can also be expressed independently in anatomically unrelated brain regions.

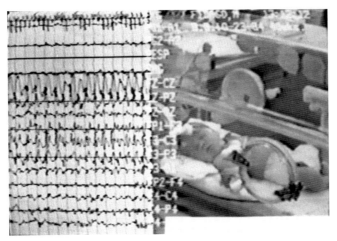

Figure 40–75. Segment of a synchronized video/electroencephalogram of a 40-week gestation, 1-day-old boy with electrographic status epilepticus noted in the left central/midline regions, after antiepileptic medication administration. Focal right shoulder clonic activity was noted only intermittently, whereas continuous electrographic seizures were documented mostly without clinical expression. This phenomenon of uncoupling of electrical and clinical seizure activity is associated with antiepileptic drug administration (see text). *(From Scher MS, Painter MJ: Controversies concerning neonatal seizures, Pediatr Clin North Am 36:290, 1989, with permission.)*

At the opposite end of the spectrum from periodic discharges, brief rhythmic discharges that are less than 10 seconds in duration have also been addressed with respect to an association with seizures and outcome (Fig. 40-76). Neonates with electrographic seizures may also exhibit these brief discharges; other neonates express only isolated discharges without seizures. Neonates with brief discharges can suffer from hypoglycemia or periventricular leukomalacia, which carries a higher risk for neurodevelopmental delay.[58]

Brainstem Release Phenomena

Based on 415 clinical seizures in 71 infants, clonic seizure activity had the best correlation with coincident electrographic seizures. "Subtle" clinical events, on the other hand, had a more inconsistent relationship with coincident EEG seizure activity, suggesting nonepileptic brainstem release phenomena for at least a proportion of such events. Functional decortication resulting from neocortical damage without coincident EEG seizures has therefore been suggested, such as with tonic posturing, as illustrated in Figure 40-72A. Newborns with nonseizure brainstem release activity may express a different functional pattern of metabolic dysfunction, detected as altered glucose uptake on single-photon emission computed tomography studies, than neonates with seizures.[3] A suggestion to document increased prolactin levels with clinical seizures has also been reported,[33] but such levels have not yet been correlated with electrographic seizures.

Subcortical Seizures and Electroclinical Dissociation

Experimental studies on immature animals also support the possibility that subcortical structures may initiate seizures, which subsequently, although intermittently, propagate to the cortical surface. Although EEG depth recordings in adults and adolescents help document subcortical seizures both with and without clinical expression, this technology is not applicable or appropriate to the neonate.

Electroclinical dissociation is one proposed mechanism by which subcortical seizures may appear only intermittently on surface-recorded EEG studies.[96] Electroclinical dissociation has been defined as a reproducible clinical event that occurs both with and without coincidental electrographic seizures. In one group of 51 infants with electroclinical seizures, 33 infants simultaneously expressed both electrical and clinical seizure phenomena. Extremity movements were more significantly associated with synchronized electroclinical seizures. However, a subset of 18 of 51 neonates (35%) also expressed electroclinical dissociation on EEG recordings. For neonates who expressed electroclinical dissociation, the clinical seizure component always preceded the electrographic seizure expression, suggesting that a subcortical focus initiated the seizure state. Some of these children also expressed synchronized electroclinical seizures, even on the same EEG record. EEG clearly is required to document the electrographic phase after the initial behavioral event.

Controversy remains over whether subcortical seizures versus nonictal functional decortication best categorizes suspect clinical behaviors without coincident EEG documentation. This dilemma should encourage the clinician to use the EEG as a neurophysiologic yardstick by which more exact seizure start points and endpoints can be assigned, before offering pharmacologic treatment with antiepileptic drugs. Neonates certainly exhibit electrographic seizures that go undetected unless EEG is used.[59] This is best shown in neonates who are pharmacologically paralyzed for ventilatory assistance, or in infants with clinical seizures that are suppressed by the use of antiepileptic drugs.[10,75,80] In one cohort of 92 infants, 60% of whom were pretreated with antiepileptic medications, 50% of neonates had electrographic seizures with no clinical accompaniment.[80] Both clinical and electrographic seizure criteria were noted for 45% of 62 preterm and 53% of 33 full-term infants. Seventeen infants were pharmacologically paralyzed when the EEG seizure was first documented. A later cohort of 60 infants, none of whom were pretreated with antiepileptic medications, included 7% with only electrographic seizures before antiepileptic drug administration,[80] and 25% who expressed electroclinical uncoupling after antiepileptic drug use.

Incidence of Neonatal Seizures

Overestimation and underestimation of neonatal seizures are consequentially reported whether clinical or electrical criteria are used. Using clinical criteria, seizure incidences ranged from 0.5% in term infants to 22.2% in preterm neonates.[69] Discrepancies in incidence reflect not only varying postconceptional ages of the study populations chosen, but also poor interobserver reliability[35] and the hospital setting in which

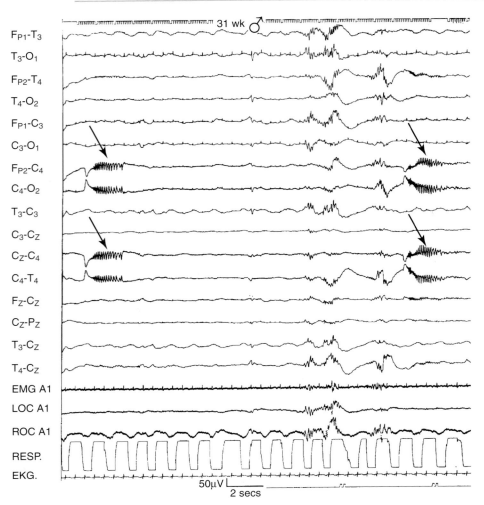

Figure 40–76. Electroencephalogram segment of a boy at 31 weeks' gestational age with repetitive brief epileptiform discharges in the right central region (*arrows*) that are less than 10 seconds in duration and do not qualify as an electrographic seizure.

the diagnosis was made. Hospital-based studies that include high-risk deliveries generally report a higher seizure incidence. Population studies[34] that include less medically ill infants from general nurseries report lower percentages. Incidence figures based only on clinical criteria without EEG confirmation include "false-positive" results, consisting of the neonates with either normal or nonepileptic pathologic neonatal behaviors. Conversely, the absence of scalp-generated EEG seizures may include a subset of "false-negative" results from subjects who express seizures only from subcortical brain regions without expression on the cortical surface. Consensus between those relying on clinical and EEG criteria is still required.

Interictal Electroencephalographic Pattern Abnormalities

Interictal EEG abnormalities (including nonictal repetitive epileptiform discharges) have important prognostic implications for both preterm and full-term infants. Severely abnormal bihemispheric patterns include the burst suppression pattern (Fig. 40-77), electrocerebral inactivity, low-voltage invariant pattern, persistently slow background pattern, multifocal sharp waves, and marked asynchrony.[9] For infants with hypoxic-ischemic encephalopathy (HIE), subclassifications of

specific EEG patterns such as burst suppression with or without reactivity may give a more accurate prediction of outcome.[89] Dysmaturity of the EEG sleep background for child's corrected age has also been an important feature to recognize; discordance between cerebral and noncerebral components of sleep state or immaturity of EEG patterns for the given postconceptional age of the infant predict a higher risk for neurologic sequelae.[75,76,93] Even focal or regional patterns have prognostic significance, such as with preterm infants who express repetitive positive sharp waves at the midline or central regions often noted with intraventricular hemorrhage and periventricular leukomalacia.[74]

Screening infants at risk for neonatal seizures with a routine EEG soon after birth allows identification of more severe interictal EEG background abnormalities that more likely predict seizure occurrence on subsequent neonatal records.[36]

Interictal EEG findings are not pathognomonic for particular etiologies, pathophysiologic mechanisms, or timing.[75] History, physical examination, and laboratory findings need to be integrated with the electrographic interpretation of both ictal and interictal pattern abnormalities for the particular child. Serial EEG studies better assist the clinician in diagnostic and prognostic interpretations.[91] As with abnormal examination findings into the second week of life, the persistence of electrographic abnormalities also raises prognostic concerns. For

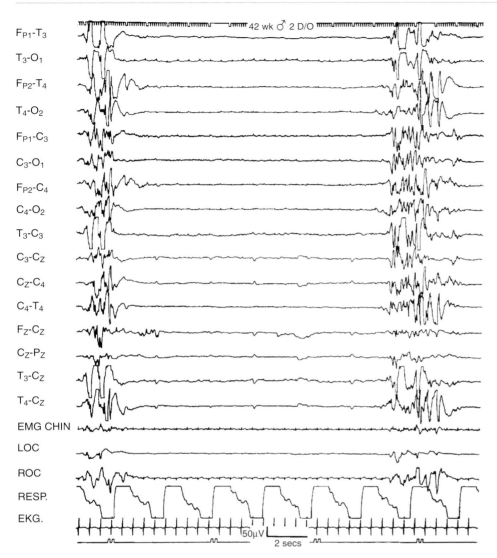

Figure 40–77. Electroencephalogram (EEG) segment of a 42-week gestation, 2-day-old boy expressing a severe interictal EEG background abnormality termed a burst suppression or paroxysmal pattern.

example, the newborn who expresses severe EEG abnormalities into the second week of life implies a greater likelihood for neurologic impairment, even despite the resolution of clinical dysfunction. Conversely, the child who rapidly recovers from a significant brain disorder, with the reemergence of normal EEG features during the first few days after birth, may experience comparatively fewer neurologic sequelae. Interictal EEG pattern abnormalities also reflect fetal brain disorders that preceded labor and delivery. The depth and severity of the neonatal brain disorder (defined by clinical and electrographic criteria) therefore may reflect chronic injury to the fetus who subsequently becomes symptomatic after a stressful intrapartum period, with or without more recent injury. (See also Part 4 of this chapter.)

MAJOR ETIOLOGIES FOR SEIZURES
Asphyxia-Related Events

See also Part 4.
Neonatal seizures are not disease specific and can be associated with a variety of medical conditions that occur before, during, or after parturition. Seizures may occur as part of an asphyxial brain disorder that is expressed after birth (termed *HIE from intrapartum stress*), or alternatively can occur as part of a more nonspecific neonatal encephalopathy from etiologies other than intrapartum asphyxia.[1,41] Importantly, neonatal seizures can also present as an isolated clinical sign from a remote antepartum disease or injury without other signs of a postnatal encephalopathy. A logistic model to predict seizures emphasizes the accumulation of both antepartum and intrapartum factors to increase the likelihood of neonatal seizure occurrence.[64] Although separately these factors had low positive predictive values, a significant cumulative risk profile included antepartum maternal anemia, bleeding, asthma, meconium-stained amniotic fluid, abnormal fetal presentation, fetal distress, and shoulder dystocia.

Hypoxia-ischemia (i.e., asphyxia) is traditionally considered the most common causal factor associated with neonatal seizures.[73,94,96] However, children suffer asphyxia either before or during parturition, and only 10% of cases of asphyxia result from postnatal causes.[4,94] When asphyxia is suspected during the labor and delivery process, biochemical confirmation can be attempted.

Intrauterine factors in the hours to days before labor can result in antepartum fetal asphyxia without later documentation of acidosis at birth or immediately before birth. Maternal illnesses such as thrombophilia or preeclampsia, or specific uteroplacental abnormalities such as abruptio placentae or cord compression may contribute to fetal asphyxial stress without providing the opportunity to document in utero acidosis at the end of parturition.[77] Antepartum maternal trauma and chorioamnionitis are additional acquired conditions that cause or contribute to intrauterine asphyxia secondary to uteroplacental insufficiency. Intravascular placental thromboses, infarction of the placenta (fetal or maternal surfaces), or umbilical cord thrombosis noted on placenta/cord examinations postnatally are additional surrogates for remote peripartum or intrapartum fetal asphyxia (see also Chapter 24). Meconium passage into the amniotic fluid may also promote an inflammatory response in the placental membranes, causing vasoconstriction and additional asphyxia. Neuroimaging, preferably with magnetic resonance imaging (MRI), may later define the destructive brain lesions that resulted from in utero asphyxia, even without HIE expressed at birth. Diffusion-weighted MRI provides a shorter time window that may or may not extend before the onset of labor or when the mother entered the hospital, depending on the length of hospitalization before birth and the postnatal age when the MRI was obtained. Therefore asphyxia-induced brain injuries may result from in utero maternal-fetal-placental diseases that later are expressed in part as neonatal seizures, independent of the biochemical marker of acidosis at birth, as well as the evolving HIE syndrome in the days after birth.[4]

Postnatal medical illnesses also cause or contribute to asphyxia-induced brain injury and seizures without HIE, after an uneventful delivery without fetal distress during labor or neonatal depression at birth. Persistent pulmonary hypertension of the newborn (PPHN), cyanotic congenital heart disease, sepsis, and meningitis are principal diagnoses.

A case-control study of term infants with clinical seizures reported a fourfold increase in the risk of unexplained early-onset seizures after intrapartum fever. All known causes of seizures were eliminated, including meningitis or sepsis. These 38 newborns, compared with 152 control subjects, experienced intrapartum fever as an independent risk factor on logistic regression that predicted seizures. The authors speculated on the role of circulating maternal cytokines that triggered "physiologic events" contributing to seizures.[40]

The American College of Obstetricians and Gynecologists[4] has published guidelines that suggest essential or collective criteria to define postasphyxial neonatal encephalopathy (i.e., HIE) after significant clinical depression noted at birth. The report acknowledges that as many as 90% of children have antepartum timing to a brain injury, with the caveat that more recent asphyxial injury may occur either in the intrapartum or peripartum periods up to 48 hours before delivery.

Postasphyxial encephalopathy refers to an evolving clinical syndrome over days after birth depression during which neonatal seizures may occur, usually in children who also exhibit severe early metabolic acidosis, hypoglycemia or hypocalcemia, and multiorgan dysfunction.[70,90] Other epiphenomena around asphyxia may contribute to seizures.

Seizures after asphyxia may be associated with trauma, intracranial hemorrhage, or other brain damage based on neurologic diagnoses besides asphyxia.

The physical examination findings of the infant with HIE and seizures include coma, hypotonia, brainstem abnormalities, and loss of fetal reflexes. Postasphyxial seizures usually occur within the first 3 days of life, depending on the length and degree of asphyxial stress during the intrapartum period.[90] An early occurrence of seizures, within several hours after delivery, sometimes suggests antepartum or peripartum occurrence of a fetal brain disorder when associated with specific fetal heart rate patterns. However, seizure onset is not a reliable indicator of timing of fetal brain injury. Earlier seizure onset, within 4 hours of birth, in encephalopathic newborns may predict a particularly adverse outcome independent of etiology for asphyxia.[21]

Asphyxia is conventionally diagnosed based on the association of several metabolic parameters with hypoxia and acidosis. The duration of asphyxia is difficult to assess based on either single or even multiple Po_2 values, and pH levels of less than 7.2 are considered of greater clinical concern for predicting HIE, although the suggested guideline of a pH of less than 7.0 is one criterion by which the clinical entity of HIE might be predicted.[4] A metabolic definition of asphyxia should also include a base deficit of less than 12 mmol/L, although specific researchers suggest a base deficit of less than 16 mmol/L because of its higher predictive power for the emergence of the HIE syndrome, including clinical seizures.[43] One caveat should always be considered before assigning a relative risk to a pH value; elevated Pco_2 values introduce a superimposed respiratory acidosis secondary to hypercarbia. Elevated Pco_2 with respiratory acidosis is comparatively less harmful to brain tissue and is more rapidly corrected by aggressive ventilatory support. Alternatively, metabolic acidosis suggests a more profound alteration of intracellular function that better predicts an evolving brain disorder, which may include seizures as part of HIE.

Low Apgar scores traditionally are associated with infants with suspected neurologic depression after delivery, with possible evolution to HIE and seizures (see also Chapter 26). Low 1- and 5-minute Apgar scores indicate the continued need for resuscitation, but only low scores at 10, 15, and 20 minutes more accurately predict sequelae. Normal Apgar scores, however, do not eliminate the possibility of severe antepartum brain injury, either from asphyxia or other causes. As many as two thirds of neonates who exhibit cerebral palsy at older ages had normal Apgar scores at birth without HIE.[57]

Placental findings may reflect disease states at any time before birth either with or without metabolic acidosis and evolving HIE after birth. Although in utero meconium passage commonly occurs in otherwise healthy newborns, meconium staining of the child's skin may be correlated with meconium-laden macrophages in placental membranes in a depressed newborn. Meconium staining through the chorionic layer to the amnion suggests a longer-standing asphyxial stress, such as over 4 to 6 hours (see also Chapter 24).

Placental weight below the 10th or above the 90th percentile suggest chronic perfusion abnormalities to the fetus. Microscopic evidence of lymphocytic infiltration, altered villous maturation, chorangiosis, and erythroblastic proliferation of placental villi each support chronic asphyxial stresses to the fetus. In a study of preterm and term neonates (23 to 42 weeks of corrected age) with EEG-confirmed seizures, a significant association between seizures and chronic (with or without acute) placental lesions was noted, increasing to a factor of 12.1 ($P < .003$) by term age. Odds ratios were not significant for infants with seizures and exclusively acute placental lesions, presumably from events closer to labor and delivery.[82]

Specific clinical findings in the depressed neonate with suspected HIE may reflect antepartum disease states.[49] Intrauterine growth restriction, hydrops fetalis, or joint contractures (including arthrogryposis) are findings that suggest remote in utero diseases that may have been associated with antepartum asphyxia and later express as intrapartum fetal distress or neonatal depression. Hypertonicity, often with cortical fisting, in a previously depressed child who rapidly recovers after a resuscitative effort also commonly reflects longer-standing fetal neurologic dysfunction before labor or the mother's admission to the hospital. Sustained hypotonia and unresponsiveness for 3 to 7 days are the expected signs of HIE after asphyxial stress during labor, with or without brain injury.

The encephalopathic newborn with depressed arousal and hypotonia nonetheless may paradoxically reflect an antepartum disease process with neonatal dysfunction or superimposed injury as a result of a problematic intrapartum period. This has been described in neurologically depressed infants with EEG seizures and isoelectric interictal EEG pattern abnormalities who are comatose and flaccid for days, requiring ventilator assistance after difficult deliveries. Children may appear neurologically depressed after asphyxial stress during the intrapartum period (i.e., low Apgar scores and metabolic acidosis). Evidence of antepartum fetal brain injury is supported by preexisting maternal disease, placental lesions, neuroimaging findings, or neuropathologic-postmortem findings. Although intrapartum asphyxial stress worsens brain injury in some children, it is impossible to differentiate neonatal encephalopathy from preexisting antepartum brain injury.

Metabolic Derangements

HYPOGLYCEMIA

Hypoglycemia is usually defined as glucose levels of 35 to 40 mg/dL (see also Chapter 49, Part 1). No clear consensus exists concerning a direct cause-and-effect relationship of hypoglycemia with seizure occurrence. Also, associated disturbances may coexist, such as hypocalcemia, craniocerebral trauma, cerebrovascular lesions, and asphyxia, which may also contribute to lowering the infant's threshold for seizures. Infants born of diabetic or toxemic mothers, particularly those who were small for gestational age, are also at risk for hypoglycemia. Jitteriness, apnea, and altered tone are clinical signs that may appear in children with hypoglycemia but are not representative of a seizure state. Cerebrovascular lesions in posterior brain regions have been reported in children with hypoglycemia. Vulnerability of brain to ischemic insults is enhanced by concomitant hypoglycemia.

HYPOCALCEMIA

Total serum calcium levels below 7.5 to 8 mg/dL generally define hypocalcemia (see also Chapter 49, Part 2). The ionized fraction is a more sensitive indicator of seizure vulnerability. As with hypoglycemia, the exact level of hypocalcemia at which seizures occur is debatable. An ionized fraction of 0.6 mg/dL or less may have a more predictable association with the presence of seizures. Hypocalcemia due to high-phosphate infant formula has been previously cited as a cause of late-onset seizures.[70] However, hypocalcemia now more commonly occurs with a variety of nonspecific problems or asphyxia, and may coexist with hypoglycemia or hypomagnesemia. Rarely, congenital hypoparathyroidism in association with other genetic abnormalities such as DiGeorge syndrome (i.e., velocardiofacial syndrome, or 22q11 deletion with cardiac and brain anomalies) must be considered. These infants may have severe congenital heart disease as well as a hypoparathyroid state with hypocalcemia and hypomagnesemia that precipitates seizures.[45] In infants with hypocalcemia of unknown etiology, the condition may be the result of maternal hypercalcemia. Ascertainment of the mother's calcium status should be considered because maternal hypercalcemia can suppress fetal parathyroid development.

HYPONATREMIA AND HYPERNATREMIA

Hyponatremia is a metabolic disturbance that may result from inappropriate secretion of antidiuretic hormone after severe brain trauma, infection, or asphyxia,[94] but is an uncommon isolated cause of neonatal seizures. (See Chapter 36.)

Hypernatremia also is a rare cause of seizures, and usually is associated with dehydration or iatrogenic disturbance of serum sodium balance by the use of IV fluids with high concentrations of sodium.

Cerebrovascular Lesions

Hemorrhagic or ischemic cerebrovascular lesions are associated with neonatal seizures, on either an arterial or venous basis.[68] (See also Parts 2 and 3 of this chapter.) Intraventricular or periventricular hemorrhage is the most common intracranial hemorrhage of the preterm infant, and has been associated with seizures in as much as 45% of a preterm population with EEG-confirmed seizures. In a cohort of newborns with clinical seizures, intraventricular hemorrhage was the predominant cause of seizures in preterm infants less than 30 weeks' gestational age.[87] Intracranial hemorrhage is usually expected within the first 72 hours of life of the preterm infant. Although intraventricular or periventricular hemorrhage may occur in otherwise asymptomatic infants, the neonate with a catastrophic deterioration of clinical status shows signs of apnea, bulging fontanelle, hypertonia, and seizures.[93] Term infants present less commonly with intraventricular hemorrhage, usually originating from the choroid plexus or thalamus.

Other sites of intracranial hemorrhage which may cause seizures include within the subarachnoid space, but is usually associated with a more favorable outcome. Subdural hematoma, whether spontaneous or with craniocerebral trauma, should always be considered, particularly when focal trauma to the face, scalp, or head has occurred; simultaneous occurrences of cerebral contusion and infarction should also be considered.

Cerebral infarction has been described in neonates with seizures and can result from events during the antepartum, intrapartum, or neonatal periods (see also Parts 2 and 3 of this chapter). Either preterm or term neonates with infarction may also present without seizure expression.[18] Seizures can also occur in otherwise healthy infants, suggesting an antepartum period when cerebral infarction occurred.[50] Aggressive use of neuroimaging during the antepartum period by fetal sonography or MRI, or within the first days after birth, may document remote brain lesions. Destructive lesions such as porencephaly require approximately 5 to 7 days before appearing radiographically. More recent intrapartum or neonatal periods during which injury occurred can be supported by the presence of early cerebral edema using diffusion-weighted MRI.[23] Cerebral infarction may also occur during the postnatal period from asphyxia, polycythemia, dehydration, or coagulopathy.

PPHN with severe and recurrent hypoxia can also be associated with cerebrovascular lesions and seizures (Fig. 40-78; see also Chapter 44). Certain infants with PPHN require extracorporeal membrane oxygenation to treat severe forms of this pulmonary disease which do not respond to traditional ventilatory and nitric oxide therapy. Radiographic documentation of brain lesions needs to be obtained before beginning extracorporeal membrane oxygenation because the anticoagulation required for this procedure may convert "bland" or ischemic infarctions to hemorrhagic forms, with greater risk for cerebral edema and herniation. Although meconium aspiration syndrome has historically been identified with an intrapartum or neonatal presentation of PPHN, in many children with this lung disease the condition reflects antepartum maternal-fetal or placental conditions that predispose the fetus to thickening of the muscular layers of the pulmonary arteries in utero, with resultant sustained increased pulmonary vascular resistance after birth.[6]

Cerebral infarction in the venous distribution of the brain may also lead to neonatal seizures.[68] Lateral or sagittal sinus thromboses after coagulopathy can occur secondary to systemic infection, polycythemia, or dehydration. Venous infarction in the deep white matter of the preterm brain also occurs in association with intraventricular hemorrhage.

Infection

See also Chapter 39.
Central nervous system infections during the antepartum or postnatal periods can be associated with neonatal seizures. Congenital infections, commonly referred to by the acronym *TORCH* (i.e., *t*oxoplasmosis, *r*ubella, *c*ytomegalovirus, and *h*erpes simplex virus), can produce severe encephalopathic damage that results in seizures, as well as more diffuse brain disorders. Other congenital infections include those caused by enteroviruses and parvoviruses. Specific infections such as neonatal herpes encephalitis have been associated with severe EEG pattern abnormalities.[56] Rubella, toxoplasmosis, and cytomegalic inclusion disease also can lead to devastating encephalitis, usually presenting with microcephaly, jaundice, body rash, hepatosplenomegaly, or chorioretinitis. Increasing lethargy and obtundation with or without seizures

may suggest the subacute presentation of encephalitis during the postnatal period. Serial spinal fluid analyses document progressively increasing protein or pleocytosis.

Bacterial infections acquired in utero or postnatally from either gram-negative or gram-positive organisms are also associated with neonatal seizures. Some organisms such as *Escherichia coli*, group B streptococci, *Listeria monocytogenes*, and mycoplasmas may produce severe leptomeningeal infiltration, with possible abscess formation and cerebrovascular occlusions. A high percentage of survivors has significant neurologic sequelae.

Central Nervous System Malformations

See also Parts 1 and 7 of this chapter.
Disorders of induction, segmentation, proliferation, migration, myelination, and synaptogenesis of neuronal components can contribute to varying degrees of malformation. Seizures may result in the newborn with malformations who experiences stress around the time of birth,[62] which presumably lowers seizure thresholds. Brain anomalies may occur as a result of either genetic causes from conception or acquired defects during the first half of gestation. Specific dysgenesis syndromes, such as holoprosencephaly and lissencephaly, are often associated with characteristic facial or body anomalies. Cytogenetic studies may document trisomies or deletion defects. Unfortunately, infants may also lack physical clues to the presence of a brain malformation. The clinician's high index of suspicion is then warranted to evaluate neonates with persistent seizures. Nine percent of 356 infants presenting with neonatal seizures had brain malformations.[87] Neuroimaging, preferably magnetic resonance techniques, documents brain dysgenesis in children who may also express severe EEG disturbances, including seizures (Fig. 40-79). Focal or regional brain malformations are rare causes of early-onset epilepsy in neonates and young infants[2]; functional imaging studies such as positron emission tomography scans[11] may identify localized areas of altered brain metabolism, which can assist in a neurosurgical approach to seizure management, even in young children who fail to respond to antiepileptic drug maintenance.[65]

Inborn Errors of Metabolism

See also Chapter 50.
Inherited biochemical abnormalities are rare causes of neonatal seizures.[46] Intractable seizures associated with elevated lactate and pyruvate levels in blood and spinal fluid may reflect specific inborn errors of metabolism. Dysplastic or destructive brain lesions, as documented on neuroimaging, may be associated with specific biochemical defects, such as glycine encephalopathy or branched-chain aminoacidopathies. Pregnancy, labor, and delivery histories for these infants are commonly uneventful. The emergence of feeding intolerance as well as increasing lethargy, stupor, coma, and seizures is an early indication of an inborn metabolic disturbance during the first few days of life. The newborn with an inherited metabolic disorder may initially present as a neurologically depressed and hypotonic child with asphyxia and seizures. Some children respond to specific dietary therapies, including vitamin supplementation, depending on the enzymatic defect.

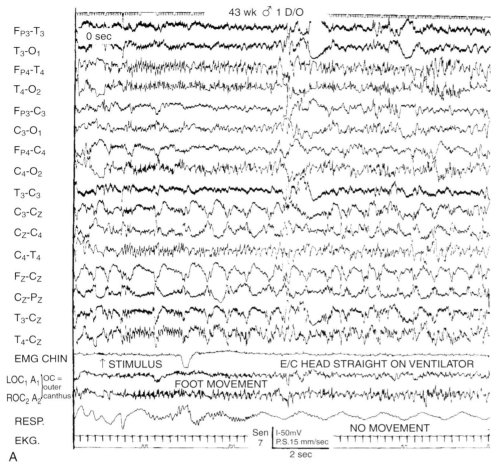

43 wk ♂ 1 D/O

FP3-T3
T3-O1
FP4-T4
T4-O2
FP3-C3
C3-O1
FP4-C4
C4-O2
T3-C3
C3-Cz
Cz-C4
C4-T4
Fz-Cz
Cz-Pz
T3-Cz
T4-Cz
EMG CHIN
LOC1 A1 OC = outer
ROC2 A2 canthus
RESP.
EKG.

0 sec

↑ STIMULUS   E/C HEAD STRAIGHT ON VENTILATOR
FOOT MOVEMENT
NO MOVEMENT

Sen 7 | I-50mV P.S.15 mm/sec

2 sec

A

Figure 40–78. A, Electroencephalogram segment of record of a 43-week gestation, 1-day-old boy with a stimulus-evoked electrographic seizure (*arrow*) without clinical accompaniments in the right temporal region. The child required ventilatory care for persistent pulmonary hypertension of the newborn (see text). B, Computed tomography scan on day 6 for the patient in A, documenting a hemorrhagic infarction in the right posterior quadrant with surrounding edema. (*From Scher MS, et al: Seizures and infarction in neonates with persistent pulmonary hypertension,* Pediatr Neurol 2:332, 1986, with permission.)

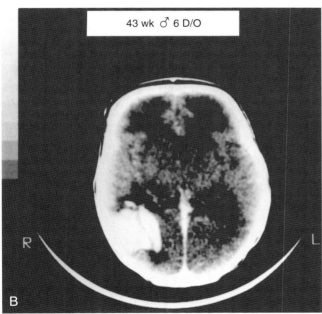

43 wk ♂ 6 D/O

R   L

B

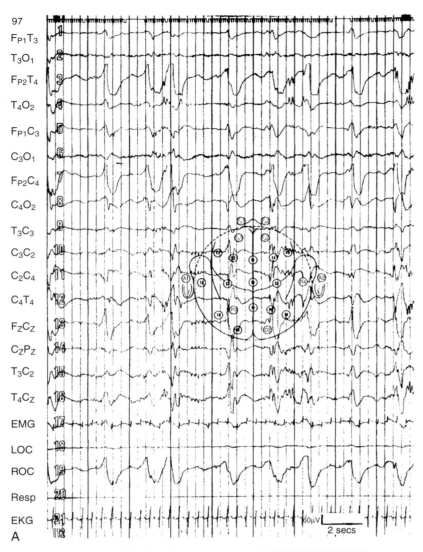

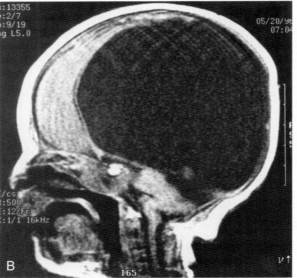

Figure 40–79. A, Electroencephalogram segment of 38-week gestation, 1-day-old infant with right hemisphere-predominant generalized electrographic seizures without clinical signs. B, Magnetic resonance image for the patient in A, demonstrating severe cerebral dysgenesis including lissencephaly, holoprosencephaly, and a small, atrophic cerebellum and brainstem. (*From Scher MS: Seizures in the newborn infant,* Clin Perinatol *24:763, 1997, with permission.*)

Specific urea cycle defects, such as ornithine transamylase or carbamoyl phosphate synthetase deficiency, may present with coma and seizures during the first 2 days of life, with marked elevations in plasma ammonia levels. These infants may respond to aggressive treatment with an exchange transfusion, dialysis, and appropriate dietary adjustments.

Vitamin B_6 or pyridoxine deficiency is a rare cause of neonatal seizures.[5] Pyridoxine acts as a cofactor in γ-aminobutyric acid synthesis, and its absence or paucity promotes seizures. The mother occasionally reports paroxysmal fetal movements.[60] The infant who is unresponsive to conventional antiepileptic medications should promptly receive an IV injection of 50 to 500 mg pyridoxine, preferably with concomitant EEG monitoring. Termination of the seizure within minutes to hours as well as resolution of EEG background disturbances suggests a pyridoxine-dependent seizure state. Prophylactic doses of pyridoxine may be needed to achieve and maintain seizure control.

Other rare causes of seizures include disorders of carbohydrate metabolism with coincident hypoglycemia,[46] as well as peroxisomal disorders, such as neonatal adrenoleukodystrophy or Zellweger syndrome. A defect in a glucose transporter protein necessary to move glucose across the blood-brain barrier has also been reported, which results in hypoglycorrhachia and seizures.[17] Such children may achieve seizure control with a ketogenic diet, but nonetheless suffer delayed development.

Molybdenum cofactor deficiency and isolated sulfite oxidase deficiencies are other rare metabolic defects that cause neonatal seizures and associated destructive changes on neuroimaging, which may resemble cerebrovascular disease or asphyxial insults.

Drug Withdrawal and Intoxication

See also Chapter 38.
Newborns born to mothers who engaged in prenatal substance use or abuse may have an increased risk for neonatal seizures. Exposure to barbiturates, alcohol, heroin, cocaine, or methadone commonly presents with neurologic findings that include tremors and irritability. Withdrawal symptoms, in addition to seizures, may occur as long as 4 to 6 weeks after birth; EEG studies are useful to corroborate such movements with coincident electrographic seizures. Certain drugs, such as short-acting barbiturates, may be associated with seizures within the first several days of life. Seizures may occur directly after substance withdrawal, or associated with longer-standing uteroplacental insufficiency promoted by chronic substance use and poor prenatal health maintenance by the mother. Careful review of placental-cord specimens may reveal chronic or acute lesions that contribute to antepartum or intrauterine asphyxia.

Inadvertent fetal injection with a local anesthetic agent during delivery may induce intoxication, which is a rare cause of seizures. Patients present during the first 6 to 8 hours of life with apnea, bradycardia, and hypotonia, and are comatose, without brainstem reflexes. If the obstetric history indicates pudendal administration of an anesthetic to the mother, a careful examination of the child's scalp or body for puncture marks is indicated. Determination of plasma levels of the suspected anesthetic agent establishes the diagnosis. Treatment consists of ventilatory support and removing the drug by therapeutic diuresis, acidification of the urine, or exchange transfusion. Antiepileptic medications are rarely indicated.

Progressive Neonatal Epileptic Syndromes

Progressive epileptic syndromes rarely present during the first month of life.[54] These children usually exhibit myoclonic or migratory seizures that are poorly controlled by antiepileptic medications, with brain malformations often demonstrable on brain imaging.[19] These neonatal epileptic syndromes are termed *early myoclonic encephalopathy* or early infantile epileptic encephalopathy (Ohtahara syndrome), and the EEG commonly documents burst suppression or markedly disorganized background rhythms. Rarely, neonates with idiopathic localization-related or partial seizures without neuroimaging abnormalities present with intractable epilepsy.

Neurocutaneous syndromes, such as incontinentia pigmenti and tuberous sclerosis, may also present during the neonatal period with symptomatic epilepsy as one clinical manifestation of these genetic disorders (see also Chapter 52). Incontinentia pigmenti is accompanied by a vesicular crusting rash that initially mimics a herpetic infection. Seizures may or may not be present. The skin lesions evolve into lightly pigmented, raised sebaceous lesions in older infants and children. Tuberous sclerosis also rarely presents with skin lesions in the newborn period. Hypopigmented lesions, initially noted under ultraviolet light, usually appear later during infancy. Two common fetal presentations of tuberous sclerosis are a cardiac tumor, usually a rhabdomyoma, or rarely a connatal brain tumor, both noted on fetal sonography. Neonatal seizures also may be the presenting feature,[51] with documentation of intracranial lesions on postnatal neuroimaging.

Benign Familial Neonatal Seizures

The autosomal dominant form of neonatal seizures is a rare genetic epilepsy that should be considered in the context of a positive family history. Infectious, metabolic, toxic, and structural causes need to be excluded before considering this entity. The genetic defect was first described on chromosome 20q,[31] specifically at the D20S19 and D20S20 loci, as well as a locus EBN2 on chromosome 8q24. By positional cloning, a potassium channel gene (KCNQ2) located on 20q13.3 was first isolated and found to be expressed in brain. A second potassium channel gene (KCNQ3) has also been described and may account for the varied phenotypic expression of seizures and outcomes.[37] Mutations in ion channels have also been implicated in Jervell and Lange-Nielsen syndromes, whose symptoms include congenital deafness and cardiac arrhythmias.[31] Infant outcomes range from excellent to guarded, depending on the persistence of seizures beyond the neonatal period. Response to antiepileptic medication is usually good, although some authors describe variable success. Further studies are needed to clarify the relationship between phenotypic and genotypic expressions of this disorder.

DIAGNOSTIC ALGORITHM

Once seizures are confirmed by EEG, the neonatologist and neurologist must place these events into the context of clinical, historical, and laboratory findings to determine the pathogenesis and timing of an encephalopathic process in the symptomatic neonate. Seizures in neonates after asphyxia support either acute intrapartum events or antepartum disease processes. The child with seizures may also express clinical and laboratory signs of evolving cerebral edema. The presence of a bulging fontanelle with neuroimaging evidence of increased intracranial pressure and cerebral edema (i.e., obliterated ventricular outline and abnormalities on diffusion-weighted MRI) strongly suggest a more recent asphyxial disease process, in or around the intrapartum period.

Hyponatremia and increased urine osmolality suggest the syndrome of inappropriate secretion of antidiuretic hormone accompanying acute or subacute cerebral edema.

Alternatively, failure to document evolving cerebral edema during the first 3 days after asphyxia, or documentation of encephalomalacia or cystic brain lesions on neuroimaging shortly after birth (i.e., even in the encephalopathic newborn), suggests a more chronic disease process and remote antepartum brain injury. Liquefaction necrosis requires 2 weeks or longer after the presumed in utero asphyxial event to produce a cystic cavity, which is then visible on neuroimaging.

Isolated seizures in an otherwise asymptomatic neonate can suggest a disease process occurring during either the postnatal or antepartum periods. Neonates present with seizures as a result of postnatal illnesses from intracranial infection, cardiovascular lesions, drug toxicity, or inherited metabolic diseases. Children with antepartum injury may express isolated seizures after in utero cerebrovascular injury on the basis of thrombolytic or embolic disease of the mother, placenta, or fetus. Fetal injury also may occur after ischemia-hypoperfusion events from circulatory disturbances, such as maternal shock, chorioamnionitis, or placental-fetal vasculopathy.[52]

Only a percentage of neonates with in utero cerebrovascular disease present with neonatal seizures. Why others remain asymptomatic until later childhood is unknown. Neonatal expression of seizures may reflect recent physiologic stress during parturition, which lowers seizure threshold in susceptible brain regions that have been previously damaged.

After a careful review of the medical histories of the mother, fetus, and newborn, determination of serum glucose, electrolytes, ammonia, lactate, pyruvate, magnesium, calcium, and phosphorus levels may diagnose correctable metabolic conditions in newborns with seizures who will not require antiepileptic medications. Spinal fluid analyses include cell count, protein, glucose, lactate, pyruvate, amino acids, and culture studies to consider central nervous system infection, intracranial hemorrhage, and metabolic disease. Metabolic acidosis on serial arterial blood gas determinations may alternatively suggest an inherited metabolic disease, particularly if intrapartum asphyxia was not judged to be severe. Absence of multiorgan dysfunction may alert the clinician to other etiologies for seizures besides intrapartum asphyxia. Signs of chronic in utero stress such as growth restriction, early hypertonicity after neonatal depression, joint contractures, or elevated

nucleated red blood cell values all suggest longer-standing antepartum stress to the fetus. Identification of genetic or syndromic conditions can contribute to the expression of neonatal encephalopathies independent of asphyxial injury.[22] Careful review of placental and cord specimens can also be extremely useful. Neuroimaging, preferably using MRI, can help locate, grade the severity of, and possibly time an insult.[38] Ancillary studies may include long-chain fatty acids and chromosomal/DNA analyses, as deemed necessary by family and clinical histories. Finally, serum and urine organic acid and amino acid determinations may be needed to delineate a specific biochemical disorder for the child with a persistent metabolic acidosis. Lysosomal enzyme studies are also occasionally considered to diagnose specific enzymatic deficiencies in children with neonatal seizures (see also Chapter 50).

TREATMENT

Rapid infusion of glucose or other supplemental electrolytes should be initiated before antiepileptic medications are considered. Severe hypoglycemia can be typically corrected by IV administration of 2 mL/kg of a 10% dextrose solution, followed by an infusion of approximately 8 to 10 mg/kg per minute and increased as needed. Persistent hypoglycemia may require more hypertonic glucose solutions. Rarely, other pharmacologic measures (e.g., diazoxide) may be needed to establish a glucose level within the normal range (see also Chapter 49, Part 1).

Hypocalcemia-induced seizures should be treated with an IV infusion of 200 mg/kg of calcium gluconate. This dosage may need to be repeated every 5 to 6 hours over the first 24 hours. Serum magnesium concentrations should also be measured because hypomagnesemia may accompany hypocalcemia; 0.2 mg/kg of magnesium sulfate should be given by IM injection. (See Chapter 49, Part 2.) Disorders of serum sodium are rare causes of neonatal seizures.

Pyridoxine dependency requires the injection of 50 to 500 mg of pyridoxine during a seizure with coincident EEG monitoring. A beneficial pyridoxine effect occurs either immediately or over the first several hours. A daily dose of 50 to 100 mg of pyridoxine should then be administered.

If the decision to treat neonates with antiepileptic medications is reached, important questions must be addressed with respect to who should be treated, when to begin treatment, which drug to use, and for how long neonates should be treated. Some authors suggest that only neonates with clinical seizures should receive medications; brief electrographic seizures need not be treated. Others suggest more aggressive treatment of EEG seizures because uncontrolled seizures potentially have an adverse effect on immature brain development.[94]

Phenobarbital and phenytoin remain the most widely used antiepileptic medications. The half-life of phenobarbital ranges from 45 to 173 hours in the neonate; the initial loading dose is recommended at 20 mg/kg, with a maintenance dose of 3 to 4 mg/kg per day. Therapeutic levels are usually suggested to range from 10 to 40 µg/mL, although there is no consensus with respect to drug maintenance.

The preferred loading dose of phenytoin is 15 to 20 mg/kg. Serum levels of phenytoin are difficult to maintain because this drug is rapidly redistributed to body tissues. Blood levels cannot be well maintained using an oral preparation.

Benzodiazepines may also be used to control neonatal seizures. The drug most widely used is diazepam. One study suggests a half-life of 54 hours in preterm infants to 18 hours in term infants. IV administration is recommended because it is slowly absorbed after an IM injection. Diazepam is highly protein bound and displacement of bilirubin from albumin is possible. Recommended IV doses for acute management should begin at 0.5 mg/kg. Deposition into muscle precludes its use as a maintenance antiepileptic medication because profound hypotonia and respiratory depression may result, particularly if barbiturates have also been administered.

Efficacy of Treatment

Studies report varying efficacy with phenobarbital or phenytoin. However, most studies apply only a clinical endpoint to seizure cessation. Coincident EEG studies are now suggested to verify the resolution of electrographic seizures because 30% of neonates may have persistent electrographic seizures after suppression of clinical seizure behaviors even after drug administration.[80] With doses of phenobarbital as high as 40 mg/kg, the rate of seizure control may be up to 85%, and the earlier administration of high-dose phenobarbital in a group of asphyxiated infants was associated with a 27% reduction in clinical seizures together with better outcome than in a group who did not receive high dosages.[25] With EEG as an endpoint to judge cessation of seizures, neither phenobarbital nor phenytoin was effective in controlling seizure activity.[61]

Assay of free or drug-bound fractions of antiepileptic drugs has been suggested to better assess both the efficacy and potential toxicity of antiepileptic drugs in pediatric populations. Drug binding in neonates with seizures has only recently been reported, and can be altered in a sick neonate with organ dysfunction. Toxic side effects may result from elevated free fractions of a drug, which adversely affect cardiovascular and respiratory function. To guard against untoward effects, evaluation of treatment and efficacy must take into account both total and free antiepileptic drug fractions, in the context of the newborn's systemic illness.

New anticonvulsant alternatives to treat seizures are being suggested such as with N-methyl-D-aspartate antagonists, and topiramate,[29,42] developed from experimental models of hypoxia-induced seizure activity in immature brain. Such models provide data regarding pharmacologic and physiologic characteristics of neuronal responses after an asphyxial stress that causes excessive release of excitotoxic neurotransmitters,[30] such as glutamate. Specific cell membrane receptors termed *metabotropic glutamate receptors* are sensitive to extracellular glutamate release and may play a role in epileptogenesis and seizure-induced brain damage. Subclasses of metabotropic glutamate receptors will prompt the investigation of novel drugs that block these membrane receptors as the mode of treatment for neonatal seizures.[39]

Other novel treatment alternatives include antiepileptic approaches with older medications such as the diuretic bumetanide. Bumetanide acts by inhibiting the excitatory action of the NKCC1, the chloride cotransporter active within the immature neuron. It has been shown that this tranporter facilitates seizures in the developing brain using an animal model.[19] Bumetanide may also enhance the action of traditional antiepileptic medications such as phenobarbitol.[20]

Innovative treatment strategies will need to consider both the mechanisms underlying seizure expression[44] as well as timing of when the brain injury occurred that subsequently caused the seizures, whether prior to or during parturition.[83]

Discontinuation of Drug Use

The clinician's decision to maintain or discontinue antiepileptic drug use depends on variable factors. Discontinuation of drugs before discharge from the neonatal unit is usually recommended so that clinical assessments of arousal, tone, and behavior will not be hampered by medication effect. However, newborns with congenital or destructive brain lesions on neuroimaging, or those with persistently abnormal results on neurologic examinations at the time of discharge, may suggest to the clinician that a slower tapering of medication is required over several weeks or months. Neonatal seizures rarely reoccur during the first 2 years of life, and prophylactic antiepileptic drug administration need not be maintained past 3 months of age, even in the child at risk. This is supported by a study suggesting a low risk of seizure reoccurrence after early withdrawal of antiepileptic drug therapy in the neonatal period.[26] Also, older infants who present with specific epileptic syndromes, such as infantile spasms, do not respond to the conventional antiepileptic drugs that were initially begun during the neonatal period. This "honeymoon period" without seizures commonly persists for many years in most children, before isolated or recurrent seizures appear.

The potential damage to the developing central nervous system by antiepileptic drugs also emphasizes the need to consider early discontinuation of these agents in the newborn period. Adverse effects on the morphology and metabolism of neuronal cells have been extensively reported from collective research performed over the last several decades.[53]

CONSEQUENCES OF NEONATAL SEIZURES

Embedded in the controversy surrounding the diagnosis of neonatal seizures is the association with altered brain development and poor neurologic outcome. The clinician must first appreciate the diverse neuropathologic processes, independent of the seizure process, associated with specific etiologies responsible for neonatal seizures and neurologic sequelae.[32] Our understanding of the underlying mechanisms responsible for brain damage in neonates with seizures is limited to a few definable factors such as central nervous system infections and severe asphyxia.

Direct effects of the seizure state also may have adverse effects on developing brain.[27] Seizures can disrupt a cascade of biochemical and molecular pathways normally responsible for the plasticity or activity-dependent development of the maturing nervous system. Seizures may disrupt the processes of cell division, migration, sequential expression of receptor formation, and stabilization of synapses, contributing to neurologic sequelae.

Experimental models of seizures in immature animals suggest less vulnerability to seizure-induced brain injury than in mature animals.[28] In adult animals, seizures alter growth of hippocampal granule cells and cause axonal and mossy fiber growth, resulting in long-term deficits in learning, memory, and behavior. A single prolonged seizure in an immature animal, on the other hand, results in less cell loss or fiber sprouting, and consequentially fewer deficits in learning, memory, and behavior. Resistance to brain damage from prolonged seizure activity, however, is age specific, as evidenced by increased cell damage after only 2 weeks of age.[71]

Repetitive or prolonged neonatal seizures increase the susceptibility of the developing brain to subsequent seizure-induced brain injury during adolescence or early adulthood from altered neuronal connectivity rather than increased cell death.[27,84] Neonatal animals subjected to status epilepticus have reduced seizure thresholds at later ages and impairments of learning, memory, and activity levels when stressed with seizures as adults. Proposed mechanisms of injury include reduced neurogenesis in the hippocampus, for example, possibly because of ischemia-induced apoptosis as well as necrotic pathways.[48] Other suggested mechanisms of injury include effects of nitric oxide synthetase inhibition on cerebral circulation, which then contributes to ischemic injury. Neonatal seizures therefore may initiate a cascade of diverse changes in brain development that become maladaptive at older ages, and increase the risk of damage after subsequent insults. Destructive mechanisms such as mossy fiber sprouting in the hippocampus or increased neuronal apoptosis may explain mutually exclusive pathways by which the immature brain suffers altered connectivity and reduced cell number, and thus is "primed" for later seizure-induced cell loss at older ages.

Because of a lack of well-designed studies, these experimental findings unfortunately are not supported by clinical investigations of outcome after neonatal seizures.[53] Better definitions of neonatal seizures of epileptic origin are needed, and the critical seizure duration required to injure brain remains controversial. Overlapping effects of underlying central nervous system injury or dysgenesis from specific etiologies versus seizure-induced brain damage make it difficult to differentiate preexisting brain lesions from the direct injurious effects of seizures themselves. The use of microdialysis probes in white and gray matter of piglet brains subjected to hypoxia indicated elevated lactate/pyruvate ratios after hypoxia, but no direct association with seizure activity.[92] These findings support the conclusion that seizures themselves may not lead to injurious metabolic dysfunction.

Aggressive use of antiepileptic medications contributes both to inaccurate estimation of seizure severity in neonates and possible medication-induced brain injury. Intractable seizures usually require the use of multiple antiepileptic medications. Such drugs impede the clinician's recognition of prolonged seizures because of the uncoupling phenomenon in which the clinical expression may be suppressed while the electrical expression of seizures continues. Clinical definitions of seizure occurrence and duration consequently underestimate seizure severity, which appears to be associated with increased risk for damage. Antiepileptic drug use also has secondary harmful effects on cardiac and respiratory function, with resultant circulatory disturbances that contribute to brain injury.[53] Finally, antiepileptic drug use may have teratogenetic effects on brain development with exposure over long periods.

PROGNOSIS

The mortality rate of infants who present with clinical neonatal seizures has declined over time. Studies of EEG-confirmed seizures documented a 50% mortality rate in preterm and a 40% rate in term infants during the 1980s; during the 1990s, the mortality rate for both groups of infants dropped below 20%. The incidence of adverse neurologic sequelae, however, remains high for approximately two thirds of survivors. Even if major neurodevelopmental sequelae such as motor deficits and mental retardation were avoided in survivors after neonatal seizures, subtle neurodevelopmental vulnerability may manifest in late teenage years as specific learning difficulties or poor social adjustment,[90] underscoring experimental findings of long-term deficits in animal populations.[27]

Prediction of outcome should also clearly consider the etiology for seizures, such as severe asphyxia, significant craniocerebral trauma, and brain infections. More accurate imaging procedures have heightened our awareness of destructive as well as congenital brain lesions with a higher risk for compromised outcome.

Interictal EEG pattern abnormalities are extremely helpful in predicting neurologic outcome in the neonate with seizures. Major background disturbances such as burst suppression (see Fig. 40-77) are highly predictive of poor outcome, particularly when persistently abnormal findings are still present on serial EEG studies into the second week of life. Ictal patterns alone may not be as accurate for predicting outcome, unless they occur in high numbers, long durations, and multifocal distribution.[47] Normal findings on interictal EEG were associated with an 86% chance of normal development at 4 years of age in 139 neonates with seizures[70]; by contrast, neonates with markedly abnormal EEG background disturbances had only a 7% chance for normal outcome. Therefore in term and preterm infants with seizures, the EEG background may be more predictive of outcome than the presence of isolated sharp-wave discharges. Even the finding of severe EEG abnormalities by single-channel spectral EEG recordings after asphyxia carries a higher risk for sequelae.

Neonates with seizures have a risk for epilepsy during childhood.[95] Based on clinical seizure criteria, epilepsy later develops in 20% to 25% of neonates with seizures. Excluding febrile seizures, the prevalence of epilepsy by 6 to 7 years of age is also estimated to be between 15% and 30% based on EEG-confirmed seizures for an inborn hospital population, two thirds of whom were preterm neonates. This is contrasted to a 56% incidence of epilepsy for an exclusively outborn neonatal population of primarily term newborns with seizures.[14] Epilepsy risk therefore reflects selection bias of specific study groups, as well as referral patterns in different hospital settings.

REFERENCES

1. Adamson SJ, et al: Predictors of neonatal encephalopathy in full term infants, *BMJ* 311:598, 1995.
2. Aicardi J: Early myoclonic encephalopathy. In Roger J, et al, editors: *Epileptic Syndromes in Infancy, Childhood, and Adolescence*, London, 1985, J. Libbey Eurotext, p 12.
3. Alfonso I, et al: Single photon emission computed tomographic evaluation of brainstem release phenomenon and seizure in neonates, *J Child Neurol* 15:56, 2000.
4. American College of Obstetricians and Gynecologists and American Academy of Pediatrics: Neonatal Encephalopathy and Cerebral Palsy: Defining the Pathogenesis and Pathophysiology, *American College of Obstetricians and Gynecologists Consensus Report*, Washington, D.C., 2003, American College of Obstetricians and Gynecologists.
5. Bejsovec M, et al: Familial intrauterine convulsions in pyridoxine dependency, *Arch Dis Child* 42:201, 1967.
6. Benitz WE, et al: Persistent pulmonary hypertension of the newborn. In Stephenson DK, Sunshine P, editors: *Fetal and Neonatal Brain Injury: Mechanisms, Management and the Risks of Practice*, 3rd ed, 2003, Cambridge University Press, p 636.
7. Biagioni E, et al: Electroclinical correlation in neonatal seizures, *Eur J Paediatr Neurol* 2:117, 1998.
8. Boylan GB, et al: Outcome of electroclinical, electrographic, and clinical seizures in the newborn infant, *Dev Med Child Neurol* 41:819, 1999.
9. Bye AME, et al: Outcome of neonates with electrographically identified seizures, or at risk of seizures, *Pediatr Neurol* 16:225, 1997.
10. Bye AME, Flanagan D: Spatial and temporal characteristics of neonatal seizures, *Epilepsia* 36:1009, 1995.
11. Chugani HT, et al: Ictal patterns of cerebral glucose utilization in children with epilepsy, *Epilepsia* 35:813, 1994.
12. Clancy RR: The contribution of EEG to the understanding of neonatal seizures, *Epilepsia* 37:S52, 1996.
13. Clancy R, Legido A: The exact ictal and interictal duration of electroencephalographic neonatal seizures, *Epilepsia* 28:537, 1987.
14. Clancy RR, Legido A: Postnatal epilepsy after EEG-confirmed neonatal seizures, *Epilepsia* 32:69, 1991.
15. Coulter DL, Allen RJ: Benign neonatal sleep myoclonus, *Arch Neurol* 39:191, 1982.
16. DaSilva O, et al: The value of standard electroencephalograms in the evaluation of the newborn with recurrent apneas, *J Perinatol* 18:377, 1998.
17. DeVivo DC, et al: Defective glucose transport across the blood-brain barrier as a cause of persistent hypoglycorrhachia, seizures, and developmental delay, *N Engl J Med* 325:703, 1991.
18. De Vries LS, et al: Infarcts in the vascular distribution of the middle cerebral artery in preterm and fullterm infants, *Neuropediatrics* 28:88, 1997.
19. Dzhala VI, et al: NKCC1 transporter facilitates seizures in the developing brain, *Nat Med* 11:1205, 2005.
20. Dzhala VI, et al: Bumetanide enhances phenobarbital efficacy in neonatal seizure model, *Ann Neurol* 63:222, 2008.
21. Ekert P, et al: Predicting the outcome of postasphyxial hypoxic-ischemic encephalopathy within 4 hours of birth, *J Pediatr* 131:613, 1997.
22. Felix JF, et al: Birth defects in children with newborn encephalopathy, *Dev Med Child Neurol* 42:803, 2000.
23. Forbes KPN, et al: Neonatal hypoxic-ischemic encephalopathy detection with diffusion-weighted MRI imaging, *AJNR Am J Neuroradiol* 21:1490, 2000.
24. Hakamada S, et al: Development of motor behavior during sleep in newborn infants, *Brain Dev* 3:345, 1981.
25. Hall RT, et al: High-dose phenobarbital therapy in term newborn infants with severe perinatal asphyxia: a randomized, prospective study with three-year follow-up, *J Pediatr* 132:345, 1998.
26. Hellström-Westas L, et al: Low risk of seizure recurrence after early withdrawal of antiepileptic treatment in the neonatal period, *Arch Dis Child* 72:F97, 1995.
27. Holmes GL, Ben-Ari Y: The neurobiology and consequences of epilepsy in the developing brain, *Pediatr Res* 49:320, 2001.
28. Huang L-T, et al: Long-term effects of neonatal seizures: a behavioral electrophysiological, and histological study, *Dev Brain Res* 118:99, 1999.
29. Jensen FE: Acute and chronic effects of seizures in the developing brain: experimental models, *Epilepsia* 40:S51, 1999.
30. Jensen FE, Wang C: Hypoxia-induced hyperexcitability in vivo and in vitro in the immature hippocampus, *Epilepsy Res* 26:131, 1996.
31. Jentsch TJ, et al: Pathophysiology of KCNQ channels: neonatal epilepsy and progressive deafness, *Epilepsia* 41:1068, 2000.
32. Keen JH, Lee D: Sequelae of neonatal convulsions: study of 112 infants, *Arch Dis Child* 48:541, 1973.
33. Kilic S, et al: Serum prolactin in neonatal seizures, *Pediatr Int* 41:61, 1999.
34. Lanska MJ, et al: A population-based study of neonatal seizures in Fayette County, Kentucky, *Neurology* 45:724, 1995.
35. Lanska MJ, et al: Interobserver variability in the classification of neonatal seizures based on medical record data, *Pediatr Neurol* 15:120, 1996.
36. Laroia N, et al: EEG background as predictor of electrographic seizures in high-risk neonates, *Epilepsia* 39:545, 1998.
37. Leppert M, Singh N: Benign familial neonatal epilepsy with mutations in two potassium channel genes, *Curr Opin Neurol* 12:143, 1999.
38. Leth H, et al: Neonatal seizures associated with cerebral lesions shown by magnetic resonance imaging, *Arch Dis Child Fetal Neonatal Ed* 77:F105, 1997.
39. Lie AA, et al: Up-regulation of the metabotropic glutamate receptor mGluR4 in hippocampal neurons with reduced seizure vulnerability, *Ann Neurol* 47:26, 2000.
40. Lieberman E, et al: Intrapartum fever and unexplained seizures in term infants, *Pediatrics* 106:983, 2000.
41. Lien JM, et al: Term early-onset neonatal seizures: obstetric characteristics, etiologic classifications, and perinatal care, *Obstet Gynecol* 85:163, 1995.
42. Liu Y, et al: Topiramate extends the therapeutic window for hypothermia-mediated neuroprotection after stroke in neonatal rats, *Stroke* 35:1460, 2004.
43. Low JA, et al: Newborn complications after intrapartum asphyxia with metabolic acidosis at term, *Am J Obstet Gynecol* 170:1081, 1994.
44. Lugli LA, et al: Neonatal seizures: monitoring and treatment. In Ramenghi, et al, editors: *Perinatal Brain Damage: From Pathogenesis to Neuroprotection*, France Montrouge, J. Libbey Eurotext,
45. Lynch BJ, Rust RS: Natural history and outcome of neonatal hypocalcemic and hypomagnesemic seizures, *Pediatr Neurol* 11:23, 1994.

46. Lyon G, et al: General aspects of hereditary metabolic diseases of the nervous system. In Lyon G, et al, editors: *Neurology of Hereditary Metabolic Diseases of Children*, 2nd ed, New York, 1996, McGraw-Hill, p 1.

47. McBride M, et al: Electrographic seizures in neonates correlate with poor neurodevelopmental outcome, *Neurology* 55:506, 2000.

48. McCabe BK, et al: Reduced neurogenesis after neonatal seizures, *J Neurosci* 21:2094, 2001.

49. McIntire DD, et al: Birth weight in relation to morbidity and mortality among newborn infants, *N Engl J Med* 340:1234, 1999.

50. Mercuri E, et al: Ischaemic and haemorrhagic brain lesions in newborns with seizures and normal Apgar scores, *Arch Dis Child* 73:F67, 1995.

51. Miller SP, et al: Tuberous sclerosis complex and neonatal seizures, *J Child Neurol* 13:619, 1998.

52. Miller V: Neonatal cerebral infarction, *Semin Pediatr Neurol* 7:278, 2000.

53. Mizrahi EM: Acute and chronic effects of seizures in the developing brain: lessons from clinical experience, *Epilepsia* 40:S42, 1999.

54. Mizrahi EM, Clancy RR: Neonatal seizures: early-onset seizure syndromes and their consequences for development, *Ment Retard Dev Disabil Res Rev* 6:229, 2000.

55. Mizrahi EM, Kellaway P: *Diagnosis and Management of Neonatal Seizures*, Philadelphia, 1998, Lippincott-Raven.

56. Mizrahi EM, Tharp BR: Characteristic EEG pattern in neonatal herpes simplex encephalitis, *Neurology* 32:1215, 1982.

57. Nelson KB, Leviton A: How much of neonatal encephalopathy is due to birth asphyxia? *Am J Dis Child* 145:1325, 1991.

58. Oliveira AJ, et al: Duration of rhythmic EEG patterns in neonates: new evidence for clinical and prognostic significance of brief rhythmic discharges, *Clin Neurophysiol* 111:1646, 2000.

59. O'Meara WM, et al: Clinical features of neonatal seizures, *J Pediatr Child Health* 31:237, 1995.

60. Osiovich H, Barrington K: Prenatal ultrasound diagnosis of seizures, *Am J Perinatol* 13:499, 1996.

61. Painter MJ, et al: A comparison of the efficacy of phenobarbital and phenytoin in the treatment of neonatal seizures, *N Engl J Med* 341:485, 1999.

62. Palmini A, et al: Prenatal events and genetic factors in epileptic patients with neuronal migration disorders, *Epilepsia* 35:965, 1994.

63. Parker S, et al: Jitteriness in full-term neonates: prevalence and correlates, *Pediatrics* 85:17, 1990.

64. Patterson CA, et al: Antenatal and intrapartum factors associated with the occurrence of seizures in the term infant, *Obstet Gynecol* 74:361, 1989.

65. Pedespan JM, et al: Surgical treatment of an early epileptic encephalopathy with suppression-bursts and focal cortical dysplasia, *Epilepsia* 36:37, 1995.

66. Pope SS, et al: *Atlas of Neonatal Electroencephalography*, New York, 1992, Raven Press.

67. Rennie JM, et al: Non-expert use of the cerebral function monitor for neonatal seizure detection, *Arch Dis Child Fetal Neonatal Ed* 89:F37, 2004.

68. Rivkin MJ, et al: Neonatal idiopathic cerebral venous thrombosis: an unrecognized cause of transient seizures or lethargy, *Ann Neurol* 32:51, 1992.

69. Ronen GM, et al: The epidemiology of clinical neonatal seizures in Newfoundland: a population-based study, *J Pediatr* 134:71, 1999.

70. Rose AL, Lombroso CT: A study of clinical, pathological, and electroencephalographic features in 137 full-term babies with a long-term follow-up, *Pediatrics* 45:404, 1970.

71. Sankar R, et al: Epileptogenesis after status epilepticus reflects age- and model-dependent plasticity, *Ann Neurol* 48:580, 2000.

72. Sarnat HB: Anatomic and physiologic correlates of neurologic development in prematurity. In Sarnat HB, editor: *Topics in Neonatal Neurology*, Orlando, FL, 1984, Grune & Stratton, p 1.

73. Sarnat HB, Sarnat MS: Neonatal encephalography following fetal distress: a clinical and encephalographic study, *Arch Neurol* 33:696, 1976.

74. Scher MS: Controversies regarding neonatal seizure recognition, *Epileptic Disord* 4:138, 2002.

75. Scher MS: Neonatal encephalopathies as classified by EEG-sleep criteria: severity and timing based on clinical/pathologic correlations, *Pediatr Neurol* 11:189, 1994.

76. Scher MS: Neurophysiological assessment of brain function and maturation: II. A measure of brain dysmaturity in healthy preterm neonates, *Pediatr Neurol* 16:287, 1997.

77. Scher MS: Prenatal contributions to epilepsy: lessons from the bedside, *Epileptic Disord* 5:77, 2003.

78. Scher MS: Pathological myoclonus of the newborn: electrographic and clinical correlations, *Pediatr Neurol* 1:342, 1985.

79. Scher MS: Stimulus-evoked electrographic patterns in neonates: abnormal form of reactivity, *Electroencephalogr Clin Neurophysiol* 103:679, 1997.

80. Scher MS, et al: Uncoupling of clinical and EEG seizures after antiepileptic drug use in neonates, *Pediatr Neurol* 28:277, 2003.

81. Scher MS, et al: Ictal and interictal durations in preterm and term neonates, *Epilepsia* 34:284, 1993.

82. Scher MS, et al: Neonates with electrically-confirmed seizures and possible placental associations, *Pediatr Neurol* 19:37, 1998.

83. Scher MS, et al: Neonatal seizure classification: a fetal perspective concerning childhood epilepsy, *Epilepsy Res* 70(suppl 1):41, 2006.

84. Schmid R, et al: Effects of neonatal seizures on subsequent seizure-induced brain injury, *Neurology* 53:1754, 1999.

85. Sexson WR, et al: Stereotypic movements after lorazepam administration in premature neonates: a series and review of the literature, *J Perinatol* 15:146, 1995.

86. Sheth RD: Electroencephalogram confirmatory rate in neonatal seizures, *Pediatr Neurol* 20:27, 1999.

87. Sheth RD, et al: Neonatal seizures: incidence, onset, and etiology by gestational age, *J Perinatol* 19:40, 1999.

88. Shuper A, et al: Jitteriness beyond the neonatal period: a benign pattern of movement in infancy, *J Child Neurol* 6:243, 1991.

89. Sinclair DB, et al: EEG and long-term outcome of term infants with neonatal hypoxic-ischemic encephalopathy, *Clin Neurophysiol* 110:655, 1999.

90. Temple CM, et al: Neonatal seizures: long-term outcome and cognitive development among "normal" survivors, *Dev Med Child Neurol* 37:109, 1995.

91. Tharp BR, et al: Serial EEGs in normal and abnormal infants with birth weights less than 1200 grams: a prospective study with long term follow-up, *Neuropediatrics* 20:64, 1989.

92. Thoresen M, et al: Lactate and pyruvate changes in the cerebral gray and white matter during posthypoxic seizures in newborn pigs, *Pediatr Res* 44:746, 1998.

93. Volpe JJ: *Neurology of the Newborn*, 4th ed, Philadelphia, 2001, WB Saunders.

94. Wasterlain CG: Controversies in epilepsy: recurrent seizures in the developing brain are harmful, *Epilepsia* 38:728, 1997.

95. Watanabe K, et al: Neonatal seizures and subsequent epilepsy, *Brain Dev* 4:341, 1982.

96. Weiner SP, et al: Neonatal seizures: electroclinical disassociation, *Pediatr Neurol* 7:363, 1991.

PART 6

Hypotonia and Neuromuscular Disease

Timothy E. Lotze and Geoffrey Miller

Clinicians who care for newborns are often required to consider the possibility that a neuromuscular disorder might be present in a hypotonic infant. When placed in the supine position, the normal full-term infant shows active movement of flexed limbs. The hips are flexed 70 to 90 degrees and abducted approximately 10 to 20 degrees. If passive extension of the legs at the knees is attempted, resistance is met when the popliteal angle is approximately 90 degrees. When the child is pulled to the sitting from the supine position, only slight head lag is present, and on reaching the sitting position, the head should wobble in the midline for a few seconds. Similarly, a predominance of flexor tone is found in the upper limbs. When the infant is held under the axillae, normal tone prevents the infant from slipping through the examiner's hands, and the infant seems to sit in the air. In horizontal suspension, the limbs are flexed, the back is straight, and the head is maintained in the midline for a few seconds. These findings need to be modified for the premature infant who shows decreasing degrees of flexor tone, depending on gestational age.[3,23]

The weak, hypotonic infant has a decrease in the expected resistance of muscle to stretch, and there is a decrease in spontaneous movement. If supine, the infant lies in a froglike position with abduction of the hips and an abnormal extension of the limbs. When pulled to a sitting position, there is head lag with a lack of compensation when the sitting position is reached. In vertical suspension, decreased tone of the shoulder girdle causes the infant to slip through the examiner's hands, and the legs are more extended than flexed. On horizontal suspension, the back hangs over the examiner's hand, and the head and limbs hang loosely. (For further details, see Chapter 27.)

DIAGNOSIS

Almost any condition that affects the central nervous system (CNS; brain or spinal cord) or peripheral nervous system of a newborn can be expressed by a reduction of tone. Furthermore, most acute or multisystem illness in neonates is accompanied by some degree of hypotonia. Therefore the examiner initially must consider whether the infant is acutely ill from sepsis, organ failure, metabolic dysfunction, or other systemic illness. If these illnesses are not present, the next step is to consider whether a primary disorder of the CNS or the peripheral nervous system is the cause. In general, a central cause leads to a reduction in tone out of proportion to the degree of muscle weakness, and the limbs demonstrate antigravity power.[25]

Although this finding is useful, there are exceptions. In some hypotonic neonates there are abnormalities in both the central and peripheral nervous systems. Examples include congenital muscular dystrophy (CMD), congenital myotonic dystrophy, acid maltase deficiency, cervical spinal cord injury, and some mitochondrial or peroxisomal disorders. In addition, some disorders that are primarily central may initially present with profound hypotonia and weakness. Examples are Prader-Willi syndrome and acute disease such as hemorrhage or infarction involving the deep central gray matter of the brain or spinal cord. Conversely, the infant with a mild congenital myopathy demonstrates some antigravity power in the limbs. Finally, hypotonia might be present in the infant without acute systemic or metabolic illness or abnormalities of the nervous system. In these children, there is an unusual degree of ligamentous laxity such as that seen in Ehlers-Danlos syndrome and osteogenesis imperfecta.

The diagnosis of a neonatal muscle disorder requires a methodical approach similar to that used in the older infant or child. A detailed family, obstetric, and delivery history should be taken. Clues to the presence of a neuromuscular disorder include polyhydramnios, a decrease in fetal movement, and malpresentation, although these conditions can be present in any pregnancy with fetal akinesia (paucity of movement). Information should be obtained about whether there was any birth trauma or asphyxia and on the condition of the infant immediately after delivery.

The general examination begins with observation. Does the infant look sick or distressed? The skin should be examined for pallor, trauma, bruising, or petechiae. Any dysmorphic features or congenital defects of the head, neck, or spine should be noted, as should weight, length, and head size and shape. Each system is then examined with a particular emphasis on respiratory rate, pattern, and diaphragmatic movement; cardiovascular status; the presence of organomegaly; the genitalia; the hips; and the presence of contractures. On neurologic examination, initial observations include the degree of alertness and whether the infant fixes or follows. Posture and spontaneous movements are noted. In particular, movement against gravity should be sought, and the examiner should observe whether movement is greater proximally or distally. When formal examination of the cranial nerves is performed, particular attention should be paid to eye movements. These can be observed as spontaneous movements, elicited by a face or a red ball or induced by gentle rotation of the head (oculovestibular reflex). A lack of fixation or following but movement with the oculovestibular reflex suggests a lesion above the brainstem. If the infant is not in severe distress and there is no possibility of cervical spine injury, the degree of hypotonia is assessed by pulling the infant to a sitting position and holding him or her in vertical and horizontal suspension. Passive movement of the joints can assess power and tone in the limbs more gently. Resistance to gentle shaking of an arm or leg (passivité) also provides a subjective assessment of tone.

During handling, cerebral dysfunction should be suspected if there is fisting or an abnormal primitive reflex. The character of the deep tendon reflexes helps distinguish between an upper or lower motor neuron lesion.* If they are abnormally brisk with clonus, then an upper motor neuron lesion is suggested. If absent, a neuropathic lesion or a severe myopathy is more likely. Assessment of sensation should be attempted because a hereditary sensory neuropathy can present during the neonatal period.[7]

Facial diplegia is a particular finding in some neuromuscular disorders and less likely in others. It can also be an early feature of severe acute basal ganglia damage. Note should be made of the infant's ability to suck and swallow, the pooling of secretions, the character of the cry, and the presence of tongue fasciculations. The latter is most often seen in acute infantile spinal muscular atrophy (SMA), but can be seen in any condition in which there is hypoglossal motor neuron damage, examples of which include storage disorders such as acid maltase deficiency, hypoxic-ischemic damage, and infantile neuronal degeneration.

NEONATAL NEUROMUSCULAR DISORDERS

See also Chapter 50.

Neonatal neuromuscular disorders are caused by lesions that affect specific parts of the neuraxis, including the anterior horn cell, peripheral nerve, neuromuscular junction, or muscle (Box 40-11). Rapid and continuing advances are being made in our understanding of the molecular genetic basis of these disorders.

There are a number of CNS conditions in which hypotonia is of sufficient severity that a neuromuscular disorder should be suspected. These are not discussed in detail here, but they include chromosomal disorders such as Prader-Willi syndrome, multiple minor congenital anomaly syndromes, and metabolic multisystem disorders.

SPINAL MUSCULAR ATROPHIES

The SMAs are predominantly autosomal recessive disorders characterized by degeneration of the anterior horn cells in the spinal cord and motor nuclei in the lower brainstem. The most frequent and best known is infantile SMA, also called *Werdnig-Hoffmann disease* (SMA type I).[38] Approximately 95% of individuals with SMA are homozygous for a deletion of exon 7 of the survival motor neuron (SMN) gene (*SMN1*) on chromosome 5q13.[59] Although the phenotype varies in severity and age of onset, the acute infantile subtype is well defined and often presents during the neonatal period. This phenotype tends to "run true" in families. Clinically, infants exhibit a severe symmetric flaccid paralysis, which is characteristically greater in the lower limbs than in the upper limbs and greater proximally than distally.

---

*An upper motor neuron lesion involves descending motor tracts in the brain and spinal cord, whereas a lower motor neuron lesion involves either the anterior horn cell, peripheral motor nerve, or muscle.

BOX 40–11 Neonatal Neuromuscular Disorders

ANTERIOR HORN CELL
Traumatic myelopathy
Hypoxic-ischemic myelopathy
Acute infantile spinal muscular atrophy
Infantile neuronal degeneration
Neurogenic arthrogryposis

CONGENITAL MOTOR AND SENSORY NEUROPATHY
Hypomyelinating neuropathy
Congenital hypomyelinating neuropathy
Charcot-Marie-Tooth disease
Dejerine-Sottas disease
Hereditary sensory and autonomic neuropathy

NEUROMUSCULAR JUNCTION
Acquired transient neonatal myasthenia
Congenital myasthenia
Infantile botulism
Magnesium toxicity
Aminoglycoside toxicity

CONGENITAL MYOPATHY
Nemaline myopathy
Central core disease
Myotubular myopathy
Multi-minicore myopathy

MUSCULAR DYSTROPHY
Congenital muscular dystrophy with merosin deficiency
Congenital muscular dystrophy without merosin deficiency
Walker-Warburg syndrome
Muscle-eye-brain disease
Fukuyama-type congenital muscular dystrophy
Congenital myotonic dystrophy
Duchenne dystrophy (Xp21-linked dystrophinopathy)
Early infantile facioscapulohumeral dystrophy

METABOLIC AND MULTISYSTEM DISEASE
Mitochondrial disorder
Peroxisomal disorder
Neonatal adrenoleukodystrophy
Cerebrohepatorenal syndrome (Zellweger syndrome)
Pompe disease (acid maltase deficiency)
Severe neonatal phosphofructokinase deficiency
Severe neonatal phosphorylase deficiency
Debrancher deficiency
Carnitine deficiency

The onset of this weakness is often identified by the mother, who experiences a decrease or loss of fetal movement during late pregnancy. Respiratory muscle function is poor in the infant. However, it is the intercostal muscles that are weak because there is relative sparing of the diaphragm. This gives rise to abdominal breathing and a later characteristic bell-shaped deformity of the chest. Deep tendon reflexes are absent or difficult to elicit. The upper cranial nerves are spared, giving rise to an infant with an alert expression, a furrowed brow, and normal eye movements. The bulbar muscles are weak, which is reflected by a weak cry, poor suck and swallow reflexes, pooling of secretions, aspiration, and tongue fasciculations. Cardiac muscle is not affected, and classic arthrogryposis is usually not a feature although rarely it can be.

Nerve conduction testing demonstrates normal or slightly decreased motor nerve conduction velocities and normal sensory nerve action potentials. Electromyography shows abnormal spontaneous activity with fibrillations and positive sharp waves as well as an increased mean duration and amplitude of motor unit action potentials, some of which are polyphasic. Serum creatine kinase activity is normal or only slightly elevated. Muscle biopsy reveals large groups of circular atrophic type 1 and 2 muscle fibers (Fig. 40-80). These fibers are interspersed among fascicles of hypertrophied type 1 fibers, which are three or four times normal size and represent fibers reinnervated by sprouting of surviving nerves.[38] This pattern might not be seen during the neonatal period, when there is often only widespread atrophy of type 1 and 2 muscle fibers, making histologic diagnosis difficult. However, a later biopsy should show evidence of reinnervation with large hypertrophied fibers and group atrophy.

The infant who presents during the neonatal period with severe acute infantile SMA characterized by profound hypotonia and weakness rarely survives beyond 1 year of age. It is the severity of weakness at the onset that determines outcome in SMA rather than the age of onset, although in most cases the earlier the onset, the greater the weakness. Artificial ventilation of an infant with severe early-onset SMA leads to an alert but completely paralyzed infant who is totally ventilator dependent.[38]

With the identification of the *SMN* gene in 1995, the diagnosis of SMA has been greatly facilitated, limiting the need for more invasive investigations. Additional understanding of the molecular genetics and protein function may provide insight into potential therapies for this otherwise fatal condition. The SMN coding region on chromosome 5q11.2-13.3 contains a telomeric and centromeric copy of the *SMN* gene, designated *SMN1* and *SMN2*, respectively. These genes are nearly identical in their coding sequence. A single nucleotide polymorphism (840C>T) in SMN2 causes disruption of normal translation.[48] The resultant protein produced by the

centromeric copy is often truncated and nonfunctional. SMN2 can produce a small amount of full-length protein, providing partial compensation for mutations in SMN1, but the majority must be produced by SMN1. A direct relationship exists between the number of copies of the SMN2 gene and the age of disease onset, with the SMA type I phenotype correlating with the lowest number of SMN2 gene copies. The exact function of SMN protein remains to be further defined, but it appears to have a critical housekeeping function in the metabolism of motor neuron cell RNA.[5]

There are a number of genetically heterogeneous SMA variants, but most of these do not present during the newborn period. Those that might, include SMA with pontocerebellar hypoplasia, X-linked SMA with arthrogryposis due to mutations in the *UBE1* gene, and SMARD1 (distal infantile SMA with diaphragm paralysis) that is due to mutations in the IGHMBP2 gene in most congenital cases.

Arthrogryposis multiplex congenita is a heterogeneous group of disorders characterized by multiple immobilized joints and degeneration of motor neurons. It is most frequently of neurogenic origin and is found in conjunction with other disorders of the CNS, genetic syndromes, or chromosomal aberrations. The neurogenic arthrogryposes are genetically heterogeneous, and both autosomal recessive and X-linked inheritance have been reported.[11,42] A subgroup of neurogenic arthrogryposis is allelic with SMA type I, and deletions of *SMN* gene have been reported.[11] These disorders are of variable severity. Some show no progression, and muscle strength can even improve. In other cases, bulbar and respiratory function is severely affected, and the prognosis is poor. In the X-linked form, there is disease progression and early death.[42]

Traumatic high cervical spinal cord injury (see Chapter 28) is a rare cause of myelopathy that can be misdiagnosed as SMA. In the absence of an asphyxial brain injury, the infant is alert with no cranial nerve signs. The myelopathy is manifested as a flaccid areflexic paralysis, which might be asymmetric. Clues to the diagnosis include evidence of trauma such as bruising or fractures and normal results on cranial nerve examination. After a few days, evidence of the myelopathy becomes more apparent with the appearance of bladder distention, priapism, and an absence of sweating below the level of the spinal lesion. A particularly useful later sign is withdrawal to a noxious stimulus in a limb that shows no spontaneous activity. Sensory testing is difficult but can be assessed by demonstrating facial grimacing to a prick on the face but no response below the neck (see Chapter 28).

In severe hypoxic-ischemic injury there can be an areflexic flaccid paralysis resulting from death of spinal motor neurons.[15] However, there are also signs of an encephalopathy and multiorgan system damage.

HEREDITARY MOTOR AND SENSORY NEUROPATHIES

The hereditary motor and sensory neuropathies are a genetically heterogeneous group of disorders with a spectrum of phenotypes that includes Charcot-Marie-Tooth disease types 1 and 2, hereditary neuropathy with liability to pressure palsies, Dejerine-Sottas syndrome, and congenital hypomyelinating neuropathy. These diseases may demonstrate an autosomal

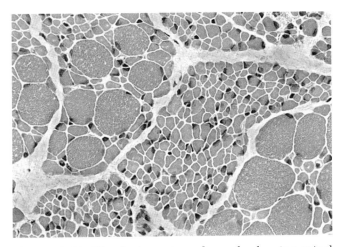

Figure 40–80. Histologic section of muscle showing spinal muscular atrophy. Groups of circular atrophic fibers are interspersed among fascicles of hypertrophied type 1 fibers. Low magnification. (*Courtesy of Hannes Vogel, MD, Baylor College of Medicine, Houston.*)

dominant, autosomal recessive, or X-linked mode of inheritance. Charcot-Marie-Tooth disease type 1 and hereditary neuropathy with liability to pressure palsies are demyelinating neuropathies, whereas Charcot-Marie-Tooth disease type 2 is an axonal disorder. Congenital onset is unusual, and these three forms of hereditary motor and sensory neuropathy most often present in the older child or young adult.[61] Congenital hypomyelinating neuropathy and Dejerine-Sottas syndrome are more often described in the infant with a congenital or early infantile onset of demyelinating neuropathy, respectively.[38,60]

Clinical manifestations vary. Affected infants are weak, hypotonic, and areflexic. The weakness is generalized, but a greater distal weakness might be detected. Arthrogryposis may be present in more severe forms. There are usually swallowing and respiratory difficulties. Sometimes facial weakness is present, but extraocular movements are usually normal. Any associated sensory loss is difficult to detect clinically. Prognosis depends on the initial degree of weakness. In some cases there is an improvement in strength.[29]

The disorders are characterized by markedly decreased motor nerve conduction velocities (typically less than 10m/s) and an elevated cerebrospinal fluid protein. Sural nerve biopsy in relatively mild cases shows varying degrees of hypomyelination with atypical onion-bulb formation. More severe cases may show complete lack of myelin.[38] These disorders result from mutations in different genes. Moreover, different mutations in the same gene causes different phenotypes (Charcot-Marie-Tooth disease type 1, Dejerine-Sottas syndrome, congenital hypomyelinating neuropathy), and, at present, the clinical phenotype cannot always be predicted on the basis of the gene mutation. Identified alleles include Schwann cell genes involved in the formation, structure, and maintenance of peripheral myelin (EGR2, PMP22, MPZ, CX32, 6JB1, PRX), neuronal genes involved in axonal transport (NEFL), and genes affecting both Schwann cell and neuronal structure (MTMR2).[58,59] Testing for these mutations is available on a clinical basis.

HEREDITARY SENSORY AND AUTONOMIC NEUROPATHIES

The hereditary sensory and autonomic neuropathies are characterized by selective involvement of peripheral sensory and autonomic neurons (Box 40-12). These disorders are

---

BOX 40–12   Hereditary Sensory and Autonomic Neuropathies

HSAN type I (hereditary sensory radicular neuropathy, autosomal dominant)
HSAN type II (congenital sensory neuropathy)
HSAN type III (Riley-Day syndrome, or familial dysautonomia)
HSAN type IV (congenital insensitivity to pain with anhidrosis)
HSAN type V (congenital insensitivity to pain with partial anhidrosis)
Progressive pan-neuropathy and hypotonia
Congenital autonomic dysfunction with universal pain loss
Familial amyloid neuropathy (autosomal dominant)

---

autosomal recessive with the exception of hereditary sensory and autonomic neuropathy type I, which is autosomal dominant. All present with varying degrees of autonomic dysfunction or insensitivity to pain and temperature.[38] In some, there is absence of the normal axonal flare response to intradermal injection of histamine. In the older child there is striking self-mutilation.

The best known of the hereditary sensory neuropathies is familial dysautonomia (Riley-Day syndrome; hereditary sensory and autonomic neuropathy type III). This disorder has a high carrier rate in individuals of Ashkenazi Jewish descent and has been mapped to chromosome 9q31-q33. Mutations in the gene for IκB kinase-associated protein (IKBKAP) account for 99% of affected individuals.[7] The clinical diagnosis of familial dysautonomia is based on five cardinal criteria: (1) absence of overflow tears, (2) absence of lingual fungiform papillae, (3) depressed patellar reflexes, (4) lack of axonal flare reaction after intradermal injection of histamine, and (5) Ashkenazi Jewish extraction. Additional clinical features typically include hypotonia, labile temperature and blood pressure, breath holding, pallor, poor feeding, failure to thrive, vomiting, loose stools, and irritability.

Treatment of these disorders is mainly supportive and survival has improved with modern medical therapies. Patients who reach adulthood continue to demonstrate slow progression of their disease. Cognition may be impaired in some forms of the disease.[6]

Clinical testing is available for familial dysautonomia. Until more molecular genetic information is available, differentiating between the other various hereditary sensory neuropathies will continue to be made by distinct characteristics of the history and examination, sensory nerve conduction and action potential size, and changes on sural nerve biopsy.[6]

NEUROMUSCULAR JUNCTION DISORDERS

Neuromuscular junction disorders are infrequent causes of weakness during the neonatal period. The principal conditions include transient acquired neonatal myasthenia, congenital myasthenia, infantile botulism, and toxic amounts of magnesium or aminoglycosides. These disorders are characterized by abnormal neuromuscular transmission, which is manifested by abnormal muscle fatigability and weakness that is sometimes permanent, particularly in the congenital forms.

Autoimmune myasthenia gravis in children and adults is caused by autoantibodies directed against neuromuscular junction proteins. In 80% of patients, acetylcholine receptor antibodies are detected in the serum. In the remaining patients, other pathologic antibodies, including those directed against muscle-specific kinase, interfere with the normal function of the acetylcholine receptor, resulting in disease.[66]

In acquired neonatal myasthenia gravis, the disease is more often active in the mother. However, she may have less obvious disease, be in remission, or not show clinical manifestations until after the pregnancy.[66] Transfer of immunoglobulin G antibodies occurs readily across the placenta. However, typical features develop in only 20% of infants born to mothers with myasthenia.[36,68] The proportion of maternal immunoglobulin G antibodies directed against the fetal type versus the adult type of acetylcholine receptor appears to have a strong influence on neonatal manifestations. Although there is no correlation between maternal antibody titers or disease severity and the development of neonatal myasthenia, there is an inverse relationship between maternal disease duration and the incidence of neonatal myasthenia. Maternal thymectomy may be protective against neonatal disease.[22]

The disorder usually presents within a few hours of birth, and onset after the third day has not been reported.[52,53] The most common presentation is generalized weakness and hypotonia.[49] Bulbar weakness is usually present, with feeding difficulties from poor sucking and swallowing, and a weak cry. Facial diplegia can be prominent, but ptosis and ophthalmoplegia are seen less frequently. Pooling of secretions and respiratory difficulties occasionally necessitate artificial ventilation. Deep tendon reflexes are normal. Assuming a correct diagnosis and management, most infants recover within a few weeks.[53] Some infants are severely affected with a history of polyhydramnios and the presence of arthrogryposis multiplex at birth.[21] Treatment is more difficult, and recovery is slower in these infants.

The diagnosis of transient neonatal myasthenia should always be suspected in the infant of a mother with active generalized acetylcholine receptor antibody-positive myasthenia gravis. When signs appear, a cholinesterase inhibitor is administered and the response gauged. To be sure of the diagnosis, an unequivocal and objective response should be chosen, such as an improvement in ventilation and oxygenation or sucking ability. IM or SC neostigmine methylsulfate in a dose of 0.15 mg/kg is the preferred diagnostic anticholinesterase agent. The drug takes effect within 15 minutes of injection and lasts 1 to 3 hours. Muscarinic side effects (diarrhea, increased tracheal secretions) might require the use of atropine in appropriate doses. Although edrophonium chloride has a more rapid onset and less intense muscarinic side effects, there is a risk of respiratory arrest.[53] When necessary, the diagnosis can be confirmed with repetitive nerve stimulation,[34] which should be performed before and after the administration of a cholinesterase inhibitor. A diagnostically positive response occurs when the amplitude of the fifth evoked compound muscle action potential is reduced by 10% or more of the amplitude of the first response, and this decrement is corrected by a cholinesterase inhibitor.[53]

The management of transient neonatal myasthenia gravis must be early and vigorous because these infants can deteriorate rapidly. Small, frequent tube feedings should be given and early ventilatory support considered. Neostigmine methylsulfate is given in a dose of 0.05 to 0.1mg/kg, IM or SC, 30 minutes before feeding. The oral dose of neostigmine is approximately 10 times the intramuscular dose and is given approximately 45 minutes before feeding. Excessive doses can cause diarrhea, increased secretions, muscle fasciculations, and cholinergic weakness. Disappearance of disease activity is monitored clinically by assessing responses to gradual decreases in the anticholinesterase dose. In addition, repetitive nerve stimulation tests can be performed as well as measurement of acetylcholine receptor antibodies. Tube feeding and artificial ventilation are usually not required for longer than 1 to 2 weeks, and the average duration of treatment is 4 weeks, with recovery in 90% of infants in less than 2 months.[53]

The congenital myasthenic syndromes are infrequent causes of neuromuscular junction failure during the neonatal period but have become increasingly recognized. They are a group of genetic disorders that are acetylcholine receptor antibody negative and are caused by either presynaptic or postsynaptic inherited defects of the neuromuscular junction. Their precise characterization requires sophisticated laboratory techniques, which are not widely available.[27] Those manifested during the neonatal period are shown in Box 40-13. Unlike acquired transient neonatal myasthenia gravis, ptosis is usually present in addition to varying degrees of ophthalmoplegia, bulbar palsy, and respiratory weakness. Fluctuating, generalized hypotonia and weakness are seen, and episodes of life-threatening apnea can occur. Exacerbations can be induced by activity, febrile illness, or other stress. The disorder often improves with age, but spontaneous exacerbations occur with a risk of sudden infant death. Arthrogryposis has been reported in one form of the disease.[27] A diagnostic response to cholinesterase inhibitors is variable but useful when positive. Some forms of the disorder, such as congenital endplate cholinesterase deficiency, are refractory to or worsened by cholinesterase inhibitors. The diagnosis is supported by a decremental response to repetitive nerve stimulation at low frequency (2 Hz). However, the low-frequency decremental response can be absent in infants with a defect in acetylcholine resynthesis or packaging, but can be induced by prolonged 10-Hz stimulation.

A number of toxic agents disturb neuromuscular transmission in the newborn. Hypermagnesemia, usually secondary to IV administration of magnesium sulfate to the mother, causes a presynaptic failure of acetylcholine release by blocking calcium release.[56] The infant shows profound generalized weakness, areflexia, and respiratory dysfunction. In addition, the CNS and smooth muscle are affected, giving rise to stupor and an ileus. Exposure to excessive amounts of aminoglycosides, particularly in conjunction with neuromuscular blockers, can be followed by prolonged weakness from a presynaptic block. Bladder, bowel, and pupillary function are affected.[68,71] Both hypermagnesemia and the neurotoxic effects of aminoglycosides are worsened by hypocalcemia.

Infantile botulism affects infants between 2 weeks and 6 months of age (see Chapter 39).[17,30,68] Unlike botulism in children and adults, which is caused by ingesting the

---

BOX 40–13   Congenital Myasthenic Syndromes Presenting during the Neonatal Period

Presynaptic defects (8%)
Choline acetyltransferase deficiency
Paucity of synaptic vesicles and reduced quantal release
Similar to Eaton-Lambert syndrome
Synaptic basal lamina-associated defects (16%)
Endplate acetylcholine esterase deficiency
Postsynaptic defects (76%)
Kinetic abnormality of acetylcholine receptor (slow- and fast-channel syndromes)
Acetylcholine receptor deficiency
Rapsyn deficiency
Plectin deficiency

exotoxin of *Clostridium* botulinum, infantile botulism occurs when the intestine is colonized by the clostridia bacteria, where they produce their toxin. This toxin causes a presynaptic cholinergic blockage that affects autonomic as well as skeletal and smooth muscle function. The disorder has a clinical spectrum. Presentation varies from mild constipation and hypotonia to unexpected death. The classic form of the disorder presents with constipation and poor feeding followed by progressive hypotonic weakness and loss of deep tendon reflexes. There is usually marked cranial nerve dysfunction, which includes pupillary paralysis and ptosis. The weakness often progresses in a descending fashion. The illness usually lasts 1 to 2 months but relapses in a small number of patients.[30] Diagnosis is made by demonstrating an incremental response to repetitive nerve stimulation at high rates (20 to 50 Hz) and by the appearance of short-duration, low-amplitude motor unit potentials on electromyography.[39] Confirmation of the diagnosis is made on isolation of the organism from the stool. Prompt treatment with human-derived botulism immunoglobulin may significantly reduce the length of time needed for clinical recovery.[55] Management is otherwise supportive.

CONGENITAL MUSCULAR DYSTROPHY

The CMDs are a variable group of autosomal recessive disorders that share the common presentation of weakness and hypotonia at birth in conjunction with a dystrophic muscle biopsy. The muscle biopsy typically shows endomysial and perimysial connective tissue proliferation, replacement of muscle by fat, and variations in muscle fiber size (Fig. 40-81). There is little evidence of necrosis or regeneration. Immunocytochemical studies help distinguish between different types.[14,51] Clinically, muscular weakness is generalized and usually involves the face. Bulbar and respiratory muscle involvement is variable but can be severe. The creatine kinase level is elevated in some types but is normal or only moderately elevated in others.[38] Arthrogryposis is a common feature.

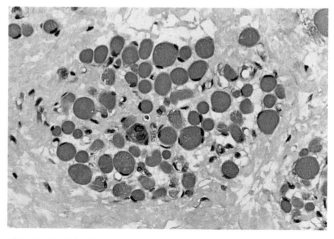

Figure 40–81. Histologic section of muscle showing congenital muscular dystrophy. The biopsy shows connective tissue proliferation, replacement of muscle by fat, and variations in fiber size. Low magnification. (*Courtesy of Hannes Vogel, MD, Baylor College of Medicine, Houston.*)

The CMDs have historically been divided into the nonsyndromic ("classic") forms, typified by normal cognition, and the syndromic forms, associated with brain malformations and mental retardation (Box 40-14). This distinction between the classic and syndromic forms has been blurred by advances in molecular genetics showing similarities between the groups and reports of classic CMD presenting with posterior pachygyria in association with cognitive defects.[41]

The classic forms are subdivided into merosin-positive and merosin-negative subtypes. The merosin-negative form accounts for nearly 50% of all CMDs. Merosin is the heavy α2 chain of the heterotrimeric protein laminin 2 (Fig. 40-82). By linking the extracellular matrix with transmuscle-membrane dystrophin-associated glycoproteins, the protein plays a critical role in myogenesis and myotubule membrane stability. It is also expressed in Schwann cells, trophoblasts, skin, and cerebral blood vessels. Mutations in the α2-laminin gene (*LAMA2*) on chromosome 6q are responsible for the disease. Mutation screening is impractical for clinical use because no single mutation predominates in this large gene. Diagnosis is best achieved with muscle biopsy showing complete absence of merosin with immunocytochemical staining.[14]

The CMDs can be classified according to the protein defect, and in many cases this can be identified by immunocytochemistry or DNA analysis.[51] Abnormalities of extracellular matrix protein defects include laminin α2–deficient CMD (MDC1A) and collagen 6A deficiencies as in Ullrich CMD (UCMD 1, 2, and 3); integrin α7 deficiency (ITGA7); abnormalities of glycosyltransferases, which lead to abnormal O-glycosylation of α-dystroglycan, and include o-mannosyltransferase 1 (POMT1), o-mannosyltransferase 2 (POMT2), o-linked mannose β1,2-N-acetyl glucosaminyl transferase (POMGnT1), fukutin, fukutin-related protein (FKRP), and Lacetylglucosaminyltransferase like protein (LARGE); and endoplasmic reticulum proteins such as selenoprotein N, which causes rigid spine syndrome (RSMD1).

The clinical presentation of merosin deficiency typifies the classic form of the CMDs. There is marked neonatal hypotonia with generalized weakness and atrophy. Although facial weakness may be present, the eye muscles are spared. Contractures occur early and affect multiple joints. Involvement of chest wall muscles results in respiratory difficulties. Cognition is usually not affected. Other clinical features of merosin

---

BOX 40–14 Congenital Muscular Dystrophies

Classic CMD
Merosin-deficient CMD
    Primary merosin deficiency
    Secondary merosin deficiency
Merosin-positive CMD
Classic CMD without distinguishing features
Rigid spine syndrome
CMD with distal hyperextensibility (Ullrich type)
CMD with mental retardation or sensory abnormalities
CMD with central nervous system abnormalities
Fukuyama CMD
Muscle-eye-brain disease
Walker-Warburg syndrome

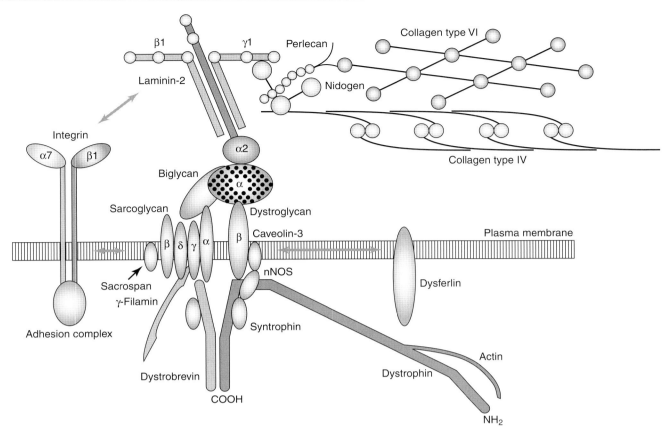

Figure 40–82. Schematic representation of the dystrophin-associated proteins and other sarcolemmal and extracellular proteins associated with congenital muscular dystrophy. nNOS, neuronal nitric oxide synthase. *(From Kirschner J, Bonnemann CG: The congenital and limb-girdle muscular dystrophies: sharpening the focus, blurring the boundaries, Arch Neurol 61:189, 2004; adapted from Jones HR, et al: Neuromuscular disorders of infancy, childhood, and adolescence: a clinician's approach. Philadelphia, 2003, Elsevier Science, with permission.)*

deficiency include a peripheral neuropathy, reflecting absence of merosin expression in Schwann cells. In addition, neuroimaging shows white matter changes, most appreciable after 6 months of age. The abnormality is best characterized by diffuse increased signal intensity on T2-weighted magnetic resonance imaging sequences. These findings are thought to correlate with lack of merosin in the cerebral vessel walls.[65] A small minority of patients show structural dysgenesis with occipital pachygyria or agyria. Epilepsy is encountered in one third of patients.[40]

Although similar in presentation, the other forms of classic CMD can be differentiated based on distinct clinical features and underlying molecular genetics. Ullrich CMD is associated with mutations in the protein subunits of type VI collagen and presents with rigidity of the spine and distal joint hyperextensibility.[19,35] Distinct from Ullrich CMD, CMD with rigid spine is associated with early rigidity of the spine and restrictive lung disease. A considerable number of these patients have been found to have mutations of the selenoprotein N gene on chromosome 1p36-p35.[47] Selenoprotein N mutations have also been described in patients with multiminicore disease, a type of congenital myopathy. The function of the protein is unknown. Mutations of the gene for fukutin-related protein on chromosome 19q13 may result in

either a severe CMD (CMD type 1C, or MDC1C) or childhood-onset limb-girdle muscular dystrophy.[40] Fukutin-related protein is a putative glycosyltransferase, and similar to the syndromic CMDs (discussed later), this form is associated with defective glycosylation of α-dystroglycan protein in the muscle membrane (see Fig. 40-82). A secondary merosin deficiency is also present on histochemical staining.[14] CMD with a partial merosin deficiency has been defined in a number of patients by biochemical studies. The partial deficiency is thought to be secondary to an underlying α-dystroglycan abnormality with abnormal binding of associated proteins. Linkage to chromosome 1q42 has been made in some of these cases.[9]

The syndromic forms of CMD are associated with brain malformations and ocular findings. The three main types are Walker-Warburg syndrome, muscle-eye-brain disease, and Fukuyama CMD. All three forms result from mutations in genes encoding distinct glycosyltransferases and related proteins involved in post-translational modification of α-dystroglycan, a pathogenetic mechanism shared by the more classic phenotype MDC1C, as previously discussed.[40] Muscle membrane integrity is compromised by the defective α-dystroglycan, which is unable to bind effectively with either extracellular laminin or transmembranous β-dystroglycan (see Fig. 40-82). Muscle biopsy immunocytochemical techniques demonstrate the abnormal α-dystroglycan expression.[14,51] In the brain, abnormal α-dystroglycan on glial scaffolds, neurons, and their processes is associated with neuronal migrational defects that include disarray of cerebral cortical layering, fusion of the cerebral hemispheres and cerebellar folia, and aberrant migration of granule cells. Disruption of the glial limitans results in cobblestone lissencephaly.[50,51]

Walker-Warburg syndrome is the most severe of the syndromic CMDs. Few infants survive for more than a few months, although prolonged survival is possible with modern medical techniques. Along with muscular dystrophy, typical features of the syndrome include cobblestone lissencephaly with agenesis of the corpus callosum, cerebellar hypoplasia, hydrocephalus, and encephalocele.[50] In contrast with other forms of lissencephaly, there is dysmyelination with the white matter appearing dark on computed tomography scan and abnormally bright on T2-weighted magnetic resonance images. Ocular findings can include cataracts, microphthalmia, buphthalmos, persistent hyperplastic primary vitreous, and Peter anomaly.[16] Some patients with Walker-Warburg syndrome have been found to have mutations in the protein O-mannosyltransferase (POMT1) gene. The gene encodes an enzyme potentially involved in the biosynthesis of specific glycans associated with dystroglycan. The lack of POMT1 mutations in many patients with Walker-Warburg syndrome suggests genetic heterogeneity.[50]

Muscle-eye-brain disease has many features in common with Walker-Warburg syndrome but is less severe.[16] Brain malformations can include cobblestone lissencephaly, absent septum pellucidum, dysgenesis of the corpus callosum, hydrocephalus, and white matter changes similar to Walker-Warburg syndrome. Eye findings include myopia, choroidal hypoplasia, optic nerve pallor, glaucoma, iris hypoplasia, cataracts, and colobomas. Newborns present with hypotonia, weakness, feeding difficulties, poor vision, and apathy. Distal contractures can be present. All infants ultimately exhibit mental retardation and seizures. In contrast to Walker-Warburg syndrome, most infants have a prolonged survival. However, independent ambulation is unusual. The development of high-amplitude visual evoked potentials by 2 years is a particular feature, and the electroencephalogram is always abnormal by 1 year of age.[26] A significant number of patients with muscle-eye-brain disease have mutations in the gene coding for the glycosyltransferase POMGnT1.[72]

Fukuyama CMD is almost entirely confined to Japan. Overall, the brain and ocular manifestations are less severe than in Walker-Warburg syndrome and muscle-eye-brain disease. A large proportion of patients have mutations of the fukutin gene on chromosome 9q31. The protein function is unknown. Muscle biopsy staining reveals absence of fukutin as well as abnormal glycosylation of α-dystroglycan.[14] In the brain, the cerebral cortex has a cobblestone appearance with pachygyria and polymicrogyria, but there are also areas with normal gyral patterns.[64] As with Walker-Warburg syndrome, partial obstruction of the subarachnoid space and hemispheric fusion are seen. Other abnormalities, which differentiate the condition from Walker-Warburg syndrome, include white matter changes, which improve with age, and only mild ventriculomegaly and cerebellar polymicrogyria. Cerebellar and pyramidal tract hypoplasia are probably not features. Eye anomalies are minor and typical of Fukuyama-type CMD. Affected infants present with generalized weakness, hypotonia, and varying degrees of muscle contractures. Facial and bulbar involvement is usually present. Seizures are frequent, and mental retardation is moderate or severe. Survival into adolescence is typical.

CONGENITAL MYOTONIC DYSTROPHY

Myotonic dystrophy is an autosomal dominant multisystem disorder of variable expression that is characterized by muscular dystrophy and myotonia in adults. In addition to involvement of muscle, many other systems are affected, including the gastrointestinal, endocrine, and skeletal systems, as well as the heart, brain, and eyes.[32,44] Two loci for the disease have been found and are characterized as DM1 and DM2. The genetic basis for DM1 is an expansion of CTG repeats in the myotonic dystrophy protein kinase (DMPK) gene on chromosome 19q13.3.[12] An amplification of greater than 45 repeats is usually associated with disease expression. DM2 is associated with a CCTG tetranucleotide expansion in the zinc finger 9 (ZNF9) gene on chromosome 3q21.[43] DM1 has a more severe clinical phenotype, with a progressively earlier onset in successive generations (genetic anticipation). Congenital myotonic dystrophy is the earliest presenting form of DM1, and it is an important cause of neonatal neuromuscular dysfunction, with an incidence of at least 1 in 3500 live births. These infants usually have greater than 1000 CTG repeats at the DMPK locus. Nuclear accumulation of the abnormal messenger RNA generated by this large repeat size is thought to cause a delay in the differentiation and maturation of skeletal muscle.[1] With rare exceptions, the disease is inherited from the mother.[73] This is related to oligospermia in male patients as well as a greater propensity for larger repeat expansions (more than 1000) during oogenesis than during spermatogenesis.[37,44] The earlier the onset of the disease in the mother and the more severe the clinical expression, the greater the risk for congenital myotonic dystrophy.[33,57] However, the disease can still be seen in offspring of only mildly affected mothers. The phenotypic variation in tissue expression is probably the result of somatic instability of the CTG repeat.[70]

At birth, affected infants frequently require resuscitation and are subject to the mortality and morbidity associated with hypoxic-ischemic encephalopathy (see Part 4 of this chapter). A history of polyhydramnios (from failure of fetal swallowing) and decreased fetal movements is frequent, and premature birth can complicate the diagnosis. Furthermore, delivery can be complicated by prolonged labor and postpartum hemorrhage because of poor uterine contractions.[32,57] Generalized weakness and hypotonia in the infant are profound, with facial diplegia and a characteristically tent-shaped triangular upper lip. Deep tendon reflexes are absent or difficult to elicit, and congenital talipes (clubfoot) is often present. Occasionally, joint contractures are more widespread.[32] There is often respiratory distress, and poor suck and swallow reflexes present the danger of aspiration. Eye movements are full, although the infant might not readily fix and follow. Poor respiratory function is due not only to muscle weakness but also to pulmonary immaturity and poor central respiratory control.[32] An elevated diaphragm on the right can be seen on radiographic examination and is probably due to the presence of the liver on that side and weak diaphragmatic muscles. Hydrops fetalis can occur in infants with cardiac failure. Laboratory investigations in general are not helpful, and the creatine kinase level is normal. The pathologic appearance of muscle differs from that in adults. The fibers are small and round with central nucleation and display poor fiber type differentiation or relatively small type 1 fibers, giving an immature appearance.[1] The typical adult features appear later. Electromyography is often noncontributory because of poor movement, although myopathic potentials can be demonstrated. Clinical and electrical myotonia are not present but appear later, during early childhood. Neuroimaging reveals ventriculomegaly, intraventricular hemorrhage, subarachnoid hemorrhage, or early periventricular leukomalacia in premature infants. The ventriculomegaly is probably of prenatal origin.[20]

Diagnosis of myotonic dystrophy is supported by clinical and electromyographic examination of the mother and confirmed by molecular genetic analysis. If the infant survives, the hypotonia and severe weakness gradually improve and are no longer evident by later childhood, although motor development is delayed. The facial diplegia with ptosis, open jaw, and triangular mouth persists, giving rise to a characteristic appearance.[32,45] Many affected infants die early, even with intensive care. There is increased mortality among infants requiring greater than 30 days of ventilation, although eventual maturation of diaphragmatic musculature allows for independent ventilation in most.[13] In most patients, mental retardation or significant learning difficulties develop.[32] Unless there is a superimposed cerebral palsy syndrome from a complication of prematurity or perinatal asphyxia, most children walk by age 3 years.[45] All patients with congenital myotonic dystrophy eventually manifest the complete spectrum of features typical of adult-onset disease.

OTHER MUSCULAR DYSTROPHIES

Severe Xp21-linked dystrophin-deficient muscular dystrophy (Duchenne type) is a degenerative muscle disorder that rarely presents during the neonatal period.[54] Information is scarce on a typical phenotype during the neonatal period. Distinguishing features are an absence of arthrogryposis, high serum creatine kinase, and regeneration or degeneration on muscle biopsy. Diagnosis is made by DNA analysis and immunoelectrophoresis or immunocytochemistry.[38]

Facioscapulohumeral muscular dystrophy is an autosomal dominant disorder that usually presents during early adolescence. Although usually a fairly benign disorder, there is intrafamilial variability, and the disease can present in early infancy.[10] The responsible abnormal gene has been assigned to the subtelomeric region of chromosome 4.[38] Affected patients have a reduction in the normal number of repeats in the DNA sequence termed *D4Z4*. In normal individuals, the EcoR1-digested DNA fragment is usually larger than 28 kilobases (kb), whereas a shorter fragment of 14 to 28 kb is detected in cases of facioscapulohumeral muscular dystrophy, correlating with the smaller number of repeats.[38] In the early infantile form of the disease, facial weakness is characteristic, and the only manifestation might be partially open eyes during sleep. Progression is variable. In some cases,

weakness is relatively mild, with later development of facial and shoulder girdle weakness. In other cases, there is early progressive weakness of the face, shoulder girdle, and ankle dorsiflexion, with loss of independent ambulation by late childhood. Bilateral sensorineural hearing loss is present in many cases. Retinal vascular abnormalities can also be found, which sometimes progress with exudation and retinal detachment. Creatine kinase levels are only moderately elevated. Biopsy of a proximal shoulder girdle muscle shows mild myopathic changes. Other pathologic findings include small, angular fibers; "moth-eaten" fibers; and cellular infiltrates, which can be extensive and appear inflammatory. Although steroids in general are not beneficial in this disorder, albuterol has shown some modest benefit.[41] Electromyography of an affected muscle reveals a myopathic pattern with short-duration, low-amplitude polyphasic potentials.

CONGENITAL MYOPATHIES

The congenital myopathies are primary muscle disorders that are present at birth. Although their expression might not be apparent during the neonatal period, infancy, or childhood, these myopathies are probably all genetically determined. Muscular dystrophies, inflammatory myopathies, muscle diseases caused by metabolic disorders, and inborn errors of metabolism are not included in this group. Congenital myopathies are usually characterized on the basis of their histologic and histochemical features. Although more than 30 different types of congenital myopathies have been described, most of these are rare and unlikely to represent clinically distinct entities. The four myopathies discussed here are relatively common and represent distinct clinical entities with unique histochemical findings.

Nemaline Myopathy

Nemaline myopathy is so called because of the characteristic rod bodies in muscle, which in longitudinal section appear threadlike (Fig. 40-83). They are best seen after modified Gomori trichrome staining of frozen sections, in which they appear red against a blue-green myofibrillar background.[14] The rod bodies are usually subsarcolemmal, and their numbers in muscle are variable and not correlated with the severity of the disease. However, intranuclear rods can be seen in the severe neonatal form of the disease. On electron microscopy, the rods appear to originate from the Z discs in conjunction with Z-disc thickening and streaming, and are composed of thin filament proteins, α-actinin, and actin. In addition to nemaline rods, muscle biopsy shows variations in fiber size, with a predominance of type 1 fibers, which are smaller than the type 2 fibers.

The disorder has a wide clinical spectrum. A severe congenital form presents with generalized weakness and hypotonia involving the face, bulbar, and respiratory muscles but clinically sparing the eye muscles.[57] Milder forms present during the neonatal period or early childhood. It is relatively nonprogressive and has a facioscapuloperoneal pattern of weakness. The face is long and thin; the palate is arched; and muscle bulk is poor. A relatively mild adult-onset form also exists. All variants can show preferential diaphragmatic weakness with a significant percentage requiring prolonged

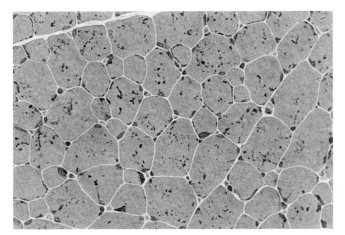

Figure 40-83. Histologic section of muscle showing nemaline myopathy. Shown are variations in fiber size. Characteristic rod bodies are seen in the muscle fibers. Low magnification. (*Courtesy of Hannes Vogel, MD, Baylor College of Medicine, Houston.*)

assisted ventilation. The severity of respiratory involvement at delivery predicts survival. Motor outcome parallels respiratory involvement in the neonatal form.[58] Cardiac involvement is rare and secondary to respiratory disease and pulmonary hypertension. Likewise, a neonatal encephalopathy is related to respiratory failure with hypoxic-ischemic injury.[58] Diagnosis is by muscle biopsy. The creatine kinase is usually normal or only slightly elevated. Electromyography in the older child usually shows myopathy, but in the newborn infant it is typically not helpful. Most cases are sporadic, although both autosomal dominant and autosomal recessive inheritance can occur. Mutations in five genes encoding for muscle thin filaments have been identified. These include α-tropomyosin (TPM3), β-tropomyosin (TPM2), α-actin (ACTA1), nebulin (NEB), and troponin T1 (TNNT1).[58,69] Mutations in the TNNT1 gene on chromosome 19q13.4 cause a severe autosomal recessive form of the disease in the Amish population that usually has a fatal outcome in the second year of life.[62] There is otherwise no correlation between mutations in the same gene, mode of inheritance, and clinical severity. In addition, there is considerable intrafamilial variation in course and outcome. Sequencing of the ACTA1 gene is clinically available.

Central Core Disease

Central core disease is an autosomal dominant disorder. Muscle biopsy reveals characteristic central cores of degenerated myofibrils in type 1 fibers, which predominate.[14] The disorder is usually mild when it presents during the neonatal period. Muscle weakness and hypotonia are usually more prominent proximally, and congenital hip dislocation is a frequent associated finding.[38] Mild delay in motor maturation occurs, and scoliosis and contractures can develop later. The gene locus responsible for almost 80% of cases has been mapped to chromosome 19q12-13.2, which is closely linked to the gene for malignant hyperthermia and the ryanodine

receptor (RYR1).[62] All affected patients are at risk for malignant hyperthermia.

Multi-Minicore Myopathy

Multi-minicore disease is characterized by multiple small areas of sarcomeric disorganization that lack oxidative activity.[28] There is a predominance of small type 1 fibers. Four homogeneous phenotypes have been defined. The classic form presents with mild proximal weakness, joint laxity, scoliosis, and respiratory insufficiency with a rigid spine. An ophthalmoplegic form is associated with facial and generalized weakness. An early onset form may result in arthrogryposis. A slowly progressive form presents with hand amyotrophy. Cardiomyopathy may occur. Both autosomal recessive and sporadic inheritance may occur.[28] Diagnosis is by muscle biopsy and mutations in the SEPN1 or RYR1 gene account for many of the cases.

Myotubular Myopathy

Myotubular myopathy presenting in the neonatal period is an X-linked recessive condition and one of the most severe congenital myopathies. It is due to mutations in the myotubularin gene (MTM1) on chromosome Xq28. The protein tyrosine phosphorylase encoded by this gene is thought to have a vital role in normal myogenesis. The myopathy is characterized pathologically by muscle fibers that contain large central nuclei and resemble fetal myotubes (Fig. 40-84).[14] This central area also lacks myofibrils and appears as a clear area with adenosine triphosphatase staining. There is a predominance of small type 1 fibers. The appearance of the muscle is not due to a general arrest in muscle development but rather is related to a persistence of fetal cytoskeletal proteins, vimentin, and desmin, which preserve the immature central portions of the nuclei.[14]

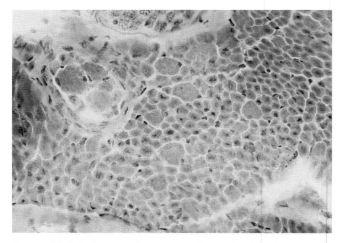

Figure 40-84. Histologic section of muscle showing myotubular myopathy. Shown are large muscle fibers with central nuclei seen primarily in small, predominantly type 1 fibers. Low magnification. (*Courtesy of Hannes Vogel, MD, Baylor College of Medicine, Houston.*)

With onset during the fetal period, there is often history of polyhydramnios. Death may occur soon after birth or within the first year of life from respiratory failure, although long-term survival is possible. Typical clinical features include generalized hypotonia with facial weakness and ophthalmoplegia. Congenital contractures may be present. Although the disease is nonprogressive in survivors, these patients remain extremely weak, wasted, and unable to sit unsupported. Female heterozygotes may exhibit early onset of limb-girdle weakness, but are usually asymptomatic.[62]

Diagnosis of the neonatal variants is initially made by muscle biopsy. Genetic analysis of the myotubularin gene is available and allows for prenatal diagnosis. The creatine kinase level is usually normal, and electromyography is not helpful.

METABOLIC AND MULTISYSTEM DISORDERS

A large number of metabolic disorders directly involve the neuromuscular system and are broadly divided into primary abnormalities of glycogen, lipid, mitochondrial, and peroxisomal metabolism.[68] Some are responsible for well-defined clinical syndromes, such as acid maltase deficiency, which causes Pompe disease, whereas others are protean in their manifestations (see Chapter 50).

Mitochondrial Myopathies

Mitochondrial myopathies are categorized according to the involved area of abnormal metabolism, as follows: (1) defects of substrate transport; (2) defects of substrate utilization and the citric acid cycle; and (3) defects of the electron transport chain and oxidative phosphorylation coupling.[68] In the newborn, defects in electron transport (respiratory chain) are those most likely to lead to prominent muscle disease. Other abnormalities of mitochondrial metabolism, such as pyruvate carboxylase and pyruvate dehydrogenase complex deficiency, are more likely to present with features of a progressive encephalopathy. The most common of the respiratory chain disorders presenting as a myopathy during the neonatal period is cytochrome-c oxidase deficiency.[38] Typically, the infant presents with profound generalized weakness, hypotonia, hyporeflexia, poor feeding reflex, respiratory difficulty, and lactic acidosis. Other features may include hepatomegaly, cardiomyopathy, renal tubular defects (de Toni-Fanconi syndrome), and macroglossia. Death occurs within a few months. A reversible form of cytochrome-c oxidase deficiency also occurs.[38] The disorder presents in a fashion similar to the severe form but improves biochemically and clinically over the next 1 to 2 years. Early diagnosis is vital to provide continuing support while improvement takes place.

A mitochondrial myopathy should be suspected in any weak infant with lactic acidosis, particularly in conjunction with multisystem involvement. The creatine kinase level can be slightly elevated, but electromyography is usually not helpful. Muscle biopsy shows nonspecific myopathic changes, ragged red fibers on Gomori trichrome staining, and an absence of histochemical staining for cytochrome-c oxidase. Electron microscopy of muscle fibers demonstrates lipid and glycogen accumulations and an increased number of large,

abnormal-looking mitochondria. The benign and severe forms are differentiated by immunohistochemical techniques, using antibodies directed against different subunits of cytochrome-c oxidase. In the fatal form, there is an absence of DNA-encoded subunit VIIa, b. In the benign form, however, both this subunit and the mitochondrial DNA-encoded subunit II are absent.[38] Cytochrome-c oxidase deficiency in Leigh syndrome (encephalopathy and magnetic resonance imaging changes) has been recently associated with mutations of SURF1, a gene located on chromosome 9q34. However, mutations have not been found in patients with cytochrome-c oxidase without Leigh syndrome.

Disorders of Glycogen Metabolism

See also Chapter 50.

Apart from acid maltase (α-glucosidase) deficiency (Pompe disease), the autosomal recessive disorders of glycogen metabolism present only rarely during the neonatal period.[68] These rare presentations occur with debrancher enzyme deficiency, phosphorylase deficiency, and phosphofructokinase deficiency.

POMPE DISEASE (TYPE II GLYCOGEN STORAGE DISEASE)

The infantile form of Pompe disease is caused by a deficiency of acid maltase (α-glucosidase). The disorder can present during the neonatal period, although clinical onset during the second month of life is more usual.[31,38] The enzyme deficiency causes glycogen accumulation in anterior horn cells of the spinal cord and in the muscles, heart, liver, and brain. Infants present with profound generalized weakness, hypotonia, hyporeflexia, impaired awareness, heart failure, and hepatomegaly. Tongue fasciculations, a large tongue, and severe bulbar weakness are often present. The chest radiograph and electrocardiogram demonstrate cardiomegaly, short PR intervals, and giant QRS complexes. The serum creatine kinase and liver enzymes are elevated and electromyography shows combinations of denervation and myopathy, including fibrillations and small polyphasic potentials. Muscle biopsy reveals vacuoles containing glycogen, which stain with periodic acid-Schiff. The gene for the α-glucosidase enzyme protein is located on chromosome 17q23-25. Diagnosis typically is made by demonstrating the enzyme deficiency in leukocytes, lymphocytes, fibroblasts, or muscle or by demonstrating mutations in both alleles. GAA is the only gene known to be associated with Pompe disease. However, there is extensive genetic heterogeneity, and common mutations are found only in ethnic groups such as Ashkenazi Jews or the Amish in Pennsylvania. Prenatal diagnosis has been successful by demonstrating enzyme deficiency in cultured amniotic cells, linkage analysis, and mutation analysis. Prognosis is usually poor, with most infants dying within the first 6 months of life. Therapy continues to be palliative despite current efforts to develop enzyme and gene therapy.[2,31]

DEBRANCHER ENZYME DEFICIENCY (TYPE III GLYCOGEN STORAGE DISEASE)

Rarely, debrancher enzyme deficiency can present during the neonatal period with hypotonia, weakness, hypoglycemia, hepatomegaly, and liver dysfunction. Muscle biopsy shows abnormal glycogen storage, and diagnosis is established by demonstration of the debrancher enzyme deficiency.[38]

McARDLE DISEASE (TYPE V GLYCOGEN STORAGE DISEASE)

There are three different isozymes of phosphorylase (liver, brain, muscle), genes of which have been cloned and localized to different chromosomes.[63] Deficiency of the muscle enzyme on chromosome 11p13 causes McArdle disease.[38] Clinical presentation occurs typically during adolescence, with exercise intolerance, cramps, and myoglobinuria. However, the disorder shows clinical variability and rarely presents during the neonatal period.[18] Infants with infantile McArdle disease are weak and hypotonic with feeding difficulties. In some infants, the weakness is extreme, contractures are present, and the outcome fatal.[46] Even in the less severe neonatal form, the weakness is slowly progressive but without significant cranial nerve dysfunction. Muscle biopsy shows variations in fiber size, absence of phosphorylase staining, and subsarcolemmal glycogen-containing vacuoles. Unlike Pompe disease, the accumulated glycogen is not membrane bound.[14] Definitive diagnosis is made by demonstrating deficiency of the muscle isozyme or by demonstrating mutations in the phosphorylase gene. Treatment for this condition remains limited. There has been some success with high-protein diets or ingestion of sucrose before exercise.[67]

PHOSPHOFRUCTOKINASE DEFICIENCY (TYPE VII GLYCOGEN STORAGE DISEASE)

Phosphofructokinase deficiency usually presents with cramps on exercise and myoglobinuria. A severe infantile form presents during the neonatal period.[4] Affected infants exhibit hypotonia, progressive weakness, and contracture formation. Some infants have seizures, cortical blindness, and mental retardation.[68] The muscle biopsy findings are similar to those of McArdle disease, with nonmembrane-bound subsarcolemmal glycogen deposits. Diagnosis is established by demonstrating a reduction of phosphofructokinase activity biochemically and histochemically.[14]

Primary Carnitine Deficiency

Primary carnitine deficiency is caused by a deficiency in the transport of carnitine from plasma into the cells of affected tissues.[38] The disorder usually presents in early childhood with a cardiomyopathy, proximal muscle weakness, or recurrent encephalopathy. Rarely, it presents during the neonatal period with weakness, hypotonia, and cardiomyopathy. Hypoketotic hypoglycemia is a clue to diagnosis.[68] Muscle biopsy shows lipid-containing vacuoles, and serum and muscle carnitine levels are low. The carnitine transporter defect can be demonstrated in cultured fibroblasts.[38]

Peroxisomal Disorders

Peroxisomal disorders can present during the neonatal period with profound hypotonia and weakness. Signs include CNS dysfunction; facial dysmorphism, as in Zellweger syndrome; hepatomegaly; cataracts; retinopathy; calcific stippling of epiphyses; and rhizomelia.[8] These disorders are discussed in Chapter 50.

REFERENCES

1. Amack JD, Mahadevan MS: Myogenic defects in myotonic dystrophy, *Dev Biol* 265:294, 2004.
2. Amalfitano A, et al: Recombinant human acid alpha-glucosidase enzyme therapy for infantile glycogen storage disease type II: results of a phase I/II clinical trial, *Genet Med* 3:132, 2001.
3. Amiel-Tison C, Gosselin J: *Neurological Development from Birth to Six Year*, Baltimore, 2001, Johns Hopkins University Press.
4. Amit R, et al: Fatal familial infantile glycogen storage disease: multisystem phosphofructokinase deficiency, *Muscle Nerve* 15:455, 1992.
5. Anderson K, Talbot K: Spinal muscular atrophies reveal motor neuron vulnerability to defects in ribonucleoprotein handling, *Curr Opin Neurol* 16:595, 2003.
6. Axelrod FB, Hilz MJ: Inherited autonomic neuropathies, *Semin Neurol* 22:381, 2003.
7. Axelrod FB: Familial dysautonomia, *Muscle Nerve* 29:352, 2004.
8. Baumgartner MR, Saudubray JM: Peroxisomal disorders, *Semin Neonatol* 7:85, 2002.
9. Brockington M, et al: Assignment of a form of congenital muscular dystrophy with secondary merosin deficiency to chromosome 1q42, *Am J Hum Genet* 66:428, 2000.
10. Brouwer OF, et al: Facioscapulohumeral muscular dystrophy in early childhood, *Arch Neurol* 51:387, 1994.
11. Burglen L, et al: Survival motor neuron gene depletion in the arthrogryposis multiplex congenita-spinal muscular atrophy association, *J Clin Invest* 98:1130, 1995.
12. Buxton J, et al: Detection of an unstable fragment of DNA specific to individuals with myotonic dystrophy, *Nature* 355:547, 1992.
13. Campbell C, et al: Congenital myotonic dystrophy: assisted ventilation duration and outcome, *Pediatrics* 113:811, 2004.
14. Carpenter S, Karpati G: *Pathology of Skeletal Muscle*, 2nd ed, New York, 2001, Oxford University Press.
15. Clancy RR, et al: Hypoxic-ischemic spinal cord injury following perinatal asphyxia, *Ann Neurol* 25:185, 1989.
16. Cormand B, et al: Clinical and genetic distinction between Walker-Warburg syndrome and muscle-eye-brain disease, *Neurology* 56:1059, 2001.
17. Cornblath DR, et al: Clinical electrophysiology of infantile botulism, *Muscle Nerve* 6:448, 1983.
18. Cornelio F, et al: Congenital myopathy due to phosphorylase deficiency, *Neurology* 33:1383, 1983.
19. Demir E, et al: Mutations in COL6A3 cause severe and mild phenotypes of Ullrich congenital muscular dystrophy, *Am J Hum Genet* 70:1446, 2002.
20. Di Costanzo A, et al: Brain MRI features of congenital- and adult-form myotonic dystrophy type 1: case-control study, *Neuromuscul Dis* 12:476, 2002.
21. Dinger J, Prager B: Arthrogryposis multiplex in a newborn of a myasthenic mother: case report and literature, *Neuromuscul Disord* 3:335, 1993.
22. Djelmis J, et al: Myasthenia gravis in pregnancy: report of 69 cases, *Eur J Obstet Gynecol* 104:21, 2002.
23. Dubowitz LMS, et al: *The Neurological Assessment of the Preterm and Fullterm Infant*, 2nd ed, London, 1999, Mac Keith Press.
24. Dubowitz V: *Muscle Biopsy: A Practical Approach*, 2nd ed, London, 1985, Baillière Tindall.

25. Dubowitz V: *The Floppy Infant*, Philadelphia, 1980, JB Lippincott.

26. Dubowitz V: Workshop report: twenty-second ENMC-sponsored workshop on congenital muscular dystrophy, *Neuromuscul Disord* 4:75, 1994.

27. Engel AG, et al: Congenital myasthenic syndromes: progress over the past decade, *Muscle Nerv* 27:4, 2003.

28. Ferreiro A, Fardeau M: 80th ENMC International Workshop on Multi-Minicore Disease: 1st International MmD Workshop 12-13th May 2000, Soestduinen, the Netherlands, *Neuromuscul Disord* 12:60, 2002.

29. Ghamdi M, et al: Congenital hypomyelinating neuropathy: a reversible case, *Pediatr Neurol* 16:71, 1997.

30. Glauser TA, et al: Relapse of infant botulism, *Ann Neurol* 28:187, 1990.

31. Hannerieke MP, et al: The natural course of infantile Pompe's disease: 20 original cases compared with 133 cases from the literature, *Pediatrics* 112:332, 2003.

32. Harper P: *Myotonic Dystrophy*, 3rd ed, London, 2001, WB Saunders.

33. Harper PS, et al: Anticipation in myotonic dystrophy: new light on an old problem, *Am J Hum Genet* 51:10, 1992.

34. Hays RM, Michaud LJ: Neonatal myasthenia gravis: specific advantages of repetitive stimulation over edrophonium testing, *Pediatr Neurol* 4:245, 1988.

35. Higuchi I, et al: Frameshift mutation in the collagen VI gene causes Ullrich's disease, *Ann Neurol* 50:261, 2001.

36. Hoff JM, et al: Myasthenia gravis: consequences for pregnancy, delivery, and the newborn, *Neurology* 61:1362, 2003.

37. Jansen G, et al: Gonosomal mosaicism in myotonic dystrophy patients: involvement of mitotic events in (CTG)n repeat variation and selection against extreme expansion in sperm, *Am J Hum Genet* 54:575, 1994.

38. Jones H, et al: *Neuromuscular Disorders of Infancy, Childhood, and Adolescence: A Clinician's Approach*, Philadelphia, 2003, Elsevier Science.

39. Jones HR, Darras BT: Acute care pediatric electromyography, *Muscle Nerve* S9:S53, 2000.

40. Kirschner J, Bonnemann C: The congenital and limb-girdle muscular dystrophies, *Arch Neurol* 61:189, 2004.

41. Kissel JT, et al: Randomized, double-blind, placebo-controlled trial of albuterol in facioscapulohumeral dystrophy, *Neurology* 57:1434, 2001.

42. Kobayashi H, et al: A gene for a severe lethal form of X-linked arthrogryposis (X-linked infantile spinal muscular atrophy) maps to human chromosome Xp11.3-q11.2, *Hum Mol Genet* 4:1213, 1995.

43. Liquori CL, et al: Myotonic dystrophy type 2 caused by a CCTG expansion in intron1 of ZNF9, *Science* 293:864, 2001.

44. Mankodi A, Thornton C: Myotonic syndromes, *Curr Opin Neurol* 15:545, 2002.

45. Miller G, Clark GD: *The Cerebral Palsies: Causes, Consequences, and Management*, Boston, 1998, Butterworth-Heinemann.

46. Milstein JM, et al: Fatal infantile muscle phosphorylase deficiency, *J Child Neurol* 4:186, 1989.

47. Moghadaszadeh B, et al: Identification of a new locus for a peculiar form of congenital muscular dystrophy with early rigidity of the spine, on chromosome 1p35-36, *Am J Hum Genet* 62:1439, 1998.

48. Monani UR, et al: A single nucleotide difference that alters splicing patterns distinguishes the SMA gene SMN1 from the copy gene SMN2, *Hum Mol Genet* 8:1177, 1999.

49. Morel E, et al: Neonatal myasthenia gravis: a new clinical and immunological appraisal on 30 cases, *Neurology* 38:138, 1988.

50. Muntoni F, et al: Defective glycosylation in congenital muscular dystrophies, *Curr Opin Neurol* 17:205, 2004.

51. Muntoni F, et al: 114th ENMC International Workshop on Congenital Muscular Dystrophy (CMD) 17-19 January 2003, Naarden, the Netherlands (8th workshop of the international consortium on CMD; 3rd workshop of the MYO-CLUSTER), *Neuromuscul Disord* 13:579, 2003.

52. Namba T, et al: Neonatal myasthenia gravis: report of two cases and review of the literature, *Pediatrics* 45:488, 1970.

53. Papazian O: Transient neonatal myasthenia gravis, *J Child Neurol* 7:135, 1992.

54. Prelle A, et al: Dystrophin deficiency in a case of congenital myopathy, *J Neurol* 239:76, 1993.

55. Reddy V, et al: Infant botulism: New York City, 2001-2002, *JAMA* 289:834, 2003.

56. Riaz M, et al: The effects of maternal magnesium sulfate treatment on newborns: a prospective controlled study, *J Perinatol* 18:449, 1998.

57. Rudnik-Schineborn S, et al: Different patterns of obstetrical complications in myotonic dystrophy in relation to the disease status of the fetus, *Am J Med Genet* 80:314, 1998.

58. Ryan MM, et al: Nemaline myopathy: a clinical study of 143 cases, *Ann Neurol* 50:312, 2001.

59. Scriver CR, et al: *The Metabolic and Molecular Basis of Inherited Disease*, 8th ed, New York, 2001, McGraw-Hill.

60. Suter U, Scherer SS: Disease mechanisms in inherited neuropathies, *Nat Rev Neurosci* 4:714, 2003.

61. Szigeti K, et al: Differentiation in congenital hypomyelinating neuropathy caused by a novel myelin protein zero mutation, *Ann Neurol* 54:398, 2003.

62. Taratuto AL: Congenital myopathies and related disorders, *Curr Opin Neurol* 15:553, 2002.

63. Tein I: Neonatal metabolic myopathies, *Semin Perinatol* 23:125, 1999.

64. Toda T, et al: The Fukuyama congenital muscular dystrophy story, *Neuromuscul Disord* 10:153, 2000.

65. Villanova M, et al: Immunolocalization of several laminin chains in normal human central and peripheral nervous system, *J Submicrosc Cytol Pathol* 29:409, 1997.

66. Vincent A, et al: Antibodies in myasthenia gravis and related disorders, *Ann N Y Acad Sci* 998:324, 2003.

67. Vissing J, Haller R: The effect of oral sucrose on exercise tolerance in patients with McArdle's disease, *N Engl J Med* 349:2503, 2003.

68. Volpe JJ: *Neurology of the Newborn*, 4th ed, Philadelphia, WB Saunders, 2001.

69. Walgren-Pettersson C, Laing NG: Report of the 83rd ENMC International Workshop: 4th Workshop on Nemaline Myopathy, 22-24 September 2000, Naarden, the Netherlands, *Neuromuscul Disord* 11:589, 2001.

70. Wong LJ, Ashizawa T, Monckton DG, et al: Somatic heterogeneity of the CTG repeat in myotonic dystrophy is age and size dependent, *Am J Hum Genet* 56:114, 1995.

71. Wright EA, McQuillen MP: Antibiotic-induced neuromuscular blockade, *Ann N Y Acad Sci* 183:358, 1971.

72. Yoshida A, et al: Muscular dystrophy and neuronal migration disorder caused by mutations in a glycosyltransferase, POMGnT1, *Dev Cell* 1:717, 2001.

73. Zeesman S, et al: Paternal transmission of the congenital form of myotonic dystrophy type 1: a new case and review of the literature, *Am J Med Genet* 107:222, 2002.

PART 7

Disorders in Head Shape and Size

Alan R. Cohen

This part focuses on conditions that result in an alteration of head size or of head shape in the newborn infant. Emphasis is on the clinical presentation, diagnostic procedures, and available treatment options.

EXAMINATION OF THE HEAD

The head is inspected for abnormalities of size and shape. The scalp is examined for the presence of a neurocutaneous signature such as a dimple, dermal sinus, hemangioma, or port wine stain. Certain mass lesions are easily detected, such as tumors of the scalp and calvaria, traumatic subperiosteal hemorrhage (the so-called cephalhematoma), and cranial dysraphic masses, such as the encephalocele.

The shape of the head is noted and the patency of the cranial sutures is ascertained. The anterior fontanelle is palpated and should be flat or slightly sunken. The anterior fontanelle is a diamond-shaped soft spot at the junction of the frontal and parietal bones, which marks the site of the future bregma, a craniometric point that denotes the junction of the metopic, coronal, and sagittal sutures. It usually closes by approximately age 18 months (range, 6 months to 2 years). It pulsates with the heartbeat and may bulge normally during crying. The mean time of closure is 16.3 months for boys and 18.8 months for girls.[2] A full or tense anterior fontanelle may signify a pathologic process associated with increased intracranial pressure. Early closure of the anterior fontanelle may be seen in microcephaly or craniosynostosis, or may be a variation of normal. The posterior fontanelle is smaller than the anterior fontanelle and bridges the parietal and occipital bones at the site of the future lambda, the craniometric point denoting the junction of the sagittal and lambdoid sutures. The posterior fontanelle usually closes by age 3 months.

The head circumference is a useful gauge of the intracranial volume, and measurement of the head circumference is of paramount importance in the neurologic examination of the newborn. A thin flexible tape measure is used to record the occipitofrontal circumference (OFC). The tape is pressed firmly against the scalp to include the most prominent portion of the occiput, which is usually at or just above the external occipital protuberance (inion) and the most prominent portion of the forehead, which is usually located just above the glabella. The OFC is plotted on a standard graph and is considered within the normal range if it is not greater than 2 standard deviations above or below the mean. The OFC provides an immediate assessment of head size and is useful for future assessment of head growth patterns. For preterm infants, gestation-adjusted age should be recorded on growth charts until 24 to 36 months.

The normal infant's OFC increases by approximately 2 cm in the first month of life and by approximately 6 cm in the first 4 months. In the healthy premature infant, there may actually be transient head shrinkage with a reduction in OFC and overriding sutures in the first days of life. This is thought to be related to water loss from the intracranial compartment.[82] This head shrinkage is maximal at approximately the third day of life, and by the second week the head circumference should be increasing.

THE SMALL HEAD

Microcephaly (Greek *mikros*, "small," *kephale*, "head") is the condition in which the size of the head, as measured by the OFC, is significantly smaller than normal. In general, microcephaly is defined as an OFC greater than two standard deviations below the mean for age and sex, although some authors use a stricter criterion of three standard deviations below the mean. Microcephaly is often, but not always, associated with intellectual retardation.

In the normal infant, the skull enlarges as a consequence of inductive pressure generated by the growing brain. Microcephaly often occurs as the consequence. *Micrencephaly* (Greek *micros*, "small," *enkephale*, "brain"), that is, the small head, is the result of a small brain. The single exception is multiple-suture craniosynostosis, the very rare disorder in which the fused skull restricts growth of the brain. The nomenclature used to categorize microcephaly has been inconsistent and confusing. On one end of the spectrum, microcephaly describes the simple finding of a small head on physical examination. On the other end, microcephaly is not a single entity, but a complex, heterogeneous group of disorders of genetic or environmental etiology characterized by abnormal brain growth.

It is helpful to categorize microcephaly as primary or secondary to distinguish disorders of brain formation from disorders characterized by destruction of already formed brain. *Primary microcephaly* describes a group of genetic or environmental insults that cause abnormalities of neuronal induction, proliferation, or migration. These insults occur sometime within the first 7 months of gestation. *Secondary microcephaly* describes a variety of insults that occur in the latter part of the third trimester or perinatal period. These insults occur after neuronal proliferation and migration and are characterized by destruction of the brain due to trauma, hypoxia-ischemia, infection, or metabolic causes. Some authors classify genetic insults as primary microcephaly and environmental insults as secondary microcephaly, but this is somewhat inaccurate because genetic and environmental factors can influence the developing brain and the already developed brain with different consequences. All classification schemes are imperfect because of overlap among the various disorders. The classification scheme here reflects both the etiology and the timing of the insult in the developing nervous system (Box 40-15).

BOX 40–15 Causes of Congenital Microcephaly

I. PRIMARY MICROCEPHALY
Disorders of brain formation; insults causing anomalies of neuronal induction, proliferation, and migration; first 7 months of gestation.

Genetic Disorders
Chromosomal anomalies

- Trisomies 13, 18, 21
- Deletion and translocation syndromes

Somatic anomalies

- Familial microcephaly (usually autosomal recessive)
- Rubinstein-Taybi syndrome
- Smith-Lemli-Opitz syndrome
- Cornelia de Lange syndrome
- Dubowitz syndrome
- Hallermann-Streiff syndrome
- Seckel syndrome
- Prader-Willi syndrome
- Aicardi syndrome
- Nijmegen breakage syndrome

Developmental Disorders (Genetic or Environmental)
Neurulation/cleavage anomalies

- Anencephaly
- Holoprosencephaly

Migrational anomalies

- Schizencephaly
- Lissencephaly
- Polymicrogyria

Environmental Disorders
Congenital infections

- Toxoplasmosis
- Rubella
- Cytomegalovirus
- Herpes simplex
- Coxsackievirus

Biochemical disorders

- Maternal diabetes mellitus
- Maternal uremia
- Maternal phenylketonuria

Environmental toxins

- Maternal malnutrition
- Hyperthermia
- Ionizing radiation
- Teratogens (phenytoin, cocaine, alcohol, carbon monoxide)

II. SECONDARY MICROCEPHALY
Destruction of already formed brain; last 2 months of third trimester or perinatal period.

Trauma
Anoxia
Infections
Metabolic disorders

III. CRANIOSYNOSTOSIS (MULTIPLE SUTURES)

Primary Microcephaly

See also Part 1 of this chapter.

Primary microcephaly describes a heterogeneous group of disorders resulting from an insult early in embryologic development that interferes with neuronal development or migration (Fig. 40-85). This broad group of disorders may have a genetic or an environmental etiology.

GENETIC DEFECTS

Primary microcephaly may occur as an isolated insult to the central nervous system or may be seen in association with chromosomal abnormalities or as a part of other well-defined multiorgan genetic syndromes. Genetic forms of primary microcephaly may be autosomal recessive, autosomal dominant, or X-linked. Of the genetic forms, autosomal recessive transmission is the most common. Like other recessive disorders, this condition occurs with increased prevalence in geographic regions with high consanguinity. Investigators have been able to study consanguineous families with homozygosity mapping to localize recessive traits.[48] Since 1998, five autosomal recessive loci for microcephaly have been mapped by molecular geneticists collaborating with clinicians working in regions where consanguinity is common.[55] Autosomal dominant microcephaly has been observed in families, often associated with normal intelligence or only mild cognitive impairment.

NEURULATION AND CLEAVAGE ANOMALIES

Anencephaly is the most devastating of all the dysraphic malformations, and occurs as a consequence of failure of the anterior neural tube to close. The insult occurs early in embryogenesis, before day 26 of gestation. Both cerebral hemispheres are absent, as is the cranial vault (Fig. 40-86). Anencephaly is a lethal condition. Infants are either stillborn or live for only a few days. The incidence of anencephaly has been decreasing.

Holoprosencephaly occurs as a consequence of failure of the prosencephalon, or embryonic forebrain, to separate and form paired telencephalic hemispheres. The hemispheres are normally cleaved at 33 days' gestation, so the insult causing holoprosencephaly must occur early. Holoprosencephaly is usually sporadic, but an autosomal dominant familial variant has been reported. The long arm of chromosome 7 (7q) is thought to be the genetic locus for holoprosencephaly.[7] Holoprosencephaly is caused by mutations in the sonic hedgehog gene (*SHH*) and other genes located on chromosome 7q. The cleavage defects produce a clinical picture of varying severity. In the most complete form, *alobar holoprosencephaly*, there is a single hemisphere of the brain and a single midline prosencephalic ventricle. Median facial defects range from a single midline eye and rudimentary nose to orbital hypotelorism, flattening of the nose, cleft lip and palate, and trigonocephaly (triangular forehead with vertical ridge along metopic suture). Neurologic findings include mental retardation, seizures, poor temperature control, and a variety of neuroendocrine disorders related to dysfunction of the anterior and posterior pituitary gland. Less severe clinical forms of the disorder include *semilobar holoprosencephaly* and *lobar holoprosencephaly*, in order of decreasing severity (Fig. 40-87).

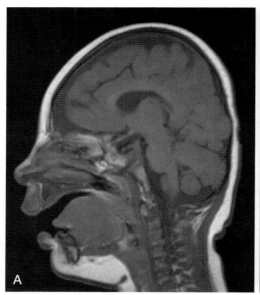
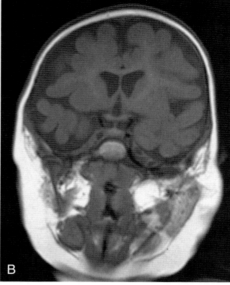

Figure 40–85. Primary microcephaly. A, T1-weighted sagittal magnetic resonance image. B, T1-weighted coronal MRI.

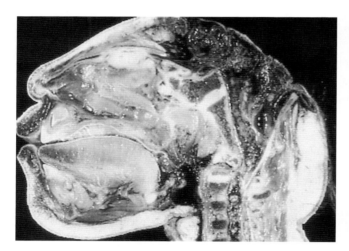

Figure 40–86. Anencephaly.

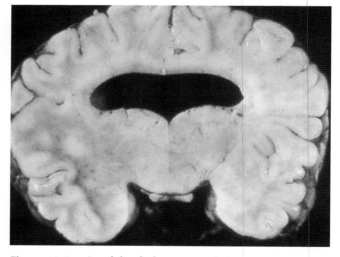

Figure 40–87. Semilobar holoprosencephaly, coronal specimen.

Other genetic causes of primary microcephaly include disorders of karyotype, including trisomies, deletions, and translocation syndromes. Among the common chromosomal abnormalities are trisomies 21, 18, and 13. Primary microcephaly may be a feature of numerous somatic disorders with normal karyotypes, including Rubinstein-Taybi syndrome, Smith-Lemli-Opitz syndrome, Cornelia de Lange syndrome, and Hallerman-Streiff syndrome (see Box 40-15). In these syndromes, characteristic dysmorphic features and patterns of other organ involvement help establish the diagnosis.

MIGRATIONAL ANOMALIES

See Part 1 of this chapter.
Neuronal migration is a radial and tangential process by which nerve cells move from their progenitor cell origin in the ventricular zone and basal forebrain to their final destination in the cerebrum. The cerebral cortex forms as the result

of neuronal migration, and anomalous gyral formation is the signature finding in all migrational disorders (Fig. 40-88). Because of this cortical disruption, seizures are the most common clinical manifestation of migrational disorders. The morphologic abnormality in *schizencephaly* is a cleft in the cerebral hemisphere, which may be unilateral or bilateral, open-lipped (walls of the cleft separated, often associated with enlargement of the lateral ventricles; Fig. 40-89) or closed-lipped. In *lissencephaly* (agyria, or "smooth brain"), the cerebral hemispheres have few or no gyri (Fig. 40-90). In *polymicrogyria*, the gyri are too numerous and too small, with a proliferation of secondary and tertiary sulci. The appearance of the cortical surface has been likened to that of a wrinkled chestnut kernel (Fig. 40-91). *Neuronal heterotopias* (brain warts) are the least severe of the migrational disorders and may stand alone or occur in association with other disturbances of migration. Agenesis of the corpus callosum,

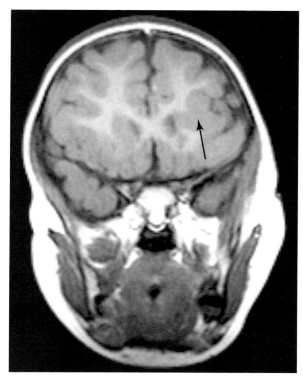

Figure 40–88. Cortical dysplasia. T1-weighted coronal magnetic resonance image shows left perisylvian cortical thickening extending to the ventricle (*arrow*).

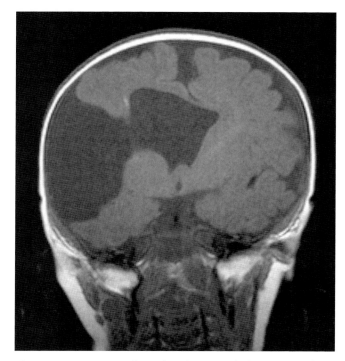

Figure 40–89. Open-lipped schizencephaly. T1-weighted coronal magnetic resonance image shows large open cleft communicating with the right lateral ventricle and absence of the septum pellucidum.

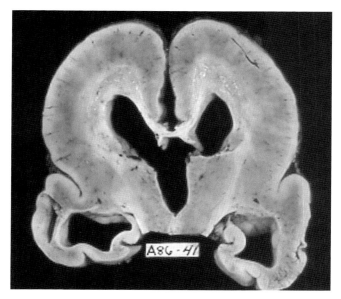

Figure 40–90. Lissencephaly, coronal specimen.

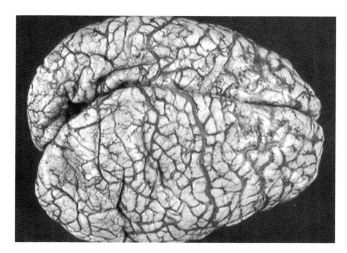

Figure 40–91. Polymicrogyria.

partial or complete, is a relatively common accompaniment in disorders of neuronal migration (Fig. 40-92). The corpus callosum is the largest of the interhemispheric commissures, and its absence may be seen in association with other midline defects, such as absence or hypoplasia of the septum pellucidum, the thin partition that divides the anterior portion of the lateral ventricles (Fig. 40-93). The triad of agenesis of the septum pellucidum, optic nerve hypoplasia, and pituitary abnormalities is called *septo-optic dysplasia,* or *DeMorsier syndrome.* Agenesis of the corpus callosum associated with cortical and subependymal gray matter heterotopias and chorioretinal lacunae was initially described by the French neurologist Jean Aicardi in 1965 (*Aicardi syndrome*).[1] This disorder, seen only in girls, is characterized by microcephaly, profound mental retardation, and seizures in the form of infantile spasms.

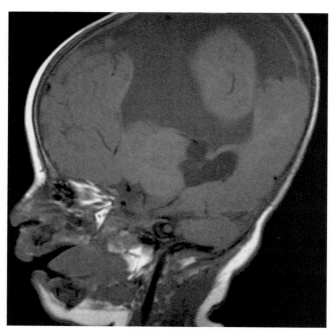

Figure 40–92. Agenesis of the corpus callosum. T1-weighted sagittal magnetic resonance image also demonstrates absence of the septum pellucidum and a large midline cerebrospinal fluid collection.

CONGENITAL INFECTIONS

See also Chapters 23 and 39.

The developing nervous system is susceptible to a variety of in utero infections. Implicated agents are collectively referred to by the acronym *TORCH* syndrome (*t*oxoplasmosis, *r*ubella, *c*ytomegalovirus, and *h*erpes simplex virus; Fig. 40-94).

BIOCHEMICAL DISORDERS

Several maternal metabolic disorders such as diabetes mellitus and uremia are associated with congenital primary microcephaly. Untreated phenylketonuria in an asymptomatic mother may be associated with microcephaly in a nonphenylketonuric infant.[49,50] Maternal malnutrition and hypertension are associated with intrauterine growth restriction and microcephaly. Teratogenic agents such as phenytoin, cortisone, cocaine, alcohol, isotretinoin, and carbon monoxide can produce microcephaly along with disorders of neuronal induction and migration. Maternal exposure to ionizing radiation has been implicated as a cause of congenital microcephaly, with earlier insults associated with more severe cases.[54]

RADIAL MICROBRAIN AND MICRENCEPHALY VERA

As our understanding of the timing of neuronal proliferation has improved, another scheme for classifying micrencephaly has been proposed. Two subgroups of micrencephaly have been postulated: *radial microbrain* and *micrencephaly vera*. This scheme is based on the work of Rakic,[63] who proposed a radial unit model to explain the major ontogenetic development of the cerebral cortex. Rakic suggested that the ependymal layer of the embryonic cerebral ventricle consists of proliferative units whose cytoarchitectonic output is translated to the expanding cerebral cortex along radial glial guides. Early symmetric division of stem cells creates these proliferative units, which behave as organized cylindrical columns containing neurons. Later asymmetric division of stem cells causes the proliferative units to enlarge, with increased numbers of neurons. Subsequent migration of the proliferative units together as columns along radial glia explains the evolution of the cerebral cortex from the primitive ventricular zone.

Radial microbrain and micrencephaly vera are disorders of micrencephaly related to impaired neuronal proliferation,

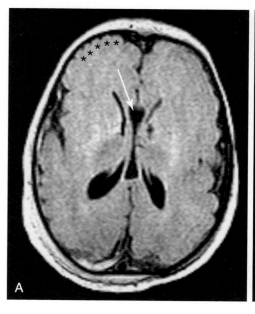
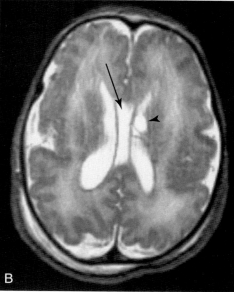

Figure 40–93. Zellweger syndrome, a peroxisomal disorder affecting the brain, kidneys, and liver. **A,** Fluid-attenuated inversion recovery (FLAIR) axial magnetic resonance image (MRI). **B,** T2-weighted axial MRI. Note the multiple migrational abnormalities including polymicrogyria (*asterisks* in **A**), subependymal cysts (*arrowhead* in **B**), cortical dysplasia, and ventricular anomalies, including a cavum septi pellucidi and cavum vergae (*arrow* in **A** and **B**).

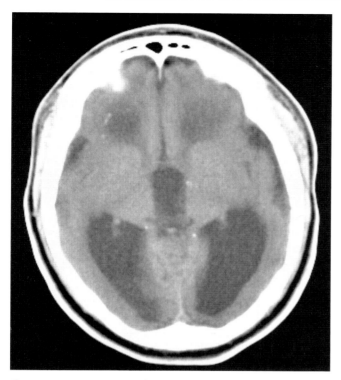

Figure 40–94. Congenital toxoplasmosis. Noncontrast computed tomography scan shows ex vacuo hydrocephalus and periventricular calcifications.

and would be categorized as forms of primary microcephaly in the conventional classification scheme. *Radial microbrain* is a rare condition described in seven cases by Evrard and colleagues,[31] in which the brain is extremely small with normal gyri and normal cortical lamination. The brain can be as small as 16 g at term (the normal newborn brain is 350 g), and in the reported cases, death has occurred in the first month. Radial microbrain is considered a genetic disorder, most likely with autosomal recessive inheritance. The pathologic finding is a marked reduction in the number of cortical neuronal columns (proliferative units), but a normal number of neurons per column. The reduced number of columns with preservation of columnar size suggests that the insult occurs early in the embryonic phase of neuronal proliferation.

Micrencephaly vera (true micrencephaly) describes a heterogeneous disorder in which the brain is well formed with a simple gyral pattern and small, but not as small as the radial microbrain. Pathologically, the number of cortical neuronal columns is normal, but the size of the columns is small because of a reduced number of neurons per column. The timing of the embryologic insult is later than that for radial microbrain, most likely between the 6th and 18th weeks of gestation. Micrencephaly vera is not a single entity and may be caused by genetic or environmental abnormalities. The distinction between radial microbrain and micrencephaly vera is of particular interest to investigators studying neuronal proliferation and the evolution of human cerebral neocortex from progenitor cells lining the embryologic ventricle.

Secondary Microcephaly

Secondary microcephaly occurs after an insult to the already developed brain. Thus, secondary microcephaly arises after neuronal induction, proliferation, and migration, typically from disorders in the last 2 months of the third trimester of pregnancy or in the perinatal period. The causes of secondary microcephaly are multifactorial and include trauma, hypoxia-ischemia, metabolic disorders, and infection (Fig. 40-95).

Craniosynostosis

Craniosynostosis, or premature fusion of one or more of the sutures of the skull, is discussed later in this chapter. Craniosynostosis causes microcephaly only rarely, when there has been premature fusion of multiple sutures. In this setting, the skull restricts growth of the brain and the infant may display irritability, lethargy, and vomiting as manifestations of increased intracranial pressure.

Evaluation and Treatment of the Small Head

A thorough history is obtained and serial measurements of the head circumference are recorded. The head circumference of both parents is measured. Laboratory investigation is tailored by the history and examination. If a congenital infection is suspected, TORCH titers can be collected from the mother and child. If a genetic disorder is suspected, karyotyping or genetic mapping can be carried out. Imaging of the brain is usually performed with computed tomography (CT) or magnetic resonance imaging (MRI). In general, CT is the optimal study to examine the bone, such as in selected cases of craniosynostosis. MRI is the optimal study to examine the architecture of the brain. Congenital microcephaly is frequently associated with significant mental retardation, sometimes with cerebral palsy and epilepsy. Appropriate supportive care as well as genetic and family counseling are important features in the management of congenital microcephaly.

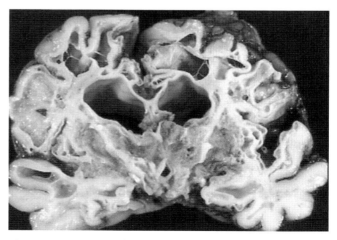

Figure 40–95. Secondary microcephaly with destruction of previously formed brain by a hypoxic-ischemic insult.

THE LARGE HEAD

Macrocephaly (Greek *makros*, "large," *kephale*, "head") is the term used to describe a large head. It is not a single disease entity, but a finding on physical examination from a variety of causes. Conventionally, macrocephaly is defined as a head circumference greater than 2 standard deviations above the mean. Evaluation should be undertaken if a single measurement of the head circumference is significantly abnormal on the growth chart or if the head circumference crosses one or more percentiles on serial examinations.

There are three general etiologies for congenital macrocephaly (Box 40-16): enlargement of the brain itself (macrencephaly), enlargement of the cerebrospinal fluid (CSF) spaces (e.g., hydrocephalus), and the presence or enlargement of other structures (e.g., brain tumor, brain abscess, intracranial hematoma).

BOX 40–16 Causes of Congenital Macrocephaly

I. ENLARGEMENT OF THE BRAIN (MACRENCEPHALY)

Isolated Macrencephaly
Familial (autosomal dominant or recessive)
Sporadic
Unilateral macrencephaly (hemimegalencephaly)

Macrencephaly and Growth Disorders
Beckwith-Wiedemann syndrome
Sotos syndrome (cerebral gigantism)
Achondroplasia

Neurocutaneous Syndromes
Neurofibromatosis type 1
Sturge-Weber disease
Tuberous sclerosis

Chromosomal Disorders
Fragile X syndrome
Klinefelter syndrome

Degenerative Disorders
Alexander disease
Canavan disease

Metabolic Disorders
Tay-Sachs disease
Generalized gangliosidoses

II. ENLARGEMENT OF THE CEREBROSPINAL FLUID SPACES

Hydrocephalus
Benign external hydrocephalus
Hydranencephaly
Dandy-Walker malformation
Arachnoid cyst

III. PRESENCE OR ENLARGEMENT OF OTHER STRUCTURES

Neoplasms
Vascular lesions (vein of Galen malformation)
Trauma (subdural hematoma, hygroma)
Infection (brain abscess, subdural empyema, effusion)

Macrencephaly

Macrencephaly (Greek *makros*, "large," *enkephalos*, "brain") literally describes enlargement or overgrowth of the brain. The term is synonymous with *megalencephaly* (Greek *megas*, "large," *enkephalos*, "brain"). Macrencephaly itself is not a single disorder. Instead, it represents a heterogeneous group of disorders resulting from abnormal proliferation of brain tissue or excessive storage of brain metabolites leading to a large or "heavy" brain. Whereas the normal infant brain weighs approximately 350 g at birth, the macrencephalic brain may weigh up to twice that amount. The neuropathologic substrates of macrencephaly have not been fully characterized. Aside from the obviously enlarged head, physical findings are varied, ranging from completely normal results on neurologic examination to severe seizures and mental retardation. The spectrum of macrencephaly is discussed in the following sections.

ISOLATED MACRENCEPHALY

Isolated macrencephaly can be familial or sporadic. Familial macrencephaly is an inherited disorder in which the head size of an otherwise normal infant is excessively enlarged. A clue to the diagnosis is the finding of an abnormally enlarged head in one or both parents. The child is born with an enlarged head that tends to remain enlarged and can sometimes grow at a rapid rate. Most children are neurologically normal or near-normal. In true familial macrencephaly, the only finding on neuroimaging studies is enlargement of the brain. Familial macrencephaly is thought to be related to another condition, so-called benign external hydrocephalus of infancy, in which there is enlargement of the extracerebral subarachnoid space (see "External Hydrocephalus," later), and one wonders whether these are really variants of the same condition. Most cases of familial macrencephaly are characterized by autosomal dominant inheritance. Infants with the rare autosomal recessive variant are more likely to be neurologically impaired, with mental retardation, seizures, and motor delay. Sporadic macrencephaly is used to describe isolated macrencephaly in an infant whose parents have normal head circumferences and for whom there is no other demonstrable etiology for brain enlargement.

MACRENCEPHALY AND GROWTH DISORDERS

Macrencephaly is sometimes associated with generalized disorders of growth. The syndrome of cerebral gigantism was described by Sotos and colleagues in 1964.[76] *Sotos syndrome* is characterized by macrencephaly along with macrosomia, enlargement of the hands and feet, and poor coordination.[28] Macrencephaly begins prenatally in 50% of cases and by 1 year in all affected children. Mental retardation is variable, but behavioral problems are significant and there is often delay in motor milestones. Midline intracranial anomalies have been described on MRI, including agenesis of the corpus callosum and septum pellucidum, as well as hypoplasia of the cerebellar vermis. Ventriculomegaly is common, with prominence of the trigone and occipital horns.[74]

Macrencephaly may be seen in association with macroglossia, macrosomia, visceromegaly, omphalocele, exophthalmos, and neonatal hypoglycemia. This condition, the *Beckwith-Wiedemann syndrome*, was described independently by John Bruce Beckwith, an American pathologist, and

Hans-Rudolf Wiedemann, a German pediatrician. Craniofacial features include a prominent occiput, large anterior fontanelle, and a ridge along the metopic suture.[40] Mental retardation, if present, is thought to be more likely a consequence of uncontrolled neonatal hypoglycemia than of malformation of the brain. Children with Beckwith-Wiedemann syndrome have an increased incidence of Wilms tumor, adrenal cortical carcinoma, and hepatoblastoma.

Achondroplasia is the most common form of dwarfism. Head enlargement in achondroplasia is sometimes a consequence of hydrocephalus and sometimes a consequence of true macrencephaly. Affected children have frontal bossing with a flattened nasal bridge, mild midface hypoplasia, as well as a short cranial base and small foramen magnum. True compression of the brainstem and cervical spinal cord are infrequent but potentially devastating. Achondroplastic children usually have normal intelligence.

NEUROCUTANEOUS SYNDROMES

The neurocutaneous syndromes, or *phakomatoses*, are each characterized in part by abnormal cellular proliferation in the central nervous system. Several of the neurocutaneous syndromes are associated with macrencephaly. *Neurofibromatosis type 1 (NF-1)* is an overgrowth syndrome that can be associated with neonatal or infantile macrencephaly. Distortion of cortical architecture has been reported, along with spongiform hamartomatous changes in the white matter, basal ganglia, brainstem, and cerebellum. Glial neoplasms are common, and optic glioma can be seen in neonates. Using quantitative MRI, Cutting and associates[24] found that brains of patients with NF-1 are significantly larger than normal, with a prevalence of macrencephaly in NF-1 of approximately 50%.

Macrencephaly may be a part of other neurocutaneous disorders, but is seen with less frequency. The *Sturge-Weber syndrome* (encephalotrigeminal angiomatosis) is a sporadic phakomatosis characterized by a facial port wine stain (nevus flammeus) and leptomeningeal vascular proliferation with cerebral cortical calcification, usually in the parietal and occipital regions. Ocular manifestations include glaucoma and buphthalmos (Greek "ox eye," also called *hydrophthalmia*: enlargement of the eye due to congenital glaucoma). Neurologic manifestations include seizures (which may be medically refractory), focal deficits of visual, language, or motor function, and developmental delay with learning disorders and mental retardation.

Tuberous sclerosis (Bourneville syndrome) is an autosomal dominant disorder affecting skin (facial angiofibromas, subungual fibromas, ash leaf spots, shagreen patches), eye (retinal hamartomas, astrocytomas), viscera (cardiac rhabdomyomas, renal angiomyolipomas, and cysts), and brain. Neurologic manifestations are characterized by the abnormal proliferation of neurons and glia. Neuropathologic findings include cortical tubers, subependymal nodules, and, occasionally, subependymal giant cell astrocytomas that can obstruct the cerebral ventricles at the foramina of Monro (Fig. 40-96). The neurologic presentation is one of seizures, cognitive impairment, and behavioral disorders.

CHROMOSOMAL DISORDERS

Fragile X syndrome is second to Down syndrome as a genetic cause of mental retardation. The genetic mutation is thought to involve unstable trinucleotide repeats, with a fragile site at

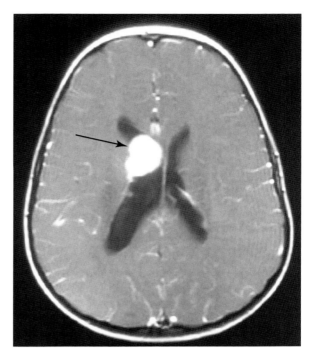

Figure 40–96. Tuberous sclerosis. An enhancing subependymal giant cell astrocytoma *(arrow)* is obstructing the right foramen of Monro, causing hydrocephalus.

the tip of the long arm of the X chromosome. The disorder predominantly affects boys. Craniofacial manifestations include macrocephaly with a prominent jaw, a long, narrow face with a prominent forehead, and prominent ears. *Klinefelter syndrome* (genotype 47 XXY) has been reported in association with macrencephaly.[13] Boys with Klinefelter syndrome may have normal intelligence, although behavioral disorders are common, along with minor disturbances in learning and development.

DEGENERATIVE DISORDERS

Canavan disease is named for Myrtelle Canavan, an American neurologist who first described the disorder in 1931. It is an autosomal recessive leukodystrophy caused by mutation in the gene for the enzyme aspartoacylase, leading to accumulations of N-acetylaspartate and deterioration of the white matter, predominantly affecting individuals of eastern European (Ashkenazi) Jewish descent. Canavan disease is a progressive cerebral spongiform degenerative disorder characterized by vacuolization of the deep layers of the cortex and the subcortical white matter. The infantile form presents in the first few months of life with hypotonia and macrencephaly. The natural history is one of mental retardation, loss of acquired motor skills, hypotonia, and acquired blindness, with death usually occurring by 3 to 4 years of age. The diagnosis can be confirmed on urine organic acid analysis by the finding of elevated levels of N-acetylaspartate. Treatment is supportive.

Alexander disease is a sporadic progressive leukodystrophy described by W. Stewart Alexander, a 20th century English pathologist. Three clinical syndromes have been described: the infantile, juvenile, and adult forms. The infantile form of the disease is the most common and is characterized by macrocephaly, developmental delay, spasticity, and seizures. Onset is at age 6 months on the average, but clinical manifestations may be seen shortly after birth. The predominant feature on cranial MRI is impairment of the white matter anteriorly, with the posterior white matter affected later. The disorder is progressive, usually leading to death within the first decade, and treatment is supportive. The pathologic finding is macrencephaly with Rosenthal fibers—spherical eosinophilic intracytoplasmic inclusion bodies in the astrocytes. Alexander disease results from a mutation in the gene for glial fibrillary acidic protein, an intermediate filament protein found in the Rosenthal fibers.[11]

METABOLIC DISORDERS

Gangliosidoses are marked by the accumulation of gangliosides (glycosphingolipids) in cellular lysosomes secondary to enzymatic deficiency states. The hallmark of the gangliosidoses is *Tay-Sachs disease* (infantile GM2 gangliosidosis), a fatal autosomal recessive disorder. Like Canavan disease, it predominantly affects individuals of Ashkenazi Jewish descent. It is caused by a deficiency of the enzyme hexosaminidase A, which leads to accumulation of the lipid GM2 ganglioside in the central nervous system. Clinical features include macrencephaly, cherry-red spots on the retinal maculae, weakness, psychomotor retardation, seizures, and blindness, leading to death in early childhood. The macular findings were described by British ophthalmologist Warren Tay in 1881 and the clinical and pathologic findings were described by American neurologist Bernard Sachs in 1887.

Macrencephaly may also be seen with other GM1 and GM2 gangliosidoses. *Sandhoff disease* is a variant of Tay-Sachs disease in which GM2 ganglioside accumulates because of deficiency of both hexosaminidase A and B. The clinical manifestations are similar to those of Tay-Sachs disease, with the addition of visceromegaly.

Enlargement of the Cerebrospinal Fluid Spaces

BACKGROUND

Macrocephaly related to enlargement of the CSF spaces occurs in relation to hydrocephalus or one of its variants. *Hydrocephalus* (Greek *hydro*, "water," *kephale*, "head") represents a pathologic accumulation of intracranial CSF usually, but not always, within the cerebral ventricles. The rate of formation of CSF for children and adults is approximately 0.3 mL/min, or 20 mL/h.[23,71] The rate of formation is lower for premature infants. Most of the CSF is produced in the ventricles by the choroid plexus in an energy-dependent active transport process. Approximately 10% to 20% of CSF production is extrachoroidal, coming from the substance of the brain and spinal cord.[69] The total volume of CSF in the newborn is approximately 50 mL, increasing to approximately 150 mL in the adult, with approximately 25 mL contained in the ventricles and the remainder in the subarachnoid space surrounding the brain and spinal cord.

Choroid plexus is present in each of the four ventricular chambers, and CSF flows from the lateral ventricles into the third ventricle through the paired intraventricular foramina of Monro, and from the third ventricle to the fourth ventricle through the narrow aqueduct of Sylvius. CSF exits the fourth ventricle through the foramina of Magendie and Luschka and circulates through the subarachnoid space, to be reabsorbed into the venous system in the arachnoid villi and pacchionian granulations, microtubular evaginations of the subarachnoid space in the venous sinuses. The granulations are most prominently located in the parieto-occipital region of the superior sagittal sinus.

In general, symptomatic hydrocephalus may develop from an imbalance between the rate of CSF formation and absorption. In practice, symptomatic hydrocephalus almost always results from an impairment in the circulation or absorption of CSF. The sole exception to this is the choroid plexus papilloma, a benign tumor which usually occurs in the atrium of the lateral ventricle in children and causes hydrocephalus in association with overproduction of CSF.

Hydrocephalus may be classified as *obstructive* or *ex vacuo*. Ex vacuo hydrocephalus, related to a reduction in the volume of cerebral tissue due to malformation or atrophy, does not cause macrocephaly. For purposes of this discussion, we consider only obstructive hydrocephalus, which is almost always related to impairment in the circulation or absorption of CSF. Obstructive hydrocephalus may be further subdivided based on the location of the obstruction. A blockage in the ventricular system that prevents CSF from entering the subarachnoid space causes noncommunicating hydrocephalus (e.g., aqueductal stenosis, atresia of the foramina of Monro, intraventricular neoplasm). In *noncommunicating hydrocephalus,* there is enlargement of the ventricular chambers rostral to the site of obstruction. A blockage outside the ventricular system that permits the ventricular CSF to communicate with the subarachnoid space but prevents absorption into the venous system causes *communicating hydrocephalus* (e.g., subarachnoid hemorrhage, meningitis).

Hydrocephalus may also be classified as congenital or acquired. Examples of congenital hydrocephalus include aqueductal stenosis, Dandy-Walker malformation, Chiari II malformation, and X-linked hydrocephalus. Examples of acquired hydrocephalus include neoplasm, posthemorrhagic hydrocephalus, and postmeningitic hydrocephalus. No classification scheme is perfect, and there is overlap among the different categories. For example, aqueductal stenosis may be congenital or acquired. In approximately 15% of cases, hydrocephalus may be idiopathic, with no definitive congenital or acquired etiology discernible.[45]

The clinical presentation of hydrocephalus depends on the status of the cranial sutures. In the newborn with open cranial sutures, macrocephaly is the presenting sign. In children over the age of 2 years, hydrocephalus usually presents with signs of increased intracranial pressure. Infantile hydrocephalus may be associated with rapid head growth, and charting may show the head circumference crossing percentiles. The fontanelles become full and tense even when the child is upright, and the cranial sutures become split. In the newborn, the cranial sutures can sometimes be slightly split in the absence of a pathologic process. A useful sign for increased intracranial pressure, usually due to hydrocephalus, is splaying of the squamosal suture, which runs horizontally above the ear between the temporal and parietal bones.

In advanced cases of hydrocephalus, the forehead is prominent, or bossed, the hair is sparse, and the skull is thin. Percussion of the head can yield a "cracked pot" sound (Macewen sign). If the cortical mantle is less than 1 cm in thickness, transillumination can demonstrate the pathologic accumulation of CSF. Unilateral or bilateral esotropia may result from paresis of the abducens nerve (cranial nerve VI), which has the longest course of all the cranial nerves. The "setting sun" sign is characterized by conjugate downward deviation of the eyes such that the sclera is seen above the iris, and is due to hydrocephalic compression of the vertical gaze center in the mesencephalic tectum. Papilledema is seen in older children and adults but is rare in children, likely because of the open cranial sutures. The presence of a prominent occipital shelf with a high-riding external occipital protuberance suggests a posterior fossa cyst or the Dandy-Walker malformation (cystic transformation of the fourth ventricle).

The simplest and safest of the neurodiagnostic imaging studies is ultrasonography (US). Cranial CT and MRI provide more anatomic detail. Prenatal imaging can be performed with US and, more recently, with MRI (Fig. 40-97).

Several etiologies of hydrocephalus in the newborn are discussed in the following sections.

AQUEDUCTAL STENOSIS

Stenosis of the aqueduct of Sylvius may be congenital or acquired and accounts for approximately 10% of cases of pediatric hydrocephalus. The cerebral aqueduct is a narrow, ependyma-lined conduit that connects the third ventricle with the fourth ventricle. At birth, the aqueduct measures approximately 0.5 mm in diameter and 3 mm in length.[30]

Stenosis of the aqueduct produces noncommunicating hydrocephalus, with enlargement of the lateral and third ventricles but a normal-sized fourth ventricle on neuroimaging studies (Fig. 40-98). Congenital aqueductal stenosis can be accompanied by forking, or branching of small aqueductal channels. Membranous obstruction of the aqueduct can result from a thin ependymal veil, often at the distal portion of the aqueduct. Aqueductal gliosis may follow perinatal hemorrhage or infection. Viral infections may cause aqueductal stenosis, and some experimental models of aqueductal stenosis are virally induced. In X-linked hydrocephalus (Bickers-Adams syndrome), aqueductal stenosis is accompanied by mental retardation and flexion-adduction abnormalities of the thumbs.[8] This disorder is caused by a mutation in the gene encoding the L1 cellular adhesion molecule, a glycoprotein at the cell surface mediating neural cell recognition.[44] Acquired aqueductal stenosis can occur as the consequence of a neoplasm. Characteristically, the tumor is a low-grade astrocytoma of the quadrigeminal plate (tectal glioma).[73] Occasionally, nontumoral stenosis of the aqueduct can occur in children with neurofibromatosis type 1.[77]

DANDY-WALKER MALFORMATION

See also Part 1 of this chapter.

The *Dandy-Walker malformation* consists of cystic transformation of the fourth ventricle, partial or complete agenesis of the cerebellar vermis, and enlargement of the posterior cranial fossa with upward displacement of the torcular herophili, transverse sinuses, and tentorium (Fig. 40-99). Enlargement of the supratentorial ventricular system may be present at birth or may develop over time. The malformation occurs in approximately 1 in 25,000 live births and is more frequent in

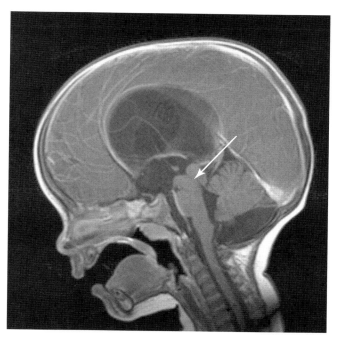

Figure 40–98. Aqueductal stenosis. T1-weighted sagittal magnetic resonance image shows noncommunicating hydrocephalus secondary to stenosis of the aqueduct of Sylvius (*arrow*). The lateral and third ventricles are enlarged, with a normal-sized fourth ventricle. An arachnoid cyst is present inferior to the cerebellum.

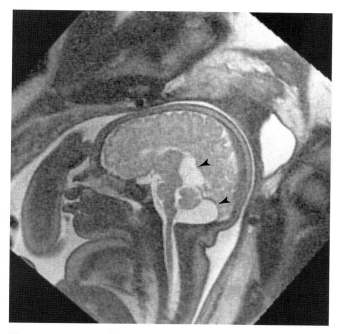

Figure 40–97. Fetal magnetic resonance image. Intrauterine sagittal view of the brain showing a quadrigeminal plate arachnoid cyst and a large cisterna magna (*arrowheads*).

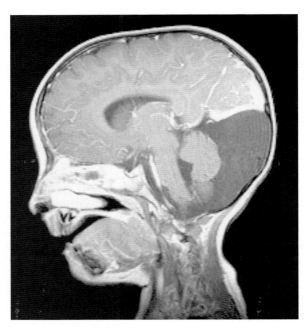

Figure 40–99. Dandy-Walker malformation. T1-weighted sagittal magnetic resonance image shows cystic transformation of the fourth ventricle with enlargement of the posterior fossa, elevation of the torcular herophili, and dysgenesis of the inferior cerebellar vermis.

girls than boys. Infants can present with macrocephaly and an enlarged posterior fossa that precedes the development of hydrocephalus.[37] Mental retardation due to associated supratentorial abnormalities is present in approximately half the cases.[15]

Most children with the Dandy-Walker malformation have hydrocephalus. MRI is useful for demonstrating other anomalies, including agenesis of the corpus callosum, absence of the septum pellucidum, heterotopias, polymicrogyria, aqueductal stenosis, and, occasionally, the presence of an occipital encephalocele or meningocele. Systemic anomalies may include cleft lip and palate, polydactyly, craniofacial malformations, and cardiac abnormalities.[70] The differential diagnosis includes the Dandy-Walker variant, in which the posterior fossa is not enlarged, and the retrocerebellar arachnoid cyst and mega cisterna magna, in which there is no hypoplasia of the cerebellar vermis.

CHIARI II MALFORMATION

See also Part 8.

The *Chiari II malformation*, described in 1896 by Hans Chiari, a pathologist from Prague, is a complex disorder occurring in almost all children with myelomeningocele. Most patients with the Chiari II malformation have hydrocephalus, either from aqueductal stenosis or a block at the outflow of the fourth ventricle, and most require treatment by placement of a diversionary extracranial ventricular shunt. Hydrosyringomyelia may also be present. Multiple associated anomalies affect the skull, dura, and central nervous system. Lückenschädel, or lacunar skull, appears as regions of calvarial thinning that are present in the fetus and usually disappear during the first year of life. The posterior cranial fossa is small with a wide foramen magnum, a low-lying tentorium, and low-lying transverse sinuses. There are often fenestrations in the falx cerebri. The hindbrain is abnormal because of a failure of the embryologic pontine flexure, with herniation of the cerebellar vermis below the foramen magnum and above the tentorial incisura, kinking of the medulla, and elongation of the fourth ventricle. The tectum is beaked and the massa intermedia is enlarged. Enlargement of the occipital horns of the lateral ventricles (colpocephaly) may occur in association with dysgenesis of the corpus callosum. The cerebral hemispheres often contain narrow, elongated gyri (stenogyria) and neuronal heterotopias. The radiographic features of the Chiari II malformation are best detected on MRI (Fig. 40-100), and many features can now be seen accurately on prenatal MRI.

The most obvious clinical manifestation of the Chiari II malformation is the presence of a myelomeningocele. Although hydrocephalus almost always accompanies the Chiari II malformation, the head may not be enlarged at birth. In fact, the head circumference may be small at birth owing to decompression of CSF into the myelomeningocele sac. Approximately 25% of infants with myelomeningocele are born with a head circumference less than the 5th percentile.[52] The head circumference may begin to expand rapidly after closure of the myelomeningocele defect.[70] Other clinical signs in infants with the Chiari II malformation are related to brainstem or cranial nerve dysfunction and include respiratory distress with inspiratory stridor, swallowing difficulties with a depressed gag response, apnea, weak cry, and quadriparesis. Hindbrain dysfunction in the Chiari II malformation may be due to compressive or ischemic factors, but also to dysgenesis of cranial nerve nuclei in the brainstem.

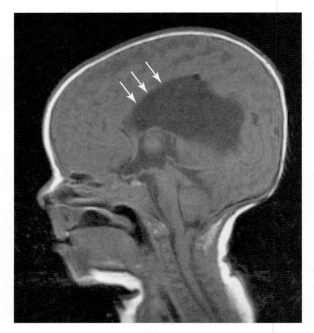

Figure 40–100. Chiari II malformation. T1-weighted sagittal magnetic resonance image shows partial agenesis of the corpus callosum (*arrows*) and multiple anomalies, including enlargement of the massa intermedia, beaking of the tectum, herniation of the cerebellum below the foramen magnum, and kinking of the medulla.

The most frequent cause of brainstem dysfunction in patients with the Chiari II malformation and shunted hydrocephalus is malfunction of the ventricular shunt.

POSTHEMORRHAGIC HYDROCEPHALUS

See also Part 3.

The subependymal periventricular germinal matrix is a site of significant cellular activity during the second and third trimester. Gelatinous in texture, it serves as a focus of neuronal and glial proliferation. The matrix has a rich vascular supply with a complex capillary bed containing large, immature, irregular vessels. After the cellular precursor activity, the germinal matrix undergoes a progressive decrease in size, and by 36 weeks' gestation it is almost completely involuted.[78]

The site of origin of intraventricular hemorrhage (IVH) in neonates is characteristically the subependymal germinal matrix (Fig. 40-101). The significant vascularity, location in the watershed zone, and paucity of vascular supportive tissue make the germinal matrix particularly susceptible to hemorrhage.[33] Neonatal IVH is thought to occur because of fluctuations in cerebral blood flow to the immature germinal matrix vasculature.[60] Because this matrix is largely involuted at term, neonatal IVH is primarily a disorder of the preterm infant. The incidence of IVH in infants weighing less than 1500 g is significant, previously estimated to be approximately 40%,[14,53,58] with most hemorrhages apparent within the first 24 hours of life. Incidence has declined markedly over the last decade (see also Part 3).

Posthemorrhagic ventriculomegaly is a common consequence of germinal matrix hemorrhage. Posthemorrhagic hydrocephalus (PHH), defined as ventriculomegaly, elevated intracranial pressure, and increasing occipitofrontal head circumference is also a consequence of germinal matrix hemorrhage. PHH occurs more commonly in infants who have sustained more severe, higher-grade hemorrhages (Fig. 40-102). Interestingly, PHH occurs less commonly in preterm infants with very low birthweight and the youngest gestational ages.[53] PHH is usually a communicating hydrocephalus, secondary to an obliterative arachnoiditis over

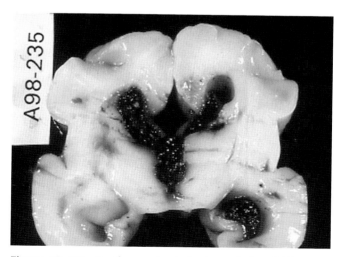

Figure 40–101. Posthemorrhagic hydrocephalus. Diffuse intraventricular hemorrhage secondary to germinal matrix bleed is seen in this coronal specimen.

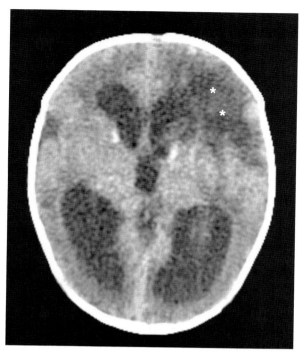

Figure 40–102. Posthemorrhagic hydrocephalus after grade IV intraventricular hemorrhage of prematurity. Computed tomography scan demonstrates enlargement of the lateral ventricles and region of left frontal encephalomalacia (*asterisks*) at the site of a parenchymal hemorrhage.

the cerebral convexities at the site of the arachnoid granulations (pacchionian villi), or at the outflow foramina of the fourth ventricle in the posterior cranial fossa. Occasionally, PHH may be a noncommunicating hydrocephalus because of obstruction of the aqueduct from intraventricular blood or blood degradation products, or subependymal scarring.

It may sometimes be difficult to differentiate posthemorrhagic ventriculomegaly from PHH. Periventricular hemorrhagic infarction may lead to encephalomalacia with relative ventriculomegaly as a consequence of volume loss. In PHH, the ventriculomegaly is often accompanied by increased head circumference and intracranial pressure. Sometimes, however, progressive hydrocephalus can develop without enlargement of the head circumference. This occurs because the immature periventricular white matter, with its paucity of myelin and excess of water, is the site of lowest resistance, allowing the ventricles to dilate before expanding the tougher dura and skull.

Treatment strategies for PHH involve a team approach. Daily neurologic examination with measurement of the OFC and weekly transfontanelle US of the brain provide useful longitudinal data to follow (Fig. 40-103). Medical therapy with acetazolamide, a noncompetitive carbonic anhydrase inhibitor, or furosemide, a loop diuretic, may provide relief, but these are usually temporizing agents. Careful monitoring of fluid and electrolyte balance is essential. Usually symptomatic hydrocephalus requires intervention with measures to remove CSF. In communicating hydrocephalus, serial lumbar punctures may be instituted. If lumbar punctures fail, or if there is noncommunicating hydrocephalus, then measures

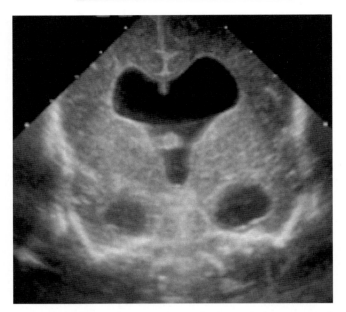

Figure 40–103. Posthemorrhagic hydrocephalus. Coronal ultrasonographic scan shows enlarged lateral ventricles and intraventricular blood.

are instituted to remove CSF from the ventricles. Such measures include ventricular taps, ventricular catheters with subgaleal reservoirs that can be tapped, ventriculosubgaleal shunts, external ventricular drains, or ventriculoperitoneal shunts. Because of the increased incidence of loculated hydrocephalus after ventricular taps, these procedures are usually reserved for infants in need of emergent CSF diversion.

POSTINFECTIOUS HYDROCEPHALUS

Communicating hydrocephalus may develop in the newborn as a consequence of arachnoidal scarring from congenital or acquired infection. Intrauterine transplacental infection (e.g., toxoplasmosis and other TORCH infections) may cause hydrocephalus due to meningoencephalitis, with pathologic changes in the subarachnoid space and cerebral parenchyma.[3,39] This may lead to the classic clinical triad of hydrocephalus, chorioretinitis, and intracranial calcification. Congenital syphilis may, on occasion, produce hydrocephalus.

Bacterial meningitis can lead to an acute acquired hydrocephalus secondary to the effects of purulent exudate in the subarachnoid space or chronic acquired hydrocephalus secondary to inflammatory fibrosis. Bacterial meningitis is a more common cause of hydrocephalus than viral meningitis. Neonates with bacterial meningitis usually have simultaneous sepsis. Among the more common causes of neonatal meningitis are group B streptococci, *Escherichia coli, Listeria monocytogenes,* and *Klebsiella pneumoniae.* In general, bacterial infection tends to obstruct the cortical subarachnoid space, whereas granulomatous infection (e.g., tuberculosis) blocks the CSF cisterns, causing a hydrocephalus secondary to basal meningitis. The incidence of postinfectious meningitis in the United States has declined on the basis of improvements in neonatal diagnosis and treatment.

EXTERNAL HYDROCEPHALUS

External hydrocephalus is a benign condition characterized by macrocephaly and widening of the subarachnoid space, particularly over the frontal lobes and in the interhemispheric fissure[36] (Fig. 40-104). The sylvian fissures may be widened. Ventricular enlargement, if present, is usually mild. The condition has also been called benign external communicating hydrocephalus of infancy, and appears related to benign familial macrocephaly, sometimes called *familial macrencephaly,* discussed earlier.

External hydrocephalus is probably a mild variant of communicating hydrocephalus caused by defective resorption of CSF at the arachnoid villi. It is a generally benign condition associated with a large, square-shaped head that may cross percentiles. A family history of macrocephaly is frequently identified.[4] Cognitive and motor development are usually normal or minimally delayed. The head size gradually levels off and the condition usually remits by age 2 to 3 years. Surgical intervention is almost never required.[70]

The condition in neonates may not always be benign. Lorch and colleagues[51] examined the natural history of graduates of the neonatal intensive care unit with macrocephaly and "benign" extra-axial fluid collections and found that they were more likely to have developmental delay and cerebral palsy than macrocephalic survivors who did not stay in the neonatal intensive care unit. They were also more likely to have bronchopulmonary dysplasia and to require the use of extracorporeal membrane oxygenation than control subjects. When the clinical course of external hydrocephalus is not benign, other disorders should be considered. Infants with a significant motor delay or movement disorder, such as choreoathetosis, should undergo further evaluation to exclude a metabolic problem such as glutaric aciduria.

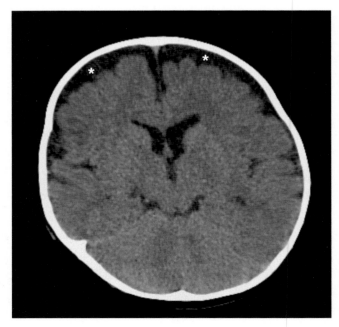

Figure 40–104. Benign external hydrocephalus of infancy. Computed tomography scan shows bifrontal extracerebral cerebrospinal fluid collections (*asterisks*).

HYDRANENCEPHALY

Hydranencephaly is a rare congenital anomaly marked by almost complete absence of the cerebral hemispheres. It is thought to occur as the result of a major in utero vascular insult during the second trimester, particularly bilateral occlusion of the carotid arteries. The brain undergoes intrauterine liquefaction and is essentially reduced to a bag of water, a meningeal sac containing CSF with a high protein content (Fig. 40-105). The diencephalon, brainstem, and posterior fossa structures are spared, and a thin occipital cortical rim may permit some visual function.

The newborn with hydranencephaly may appear neurologically normal at birth because of the normally functioning thalami and brainstem. Difficulty with visual fixing and following may be appreciated. The head size may be normal or even small at birth but can enlarge rapidly owing to malabsorption of the proteinaceous CSF. On occasion, the diagnosis of hydranencephaly is made after several months because of failure to achieve developmental milestones.

Significant macrocephaly may be treated with a ventriculoperitoneal shunt. The decision to shunt can be difficult because shunting is primarily done for social reasons and does not lead to an improved level of neurologic function. The long-term outcome for infants with hydranencephaly is poor, and most do not live for more than 1 or 2 years.

Hydranencephaly can be diagnosed by US, although CT and MRI are more accurate (Fig. 40-106). Hydranencephaly is distinguished from anencephaly by the presence of intact meninges and skull. It is important to distinguish between hydranencephaly and advanced hydrocephalus, which may have a similar clinical and radiographic presentation. The compressed cerebral mantle in hydrocephalus can expand, sometimes dramatically, after ventricular shunt placement.

INTRACRANIAL CYSTS

Intracranial cysts are rare causes of congenital macrocephaly. Arachnoid cysts arise from a duplication of the arachnoid membrane and are most commonly located in the middle cranial fossa, with up to 50% of intracranial arachnoid cysts located in this region (Fig. 40-107). They occur more frequently in boys than girls, and more often on the left side than the right. Arachnoid cysts may also be seen in the suprasellar area, over the cerebral convexity, and in the posterior fossa. Some cysts, such as suprasellar arachnoid cysts, may obstruct the ventricular system and cause hydrocephalus. Symptomatic arachnoid cysts are treated with fenestration or shunting procedures.

Neuroepithelial cysts are benign developmental cysts believed to have a neuroectodermal origin. Choroid plexus cysts are the most common of the neuroepithelial cysts. They are usually asymptomatic, can be diagnosed on prenatal US, and may involute spontaneously. Occasionally choroid plexus cysts can obstruct CSF flow in the ventricles and cause hydrocephalus. Intraventricular cysts may form in relation to the septum pellucidum, a midline ependyma-lined structure

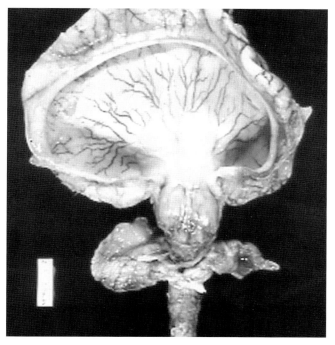

Figure 40–105. Hydranencephaly secondary to intrauterine liquefactive necrosis, sagittal specimen.

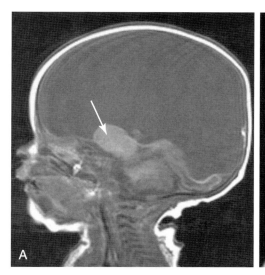
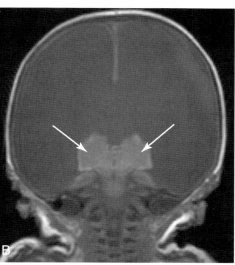

Figure 40–106. Hydranencephaly. T1-weighted sagittal (A) and coronal (B) magnetic resonance images show almost complete absence of the cerebral hemispheres, with preservation of the thalami (*arrows*) and hindbrain.

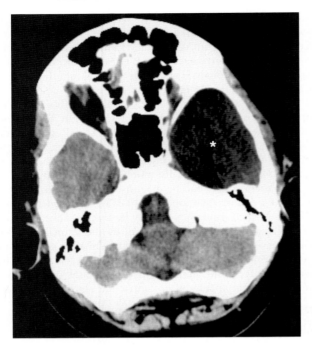

Figure 40–107. Arachnoid cyst. Computed tomography scan shows large arachnoid cyst (*asterisk*) of the left middle cranial fossa.

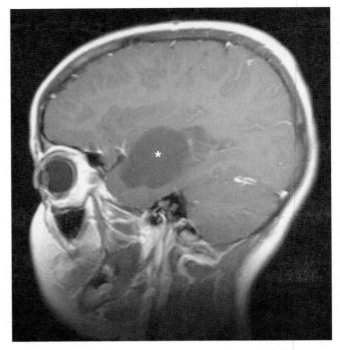

Figure 40–108. Dysembryoplastic neuroepithelial tumor, a low-grade primary neoplasm of the right temporal lobe (*asterisk*). T1-weighted sagittal contrast-enhanced magnetic resonance image.

that separates the two lateral ventricles. In the embryo a cavity or cavum is present between the leaves of the septum pellucidum. This cavum of the septum pellucidum usually involutes shortly after birth but can persist asymptomatically in 20% of the population. Rarely, an intraventricular cavum septum pellucidum cyst develops that may obstruct the foramina of Monro and cause hydrocephalus. Even more rarely, a cyst of the cavum vergae, the posterior extent of the septum pellucidum, can enlarge and obstruct the foramina of Monro.

Presence or Enlargement of Other Structures

NEOPLASMS

Brain tumors in the neonate are uncommon. The most common presenting sign, regardless of histology, is macrocephaly, and most tumors are quite large.[80] Isaacs[38] reviewed 250 cases of fetal and neonatal brain tumors from the literature and found a survival rate of 28%. In children younger than 1 year of age, the preponderance of brain tumors is located supratentorially.[32] Slow-growing tumors such as the choroid plexus papilloma, low-grade astrocytoma, and ganglioglioma have the most favorable prognosis (Fig. 40-108). Rapidly growing tumors such as the primitive neuroectodermal tumor (Fig. 40-109) and malignant teratoma have a much poorer prognosis.

VASCULAR LESIONS

Rarely, macrocephaly in the newborn may be secondary to a *vein of Galen malformation*. Named for Claudius Galen of Pergamon, who described the deep venous system, this vascular

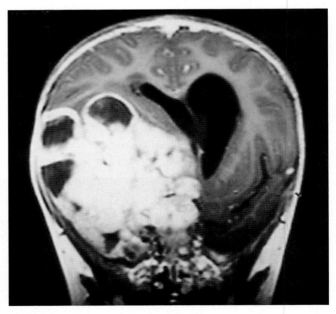

Figure 40–109. Large primitive neuroectodermal tumor of the right temporal lobe shown deforming the brain on a contrast-enhanced, T1-weighted coronal magnetic resonance image.

malformation arises in the first trimester of pregnancy as a persistent embryonic promesencephalic vein of Markowski.

The clinical presentation of a vein of Galen malformation in the neonate is dramatic. Massive shunting of blood through the arteriovenous fistula produces a refractory, high-output congestive heart failure. Cerebral venous hypertension and vascular steal lead to cerebral ischemia and infarction. A loud intracranial bruit can be auscultated at the vertex. Hydrocephalus may cause progressive head enlargement, occasionally requiring early shunting. Macrocephaly with seizures and developmental delay is a more common presentation in the infant than the newborn. Treatment is directed at endovascular obliteration of the fistula. The morbidity and mortality of the neonatal vein of Galen malformation remain high.

TRAUMA

See also Chapter 28.

Traumatic intracranial hemorrhage can lead to macrocephaly before the sutures are closed. The most common cause of traumatic macrocephaly in the neonate is subdural hematoma due to birth trauma. The hematoma is often located posteriorly, in relation to the tentorium ("tentorial tear"). The differential diagnosis includes postnatal trauma, including nonaccidental trauma, and bleeding diathesis (Fig. 40-110). The head circumference can increase rapidly, with a full anterior fontanelle. Consciousness may be impaired, with abnormal posturing and seizures. Diagnosis is best confirmed by CT. Subdural hematomas in the neonate may be unilateral or bilateral. Treatment may require craniotomy for acute bleeds. Subacute or chronic bleeds may be evacuated through a burr hole, sometimes with placement of a subdural drain or shunt.

INFECTION

Brain abscess is a rare cause of macrocephaly in the neonate. Risks factors include cyanotic congenital heart disease, pulmonary arteriovenous shunts, and impaired host defenses (e.g.,

congenital immunodeficiency states, human immunodeficiency virus infection). Brain abscess may develop from a contiguous otologic or paranasal sinus focus. The clinical presentation is one of systemic illness with elevated intracranial pressure and focal neurologic dysfunction related to location of the abscess. Causative organisms are most commonly aerobic and anaerobic streptococci. Other organisms include staphylococci, gram-negative bacilli, and anaerobes such as *Bacteroides*. Brain abscess is an infrequent complication of meningitis due to *Citrobacter diversus* or *Proteus mirabilis*. Diagnosis is made by CT or MRI, and treatment consists of antimicrobial therapy along with surgical drainage. Antiepileptic medication and corticosteroids are commonly used. It is essential to carry out a search for the underlying cause of the abscess.

Rarely, pyogenic infection occurs in the subdural space as the so-called subdural empyema. The presentation is similar to brain abscess and surgical drainage is an essential part of the treatment.

THE ABNORMALLY SHAPED HEAD

The two most common causes of a misshapen head in infancy are craniosynostosis and deformational plagiocephaly (Box 40-17). The former condition usually requires surgical correction and the latter condition is treated nonsurgically.

Craniosynostosis

Craniosynostosis (Greek *kranion*, "skull," syn, "together," *osteon*, "bone") is a disorder marked by the premature fusion of one or more of the sutures of the skull. Premature cranial suture fusion leads to an abnormally shaped head and, sometimes, facial dysmorphism as well. Occasionally, particularly in cases of multiple suture fusion, craniosynostosis can lead to increased intracranial pressure and neurocognitive impairment (Fig. 40-111). Craniosynostosis is classified as *nonsyndromic* when there is isolated fusion of one or more sutures

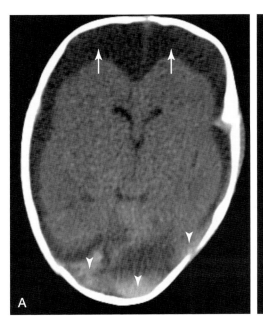

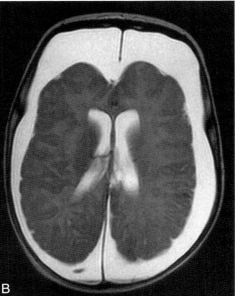

Figure 40-110. Nonaccidental trauma with bilateral subdural hematomas. **A,** Computed tomography scan shows bilateral frontal chronic subdural hematomas (*arrows*) and bilateral occipital acute subdural hematomas (*arrowheads*). **B,** T2-weighted axial magnetic resonance image, same patient, shows the extensive bilateral subdural hematomas.

BOX 40–17 Causes of Abnormal Head Shape

I. CRANIOSYNOSTOSIS

Nonsyndromic
Sagittal synostosis
Unilateral coronal synostosis
Bilateral coronal synostosis
Metopic synostosis

Syndromic
Crouzon syndrome
Apert syndrome
Pfeiffer syndrome
Saethre-Chotzen syndrome

II. DEFORMATIONAL PLAGIOCEPHALY

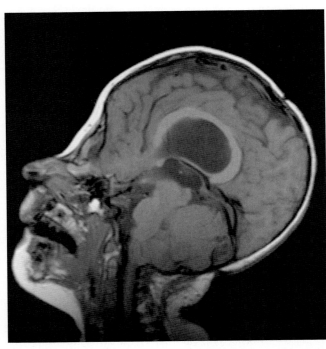

Figure 40–111. Brachyturricephaly secondary to multiple-suture synostosis, T1-weighted sagittal magnetic resonance image. Note the towering head. A basal frontal encephalocele is present with inferior herniation of the frontal lobes into the sphenoid sinus.

without associated anomalies and as *syndromic* when there is phenotypic expression of associated craniofacial, skeletal, and extraskeletal malformations. Craniosynostosis is also classified as *primary* or *secondary*. Most cases of craniosynostosis, whether nonsyndromic or syndromic, are due to primary closure of one or more cranial sutures. Occasionally, craniosynostosis may be secondary to systemic disorders, such as rickets, hyperthyroidism, polycythemia vera, and thalassemia.

In general, the bones of the skull vault grow perpendicular to the cranial sutures, and premature suture fusion restricts bone growth in the plane perpendicular to the fused suture (Virchow's law).[81] Other factors contribute to alterations in head shape, including compensatory bone growth at perimeter sutures, associated premature fusion of sutures at the cranial base in some cases, and mechanical factors such as increased intracranial pressure.

The etiopathogenesis of craniosynostosis is multifactorial. Intrauterine growth constraint, oligohydramnios, and abnormal lodging of the fetal head in the pelvis have been reported.[19,34] The timing of cranial suture fusion is a complex process. The dura signals the cranial sutures to remain patent until brain growth is complete. Alterations in the orchestration of these signals can lead to craniosynostosis. Advances in molecular genetics have implicated defects in fibroblast growth factor receptors (FGFRs) in many cases of craniosynostosis. Fibroblast growth factors are polypeptides whose binding to specialized receptors stimulates tyrosine kinase phosphorylation signaling pathways to direct cell growth and differentiation. Mutations in FGFRs have been found in syndromic and nonsyndromic forms of craniosynostosis. An FGFR2 mutation has been identified in Crouzon syndrome and in Apert syndrome (discussed later). FGFR1 and FGFR2 mutations have been identified in Pfeiffer syndrome. FGFR mutations have also been reported in nonsyndromic craniosynostosis. FGFR3 mutations have been isolated in some cases of nonsyndromic unisutural synostosis.[35,64]

The diagnosis of craniosynostosis is usually made on clinical criteria (Table 40-9). In cases of single suture involvement, skull radiographs confirm the diagnosis by showing sclerosis along all or part of the fused suture and compensatory changes. For complex cases, CT or three-dimensional CT scanning can help to delineate the pathologic process.

NONSYNDROMIC CRANIOSYNOSTOSIS

Sagittal Craniosynostosis

Premature fusion of the sagittal suture is the most common type of craniosynostosis. The prevalence has been estimated at approximately 1 per 1000 live births with a male-to-female

TABLE 40–9 Abnormal Head Shapes

Term	Definition	Fused Suture
Scaphocephaly	Boat head	Sagittal
Dolichocephaly	Long head	Sagittal
Clinocephaly	Saddle head	Sagittal
Brachycephaly	Short head	Bilateral coronal or lambdoid
Plagiocephaly	Oblique head	Unilateral coronal or lambdoid (or may be deformational)
Trigonocephaly	Triangular head	Metopic
Turricephaly	Towering head	Multiple
Acrocephaly	Peaked head	Multiple
Oxycephaly	Pointed head	Multiple
Hypsicephaly	High head	Multiple
Kleeblattschädel	Cloverleaf head	Multiple

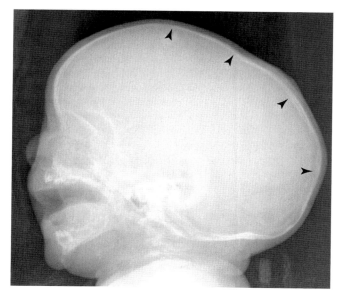

Figure 40–112. Sagittal synostosis. Skull radiograph shows fusion of the sagittal suture (*arrowheads*) with scaphocephaly and frontal bossing.

ratio of 4:1.[10] Sagittal synostosis is usually a sporadic disorder, but up to 10% of cases may be familial, with autosomal dominant inheritance.[47,59]

Infants with sagittal synostosis have a narrow, elongated head with a ridge along the sagittal suture (Fig. 40-112). The craniometric finding is described as scaphocephaly (Greek *skaphe*, "boat," *kephale*, "head") or dolichocephaly (Greek *dolichos*, "long"; see Table 40-9). The parietal diameter is narrow, often with compensatory changes that include frontal bossing, temporal hollowing, and an occipital protuberance (Fig. 40-113). Results of the neurologic examination are most often normal, although some investigators have reported coexistent findings including neurodevelopmental sequelae and even increased intracranial pressure (usually found only in association with multiple-suture synostosis).[41,66,79]

Numerous operative procedures are available for the correction of sagittal craniosynostosis. The surgical outcome is affected by age, with better results, in general, if the correction is performed early, before the age of 6 months.[10] Early correction allows the surgeon to take advantage of rapid brain growth in remodeling the skull—the brain weight triples in the first year of life. The major surgical risk associated with sagittal synostectomy, and for all forms of craniosynostosis surgery, is blood loss.

Unilateral Coronal Craniosynostosis

Premature fusion of one coronal suture produces a characteristic presentation of anterior plagiocephaly (Greek *plagio*, "oblique," *kephale*, "head") with flattening of the ipsilateral forehead and compensatory bossing of the contralateral forehead (Fig. 40-114). A ridge is palpable along the fused suture. The orbit on the affected side is shallow and the zygoma is foreshortened. The superolateral margin of the ipsilateral orbit is drawn upward and backward toward the elevated sphenoid wing, giving rise to the typical "harlequin" deformity on skull radiographs (Fig. 40-115). Facial asymmetry is frequent, often with ipsilateral deviation of the nasal root, contralateral deviation of the nasal tip, and vertical orbital

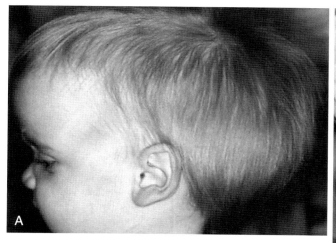
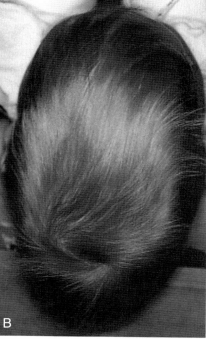

Figure 40–113. Sagittal synostosis, with scaphocephaly, frontal bossing, and protuberance at the occiput. A, Side view. B, Top view.

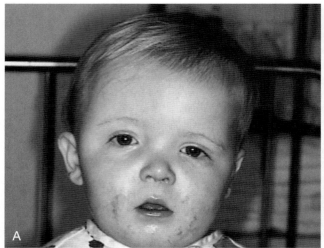

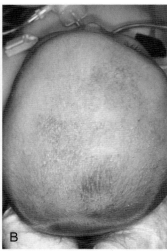

Figure 40–114. Unilateral right coronal synostosis. Note the facial asymmetry, ipsilateral frontal flattening, and vertical orbital dystopia with inferior displacement of the contralateral orbit. **A,** Front view. **B,** Top view.

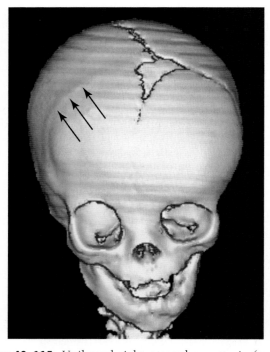

Figure 40–115. Unilateral right coronal synostosis *(arrows)* on three-dimensional computed tomography scan. The ipsilateral orbit is drawn upward and backward (harlequin eye).

dystopia with inferior displacement of the contralateral orbit. There is a slight female predominance.

Although considered a form of simple synostosis due to premature fusion of a single suture, unilateral coronal synostosis is often associated with fusion of other sutures at the cranial base, including the sphenozygomatic, sphenofrontal, and sphenoethmoidal sutures. These sutures constitute the "coronal ring" and interact with one another to affect growth of the anterior cranial fossa.

Surgical correction consists of craniotomy for anterior cranial vault reconstruction, which is usually carried out bilaterally because of the significant side-to-side asymmetry.

The orbital bar is advanced as a "mortise and tenon" bone graft, with surgery facilitated by the introduction of absorbable plates and screws. Variable aesthetic results may be related to the heterogeneous presentation of unicoronal synostosis and the degree of involvement of sutures at the base of the coronal ring.[25]

Bilateral Coronal Craniosynostosis

Bilateral coronal craniosynostosis causes brachycephaly (Greek *brachy*, "short," *kephale*, "head") with palpable ridges over both coronal sutures. The head is foreshortened in the anteroposterior plane, often associated with compensatory widening and increased height (turricephaly; Fig. 40-116). As with unilateral coronal synostosis, there is a female predominance. Surgical repair is similar to that for unicoronal synostosis, with bifrontal craniotomy and orbital bar advancement.

Although bicoronal synostosis may be nonsyndromic, all children with brachycephaly due to premature fusion of the coronal sutures should undergo evaluation to rule out associated malformations. This is because premature fusion of both coronal sutures is the most common pattern observed in syndromic craniosynostosis.

Metopic Craniosynostosis

Premature fusion of the metopic suture accounts for approximately 10% to 20% of patients referred for evaluation of craniosynostosis.[21] As in sagittal synostosis, there is a male predominance. The clinical presentation is trigonocephaly (Greek *trigonon*, "triangle," *kephale*, "head"), which is a characteristic triangular head with a vertical keel over the forehead along the fused metopic suture (Fig. 40-117). The volume of the anterior cranial vault is small, often with associated hypotelorism, elevation of the lateral canthi, and temporal hollowing. A compensatory finding is widening of the biparietal diameter.

Metopic synostosis may occur as an isolated finding without associated neurologic abnormalities, or it may occur with intracranial anomalies including holoprosencephaly and agenesis of the corpus callosum. Infants with mild cranial deformities can be treated nonoperatively.

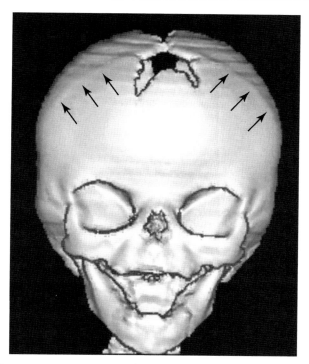

Figure 40–116. Bicoronal synostosis *(arrows)*. Three-dimensional computed tomography scan shows brachyturricephaly.

Significant trigonocephaly usually requires surgical correction by bifrontal craniotomy and orbital bar advancement, which is usually carried out at approximately 6 months of age.

SYNDROMIC CRANIOSYNOSTOSIS

The craniofacial syndromes are relatively rare and often complex. Treatment has been aided by the formation of multidisciplinary craniofacial centers using a coordinated team approach. The craniofacial team includes specialists in anesthesiology, audiology, child life, critical care, developmental therapeutics, genetics, neurosurgery, nursing, occupational therapy, ophthalmology, oral surgery, orthodontics, otolaryngology, dentistry, pediatrics, plastic surgery, social work, and speech therapy.

Surgical correction of syndromic craniosynostosis is carried out by a craniofacial team that includes a pediatric neurosurgeon, plastic surgeon, and anesthesiologist. Surgery is directed at expanding the craniofacial skeleton and may include anterior cranial vault (fronto-orbital) expansion, posterior cranial vault expansion, and sometimes combined anterior and posterior cranial vault expansion.

The more common forms of syndromic craniosynostosis are discussed in the following paragraphs.

Crouzon Syndrome

Crouzon syndrome, or craniofacial dysostosis, was originally described by Octave Crouzon, a French neurologist, in 1912.[22] The incidence of Crouzon syndrome is approximately 1 in 25,000 births, with an autosomal dominant mode of inheritance. Approximately half of the cases of Crouzon syndrome are familial. The rest arise as spontaneous mutations, with the suggestion that advanced paternal age at conception is implicated in some instances.[46] A mutation of the FGFR2 gene has been identified in more than half the cases.

The clinical presentation of Crouzon syndrome is variable. Typical features include brachycephaly with exophthalmos and maxillary hypoplasia (Fig. 40-118). Subluxation of the globes can occur in advanced cases. The head shape is determined by the degree of premature cranial suture fusion. Craniosynostosis is usually not present at birth but evolves during the first year of life. The coronal sutures are fused in almost all cases. The lambdoid and sagittal sutures may also fuse prematurely, and there is often premature fusion of the basilar synchondrosis. Other facial features include strabismus, parrot-beak nose, small nasopharynx, arched palate, and mandibular prognathism. Extracranial features include fusion of cervical vertebrae, ankylosis of the elbows, and radial head subluxation. Hydrocephalus may occur, although mental retardation is infrequent. A crowded hypoplastic posterior fossa with herniation of the cerebellar tonsils below the foramen magnum

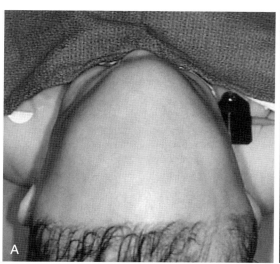
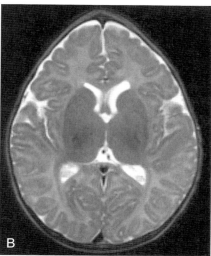

Figure 40–117. Trigonocephaly secondary to premature fusion of the metopic suture. **A,** Top view. **B,** T2-weighted axial magnetic resonance image.

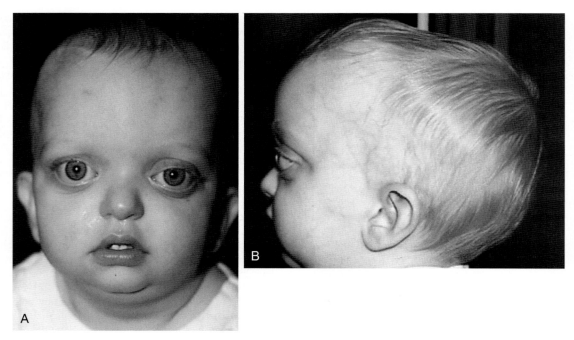

Figure 40–118. Crouzon syndrome (craniofacial dysostosis) with brachyturricephaly, exophthalmos, and maxillary hypoplasia. **A,** Front view. **B,** Side view.

(Chiari-like malformation) has been attributed to early fusion of the lambdoid sutures.[18]

Apert Syndrome

Apert syndrome, or acrocephalosyndactyly type 1, was originally described by the French pediatrician, Eugene Apert, in 1906, based on his observations of one personal case and several other cases published earlier.[5] The prevalence of Apert syndrome has been estimated to be 1 in 55,000 births.[67] Although autosomal dominant transmission has been described, most cases are sporadic, with advanced paternal age considered to be a risk factor.[68] Mutations tend to involve the *FGFR2* gene.[56]

Apert syndrome is characterized by the clinical triad of craniosynostosis, maxillary hypoplasia, and symmetric syndactyly of the hands and feet (Fig. 40-119). There is brachyturricephaly with a flattened occiput. Unlike Crouzon syndrome, the craniofacial anomalies are usually present at birth. Similar to Crouzon syndrome, the craniofacial appearance is determined by which sutures fuse prematurely. The coronal sutures are fused with a widely open anterior fontanelle and metopic suture. The lambdoid sutures are often prematurely fused, as are sutures at the cranial base. There is occasional premature fusion of the sagittal suture.

The cerebral ventricles are often enlarged, and widening of the subarachnoid spaces may be seen. The ventriculomegaly is often nonprogressive but may on occasion lead to frank hydrocephalus with increased intracranial pressure. Malformations of the corpus callosum and septum pellucidum have been described. Mental retardation is common. Mental retardation in Apert syndrome has been shown to correlate with anomalies of the septum pellucidum. Ventriculomegaly and corpus callosum anomalies, on the other

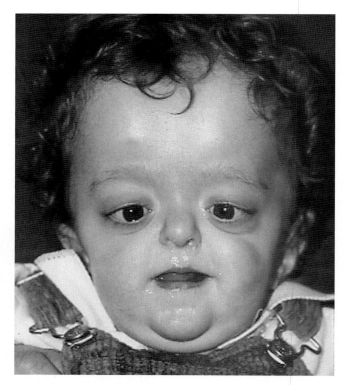

Figure 40–119. Apert syndrome (acrocephalosyndactyly type 1). There is brachyturricephaly, maxillary hypoplasia, hypertelorism with downsloping of the palpebral fissures, and a depressed nasal bridge. The child also has symmetric syndactyly of the hands and feet.

hand, appear to have no influence on intellectual achievement in patients with Apert syndrome.[67] As in Crouzon syndrome, cerebellar tonsillar herniation appears to be a function of a small posterior cranial fossa secondary to premature fusion of the lambdoid sutures.

Ocular hypertelorism (wide separation of the eyes) is present with proptosis and downward slanting of the palpebral fissures (antimongoloid slant).[17] Unlike in Crouzon syndrome, orbital subluxation is rare. Other craniofacial findings include maxillary hypoplasia with a high arched and occasionally cleft palate, relative prognathism with dental malocclusion, and low-set ears with eustachian tube abnormalities. The nose is short and beaked with a small nasopharynx and frequent associated respiratory complications.

The most distinguishing feature of Apert syndrome is symmetric polysyndactyly of the hands and feet, usually involving the second, third, and fourth digits. The syndactyly is both cutaneous and osseous. Other extracranial features may include finger duplication, short humerus, fusion of cervical vertebrae, and scoliosis.

Pfeiffer Syndrome

Pfeiffer syndrome, or acrocephalosyndactyly type 5, was described in 1964 by Rudolf Pfeiffer, a German geneticist who observed members of three generations of a family who had craniosynostosis, broad thumbs and great toes, and variable syndactyly of other digits.[62] Although Pfeiffer syndrome bears similarities to Crouzon and Apert syndromes, it appears to be a distinct disorder, with autosomal dominant inheritance or sporadic presentation. Mutations have been described on the *FGFR1* and *FGFR2* genes. Pfeiffer syndrome is rare, with an estimated incidence of 1 in 200,000 live births.[6]

The Pfeiffer phenotype shares features with Crouzon and Apert syndrome, including brachyturricephaly, exorbitism, maxillary hypoplasia, and mandibular prognathism. The coronal sutures are fused, with variable fusion of multiple sutures, including lambdoid, sagittal, metopic, and frontosphenoidal. Convolution markings on the inner surface of the skull can signify increased intracranial pressure (Fig. 40-120). Hydrocephalus may develop. The nose is beaked with a depressed nasal bridge, and the palate is high and arched with

a bifid uvula. The thumbs and great toes are broad, short, and medially deviated. Syndactyly of the hands and feet is sometimes present.

Patients with Pfeiffer syndrome have been differentiated into three groups.[20] Type I Pfeiffer syndrome is the classic form that was described by Pfeiffer and is associated with normal intellect and a favorable prognosis. Types II and III are associated with severe central nervous system abnormalities, mental retardation, and developmental delay. Type III has the poorest prognosis and is differentiated from type II by the presence of a cloverleaf deformity of the skull.

Cloverleaf skull, or *kleeblattschädel*, describes a trilobar skull shape associated with multiple-suture synostosis. Kleeblattschädel is a descriptive term rather than a unique craniofacial syndrome. It represents the most severe form of multiple-suture craniosynostosis and has been reported in a variety of disorders, including Crouzon and Apert syndromes. It is seen most commonly in Pfeiffer syndrome type III. There is invariably hydrocephalus and increased intracranial pressure. The coronal, metopic, and lambdoid sutures are prematurely fused. The characteristic trefoil appearance is the result of brain herniating through the patent sagittal and squamosal sutures.

Saethre-Chotzen Syndrome

This craniofacial syndrome was described independently by Haakon Saethre, a Norwegian psychiatrist, in 1931, and F. Chotzen, a German psychiatrist, in 1932.[27,72] Saethre-Chotzen syndrome, or acrocephalosyndactyly type 3, is usually transmitted by autosomal dominant inheritance, with some cases occurring sporadically. Mutations of the *TWIST* gene, which maps to the short arm of chromosome 7 (7p21-22), have been identified.[12,29]

Clinical manifestations of Saethre-Chotzen syndrome include brachycephaly, maxillary hypoplasia, ptosis, hypertelorism, low-set hairline, small, round, angulated ears, and occasionally a beaked nose. There may be premature fusion of one or both coronal sutures, with metopic and lambdoid suture fusion found in some cases. Some individuals may have syndactyly of the second and third fingers, brachydactyly, and broad great toes. Intelligence is usually normal.

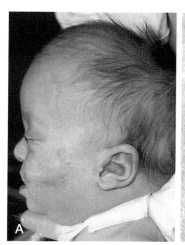 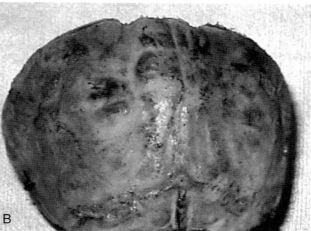

Figure 40–120. Pfeiffer syndrome (acrocephalosyndactyly type 5). **A,** Side view. There is brachyturricephaly, maxillary hypoplasia, and choanal atresia (note indwelling tracheostomy). The child also has broad thumbs and great toes. **B,** Undersurface of the skull at craniofacial reconstruction. Note the convolutional markings from increased intracranial pressure.

Deformational Plagiocephaly

DIAGNOSIS

Cranial asymmetry due to flattening of the occiput is a common condition that is seen with increased frequency in pediatric neurosurgical practices. In neurosurgical practice, cranial asymmetry due to occipital flattening may be the single most common cause for referral. The cranial asymmetry is usually due to mechanical factors and goes by a number of names, including *occipital plagiocephaly, deformational plagiocephaly, positional molding,* and *nonsynostotic occipital plagiocephaly.*

Posterior plagiocephaly is almost always deformational and rarely related to premature fusion of the lambdoid suture. Anterior plagiocephaly, on the other hand, is most commonly due to unilateral coronal synostosis (discussed previously). The incidence of true lambdoid synostosis is very low, estimated to occur in only approximately 3% of patients with craniosynostosis.[59,65]

The prevalence of deformational plagiocephaly has increased dramatically since 1992, when the American Academy of Pediatrics instituted the "back to sleep" program.[43,83] The prone position has been linked with the sudden infant death syndrome, and placing infants on their backs has led to a significant reduction in the frequency of this syndrome. The tradeoff has been an increase in the diagnosis of deformational plagiocephaly, with one institution reporting a sixfold annual increase in referrals to their center beginning in 1992, compared with the previous 13 years.[42]

The diagnosis of deformational plagiocephaly is usually made on the history and confirmed by the physical examination. Typically, the infant has a normal, rounded head at birth. After several weeks or months, the head assumes the shape of a parallelogram. Usually, the child has been lying on his or her back with the head favoring one direction. The parallelogram shape is best seen by examining the head from above. There is unilateral flattening of the occiput with an ipsilateral frontal prominence, creating a characteristic "windswept" appearance. The ipsilateral ear is displaced forward, but both ears are in the same horizontal plane (Fig. 40-121). Radiographic confirmation is unnecessary in typical cases. When skull films are obtained, they usually show patent lambdoid sutures,

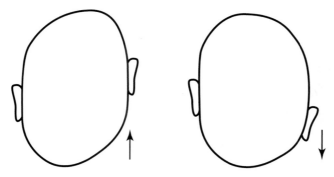

Figure 40–121. Deformational plagiocephaly (left) with right occipital flattening and anterior displacement of the ipsilateral ear. Right lambdoid synostosis (right) with right occipital flattening and posterior and inferior displacement of the ipsilateral ear.

sometimes with associated perisutural sclerosis. Perisutural sclerosis has no diagnostic value because in true lambdoid synostosis the suture is obliterated radiographically.[59] A common CT finding in deformational plagiocephaly is prominent extra-axial CSF collections (widening of the subarachnoid spaces).[26]

Deformational plagiocephaly is differentiated from true lambdoid synostosis by several features. Statistically, true lambdoid synostosis occurs much more infrequently. Lambdoid synostosis is more likely to cause occipital flattening at the time of birth. Lambdoid synostosis, like deformational plagiocephaly, causes ipsilateral occipital flattening, but in lambdoid synostosis the ipsilateral ear is drawn posteriorly and inferiorly compared with the contralateral ear, and the skull shape is that of a rhomboid rather than a parallelogram. The degree of frontal asymmetry in lambdoid synostosis is less than in deformational plagiocephaly, and the frontal bossing tends to be contralateral rather than ipsilateral. The foramen magnum is drawn toward the fused suture in lambdoid synostosis and appears normal in deformational plagiocephaly. A ridge is sometimes, but not always, palpable along the fused suture in lambdoid synostosis.

Deformational plagiocephaly may be associated with multiple forces acting on the skull. Prenatal factors include uterine abnormalities such as a bicornuate uterus, uterine crowding due to a large fetus, twinning, or a pelvic lie. Postnatal factors include behavioral perseverance (child favors a particular position), torticollis with shortening or contracture of the sternocleidomastoid or trapezius muscles, head tilt from trochlear nerve palsy, and congenital vertebral disorders such as hemivertebrae or Klippel-Feil syndrome.[27]

TREATMENT

Management strategies for deformational plagiocephaly include preventive counseling, exercises and mechanical adjustments, skull-molding helmets, and surgery.

To prevent deformational plagiocephaly, parents should be instructed to alternate the head position when the newborn infant is put down to sleep in the supine position. Alternately placing the left occiput down and the right occiput down helps protect against cumulative deformational forces at a time when the skull is maximally deformable. The general principle is to avoid continuous pressure at one site. Prone positioning can be used when the infant is awake and under observation ("tummy time"). If plagiocephaly develops, the same principles of repositioning can be used. The position of the crib can be changed to reorient the infant to activity in the room.

Neck range-of-motion exercises are recommended, particularly if there is underlying torticollis. The stretching exercises are usually carried out for several months. They can be performed under supervision of the parents, sometimes with input from a physical therapist. It is recommended that the exercises be done frequently, in groups of three repetitions per exercise, at every diaper change. To stretch the sternocleidomastoid muscle, one hand is placed on the infant's chest and the other rotates the head such that the chin touches the shoulder for approximately 10 seconds. The head is then rotated in the opposite direction. To stretch the trapezius muscle, the head is tilted such that the ear touches one shoulder for approximately 10 seconds. This is repeated for the other side.[61] Most cases of deformational plagiocephaly show some improvement with a regimen of repositioning and exercise. Once the infant begins to sit and spends less time in the recumbent position, further brain growth helps to reshape the head. The process by which the head becomes more rounded is usually slow and goes on for many months. Residual occipital flattening, if it is mild, is often masked by the growth of hair.

Skull-molding helmets can be used to reshape the head. These helmets, or headbands, are lightweight devices that are worn for most of the day, and are designed to place pressure on the prominent areas. Such external orthotic devices tend to work best in younger infants, whose skulls are thinner and more malleable. Headbands have been used to treat deformational plagiocephaly, with reports of improvement in anthropometrically measured cranial asymmetry.[68] Others, however, have reported similar improvement in cranial vault asymmetry using a regimen of aggressive repositioning and exercise only.[57] Exercise and repositioning can be used to treat most cases of mild to moderate deformational plagiocephaly, and headband can be used as therapy for more severe cases.

Surgery for posterior plagiocephaly is usually reserved for selected cases caused by premature fusion of one lambdoid suture (true lambdoid synostosis). Bilateral posterior cranial vault reconstruction gives results that are superior to simple unilateral strip craniectomy or unilateral craniotomy. Very infrequently there is a role for surgery in severe cases of deformational plagiocephaly refractory to nonsurgical measures.

REFERENCES

1. Aicardi J, et al: Spasms in flexion, callosal agenesis, ocular abnormalities: a new syndrome, *Electroencephalogr Clin Neurophysiol* 19:609, 1965.

2. Aisenson M: Closing of the anterior fontanelle, *Pediatrics* 6:223, 1950.

3. Altschuler G: Toxoplasmosis as a cause of hydrocephaly, *Am J Dis Child* 125:251, 1973.

4. Alvarez L, et al: Idiopathic external hydrocephalus: a natural history and relationship to benign familial macrocephaly, *Pediatrics* 77:901, 1986.

5. Apert E: De l'acrocephalosyndactylie, *Bull Med Soc Paris* 23:1310, 1906.

6. Arnaud E, et al: Craniofacial anomalies, In Choux M, et al, editors: *Pediatric Neurosurgery*, Edinburgh, 1999, Churchill Livingstone, p 323.

7. Benzacken B, et al: Different proximal and distal rearrangements of chromosome 7q associated with holoprosencephaly. *J Med Genet* 35:614, 1998.

8. Bickers D, Adams R: Hereditary stenosis of the aqueduct of Sylvius as a cause of congenital hydrocephalus, *Brain* 72:246, 1949.

9. Blanc C: Apert's syndrome (a type of acrocephalosyndactyly): observations on a British series of thirty-nine cases, *Ann Hum Genet* 24:151, 1960.

10. Boop F, et al: Outcome analysis of 85 patients undergoing the pi procedure for correction of sagittal synostosis, *J Neurosurg* 85:50, 1996.

11. Brenner M, et al: Mutations in GFAP, encoding glial fibrillary acidic protein, are associated with Alexander disease, *Nat Genet* 27:117, 2001.

12. Brueton L, et al: The mapping of a gene for craniosynostosis: evidence for a linkage of Saethre-Chotzen syndrome to distal chromosome 7p, *J Med Genet* 29:681, 1992.

13. Budka H: Megalencephaly and chromosomal anomaly, *Acta Neuropathol (Berlin)* 15:263, 1978.

14. Burstein J, et al: Intraventricular hemorrhage and hydrocephalus in premature newborns: a prospective study with CT, *Am J Radiol* 132:631, 1979.

15. Carmel P, et al: Dandy Walker syndrome: clinicopathological features and re-evaluation of modes of treatment, *Surg Neurol* 8:132, 1977.

16. Casey P, et al: Growth status and growth rates of a varied sample of low birth weight, preterm infants: a longitudinal cohort from birth to three years of age, *J Pediatr* 119:599, 1991.

17. Chotzen F: Eine eigenartige familiare Entwicklingsstorung (Akrocephalosyndactylie, Dysostosis craniofacialis und Hypertelorismus), *Monatschr Kinderheilkd* 55:97, 1932.

18. Cinalli G, et al: Chronic tonsillar herniation in Crouzon's and Apert's syndromes: the role of premature synostosis of the lambdoid suture, *J Neurosurg* 83:575, 1995.

19. Cohen M: Etiopathogenesis of craniosynostosis, *Neurosurg Clin North Am* 2:507, 1991.

20. Cohen M: Pfeiffer syndrome update: clinical subtypes and guidelines for differential diagnosis, *Am J Med Genet* 45:300, 1993.

21. Collmann H, et al: Consensus: trigonocephaly, *Childs Nerv Syst* 12:664, 1996.

22. Crouzon O: Dysostose cranio-faciale hereditaire, *Bull Soc Med Hop Paris* 33:545, 1912.

23. Cutler R, Page L, Galicich J: Formation and absorption of cerebrospinal fluid in man, *Brain* 91:707, 1968.

24. Cutting L, et al: Relationship of cognitive functioning, whole brain volumes, and T2-weighted hyperintensities in neurofibromatosis-1, *J Child Neurol* 15:157, 2000.

25. Di Rocco C, Velardi F: Nosographic identification and classification of plagiocephaly, *Childs Nerv Syst* 4:9, 1988.

26. Dias M, et al: Occipital plagiocephaly: deformation or lambdoid synostosis? I: Morphometric analysis and results of unilateral lambdoid craniectomy, *Pediatr Neurosurg* 24:61, 1996.

27. Dias M, Klein D: Occipital plagiocephaly: deformation or lambdoid synostosis? Part II: A unifying theory regarding pathogenesis, *Pediatr Neurosurg* 24:69, 1996.

28. Dodge P, et al: Cerebral gigantism, *Dev Med Child Neurol* 25:248, 1983.

29. El Ghouzzi V, et al: Mutations of the TWIST gene in the Saethre-Chotzen syndrome, *Nat Genet* 15:42, 1997.

30. Emery J, Staschak M: The size and form of the cerebral aqueduct in children, *Brain* 95:591, 1972.

31. Evrard P, et al: Abnormal development and destructive processes of the human brain during the second half of gestation. In Evrard P, Minkowski A, editors: *Developmental Neurobiology*, Nestle Nutrition Workshop Series, 12, New York, 1989, Raven Press, p 1.

32. Geyer J: Infant brain tumors, *Neurosurg Clin North Am* 3:781, 1992.

33. Goddard-Finegold J: Periventricular, intraventricular hemorrhages in the preterm newborn: update on pathologic features, pathogenesis, and possible means of prevention, *Arch Neurol* 41:766, 1984.

34. Graham J, Smith D: Metopic craniosynostosis as a consequence of fetal head constraint: two interesting experiments of nature, *Pediatrics* 65:1000, 1980.

35. Gripp K, et al: Identification of a genetic cause for isolated unilateral coronal synostosis: a unique mutation in the fibroblast growth factor receptor 3, *J Pediatr* 132:714, 1998.

36. Handique S, et al: External hydrocephalus in children, *Ind J Radiol* 12:197, 2002.

37. Hirsch J, et al: The Dandy-Walker malformation: a review of 40 cases, *J Neurosurg* 61:515, 1984.

38. Isaacs H: Perintal brain tumors: a review of 250 cases, *Pediatr Neurol* 27:249, 2002.

39. Johnson R: Hydrocephalus and viral infections, *Dev Med Child Neurol* 17:807, 1975.

40. Jones K: *Recognizable Patterns of Human Malformation*, Philadelphia, 1997, WB Saunders.

41. Kaiser G: Sagittal synostosis: its clinical significance and the results of three different methods of craniectomy, *Childs Nerv Syst* 4:223, 1988.

42. Kane A, et al: Observations on a recent increase of plagiocephaly without synostosis, *Pediatrics* 97:877, 1996.

43. Kattwinkel J, et al: Positioning and SIDS, *Pediatrics* 89:1120, 1992.

44. Kenwrick S, et al: Neural cell recognition molecule L1: relating biological complexity to human disease mutations, *Hum Mol Genet* 9:879, 2000.

45. Kirkpatrick M, et al: Symptoms and signs of progressive hydrocephalus, *Arch Dis Child* 64:124, 1989.

46. Kreiborg S: Crouzon syndrome, *Scand J Plast Reconstr Surg Suppl* 18:1, 1981.

47. Lajeunie E, et al: Genetic study of scaphocephaly, *Am J Med Genet* 62:282, 1996.

48. Lander E, Botstein D: Homozygosity mapping: a way to map human recessive traits with the DNA of inbred children, *Science* 236:1567, 1987.

49. Lenke R, Levy H: Maternal phenylketonuria and hyperphenylalaninemia, *N Engl J Med* 303:1202, 1980.

50. Lenke R, Levy H: Maternal phenylketonuria: results of dietary therapy, *Am J Obstet Gynecol* 142:548, 1982.

51. Lorch S, et al: "Benign" extra-axial fluid in survivors of neonatal intensive care, *Arch Pediatr Adolesc Med* 158:178, 2004.

52. McLone D, Knepper P: The cause of Chiari II malformation: a unified theory, *Pediatr Neurosci* 15:1, 1989.

53. Ment L, et al: Posthemorrhagic hydrocephalus: low incidence in very low birth weight neonates with intraventricular hemorrhage, *J Neurosurg* 60:343, 1984.

54. Miller R, Blot W: Small head after in utero exposure to atomic radiation, *Lancet* 2:784, 1972.

55. Mochida G, Walsh C: Molecular genetics of human microcephaly, *Curr Opin Neurol* 14:151, 2001.

56. Moloney D, et al: Apert syndrome results from mutations of FGFR2 and is allelic with Crouzon syndrome, *Nat Genet* 9:165, 1995.

57. Moss S: Nonsurgical nonorthotic treatment of occipital plagiocephaly: what is the natural history of the misshapen neonatal head? *J Neurosurg* 87:667, 1997.

58. Papile L, et al: Incidence and evolution of the subependymal intraventricular hemorrhage: a study of infants with birth weights less than 1500 grams, *J Pediatr* 92:529, 1978.

59. Park T, Robinson S, editors: *Nonsyndromic craniosynostosis*, Philadelphia, 2001, WB Saunders.

60. Perlman J, et al: Reduction in intraventricular hemorrhage by elimination of fluctuating cerebral blood flow velocity in preterm infants with respiratory distress syndrome, *N Engl J Med* 312:55, 1985.

61. Persing J, et al: Prevention and management of positional skull deformities in infants. American Academy of Pediatrics clinical report, *Pediatrics* 112:199, 2003.

62. Pfeiffer R: Dominant erbliche Akrocephalosyndactylie, *Z Kinderheilkd* 90:301, 1964.

63. Rakic P: Specification of cerebral cortical areas, *Science* 241:170, 1988.

64. Reardon W, et al: Craniosynostosis associated with FGFR3 pro250arg mutation results in a range of clinical presentations including unisutural sporadic craniosynostosis, *Med J Genet* 34:632, 1997.

65. Rekate H: Occipital plagiocephaly: a critical review of the literature, *J Neurosurg* 89:24, 1998.

66. Renier D, et al: Intracranial pressure in craniosynostosis, *J Neurosurg* 57:370, 1982.

67. Renier D, et al: Prognosis for mental function in Apert's syndrome, *J Neurosurg* 85:66, 1996.

68. Ripley C, et al: Treatment of positional plagiocephaly with dynamic orthotic cranioplasty, *J Craniofac Surg* 5:150, 1994.

69. Rosenberg D, et al: The rate of CSF formation in man: preliminary observations on metrizamide washout as a measure of CSF bulk flow, *Ann Neurol* 2:503, 1977.

70. Roth P, Cohen A: Management of hydrocephalus in infants and children. In Tindall G, et al, editors: *The Practice of Neurosurgery*, Baltimore, 1996, Williams & Wilkins, p 2707.

71. Rubin R, et al: The production of cerebrospinal fluid in man and its modification by acetazolamide, *J Neurosurg* 25:430, 1966.

72. Saethre H: Ein Beitrag zum Turmschaedelproblem (Pathogenese, Erblichkleit und Symptomologie), *Dtsch Z Nervenheilkd* 117:533, 1931.

73. Sanford R, et al: Pencil gliomas of the aqueduct of Sylvius, *J Neurosurg* 57:690, 1982.

74. Schaefer G, et al: The neuroimaging findings in Sotos syndrome, *Am J Med Genet* 60:480, 1997.

75. Sherry B, et al: Evaluation of and recommendations for growth references for very low birth weight (≤1500 gm) infants in the United States, *Pediatrics* 111:750, 2003.

76. Sotos J, et al: Cerebral gigantism in childhood: a syndrome of excessively rapid growth and acromegalic features and a nonprogressive neurologic disorder, *N Engl J Med* 271:109, 1964.

77. Spadaro A, et al: Nontumoral aqueductal stenosis in children affected by von Recklinghausen's disease, *Surg Neurol* 26:487, 1986.

78. Szymonowicz W, et al: Ultrasound and necropsy study of periventricular hemorrhage in preterm infants, *Arch Dis Child* 59:637, 1984.

79. Thompson D, et al: Intracranial pressure in single suture craniosynostosis, *Pediatr Neurosurg* 22:235, 1995.

80. Tomita T, McLone D: Brain tumors during the first 24 months of life, *Neurosurgery* 176:913, 1985.

81. Virchow R: Uber den Cretinismus, Namentlicht in Franken, und uber pathologische Schadelformen, *Ver Phys Med Gesellsch Wurzburg* 2:230, 1851.

82. Williams J, et al: Postnatal head shrinkage in small infants, *Pediatrics* 59:619, 1977.

83. Willinger M, et al: Infant sleep position and risk for sudden infant death syndrome: report of meeting held January 13 and 14, 1994, National Institutes of Health, Bethesda, MD, *Pediatrics* 93:814, 1994.

PART 8

Myelomeningocele

Alan R. Cohen and Michele C. Walsh

DEFINING ANATOMY

A midline bony defect in the neural arches is present, usually involving several vertebrae in the lumbosacral region. Meninges, nerve roots of the cauda equina, and neural tissue, including dysplastic spinal cord, may protrude into a cystic structure over the lower back, which may or may not be covered by skin. Rarely, the neural structures herniate anteriorly into the retroperitoneal space. Myelomeningoceles are almost always associated with the Chiari II malformation.

EMBRYOLOGY AND PATHOGENESIS

Whether the primary pathogenesis is due to failure of closure of the bony elements, a disorder of neural induction, or reopening of a transiently closed posterior neuropore at 28 days' gestation, is an unresolved issue.[2] Risk of myelomeningocele in humans and experimental animals is increased with folic acid deficiency and exposure of the embryo to excessive retinoic acid or vitamin A. Many neural tube defects can be prevented by preconceptional folic acid supplementation of 0.4 mg per day.[4] Although the condition is not a direct mendelian trait, mothers with one affected infant are at higher risk for another than the control population and should receive 4 mg per day of folic acid. This malformation involves all ethnic groups but is higher in some populations such as the Irish.

Specific Types

See also Chapter 11.

A *meningocele* is a cystic dilation of the meninges associated with spina bifida and a defect in the overlying skin. The spinal cord and nerve roots are normal in their structure and position in the spinal canal. Accordingly, infants with meningoceles typically do not show neurologic deficits.

A *myelomeningocele* is a lesion identical to the meningocele but with associated abnormalities in the structure and position of the spinal cord. A myelomeningocele results from failure of primary neurulation. The neural tube does not fuse dorsally, leaving an open neural placode, similar to an open book. The majority of myelomeningoceles are located in the low thoracolumbar spine or more distally. Affected infants typically show neurologic deficits below the level of the lesion. Emerging evidence suggests that in addition to failure of neural tube closure, a primary disruption of brain development may be involved.[1,3]

Spina bifida occulta refers to a nonfusion of one or more of the posterior arches of the spine, usually in the lumbosacral region. A frequent abnormality found at L5 in 30% of adults, the lesion is of neurologic consequence only when associated with underlying abnormalities such as tethering

of the spinal cord. This condition comprises a low-lying conus below L1/L2, best diagnosed by MRI. It may require prophylactic surgery as growth provides traction. Significant associated abnormalities usually are signaled by the presence of a neurocutaneous signature such as a hemangioma, a patch of abnormal hair, a dimple, or a lipoma in the lumbosacral area. Underlying lesions can include diastematomyelia (split cord malformation), spinal lipomas, dermoids, and dermal sinuses.

CLINICAL EXPRESSION

The extent of neural tissue involvement in the myelomeningocele determines the severity of the deficit in motor and sensory function involving the lower extremities and the presence of involvement of bladder and bowel functions (Table 40-10). Many infants with lesions at the L5 to S1 level ultimately will ambulate, with or without short leg braces. Although the ability to predict later function from the level of early neurologic function has been shown to be only modestly accurate, long-term outcomes of patients with myelomeningocele are favorable. In a longitudinal 25-year study of 220 consecutive patients with myelomeningocele, 78% had hydrocephalus treated with ventricular peritoneal shunts.[7] Sixty-three percent required one or more shunt revisions. A tethered cored ultimately developed in 40 (20%) patients. Over a 25-year follow-up period, there were 5 (2%) deaths, and 18 patients (9%) with severe neurologic morbidity. Ninety-seven percent of survivors with an initial lesion below L2 were functioning independently, attending regular schools, and achieved "social continence." In a separate report studying 50 teenagers with myelomeningocele, 21 patients were dependent on wheelchairs. Overall, this group described diminished health-related quality of life, specifically regarding emotional well-being, self-esteem, and peer relations.[5]

Infants with lesions at L3 to L4 might be ambulatory with the assistance of long leg braces and crutches. These infants are prone to paralytic hip dislocation. Infants with lesions at L1 to L2 or higher are completely paraplegic with no functional ambulatory ability (Table 40-11).

Hydrocephalus is a frequent associated complication of myelodysplasia. In general, the more rostral the presence of the myelomeningocele, the more likely hydrocephalus will exist, as a consequence of either the Chiari II malformation or aqueductal stenosis.

TREATMENT

A newborn with a myelomeningocele presents the clinician with difficult decisions about what to tell parents and whether to close the spinal defect surgically. Surgery should be undertaken within the first 72 hours after birth to prevent further deterioration of the spinal cord and nerve roots, and to prevent infection (meningitis). Fetal therapy of myelomeningocele is discussed in Chapter 11.

Factors that influence surgical planning include size and location of the lesion, the technical feasibility of surgical closure, the prognosis for ambulation, the presence or absence of associated abnormalities (hydrocephalus, kyphosis, or other major structural abnormalities), the availability of

TABLE 40–10 Motor Examination of Lower Extremities in Children with Meningomyeloceles

Movement	SPINAL SEGMENT		
	Lumbar	Sacral	Muscle
Hip			
Flexion	1, 2, 3, 4		Iliopsoas, rectus femoris
Adduction	2, 3, 4		Adductors
Abduction	4, 5	1	Gluteus medius
Extension	4, 5	1, 2	Gluteus maximus, obturator
Knee			
Extension	2, 3, 4		Quadriceps
Flexion	5	1, 2	Hamstrings
Foot			
Dorsiflexion	4, 5	1	Tibialis anterior
Plantar flexion	5	1, 2	Soleus, gastrocnemius

TABLE 40–11 Deficit and Prognosis of Meningomyeloceles Related to Site of Lesion

Motor/Sensory Level	Maximum Motor Deficit	Prognosis for Ambulation	Risk of Hydrocephalus
L5-S1	Dorsiflexion and plantar flexion of feet, weakness of glutei	Will ambulate with or without short leg braces; outlook good	60%
L3-L4	Involvement of quadriceps and hamstrings, plus above	May be able to ambulate with long leg braces and crutches; paralytic hip dislocation	86%
L1 and L2 or above	Complete paraplegia	No functional ambulation	96%

personnel and a facility to provide adequate care for the infant, the infant's family structure, and the attitudes of the family toward the defect and its consequences. The usual decision is to proceed with early surgical closure of the spinal defect, followed by placement of a ventriculoperitoneal shunt if hydrocephalus is present (see Part 7 of this chapter). Thereafter, the infant requires long-term neurosurgical, orthopedic, and urologic follow-up to maintain shunt stability, promote ambulation if possible, and minimize the untoward effect of multiple urinary tract infections. In the past, infants with an associated severe chromosomal malformation (e.g., trisomy 18) were not repaired. Currently, most infants are offered palliative surgical care to correct the defect. This facilitates discharge and eases the family's burden of caring for these infants at home.

REFERENCES

1. Chiaretti A, Ausili E, Di Rocco C, et al: Neurotrophic factor expression in newborns with myelomeningocele: preliminary data, *Eur J Paediatr Neurol* 12:113, 2008.
2. Finnell RH, Gould A, Spiegelstein: Pathobiology and genetics of neural tube defects, *Epilepsia* 44:14, 2003.
3. Juranek J, Fletcher JM, Hasan KM, et al: Neocortical reorganization in spina bifida, *Neuroimage* 40:1516, 2008.
4. Kilbar Z, Capra V, Gros P: Toward understanding the genetic basis of neural tube defects, *Clin Genet* 71:295, 2007.
5. Müller-Godeffroy E, Michael T, Poster M, et al: Self-reported health-related quality of life in children and adolescents with myelomeningocele, *Dev Med Child Neurol* 50:456, 2008.
6. Seitzberg A, Lind M, Biering-Sorensen F: Ambulation in adults with myelomeningocele, Is it possible to predict the level of ambulation in early life? *Childs Nerv Syst* 24:231, 2008.
7. Talamonti G, D'Aliberti G, Collice M: Myelomeningocele: long-term neurosurgical treatment and follow-up in 202 patients, *J Neurosurg* 107:368, 2007.

CHAPTER 41

Follow-up for High-Risk Neonates

Deanne Wilson-Costello and Maureen Hack

Advances in obstetric and neonatal care have been responsible for the improved survival of high-risk neonates. A major concern persists, however, that newer therapies may result in an increased number of permanently disabled infants. The earliest follow-up studies of preterm infants after the introduction of modern methods of neonatal intensive care in the 1960s described a decrease in adverse neurodevelopmental sequelae compared with that of the preceding era.[76] During the 1980s and 1990s, there was a continued decrease in mortality, and thus the absolute number of both healthy and neurologically impaired survivors increased.[22,72,73] Furthermore, the survival of increasing numbers of extremely immature infants with low birthweight resulted in a relatively high disability rate in the subpopulation of infants born weighing less than 750 g or born at less than 26 weeks' gestation.[33,37,105] Since 2000, mortality rates for infants with very low birthweight have leveled off. Several studies suggest declining rates of neurodevelopmental impairment, including cerebral palsy.[74,78,101]

Conditions of presumed genetic and prenatal origin account for more children with neurodevelopmental dysfunction than disorders arising out of the perinatal period. Infants who are at highest risk for later neurodevelopmental problems resulting from perinatal sequelae include those who had severe asphyxia, severe intracranial hemorrhage, infarction or periventricular leukomalacia, meningitis, seizures, respiratory failure resulting from pneumonia, persistent fetal circulation or severe respiratory distress syndrome, and multisystem congenital malformations, as well as children born with extremely low birthweight or at extremely early gestational age (Boxes 41-1 and 41-2). The rates of health problems and neurodevelopmental sequelae increase with decreasing birthweight and gestation (Tables 41-1 and 41-2).

Follow-up programs should be an integral extension of every neonatal intensive care unit. Specialized care must be made available for problems of growth, development, and chronic disease and is best provided within the setting of a neonatal follow-up program. The follow-up care should, if possible, initially be provided by the neonatologist together with the family pediatrician. If there are developmental or neurologic problems, the child should also be referred to a subspecialist or a child development center.

The initial continuity of care is important to reassure the family that the same personnel responsible for the life-saving decisions are continuing to assume responsibility for the child's adaptation into home life. Furthermore, even if the neonatal staff members do not continue the follow-up after infancy or early childhood, they will benefit greatly by maintaining contact with the infants leaving the nursery and recognizing the sequelae of prematurity. Growth (weight, height, and head circumference), neurologic development, psychomotor and cognitive development, vision, and hearing all should be sequentially assessed.

In planning neonatal follow-up programs, various options are possible.[8] These depend on the available resources. A minimal requirement for the clinical monitoring of outcomes is a periodic assessment of growth and neurosensory development during the first 2 years of life. The ideal is a comprehensive program involving all aspects of care, including well-baby care, evaluation of outcome, social and educational intervention, and therapy when needed. A home nurse visiting program, especially during the early postdischarge period, and parent support groups for selected high-risk conditions (e.g., children with chronic lung disease) also should be considered. There is evidence that educational enrichment during infancy and early childhood might improve the outcome of high-risk and preterm infants, especially those from socioeconomically deprived groups.[51]

Outcomes from different units might not be comparable because they are heavily influenced by the demographic and socioeconomic profile of the parents, the incidence of extreme prematurity, a selective treatment or admission policy, the percentage of inborn patients at any center, and the rate of follow-up.[96] Intercenter differences in neonatal sequelae and outcome are well described.[34,99] Regional results therefore reflect a more accurate picture of outcome because

---

BOX 41-1 Factors Affecting Outcome of the Infant with Very Low Birthweight

Birthweight <750 g or <25 weeks' gestation
Periventricular hemorrhage (grades III and IV) or infarction
Periventricular leukomalacia
Persistent ventricular dilation
Neonatal seizures
Chronic lung disease
Neonatal meningitis
Subnormal head circumference at discharge
Parental drug abuse
Poverty and parental deprivation
Coexisting congenital malformation

BOX 41-2 Factors Affecting Outcome of the Term Infant

Birth depression or asphyxia
Persistent fetal circulation
Meningitis
Intrauterine growth failure
Intrauterine infections
Symmetric growth restriction (microcephaly)
Major congenital malformations
Neonatal seizures
Extracorporeal membrane oxygenation (ECMO) and nitric oxide therapy
Persistent hypoglycemia
Severe hyperbilirubinemia

TABLE 41-1 Birthweight-Specific Neurodevelopmental Outcomes

Variable	BIRTHWEIGHT (kg)			
	<1	1-1.49	1.5-2.49	≥2.5
Neurologic abnormality (%)	20	15	8	<5
Cerebral palsy (%)	>5	4	2	<0.4
Intelligence				
Mean IQ	88	96	96	103
IQ < 70 (%)	13	5	5	0-3
Behavioral problems (%)	29	28	29	21

IQ, intelligence quotient.
Data from Hack M, et al: Long-term developmental outcomes of low birth weight infants, *Future Child* 5:176, 1995.

TABLE 41-2 Health Outcomes by Birthweight at 8 Years

Variable	BIRTHWEIGHT (kg)			
	<1	1-1.49	1.5-2.49	≥2.5
Asthma (%)	17	18	12	11
Rehospitalization, previous year (%)	7	7	5	2
Limitation of >1 activity of daily living because of health (%)	46	34	27	17

Data from Hack M, et al: Long-term developmental outcomes of low birth weight infants, *Future Child* 5:176, 1995.

Any evaluation of the outcome studies of high-risk infants must include the population status (inborn, outborn, or regional) and the choice of a comparison group that includes either a normal birthweight group or infants within a similar birthweight or gestational age range who do not have the condition or therapy under study. It also is essential to control for sociodemographic factors such as maternal marital status, ethnicity, and education and to consider possible genetic factors when evaluating cognitive outcome or school performance.

Consideration of neonatal mortality is important for judging the aggressiveness and level of neonatal care, which might influence the quality of outcome of the survivors.[59] Other factors to be considered are the rate of loss of infants to follow-up, the neonatal and postdischarge death rate, the age at follow-up, and the method of follow-up.[102] Two years is the earliest age to get a fairly reliable assessment of neurodevelopmental outcome. At age 4 to 5 years, cognitive function and language can be better measured, and follow-up to age 7 to 9 years allows an assessment of subtle neurologic and behavioral dysfunction and school academic performance (Fig. 41-1).[35,43,94]

Because it is impossible to provide ongoing high-risk follow-up care for all infants treated in the neonatal intensive care unit, specific criteria have been proposed to identify children at greatest risk for sequelae.[11] Traditionally, follow-up programs primarily targeted children with birthweight of less than 1500 g or gestational age of less than 32 weeks. However, more recent therapies, such as inhaled nitric oxide and extracorporeal membrane oxygenation, have increased the demand for highly specialized follow-up clinics for term infants with persistent pulmonary hypertension, meconium aspiration, and sepsis.

In addition, a growing number of infants with major congenital malformations such as congenital diaphragmatic hernia now survive the neonatal period to require intensive ongoing follow-up support. University-affiliated follow-up programs could select additional candidates for follow-up in the high-risk clinic on the basis of participation in specific research studies. Because of the significant costs associated with evaluating all eligible follow-up patients in the clinic setting, parent and teacher questionnaires have been suggested. These

they include all infants born in an area. This is the ideal situation, but such studies are rarely available in the United States. Individual centers should be aware of their own patients' social risk factors and rates of neonatal morbidity and, if possible, maintain their own follow-up outcome data.

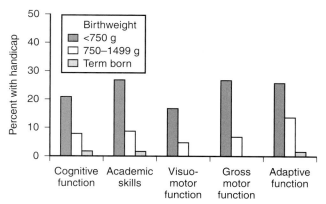

Figure 41–1. Percentage of 6- to 7-year-old children born from 1982 to 1986 by birthweight (<750 g, 750-1499 g, and term born) with subnormal functioning. Subnormal functioning was defined as a standard score of <70 for cognitive function, academic skills, visuomotor function, and adaptive function and a score of <30 for gross motor function. (*Data from Hack M, et al: School-age outcomes in children with birth weights under 750 grams, N Engl J Med 331:753, 1994.*)

questionnaires typically provide a checklist of various individual measures of health status and disability (Box 41-3).[52]

MEDICAL PROBLEMS

Neonatal medical complications include chronic lung disease, intraventricular hemorrhage, retinopathy of prematurity, hearing loss, increased susceptibility to infections, and sequelae of necrotizing enterocolitis. These in turn can contribute to multiple rehospitalizations after discharge, poor physical growth, and an increase in postneonatal deaths. Children with neurologic sequelae such as cerebral palsy and hydrocephalus have a higher rate of rehospitalization for conditions such as shunt complications, orthopedic correction of spasticity, and eye surgery. Furthermore, a high percentage of children with chronic lung disease, extreme prematurity, or both, require rehospitalization during their first year.

Although the incidence of severe bronchopulmonary dysplasia has decreased in recent years, some children require home oxygen and other medications such as diuretics or bronchodilators after discharge. They are prone to recurrent respiratory infections, poor nutrition, and growth failure related to their chronic lung disease and thus require multispecialty follow-up, including neonatal, developmental, nutrition, and pulmonary specialists. The medical complications of prematurity tend to diminish after the second year of life, although airway reactivity and asthma may persist.

Physical Growth

Intrauterine or neonatal growth restriction, or both, occur commonly in preterm infants. The poor neonatal growth is related to inadequate nutrition during the acute phase of neonatal disease, feeding intolerance, and chronic medical sequelae that result in increased calorie requirements. These

---

BOX 41–3 | **Suggested Criteria for Severe Disability at Age 2 Years**

MALFORMATION
Impairs the performance of daily activities

NEUROMOTOR FUNCTION
Unable to sit
Unable to use hands to feed
Unable to control head movement (or no head control)

SEIZURES
More than 1 per month despite treatment

AUDITORY FUNCTION
Hearing impaired despite aids

COMMUNICATION
Unable to comprehend
Unable to produce more than five recognizable sounds

VISUAL FUNCTION
Blind or sees light only

COGNITIVE FUNCTION
About 12 months behind at 2 years

OTHER PHYSICAL DISABILITY

Respiratory
■ Requires continual oxygen therapy
■ Requires mechanical ventilation

Gastrointestinal Function
■ Requires tube feeding
■ Requires parenteral nutrition

Renal Function
■ Requires dialysis

Growth
■ Height or weight more than 3 standard deviations below mean for age

From Johnson A: Follow up studies: a case for a standard minimum data set, *Arch Dis Child* 76:F61, 1997.

---

include chronic lung disease, recurrent infections, and malabsorption secondary to necrotizing enterocolitis. The use of postnatal steroids may also contribute to growth failure. Catch-up growth may occur later in infancy and childhood. Poor feeding in chronically ill or neurologically impaired children may also affect neonatal growth. The parents' size contributes to the eventual growth outcome.

Intrauterine and neonatal brain growth failure and lack of later brain catch-up growth can affect cognitive functioning.[31] Many infants with very low birthweight who are small for gestational age also have subnormal head growth, and brain growth failure can occur during the neonatal period. Catch-up brain growth can occur during infancy in infants with very low birthweight who are either appropriate or small for gestational age; however, as many as 10% of infants with very low birthweight who are appropriate for gestational age and 25% who are small for gestational age still have a subnormal head size at 2 to 3 years of age that persists at school age. Poor growth attainment is especially apparent in the child with an extremely low birthweight or gestational age (Fig. 41-2).

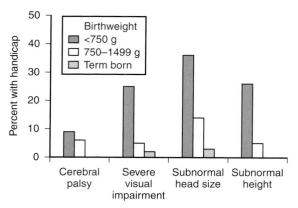

Figure 41–2. Percentage of 6- to 7-year-old children born from 1982 to 1986 by birthweight group (<750 g, 750-1499 g, and term born), with each of four major impairments. Cerebral palsy was defined to include hemiplegia, diplegia, or quadriplegia. Visual impairment includes unilateral or bilateral blindness or visual acuity of <20/200 without glasses in at least one eye. Subnormal head size and height are <2 standard deviations below the mean for the child's age. (*Data from Hack M, et al: School-age outcomes in children with birth weights under 750 grams,* N Engl J Med 331:753, 1994.)

Growth after discharge is a good measure of physical, neurologic, and environmental well-being. To promote optimal catch-up growth of high-risk infants, neonatal nutrition must be maximized. This is especially important because catch-up of head circumference occurs only during the first 6 to 12 months after the expected date of delivery.[31] During recent years, increased-calorie postdischarge formulas have been introduced. These formulas have been associated with improved growth to 9 months. Reports of osteopenia or rickets of prematurity have increased with the improved survival of extremely premature infants whose birth precedes the period of greatest in utero mineral accretion. Although rickets of prematurity appears to be a self-resolving disease, postdischarge formulas with higher calcium and phosphorus content have enhanced growth and bone mineral accretion among preterm infants.[75]

NEURODEVELOPMENTAL OUTCOME
Transient Neurologic Problems

A high incidence of transient neurologic abnormalities, ranging from 40% to 80%, occurs in high-risk infants. These include abnormalities of muscle tone such as hypotonia or hypertonia (occurring as poor head control at 40 weeks' postconceptional age), poor back support at 4 to 8 months, or a slight increase in muscle tone of the upper extremities. Because some degree of physiologic hypertonia normally exists during the first 3 months, it may be difficult to diagnose the early developing spasticity related to cerebral palsy.[27]

Children who will later develop cerebral palsy often initially have hypotonia (poor head control and back support) and only later develop spasticity of the extremities. Spasticity during the first 3 to 4 months is, however, a poor prognostic

sign. Persistence of primitive reflexes also might be a sign of early cerebral palsy. Although mild hypotonia or hypertonia persisting at 8 months usually resolves by the second year, it might indicate later subtle neurologic dysfunction.[20]

Major Neurologic Sequelae

Major neurologic sequelae can usually be diagnosed during the latter part of the first year of life or even earlier if they are very severe. Major neurologic disability is usually classified as cerebral palsy (spastic diplegia, spastic quadriplegia, or spastic hemiplegia or paresis), hydrocephalus (with or without accompanying cerebral palsy or sensory deficits), blindness (usually caused by retinopathy of prematurity), seizures, or deafness (Box 41-4). The intellectual outcome can differ greatly according to neurologic diagnosis. For example, children with spastic quadriplegia usually have severe developmental delay, whereas children with spastic diplegia or hemiplegia may have better mental functioning. Cognitive function is not well measurable until after 2 to 3 years of age, especially among neurologically impaired children.

Most neurologic problems either resolve or become permanent during the second year of life. During the second year, the environmental effects of maternal education and social class begin to play a major role in the various cognitive outcome measures. Further problems could emerge during the school-age years. These include subtle motor, visual, and behavioral difficulties even among children with normal intelligence.[92] These are best diagnosed and treated in a psychological and educational, rather than a medical, follow-up setting.

Cerebral palsy, an umbrella term that refers to "a group of non-progressive, but often changing, motor impairment syndromes secondary to lesions of the developing brain" occurs about 70 times more frequently among infants with extremely low birthweight than among controls with normal birthweight.[66] Risk factors include periventricular echolucencies noted on cranial ultrasound, intrauterine and neonatal infection, hypotension, severe respiratory distress,

BOX 41–4	Types of Neurologic Dysfunction in Children Who Were High-Risk Neonates

Motor deficits
Spastic diplegia
Spastic quadriplegia
Spastic hemiplegia
Mental retardation
Seizures
Hearing deficits
Visual abnormalities
Eye motility dysfunction
Posthemorrhagic hydrocephalus
Visuomotor deficits
Learning deficits
Subtle neurologic dysfunction
Hyperactivity
Poor attention

hypothyroxinemia, postnatal corticosteroid exposure, and multiple gestation.[15,24,29,30] Despite these identified factors, most cerebral palsy cases, especially among term infants, do not have a readily identifiable cause. Protective factors could include maternal antenatal corticosteroid therapy, preeclampsia, and antenatal magnesium sulfate.[24,62] Although birth asphyxia has been identified as a frequent cause of cerebral palsy among term infants, low Apgar scores have correlated poorly with cerebral palsy for preterm infants.[21]

Epidemiologic studies of cerebral palsy rates have been hampered by disagreement over both the specific diagnostic criteria used and the age at which a diagnosis should be made. Most of the cases of cerebral palsy among preterm children pertain to children with spasticity rather than to the athetotic or dyskinetic types of cerebral palsy. These include the subtypes with bilateral (diplegia, quadriplegia) or unilateral (hemiplegia) spasticity. Diplegia and hemiplegia are the most common types of cerebral palsy seen in preterm children. Children with global hypotonia are usually not included in the diagnosis of cerebral palsy. Cerebral palsy was previously defined as mild, with no loss of function and independent walking; moderate, with functional disabilities requiring assistance for walking with aids or walkers; and severe, nonambulatory, requiring a wheelchair. Cerebral palsy was alternatively labeled *disabling* or *nondisabling* to incorporate a crude measure of functional impairment.[71] With the exception of these descriptive terms, there was no reliable measure of the severity of motor disability or consideration of other cognitive or neurosensory problems associated with cerebral palsy. In 2004, an international workshop on the definition and classification of cerebral palsy proposed inclusion not only of motor disorders but also of other associated deficits that may coexist, including seizures and cognitive, perceptual, sensory (visual and hearing), and behavioral impairments.[6] The 2004 classification also includes anatomic and radiologic findings and causation and timing of the lesion. Very few reports to date include this new definition. In the future, its use should improve the classification of children with cerebral palsy and facilitate studies of trends in the rates of cerebral palsy and its correlates.

The diagnosis of cerebral palsy is usually delayed until motor development has been established. The minimal age before a definitive diagnosis can be made should be at least 3 years and preferably 5 years of age. This is because in some cases, the neurologic findings may decrease or disappear by 5 years of age, and in other mild cases, the findings may only become apparent later.[67,86] The longest study of trends in the rates of cerebral palsy has been that of Hagberg and colleagues. They have monitored the rates in western Sweden in a series of nine reports from 1954 until the most recent period of 1995 to 1998.[45,48] During the 1950s, very few of the children with cerebral palsy in the western Swedish register were born before 28 weeks' gestation, whereas by 1995 to 1998, 20% to 25% of these children were born at this extremely low gestation, evidence of the increase in survival of these infants. Survival increased progressively during the periods of study. Overall, the prevalence of cerebral palsy among preterm infants decreased between the periods 1954 to 1958 and 1967 to 1970, partly owing to discontinuation of various iatrogenic therapies such as prolonged starvation and discontinuation of limitation of oxygen thought to cause retinopathy of prematurity. After the introduction of methods of neonatal intensive care and the increase in survival of infants of extremely low birthweight and gestation, the rates of cerebral palsy increased by 1987 to 1990, with an increase in cases with severe multiple handicaps. Similar trends were noted by others.[16] The prevalence then decreased significantly by 1995 to 1998 (Fig. 41-3). Most recently, several other reports have suggested similar decreases in the rates of cerebral palsy.[74,78,101]

Assessment of Functional Outcomes

One of the most widely used tools to classify gross motor function for children with cerebral palsy is the Gross Motor Function Classification System (GMFCS) introduced by Palisano.[7,70] This tool defines motor function on the basis of self-initiated movement with particular emphasis on sitting, walking, and mobility using a five-level classification system in which criteria meaningful to daily living distinguish the levels. Distinctions are based on functional limitations, the need for hand-held mobility devices such as walkers, crutches, or wheeled mobility,

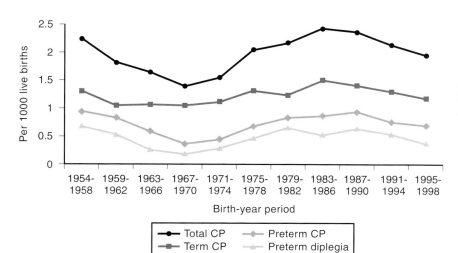

Figure 41-3. Crude prevalence of cerebral palsy (CP) per 1000 live births, 1954 to 1994. (*Data from Himmelmann K, et al: Changing panorama of cerebral palsy in Sweden. IX. Prevalence and origin in the birth year period 1995-98,* Acta Paediatr 94:287, 2005.)

and to a much lesser extent, quality of movement. Because classification of motor function is dependent on age, separate descriptions are applied over a variety of age ranges. The focus of GMFCS is on determining which level best represents the child's present abilities and limitations. Emphasis is placed on usual performance in home, school, and community settings rather than on what the children can do as their best capability. An example of the classification system used for toddlers is presented in Figure 41-4.

Other measures used in examining functional outcomes include limitations in activities of daily living, such as difficulty feeding, dressing, and toileting, as well as the inability to play with other children. Most of these functions are applicable only after 2 years of age.

The functional measures of outcome that focus on the consequences of the various diverse medical, behavioral, and cognitive disorders resulting from prematurity are more suited for planning services for children with special health care needs.[82] Additional measures that can be used include the assessment of the overall health status of the child, the Child Health and Illness Profile, and the QUICCC (Questionnaire for Identifying Children with Chronic Conditions) and measures of the quality of life of the child.[56,79,87,88]

Children with a birthweight of less than 750 g or gestational age younger than 26 weeks have higher rates of functional limitations, greater compensatory dependence, and an increased need for services compared with those with a birthweight of greater than 750 g.[36,41] Recent data from Europe indicate that increased survival of infants with a birthweight of ≤750 g coincided with slightly greater impaired neurodevelopmental outcome at 2 years of age. Small-for-gestational-age infants are especially at risk.[15a] With the exception of a few children (3% to 5%) with severe disability, the major needs for services are those related to special education for the various academic learning and behavioral problems in school. Although reports by Saigal and associates and others note an acceptable quality of life for most adolescents and young adults who were born preterm, even for those with disability, educational and behavioral problems persist into adolescence and young adulthood.[10,79]

Timing of Follow-up Visits

The initial follow-up visit should be 7 to 10 days after discharge from the neonatal nursery. This is important for evaluating how the child is adapting to the home environment. A clinic visit at about 4 to 6 months of corrected age is important for documenting problems of inadequate catch-up growth and severe neurologic abnormality that might require intervention or occupational and physical therapy. Eight to 12 months of corrected age is a good time to identify the suspicion or presence of cerebral palsy or other neurologic abnormality. It also is an excellent time for the first developmental assessment to be performed, usually the Bayley Scales of Infant Development, because the children show little stranger anxiety at this age and are most cooperative.

By 18 to 24 months of age, most transient neurologic findings will have resolved, and the neurologically abnormal child will be showing some adaptation, with improving functional ability. Most potential catch-up growth will have occurred. At the same time, the cognitive and language scales of the Bayley Scales of Infant Development provide some assessment of the child's cognitive functioning.

At 3 years, other measures of cognitive function can be performed that better validate the child's mental abilities. Language is well measurable at this age. From 4 years of age, more subtle neurologic, visuomotor, and behavioral difficulties are measurable. These difficulties can affect school performance, even in children who have normal intelligence.[32,33,37,68]

GROSS MOTOR FUNCTION

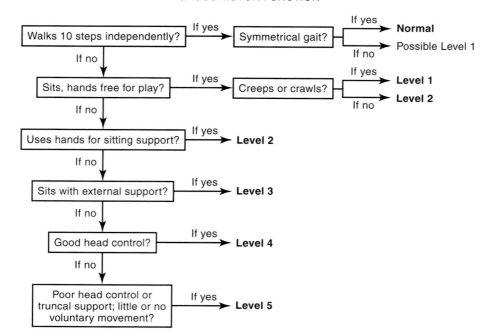

Figure 41-4. Gross motor function classification system for toddlers. (*Data from Palisano RJ, et al: Development and reliability of a system to classify gross motor function in children with cerebral palsy, Dev Med Child Neurol 39: 214, 1997.*)

Developmental and Neurologic Testing

The neurologic examination during infancy is largely based on changes in muscle tone that occur during the first year of life. The examination developed by Amiel-Tison measures the progressive increase in active muscle tone (head control, back support, sitting, standing, walking) together with the concomitant decrease in passive muscle tone. This also documents visual and auditory responses and some primitive reflexes. This method gives a qualitative assessment of neurologic integrity, which is defined as normal, suspect, or abnormal. A conventional neurologic examination should be performed thereafter, together with the Amiel-Tison method for early childhood.[2,3]

The Bayley Scales of Infant Development is the most commonly used tool for monitoring early cognitive and motor development for high-risk infants. During the past 25 years, longitudinal follow-up programs have used this assessment tool to evaluate early outcomes. It is also used clinically to identify infants who might benefit from interventional services. The scales were developed for children aged 1 month to 3½ years of age. The first and second editions of the Bayley Scales were divided into three subtests or scales (mental, motor, and behavior) and provided a Mental Developmental Index and Psychomotor Developmental Index (PDI) with a mean of 100 and a standard deviation of 15. The Mental Development Index and Psychomotor Development Index scores have long served as useful tools for neonatal outcomes research. The 1992 revision yielded lower scores for survivors than those described for children born during the 1980s and early 1990s and tested with the original Bayley Scale.[102]

In 2006, the most recent iteration of the Bayley Scales, the third edition, was introduced. A major driving force for the revision was to provide additional scales to fulfill the requirements of federal and state mandates regarding five major areas of development for early childhood assessment from birth through 3 years of age. As a result, the newest version contains five scales: cognitive, language, motor, social-emotional, and adaptive behavior, the latter two in the form of parent questionnaires. Thus, the third edition of the Bayley Scale does not generate a "mental developmental index" but rather separate cognitive and language scores. Preliminary evaluations have suggested improved early cognitive outcomes for preterm infants using the third edition of the Bayley Scale.

It is not clear that infant tests measure the same constructs as intelligence tests that are administered to older children and adults. Infant tests are seen as a description of current functioning and thus are not predictive. Generally, infant tests have not been shown to have long-term validity, especially for some clinical subgroups. The poor prediction is considered to result from difficulties in infant testing, measurement error, changes in function of the child, and environmental influences that become more evident after 2 years of age. Several recent studies of children with extremely low birthweight have reported significantly lower rates of intellectual impairment at school age than during early childhood.[40,98]

The Ages and Stages Questionnaire may be used as a screening tool for children aged 3 months to 5 years to identify developmental delays.[14] The tool uses parents as the source of information about child development and has been successful in identifying cognitive and motor delays in the follow-up of premature infants and those with hypoxic ischemic encephalopathy.[37,83] However, it does not give a quantitative assessment and thus cannot be used to quantify outcome in specific high-risk populations. The Wechsler Scales may be used with prekindergarten and school-age children. The Wechsler Intelligence Scale for Children, third edition, is probably the most commonly used instrument for school-age assessment. The Kaufman Test was standardized on a 2½- to 10-year-old population and is less heavily weighted by verbal items than other tests.

Ophthalmologic testing should be performed in all high-risk children (see Chapter 53). If the results are abnormal, repeat examinations should be done at the discretion of the ophthalmologist. All children should have a repeat eye examination between 12 and 24 months of age (see Chapter 53, Part 3, for specific examination timetables).

Hearing should be screened before discharge from the neonatal intensive care nursery. Most hearing screening programs use the otoacoustic emissions test, in which a small earphone and microphone are inserted into the infant's ears. When sounds are played, a normally functioning ear will create an echo that can be picked up by the microphone. In a baby with hearing loss, no echo can be detected. Otoacoustic emissions can reliably detect hearing losses above 1500 Hz, but only in the presence of outer hair cell dysfunction. Auditory brainstem response testing may be used for infants who fail the initial hearing screen. The auditory brainstem response test uses electrodes to detect brainwaves. As sounds are played, the test measures the brain's response. The test can detect improper functioning in the inner ear, acoustic nerve, and auditory brainstem pathways associated with hearing. It can detect hearing sensitivity from 1000 to 8000 Hz (see Chapter 42). Hearing should be reexamined at 12 to 24 months because hearing loss can appear later as a sequela of ototoxic drugs such as diuretics. In addition, late-onset hearing loss can occur secondary to cytomegalovirus infection in the newborn period. Hearing loss related to middle ear infections can also occur after the neonatal period and during the first 2 years of life.

SCHOOL-AGE OUTCOME

Measuring school-age outcomes is an important landmark in longitudinal follow-up. Most of the school-age outcome studies of very premature children have compared these premature survivors with children of normal birthweight, documenting significantly more major and subtle neurologic dysfunction, lower intelligence, poorer performance on tests of language and academic achievement, and more behavioral difficulties than control groups of children with normal birthweight who have similar race, gender, and sociodemographic backgrounds.[4,5,35] When only those children with normal intelligence who are free of major neurologic impairment are considered, some of these differences disappear. However, significant differences in tests of visuomotor function and mathematics continue.[93] There also are behavioral differences that interfere with the child's attention and ability to complete a task (Fig. 41-5).[9,43]

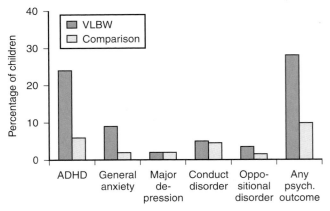

Figure 41–5. Psychiatric (psych.) outcomes in adolescent children who had very low birth-weight (VLBW). ADHD, attention deficit hyperactivity disorder. (*Data from Botting N, et al: Attention deficit hyperactivity disorders and other psychiatric outcomes in very low birthweight children at 12 years,* J Child Psychol Psychiatry 38:931, 1997.)

Few studies have compared school-age outcomes among premature infants over time. One study comparing survivors of very low birthweight born in the early 1980s with those born in the mid-1990s suggests that, despite improved survival rates, mean intelligence scores did not differ.[46] Another study of survivors at 8 years of age documents lower rates of disability for children with extremely low birthweight born in the 1990s compared with the early 1980s.[23]

In terms of their overall health status, extremely preterm children have many more functional limitations and compensatory dependency needs and require many more services above routine than term-born children.[41] These differences persist even when children with neurosensory impairments are excluded. Although most children with very low birthweight remain in the regular school system, many have difficulty coping with the demands of school learning and require more special education and remedial therapy.[68,103] The problems that appear to be most related to academic success in addition to cognition fall within the psychological and psychiatric domains and include deficits in attention, memory, and behavior. Most preterm children who are free from major disability are functioning within the low-normal range on intelligence quotient tests. Sociodemographic and environmental factors may contribute more to the differences in cognitive outcomes than biologic risk factors, with social risks becoming more pronounced as the children age. Structural brain abnormalities detected by magnetic resonance imaging and involving the lateral ventricles, corpus callosum, and white matter are more common among preterm survivors than among controls. These findings provide an anatomic basis for these neurodevelopmental problems.[90]

YOUNG ADULT OUTCOMES

Information on the young adult outcomes of the initial survivors of neonatal intensive care has now been reported from around the developed world.* The studies have differed with

regard to whether they were regional or hospital based and the birthweight group, rate of survival, sociodemographic status, and types of outcome studied. Despite these differences, the overall results suggest that neurodevelopmental and growth sequelae of prematurity persist into young adulthood. Traditionally, educational attainment, employment, independent living, marriage, and parenthood have been considered as markers of successful transition to adulthood. When compared with controls with normal birthweight, young adults with very low birthweight have poorer educational achievement, more chronic illnesses such as asthma or cerebral palsy, and less physical activity.[42] Higher rates of obesity among females have also been reported. In terms of brain structure, diffuse abnormalities including reduction in gray and white matter volume, increased ventricular volume, thinning of the corpus callosum, and periventricular gliosis have all been reported among young adults born prematurely.[1,26,84] The impact of these structural differences on brain function is uncertain; however, cognitive and behavioral differences have been reported. In general, young adults with very low birthweight report less risk taking. Fewer females born at very low birthweight have ever dated or been involved in an intimate relationship. In addition, pregnancy and childbirth rates are lower for young women with very low birthweight. Alcohol and marijuana use also tend to be less prevalent among the former preterm adults.[38,42] Although the information varies, there is currently no clear evidence of an increase in attention deficit hyperactivity disorder or psychosis among adult preterm survivors. However, there is some evidence for an increase in anxious, withdrawn, and depressed symptoms, predominantly among women. This may affect both the development of adult social interactions and the formation of permanent relationships and predispose to further psychopathology later in life.[12,39,44]

The adult outcomes described to date pertain mainly to preterm infants born in the 1970s and early 1980s, a time when neonatal mortality was high and few extremely immature infants survived. Despite statistically significant differences in most outcomes measured, including educational achievement, health status, and socialization, most preterm survivors born during the early years of neonatal intensive care do well and live fairly normal lives. In fact, studies have demonstrated similar self-esteem, overall health satisfaction, and quality of life compared with adults with normal birthweight.[17,80,95,108]

Researchers in Sweden and Norway have recently used their excellent national longitudinal databases to examine the adult outcomes over the complete spectrum of gestational age, ranging from 23 weeks to term gestation, thus allowing for the examination of the relative outcomes of extremely preterm, late preterm, and term-born children.[58,60,65,91] These national studies, which link birth data to later outcomes, also have the advantage of including all the subjects of interest with very little loss to follow-up. Outcomes reported from these national databases pertain to health, functional, educational, and developmental outcomes of importance to society, but provide very little in depth analyses of the correlates and predictors of specific outcomes. The two major predictors

---

*References 13,17,41,80,95,108.

of adult outcomes are lower gestational age, which reflects perinatal injury, and family sociodemographic status, which reflects both genetic and environmental effects.

CHILDREN BORN AT THE THRESHOLD OF VIABILITY

With advanced perinatal care, survival at a birthweight of less than 750 g increased from 32% to 46% in the early 1990s to 55% to 67% more recently.[25,49,50,89] Evaluating the outcomes of these infants born at the threshold of viability raises one of the most difficult problems for obstetricians and pediatricians. Published outcome reports derive from a range of populations including those from single tertiary centers with selected patients and others based on geographically defined areas. Furthermore, survival and morbidity are defined differently in different studies and show wide variation. Outcome data by gestational age are sparse and exquisitely dependent on many other covariables. For example, a recent evaluation of 2-year outcomes for infants enrolled in the Neonatal Research Network of the National Institute of Child Health and Human Development and born between 22 and 25 weeks' gestation reported a 51% survival rate, with 61% experiencing death or profound impairment. In multivariable analyses, exposure to antenatal corticosteroids, female sex, singleton birth, and a higher birthweight were each associated with reductions in the risk for death or profound impairment, similar to those associated with a 1-week increase in gestational age.[97]

The largest population-based study of infants born between 20 and 25 weeks' gestation is the EPICure study from the United Kingdom and Ireland. The major morbidities influencing later development included chronic lung disease, severe brain injury, and severe retinopathy of prematurity.[18] In addition to severe brain insult and chronic lung disease, factors reported to correlate with later poor outcome include male sex, maternal chorioamnionitis, postnatal steroid exposure, neonatal sepsis, transient hypothyroxinemia, and jaundice.[37,69,77,93,100,106]

School-age follow-up of the EPICure cohort at 6 years revealed cognitive impairment in 21% of the children, severe disability in 22%, and disabling cerebral palsy in 12%.[61] In terms of overall function, the EPICure children demonstrated school difficulties, language problems, poor respiratory health, and a variety of pervasive behavioral problems, including attention deficit, hyperactivity, and social-emotional problems.[47,81,104] At age 11 years, the EPICure survivors continued to demonstrate cognitive impairment with specific problems in reading and mathematics. Fifty-seven percent required special educational services.[54] Similar results have been reported at school age for a regional cohort of children born weighing less than 1000 g or before 28 weeks' gestation in Australia.[4,19]

A review of the world literature on survivors of a birthweight of less than 750 g or before 26 weeks' gestation reveals that during early childhood, the rates of severe neurosensory disability range from 9% to 37%, with cerebral palsy occurring in 5% to 37%, blindness in 2% to 25%, and deafness in 0% to 7%. Subnormal cognitive function is noted in 15% to 47% of survivors.[36] This population of children thus represents a subgroup of preterm children who are at the highest risk for poor school performance.

EARLY INTERVENTION

In response to the concern for the adverse developmental and scholastic outcomes among preterm infants, the Infant Health and Development Program undertook a multicenter randomized trial to assess the benefit of a comprehensive early intervention program. The program, which provided intensive educational enrichment to preterm infants with low birthweight, improved the intelligence quotient scores of the children at 3 years of age; however, children of the lowest birthweight (<1000 g) and thus at greater biologic risk were less responsive to the intervention.[51] Subsequent follow-up of the cohort at age 8 years demonstrated only minimal effects of the intervention on cognitive status, school achievement, or behavior.[63] Additional studies of the impact of early intervention on childhood outcomes have yielded mixed results.[28,53,55,107] A meta-analysis of 16 studies, including 6 randomized controlled trials of early intervention programs, suggests improved cognitive outcomes in infancy and preschool, but no significant impact at school age.[85] Recently, the late adolescent outcomes of children enrolled in the Infant Health and Development Program were reported, suggesting slight improvements in mathematics, vocabulary, and behavior among those who received early intervention; however, these improvements were noted only among the larger preterm children.[64] Physical and occupational therapy have not been shown in randomized, controlled trials to significantly improve outcomes. Despite these findings, early intervention programs can provide educational support to parents and are considered beneficial, especially for children from deprived homes.

REFERENCES

 1. Allin M, et al: Effects of very low birthweight on brain structure in adulthood, *Dev Med Child Neurol* 46:46, 2004.
 2. Amiel-Tison C, et al: *Neurologic examination of the infant and newborn*, New York, 1983, Masson Publishing.
 3. Amiel-Tison C, et al: Follow-up studies during the first five years of life: a pervasive assessment of neurologic function, *Arch Dis Child* 64:496, 1989.
 4. Anderson P, et al: Neurobehavioral outcomes of school-age children born extremely low birth weight or very preterm in the 1990's, *JAMA* 289:3264, 2003.
 5. Anderson P, et al: Executive functioning in school-aged children who were born very preterm or with extremely low birth weight in the 1990's, *Pediatrics* 114:50, 2004.
 6. Bax M, et al: Proposed definition and classification of cerebral palsy, April 2005. *Dev Med Child Neurol* 4:571, 2005.
 7. Beckung E, et al: Correlation between ICIDH handicap code and Gross Motor Function Classification System in children with cerebral palsy, *Dev Med Child Neurol* 42:669, 2000.
 8. Bernbaum JC, et al: *Primary Care of the Preterm Infant*, St. Louis, 1991, Mosby-Year Book.
 9. Bhutta AT, et al: Cognitive and behavioral outcomes of school-aged children who were born preterm: a meta-analysis, *JAMA* 288:728, 2002.
10. Bjerager M, et al: Quality of life among young adults born with very low birthweights, *Acta Paediatr Scand* 84:1339, 1995.
11. Blackman J: *Warning signals: basic criteria for tracking at-risk infants and toddlers*, Washington, D.C., 1986, National Center for Clinical Infant Programs.

12. Botting N, et al: Attention deficit hyperactivity disorders and other psychiatric outcomes in very low birth-weight children at 12 years, *J Child Psychol Psych* 38:931, 1997.

13. Brandt I, et al: Catch-up growth of head circumference of very low birth weight, small for gestational age preterm infants and mental development to adulthood, *J Pediatr* 142:463, 2003.

14. Bricker D, et al: Ages and Stages Questionnaires (ASQ): *A parent-completed, child monitoring system,* 2nd ed, 1999, Paul H. Brooks Publishing.

15. Briet JM, et al: Neonatal thyroxine supplementation in very preterm children: developmental outcome evaluated at early school age, *Pediatrics* 107:712, 2001.

15a. Claas MJ, Bruinse HW, Koopman C, et al: Two-year neurodevelopmental outcome of preterm born children ≤750 g at birth, *Arch Dis Child Fetal Neonatal Ed* first published online June 7, 2010 as doi:10.1136/adc.2009.174433.

16. Colver AF, et al: Increasing rates of cerebral palsy across the severity spectrum in north-east England 1964-1993, *Arch Dis Child Fetal Neonatal Ed* 83:F7, 2000.

17. Cooke RW: Health, lifestyle and quality of life for young adults born very preterm, *Arch Dis Child* 89:201, 2004.

18. Costeloe K, et al: The EPICure study: outcomes to discharge from hospital for infants born at the threshold of viability, *Pediatrics* 106:659, 2000.

19. Davis NM, et al: Developmental coordination disorder at 8 years age in a regional cohort of extremely low birthweight or very preterm infants, *Dev Med Child Neurol* 49:325, 2007.

20. D'Eugenio DB, et al: Developmental outcome of preterm infants with transient neuromotor abnormalities, *Am J Dis Child* 147:570, 1993.

21. Dite GS, et al: Antenatal and perinatal antecedents of moderate and severe spastic cerebral palsy, *Aust N Z J Obstet Gynaecol* 38:377, 1998.

22. Doyle LW, et al: Evaluation of neonatal intensive care for extremely low birthweight infants in Victoria over two decades, *Pediatrics* 113:505, 2004.

23. Doyle LW, et al: Improved neurosensory outcome at 8 years of age of extremely low birth weight children born in Victoria over 3 different eras, *Arch Dis Child Fetal Neonatal Ed* 17:1, 2005.

24. Dunin-Wasowicz D, et al: Risk factors for cerebral palsy in very low-birthweight infants in the 1980s and 1990s, *J Child Neurol* 15:417, 2000.

25. Fanaroff AA, et al: Very-low-birth-weight outcomes of the National Institute of Child Health and Human Development Neonatal Research Network, May 1991 through December 1992, *Am J Obstet Gynecol* 173:1423, 1995.

26. Fearon P, et al: Brain volumes in adult survivors of very low birth weight: a sibling-controlled study, *Pediatrics* 114:367, 2004.

27. Georgieff MK, et al: Abnormal truncal muscle tone as a useful, early method for developmental delay in low birth weight infants, *Pediatrics* 77:659, 1986.

28. Glazebrook C, et al: Randomized trial of a parenting intervention during neonatal intensive care, *Arch Dis Child Fetal Neonatal Ed* 92:F438, 2007.

29. Gray PH, et al: Maternal antecedents for cerebral palsy in extremely preterm babies: a case-control study, *Dev Med Child Neurol* 43:580, 2001.

30. Grether JK, et al: Intrauterine exposure to infection and risk of cerebral palsy in very preterm infants, *Arch Pediatr Adolesc Med* 157:26, 2003.

31. Hack M, et al: Effects of very low birth weight and subnormal head size on cognitive abilities at school age, *N Engl J Med* 325:231, 1991.

32. Hack M, et al: The effect of very low birth weight and social risk on neurocognitive abilities at school age, *J Dev Behav Pediatr* 13:412, 1992.

33. Hack M, et al: School-age outcomes in children with birth weights under 750 g, *N Engl J Med* 331:753, 1994.

34. Hack M, et al: Very low birthweight outcomes of the NICHD Neonatal Network, November 1989-October 1990, *Am J Obstet Gynecol* 172:457, 1995.

35. Hack M, et al: Long-term developmental outcomes of low birth weight infants, *Future Child* 5:176, 1995.

36. Hack M, et al: Functional limitations and special health care needs of 10- to 14-year-old children with birth weights under 750 grams, *Pediatrics* 106:554, 2000.

37. Hack M, Fanaroff AA: Outcomes of children of extremely low birthweight and gestational age in the 1990s, *Semin Neonatol* 5:89, 2000.

38. Hack M, et al: Outcomes in young adulthood for very-low-birth-weight infants, *N Engl J Med* 346:149, 2002.

39. Hack M, et al: Behavioral outcomes and evidence of psychopathology among very low birth weight infants at age 20 years, *Pediatrics* 114:932, 2004.

40. Hack M, et al: Poor predictive validity of the Bayley Scales of Infant Development for cognitive function of extremely low birth weight children at school age, *Pediatrics* 116:333, 2005.

41. Hack M, et al: Chronic conditions, functional limitations, and special health care needs of school-aged children born with extremely low-birth-weight in the 1990's, *JAMA* 294:318, 2005.

42. Hack M: Young adult outcomes of very-low-birth-weight children, *Semin Fetal Neonatal Med* 11:127, 2006.

43. Hack M, et al: Behavioral outcomes of extremely low birth weight children at age 8 years, *J Dev Behav Pediatr* 30:122, 2009.

44. Hack M: Adult outcomes of preterm children, *J Dev Behav Pediatr* 2009;30:460-7.

45. Hagberg B, et al: Changing panorama of cerebral palsy in Sweden. VIII. Prevalence and origin in the birth year period 1991-94, *Acta Paediatr* 90:271, 2001.

46. Hansen BM, et al: Is improved survival of very-low birth-weight infants in the 1980's and 1990's associated with increasing intellectual deficit in surviving children? *Dev Med Child Neurol* 46:812, 2004.

47. Hennessy EM, et al: Respiratory health in pre-school and school age children following extremely preterm birth, *Arch Dis Child* 93:1037, 2008.

48. Himmelmann K, et al: The changing panorama of cerebral palsy in Sweden. IX. Prevalence and origin in the birth-year period 1995-1998, *Acta Paediatr* 94:287, 2005.

49. Horbar JD, et al: Predicting mortality risk for infants weighing 501 to 1500 grams at birth: a National Institute of Health Neonatal Research Network report, *Crit Care Med* 21:12, 1993.

50. Horbar JD, et al: Trends in mortality and morbidity for very low birth weight infants, 1991-1999, *Pediatrics* 110:143, 2002.

51. Infant Health and Development Program: Enhancing the outcomes of low-birth-weight premature infants, *JAMA* 263:3035, 1990.

52. Johnson A: Follow up studies: a case for a standard minimum data set, *Arch Dis Child* 76:F61, 1997.

53. Johnson S, et al: Randomised trial of parental support for families with very preterm children: outcome at 5 years, *Arch Dis Child* 90:909, 2005.

54. Johnson S, et al: Academic attainment and special educational needs in extremely preterm children at 11 years of age: the EPICure Study, *Arch Dis Child Fetal Neonatal Ed* 2009;94:F283-9.

55. Kaaresen PI, et al: A randomized controlled trial of an early intervention program in low birth weight children: outcome at 2 years, *Early Hum Dev* 84:201, 2008.

56. Landgraf JM, et al: *Child health questionnaire user's manual*, Boston, 1996, Health Institute, New England Medical Center.

57. Lindsay NM, et al: Use of the Ages and Stages Questionnaire to predict outcome after hypoxic-ischaemic encephalopathy in the neonate, *J Paediatr Child Health* 44:590, 2008.

58. Lindstrom K, et al: Preterm infants as young adults: a Swedish national cohort study, *Pediatrics* 120:70: 2007.

59. Lorenz JM, et al: A quantitative review of mortality and developmental disability in extremely premature newborns, *Arch Pediatr Adolesc Med* 152:425, 1998.

60. Lundgren EM, et al: Intellectual and psychological performance in males born small for gestational age with and without catch-up growth, *Pediatr Res* 50:91, 2001.

61. Marlow N, et al: Neurologic and developmental disability at six years of age after extremely preterm birth, *N Engl J Med* 352:9, 2005.

62. Marret S, et al: Is it possible to protect the preterm infant brain and to decrease later neurodevelopmental disabilities? *Arch Pediatr* 15:S31, 2008.

63. McCarton CM, et al: Results at age 8 years of early intervention for low-birth-weight premature infants: The Infant Health Development Program, *JAMA* 277:126, 1997.

64. McCormick M, et al: Early Intervention in low birth weight premature infants: results at 18 years of age for the Infant Health and Development Program, *Pediatrics* 117:771, 2006.

65. Moster D, et al: Long-term medical and social consequences of preterm birth, *N Engl J Med* 359:262, 2008.

66. Mutch L, et al: Cerebral palsy epidemiology: where are we now and where are we going? *Dev Med Child Neurol* 34:547, 1992.

67. Nelson KB, et al: Children who "outgrew" cerebral palsy, *Pediatrics* 69:529, 1982.

68. Ornstein M, et al: Neonatal follow-up of very low birthweight/extremely low birthweight infants to school age: A critical overview, *Acta Paediatr Scand* 80:741, 1991.

69. O'Shea TM, et al: Intrauterine infection and the risk of cerebral palsy in very low-birthweight infants, *Paediatr Perinat Epidemiol* 12:72, 1998.

70. Palisano RJ, et al: Development and reliability of a system to classify gross motor function in children with cerebral palsy, *Dev Med Child Neurol* 39:214, 1997.

71. Paneth N, et al: Reliability of classification of cerebral palsy in low birthweight children in four countries, *Dev Med Child Neurol* 45:628, 2003.

72. Piecuch RE, et al: Outcome of extremely low birth weight infants (500 to 999 grams) over a 12-year period, *Pediatrics* 100:633, 1997.

73. Piecuch RE, et al: Infants with birth weight 1,000-1,499 grams born in three time periods: has outcome changed over time? *Clin Pediatr* 37:537, 1998.

74. Platt MJ, et al: Trends in cerebral palsy among infants of very low birthweight (<1500 grams) or born prematurely (<32 wk) in 16 European centres, *Lancet* 369:43, 2007.

75. Pohlandt F: Prevention of postnatal bone demineralization in very low-birth-weight infants by individually monitored supplementation with calcium and phosphorus, *Pediatr Res* 35:125, 1994.

76. Rawlings G, et al: Changing prognosis for infants of very-low-birthweight, *Lancet* 1:516, 1971.

77. Reuss ML, et al: The relation of transient hypothyroxinemia in preterm infants to neurologic development at two years of age, *N Engl J Med* 334:821, 1996.

78. Robertson CMT, et al. Changes in the prevalence of cerebral palsy for children born very prematurely within a population-based program over 30 years, *JAMA* 297:2733, 2007.

79. Saigal S, et al: Self-perceived health status and health-related quality of life of extremely low-birth-weight infants at adolescence, *JAMA* 276:453, 1996.

80. Saigal S, et al: Transition of extremely low-birth-weight infants from adolescence to young adulthood: comparison with normal birth-weight controls, *JAMA* 295:667, 2006.

81. Samara M, et al: Pervasive behavior problems at 6 years of age in a total-population sample of children born ≤ 25 weeks of gestation, *Pediatrics* 122:562, 2008.

82. Schreuder AM, et al: Standardised method of follow-up assessment of preterm infants at the age of 5 years: Use of the WHO classification of impairments, disabilities, and handicaps. Report from the Collaborative Project on Preterm and Small for Gestational Age Infants (POPS) in the Netherlands, 1983, *Paediatr Perinat Epidemiol* 6:363, 1992.

83. Skellern CY, et al: A parent-completed developmental questionnaire: follow-up of ex-premature infants, *J Paediatr Child Health* 37:125, 2001.

84. Skranes JS, et al: Cerebral MRI findings in very-low-birth-weight and small-for-gestational-age children at 15 years of age, *Pediatr Radiol* 35:758, 2005.

85. Spittle AJ, et al: Early developmental intervention programs post hospital discharge to prevent motor and cognitive impairments in preterm infants, *Cochrane Database Syst Rev* 18: CD005495, 2007.

86. Stanley F, et al: Cerebral palsies: epidemiology and causal pathways. In *Clinics in Developmental Medicine*, No. 151, London, 2000, Mac Keith Press.

87. Starfield B, et al: The adolescent child health and illness profile: A population-based measure of health, *Med Care* 33:553, 1995.

88. Stein REK, Jessop DJ: Functional Status II (R): a measure of child health status, *Med Care* 28:1041, 1990.

89. Stevenson DK, et al: Very low birth weight outcomes of the National Institute of Child Health and Human Development Neonatal Research Network, January 1993 through December 1994, *Am J Obstet Gynecol* 179:1632, 1998.

90. Stewart AL, et al: Brain structure and neurocognitive and behavioral function in adolescents who were born very preterm, *Lancet* 353:1653, 1999.

91. Swamy GK, et al: Association of preterm birth with long-term survival, reproduction and next generation preterm birth, *JAMA* 299:1429, 2008.

92. Taylor HG, et al: Achievement in <750 gm birth weight children with normal cognitive abilities: Evidence for specific learning disabilities, *J Pediatr Psychol* 20:703, 1995.

93. Taylor HG, et al: Predictors of early school age outcomes in very low birth weight children, *J Dev Behav Pediatr* 19:235, 1998.

94. Taylor HG, et al: Mathematic deficiencies in children with very low birth weight or very preterm birth, *Dev Disabil Res Rev* 15:52, 2009.

95. Tideman E, et al: Longitudinal follow-up of children born preterm: somatic and mental health, self-esteem and quality of life at age 19, *Early Hum Dev* 61:97, 2001.

96. Tin W, et al: Outcome of very preterm birth: children reviewed with ease at 2 years differ from those followed up with difficulty, *Arch Dis Child Fetal Neonat Ed* 79:F83, 1998.

97. Tyson JE, et al: Intensive care for extreme prematurity-moving beyond gestational age, *N Engl J Med* 358:1672, 2008.

98. Victorian Infant Collaborative Study Group: Neurosensory outcome at 5 years and extremely low birthweight, *Arch Dis Child Fetal Neonatal Ed* 73:F143, 1995.

99. Vohr BR, et al: Center differences and outcomes of extremely low birth weight infants, *Pediatrics* 113:781, 2004.

100. Wilson-Costello D, et al: Perinatal correlates of cerebral palsy and other neurologic impairment among very low birth weight children, *Pediatrics* 102:1, 1998.

101. Wilson-Costello D, et al: Improved neurodevelopmental outcomes for extremely low birth weight infants in 2000-2002, *Pediatrics* 119:37, 2007.

102. Wolke D, et al: The cognitive outcome of very preterm infants may be poorer than often reported: an empirical investigation of how methodological issues make a big difference, *Eur J Pediatr* 153:906, 1994.

103. Wolke D, et al: Cognitive status, language attainment, and rereading skills of 6-year-old very preterm children and their peers: The Bavarian Longitudinal Study, *Dev Med Child Neurol* 41:94, 1999.

104. Wolke D, et al: Specific language difficulties and school achievement in children born at 25 weeks of gestation or less, *J Pediatr* 152:256, 2008.

105. Wood NS, et al: Neurologic and developmental disability after extremely preterm birth, *N Engl J Med* 343:378, 2000.

106. Wood NS, et al: The EPICure study: associations and antecedents of neurological and developmental disability at 30 months of age following extremely preterm birth, *Arch Dis Child Fetal Neonatal Ed* 90:F134, 2005.

107. Zhang GQ, et al: Neurodevelopmental outcome of preterm infants discharged from NICU at 1 year of age and the effects of intervention compliance on neurodevelopmental outcome, *Zhongguo Dang Dai Er Ke Zhi* 9:193, 2007.

108. Zwicker JG, et al: Quality of life of formerly preterm and very low birth weight infants from preschool age to adulthood: a systematic review, *Pediatrics* 121:e366, 2008.

CHAPTER 42

Hearing Loss in the Newborn Infant

Betty Vohr

BACKGROUND

Tremendous progress has been made during the past 15 years in the identification of hearing loss in newborns. The National Institutes of Health issued a "Consensus Statement on Early Identification of Hearing Impairment in Infants and Young Children in 1993."[33] The statement concluded that all infants admitted to the neonatal intensive care unit (NICU) should be screened for hearing loss before hospital discharge and that universal hearing screening should be implemented for all infants within the first 3 months of life. At the time of the National Institutes of Health consensus statement, only 11 hospitals in the United States were screening more than 90% of their newborn infants. In the United States, the percentage of infants screened for hearing loss increased significantly from 46% in 1999 to 93% in 2006.[10]

The percentage of infants who fail the screening process is about 2.1% (range, 0.3% to 6.5%), and rates of permanent hearing loss subsequently diagnosed by comprehensive audiology testing range from 1 to 3 per 1000, making congenital hearing loss the most common birth defect diagnosed as a result of the newborn screening process.[10] Undetected, hearing loss negatively affects communication development, academic achievement, literacy, and social and emotional development,[28,29] whereas early identification and intervention, particularly within the first 6 months of life, clearly provide benefit for communication development in infants.[50] There is accumulating evidence that the brain may be optimally responsive to language input early in life.[42,43]

Based on these findings, the Joint Committee on Infant Hearing 2000 and 2007 Position statements[21,22] published the 1-3-6 recommendation to maximize the outcomes of infants with all degrees of hearing loss: All infants should be screened for hearing loss no later than 1 month of age, and infants who do not pass the screen should have a comprehensive evaluation by an audiologist no later than 3 months of age for confirmation of hearing status. Infants with confirmed hearing loss should receive appropriate intervention no later than 6 months of age from professionals with expertise in hearing loss and deafness in infants and young children.

NORMAL HEARING AND HEARING LOSS

The ear consists of outer, middle, and inner components. The external ear includes the pinna and the outer ear canal. Sounds waves travel through the air and are conducted through the outer ear canal to the tympanic membrane, where vibrations enter the middle ear and are amplified and transmitted through the ossicles to the fluid within the cochlea (inner ear). Sound waves in the inner ear are transmitted through the fluid and stimulate both the outer and inner hair cells of the cochlea. The outer hair cells respond to sound energy by producing an echo of sounds called *otoacoustic emissions*, and the inner hair cells act by converting mechanical energy into electrical energy transmitted to the cochlear branch of the eighth cranial nerve, the brainstem, and finally the auditory cortex for perception of the meaning of sounds. In normal hearing individuals, all components of the pathway are intact and functioning. Blockage of sound conduction in the outer or middle ear may result in either a transient (fluid or debris) or permanent (anatomic abnormality such as atresia or microtia) conductive hearing loss. Failure of sound transmission within the cochlea, outer and inner hair cells, and eighth cranial nerve are a manifestation of sensorineural hearing loss, whereas pathology of the inner hair cells and eighth cranial nerve with intact outer hair cells is characteristic of neural hearing loss, also referred to as *auditory neuropathy* or *auditory dyssynchrony*.

Hearing loss can be classified as bilateral or unilateral and as mild, moderate, severe, or profound. The types of hearing loss that can be identified at birth are shown in Table 42-1. Types of permanent hearing loss that can be identified with newborn screening include sensorineural, neural, and conductive. Transient conductive hearing loss may also be present, especially in infants who have been hospitalized in an

TABLE 42–1 Types of Hearing Loss

Type	Characteristics
Sensorineural	Pathology involving cranial nerve VIII and outer hair cells and inner hair cells of the cochlea that impairs neuroconduction of sound energy to the brainstem
Permanent conductive	Anatomic obstruction of the outer ear (atresia) or middle ear (fusion of ossicles) that blocks transmission of sound
Neural or auditory neuropathy or auditory dyssynchrony	Pathology of the myelinated fibers of cranial nerve VIII or the inner hair cells that impairs neuroconduction of sound energy to the brainstem. The function of the outer hair cells remains intact.
Transient conductive	Debris in the ear canal or fluid in the middle ear that blocks the passage of sound waves to the inner ear
Mixed hearing loss	A combination of sensorineural or neural hearing loss with transient or permanent conductive hearing loss

NICU. Mixed hearing loss is a combination of permanent hearing loss and transient conductive hearing loss.

TESTS FOR HEARING LOSS

Screening and hearing diagnostic tests are shown in Table 42-2. Physiologic tests include those that measure electrical activity or reflexes and include OAE and auditory brainstem response (ABR) testing. These tests do not require an active response from the infant and can be performed when asleep. OAE screen measurements are obtained using a sensitive microphone within a probe inserted into the ear canal that records the sound produced by the outer hair cells of a normal cochlea in response to a sound stimulus. Abnormal outer and middle ear function due to blockage or background noise may interfere with recording OAEs. Automated auditory brainstem response (AABR) for screening and ABR for diagnostic testing are obtained from surface electrodes that record neural activity in the cochlea, outer and inner hair cells, auditory nerve, and brainstem in response to a click stimulus. In AABR, a predetermined algorithm provides an automated pass-or-fail response to the presence or absence of wave 5 on the ABR. Both OAE and ABR detect sensorineural and conductive hearing loss. A false-positive fail screen for permanent hearing loss may result from outer or middle ear dysfunction, including the presence of a transient conductive hearing loss (fluid or debris) or noise interference. OAEs cannot be used to screen for neural hearing loss because pathology in this disorder involves the inner hair cells, eighth cranial nerve, and brainstem with intact outer hair cells. Infants with neural hearing loss will therefore fail ABR but pass OAE. The Joint Committee on Infant Hearing 2007 states that infants cared for in the NICU for greater than 5 days are at highest risk for neural hearing loss and therefore should only be screened with AABR.[22] Some hospitals use a two-step screen with both AABR and OAE.

Tympanometry (immittance) testing is used to assess the peripheral auditory system, including the function, intactness, and mobility of the tympanic membrane, the pressure in the middle ear, and the mobility of the middle ear ossicles. A probe is placed in the inner ear, and air pressure is changed to assess the movement of the tympanic membrane. The tympanogram shows the response of the tympanic membrane in response to the pressure stimulus: a type A curve is considered a normal response. A completely flat response may be reflective of fluid in the middle ear or perforation of the tympanic membrane. Tympanometry is not used for screening.

Behavioral tests include vision reinforcement audiometry (VRA), which is appropriate for rested alert infants with a developmental age of at least 6 months. The infant must have the functional capability of turning to sounds. For administration of VRA, the infant sits on the mother's lap in a sound booth, earphones are inserted, and the infant is conditioned to turn to sounds that are paired to animated toys that appear either to the right or left side. Traditional behavioral testing is used for toddlers at least 2½ years of age. Children respond by placing a block in a box each time they hear a sound.

For confirmation of an infant's hearing status, a test battery is required to cross-check results of both the physiologic measures and the behavioral measures.[19] The purposes of the audiologic test battery are to assess the integrity of the auditory system, to estimate hearing sensitivity across the frequency range, and to determine the type of loss. Infants who fail a newborn screen should have a diagnostic assessment as soon as possible after the newborn screen and not later than 3 months of age.

EARLY INTERVENTION SERVICES

There is a body of evidence supporting the importance of early enrollment in early intervention services to improve the outcomes of children with hearing loss. Before universal hearing screening, children with severe to profound hearing loss were identified at 24 to 30 months of age and subsequently demonstrated significant delays in communication, language, and literacy.[28,29] The Colorado study first reported that children with hearing loss who received intervention services before 6 months of age had speaking, sign, or total communication language scores comparable with hearing children at 3 years of age.[50] A second report demonstrated that at 12 months, children with hearing loss who were enrolled in early intervention at 3 months or younger had

TABLE 42–2 Tests for Hearing Screening and Diagnosis

Test	Mechanism	Type of Hearing Loss Detected
Otoacoustic emissions (OAE) screen	OAE tests represent a response of the outer hair cells in the cochlea to a sound stimulus; the hair cells produce echo-like responses that can be detected and recorded with a high-sensitivity microphone. Automated equipment is available.	Sensorineural Conductive
Automated auditory brainstem response screen	Automated auditory brainstem response screen tests based on threshold algorithms have become standard for screening.	Sensorineural Conductive Neural
The following physiologic and behavioral tests are used as part of a diagnostic battery:		
Auditory brainstem response diagnostic	Auditory brainstem response potentials are a reflection of electrical activity in cranial nerve VIII and auditory brainstem pathway that can be detected with scalp electrodes to produce an auditory brainstem response.	Sensorineural Conductive Neural
Tympanometry battery	This measure of middle ear function is part of the battery for all children. For infants younger than 6 months, a high-frequency probe tone of 1000 Hz is indicated.	Conductive
Vision reinforcement audiometry (>6 months of age) Conditioned audiometry response (>2.5 years of age)	Observations of the infant's behavioral responses to sounds	Sensorineural Conductive Neural
Standard audiometry (>4.5 years of age)	Observation of the child's behavioral responses to a task in response to sounds	Sensorineural Conductive Neural

significantly higher scores for number of words understood, words produced, early gestures, later gestures, and total gestures compared with children enrolled after 3 months of age.[49] The Joint Committee on Infant Hearing 2007 recommends that infants with all degrees of unilateral or bilateral hearing loss need to be referred to Early Intervention Services at the time of diagnosis and receive services no later than 6 months of age. These services should be provided by professionals who have expertise in hearing loss, including educators of the deaf, speech-language pathologists, and audiologists.

ETIOLOGY OF HEARING LOSS

It is estimated that at least 50% of congenital hearing loss is hereditary. Nearly 400 syndromes and hundreds of genes associated with hearing loss have been identified.[9,18,31,32] Genetic hearing loss is about 30% syndromic and 70% nonsyndromic. Among children with nonsyndromic hearing loss, 75% to 85% of cases are autosomal recessive (DFNB), 15% to 24% are autosomal dominant (DFNA), and 1% to 2% are X-linked (DNF). Therefore, most infants with hearing loss have nonsyndromic autosomal recessive hearing loss and are born to hearing parents. A single gene, GJB2, which encodes connexin 26, a gap-junction protein expressed in the connective tissues of

the cochlea, accounts for up to 50% of all cases of profound nonsyndromic hearing loss. More than 100 mutations of GJB2 have been identified. A single GJB2 mutation, 35delG, accounts for up to 70% of the mutations. The etiology of hearing loss will be reviewed relative to the risk factors for hearing loss published by the Joint Committee on Infant Hearing 2007 (Box 42-1).

RISK FACTORS

The first two risk factors are obtained by parent report. Parents may not be aware of a family history of hearing loss or of syndromes associated with hearing loss until discussing the possibility with relatives. If a family history of hearing loss is reported for an infant who passes the screen, ongoing surveillance is indicated with at least one follow-up audiologic assessment by 24 to 30 months of age. All families with an infant with hearing loss, regardless of family history of hearing loss, will benefit from a genetics consultation. Risk factor 2, caregiver concern regarding hearing, speech, language, or developmental delay in the first 2 to 3 years of life,[37] has also been shown to be associated with an increased risk for late-onset or progressive hearing loss not detected in a newborn screen. It is important to remember that the rate of hearing loss doubles between birth and school age

---

BOX 42–1 **Risk Factors Associated with Permanent Congenital, Delayed Onset, or Progressive Hearing Loss**

1. Caregiver concerns* regarding hearing, speech, language, or developmental delay
2. Family history of permanent hearing loss*
3. Neonatal intensive care for >5 days, including any of the following: extracorporeal membrane oxygenation,* assisted ventilation, exposure to ototoxic medications (gentamicin and tobramycin) or loop diuretics (furosemide, Lasix), and, regardless of length of stay, hyperbilirubinemia requiring exchange transfusion
4. In utero infections, such as cytomegalovirus,* herpesvirus, rubella, syphilis, and toxoplasmosis
5. Craniofacial anomalies, including those that involve the pinna, ear canal, ear tags, ear pits, and temporal bone anomalies
6. Physical findings, such as white forelock, that are associated with syndromes known to include a sensorineural or permanent conductive hearing loss
7. Syndromes associated with hearing loss or progressive or late-onset hearing loss,* such as neurofibromatosis, osteopetrosis, and Usher syndrome. Other frequently identified syndromes include Waardenburg, Alport, Pendred, and Jervell and Lange-Nielsen syndromes.
8. Neurodegenerative disorders* such as Hunter syndrome or sensory motor neuropathies such as Friedrich ataxia or Charcot-Marie-Tooth disease
9. Culture-positive postnatal infections* associated with sensory neural hearing loss including confirmed bacterial and viral (especially herpesviruses and varicella) meningitis
10. Head trauma, especially basal skull or temporal bone fracture, that requires hospitalization
11. Chemotherapy*

*Risk factors that are of greater risk for delayed onset or progressive hearing loss.

---

from 2 to 3 per 1000 in newborns to about 7 per 1000 at school age,[20] and, therefore, caregiver concern should prompt a referral for further evaluation.

Medical complications are associated with 40% of childhood permanent hearing loss. Risk factor 3 includes infants requiring neonatal intensive care for greater than 5 days, *and any of the following morbidities regardless of length of stay*: extracorporeal membrane oxygenation, assisted ventilation, exposure to ototoxic medications (gentamicin and tobramycin) or loop diuretics (furosemide or Lasix), and hyperbilirubinemia requiring exchange transfusion.[14,37,38] Risk factor 4 includes in utero infections such as cytomegalovirus, herpes, rubella, syphilis, and toxoplasmosis.[14-16,26,32,36] Cytomegalovirus remains the most common medical cause of both early- and delayed-onset hearing loss in infants and children.[16] Most infants with congenital cytomegalovirus infection have no clinical findings at birth, and the diagnosis goes unrecognized.

Risk factors 5 to 8 are all associated with congenital abnormalities or syndromes. Risk factor 5 includes craniofacial anomalies, such as those involving the pinna, ear canal, ear tags, ear pits, and temporal bone anomalies.[11] These defects are common in both the well-baby nursery and the NICU. Many of these findings reflect abnormalities in the embryologic development of the ear. The external ear, middle ear, and eustachian tube develop from the branchial apparatus beginning at the fourth week of gestation. The pinna arises from the coalescence of the first and second arch tissues of the first branchial cleft, which will become the external auditory canal. The eustachian tube and middle ear space develop from the first pharyngeal pouch, and the ossicles from the mesoderm of the first and second arches. The inner ear develops from surface ectoderm and neuroectoderm beginning in the third week of gestation, with the cochlea, semicircular canals, utricle, and saccule formed by 15 weeks. The inner ear reaches adult size by 23 weeks. Risk factor 6 includes visible physical findings such as white forelock, which is associated with Waardenburg syndrome.

Risk factor 7 includes syndromes associated with hearing loss or progressive or late-onset hearing loss such as neurofibromatosis, osteopetrosis, and Usher syndrome.[38] Usher syndrome is the most common cause of autosomal recessive syndromic hearing loss (4% to 6% of children with hearing loss). Affected individuals develop vestibular problems secondary to progressive retinitis pigmentosa and become blind with increasing age. Subtypes are associated with either mild to severe or severe to profound hearing loss. Early diagnosis is critical because a visual means of communication is not an option for a child who will become blind with increasing age. Other frequently identified syndromes include Waardenburg, Pendred, Jervell and Lange-Nielsen, and Alport syndromes.[31] The most common autosomal dominant syndrome is Waardenburg syndrome. It occurs in 1% to 4% of children with hearing loss. Children have sensorineural or permanent conductive hearing loss and associated heterochromia iridis. Pendred syndrome is the second most common autosomal recessive cause of syndromic hearing loss. It is characterized by severe to profound hearing loss and euthyroid goiter, which presents during adolescence or later. An abnormality called Mondini dysplasia or dilated vestibular aqueduct, which is diagnosed by computed tomography examination of the temporal bones, is associated with Pendred syndrome. Jervell and Lange-Nielsen syndrome is characterized by prolongation of the QT segment on electrocardiogram and is associated with sudden infant death and syncope. Children with QT prolongation should be seen in consultation by cardiology for management. Branchio-otorenal syndrome is autosomal dominant and occurs in 2% of hearing loss. It is characterized by preauricular pits, malformed pinnae, branchial fistulas, and renal anomalies. Alport syndrome is X-linked or autosomal recessive, occurs in 1% of children with hearing loss, and is associated with progressive hearing loss

Risk factor 8 consists of neurodegenerative disorders such as Hunter syndrome or sensory motor neuropathies such as Friedreich ataxia and Charcot-Marie-Tooth syndrome.[38]

Risk factor 9 is culture-positive postnatal infections and includes confirmed bacterial and viral (especially herpesviruses and varicella virus) meningitis. Meningitis is associated with an increased incidence of sensorineural hearing loss.[3,6,7,38]

Risk factors 10 and 11 are risk factors encountered after discharge. Serious head trauma, especially basal skull or temporal bone fractures requiring hospitalization, is a risk factor for hearing loss in childhood.[25,51] Although rare in children, chemotherapy for leukemia or cancer remains a risk factor, which in some cases is reversible.[5] Box 42-1 identifies the risk factors associated with delayed-onset hearing loss. Although all children with a risk factor should have at least one follow-up visit with an audiologist, children with increased risk for delayed-onset hearing loss may require more frequent assessments.

MEDICAL WORKUP FOR HEARING LOSS AND CARE COORDINATION

A physician visit should be scheduled with the family as soon as a diagnosis of hearing loss is made to discuss the audiologist's report, provide information on community resources, and provide support for the family during a period of stress. During the postdiagnosis appointment with the family, the physician reviews the pregnancy, neonatal, and family history for hearing loss, reexamines the child for evidence of any craniofacial abnormalities or a syndrome associated with hearing loss, and discusses the benefits of early intervention services and amplification. The primary care physician, therefore, needs to be aware of community resources and support the family choice of early intervention program and mode of communication.

Every infant with confirmed hearing loss should be evaluated by an otolaryngologist with knowledge of pediatric hearing loss. The otolaryngologist conducts a comprehensive assessment to determine the etiology of hearing loss and provides recommendations and information to the family, audiologist, and primary care provider on candidacy for amplification, assistive devices, and surgical intervention, including reconstruction, bone-anchored hearing aids, and cochlear implantation.

Because of the prevalence of hereditary hearing loss, all families of children with confirmed hearing loss should be offered a genetics evaluation and counseling. This evaluation can provide families with information on etiology, prognosis, associated disorders, and the likelihood of hearing loss in future offspring. The geneticist will review the family history for specific genetic disorders or syndromes, examine the child, and complete genetic testing for syndromes or gene mutations for nonsyndromic hearing loss such as *GJB2* (connexin 26).[41]

Additional referrals may be made at that time for a developmental assessment or other indicated specialty evaluation. Because 30% to 40% of children with confirmed hearing loss have comorbidities or other disabilities, the primary care physician should closely monitor developmental milestones and initiate referrals related to suspected disabilities as needed.[23] Because of the association of hearing loss with vision impairments and the importance of vision for children with hearing loss, it is recommended that each child with a permanent hearing loss have at least one examination to assess visual acuity by an ophthalmologist experienced in evaluating infants.

MIDDLE EAR DISEASE

Otitis media with effusion (OME) is highly prevalent among young children, and about 90% of children have an episode of OME before starting school.[45] Middle ear status should be monitored closely in children with permanent hearing loss because the presence of middle ear effusion can further compromise hearing. Recommendations related to diagnosis of OME include examination with a pneumatic otoscope and documentation of laterality, duration of effusion, and severity of symptoms. Although about 40% to 50% of children with OME do not have symptoms,[39] some children may have associated balance problems.[17] Medical management of OME in children with permanent hearing loss may include hearing testing, amplification adjustment, and tympanostomy tubes. Most OME is self-limited,[40] and 75% to 90% of cases spontaneously resolve in 3 months. Therefore, a 3-month period of observation is recommended. Evidence suggests that no benefit is derived from the use of antihistamines or decongestants in children.

Children with persistent OME (≥4 months' duration) with associated persistent hearing loss or structural injury to the tympanic membrane or middle ear become candidates for surgical intervention with tympanostomy. Tympanostomy has been shown to be associated with decreases in middle ear effusion and improved hearing.

COMMUNICATION OPTIONS

One of the important decisions that the family needs to make for the child is the communication mode that will work optimally for the child and family. There are five options. Auditory oral communication encourages the use of residual hearing and amplification with visual support (speech reading), and the goal is spoken language. Auditory verbal communication is based on listening skills alone, and the goal is spoken language. Cued speech uses a visual communication system that combines listening with eight hand shapes in four placements near the face and supports spoken language. Total communication combines all means of communication and encourages simultaneous use of speech and sign. Deaf children learn American Sign Language, and English is learned as a second language once American Sign Language is mastered. The choice of communication option for the family may change over time depending on the progress of the child and the degree of hearing loss. For example, for an infant born with a profound hearing loss, the family may initially choose total communication but, after a cochlear implant at 12 months of age, may use predominantly auditory verbal or auditory oral communication.

HEARING AIDS, FREQUENCY MODULATED SYSTEMS, AND COCHLEAR IMPLANTS
Hearing Aids

Hearing aids are compact and worn either in-the-ear (ITE) or behind-the-ear (BTE), and can be fitted on an infant in the first month of life. The main components are the microphone that picks up sounds and the amplifier. The audiologist uses computer programming to adjust the sound for an individual child's needs. If the child has different degrees of hearing loss at different frequencies, the audiologist adjusts the gain (loudness) by frequency. Normal speech range is from 500 to 2000 Hz. Ear molds are made from an impression of the child's ear. As a young infant grows, the ear molds may need to be replaced every 6-8 weeks.

Frequency Modulated Systems

Frequency modulated (FM) systems were developed for individuals with hearing loss to hear better in noisy environments. An FM system consists of a microphone and a receiver. A small radio transmitter is attached to a microphone and a small radio receiver. A parent or teacher wears the FM transmitter and microphone while the child wears the FM receiver. The FM transmitter sends a low-power radio signal to the FM receiver that needs to be within 50 feet of the transmitter. The FM receiver gets the signal from the microphone and sends it to a personal hearing aid or cochlear implant. Listening to the FM signal is similar to listening to speech only inches away. FM systems can be used in a variety of situations, including in the home, while shopping, or at school.

Cochlear Implants

According to the U.S. Food and Drug Administration, 30,000 children in the United Sates had received cochlear implants by the end of 2009. Candidacy criteria for pediatric cochlear implantation currently is 18 months or older for children with severe to profound bilateral sensorineural hearing loss and 12 to 18 months for children with profound hearing loss. In cases of deafness due to meningitis, implants may be placed early in the first year of life. A lack of benefit in the development of auditory skills with amplification needs to be demonstrated for eligibility for an implant. Children up to 7 years of age appear to derive the greatest benefit from a cochlear implant for the development of speech.[44]

Because of an increased risk for bacterial meningitis, it is recommended that physicians monitor all patients with cochlear implants, particularly children whose implants have a positioner,[7,34] for middle ear and other infections. *Streptococcus pneumoniae* is the most common pathogen causing meningitis in cochlear implant recipients.[27,46] All children with cochlear implants should be vaccinated according to the American Academy of Pediatrics high-risk schedule.

CONTINUED SURVEILLANCE

The Joint Committee on Infant Hearing 2007[22] has new recommendations for ongoing surveillance in the medical home for all infants with and without risk factors for hearing loss. Regular surveillance of developmental milestones, auditory skills, parental concerns, and middle ear status should be performed in the medical home, consistent with the American Academy of Pediatrics periodicity schedule.[2] All infants should have an objective standardized screen of global development with a validated screening tool at 9, 18, and 24 to 30 months of age or at any time if the health care professional or family

has concern.[22] Language screens that can be used in the primary care setting include the Early Language Milestone Scale,[12] the MacArthur Communicative Development Inventory,[13] the Language Development Survey,[35] and Ages and Stages.[8]

Infants who do not pass the speech-language portion of a global screening or for whom there is a concern regarding hearing or language should be referred for speech-language evaluation and audiology assessment. This recommendation was implemented because of the known increase in the number of children identified with hearing loss between the newborn screen and school age. This is related to three factors: mild hearing loss is missed with newborn screening tools, there is delayed onset or progressive hearing loss such as that associated with cytomegalovirus, and there is late-onset hearing loss secondary to trauma or chemotherapy. Infants with OME may have transient hearing loss and associated language delays.

STRESS AND IMPACT ON THE FAMILY

Parents perceive varying degrees of stress when they are informed that their infant has failed a newborn hearing screen. Although the screen result may be either a false-positive or a true fail, most parents will have some increase in worry until their infant is rescreened. NICU infants have higher false-positive rates and higher fail rates than well-baby nursery infants. In one study[47] of well-baby nursery infants, parents reported increased "worry" at 2 to 8 weeks of age when they returned for the rescreen. Mothers who were more informed about hearing screening experienced decreased worry. Physicians who understand the screening process can support the family whose infant fails the screen, encourage the family to return for the rescreen, and follow-up with the family about the rescreen results. A second study[48] reported that mothers of infants with a false-positive screen did not report increased levels of stress or impact at 12 to 16 months or at 18 to 24 months. In addition, greater family resources were protective against persistent stress, whereas NICU stay contributed to prolonged stress.[48]

There is a continuum of increasing stress for families whose infants are identified with loss that increases as they progress though the hearing screen fail, rescreen fail, diagnostic fail, and intervention process.[24] Perception of stress at the time of diagnosis varies significantly among parents. Parents who are culturally deaf may have anticipated the diagnosis and be totally comfortable with it. Hearing parents of children diagnosed with a hearing loss perceive greater stress, which is, in part, related to the fear of disability.[1,4,24,47] About 95% of children with congenital hearing loss are born to hearing parents. Prompt sharing of diagnostic test results with the family and physician and referral to early intervention services by the audiologist on the day of diagnosis may facilitate the provision of needed information and support to parents to mediate stress.

If the physicians become aware of financial difficulties experienced by the family, the case manager from Part C Early Intervention should be alerted to assist the family to identify resources such as a hearing aid loaner program, Social Security benefit, Katie Beckett Program, or eligibility for Medicaid. The physician may also facilitate referrals to parent support groups such as Hands and Voices and Family Voices. Because half of the children identified with congenital hearing loss had been in an NICU, and about 40% of children with permanent hearing loss have other disabilities, these children may require the resources of a number of different medical and educational disciplines, adding to both the financial and emotional burden.[23,30]

In summary, infants born in 2010 with congenital hearing loss who have early identification, amplification, and intervention have enhanced opportunities for successful communication and academic achievement.

REFERENCES

1. Abdala deUzcategu C, Yoshinaga-Itano C: Parents' reactions to newborn hearing screening, *Audiology Today* 9(1):24, 1997.
2. American Academy of Pediatrics: Policy statement: identifying infants and young children with developmental disorders in the medical home: an algorithm for developmental surveillance and screening, *Pediatrics* 118:405, 2006.
3. Arditi M, et al: Three-year multicenter surveillance of pneumococcal meningitis in children: clinical characteristics, and outcome related to penicillin susceptibility and dexamethasone use, *Pediatrics* 102:1087, 1998.
4. Barringer D, Mauk G: Survey of parents' perspectives regarding hospital-based newborn hearing screening, *Audiology Today* 1:18, 1997.
5. Bertolini P, et al: Platinum compound-related ototoxicity in children: long-term follow-up reveals continuous worsening of hearing loss, *J Pediatr Hematol Oncol* 26:649, 2004.
6. Bess FH: Children with unilateral hearing loss, *J Acad Rehabilitative Audiol* 15:131, 1982.
7. Biernath KR, et al: Bacterial meningitis among children with cochlear implants beyond 24 months after implantation, *Pediatrics* 117:284, 2006.
8. Bricker D, Squires J: *Ages and stages questionnaires: a parent-completed, child-monitoring system*, Baltimore, MD, 1999, Paul H. Brookes.
9. Brookhouser PE, et al: Fluctuating and/or progressive sensorineural hearing loss in children, *Laryngoscope* 104:958, 1994.
10. Centers for Disease Control and Prevention. Early Hearing Detection and Intervention (EHDI) Program (website). www.cdc.gov/ncbddd/ehdi. Accessed May, 2010.
11. Cone-Wesson B, et al: Identification of neonatal hearing impairment: infants with hearing loss, *Ear Hear* 21:488, 2000.
12. Coplan J: *Early language milestone scale*, 2nd ed, Austin, TX, 1993, Pro-ed.
13. Fenson L, Dale PS, Reznick JS, et al: *The McArthur communicative development inventories: user's guide and technical manual*, San Diego, 1993, Singular: Thomson Learning.
14. Fligor BJ, et al: Factors associated with sensorineural hearing loss among survivors of extracorporeal membrane oxygenation therapy, *Pediatrics* 115:1519, 2005.
15. Fowler K, et al: The outcome of congenital cytomegalovirus infection in relation to maternal antibody status, *N Engl J Med* 326:663, 1992.
16. Fowler KB, et al: Progressive and fluctuating sensorineural hearing loss in children with asymptomatic congenital cytomegalovirus infection, *J Pediatr* 130:624, 1997.
17. Golz A, et al: Evaluation of balance disturbances in children with middle ear effusion, *Int J Pediatr Otorhinolaryngol* 43:21, 1998.
18. Gorlin RJ, et al: *Hereditary hearing loss and its syndromes*. NY, 1995 Oxford University.
19. Jerger JF, Hayes D: The cross-check principle in pediatric audiometry, *Arch Otolaryngol* 102:614, 1976.
20. Johnson JL, et al: A multisite study to examine the efficacy of the otoacoustic emission/automated auditory brainstem response newborn hearing screening protocol: introduction and overview of the study, *Am J Audiol* 14:S178, 2005.
21. Joint Committee on Infant Hearing. Year 2000 position statement: principles and guidelines for early hearing detection and intervention programs, *Am J Audiol* 9:9, 2000.
22. Joint Committee on Infant Hearing. Year 2007 position statement: principles and guidelines for early hearing detection and intervention programs, *Pediatrics* 120:898, 2007.
23. Karchmer MA, Allen TE: The functional assessment of deaf and hard of hearing students, *Am Ann Deaf* 144:68, 1999.
24. Kurtzer-White E, Luterman D: Families and children with hearing loss: grief and coping, *Ment Retard Dev Disabil Res Rev* 9:232, 2003.
25. Lew HL, et al: Brainstem auditory-evoked potentials as an objective tool for evaluating hearing dysfunction in traumatic brain injury, *Am J Phys Med Rehabil* 83:210, 2004.
26. Madden C, et al: Audiometric, clinical and educational outcomes in a pediatric symptomatic congenital cytomegalovirus (CMV) population with sensorineural hearing loss, *Int J Pediatr Otorhinolaryngol* 69:1191, 2005.
27. Manruqie M, et al: Advantages of cochlear implantation in prelingual deaf children before 2 years of age when compared with later implantation, *Laryngoscope* 114:1462, 2004.
28. Mayne AM, et al: Expressive vocabulary development of infants and toddlers who are deaf or hard of hearing, *Volta Rev* 100:1, 1998.
29. Mayne AM, et al: Receptive vocabulary development of infants and toddlers who are deaf or hard of hearing, *Volta Rev* 100:29, 1998.
30. Mitchell RE: National profile of deaf and hard of hearing students in special education from weighted survey results, *Am Ann Deaf* 149:336, 2004.
31. Nance WE: The genetics of deafness, *Ment Retard Dev Disabil Res Rev* 9:109, 2003.
32. Nance WE, et al: Importance of congenital cytomegalovirus infections as a cause for pre-lingual hearing loss, *J Clin Virol* 35:221, 2006.
33. National Institutes of Health: Early Identification of Hearing Impairment in Infants and Young Children: NIH Consensus Development Conference Statement, Bethesda, MD: 1993, National Institutes of Health. http://consensus.nih.gov/1993/1993HearingInfantsChildren092html.htm. Accessed January 24, 2007.
34. Reefhuis J, et al: Risk of bacterial meningitis in children with cochlear implants, *N Engl J Med* 349:435, 2003.
35. Rescoria L: The Language Development Survey: a screening tool for delayed language in toddlers, *J Speech Hear Dis* 54:587, 1989.
36. Rivera L, et al: Predictors of hearing loss in children with symptomatic congenital cytomegalovirus infection, *Pediatrics* 110:762, 2002.
37. Roizen NJ: Etiology of hearing loss in children. Nongenetic causes, *Pediatr Clin North Am* 46:49, 1999.
38. Roizen NJ: Nongenetic causes of hearing loss, *Mental Retard Dev Disabil Res Rev* 9:120, 2003.
39. Rosenfeld RM, et al: Quality of life for children with otitis media, *Arch Otolaryngol Head Neck Surg* 123:1049, 1997.

40. Rosenfeld RM, Kay D: Natural history of untreated otitis media, *Laryngoscope* 113:1645, 2003.

41. Santos RL, et al: Hearing impairment in Dutch patients with connexin 26 (GJB2) and connexin 30 (GJB6) mutations, *Int J Pediatr Otorhinolaryngol* 69:165, 2005.

42. Sharma A, et al: A sensitive period for the development of the central auditory system in children with cochlear implants: implications for age of implantation, *Ear Hear* 23:532, 2002.

43. Sharma A, et al: Central auditory maturation and babbling development in infants with cochlear implants, *Arch Otolaryngol Head Neck Sur* 130:511, 2004.

44. Sharma A, et al: The influence of a sensitive period on central auditory development in children with unilateral and bilateral cochlear implants, *Hear Res* 203:134, 2005.

45. Tos M: Epidemiology and natural history of secretory otitis, *Am J Otol* 5:459, 1984.

46. Uchanski R, Geers A: Acoustic characteristics of the speech of young cochlear implant users: a comparisons with normal-hearing age-mates, *Ear Hear* 24:90S, 2003.

47. Vohr BR, et al: Maternal worry about neonatal hearing screening, *J Perinatol* 21:15, 2001.

48. Vohr BR, et al: Results of newborn screening for hearing loss: effects on the family in the first 2 years of life, *Arch Pediatr Adolesc Med* 162:205, 2008.

49. Vohr B, et al: Early language outcomes of early-identified infants with permanent hearing loss at 12 to 16 months of age, *Pediatrics* 122:535, 2008.

50. Yoshinaga-Itano C: Levels of evidence: universal newborn hearing screening (UNHS) and early hearing detection and intervention systems (EHDI), *J Commun Disord* 37:451, 2004.

51. Zimmerman WD, et al: Peripheral hearing loss following head trauma in children, *Laryngoscope* 103:87, 1993.

CHAPTER 43

Neurobehavioral Development of the Preterm Infant

Heidelise Als and Samantha Butler

Swiftly the brain becomes an enchanted loom, where millions of flashing shuttles weave a dissolving pattern, always a meaningful pattern though never an abiding one
— *Sir Charles Sherrington, 1940,*
Man on His Nature, p. 178

About 13 million preterm deliveries occur per year around the world, with an overall incidence of about 9%.[67] In developed regions of the world, the incidence varies from 5% to 12%; it may be as high as 40% in less developed, poor areas.[24,48] Prematurity rates are steadily rising, especially in Western countries, with the advent of extensive infertility treatment and women's increased age at child bearing. For reasons of generational poverty and stress associated with discrimination, as well as lack of ready access to health care, the incidence stands at an all-time high of 18% for African-American families. Given significant advances in perinatology and neonatology in industrialized countries, survival rates have dramatically increased, even for infants with very low and extremely low birthweights. Today, more than 90% of infants born after 28 weeks' gestation. For infants born at 23 weeks, the probability of intact survival, that is, discharge home free of major disabilities, is less than 10%; it is less than 25% at 24 weeks and 35% at 25 weeks. Not until 26 weeks is the rate more than 50%.

Although infants born very early make up only a small percentage of births, they add disproportionately to the mortality, morbidity, and cost of medical care and of long-term disability services.[50,51,65] Preterm-born infants experience a range of adverse physical, behavioral, and mental health problems. Previously, it was believed that in the absence of major complications (e.g., large intraventricular hemorrhages, significant chronic lung disease, severe intrauterine growth restriction, necrotizing enterocolitis), preterm-born

children would "catch up" over time. However, this is not the case. Recent research suggests that as preterm-born infants mature, they remain increasingly disadvantaged on many measures of cognitive function and mental processing. This is evidenced by problems related to academic achievement, behavior regulation, and social and emotional adaptation.[35,53,60] Prematurity is increasingly understood as a life-long condition.[16]

Not only to ensure survival, but also to foster best development of the increasing numbers of preterm infants, an understanding of their neurodevelopmental course is critical. This chapter provides a framework for the understanding and assessment of the preterm infant's neurobehavioral development as well as for the delivery of care from a neurodevelopmental perspective.

A NEURODEVELOPMENTAL FRAMEWORK

Preterm infants are fetuses who develop in extrauterine settings at a time when their brains are growing more rapidly than ever in their life span. They expect three securely inherited environments, namely their mother's womb, their parent's body, and their family and community's social group.[36] However, given medical and other complications, they are removed from the protective womb environment at this highly vulnerable phase of development. Prematurely born infants require care available only in the specialized, medical technological environments of newborn intensive care units (NICUs) and special care nurseries. Infants in these unexpected, yet medically necessary, environments are at high risk for organ impairments, the most devastating of which include chronic lung disease or bronchopulmonary dysplasia, intraventricular hemorrhage, retinopathy of prematurity, and necrotizing enterocolitis. Aside from such impairments, the mismatch of the fetal brain's expectation and the characteristics of the intensive or special care nursery provide significant challenges, which influence the infant's neurophysiologic, neuropsychological, psychoemotional, and psychosocial development. The fetus, and in turn the premature infant, expects total cutaneous-somesthetic input from amniotic fluid and kinesthetic input from the continuously reactive amniotic sac, which ensures mutual extensor-flexor modulation for head, trunk, and extremities. Fetal infants expect maternal diurnal rhythms to entrain differentiating states of consciousness and muted inputs to ready the primary senses of audition, olfaction, and gustation. Parental disruption of the expected emotional and physical preparation of pregnancy further adds to the challenge for preterm infants and parents. Even medically healthy preterm infants show an increase in later developmental difficulties, such as learning disabilities, lower intelligence quotients, executive function and attention deficit disorders, lower thresholds to fatigue, visual motor impairments, spatial processing disturbances, language comprehension and speech problems, emotional vulnerabilities, difficulties with self-regulation and self-esteem, and significant school performance deficits.[34] It appears that development in the extrauterine environment leads to different and potentially maladaptive developmental trajectories.

It is important to ask how to ensure these infants' smooth and balanced functioning outside of the womb. Realignment and emergence of the next developmental agenda best occur on the background of well-integrated functioning. This avoids reinforcement of costly maladaptive defense behaviors that all too readily spiral into vicious cycles of increasing distortion and disorganization, which in turn modify both

brain structure and function.[6,8] It is not surprising that many of these infants later experience behavioral and neurologic difficulties. Understanding the neurodevelopmental expectations of the fetal infant provides a basis for modification of traditionally delivered newborn intensive care, which inadvertently increases stress and challenges the vulnerable preterm nervous system, and therewith the preterm child.

BRAIN-ENVIRONMENT INTERACTION

The environment influences the development of the fetal brain through the various senses of the infant, including the visual, auditory, cutaneous, tactile, somesthetic, kinesthetic, olfactory, and gustatory senses. Increasingly, animal and human studies indicate the importance of sensory information and experience in the womb for the complexity of fetal brain development. The sensory environment outside the womb presents stark contrasts and fully unexpected challenges to the fetal brain and may lead to malfunction and distortion of brain development and therewith neurobehavioral dysfunction. Human cortex begins development at about the sixth week of gestation, when the embryo is less than 1.5 cm in length, with the arrival of primitive corticipetal fibers, followed by the establishment of a superficial, primordial plexiform lamina. Cortical layer I, part of this plexiform lamina, appears to be necessary for the subsequent inside-out formation of the cortical plate, which represents the actual mammalian neocortical gray matter, and appears to play a significant role in the overall structural organization of the mammalian cerebral cortex. It controls the migration of all future neurons regardless of size, cortical location, or functional role.[49] Figure 43-1A presents these early

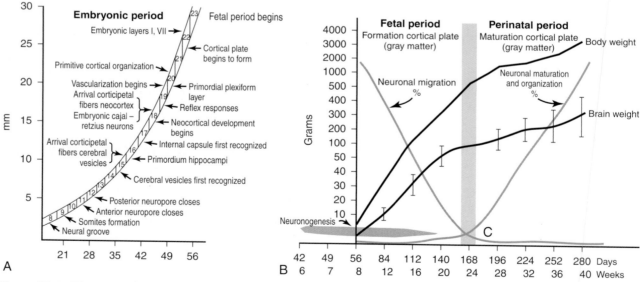

Figure 43–1. The major developmental events of the embryonic (**A**), fetal (**B**), and perinatal (**C**) periods of the prenatal ontogenesis of the human cerebral cortex. The embryonic period is characterized by the appearance of the cerebral vesicles, the arrival of the first corticipetal fibers, and the establishment of the primordial plexiform layer before the formation of the cortical plate. The fetal period is characterized by the process of neuronal migration and the inside-out formation of the cortical plate. The perinatal period is characterized by the ascending neuronal differentiation and maturation of the cortical plate (gray matter). (*Reprinted with permission from Marin-Padilla M: Pathogenesis of late-acquired leptomeningeal heterotopias and secondary cortical alterations: a Golgi study. In Galaburda AM, editor: Dyslexia and development. Cambridge, MA, 1993, Harvard University Press.*)

stages of cortical formation. By 6 weeks, the superficial musculature of the embryo is highly developed,[16] and cutaneous innervation and sensitivity are well on their way.[38] It begins with sensitivity in and about the mouth and extends to the nose and chin, eyelids, palms of the hands, genitalia, and the soles of the feet. Feedback loops are set up and dynamically construct the highly complex human central nervous system. Throughout development, a disproportionately large area of somatosensory cortex, dedicated to the earliest innervated surface regions, supports their specific evolutionary significance. It is these regions that appear difficult to satisfy and inhibit behaviorally in the fetal infant outside the womb.[1] Preterm infants brace with their feet, grasp with hands and feet, bring their hands to their mouths, search with mouth and tongue, suck, and make strong efforts to tuck themselves into flexion. This is especially apparent in the first 24 to 48 hours after delivery, before exhaustion leads to flaccidity.

Sixty years ago, Gesell and Armatruda[30] documented the organized specificity of very early fetal behavior. They showed specific turning away to a hair probe touch, whereas exploratory approach movements appeared to dominate in spontaneous undisturbed activity. This early appearance of the avoidance and approach continuum is in keeping with Denny-Brown's[26] model of motor system development, which involves gradual differentiation and integration of the dual antagonist extensor and flexor, that is, avoidance and approach movements. The differentiating spontaneous movement repertoire of the fetus is increasingly documented by ultrasound studies and indicates flexor-extensor adjustments; complex grasping and release sequences; interaction with the continuously available, pliable, and moving umbilical cord; exploration of face, neck, and head; sucking; holding on with one hand to the other; stepping; clasping one foot against the other; and so forth (Fig. 43-2).

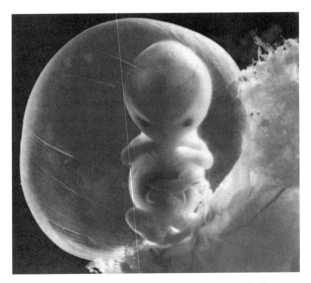

Figure 43–2. Seven weeks old, nearly an inch long, and weighing about 2 g: spontaneous exploratory behavior. *(Reproduced with permission from Als H, et al: Individualized behavioral and environmental care for the very low birth weight preterm infant at high risk for bronchopulmonary dysplasia: neonatal intensive care unit and developmental outcome, Pediatrics 78:1123, 1986, Copyright © 1986 by the AAP.)*

Such patterns set up increasingly complex feedback loops and generate the species—specifically complex human brain cytoarchitecture, with its enormously increased frontal-cortical systems.

Each of the millions of neurons in human cerebral cortex originates in the germinal lining of the ventricular system. In its prime, the germinal matrix releases as many as 100,000 cortical neurons per day, each of which migrates through the entire thickness of cortex to a specific location. These migrations occur in waves. They begin at about 8 postovulatory weeks and gradually tail off around 24 weeks of pregnancy, as Figure 43-1B shows, when neuronal maturation and organization increases dramatically, as Figure 43-1C indicates. Much of neuronal maturation and organization for the preterm infant occurs in the interaction with the extrauterine rather than the intrauterine environment. Each of the estimated 100 billion total human neurons, once migrated to their respective locations, develops dendritic and axonal interconnections with an average of 100 other cells. Although the first synaptic contacts are established as early as 7 weeks after conception, new cortical cells are generated at a low rate up until and beyond 40 weeks, and synapses continue to be established richly until age 5 years, more slowly, at least until age 18 years, and as now known, throughout the life span.[66] As cells become larger and more elaborately connected, more and more sulci and gyri develop, and different brain areas organize for different functions. A marked increase in the number of gyri occurs at the end of the second trimester and correlates with a concurrent growth spurt of the brain in terms of weight and a change in head contour from oval to prominent biparietal bossing. This is also the time when fetal behavior becomes increasingly complex with increased sucking on fingers or hand, grasping, extension and flexion rotations, increasingly discernible sleep and wake periods, and reactions to sound. Myelin, a fatty sheath somewhat like insulation, deposits around the axons and allows faster and highly repetitive conduction of impulses. It serves mainly to accommodate the increased length of the neuronal tracks with growth. Myelination occurs with peak activity around term birth and continues significantly until age 9 years and perceptibly into the 40s. Concurrent with the processes of cell differentiation, myelination, and neurobehavioral differentiation, neurochemical development occurs. Passage of impulses or messages between cells occurs by chemical neurotransmitters, which often are released only if up to four or five different regulatory systems co-occur in specific configurations. More than two dozen neurotransmitters have so far been identified, and no doubt there are many more. The sensitivities and densities of neurotransmitter receptors vary widely from brain region to region. Experience influences receptor development. Brain and sensory organs are interdependent for structural and functional development. The vulnerability of the support structure tissue adds to the picture of sensitivity and fragility of the preterm brain and the consequent sensitivity in overall functioning. Up to 50% of preterm infants born before 32 weeks' gestation have some degree of brain hemorrhage, and the incidence increases with the reduction in gestational age.[66]

Animal models have provided substantial evidence for the fine-tuned specificity of environmental inputs necessary for support of normal cortical ontogenesis in the course of sensitive periods of brain development and in the absence of focal lesions. The mechanisms implicated, when expected inputs are not forthcoming, are largely active inhibition of developing pathways consequent to overactivation of prematurely functional pathways, mediated by the endorphin system. Further support for a brain-based formulation of understanding preterm functioning comes from the Goldman-Rakič[64a] research team, who showed that the specific connection systems developed in primates involve not only competition between axon terminals, and trophic feedback between presynaptic and postsynaptic cells, but also dynamic modification of connection at long distances due to functional activity. They concluded that changes in activity of distant yet synaptically related structures, which reduce or change specific input to cortex, affect subsequent developmental events, and provide the setting for new cell relations, the net outcome of which are unique cerebral cytoarchitectonic and chemoarchitectonic maps. Changes induced in mid-gestation in monkey thalamic fiber projections have yielded the formation of hybrid cortex, indicating that during rapid brain development, new cytoarchitectonic regions may arise by altered interactions, depending on unique combinations of intrinsic properties of the cortical neurons and afferent fibers involved.[66] Furthermore, differential cell death and other regressive events, which begin at about 24 weeks' gestation with the tailing off of cell migration, appear to be of key importance in sculpting developing cortex. These normally occurring regressive events are timed to be directly affected by the condition of premature birth. Of interest in this regard is also the function of subplate neurons, which are born in the generative zones and migrate to the primitive marginal zone before generation. The next step is migration of the neurons of the cortical plate themselves.[66] Subplate neurons provide a site for synaptic contact for axons that ascend from the thalamus and other cortical sites, termed *waiting* thalamocortical and corticocortical afferents, because their neuronal targets in the cortical plate have not yet arrived or differentiated. These subplate neurons establish a functional synaptic link between waiting afferents and their cortical targets. They guide ascending axons to their targets. When the subplate neurons are experimentally eliminated, thalamocortical afferents destined for overlying cortex fail to move superiorly into the cortex at the appropriate site and continue to grow aimlessly in the subcortical region.[66] Thus, subplate neurons are strongly involved in cerebral cortical organization. Furthermore, their descending axon collaterals guide the initial projections from cerebral cortex toward subcortical targets and toward other cortical sites. The subplate neuron layer in frontal human cortex reaches its peak at 32 to 34 weeks of gestation. This is a time that the preterm infant spends outside of the womb and experiences quite unexpected sensory inputs to primary cortical areas, such as visual cortex and somatosensory and auditory cortex. Visual cortex in the womb receives neither light, color, nor pattern input. The somatosensory and auditory cortex in the womb receives inputs, yet of a quite different kind from that outside the womb.

It seems warranted to hypothesize that messages transmitted from primary cortical regions to other cortical areas, including frontal cortex, are quite different for the preterm infant in the NICU than they would be for the fetus in the womb. It is also likely that waiting and regressive events are modified when the brain finds itself in unusual sensory circumstances, such as outside of the womb too early, and that cells are preserved, which might otherwise be eliminated, and cells are eliminated, which might otherwise be preserved. Monkeys delivered experimentally prematurely, while unchanged in visual cortical cell number, show significantly different visual cortical synapse formations in terms of size, type, and laminar distribution, compared with term monkeys tested at comparable post-term ages. The extent of difference correlates with the degree of prematurity.[20,21] Thus, although some events influence neuronal migration per se, other events, including difference in sensory input, appear to alter corticocortical connectivities and lead to unique cytoarchitectures and chemoarchitectures of cerebral cortex. This supports the finding that preterm infants show brain-based differences in neurofunctional performance. Premature activation of cortical pathways appears to inhibit later differentiations and interfere with appropriate development and sculpting, especially of cross-modal and frontal connection systems implicated in complex mental processing, as well as attention processes and self-regulation. Furthermore, corpus callosum differences have also been documented in preterm children studied at school age.[65]

In the term child, axonal and dendritic proliferation and the massive increase in outer layer cortical cell growth and differentiation lead to the enormous gyri and sulci formation of the human brain. This occurs in an environment of mother-mediated protection from environmental perturbations. It relies on a steady supply of nutrients, temperature control, and the presence of multiple regulating systems, including maternal-fetal chronobiologic and affective rhythms. The traditional NICU environment involves sensory overload and stands in stark mismatch to the developing nervous system's expectation.[14] Prolonged diffuse sleep states, unattended crying, supine positioning, routine and excessive handling, loud ambient sounds, lack of opportunity for sucking, and poorly timed social and caregiving interactions all exert deleterious effects on the immature brain and alter its subsequent development. How does one estimate the potential effects for the individual infant's nervous system moving too early from the relative equilibrium of the intrauterine aquatic econiche of the mother to the extrauterine terrestrial environment of the NICU?

A MODEL FOR OBSERVING THE PRETERM INFANT'S BEHAVIOR

According to Denny-Brown,[26] underlying the developing nervous system's striving for smoothness of integration is the tension between two basic antagonists of behavior, namely the exploratory and the avoiding response. The two dimensions are released simultaneously and stand in conflict with one another. If a threshold of organization-appropriate stimulation is passed, one may abruptly switch into the other. These two poles of behavior are basic to all functioning. This is demonstrated by the existence of somatosensory cortex single cells, which on stimulation produce toward or avoidance movements of the total body. The same principle operates in the gradual specialization of central arousal processes, which lead to functionally adaptive action patterns in altricial animals, such as suckling, nipple-grasping, huddling, and others. The principle of dual antagonist integration is helpful when assessing preterm infants' behavioral thresholds from integration to stress. In the well-integrated performance, the two antagonists of toward and avoidance modulate each other in bringing about an adaptive response. When an input is compelling to the fetal infant and matches interest and internal readiness, the infant will approach the input, react to and interact with it, seek it out, and become sensitized to it. When the input overloads the infant's neuronal network circuitry, the infant will defend against it, actively avoid the input, and withdraw from it. Both response patterns mutually modulate one another. For instance, the animate face of the interacting caregiver draws in the term newborn. As the infant's attention intensifies, eyes widen, eyebrows rise, mouth shapes toward the interacter, and fingers open and close softly. If the dampening processes of this intensity are poorly established, as in the preterm infant, the whole head may move forward; arms, legs, fingers, and toes extend toward the interacter; the mouth may shape forward; the wide-eyed gaze may trigger the visceral system; and the infant may hiccough or vomit. The response, which in the term infant is largely confined to face and hands, in the preterm infant may involve the entire body in an overly generalized way.

The overriding issue for preterm-born newborns is the integration of autonomic functions, such as respiration, heart rate, temperature control, digestion, and elimination, with the functioning of a motor system, which seeks to explore, contain itself, tuck into flexion, expand and extend, rotate, somersault, bring the hand to the mouth and suck, and grasp the umbilical cord. The motor system expects the cutaneous input of the amniotic fluid and amniotic sac wall, which support flexor-extensor balance. Preterm infant state organization no longer is supported by the maternal sleep-wake and rest-activity cycles, nor by the maternal hormonal, affective, and nutritional cycles. The model for observation and assessment of preterm infants' subsystem differentiation, termed synactive,[1] highlights the simultaneity of the subsystems in negotiation with one another and with the current environment. Systems continually open up and transform to new levels of more differentiated integration, from which the next steps of differentiation press to actualization.[1] To paraphrase Erikson (1962), self-actualization is participation with the world and interaction with another with a "minimum of defensive maneuvers and a maximum of activation; a minimum of idiosyncratic distortion and a maximum of joint validation."

BEHAVIORAL LANGUAGE OF THE PRETERM INFANT

Observation of preterm infants' behavior provides the base for estimation of the fetal infant brain's expectation for input, for inference of the infant's developmental goals for co-regulatory support, and for assessment of the infant's current functional competence. The formulation of observation and assessment is conceptually based in a combination of knowledge of fetal brain and behavior development, of term developmental functioning in negotiating the altered environment-fetus transaction, and of the individual-specific strategies employed by each infant. The behavior of the infant offers a common channel of expression of all three components and provides a base for inference of appropriate environment and care.[1]

Even fragile infants and those born very early display reliably observable behaviors in the form of autonomic and visceral responses, such as respiration patterns, color fluctuations, spitting, gagging, hiccoughing, and bowel movement strains. Infants also show observable movement patterns, postures, and tone of trunk, extremities, and face, exhibited in finger splays, arching, and grimacing, among others. Furthermore, the infants' levels of awareness, referred to as states, such as sleeping, wakefulness, and aroused upset, allow for valuable information. This makes possible an observation and assessment approach geared to documentation and understanding of such behaviors as evidence of stress and of competence and goal strivings. Such an approach provides the base for formal training and education in reading and assessment of the infant, with inference to reduce stress, support behavioral competence, and improve development.

The infant's vocabulary is identifiable along the lines of the three main systems outlined, the autonomic system, the motor system, and the state system, with special emphasis on the attention system. The infant's continued communication along these subsystem lines indicates whether what is currently going on around and within the infant is supportive of the infant's own goal strivings or is taxing, demanding, and potentially stressful for the infant.[1] Behavioral communications associated with each of the systems are delineated further in terms of various subchannels of communication within each system. Table 43-1 outlines the systems and their channels.

The autonomic system's efforts are observable in the infant's breathing patterns, color fluctuation, and visceral stability or instability. Simultaneously, the infant's motor system efforts are

TABLE 43-1   Channels of Communication

Autonomic System	Motor System	State System
Respiration pattern	Tone	Robustness of states
Color	Postural repertoire	Range of states
Visceral stability	Movements	Transition patterns

Adapted from Als H: Reading the premature infant. In Goldson E, editor: *Nurturing the premature infant: developmental interventions in the neonatal intensive care nursery.* New York, 1999, Oxford University Press, p 18.

observable in the infant's maintenance of body tone as well as postural repertoire and movement patterns. State organization is observable in the infant's range of states available, the robustness and modulation of the available states, and the patterns of transition from state to state. To document an infant's ongoing communication, a methodology was developed for the recording of detailed observations of infants' naturalistically occurring behaviors in the NICU. The continuous time sampling method uses 2-minute time epochs as recording intervals. Figure 43-3 shows the behavior observation sheet, which is designed for use by trained observers at the infant's bed or care site. The infant is observed typically for about 20 minutes before a caregiver interacts with the infant, then throughout the duration of caregiving interaction, whether it is vital sign taking, suctioning, diaper change, or feeding, and then for at least 20 minutes after the caregiving interaction. Such an observation, especially if repeated over time, yields information regarding an infant's robustness and development as the infant attempts to integrate and make the best use of the care provided. The observations are used as the basis for

OBSERVATION SHEET Name: _____ Date: _____ Sheet Number _____

Left panel — Time: ____

		0-2	3-4	5-6	7-8	9-10
Resp:	Regular					
	Irregular					
	Slow					
	Fast					
	Pause					
Color:	Jaundice					
	Pink					
	Pale					
	Webb					
	Red					
	Dusky					
	Blue					
	Tremor					
	Startle					
	Twitch Face					
	Twitch Body					
	Twitch Extremities					
Visceral/Resp:	Spit up					
	Gag					
	Burp					
	Hiccough					
	BM Grunt					
	Sounds					
	Sigh					
	Gasp					
Motor:	Flaccid Arm(s)					
	Flaccid leg(s)					
	Flexed/Tucked Arms Act.					
	Flexed/Tucked Arms Post.					
	Flexed/Tucked Legs Act.					
	Flexed/Tucked Legs Post.					
	Extend Arms Act.					
	Extend Arms Post.					
	Extend Legs Act.					
	Extend Legs Post.					
	Smooth Mvmt Arms					
	Smooth Mvmt Legs					
	Smooth Mvmt Trunk					
	Stretch/Drown					
	Diffuse Squirm					
	Arch					
	Tuck Trunk					
	Leg Brace					
Face:	Tongue Extension					
	Hand on Face					
	Gape Face					
	Grimace					
	Smile					

Right panel — Time: ____

		0-2	3-4	5-6	7-8	9-10
State:	1A					
	1B					
	2A					
	2B					
	3A					
	3B					
	4A					
	4B					
	5A					
	5B					
	6A					
	6B					
	AA					
Face (cont.):	Mouthing					
	Suck Search					
	Sucking					
Extrem.:	Finger Splay					
	Airplane					
	Salute					
	Sitting On Air					
	Hand Clasp					
	Foot Clasp					
	Hand to Mouth					
	Grasping					
	Holding On					
	Fisting					
Attention:	Fuss					
	Yawn					
	Sneeze					
	Face Open					
	Eye Floating					
	Avert					
	Frown					
	Ooh Face					
	Locking					
	Cooing					
	Speech Mvmt.					
Posture:	(Prone, Supine, Side)					
Head:	(Right, Left, Middle)					
Location:	(Crib, Incubator, Held)					
Manipulation:						
	Heart Rate					
	Respiration Rate					
	TcPO$_2$					

2002-02 1M (12/83)   H Als 1981

Figure 43-3. Behavior observation sheet. (*From Als H, et al: Individualized behavioral and environmental care for the very low birth weight preterm infant at high risk for bronchopulmonary dysplasia: neonatal intensive care unit and developmental outcome,* Pediatrics 78:1123, 1986.)

caregiving suggestions and modifications in the adaptation of the environment's structure as well as the infant's individualized care plan.

As a rule, extension and diffuse behaviors are thought to reflect stress; flexion and well-modulated behaviors are thought to reflect self-regulatory competence. Regular respirations; pink color; smooth but not overly flexed active tone in arm, leg, and trunk position; smooth movements of arms, legs, and trunk; efforts and successes at tucking the trunk into flexion and bracing the legs all reflect self-regulatory competence. In the very young infant, hand-on-face behavior and mouthing may reflect stability; if overly frequent, however, this may indicate stress if not seizure activity. Suck-searching and sucking; hand clasp and foot clasp; hand-to-mouth efforts, grasping and holding on; face opening; frowning, ooh face, locking, cooing, and speech movements; heart rate between 120 and 160 beats per minute; breathing rate between 40 and 60 breaths per minute; and oxygen saturation (Sao$_2$) between 92% and 96% are typically read as effective self-regulation. *Stress and a low threshold to react* reflect great sensitivity. This is seen in irregular breathing, that is, slow or fast breathing and breathing pauses; color other than pink, that is, pale, webbed and mottled, red, dusky, grey or blue; tremors, startles, and twitches; visceral signs such as spit up, gags, hiccoughs, bowel movement grunts, passing gas, sounds, gasps, and sighs; flaccidity of arms, legs, and trunk; frequent extensor movement of arms and legs; stretch-drown behavior, frequent squirming, arching; frequent tongue extensions, gape face, and frequent grimacing; finger splays, airplane postures, salutes, sitting on air, and frequent fisting; fussing; frequent yawning, sneezing, and eye floating; frequent eye averting; heart rate less than 120 or greater than 160 beats per minute; respiratory rate of less than 40 or greater than 60 breaths per minute; and Sao$_2$ of less than 92% or higher than 96%.

The behavioral description of the infant's functioning in the course of an interaction observed and when anchored in the infant's current medical and family history provides the empirical basis from which to estimate the infant's current developmental goals. For instance, the infant may actively seek to pull himself or herself into flexion; seek to grasp and to tuck legs and feet into bedding and against the wall or surface of the incubator as if attempting to find boundaries and confinement; seek to bring hand and fingers to and into the mouth in order to suck; make efforts to breathe smoothly *with* rather than against the respirator, only to be interrupted repeatedly by the fixed respirator rate setting; attempt to settle back into sleep and restfulness after being care for, and thwarted repeatedly by ongoing sounds from alarms, faucets, voices, equipment being moved about, and so forth. On the basis of the goals inferred from the infant's behaviors observed, the next step is the exploration of supportive opportunities in terms of the environment and the delivery of care to enhance the infant's well-being and sense of competence and effectiveness, and therewith, development. Such considerations begin with appropriate support and nurturance of the infant's parents and family. Family members are understood as the primary co-regulators of the infant's development. They include an atmosphere and ambiance of care, nurturance, and respect for infant and family in the NICU environment; the organization and layout of the infant's care space; the structuring and delivery of specific medical and nursing care procedures and specialty care indicated; and an overall safeguarded and assured developmental perspective on care and environment provided. This is more fully described elsewhere.[2] Key points of the Newborn Individualized Developmental Care and Assessment Program (NIDCAP), are highlighted here.

Assurance of the parents' well-being as the infant's primary nurturers is important. The sensitization to the NICU environment in light of the family's key role is essential. Parents' attunement is exquisite in terms of the emotional ambiance of the setting, in which their immature infant lives and receives care. Parents find disturbing casual staff conversations; off-handed interactions; socializing of staff with one another; being talked over and about; conflict-ridden staff interactions, and so forth. All these activities indicate poor understanding of the parents' important role in the lives and care of their infants. Parents seek a respectful and supportive, professionally consistent environment, which instills a sense of trust through accountability and reliability. The infant's care space is often the infant's home for 3 or 4 months. Its organization and layout present a critical opportunity for support and nurturance of infant and family. Questions to ask include the following: Is the care area quiet, protected from traffic and activity not related to the infant's care? Is the infant's medical chart available to the family at all times? Is there individual and adjustable lighting for each infant's care area? Is there a telephone at each bedside for the family's outgoing calls? Is the family encouraged and guided to arrange, decorate, and personalize the care space, supportive of the infant's development and reflective of the family? Are there opportunities and furniture appropriate for the parents and siblings to be with the child at the bed space? Is staff knowledgeable and skilled in postpartum parent support, including care and comfort for the mother who breastfeeds her infant? Are there provisions for the family's opportunity for rooming with the infant in the NICU? Are there appropriate interpreter services available for all the languages presented by the parents in the NICU?

The infant's care involves many procedures, examinations, and therapeutic interventions delivered by staff from various disciplines. Structure and delivery of specific medical care procedures and specialty care as indicated must be carried out in a developmental perspective that permeates all care and environmental aspects. Primary care is of great importance in this model. It provides consistency of staffing, ensures continuity in care, and fosters intimate knowledge of infant and family. A primary care model effectively uses infants' communications as a basis for individualized care planning and care delivery. Parents are active members of the primary team and participate in rounds, care conferences, decision making, and care implementation. A developmental professional is important in supporting the specialty disciplines in maintaining a developmental perspective in all care planning and delivery. Figure 43-4 conceptualizes the developmental synactive model of care delivery, with focus on infant and family. The immediate safeguard of developmental structuring of care is the primary nursing team in collaboration with the primary physician, supported by specialists, such as respiratory, occupational, and physical therapists and social workers, among others, as indicated. A professional with a developmental specialty background and a nurse clinician

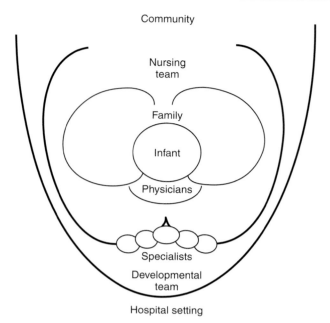

Figure 43–4. Developmental care model in the newborn intensive care unit. *(From Als H: Reading the preterm infant. In Goldson E, et al, editors: Nurturing the premature infant: developmental interventions in the neonatal intensive care nursery. New York, 1999, Oxford University Press, p 18.)*

form an effective team for provision of continued support for the caregivers' developmental perspective and collaboration. Qualifications for the developmental discipline professional include background and training in developmental and clinical pediatric or child psychology with specialization in NICU work in order to collaborate appropriately with the nurse clinician. Jointly they provide appropriate developmental support to the primary care teams in delivering supportive, individualized care in a developmental framework that encompasses infants and families.

TESTING THE VALIDITY OF NIDCAP

The NIDCAP Federation International is the professional organization that safeguards all NIDCAP training and professional certification in the NIDCAP approach to care.

The study of NIDCAP, which is based on reading the preterm infant's behavioral cues, is challenging. NIDCAP is theory driven and relationship based and requires systems integration. Its hardware and technology-free nature make adoption more difficult. The essence of developmental care lies in the continuous resourceful modification of care adapted to the individual infant's competence and vulnerabilities. It requires an open mind for "doing, learning, and coming to know."[31] Common misunderstandings of developmental care include minimal stimulation (fully covered incubators, protection from all visual and auditory contact, and clustered care of rapid routines at set intervals), and the developmental decoration approach to care (pretty nests and incubator covers; indirect lighting; whisper zones; yet routinized care as before). The change that developmental care requires is internal: a shift in

mind and attitude, a "seeing anew." Further challenges exist for cultures and systems in which reflection and relationship-based processes are alien and in which medical professionals have ultimate authority for all decisions. Nurseries may differ in financial and leadership stability, staff relationships, patient census, staff-to-patient ratios, family characteristics, history, tradition and culture, organizational, communication and conflict resolution styles, and their distinctive competencies.[31] Yet the hopes and expectations of infants and families remain the same worldwide. Combining best technology and intensive care with the most sensitive, individualized, developmental care is a demanding responsibility. The NIDCAP training program (www.NIDCAP.org) focuses on education and training of multidisciplinary professional teams in NICUs. These in turn support, educate, and mentor all direct caregivers in the nursery in individualizing care and in fully integrating the parents.[45,70]

The several historical phase-lag trials that have studied NIDCAP are criticized for the possibility of contamination of the results by uncontrolled intervening variables. The preferred design is understandably that of randomized controlled trials. Trials of developmental interventions require large NICUs to provide simultaneous control and experimental group subjects. Staff must understand behavioral research. Cross-contamination of caregiver-implemented interventions is unavoidable; experimental effects must exceed contamination effects. Developmental care research requires experienced professionals, superb nursing and neonatology leadership, and extensive research expertise to safeguard the fidelity of the intervention implementation, the acquisition of complex databases, and the analysis of large data sets. Developmental research is highly labor intensive. Result generalizability is limited to study population and NICU characteristics.

Six randomized controlled trials[6,8,9,22,29,68] have investigated the effectiveness of developmental care. One incomplete and negative review[41] aside, results provided consistent evidence in infants 29 weeks' postmenstrual age and younger at birth, of improved lung function, feeding behavior, and growth, reduced length of hospitalization, and improved neurobehavioral and neurophysiologic functioning. A study of infants 28 to 32 weeks' postmenstrual age at birth[6] showed enhanced brain fiber tract development in frontal lobe and internal capsule. Figure 43-5 depicts the four electroencephalogram (EEG) coherence factor maps, which demonstrate for the intervention group increased coherence between left frontal regions and occipital and parietal regions (factors 7, 10, and 19), whereas midline central to occipital coherence was reduced (factor 11). Thus, developmental care intervention brought about changes in functional connectivity between brain regions, with preferential enhancement of frontal to occipital coherence (long distance coherences—newly emerging competencies) and pruning of central to occipital coherence (short distance coherence—already well-integrated competence). Moreover, Figure 43-6 shows the significantly enhanced white matter fiber tracts in an experimental group infant at 2 weeks' corrected age when compared with a control group infant from this study. The findings suggest more advanced white matter development in the frontal region and the internal capsule. In addition to the medical advantages for the infants born at 29 weeks' postmenstrual age or younger described earlier, a three-center trial[8] of such

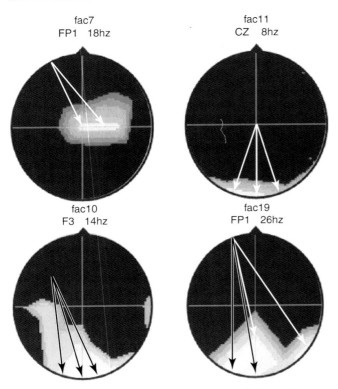

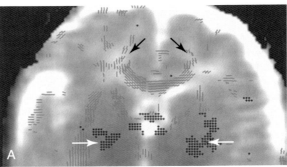

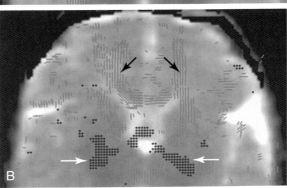

Figure 43–5. See color insert. Electroencephalographic coherence measures at 2 weeks' corrected age, control versus experimental group infants. Four heads, each corresponding to a utilized coherence factor, *top view, scalp left to image left.* Each shows the maximal loadings (correlations) of original coherence variables on the indicated factor. An index electrode and frequency are printed above each head. *Colored regions* indicate location, magnitude, and sign (*red,* positive; *blue,* negative) of maximally loading coherences on the factor. *Arrows* also illustrate coherence variables; however, *arrow color* compensates for signs of factor loadings on subsequent statistically derived canonical variates, thus illustrating how original coherence variables differ between experimental (*red,* increased; *green,* decreased) and control infants. (*From Als H, et al: Early experience alters brain function and structure,* Pediatrics 113:847, 2004. Copyright © 2004 by the AAP.)

Figure 43–6. See color insert. Comparison of control and experimental group infants, at 2 weeks' corrected age, with magnetic resonance imaging and diffusion tensor imaging. Examples of diffusion tensor maps from identical axial slices through the frontal lobes of a representative control (**A**) and an experimental group (**B**) infant obtained at 2 weeks' corrected age. In each example, the principal eigenvectors (shown in *red* and *black*) overlie the apparent diffusion coefficient (ADC) map to show anisotropy in white matter. The *red lines* denote eigenvectors located within the plane of the image, and the *black dots* indicate eigenvectors oriented mostly perpendicular to the image plane. The ratio E1/E3 has been used as a threshold to show only eigenvectors at those voxels where E1/E3 exceeds a threshold value of 1.3 in both images. Note the greater anisotropy of white matter found in the experimental infant (**B**) compared with the control infant (**A**), at the posterior limbs of the internal capsule (*white arrows* in **A** and **B**) and the frontal white matter adjacent to the corpus callosum (*black arrows* in **A** and **B**). The greater anisotropy found in the experimental infant (**B**) suggests more advanced white matter development in these regions than is found in the control infant (**A**). (*Reproduced with permission from Als H, et al: Early experience alters brain function and structure,* Pediatrics 113:847, 2004. Copyright © 2004 by the AAP.)

infants, from two transport and one inborn NICU, also showed positive results in infant and parent social emotional functioning, which included significantly lower parental stress, enhanced parental competence, and higher infant individualization.

Furthermore, recent research with fragile preterm infants (<1500 g) has demonstrated that even routine caregiving procedures that are performed frequently every day, such as diaper changes and breathing tube adjustments, are associated with major circulatory fluctuations, which increase the risk for brain injury.[47] Thus, research that demonstrates decreased pain scores, fewer hypoxic events, increased heart rate stability, and increased brain oxygenation during individualized nursing and caregiving events, such as individually adapted weighing and diaper changes,[23,64] become more

important and provide invaluable evidence for the critical necessity of developmental care. Infants who received developmental care showed faster recoveries from procedures, and their parents reported an increase in their feelings of closeness with their preterm infant.[42]

The durability of NIDCAP effectiveness beyond the newborn period has been demonstrated in several studies. Infants who received NIDCAP in the NICU showed better Bayley mental and psychomotor developmental indexes at 3, 5,[56] and 9 months' corrected age,[9,10] as well as improved attention, interaction, cognitive planning, affect regulation, fine and gross motor modulation, and communication. A review of developmental care in the NICU for children born at less than 2000 g showed benefits that were sustained until 2 years of age.[17] At 3 years' corrected age, a Swedish study[43] documented better auditory processing and speech (Griffith Developmental Scales), fewer behavior symptoms, and better mother-child communication. At 6 years' corrected age,[69] the study showed higher survival rates without developmental disabilities.

Thus, developmental care is evidence based. It saves NICU and education system costs. NIDCAP training requires financial and staff time investment, yet is highly cost effective, given the documented care cost reductions of $4000 to $12,000 per developmental care infant. Because developmental care is in direct keeping with family-centered care, it promises to become the standard of care for future NICUs. The individualized approach requires continued NICU leadership support, aside from staff training, education, and role redefinition. All NICU work involves human interaction at many levels and in the complex interface of physical and emotional vulnerability. At its core is the tiny, immature, dependent, highly sensitive, and rapidly developing fetal infant and this infant's hopeful, open, and vulnerable parents. Infant and parents trust in, and count on, the caregiver's knowledge and skill and foremost the caregiver's sustained educated attention and emotional attunement and investment. Therein lay the challenge and the opportunity of developmental NICU care. Figures 43-7, 43-8,[3] and 43-9 show images of individualized developmental care in the NICU.

The results of developmental care are consistent with the underlying conceptual basis of the individualized brain-based developmental approach described, which views infants as active participants and structurers of their development, who seek continued regulatory support during initial stabilization and their developmental progression. Individualized care delivered by the infants' parents in collaboration with their professional care teams provides an extrauterine environment that supports overall infant and parent development. Preterm birth triggers the premature onset of sensitive

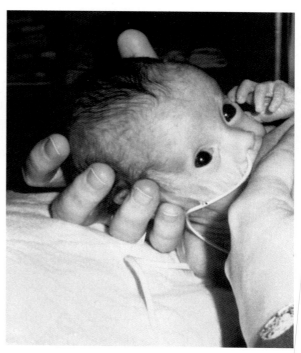

Figure 43–8. Shiny-eyed, now 30-week preterm infant born at 25 weeks, nibbling on the breast while gavage feeding. (*From Als H: Individualized, family-focused developmental care for the very low birthweight preterm infant in the NICU. In Friedman SL, Sigman MD, editors:* Advances in applied developmental psychology *(vol 6), Norwood, NJ, 1992, Ablex.*)

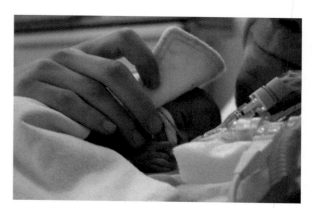

Figure 43–9. Former 26-week preterm infant, now 28 weeks, cared for and relaxing in skin-to-skin contact with her father.

periods. Preterm infants, who receive developmental care delivered in accordance with their own goals, show much reduced costs of such triggering and much improved functioning. This appears as a result of the individually attuned co-regulatory and continuous adaptation of the extrauterine sensory experiences in the nursery to the expectations of the rapidly developing brain.

In summary, reading and trusting the preterm infant's behavior as meaningful communication moves traditional newborn intensive care delivery into a collaborative, relationship-based

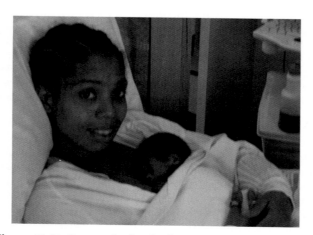

Figure 43–7. One week after birth, a 32-week preterm infant is held and cared for in skin-to-skin contact with her mother.

neurodevelopmental framework. It leads to respect for infants and families as mutually attuned to, and invested in, one another and as active structurers of their own development. It sees infants, parents, and professional caregivers engaged in continuous co-regulation with one another, and in turn in co-regulation with their physical and social environments. It highlights the importance of mutually supportive efforts to realize developmental and individual-specific expectations for the increased differentiation and modulation toward mutually shared goals. In turn, it improves outcome.

DIRECT ASSESSMENT OF PRETERM INFANTS' BEHAVIOR

Systematic, direct assessment of newborn functioning is more common in medical practice than is detailed naturalistic behavioral observation. Direct assessment of the newborn stems from two schools of thought, a more neurologically oriented mode of newborn assessment derived from the model of assessing adult neurologic status and a behaviorally, psychologically oriented mode of assessment derived primarily from psychological laboratory procedures for the study of specific newborn functions. These distinctions at times have led to confusion and artificial separation of aspects of newborn functioning, based largely on a misconception of separateness of neurologic and psychological functioning. More recently, there have been various efforts to combine the neurologic and behavioral aspects into more comprehensive assessments and to address the issues of preterm functioning. The goals of the neurologic assessment of the newborn typically are threefold: first, a diagnosis of a suspected neurologic problem; second, the evaluation of a known neurologic problem or pathologic process; third, the long-term prognosis for a newborn who recovers from a neurologic insult or who is judged at risk due to nonoptimal circumstances in pregnancy, labor, or delivery. The main focus for assessment of newborn neurologic functioning has been the assessment of a variety of reflexes. Peiper[57] was one of the first to describe extensively the reflex and behavioral repertoire of the newborn. His work provides a wealth of detailed information. McGraw[52] published studies specifically on newborn and infant neuromotor development. The French neurologic school under the leadership of André-Thomas and St.-Anne Dargassies brought out the first systematic neurologic examination of the newborn, translated into English in 1960.[62] It focuses on the normal infant's responses, and aside from a survey of the family history, pregnancy, delivery, birth conditions, and placenta, it includes an assessment of tone, reflexes (obligatory and more simple responses), and reactions (flexible and more complex responses). These clinicians for the first time presented a definite examination schedule in assessing the newborn. Prechtl and Beintema[59] developed the most popular examination published in English; Prechtl alone[58] published a second edition. The first part consists of observational assessment of resting posture, spontaneous motor activity, tremor, skin, respiratory rate, body temperature, body weight, skull (fontanelles, head circumference), face, and eyes. A second section includes sequential observation throughout the examination period, with state, postural, and movement assessment. In the Prechtl examination, the

infant's state is continuously monitored and, if necessary, modified. For many of the elicited reflexes, the manual includes a statement about their clinical significance; for a number of them, their significance is unknown. The examination takes about 20 to 40 minutes, depending on how easily the infant is pacified. It involves some very taxing maneuvers, for example, three different types of Moro elicitations and the elicitation of the corneal reflex. Three parameters, the reactivity dimension (hyperexcitability or hypoexcitability), the stability dimension (easy or difficult to pacify), and the attention paid to asymmetry are of particular value in gaining a fuller understanding of the integrative intactness of the newborn. The examination systematizes the assessment of a diverse set of infant skills. Formal validity and reliability studies are not available. In the search for a simpler yet integrative assessment of functioning of the newborn's immediate postparturition status, Apgar[15] proposed a screening rating of 0 to 2 for five parameters, including heart rate, respiratory effort, reflex irritability, muscle tone, and color. This covers three aspects of autonomic system viability and two aspects of baseline intactness of the motor system. They are rated at 1, 5, and 10 minutes after delivery, often by the attending anesthesiologist or the obstetrician. Reliability training is not typically practiced. Nevertheless, the Apgar score shows considerable validity when extreme scores are examined. The probability of neonatal deaths is essentially nil with ratings of 8 or better and is very high with ratings of 0 to 3. There are no studies that assess the predictive significance of the change in Apgar scores from 1 to 5 to 10 minutes, although clinically, this appears the most often used index for immediate treatment and for relative confidence in the newborn's well-being. The use of the Apgar score for prediction in preterm infants is controversial. Nevertheless, used in context with other parameters of perinatal well-being, the Apgar score has held up across decades as a clinically valuable early descriptor. Organismic psychologists have long held that *observable behavior* is an expression of underlying neurologic status and brain function and that behavior may be used to identify specific brain lesions or diagnose more diffuse brain compromise. Such psychologists have widened the traditional medical perspective on the newborn to a broader developmental perspective. Approaches typically involve sampling from complex behaviors beyond the reflex repertoire.

Graham[32] developed the first behavioral assessment of the newborn with the goal of differentiating normal infants from brain-injured infants. The medical literature refers to her examination as a neurologic assessment, the psychological literature as a behavioral assessment. The examination includes pain threshold assessment to electric shock; motor responses including prone position, crawl, and defensive response; visual attention capacities such as object fixation and pursuit; and integrative parameters such as irritability and muscle tension. A standardization and validation study[33] identified reliable mean differences in a group of 30 normal term newborns compared with a group of 81 traumatized term newborns, with conditions of anoxia, mechanical trauma, infection, and medical disease. Nonetheless, predictive validity to ages 3 and 7 years was not encouraging. Rosenblith in 1961[59a] modified the Graham scale; she deleted the pain threshold test and divided the rest of the examination into two subscores, a motor score and a tactile adaptive score. Furthermore, she established two sensory scales, one to assess auditory responses and one to assess vision. She rated best rather than average performance in an effort to overcome behavioral instability in the newborn. Predictive validity studies showed low-level significance with 8-month Bayley measures. The Brazelton Neonatal Behavioral Assessment Scale[18,19,58] is a comprehensive behavioral assessment of the term newborn that incorporates and largely extends parameters assessed in the Graham-Rosenblith scales. It grew out of the collaboration of pediatrics (Brazelton) and psychology (Freedman) and was published as the Cambridge Newborn Behavioral and Neurological Scales. It was subsequently modified further in collaboration with psychologists Sameroff, Horowitz, Tronick, and Koslowski. Its main goal is the assessment of individuality in the spectrum of healthy term newborns. Therefore, in addition to assessing in a screening mode the basic reflex repertoire of the infant, it focuses on motor system integration, state regulation, and attention-interactive capacities, as well as reactivity, and on consoling capacities as measured in cuddliness, consolability, peak of excitement, rapidity of buildup to crying, and irritability. The adequacy of reflex performance is scored on four-point scales; the behavioral dimensions are rated on 26 nine-point behaviorally defined scales. Like the Graham-Rosenblith scales, the Brazelton Neonatal Behavioral Assessment Scale measures best performance. Extensive training is required to elicit the newborn's performance reliably and to score accurately the behavior observed. Training centers to achieve expertise in the use of the Brazelton scale have been established in Boston and other cities in the United States and in many countries around the world through the Brazelton Institute (Children's Hospital, Boston). Training is available to members of various medical, paramedical, psychological, and educational disciplines. Since publication, the Brazelton scale has received much attention and use in clinical and research areas. It provides an interactive approach and attends to more complex organizational parameters of functioning than do most other newborn assessments. The later editions have added supplemental items, which further qualify the behavior of the newborn. These are derived from the Neonatal Behavioral Assessment with Kansas supplements (1978)[37] and the Assessment of Preterm Infants' Behavior.[11]

The Brazelton Neonatal Behavioral Assessment Scale is distinguished from other newborn assessments in its use as an intervention with parents and medical staff. Employed in this manner, it is intended to improve and enhance the caregiver's attitude to and interaction with the infant. The intervention efforts with parents have involved low-risk and high-risk situations as well as term and preterm infants. Nugent and Brazeton give a clinical description of the use the scale in this manner.[55] The success of this work may well be related to the fact that the Brazelton assessment focuses on interactive and highly individualized parameters of newborn functioning. This focus enhances the caregiver's perception of the newborn as a competent, autonomous being. The use of the scale exerts a major impact on pediatric care delivery. Research use is extensive.

Scanlon and colleagues attempted to answer the need for a brief and easily administered neurobehavioral examination of the newborn for the study of obstetric medication effects. The resultant Early Neonatal Neurobehavioral Scale (ENNS)[61]

combines several items from the Brazelton scale[18] and the neurologic examination of Prechtl and Beintema.[59] The testing sequence is designed to arouse the infant to maximal activation during the course of the examination. Tests involve physical manipulation and disturbing, aversive stimuli, such as measures of muscle tone or pinprick. These are performed before the measures of integrative neurologic function. The central theme of the ENNS is the assessment of response decrement with repeated elicitation, which is seen as an index of cortical functioning as distinct from subcortical motor functions supposedly traditionally assessed in neurologic examinations of the newborn. Furthermore, Scanlon and coworkers consider response decrement as independent of state arousal. The sequence of ENNS items moves from repeated pinpricks (12) to pull-to-sit, arm recoil, assessment of trunk tone, general body tone, rooting response, sucking, response to repeated Moro maneuvers (12), placing response, and the general observation of alertness, followed by an overall rating of the newborn's functioning. The ENNS takes between 5 and 7 minutes to administer and requires training, yet background in neurology or psychology is not required. It is a repetitive, rapid, and partial screen of central nervous system integrity.

The Amiel-Tison assessment,[13] the Neurologic and Adaptive Capacity Score, based on the French school led by St.-Anne Dargassies and Minkowski, is geared to the detection and differentiation of drug depression from perinatal asphyxia and birth trauma and, furthermore, to the prediction of later outcome. In Amiel-Tison's view, subtle imbalances of extensor and flexor tone of the neck muscles and the upper extremities are related to perinatal asphyxia or mild birth trauma, whereas general mild hypotonia, mediocre primary reflex responses, and absent or poor habituation to repeated stimuli are more frequently related to drug depression. Amiel-Tison incorporates items from Scanlon's ENNS and from the Brazelton scale and contends that both tests have shortcomings. She considers the Brazelton too complicated and time consuming and the ENNS too noxious and lacking the assessment of motor tone, which Amiel-Tison considers diagnostic. Her examination yields a single total score, a feature desired by many clinicians. The differentiating and predictive value of the Neurologic and Adaptive Capacity Score remains to be determined. Attention to active tone is clearly important. The speed and selectiveness of the items, together with the global nature of scoring (0, 1, 2), does not recommend the assessment for the evaluation of subtle neurointegrative differences, restricting its use to relatively vigorous term infants.

OVERVIEW OF PRETERM NEWBORN NEUROBEHAVIORAL ASSESSMENTS

Several tests have been developed specifically for the assessment of preterm functioning. The Albert Einstein Neonatal Neurobehavioral Assessment Scale[25] has as its goal a parsimonious, reliable, yet comprehensive evaluation of neurologic and behavioral organization of both the preterm and full term newborn. The 30- to 45-minute examination assesses performance on 20 specific behavioral test items and yields additional ratings on four summary scales. Like the Brazelton scale, the test pays attention to the state of the infant. Administration directions are identical to those of the

Brazelton scale. Of the 20 specific behavioral items, 13 are directly derived from the Brazelton scale, 4 are drawn from Prechtl's examination, and 1 is derived from the Dubowitz Assessment of Gestational Age[27] and is described in Amiel-Tison's examination described previously. All scales are four-point scales. Despite the instruction to work for optimal performance, the administration directions per item are highly specific and preclude optimal performance. High-risk preterm infants assessed approximately at term-equivalent age did significantly more poorly than term infants on all orientation items, a number of the reflex items tested, active mobility, passive tone, and the summary items of state profile and latency to consolation. When low-risk preterm and healthy infants were compared at term, there was greater similarity than dissimilarity between the two groups. Comparison of high-risk term and preterm infants with low-risk term and preterm groups with the Einstein scale showed that term asphyxiated newborns and those who were small for gestational age had the most abnormal responses. Predictive validity of the Einstein scale has been shown to improve from 1 to 3 years of age.

The Dubowitz Neurological Assessment of the Preterm and Fullterm Newborn Infant draws primarily from the earlier assessment of gestational age,[27] supplemented by Prechtl and Beintema items,[59] items from St.-Anne Dargassies[63] and items from the Brazelton Neonatal Behavioral Assessment Scale.[18] This compilation of items was pretested with a newborn population of about 500 infants, including preterm and term. A chart with four- to five-point range descriptors and stick-figure newborn drawings facilitates scoring of some 32 items of newborn functioning. According to the authors, the examination does not require particular experience or expertise in neonatal neurology. Performance time is 10 to 15 minutes. A cautionary note is indicated regarding use of this stressful examination for infants born with very low birthweight and very early.

This caution also applies to the Neurobehavioral Assessment of the Preterm Infant.[44] Few assessments have undergone as thorough a design and item evaluation process as this assessment. Korner and associates detail the process of item development, reliability, and validity. The test's goal is to document weekly change in neurobehavioral functioning from 32 weeks to term age. Test items include motor development, vigor, scarf sign, popliteal angle, alertness and orientation, percent asleep ratings, irritability, and vigor of crying. Despite rigorous test development, the testing items lack a unifying theoretical construct and have not shown predictive validity or reliability in differentiation of subgroups or intervention effects.

The most recent combination of neurological, maturational, and behavioral items is the Neonatal Intensive Care Unit Network Neurobehavioral Scale.[46] This scale assesses and scores the full range of infant neurobehavioral performance. It assesses infant stress, abstinence and withdrawal behaviors, neurologic functioning, and features of gestational age assessment. It attempts to provide a comprehensive evaluation of the neurobehavioral performance of the high-risk and substance-exposed infant during the perinatal period. Its use is applicable for a great variety of infants of varying histories and gestational ages, as long as the infants are stable. The Neonatal Intensive Care Unit Network Neurobehavioral Scale follows a standardized administration format that removes the examiner from the behavior assessed. The order of items is strictly specified. If the infant is in the wrong state for an item, the item is skipped. There are, furthermore, specific guidelines for when and how to console the infant. The test provides an estimate of how an infant at a particular time responds to a standardized set and sequence of events. This shortens the examination's administration. Training required is brief and quite simple. There is little need for judgment. Skill to elicit best performance is not required. As such, the Neonatal Intensive Care Unit Network Neurobehavioral Scale resembles more the Neurobehavioral Assessment of the Preterm Infant than the Brazelton scale. It lacks a theoretical conceptual framework, and is purposely not a relationship-based interactive assessment. This makes it questionable for the fair assessment of the newborn infant, who is neuroessentially social.

A detailed review of several of the previously referenced newborn assessments appears in a special edition of the journal *Mental Retardation and Developmental Disabilities Research Reviews*.[5]

THE ASSESSMENT OF PRETERM INFANTS' BEHAVIOR

The specificity and organization of preterm and full-term infants' behavioral functioning is assessed most comprehensively in the Assessment of Preterm Infants' Behavior (APIB). The APIB is designed to observe the infant's threshold to disorganization, functional stability, and ability to recover from disorganization as measured in degree of differentiation and modulation of the balanced subsystems.[5,11,12] The main objective of the APIB is the assessment of infant individuality and competence, based on observation of the behavioral subsystems in interaction with each other and with the environment. The goal is to determine the infant's reactivity and thresholds from modulation to disorganization in the face of varied environmental challenges.

The test items of the Brazelton scale[18] are organized into six increasingly vigorous packages of questions posed to the infant. Each package presents the infant with increasingly challenging, complex interactions and quantifies the infant's behavioral organizational response patterns. Stimuli presented in the initial packages are distal in nature. For example, while the infant is sleeping, the response to repeated light from a flashlight or to the repeated sound of a rattle is noted. As the examination progresses, the stimuli become proximal in nature and involve cutaneous tactile, kinesthetic, and vestibular inputs. For example, responses to cutaneous input to the face are noted as well as responses to movement of the limbs and trunk, as elicited for instance in the pull-to-sit or stepping maneuvers. The sixth package engages the infant to attend to, localize, or visually track a variety of animate and inanimate sounds and sights related to objects and the examiner's face and voice. The organization of the autonomic, motor, state and self-regulatory subsystems are scored on nine-point rating scales before, during, and after each of the six packages. Because package six requires focused alertness, the attention-interaction subsystem is additionally scored before, during, and after this package. A measure of the amount of examiner facilitation is included for each package to assess the amount of examiner-supplied environmental support necessary to help the infant maintain or regain subsystem integration while responding to the questions of the examination.

The APIB scores reflect the infant's organization of the five subsystems in the course of the interactive assessment and the amount of examiner facilitation required; together, they are referred to as *system scores*. These system scores represent an innovative component of newborn assessment. They focus on the simultaneity of subsystems in their interplay and in turn their respective interplay with the environment, as based in the synactive theory of development.[18] For the traditional newborn examiner, this component of the APIB is the most challenging because it requires a dynamic perspective of neurodevelopment, human evolution, and self-constructing neurologic and pediatric thinking and education. Training in the assessment encompasses background teaching in neurodevelopment and human evolution.

In addition to the system scores, each of the responses elicited in the course of the APIB dialogue with the infant is assessed along various dimensions. Overall, the APIB yields 285 raw scores, which are reduced to 32 a priori summary scores. Most of the APIB raw scores are scored on one- to nine-point scales, with 1 representing well-organized behavior and 9 representing poorly organized behavior. The remaining APIB raw scores are scored on zero- to three-point scales, in which a score of 0 reflects absence of a response, and a score of 3 an obligatory, hyperreactive response.

APIB summary scores are obtained by averaging specified APIB raw scores. For the subgroup of APIB raw scores referred to as system scores, each system summary score remains scaled from one to nine, in which 1 represents well-organized behavior and 9 represents poorly organized behavior. The remaining nine-point APIB raw scores are converted to summary scores with reversed scale direction, in which 1 represents disorganized behavior and 9 represents well-organized behavior. The APIB raw scores, which use zero- to three-point scaling, yield summary scores on a similar zero- to three-point scale, in which 0 indicates that a response was not obtained and 3 indicates an obligatory, hyperreactive, or too frequently observed response.

The APIB requires extensive training by a certified APIB trainer. Ninety percent inter-rater reliability is the established minimal criterion for use of the APIB. APIB test-retest reliability across 4 weeks (40 to 44 weeks) for system scores and cluster-analyzed profile groups is highly stable.[7]

For psychological tests, four categories of validity are required: predictive, concurrent, content, and construct validity. APIB predictive validity has been established with a behavioral assessment known as the Kangaroo Box Paradigm and the Bayley Scales of Infant Development, based on a sample of 160 healthy preterm and term infants restudied at 9 months.[10] A second study reports predictive validity to neuropsychological testing at 5 years of age as well as to the Kangaroo Box Paradigm at 5 years of age.[7] Concurrent validity has been established in a study comparing APIB scores and quantified EEG with topographic mapping performed at the same age point. Similarly, unrestricted spectral coherence of brain electrical activity was highly correlated with APIB behavioral factor scores in a study of 312 newborn infants with varying gestational ages. All infants were examined

2 weeks after expected term due date.[28] Brain structural assessment with magnetic resonance imaging,[39,40] as well as with magnetic resonance diffusion tensor imaging,[6,39] also showed significant correlation to APIB behavioral scores. All studies implicated frontal lobe parameters as associated with attention system scores and overall APIB system modulation. This points to a differential vulnerability of frontal systems in the early-born preterm population. Content validity refers to the degree that test items sample what the test purports to measure. This is important in order to allow valid inferences from test results. APIB subsystem scales operationalize the behavioral constructs measured by the APIB. Whether the specific behavioral items selected as indicative of subsystem function truly sample subsystem function must be addressed in future studies of the APIB's relationship to other measures of the same construct. Such measures are not available at this time. Related to content validity is construct validity. There are several ways to establish construct validity. One way is by comparison of test scores for groups of subjects that are known to differ, or by comparison of subjects that are theorized to perform differently. The APIB distinguishes well between groups of infants that differ on various dimensions. These include differences in gestational age and in degree of illness.[28] Another method of assessing construct validity occurs when the theory suggests how an intervention should alter behavior relevant to the construct. All intervention studies reported to date and based in the synactive theory of development have demonstrated that intervention group infants, compared with control group infants, showed significantly improved functioning as measured with the APIB. This supports high construct validity. Overall, it appears that the APIB has good test properties, especially compared with some of the other newborn assessments reviewed previously.[6-10,54]

The past four decades thus have seen much work devoted to the development of assessments that capture the neurobehavioral repertoire of the preterm infant. Earlier assessments were often compilations of reflex behaviors and ignored organizational capacities and competencies. Although the work of Graham and Rosenblith set the stage for later neurobehavioral assessment, Brazelton was the first to emphasize the individual competencies of the term newborn. The APIB has taken neurobehavioral assessment a step further by articulation of the behavioral organization constructs of differentiation and modulation of functioning. The APIB is based in comprehensive developmental theory, which makes APIB results cohesive and interpretable in a neurodevelopmental dynamic framework.

The implications of the preterm assessments presented, especially those of the APIB, suggest that even when the physical health of the preterm infant is ensured, premature birth itself appears to contribute to behavioral and electrophysiologic differences in functioning. Preterm infants emerge as more sensitive and easily disorganized and have much greater difficulty with self-regulation. Their motor systems show poor modulation, and their autonomic reactivity is more costly. Their brain function, especially of association cortical and, in particular, frontal lobe regions, reflects these differences. The differences appear to hold up across time into school age. Poorer state and attention scores are more typical of preterm infants than healthy term infants.

They are more difficult to bring to alertness; they are more likely to move from sleep states into uncontrolled crying; and they show more stress with state transition. They muster often only strained alertness, diffuse protest, and diffuse sleep. They require more facilitation for state maintenance and self-regulation. They are likely to exhibit attention difficulties and distractibility in later infancy and school age, even in the face of normal intelligence. The attention measures show the strongest correlations with EEG coherence factor.[28] Clinical experience with older children indicates that difficulties in concentration and problems with attention are frequent in former preterm children, even those spared significant medical sequelae. Attention regulation problems are also the most common subtle neurologic residua after recovery from even very mild encephalopathy. Similarly, mild reduction of clinical EEG background voltages is a subtle residuum of anoxic encephalopathy, toxic, or metabolic derangement. Thus, the finding of significant reduction of EEG spectral content as the legacy of prematurity takes on added significance.

The prominent frontal region involvement, as identified by EEG spectral coherence measures, and found in even healthy preterm infants, is of interest given the known association of attention disorders with frontal dysfunction. The frontal lobe may be relatively more sensitive to subtle insult than other regions. Thus, the simple fact of premature extrauterine experience may have important consequences. The extrauterine multisensory experience before term may trigger sensitive periods at a time when the infant is not in a position to incorporate appropriately such sensory influences, thereby inducing altered subsequent neural development. Follow-up at 8 years corrected age appears to indicate that the earliest born preterm infants exhibit extraordinary variability of cognitive processing. Figure 43-10 shows the example of an early born, medically healthy child's performance profile on a number of the neuropsychological subtests.[4,70] Although this child shows both a verbal and performance intelligence quotient both of 115 (i.e., a standard deviation above the mean

for age), this child had great difficulty in the second-grade classroom. The child's subtest profile indicates extraordinarily high performance on several subtests; for example, Similarities (Wechsler Intelligence Scale for Children, Revised) and Gestalt Closure (Kaufman Assessment Battery for Children) are 3 standard deviations above the mean, which is in the very superior or gifted range, whereas other subtests show performance at or below a standard deviation below the mean for age, in the dull normal to borderline range. These include Arithmetic (Wechsler Intelligence Scale for Children, Revised), Matrix Analogies (Kaufman Assessment Battery for Children), and the Rey-Osterreith Complex Figure Test-Recall condition. Subdomain discrepancy with valleys of disability is typical for children with brain lesions. Yet, such children do not show the extraordinary peaks of excellence seen in presumably focally brain-intact, yet very early born, preterm infants. This performance picture appears to indicate brain reorganization rather than lesion, owing to very early difference in brain-environment interaction. This difference appears to accentuate differentially the development of certain brain systems, which are ready to take advantage of the extrauterine challenge, whereas it inhibits other brain systems, which expect intrauterine inputs for several more months.

SUMMARY

Intrauterine and extrauterine environments appear to influence brain development differentially. Provision of co-regulatory, neurodevelopmental support and care for the preterm infant understood as biologically evolved in a neuroregulatory family system may enhance neurobehavioral, neuroelectrophysiologic, and family functioning not only for high-risk but also for medically low-risk preterm infants.

During the perinatal period from 24 weeks' gestation to the time of term birth, the human cortex appears particularly vulnerable because its neurons are undergoing significant structural and functional transformations in response to

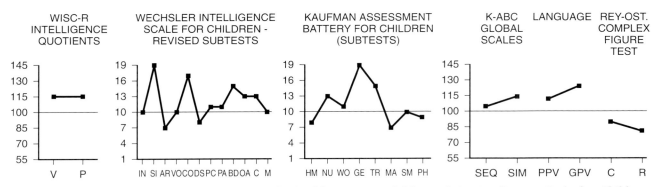

Figure 43-10. Test profile of early-born, medically healthy preterm child. Wechsler Intelligence Scale for Children, Revised (WISC-R) Intelligence Quotients: P, performance IQ; V, verbal IQ. WISC-R Subtests: AR, arithmetic; BD, block design; CO, coding; DS, digit span; IN, information; M, mazes; OA, object assembly; PA, picture arrangement; PC, picture completion; SI, similarities; VO, vocabulary. Kaufman Assessment Battery for Children (K-ABC) Subtests: GE, gestalt closure; HM, hand movements; MA, matrix analogies; NU, number recall; PH, photo series; SM, similarities; TR, triangles; WO, work order. K-ABC Global Scales: SEQ, sequential processing; SIM, simultaneous processing. Language: GPV, Gardner One-Word Picture Vocabulary Test, Revised; PPV, Peabody Picture Vocabulary Test, Revised Rey-Osterrieth Complex Figure: C, copy; R, recall. (*From Als H: The preterm infant: A model for the study of fetal brain expectation. In Lecanuet J-P, et al, editors:* Fetal development: a psychobiological perspective, *Hillsdale, NJ, 1995, Lawrence Erlbaum.*)

incoming fibers. To achieve its complex organization, the cerebral cortex must be subject to significant developmental constraints. Disruptions through injury or violation in evolved expectancy of input may well result in disturbance of the cortex's anatomic and neurochemical integrity and therewith challenge the normal developmental constraints of the still-growing cortex. Thus, the neurofunctional differences observed in preterm infants may represent secondary modifications and readaptations to locally disturbed cortical developments. The differential vulnerability of the frontal lobe system is of particular importance in designing preventive and ameliorative brain-nurturing environments and care provision. The frontal lobe is the human's most species-specific lobe of the brain, evolved most recently, is most complexly organized, and is critically important for complex planning and communication. The frontal lobe is necessary to foresee and predict outcome without trial-and-error action sequences. It inhibits impulsive stimulus reactions and supports reflective analysis of complex, multidimensional, open-ended situations. It supports delay of gratification and suspension of judgment and action, whereas it affords sustained inquiry in the face of ambiguity and uncertainty. It diffuses pressure toward solutions but maintains initiative and goal orientation. In addition, it supports decision power and prioritization. This uniquely human species survival organ of the cortex appears to be simultaneously the most easily damaged or altered. In the "good-enough" term situation, it appears to be nurtured in the social-emotional communicative matrix of good-enough parenting in good-enough social groups. In unexpected situations, such as in preterm circumstances, it requires special attention for preventive and ameliorative care.

Social contexts have evolved in the course of human phylogeny, are specific and fine-tuned, and provide good-enough environments for the human cortex to unfold, initially in the womb, then outside the womb. They ensure the continuation of human evolution. With the advances in medical technology, even very immature nervous systems survive and develop outside the womb. However, the social contexts of traditional special care nurseries often bring with them less than adequate support for immature nervous systems, leading to maladaptations and disabilities, yet also perhaps to accelerations and extraordinary abilities. Detailed observation of the behavior of the fetus who is displaced from the uterus into the NICU provides the opportunities to estimate and infer appropriate environmental and social contexts, sufficiently astute to support the highly sensitive and vulnerable nervous systems of preterm infants in their developmental progressions.

The information presented here indicates that an individualized, behavioral-developmental approach to care improves outcome not only medically but also behaviorally, neurophysiologically, and in terms of brain structure. Such an approach emphasizes from early on the infant's own strengths and apparent developmental goals and institutes support for self-regulatory competence and achievement of these goals. The results indicate that increase in support to behavioral self-regulation improves developmental outcome, perhaps by prevention of active inhibition of central nervous system pathways due to inappropriate inputs during a highly sensitive period of brain development. Developmentally appropriate care is associated with improved cortical and specifically frontal lobe development. Adaptations of environment and care are productive when based on the astute observation and direct assessment of individual infants' current behavior and on the interpretation of behavior in a framework of regulatory efforts toward self-set goals of continued differentiation and self-construction. The results support the formulation of highly specific brain expectations during early development, and neurodevelopmental care emerges as neonatology's new frontier.

ACKNOWLEDGMENTS

Supported by grant sponsor NIH/ NICHD, grant numbers R01 HD047730 and R01 HD046855 (H. Als); grant sponsor U.S. Department of Education/OSEP, grant number H324CO40045 (H. Als); grant sponsor I. Harris Foundation (H. Als); and grant sponsor NIH/MRDDRC, grant number P01HD18655 (M. Greenberg).

REFERENCES

1. Als H: Toward a synactive theory of development: promise for the assessment of infant individuality, *Inf Mental Health J* 3:229, 1982.
2. Als H: Reading the premature infant, In Goldson E, editor: *Developmental interventions in the neonatal intensive care nursery.* New York, 1999, Oxford University Press, pp 18–85.
3. Als H: Individualized, family-focused developmental care for the very low birthweight preterm infant in the NICU. In Friedman SL, Sigman MD, editors: *Advances in applied developmental psychology*, Vol 6, Norwood, NJ, 1992, Ablex Publishing Company, pp 341–388.
4. Als H: The preterm infant: a model for the study of fetal brain expectation. In Lecanuet J-P, et al, editor: *Fetal development: a psychobiological perspective.* Hillsdale, NJ, 1995, Lawrence Erlbaum Publishers, pp 439–471.
5. Als H, et al: The assessment of preterm infants' behavior (APIB): Furthering the understanding and measurement of neurodevelopmental competence in preterm and fullterm infants, *Ment Retard Develop Disabil Res Rev* 11:94, 2005.
6. Als H, et al: Early experience alters brain function and structure, *Pediatrics* 113:846, 2004.
7. Als H, et al: Continuity of neurobehavioral functioning in preterm and fullterm newborns. In Bornstein MH, Krasnegor NA, editors: *Stability and continuity in mental development.* Hillsdale, NJ, 1989, Lawrence Erlbaum, pp 3–28.
8. Als H, et al: A three-center randomized controlled trial of individualized developmental care for very low birth weight preterm infants: medical, neurodevelopmental, parenting and caregiving effects, *J Dev Behav Pediatr* 24:399, 2003.
9. Als H, et al: Individualized developmental care for the very low birthweight preterm infant: medical and neurofunctional effects, *JAMA* 272:853, 1994.
10. Als H, et al: Individualized behavioral and environmental care for the very low birth weight preterm infant at high risk for bronchopulmonary dysplasia: neonatal intensive care unit and developmental outcome, *Pediatrics* 78:1123, 1986.
11. Als H, et al: Manual for the assessment of preterm infants' behavior (APIB). In Fitzgerald HE, et al, editor: *Theory and research in behavioral pediatrics.* Vol 1. New York, 1982, Plenum Press, pp 65–132.

12. Als H, et al: Towards a research instrument for the assessment of preterm infants' behavior. In Fitzgerald HE, et al, editor: *Theory and research in behavioral pediatrics.* Vol 1. New York, 1982, Plenum Press, pp 35–63.

13. Amiel-Tison C: Neurological evaluation of the maturity of newborn infants, *Arch Dis Child* 43:89, 1968.

14. Anand KJS, Scalzo FM: Can adverse neonatal experiences alter brain development and subsequent behavior? *Biol Neonat* 77:69, 2000.

15. Apgar V: A proposal for a new method of evaluation of the newborn infant, *Anesth Anal* 32:260, 1953.

16. Behrman RE, Stith Butler A: *Preterm birth: causes, consequences, and prevention.* Washington, D.C., 2007, The National Academies Press.

17. Bonnier C: Evaluation of early stimulation programs for enhancing brain development, *Acta Paediatr* 97:853, 2008.

18. Brazelton TB: *Neonatal behavioral assessment scale.* London, 1973, Heinemann.

19. Brazelton TB, Nugent JK: *Neonatal behavioral assessment scale.* Vol 137. 3rd ed London, 1995, Mac Keith Press.

20. Bourgeois JP, et al: Synaptogenesis in visual cortex of normal and preterm monkeys: evidence for intrinsic regulation of synaptic overproduction, *Proc Nat Acad Sci U S A* 86:4297, 1989.

21. Bourgeois J: Synaptogenesis, heterochrony and epigenesis in the mammalian neocortex, *Acta Paediatr Suppl* 422:27, 1997.

22. Buehler DM, et al: Effectiveness of individualized developmental care for low-risk preterm infants: behavioral and electrophysiological evidence, *Pediatrics* 96:923, 1995.

23. Catelin C, et al: Clinical, psychological, and biologic impact of environmental and behavioral interventions in neonates during a routine nursing procedure, *J Pain* 6:791, 2005.

24. Creasy RK: Preventing preterm birth, *N Engl J Med* 5:669, 1991.

25. Daum C, et al: *The Albert Einstein neonatal neurobehavioral scale manual.* Bronx, NY, 1977, Albert Einstein College of Medicine.

26. Denny-Brown D: *The basal ganglia and their relation to disorders of movement.* Oxford, 1962, Oxford University Press.

27. Dubowitz L, et al: Clinical assessment of gestational age in the newborn infant, *J Pediatr* 77:1, 1970.

28. Duffy FH, et al: Infant EEG spectral coherence data during quiet sleep: unrestricted Principal Components Analysis. Relation of factors to gestational age, medical risk, and neurobehavioral status, *Clin Electroencephalography* 34:54, 2003.

29. Fleisher BF, et al. Individualized developmental care for very-low-birth-weight premature infants, *Clin Pediatr* 34:523, 1995.

30. Gesell A, Armatruda C: *The embryology of behavior.* Westport, CT, 1945, Connecticut Greenwood Press.

31. Gilkerson L, Als H: Role of reflective process in the implementation of developmentally supportive care in the newborn intensive care unit, *Inf Young Child* 7:20, 1995.

32. Graham F: Behavioral differences between normal and traumatized newborns: I. The test procedures, *Psychol Monogr (Gen Appl)* 70:1, 1956.

33. Graham F, et al: Behavioral differences between normal and traumatized newborns: II. Standardization, reliability, and validity, *Psychol Monogr (Gen Appl)* 70:17, 1956.

34. Hack M, et al: Outcomes in young adulthood for very-low-birth-weight infants, *N Engl J Med* 346:149, 2002.

35. Hack M, et al: Chronic conditions, functional limitations, and special health care needs of school-aged children born with extremely low-birth-weight in the 1990s, *JAMA* 294:318, 2005.

36. Hofer MA: Early social relationships: a psychobiologist's view, *Child Dev* 58:633, 1987.

37. Horowitz FD, et al: Stability and instability in the newborn infant: the quest for elusive threads. Monographs, *Soc Res Child Dev* 43:29, 1978.

38. Humphrey T: Some correlations between the appearance of human fetal reflexes and the development of the nervous system, *Prog Brain Res* 4:93, 1964.

39. Hüppi PS, et al: Microstructural changes in brain development in premature infants with intrauterine growth restriction (IUGR): a voxel-based analysis of diffusion tensor imaging, *Pediatr Res* 55:582A, 2004.

40. Hüppi P, et al: Structural and neurobehavioral delay in postnatal brain development of preterm infants, *Pediat Res* 39:895, 1996.

41. Jacobs S, et al: The newborn individualized developmental care and assessment program is not supported by meta-analyses of the data, *J Pediatr* 140:699, 2002.

42. Kleberg A, et al: Mothers' perception of Newborn Individualized Developmental Care and Assessment Program (NIDCAP) as compared to conventional care, *Early Hum Devel* 83:403, 2007.

43. Kleberg A, et al: Developmental outcome, child behavior and mother-child interaction at 3 years of age following Newborn Individualized Developmental Care and Intervention Program (NIDCAP) intervention, *Early Hum Dev* 60:123, 2000.

44. Korner AF, et al: Establishing the reliability and developmental validity of a neurobehavioral assessment for preterm infants: a methodological process, *Child Dev* 62:1200, 1991.

45. Lawhon G, Hedlund R: Newborn individualized developmental care and assessment program training and education, *J Perinat Neonat Nurs* 22:133, 2008.

46. Lester BM, Tronick EZ: The Neonatal Intensive Care Unit Network Neurobehavioral Scale (NNNS), *Pediatrics* 2004;113:676–678.

47. Limperopoulos C, et al: Cerebral Hemodynamic Changes During Intensive Care of Preterm Infants, *Pediatrics* 122:1006, 2008.

48. Lockwood CJ, Kuczynski E: Risk stratification and pathological mechanisms in preterm delivery, *Pediatr Perinatal Epidemiol* 15:78, 2001.

49. Marin-Padilla M: Pathogenesis of late-acquired leptomeningeal heterotopias and secondary cortical alterations: a Golgi study. In Galaburda AM, editor: *Dyslexia and development.* Cambridge, MA, 1993, Harvard University Press, pp 64–89.

50. McCormick MC: Has the prevalence of handicapped infants increased with improved survival of the very low birthweight infant? *Clin Perinatol* 20:263, 1993.

51. McGrath JM: Developmentally supportive caregiving and technology in the NICU: Isolation or merger of intervention strategies? *J Perinat Neonatal Nurs* 14:78, 2000.

52. McGraw MB: *The neuromuscular maturation of the human infant.* New York, 1943, Columbia University Press.

53. Mercuri E, et al: Neonatal cerebral infarction and neuromotor outcome at school age, *Pediatrics* 113:95, 2004.

54. Mouradian LE, Als H: The influence of neonatal intensive care unit caregiving practices on motor functioning of preterm infants, *Am J Occup Ther* 48:527, 1994.

55. Nugent JK, Brazelton TB: Preventive intervention with infants and families: the NBAS model, *Inf Mental Health J* 10:84, 1989.

56. Parker SJ, et al: Outcome after developmental intervention in the neonatal intensive care unit for mothers of preterm infants with low socioeconomic status, *J Pediatr* 120:780, 1992.

57. Peiper A: *Die Hirntätigkeit des Säuglings.* Berlin, 1928, Springer.
58. Prechtl HFR: *The neurological examination of the full-term infant: a manual for clinical use.* 2nd edition ed, Philadelphia, 1977, Lippincott.
59. Prechtl H, Beintema D: *The neurological examination of the full-term newborn infant; a manual for clinical use.* London, 1964, Spastics Society Medical Education and Information Unit.
59a. Rosenblith J: *The modified Graham behavior test for neonates: test retest reliability, normative data, and hypotheses for future work, Biol Neonatol* 3:174, 1961.
60. Saigal S, et al: Transition of extremely low-birth-weight infants from adolescence to young adulthood: comparison with normal birth-weight controls, *JAMA* 295:667, 2006.
61. Scanlon JW, et al: Neurobehavioral responses of newborn infants after maternal epidural anesthesia, *Anesthesia* 30:121, 1974.
62. St.-Anne Dargassies S: Methode d'examen neurologique due nouveau-ne, *Études neonatales* 3:101, 1954.
63. St.-Anne Dargassies S: Neurodevelopmental symptoms during the first year of life. I: Essential landmarks for each key age, *Dev Med Child Neurol* 14:235, 1972.
64. Sizun J, et al: Developmental care decreases physiologic and behavioral pain expression in preterm neonates, *J Pain* 3:446, 2002.
64a. Schwartz ML, Goldman-Rakic P: Development and plasticity of the primate cerebral cortex, *Clin Perinatol* 17:83, 1990.
65. Vohr BR, et al: Neurodevelopmental and functional outcomes of extremely low birth weight infants in the national institute of child health and human development neonatal research network, 1993–1994, *Pediatrics* 105:1216, 2000.
66. Volpe JJ: *Neurology of the newborn*, 4th ed. Philadelphia, 2001, WB Saunders.
67. Villar J, et al: Characteristics of randomized controlled trials included in systematic reviews of nutritional interventions reporting maternal morbidity, mortality, preterm delivery, intrauterine growth restriction and small for gestational age and birth weight outcomes, *J Nutr* 133:1632, 2003.
68. Westrup B, et al: A randomized controlled trial to evaluate the effects of the Newborn Individualized Developmental Care and Assessment Program in a Swedish setting, *Pediatrics* 105:66, 2000.
69. Westrup B, et al: Preschool outcome in children born very prematurely and cared for according to the Newborn Individualized Development Care and Assessment Program (NIDCAP). Developmentally supportive neonatal care: a study of the Newborn Individualized Developmental Care and Assessment Program (NIDCAP) in Swedish settings, *Stockholm: Repro Print AB* VI:1, 2003.
70. Westrup B: Newborn Individualized Developmental Care and Assessment Program (NIDCAP): family-centered developmentally supportive care, *Early Hum Dev* 83:443, 2007.

CHAPTER 44

The Respiratory System

PART 1

Lung Development and Maturation
Alan H. Jobe

A BRIEF HISTORY

An understanding of lung development and maturation is central to the care of preterm infants because lung function is so critical to survival of the preterm. Although von Neergaard reported the presence of air-fluid interfaces in lungs in 1929, there was no substantial increase in the understanding of lung immaturity until Pattle and Clements noted the presence of surfactant in pulmonary edema foam and lung extracts. Avery and Mead in 1959 correlated respiratory failure with decreased surfactant levels in saline extracts from the lungs of infants with respiratory distress syndrome (RDS).[2] Once the association between atelectasis with hyaline membranes and surfactant levels was appreciated, a large international research effort focused on the surfactant system. The first direct clinical benefit was identified in 1971 when the lecithin-sphingomyelin (L-S) ratio using amniotic fluid was used to predict lung immaturity and the risk for RDS in preterm infants.[16] The usefulness of phosphatidylglycerol measurements for lung maturity testing was appreciated by 1976.[18] The development of continuous positive airway pressure to maintain functional residual capacity (FRC) for infants with RDS was the initial progress with respiratory support. Liggins and Howie first reported a decreased incidence in RDS with maternal corticosteroid treatments in 1972.[34] The feasibility of surfactant treatment for lung immaturity was demonstrated in animal models in the 1970s, primarily by Enhörning and Robertson, and surfactant was successfully used in humans by Fujiwara and colleagues in 1980. This research resulted in the development of perhaps the two most effective treatments in neonatology—antenatal corticosteroids and postnatal surfactant for RDS. This progress in the application of research to the pulmonary care of the infant will no doubt continue as molecular and cell biologic observations improve the general understanding of lung development.[49] A major interest for the future is the prevention of chronic lung disease (CLD) in infants who are very preterm.

LUNG STRUCTURAL DEVELOPMENT
Embryonic Period

The lung first appears as a ventral bud off the esophagus just caudal to the laryngotracheal sulcus.[10] The grooves between the lung bud and the esophagus deepen, and the bud elongates within the surrounding mesenchyme and divides to form the main stem bronchi (Fig. 44-1). Subsequent dichotomous branching gives rise to the conducting airways. The branching of the endodermal endothelium is controlled by the underlying mesenchyme because removal of the mesenchyme stops branching. Transplantation of the mesenchyme from a branching airway to more proximal airway structures induces budding in the new location.

The commitment of endodermal cells to epithelial cell lineages requires the expression of families of transcription factors that include thyroid transcription factor-1, forkhead gene family members, and others.[48] At least 15 homeobox domain-containing genes (*HOX* genes) also contribute to lung morphogenesis. Multiple other growth and differentiation factors, such as retinoic acid and the fibroblast growth factor family members (FGF)-7 and FGF-10 and their receptors are temporally and spatially expressed and are critical to early lung morphogenesis and subsequent development. Genetic ablation of these transcription and growth factors, among others, causes lung developmental abnormalities that range from tracheoesophageal fistula and altered branching morphogenesis to severe lung hypoplasia and complete aplasia of the lungs. Lobar airways are formed by about 37 days, with progression to segmental airways by 42 days and subsegmental bronchi by 48 days in the human fetus. The pulmonary vasculature branches off the sixth aortic arch to form a vascular plexus in the mesenchyme of the lung bud. Major regulators of vascular development are vascular endothelial growth factor and its receptors in the mesenchyme. Vascular development additionally requires extracellular matrix (fibronectin, laminin, type IV collagen) and other growth factors such as platelet-derived growth factor. The pulmonary artery can be identified by about 37 days, and venous structures appear somewhat later. Abnormalities in early lung embryogenesis cause tracheoesophageal syndromes, branching morphogenesis abnormalities, and aplasia.

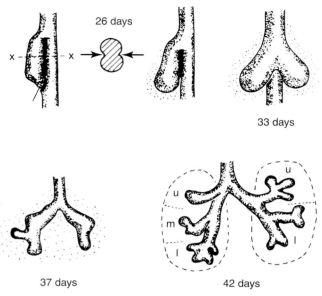

Figure 44–1. Embryonic lung development. At 26 days the lung first appears as a protrusion of the foregut. By 33 days the lung bud has branched, and by 37 days the prospective main bronchi are penetrating the mesenchyme. Airways to the lobar and initial segmental bronchi have formed by 42 days. *(Modified from Burri PW: Development and growth of the human lung. In Fishman AP, Fisher AB, editors:* Handbook of physiology: the respiratory system, *Bethesda, MD, 1985, American Physiologic Society, p 1, with permission.)*

Pseudoglandular Stage

The 15 to 20 generations of airway branching occur in the pseudoglandular period of lung development from about the 7th to the 18th week (Fig. 44-2). All airway branching to the level of the future alveolar ducts is complete. The developing airways are lined with simple cuboidal cells that contain large amounts of glycogen. There is some epithelial differentiation with the appearance of neuroepithelial bodies and cartilage by 9 to 10 weeks. Ciliated cells, goblet cells, and basal cells are in the proximal airways by 13 weeks. In general, epithelial differentiation is centrifugal in that the most distal tubules are lined with undifferentiated cells with progressive differentiation of the more proximal airways. Regulators of branching morphogenesis are FGF-10 and FGF-7 as well as endothelial growth factor, transforming growth factor-α, and other growth factors.[45] Upper lobar development occurs earlier than lower lobe development in animals, and a similar pattern of development probably occurs in humans. Early in the pseudoglandular stage, the airways are surrounded by a loose mesenchyme through which loose capillaries randomly spread. Pulmonary arteries grow in conjunction with the airways, with the principal arterial pathways being present by 14 weeks. Pulmonary venous development occurs in parallel but with a different pattern that demarcates lung segments and subsegments. By the end of the pseudoglandular stage, airways, arteries, and veins have developed in the pattern corresponding to that found in the adult.

Canalicular Stage

The canalicular stage between 16 and 25 weeks' gestation represents the transformation of the previable lung to the potentially viable lung that can exchange gas (Fig. 44-3).[50] The bronchial tree has completely branched and respiratory bronchioles are forming. The three major events during this stage are the appearance of the acinus, epithelial differentiation with the development of the potential air-blood barrier, and the start of surfactant synthesis within recognizable type II cells.[10] The acinus in the mature lung is the tuft of airways and alveoli originating from a terminal bronchiole that includes about six generations of respiratory bronchioles, and alveolar ducts that alveolarize with maturation. This saccular branching is the critical first step for the development of the future gas exchange surface of the lung. The mesenchyme surrounding the airways becomes more vascular and more closely approximated to the airway epithelial cells (Fig. 44-4). Capillaries initially form as a double capillary network between future airspaces and subsequently fuse to form a single capillary. With fusion of the vascular and epithelial basement membranes, a structure comparable to the adult air-blood barrier forms. If the double capillary network fails to fuse, the infant will have severe hypoxemia resulting from alveolar-capillary dysplasia. The total surface area occupied by the air-blood barrier begins to increase exponentially toward the end of the canalicular stage with a resultant fall in the mean wall thickness and with an increased potential for gas exchange.

Epithelial differentiation is characterized by proximal to distal thinning of the epithelium by transformation of cuboidal cells into thin cells that line tubes. The tubes grow both in length and in width with attenuation of the mesenchyme, which is simultaneously becoming vascularized. During the canalicular stage, many of the cells would best be characterized as intermediary cells, because they are neither mature type I nor type II epithelial cells.[10] These epithelial cells develop attenuated extensions as well as some characteristics of mature type II cells such as lamellar bodies, supporting the concept that type I cells are derived from type II cells or intermediary cells that then further differentiate into type I cells. After about 20 weeks in the human fetus, cuboidal cells rich in glycogen begin to have lamellar bodies in their cytoplasm. The transcription factors TTF-1, FOXa1, FOXa2, and GATA 6 mediate type II cell differentiation.[48] The glycogen in type II cells provides substrate for surfactant synthesis as the lamellar body content increases. In the adult human lung, the thin type I cells occupy about 93% of the alveolar surface versus 7% for type II cells.[13] About 8% of the lung cells are type I cells and about 16% of lung cells are type II cells.

Saccular and Alveolar Stages

The saccular stage encompasses the period of lung development during the potentially viable stages of prematurity from about 25 weeks to term. The terminal sac or saccule is the distal airway structure that is elongating, branching, and widening until alveolarization is completed. Alveolarization is initiated from the terminal saccules by the appearance of septa in association with capillaries, elastin fibers, and collagen fibers (see Fig. 44-4). Shallow alveolar structures with crests (or septa) with elastin at the free margin of the crests

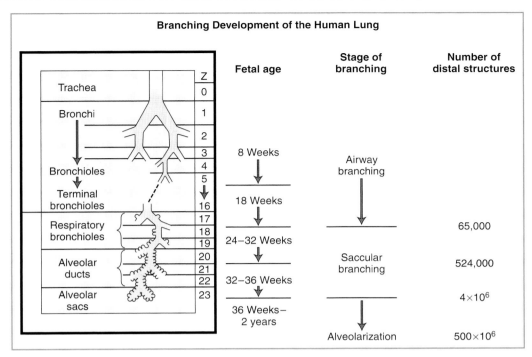

Figure 44-2. Airway branching, fetal age, and number of branches during lung development. Airway branching results in about 16 generations of airways by about 18 weeks' gestation. Branching of distal saccular structures yields respiratory bronchioles and alveolar ducts in the saccular lung by about 32 weeks' gestation. Alveolarization continues from 32 to 36 weeks until 2 years of age. (*Modified from Burri PW: Development and growth of the human lung. In Fishman AP, Fisher AB, editors:* Handbook of physiology: the respiratory system, *Bethesda, MD, 1985, American Physiology Society, p 1.*)

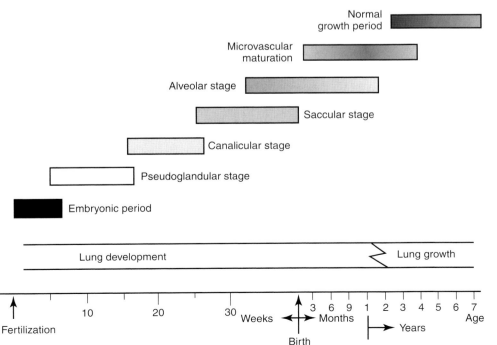

Figure 44-3. Timetable for lung development. The period of lung development continues to 1 to 2 years of age. The timing of the saccular and alveolar stages and the period of microvascular maturation overlap with indeterminate initiation and endpoints. (*Modified from Zeltner TB, Burri, PH: The postnatal development and growth of the human lung: II. Morphology,* Respir Physiol *67:269, 1987, with permission from Elsevier Science.*)

Capillaries

Alveolar septation

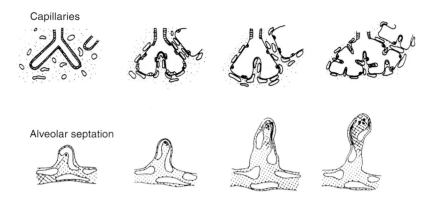

Figure 44–4. Development of alveolar septa and capillaries. An alveolar septum is identified by the epithelium folding over elastic fibers with subsequent elongation of the septum. Capillaries arrange themselves around epithelial tubes. The double-capillary network becomes progressively more closely associated with the epithelium of the developing airspace with subsequent loss of the double-capillary network. (*Modified from Burri PW: Development and growth of the human lung. In Fishman AP, Fisher AB, editors:* Handbook of physiology: the respiratory system, *Bethesda, MD, 1985, American Physiologic Society, p 1, with permission.*)

can be identified by 28 weeks' gestation in the human.[21] Alveolar number increases from about 32 weeks' gestation, and the term human lung contains between about 50 and 150 million alveoli.[21,32] For comparison, the adult human lung has about 500 million alveoli.[40] The most rapid rate of accumulation of alveoli occurs between 32 weeks' gestational age and the first months after term delivery (Fig. 44-5). The potential lung gas volume and surface area increases from about 25 weeks' gestation to term. This increase in lung volume, and the surface area of sacculi establishes the anatomic

potential for gas exchange and thus for fetal viability. There is a wide range of lung volumes and surface areas at a given gestational age. Therefore the gas exchange potential of different fetuses at the same gestational age will be determined in part by the structural development of the lung.

Alveolarization progresses rapidly from late fetal to early neonatal life and may be complete by 1 to 2 years after birth (see Fig. 44-5). A number of factors that can stimulate or interfere with alveolarization have been identified (Box 44-1).[31] Chronic mechanical ventilation of preterm animals using

Figure 44–5. Increases in surface area and alveoli with development. **A,** The large increase in lung surface area does not occur until after the saccular lung begins to alveolarize. **B,** Alveolar number and weekly rate of accumulation of alveoli are expressed as a percentage of the adult number of alveoli. The curves assume that the term infant has 30% of the adult number of alveoli. (**A,** *Redrawn from Langston C, et al: Human lung growth in late gestation and in the neonate,* Am Rev Respir Dis *129:607, 1984.* **B,** *Idealized curves based on Langston C, et al: Human lung growth in late gestation and in the neonate,* Am Rev Respir Dis *129:607, 1984, and Hislop AA, Wigglesworth JS, Desai R: Alveolar development in the human fetus and infant,* Early Hum Dev *13:1, 1986.*)

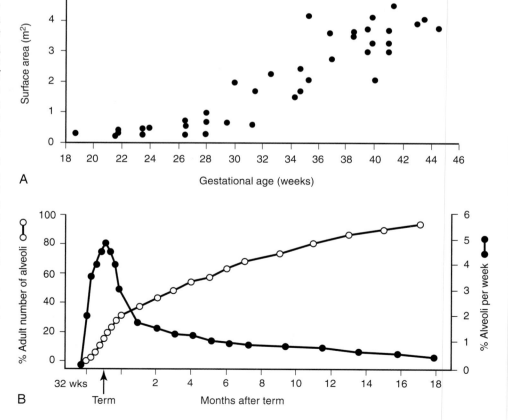

BOX 44-1   Modulators of Alveolarization

FACTORS THAT DELAY OR INTERFERE WITH ALVEOLARIZATION
Mechanical ventilation
Antenatal and postnatal glucocorticoids
Proinflammatory mediators
Hyperoxia or hypoxia
Poor nutrition

FACTORS THAT STIMULATE ALVEOLARIZATION
Vitamin A (retinoids)
Thyroxin

modest tidal volumes and low oxygen exposures interrupts both alveolarization and vascular development (Fig. 44-6).[11] Mechanical ventilation of the saccular lung disrupts elastin at the developing crests and induces an "arrest in development" characterized by lack of secondary crest formation and resulting in fewer and larger alveoli without much fibrosis or inflammation (Fig. 44-7).[6] Preterm infants who have died after long-term ventilation or after the development of bronchopulmonary dysplasia (BPD) also have decreased alveolar numbers and an attenuated microvasculature with less prominent airway injury and fibrosis than in the past.[4] Factors that likely contribute to this arrest of lung development include many of the components of care of preterm infants. Antenatal glucocorticoid treatments in monkeys and sheep cause thinning of the interstitium and an increased surface area for gas exchange with delayed alveolar septation. Postnatal glucocorticoid treatments of the saccular lung also interrupt alveolarization and capillary development. Hyperoxia or hypoxia and poor nutrition can interfere with alveolarization. In transgenic mice, overexpression of proinflammatory mediators in the pulmonary epithelium interferes with alveolar development. Antenatal lung inflammation associated with chorioamnionitis in sheep causes delayed alveolar and microvascular development.[31] Multiple factors may contribute to

delayed alveolarization in preterm infants. Because lung growth following the completion of alveolarization is by increase in airway and alveolar size, any event that decreases alveolar number could impact lung function as the individual ages.

PULMONARY HYPOPLASIA

Pulmonary hypoplasia is a relatively common abnormality of lung development with a number of clinical associations and anatomic correlates.[33] Primary pulmonary hypoplasia is unusual and is likely caused by abnormalities of the transcription factors and growth factors that regulate early lung morphogenesis such as thyroid transcription factor-1 and FGF family members.[48] Severe forms of acinar aplasia that probably result from abnormal regulation of lung growth and development have been reported. Secondary pulmonary hypoplasia is associated with either a restriction of lung growth or the absence of fetal breathing (Box 44-2). Any reduction of the chest cavity by a mass, effusion, or external compression can impact lung growth. Lung hypoplasia can be minimal or severe. Severe pulmonary hypoplasia associated with renal agenesis and prolonged oligohydramnios is characterized by a decrease in lung size and cell number together with narrow airways, a delay of epithelial differentiation, and surfactant deficiency. Relatively short-term oligohydramnios caused by ruptured membranes in the 16th to 28th week of gestation also can result in pulmonary hypoplasia, the magnitude in general correlating with the severity and length of the oligohydramnios. Infants with congenital diaphragmatic hernia have more severe hypoplasia on the ipsilateral side than on the contralateral side, although the contralateral lung also may be hypoplastic. The lungs have fewer and smaller acinar units, delayed epithelial maturation, and an associated surfactant deficiency. In experimental models, tracheal occlusion in late gestation can reverse much of the pulmonary hypoplasia resulting from diaphragmatic hernia, but the occlusion induces a decrease in type II cells and surfactant deficiency.[30]

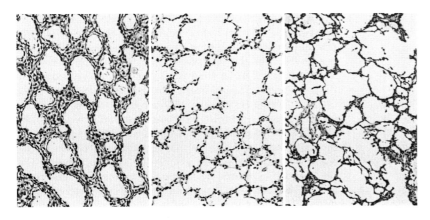

Figure 44-6. Tissue from lungs of ventilated preterm baboons. *Left,* The lung of a 125 days' gestation fetal baboon has rounded saccular structures with thick walls (×170). *Center,* Lung from a term baboon (186 days' gestation) with airspaces that are a mixture of saccular and alveolar structures (×170). *Right,* Lung tissue from a preterm baboon delivered at 125 days' gestation and ventilated for 30 days demonstrates enlarged airspaces with increased interstitial cellularity (×70). The ventilated lung has larger airspaces even though the photomicrograph is at a 2.4-fold lower magnification. *(Modified from Coalson JJ, et al: Neonatal chronic lung disease in extremely immature baboons, Am J Respir Crit Care Med 160:1333, 1999, with permission. Copyright © 1999 American Lung Association.)*

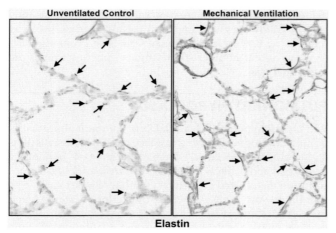

Unventilated Control	Mechanical Ventilation

Elastin

Figure 44–7. See color insert Changes in elastin distribution in lungs of 5-day-old mice ventilated for 24 hours with 40% oxygen. Lung sections from controls (*left*) demonstrate elastin with Hart stain at the tips of developing septa. In contrast, the ventilated lungs (*right*) have more elastin without the focal distribution in the distal airspaces. (*Reprinted with permission from Bland RD, et al: Mechanical ventilation uncouples synthesis and assembly of elastin and increases apoptosis in lungs of newborn mice. Prelude to defective alveolar septation during lung development? Am J Physiol Lung Cell Mol Physiol 294:L3, 2008.*)

BOX 44–2   Clinical Associations of Pulmonary Hypoplasia

THORACIC COMPRESSION
Renal agenesis (Potter syndrome)
Urinary tract outflow obstruction
Oligohydramnios before 28 weeks' gestational age
Extra-amniotic fetal development

DECREASED INTRATHORACIC SPACE
Diaphragmatic hernia
Pleural effusions
Abdominal distention sufficient to limit chest volume
Thoracic dystrophies
Intrathoracic masses

DECREASED FETAL BREATHING
Intrauterine central nervous system damage
Fetal Werdnig-Hoffmann syndrome
Other neuropathies and myopathies

OTHER ASSOCIATIONS
Primary pulmonary hypoplasia
Trisomy 21
Multiple congenital anomalies
Erythroblastosis fetalis

FETAL LUNG FLUID

The fetal airways are filled with fluid until delivery and the initiation of ventilation. Most of the information concerning quantitative aspects of fetal lung fluid is from the fetal lamb with sonographic and pathologic correlates available for the human. The fetal lung close to term contains enough fluid to maintain the airway fluid volume at about 40 mL/kg of body weight, which is somewhat larger than the FRC once air breathing is established.[35] The composition of fetal lung fluid is unique relative to other fetal fluids in the fetal sheep and most other mammalian species.[24] The chloride content is high (157 mEq/L), whereas the bicarbonate and protein contents are very low. In contrast, the bicarbonate and chloride concentrations in fetal lung fluid from the rhesus monkey are not different from plasma values, demonstrating species differences in ion composition of fetal lung fluid. The electrolyte composition is maintained by transepithelial chloride secretion with bicarbonate reabsorption. Fetal lung fluid contains little protein because the fetal epithelium is quite impermeable to protein. Active transport of Cl^- from the interstitium to the lumen yields a production rate for fetal lung fluid of 4 to 5 mL/kg per hour. Assuming the fetus is 3 to 4 kg, the daily production of fetal lung fluid is about 400 mL per day. Fetal lung fluid flows intermittently up the trachea with fetal breathing movements, and some of this fluid is swallowed while the rest mixes with the amniotic fluid. The pressure in the fetal trachea exceeds that in the amniotic fluid by about 2 mm Hg, maintaining an outflow resistance and the fetal lung fluid volume. The secretion of fetal lung fluid seems to be an intrinsic metabolic function of the developing lung epithelium because changes in vascular hydrostatic pressures, tracheal pressures, and fetal breathing movements do not greatly alter fetal lung fluid production rates.

Although normal amounts of fetal lung fluid are essential for normal lung development, its clearance is equally essential for normal neonatal respiratory adaptation.[39] Fetal lung fluid production can be completely stopped at term by vascular infusions of epinephrine at concentrations that approximate the levels of epinephrine present during labor. The epinephrine-mediated reversal of fetal lung fluid flux from secretion to reabsorption does not occur in the preterm lung. However, epinephrine-mediated clearance can be induced by pretreatment of fetal sheep with the combination of corticosteroid and triiodothyronine. Inhibition of prostaglandin synthesis with indomethacin in the fetus reduces the production of fetal lung fluid and urine. Fetal lung fluid production and fetal lung fluid volumes are maintained in the fetal sheep until the onset of labor. During active labor and delivery, fetal lung fluid volumes decrease, leaving about 35% of the fetal lung fluid to be absorbed and cleared from the lungs with breathing. Most of the fluid moves rapidly into the interstitial spaces and subsequently into the pulmonary vasculature, with less than 20% of the fluid being cleared by pulmonary lymphatics. The clearance of the fluid from the interstitial spaces occurs over many hours. Fluid clearance after birth results from active sodium transport via the epithelial sodium channel (ENaC), which can be blocked with amiloride.[22] See also chapter 34 Genetic ablation of the α subunit of the ENaC causes death in newborn mice because fetal lung fluid is not cleared from the lungs (Fig. 44-8). Glucocorticoids upregulate the messenger

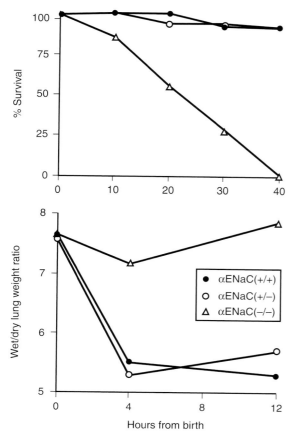

Figure 44–8. Ablation of the function of the α-epithelial sodium channel (ENaC) subunit prevents water clearance as indicated by the lack of decrease in the lung wet-to-dry weight ratio and results in neonatal death in mice. *(Redrawn from Hummler E, et al: Early death due to defective neonatal lung liquid clearance in α-ENaC–deficient mice,* Nat Genet *12:325, 1996, with permission.)*

RNA (mRNA) for the EnaC subunits in the fetal human lung. Transient respiratory difficulties in many infants result from delayed clearance of fetal lung fluid.

SURFACTANT METABOLISM

Composition

Surfactant recovered from lungs of all mammalian species by alveolar wash procedures contains 70% to 80% phospholipids, about 10% protein, and about 10% neutral lipids, primarily cholesterol (Fig. 44-9). The phosphatidylcholine species of the phospholipids represent about 60% by weight of the surfactant and about 80% of the phospholipids. The composition of the phospholipids in surfactant is unique relative to the lipid composition of lung tissue or other organs. About 60% of the phosphatidylcholine species are saturated, meaning that both fatty acids esterified to the glycerol-phosphorylcholine backbone are predominantly the 16-carbon saturated fatty acid, palmitic acid. Most other phosphatidylcholine species in surfactant have a fatty acid with one double bond in the 2 position

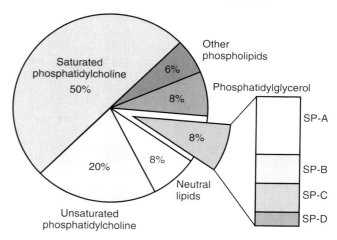

Figure 44–9. Composition of surfactant. The major component is saturated phosphatidylcholine. The surfactant proteins contribute about 8% to the mass of surfactant.

of the molecule. Saturated phosphatidylcholine is the principal surface-active component of surfactant, and much less saturated phosphatidylcholine is present in lipid fractions of lung not associated with surfactant metabolism. Thus saturated phosphatidylcholine can be used as a relatively specific probe of surfactant metabolism. The acidic phospholipid, phosphatidylglycerol, is present in surfactant in small amounts that vary between 4% and 15% of the phospholipids in different species (Table 44-1). Surfactant phospholipids from the immature fetus or newborn contain relatively large amounts of phosphatidylinositol, which then decrease as phosphatidylglycerol appears with lung maturity.[18] The switch from phosphatidylinositol to phosphatidylglycerol probably results from a fall in the circulating and lung tissue pools of free inositol in the fetus during late gestation. Phosphatidylglycerol is a convenient marker for lung maturity. The surfactant from the preterm lung is qualitatively inferior relative to surfactant from the mature lung when tested for in vivo function than is surfactant from term newborns.[26]

TABLE 44–1	Changes in Surfactant with Development	
Variables	Immature Lung	Mature Lung
Type II cells		
Glycogen lakes	High	Gone
Lamellar bodies	Few	Many
Microvilli	Few	Many
Surfactant composition		
Sat PC/Total PC	0.6	0.7
Phosphatidylglycerol (%)	<1	10
Phosphatidylinositol (%)	10	2
Surfactant Protein A (%)	Low	5
Surfactant function	Decreased	Normal

Four surfactant-specific proteins have been identified and their functions in part elucidated.[49] SP-A is a water-soluble collectin coded on human chromosome 10. The 24-kDa protein is heavily glycosylated in the carboxy-terminal region with blood group antigen as well as other carbohydrate moieties to yield a protein of about 36 kDa. SP-A has a number of isoforms because of the variable glycosylation. This protein has a collagen domain that permits SP-A monomers to form a collagen-like triple helix that then aggregates to form a multimeric protein with a molecular size of 650 kDa. SP-A contributes to the biophysical properties of surfactant primarily by decreasing protein-mediated inhibition of surfactant function. Mice that lack SP-A have no tubular myelin but have normal lung function and surfactant metabolism indicating that SP-A is not critical to regulation of surfactant metabolism. The major function of SP-A is as an innate host defense protein and as a regulator of inflammation in the lung. SP-A can both suppress and activate macrophage function under different test situations. SP-A binds to multiple pathogens such as group B streptococcus, *Staphylococcus aureus*, and herpes simplex type 1. The protein facilitates phagocytosis of pathogens by macrophages and their clearance from the airspace. SP-A can prevent influenza virus infection and decrease the inflammation caused by adenovirus. Patients with a deficiency of SP-A have not been identified. SP-A levels are low in surfactant from preterm lungs and increase with corticosteroid exposure. SP-A is not in surfactants used for treatment of RDS.

SP-B and SP-C are two small hydrophobic proteins that are extracted with the lipids from surfactant by organic solvents. These proteins contribute about 2% to 4% to the surfactant mass.[49] The SP-B gene is on human chromosome 2, and the primary translation product is 40 kDa. The protein is clipped to become an 8-kDa protein in the type II cell before it enters lamellar bodies for cosecretion with the phospholipids. SP-B facilitates surface absorption of lipids and the development of low surface tensions on surface area compression. Animals with antibodies to SP-B develop respiratory failure, and infants with a genetic absence of SP-B have lethal RDS after term birth. The genetic absence of SP-B is most frequently caused by a two base-pair insertion (121 ins 2) resulting in a frame-shift and premature termination signal resulting in a complete absence of SP-B. Multiple other mutations resulting in complete or partial SP-B deficiencies have been described.[38] (See also Part 3 of this chapter.) About 15% of term infants dying of a syndrome similar to RDS have SP-B deficiency. The lack of SP-B causes a loss of normal lamellar bodies in type II cells, a lack of SP-C, and the appearance of incompletely processed SP-C in the airspaces. These pro-SP-C forms are diagnostic of SP-B deficiency. Respiratory failure develops in mice that have less than about 20% of the normal amount of SP-B.

The SP-C gene is on chromosome 8, and its primary translation product is a 22-kDa protein that is processed to an extremely hydrophobic 4-kDa protein that is associated with lipids in lamellar bodies.[49] The mRNA for SP-C appears in cells lining the developing airways from early gestation. With advancing lung maturation, the mRNA for SP-C becomes localized only to type II cells. The sequence and cellular localization of the protein have been remarkably conserved across species; however, mice that lack SP-C have normal lung and surfactant function at birth. However, the mice develop progressive interstitial lung disease and emphysema as they age. Infants with a progressive interstitial lung disease resulting from a lack of SP-C are being reported, as are large kindreds of patients with the onset of interstitial lung disease at variable ages.[38] These patients generally do not have genetic alterations in the coding region of the protein, but do have dominant negative mutations that disrupt the processing of SP-C. The misprocessed SP-C results in SP-C deficiency in the airspaces and seems to also injure the type II cell. SP-B and SP-C probably work cooperatively to optimize rapid adsorption and spreading of phospholipids on a surface and to facilitate the development of low surface tensions on surface area compression. Surfactants prepared by organic solvent extraction of natural surfactants or from lung tissue contain SP-B and SP-C, but lack SP-A. Such surfactants are similar to natural surfactants when evaluated for in vitro surface properties or for function in vivo. Surfactant recovered from preterm animals has low amounts of SP-B and SP-C, which may, in part, explain its poor function.

The true incidences of genetic abnormalities of the surfactant system are not well known. A recent report of more than 300 term infants with severe RDS found about 14% had SP-B deficiency, and some infants had a new deficiency of the ATP-binding cassette transporter gene—ABCA3.[7] This ABCA3 gene product is localized to lamellar bodies and functions as a lipid transporter. This clinical presentation is very much like SP-B deficiency. Some of the lethal RDS in term infants is explained by mutations in genes essential for surfactant metabolism. However, other infants probably have yet to be identified mutations in genes that disrupt other aspects of lung development as explanations for their respiratory failure.

SP-D is a hydrophilic protein of 43 kDa that is a collectin with structural similarities to SP-A.[49] It has a collagen-like domain as well as a glycosylated region that gives it lectin-like functions. This protein is synthesized by type II cells and Clara cells as well as in other epithelial sites in the body. Like the other SPs, its expression is developmentally regulated by glucocorticoids and inflammation. SP-D is a large multimer that functions as an innate host defense molecule by binding pathogens and facilitating their clearance. The absence of SP-D results in increased surfactant lipid pools in the airspaces and emphysema but no major deficits in surfactant function in mice. No humans with SP-D deficiency have been described.

Synthesis and Secretion

The type II cell is responsible for the major pathways involved in surfactant metabolism (Fig. 44-10). The synthesis and secretion of surfactant is a complex sequence of biochemical synthetic events that results in the release by exocytosis of the lamellar bodies to the alveolus. The basic pathways for the synthesis of phospholipids are common to all mammalian cells. Specific enzymes within the endoplasmic reticulum use glucose, phosphate, and fatty acids as substrates for phospholipid synthesis. The uniqueness of a phospholipid is determined by the character of the fatty acid side chains esterified to the glycerol carbon backbone and by the head group (e.g., choline, glycerol, and inositol) linked to the phosphate. Although the overall synthetic pathways are

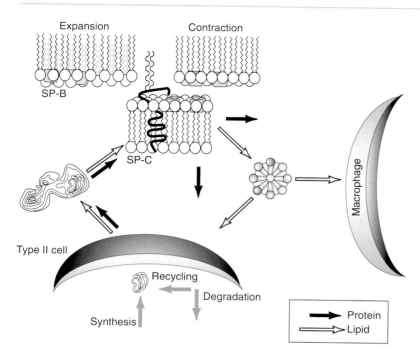

Figure 44–10. Surfactant metabolism in the type II cell in the alveolus. The lipid-associated surfactant proteins B (SP-B) and SP-C (*solid arrows*) track with the lipid from synthesis to secretion and surface film formation. The small vesicular forms of surfactant do not contain SP-B or SP-C.

known, the details of how the components of surfactant condense with SP-B and SP-C to form the surfactant lipoprotein complex within lamellar bodies remain obscure. Ultrastructural abnormalities of type II cells with SP-B deficiency and ABCA3 deficiency in term infants indicate that these gene products are critical to lamellar body formation.[7] If SP-B is absent, lamellar bodies are abnormal and SP-C is not processed correctly. Surfactant secretion can be stimulated by a number of mechanisms. Type II cells respond to β-agonists with increased surfactant secretion. Purines such as adenosine triphosphate are potent stimulators of surfactant secretion and may be important for surfactant secretion at birth. Surfactant secretion also is stimulated by mechanical stretch such as with lung distention and hyperventilation. The surfactant secretion that occurs with the initiation of ventilation following birth probably results from the combined effects of elevated catecholamines and lung stretch.

Surfactant Pool Sizes

Following the observation of Avery and Mead that saline extracts of the lungs of infants with RDS had high minimum surface tensions,[2] decreased alveolar and tissue surfactant pools were demonstrated in preterm animals. Increasing surfactant pool sizes correlate with improving compliances during development, although other factors such as structural maturation also influence compliance. Infants with RDS have surfactant pool sizes on the order of about 5 mg/kg of body weight. Preterm lambs with RDS can be managed with continuous positive airway pressure if their surfactant pool sizes exceed about 4 mg/kg. The quantity of surfactant recovered from the airspaces of infants with RDS is not much less than the amount of surfactant found in the alveoli of healthy adult animals or humans. However, much less surfactant is recovered from preterms than healthy term animals, who have surfactant pool sizes of about 100 mg/kg of body weight.[26]

The large amount of surfactant in amniotic fluid in the human at term indicates that the term human fetal lung also has large pool sizes. Both the quantity and the quality of the surfactant from the preterm together with surfactant inhibition contribute to the deficiency state. The clinical observations that many preterm infants and animals respond remarkably to surfactant treatment supports the conclusion that in many infants surfactant deficiency is the primary problem. The endogenous pool sizes of surfactant that are sufficient for good lung function are lower than for treatment doses of surfactant, probably because the endogenous surfactant is optimally distributed and treatment doses of surfactant are not distributed uniformly at the alveolar level.

The rate of increase in the pool size of alveolar surfactant after preterm birth has been measured in ventilated preterm monkeys recovering from RDS (Fig. 44-11).[23] The surfactant pool size increased toward the 100 mg/kg value measured in term monkeys within 3 to 4 days. Although there is no comparable quantitative information for the human, Hallman and colleagues[19] measured the concentration of saturated phosphatidylcholine in airway suction samples from infants recovering from RDS and compared the results with values for infants without RDS and for surfactant-treated infants. The concentration of saturated phosphatidylcholine increased over a 4- to 5-day period to become comparable with values for normal or surfactant-treated infants. This slow increase in pool size is consistent with a clinical course of RDS of 3 to 5 days. The explanation for why surfactant pool sizes increase slowly after preterm birth is apparent from measurements of the kinetics of surfactant secretion and clearance in the newborn (Figs. 44-12 and 44-13). Following the intravascular injection of radiolabeled precursors of surfactant phosphatidylcholine, incorporation into lung phosphatidylcholine is rapid. However, there are long time delays between synthesis and the movement of surfactant components from the endoplasmic reticulum through the Golgi apparatus to

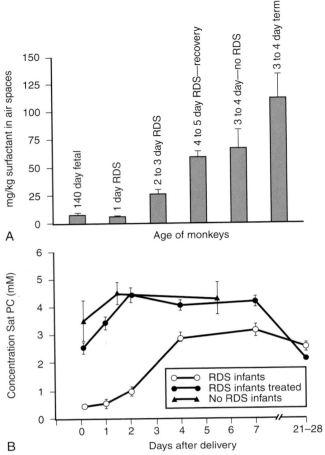

Figure 44–11. Changes in surfactant pool sizes with resolution of respiratory distress syndrome (RDS). **A,** The amount of surfactant recovered by alveolar lavage from monkeys with RDS and cared for with mechanical ventilation is shown relative to age and stage of the disease. **B,** The concentrations of saturated phosphatidylcholine (Sat PC) in airway samples from infants with RDS, infants with RDS treated with surfactant, and infants without RDS are graphed relative to age from birth. The concentration of Sat PC approached values for healthy preterm infants by 4 to 7 days. (**A,** *Data from Jackson JC, et al: Surfactant quantity and composition during recovery from hyaline membrane disease,* Pediatr Res *20:1247, 1986;* **B,** *Data drawn from Hallman M, et al: Surfactant protein A, phosphatidylcholine, and surfactant inhibitors in epithelial lining fluid: correlation with surface activity, severity of respiratory distress syndrome, and outcome in small premature infants,* Am Rev Respir Dis *144:1376, 1991.)*

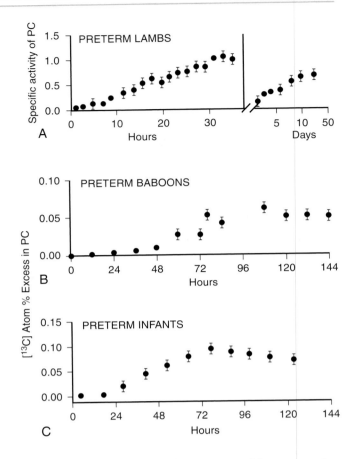

Figure 44–12. Time course of appearance of de novo synthesized surfactant phosphatidylcholine (PC) in the airways. **A,** Labeling of saturated phosphatidylcholine (Sat PC) in airway samples of ventilated preterm lambs given a single intravascular injection of [³H]palmitic acid at birth and not treated with surfactant until about 38 hours of age. The discontinuity in the curve demonstrates the fall in the specific activity after treatment with surfactant (shown in days). **B,** Labeling of PC in airway samples of preterm surfactant-treated baboons that were ventilated for 6 days. The animals received [¹³C]glucose by intravascular infusion for the first 24 hours of age, and the [¹³C] in PC is expressed as [¹³C]atom % excess. **C,** Labeling of PC in airway samples of preterm surfactant-treated mechanically ventilated infants with respiratory distress syndrome after intravascular infusion of [¹³C]glucose for the first 24 hours of life. The label in the PC is expressed as atom % excess. (**A,** *Data redrawn from Jobe AH, et al: Saturated phosphatidylcholine secretion and the effect of natural surfactant on premature and term lambs ventilated for 2 days,* Exper Lung Res *4:259, 1983;* **B,** *Data redrawn from Bunt JE, et al: Metabolism of endogenous surfactant in premature baboons and effect of prenatal corticosteroids,* Am J Respir Crit Care Med *160:1481, 1999;* **C,** *Data redrawn from Bunt JE, et al: The effect in premature infants of prenatal corticosteroids on endogenous surfactant synthesis as measured with stable isotopes,* Am J Respir Crit Care Med *162:844, 2000.)*

lamellar bodies for eventual secretion. The time lag from surfactant phospholipid synthesis to peak secretion of labeled surfactant is about 30 hours in ventilated preterm lambs with RDS.[28] These measurements of synthesis and secretion in animals were made using radiolabeled precursors of phosphatidylcholine and pulse labeling techniques not possible in preterm infants. However, phosphatidylcholine secretion was measured in preterm baboons and human infants with RDS using intravascular infusions of the precursors glucose and

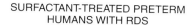

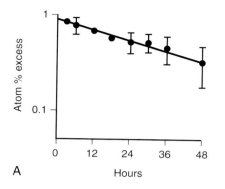

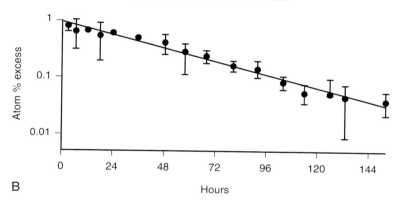

Figure 44–13. Time course for disappearance of surfactant from the airspace. **A,** Curve for decrease in atom % excess in airway samples for [^{13}C]dipalmitoylphosphatidylcholine-labeled surfactant used to treat preterm ventilated infants with respiratory distress syndrome. The atom % excess in the initial surfactant dose given after delivery fell exponentially for 48 hours. **B,** A second dose given at about 2 days of age resulted in a similar curve. (*Data redrawn from Torresin M, et al: Exogenous surfactant kinetics in infant respiratory distress syndrome: a novel method with stable isotopes,* Am J Respir Crit Care Med *161:1584, 2000.*)

palmitic acid labeled with stable isotopes.[8,9] The secretion kinetics of the stable isotopically labeled phosphatidylcholine are similar to the preterm lambs. There were lags of about 20 hours before glucose-labeled phosphatidylcholine was detected in the airway samples and peak enrichment of the stable isotope occurred at about 70 hours. There were delays between synthesis and secretion and the interval to peak airway accumulation of endogenously synthesized surfactant lipid is long in the preterm human.[12] In preterm ventilated baboons developing CLD, the percentage of the phospholipid that is secreted after synthesis is low relative to values measured in newborn or adult animals despite high accumulations of surfactant lipids in lung tissue.[44] The animals have an abnormality of processing and secretion of surfactant despite surfactant deficiency.

The slow secretion and alveolar accumulation of surfactant are balanced in the term and preterm lung by slow catabolism and clearance. Trace amounts of radiolabeled surfactant phospholipid given into the airspaces of term lambs are cleared from the lung with a half-life on the order of 6 days. The half-life measurements for infants with RDS made with stable isotope yield values of 3 to 5 days (see Fig. 44-13).[46] This slow lung clearance is in striking contrast to the more rapid catabolism characteristic of the adult lung with half-life values on the order of 12 hours. Preterm ventilated baboons that are developing CLD degrade a treatment dose of surfactant more

rapidly with a half-life of about 2 days, suggesting that surfactant catabolic rates increase with lung injury.[44] Trace or treatment doses of radiolabeled surfactant given into the airspaces do not remain static in the airspaces. The surfactant phospholipids move from the airspaces back to type II cells, where they are taken up by an endocytotic process into multivesicular bodies. In the term and preterm lung, about 90% of the phospholipids are recycled back to lamellar bodies and resecreted to the airspace. In the adult lung, this process is perhaps only 50% efficient. The phospholipids are recycled as intact molecules without degradation and resynthesis.

The metabolic characteristics of surfactant phospholipids in the preterm are favorable for surfactant treatment strategies.[26] Alveolar and tissue pool sizes are small, and the rate of accumulation is slow. Treatment acutely increases both the alveolar and tissue pools because the exogenously administered saturated phosphatidylcholine is taken up into type II cells and processed for resecretion. The surfactants used clinically are not equivalent in function to native surfactant in the mature lung. However, within hours following surfactant treatment of preterm animals the surfactant recovered by alveolar wash has improved function, indicating that the preterm lung, if uninjured, can rapidly transform surfactant used for treatment with poor function to a good surfactant. Also of benefit is the slow catabolic rate of the lipid components of surfactant. This characteristic of the system means that the surfactant used for treatment remains in the lungs and is not rapidly degraded. Infants treated with surfactant can be extubated earlier if they maintain higher surfactant pool sizes.[47] Treatment doses of surfactant do not feedback-inhibit the endogenous synthesis of saturated phosphatidylcholine or the SPs. No adverse metabolic consequences of surfactant treatment on the endogenous metabolism of surfactant or other lung functions have been identified.

There is less information about the metabolism of the SPs in the preterm lung. SP-A, SP-B, and SP-C all seem to be recycled to some degree from the airspace back into lamellar bodies for resecretion with surfactant.[26] All three proteins have alveolar clearance kinetics that are similar to saturated phosphatidylcholine in the preterm lung. Therefore the critical surfactant components are conserved by recycling. The presumed function of the recycling pathways is to reassemble the components to regenerate biophysically active surfactant. SP-B and SP-C enter the lamellar bodies during their biogenesis in parallel with the phospholipids. In contrast, de novo synthesized SP-A is secreted independently of the lamellar bodies. This protein then associates with the phospholipids to form tubular myelin in the airspace. It is then recycled via lamellar bodies but with a lower efficiency than is saturated phosphatidylcholine. In the preterm ventilated baboon developing BPD, SP-A accumulates in high amounts in lung tissue and is minimally secreted, a pattern similar to that of phosphatidylcholine. Lung injury of the preterm results in abnormalities in surfactant metabolism and function.

Alveolar Life Cycle of Surfactant

After secretion as lamellar bodies, surfactant goes through a series of form transitions in the airspace.[26] The lamellar bodies "unravel" to form an elegant structure called *tubular myelin*. This lipoprotein array has SP-A at the corners of the lattice and requires at least SP-A, SP-B, and the phospholipids for its unique structure. Tubular myelin and other surfactant lipoprotein arrays are believed to be the reserve pool in the fluid hypophase for the formation of the surface film within the alveolus and small airways. Area compression of this film then squeezes out unsaturated lipid and some protein components of surfactant with concentration of saturated phosphatidylcholine in the surface film. New surfactant enters the surface film and "used" surfactant leaves in the form of small vesicles, which then are cleared from the airspaces. The major difference in composition between the surface-active tubular myelin and loose lipid arrays and the small vesicular forms is that the small forms contain little SP-A, SP-B, or SP-C. Although a complete surfactant contains multiple lipid and protein components, all of the components are not essential for biophysical function. Surfactants for treatment probably work well despite lacking some components of native surfactant.

Just preceding and following birth, lamellar bodies are secreted to yield an alveolar pool that is primarily lamellar bodies and tubular myelin. This surfactant then begins to function with aeration of the lung. As the newborn goes through neonatal transition, the percentage of surface active forms falls as the small vesicular forms increase. At equilibrium approximately 50% of the surfactant in the airspaces is in a surface-active form and 50% is in the inactive vesicular form. The vesicular forms of surfactant are believed to be the pools used for recycling of the phospholipid components of surfactant. The total surfactant pool size is not equivalent to the amount of active surfactant. In the preterm, conversion from surface active to inactive surfactant forms occurs more rapidly, probably because less SP is present. Pulmonary edema can further accelerate the process with the net result being a depletion of the surface active fraction of surfactant despite normal or high total surfactant pool sizes.

PHYSIOLOGIC EFFECTS OF SURFACTANT IN THE PRETERM LUNG

Alveolar Stability

Although alveoli have been traditionally considered to be independent spheres on which surfactant acts to stabilize their size, alveoli are polygonal in shape with flat surfaces and curvatures where the walls intersect. Furthermore, alveoli are interdependent in that their structure is determined by the shape and elasticity of neighboring alveolar walls. The forces acting on the pulmonary microstructure are chest wall elasticity, lung tissue elasticity, and surface tensions of the air-fluid interfaces in the small airways and alveoli. At functional residual capacity, the alveolus is open to atmospheric pressure. Although the surface tension of surfactant decreases with surface area compression and increases with surface area expansion, the surface area of an alveolus changes very little with tidal breathing. The low surface tensions resulting from surfactant help prevent alveolar collapse and keep interstitial fluid from entering the alveolus. Surfactant also keeps small airways from filling with fluid and causing luminal obstruction.[15] If alveoli collapse or fill with fluid, the shape of adjacent alveoli will change, which may result in distortion, overdistention, or collapse. When positive pressure is applied to a surfactant-deficient lung, the more normal alveoli tend to overexpand and the less normal (i.e., less surfactant) alveoli collapse, generating a nonhomogeneously inflated lung (Fig. 44-14).[41] Surfactant treatment can normalize alveolar size.

Pressure-Volume Curves

The effects of surfactant on the preterm surfactant-deficient lung are demonstrated by pressure-volume relationships during quasi-static inflation and deflation.[42] Preterm surfactant-deficient rabbit lungs do not begin to inflate until pressures exceed 25 cm H_2O (Fig. 44-15). The pressure needed to open a lung unit is related to the radius of curvature and surface tension of the meniscus of fluid in the airspace leading to the lung unit. In the collapsed lung, there are many different collapsed units with different radii. The units with larger radii and lower surface tensions "pop" open first because, with partial expansion, the radius increases and the forces needed to finish opening the unit decrease. The movement of fluid with high surface tensions in the airways causes very high sheer forces that can disrupt the airway epithelium.[27] With surfactant treatment, the fluid menisci in the airways have lower surface tensions that decrease the opening pressure from about 25 to 15 cm H_2O in this example with preterm rabbit lungs. The subsequent inflation is more uniform as

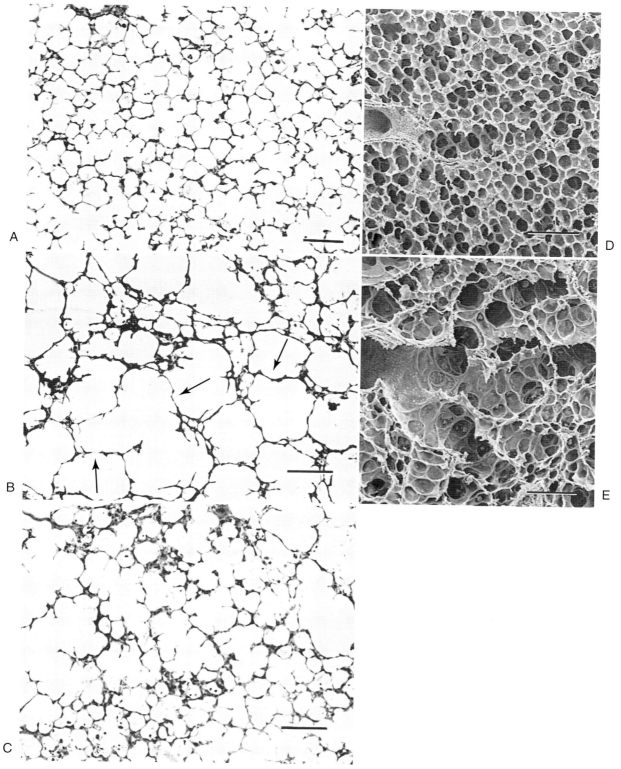

Figure 44–14. Ventilation of the preterm lamb lungs for 24 hours results in nonuniform alveolar inflation and dilation of alveolar ducts. Light microscopy in frames on left demonstrates uniform alveolar sizes in fetal lungs that have not been ventilated (**A**), dilated ducts and shallow alveoli (*arrows*) after 24 hours of ventilation (**B**), and a more normal-appearing lung following surfactant treatment at birth and ventilation for 24 hours (**C**). Scanning electron microscopy in the frames on the right taken at the same magnification demonstrates alveoli of uniform size in the unventilated lung (**D**) and dilated alveolar ducts with flattening of some alveoli and compression of others creating microatelectasis (**E**). Bar is 160 m. (*Modified from Pinkerton KE, et al: Lung parenchyma and type II cell morphometrics: effect of surfactant treatment on preterm ventilated lamb lungs, J Appl Physiol 77:1953, 1994, with permission.*)

Figure 44–15. Pressure-volume relationships for the inflation and deflation of surfactant-deficient and surfactant-treated preterm rabbit lungs. The control lungs are from 27-day preterm rabbits. Surfactant deficiency is indicated by the high opening pressure, the low maximal volume at a distending pressure of 35 cm H_2O, and the lack of deflation stability at low pressures on deflation. In contrast, treatment of 27-day preterm rabbits with a natural surfactant alters the pressure-volume relationships. (*From Creasy RK, et al, editors:* Creasy & Resnik's maternal-fetal medicine, *6th ed, Philadelphia, 2009, Elsevier, p 201.*)

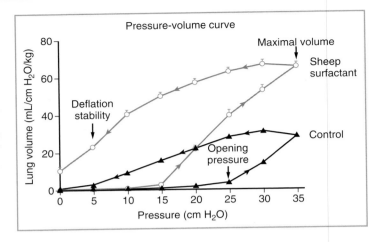

more units open at lower pressures, resulting in less epithelial injury and overdistention of the open units.

A particularly important effect of surfactant on the surfactant-deficient lung is the increase in maximal volume at maximal pressure. In the example in Figure 44-15, maximal volume at 35 cm H_2O is increased about 2.5-fold by surfactant treatment to a volume that is similar to that achieved in a term newborn rabbit lung. Pressures greater than 35 cm H_2O in control lungs result in lung rupture with little further volume accumulation. The opening pressures of many distal lung units in the surfactant-deficient lung exceed 35 cm H_2O and exceed the rupture pressure of the preterm lung. This volume difference resulting from surfactant treatment is lung volume that improves gas exchange because it is primarily parenchymal gas volume. Lung volume recruitment can be achieved rapidly with surfactant treatment. Another important effect of surfactant is the stabilization of the lung on deflation. The surfactant-deficient lung collapses at low transpulmonary pressures, whereas the surfactant-treated lung retains about 40% of the lung volume on deflation to 5 cm H_2O. This retained volume is equivalent to the total volume of the surfactant-deficient lung at 30 cm H_2O and demonstrates how surfactant treatments increase the functional residual capacity of the lung.

Dynamic lung mechanics also are altered by surfactant treatments. Time constants for deflation increase, resulting in less effective lung emptying. The clinical correlate is that a surfactant treatment may increase the FRC of infants with RDS by two mechanisms: the improved deflation stability and the longer expiratory time constant. The consistent initial response of infants with RDS to surfactant treatments is a rapid improvement in oxygenation, whereas improvements in PCO_2, compliance, and therefore ventilatory support variables tend to change more gradually. The explanation for improved oxygenation without changes in ventilation results from the acute increase in lung volumes following surfactant treatments.

LUNG MATURATION AND LUNG MATURITY TESTING
Surfactant Appearance with Development

Lamellar bodies first appear within type II cells by 20 to 24 weeks' gestation in the human fetus, and the amount of saturated phosphatidylcholine increases in lung tissue to term. This early presence of surfactant within human fetal lung tissue is consistent with the clinical experience that some infants born as early as 24 weeks' gestation have little lung disease. Lung maturity in the human fetus is generally present after 35 weeks' normal gestation. Therefore, an 11-week window of "early maturation" is possible for the human, at least in part because the surfactant synthetic and storage machinery is present and inducible in the human early in gestation.

The tests for fetal lung maturation depend on amniotic fluid composition reflecting the status of surfactant in the fetal lung. The lung secretes fetal lung fluid and any surfactant released into that lung fluid throughout late gestation. The flow of fluid out of the lung is episodic, and the balance between swallowing or loss of fetal lung fluid to the amniotic cavity is controlled by the larynx. The amniotic fluid can be characterized as the fetal cesspool, containing all fetal excretions as well as desquamated cells and other biologic matter. In normal pregnancies any test of gestational age or general fetal maturation, independent of which organ is targeted, correlates well with the degree of fetal lung maturity because maturational events are normally linked closely with gestational age. A remarkable aspect of the human fetus is the extraordinary inducibility of lung maturation at gestational ages as early as 24 weeks. Tests of lung maturation have been developed to identify fetuses with early lung maturation.

The L-S ratio introduced by Gluck and associates in 1971 remains the standard against which other tests are compared.[16] It depends on the flow of fetal lung fluid into the amniotic fluid being sufficient to change amniotic fluid phospholipid composition in a timely manner relative to the fetal lung maturation. The results are expressed as the ratio of a lecithin (phosphatidylcholine) fraction (cold acetone precipitated to enrich for saturated phosphatidylcholine) to sphingomyelin. Sphingomyelin is a membrane lipid and is a nonspecific component of amniotic fluid not related to lung maturation. The sphingomyelin content per milliliter of amniotic fluid tends to fall from about 32 weeks' gestational age to term, whereas the lecithin content, a large part of which is from the fetal lung, increases. The use of the lecithin measurement standardized against an internal control, sphingomyelin, will correct for changes in amniotic fluid volume. A value of 2 is achieved by 35 weeks' gestation in the normal fetus. Empirically, RDS is unlikely if the L-S ratio is 2 or greater.[16] Values of 1.5 to 2 are "immature"; however, the risk of RDS is low. The incidence of RDS is high for ratios less than 1.

Surfactant from the mature lung contains other lipids and the SPs, each of which has a unique developmental profile as surfactant composition changes with development.[18] Phosphatidylglycerol normally appears in amniotic fluid at the time of lung maturity at about 35 weeks' gestation. Phosphatidylglycerol is absent from the amniotic fluid or tracheal aspirates of infants with RDS, and it appears in the lungs as the disease resolves. Phosphatidylglycerol can be detected before 30 weeks' gestation in infants with early lung maturation. Phosphatidylglycerol is present in appreciable amounts only in lung tissue and surfactant. Therefore phosphatidylglycerol can be measured in amniotic fluid contaminated with blood or meconium. Numerous other tests for lung maturity have been developed. The TDx-FLM assay of the ratio of amniotic fluid surfactant to albumin seems to be equivalent to the L-S ratio for the prediction of RDS.[5] Clinical tests are less frequently used in clinical practice than in the past because virtually all women at risk of preterm delivery are treated with antenatal corticosteroids and the clinical decision to deliver a preterm seldom includes considerations of fetal lung maturation.

Although surfactant deficiency is the hallmark of RDS, other aspects of lung immaturity cause lung disease and morbidity. Lung structural immaturity may be clinically significant if the alveolar surface area has not developed sufficiently to sustain life or if airway immaturity results in pulmonary interstitial emphysema (PIE) and other severe air leak syndromes. The preterm lung is susceptible to oxidant damage and BPD if protective mechanisms have not developed. The surfactant deficiency component of lung immaturity can be corrected by surfactant treatment. Therefore the presence of surfactant may be a less critical factor in the clinical decision about whether to deliver preterm infants than in the past.

All tests of lung maturation are based on the premise that amniotic fluid accurately reflects the degree of differentiation of the type II cell population in the fetal lung. When the complexities of the pathway from surfactant synthesis in the fetal lung to its arrival in the amniotic fluid are considered, together with the multiple known effectors of the pathway, it is surprising that these tests are predictive in the evaluation of complicated pregnancies (Fig. 44-16). Amniotic fluid phospholipids are far downstream both in distance and time from the type II cell. As a generalization, developing animals require several days to process surfactant phospholipids from synthesis to secretion. Surfactant secretion and the flow of fetal lung fluid are influenced by preterm labor and delivery. The occurrence of preterm labor implies stress and elevated fetal catecholamine, cortisol, and prostaglandin levels. Epinephrine and selected prostaglandins cause surfactant secretion and decrease the flow of fetal lung fluid. Although the increased secretion should ultimately increase the L-S ratio, the secreted surfactant might not reach the amniotic fluid if fetal lung fluid ceased to flow. Changes in fetal breathing movements and fetal swallowing patterns also disrupt the normal egress of fetal lung fluid into the amniotic fluid. Finally, little is known about the turnover of surfactant phospholipids

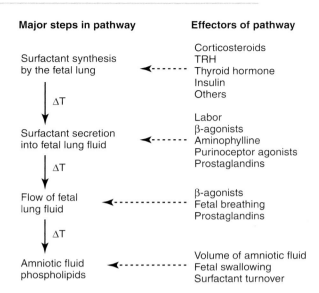

Figure 44–16. Pathway of surfactant from the fetal lung to amniotic fluid. The time relationships between surfactant synthesis and secretion and the amniotic fluid are not known even for the normal fetus. The figure indicates some of the factors that can modulate the events. (*From Jobe A: Evaluation of fetal lung maturity. In Creasy RK, et al, editors:* Maternal-fetal medicine: principles and practice, *Philadelphia, 1994, WB Saunders, p 423, with permission.*)

in amniotic fluid. Given the physiology and the complications introduced by pregnancy abnormalities and preterm labor, it is surprising that lung maturity tests usually are consistent with newborn outcomes.

Induced Lung Maturation

Numerous clinical trials have documented that maternal corticosteroid treatments decrease the incidence of RDS by about 50%, and those infants with RDS tend to have less severe disease.[43] The decreased incidence of RDS needs to be interpreted within the context of maturational phenomena that occur spontaneously in the preterm. Most infants destined to deliver at term do not have mature lungs until about 36 weeks' gestational age. However, only about 50% of infants born at 30 weeks' gestational age have RDS. Although the incidence of RDS increases as gestational age decreases, some infants at 24 to 25 weeks' gestational age have functional lung maturity. This spontaneous early lung maturation in the human fetus is believed to result from stress-induced maturation events that can be maternal, placental, or fetal in origin. Although specific abnormalities related to prematurity have been associated with early maturation, recent epidemiologic data do not support induced lung maturation with fetal growth restriction, preeclampsia, or prolonged preterm rupture of membranes. The changing epidemiology probably results from the more frequent use of antenatal glucocorticoids and a change in obstetric practices to delay preterm delivery as long as possible. Chronic infection and fetal exposure to inflammation is frequent in those pregnancies with preterm labor between 22 and 30 weeks' gestation.[17] Histologic chorioamnionitis was associated with a decreased incidence of RDS, and in experimental models, bacterial endotoxin or the proinflammatory cytokine interleukin-1 (IL-1) induces lung maturation when given by intra-amniotic injection.[31] Fetal proinflammatory exposures induce striking increases in surfactant and improvements in postnatal lung function after preterm delivery of lambs without increasing fetal cortisol levels. Therefore fetal exposure to inflammation may have the short-term benefit of decreasing RDS, but longer term effects such as increased incidences of BPD and periventricular leukomalacia are concerning. Prematurity cannot be considered a normal condition. It is useful to think of the infant with RDS as the normal unstressed preterm, whereas the preterm without RDS has experienced a stress sufficient to induce lung maturation.

The events resulting in spontaneous early lung maturation in the human have not been well characterized. Explants of human lung at 14 to 20 weeks' gestational age differentiate in organ culture in the absence of hormonal stimuli, and agents such as corticosteroids and thyroid hormones accelerate maturation.[36] Several agents, such as insulin and transforming growth factor-β, tend to block lung maturation, and androgens delay maturation. Because about half of corticosteroid-treated fetuses do not seem to respond, it is reasonable to propose that fetal lung maturation normally is suppressed in favor of growth. If this suppression is released by stress-related signals, then the lung is susceptible to either endogenously mediated maturational signals or to exogenous effectors. Corticosteroids are one of the categories of agents that can influence lung maturation; however, many other agents also can influence lung maturation. The inducing agents can act additively or synergistically in terms of both the timing and the magnitude of the response in experimental models.

The responses of the fetal lung to corticosteroids are multiple and impact many different systems that could influence the clinical outcome. The particular response depends on species, corticosteroid dose, and gestational age.[25] In general, corticosteroids induce lung structural maturation by increasing the surface area for gas exchange as is reflected by lung volume measurements. Type II cell maturation has been noted primarily in vitro. Biochemical markers of maturation include glycogen loss from type II cells, increased fatty acid synthesis, increased β-receptors, and increased choline incorporation into surfactant phosphatidylcholine. In vivo, animals demonstrate improved lung function and survival. Corticosteroid treatment also decreases the tendency of the preterm lung to develop pulmonary edema. Although the primary effect of corticosteroids on the fetal lung is generally considered to be induction of surfactant synthesis, effects on enzymes in the synthetic pathway have not been consistently demonstrated, and surfactant pool sizes do not increase until more than 4 days after maternal glucocorticoid treatments in sheep.[25] Lung function can improve following corticosteroid treatments even if surfactant is not increased because of changes in lung structure. In preterm animal models, corticosteroid treatment changes the dose-response curve such that less surfactant is needed to cause larger clinical responses.

Because of increased lung volume, corticosteroid-treated fetuses also have improved responses to postnatal surfactant. There are additive or synergistic effects between the corticosteroid-exposed lungs and surfactant treatments.

Antenatal corticosteroid treatment is now the standard of practice for pregnancies at risk of preterm delivery.[43] This therapy is effective and safe, although there is not long-term follow-up data for infants born before 28 weeks' gestation. Repetitive courses of antenatal glucocorticoids have been given at 7- to 10-day intervals, a practice based on the suggestion that the fetal benefit was lost after this interval.[25] Maternal glucocorticoid treatments at 7-day intervals in sheep cause fetal growth restriction but augment lung maturation. Randomized trials in women at risk for preterm delivery demonstrate modest benefit, but there is some concern about longer-term outcomes, especially for infants exposed to four or more antenatal doses of antenatal corticosteroids.[14] There is presently insufficient information for a strong recommendation about the use of repeated corticosteroid treatments.

The only other lung maturation strategy that has been extensively evaluated clinically is the combination of corticosteroids and thyrotropin-releasing hormone (TRH). Thyroid axis hormones induce lung maturation and can act synergistically with corticosteroids in vitro. Thyroid hormones do not cross the human placenta efficiently, but the tripeptide TRH crosses to the fetal circulation and increases fetal thyroid hormone levels. Unfortunately, when evaluated in large randomized, controlled trials, TRH demonstrated no benefit and possible risks were identified.[1] Therefore, the use of TRH to supplement antenatal corticosteroid therapy is not recommended.

As noted earlier, fetal exposure to chorioamnionitis also can induce lung maturation. In experimental models, intra-amniotic endotoxin, or IL-1 will induce more striking lung maturation than will maternal corticosteroid treatments (Fig. 44-17).[3,29] The inflammatory mediators trigger lung maturation by direct contact with the fetal lung and induce a modest lung inflammation/injury response that resolves with large improvements in lung mechanics and increased surfactant lipid and protein pool sizes. Of clinical relevance, the maturational effects of maternal corticosteroids and chorioamnionitis seem to be additive for induced lung maturation.[37] The corticosteroids can suppress inflammation initially, but the inflammatory response is amplified in the fetal sheep at later times, perhaps because corticosteroids mature fetal innate immune responses. In clinical practice, ruptured membranes, a surrogate for chorioamnionitis, are not a contraindication to maternal corticosteroid treatment.[20]

This chapter focuses on the lung. However, maturation of other organs occurs in parallel in most fetuses. Other organs also are sensitive to corticosteroids and other agents. Maternal corticosteroid treatments not only decrease the incidence and severity of RDS but also decrease the incidence of patent ductus arteriosus, intraventricular hemorrhage, and necrotizing enterocolitis and increase kidney tubular function and postnatal blood pressure. Therefore, strategies to optimize maturation of the fetus at risk for preterm delivery target not only the lung but also other organs.

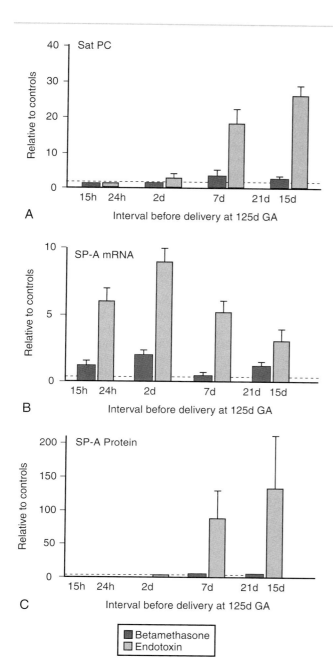

Figure 44–17. Intra-amniotic endotoxin increases the amount of saturated phosphatidylcholine (Sat PC) and SP-A more than maternal betamethasone in preterm fetal sheep. **A,** Although maternal betamethasone increased alveolar Sat PC 7 days and 21 days after treatment, the responses were less than for the fetal response to intra-amniotic endotoxin. **B,** SP-A mRNA increased more and stayed elevated following intra-amniotic endotoxin than in response to maternal betamethasone. **C,** Endotoxin exposure caused large increases in SP-A protein in the alveolar lavage. *(Data redrawn from Ballard PL, et al: Glucocorticoid regulation of surfactant components in immature lambs,* Am J Physiol *273:L1048, 1997; Zeltner TB, Burri PH: The postnatal development and growth of the human lung. II. Morphology,* Respir Physiol *67:269, 1987; and Tan RC, et al: Developmental and glucocorticoid regulation of surfactant protein mRNAs in preterm lambs,* Am J Physiol *277:L1142, 1999.)*

REFERENCES

1. ACTOBAT: Australian collaborative trial of antenatal thyrotropin-releasing hormone (ACTOBAT) for prevention of neonatal respiratory disease, *Lancet* 345:877, 1995.
2. Avery ME, Mead J: Surface properties in relation to atelectasis and hyaline membrane disease, *Am J Dis Child* 97:517, 1959.
3. Ballard PL, Ning Y, Polk D, et al: Glucocorticoid regulation of surfactant components in immature lambs, *Am J Physiol* 273:L1048, 1997.
4. Baraldi E, Filippone M: Chronic lung disease after premature birth, *N Engl J Med* 357:1946, 2007.
5. Bender TM, Stone LR, Amenta JS: Diagnostic power of lecithin/sphingomyelin ratio and fluorescence polarization assays for respiratory distress syndrome compared by relative operating characteristic curves, *Clin Chem* 40:541, 1994.
6. Bland RD, Ertsey R, Mokres LM, et al: Mechanical ventilation uncouples synthesis and assembly of elastin and increases apoptosis in lungs of newborn mice. Prelude to defective alveolar septation during lung development? *Am J Physiol Lung Cell Mol Physiol* 294:L3, 2008.
7. Bullard JE, Wert SE, Nogee LM: ABCA3 deficiency: neonatal respiratory failure and interstitial lung disease, *Semin Perinatol* 30:327, 2006.
8. Bunt JE, Carnielli VP, Darcos Wattimena JL, et al: The effect in premature infants of prenatal corticosteroids on endogenous surfactant synthesis as measured with stable isotopes, *Am J Respir Crit Care Med* 162:844, 2000.
9. Bunt JE, Carnielli VP, Seidner SR, et al: Metabolism of endogenous surfactant in premature baboons and effect of prenatal corticosteroids, *Am J Respir Crit Care Med* 160:1481, 1999.
10. Burri PH: Structural aspects of prenatal and postnatal development and growth of the lung. In McDonald JA, editor: *Lung growth and development*, New York, 1997, Marcel Dekker.
11. Coalson JJ, Winter VT, Siler-Khodr T, et al: Neonatal chronic lung disease in extremely immature baboons, *Am J Respir Crit Care Med* 160:1333, 1999.
12. Cogo PE, Carnielli VP, Bunt JE, et al: Endogenous surfactant metabolism in critically ill infants measured with stable isotope labeled fatty acids, *Pediatr Res* 45:242, 1999.
13. Crapo JD, Barry BE, Gehr P, et al: Cell number and cell characteristics of the normal human lung, *Am Rev Respir Dis* 126:332, 1982.
14. Crowther CA, Doyle LW, Haslam RR, et al: Outcomes at 2 years of age after repeat doses of antenatal corticosteroids, *N Engl J Med* 357:1179, 2007.
15. Enhorning G, Duffy LC, Welliver RC: Pulmonary surfactant maintains patency of conducting airways in the rat, *Am J Respir Crit Care Med* 151:554, 1995.
16. Gluck L, Kulovich MV, Borer RC Jr, et al: The interpretation and significance of the lecithin-sphingomyelin ratio in amniotic fluid, *Am J Obstet Gynecol* 120:142, 1974.
17. Goldenberg RL, Hauth JC, Andrews WW: Intrauterine infection and preterm delivery, *N Engl J Med* 342:1500, 2000.
18. Hallman M, Kulovich M, Kirkpatrick E, et al: Phosphatidylinositol and phosphatidylglycerol in amniotic fluid: indices of lung maturity, *Am J Obstet Gynecol* 125:613, 1976.
19. Hallman M, Merritt TA, Akino T, et al: Surfactant protein-A, phosphatidylcholine, and surfactant inhibitors in epithelial lining fluid—correlation with surface activity, severity of

respiratory distress syndrome, and outcome in small premature infants, *Am Rev Respir Dis* 144:1376, 1991.

20. Harding JE, Pang J, Knight DB, et al: Do antenatal corticosteroids help in the setting of preterm rupture of membranes? *Am J Obstet Gynecol* 184:131, 2001.

21. Hislop AA, Wigglesworth JS, Desai R: Alveolar development in the human fetus and infant, *Early Hum Dev* 13:1, 1986.

22. Hummler E, Barker P, Gatzy J, et al: Early death due to defective neonatal lung liquid clearance in alpha- ENaC-deficient mice, *Nat Genet* 12:325, 1996.

23. Jackson JC, Palmer S, Truog WE, et al: Surfactant quantity and composition during recovery from hyaline membrane disease, *Pediatr Res* 20:1243, 1986.

24. Jain L, Eaton DC: Physiology of fetal lung fluid clearance and the effect of labor, *Semin Perinatol* 30:34, 2006.

25. Jobe AH: Animal models of antenatal corticosteroids: clinical implications, *Clin Obstet Gynecol* 46:174, 2003.

26. Jobe AH: Why surfactant works for respiratory distress syndrome, *Neo Reviews* 7:e95, 2006.

27. Jobe AH, Hillman NH, Polglase G, et al: Injury and inflammation from resuscitation of the preterm infant, *Neonatology* 94:190, 2008.

28. Jobe AH, Ikegami M, Glatz T, et al: Saturated phosphatidylcholine secretion and the effect of natural surfactant on premature and term lambs ventilated for 2 days, *Experimental Lung Res* 4:259, 1983.

29. Jobe AH, Newnham JP, Willet KE, et al: Endotoxin induced lung maturation in preterm lambs is not mediated by cortisol, *Am J Respir Crit Care Med* 162:1656, 2000.

30. Khan PA, Cloutier M, Piedboeuf B: Tracheal occlusion: a review of obstructing fetal lungs to make them grow and mature, *Am J Med Genet C Semin Med Genet* 145C:125, 2007.

31. Kramer BW, Kallapur S, Newnham J, et al: Prenatal inflammation and lung development, *Semin Fetal Neonatal Med* 14:2, 2009.

32. Langston C, Kida D, Reed M, et al: Human lung growth in late gestation and in the neonate, *Am Rev Respir Dis* 129:607, 1984.

33. Liggins GC: Growth of the fetal lung, *J Dev Physiol* 6:237, 1984.

34. Liggins GC, Howie RN: A controlled trial of antepartum glucocorticoid treatment for prevention of RDS in premature infants, *Pediatrics* 50:515, 1972.

35. Lines A, Hooper SB, Harding R: Lung liquid production rates and volumes do not decrease before labor in healthy fetal sheep, *J Appl Physiol* 82:927, 1997.

36. Mendelson CR, Boggaram V: Hormonal and developmental regulation of pulmonary surfactant synthesis in fetal lung, *Baillieres Clin Endocrinol Metab* 4:351, 1990.

37. Newnham JP, Moss TJ, Padbury JF, et al: The interactive effects of endotoxin with prenatal glucocorticoids on short-term lung function in sheep, *Am J Obstet Gynecol* 185:190, 2001.

38. Nogee LM: Alterations in SP-B and SP-C expression in neonatal lung disease, *Annu Rev Physiol* 66:601, 2004.

39. O'Brodovich H, Yang P, Gandhi S, et al: Amiloride-insensitive Na+ and fluid absorption in the mammalian distal lung, *Am J Physiol Lung Cell Mol Physiol* 294:L401, 2008.

40. Ochs M, Nyengaard JR, Jung A, et al: The number of alveoli in the human lung, *Am J Respir Crit Care Med* 169:120, 2004.

41. Pinkerton KE, Lewis JF, Rider ED, et al: Lung parenchyma and type II cell morphometrics: effect of surfactant treatment on preterm ventilated lamb lungs, *J Appl Physiol* 77:1953, 1994.

42. Rider ED, Jobe AH, Ikegami M, et al: Different ventilation strategies alter surfactant responses in preterm rabbits, *J Appl Physiol* 73:2089, 1992.

43. Roberts D, Dalziel S: Antenatal corticosteroids for accelerating fetal lung maturation for women at risk of preterm birth, *Cochrane Database Syst Rev* 3:CD004454, 2006.

44. Seidner SR, Jobe AH, Coalson JJ, et al: Abnormal surfactant metabolism and function in preterm ventilated baboons, *Am J Respir Crit Care Med* 158:1982, 1998.

45. Shannon JM, Hyatt BA: Epithelial-mesenchymal interactions in the developing lung, *Annu Rev Physiol* 66:625, 2004.

46. Torresin M, Zimmermann LJ, Cogo PE, et al: Exogenous surfactant kinetics in infant respiratory distress syndrome: a novel method with stable isotopes, *Am J Respir Crit Care Med* 161:1584, 2000.

47. Verlato G, Cogo PE, Balzani M, et al: Surfactant status in preterm neonates recovering from respiratory distress syndrome, *Pediatrics* 122:102, 2008.

48. Whitsett JA, Matsuzaki Y: Transcriptional regulation of perinatal lung maturation, *Pediatr Clin North Am* 53:873, 2006.

49. Whitsett JA, Weaver TE: Hydrophobic surfactant proteins in lung function and disease, *N Engl J Med* 347:2141, 2002.

50. Zeltner TB, Burri PH: The postnatal development and growth of the human lung. II. Morphology, *Respir Physiol* 67:269, 1987.

> ## PART 2
>
> # Assessment of Pulmonary Function
>
> *Waldemar A. Carlo and Juliann M. Di Fiore*

Most neonates requiring intensive care present with respiratory symptoms. Although standard techniques for assessing pulmonary function can be applied in a healthy infant, special limitations and problems are encountered in very small or sick neonates. Methods have been developed to evaluate pulmonary function in neonates with suspected abnormalities of the cardiopulmonary system. This section presents a practical and clinical approach to disordered cardiopulmonary function and attempts to help distinguish between heart and lung disease.

CLINICAL OBSERVATIONS

Five common physical signs relay indirect information regarding pulmonary function: respiratory rate, retractions, nasal flaring, grunting, and cyanosis.

Respiratory Rate

Precise monitoring of respiratory rate is invaluable as deviations from the normal respiratory patterns have been observed with mechanical pulmonary dysfunction, acid-base imbalances, and arterial blood gas abnormalities. During spontaneous breathing, infants can only achieve successful gas exchange within a limited range of respiratory rates. At low rates, decreased alveolar minute ventilation may occur, while at high rates and corresponding low tidal volumes (V_T), a large proportion of the minute ventilation is wasted in ventilating dead space.

Infants may also adjust the respiratory rate to minimize work of breathing. The total work of breathing consists of elastic and resistive components. The elastic component represents the work required to stretch the lungs and chest wall during a tidal inspiration, and the resistive component is the work required to overcome friction caused by lung tissue movement and gas flow through the airways. Healthy infants rely on approximate respiratory rates of 40 to 60 breaths per minute and tidal volumes of 6 to 7 mL/kg. Infants with stiff lungs, such as those with respiratory distress syndrome (RDS), attempt to compensate for the increased workload with rapid shallow breathing, while patients with increased resistance (e.g., subglottic stenosis) usually exhibit slower and deeper breathing (Fig. 44-18).

Retractions

The neonatal chest wall is extremely compliant, and substernal, subcostal, and intercostal retractions are readily observable even with a relatively minor derangement in lung mechanics. Retractions are caused by negative intrapleural pressure–generated contraction of the diaphragm and other respiratory muscles and the mechanical properties of the lungs and chest wall. In neonates with respiratory distress, retractions become more apparent as the lungs become stiffer.

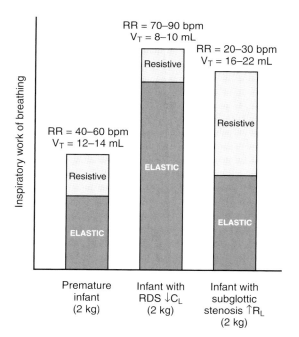

Figure 44–18. Relative contributions of the elastic and resistive components of the work of breathing in infants with normal pulmonary function, decreased lung compliance (C_L), and increased lung resistance (R_L). RDS, respiratory distress syndrome; RR, respiratory rate; V_T, tidal volume.

Apart from their characteristic appearance in RDS and other pulmonary diseases, severe retractions can signal complications of respiratory disease such as airway obstruction, misplacement of an endotracheal tube, pneumothorax, or atelectasis (see Part 4). Decreased retractions in the presence of adequate inspiratory effort suggest that lung compliance is improving.

Nasal Flaring

Nasal flaring is another sign of respiratory distress often observed in infants. The dilation of nostrils produced by contraction of the alae nasi muscles results in a marked reduction in nasal resistance. Because newborns are preferential nose breathers, and because nasal resistance contributes substantially to total lung resistance, nasal flaring markedly decreases the work of breathing. Nasal flaring is occasionally observed in the absence of other signs of respiratory distress, particularly during feeding and active sleep. Activation of other respiratory muscles, such as the genioglossus (tongue) and the laryngeal muscles, is also important for optimal function of the upper airways. The genioglossus muscle protrudes the tongue and, in part, maintains pharyngeal patency while the laryngeal muscles move the vocal cords and regulate airflow, particularly during expiration.

Grunting

With normal breathing, the vocal cords abduct to enhance inspiratory flow. In some respiratory disorders neonates attempt to close (adduct) their vocal cords during expiration. Expiration through partially closed vocal cords produces the grunting sound. During the initial phase of expiration, the infant closes the glottis, holds gas in the lungs, and produces an elevated transpulmonary pressure in the absence of airflow. During the last part of the expiratory phase, gas is expelled from the lungs against partially closed vocal cords, causing an audible grunt. During the expiratory phase, when the vocal cords are partially or completely closed, the ventilation-perfusion ratio ($\dot{V}/\dot{Q}$) is enhanced because of increased airway pressure and lung volume.

Grunting may be either intermittent or continuous, depending on the severity of lung disease. Grunting can maintain functional residual capacity (FRC) and partial pressure of arterial oxygen (Pao_2) equivalent to the application of 2 or 3 cm H_2O of continuous distending pressure. Because endotracheal intubation abolishes grunting, maintenance of lung volume with positive end-expiratory pressure (PEEP) is important following intubation.

Cyanosis

Central cyanosis, best observed by examining the tongue and oral mucosa, is an important indicator of impaired gas exchange. Clinical detection of cyanosis depends on the total amount of desaturated hemoglobin. Thus patients with anemia may have a low Pao_2 without clinically detectable cyanosis, and patients with polycythemia may be clinically cyanotic despite a normal Pao_2. Peripheral cyanosis may be normal in neonates but also occurs in situations of decreased cardiac output. The clinical features of cyanosis and their significance are discussed in detail in Chapter 45.

BLOOD GAS MEASUREMENTS

Maintaining optimal gas exchange is the primary function of the lung. Thus pulmonary evaluations should include blood gas estimates in addition to measurements of pulmonary mechanics. Both invasive and noninvasive blood gas measurements are available in the infant population. Blood gas measurements are the most widely used clinical method for assessing pulmonary function in neonates and form the basis for diagnosis and management of cardiorespiratory disease. Changes in partial pressure of alveolar oxygen (P_{AO_2}) and P_{ACO_2} can identify disordered pulmonary function in various clinical situations. P_{AO_2} and P_{ACO_2} values depend on the composition and volume of alveolar gas, the composition and volume of the mixed venous blood, and the mechanisms of pulmonary gas exchange impairment. Alveolar gas composition can be obtained from the equation

$$P_{AO_2} = P_{IO_2} - \frac{P_{ACO_2}}{R}\left[F_{IO_2} + \frac{1 - F_{IO_2}}{R}\right]$$

where P_{IO_2} is partial pressure of inspired oxygen (P_{IO_2} = $F_{IO_2} \times$ [barometric pressure − water vapor pressure]). At sea level, barometric pressure is 760 mm Hg; at 100% humidity, water vapor pressure is 47 mm Hg. P_{ACO_2} is the partial pressure of alveolar carbon dioxide, and R is the respiratory quotient (usually 0.8). The mechanisms of pulmonary gas exchange impairment include $\dot{V}/\dot{Q}$ mismatch, shunt, hypoventilation, and diffusion limitation. Appropriate matching of the alveolar gas with the mixed venous blood yields optimal gas exchange. Mixed venous blood composition and volumes are determined by the arterial blood gas content, cardiac output, oxygen consumption, and carbon dioxide production.

Techniques of blood gas determination in infants with RDS are discussed in Part 3. Gas exchange during assisted ventilation is discussed in Part 4. Acid-base physiology is discussed in Chapter 36.

Partial Pressure of Arterial Oxygen

Depending on the efficacy of gas exchange, the alveolar oxygen partial pressure (tension) tends to equilibrate with the mixed venous blood, resulting in the Pa_{O_2}, which determines the degree of oxygen saturation of hemoglobin. In addition to its chemical combination with hemoglobin, oxygen is also dissolved in plasma and red blood cells (RBCs). Most of the oxygen in whole blood is bound to hemoglobin (measured clinically as oxygen saturation), whereas the amount of dissolved oxygen is only a small fraction of the total quantity carried in whole blood.

The quantity of oxygen bound to hemoglobin depends on the Pa_{O_2} and the oxygen dissociation curve (Fig. 44-19). The blood is almost completely saturated at a Pa_{O_2} of 90 to 100 mm Hg. The flattening of the upper portion of the S-shaped dissociation curve makes it virtually impossible to estimate oxygen tension greater than 60 to 80 mm Hg by using arterial oxygen saturation alone. The dissociation curve of fetal hemoglobin (compared with adult hemoglobin) is shifted to the left, and at any Pa_{O_2} less than 100 mm Hg, fetal blood binds more oxygen. The shift appears to be the result of the lower affinity

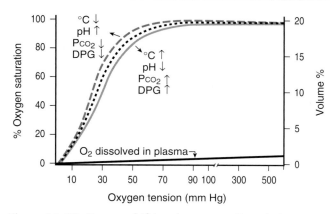

Figure 44–19. Factors shifting the oxygen dissociation curve of hemoglobin. (Fetal hemoglobin is shifted to the left.) (*From Martin RJ, et al: Respiratory problems. In Klaus M, et al, editors: Care of the high-risk neonate, Philadelphia, 1993, WB Saunders, p 228, with permission.*)

of fetal hemoglobin for 2,3-diphosphoglycerate. Note that pH, Pa_{CO_2}, temperature, and diphosphoglycerate content influence the position of the dissociation curve.

Arterial oxygen content (Ca_{O_2}) is the sum of hemoglobin-bound and dissolved oxygen, as described by the following equation:

$$Ca_{O_2} = (1.37 \times Hb \times Sa_{O_2}) + (0.003 \times Pa_{O_2})$$

where the arterial oxygen content is in mL/100 mL of blood, 1.37 is the approximate amount of oxygen (in milliliters) bound to 1g of hemoglobin at 100% saturation, Hb is hemoglobin concentration (g/100 mL), Sa_{O_2} is the percentage of hemoglobin bound to oxygen, and 0.003 is the solubility factor of oxygen in plasma (mL/mm Hg). In this equation, the first term ($1.37 \times Hb \times Sa_{O_2}$) is the amount of oxygen bound to hemoglobin. The second term ($0.003 \times Pa_{O_2}$) is the amount of oxygen dissolved in plasma and red blood cells.

Most of the oxygen in the blood is carried by hemoglobin. For example, if an infant has a Pa_{O_2} of 80 mm Hg, an Sa_{O_2} of 99%, and a hemoglobin concentration of 15 g/100 mL, Ca_{O_2} is the sum of oxygen bound to hemoglobin ([$1.37 \times 15 \times 99$]/100 = 20.3 mL) plus the oxygen dissolved in plasma (0.003×80 = 0.24 mL). In this example, just over 1% of oxygen in blood is dissolved in plasma and almost 99% is carried by hemoglobin.

The partial pressure of oxygen in arterial blood not only depends on the ability of the lungs to transfer oxygen as determined by alveolar ventilation but also is largely influenced by the $\dot{V}/\dot{Q}$. For normal gas exchange, the ventilation and perfusion should be proportional. The ratio should be very close to 1:1; that is, for every milliliter of gas that passes the alveoli, there should be a proportional volume of blood in the pulmonary capillary bed. If the $\dot{V}/\dot{Q}$ is decreased (as in RDS), only partial oxygenation and CO_2 removal from the mixed venous blood will occur. Oxygen supplementation can largely overcome the hypoxemia when the $\dot{V}/\dot{Q}$ is decreased. If the $\dot{V}/\dot{Q}$ is high, as in overventilation, partial pressure of oxygen is increased slightly.

The mechanism of shunt becomes evident when blood bypasses the alveoli, as occurs in congenital cyanotic heart disease, persistent fetal circulation, or atelectasis. Oxygen supplementation does not prevent the hypoxemia produced by such a shunt. Hypoventilation (e.g., due to apnea) is a common cause of hypoxemia. Diffusion limitation can affect oxygenation slightly, but this mechanism is not a common cause of severe hypoxemia in neonates. Hypoxemia due to either hypoventilation or diffusion limitation usually can be treated easily with oxygen supplementation.

Three indexes can be used to estimate the degree of oxygenation derangement (see also Part 8). The *arterial-alveolar oxygen tension ratio* (PaO_2/PAO_2 or a/AO_2 ratio) has no units, decreases with worsening oxygenation, and can be obtained from the equation

$$P(a/A)O_2 = \frac{PaO_2}{PiO_2 - \frac{PACO_2}{R}\left[FiO_2 + \left(\frac{1 - FiO_2}{R}\right)\right]}$$

where R is the respiratory quotient. Because $[FiO_2 + (1 - FiO_2)/R]$ approximates 1.0 and $PACO_2$ approximates $PaCO_2$, the equation can be simplified as follows:

$$P(a/A)O_2 \sim \frac{PaO_2}{PiO_2 - \frac{PaCO_2}{R}}$$

The *alveolar-arterial oxygen tension gradient* ($PAO_2 - PaO_2$ or $AaDO_2$) is expressed in millimeters of mercury, increases with worsening oxygenation, and can be obtained from the equation

$$P(A-a)O_2 = PiO_2 - PACO_2\left[FiO_2 + \left(\frac{1 - FiO_2}{R}\right)\right] - PaO_2$$

or

$$P(A-a)O_2 \cong PiO_2 - \frac{PACO_2}{R} - PaO_2$$

The *oxygenation ratio* is expressed in millimeters of mercury, decreases with worsening oxygenation, and can be obtained from the equation

$$\text{Oxygenation ratio} = \frac{PaO_2}{FiO_2}$$

The oxygenation ratio is less often used because it is subject to inaccurate assessment of the oxygenation derangement when $PaCO_2$ varies markedly.

Often it is necessary to correct the degree of oxygenation for the ventilatory support because oxygenation is strongly influenced by mean airway pressure ($\bar{P}aw$) during assisted ventilation. The oxygenation index (OI) is useful under these circumstances. The OI, which increases with worsening oxygenation or increasing $\bar{P}aw$, has units of centimeters of water per millimeters of mercury and can be obtained by the equation

$$OI = \frac{\bar{P}aw \times FiO_2}{PaO_2} \times 100$$

Partial Pressure of Arterial Carbon Dioxide

$PaCO_2$ is an important measure of pulmonary function in neonatal respiratory disease. Mechanisms responsible for impairment of pulmonary exchange of CO_2 include hypoventilation, $\dot{V}/\dot{Q}$ mismatch, and shunt. In addition, an increase in dead space, as occurs with alveolar overdistention or gas trapping, impairs CO_2 elimination. Because of the high solubility coefficient of CO_2, diffusion limitation rarely affects CO_2 exchange. As tissue levels of CO_2 increase above those of arterial blood, molecules diffuse into the capillaries and are transported in RBCs and plasma. Unlike the S-shaped dissociation curve for O_2, the relationship between CO_2 tension and content is almost linear over the physiologic range.

The initiation of ventilation with the first breath after normal delivery results in a rapid fall in $PaCO_2$ within minutes of birth. PaO_2 rises rapidly to levels of 60 to 90 mm Hg, although some degree of mismatching of $\dot{V}/\dot{Q}$ is evident in the first 1 to 2 hours of life. This is believed to be the result of intracardiac and pulmonary right-to-left shunting. More recent data in larger groups of infants have characterized the increase in oxygenation following birth by way of pulse oximetry, allowing for further differentiation between preductal and postductal levels (Fig. 44-20).[58] The speed with which pulmonary ventilation and perfusion are uniformly distributed is an indication of the neonate's remarkable capacity for maintaining homeostasis.

Noninvasive Blood Gas Measurements (See also Chapter 31)

CARBON DIOXIDE

Noninvasive estimates of CO_2 by end tidal or transcutaneous detectors provide a reasonable alternative to frequent blood gas sampling, allowing for continuous monitoring of CO_2

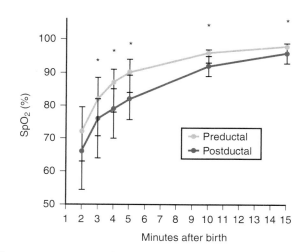

Figure 44–20. A rapid postnatal rise in oxygenation occurs during the normal fetal to neonatal transition. Preductal and postductal levels measured by way of pulse oximetry showed significantly lower postductal than preductal levels at 3, 4, 5, 10, and 15 minutes. *$P < .05$. (*Mariani, et al: Pre-ductal and post-ductal O_2 saturation in healthy term neonates after birth,* J Pediatr 150:418, 2007.)

over prolonged periods of time. End-tidal has been shown to correlate well with arterial blood gases in term and preterm infants without pulmonary disease and can be useful for detection of rapid changes in exhaled CO_2 because data are displayed on a breath-by-breath basis.[62] However, with small tidal volumes and high respiratory rates it may underestimate the true alveolar gas in neonates. Transcutaneous CO_2 detectors have been shown to be superior to end-tidal CO_2 in ill neonates.[62] Yet sensor preparation, taping, and the need for changes in sensor location may limit its usefulness. Despite the limitations of end-tidal and transcutaneous monitoring of CO_2, these methods provide critically important continuous information pertaining to changes in the respiratory system and minimize the need for blood gas analysis.

OXYGEN

Maintenance of oxygenation in an acceptable range requires constant monitoring that is not possible with intermittent blood gas measurements. This has led to the widespread implementation of pulse oximetry as a means of continuous noninvasive O_2 monitoring. See also part 3 Pulse oximetry measures the amount of hemoglobin molecules that are loaded with oxygen. It has a rapid response time and can be used as an estimate of PaO_2 for detecting short intermittent hypoxic episodes. However, as shown by the oxyhemoglobin dissociation curve (see Fig. 44-20), oxygen saturation levels should remain below 95% in infants requiring supplemental O_2 because hyperoxic values of PaO_2 cannot be distinguished beyond that range. With no current standards, ongoing multicenter trials are attempting to establish the optimal range for oxygenation in infants. Excessive levels of oxygen can result in retinopathy of prematurity, while low levels may increase vulnerability to intermittent hypoxic episodes. Recent data have shown a lower target range of oxygenation (85-89%), as compared with a higher range (91-95%), resulted in an increase in mortality and a substantial decrease in severe retinopathy.[81a] Completion of the multicenter trials should result in identification of these high and low alarm settings to minimize both hyperoxia and hypoxia in the preterm population. As results of these trials become published, implementation guidelines of the new standards will be needed; studies have shown varying levels of success in maintaining saturation values within a given range.[41,51] Studies combining pulse oximetry with automated adjustments in FiO_2 show promise in maintaining oxygen levels within the desired range, minimizing both hyperoxic and hypoxic events that are detrimental in this infant population.[17]

Hyperoxia-Hyperventilation Test

The hyperoxia test aids in differentiating between primary lung disease and congenital heart disease with right-to-left shunting. The test is performed by placing the infant in 100% oxygen for 5 to 10 minutes followed by monitoring oxygenation by arterial blood gas or noninvasive measures (see Part 3). In patients with primary lung disease, oxygen should diffuse into the poorly ventilated areas and improve oxygenation by 5 to 10 minutes of oxygen exposure. Persistent hypoxemia after this time period would suggest the presence of right-to-left shunting.

A modification of the hyperoxia test combining hyperoxia with hyperventilation can be used to distinguish between structural congenital heart disease and primary (or persistent)

pulmonary hypertension of the newborn (PPHN), both of which have right-to-left shunting. Inhalation of 100% oxygen improves oxygenation in some patients with PPHN. In response to hyperventilation with 100% oxygen ($PaCO_2$ 25 to 30 mm Hg), more infants with PPHN achieve PaO_2 levels higher than 100 mm Hg. In contrast, patients with anatomically fixed right-to-left shunting rarely generate a PaO_2 well above 40 to 50 mm Hg, even with inhalation of 100% oxygen and hyperventilation (see Chapter 45).

Evaluation of Shunting

Desaturated blood from the right side of the heart enters the main pulmonary artery and crosses the ductus to the descending aorta when right-to-left ductal shunting occurs. Because the ductus almost always enters the aorta after the origin of the right subclavian and carotid arteries, blood arriving at these two sites is well oxygenated, whereas blood samples from the aorta and usually the left subclavian artery are less oxygenated if there is a right-to-left ductal shunt. Thus preductal gases can be obtained from the right radial artery, whereas blood in the descending aorta, and usually the left radial artery, is of postductal origin. Alternatively, placement of two pulse oximeters (one on the right hand and the other on the left hand or either foot) accomplishes the same effect in differentiating preductal and postductal PaO_2 or oxygen saturation.

Patients with PPHN sometimes have right-to-left shunting through the foramen ovale and the ductus arteriosus. Ductal shunting can be demonstrated by the presence of a simultaneous oxygenation gradient between preductal and postductal arterial blood, whereas foramen ovale shunting affects both preductal and postductal oxygenation. Echocardiography can be used to confirm foramen ovale and ductal shunts.

PHYSIOLOGIC MEASUREMENTS

Tests of cardiopulmonary function performed on sick neonates can assist in diagnosis and treatment. Radiographic evaluation of the chest is an integral part of the diagnostic evaluation of respiratory disorders and is discussed in Chapter 37. Measurements of central venous and pulmonary artery pressures could indirectly give useful information regarding pulmonary function but are rarely available in the clinical neonatal setting. Knowledge of pulmonary mechanics may be useful in identifying disease entities and guide treatments, while plots of airflow, volume, and pressure may provide additional information on a breath-by-breath basis.

Airflow

Many devices are available for estimating airflow in infants. Noninvasive devices can be used for extended periods, yielding qualitative measurements of airflow that are sufficient for cardiorespiratory monitoring. These include devices to estimate chest wall expansion using impedance, strain gauges, or respiratory inductance plethysmography and devices to estimate airflow at the nose by application of a thermistor or end-tidal CO_2 detector. These devices can give approximations of tidal volume and information regarding the presence or absence of airflow and, used in conjunction, can distinguish central from obstructive apnea.

Precise quantitative measurements of airflow needed for analysis of pulmonary mechanics require an alternative group of devices placed at the nose such as a pneumotachometer or hot-wire anemometer. The pneumotachometer is the gold standard for quantitative measurement of airflow. To accurately measure flow, all air must pass through the pneumotachometer. In a ventilated patient, the pneumotachometer can be attached to an endotracheal tube with leaks minimized by repositioning the infant, using a cuffed tube, or applying gentle pressure to the neck. In a spontaneously breathing infant, the pneumotachometer must be incorporated into a nasal or oral mask that is tightly sealed around the patient's nose and mouth.[2] The hot-wire anemometer may also become an alternate choice in the measurement of pulmonary mechanics as improvements in hot-wire anemometer design continue in terms of accuracy and response time.[73] After reliable measures of flow are acquired, the flow signal is integrated to calculate volume.

Lung Volume

The total volume of gas in the lungs and airways can be measured and subdivided into various volumes (Fig. 44-21). The size of the lung compartments is related to the height, weight, and surface area of the subjects. FRC is the volume of gas in the lungs that is in direct communication with the airways at the end of expiration. The volume of gas in the FRC serves as an oxygen storage compartment in the body and a buffer so that large changes in alveolar gas tension are reduced. Helium dilution and nitrogen washout techniques have been adapted to measure FRC in infants.[33,34,75] The helium dilution technique uses the equilibration between a known volume and concentration of helium and the lung volume to be measured. After gas mixing and equilibration, FRC is calculated using the

initial and final concentration of the helium and the initial volume of helium. Similarly, FRC can be estimated by measuring the volume of nitrogen washout from the lungs when nitrogen-free gas is inhaled.

Thoracic gas volume is the total volume of gas in the thorax at the end of expiration and, in contrast to FRC, includes gas that is not in communication with the airways (e.g., gas in pulmonary interstitial emphysema [PIE]). Thoracic gas volume is calculated by measuring pressure and volume changes during respiratory efforts against an occluded airway while the infant is inside a body plethysmograph.[57,70] With an inspiratory effort, the gas in the lungs expands, the lung volume increases, and the pressure or volume in the box increases. Because the product of pressure and volume is constant, the pressure changes in the box can be used to determine the lung volume changes, which, when analyzed with the pressure changes in the airway, yield the thoracic gas volume.

Tidal volume, the volume of gas in and out of the lungs during a single breath, can be measured either with a pneumotachometer or a plethysmograph. *Vital capacity* (the total gas capacity of the lungs) cannot be measured in infants because of lack of cooperation, but crying vital capacity, the V_T during crying, can be obtained.

One of the principal functions of the first breaths is to transform the fluid-filled fetal lung from a gasless organ to one with an appropriate FRC (see Chapter 26). The ability of the lungs to maintain a volume of gas at end-expiration depends on two factors. One is the chest wall, which acts as a support for the lungs, and the other is surfactant, which stabilizes the expanded alveoli. These two factors are not well developed in the premature infant.

The mechanisms responsible for initiation of breathing probably include both environmental and physiologic stimuli.

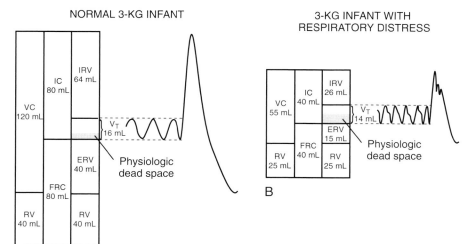

Figure 44–21. Partitioning of lung volumes and other measures of pulmonary function in a normal infant (**A**) and in an infant with respiratory distress syndrome (**B**).VC - Vital Capacity, RV - Residual Volume, IC - Inspiratory Capacity, FRC - Functional Residual Capacity, IRV - Inspiratory Reserve Volume, ERV - Expiratory Reserve Volume, VT - Tidal Volume. (*From Avery M, et al, editors:* The lung and its disorders in the newborn infant, *Philadelphia, WB Saunders, 1981, with permission.*)

36	Respiratory rate/minute	70
0.3	Dead space/tidal volume ratio	0.6
5	Intraesophageal pressure diff. (cm H_2O)	18
4.4	Compliance (mL/cm H_2O)	1.0
29	Resistance (cm H_2O/liter/sec)	23
40	Total work/breath (gm cm)	111
1440	Total work/minute (gm cm)	7770

After delivery the infant is exposed to cold and tactile environment. In addition, interactions occur between pH, P_{O_2}, and P_{CO_2}, whose contributions to inducing breathing in the human neonate have yet to be determined. Once initiated, the negative intrathoracic pressure of the first breath must overcome the effects of viscosity of fluid in the airway, surface tension, and tissue resistance. Radiographic studies of the lung indicate that inflation with air occurs immediately with the first breath. Transient retention of lung fluid might underlie transient tachypnea of the newborn (see Part 4). FRC is rapidly established, with little change throughout the first week of life.

Dead space, the portion of V_T not involved in gas exchange, varies with the incidence of areas of high $\dot{V}/\dot{Q}$. The dead space is divided into several compartments. *Anatomic dead space* is the airway volume not involved in gas exchange and is made up of the air passage from nares to terminal bronchioles. *Alveolar dead space* is the volume of gas in alveoli that are well ventilated but underperfused. Physiologic dead space is the sum of anatomic and alveolar dead space. In the normal newborn, physiologic dead space is 6 to 8 mL; smaller values are obtained in premature infants. The relationship of dead space to V_T is normally about 0.3. It is important to minimize the dead space added by apparatus for assisted ventilation or measurement of lung function to prevent rebreathing and inadvertent accumulation of carbon dioxide.

Pressures

Measurements of pressure that produce lung inflation are essential for pulmonary function testing. There are two ways to measure pressure, with the location of the measurement defining the system. Pressure can be determined by placing an esophageal balloon or catheter into the distal third of the esophagus. This measurement reflects pleural or alveolar pressure and is referred to as *transpulmonary pressure*. Transmission of pleural pressure can be compromised by chest wall distortion, which is common in preterm infants.[52] This problem can be resolved by catheter placement above the cardia but below the carina, which has been shown as a reliable measure of esophageal pressure transmission, independent of chest wall distortion.[18] The accuracy of this measurement should be verified by demonstrating the absence of a pressure gradient between the airway and esophageal pressure tracings during airway occlusion.

In the case of mechanically ventilated patients, pressure can be measured at the airway opening. This reflects pressure of the entire respiratory system. This is equivalent to pleural or alveolar pressure plus the pressure component due to the chest wall and is known as *transrespiratory pressure*. Because transrespiratory pressure and corresponding measurements of respiratory mechanics will be greater than those using transpulmonary pressure, it is important to clarify the type of pressure measurement when making comparisons between studies.

Respiratory Mechanics

There are many algorithms for calculating resistance and compliance that include the Mead-Whittenberger technique, linear regression, nonlinear regression, the linear portion of the flow curve, and the occlusion technique. The most commonly used algorithm in commercial devices for infants is the multiple linear regression technique also known as the *equation of motion* or *the Rhor equation*.

The *equation of motion* defines the relationship between pressure, flow, volume, and the elastic, resistive, and inertial components of the respiratory system. It is represented as

$$P = \frac{1}{C} \times V + R \times \dot{V} + I \times \ddot{V}$$

where P is the pressure that produces lung inflation, C is compliance, V is volume, R is resistance, $\dot{V}$ is flow, I is inertance, and $\ddot{V}$ is acceleration. As the inertial component is considered negligible for clinical considerations, the equation of motion is further simplified with the inertial component often dropped from the equation. This equation assumes a linear relationship which is not the case in the preterm infant. Yet, although not optimal, as nonlinear models have not lead to improvements in clinically applicable values for respiratory mechanics, the equation of motion continues to be the mode of choice in the clinical and research setting.

Although the equation of motion allows for the simultaneous calculation of compliance and resistance, these parameters can also be analyzed independently with known measurements of flow, volume, and pressure (transpulmonary or transrespiratory).[50,66]

Compliance

Compliance is a measure of elasticity or distensibility (e.g., of the lungs, chest wall, or respiratory system) and is defined as

$$\text{Compliance} = \frac{\Delta \text{Volume}}{\Delta \text{Pressure}}$$

Elastance is the reciprocal of compliance. In neonates, lung compliance is the most important component because the chest wall is very distensible. Lung compliance is low at the initiation of the first breath even in normal newborns. With the establishment of breathing and with gradual clearance of lung fluid during the first 3 to 6 hours after birth, FRC increases with concomitant improvement in lung compliance. Pathophysiologic factors that can increase the amount of fluid or impede the clearance of lung fluid could delay this improvement. The variability of compliance values in the first 2 hours after birth, in part the result of physiologic variation, could account for the frequent observations of higher respiratory rates in some infants during this period.

In distressed infants in whom lung compliance is markedly reduced, the compliant chest wall poses a disadvantage in that, as the infant attempts to increase negative intrathoracic pressure, the chest wall collapses (retracts). In addition, the more compliant neonatal airways could predispose the preterm infant to airway collapse during expiration and result in distal gas trapping.

Lung compliance is a measure of the intrinsic elasticity of pulmonary tissue and is measured either dynamically or statically depending on the absence or presence of relaxation of the respiratory muscles. Dynamic lung compliance can be measured during spontaneous breathing using devices to measure V_T and esophageal pressure as described earlier.

With this method, dynamic lung compliance is calculated by dividing the change in V_T by the corresponding change in esophageal pressure at points of no airflow (e.g., between end-inspiration and end-expiration). This is represented by the line drawn from point C to point A in Figure 44-22. End-inspiration and end-expiration are used as quasistatic points of reference for pressure equilibration. At high respiratory rates or increased levels of resistance, pressure does not equilibrate between these two points resulting in an underestimation of the true compliance under these circumstances.

Alternatively, static lung compliance can be calculated between points of no flow when the respiratory muscles are relaxed by employing occlusion of the airway. This allows for complete equilibration of pressure throughout the system. During the occlusion, static respiratory system compliance can be calculated by dividing the total exhaled volume by the pressure change during the occlusion minus the pressure at end-expiration (Fig. 44-23).[64] An important advantage of this technique is that it does not require an esophageal balloon to measure pressure.

Both dynamic and static compliance, using a single occlusion, assume that compliance is constant throughout the breath. This may not be the case during periods of lung disease or overdistention of the lung during mechanical ventilation. Under these conditions, dynamic compliance underestimates the true compliance. True changes in compliance throughout a breath can be determined by expanding the single occlusion technique to include multiple brief interruptions during the expiratory phase of a breath, also known as the *multiple-interruption technique* (Fig. 44-24).[15,28,76] Using this technique, a decrease in compliance can be seen with increasing pressure as the lung becomes overdistended. In mechanically ventilated infants, compliance measurements should be acquired at the same PEEP and peak inspiratory pressure (PIP) to obtain values at the same section of the pressure-volume curve.

Because lung elasticity depends on lung volume, changes in FRC can alter lung compliance. The degree of elasticity corrected for lung volume or patient size is called specific compliance.[35] Whereas specific lung compliance in the normal neonate (1 to 2 mL/cm H_2O per kilogram) is comparable

to that of the adult when corrected for unit body weight, compliance of the chest wall is relatively much higher in infants.

In addition to compliance, expiratory occlusion can also be used to determine the lung volume above the relaxation volume of the respiratory system (see Fig. 44-23). Expiratory volume clamping is a modification of the occlusion technique in which exhalation is prevented during several breaths at increasing lung volumes.[40] After plotting the corresponding volumes and pressures acquired during each occlusion, the slope of the function represents the compliance of the respiratory system. In addition, the intercept along the volume axis represents the resting volume of the respiratory system.

Resistance

Pulmonary resistance is a measure of the friction encountered by gas flowing through the nasopharynx, trachea, and bronchi and by tissue moving against tissue. The basic definition of resistance states

$$\text{Resistance} = \frac{\Delta \text{Pressure}}{\Delta \text{Flow}}$$

Conductance is the reciprocal of resistance. Resistance depends on the airway caliber, tissue properties, and flow rate. In the full-term infant pulmonary resistance is around 30 cm H_2O/L per second, approximately six times higher than that in the adult. Both airway resistance (the resistance caused by the airways) and viscous resistance (the resistance caused by tissues) contribute to total pulmonary resistance. Because of the high resistance in infants, respiratory apparatus with low added resistance should be used. An apparatus with a high resistance alters the same variables that are measured. A major site of airway resistance in the neonate is the upper airway, particularly the nares. The high resistance of the upper airway limits the ability to detect small changes in pulmonary resistance.

The pressure-volume and flow-volume loops generated from these waveforms can be used to calculate resistance. For

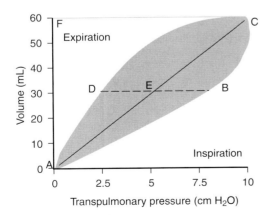
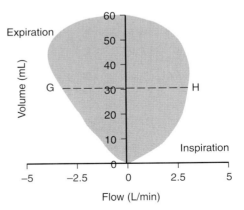

Figure 44–22. Dynamic lung compliance can be calculated as the Δ volume/Δ pressure as shown by the slope of line AC. Work of breathing is represented as the area inside the section drawn by ABCFA. Resistance can be calculated as the change in pressure, shown by the difference between points D and B, divided by the change in flow, shown by the difference between points G and H at the same mid-volume points.

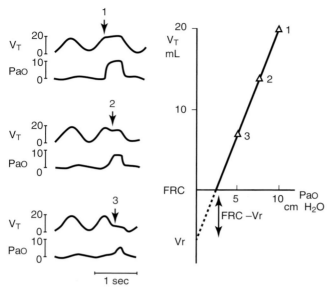

Figure 44–23. Schematic representation (from actual records) of the changes in lung volume (V_T in milliliters) and airway pressure (Pao in cm H_2O) during one spontaneous breath and occlusion of the airways during the expiratory phase of the following breath in a ventilated infant. In the three examples shown, occlusion is performed (from top to bottom) at end-inspiration, in the first third of expiration, and in the last third of expiration. After the occlusions (indicated by *arrows*), Pao gradually rises to a plateau, corresponding to the recoil value of the respiratory system at that lung volume. *Right,* Plot of the changes in lung volume above the end-expiratory level (FRC) against the corresponding changes in Pao as obtained in the left panel. The slope of the function represents the compliance of the respiratory system, the intercept on the Pao axis represents the internal recoil of the respiratory system at FRC, and the intercept of the V_T axis represents the resting volume of the respiratory system (Vr). *(From Mortola JP, et al: Measurements of respiratory mechanics in the newborn: a simple approach, Pediatr Pulmonol 3:123, 1987. Reprinted with permission of Wiley-Liss, Inc., a subsidiary of John Wiley & Sons, Inc.)*

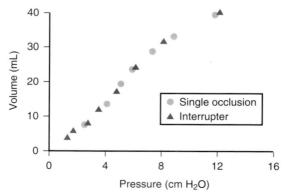

Figure 44–24. A typical example of the volume-pressure relationships obtained with both the interrupter and single occlusion techniques. Each point represents the compliance at that particular volume within the breath.

example, as shown in Fig. 44-22, the Mead-Whittenberger technique assesses resistance at midvolume by dividing the change in pressure between points D and B by the change in flow between points G and H. Resistance can be measured at additional volumes throughout the breath by using the occlusion or multiple-interruption technique as described earlier. In this case, resistance is calculated by dividing the pressure during the occlusion by the flow immediately preceding the occlusion (Fig. 44-25). These points of pressure and flow can be plotted to represent resistance over a range of volumes throughout the breath.[28] Furthermore, this technique can be used to partition the components of resistance into those due to airflow and those due to viscous tissue resistance.

At this point, three modes of calculating resistance have been discussed: the equation of motion, the Mead-Whittenberger technique, and the multiple-interrupter technique. The equation of motion uses linear regression to acquire the best fit corresponding to an average overall resistance for that breath. The Mead-Whittenberger technique gives the resistance for that same breath at only one point in time, midvolume (Fig. 44-26). The multiple-interrupter technique can be used to reveal changes in resistance within the breath by plotting the pressure and flow for each occlusion. These are important considerations when calculating resistance in that these techniques may result in different values of resistance for the same breath.

To understand why multiple techniques may result in conflicting values of resistance for the same breath, knowledge of flow patterns is needed. During periods of low pressure, the corresponding flow regimen is laminar and the assumption that resistance is constant throughout the breath holds true (see Fig. 44-26). Under these conditions the deviation amongst techniques is minimized. As the pressure increases further, the flow regimen changes from laminar to turbulent. At this point, the corresponding increase in flow is diminished. Further increases in pressure will reach the point of flow limitation where no additional increase in flow occurs. This is a common occurrence in both spontaneously breathing infants with lung disease and mechanically ventilated infants. During a turbulent flow regimen, resistance is no longer constant throughout the breath and is dependent on the technique used. These discrepancies in resistance values, due to various techniques and flow regimens, have severely limited the application of resistance as a diagnostic tool in the clinical setting.

Time Constant

The *time constant* of the respiratory system is the duration (expressed in seconds) necessary for a step (e.g., pressure or volume) change to partially equilibrate throughout the lungs. A duration equivalent to one time constant allows for 63% of the equilibration of the change. Although one time constant is not a very useful parameter in the clinical environment, five time constants are equivalent to the amount of time needed for 99% equilibration of the system. This value can be useful in areas of patient care such as mechanical ventilation (see Part 4).

The time constant of the respiratory system can be obtained from the flow-volume plot acquired during a passive exhalation. With this plot, the slope during the expiratory

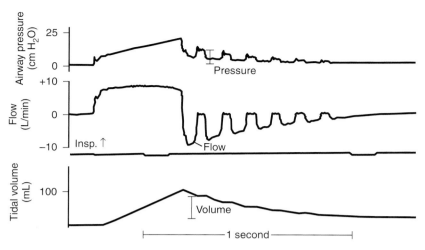

Figure 44–25. Illustration of data collected with the interrupter technique. The top channel is airway pressure proximal to the interrupter valve. The middle and bottom channels represent flow and volume, respectively. Compliance is calculated by dividing the volume above the end-expiratory level by the pressure during the occlusion. Resistance is calculated by dividing this pressure by the flow that preceded the interruption.

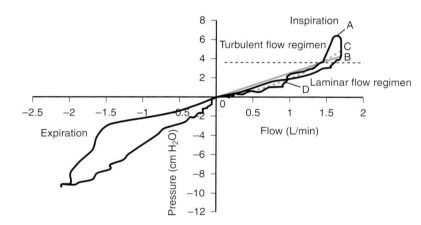

Figure 44–26. During a laminar flow regimen, resistance is constant throughout the breath and discrepancies between various techniques of measuring resistance are minimized. As the flow regimen changes from laminar to turbulent, resistance is no longer constant throughout the breath and becomes flow dependent. During this time, values of resistance between various techniques begin to diverge: Mead-Whittenberger (20 cm H_2O/L/sec; **A**), linear regression (152 cm H_2O/L/sec; **B**), nonlinear regression (32 cm H_2O/L/sec; **C**), and the linear portion of the curve (106 cm H_2O/L/sec; **D**). *(Reproduced with permission from Di Fiore JM, et al: Respiratory function in infants. In Haddad G, et al, editors:* Basic Mechanisms of Pediatric Respiratory Disease, *Toronto, 2002, BC Decker, p 165.)*

phase of the breath is equivalent to the time constant of the respiratory system (Fig. 44-27). Calculation of the time constant using the flow volume curve assumes that the slope is linear throughout expiration. Flow limitation—as may occur with bronchoconstriction during expiration, postinspiratory activity of the respiratory muscles, or laryngeal adduction—can be identified by convexity toward the volume axis.[82] In this case, calculations of a single time constant are no longer valid. Although a numerical value for time constant cannot be accurately determined under these conditions, X-Y plots of flow and volume can be used to characterize pulmonary function. Normal and abnormal flow-volume loops can be used to identify infants with airflow limitation patterns (Fig. 44-28).[11,20,39] The maximal expiratory flow volume relationship can be measured in infants without the needed patient cooperation by using technology that produces a forced expiration. A respiratory jacket or cuff placed around the chest and abdomen can be suddenly inflated at the end of lung inflation to produce rapid thoracoabdominal compression and forced expiratory flow.[81] Alternatively, sudden exposure of the inflated lung to a negative pressure at the airway opening can be used to produce a forced deflation.[65] During this maneuver, peak expiratory flow, maximal flow

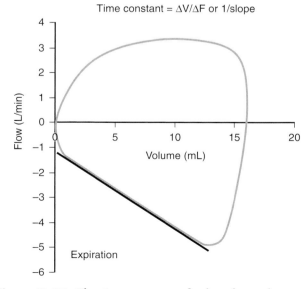

Figure 44–27. The time constant of a breath can be represented by the change in volume divided by the change in flow during the expiratory phase of the breath.

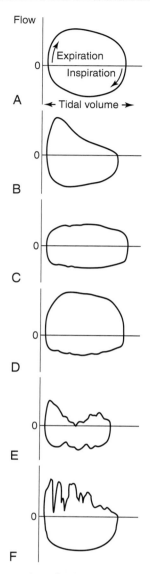

Figure 44–28. Examples of relationships between tidal flow and volume. Normal lemon-shaped loop (**A**); ski-slope loop observed with expiratory airflow limitation as seen in babies with bronchopulmonary dysplasia (BPD) (**B**); cigar-shaped loops observed in babies with extrathoracic airway obstruction with inspiratory and expiratory air flow limitation as seen in babies with subglottic stenosis or narrow endotracheal tubes (**C**); bun-shaped loop observed in babies with intrathoracic inspiratory airflow limitation as seen in babies with intraluminal obstruction (close to the carina) or an aberrant vessel compressing the trachea (**D**); crumpled loop as observed in babies with unstable airways or tracheomalacia (**E**); mountain-peaks loop is usually suggestive of an erratic airflow limitation as seen with airway secretions (**F**).

at FRC, and the patterns of flow-volume curves can be measured using a pneumotachograph. Flow-volume curves can be used to evaluate intrathoracic airway abnormalities and can detect flow limitation missed by the passive expiratory techniques.[81]

The time constant of the respiratory system can also be calculated without the use of the flow-volume curve using the relationship between the time constant, resistance, and compliance (see Part 4):

$$\text{Time Constant} = \text{Resistance} \times \text{Compliance}$$

Because both compliance and resistance are affected by different volumes and flows or by pulmonary disease, pulmonary mechanics change throughout the respiratory cycle and a single time constant may not always accurately represent lung mechanics.[71,79] However, for clinical purposes, linearity is assumed, and single values of compliance, resistance, and time constant usually suffice.[42]

Work of Breathing

The work of breathing is a measure of the energy expended in inflating the lungs and moving the chest wall. In general terms, work is the cumulative product of pressure and the volume of gas moved at each instant. In the normal infant, total pulmonary work has been determined to equal an average value of 1440 g/cm per minute. In an infant with respiratory distress, the total pulmonary work can increase as much as sixfold. This becomes most important when considered in terms of the oxygen cost of breathing. The neonate requires a higher caloric expenditure to breathe than does the adult, and the distressed infant requires an even higher caloric expenditure for this function. In the full-term infant, the work of breathing is minimal when the infant has a respiratory rate of 30 breaths per minute.

The pressure-volume and flow-volume loops generated from these waveforms can be used to calculate work of breathing as represented by the area inside the section drawn by ABCFA in Figure 44-22.

Limitations

Before any measurements of pulmonary function can be made, a clear understanding of equipment performance is needed. Although beyond the scope of this chapter, a clear adherence to these guidelines is imperative to ensure that lung function measurements can be performed with an acceptable degree of safety, precision, and reproducibility.[29] Once data are acquired, there are a multitude of algorithms for measuring pulmonary mechanics available. As no algorithm is ideal, standards are available addressing a range of issues from equipment criteria[29,30] to testing procedures.[9,63,77,79] A review of the techniques for measuring pulmonary mechanics and function has been published by the American Thoracic Society and the European Respiratory Society.[1]

Because various algorithms yield different results for the same breath, a wide range of published values for any given patient population has resulted, making it extremely difficult to define ranges for comparison between normal and diseased states. Compounding the issue is the large intrasubject variability of compliance and resistance.[38] In preterm infants, variability has been shown to range from 11% to 14% for compliance and 22% to 32% for resistance during spontaneous breathing with less variability (8% to 15% for compliance and 13% to 21% for resistance) during mechanical ventilation.

This is most likely due to muscle relaxation, and reduced fluctuations in respiratory rate and tidal volume compared with spontaneous respiration.

During mechanical ventilation, leaks around the endotracheal tube, a common occurrence in the neonatal intensive care unit setting, can result in overestimation of resistance and underestimation of elastance.[49] This error is minimized during the expiratory phase of the breath. A leak of less than 10% to 20% between the inspiratory and expiratory volume is generally considered acceptable to obtain reliable measurements of resistance and compliance.[49,54] Given these limitations, measurements of resistance and compliance during the expiratory phase of mechanical breaths with a leak of less than 10% should give the most precise and reproducible values.

Additional confounders that affect respiratory mechanics include sleep state,[69] posture,[10,16] endotracheal tube size,[56] FRC,[36] laryngeal braking,[36] gender,[80] race,[80] and respiratory patterns.[31] Errors in data calculation or interpretation can also occur if there are no compensatory modifications in mechanical ventilator settings in response to changes in lung function. For example, improvements in compliance at low pressures using the interrupter technique have been found in response to surfactant with no change in dynamic compliance.[14] This can occur due to overdistension of the lung as compliance improves in response to therapy if PIP is not decreased accordingly. As pressure-volume and flow-volume curves become more readily available on mechanical ventilators, they may become a useful tool, with or without measurements of respiratory mechanics, in distinguishing changes in pulmonary function. Figure 44-29 shows a simulation of a pressure-volume curve for a mechanically ventilated infant before and after surfactant administration with no change in peak inspiratory pressure. A numerical representation for dynamic compliance would show no change in compliance in response to surfactant administration. In contrast, visualization of the graph reveals improvement in compliance at low pressures but overdistension of the lung at high pressures as the peak inspiratory pressure was not decreased.

CLINICAL APPLICATIONS

Even with these limitations, information about pulmonary mechanics may be useful for diagnosis and management of acute or chronic pulmonary disorders.[32,59,78] The goal of clinical care in terms of respiratory support is to optimize oxygenation and CO_2 elimination with the lowest possible ventilator settings to minimize lung injury. The use of pulmonary function testing can be a valuable tool in achieving this goal and reducing the incidence of barotrauma.[72] Visualization of pressure-volume curves and measurements of compliance can be used to assist in identification of excessive PIP or PEEP leading to lung overdistension[21,26,68] and to distinguish between alveolar collapse and overdistension to assist in determining the most advantageous PEEP.[4,8] High compliance and low resistance have also been shown to be associated with the likelihood of extubation success in infants recovering from RDS.[7]

Pulmonary function measurements have been used to assess mechanical effects of pharmacologic interventions. To optimize the response, changes in resistance have been used to compare treatment modalities with the meter-dosed inhaler and ultrasonic nebulizer being shown as superior modes of bronchodilator administration.[27] Although surfactant results in rapid improvement of gas exchange, early beneficial effects on respiratory mechanics have been shown in some studies[22,47,67] with other results not evident until 24 hours after dosing.[12,19] There has been interest in the effect of nitric oxide (NO) on respiratory mechanics and the incidence of chronic lung disease.[6,48,74] Although beneficial effects of NO are dependent on dose, time of administration, and disease severity,[6] there is currently no evidence that NO leads to improvement in respiratory mechanics.[3,23] However, infants who received inhaled NO for PPHN had maximal expiratory flows comparable to those who were treated with extracorporeal membrane oxygenation (ECMO) but lower flows than control subjects.[45] Furthermore, inhaled NO to prevent BPD has resulted in decreased need for bronchodilator therapy at 1 year of age.[43] Both postnatal and antenatal steroid use enhance lung function.[5,60] Recent data have shown the relevance of timing of treatment, with a diminished response to antenatal steroids if delivery occurs more than 7 days after therapy.[61] Lastly, diuretic administration has been shown to enhance lung function.[25,46] Interestingly, improvements in resistance and compliance did not always correlate with better oxygenation.[25]

Respiratory mechanics have also been employed in longitudinal studies to evaluate the clinical course of pulmonary diseases. The occurrence of meconium aspiration syndrome during infancy has been associated with alveolar hyperinflation and airway hyperreactivity to exercise at 7 ± 2 years of age.[24] Measurements of pulmonary mechanics at 1 year follow-up showed no difference between survivors in

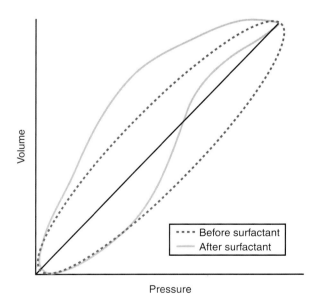

Figure 44–29. A representation of the change in compliance in response to surfactant administration. Note that dynamic compliance, as represented by the line, reflects no change. In contrast, visualization of the graph shows improvement in compliance at low volumes and overdistension of the lung, indicating the need to decrease peak inspiratory pressure.

trials of high-frequency ventilation versus conventional ventilation.[44,83] Hypoxemic respiratory failure has been linked with an increased risk for impaired pulmonary function, particularly in the presence of congenital diaphragmatic hernia or ECMO.[55] Decreases in FRC, compliance, and conductance have been shown to be predictive of BPD,[13,37,53] with gradual improvements in this cohort as the lungs grow.[35] Because BPD is a manifestation of prolonged oxygen exposure or barotrauma, pulmonary function measurements and graphical displays may be most helpful in this area to minimize ventilator settings and duration of ventilatory support.

Even with the current limitations in methodology and confounders in the area of pulmonary function, diagnostic evaluations can be a useful tool in neonatal patient care. Ideally clinical evaluation should include both numerical values for resistance and compliance in addition to visualization of flow-volume, pressure-volume, and pressure-flow curves. Application of these tools for pulmonary function measurements should complement clinical assessment in the care of infants with pulmonary disorders.

REFERENCES

1. American Thoracic Society and the European Respiratory Society: Respiratory mechanics in infants: physiologic evaluation in health and disease, *Am Rev Respir Dis* 147:474, 1993.

2. Anderson JV, et al: An improved nasal mask pneumotachograph for measuring ventilation in neonates, *J Appl Physiol* 53:1307, 1982.

3. Athavale K, et al: Acute effects of inhaled nitric oxide on pulmonary and cardiac function in preterm infants with evolving bronchopulmonary dysplasia, *J Perinatol* 24:769, 2004.

4. Aufricht C, et al: Quasi-static volume-pressure curve to predict the effects of positive end-expiratory pressure on lung mechanics and gas exchange in neonates ventilated for respiratory distress syndrome, *Am J Perinatol* 12:67, 1995.

5. Avery GB, et al: Controlled trial of dexamethasone in respirator-dependent infants with bronchopulmonary dysplasia, *Pediatrics* 75:106, 1985.

6. Ballard RA, et al: Inhaled nitric oxide in preterm infants undergoing mechanical ventilation, *N Engl J Med* 355:343, 2006.

7. Balsan MJ, et al: Measurements of pulmonary mechanics prior to the elective extubation of neonates, *Pediatr Pulmonol* 9:238, 1990.

8. Bartholomew KM, et al: To PEEP or not to PEEP? *Arch Dis Child* 70:F209, 1994.

9. Bates JHT, et al, on behalf of the ERS/ATS Task Force on Standards for Infant Respiratory Function Testing: Tidal breath analysis for infant pulmonary function testing, *Eur Respir* 16:1180, 2000.

10. Bhat RY, et al: Effect of posture on oxygenation, lung volume, and respiratory mechanics in premature infants studied before discharge, *Pediatrics* 112:29, 2003.

11. Bhutani VK, Sivieri EM: Clinical use of pulmonary mechanics and waveform graphics, *Clin Perinatol* 28:487, 2001.

12. Bhutani VK, et al: Pulmonary mechanics and energetics in preterm infants who had respiratory distress syndrome treated with synthetic surfactant, *J Pediatr* 120:S18, 1992.

13. Bhutani VK, et al: Relative likelihood of bronchopulmonary dysplasia based on pulmonary mechanics measured in preterm neonates during the first week of life, *J Pediatr* 120:605, 1992.

14. Bjorklund LJ, et al: Changes in lung volume and static expiratory pressure-volume diagram after surfactant rescue treatment of neonates with established respiratory distress syndrome, *Am J Respir Crit Care Med* 154:918, 1996.

15. Carlo WA: Validation of the interrupter technique in normal and surfactant deficient lungs. In Bhutani VK, et al, editors: *Neonatal Pulmonary Function Testing*, Ithaca, NY, 1988, Perinatology Press, p 35.

16. Carlo WA, et al: Neck and body position effects on pulmonary mechanics in infants, *Pediatrics* 84:670, 1989.

17. Claure N, et al: Close-loop controlled inspired oxygen concentration for mechanically ventilated very low birth weight infants with frequent episodes of hyperoxemia, *Pediatrics* 107:1120, 2001.

18. Coates AL, et al: An improved nasal mask pneumotachometer for measuring ventilation in neonates, *J Appl Physiol* 53:1307, 1982.

19. Couser RJ, et al: Effects of exogenous surfactant therapy on dynamic compliance during mechanical breathing in preterm infants with hyaline membrane disease, *J Pediatr* 116:119, 1990.

20. Cullen JA, et al: Pulmonary function testing in the critically ill neonate: Part II: Methodology, *Neonatal Netw* 13:7, 1994.

21. da Silva WJ, et al: Role of positive end-expiratory pressure changes on functional residual capacity in surfactant-treated preterm infants, *Pediatr Pulmonol* 18:89, 1994.

22. Davis JM, et al: Changes in pulmonary mechanics after the administration of surfactant to infants with respiratory distress syndrome, *N Engl J Med* 319:476, 1988.

23. Di Fiore, et al: The effect of inhaled nitric oxide on pulmonary function in preterm infants, *J Perinatol* 27:766, 2007.

24. Djemal N, et al: Pulmonary function in children after neonatal meconium aspiration syndrome, *Arch Pediatr* 15:105, 2008.

25. Englehardt B, et al: Short- and long-term effects of furosemide on lung function in infants with bronchopulmonary dysplasia, *J Pediatr* 109:1034, 1986.

26. Fisher JB, et al: Identifying lung overdistention during mechanical ventilation by using volume-pressure loops, *Pediatr Pulmonol* 5:10, 1988.

27. Fok TF, et al: Delivery of salbutamol to nonventilated preterm infants by metered-dose inhaler, jet nebulizer, and ultrasonic nebulizer, *Eur Respir J* 12:159, 1998.

28. Freezer NJ, et al: Effect of volume history on measurements of respiratory mechanics using the interrupter technique, *Pediatr Res* 33:261, 1993.

29. Frey U, et al, on behalf of the ERS/ATS Task Force on Standards for Infant Respiratory Function Testing: Specifications for equipment used for infant pulmonary function testing, *Eur Respir* 16:731, 2000.

30. Frey U, et al, on behalf of the ERS/ATS Task Force on Standards for Infant Respiratory Function Testing: Specifications for signal processing and data handling used for infant pulmonary function testing, *Eur Respir* 16:1016, 2000.

31. Galal MW, et al: Effects of rate and amplitude of breathing on respiratory system elastance and resistance during growth of healthy children, *Pediatr Pulmonol* 25:270, 1998.

32. Gappa M, et al: Lung function tests in neonates and infants with chronic lung disease, *Pediatr Pulmonol* 41:291, 2006.

33. Gaultier C: Lung volumes in neonates and infants, *Eur Respir J* 4:130S, 1989.

34. Gerhardt T, et al: Functional residual capacity in normal neonates and children up to 5 years of age determined by an N2 washout method, *Pediatr Res* 20:688, 1986.

35. Gerhardt T, et al: Serial determination of pulmonary function in infants with chronic lung disease, *J Pediatr* 110:448, 1987.

36. Gerhardt TO, et al: Measurement of pulmonary mechanics in the NICU: Limitations to its usefulness, *Neo Respir Dis* 5:1, 1995.

37. Goldman SL, et al: Early prediction of chronic lung disease by pulmonary function testing, *J Pediatr* 102:613, 1983.

38. Gonzalez A, et al: Intrasubject variability of repeated pulmonary function measurements in preterm ventilated infants, *Pediatr Pulmonol* 21:35, 1986.

39. Greenspan JS, et al: Pulmonary function testing in the critically ill neonate, Part I: An overview, *Neonatal Network* 13:9, 1994.

40. Grunstein MM, et al: Expiratory volume clamping: a new method to assess respiratory mechanics in sedated infants, *J Appl Physiol* 62:2107, 1987.

41. Hagadorn JI, et al: Achieved versus intended pulse oximeter saturation in infants born less than 28 weeks' gestation: the AVIOx study, *Pediatrics* 188(4):1574, 2006.

42. Haouzi P, et al: Respiratory mechanics in spontaneously breathing term and preterm neonates, *Biol Neonate* 60:350, 1991.

43. Hibbs AM, Walsh MC, Martin RJ, et al: One-year respiratory outcomes of preterm infants enrolled in the nitric oxide (to prevent) chronic lung disease trial, *J Pediatr* 153-525, 2008.

44. The HIFI Study Group: High frequency oscillatory ventilation compared with conventional mechanical ventilation in treatment of respiratory failure in preterm infants: assessment of pulmonary function at 9 months of corrected age, *J Pediatr* 116:933, 1990.

45. Hoskote AU, et al: Airway function in infants treated with inhaled nitric oxide for persistent pulmonary hypertension, *Pediatr Pulmonol* 43:224, 2008.

46. Kao LC, et al: Oral theophylline and diuretics improve pulmonary mechanics in infants with bronchopulmonary dysplasia, *J Pediatr* 111:439, 1987.

47. Kelly E, et al: Compliance of the respiratory system in newborn infants pre- and post-surfactant replacement therapy, *Pediatr Pulmonol* 15:225, 1993.

48. Kinsella JP, et al: Early inhaled nitric oxide therapy in premature newborns with respiratory failure, *N Engl J Med* 355:354, 2006.

49. Kondo T, et al: Respiratory mechanics during mechanical ventilation: a model study on the effects of leak around a tracheal tube, *Pediatr Pulmonol* 24:423, 1997.

50. Lanteri CJ, et al: Measurement of dynamic respiratory mechanics in neonatal and pediatric intensive care: the multiple linear regression technique, *Pediatr Pulmonol* 19:29, 1995.

51. Laptook AR, et al: Pulse oximetry in very low birth weight infants: can oxygen saturation be maintained in the desired range? *J Perinatol* 26:337, 2006.

52. LeSouef PN, et al: Influence of chest wall distortion on esophageal pressure, *J Appl Physiol* 55:353, 1983.

53. Lui K, et al: Early changes in respiratory compliance and resistance during the development of bronchopulmonary dysplasia in the era of surfactant therapy, *Pediatr Pulmonol* 30:282, 2000.

54. Main E, et al: The influence of endotracheal tube leak on the assessment of respiratory function in ventilated children, *Intensive Care Med* 27:1788, 2001.

55. Majaesic CM, et al: Clinical correlations and pulmonary function at 8 years of age after severe neonatal respiratory failure, *Pediatr Pulmonol* 42:829, 2007.

56. Manczur T, et al: Resistance of pediatric and neonatal endotracheal tubes: influence of flow rate, size and shape, *Crit Care Med* 28:1595, 2000.

57. Marchal F, et al: Thoracic gas volume at functional residual capacity measured with integrated flow plethysmograph in infants and young children, *Eur Respir J* 4:180, 1991.

58. Mariani, et al: Pre-ductal and post-ductal O2 saturation in healthy term neonates after birth, *J Pediatr* 150:418, 2007.

59. McCann EM, et al: Pulmonary function in the sick newborn infant, *Pediatr Res* 21:314, 1987.

60. McEvoy C, et al: Functional residual capacity and passive compliance measurements after antenatal steroid therapy in preterm infants, *Pediatr Pulmonol* 31:425, 2001.

61. McEvoy C, et al: Decreased respiratory compliance in infants less than or equal to 32 weeks gestation, delivered more than 7 days after antenatal steroid therapy, *Pediatrics* 121:e1032, 2008.

62. Molloy, et al: Are carbon dioxide detectors useful in neonates? *Arch Dis Child Fetal Neonatal Ed* 91:F295, 2006.

63. Morris MG, et al, on behalf of the ERS/ATS Task Force on Standards for Infant Respiratory Function Testing: The bias flow nitrogen washout technique for measuring the functional residual capacity in infants, *Eur Respir* 17:529, 2001.

64. Mortola JP, et al: Measurements of respiratory mechanics in the newborn: a simple approach, *Pediatr Pulmonol* 3:123, 1987.

65. Motoyama EK, et al: Early onset of airway reactivity in premature infants with bronchopulmonary dysplasia, *Am Rev Respir Dis* 136:50, 1987.

66. Nelson M, et al: Basic neonatal respiratory disorders. In Donn SM, editor: *Neonatal and pediatric pulmonary graphics: principles and clinical applications,* Armonk, NY, 1008, Futura, p 253.

67. Nikischin W, et al: Improvement in respiratory compliance after surfactant therapy evaluated by a new method, *Pediatr Pulmonol* 29:276, 2000.

68. Philips J, et al: Effect of positive end-expiratory pressure on dynamic respiratory compliance in neonates, *Biol Neonate* 38:270, 1980.

69. Pratl B, et al: Effects of sleep stages on measurements of passive respiratory mechanics in infants with bronchiolitis. *Pediatr Pulmonol* 27:273, 1999.

70. Quanjer PH, et al: Standardization of lung function tests in paediatrics, *Eur Respir J* 4:121S, 1989.

71. Ratjen F, et al: Effect of changes in lung volume on respiratory system compliance in newborn infants, *J Appl Physiol* 67:1192, 1989.

72. Rosen WC, et al: The effects of bedside pulmonary mechanics testing during infant mechanical ventilation: a retrospective analysis, *Pediatr Pulmonol* 16:147, 1993.

73. Scalfaro P, et al: Reliable tidal volume estimates at the airway opening with an infant monitor during high-frequency oscillatory ventilation, *Crit Care Med* 29:1925, 2001.

74. Schreiber MD, et al: Inhaled nitric oxide in premature infants with the respiratory distress syndrome, *N Engl J Med* 349:2099, 2003.

75. Sivan Y, et al: An automated bedside method measuring functional residual capacity by N2 washout in mechanically ventilated children, *Pediatr Res* 28:446, 1990.

76. Sly PD, et al: Noninvasive determination of respiratory mechanics during mechanical ventilation of neonates: a review of current and future techniques, *Pediatr Pulmonol* 4:39, 1988.

77. Sly PD, et al, on behalf of the ERS/ATS Task Force on Standards for Infant Respiratory Function Testing: Tidal forced expirations, *Eur Respir* 16:741, 2001.

78. Stenson BJ, et al: Randomized controlled trial of respiratory system compliance measurements in mechanically ventilated neonates, *Arch Dis Child Fetal Neonatal Ed* 78:F15, 1998.

79. Stocks J, et al: The numerical analysis of pressure-flow curves in infancy, *Pediatr Pulmonol* 1:19, 1985.

80. Stocks J, et al: Influence of ethnicity and gender on airway function in preterm infants, *Am J Respir Crit Care Med* 156:1855, 1997.

81. Stocks J, et al, on behalf of the ERS/ATS Task Force on Standards for Infant Respiratory Function Testing: Plethysmographic measurements of lung volume and airway resistance, *Eur Respir* 17:302, 2001.

81a. SUPPORT Study Group of the Eunice Kennedy Shriver NICHD Neonatal Research Network: Target Ranges of oxygen saturation in extremely preterm infants, *New Eng J Med* 362:1959, 2010.

82. Tepper RS, et al: Expiratory flow limitation in infants with bronchopulmonary dysplasia, *J Pediatr* 109:1040, 1986.

83. Thomas MR, et al: Pulmonary function at follow-up of very preterm infants from the United Kingdom oscillation study, *Am J Respir Crit Care Med* 169:868, 2004.

PART 3

Pathophysiology and Management of Respiratory Distress Syndrome

Aaron Hamvas[*]

Enormous strides have been made in understanding the pathophysiology of respiratory distress syndrome (RDS) and more particularly the role of surfactant in its cause. Nevertheless, RDS, formerly referred to as hyaline membrane disease, remains a dominant clinical problem encountered among preterm infants.[3] The greatly improved outcome in RDS can be attributed primarily to the introduction of pharmacologic acceleration of pulmonary maturity and the development of surfactant replacement therapy.[9,29]

Because more of the sickest, most immature infants are surviving, the incidence of complications in the survivors of RDS remains significant. These include intracranial hemorrhage, patent ductus arteriosus (PDA), pulmonary hemorrhage, sepsis, and bronchopulmonary dysplasia (BPD), as discussed elsewhere in this textbook. It is often impossible to determine whether these disorders are the sequelae of RDS, of its treatment, or of the underlying prematurity. In this section the clinical features and evaluation of infants with RDS are discussed, and therapeutic approaches other than assisted ventilation are outlined.

[*]Ricardo J. Rodriguez, Richard J. Martin, and Avroy A. Fanaroff contributed to previous editions of this chapter.

INCIDENCE

RDS is one of the most common causes of morbidity in preterm neonates, although lack of a precise definition in infants with very low birthweight necessitates cautious interpretation of statistics regarding incidence, mortality, and outcome. The diagnosis can be established pathologically or by biochemical documentation of surfactant deficiency; nonetheless, most series refer only to a combination of clinical and radiographic features. Without biochemical evidence of surfactant deficiency, it is difficult to clinically diagnose RDS in infants with extremely low birthweight. The term *respiratory insufficiency of prematurity* has been widely used in some centers for infants who need oxygen and ventilator support in the absence of typical radiographic evidence of RDS.

RDS occurs throughout the world and has a slight male predominance. The greatest risk factors appear to be young gestational age and low birthweight (Fig. 44-30); however, late preterm delivery (35 to 36 weeks) or elective delivery in the absence of labor are becoming increasingly prominent as risk factors.[23] Other risk factors include maternal diabetes and perinatal hypoxia-ischemia. The NICHD Neonatal Research Network reported that 44% of infants between 501 and 1500 g were noted to have RDS, including 71% between 501 and 750 g, 55% between 751 and 1000 g, 37% between 1001 and 1250 g, and 23% between 1251 and 1500 g.[10]

PHARMACOLOGIC ACCELERATION OF PULMONARY MATURATION

In the early 1970s, while studying the effects of steroids on premature labor in lambs, Liggins noticed the lack of RDS and increased survival in preterm animals prenatally exposed to steroids. The effects of various catecholamines as well as aminophylline and thyroid hormone have been studied; however,

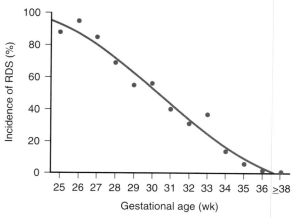

Figure 44–30. Relationship between gestational age at birth and the incidence of respiratory distress syndrome (RDS). (*From Robertson PA, et al: Neonatal morbidity according to gestational age and birth weight from five tertiary care centers in the United States, 1983 through 1986, Am J Obstet Gynecol 166:1629, 1992, with permission.*)

the most successful method to induce fetal lung maturation is prenatal corticosteroid administration.[31]

If premature delivery of any infant appears probable or necessary, lung maturity can be hastened pharmacologically. Accelerated lung maturation occurs with physiologic stress levels of corticosteroids, via receptor-mediated induction of specific developmentally regulated proteins, including those associated with surfactant synthesis. Steroids, when administered to the mother at least 24 to 48 hours before delivery, decrease the incidence and severity of RDS. Corticosteroids appear to be most effective before 34 weeks of gestation and when administered at least 24 hours and no longer than 7 days before delivery. Because corticosteroid therapy for less than 24 hours is still associated with significant reductions in neonatal mortality, RDS, and intraventricular hemorrhage (IVH), antenatal steroids should always be considered unless immediate delivery is anticipated.[1] The use of antenatal corticosteroids before 24 weeks' or after 34 weeks' gestation remains controversial.

Less clear are the effects of repeated courses of antenatal corticosteroids on the short- and long-term outcomes of preterm infants. Decreased fetal growth and poorer neurodevelopmental outcomes have been reported in retrospective clinical studies.[4] Therefore, until prospective data are available, caution should be exercised with the widespread use of multicourse therapy.

Concern about the possibility of increased infection in mother or infant appears to be unfounded. Indeed, even when corticosteroids are administered to women with prolonged rupture of membranes, there is no evidence of increased risk of infection, and the neuroprotective effects of corticosteroids are still evident. Maternal steroids may induce an increase in total leukocyte and immature neutrophil counts in the infant, which should be considered if neonatal sepsis is suspected.

There is proven benefit from the combined use of prenatal corticosteroids and postnatal surfactant therapy in preterm infants (see also Surfactant Therapy later in this section). Their effects appear to be additive in improving lung function. Antenatal steroids induce structural maturation of the lung, as evidenced by physiologic and morphometric techniques, that is not secondary to increases in alveolar surfactant pool sizes.[25] These structural changes translate into improved physiologic properties of the lung such as increased lung volume, increased lung compliance, and increased response to exogenous surfactant treatment.

Antenatal corticosteroids appear to reduce the incidence of other comorbidities associated with prematurity including intracranial hemorrhage and necrotizing enterocolitis.[1,30] The beneficial effect on intracranial hemorrhage does not correlate directly with improved pulmonary morbidity and may be secondary to stabilization of cerebral blood flow or a steroid-induced maturation of vascular integrity in the germinal matrix, or both.

In the 1990s, the observation that thyroid hormone could augment lung development and surfactant production in vitro prompted trials of antenatally administered thyrotropin-releasing hormone (TRH). However, these trials failed to demonstrate a benefit and raised concerns for adverse consequences on neurodevelopment, thereby significantly dampening enthusiasm for this therapy.

PATHOPHYSIOLOGY

The lungs of infants who succumb from RDS have a characteristic uniformly ruddy and airless appearance, macroscopically resembling hepatic tissue. On microscopic examination, the striking feature is diffuse atelectasis such that only a few widely dilated alveoli are readily distinguishable (Fig. 44-31). An eosinophilic membrane lines the visible airspaces that usually constitute terminal bronchioles and alveolar ducts. This characteristic membrane (from which the term *hyaline membrane disease* is derived) consists of a fibrinous matrix of materials derived from the blood and contains cellular debris derived from injured epithelium. The recovery phase is characterized by regeneration of alveolar cells, including the type II cells, with a resultant increase in surfactant activity.

The development of RDS begins with impaired or delayed surfactant synthesis and secretion followed by a series of events that may progressively increase the severity of the disease for several days (Fig. 44-32). Surfactant synthesis is a dynamic process that depends on factors such as pH, temperature, and perfusion, and may be compromised by cold stress, hypovolemia, hypoxemia, and acidosis. Other unfavorable factors, such as exposure to high inspired oxygen concentration and the effects of barotrauma and volutrauma from assisted ventilation, can trigger the release of proinflammatory cytokines and chemokines and further damage the alveolar epithelial lining, resulting in reduced surfactant synthesis and function. The leakage of proteins such as fibrin in the intra-alveolar space further aggravates surfactant deficiency by promoting surfactant inactivation. Deficiency of surfactant and the accompanying decrease in lung compliance lead to alveolar hypoventilation and ventilation-perfusion $(\dot{V}/\dot{Q})$ imbalance.

Severe hypoxemia and systemic hypoperfusion result in decreased oxygen delivery with subsequent lactic acidosis secondary to anaerobic metabolism. Hypoxemia and acidosis also result in pulmonary hypoperfusion secondary to pulmonary vasoconstriction, and the result is a further aggravation of hypoxemia due to right-to-left shunting at the level of the ductus arteriosus and foramen ovale and within the lung itself.

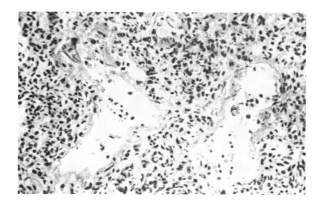

Figure 44–31. Histologic appearance of the lungs in an infant with respiratory distress syndrome. Note the marked atelectasis and so-called hyaline membranes lining the dilated alveolar ducts.

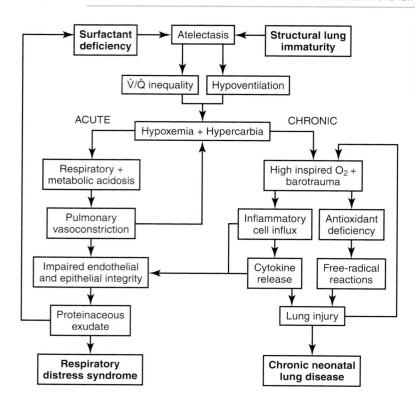

Figure 44–32. Schematic representation of the complex series of acute and chronic events that lead to neonatal respiratory distress syndrome and the accompanying lung injury secondary to therapeutic intervention in these infants.

The relative roles of surfactant deficiency and pulmonary hypoperfusion in the overall clinical picture of RDS vary somewhat with each patient. The natural history of RDS is now almost invariably altered by a combination of exogenous surfactant therapy and assisted ventilation.

Heritability of Respiratory Distress Syndrome

A genetic contribution to the risk of RDS has been suggested in twin studies where the concordance of RDS in monozygotic twins is greater than that of dizygotic twins and with isolated reports of recurrence in families.[27,33] With the application of molecular techniques, the contribution of genetic variations (polymorphisms, mutations) to the pathogenesis of respiratory disorders in newborns has rapidly emerged.[7]

Mutations in genes encoding surfactant protein-B (*SFTPB*), surfactant protein-C (*SFTPC*), and the adenosine triphosphate (ATP)-binding cassette subfamily A, member 3 (*ABCA3*) represent rare monogenic causes of RDS.[6,18] Inherited surfactant protein-B (SP-B) deficiency is a recessive disorder that presents as severe respiratory failure in the immediate newborn period and is unresponsive to standard intensive care interventions. With a disease frequency of approximately 1 per million live births, the absence of SP-B, the presence of an incompletely processed proSP-C, and a generalized disruption of surfactant metabolism cause surfactant dysfunction and the clinical syndrome. Dominant mutations in *SFTPC* typically result in interstitial lung disease in infants older than 1 month of age, although an "RDS-like" presentation has been described. The accumulation of misfolded proSP-C within cellular secretory pathways results in activation of cell stress responses and apoptosis and impaired surfactant function. The frequency of

disease due to recessive mutations in *ABCA3* in the population is unknown although initial studies suggest that *ABCA3* deficiency may be the most common of these disorders of surfactant homeostasis. Over 150 mutations in *ABCA3* have been identified in association with lethal RDS in newborns and with chronic respiratory insufficiency in children. Even though the exact role of *ABCA3* in surfactant metabolism remains unknown, data from humans and mice suggest that *ABCA3* mediates phosphatidylcholine (PC) and phosphatidylglycerol (PG) transport into lamellar bodies, and thus dysfunction of phospholipid transport into the lamellar body leads to reduced surfactant function.[11,15] One variant, a substitution of valine for glutamic acid in codon 292 (E292V) has been found in approximately 0.4% of the general population and in 4% of a cohort of preterm and term infants with RDS, suggesting that this variant may be a genetic modifier for the risk or severity of respiratory disease in susceptible individuals.[14]

Large-scale genotyping and resequencing efforts have failed to identify an unequivocal contribution of rare or common variants in the surfactant protein-B or -C genes to RDS in newborns, suggesting that if these genes play a role in RDS, it is likely to be through interactions with variants in other lung-associated genes.[17] High throughput resequencing methods and novel statistical approaches will be necessary to detect these interactions between rare and common variants in pathways that influence lung development and respiratory transition in the newborn period.[48]

CLINICAL FEATURES

The classic clinical presentation of RDS includes grunting respirations, retractions, nasal flaring, cyanosis, and increased oxygen requirement, together with diagnostic radiographic findings and onset of symptoms shortly after birth. The respiratory rate is usually regular and increased well above the normal range of 30 to 60 breaths per minute. These patients usually show progression of symptoms and require supplemental oxygen. The presence of apneic episodes at this early stage is an ominous sign that could reflect thermal instability or sepsis but more often is a sign of hypoxemia and respiratory failure. This characteristic picture is modified in many infants with low birthweight as a result of the early administration of exogenous surfactant and immediate assisted ventilation.

Retractions are prominent and are the result of the compliant rib cage collapse on inspiration as the infant generates high intrathoracic pressures to expand the poorly compliant lungs. The typical expiratory grunt is an early feature of the clinical course and may subsequently disappear. It is believed to result from partial closure of the glottis during expiration and in this way acts as a means of trapping alveolar air and maintaining functional residual capacity (FRC). Although these signs are characteristic for neonatal RDS, they can result from a wide variety of nonpulmonary causes, such as hypothermia, hypoglycemia, anemia, or polycythemia; furthermore, such nonpulmonary conditions can complicate the clinical course of RDS.

Cyanosis is a consequence of right-to-left shunting in RDS and is typically relieved by administering a higher concentration of oxygen and ventilatory support. Impaired cardiac output resulting from respiratory effort that is asynchronous with the ventilator may further impede oxygen delivery and lead to poor peripheral perfusion or cyanosis. The consistency of the arterial wave form with invasive blood pressure monitoring or the pulse signal with oxygen saturation monitoring can provide information about the effectiveness of cardiac output. Acrocyanosis of the hands and feet is a common finding in normal infants and should not be confused with central cyanosis, which always must be investigated and treated. Peripheral edema, often present in RDS, is of no particular prognostic significance unless it is associated with hydrops fetalis.

During auscultation of the chest, breath sounds are widely transmitted and cannot be relied upon to reflect pathologic conditions. Nonhomogeneous aeration plus elevated endogenously or exogenously generated intrathoracic pressures can cause pulmonary air leaks. Thus unilaterally decreased breath sounds (with mediastinal shift to the opposite side) or bilaterally decreased air entry could indicate pneumothorax, and immediate transillumination must be performed. Chest radiography is also needed to confirm endotracheal tube placement if air entry sounds asymmetric. The murmur of a PDA is most often audible during the recovery phase of RDS, when pulmonary vascular resistance has fallen below systemic levels and there is left-to-right shunting. Distant, muffled heart sounds should alert one to the possibility of pneumopericardium. Percussion of the chest is of no diagnostic value in preterm infants.

A constant feature of RDS is the early onset of clinical signs of the disease. Most infants present with signs and symptoms either in the delivery room or within the first 6 hours after birth. Inadequate observation can lead to the impression of a symptom-free period of several hours. The uncomplicated clinical course is characterized by a progressive worsening of symptoms with a peak severity by days 2 to 3 and onset of recovery by 72 hours. Surfactant therapy often greatly shortens this course. When the disease process is severe enough to require assisted ventilation or is complicated by the development of air leaks, significant shunting through a PDA, or early signs of BPD, recovery can be delayed for days, weeks, or months (see Fig. 44-32). In the most affected patients, the transition from the recovery phase of RDS to BPD is clinically imperceptible.

RADIOGRAPHIC FINDINGS

See also Chapter 37.

The diagnosis of RDS is based on a combination of the previously described clinical features, evidence of prematurity, exclusion of other causes of respiratory distress, and characteristic radiographic appearance. The typical radiographic features consist of a diffuse reticulogranular pattern, giving the classic ground-glass appearance, in both lung fields with superimposed air bronchograms (Fig. 44-33). Although the radiologic appearance of RDS is typically symmetric and homogeneous, asymmetry has also been described, especially if surfactant therapy has been administered preferentially to one side.

The reticulogranular pattern is primarily caused by alveolar atelectasis, although there may be some component of pulmonary edema. The prominent air bronchograms represent aerated bronchioles superimposed on a background of nonaerated alveoli. An area of localized air bronchograms may be normal in the left lower lobe overlying the cardiac silhouette, but in RDS they are widely distributed, particularly in the upper lobes. In the most severe cases, a complete whiteout of the lungs can be observed with total loss of heart borders. Heart size is typically normal or slightly increased. Cardiomegaly may herald the development of congestive cardiac failure from a PDA. After the administration of exogenous surfactant therapy, the chest radiograph usually shows improved aeration of the lungs bilaterally; however, asymmetric clearing of the lungs may occur.

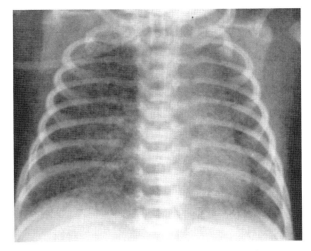

Figure 44–33. Typical radiographic appearance of respiratory distress syndrome with reticulogranular infiltrate and air bronchograms.

The radiographic appearance of RDS, typical or atypical, cannot be reliably differentiated from that of neonatal pneumonia, which is most commonly caused by group B streptococci. This problem has been the major reason for the widespread use of antibiotics in the initial management of infants with RDS. Infants with RDS reportedly have a larger thymic silhouette than infants of comparable size without RDS. This supports the theory that patients with RDS have had reduced exposure to endogenous corticosteroids during fetal life.

Echocardiographic evaluation of infants with RDS may be of value in the diagnosis of a PDA to quantitate elevations in pulmonary artery pressure, to assess cardiac function, and to exclude congenital heart disease (e.g., obstructed total anomalous pulmonary venous return).

TREATMENT

Therapy for RDS includes careful application of general supportive measures supplemented by surfactant therapy and specific means of controlling and assisting ventilation. Close and detailed supervision of small infants requires a dedicated, trained staff experienced in problems specific to the newborn and skillful in the unique technical procedures involved, such as assessment of neonatal blood gases.

Positive Pressure Ventilation

See Part 4.
Delivery of distending pressure to maintain airway and alveolar expansion through invasive and noninvasive means is the mainstay of treatment for RDS. The most common approaches of invasive mechanical ventilation via an endotracheal tube use a time-cycled, pressure-limited mode or volume-controlled mode with synchronized ventilated breaths. Alternatively, high-frequency jet ventilation or high-frequency oscillatory ventilation is used both as a primary means of ventilation as well as rescue when conventional ventilation has failed. Increasing enthusiasm for nasal continuous positive airway pressure (CPAP) to deliver positive pressure has demonstrated that many premature infants can be successfully managed without intubation or with intubation only for surfactant administration.[32,44]

Surfactant Therapy

No intervention in the past 20 years has had more impact on the care of newborns with RDS than surfactant replacement therapy, which was first introduced in 1990. A thorough history of the development of surfactant replacement therapy can be found in reference 16. The discovery that surfactant deficiency was key in the pathophysiology of RDS led several investigators to administer artificial aerosolized phospholipids to infants with RDS. In these early studies, only limited therapeutic success was encountered. In contrast, animal models in which natural surfactant compounds were used yielded more promising results.

Because intact lung preparations were not available in Japan, Fujiwara and coworkers developed a mixture of both natural and synthetic surface-active lipids for use in humans.[12] Such a mixture might also afford alveolar stability with less potential risk for a reaction to foreign protein than would be the case

with exclusively natural surfactant. When administered to an initial group of 10 preterm infants with severe RDS who were not improving despite artificial ventilation, a single 10-mL dose of surfactant instilled into the endotracheal tube resulted in a dramatic decrease in inspired oxygen and ventilator pressures. None of the infants in this uncontrolled series subsequently succumbed from RDS. Recovery, however, was complicated by clinical evidence of a PDA in nine of the infants, possibly the result of a prompt fall in pulmonary vascular resistance with the resultant left-to-right shunting after surfactant therapy.

Multiple studies have employed various combinations of prevention (delivery room administration) and rescue (administration for established RDS) protocols using synthetic and mixed natural-synthetic preparations.[24,41,42] Synthetic-only preparations used protein-free synthetic phospholipid products which contain alcohol to act as a spreading agent for dipalmitoyl phosphatidylcholine at the air-fluid-alveolar interface.[35] The mixed-surfactant preparations contain extracts of calf lung lavage or minced bovine or porcine lung. Direct comparison between synthetic and natural preparations has revealed a more rapid physiologic response after natural (protein-containing) preparations as manifested by the ability to lower inspired oxygen and ventilator pressures.[41] Comparison of natural surfactants has shown modest differences in oxygenation during the first few hours after treatment, without a significant effect on morbidity or mortality. Despite differences in their chemical composition and manufacturing methods, formulations currently approved by the U.S. Food and Drug Administration demonstrate comparable clinical efficacy.

All regimens of surfactant therapy appear to decrease the incidence of air leaks and improve oxygenation of ventilated preterm infants. More strikingly, mortality from RDS, and even overall mortality of ventilated preterm infants, is significantly reduced, especially when multidose surfactant therapy is used for these infants. Early selective surfactant administration (within 2 hours after birth) given to infants with RDS requiring assisted ventilation leads to decreased risk of pneumothorax and pulmonary interstitial emphysema and a decreased risk of neonatal mortality and chronic lung disease compared with delaying treatment until RDS is well established. Furthermore, this strategy does seem to reduce the need for subsequent retreatment and the requirement for supplemental oxygen and mechanical ventilation.[34,42] However, it is unclear whether a preventive dose administered endotracheally in the delivery room (prophylactic) has any advantage over treatment given after the patient has been resuscitated and stabilized (early treatment).[22] Such preventive therapy is only relevant for very immature infants who are most likely to develop significant lung disease, but this therapy is potentially prone to administration errors related to suboptimal endotracheal tube placement or the unnecessary treatment of many babies who were not destined to develop RDS. Furthermore the SUPPORT trial demonstrated that 17% of extremely low birthweight infants may never need intubation.[44a]

The dramatic improvement in oxygenation is not accompanied by an immediate improvement in $PaCO_2$ if ventilator settings remain unchanged more than 30 minutes after surfactant therapy. These data strongly suggest that enhanced matching of ventilation and perfusion is the primary mechanism whereby surfactant dramatically improves PaO_2 in preterm infants with RDS. Consistent with the failure of $PaCO_2$

to improve rapidly are observations that lung compliance does not improve rapidly after surfactant therapy. Dramatic improvement in oxygenation after surfactant therapy does correlate with an increase in lung volume and resultant stabilization of FRC. This improvement occurs despite the failure of lung compliance to increase rapidly and suggests that surfactant therapy might induce regional overdistention of alveoli. However, if lung compliance is measured on spontaneous rather than ventilator breaths, or if ventilator pressures are promptly lowered in response to the increase in PaO_2 induced by surfactant therapy, then an increase in compliance in response to surfactant can be seen.[8] In contrast with the impressive improvement in mortality, the incidence of BPD, IVH, sepsis, and symptomatic PDA appears unaltered in most studies.[24] Of particular interest is the failure of surfactant therapy to significantly reduce the incidence of BPD. Although individual studies have shown a decreased incidence of BPD, these results have not been substantiated by meta-analysis of large randomized trials. This could be a consequence of the enhanced survival caused by surfactant administration to infants who are very preterm. Furthermore, many infants who are preterm develop BPD without antecedent RDS.

Data from the early trials suggested slightly higher pulmonary hemorrhage rates in association with surfactant therapy in the smallest and most immature infants. However, these findings have not been consistent throughout the literature, and controversy still exists. Pulmonary hemorrhage has been reported in up to 6% of preterm infants treated with exogenous surfactant and typically occurs in the first 72 hours of life.[13] Generally, an acute deterioration in oxygenation and ventilation accompanied by variable degrees of cardiovascular compromise constitute the typical clinical findings. One of the major hurdles encountered in defining the magnitude of the problem has been the lack of precise diagnostic criteria. In surfactant-treated infants, there tends to be extensive intra-alveolar hemorrhage, in contrast to infants not exposed to surfactant therapy, in whom hemorrhages occur as interstitial hemorrhage and localized hematomas. The improvement in lung compliance after surfactant therapy probably promotes an increase in left-to-right shunt through the PDA. The increase in pulmonary blood flow results in pulmonary congestion and elevated capillary pressure. Stress failure of alveolar capillaries and their supporting epithelial tissues leads to intra-alveolar hemorrhagic pulmonary edema. In the large randomized, controlled trial of prophylactic indomethacin for prevention of IVH, despite a significant reduction in PDA in the treated group, the incidence of pulmonary hemorrhage did not change (Box 44-3).[37] A follow-up study of infants who developed pulmonary hemorrhage after surfactant administration showed no difference in the incidence of BPD, necrotizing enterocolitis, or intracranial hemorrhage. Furthermore, the neurodevelopmental outcome assessed by the Bayley Mental Developmental Index at 20 months of age was also similar.[45] Thus, although the role of PDA in the pathogenesis of pulmonary hemorrhage has not been conclusively demonstrated, a PDA is a frequent contributing factor.

Some infants do not exhibit the anticipated favorable response to surfactant therapy. The need for a high oxygen concentration and ventilatory pressures during the early stages

---

BOX 44–3 Surfactant Therapy for Respiratory Distress Syndrome

RESOLVED

Improved mortality from respiratory distress syndrome (RDS)

Greatest benefit when antenatal corticosteroids are also employed

Exogenous surfactant does not inhibit endogenous surfactant synthesis

Retreatment may be required in severe RDS

Major component for lowering surface tension: phosphatidylcholine

Endotracheal intubation required for administration of fluid suspension

Improvement in oxygenation, functional residual capacity, and lung compliance

Protein-containing preparations show a faster therapeutic response

Decrease in incidence of air leaks

Prophylactic or early use beneficial in infants with extremely low birthweight (<29 weeks' gestation)

Efficacy of surfactant therapy, early extubation, nasal continuous positive airway pressure strategy

UNRESOLVED

Factors predicting likelihood of success of an initial CPAP-based strategy

Optimal ventilatory strategy to maximize surfactant response

Effect on incidence and severity of bronchopulmonary dysplasia

Role of surfactant proteins as modulator of the immune system and inflammatory response

Role for recombinant surfactant protein-based preparations

---

of RDS has been identified as a risk factor for an inadequate response. Animal studies have shown that even a few large tidal volume breaths in a surfactant-deficient lung are associated with alveolar accumulation of protein-rich edema fluid and decreased response to surfactant treatment.[21] Thus, it is unclear if lack of response is secondary to the initial severity of the disease or to the damage induced by short periods of aggressive ventilation prior to surfactant replacement. Furthermore, reactive oxygen species in preterm infants with poorly developed antioxidant defenses (i.e., superoxide dismutase, catalase, and reduced glutathione) may inactivate endogenous and exogenous surfactants. Finally, intrauterine inflammation or genetically determined factors may disrupt lung development or endogenous surfactant metabolism thereby influencing response to surfactant therapy.

Data from large numbers of infants in the United States and Europe indicate no adverse effects on physical growth, respiratory symptoms, or neurodevelopmental outcome. In a systematic review of randomized, controlled trials, surfactant treatment was associated with a reduction in the combined outcomes of death or severe disability at 1 year of age.[40] Furthermore, this improvement in mortality and morbidity induced by surfactant therapy is accompanied by significant cost savings.[38]

Despite the efficacy of currently available surfactant preparations, attempts to enhance these preparations continue. Although no adverse immunologic consequences of foreign tissue protein administration have been reported in the recipients of natural surfactant therapy, concerns for transmitted disease prompt the desire to develop synthetic, non-animal based products. Preparations that contain synthetic peptides that mimic the biophysical properties of SP-B or SP-C have been studied in newborns (SP-B) and adults (SP-C) but have not found their way into general use.[26,43] SP-A and SP-D, while not essential for surface-lowering activity, could play a significant role in the lung's innate immune response and modulation of inflammation. It is not yet known whether the use of purified SP-A or recombinant SP-D has a therapeutic role in neonatal lung disease. The combination of a new generation of surfactants along with a gentler ventilatory approach could hold the key to optimal pulmonary outcomes in the future.

Inhaled Nitric Oxide Therapy

Inhaled nitric oxide, currently approved for treatment of hypoxic respiratory failure in near-term and full-term infants, has been proposed as a potential intervention in premature infants at risk for development of BPD. Although trials have suggested short-term benefits in improved survival without BPD and decreased use of bronchodilators and steroids in the first year, the impact on longer-term neurodevelopmental outcome is unknown. Further evaluation of the short-term and long-term effects of this intervention is needed, especially as several trials have failed to show benefit in preterm infants (See Part 8).[19]

Assessment of Blood Gas Status

See also Part 2.
The ability to accurately monitor gas exchange is essential in all cases of neonatal respiratory disease. In its most basic form this involves intermittent arterial sampling, usually via an indwelling umbilical arterial catheter or, less commonly, a peripheral (e.g., radial) arterial line. Infants with acute respiratory distress requiring a significantly increased inspired oxygen concentration or assisted ventilation should have blood gases sampled every 4 hours or more often as their clinical condition dictates.

In infants with RDS, partial pressure of arterial oxygen (PaO_2) is customarily maintained between 50 and 80 mm Hg, $PaCO_2$ in the 40 to 55 mm Hg range, and pH at least 7.25, although in the most immature infants, these ranges have been relaxed to minimize oxygen supplementation and the degree of ventilatory support in an effort to decrease oxygen- and ventilation-associated morbidity.[2,23] Analysis of continuous in-line arterial blood gases and electrolytes has been introduced in neonatal intensive care units. This promising technology offers advantages over intermittent sampling: less handling of the critically ill patient, fewer breaks in the line that could introduce infection, and continuous evaluation of therapeutic maneuvers.[49] In conjunction with continuous noninvasive monitoring of oxygen saturation, it is possible to rapidly identify clinical deterioration, expedite weaning, and minimize morbidity from oxygen toxicity or hypocarbia. Moreover, the need for blood sampling is substantially decreased, which can decrease the incidence of iatrogenic anemia and the need for blood transfusions.

One should bear in mind that a normal arterial oxygen tension or saturation does not ensure adequate tissue oxygen delivery, because oxygen delivery is dependent on cardiac output and oxygen content of the blood. Therefore, interpretation of gas exchange should always be correlated with a thorough clinical assessment.

ARTERIAL SAMPLING

Umbilical catheterization should be performed by an experienced operator and under strict surgical aseptic technique. Once the umbilical arteries have been identified by their anatomic characteristics, one of the vessels is dilated with the use of an iris forceps. The catheter is then gently advanced to a predetermined length that will place its tip at a high (T6-T8) or at a low (L3-L4) position. Several methods have been developed to estimate the length of catheter to be inserted to achieve proper placement; however, radiologic confirmation of catheter position is still imperative.

Although umbilical artery catheters still form the basic means of arterial sampling in infants with RDS, the list of catheter-related complications is formidable. The most common visible problem from an umbilical or radial line is blanching or cyanosis of part or all of a distal extremity or the buttock area, resulting either from vasospasm or a thrombotic or embolic incident. This complication may be reduced in the case of an umbilical catheter by high placement, with the catheter tip at the level of T7 or T8 as opposed to lower placement at L3 or L4 just above the aortic bifurcation.

Tyson and associates observed thromboatheromatous complications resulting from umbilical artery catheters in 33 of 56 neonates at autopsy.[46] Hypertension can result if a renal artery is involved. A rare complication of indwelling arterial umbilical catheters is aneurysmal dilation with dissection of the abdominal aorta, which can be diagnosed by careful ultrasound examination. Passage of a catheter beyond the origin of the superior mesenteric artery might increase the risk of necrotizing enterocolitis. Retrograde blood flow into the proximal aorta can occur during flushing of radial and umbilical artery lines and result in transient blood pressure elevation; therefore, routine flushing should be performed with a small volume over a period of several seconds.

Small amounts of heparin added to the continuous infusion appear to reduce the risk of arterial thrombi. Use of siliconized catheters is associated with decreased thrombogenicity. Catheter-associated thrombosis may be further reduced by limiting the number of days these catheters remain in place. All these complications illustrate the importance of applying rigid criteria for the insertion and removal of indwelling arterial catheters and the need for less hazardous methods of monitoring blood gases.

If a peripheral arterial catheter is to be used, an Allen test should be performed prior to the insertion of a radial artery line to establish the presence of adequate collateral circulation to the fingers.

NONINVASIVE MONITORING: PULSE OXIMETRY

Risk of infection and other complications have prompted early umbilical line removal and increased the reliance on noninvasive methods for measuring gas exchange. Pulse oximetry is a well-established technique for indirectly determining oxygenation in a noninvasive and continuous manner. For infants with mild respiratory distress, pulse oximetry is extremely valuable and could make an umbilical arterial catheter unnecessary, as long as intermittent assessments of pH and P_{CO_2} are made. Generally this is not the case in infants with moderate or severe respiratory disease in whom noninvasive measurement remains an important adjunct rather than a substitute for arterial blood gas sampling.

Continuous noninvasive measurement of arterial hemoglobin oxygen saturation (pulse oximetry) has gained widespread acceptance. Pulse oximetry typically employs a microprocessor-based pulse oximeter consisting of a light-emitting probe attached to a distal extremity of the infant. Oxygen saturation is computed from the light absorption characteristics of the pulsatile flow (containing both oxygenated and nonoxygenated hemoglobin) as it passes beneath the probe. The monitor readings closely correlate with saturation measurements obtained from arterial samples (see also Part 2).

The major disadvantage of pulse oximetry is that changes in saturation are small on the flat portion of the hemoglobin dissociation curve at Pa_{O_2} values greater than about 60 mm Hg (depending on the fetal hemoglobin content and other factors affecting position of the hemoglobin dissociation curve). This is not a substantial problem in infants with BPD when oxygen saturation is generally maintained in the high 80s to mid 90s, and these infants are unlikely to be at risk for hyperoxemia. On the other hand, significant decreases in severe forms of retinopathy of prematurity have been seen when oxygen saturation limits are constrained between 85% and 92%; thus oxygen supplementation is more restricted.[20] However, significant variability in even resting oxygen saturations in some infants provides a significant challenge to administer the appropriate amount of oxygen to remain within these constraints.

Pulse oximeters are technically easy to use, do not require calibration or heating of the skin, and provide immediate data on arterial oxygenation. However, this ease of use can allow misinterpretation of potentially erroneous measurements.[36] Placement must not be associated with excess pressure, and peripheral perfusion must be adequate, although pulse oximeters are less dependent on peripheral perfusion than the previously widely used transcutaneous Pa_{O_2} probes. Pulse oximeters are quite sensitive to sudden changes in background signal such as those due to body movements. It is therefore important to ensure that the pulsatile waveforms, from which oxygen saturation is derived, are not distorted. This is typically done by comparing pulse rate from the oximeter with heart rate obtained from a cardiorespiratory monitor; these values should be identical. Newer signal extraction technology has significantly improved the accuracy and reliability of pulse oximetry measurements.

A major effect of pulse oximetry has been the ability to rapidly optimize respiratory care and drastically reduce the time required to determine optimum inspired oxygen concentrations, levels of CPAP, and respirator settings. Other benefits include the ability to assess responses to all procedures, including surfactant instillation, as well as excessive handling. Complications such as pneumothorax, endotracheal tube dislodgement, disconnection from oxygen supply, and respirator malfunction are rapidly recognized so that

immediate corrective treatment can be initiated. Episodes of hypoxemia or desaturation can occur spontaneously or accompany feeds and have complex etiologies, as discussed elsewhere in this text. Noninvasive monitoring of oxygenation allows such episodes to be identified and their relationship to apnea and bradycardia recorded.

NONINVASIVE CARBON DIOXIDE MONITORING

Although not used as universally as pulse oximetry, noninvasive methods for monitoring carbon dioxide levels can also provide an important adjunct to blood gas monitoring. Capnography has become the standard of care in resuscitation situations for accurately and rapidly demonstrating that the endotracheal tube is in the airway (see also Chapter 26, Part 2). End-tidal CO_2 monitoring, though routinely used during anesthesia, is useful for following trends, but is not always reliable in very low birthweight infants. Transcutaneous P_{CO_2} monitoring is also useful for monitoring trends, especially when trying to optimize the ventilatory settings when initiating conventional or high-frequency ventilation. The association of Pa_{CO_2} levels of less than 30 mm Hg with periventricular leukomalacia in premature newborns demonstrates the need for careful CO_2 monitoring.[39]

General Measures

THERMOREGULATION

Infants with respiratory difficulty require an optimal thermal environment to minimize oxygen consumption and oxygen requirements. Infants who are hypoxic lose the ability to increase metabolic rate when they are cold stressed, and a fall in body temperature may be noted. Thus, meticulous attention must be paid to the temperature and humidity of the infant's environment and inspired air so that the appropriate neutral thermal environment can be maintained.

FLUID, ELECTROLYTES, AND NUTRITION

See also Chapters 35 and 36.

The importance of nutritional support for infants with RDS cannot be overemphasized. The ability to supply an adequate caloric intake to the critically ill infant receiving respiratory assistance is facilitated by intravenous glucose, amino acid, and lipid solutions. Premature infants receiving as little as 60 cal/kg per day, with 10% of the calories provided as protein, could remain in positive nitrogen balance. It is now common practice to start administration of an amino acid–glucose solution by the first day of life, especially for infants weighing less than 1000 g and receiving mechanical ventilation. Small-volume gavage feedings of breast milk or formula should be initiated as early as feasible.

Fluid balance must be closely watched because overenthusiastic attention to calories can cause fluid overload and perhaps contribute to the development of a clinically significant PDA. Maintenance fluid requirements usually begin at 60 to 80 mL/kg per day as a 10% dextrose solution and increase gradually to 120 mL/kg per day by the fifth day of life. However, these fluid requirements are greatly modified by many additional factors, particularly the high insensible water loss experienced by many infants with very low birthweight under radiant warmers or phototherapy and the limited concentrating ability of immature kidneys (see Chapter 36). In a prospective study using sequential analysis, Bell and associates showed that the risk of a PDA with congestive heart failure was greater in infants receiving a high-fluid volume regimen (169 ± 20 mL/kg per day) than in those on a low-volume regimen (122 ± 14 mL/kg per day). In the high-volume group, 35 (41%) of 85 developed murmurs consistent with a PDA, and 11 of these were associated with congestive heart failure. In contrast, only 9 (11%) of the 85 infants in the low-volume group had a PDA murmur, and congestive heart failure developed in 2. More cases of necrotizing enterocolitis also were observed in the high-volume group.[5] These results, together with other data, indicate that limitation of fluid intake could possibly reduce the risk of PDA, necrotizing enterocolitis, and even BPD, although routine or prophylactic diuretic therapy cannot be recommended. Fluid therapy in infants with RDS is thus a critical aspect of care.

In infants with extremely low birthweight, especially during the first few days of life, free water depletion due to high insensible water losses could lead to hypernatremic dehydration. Later, usually after the first week of life, the renal inability to conserve salt, a low sodium intake, overzealous use of diuretics, or the osmotic diuresis associated with hyperglycemia can precipitate hyponatremia, particularly in infants weighing less than 1000 g. Maintenance of sodium balance usually is achieved by administering 2 to 4 mEq/kg per day of sodium, commencing at 48 to 72 hours, and closely monitoring serum sodium levels. Potassium balance is accomplished by adding 1 to 2 mEq/kg per day to the intravenous infusion from the second day of life, as long as normal renal function and diuresis are present. In the more immature infant, non-oliguric hyperkalemia might be present secondary to a shift of intracellular potassium to the extracellular space due to an immature Na^+, K^+-ATPase pump. Thus serum electrolytes should be monitored sequentially to determine proper adjustments of fluid therapy.

ACID-BASE THERAPY

A change in acid-base balance should prompt a rapid determination of the type of imbalance, respiratory or metabolic, and a thorough evaluation of the cause. Acidosis, respiratory or metabolic, especially when coupled with hypoxia, can cause pulmonary arterial vasoconstriction and ventilation-perfusion abnormalities, decreased cardiac output, or both. Metabolic acidosis is most often encountered when the infant was depressed at birth and required resuscitation. A subsequent metabolic acidosis out of proportion to the degree of respiratory distress might signify hypoperfusion, sepsis, or an IVH. Metabolic acidosis occurring at any time typically improves with sodium bicarbonate administration, as long as there are no signs of respiratory failure that might hinder elimination of carbon dioxide. Sodium bicarbonate is hypertonic and thus should be administered slowly and judiciously. Rapid infusions may increase blood osmolality and predispose to intracranial hemorrhage or hepatic necrosis (if administered through an umbilical venous catheter with the tip in the liver).

Respiratory acidosis requires assisted ventilation. Administration of sodium bicarbonate to infants with respiratory acidosis is not indicated and could further increase the Pco_2. For infants in respiratory acidosis, alkali therapy should be withheld until some form of assisted ventilation has been initiated. If this fails to improve oxygenation and raise the pH, sodium bicarbonate may be administered while continuing with assisted ventilation and always attempting to determine the cause of the acidosis. In recent years, the administration of sodium bicarbonate has been increasingly challenged, and its role in treating metabolic acidosis in neonates is very limited.

CARDIOVASCULAR MANAGEMENT

Comprehensive management of patients with RDS includes a close evaluation and monitoring of the cardiovascular system. An in-depth understanding of the physical and physiologic interactions between the cardiovascular and pulmonary systems in the mechanically ventilated patient is paramount. For example, after surfactant administration, with the improvement in the mechanical properties of the lungs, an unrecognized overdistention of the lungs by excessive mechanical ventilation support can decrease systemic venous return to the heart that results in a decrease in cardiac output. Radiographically, a typical squeezed-heart silhouette and flattened diaphragm are found. A thorough clinical evaluation should include sequential assessment of vital signs, peripheral pulses, capillary refill, and urine output as surrogate markers of adequate cardiac output.

Myocardial dysfunction secondary to birth asphyxia may be present and could lead to decreased peripheral perfusion with lactic acidemia and metabolic acidosis. Systemic hypotension is common in the early stages of RDS; thus continuous monitoring of systemic blood pressure by means of an indwelling arterial catheter is of utmost importance in the moderately to severely ill infant. Noninvasive intermittent monitoring of systemic blood pressure should be reserved for the mildly affected neonate. Judicious use of crystalloids for intravascular expansion and vasopressor support are often indicated. In patients with persistent hypotension not responsive to fluid therapy or catecholamines, serum cortisol levels should be measured and treatment with stress doses of hydrocortisone should be considered.

Failure of the ductus arteriosus to close is a common complication in infants with RDS and has been linked to the development of necrotizing enterocolitis and BPD. Clinically, the presence of a PDA is heralded by a widened pulse pressure, an active precordium, and bounding peripheral pulses. A heart murmur on the left subclavicular area and the back is often present. On the chest radiograph, cardiomegaly might signal the presence of a hemodynamically significant PDA with congestive heart failure. With clinical suspicion, a confirmatory echocardiogram, which should demonstrate evidence of pulmonary overcirculation, such as left atrial enlargement, is usually obtained before proceeding with the pharmacologic closure of the ductus arteriosus with a prostaglandin synthesis inhibitor such as indomethacin or ibuprofen.[47] Fluid restriction, vasopressors, and a loop diuretic (e.g., furosemide) may be indicated for the medical management of a hemodynamically significant PDA with congestive heart failure.

ANTIBIOTICS

Neonatal pneumonia (most commonly caused by group B streptococci) can be indistinguishable from RDS both clinically and radiographically. Such infection usually is acquired around the time of delivery either through ascending infection or passage through a colonized genital tract. The potentially fulminant course of neonatal pneumonia, especially in preterm infants, and the difficulty in distinguishing it from RDS have led to the recommendation that all infants with significant respiratory distress receive antibiotics after appropriate cultures.

Prenatal features suggestive of neonatal infection include maternal fever, prolonged rupture of membranes, and clinical evidence of chorioamnionitis. The suspicion for bacterial infection is raised by a history of maternal genital colonization with group B streptococci, especially in an inadequately treated mother. In recent years pneumonia or sepsis from gram negative organisms, such as E. Coli, may pose an even greater risk.

In the newborn, persistent hypotension, metabolic acidosis, early onset of apnea, neutropenia, and neutrophilia accompanied by an increase in immature cells (left shift) are clinical findings suggestive of systemic infection. Nonetheless, the absence of these features does not exclude the diagnosis of pneumonia. A penicillin combined with an aminoglycoside is the antibiotic regimen of choice and should be discontinued after 48 hours if cultures are negative. Appropriate gram negative organism coverage must be a consideration.

BLOOD TRANSFUSION

In the acutely ill newborn with RDS, mild anemia, which is usually well tolerated by asymptomatic preterm infants, can significantly decrease oxygen content of blood and tissue oxygen delivery. During the first few days of life, anemia is usually the result of excessive blood extraction for laboratory determinations. In-line blood gas and chemistry analyzers and microsampling techniques have significantly decreased the volume of blood required for testing. This decrease should translate into a decrease in blood loss and transfusion requirements.

It is customary to maintain a venous hematocrit of at least 35% to 40% during the acute phase of RDS to support an adequate oxygen-carrying capacity because, in the presence of anemia, most infants do not manifest any signs of impaired oxygen-carrying capacity. Thus the potential risks of blood replacement, including transmission of infectious agents, blood group antigen exposure, or rarely iron overload, should be carefully considered.

Administration of recombinant human erythropoietin over the first 6 weeks of life for preventing anemia in infants with extremely low birthweight during the acute phase of RDS remains controversial.[28]

Despite substantial improvements in the treatment of RDS, prevention of premature birth is still an ultimate goal and will have significant impact on the prevention of RDS. In the meantime, understanding the interactions of the intrauterine environment and genetic determinants of lung development to the pathogenesis of RDS is essential to develop mechanism-specific interventions.

REFERENCES

1. *Report of the consensus development conference on the effect of corticosteroids for fetal maturation on perinatal outcomes,* Bethesda, MD, National Institute of Child Health and Human Development, Office of Medical Applications of Research, National Institutes of Health, February 28, 1994 to March 2, 1994 NIH Pub No. 95-3784, 1994.

2. Askie LM, Henderson-Smart DJ: Restricted versus liberal oxygen exposure for preventing morbidity and mortality in preterm or low birth weight infants, *Cochrane Database of Systematic Reviews* 4:CD001077, 2001.

3. Avery ME, et al: Surface properties in relation to atelectasis and hyaline membrane disease, *Am J Dis Child* 97:517, 1959.

4. Banks BA,, et al: Multiple courses of antenatal corticosteroids and outcome of premature neonates, *Am J Obstet Gynecol* 181:709, 1999.

5. Bell EF, et al: Effect of fluid administration on the development of symptomatic patent ductus arteriosus and congestive heart failure in premature infants, *N Engl J Med* 302:598, 1980.

6. Bullard JE, et al: ABCA3 deficiency: neonatal respiratory failure and interstitial lung disease, *Semin Perinatol* 30:327, 2006.

7. Cole FS, et al: Genetic disorders of neonatal respiratory function, *Pediatr Res* 50:157, 2001.

8. Davis JM, et al: Changes in pulmonary mechanics after the administration of surfactant to infants with respiratory distress syndrome, *N Engl J Med* 319:476, 1988.

9. Engle WA: American Academy of Pediatrics Committee on Fetus and Newborn. Surfactant-replacement therapy for respiratory distress in the preterm and term neonate, *Pediatrics* 121:419, 2008.

10. Fanaroff AA, et al: Trends in neonatal morbidity and mortality for very low birthweight infants, *Am J Obstet Gynecol* 196:147e1, 2007.

11. Fitzgerald ML, et al: ABCA3 inactivation in mice causes respiratory failure, loss of pulmonary surfactant, and depletion of lung phosphatidylglycerol, *J Lipid Res* 48:621, 2007.

12. Fujiwara T, et al: Artificial surfactant therapy in hyaline membrane disease, *Lancet* 1:55, 1980.

13. Garland J, et al: Pulmonary hemorrhage risk in infants with a clinically diagnosed patent ductus arteriosus: a retrospective cohort study, *Pediatrics* 94:719, 1994.

14. Garmany TH, et al: Population and disease-based prevalence of the common mutations associated with surfactant deficiency, *Pediatr Res* 63:645, 2008.

15. Garmany TH, et al: Surfactant composition and function in patients with abca3 mutations, *Pediatr Res* 59:801, 2006.

16. Halliday HL: Surfactants: past, present and future, *J Perinatol* 28:S47, 2008.

17. Hamvas A, et al: Comprehensive genetic variant discovery in the surfactant protein B gene, *Pediatr Res* 62:170, 2007.

18. Hamvas A: Inherited surfactant protein-B deficiency and surfactant protein-C-associated disease: clinical features and evaluation, *Semin Perinatol* 30:316, 2006.

19. Hibbs AM, et al: One-year respiratory outcomes of preterm infants enrolled in the nitric oxide (to prevent) chronic lung disease trial, *J Pediatr* 153:525, 2008.

20. Higgins RD, et al: Executive summary of the workshop on oxygen in neonatal therapies: controversies and opportunities for research, *Pediatrics* 119:790, 2007.

21. Hillman NH, et al: Brief, large tidal volume ventilation initiates lung injury and a systemic response in fetal sheep, *Am J Respir Crit Care Med* 176:575, 2007.

22. Horbar JD, et al: Timing of initial surfactant treatment of infants 23 to 29 weeks' gestation: is routine practice evidence based? *Pediatrics* 113:1593, 2004.

23. Jain L: Respiratory morbidity in late-preterm infants: prevention is better than cure! *Am J Perinatol* 25:75, 2008.

24. Jobe AH: Pulmonary surfactant therapy, *N Engl J Med* 328:861, 1993.

25. Jobe AH, et al: Beneficial effects of the combined use of prenatal corticosteroids and postnatal surfactant on preterm infants, *Am J Obstet Gynecol* 168:508, 1993.

26. Kattwinkel J: Synthetic surfactants: the search goes on, *Pediatrics* 115:1075, 2005.

27. Khoury MJ, et al: Recurrence of low birth weight in siblings. *J Clin Epidemiol* 42:1171, 1989.

28. Kotto-Kome AC, et al: Effect of beginning recombinant erythropoietin treatment within the first week of life, among very-low-birth-weight neonates, on 'early' and 'late' erythrocyte transfusions: a meta-analysis, *J Perinatol* 24:24, 2004.

29. Kwang-Sun L, et al: Trend in mortality from respiratory distress syndrome in the United States, 1970-1995, *J Pediatr* 134:434, 1999.

30. Leviton A, et al: Antenatal corticosteroids appear to reduce the risk of postnatal germinal matrix hemorrhage in intubated low birth weight newborn, *Pediatrics* 91:1083, 1993.

31. Liggins GC: A controlled trial of antepartum glucocorticoid treatment for prevention of the respiratory distress syndrome in premature infants, *Pediatrics* 50:515, 1972.

32. Morley CJ, et al: Nasal CPAP or intubation at birth for very preterm infants, *N Engl J Med* 358:700, 2008.

33. Myrianthopoulos NC, et al: Respiratory distress syndrome in twins, *Acta Genet Med Gemellol* 20:199, 1971.

34. OSIRIS Collaborative Group: Early versus delayed neonatal administration of a synthetic surfactant-the judgment of OSIRIS, *Lancet* 340:1363, 1992.

35. Phibbs RH, et al: Initial clinical trial of Exosurf, a protein-free synthetic surfactant, for the prophylaxis and early treatment of hyaline membrane disease, *Pediatrics* 88:1, 1991.

36. Poets CF, et al: Noninvasive monitoring of oxygenation in infants and children: practical considerations and areas of concern, *Pediatrics* 93:737, 1994.

37. Schmidt B, et al: Long term effects of indomethacin prophylaxis in extremely low birth weight infants, *N Engl J Med* 344:1966, 2001.

38. Schwartz RM, et al: Effect of surfactant on morbidity, mortality, and resource use in newborn infants weighing 500 to 1500 g, *N Engl J Med* 330:1476, 1994.

39. Shankaran S, et al: Cumulative index of exposure to hypocarbia and hyperoxia as risk factors for periventricular leukomalacia in low birth weight infants, *Pediatrics* 118:1654, 2006.

40. Sinn JK, et al: Developmental outcome of preterm infants after surfactant therapy: systematic review of randomized controlled trials, *J Paediatr Child Health* 38:597, 2002.

41. Soll RF, Blanco F: Natural surfactant extract versus synthetic surfactant for neonatal respiratory distress syndrome, *Cochrane Database Syst Rev* (2):CD000144, 2001.

42. Soll RF, Morley CJ: Prophylactic versus selective use of surfactant in preventing morbidity and mortality in preterm infants, *Cochrane Database Syst Rev* (2):CD000510, 2001.

43. Spragg RG, et al: Effect of recombinant surfactant protein c-based surfactant on the acute respiratory distress syndrome, *N Engl J Med* 351:884, 2004.

44. Stevens TP, et al: Early surfactant treatment with brief ventilation vs selective surfactant and continued mechanical ventilation for preterm infants with or at risk of respiratory distress syndrome, *Cochrane Database Syst Rev* (3) CD003063, 2004.

44a. SUPPORT Study Group of the Eunice Kennedy Shriver NICHD Neonatal Research Network. Early CPAP versus surfactant in extremely preterm infants, *N Engl J Med* 362:1970, 2010.

45. Tomaszewska M, et al: Pulmonary hemorrhage: clinical course and outcomes among very low-birth-weight infants, *Arch Pediatr Adolesc Med* 153:715, 1999.

46. Tyson JE, et al: Thromboatheromatous complications of umbilical arterial catheterization in the newborn period, *Arch Dis Child* 51:744, 1976.

47. Van Overmeire B, et al: A comparison of ibuprofen and indomethacin for closure of patent ductus arteriosus, *N Engl J Med* 343:674, 2000.

48. Whitsett JA, et al: Genetic disorders influencing lung formation and function at birth, *Hum Mol Genet* 13:R207, 2004.

49. Widness JA, et al: Clinical performance of an in-line point-of-care monitor in neonates, *Pediatrics* 106:497, 2000.

PART 4

Assisted Ventilation and Its Complications

Steven M. Donn and Sunil K. Sinha

Mechanical ventilation has been used to treat neonatal respiratory failure for nearly a half century. The earliest applications began as modifications of adult ventilators, treating babies of modest size and prematurity by today's standards.[21] Most devices were time-cycled, pressure-limited ventilators. Landmark advances in respiratory care occurred in the 1970s. Antenatal corticosteroids were shown to enhance fetal lung maturity, and transcutaneous oxygen monitoring taught much about the vulnerability of the preterm infant. The 1980s brought pulse oximetry and high-frequency ventilation (HFV), which greatly expanded the therapeutic armamentarium. The surfactant replacement era began in the 1990s and was accompanied contemporaneously by patient-triggered ventilation, real-time pulmonary graphics, and a host of pharmacologic agents. Finally, in the new millennium, the microprocessor was incorporated into neonatal ventilators to greatly expand capabilities, monitoring, safety, and efficacy. This technological revolution has extended survival to infants born extremely prematurely as well as those with severe pulmonary disease that was heretofore lethal.

Mechanical ventilation can now be provided in many permutations. Clinicians can alter target variables, waveforms, cycling mechanisms, and modes simply by adjusting a dial. This has led to the development of disease-specific strategies to deal with the wide spectrum of neonatal respiratory failure. Similar to the rapidity of change in the computer industry, advances have been rapid and are often introduced into clinical practice without much of an evidence base, causing further confusion and consternation. This chapter reviews the classification and principles of both noninvasive ventilation and mechanical ventilation, with an emphasis on nomenclature and terminology.

CONTINUOUS POSITIVE AIRWAY PRESSURE AND NONINVASIVE VENTILATION

Although mechanical ventilation is the primary treatment for respiratory failure in most preterm babies, there is a concern that it is a major contributor to lung injury. This has led to a growing interest in noninvasive forms of respiratory support in the belief that this will reduce the need for mechanical ventilation and its associated complications. The two major types of noninvasive neonatal respiratory support modalities are continuous positive airway pressure (CPAP) and nasal intermittent positive pressure ventilation (NIPPV). One other form of noninvasive respiratory support is continuous negative extra thoracic pressure (CNEP) but its use has been largely abandoned.

Physiology of Continuous Positive Airway Pressure

When used to treat respiratory distress syndrome (RDS), CPAP prevents collapse of the alveoli at end expiration, maintaining some degree of alveolar inflation. It thus decreases the work of breathing in accordance with LaPlace's law, in which the pressure required to overcome the collapsing forces generated by surface tension is reduced because the radius of curvature is greater when the alveolus is partially inflated. In this way, CPAP helps maintain functional residual capacity (FRC) and facilitate gas exchange.

CPAP also helps maintain upper airway stability by stenting the airway and decreasing obstruction. It may also augment stretch receptors and decrease diaphragmatic fatigue, and thus be useful in treating apnea of prematurity.

Complications of Continuous Positive Airway Pressure

Excessive CPAP may contribute to lung overinflation and increase the risk for air leaks. It can increase intrathoracic pressure and decrease venous return and cardiac output. If set too high, CPAP may result in carbon dioxide retention and impaired gas exchange. Gastric distention is a commonly encountered problem and can be at least partially alleviated by placement of an orogastric tube.

Care must be taken to avoid soft tissue injury, particularly to the nasal mucosa, nasal septum, and philtrum. Complications may also be associated with the fixation devices. Earlier reports of cerebellar hemorrhage associated with occipital fixation led to the virtual abandonment of CPAP for nearly two decades.

Nasal Continuous Positive Airway Pressure

CPAP is a form of continuous distending pressure (CDP), which is defined as the maintenance of increased transpulmonary pressure during the expiratory phase of respiration. When positive pressure is applied to the airways of spontaneously breathing infants, it is called continuous positive airway pressure, whereas distending pressure applied to a mechanically ventilated infant is called positive end-expiratory pressure (PEEP). Thus both CPAP and PEEP are types of CDP

(although not technically a form of ventilation), which provide low-pressure distention of the lungs and prevent the collapse of alveoli at the end of expiration. CDP helps maintain FRC and thus facilitates gas exchange throughout the respiratory cycle. CPAP also supports the breathing of premature infants in a number of other ways including abolition of upper airway occlusion and decreasing upper airway resistance, enhancement of diaphragmatic tone and activity, improvement in lung compliance and decrease in lower airway resistance, increase in tidal volume delivery by improving pulmonary compliance, conservation of surfactant at the alveolar surface, and reduction in alveolar edema.[52]

CPAP may be administered invasively through an indwelling endotracheal tube, or it may be provided noninvasively using a variety of different nasal interfaces. This is referred to as nasal CPAP (NCPAP). Long nasopharyngeal tubes are still used in some centers but have the disadvantage of high resistance and therefore a large reduction in delivered pressure. They are also difficult to suction. Single nasal prongs are usually cut from endotracheal tubes and passed 1 to 2 cm into one nostril with about 3 cm residing externally. Although resistance is usually less than with nasopharyngeal tubes, it is still high with this device and there is a loss of pressure from the other nostril. Nasal masks are now used in the belief that they reduce trauma to the nostrils. However, it is often difficult to produce a good seal without undue pressure, which may still cause injury in the region between the nasal septum and the philtrum. Short binasal prongs are available in several designs; all have two short tubes that provide the least resistance of any other nasal interface. Current meta-analysis shows that short binasal prongs are more effective at maintaining extubation and preventing reintubation than single nasal prongs.[22]

Methods of Generating Continuous Positive Airway Pressure

See Box 44-4.

The gas mixture delivered by CPAP is derived from either continuous or variable flow. Continuous flow CPAP consists of gas flow generated at a source and directed against the resistance of the expiratory limb of the circuit. Ventilator-derived CPAP and bubble or underwater CPAP are examples of continuous flow devices, whereas infant flow drivers (flow-driven CPAP) and Benveniste valve CPAP are examples of variable-flow devices.

Flow-Driven Continuous Positive Airway Pressure

Flow-driven CPAP is a prototype of variable-flow CPAP. It uses a dedicated flow driver and gas generator with a fluidic-flip mechanism to deliver variable-flow CPAP. The principle is the Bernoulli effect, which directs gas flow toward each nostril, and the Coanda effect, which causes the inspiratory flow to flip and leave the generator chamber via the expiratory limb during exhalation. This assists spontaneous breathing and reduces the work of breathing by lowering expiratory resistance and maintaining stable airway pressure. Flow-driven CPAP can be delivered using binasal prongs or a nasal mask.

BOX 44–4	Methods of Providing Continuous Positive Airway Pressure

Ventilator-derived CPAP
Flow-driven CPAP
Bubble (underwater) CPAP
High-flow nasal cannula CPAP

BOX 44–5	Clinical Indications for Continuous Positive Airway Pressure

Delivery room resuscitation
Management of respiratory distress syndrome
Postextubation support
Apnea
Mild upper airway obstruction

Bubble Continuous Positive Airway Pressure

Underwater bubble continuous positive airway pressure (BCPAP) is a continuous flow system used since the early 1970s. In this method, the blended gas is heated and humidified, and then delivered to the infant through a secured low-resistance nasal prong cannula. The distal end of the expiratory tubing is immersed underwater and the CPAP pressure generated is equal to the depth of immersion of the CPAP probe. It has also been proposed that chest vibrations produced by the bubbling may contribute to gas exchange. BCPAP is an effective and inexpensive option to provide respiratory support to premature babies. In a recent randomized, controlled trial, BCPAP was found to be at least as effective as flow-driven CPAP in postextubation management of babies with respiratory distress syndrome.[41]

Ventilator-derived CPAP is another conventional way to administer continuous flow CPAP. The CPAP is increased or decreased by varying the ventilator's expiratory orifice diameter. The exhalation valve works in conjunction with other controls, such as flow control and pressure transducers, to maintain the CPAP at the desired level.

High-Flow Nasal Cannula

Flow of gas in excess of 2 L/min through a small nasal cannula provides some degree of CPAP. Because it is easy to use, utilization of this technique has increased in many units. However, the major problem with this technique is that the CPAP level is usually not measurable in clinical practice and has been shown to be highly variable depending on the leak at the nose or mouth.[52] Nasal leaks are indeed problematic, because the nasal cannula fits loosely in the nostrils. The reintubation rate in babies receiving high-flow nasal cannula CPAP is significantly higher compared with rates for NCPAP. A recently introduced device, which provides CPAP by using heated and humidified gas at very high flow rates (e.g., 7 L/min) had some degree of popularity until problems with infection and air leak were found.

Clinical Indications for Continuous Positive Airway Pressure in Newborns

See Box 44-5.

The clinical use of NCPAP in the neonate falls into one of several groups: (1) early use in resuscitation, (2) management of RDS, (3) postextubation care, (4) treatment of apnea, and (5) management of mild upper airway obstruction.

The only randomized trial of CPAP for resuscitation of newborns was conducted by Finer and colleagues in 2004. About 50% of infants required intubation for resuscitation, which was not affected by the use of CPAP or PEEP. The need for intubation was mostly dependent upon gestational age,

with 100% of infants at 23 weeks and only 18% of infants at 27 weeks requiring intubation. By 7 days of age, 80% of infants had required intubation.[35]

With respect to the management of RDS, most of the available data arose from observational studies and suggest that CPAP may obviate the need for surfactant and avoid intubation in some babies. Most of the data are from the era preceding both surfactant and the widespread use of antenatal steroids. Since then, there have been a number of controlled trials, but they are either small in number or have used different protocols, making it difficult to derive meaningful conclusions. A recent multicenter international randomized trial suggests that NCPAP may be an acceptable alternative to endotracheal intubation in the delivery room but a number of issues remain unresolved.[53] Pneumothorax developed in three times as many babies receiving CPAP than in those who were intubated. Longer-term outcome data of the studied infants are not yet available. An alternative strategy of intubation, surfactant administration, and rapid extubation to NCPAP has shown equivalent outcomes to a prophylactic surfactant strategy. The SUPPORT study demonstrated that a purely CPAP-based strategy could be effective in very immature babies.[73a]

CPAP is an established method of providing respiratory support following extubation from mechanical ventilation. Multiple studies confirm that postextubation CPAP enhances the success rate of extubation and decreases the need for reintubation.[17,18]

Practical Problems of Nasal Continuous Positive Airway Pressure

Despite its widespread use, a number of problems still persist.[34] Nasal prongs rarely fit tightly into the nostrils, thus resulting in gas leak and inability to maintain a baseline pressure. The set CPAP level is rarely maintained in the pharynx. The best way to reduce nose leak is to ensure that the prongs are of sufficient size to snugly fit the nostrils without making them blanch. A chin strap can be used to reduce leaks around the mouth, but it is not simple to use in practice.

Nasal trauma is also a common problem with NCPAP. It is mostly caused by incorrect positioning of the prongs. To prevent injury, the nasal device must not be pushed up against the columella. Selection of appropriate size prongs, constant nursing vigilance, and attention to correct positioning are necessary to prevent nasal injury during NCPAP.

Noninvasive Nasal Ventilation

Methods of noninvasive ventilation include nasal intermittent positive pressure ventilation (NIPPV), synchronized nasal intermittent positive pressure ventilation (SNIPPV), and synchronized bilevel CPAP (SiPAP). In all of these modalities, ventilator inflations augment NCPAP while PEEP, peak inspiratory pressure (PIP), respiratory rate, and inspiratory time can all be manipulated. Terminology used to describe NIPPV is not standardized and may be confusing. SiPAP, a form of NIPPV, is also termed *biphasic* or *bilevel nasal CPAP*. There are no clinical trials to confirm that a bilevel approach to noninvasive respiratory support with SiPAP is more beneficial than the conventional NCPAP.

The mechanism of action of NIPPV remains unclear. It is not known whether mechanical inflations during NIPPV are transmitted to the lungs; clinical studies show contradictory results. Other trials also found no differences in tidal volume or minute volume when comparing NCPAP with SNIPPV. Similarly, there are conflicting reports on work of breathing, pulmonary mechanics, and thoracoabdominal synchrony during comparisons of NCPAP with SNIPPV.[20] The availability of synchronized NIPPV has decreased because the sole device capable of providing it has been withdrawn from the market.

Clinical Indications for Nasal Intermittent Positive Pressure Ventilation

Several studies have compared nonsynchronized NIPPV with NCPAP for treatment of apnea in premature infants, but showed no advantage of NIPPV over NCPAP. Trials have also compared SNIPPV with NCPAP following extubation and found a significant reduction in extubation failure using SNIPPV. Studies have also assessed NIPPV as a primary strategy to treat RDS while avoiding intubation. These studies reported improved carbon dioxide removal, reduced apnea, and shorter duration of ventilation in the NIPPV group. Nonetheless, these are small studies, and they used sufficiently different protocols to prevent generalizable conclusions. Moreover, the understanding of, and evidence for, NIPPV is limited. Large controlled studies are needed to resolve this conundrum.

INDICATIONS FOR ASSISTED VENTILATION

Mechanical ventilation is intended to take over or assist the work of breathing in babies who are unable to support effective pulmonary gas exchange on their own. The causes for respiratory insufficiency may be pulmonary, such as respiratory distress syndrome or meconium aspiration syndrome, extrapulmonary, such as airway obstruction or compression, or neurologic, such as central apnea or neuromuscular disease. Respiratory failure may also accompany other system derangements, including sepsis or shock.

Indications for assisted ventilation may be thought of as absolute and relative (Box 44-6). Absolute indications include entities encountered in the delivery room, such as the failure to establish spontaneous breathing despite bag and mask ventilation, persistent bradycardia despite positive pressure ventilation by mask, or the presence of major anomalies, such as diaphragmatic hernia or severe hydrops fetalis, wherein there is a high likelihood of immediate respiratory failure. In the neonatal intensive care unit, sudden respiratory or cardiac collapse with apnea and bradycardia unresponsive to mask ventilation and massive pulmonary hemorrhage are two examples of absolute indications.[39]

BOX 44-6   Indications for Assisted Ventilation

ABSOLUTE INDICATIONS
Failure to initiate or sustain spontaneous breathing
Persistent bradycardia despite bag-mask ventilation
Presence of major airway or pulmonary malformations
Sudden respiratory or cardiac collapse with apnea/
  bradycardia

RELATIVE INDICATIONS
High likelihood of subsequent respiratory failure
Surfactant administration
Impaired pulmonary gas exchange
Worsening apnea unresponsive to other measures
Need to maintain airway patency
Need to control carbon dioxide elimination

Relative indications may be based on clinical judgment, such as intubating very preterm babies for prophylactic or early surfactant administration, or they may be based on an objective assessment of impaired gas exchange as evidenced by abnormal blood gases. Various recommendations exist to define respiratory failure severe enough to warrant assisted ventilation. In general, the easiest of these is the so-called 50-50 rule, wherein hypoxemia is defined as a failure to maintain an arterial oxygen tension of 50 mm Hg with a fraction of inspired oxygen of 0.5 (50%) or greater and hypercapnia is defined as an arterial carbon dioxide tension greater than 50 mm Hg. Some have suggested that the arterial carbon dioxide tension criterion should be coupled with a pH value, such as less than 7.25. Additional relative indications for assisted ventilation include the stabilization of infants who are at risk for sudden deterioration, such as preterm infants with apnea unresponsive to CPAP or methylxanthines, severe systemic illness, such as sepsis, the need to maintain airway patency, such as meconium aspiration syndrome or tracheobronchomalacia, or the need to maintain control of carbon dioxide elimination, such as persistent pulmonary hypertension or following severe hypoxic-ischemic brain injury.

GENERAL PRINCIPLES OF ASSISTED VENTILATION
Oxygenation

The two major factors responsible for oxygenating the blood are the fraction of inspired oxygen and the pressure to which the lung is exposed (Box 44-7). The role of inspired oxygen can be understood from the alveolar gas equation

---

BOX 44-7   Determinants of Oxygenation

Fraction of inspired oxygen
Mean airway pressure
Positive end-expiratory pressure (PEEP)
Peak inspiratory pressure (PIP)
Inspiratory time
Frequency
Gas flow rate

(see Part 2 of this chapter). Oxygenation is also proportional to mean airway pressure (mean Paw), which is the average pressure applied to the lungs during the respiratory cycle and is represented by the area under the curve for the pressure waveform. Inflation of the lung exposes more of the pulmonary surface area to alveolar gas. Thus, those factors that increase mean airway pressure will, up to a certain point, improve oxygenation (Fig. 44-34).[13]

The most direct impact comes from PEEP because it is applied throughout the respiratory cycle. PEEP is the baseline pressure, the lowest level to which airway pressure falls. It is used to take advantage of LaPlace's law, by maintaining some degree of alveolar inflation during expiration, thus reducing the pressure necessary to further inflate the alveolus during inspiration. There is a 1:1 relationship between PEEP and mean Paw: For every cm H_2O increase in PEEP, there is a cm H_2O increase in mean Paw. Excessive PEEP is potentially harmful. It may overdistend the alveoli, increasing the risk of air leaks; it may impede venous return and cardiac output; it may decrease the amplitude, leading to carbon dioxide retention (see later).[11]

PIP also increases the mean Paw, but this is proportional to the inspiratory time (T_1) or duration of positive pressure. PIP is the driving pressure and establishes the upper limit of the amplitude. Excessive PIP poses many of the same risks as excessive PEEP, including hyperinflation (overdistention) of the lung, leading to excessive stretch of the alveolar units (barotrauma or volutrauma); high intrathoracic pressure with decreased venous return and cardiac output; and air leaks. Additionally, if PIP, PEEP, or both are inadequate, there may be alveolar atelectasis and resultant damage to the lung from cyclic opening and closing of lung units, a process referred to as *atelectrauma*.[16]

Mean Paw is also affected by T_1 and the duration of positive pressure. As T_1 increases, the mean Paw also increases if all other parameters are held constant. Similarly, on machines in which the inspiratory/expiratory (I/E) ratio is adjusted, mean Paw increases as the inspiratory phase is lengthened or the expiratory phase is shortened. If the T_1 is too long, however, there is an increased risk of gas trapping, inadvertent PEEP, and air leak. If it is too short, there may be inadequate lung expansion, air hunger, and patient-ventilator asynchrony, leading to inefficient gas exchange.

Changes in the ventilator rate have a slight effect on mean Paw. At faster rates, the mean Paw rises, because there are more breaths delivered per minute, and the cumulative area under the curve per unit of time increases. Rapid rates may result in incomplete emptying of the lung, with gas trapping, inadvertent PEEP, and lung hyperinflation.

Finally, circuit gas flow also impacts mean Paw. If the T_1 is held constant, more volume (and hence higher pressure) is delivered as flow is increased. If the flow is set too high, turbulence, incomplete emptying of the lung, inadvertent PEEP, and hyperinflation may occur.[63] If the flow is set too low, air hunger and asynchrony result. The injurious effects of improper airway flow have been referred to as *rheotrauma*.[25]

Ventilation

Ventilation refers to carbon dioxide removal. Its two primary determinants are tidal volume and frequency (Box 44-8).[11] Tidal volume is determined by the amplitude of the mechanical breath, or the difference between the peak (PIP) and baseline (PEEP) pressures. During conventional mechanical (CMV) ventilation, carbon dioxide removal is the product of tidal volume and frequency. Clinically, this is usually expressed as the minute volume, or mL/kg/min of exhaled gas. It is also important to consider the contribution of spontaneous breathing to minute ventilation (which is not always measured), and that pulmonary bloodflow is also a key element in carbon dioxide removal, as well as oxygenation. During HFV, carbon dioxide removal is the product of frequency and the *square* of the tidal volume.[8] Thus small changes in amplitude may have a profound effect on arterial carbon dioxide tension (see later).

Control of ventilation during patient-triggered ventilation requires an understanding of the physiology of gas exchange. Most newborns have intact chemoreceptors and seek to maintain normocapnia. This is accomplished by adjustments in minute ventilation. Thus if the clinician sets the amplitude too low, the baby compensates by increasing the spontaneous (and hence, triggered) breathing rate. Conversely, if the

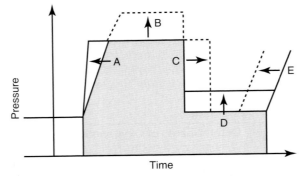

MEAN AIRWAY PRESSURE FACTORS

Figure 44–34. Graphic representation of determinants of mean airway pressure. The mean airway pressure is the area under the curve (*shaded*). Note the effects of increasing the rise time (*A*), peak inspiratory pressure (*B*), inspiratory time (*C*), and positive end-expiratory pressure (*D*), and of decreasing the expiratory time (*E*).

BOX 44–8 Determinants of Alveolar Ventilation

MINUTE VOLUME
Tidal volume
Amplitude (PIP − PEEP)
Frequency

For Conventional Ventilation

Minute Volume = Frequency × Tidal Volume

For High-Frequency Ventilation

Minute Volume = Frequency × (Tidal Volume)^2

EXPIRATORY TIME (OR I/E RATIO)

amplitude is set too high, the infant's hypercapnic drive is abolished and the baby "rides" the ventilator rate.[27]

Carbon dioxide tension is affected by minute ventilation, which in turn is the product of tidal volume and frequency during CMV. Of these two parameters, adjustment in tidal volume (by adjusting the amplitude) has a more predictable effect on minute ventilation.[11]

Time Constant

Use of mechanical ventilators requires an understanding of the pulmonary time constant. The pulmonary time constant refers to the time required to allow pressure and volume equilibration of the lung (see Part 2). Mathematically, the time constant is the product of compliance and resistance. When the lung is stiff (low compliance) and has limited expansibility, such as occurs during RDS, it takes less time to fill and empty than it does at higher compliance. This pattern is clinically illustrated by observing the spontaneous breathing pattern of an infant with RDS not requiring assisted ventilation. Early on, when compliance is poor, the baby breathes rapidly and takes shallow breaths. As the disease process remits, compliance improves, and the baby breathes more slowly and takes deeper breaths.

If expiratory time is set at one time constant, approximately 63% of the change in pressure or volume occurs; if it is lengthened to three time constants, changeover increases to 95%, and at a five time constant length, it approaches 99%. Thus setting the expiratory time at less than three to five times the length of the time constant increases the risk of gas trapping and potentially inadvertent PEEP and alveolar rupture.[12]

Classification of Mechanical Ventilators

Over the past decade, newer mechanical ventilation devices based on sound physiologic principles have been introduced into neonatal practice. The proliferation of devices and techniques has caused confusion about nomenclature and classification, which are frequently device specific. In a general sense, mechanical ventilators can be divided into two groups, those that deliver physiologic tidal volumes, often referred to as *conventional mechanical ventilators*, and those that deliver tidal volumes that are less than physiologic dead space, referred to as *high-frequency devices*.

Among conventional mechanical ventilators, it is advisable to use a simple hierarchical classification to describe devices according to the variables they use (Fig. 44-35). These variables fall into two categories, those that control the type of ventilation (called *ventilatory modalities*) and those that determine the breath type (called *ventilatory modes*).[10,14,37]

Control Variables (Ventilatory Modalities)

At any one time, the ventilator can control only a single variable: time, pressure, or volume. However, the same ventilatory device can operate using different control variables at different times. Ventilatory modalities can target either pressure or volume as the primary variable. Because volume is the integral of flow, volume- and flow-controlled ventilation are actually the same. When pressure is controlled, volume fluctuates according to the compliance of the lungs; conversely, when volume is controlled, pressure fluctuates as a function of compliance.[76]

Phase Variables (Ventilatory Modes)

The mechanical breaths delivered by the ventilator have four phases and more than one variable can be used to design the type of breath to suit the underlying lung mechanics or pathophysiology. The first of these is the variable that initiates or triggers inspiration (trigger). The second is the variable that is used to limit the inspiratory gas flow (limit). The third is the variable that changes inspiration to expiration and vice versa (cycle). The final is the variable that maintains the baseline pressure during expiration (PEEP).[76]

A number of variables can be used to trigger a breath. In the past, most neonatal ventilators used time to start inspiration. The clinician programmed either a set inspiratory time or ventilator rate and inspiratory/expiratory ratio, and the exhalation valve would open and close according to the lapse of time. More recently, other triggering variables have been introduced, allowing for the synchronization of the onset of mechanical breaths to spontaneous breathing. The clinician can set a threshold flow or pressure, above which the ventilator initiates a mechanical breath. These variables are used as a surrogate for spontaneous effort and include pressure or flow, with time as a backup. Most present ventilators use flow-triggering devices because this requires less effort to trigger and is thus associated with less work of breathing.[26]

The limit variable restricts the expiratory flow to a preset value. Traditionally, pressure has been used as a limit variable, but volume and flow are other variables that can limit inspiratory flow. True volume limitation is difficult to achieve

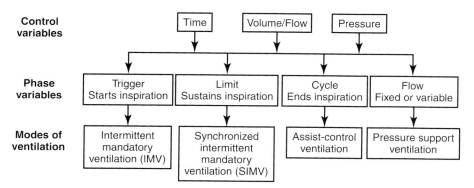

Figure 44–35. Hierarchical classification of conventional mechanical ventilators.

because cuffed endotracheal tubes are not used, and there is almost always some degree of volume loss around the endotracheal tube.

The cycling mechanism is the variable used to end inspiration. Most neonatal ventilators, including high-frequency ventilators, are time-cycled, but changes in airway flow may also be used to end the inspiratory phase.[26] Termination of inspiration occurs when decelerating inspiratory flow has reached a preset percentage of peak inspiratory flow. At this point, the exhalation valve opens and expiration begins. Flow cycling more accurately mimics the physiologic breathing pattern and allows for the mechanical breath to be fully synchronized to the spontaneous breath during both inspiration and expiration. Changes in transthoracic electrical impedance that occur during spontaneous respiration can also be used to generate a trigger signal.[68] Thus triggering during both active inspiration and active expiration can achieve total synchronous breathing between the baby and the ventilator.

Modes of Ventilation

Using different phase variables, which are interchangeable, a variety of ventilatory modes can be generated, which are applicable to both pressure- and volume-controlled modalities. The commonly used ventilatory modes are intermittent mandatory ventilation (IMV), synchronized intermittent mandatory ventilation (SIMV), assist/control (A/C) ventilation, and pressure support ventilation (PSV).[42] Figure 44-36 is a graphic comparison of IMV and SIMV demonstrating the effects of asynchronous ventilation.

INTERMITTENT MANDATORY VENTILATION

IMV delivers mechanical breaths at a rate set by the clinician. Breaths are provided at regular intervals and are not influenced by spontaneous breathing. The baby may breathe spontaneously with, between, or even against the mechanical breath, supported only by PEEP, and patient-ventilator dyssynchrony can be a major problem, resulting in a wide variability in delivered tidal volume. Efforts to reduce dyssynchrony include increasing the rate to override the spontaneous drive and "capture" the baby, generous use of sedatives, and, in some instances, the administration of skeletal muscle relaxants.

SYNCHRONIZED INTERMITTENT MANDATORY VENTILATION

Synchronized intermittent mandatory ventilation (SIMV) is a mode in which the onset of mechanical breaths is synchronized to the onset of spontaneous breaths if the patient begins to breathe within a timing window. As a result, mechanical breaths are not delivered as regularly as in IMV, but vary slightly according to the baby's own breathing pattern. In between the mechanical breaths, the baby may breathe spontaneously, but again, the spontaneous breaths are supported only by PEEP unless pressure support is used (see later). In time-cycled SIMV, synchrony between mechanical and spontaneous breathing occurs only during inspiration, because the inspiratory time for both mechanical and spontaneous breaths may be different. This discrepancy can be offset by using flow cycling, in which synchrony occurs during both inspiration and expiration.

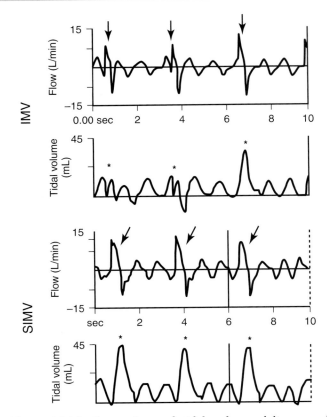

Figure 44–36. Comparison of tidal volume delivery and flow during intermittent mandatory ventilation (IMV) and synchronized intermittent mandatory ventilation (SIMV). Note the tremendous variability in delivered tidal volume (noted by *asterisks*) during IMV breaths (*vertical arrows*) as compared to SIMV breaths (*diagonal arrows*). Dyssynchronous breathing during IMV leads to inefficient gas exchange.

ASSIST/CONTROL

In the A/C mode, the ventilator delivers a mechanical breath each time the patient's inspiratory effort exceeds the preset threshold criterion. When the patient triggers the ventilator to deliver a mechanical breath, the breath is said to be *assisted*. This mode also provides the safety of a guaranteed minimal mechanical breath rate (the control rate, set by the operator) in case no patient effort occurs or is detected. A/C breaths can be time-cycled or flow-cycled. During A/C ventilation, as long as the baby breathes above the control rate, lowering the control rate has no effect on the total respiratory rate, and thus the reduction of pressure should be the primary weaning strategy (see later).[62]

PRESSURE SUPPORT VENTILATION

Pressure support ventilation was developed to help intubated patients overcome the imposed work of breathing created by the narrow lumen (high resistance) endotracheal tube, circuit dead space, and demand valve (if one is being used). It is, however, a *spontaneous* breath mode. Spontaneous breaths that exceed the trigger threshold result in the delivery of additional inspiratory pressure to a limit set by the clinician.

These breaths are flow-cycled, but for safety purposes they may be time-limited. PSV is most commonly used in conjunction with SIMV to support spontaneous breathing between SIMV breaths with something more substantial than PEEP (Fig. 44-37). If the pressure limit of the PSV breath is adjusted to provide a full tidal volume breath, it is referred to as PS_{max}. If the pressure applied is just enough to overcome the imposed work of breathing, it is referred to as PS_{min}. PSV is a relatively new neonatal mode and is being actively explored. It appears that it is most commonly used as a weaning strategy with low-rate SIMV.[60]

Pressure-Targeted Modalities

Pressure-targeted modalities are characterized by limiting the amount of pressure that can be delivered during inspiration. The clinician sets the maximum pressure and the ventilator does not exceed this level. The volume of gas delivered to the baby varies according to lung compliance and the degree of synchronization between the baby and the ventilator. If compliance is low, less volume is delivered than if compliance is high.[61] In IMV, tidal volume fluctuates depending on whether the baby is breathing with the ventilator or against it.

There are three main pressure targeted modalities: pressure-limited ventilation (PLV), pressure control ventilation (PCV), and pressure support ventilation (PSV), which is also a mode. All three are pressure-limited. Some devices allow both PLV and PCV to be time- or flow-cycled. PSV is flow-cycled but time-limited. Inspiratory flow during PLV is continuous and is set by the clinician. During both PCV and PSV, inspiratory flow is variable and is related to lung mechanics and patient effort. It accelerates rapidly early in inspiration, then decelerates quickly, producing a characteristic waveform.[23] Some devices allow modulation of the accelerating portion by offering an adjustable rise time. This enables "fine tuning" of flow to avoid pressure overshoot or flow starvation and helps achieve optimal hysteresis of the pressure-volume loop.

PLV has been used to treat neonatal respiratory failure for almost a half century. It was developed from adult ventilators by adding continuous flow to the bias circuit to allow the baby to have a fresh source of gas from which to breathe between mechanical breaths. It is relatively easy to use and was presumed to be safe because the delivered inspiratory pressure could be limited, thus reducing the risks associated with barotrauma. Although the inspiratory pressure is very consistent on a breath-to-breath basis, the delivered tidal volume fluctuates. In the postsurfactant era, lung compliance may vary considerably following the administration of surfactant, and unless the clinician is vigilant, increasing tidal volume can lead to overexpansion and volutrauma.

PCV was recently introduced into neonatal ventilators. It differs from PLV primarily in the manner in which flow is regulated. This produces a waveform that accelerates then decelerates rapidly. A rapid rise in flow early in inspiration leads to earlier pressurization of the ventilator circuit and delivery of gas to the baby early in inspiration. Intuitively, this should be beneficial in disease states characterized by homogeneity and the need for a higher opening pressure, such as RDS. Variable flow should be advantageous when resistance is high, such as when a small endotracheal tube is used. The relative novelty of PCV has thus far precluded adequate comparison to PLV.

Both PLV and PCV are used as mandatory modes (IMV, SIMV) or A/C. PSV is a spontaneous mode; that is, it is applied to spontaneous breaths the baby takes between mandatory mechanical breaths to support spontaneous breathing and overcome the imposed work of breathing created by the narrow lumen endotracheal tube, circuit dead space, and

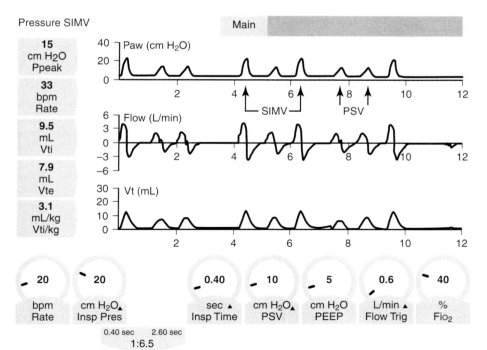

Figure 44-37. Graphic representation of the combined use of synchronized intermittent mandatory ventilation (SIMV) and pressure support ventilation (PSV), in which additional inspiratory pressure is applied to spontaneous breaths to help overcome the imposed work of breathing.

demand valve (if one is used). Because it is patient-triggered and flow-cycled, it is completely synchronized to the baby's own breathing; thus the baby controls the rate and the inspiratory time. The clinician sets the pressure level to augment spontaneous breathing. PSV can be used in conjunction with SIMV, or in patients with reliable respiratory drive, it may be used as a primary modality.[24] There is an evolving body of evidence that PSV is both safe and efficacious.* Still to be determined is the best way to apply PSV as a weaning tool. Table 44-2 compares the characteristics of pressure-targeted modalities.

Volume-Targeted Modalities

Broadly speaking, volume-targeted ventilation can be provided in several ways. Volume controlled ventilation (VCV), targets a set tidal volume, which is delivered irrespective of lung compliance or the pressure required to deliver it (pressure may be limited for safety reasons). Hybrid ventilators are essentially pressure-targeted but aim to deliver the tidal volume within a set range using computer-controlled feedback mechanisms. Finally, standard pressure-targeted ventilation can function in a quasi volume-targeted capacity if strict and vigilant attention is paid to volume delivery.[19]

VOLUME-CONTROLLED VENTILATION

The first ventilator designed specifically for volume-targeted ventilation in infants was the Bourns LS 104-150, which was modified from an adult ventilator. Because of many problems, including a high trigger sensitivity, long response times, and lack of continuous flow during spontaneous breathing, limited rate, poor circuit design, and the inability to measure the small tidal volumes, this device (and VCV) fell out of favor in the early 1980s. Technological advances in the 1990s enabled reintroduction of VCV to neonatal and pediatric patient populations. The new ventilators incorporate sophisticated devices to trigger, deliver, and accurately measure the tiny tidal volumes required by infants weighing as little as 500 g.

VCV for newborns differs from "adult" volume-cycled ventilation, in which inspiration is terminated and the machine is cycled into expiration when the specific target tidal volume has been delivered. However, the use of uncuffed endotracheal tubes in newborns results in some degree of gas leak around the tube and precludes the ability to cycle based on a true delivered tidal volume. Thus *volume cycling* is a misnomer in neonatal ventilation, and the terms *volume-controlled, volume-targeted,* or

volume-limited better describe this modality. Many current ventilators provide the option of using a leak compensation algorithm to at least partially offset this problem.

During VCV, there is also a discrepancy between the volume of gas leaving the ventilator and that reaching the proximal airway which results from compression of gas within the ventilator circuit. This is referred to as compressible volume loss, which is greatest when pulmonary compliance is lowest. The use of semirigid circuits may help offset this. Compressible volume is also affected by humidification. It is, therefore, critical that the delivered tidal volume is measured as close to the proximal airway as possible.

The principal feature of VCV is that it delivers the set tidal volume regardless of the underlying lung compliance by automatically adjusting the PIP (Fig. 44-38). Another important feature of VCV that differentiates it from PLV is the way that gas is delivered during the inspiratory phase.[74] In traditional VCV, a square flow waveform is generated and peak volume and pressure delivery are achieved at the end of inspiration (Fig. 44-39). These may be thought of as "back end" loaded breaths. In comparison, in PLV, the gas flow pattern accelerates rapidly, then decelerates, resulting in the achievement of peak pressure and volume delivery early in inspiration. This produces a "front end" loaded breath. Because these are very different, certain disease states might be more amenable to one form than the other.

Detractors of VCV have argued that, unlike the limited pressure used in PLV, VCV may use a high inflation pressure to deliver the preset volume in cases of decreased compliance. This anxiety in the past arose because of the perceived risks of barotrauma and its consequences associated with high PIP. However, because it has become clear that it is not necessarily the high pressure but rather the excessive tidal volume (volutrauma) that causes lung injury,[31] attention to controlling tidal volume delivery has become an essential part of neonatal ventilation. It should also be realized that high peak pressure associated with fixed-flow delivery in VCV is a reflection of proximal airway pressure rather than alveolar pressure. When the compliance of the patient's lungs improves (increases), the ventilator generates less pressure to deliver the same tidal volume, thus leading to an automatic reduction of the PIP. It is also a misconception that pressure-limited ventilation of infants is superior to VCV because it maintains a constant airway pressure in the presence of leaks around uncuffed endotracheal tubes. The reasoning seems to be that constant pressure implies that the delivered volume remains constant, but this is not true in that leaks around the uncuffed endotracheal tube also occur with PLV. Some VCV devices provide a way to compensate for leaks by adding

*References 10, 14, 37, 40, 45, 59.

TABLE 44-2	**Characteristics of Pressure-Targeted Modalities**		
Parameter	Pressure-Limited	Pressure Control	Pressure Support
Limit variable	Pressure	Pressure	Pressure
Inspiratory flow	Fixed	Variable	Variable
Cycle mechanism	Time or flow*	Time or flow*	Flow (time-limited)

*Device specific; not available on all machines.

PRESSURE VS. VOLUME
(CONTROL VARIABLES)

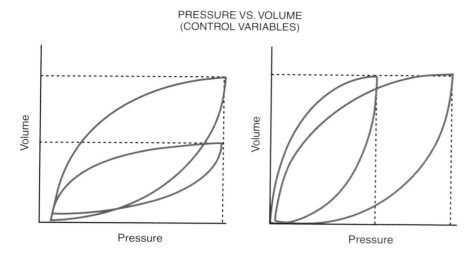

Figure 44–38. Responses to changes in compliance in pressure versus volume-targeted ventilation. In pressure-targeted ventilation, change in pulmonary compliance results in a change in delivered tidal volume, whereas pressure remains constant (left). In volume-targeted ventilation, changes in compliance result in a change in pressure, while delivered tidal volume remains constant (right).

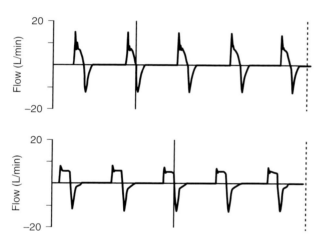

Figure 44–39. Flow waveforms for pressure-targeted *(top)* and volume-targeted *(bottom)* ventilation. Pressure-targeted ventilation produces a spiked waveform with rapid acceleration and deceleration of flow, producing peak pressure and volume delivery early in inspiration. Volume-targeted ventilation produces a characteristic "square wave," with constant or plateau flow. This results in peak pressure and volume delivery at the end of inspiration.

additional flow to the circuit to automatically maintain a stable baseline pressure.

VCV, like PLV, can be provided as IMV, SIMV, and A/C ventilation. It may also be combined with PSV during SIMV and even A/C in some devices.[61]

Hybrid Volume Targeted Ventilation

Some newer devices use a blended approach to volume targeting. They are primarily pressure-targeted ventilators but involve computerized servocontrolled ventilation, in which a ventilator algorithm adjusts the rise and fall of pressure to produce tidal volume delivery within a set range. These include Volume Guarantee (VG), Pressure Regulated Volume Control (PRVC), and Volume Assured Pressure Support (VAPS). VG and PRVC use the tidal volume of previous

breaths as a reference, but follow-up adjustments in PIP take place on four to six breath averages. VAPS makes intrabreath adjustments of pressure, inspiratory time, or both until the desired volume has been provided. These hybrid forms try to achieve the same goal, the optimization of tidal volume delivery, although each has a different mechanism. Clinicians must familiarize themselves with the specific features of individual machines in order to maximize safety and efficacy.

VOLUME GUARANTEE VENTILATION

VG ventilation is a commonly used form of volume targeting.[46] It is a dual-loop, synchronized, pressure-targeted modality of ventilation with microprocessor-based adjustments in pressure to ensure adequate tidal volume delivery. The operator chooses a target tidal volume and selects a pressure limit up to which the inspiratory pressure (the working pressure) may be adjusted. The machine uses the exhaled tidal volume of the previous breath as a reference to adjust the working pressure up or down over the next few breaths to achieve the target volume. The auto-feedback mechanism is an improvement in design but has some limitations. For example, as adjustments to PIP are made in small increments to avoid overcompensation, and as adjustments are based on the exhaled tidal volumes, the delivered tidal volume may not compensate for large breath-to-breath fluctuations in the presence of large leaks. Moreover, as catch-up adjustments in pressures occur every few breaths, it may not work if the ventilator rate is set at low levels such as those used during weaning. In this context, the term "guarantee" is somewhat misleading.

VG can only be used in conjunction with patient-triggered modes, that is, A/C, SIMV, and PSV. The inspiratory pressure is set at the upper desired pressure limit. If this pressure is reached and the set tidal volume has not been delivered, an alarm sounds. Automatic pressure changes are made in increments to avoid overcompensation. No more than 130% of the target tidal volume is supposed to be delivered. The usual starting target is a tidal volume of 4 to 5 mL/kg. The pressure limit is set approximately 15% to 20% above the peak pressure needed to constantly deliver the target tidal volume. Most infants can be extubated when they consistently maintain tidal volume at or above the target value with delivered

PIP less than 10 to 12 cm H_2O and with good sustained respiratory effort.

PRESSURE-REGULATED VOLUME CONTROL VENTILATION

PRVC is another modality of ventilation that attempts to combine the benefits of PLV and VCV.[9] It is a flow-cycled modality that offers the variable flow rate of pressure control ventilation with a targeted tidal volume. Like VG, PRVC is also a form of closed loop ventilation in which pressure is adjusted according to the tidal volume delivered. The clinician selects a target tidal volume and the maximum pressure allowed to deliver the tidal volume. The microprocessor of the ventilator attempts to use the lowest possible pressure with a decelerating flow waveform to deliver the set tidal volume. The first breath is delivered at 10 cm H_2O above PEEP and is used as a test breath to enable the microprocessor to calculate the pressure needed to deliver the selected tidal volume based on the patient's compliance. The next three breaths are delivered at a pressure of 75% of the calculated pressure needed. If the targeted tidal volume is not achieved, the inspiratory pressure is increased by 3 cm H_2O for each breath until the desired tidal volume is reached. If targeted tidal volume is exceeded, the inspiratory pressure is decreased by 3 cm H_2O. Inspiratory pressure is regulated by the ventilator between the PEEP level and 5 cm H_2O below the clinician-set upper pressure limit. In PRVC, the pressure is adjusted based on the average of four breaths, so variations in delivered tidal volume still occur.

VOLUME ASSURED PRESSURE SUPPORT VENTILATION

VAPS is a hybrid modality of ventilation that optimizes two types of inspiratory flow patterns (VAPS = PSV + VCV), thus combining the advantages of both pressure and volume ventilation within a single breath and on a breath-to-breath basis.[6] It is best described as *variable flow volume ventilation.* VAPS can be used in either A/C or SIMV modes, or alone in babies with reliable respiratory drive. Spontaneous breaths begin as PSV breaths. The ventilator measures the gas volume delivered when the inspiratory flow has decelerated to the minimal set value. As long as the delivered volume exceeds the desired level (set by the clinician), the breath behaves like a pressure support breath and is flow-cycled. If the preset tidal volume has not been achieved, the breath transitions to a volume-controlled breath; the set flow persists and the inspiratory time is prolonged (and pressure may increase slightly) until the desired volume is reached. VAPS can be used both in the acute phase of respiratory illness, wherein the patient requires a substantial level of ventilatory support, and when a patient is being weaned from the ventilator, especially in the face of unstable ventilatory drive. The optimal flow acceleration varies with patient dynamics, patient demand, and patient circuit characteristics. Pulmonary graphics are an essential tool for making the appropriate adjustments with VAPS.

VOLUME SUPPORT VENTILATION

Volume support ventilation (VSV) is another hybrid modality combining features of PSV and PRVC.[9] It is intended for patients who are breathing spontaneously with sufficient respiratory drive. Similar to PRVC, breath rate, tidal volume, and minute volume are preselected by the clinician; however, inspiratory time is determined by the patient. Like PRVC, the ventilator algorithm increases or decreases the pressure limit by no more than 3 cm H_2O at a time. Adjustments are made in sequential breaths until the target tidal volume is achieved. The flow, pressure, and volume graphics for a volume-supported breath are similar to those of pressure-supported breaths; however, evidence for efficacy of volume support can only be assessed by evaluating sequential graphic presentations over time, as in PRVC. The tidal volume waveform increases in a stepwise fashion until the targeted volume is reached.

PRESSURE AUGMENTATION

Pressure augmentation is a hybrid modality that offers the benefit of matching the patient's flow demand while guaranteeing a minimal tidal volume. Pressure augmentation differs from PRVC in the following ways: (1) the preset tidal volume is only a minimum and the patient can breathe above this level, (2) the minimum tidal volume is guaranteed by adjustment in flow rather than pressure, which is fixed at a preselected level, and (3) adjustment to flow is made within each breath rather than several sequential breaths. Pressure augmentation is interactive with the patient and is dependent upon the patient's flow demand and lung dynamics. Pressure augmentation can be used in either the A/C or SIMV modes, where volume-controlled breaths are selected.

SUGGESTED VENTILATORY MANAGEMENT GUIDELINES

Initiation of pressure targeted ventilation is aimed at achieving adequate pulmonary gas exchange at the least possible pressure. Selection of pressure limited or pressure control ventilation should be based on the pathophysiology of the respiratory failure. When the lungs are very stiff (poor compliance), such as in RDS, and there is a need for a high opening pressure, pressure control may be advantageous because of the rapid pressurization of the ventilator circuit and delivery of gas flow early in inspiration. If parenchymal disease is less heterogeneous, pressure-limited ventilation with slower inspiratory flow may be safer. Rapidly moving gas preferentially ventilates the more compliant areas of the lung, perhaps contributing to ventilation-perfusion mismatch.

Pressure should be adequate to cause a visible rise in the chest wall during inspiration, and adequate breath sounds should be appreciated on auscultation. If measured, tidal volumes should be 4 to 7 mL/kg in preterm infants and 5 to 8 mL/kg in term infants.[55] PEEP is generally initiated at 4 to 6 cm H_2O, although higher levels are sometimes necessary. The selection of a mode is usually based on personal preference, although A/C offers the most support. The rate should be adjusted to normalize minute ventilation and achieve normocapnia.

The inspiratory time should be chosen according to the pulmonary time constant. Small babies with stiff lungs generally require short inspiratory times, which are proportional to birthweight,[70] Care must be taken to avoid gas trapping (see later).

The circuit (bias) flow rate should be adjusted to ensure that it is adequate to meet the PIP within the allotted inspiratory time, but it should not be too high or it may cause turbulence, inefficient gas exchange, inadvertent PEEP, and lung overdistention.

Brief summaries of the clinical management protocol for VCV and VG are listed in Table 44-3. In VCV (see Table 44-3), ventilation is generally initiated in the A/C mode using a desired inspiratory tidal volume of 4 to 8 mL/kg (measured at the proximal endotracheal tube) as the reference range to achieve the target blood gases. However, for monitoring and further adjustments in tidal volume delivery, expired tidal volume should be used as the reference as it provides a more accurate measurement of the gas delivery to the lungs. To start weaning, a combination of low rate SIMV (6 to 20 breaths/min) and PSV to augment spontaneous breathing seems best, because it compensates for the imposed work of breathing. In the beginning, the amount of pressure support should deliver a full tidal volume breath (PS_{max}) and with further improvement in spontaneous breathing, the PSV support can be reduced sequentially until a tidal volume of 3 to 4 mL/kg is reached (PS_{min}). Most babies can be extubated from this level of support if they are showing regular respiratory drive.

In VG, the initial ventilation is started in the synchronized intermittent positive pressure ventilation (SIPPV) mode with a trigger sensitivity set at 1. This may need subsequent adjustment to reduce the effect of leak-induced auto-triggering. The starting tidal volume reference range is 4 to 6 mL/kg, which can be adjusted based on blood gas analyses. It takes between six and eight breaths to reach the targeted tidal volume; the exact number depends upon the respiratory rate. If the PIP being used to deliver the desired tidal volume is several cm H_2O below P_{INSP} (where P_{INSP} is the maximum allowed pressure), then the set P_{INSP} may be left as is. This extra available peak pressure can be used by the ventilator if lung compliance decreases (or resistance increases, endotracheal tube leak increases, or respiratory effort decreases). If the PIP used by the ventilator is close to or equal to the set P_{INSP}, the set P_{INSP} should be increased by at least 4 to 5 cm H_2O. This allows the ventilator some leeway to deliver the desired tidal volume in the event that compliance decreases. Once appropriate levels of tidal volume have been established, weaning should be an "automatic" process, with the amount of pressure deployed by the ventilator to provide the set tidal volume decreasing as the infant recovers. When the peak airway pressure used is very low, the infant may be ready for extubation.[46]

WEANING INFANTS FROM ASSISTED VENTILATION

Weaning is the process in which the work of breathing is shifted from the ventilator to the patient (see Box 44-9). Signs that an infant is ready to be weaned include improved gas exchange, more spontaneous breathing, and greater assumption of the work of breathing by the baby.[29] The most common reason for failure to wean is failure to wean!

There are physiologic requisites for weaning. First, the baby must have adequate spontaneous drive to sustain alveolar ventilation. This can be assessed by observation (how easily the baby appears to be breathing), and measurement of

TABLE 44–3	Suggested Methods for Using Volume-Controlled Ventilation
Initial Mode	Start in volume-assist control mode. Adjust volume at the machine to deliver 4 to 6 mL/kg (measured at proximal endotracheal tube).
Time limit (A/C)	Use flow to adjust inspiratory time to 0.25 to 0.4 second.
Target ABG range	pH: 7.25 to 7.4 Pco_2: 40 to 60 mm Hg Po_2: 50 to 80 mm Hg
Weaning	Wean by reducing volume as tolerated but continue in A/C with control rate to ensure normocapnia and tidal volume delivery at 4 to 6 mL/kg. Switch to SIMV/PS when control rate is less than 30 breaths/min. Load with a methylxanthine.
Weaning to extubation	Decrease SIMV rate to 10 to 20 breaths/min. Decrease pressure support to maintain tidal volume at 3 to 4 mL/kg.
Trial of extubation	Consider when pressure has been weaned to provide 3 to 4 mL/kg tidal volume and baby is breathing spontaneously at low rate SIMV.

ABG, arterial blood gas; A/C, assist/control; SIMV, synchronized intermittent mandatory ventilation.

BOX 44–9 Weaning from Assisted Ventilation

PHYSIOLOGIC REQUISITES
Adequate spontaneous drive
Overcome respiratory system load

ELEMENTS OF WEANING
Maintenance of alveolar ventilation
    Tidal volume
    Frequency
Assumption of work of breathing
Nutritional aspects

IMPEDIMENTS TO WEANING
Infection
Neurologic/neuromuscular dysfunction
Electrolyte imbalance
Metabolic alkalosis
Congestive heart failure
Anemia
Sedatives/analgesics
Nutrition (inadequate calories or excessive non-nitrogen calories)

tidal volume and frequency, and thus calculation (or measurement) of minute ventilation. Second, the baby must be able to overcome the respiratory system load, which can be defined as the forces necessary to overcome the elastic and resistive properties of the lungs and airways.[29] In addition, there are defined elements of weaning (see Box 44-9). Tidal volume determinants include amplitude, inspiratory time gas flow rate, and pulmonary compliance. Frequency determinants include chemoreceptor function, and carbon dioxide production, as well as acid-base balance. Minute ventilation is determined by the product of tidal volume and frequency, and both spontaneous and mechanical components need to be evaluated. The work of breathing refers to the force or pressure necessary to overcome those forces that oppose gas flow and expansion of the lung during inspiration. It may be estimated by the product of pressure and volume or graphically as the integral of the pressure-volume loop; it is thus proportional to compliance, but it may also be elevated if there is increased resistance. It is an indirect measurement of energy expenditure or oxygen consumption. Finally, there are nutritional aspects. Adequate calories need to be provided to fuel the work of breathing and avoid catabolism. However, an excess of nonnitrogen calories may increase carbon dioxide production and impede weaning.[75]

Clinicians should also recognize impediments to successful weaning (see Box 44-9). These should be avoided or treated, if present, to provide the best possible chance for the baby to be successfully weaned and extubated. Adjunctive therapies, including corticosteroids, diuretics, and bronchodilators are often used to facilitate weaning, but only methylxanthines have sufficient evidence to be recommended.[5,43]

Weaning Strategies

Because infants are placed on assisted ventilation for differing reasons and because different primary strategies are used for the different causes of respiratory failure, it is nearly impossible to design a "one size fits all" strategy. It has become even more confusing in the era of patient-triggered ventilation. In earlier times, when IMV was the only available mode, the usual strategy was to sequentially lower the rate and allow the baby to assume a greater burden of gas exchange by spontaneous breathing. During triggered ventilation, as long as the baby breathes above the control rate, lowering the ventilator rate has no effect on gas exchange.

In general, it is probably best to reduce the potentially most harmful parameter first. With the exception of HFOV, it is best to limit changes to one parameter at a time to better assess its impact on the baby's respiratory status. Avoid changes of a large magnitude, and be sure to document the baby's responses to changes, so that subsequent care providers can continue or adjust the plan.

Weaning and Ventilator Modes

For A/C ventilation, the primary strategy should be to decrease the PIP. The PIP should be adjusted to keep tidal volume and P_{CO_2} in a reasonable range. If it is reduced too much, and if alveolar ventilation is inadequate, it is reflected by an increase in the spontaneous (and hence, mechanical) ventilator rate. It has also been suggested that

increasing the assist sensitivity to increase the patient effort to trigger might be an alternative method, but there are no data to date to support this. Babies may be extubated directly from A/C, or they may be switched to SIMV or low rate SIMV with PS.

SYNCHRONIZED INTERMITTENT MANDATORY VENTILATION

The goal of weaning in SIMV is to maintain minute ventilation while reducing the level of mechanical support. This can be accomplished by reductions in either the PIP or the SIMV rate, using the spontaneous rate as the monitored variable. As the SIMV rate is lowered, the baby may require additional support of spontaneous breathing to overcome the imposed work of breathing, either by increasing the PEEP, flow rate, or inspiratory time, or by adding PSV.

SYNCHRONIZED INTERMITTENT MANDATORY VENTILATION AND PRESSURE SUPPORT VENTILATION

The combined use of SIMV and PSV is analogous to A/C ventilation, except that changes can be made independently. Physiologic studies have demonstrated that if spontaneous breaths are fully supported with PSV (sufficient pressure to deliver a full tidal volume breath), lower SIMV rates can be used and weaning is faster.[40] In addition, the PSV breaths are fully synchronized because they are patient-triggered and flow-cycled. If babies demonstrate reliable respiratory drive, PSV can even be used alone as a weaning strategy, with extubation occurring when the delivered tidal volumes are in the 3- to 5-mL/kg range.

ASSESSMENT FOR EXTUBATION

In the past, predictive indices, such as blood gas or pulmonary mechanics testing, have not been adequately sensitive or specific in assessing readiness for extubation.[3,67] Part of the problem is not knowing what will happen to the airway once the endotracheal tube is removed, and obstructive apnea is common. More recently, attention to spontaneous breathing while receiving only endotracheal CPAP has been shown to have a high positive predictive value for successful extubation. This can be accomplished by examining the relationship of spontaneous to mechanical ventilation,[36,77] or simply by observing patient stability during a 10-minute period of CPAP.[44]

Postextubation Care

The care of the infant after extubation usually reflects clinician or institution preference. Most infants are extubated and placed on some form of continuous pressure provided by either nasal CPAP or nasal cannula, with or without supplemental oxygen. Most clinical trials support the use of CPAP to avoid postextubation failure.[18] Prone positioning has also been shown to improve gas exchange, perhaps by stabilizing the chest wall and allowing abdominal viscera to fall away from the diaphragm. Postextubation stridor is a relatively common occurrence from narrowing of the upper airway from swelling. It is usually transient, but it may require reintubation. Some affected infants benefit from inhalational sympathomimetics or a short course of corticosteroids.

HIGH-FREQUENCY VENTILATION

HFV refers to a form of assisted ventilation in which the delivered gas volumes are less than the anatomic dead space volume and are provided to the patient at very rapid rates. During HFV, carbon dioxide removal is the product of frequency and the square of the tidal volume, and thus the pressure required to set the amplitude can be considerably less than that used during conventional mechanical (tidal) ventilation (CMV). In addition, because the inspiratory times are much shorter, the duration of positive pressure is less and the alveoli are potentially exposed to less barotrauma. Because carbon dioxide removal can be achieved at lower amplitudes compared to conventional ventilation, HFV allows the clinician to use a higher PEEP with a wider degree of safety.[8] The two most commonly used forms of HFV are high-frequency jet ventilation (HFJV) and high-frequency oscillatory ventilation (HFOV) (Table 44-4).

HFV has been used to treat lung conditions that have been challenging for CMV, including air leaks, refractory hypoxemia, and respiratory insufficiency after cardiac surgery. It also differs from CMV in not trying to mimic normal spontaneous breathing, and because of its unique flow characteristics, it provides a different pattern of gas distribution within the lungs, where airway resistance, and not compliance, is the major determinant of gas distribution. Because gas flow is more rapid during HFV than during CMV, the gas flow profile is more laminar or parabolic. Thus inspiratory gas tends to remain in the center of the airways, enabling it to penetrate more deeply into the lung and to bypass airway disruptions, such as bronchopleural or tracheoesophageal fistulas,[30] or other thoracic air leaks, such as pneumothorax or pulmonary interstitial emphysema.[48]

Although the basic principles of mechanical ventilation are essentially the same for HFV as for CMV, HFV enables better uncoupling of oxygenation and ventilation. During CMV, adjustments made to improve oxygenation often adversely affect ventilation, and vice versa. This phenomenon is much less apparent during HFV, particularly during oscillatory ventilation.

Although both HFJV and HFOV have been in use for more than 20 years, there is a relative paucity of evidence for either modality. A recent thorough review by Lampland and Mammel summarizes the clinical evidence to date.[50]

High-Frequency Jet Ventilation

HFJV involves pulses of high-velocity gas injected directly into the upper airway, either by a special endotracheal tube adapter (proximally) or a specialized triple lumen endotracheal tube (distally). It is used in tandem with a conventional ventilator, which provides PEEP and can be used to deliver "sigh" breaths and maintain lung expansion.

HFJV is similar to CMV in that inspiration is active and expiration is passive, meaning that exhaled gas flow results from the elastic recoil of the lungs. Theories of gas exchange during HFJV suggest that there may be some facilitation of expiratory gas flow by countercurrent energy imparted by the inspiratory flow. HFJV rates range from 240 to 660 breaths/min, and most commonly rates of 360 to 450 are used in clinical practice. Inspiratory time is usually set at 0.02 second (20 msec). Gas volumes delivered during HFJV are considerably smaller than those delivered during CMV.[47]

Different strategies for using HFJV have been proposed for different diseases. A "low-pressure" strategy is adopted for conditions in which air leak is the predominant pathophysiology. Here, the use of lower PIP allows for healing. If oxygenation is problematic, higher PEEP or more CMV support can be offered. The "optimal volume" strategy is used for conditions in which there is a tendency for the alveoli to collapse, such as RDS. HFJV is used to optimize the lung volume and improve ventilation/perfusion matching. Clinicians must be aware that because two ventilators are being used, there are usually two oxygen blenders, and both must be adjusted when a change in the fraction of inspired oxygen is made.

Clinical experience has demonstrated that HFJV is superior to rapid rate IMV in the management of preterm infants with pulmonary interstitial emphysema.[48] HFJV has also been used to treat other types of intractable air leaks, such as esophageal atresia/tracheoesophageal fistula complicated by RDS.[30] One trial comparing HFJV with IMV for the early management of RDS showed less oxygen dependency at discharge when HFJV was used.[49]

High-Frequency Oscillatory Ventilation

HFOV is another form of HFV. Its major distinguishing feature is the addition of active exhalation, whereby removal of exhaled gas is facilitated by negative pressure applied during expiration. Typical rates vary between 8 and 15 Hz (480 and 900 breaths/min). Depending upon the nature of the device, I/E ratios vary from 1:1 to 1:2, and the clinical implication is that inspiratory times and tidal volumes are very short and small, respectively.

The general principles of mechanical ventilation also apply to the oscillator. Mean Paw is used to inflate the lung and recruit alveoli for oxygenation. This may be thought of as continuous distending pressure, in that the lung remains inflated throughout the respiratory cycle. Ventilation is

TABLE 44–4	Characteristics of High-Frequency Ventilation	
	High-Frequency Jet Ventilation	High-Frequency Oscillatory Ventilation
Rate	360 to 450 breaths/min	480 to 900 breaths/min
Inspiratory time	20 msec	10 to 20 msec
Exhalation	Passive	Active
Tandem CMV	Yes	No
Gas delivery	High-velocity injector	Piston

accomplished by adjusting the amplitude, which in turn regulates gas delivery during inspiration and gas removal during expiration.

HFOV has been used both as a primary device for the initial treatment of respiratory failure, and as a rescue strategy for infants who fail to respond to CMV. Some centers prefer to wean and extubate directly from HFOV, whereas others prefer to transition to and wean from CMV. HFOV appears to be the best way to deliver inhaled nitric oxide because of its ability to recruit lung volume and match ventilation and perfusion.

The major drawback to HFOV is the inability to monitor the baby as closely as is possible with CMV. Proper settings are verified by blood gases, the degree of lung expansion on the chest radiograph, and by an assessment of chest wall movement during HFOV, referred to as the "chest wiggle factor." Because intrathoracic pressure can be high, close attention needs to be paid to cardiac output and perfusion. In addition, care must be taken to avoid gas trapping in babies requiring a high amplitude for adequate ventilation, which can result in the collapse of the smaller airways, described as "choke points," during active exhalation.[15]

MONITORING OF VENTILATED INFANTS

Babies requiring assisted ventilation require close monitoring to assess underlying lung pathology, response to treatment, and surveillance for associated complications. Monitoring may be considered in five broad categories: (1) clinical evaluation, (2) assessment of gas exchange, (3) chest imaging, (4) pulmonary function and pulmonary mechanics testing, and (5) extrapulmonary monitoring to screen for complications known to contribute to neonatal mortality and morbidity.

Clinical Evaluation

Clinical examination of the cardiorespiratory system includes observations for general physical condition, chest wall movement, equality of air entry, and the presence of abnormal sounds such as rales, rhonchi, or heart murmurs. The clinician must evaluate the interaction between positive pressure ventilation and the baby's spontaneous breaths to detect dyssynchrony, which can interfere with gas exchange and lead to gas trapping and air leaks. Rapid shallow breathing and the presence of subcostal/intercostal retractions in ventilated babies may suggest air hunger or increased work of breathing, which can be corrected by adjustments of ventilator parameters. A hyperactive precordium, tachycardia, easily felt peripheral pulses, and the presence of a cardiac murmur appearing on day 2 or 3 suggest a left-to-right shunt through a patent ductus arteriosus (PDA). In contrast, right-to-left shunting causing cyanosis (and desaturation on pulse oximetry) suggests persistent pulmonary hypertension of the newborn. Assessment of cardiac function, blood pressure, and tissue perfusion is an important part of evaluation because these directly affect respiratory status. Blood pressure measurements should be interpreted in conjunction with other indices of tissue perfusion, such as capillary refill time, acid-base status, urinary output, and echocardiographic evaluation of myocardial contractility and cardiac output. Bedside transillumination by a bright fiberoptic light

source applied to the chest wall is a useful and effective way to detect pneumothorax, pneumomediastinum, and pneumopericardium, which may require urgent attention. Other systemic clinical evaluation includes examination of abdomen for tenderness or distention and an assessment of the neurologic status by assessing tone, posture, and movement.

Assessment of Gas Exchange
BLOOD GASES AND ACID-BASE BALANCE

Clinical interpretation of blood gases alone conveys relatively little information and must be interpreted in a clinical context, taking into account factors such as the work of breathing, recent trends, and the stage of illness. For example, a $PaCO_2$ of 65 mm Hg is a genuine source of concern in an infant in the first few hours of life but may be perfectly acceptable in an infant on long-term ventilation for bronchopulmonary dysplasia (BPD). There is also a wide range of "normal" blood gas values, depending upon gestational age, postnatal age, source (arterial, venous, or capillary), and disease state. In most infants with respiratory disease, the goal is not to make blood gases entirely normal, but to keep them within a target range appropriate for the clinical status.

Analysis of gas exchange also requires an understanding of respiratory physiology. Oxygenation is dependent on ventilation-perfusion matching, whereas movement of CO_2 from the blood into the alveoli is dependent on alveolar ventilation (the product of alveolar tidal volume and respiratory rate). The pH of arterial blood is determined primarily by $PaCO_2$, lactic acid (produced by anaerobic metabolism), and buffering capacity, particularly serum or plasma bicarbonate and plasma hemoglobin concentration.

Arterial blood gases remain the gold standard for assessment, but analysis can only be performed intermittently. Moreover, arterial catheters are invasive and intermittent arterial sampling requires skill and is painful for the patient. These limitations have led to increasing acceptance of noninvasive techniques, such as transcutaneous oxygen monitoring ($TcPO_2$) and oxygen saturation monitoring using pulse oximetry. There are no data to show that any one method is superior. A $TcPO_2$ value of more than 80 mmHg is associated with a higher incidence of retinopathy of prematurity. A correlation between $TcPO_2$ and pulse oximetry (SpO_2) showed that oxygen saturation above 92% carries a risk of hyperoxia and thus an increased risk of ROP in preterm babies receiving supplemental oxygen.[66] One disadvantage of pulse oximetry is that it is not reliable in cases of severe hypotension or marked edema. Pulse oximeters measure either functional saturation or fractional saturation, which are device-specific. Before interpreting an SpO_2 reading, the quality of signal should be assessed by observing the accompanying arterial pulse waveform. (See part 2)

The ventilatory parameters that affect oxygenation include FiO_2, PIP, PEEP, inspiratory time, tidal volume, and flow rate. Persistent hypoxemia despite appropriate adjustments in ventilatory parameters may indicate inadequate pulmonary bloodflow or perfusion, or right-to-left shunting. Another important factor which affects arterial oxygen tension is altitude and this is relevant to air transport of sick babies.

Transcutaneous partial pressure of carbon dioxide ($TcPCO_2$) can be measured noninvasively and continuously using a special skin electrode. One of the factors influencing measurements is sensor temperature, which is optimal at 42°C. If $TcPCO_2$ is used in combination with a $TcPCO_2$ sensor, a sensor temperature of 44°C can be used without jeopardizing the precision of the $TcPCO_2$ measurement. $TcPCO_2$ measurements are relatively independent of sensor site and skin thickness. $TcPCO_2$ may be falsely high in severe shock and its precision may be affected if $Paco_2$ is more than 45 mmHg or if arterial pH is less than 7.30, but there is no systemic overestimation or underestimation of $Paco_2$ under these conditions. Sensitivity of $TcPCO_2$ in detecting hypercapnia and hypocapnia is 80% to 90%.

Base Deficit

In the healthy term infant, the base deficit is usually 3 to 5 mEq/L. However, base deficit can vary significantly. In patients with a base deficit between 5 and 10 mEq/L, assuming reasonable tissue perfusion, no acute intervention is generally needed. However, a base deficit greater than 10 mEq/L should prompt a careful assessment of the infant for evidence of hypoperfusion. In most cases, correcting the underlying cause of metabolic acidosis is far more effective and less dangerous than administering sodium bicarbonate.

Capnometry or End-Tidal Carbon Dioxide Monitoring

$ETCO_2$ is an alternative method of measuring carbon dioxide and is called capnometry. Depending on the gas sampling technique, devices are either mainstream or sidestream capnometers. Capnometry measurements are less reliable than $TCPCO_2$ monitoring especially when the ventilation/perfusion relationship is not uniform within the lungs, as in infants with RDS or persistent pulmonary hypertension of the newborn.

Partial pressure of CO_2 is affected by minute ventilation, which in turn is the product of tidal volume and frequency during CMV. Of these two parameters, adjustment in tidal volume (by adjusting the amplitude) has a more predictable effect on minute ventilation changes.

Radiography and Other Chest Imaging

Chest radiography is the most commonly used imaging modality on neonatal intensive care units, both for diagnosing and following the course of a disease process. However, the specificity of chest radiography is poor and should always be interpreted in context with clinical information. The findings on chest radiographs are mostly suggestive of pathology and are not always diagnostic.

Ultrasound is a very popular imaging modality because of its portability and scope of repeated examination without any ionizing radiation. Although use of ultrasound for diagnosis of primary respiratory disorders is limited, it can be used to evaluate diaphragmatic excursion and position in suspected cases of phrenic nerve paresis or paralysis.

Computed tomography and magnetic resonance imaging have limited use in neonatal intensive care units because of practical difficulties but are helpful in certain conditions such as congenital cystic adenomatoid malformation, pulmonary sequestration, or complex congenital heart disease when there is insufficient information from echocardiography (e.g., total anomalous pulmonary venous return). Color Doppler echocardiography is now routinely used for assessment of cardiac function and hemodynamic assessment, which may impact the respiratory status in ventilated infants.

Real-Time Pulmonary Graphic Monitoring

Real-time graphic analysis of pulmonary mechanics in infants receiving assisted ventilation has emerged as a valuable tool to aid clinical decision making. A working knowledge of pulmonary mechanics also improves understanding of pulmonary physiology and pathophysiology. Pulmonary mechanics monitoring consists of measurements of several parameters, which define different aspects of lung function. Specifically, clinicians are interested in the *pressure* necessary to cause a *flow* of gas to enter the airway and increase the *volume* of the lungs. From these variables, several other measures of pulmonary mechanics can also be derived, such as pulmonary *compliance* (Fig. 44-40) and *resistance*, and resistive work of breathing (energetics). From this information, displayed as either numerical values or graphic representations, useful information can be obtained and used for diagnosing specific lung pathology, evaluating the disease progression, and determining therapeutic interventions. Besides assessment of acute respiratory distress and evaluation of mechanical ventilation, other potential benefits of pulmonary graphics include assessment of suitability for weaning and the objective determination of the efficacy of pharmacologic treatments. (See Part 2.)

The two representations of pulmonary graphics most commonly used in clinical practice are waveforms and loops. Both patterns display the relationships between pressure, volume, flow, and time.

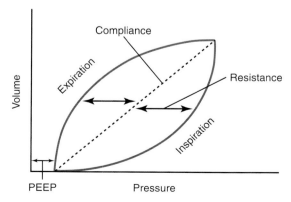

Figure 44–40. Schematic representation of a pressure-volume loop denoting the relationship of pressure, volume, and time.

VOLUME AND PRESSURE WAVEFORMS

Measurement of tidal volume is becoming increasingly important in ventilatory management. The desired inspiratory tidal volume for a ventilated breath ranges from 4 to 7 mL/kg; for spontaneous breaths, a tidal volume of 3 to 4 mL/kg generally indicates suitability for weaning or extubating. Minute ventilation (tidal volume × frequency) is another predictor of weaning, especially in small infants who have short inspiratory times and a higher frequency. Normal values are generally between 240 and 360 mL/kg/min. Breath-to-breath variability and longer term trends are useful in selecting the mode and modality of ventilation and designing individualized strategies based on pulmonary pathophysiology.

FLOW WAVEFORM

Flow is the volume of gas delivered per unit of time. Inspiratory flow is plotted above (positive) and expiratory flow is plotted below the abscissa (negative). The duration and shape of the inspiratory and expiratory flow waveforms are affected by many factors including type of ventilation, I/E ratio, impedance and resistance to gas flow (Fig. 44-41), and the effect of therapeutic agents, such as bronchodilators. The flow waveform can be used to determine if gas trapping is present (Fig. 44-42).

PULMONARY MECHANICS (LOOPS)

Loops are commonly used to demonstrate correlations between airway pressure and volume, and airflow and lung volume. Pressure-volume (P-V) loops graphically depict the correlation between the ventilator inspiratory pressure and the volume of gas entering the lungs on a breath-to-breath basis. A line connecting the points of zero flow (the changeover from expiration to inspiration) is the compliance axis and the slope of this line reflects pulmonary compliance (a measure of the change in volume per unit of added pressure). An estimate of compliance can be made by looking at the slope of the compliance axis; a 45-degree slope indicates a compliance of 1.0. If this slope is more toward vertical, compliance is improving, and conversely, if the axis moves nearer to horizontal, compliance is decreasing. (See also Part 2 of this chapter.)

Increased resistance, as is seen in conditions like meconium aspiration syndrome and BPD, causes a bowing around the compliance line, and is an indirect measure of the work of breathing, which can be estimated by the P-V loop and the area to its left, as measured from the highest point. The P-V loop may also be used to determine the optimal PEEP. Pressure-volume loops that appear "boxlike" indicate the need for a higher opening pressure, and the shape can be normalized by increasing the PEEP and PIP. Another potentially dangerous condition, lung hyperinflation, can also be detected graphically (Fig. 44-43).

Another valuable measurement is resistance. This can be assessed by observing the flow-volume (F-V) loop, which graphically displays the relation between change in volume and change in airflow (Fig. 44-44). A normal flow volume loop should be rounded or oval and should appear symmetrical with respect to the abscissa. Identification and measurement of endotracheal tube leak is possible with graphic monitoring. Increased resistance, and turbulent gas flow from excessive condensation in the ventilator circuit or secretions in the airway can also be identified by the appearance of a noisy flow signal.

Graphic monitoring is largely pattern recognition and should be used to trend data. Appropriate scaling of axes is crucial to proper interpretation. However, if properly calibrated, the real-time breath-to-breath view of pulmonary mechanics and respiratory waveforms allows the clinicians to fine-tune ventilator settings and provides constant surveillance

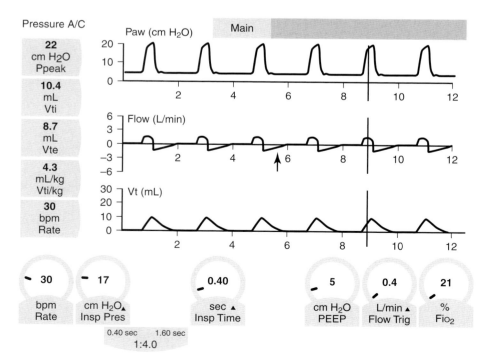

Figure 44–41. Flow waveform center tracing demonstrating high expiratory resistance. Note the decreased peak expiratory flow and the prolonged time to return to baseline (*arrow*).

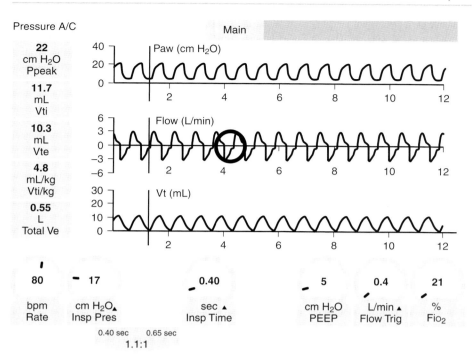

Pressure A/C

22 cm H₂O Ppeak	
11.7 mL Vti	
10.3 mL Vte	
4.8 mL/kg Vti/kg	
0.55 L Total Ve	

80	17	0.40	5	0.4	21
bpm Rate	cm H₂O▲ Insp Pres	sec ▲ Insp Time	cm H₂O PEEP	L/min ▲ Flow Trig	% Fio₂

0.40 sec   0.65 sec
1.1:1

Figure 44–42. Flow waveform showing gas trapping *(circle)*. Note that the expiratory portion of the flow waveform fails to reach the baseline (zero flow state) before the next breath is initiated.

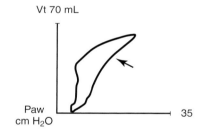

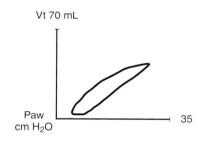

Figure 44–43. Pressure-volume loops. The loop on the left shows hyperinflation. Note the upper inflection point *(arrow)*. Above this point, incremental pressure is producing less change in lung volume per unit pressure than below it. On the right, peak inspiratory pressure has been reduced and the loop shows normal hysteresis.

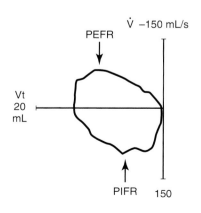

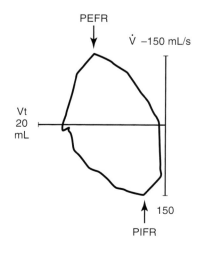

Figure 44–44. Flow-volume loops. On the left, increased resistance produces a smaller loop, with decreased peak inspiratory flow rates (PIFR) and peak expiratory flow rates (PEFR), denoted by *arrows*. On the right, successful treatment with a bronchodilator decreased resistance and improved both PIFR and PEFR.

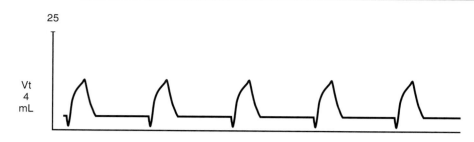

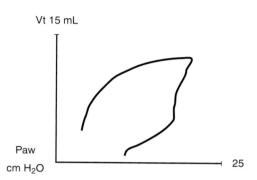

Figure 44–45. Large endotracheal tube leak. Note that the pressure-volume loop (bottom) fails to close, and the volume waveform fails to reach zero (top).

for many potential complications such as gas trapping and lung overdistention before they become clinically apparent. Endotracheal tube leaks may also be detected graphically (Fig. 44-45).

COMPLICATIONS OF ASSISTED VENTILATION

See Box 44-10.

Airway

Placement of an endotracheal tube into the airway can potentially damage the mucosal and submucosal tissues causing injury which can obstruct gas exchange, lead to other functional disabilities, and create cosmetic deformities. Some of these are idiosyncratic, while others relate to the duration of ventilation, frequency of intubations, and associated complications such as infection.

UPPER AIRWAY

Procedural complications of endotracheal intubation are generally traumatic in nature and result from mechanical damage to structures in the nasopharynx or oropharynx, trachea, and larynx. These injuries include superficial mucosal erosion, damage to the alveolar ridge (with subsequent dental problems),[54] perforation of the esophagus[65] or trachea,[69] injury to the vocal cords,[78] and injury related to fixation devices such as tape. Long-term nasotracheal intubation may cause

erosion of the nasal septum and nasal deformities.[38] Acquired palatal grooves[33] and even cleft palate[32] have been described after long-term orotracheal intubation.

TRACHEA

Less serious problems, which tend to resolve spontaneously over time, include tracheal and laryngeal mucosal metaplasia, subglottic cysts, tracheal enlargement, and tracheobronchomalacia. Subglottic stenosis is a life-threatening condition generally requiring tracheostomy. Its etiology is still not completely understood, but associations have been demonstrated for duration of intubation, number of intubations, and the degree of prematurity.[71] Necrotizing tracheobronchitis was another highly lethal acquired entity.[7] This disorder was seen most commonly in the early days of HFJV and was thought to be related to the effects of insufficient humidification of inspired gas. It has all but disappeared since refinements were made in humidification systems.

Lungs

VENTILATOR-ASSOCIATED PNEUMONIA

Ventilator-associated pneumonia (VAP) is a disease entity defined as pneumonia characterized by the presence of new and persistent focal radiographic infiltrates in a ventilated infant appearing more than 48 hours after admission to the neonatal intensive care unit. (See Part 4.)

VAP is a commonly observed complication in babies requiring mechanical ventilation. It results from either

---

BOX 44–10   Complications of Assisted Ventilation

AIRWAY
Upper airway
   Trauma
   Abnormal dentition
   Esophageal perforation
   Nasal septal injury (nasotracheal tubes)
   Acquired palatal groove (orotracheal tubes)
Trachea
   Tracheal and laryngeal mucosal metaplasma
   Subglottic cysts
   Tracheal enlargement
   Tracheobronchomalacia
   Tracheal perforation
   Vocal cord paralysis/paresis
   Subglottic stenosis
   Necrotizing tracheobronchitis

LUNGS
Ventilator-associated pneumonia
Air leaks
   Pneumomediastinum
   Pneumothorax
   Subcutaneous emphysema
   Pulmonary interstitial emphysema
   Pneumopericardium
   Pneumoperitoneum (transdiaphragmatic)
Ventilator induced lung injury
Chronic lung disease/bronchopulmonary dysplasia

MISCELLANEOUS
Imposed work of breathing
Patent ductus arteriosus

NEUROLOGIC
Intraventricular hemorrhage
Periventricular leukomalacia
Retinopathy of prematurity

---

dissemination of microorganisms from colonized mucosal sites or aspiration of gastric contents. Repeated and prolonged endotracheal intubation, as well as suctioning, can disrupt mucosal integrity and promote dissemination. Occasionally microorganisms may be transmitted from contaminated equipment. The reported incidence of VAP is 6.5 cases per 1000 ventilator days. A number of risk factors and associations have been identified, including prematurity; use of corticosteroids, H2 blockers, antacids, and proton pump inhibitors; overcrowding, understaffing; and inadequate disinfection of equipment.

VAP should be suspected in a ventilated infant if there is deterioration in the respiratory status unexplained by other events or conditions. Blood cultures may or may not be positive in infants with VAP. Sepsis and pneumonia should also be considered when there is unexplained temperature instability, hyperglycemia, hypoglycemia, acidosis, feeding intolerance, or abdominal distention. Radiographic findings are nonspecific and may be difficult to distinguish from chronic lung disease in the older baby. Bacterial and fungal pathogens are the most common agents. Tracheal aspirates for culture are not helpful in diagnosis of pneumonia and may merely reflect colonization. Laboratory investigations, such as abnormal blood counts and elevated acute phase reactants, such as C-reactive protein, suggest the diagnosis of sepsis or pneumonia.[58]

Management of VAP includes broad-spectrum antibacterial or antifungal agents, hemodynamic support, and provision of adequate nutrition. Respiratory support should be maintained as necessary. If hypoxemia is refractory despite maximal ventilatory support, consideration should be given to use of inhaled nitric oxide or extracorporeal membrane oxygenation for term and late preterm infants, if they meet criteria. Benefit from the use of additional surfactant is unproven but anecdotal reports suggest efficacy with preparations that contain surfactant proteins A and D. A recent study by Aly and associates suggests that more frequent positioning of babies on their sides, as opposed to supine, may decrease the incidence of VAP.[1]

AIR LEAKS

Thoracic air leaks are collections of pulmonary gas residing outside the pulmonary airspaces. They include pneumothorax, pneumomediastinum, pneumopericardium, pulmonary interstitial emphysema (PIE), pneumoperitoneum, and subcutaneous emphysema. Pneumothorax often results from high inspiratory pressure and unevenly distributed ventilation. The ventilator parameters that are conducive to the development of pneumothorax include (1) a prolonged inspiratory time or an inversed I/E ratio, (2) high PIP or mean Paw, (3) high flow rates, and (4) patient-ventilator asynchrony. There is also higher incidence of pneumothorax in the presence of certain disease conditions such as meconium and other aspiration syndromes, cystic fibrosis, and pulmonary hypoplasia, which are characterized by uneven lung compliance and alveolar overdistention. (See Part 4.)

Pneumothorax in patients receiving positive pressure ventilation can manifest in three ways: (1) asymptomatic, where it is first detected on a routine chest radiograph without or with subtle clinical signs; (2) deterioration in laboratory or bedside monitoring findings, without an obvious change in the patient's clinical condition, but is suspected because of worsening blood gases and increasing ventilatory requirements; and (3) acute clinical deterioration with tension, which is the most common presentation in ventilated infants. Infants with tension pneumothorax present with agitation and increasing respiratory distress, hypotension, and other signs of cardiovascular collapse. Auscultation of the chest reveals diminished or absent breath sounds on the affected side, with a contralateral shift of heart sounds and the point of maximum impulse. Breath sounds on the contralateral side may also be decreased as tension worsens and compresses the unaffected lung. Arterial blood gases may show respiratory or mixed acidosis and hypoxemia. Transillumination reveals increased transmission of light on the involved side. Chest radiography is confirmatory. Tension pneumothorax is a medical emergency and requires prompt treatment. Needle aspiration (thoracentesis) can be used as a temporizing measure, but generally needs to be followed by placement of a chest tube (thoracostomy) for resolution. Smaller gas collections may resolve spontaneously without further intervention but are likely to recur with ongoing mechanical ventilation.

The incidence of pneumothorax has diminished over the years. This may be related to a number of factors including antenatal corticosteroid treatment, surfactant therapy, and the increased use of prenatal ultrasound, which has enabled the diagnosis of conditions like congenital diaphragmatic hernia/pulmonary hypoplasia with predisposition to pneumothorax. Various ventilatory strategies have also been employed to reduce the risks of air leak. Rapid rate IMV (more than 60 breaths/min) has been used to decrease inspiratory time and the duration of positive pressure (and hence tidal volume), and to produce less asynchronous breathing. However, rapid rate ventilation can also cause inadvertent PEEP and gas trapping. Synchronized ventilation, such as SIMV or A/C, may reduce the incidence of air leak by avoiding patient-ventilator asynchrony. The use of flow cycling enables complete synchronization, even during expiration. In rare instances, neuromuscular paralysis may be needed when a patient is actively "fighting" the ventilator despite adequate sedation.

Pulmonary interstitial emphysema often precedes the development of pneumothorax and can be localized or widespread throughout one or both lungs. It develops when the most compliant portion of the terminal airway ruptures, allowing gas to escape into the interstitial space. Gas may accumulate in the interstitium, compressing both the airway and adjacent alveoli. PIE alters pulmonary mechanics by decreasing compliance, increasing resistance, contributing to gas trapping, and increasing ventilation-perfusion mismatch. PIE also impedes pulmonary blood-flow. Diagnosis is based on the chest radiograph, which shows fine linear or radial radiolucencies. Unilateral PIE that is less severe may respond to decubitus positioning. Left-sided PIE may be alleviated by selective intubation of the right main bronchus if the infant can tolerate single lung ventilation. Management of generalized PIE should aim to reduce inspiratory time and pressure. An often used strategy is to increase the PEEP in an attempt to stent the airways and allow more complete emptying of the alveoli during expiration. Alternatively, HFJV has been shown to decrease time to resolution and to improve survival in infants with very low birthweight, compared with rapid rate IMV.[48]

Pneumomediastinum is usually of little clinical importance and usually does not need to be drained. However, its presence should alert the clinician of an increased risk for subsequent symptomatic air leaks. Symptomatic infants are often placed in 100% oxygen for up to 24 hours (nitrogen washout). Although this may make the infant more comfortable and potentially decrease the air leak, there is no evidence to support the practice.

Pneumopericardium occurs when air from the pleural space or mediastinum enters the pericardial sac through a defect that is often located at the reflection near the ostia of pulmonary veins. The diagnosis should be suspected from rapid clinical deterioration, which includes respiratory compromise and cardiovascular collapse, with a narrow pulse pressure and diminished perfusion. It can be diagnosed by transillumination and confirmed by radiography, which shows the air completely encircling the heart. Cardiac tamponade is a life-threatening event and requires immediate drainage. Needle aspiration (pericardiocentesis) via the subxiphoid route may be used to drain the air as a temporizing measure, but a pericardial drain is usually necessary. The majority of cases occur in infants ventilated with high PIP, high mean Paw, and long inspiratory time.

Pneumoperitoneum usually results from rupture or perforation of an abdominal viscus, but on rare occasions, gas from a thoracic leak can dissect transdiaphragmatically to an abdominal location. Recognition of this phenomenon can avoid an unnecessary laparotomy. A sample of the abdominal gas may be aspirated by abdominal paracentesis and analyzed for its oxygen concentration (if the baby is receiving more than room air). If the FiO_2 is greater than 0.21, the likely source is thoracic.

VENTILATOR-INDUCED LUNG INJURY

Despite the introduction of newer ventilatory techniques, which are based on sound physiologic principles, the incidence of chronic lung disease remains unacceptably high among babies who require mechanical ventilation, particularly for those born extremely prematurely. Chronic lung disease is multifactorial and involves a number of overlapping factors, such as prematurity, oxidant injury, inflammation, and injury related to mechanical ventilation, referred to as ventilator-induced lung injury (VILI).

Various terms, such as the pulmonary injury sequence, have been used to describe the individual components of VILI (Fig. 44-46); these are probably inter-related and likely to act synergistically to damage the developing lung as part of a pulmonary injury sequence.[2] Barotrauma, or excessive pressure, may disrupt airway epithelium and alveoli. Volutrauma refers to injury related to overdistention or stretching of the lung units by delivering too much gas. Atelectrauma refers to the damage caused by the repetitive opening and closing of the lung units (the cycle of recruitment and subsequent derecruitment). Biotrauma is a collective term to describe infection and inflammation, as well as the role of oxidative stress on the delicate tissue of the developing lung. Rheotrauma refers to damage evoked by inappropriate airway flow. If flow is excessive, inefficient gas exchange, inadvertent positive-end-expiratory pressure (PEEP), turbulence, and lung overinflation may occur. On the other hand, if flow is inadequate, it may lead to air hunger (flow starvation) and increased work of breathing. The cumulative effects of both endogenous and exogenous insults to the developing lung are a reduction in alveolarization and diminished pulmonary surface area capable of effective gas exchange.

With the introduction of newer techniques of mechanical ventilation in newborns, including pulmonary graphic monitoring, clinicians have now initiated strategies to avoid VILI. Monitoring of tidal volume delivery, irrespective of whether the target variable is volume or pressure, has become much more important in recent years. Indeed, delivering a physiologic tidal volume during conventional ventilation seems prudent. Of equal importance is the ability to customize ventilator settings to the specific needs of the patient.[28]

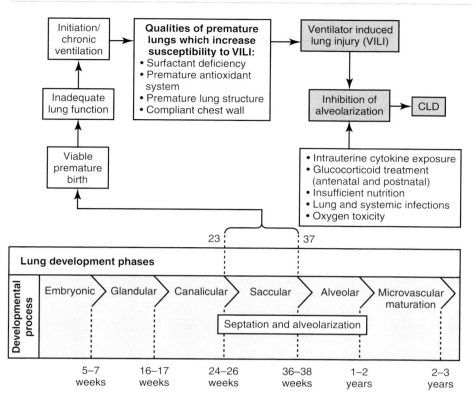

Figure 44–46. Pulmonary injury sequence leading to ventilator-induced lung injury and chronic lung disease. *(From Attar MA, Donn SM: Mechanisms of ventilator-induced lung injury in premature infants, Semin Neonatol 7:353, 2002. Copyright, Elsevier Science Ltd, with permission.)*

CHRONIC LUNG DISEASE (BRONCHOPULMONARY DYSPLASIA)

See also Part 7.

Despite high use of antenatal steroids, surfactant replacement therapy, and newer ventilation techniques, chronic lung disease remains the major problem of neonatal intensive care. Bronchopulmonary dysplasia is a severe form of chronic lung disease and is characterized by presence of chronic respiratory insufficiency and a supplemental oxygen requirement, and an abnormal chest radiograph at 36 weeks' postmenstrual age. When Northway and colleagues originally described BPD in 1967, the affected infants ranged from 32 to 39 weeks' gestation and weighed 1474 to 3204 g at birth. Most had required high airway pressures and significant concentrations of supplemental oxygen. Their chest radiographs showed typical overinflation and cystic emphysema. A quarter of a century later, the demographics of BPD have changed. It occurs in more immature and very low birth weight babies who required only modest supplemental oxygen and ventilatory support. Their chest radiographs are also different and are characterized by diffuse haziness and a fine, lacy pattern. Infants with the "new" BPD do not seem to have had typical RDS, and many do not require ventilation during the first few days of life.[4]

Because BPD is associated with mechanical ventilation, some have advocated for the avoidance of assisted ventilation and the alternative use of noninvasive respiratory support such as NIPPV or NCPAP. This hypothesis is presently undergoing clinical evaluation. Attempts have also been made to use "gentler" ventilation by allowing "permissive hypercapnia" as a protective lung strategy.[51] The rationale for permissive hypercapnia is that by using less ventilation, there may be less volutrauma, a reduction of the duration of positive-pressure ventilation, and decreased alveolar ventilation. Whereas the secondary goals appear to be achievable, this approach has thus far failed to show a reduction in the incidence of BPD. In addition, it is very difficult to accomplish in the era of patient-triggered ventilation, because the baby with intact chemoreceptors increases his minute ventilation to try to achieve normocapnia.

There is compelling evidence that excessive tidal volume causes lung injury, so targeting tidal volume in a normal range (4 to 7 mL/kg) is gaining support within the neonatal community. In a recently published randomized clinical trial, babies receiving volume controlled ventilation were shown to have a trend toward reduction in chronic lung disease compared to those managed with pressure-limited ventilation.[65] A 20-month follow-up study of these infants also showed a reduced frequency of respiratory symptoms and need for treatment in the babies who had received volume-controlled ventilation.[64]

HFV is often used as an alternative to conventional ventilation and there is a large pool of data, both from animal and human studies, suggesting that this form of ventilation may have advantage over conventional tidal ventilation in reducing lung injury. However, the cumulative evidence from clinical trials does not show a reduction in CLD.[72]

Clinical investigation has not yet demonstrated a beneficial effect from any form of ventilation in preventing lung injury associated with mechanical ventilation. This may be the result of a number of other factors, including the underlying immaturity of the lung itself, which is more susceptible to the damaging effects of extrinsic factors.

MISCELLANEOUS COMPLICATIONS

Imposed Work of Breathing

Infants placed on mechanical ventilation assume additional burdens of breathing. First, there is an increase in airway resistance because of the placement of the narrow lumen endotracheal tube. Resistance to airflow is proportional to the fourth power of the radius of the tube and is linearly related to tube length. Second, there is an increase in dead space created by tubing and connectors. Finally, if a demand system is used, there is effort required to open the demand valve. Collectively, these have been referred to as the imposed work of breathing, primarily affecting spontaneous breaths taken by the baby between mechanical breaths. These spontaneous breaths are supported only by PEEP, unless the baby is receiving assist/control or pressure support ventilation, which was developed to overcome the imposed work of breathing and enhance patient comfort and endurance.

Patent Ductus Arteriosus

See also Chapter 45.

Patency of the ductus arteriosus (PDA) is a common problem in preterm infants. Its incidence varies inversely with gestational age and may be as high as 60% in infants less than 28 weeks' gestation. Its relationship to lung disease and mechanical ventilation is well established. Preterm infants have an immature closure mechanism, decreased sensitivity to normal constrictors, such as oxygen tension, and increased sensitivity to prostaglandin E$_2$, all of which promote patency. Other factors that have been associated with a PDA include severe lung disease, exogenous surfactant therapy, phototherapy, high fluid administration, early use of furosemide, and lack of antenatal glucocorticoid exposure.

The pathophysiologic effects of a PDA are determined by the direction of shunting. When pulmonary vascular resistance is high, such as with early RDS or meconium aspiration syndrome, shunting is in a right-to-left direction, resulting in mixing of deoxygenated and oxygenated blood and resultant hypoxemia. When pulmonary vascular resistance is less than systemic vascular resistance, shunting is left-to-right. Overperfusion of the lungs can alter pulmonary mechanics, causing a need for higher levels of supplemental oxygen and ventilatory support and an increase in the cardiac work load. A diastolic steal may also occur, reducing bloodflow to organs and increasing the risk of ischemic complications. Persistent PDA is also associated with increased risks for apnea, BPD, congestive heart failure, and impaired weight gain. Diagnosis and treatment of PDA is discussed in detail in Chapter 45.

Neurologic Complications

INTRAVENTRICULAR HEMORRHAGE AND PERIVENTRICULAR LEUKOMALACIA (See Ch. 40)

Premature babies requiring mechanical ventilation are at increased risk of brain injuries. The spectrum of brain injuries observed in these infants includes periventricular-intraventricular hemorrhage (PV-IVH) and periventricular leukomalacia (PVL). The main reason for the increased susceptibility to hemorrhagic or ischemic brain injuries is the unique anatomic and physiologic immaturity of brain. Absent or reduced auto-regulation of cerebral bloodflow creates pressure-passive cerebral circulation and thus renders the brain prone to damage during periods of systemic hypotension and hypertension. Cerebral circulation (and auto-regulation) is also affected by changes in Paco$_2$ and to a lesser extent pH. A rise in Paco$_2$ (hypercapnia) during the first three to four days of life is a recognized risk factor for PV-IVH. Conversely, hypocapnia (Pco$_2$ less than 35 mm Hg) is potentially dangerous, as it may cause cerebral ischemia and PVL, especially if Paco$_2$ decreases rapidly as can sometimes occur with the institution of HFV. Another recognized risk factor for PV-IVH is the fluctuation in cerebral bloodflow observed in babies who fight the ventilator (asynchronous breathing). The use of high PIP or PEEP can result in lung overdistention leading to increased central venous pressure, which is transmitted to cerebral veins. Increased intrathoracic pressure can also decrease venous return to the heart and thus reduce cardiac output. Additional threats to central nervous system function may come from a PDA, with right-to-left shunting, from focal or systemic infections, which initiate the inflammatory responses associated with white matter damage, and from pneumothorax or PIE, which may also aggravate respiratory failure and hemodynamic function. Concerns also exist that cerebral perfusion may be jeopardized during routine procedures, such as endotracheal tube suctioning or reintubation.

RETINOPATHY OF PREMATURITY

See also Chapter 53.

Retinopathy of prematurity (ROP) is a condition confined to the developing retinal vessels in very premature infants. The major risk factors for ROP are the degree of prematurity and high arterial oxygen content. There is higher incidence of ROP in babies with low birthweight who require mechanical ventilation and supplemental oxygen. Hyperoxia, hypoxemia, and fluctuations of arterial oxygen content, even within the normal range, have all been implicated as etiologic factors. Many other risk factors have also been suggested, including vitamin E deficiency, exchange transfusions, necrotizing enterocolitis, treatment for PDA, and other complications of prematurity. Despite meticulous neonatal care, ROP is not entirely preventable. Maintaining arterial oxygen tension between 60 to 80 mm Hg and pulse oximetry between 88% and 92% has been shown to reduce the incidence of ROP in babies who receive oxygen treatment. Nonetheless, the ideal level of oxygen saturation in ventilated preterm babies remains unknown. Ongoing large clinical trials are exploring this.[73b]

REFERENCES

1. Aly H, Badawy M, El-Kohly A, et al: Randomized, controlled trial on tracheal colonization of ventilated infants: can gravity prevent ventilator-associated pneumonia? *Pediatrics* 122:770, 2008.
2. Attar MA, Donn SM: Mechanisms of ventilator-induced lung injury in premature infants, *Semin Neonatol* 7:353, 2002.

3. Balsan MJ, Jones JG, Watchko JF, Guthrie RD: Measurements of pulmonary mechanics prior to the elective extubation of neonates, *Pediatr Pulmonol* 9:238, 1990.

4. Bancalari E: Changes in the pathogenesis and prevention of chronic lung disease of prematurity, *Am J Perinatol* 18:1, 2001.

5. Barrington KJ, Finer NN: A randomized, controlled trial of aminophylline in ventilatory weaning of premature infants, *Crit Care Med* 21:846, 1993.

6. Becker MA, Donn SM: Bird VIP Gold ventilator. In Donn SM, Sinha SK, editors: *Manual of neonatal respiratory care,* 2nd ed, Philadelphia, 2006, Mosby-Elsevier, pp 249-255.

7. Boros SJ, Mammel MC, Lewallen PK, et al: Necrotizing tracheobronchitis: a complication of high-frequency ventilation, *J Pediatr* 109:95, 1986.

8. Bunnell JB: High-frequency ventilation: general concepts. In Donn SM, Sinha SK, editors: *Manual of neonatal respiratory care,* 2nd ed, Philadelphia, 2006, Mosby-Elsevier, pp 222-230.

9. Buschell MK: Servo-I ventilator. In Donn SM, Sinha SK, editors: *Manual of neonatal respiratory care,* 2nd ed, Philadelphia, 2006, Mosby-Elsevier, pp 273-278.

10. Carlo WA, Ambalavanan N, Chatburn RL: Classification of mechanical ventilation devices. In Donn SM, Sinha SK, editors: *Manual of neonatal respiratory care,* 2nd ed, Philadelphia, 2006, Mosby-Elsevier, pp 74-80.

11. Carlo WA, Ambalavanan N, Chatburn RL: Ventilator parameters. In Donn SM, Sinha SK, editors: *Manual of neonatal respiratory care,* 2nd ed, Philadelphia, 2006, Mosby-Elsevier, pp 81-85.

12. Carlo WA, Chatburn RL: Assisted ventilation of the newborn. In Carlo WA, Chatburn RL, editors: *Neonatal respiratory Care,* 2nd ed, Chicago, 1988, Year Book Medical Publishers, pp 320-46.

13. Carlo WA, Greenough A, Chatburn RL: Advances in mechanical ventilation. In Boynton BR, Carlo WA, Jobe AH, editors: *New therapies for neonatal respiratory failure: a physiologic approach,* Cambridge, UK, 1994, Cambridge University Press, pp 131-151.

14. Chatburn RL: Classification of mechanical ventilators. In Branson RD, Hess DR, Chatburn RL, editors: *Respiratory care equipment,* Philadelphia, 1995, JB Lippincott, pp 264-293.

15. Clark RH, Gerstmann DR: High-frequency oscillatory ventilation. In Donn SM, Sinha SK, editors: *Manual of neonatal respiratory care,* 2nd ed, Philadelphia, 2006, Mosby-Elsevier, pp 237-246.

16. Clark RH, et al: Lung injury in neonates: causes, strategies for prevention, and long-term consequences, *J Pediatr* 139:478, 2001.

17. Courtney SE, Barrington KJ: Continuous positive airway pressure and noninvasive ventilation, *Clin Perinatol* 34:73, 2007.

18. Davis PG, Henderson-Smart DJ: Nasal continuous positive airway pressure immediately after extubation for preventing morbidity in preterm infants, *Cochrane Database Syst Rev* 2:CD000143, 2003.

19. Davis PG, Morley C: Volume control: a logical solution to volutrauma, *J Pediatr* 149:290, 2006.

20. Davis PG, Morley CJ, Owen LS: Non-invasive respiratory support of preterm neonates with respiratory distress: continuous positive airway pressure and nasal intermittent positive pressure ventilation, *Semin Fetal Neonatal Med* 10:1, 2008.

21. Delivoria-Papadopoulis M, Swyer PR: Assisted ventilation in terminal hyaline membrane disease, *Arch Dis Child* 39:481, 1964.

22. DePaoli AG, Morley CJ, Davis PG, et al: In vitro comparison of nasal continuous positive airway pressure devices for neonates, *Arch Dis Child Fetal Neonatal Ed* 87:F42, 2002.

23. Donn SM: Pressure control ventilation. In Donn SM, Sinha SK, editors: *Manual of neonatal respiratory care,* 2nd ed, Philadelphia, 2006, Mosby-Elsevier, pp 210-211.

24. Donn SM, Becker MA: Special ventilation techniques and modalities I: patient-triggered ventilation. In Goldsmith JP, Karotkin EH, editors: *Assisted ventilation of the neonate,* 4th ed, Philadelphia, 2003, WB Saunders, pp 203-218.

25. Donn SM, Sinha SK: Advances in neonatal ventilation. In Kurjak A, Chervenak F, editors: *Textbook of perinatal medicine,* 2nd ed, London, 2006, Taylor & Francis Medical Books, pp 39-48.

26. Donn SM, Sinha SK: Controversies in patient-triggered ventilation, *Clin Perinatol* 25:49, 1998.

27. Donn SM, Sinha SK: Invasive and noninvasive neonatal mechanical ventilation, *Respir Care* 48:426, 2003.

28. Donn SM, Sinha SK: Minimising ventilator induced lung injury in preterm infants, *Arch Dis Child Fetal Neonatal Ed* 91:F226, 2006.

29. Donn SM, Sinha SK: Weaning and extubation. In Donn SM, Sinha SK, editors: *Manual of neonatal respiratory care,* 2nd ed, Philadelphia, 2006, Mosby-Elsevier, pp 375-382.

30. Donn SM, Zak LK, Bozynski MEA, et al: Use of high-frequency jet ventilation in the management of congenital tracheoesophageal fistula associated with respiratory distress syndrome, *J Pediatr Surg* 25:1219, 1990.

31. Dreyfuss D, Saumon G: Barotrauma is volutrauma, but which volume is the one responsible? *Intensive Care Med* 18:139, 1992.

32. Duke PM, Coulson JD, Santos JI, Johnson JD: Cleft palate associated with prolonged orotracheal intubation in infancy, *J Pediatr* 89:990, 1976.

33. Erenberg A, Nowak AJ: Palatal groove formation in neonates and infants with orotracheal tubes, *Am J Dis Child* 138:974, 1984.

34. Finer NN: Nasal cannula use in the preterm infant: oxygen or pressure? *Pediatrics* 116:1216, 2005.

35. Finer NN, Carlo WA, Duara S, et al: Delivery room continuous positive airway pressure/positive end-expiratory pressure in extremely low birth weight infants: a feasibility trial, *Pediatrics* 114:651, 2004.

36. Gillespie LM, White SD, Sinha SK, Donn SM: Usefulness of the minute ventilation test in predicting successful extubation in newborn infants: a randomized controlled trial, *J Perinatol* 23:205, 2003.

37. Goldsmith JP, Karotkin EH: Introduction to assisted ventilation. In Goldsmith JP, Karotkin EH, editors: *Assisted ventilation of the neonate,* 4th ed, Philadelphia, 2003, WB Saunders, pp 1-14.

38. Gowder K, Bull MJ, Schreiner RL, et al: Nasal deformities in neonates, *Am J Dis Child* 134:954, 1980.

39. Greenough A, Milner AD: Indications for mechanical ventilation In Donn SM, Sinha SK, editors: *Manual of neonatal respiratory care,* 2nd ed, Philadelphia, 2006, Mosby-Elsevier, pp 303-304.

40. Gupta S, Sinha SK, Donn SM: The effect of two levels of pressure support ventilation on tidal volume delivery and minute ventilation in preterm infants, *Arch Dis Child Fetal Neonatal Ed* 94: F80, 2009.

41. Gupta S, Sinha SK, Tin W, Donn SM: A randomized controlled trial of post-extubation Bubble CPAP vs Infant Flow Driver CPAP in preterm infants with respiratory distress syndrome, *J Pediatr* 154:645, 2009.

42. Hagus CK, Donn SM: Pulmonary graphics: basics of clinical application. In Donn SM, editor: *Neonatal and pediatric pulmonary graphic analysis: principles and clinical applications,* Armonk, NY, 1998, Futura Publishing, pp 81-127.

43. Henderson-Smart DJ, Davis PG: Prophylactic methylxanthines for extubation in preterm infants. *Cochrane Database Syst Rev* 1:CD000139, 2003.

44. Kamlin CO, Davis PG, Argus B, et al: A trial of spontaneous breathing to determine readiness for extubation in very low birth weight infants: a prospective evaluation, *Arch Dis Child Fetal Neonatal Ed* 93:305, 2008.

45. Keszler M: Pressure support ventilation and other approaches to overcome the imposed work of breathing, *Neoreviews* 7:e226, 2006.

46. Keszler M, Abubakar KM: Volume guarantee ventilation, *Clin Perinatol* 34:107, 2007.

47. Keszler M: Bunnell Life Pulse high-frequency jet ventilator. In Donn SM, Sinha SK, editors: *Manual of neonatal respiratory care,* 2nd ed, Philadelphia, 2006, Mosby-Elsevier, pp 286-287.

48. Keszler M, Donn SM, Bucciarelli RL, et al: Multicenter controlled trial comparing high-frequency jet ventilation and conventional mechanical ventilation in newborn infants with pulmonary interstitial emphysema, *J Pediatr* 119:85, 1991.

49. Keszler M, Modanlou HD, Brudno S, et al: Multicenter controlled trial of high-frequency jet ventilation in preterm infants with uncomplicated respiratory distress syndrome, *Pediatrics* 100:593, 1997.

50. Lampland AL, Mammel MC: The role of high-frequency ventilation in neonates: evidence-based recommendations, *Clin Perinatol* 34:129, 2007.

51. Mariani G, Cifuentes J, Carlo WA: Randomized trial of permissive hypercapnia in preterm infants, *Pediatrics* 104:1082, 1999.

52. Morley CJ, Davis PG: Continuous positive airway pressure: scientific and clinical rationale, *Curr Opin Pediatr* 20:119, 2008.

53. Morley CJ, Davis PG, Doyle LW, et al, COIN Trial Investigators: Nasal CPAP or intubation at birth for very preterm infants, *N Engl J Med* 358:700, 2008.

54. Moylan FMB, Seldin EB, Shannon DC, Todres ID: Defective primary dentition in survivors of neonatal mechanical ventilation, *J Pediatr* 96:106, 1980.

55. Nicks JJ: Neonatal graphic monitoring In Donn SM, Sinha SK, editors: *Manual of neonatal respiratory care,* 2nd ed, Philadelphia, 2006, Mosby-Elsevier, pp 134-147.

56. Nicks JJ, Becker MA, Donn SM: Bronchopulmonary dysplasia: response to pressure support ventilation, *J Perinatol* 14:495, 1994.

57. Osorio W, Claure N, D'Ugard C, et al: Effects of pressure support during an acute reduction of synchronized intermittent mandatory ventilation in preterm infants, *J Perinatol* 25:412, 2005.

58. Parravicini E, Polin RA: Pneumonia in the newborn infant. In Donn SM, Sinha SK, editors: *Manual of neonatal respiratory care,* 2nd ed, Philadelphia, 2006, Mosby-Elsevier, pp 310-324.

59. Reyes ZC, Claure N, Tauscher MK, et al: Randomized, controlled trial comparing synchronized intermittent mandatory ventilation and synchronized intermittent mandatory ventilation plus pressure support in preterm infants, *Pediatrics* 118:1409, 2006.

60. Sarkar S, Donn SM: In support of pressure support, *Clin Perinatol* 34:117, 2007.

61. Serlin SP, Dailey WJR: Tracheal perforation in the neonate: a complication of endotracheal intubation, *J Pediatr* 86:596, 1975.

62. Servant G, Nicks JJ, Donn SM, et al: Feasibility of applying flow synchronized ventilation to very low birthweight infants, *Respir Care* 37:249, 1992.

63. Sherman JM, Lowitt S, Stephenson C, Ironson G: Factors influencing the development of acquired subglottic stenosis in infants, *J Pediatr* 109:322, 1986.

64. Singh J, Sinha SK, Alsop E, et al: Long term follow-up of VLBW infants from a neonatal volume vs pressure mechanical ventilation trial, *Arch Dis Child Fetal Neonatal Ed* 94:F360, 2009.

65. Singh J, Sinha SK, Clarke P, et al: Mechanical ventilation of very low birth weight infants: is volume or pressure a better target variable? *J Pediatr* 149:308, 2006.

66. Singh J, Sinha SK, Donn SM: Volume-targeted ventilation of newborns, *Clin Perinatol* 34:93, 2007.

67. Sinha SK, Donn SM: Difficult extubation in babies receiving assisted mechanical ventilation, *Arch Dis Child Educ Pract Ed* 91:ep42, 2006.

68. Sinha SK, Donn SM: Newer forms of conventional ventilation of preterm newborns, *Acta Paediatrica* 97:1338, 2008.

69. Sinha SK, Donn SM: Volume-controlled ventilation. In Goldsmith JP, Karotkin EH, editors: *Assisted ventilation of the neonate,* 4th ed, Philadelphia, 2003, WB Saunders, pp 171-182.

70. Sinha SK, Donn SM: Weaning infants from mechanical ventilation: art or science? *Arch Dis Child* 83:F64, 2000.

71. Sivieri E, Bhutani VK: Pulmonary mechanics. In Donn SM, Sinha SK, editors: *Manual of neonatal respiratory care,* 2nd ed, Philadelphia, 2006, Mosby-Elsevier, pp 50-60.

72. Stark AR: High-frequency oscillatory ventilation to prevent bronchopulmonary dysplasia—are we there yet? *N Engl J Med* 347:682, 2002.

73. Stein RT, Wall PM, Kaufman RA, et al: Neonatal anterior esophageal perforation, *Pediatrics* 60:744, 1977.

73a. SUPPORT Study Group of the Eunice Kennedy Shriver NICHD Neonatal Research Network: Early CPAP versus surfactant in extremely preterm infants, *N Engl J Med* 362:1970, 2010.

73b. SUPPORT Study Group of the Eunice Kennedy Shriver NICHD Neonatal Research Network: Target ranges of oxygen saturation in extremely preterm infants, *N Engl J Med* 362:1959, 2010.

74. Tin W, Gupta S: Optimum oxygen therapy in preterm babies, *Arch Dis Child Fetal Neonatal Ed* 92:F143, 2007.

75. Veness-Meehan K, Richter S, Davis JM: Pulmonary function testing prior to extubation in infants with respiratory distress syndrome, *Pediatr Pulmonol* 9:2, 1990.

76. Visveshwara N, Freeman B, Peck M, et al: Patient-triggered synchronized assisted ventilation of newborns: report of a preliminary study and 3 years' experience, *J Perinatol* 11:347, 1991.

77. Wilson BJ Jr, Becker MA, Linton ME, Donn SM: Spontaneous minute ventilation predicts readiness for extubation in mechanically ventilated preterm infants, *J Perinatol* 18:436, 1998.

78. Wohl DL: Traumatic vocal cord avulsion injury in a newborn, *J Voice* 10:106, 1996.

PART 5

Respiratory Disorders in Preterm and Term Infants

Jalal M. Abu-Shaweesh*

> *And whomsoever God wills to let go astray, He causes his chest*
> *to be tight and constricted, as if he were climbing unto the skies.*
> *Holy Quran, Al-An'am chapter, 6:125.*

Multiple pathophysiologic mechanisms can present with pulmonary manifestations in term and preterm infants. The clinical picture is most commonly dominated by respiratory distress, which presents as tachypnea, grunting, flaring, retractions, cyanosis, and hypoxemia. However, apnea and hypoventilation are also common. In preterm infants, these manifestations are commonly associated with respiratory distress syndrome (RDS) as discussed in Part 3. Nonpulmonary etiologies of respiratory distress include, thermal instability, circulatory problems, cardiac disease, neuromuscular disorders, sepsis, anemia or polycythemia, and methemoglobinemia (Box 44-11). This section presents an overview of the many other respiratory disorders that can affect preterm and term infants.

FETAL AND NEONATAL BREATHING

Although many aspects of the regulation of breathing in humans and mammals have been explored in the past century, more questions have yet to be answered. Breathing results in the exchange of Pa_{O_2} and Pa_{CO_2} between the lungs and the environment, maintaining homeostasis and control of blood pH. At the same time, energy-consuming breathing movements are present in utero, where such gas exchange is not possible. Maturation of breathing is a continuous process that bridges fetal and neonatal life. Many features of immature fetal breathing responses are present to a lesser degree in the neonate.

FETAL BREATHING

Fetal breathing activity has been described in many species and is identified very early in gestation. Breathing activity in the human fetus can be detected using ultrasound by 11 weeks' gestation. The placenta is the site of gas exchange in utero; however, fetal breathing movement (FBM) is important in enhancement of lung growth and development, and decreased diaphragmatic activity has been associated with pulmonary hypoplasia. In addition, FBM has been shown to significantly increase fetal cardiac output and bloodflow to a number of vital organs including the heart, brain, and placenta. FBM changes from early continuous movement that seems to originate from the spinal cord to a phasic pattern that occurs only during rapid eye movement (REM) in the third trimester with total cessation of breathing during non-REM sleep, possibly secondary to descending inhibitory pontine input to the medullary rhythm-generating center. The mechanisms underlying loss of phasic FBM and establishment of continuous breathing after birth are not clear.

---

*Richard J. Martin and Martha Miller contributed to previous editions of this chapter.

BOX 44–11   Classification of Extrapulmonary Causes of Respiratory Distress

NEUROMUSCULAR DISORDERS (CHAPTER 40)
Central nervous system: asphyxia, hemorrhage, malformations, drugs, infection
Spinal cord: cord injury, spinal muscular atrophy
Nerves: phrenic nerve injury, cranial nerve palsy
Neuromuscular plate: myasthenia gravis
Muscular: dystrophies

OBSTRUCTIVE-RESTRICTIVE DISORDERS
Airway obstruction (Part 6)
- Intrinsic: choanal atresia, floppy epiglottis, laryngeal web, cord paralysis, laryngospasm, malacia, tracheal stenosis
- Extrinsic: tubes, secretions, Pierre Robin syndrome, macroglossia, goiter, vascular ring, cystic hygroma, mediastinal and cervical masses
Rib cage abnormalities
- Thoracic dystrophies
- Rickets and bone disease
- Fractures
- Pectus excavatum

DIAPHRAGMATIC DISORDERS
Congenital eventration
Abdominal distention

HEMATOLOGIC DISORDERS (CHAPTER 46)
Anemia
Polycythemia
Methemoglobulinemia

METABOLIC DISORDERS (CHAPTER 49)
Hypoglycemia
Hypocalcemia
Metabolic acidosis

CARDIOVASCULAR DISORDERS (CHAPTER 45)
Increased pulmonary flow
- Patent ductus arteriosus
- Ventricular septal defect
- Transposition of the great arteries
- Truncus arteriosus

Decreased pulmonary flow
- Persistent pulmonary hypertension
- Pulmonary atresia
- Tetralogy of Fallot
- Tricuspid atresia

Cardiomegaly
- Tricuspid atresia
- Ebstein anomaly
- Left heart obstruction (e.g., coarctation, mitral atresia, total anomalous pulmonary venous return)

Hypotension

MISCELLANEOUS (CHAPTERS 30, 39)
Sepsis
Pain
Hypothermia
Hyperthermia

However, several factors have been implicated, including serotonin, γ-aminobutyric acid (GABA), corticotrophin-releasing factor, and prostaglandins.[2]

Fetal hypercapnia increases the incidence and depth of FBM only during REM sleep, although it does not affect breathing frequency. This response is present from 24 weeks' gestation with an increase in CO_2 sensitivity with advancing gestational age. In contrast, fetal hypocapnia causes a decrease or disappearance of FBM, which implies that baseline CO_2 level is essential for the presence of FBM. Although the fetus lives in a relatively hypoxemic condition (PaO_2 23-27 mm Hg), oxygen delivery in utero is adequate because it matches oxygen consumption and allows for fetal activity and growth. Unlike adults, the fetus responds to hypoxia by a decrease in breathing activity. The cause of this hypoxic ventilatory depression in utero appears to be central in origin. Brainstem transection or lesions in the lateral upper pons allow acute hypoxemia to stimulate FBM even in the absence of the carotid bodies. This is consistent with the concept that hypoxic depression is the result of descending pontine or suprapontine inhibition. Unlike the fetal breathing response to hypercapnia, the hypoxic response is "logical" in the sense that an increase in breathing in response to hypoxia would be counterproductive.

POSTNATAL DEVELOPMENT OF BREATHING RESPONSES

Although better developed than the fetal pattern, breathing in the neonate is still immature. This immaturity is manifested in almost all aspects of respiratory control from peripheral afferent input, to central respiratory output and respiratory muscle responses. Moreover, preterm infants exhibit more pronounced immaturity of respiratory control than term infants, the net result of which is a high incidence of apnea and bradycardia. There seems to be an overriding inhibitory influence of central origin in the control of breathing in the neonate. This is manifested by a decrease in the breathing response to CO_2, a paradoxical response to hypoxia, an exaggerated reflex apnea, and irregularities of breathing pattern manifested by periodic breathing, apnea, and tachypnea. The origin of this inhibitory effect on neonatal breathing could be secondary to increased inhibitory pathways, decreased excitatory pathways, or a combination of the two.

Neonatal Breathing Pattern

Neonatal respiratory activity is characterized by irregularity and spontaneous changes in the breathing pattern between eupnea, apnea, periodic breathing, and tachypnea. Respiratory frequency, often inversely proportional to body weight, may be quite variable in the preterm infant. Periods of slow respiratory frequency in the human neonate are secondary to prolongation of expiratory time (T_E) while inspiratory time (T_I) remains relatively unchanged during development. Extreme prolongation of T_E results in respiratory pauses and apnea, which occur frequently in preterm and, to a lesser extent, in term neonates. The incidence of central apnea decreases with advancing gestational age, occurring in almost all infants weighing less than 1000 g at birth, until 43 to

44 weeks' corrected gestational age when the incidence is comparable to that of a term neonate. Paradoxical inward movement of the rib cage during inspiration is common especially in preterm infants. The mechanisms behind this paradoxical movement are related to a combination of a highly compliant rib cage and diminished intercostal muscular tone, opposed by diaphragmatic contraction. The muscular effort required to produce a tidal volume during these paradoxical movements is substantially greater than during "normal" breathing, which further hinders an already immature breathing pattern in the neonate.

Hypercapnia and Acidosis

Small increase in arterial PCO_2 or central acidosis increases ventilation dramatically. The ventilatory response to CO_2 is the net result of activation of both peripheral and central chemoreceptors. The contribution of the peripheral chemoreceptors, mainly through the carotid body, is 10% to 40% of the total hypercapnic response. Central chemoreceptors originally thought to be confined to the ventrolateral medulla have been found to be widely spread in the brainstem, including retrotrapezoid nucleus, the region of the nucleus tractus solitarius, the region of the locus coeruleus, the rostral aspect of the ventral respiratory group, and the medullary raphe.[53] Other sites of chemoreception include the fastigial nucleus of the cerebellum and the pre-Botzinger complex. The ventilatory response to CO_2 is impaired in preterm infants when compared with term newborns and adults; however, it increases with advancing postnatal and gestational age. Unlike adults, preterm infants and newborn animals were not able to increase breathing frequency in response to CO_2 while tidal volume increased appropriately.[1] Possible mechanisms for this impaired response to CO_2 include changes in the mechanical properties of the lung, maturation in the peripheral or central chemoreceptors, or changes in the central integration of chemoreceptor or other neuronal signals. Multiple studies have indicated a central origin for the attenuated CO_2 response in preterm babies, in particular those with apnea. However, a cause-and-effect relationship between apnea of prematurity and the attenuated response to CO_2 has not been clearly established, and both might simply represent facets of a decreased respiratory drive.

Hypoxia

Unlike adults who express a sustained response to hypoxia, the neonatal hypoxic ventilatory response is biphasic with an initial increase in ventilation that lasts 1 to 2 minutes, followed by a decline that reaches below baseline ventilation in preterm infants (Fig. 44-47). This late decline has been traditionally termed *hypoxic ventilatory depression*. While the increase in tidal volume is sustained, breathing frequency decreases during hypoxic exposure, thus contributing most to the biphasic response. The increase in ventilation occurs through activation of peripheral chemoreceptors located primarily in the carotid body and is eliminated by carotid body denervation. During development, the initial rise increases while the late depression decreases with advancing postnatal age; however, hypoxic ventilatory depression persisted in convalescing preterm neonates at 4 to 6 weeks of age.[50] Several mechanisms have been postulated to explain

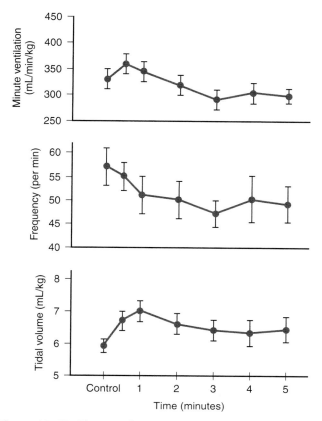

Figure 44–47. The ventilatory response to 15% hypoxia in 4- to 6-week-old preterm infants. (*From Martin RJ et al: Persistence of the biphasic ventilatory response to hypoxia in preterm infants, J Pediatr 132:960, 1998, with permission.*)

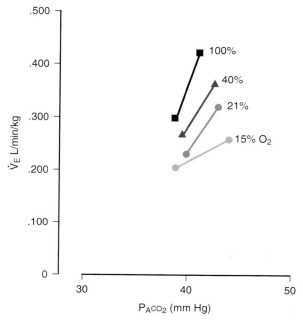

Figure 44–48. Steady-state carbon dioxide response curves at different inspired oxygen concentrations. The more hypoxic the infant, the flatter the response to carbon dioxide. (*From Rigatto H et al: Effects of O_2 on the ventilatory response to CO_2 in preterm infants, J Appl Physiol 30:896, 1975, with permission.*)

the pathogenesis of the late depression, including a time-dependent decrease in carotid body stimulation, hypocapnea secondary to the initial hyperventilation, and a decrease in metabolism. Increasing evidence, however, suggests a central origin for hypoxic ventilatory depression, probably through interaction of multiple neurotransmitters, including adenosine, GABA, and endorphins, or through descending inhibitory pontine tracts. Consistent with these findings is the observation that a progressive decrease in inspired oxygen concentration causes a significant flattening of carbon dioxide responsiveness in preterm infants (Fig. 44-48).

Laryngeal and Pulmonary Afferent Reflexes

Stimulation of the laryngeal mucosa, either chemically (water, ammonium chloride, or acidic solutions) or mechanically, causes inhibition of breathing and apnea in neonates and newborn animals. This reflex-induced apnea, known as the *laryngeal chemoreflex* (LCR), is usually associated with glottic closure, swallowing, bradycardia, and hypotension, and has been shown to undergo maturational changes with age. Preterm infants express an exaggerated LCR as evidenced by prolonged apnea response to instilling saline in the oropharynx. The mechanisms underlying such maturational change in reflex-induced apnea are not known, but seem to be related to a decrease in central neural output or a dominance

of inhibitory pathways. The inhibitory neurotransmitters adenosine and GABA have both been implicated where blockade of $GABA_A$ receptors prevented and activation of adenosine A_{2A} exaggerated the LCR.[3]

Lung afferents play an important role in regulating respiratory timing and may play a role in apnea of prematurity. Stimulation of pulmonary stretch receptors through increasing lung volume causes shortening of inspiratory time, prolongation of expiratory time, or both. This reflex is known as the *Hering-Breuer reflex*. The decrease in respiratory frequency and prolongation of expiratory time following institution of nasal continuous positive airway pressure (CPAP) is mediated through activation of this reflex. This probably serves to prevent lung overdistention on CPAP. The Hering-Breuer deflation reflex is activated on deflation of the lung and results in inspiratory augmentation. However, unlike term infants, preterm infants are less likely to initiate breathing and tend to have respiratory pauses on deflation of the lung, thus making them less likely to recover from an apnea.

Neurotransmitters and Neuromodulators

There are limited data regarding the balance of excitatory and inhibitory neurotransmitters during development of respiratory control. Because invasive studies cannot be performed in newborn infants, most studies on the relationship of neurotransmitters to respiratory control are based on the effect of these substances or their inhibitors on the breathing responses to hypoxia, hypercapnia, and reflex apnea in animal models. The most widely studied neurotransmitters in relation to disturbances in control of breathing include adenosine, GABA, prostaglandins, endorphins, and serotonin.

GABA is the major inhibitory neurotransmitter in the central nervous system (CNS). GABA has been implicated in the attenuated ventilatory responses to hypoxia, hypercapnia, and LCR. Blocking $GABA_A$ receptors prevented hypoxic ventilatory depression and the decrease in breathing frequency in response to CO_2 and attenuated the LCR. Both structural and functional differences in $GABA_A$ receptors have been observed during development. $GABA_A$ receptors are hetero-oligomers assembled from five subunits. During embryonic and early postnatal development, the brainstem has a much higher $GABA_A$ receptor density than does the adult brainstem and the "mix" of $GABA_A$ receptor subunits differs from that in adults. Therefore, GABA has the potential to play a key role in the vulnerability of preterm infants to disturbed breathing, including apnea of prematurity. Of interest is the observation that GABA may switch from an excitatory to inhibitory neurotransmitter during the transition from fetal to neonatal life.

Adenosine is a product of ATP that is ubiquitous to most brain tissue as well as the cerebrospinal fluid (CSF). Adenosine is known to depress neural function and respiration, and its level has been shown to increase during hypoxia in brain tissue, CSF, and plasma. Furthermore, adenosine antagonists reversed hypoxic depression in anesthetized newborn piglets. The role of adenosine in apnea of prematurity is suggested by the ability of the methylxanthines, theophylline, and caffeine, which are nonspecific adenosine receptor inhibitors, to decrease the incidence of apnea of prematurity. However, the exact mechanism and location of action of adenosine, as well as the interaction of adenosine with other neurotransmitters, remain to be identified. Adenosine receptors may be inhibitory (A_3) or excitatory (A_{2B}). Recent reports have documented an interaction between adenosine and GABA in the regulation of breathing. Blockade of $GABA_A$ receptors abolished the inhibition of phrenic activity and the exaggerated LCR induced by adenosine A_{2A} agonist. Furthermore, A_{2A} receptors were found to colocalize on GABAergic neurons in the medulla oblongata of both piglets and rats. These data suggest that the mechanism of action of methylxanthines in the prevention of apnea of prematurity is through central blockade of either inhibitory A_1 receptors or excitatory A_2 adenosine receptors on GABAergic neurons.[3] In either case, respiratory inhibition is diminished.

Exogenous endorphin and enkephalin analogues have been shown to produce a consistent decrease in respiration in fetal and neonatal animals. Endorphin levels are elevated in the human neonate at birth and endogenous opioids were found to modulate the hypoxic ventilatory response in newborn infants and animals. Furthermore, the opioid antagonist naloxone produced an improvement in apnea and periodic breathing in infants in whom β-endorphin–like immunoreactivity in the CSF was elevated. Although these data support a role for opioids in respiratory control in neonates, the effect of anesthesia in such studies and the interaction of opioids with other inhibitory neurotransmitters need to be clarified. Infusion of prostaglandin E_1 (PGE_1) produces respiratory depression in 12% of infants during treatment for congenital heart disease. PGE_1 has been shown to decrease and indomethacin has been shown to enhance phrenic activity in newborn piglets.

Although the involvement of serotonin in respiratory control is well established, the nature of this involvement is complex. Both activation and inhibition of breathing have been described with different doses, routes of administration, and peripheral versus central effects. The different responses may be due, in part, to the effect on different subtypes of serotonin receptors preferentially expressed on respiratory neurons. Serotonin has been implicated as a regulatory factor in the production of apneusis. Blocking $5-HT_{1A}$ receptors has been shown to reverse apneustic breathing, which might result during hypoxia or ischemia. There is increasing evidence to suggest an important role for serotonergic neurons in the raphe nuclei in maturation of central chemoreception. This has been highlighted by findings in cohorts of sudden infant death syndrome (SIDS) victims (Japanese, African-American, and whites) in whom there was a significant positive association with the presence of a homozygous gene that encodes for the long allele of the 5-HT transporter promoter (5-HTT), as well as the long allele itself. In both studies, SIDS victims were more likely than control subjects to express the long allele of 5-HTT, as well as to miss the short allele of 5-HTT.[69] Therefore it is possible that a delay in maturation of serotonergic neurons or overexpression of the long allele for 5-HTT in the arcuate nucleus as well as in other respiratory groups might contribute to lack of respiratory responses to a stressful condition. This may be an underlying mechanism in the pathogenesis of SIDS.

Role of Astrocytes

It is becoming obvious that astrocytes play an important role in neural transmission. Astrocytes are able to release chemical transmitters including adenosine, D-serine, and glutamate, which play a role in synchronizing neuronal activity and modulating synaptic transmission. The role of astrocytes in modulation of respiration is suggested by the findings that application of methionine sulfoximine (MS), an inhibitor of glutamate release from astrocytes, in vitro to medullary slices diminished respiratory-related rhythm in the rostral medulla oblongata and decreased respiratory frequency in vivo in rats.[71]

APNEA OF PREMATURITY
Definition and Epidemiology

Apnea of prematurity has been defined most widely as cessation of breathing in excess of 15 seconds and typically accompanied by desaturations and bradycardia. Shorter episodes of apnea may also be accompanied by significant bradycardia or hypoxia. Whereas brief respiratory pauses of less than 10 seconds in duration can occur in conjunction with startles, movement, defecation, or swallowing during feeding, these short pauses are self-limited and not typically associated with bradycardia or hypoxemia. Prolonged desaturation episodes have also been reported in the absence of apnea or bradycardia, both in healthy preterm infants and more frequently in infants with chronic lung disease. These episodes might represent obstructive apnea, hypoventilation, or intrapulmonary right-to-left shunting. Although the significance of such episodes is unclear, recurrent hypoxemia has been associated with retinopathy of prematurity, necrotizing enterocolitis, and periventricular leukomalacia.

Apnea is traditionally classified into three categories based on the presence or absence of obstruction of the upper airways. These include central, obstructive, and mixed apnea. Central apnea is characterized by total cessation of inspiratory efforts with no evidence of obstruction. In obstructive apnea, the infant tries to breathe against an obstructed upper airway resulting in chest wall motion without nasal airflow throughout the entire apnea. Mixed apnea consists of obstructed respiratory efforts usually following central pauses (Fig. 44-49) and is probably the most common type of apnea followed in decreasing frequency by central and obstructive apnea. The site of obstruction in the upper airways is mostly in the pharynx; however, it may also occur at the larynx and possibly at both sites.

The incidence of apnea of prematurity is inversely related to gestational age and occurs in the vast majority of infants with extremely low birthweight. Apnea may occur from the first day of life in infants without RDS but may be delayed until several days in infants with RDS. The precise incidence of apnea depends on the diagnostic criteria employed; even so, the frequency and duration of apnea decrease with advancing postnatal age. Apnea is not exclusively confined to preterm babies in that healthy term infants were also found to have apnea exceeding 20 seconds on home monitoring.

Pathogenesis

Apnea of prematurity is a developmental disorder that probably reflects *physiologic* rather than *pathologic* immaturity of respiratory control (Table 44-5). However, despite major advances in our understanding of the control of breathing over the last decade, the exact mechanisms responsible for apnea in premature infants have not been clearly identified. This is clearly understandable in view of the limitations of studying human infants and the lack of an animal model that exhibits spontaneous apnea. Therefore most of our knowledge is derived from both physiologic studies in preterm infants and studies in immature animals. Immaturity of breathing responses in preterm infants affects all levels of respiratory control, including central and peripheral chemosensitivity, as well as inhibitory pulmonary afferents. This immaturity is manifested by impaired ventilatory responses to hypoxia and hypercapnia, and an exaggerated inhibitory response to stimulation of airway receptors, as described previously. Although a cause-and-effect relationship has not been documented for disturbed control of breathing and the occurrence of apnea in preterm infants, strong associations are very well established. Histologically, immaturity of the preterm brain is manifested by a decreased number of synaptic connections, dendritic arborizations, and paucity of myelin. Functionally, auditory evoked responses are impaired in infants with apnea when

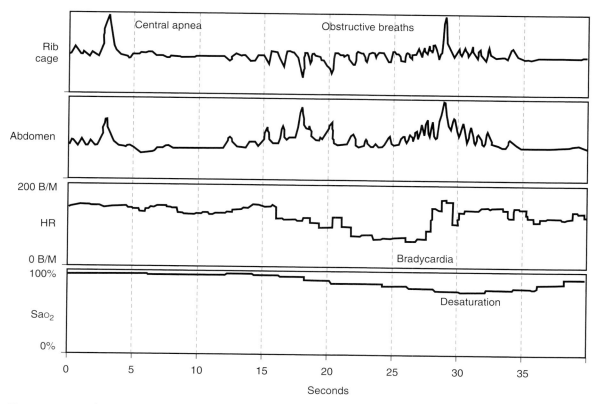

Figure 44–49. Characteristic mixed apnea of approximately 20 seconds' duration commencing with a central component and prolonged by obstructed inspiratory efforts. In the absence of simultaneous measurement of rib cage and abdominal motion as occurs during routine impedance monitoring of chest wall motion, the obstructed inspiratory efforts would not be recognized. As noted in this tracing, bradycardia and desaturation are secondary to the cessation of effective ventilation during the mixed apnea. B/M, beats per minute; HR, heart rate; SaO_2, arterial oxygen saturation.

TABLE 44-5	Factors Implicated in the Pathogenesis of Apnea of Prematurity	
Central Mechanisms	**Peripheral Reflex Pathways**	**Others**
Decreased central chemosensitivity	Decreased carotid body activity	Genetic predisposition
Hypoxic ventilatory depression	Increased carotid body activity	Sepsis and cytokines
Upregulated inhibitory neurotransmitters, GABA, adenosine	Laryngeal chemoreflex Excessive bradycardic response to hypoxia	Bilirubin

From Abu-Shaweesh JM, Martin RJ: Neonatal apnea: what's new? *Pediatr Pulmonol* 43:937, 2008, with permission.

compared with matched preterm control subjects, indicating delay in brainstem conduction time. Interestingly, this delay improves after treatment with aminophylline, signifying a functional rather than an anatomic immaturity.

The impairment of central chemosensitivity in preterm neonates is evident by the flat ventilatory response to CO_2 when compared with that in term neonates or adults. This impairment of hypercapnic ventilatory response is more pronounced in preterm neonates with apnea when compared with their controls without apnea. In other words, at the same level of CO_2 and for the same degree of change in alveolar CO_2, minute ventilation in babies with apnea is decreased (Fig. 44-50). Whereas exposure to hyperoxia silences the carotid body and may induce apnea, hypoxic ventilatory depression does not seem to contribute to the initiation of apnea because most infants are not hypoxic before apnea occurs. However, once apnea occurs it might prolong apnea and delay its recovery.

The peripheral chemoreceptors are located primarily in the carotid body and are responsible for stimulating breathing in response to hypoxia. Both enhanced and reduced peripheral chemoreceptor function may lead to apnea, bradycardia, or desaturations in the premature infant. In utero, the carotid chemoreceptor O_2 sensitivity is adapted to the normally low PaO_2 of the mammalian fetal environment (23 to 27 mm Hg). In response to the fourfold increase in PaO_2 with the establishment of air breathing, the peripheral chemoreceptors are silenced. This is followed by gradual increase in hypoxic chemosensitivity, although the mechanisms underlying this

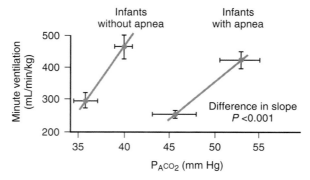

Figure 44-50. The ventilatory response to carbon dioxide has a decreased slope in infants with apnea. (*From Gerhardt T et al: Apnea of prematurity: I. Lung function and regulation of breathing,* Pediatrics 74:58, 1984. *Reproduced by permission of* Pediatrics.)

maturation are not completely clear.[13] A similar developmental profile has been described for both preterm and term infants. However, the contribution of immaturity of the peripheral chemoreceptors to apnea of prematurity is not clear. Maturation of peripheral arterial chemosensitivity is more or less complete by 2 weeks after birth in human infants whether the infant is term or preterm. Significant and prolonged apnea, however, can persist for many weeks to months in the most premature infants. Excessive peripheral chemoreceptor sensitivity in response to repeated hypoxia as seen in babies with bronchopulmonary dysplasia may also destabilize breathing patterns in the face of significantly fluctuating levels of oxygenation. Data in rat pups indicate that conditioning with intermittent hypoxic exposures results in facilitation of carotid body sensory discharge in response to subsequent hypoxic exposure. Furthermore, preterm infants with high frequency of apnea were found to have increased carotid body activity.[54] Hypoxia can also inhibit metabolism in the preterm infant and decrease CO_2 level, narrowing the difference between baseline CO_2 and apneic threshold CO_2 (CO_2 level below which apnea occurs). The baseline $PaCO_2$ in both preterm and term infants was found to be only 1 to 1.3 mm Hg above the apneic threshold.[39] The closeness of the apneic threshold to baseline CO_2 together with excessive activation of the carotid body might allow small oscillations of CO_2 in response to mild hyperventilation, startles, or stimulation to cause apnea. Clearly, much remains to be learned about both the short- and long-term consequences of intermittent hypoxic episodes during early development.

While laryngeal chemoflex (LCR) is thought to be an important contributor to apnea, bradycardia, and desaturation episodes associated with feeding and gastroesophageal reflux in preterm babies, the relationship of LCR to apnea of prematurity is less clear. The association of both apnea of prematurity and LCR with swallowing movements, as well as the observation of glottic closure and swallowing in fetal lambs during spontaneous apnea, points to the possibility of a common neural network controlling both disorders. Furthermore, similar to apnea of prematurity, LCR matures with advancing gestational age and is thought to be exaggerated in immature newborns and animals secondary to decreased central neural output or a dominance of inhibitory pathways.[4]

Bradycardia is a prominent feature in preterm infants with apnea. The mechanism underlying bradycardia associated with apnea in preterm infants is not clear, although it has been postulated that bradycardia during apnea might be related to hypoxic stimulation of the carotid body chemoreceptors, especially in the absence of lung inflation (Fig. 44-51). On the

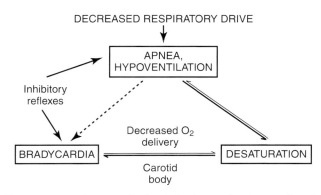

Figure 44–51. Proposed physiologic mechanisms whereby apnea induces reflex bradycardia. This can occur secondary to hypoxemia in the absence of lung inflation or by stimulation of upper airway inhibitory afferents. *(From Martin RJ, Fanaroff AA: Neonatal apnea, bradycardia or desaturation: does it matter?* J Pediatr *132:758, 1998, with permission.)*

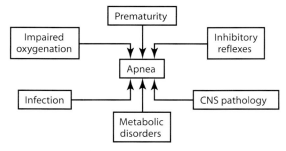

Figure 44–52. Specific contributory causes of apnea. CNS, central nervous system. *(From Martin RJ et al: Pathogenesis of apnea in preterm infants,* J Pediatr *109:733, 1986, with permission.)*

other hand, bradycardia occurs simultaneously with apnea during stimulation of laryngeal receptors suggesting a central mechanism for the production of both. The interaction between central respiratory and cardiovascular centers in the production of bradycardia in association with apnea of prematurity clearly needs further investigation.

The effect of genetic variability on regulation of breathing and apnea is suggested by the finding of a mutation in the *PHOX2B* gene in patients with congenital central hypoventilation. Similar to preterm infants with apnea, these children are characteristically symptomatic during the initial months of life and demonstrate absent or extremely reduced ventilatory responses to CO_2 and hypoxia even though no obvious brain, muscular, cardiac, or pulmonary lesions are apparent.[28] Tamim and colleagues found a higher incidence of apnea of prematurity in infants born to first-degree consanguineous parents than in other infants.[66] These findings raise the possibility of a role for developmentally regulated genes that might contribute to the vulnerability of preterm neonates to apnea. Further studies are clearly needed to explore the role of genetics in the pathogenesis of apnea of prematurity.

Clinical Associations

Apnea can be the presenting sign or may accompany multiple disorders that affect the preterm infant. A thorough consideration of possible causes is always warranted, especially when there is an unexpected increase in the frequency of episodes of apnea and/or bradycardia (Fig. 44-52). CNS disorders, particularly intracranial hemorrhage, hypoxic ischemic encephalopathy, and malformations can precipitate apnea in the preterm infant. Upper spinal cord trauma or malformations should be considered in an otherwise healthy infant presenting with apnea at birth.

Consideration of neonatal sepsis as a potential trigger for apnea of prematurity is widely known. Only recently has insight into a novel underlying mechanism emerged. In rat pups, systemic administration of the cytokine IL-1β inhibited respiratory activity, both at rest and in response to hypoxia, and this respiratory inhibition was diminished by prior block-

ade of prostaglandin synthesis with indomethacin. In subsequent work from the same group of investigators, evidence was presented for IL-1β binding to IL-1 receptors on vascular endothelial cells of the blood-brain barrier during a systemic immune response. Activation of the IL-1 receptor, in turn, induces synthesis of prostaglandin E_2, which is released into respiratory-related regions of the brainstem, resulting in respiratory depression.[31] New-onset apnea or increase in baseline incidence of apnea should prompt appropriate workup for sepsis and possibly antibiotic therapy. In the older infant, the presentation of respiratory syncytial virus (RSV) and other viral infections is sometimes heralded by apnea.

Anemia, another frequent problem in preterm infants, whether iatrogenic or secondary to bleeding, is a potential precipitating factor. Blood transfusions can improve irregular breathing patterns in preterm infants, although the limited benefit and potential risk of blood transfusion have limited its use as treatment for apnea. Other disease states that may precipitate apnea include metabolic disorders such as hypoglycemia, hypocalcemia, and electrolyte imbalance. Temperature instability and metabolic acidosis may be associated with apnea, although there is always the risk that sepsis is the underlying cause. Medications including opiates, benzodiazepines, magnesium sulfate, and PGE_1 can all precipitate apnea.

Gastroesophageal Reflux and Neonatal Apnea

Gastroesophageal reflux (GER) is often incriminated in causing neonatal apnea. Despite the frequent coexistence of apnea and GER in preterm infants, investigations of the timing of reflux in relation to apneic events indicate that they are rarely temporally related. Furthermore, when apnea and reflux coincide, there is no evidence that GER prolongs the concurrent apnea. Although physiologic experiments in animal models reveal that reflux of gastric contents to the larynx induces reflex apnea, there is no clear evidence that treatment of reflux will affect the frequency of apnea in most preterm infants. Therefore, pharmacologic management of reflux with agents that decrease gastric acidity or enhance gastrointestinal motility generally should be reserved for preterm infants who exhibit signs of emesis or regurgitation of feedings, regardless of whether apnea is present. Most recent studies have employed multichannel intraluminal impedance in addition to monitoring esophageal pH. This allows respiratory pauses to be correlated with both acidic and nonacidic bolus events in the esophagus and has allowed postprandial (nonacid) events to be carefully characterized. Currently available data with this new technique also do not readily support a clear relationship between gastroesophageal reflux and apnea in preterm infants, again raising doubts about the efficiency of widespread antireflux medication use in this population.[64]

Continuous Positive Airway Pressure Therapy

CPAP therapy at 4 to 6 cm H_2O has been used safely and effectively for more than 35 years. Because longer episodes of apnea frequently involve an obstructive component, CPAP appears to be effective by splinting the upper airway with positive pressure and decreasing the risk of pharyngeal or laryngeal obstruction. CPAP also benefits apnea by increasing functional residual capacity, thereby improving oxygenation status. At a higher functional residual capacity, time from cessation of breathing to desaturation and resultant bradycardia is prolonged. High-flow nasal cannula therapy has been suggested as an equivalent treatment modality that may allow CPAP delivery while enhancing mobility of the infant. This approach is widely taken, although it has not been well studied. In fact, considerable questions have been raised about the safety and efficacy of devices that provide relatively unregulated high flow as a means of CPAP delivery. While the mode of delivery for low CPAP in preterm infants will continue to be refined, CPAP use for ventilatory support and treatment of apnea is more widely used than ever in neonatal intensive care (see also Part 4).

Xanthine Therapy

Methylxanthines have been the mainstay of pharmacologic treatment of apnea of prematurity for more than 30 years. Both theophylline and caffeine are used, and both have multiple physiologic and pharmacologic mechanisms of action. Xanthine therapy increases minute ventilation, improves CO_2 sensitivity, decreases hypoxic depression of breathing, enhances diaphragmatic activity, and decreases periodic breathing. The precise pharmacologic basis for these actions, which are mediated by an increase in respiratory neural output, is still under investigation, although competitive antagonism of adenosine receptors is a well-documented effect of xanthines. While adenosine acts as an inhibitory neuroregulator in the CNS via activation of adenosine A_1 receptors, an effect on adenosine A_{2A} receptors' activation of GABAergic neurons, described earlier, might also play a role. The methylxanthines have some well-documented acute adverse effects. Toxic levels may produce tachycardia, cardiac dysrhythmias, feeding intolerance, and infrequently, seizures, although these effects are seen less commonly with caffeine at the usual therapeutic doses. Mild diuresis is caused by all methylxanthines. The observation that xanthine therapy causes an increase in metabolic rate and oxygen consumption of approximately 20% suggests that the caloric demands may be increased with this therapy at a time when nutritional

intake already is compromised. A large international multicenter clinical trial has been completed in which preterm infants were randomized to caffeine versus placebo therapy. This study was designed to test short- and long-term safety of this therapy. Initial evaluation of the findings has revealed a significant reduction in the postmenstrual ages at which both supplemental oxygen and endotracheal intubation were needed. Subsequent reports of neurodevelopmental outcome are also very encouraging with evidence for a significant decrease in cerebral palsy and cognitive delay in the caffeine treated group.[62] This finding raises interesting questions regarding possible mechanisms underlying this beneficial effect of caffeine on neurodevelopmental outcome (Fig. 44-53). These include the observation in animal models that loss of the adenosine A_1 receptor gene or caffeine administration are protective against hypoxia-induced loss of brain white matter and ventriculomegaly.[10] Furthermore, caffeine was found to increase amplitude and periods of continuity of EEG in preterm infants.[65a] While caffeine clearly decreases apneic episodes in preterm infants, the effect of caffeine on hypoxemic episodes is unclear; earlier data have not shown a clear benefit, making this worthy of further study.

Other Therapeutic Approaches

Any approach to nursing care that optimizes the infants' well-being is clearly highly desirable. "Kangaroo" care, or skin-to-skin nursing, has achieved widespread acceptance for stable infants, and provides an opportunity for greater parental involvement. Although the advocates of this approach have suggested a decrease in apnea rates, recent data have not supported this impression. Meanwhile, research on the biologic basis of sleep and awake states needs to be translated into preventive strategies for apnea.[46] There is considerable interest in identifying the optimal target oxygen saturation (e.g., 85% to 89% versus 91% to 95%) for preterm infants, and this issue is not yet resolved. One might anticipate that desaturation accompanying apnea will be greater at lower baseline SaO_2, but this has not been well documented. It has

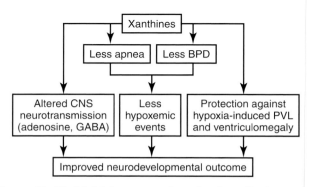

Figure 44–53. Multiple proposed mechanisms for improved neurodevelopmental outcome associated with xanthine therapy for apnea of prematurity. BPD, bronchopulmonary dysplasia; CNS, central nervous system; GABA, γ-aminobutyric acid; PVL, periventricular leukomalacia. (*From Abu-Shaweesh JM, Martin RJ: Neonatal apnea: what's new? Pediatr Pulmonol 43:937, 2008, with permission.*)

also been assumed, although unproven, that enhanced oxygen-carrying capacity, as with red blood cell transfusion, may decrease the likelihood of hypoxia-induced respiratory depression and resultant apnea. A novel approach is supplementation of inspired air with a very low concentration of supplemental CO_2 to increase respiratory drive. While of great interest from a physiologic perspective, and likely to be successful in decreasing apnea, it is doubtful that this would gain widespread clinical acceptance.

Resolution and Consequences of Apnea of Prematurity

Apnea of prematurity generally resolves by about 36 to 40 weeks' postconceptional age. However, in more immature infants, apnea frequently persists beyond this time. Data indicate that cardiorespiratory events in such infants return to the baseline "normal" level at about 43 to 44 weeks' postconceptional age. In other words, beyond 43 to 44 weeks' postconceptional age, the incidence of cardiorespiratory events in preterm infants does not significantly exceed that in term babies. For a subset of infants, the persistence of cardiorespiratory events may delay hospital discharge. In these infants, apnea longer than 20 seconds is rare; rather, these infants exhibit frequent bradycardia to less than 70 or 80 beats per minute with short respiratory pauses.[22] The reason some infants exhibit marked bradycardia with short pauses is unclear, but data suggest a vagal phenomenon and benign outcome. For a few of these infants, home cardiorespiratory monitoring, until 43 to 44 weeks' postconceptional age is offered in the United States as an alternative to a prolonged hospital stay.

The problem of correlating apnea with outcome is compounded by the fact that nursing reports of apnea severity may be unreliable, and impedance monitoring techniques fail to identify mixed and obstructive events. Despite these reservations, data suggest a link between the number of days that apnea and assisted ventilation were recorded during hospitalization and impaired neurodevelopmental outcome. A relationship between delay in resolution of apnea and bradycardia beyond 36 weeks' corrected age and a higher incidence of unfavorable neurodevelopmental outcome has also been recently shown.[57] Finally, a high number of cardiorespiratory events recorded after discharge via home cardiorespiratory monitoring appears to correlate with less favorable neurodevelopmental outcome. Future studies might better focus on the incidence and severity of desaturation events, in that techniques for long-term collection of pulse oximeter data are now more advanced. Furthermore, it is likely that recurrent hypoxia is the detrimental feature of the breathing abnormalities exhibited by preterm infants. For example, neonatal mice exhibiting hyperoxia-induced lung injury and exposed to intermittent hypoxia exhibit neurofunctional handicap when compared with normoxic mice with lung injury not subjected to intermittent hypoxia. Former preterm infants appear to be at greater risk of later sleep-disordered breathing, and recent data link xanthine use for apnea of prematurity with later sleep-disordered breathing. Recurrent episodes of desaturation during early life and resultant effects on neuronal plasticity related to peripheral or central respiratory control mechanisms may

serve as the underlying mechanisms for such a putative relationship.

Apnea and Sudden Infant Death Syndrome

The apparent lack of a relationship between persistent apnea of prematurity and SIDS has become clearer in recent years. In fact, no clinical evidence reliably links a physiologic ventilatory control abnormality to SIDS. SIDS continues to be the leading cause of postneonatal mortality with a peak incidence at 2 to 3 months of age and during winter months. SIDS continues to be a diagnosis of exclusion and in 2004 an expert panel defined SIDS as "the sudden and unexpected death of an infant under 1 year of age, with onset of the lethal episode apparently occurring during sleep, that remains unexplained after a thorough investigation including performance of a complete autopsy, and review of the circumstances of death and the clinical history." Certain risk factors have been consistently identified such as nonsupine sleep position, sleeping on a soft surface, maternal smoking during pregnancy, overheating, late or no prenatal care, young maternal age, preterm birth and/or low birthweight, male gender, and African American, American Indian, or Alaska native race. The use of pacifier has been associated with a protective effect on the occurrence of SIDS (odds ratio [OR], 0.39; 95% confidence interval [CI], 0.31-0.50).[30] Malloy and associates have shown that the mean postconceptional age at which SIDS occurs in preterm infants is younger than that of term infants. Clinically significant apnea has resolved by that postnatal age (Fig. 44-54).[49] The incidence of SIDS has decreased by more than half with the introduction of the international campaign to avoid all sleep positions except supine. However, the relative contribution of other risk factors including maternal smoking and socioeconomic factors to the incidence of SIDS increased during the same period (Fig. 44-55),[25] emphasizing the need for targeting these factors in order to further decrease the risk of SIDS.

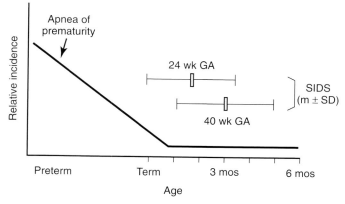

Figure 44–54. Schematic representation of the timing of sudden infant death syndrome (SIDS) in term (40 weeks' gestation) and very preterm (24 weeks' gestation) infants, in relation to the decline in incidence of apnea of prematurity. It would appear that apnea has largely resolved by 44 weeks' postconceptional age, which is prior to the peak incidence of SIDS at all gestational ages (GA).

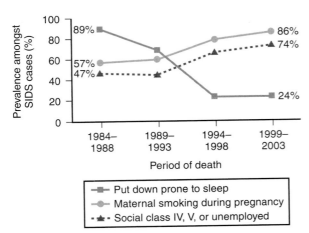

Figure 44–55. The prevalence of risk factors among victims of sudden infant death syndrome with the Back to Sleep campaign. Social class IV, semi-skilled occupation Social class V, unskilled occupation (*Adapted from Fleming P, Blair PS: Sudden infant death syndrome and parental smoking*, Early Hum Dev 83:721, 2007, with permission.)

The triple risk hypothesis has been widely adapted as an explanation for the pathophysiology of SIDS. It states that SIDS occurs in vulnerable at-risk infants during a developmental duration of risk and is precipitated by an acute insult. Vulnerability of SIDS victims may come from the environmental risk factors mentioned earlier, together with alcohol consumption during pregnancy, especially in Native Americans, as well as a genetic predisposition that includes the abnormalities of the serotonin system described previously. The peak incidence of SIDS (1 to 6 months of age) constitutes the developmental duration of risk, and the actual final insult might include apnea, asphyxia, or the LCR described previously.

DEVELOPMENTAL LUNG DISEASES
Pulmonary Agenesis/Hypoplasia

Abnormal lung development varies from complete agenesis of one lung or lobe of a lung to mild lung hypoplasia. It can also be classified as primary or secondary. Complete agenesis of the lung is usually unilateral, although dysgenesis of the other lung might also be present. While lung agenesis can be an isolated finding, it is commonly associated with other congenital malformations including renal, vertebral, cardiac, and gastrointestinal, as well as malformations of the first and second arch derivatives and radial ray defects. As a result, it was suggested that pulmonary agenesis may occur as an alternate to tracheoesophageal fistula in the VACTERL (V, vertebral anomalies; A, anal atresia; C, cardiac defect; TE, tracheoesophageal fistula; R, renal abnormalities; L, limb abnormalities) sequence or as part of the Goldenhar anomaly. In a review of 71 cases of lung agenesis, the defect was unilateral in 90% of the cases (49% on the right and 41% on the left) and bilateral in 10% of the cases.[20] There is usually compensatory hypertrophy of the contralateral lung with herniation to the affected hemithorax. Diagnosis is confirmed on antenatal ultrasound by the presence of mediastinal shift in the absence of diaphragmatic hernia. Antenatal echocardiogram reveals

total absence of the pulmonary artery or one of its branches on the affected side. Magnetic resonance imaging (MRI) examination can confirm the diagnosis, evaluate the size of the remaining lung, and evaluate the presence of other congenital malformations.

Unilateral or bilateral pulmonary hypoplasia is classified as *primary*, caused by intrinsic failure of normal lung development, or *secondary*, caused by multiple pathologic processes that interfere with normal lung development. Pulmonary hypoplasia is present in up to 33% of patients with oligohydramnios and can be associated with a high mortality rate (55% to 100%) depending on the severity of hypoplasia. (See also Chapter 22.) The pathophysiology of secondary pulmonary hypoplasia includes (1) oligohydramnios secondary to renal malformations, prolonged early amniotic fluid leak, placental abnormalities, or intrauterine growth restriction, (2) space-occupying lesions compressing the lungs and preventing normal growth as seen with congenital diaphragmatic hernia, cystic lung disease, or cardiac malformations with extreme cardiomegaly (e.g., tricuspid atresia or Ebstein anomaly), and (3) absence or abnormal diaphragmatic activity (that is essential for lung development) resulting from central or peripheral nervous disorders or musculoskeletal disease. Antenatal diagnoses can be achieved using different ultrasonography measurements including thoracic circumference (TC) corrected for gestational age or femur length, TC/abdominal circumference ratio, and *thoracic/heart area*. Recently, measurement of lung volume using three-dimensional ultrasound corrected for gestational age carried the best diagnostic accuracy versus three-dimensional ultrasound measurements. In addition to evaluation of the size of the lung, MRI can also diagnose associated anomalies that might be contributing to hypoplasia. Pathologic examination of the hypoplastic lung can show low ratio of lung to body weight, low DNA content, or decreased radial alveolar count. Peripheral bronchioles are decreased in number, as are the pulmonary arterioles, which often exhibit hypertrophy of medial smooth muscle, thus predisposing to persistent pulmonary hypertension.

After delivery, diagnosis of infants with unilateral pulmonary agenesis can be suspected by decreased breath sounds and displacement of the mediastinum to the affected side. Some breath sounds, however, may be audible over the affected side if a portion of normal lung has herniated across the midline. The radiographic appearance of a radiopaque hemithorax helps confirm the diagnosis, and accompanying vertebral defects are not uncommon (Fig. 44-56). Treatment is largely supportive, and prognosis depends on the presence or absence of other anomalies.

Secondary pulmonary hypoplasia is most commonly encountered in oligohydramnios and congenital diaphragmatic hernia (CDH). Survival of these infants depends on the degree to which lung growth is restricted and the underlying cause of hypoplasia. It is not uncommon for these patients to present with severe respiratory distress associated with bilateral pneumothorax. Patients with pulmonary hypoplasia secondary to prolonged premature rupture of membranes (PPROM) starting in the second trimester have recently been shown to have a better prognosis than initially expected. In a review of 98 deliveries with PPROM starting at 20 weeks' gestation, survival using modern neonatal therapies was 70% and medical history was not helpful

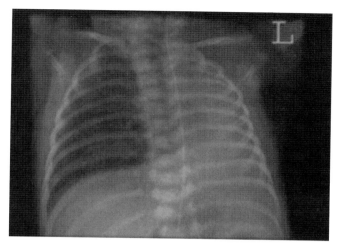

Figure 44–56. Unilateral left lung agenesis. *(From Greenough et al: Greenough A, Ahmed J, Broughton S: Unilateral pulmonary agencies, J Perinat Med 34:80, 2006. Perinat Med 34:80, 2006, with permission.)*

in predicting survival.[24] Both human and animal studies have shown that some of these infants who present with early severe respiratory failure consistent with pulmonary hypoplasia may benefit from inhaled nitric oxide (iNO). This treatment should be used with caution in premature infants, as some might have a dramatic response to iNO causing a rapid and extreme increase in PaO_2. Unlike term neonates, these babies usually do not show rebound persistent pulmonary hypertension (PPHN), and fast weaning of the inspired oxygen should be attempted.

Congenital Diaphragmatic Hernia (see Part 8)

Congenital diaphragmatic hernia occurs as a result of displacement of abdominal contents into the chest cavity through posterolateral or central diaphragmatic defects causing Bochdalek and Morgagni hernias, respectively. The incidence is between 1 in 2200 to 4000 live births, and it occurs most commonly on the left side (85%), while bilateral hernias are rare (1%) and mostly fatal. CDH is commonly associated with multiple congenital anomalies including cardiac, urogenital, chromosomal, syndromic, and musculoskeletal. The reported incidence of associated malformations varies between 20% and 60% depending on the method of diagnosis, the inclusion of autopsy cases or aborted fetuses, and whether extensive evaluation was performed. In a recent review of 3062 patients with CDH, the Congenital Diaphragmatic Hernia Study Group reported an incidence of 28% of severe malformations (major cardiac, syndromal and chromosomal disorders) in patients who did not undergo surgical repair secondary to unsalvageable hernia compared with 7% in repaired patients.[16] This emphasizes the importance of adequate evaluation of associated malformations in patients with CDH.

The underlying pathophysiology of CDH is that of pulmonary insufficiency and PPHN secondary to pulmonary hypoplasia, lower number of alveoli, and airway and vascular muscular hypertrophy associated with compression by abdominal contents. Pulmonary hypoplasia may also have a primary

developmental component, in that animal models have confirmed that developmental regulation of the lung and diaphragm are controlled by some of the same genes. The severity of CDH is related mostly to the degree of hypoplasia, which depends on the size of the defect,[16] the presence of the liver in the chest, and how early in gestation the abdominal contents were displaced. In a review of reports from 13 tertiary centers, 56% of CDH cases were diagnosed antenatally. Antenatal diagnosis is associated with a poor prognosis, and the data suggest that infants with a prenatal diagnosis had a better chance of survival if they were born in a tertiary center.[48] Several antenatal parameters have been evaluated for their ability to predict survival and morbidity in isolated CDH, including lung area to head circumference ratio (LHR), lung to chest transverse diameter ratio, the presence of fetal liver in the chest, estimated fetal lung volume by MRI and three-dimensional ultrasound corrected for body weight or gestational age, and size of pulmonary artery.[34] Even though most of these studies have reported lower values of lung volume assessment in patients with CDH when compared with standard measurements, the ability of these parameters to predict survival has not been consistent. This is mostly secondary to small number of patients in each series, challenges in measurement consistency, absence of standardized measurement and lack of correlation with actual lung volume, and inconsistent measures for survival or morbidity. Nevertheless, in a recent multicenter study involving 184 patients with isolated left CDH, there were no survivors in this large cohort in patients with liver herniation and LHR less than 0.8, and only 3 of 27 infants (11%) with LHR less than 1 survived. In comparison, survival was 58% (11 of 19) in fetuses with LHR greater than 1 and without liver herniation.[37] Even though the data from MRI and three-dimensional ultrasound studies look promising, they need further validation in larger group of patients. Postnatal factors associated with increased mortality and morbidity include low 5-minute Apgar score (0-3), size of the diaphragmatic defect (OR,14 for mortality with agenesis of the diaphragm), and need for patch repair.[16]

The clinical presentation of patients with CDH can vary from asymptomatic in mild cases to severe respiratory failure at birth. Diagnosis should be suspected in previously undiagnosed patients by the presence of severe respiratory distress, cyanosis, scaphoid abdomen, and failure to improve with ventilation. Physical examination reveals absence of air entry on the affected side with displacement of heart sounds to the contralateral side. Sometimes bowel sounds can be heard over the chest cavity. Once the diagnosis is made or suspected, patients should be immediately intubated and an orogastric tube placed to evacuate the stomach. Hyperventilation and escalation of peak inspiratory pressure (PIP) should be avoided (see later). Chest radiograph shows the presence of bowel loops in the affected chest cavity with shifting of the heart to the contralateral side (Fig. 44-57). If the stomach is included in the hernia, the tip of orogastric tube will overlie the affected chest cavity. The presence of liver in the chest is suspected by deviation of the umbilical venous line. Late presentation of Bochdalek hernia occurs in 5% to 10% of cases. These patients can be asymptomatic at birth and usually present later in life with respiratory or gastrointestinal symptoms. High index of suspicion is needed in these cases to prevent unwarranted and potentially dangerous interventions like insertion of a chest

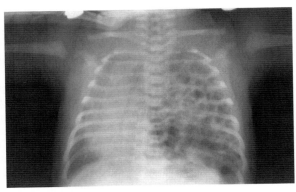

Figure 44–57. Left-sided diaphragmatic hernia in a 1-day-old term infant.

tube for suspected pleural effusion or pneumothorax. Diagnosis can be made after nasogastric tube insertion, contrast upper gastrointestinal study, or chest computed tomography (CT) scan. Prognosis for cases with late presentation is excellent once the correct diagnosis is made.

Improved survival has been reported recently using a consistent approach in the management of CDH that can be facilitated by the development of multidisciplinary standardized treatment guidelines, including input from neonatology, pediatric surgery, extracorporeal membrane oxygenation (ECMO) specialists, and respiratory therapy (Box 44-12). Predetermined criteria for the use of ECMO and an underlying "protect the

---

BOX 44–12 **Management of Congenital Diaphragmatic Hernia**

RESOLVED ISSUES

There is a high incidence of associated malformations.
Delivery at a tertiary center improves survival for antenatally diagnosed cases.
Agenesis of the diaphragm and herniation of the liver are poor prognostic signs.
Multidisciplinary approach using gentle ventilation improves outcome.
Survivors need long-term follow-up and management of associated complications.

UNRESOLVED ISSUES

The utility of antenatal ultrasound and magnetic resonance imaging markers to predict survival
The role of antenatal steroids, surfactant, and inhaled nitric oxide in management
Surgical approach
Benefit of extracorporeal membrane oxygenation (ECMO) and use of chest tube

RECOMMENDATIONS

Accept preductal saturations ≥ 85%, $PaCO_2$ ≤ 65, and pH ≥ 7.25.
Identify preset ventilatory limits not to be exceeded.
Use of high-frequency oscillatory ventilation if CMV, conventional mechanical ventilation fails
Use of ECMO per preset criteria
Delay surgery until persistent pulmonary hypertension improves.

---

lung" strategy are essential components in the care of these infants and can be as important as the specific medical interventions chosen. Whereas animal studies have suggested lung immaturity and surfactant deficiency in animal models of CDH, the use of antenatal steroids and surfactant replacement has not been shown to be beneficial. On the contrary, a bolus dose of surfactant may be associated with sudden irreversible decompensation that requires ECMO. A recent systematic review of strategies associated with improved survival among infants with CDH in 13 centers that cared for at least 20 patients and reported a survival rate of 75% or more has described multiple successful treatment strategies associated with this improved survival.[48] Although these centers used different mechanical ventilation strategies, most of these targeted the use of gentle ventilation or permissive hypercapnia. The basic elements of this treatment strategy are:

1. Setting ventilatory pressure limits that should not be exceeded to prevent lung damage secondary to volutrauma. The pressure limits varied in different centers between 20 to 25 and 30 to 35 cm H_2O for PIP and 12 to 18 cm H_2O for mean airway pressure.
2. Accepting preductal saturations of greater than or equal to 85%, regardless of postductal saturation, and higher $PaCO_2$ levels of less than or equal to 65 with pH of at least 7.25 as long as there is evidence of adequate tissue perfusion and oxygenation evaluated by pH and lactate levels.
3. Instituting high-frequency oscillatory ventilation (HFOV) or high-frequency positive pressure ventilation once the preset limit failed to achieve adequate saturations or $PaCO_2$ levels, although HFOV was used by some as the primary mode of ventilation.
4. Even though iNO might produce short-term benefits, the routine use of iNO is not supported by current data and might actually be associated with worse outcome.
5. Using ECMO as rescue therapy with variable indications in different centers including persistent oxygenation index (OI) above 40, persistent hypoxemia, or failure of ventilatory management to support oxygenation, ventilation, or tissue perfusion.
6. Delaying surgical repair until physiologic stabilization and improvement of PPHN.

Questions regarding the use of chest tubes, repair on or off ECMO, and benefits of various options for surgical reconstruction of large defects remain to be answered.

The overall survival using this approach in the management of 763 infants with symptomatic CDH was 79%, while that for isolated CDH was 85%. Survival was approximately 70% and 90% for patients with isolated CDH with and without need for ECMO, respectively. Mortality was generally attributed to the presence of additional anomalies, iatrogenic lung injury, severe pulmonary hypoplasia or PPHN, and bleeding complications among ECMO-treated infants. However, the survival data might underestimate hidden mortality secondary to termination, rate of diagnosis, and referral pattern for outborn patients. Infants born with CDH have multiple long-term morbidities affecting the pulmonary, gastrointestinal, and skeletal systems. Respiratory complications include pulmonary vascular abnormalities presumably causing pulmonary hypertension, a higher incidence of obstructive airway disease, and a restrictive lung function pattern. Gastroesophageal reflux disease sometimes in combination with failure to thrive is a well-recognized complication in patients with CDH and several patients require antireflux surgery. It is unknown whether GERD has an effect on pulmonary function in this population. Pulmonary hypoplasia and PPHN predispose children born with CDH to a high risk for hypoxemia, which may result in neurodevelopmental delay. Chest wall deformities and scoliosis are more common among CDH patients, although deformities are mild and surgery is rarely required.[55] These data emphasize the need for multidisciplinary team approach in the postoperative management and follow-up of all survivors of CDH.

Capillary Alveolar Dysplasia

Capillary alveolar dysplasia (CAD) is a rare fatal pulmonary disease that usually presents in the newborn period with severe hypoxemia and PPHN unresponsive to treatment. Although the disease is mostly sporadic, reports of multiple affected siblings in subsets of families suggest an autosomal recessive inheritance. CAD is a pathologic diagnosis that is mostly identified at autopsy while 10% can be diagnosed with antemortem lung biopsy. Histologically, CAD is characterized by paucity of capillaries proximal to the alveolar epithelium, anomalous distended pulmonary veins within the bronchovascular bundle instead of the interlobular septa, and immature alveolar development with medial thickening of small pulmonary arteries and muscularization of the arterioles. These characteristic findings are diffuse in 85% of patients and patchy in the rest. While the mechanisms underlying PPHN are not clear, they are probably related to capillary hypoplasia, impaired pulmonary bloodflow secondary to discontinuity of capillaries, and pulmonary veins and reactive pulmonary vasoconstriction mediated by hypoxia that might respond transiently to pulmonary vasodilators.[63] Multiple other congenital nonlethal malformations might be associated with CAD. These include gastrointestinal (30%), cardiac (30%), renal (23%), right-left asymmetry as well as CDH, and phocomelia.

Most patients with CAD present within the first few hours of life. These infants are usually born at term and have appropriate size and normal Apgar scores. Although these babies might be asymptomatic at delivery, respiratory distress, cyanosis, and hypoxemia progress quickly to respiratory failure in more than half of these patients within hours after delivery. About 14% of these patients do not present with symptoms until 2 to 6 weeks of life. Treatment is always unsatisfactory. Although transient response to iNO might be observed, this is usually short lasting. PPHN is not responsive to medical treatment and the disease progression is that of a fulminant course and rapid progression to death, although there are reports of survival beyond the neonatal period. High index of suspicion and diagnostic lung biopsy are required to avoid the use of more invasive and futile treatments, including ECMO.

Congenital Pulmonary Lymphangiectasia

Congenital pulmonary lymphangiectasia (CPL) is a rare disorder of term neonates although presentation in preterm infants has been described. Most cases of CPL are sporadic with predilection for male involvement (2:1). However, familial presentations suggestive of autosomal recessive inheritance have been described. CPL is classified as primary or secondary. Primary CPL can present as a diffuse or localized primary pulmonary developmental defect or as a part of more generalized lymphatic involvement. Patients with generalized lymphangiectasia tend to have less severe pulmonary involvement. Secondary cases of CPL are mostly seen with cardiac malformations associated with obstructed pulmonary venous return including total obstructed anomalous pulmonary venous return, hypoplastic left heart syndrome, and cor triatrium. CPL has also been described in multiple syndromes including Noonan, Down, and Ullrich-Turner. The characteristic pathologic finding of CPL is pulmonary lymphatic dilation in the subpleural, interlobar, perivascular, and peribronchial lymphatics.

The etiology of CPL is not clear but is thought to be secondary to failure of regression of lymphatics that occurs normally between 16 and 20 weeks' gestation. Recently, multiple genes have been found to be involved in lymphatic development, including *FOXC2*, vascular endothelial growth factor 3, and integrin $\alpha9\beta1$ genes. Mice homozygous for a null mutation in the integrin $\alpha9$ subunit gene died of respiratory failure due to bilateral chylothorax within 6 to 12 days after birth with pathologic features similar to those in CPL. Patients with CPL usually present with intractable respiratory failure, cyanosis, and hypoxia associated with bilateral chylothorax in the first few hours of life, although diagnosis can be delayed for several weeks in cases of unilobar involvement. Nonimmune hydrops is also a well-recognized presentation in patients with CPL. Examination of the pleural fluid shows characteristic findings of chylothorax with lymphocytosis, although elevated triglycerides might be absent in nonfed infants (see later). Chest radiograph reveals hyperinflation of the lung with bilateral interstitial infiltrates and bilateral pleural effusions. High-resolution computed tomography demonstrates diffuse thickening of the peribronchovascular interstitium and the septa surrounding the lobules. Definitive diagnosis is made by lung biopsy showing the characteristic features, although differentiation from lymphangiomatosis can be difficult.[11]

Treatment is mostly supportive. Intubation and mechanical ventilation, drainage of pleural and peritoneal effusions, correction of hypoxia, acidosis, and shock might be needed in the delivery room for stabilization. Persistent chylothorax might require chest tube placement. Genetic therapy involving VEGF might be promising in patients with severe involvement. Prognosis appears to depend on the severity of symptoms in the immediate newborn period. Although traditionally thought to be fatal, there are recent reports of survival in some patients who present in the immediate neonatal period with respiratory failure, chylothorax, and hydrops fetalis. Later presentation carries a better prognosis with the possibility of spontaneous resolution, although respiratory morbidity might be common.

Chylothorax

Chylothorax or the accumulation of lymph fluid in the pleural cavity is the commonest cause of clinically significant pleural effusion in neonates and can be congenital or acquired. Congenital chylothorax can be seen in association with multiple congenital malformations that result in poor development or obstruction of the lymphatic system. These include pulmonary lymphangiectasia, lymphangiomatosis, congenital heart disease (CHD), mediastinal masses, or chromosomal anomalies. Acquired chylothorax is most commonly associated with trauma during thoracic surgery for CHD or CDH, but can also occur secondary to increase in venous pressure in patients with venous thrombosis. Significant antenatal chylothorax accumulation can impair lung development and cause pulmonary hypoplasia. The rate of lymph drainage is about 1 mL/kg per hour, most of which is reabsorbed by lymphatic capillaries into the thoracic duct. Flow is increased by physical activity and by enteral feeding. Chylothorax is usually unilateral and more commonly affects the right side.

Clinical presentation is that of respiratory distress secondary to lung compression, pulmonary hypoplasia, or symptoms of the underlying pulmonary or cardiac disease. Significant loss of lymphatic fluid postnatally can result in malnutrition secondary to fatty acid, triglyceride and protein loss, and infection secondary to loss of immunoglobulins and lymphocytes. Physical examination is significant for decreased breath sounds on the affected side with shifting of the cardiac apex to the contralateral side. Chest radiograph shows pleural effusion, compression of the lung on the affected side, and displacement of the heart to the opposite side. Diagnosis is established by analysis of the pleural fluid. In babies with established feeding, chylothorax appears milky with opaque color; however, in nonfed neonates it is clear. Lymphatic fluid is rich in triglycerides (more than 1.1 mmol/L), protein, and cells (more than 1000 cells/μL) with more than 80% lymphocytes.

Treatment is mostly supportive while awaiting resolution of the effusion. Mechanical ventilation and drainage of the chylothorax might be needed in patients with large effusions, and nutritional support using total parenteral nutrition is essential. Feeding, once started, with formulas containing high percentage of medium chain triglycerides (MCTs) is recommended because lymphatics are not needed for MCT absorption. However, this approach does not appear to significantly reduce the triglyceride and fatty acid content of the fluid accumulating in the pleural space. Intravenous immunoglobulin administration should be considered in patients with recurrent infections, especially if hypogammaglobulinemia is present. In most cases spontaneous resolution occurs within 4 to 6 weeks. Several treatment strategies have been described for cases with persistent chylothorax, including pleurodesis, ligation of the thoracic duct, and pleuroperitoneal shunt. Whereas povidone-iodine pleurodesis has been used successfully in persistent chylothorax, it has also been associated with renal failure. There is growing evidence from uncontrolled case studies suggesting a markedly positive effect of somatostatins and in particular octreotide in the treatment of chylothorax with minimal side effects. In the absence of a controlled trial evaluating safety and efficacy, this therapy should be reserved for persistent and severe cases and not as first line of treatment.[60]

Congenital Cystic Pulmonary Malformations

Congenital cystic lung disease comprises a broad spectrum of rare but clinically significant developmental abnormalities, including congenital cystic adenomatoid malformation (CCAM), bronchopulmonary sequestration (BPS), bronchogenic cyst (BC), and congenital lobar emphysema (CLE). These lesions were originally thought to be separate entities. However, the description of coexistence of multiple lesions (bronchogenic cyst, CCAM, and extralobar BPS) in the same patient suggests a common embryologic origin for these malformations. Blood supply to early bronchial buds is provided by primitive systemic capillaries that regress as pulmonary arterial blood supply becomes dominant. Interruption of tracheobronchial and vascular development at different sites and during different stages of lung growth would determine the congenital lesion produced as well as its blood supply.

CONGENITAL CYSTIC ADENOMATOID MALFORMATION

CCAM constitutes multiple different hamartomatous lesions arising from the abnormal branching of immature bronchial tree. The term *congenital pulmonary adenomatoid malformation* (CPAM) has been proposed to substitute for CCAM because only two types of CCAM are cystic. CCAM is the most common congenital cystic lung disease occurring in 1 in 25,000 to 30,000 live births and more commonly in males. It affects both lungs equally, and is most commonly unilobar with predilection to affecting lower lung lobes. Unlike BPS, it is connected with the tracheobronchial tree and has pulmonary blood supply (Table 44-6). Different classifications have been proposed for CCAM, including types 1-3 based on

TABLE 44–6 Characteristics of Congenital Cystic Adenomatoid Malformation Versus Bronchopulmonary Sequestration

	Congenital Cystic Adenomatoid Malformation	Bronchopulmonary Sequestration
Classification	Types 0-4, microcystic and macrocystic	Intralobar and extralobar
Connection to tracheobronchial tree	Yes	No
Systemic blood supply	No	Yes
Associated malformation	Common	Less common
Location	Either lower lobe	Left lower lobe
Malignant transformation	Yes	Yes
Spontaneous regression of antenatally diagnosed cases	11%	75%

histopathologic findings, expanded later to include types 0-4, and microcystic versus macrocystic based on gross anatomy and antenatal ultrasound appearance. Whereas the latter classification has poor correlation with histologic features, it has a much better prognostic value than the earlier classification with microcystic lesions (cysts less than 5 mm) having poorer prognosis than macrocystic lesions (greater than 5 mm). Type 1 CCAM is the most common (50% to 65%) and consists of large cysts surrounded by multiple small cysts and is rarely associated with congenital malformations. Type 2 (10% to 40%) consists of multiple small cysts (0.5 to 2 cm) and is associated with cardiac, renal, and chromosomal abnormalities, whereas type 3 (5% to 10%) consists of multiple smaller cysts (rarely more than 0.2 cm) or solid mass that is associated with significant risk of hydrops and polyhydramnios resulting from caval obstruction and cardiac compression secondary to mediastinal shift.[65]

Clinical presentation varies. Fifteen percent of CCAM patients are stillborn and have a high incidence of associated anomalies. Of liveborn infants, 80% present with respiratory distress in the neonatal period while less than 10% present after the first year of life with recurrent pneumonia, lung abscess, failure to thrive, pneumothorax, or malignancy. With the advancement of ultrasonography, more cases of CCAM have been diagnosed antenatally. Second trimester ultrasound can identify the presence of echogenic pulmonary masses with mediastinal shift, hydrops, or polyhydramnios; assess the size of the lung and evidence of hypoplasia; and diagnose associated malformations. Fetal echocardiogram might diagnose cardiac malformations as well as identify the origin of the blood supply. High-resolution ultrasonography or fetal MRI can differentiate CCAM from other lesions, including BPS, BC, congenital emphysema, CDH, or enteric duplication. The natural history of CCAM is variable. Up to 40% undergo rapid growth and enlargement causing compression of the adjacent lung and heart with mediastinal shift, cardiac failure, and hydrops, whereas 11% undergo spontaneous regression. Maximum CCAM growth is achieved by 28 weeks' gestation and decrease in size can start afterward. Most cases of spontaneous regression usually occur in type 3 lesions and are not limited to small or mild cases, in fact, cases of CCAM associated with hydrops have been described to undergo spontaneous improvement and regression. These cases do not actually "disappear" but become isoechogenic with the adjacent lung tissue and cannot be differentiated by ultrasound or postnatal chest radiograph. However, fetal MRI or postnatal chest CT will identify these lesions (Fig. 44-58).

Despite reported cases of spontaneous resolution, the presence of hydrops in CCAM patients is the single most important poor prognostic factor associated with high mortality. Fetal surgery using thoracoamniotic shunting or open fetal surgery has been associated with 60% and 70% survival, respectively. (See also Chapter 11.) Patients who are not suitable for surgery might benefit from antenatal steroids which were shown to decrease the size of CCAM lesions. The EXIT procedure should be considered in patients with significant mediastinal shift and cardiac compression at time of delivery.[9]

There is consensus on the need for surgical excision in treating symptomatic CCAM patients. In most cases, lobectomy or segmental excision might be adequate. However,

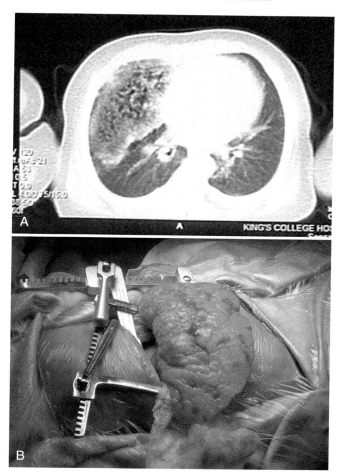

Figure 44–58. See color insert. A, Computed tomography scan showing right-sided microcystic congenital cystic adenomatoid malformation (CCAM). B, Lung resection of predominantly solid and small cysts (type 2) CCAM. *(Adapted from Stanton M, Davenport M: Management of congenital lung lesions, Early Human Dev 82:289, 2006, with permission.)*

pneumonectomy or multiple excisions might be needed in multilobar or bilateral lesions. In hybrid cases with associated BPS, special attention to identify and ligate the systemic blood supply is needed. The treatment of asymptomatic patients continues to be controversial between expectant management versus elective resection. However, the majority opinion seems to favor elective resection at 2 to 6 months of age secondary to the associated later complications, including recurrent pneumonia and malignancy. Following successful resection, the long-term functional outcome of children with CCAM is excellent with no physical limitations or increased risk for infection, although RSV immunoglobulin prophylaxis is advised in these patients.[9]

BRONCHOPULMONARY SEQUESTRATION

BPSs are microscopic cystic masses of nonfunctioning lung tissue that are usually supplied by the systemic circulation. The origin of sequestrations is believed to be an accessory lung bud that forms distal to the normal lung and migrates caudally with the esophagus. Two forms are recognized: intralobar sequestration (ILS) and extralobar sequestration (ELS). If the accessory bud arises before establishment of the pleura, it is contained within the normal lung (ILS); if it arises afterward, it has its own pleural covering and is completely separated from the normal lung (ELS). Like CCAM, sequestrations can be associated with multiple congenital malformations including chest wall, cardiac, gastrointestinal, and vertebral anomalies. ILS is usually asymptomatic in the neonatal period and can be diagnosed on routine antenatal ultrasonography. ELS can be asymptomatic or can present with pneumonia, atelectasis, bleeding, or high-output cardiac congestive heart failure secondary to the systemic arteriovenous blood shunting. Both forms are more common in the left lower chest and 10% of ELS are intra-abdominal. In 20% of patients with ELS, systemic blood supply originates from the infradiaphragmatic aorta. Large thoracic lesions can cause mediastinal shift and present with hydrops, although this presentation is very uncommon. Intra-abdominal ELS does not cause hydrops or pulmonary hypoplasia, although it may cause polyhydramnios secondary to gastrointestinal obstruction.[15]

On antenatal ultrasound, sequestrations appear as well-defined, echodense, homogeneous masses, and the diagnosis is confirmed by the documentation of systemic blood supply by color Doppler. If unclear, ultrafast MRI can establish the systemic blood supply, define the lesion, and identify other associated malformations. ELS can be differentiated from ILS if surrounded by pleural effusion. Intra-abdominal ELS appears as a suprarenal solid mass and should be differentiated from other suprarenal masses including neuroblastoma and mesoblastic nephroma. Antenatal or postnatal echocardiography can show associated cardiac malformation. BPS appears on chest radiograph as a posterior thoracic mass mostly on the left. Chest CT scan or even MRI might be needed to further delineate systemic blood supply.

Fetuses diagnosed antenatally with BPS should be delivered at a tertiary center where appropriate management of severe respiratory compromise and pulmonary hypertension is available. Following supportive care with appropriate respiratory management, symptomatic patients should be treated with surgical excision. However, this should be deferred until after stabilization in patients with severe PPHN. Up to 60% of right-sided ILS had anomalous pulmonary venous return, and accurate identification of arterial and venous supply is essential to prevent ligation of pulmonary vessels. Asymptomatic patients should undergo elective resection to prevent complications of malignancy or infection.[18]

Up to 75% of antenatally diagnosed BPS undergo spontaneous resolution. This is thought to be secondary to infarction associated with an overgrown blood supply or torsion, or due to decompression in the tracheobronchial tree. Untreated BPS cases associated with hydrops are uniformly fatal. Several fetal surgeries have been proposed including thoracoamniotic shunt for decompression of pleural effusion, surgical excision, or EXIT procedure.[18] Long-term complications of patients with resected BPS include gastroesophageal reflux disease, asthma, chest wall malformations, and pneumonia.

BRONCHOGENIC CYST

BCs consist mostly of a single cyst lined by respiratory epithelium and covered with elements of tracheobronchial tree including cartilage and smooth muscle. BCs originate from an abnormal budding of the ventral surface of the primitive foregut without undergoing further branching, resulting in a blind cyst that may or may not communicate with the airways. While cysts are mostly found centrally in the mediastinum, budding that starts late in gestation might originate from the distal airways generating peripheral cysts embedded within normal lung tissue. Potential locations for a BC include cervical, paratracheal, subcarinal, hilar, mediastinal, and intrapulmonary. Less common ectopic sites include paravertebral, paraesophageal, and pericardial locations.

In the neonatal period, most patients with BC are asymptomatic, and diagnosis is made on prenatal ultrasound or incidentally on a chest radiograph after birth. Symptoms, if present, are secondary to mass effect on airways, gastrointestinal tract, or the cardiovascular system. Even though major airway obstruction is uncommon, subcarinal lesions can present with severe obstruction. On the other hand, obstruction of smaller airways can cause air trapping, overdistention, and a clinical picture similar to that of congenital labor emphysema. Undiagnosed cases in the neonatal period usually present in older children or adults with pneumonia, hemoptysis, pneumothorax, dysphagia, or signs of caval obstruction.

Lesions diagnosed on prenatal ultrasound can be further differentiated from other cystic lesions by prenatal MRI. Postnatally, fluid-filled BCs can appear on chest radiograph as radiopaque areas. If connected to the airway, an air-fluid level may be seen. CT scan is the study of choice before undergoing surgery and provides a thorough characterization of the lesion and its relation to mediastinal structures.

Treatment of all cases of BCs is complete surgical excision. In symptomatic patients, this is performed after immediate clinical stabilization. Simple aspiration should be considered in patients with severe compromise as a temporizing measure, but complete resection is subsequently required. In asymptomatic newborns, surgery can be done electively at a few months of age. Patients who undergo resection of a BC have an excellent outcome. Life-threatening complications before surgery develop in a few patients who have a poor outcome. There are no long-term complications related to the resection of a BC.[43]

CONGENITAL LOBAR EMPHYSEMA

CLE is a rare anomaly of the lung that is characterized by postnatal overdistention of one or more segments or lobes of the lung. The mechanism underlying CLE is that of intrinsic or extrinsic obstruction of the airways causing air trapping, overdistention, and subsequent emphysema. Multiple mechanisms have been described to explain the development of CLE including dysplastic bronchial cartilage, inspissated mucus, aberrant cardiopulmonary vasculature, and infection. In half of the cases no underlying pathology is identified. The left upper lobe is most frequently affected (42%), followed by right middle lobe (35%) and the right upper lobe (21%). The lower lobes are involved in 1% of the cases. CLE is three times as common in males.

Patients usually present in the neonatal period with respiratory distress; however, later presentations have been described. The severity of the clinical picture depends on the size of the CLE and the degree of compression of the normal lung. Physical examination might be indistinguishable from pneumothorax with decreased air entry, bulging of the affected hemithorax, and in severe cases, shifting of the apical heartbeat to the contralateral side. CLE can be detected at midgestation using a combination of ultrasonography and ultrafast fetal MRI, although differentiation from CCAM might be difficult. Diagnosis is usually made by chest radiograph that may show an early opaque mass due to delayed clearance of lung fluid followed by a hyperlucent overexpanded area of lung with atelectasis of the adjacent lobes of the lung, depression of the diaphragm, and mediastinal shift to the opposite side (Fig. 44-59). The distinction of CLE from pneumothorax is essential to prevent attempted aspiration and potential development of tension pneumothorax. The presence of alveolar air markings throughout the emphysematous area is supportive of CLE. The emphysematous segment may also herniate anterior to the heart and great vessels. CT scan of the chest is a useful adjunct. Treatment of CLE depends on the severity of symptoms. Conservative and supportive management should be considered in milder cases. Surgical resection of the affected area should be considered in patients with life-threatening progressive pulmonary insufficiency from compression of the adjacent normal lung. Once the emphysematous area is resected, the long-term prognosis is excellent.[42]

Pulmonary Arteriovenous Malformation

Intrapulmonary arteriovenous malformation is a rare vascular anomaly of the lung that is associated with cyanosis and may lead to significant morbidity. It can be associated with skin hemangiomas and present with cyanosis not responding to medical management. Antenatal diagnosis of intrapulmonary arteriovenous malformations is possible and allows early treatment. Postnatal diagnosis is confirmed by angiography. Treatment is by surgical resection, although successful management with resolution of intrapulmonary shunting has been described using transcatheter occlusion with multiple coils.[38]

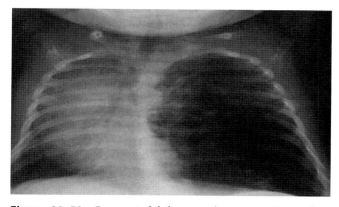

Figure 44–59. Congenital lobar emphysema with marked tracheal and mediastinal shift, in a patient who required emergency lobectomy. (*From Shanmugam G et al: Congenital lung malformations—antenatal and postnatal evaluation and management,* Eur J Cardiothorac Surg 27:45, 2005, with permission.)

ACQUIRED NEONATAL PULMONARY DISEASES

Meconium Aspiration Syndrome

Meconium is comprised of desquamated fetal intestinal cells, bile acids, minerals, enzymes including alpha$_1$ antitrypsin and phospholipase A$_2$, as well as swallowed amniotic fluid, lanugo, skin cells, and vernix caseosa. Antenatal passage of fetal intestinal contents into the amniotic fluid is common at 15 weeks' gestation; however, the incidence decreases with increasing gestational age, and becoming very infrequent by 34 weeks' gestation.

Meconium staining of amniotic fluid (MSAF) occurs in 5% to 24% of normal pregnancies (mean 13%). Risk factors for MSAF include postmaturity (gestational age beyond 41 weeks), small for gestational age (SGA), fetal distress, and compromised in utero conditions including placental insufficiency and cord compression. The latter is evident by the observation that 20% to 30% of infants born through MSAF are depressed at birth with an Apgar score of 6 or less at 1 minute. The mechanisms underlying MSAF are not clear; however, there is evidence of increased parasympathetic activity causing increased peristalsis and relaxation of the anal sphincter secondary to enhanced vagal output during cord compression. Recently, corticotrophin releasing factor, a known mediator of colonic motility, has been implicated in the pathogenesis of hypoxia-induced MSAF in a rat model.[44]

Meconium aspiration syndrome (MAS) has been defined as respiratory distress in an infant born through MSAF whose symptoms cannot be otherwise explained. This definition correctly implies that respiratory distress might occur in infants born through MSAF for a variety of reasons other than MAS. Infants born through MSAF were found to have a 100-fold increase in the likelihood of developing respiratory distress than those born through clear amniotic fluid, even in those with normal fetal heart tracing and Apgar scores. MAS occurs in only 5% of patients born through MSAF, although the case-fatality rate of affected infants remains high at 5% to 40%. The incidence of MAS had decreased recently secondary to improved obstetric standards, especially secondary to a decrease in number of deliveries beyond 41 weeks' gestation in developed countries. Two large recent studies from the United States and Australia/New Zealand confirmed that the incidence of MAS increases with increasing GA for infants between 37 and 41 weeks in a study cohort involving more than 14 million babies. The incidence of MAS (USA) and MAS requiring intubation (AUS) in this cohort increased twofold to threefold at 41 weeks' gestation compared with neonates born at an earlier gestation.[21,73]

PATHOPHYSIOLOGY

During normal fetal breathing, pulmonary fluid moves predominately outward from the airways into the oropharynx. However, severe asphyxia in utero can induce gasping and aspiration of amniotic fluid and particulate matter into the large airways. The meconium inhaled by the fetus may be present in the trachea or larger bronchi at delivery. Meconium and squamous epithelium can also be found as far as the alveoli in stillborn infants, and it is widely recognized that meconium aspiration can occur antenatally. After air breathing has commenced, especially if accompanied by gasping respirations, there is a rapid distal migration of meconium within the lung. Thick meconium, nonreassuring fetal heart tracing, low Apgar score at 5 minutes, instrumental delivery, especially emergency cesarean section, and planned home delivery are associated with increased risk for development of MAS.[21,40] The presence of such risk factors in a depressed infant born through MSAF should alert the treating physicians that vigorous postnatal therapeutic intervention should be pursued.

The mechanisms involved in the development of MAS reflect the cumulative effect of aspiration of MSAF in an already compromised infant. Therefore, the underlying pathology is that of fetal compromise, discussed elsewhere, and pulmonary injury secondary to aspiration of meconium. Meconium aspiration causes injury to lung tissues through a variety of mechanisms including complete or partial obstruction of airways, sepsis, inflammation, complement activation and cytokine production, inhibition of surfactant synthesis and function, apoptosis of epithelial cells, and increased pulmonary vascular resistance (Fig. 44-60).

Aspiration of meconium particles can result in complete or partial obstruction of the airways. Complete obstruction causes collapse of the lung area distal to the obstruction and subsequent atelectasis. The effect of partial obstruction, however, has been traditionally thought of as a ball-valve effect, wherein air can enter during inspiration but is unable to escape during expiration. The resultant trapped air and overdistention increase the incidence of air leaks, including pneumothorax, which can occur in as many as 15% to 30% of affected infants.

The various components of meconium have been shown to induce inflammation and cytokine activation in different studies. Within hours, neutrophils and macrophages are found in the alveoli, larger airways, and the lung parenchyma. This is associated with activation of proinflammatory cytokines, tumor necrosis factor TNF-α, γ-interferon, and interleukins (IL) 1β, IL-6, and IL-8. Furthermore, meconium was found to activate the lectin and alternative complement pathways, and administration of complement 1 inhibitors efficiently reduced the level of these proinflammatory factors, thus adding a potential therapeutic target for the treatment of MAS.[61] Meconium has also been shown to cause apoptosis of pulmonary epithelial cells through a caspase-3 mechanism.

Meconium has been shown to decrease synthesis and activity of surfactant in in vitro and in vivo animal and human studies. The exact mechanism is not clear; however, bile acids and secretary phospholipase A_2, both of which are components of meconium, have been implicated. Meconium has also been shown to displace surfactant from the alveolar surface, decreasing its ability to decrease surface tension. Decreased surfactant availability might result in increased surface tension with atelectasis, decreased lung compliance and lung volume, and subsequent hypoxia.[35]

Severe persistent pulmonary hypertension often complicates cases of MAS. The mechanism of pulmonary vasoconstriction in these patients is not clear. Pulmonary artery vasoconstriction induced by fetal and neonatal hypoxia most likely play a major role. The direct effect of meconium on pulmonary vasculature is controversial. In vitro studies observed relaxation of tracheal and pulmonary vasculature smooth muscles in response to meconium exposure in rats. On the other hand, in vivo administration of meconium caused increased contractility of vascular and tracheal smooth muscles suggesting that meconium induces pulmonary vasoconstriction through lung release of pulmonary vasoconstrictor humoral factors. The potent vasoconstrictors thromboxane A_2 and angiotensin II, as well as cytokines, have been implicated in this mechanism.

CLINICAL FEATURES

The infant with MAS often exhibits the classic signs of postmaturity with evidence of weight loss, cracked skin, and long nails, together with heavy staining of nails, skin, and umbilical cord with a yellowish pigment. These infants often are depressed at birth. In fact, the initial clinical picture can be dominated by neurologic and respiratory depression secondary to the hypoxic insult precipitating the passage of meconium. Respiratory distress with cyanosis, grunting, flaring, retractions, and marked tachypnea soon ensues.

Characteristically, the chest acquires an overinflated appearance, and rales can be audible on auscultation. The chest radiograph shows coarse, irregular pulmonary densities with areas of diminished aeration or consolidation (Fig. 44-61). If such infiltrates are a manifestation of retained lung fluid, they would be expected to clear within 24 to 48 hours. Pneumothorax and pneumomediastinum are common in infants with severe MAS. Hyperinflation of the chest and flattening of the diaphragm secondary to air trapping are sometimes noted on chest radiograph. Cardiomegaly also might be detected, possibly as a manifestation of the underlying perinatal hypoxia.

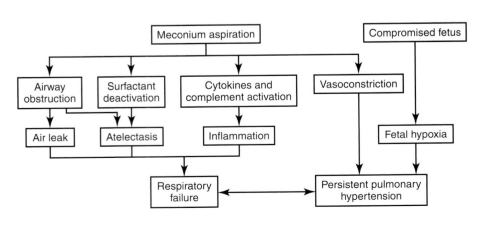

Figure 44–60. Pathophysiology of meconium aspiration syndrome.

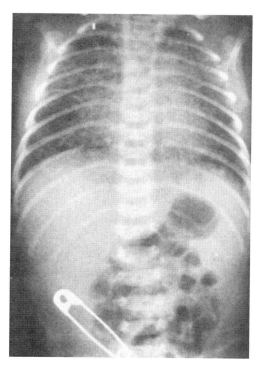

Figure 44–61. Chest radiograph showing multiple linear streaks of meconium aspiration pneumonia.

BOX 44–13 Management of Meconium Aspiration Syndrome

DELIVERY ROOM

Women at risk should deliver in a center where immediate neonatal care is available.

Meconium aspiration can develop in utero.

Amnioinfusion for meconium staining of amniotic fluid (MSAF) in the setting of standard peripartum surveillance is not routinely indicated.

Suctioning via endotracheal tube is indicated for depressed infants before stimulation.

NEONATAL INTENSIVE CARE UNIT

Surfactant administration may be beneficial.

Inhaled nitric oxide is indicated for associated persistent pulmonary hypertension.

UNRESOLVED ISSUES

The use of amnioinfusion for MSAF when routine surveillance is not available, such as in developing countries

Routine suctioning of the oropharynx at the perineum

The administration of surfactant as a bolus versus lavage

The utility of anti-inflammatory agents

Arterial blood gases characteristically reveal hypoxemia with evidence of right-to-left shunting. Hyperventilation can result in respiratory alkalosis, although infants with severe disease usually have a combined respiratory and metabolic acidosis secondary to hypoxia and respiratory failure. One should be alert to the possible development of PPHN, which frequently accompanies MAS and can contribute substantially to morbidity.

MANAGEMENT

In the Delivery Room

Successful management of patients with MAS depends on close observation during and immediately following labor in at-risk mothers as well as aggressive intervention in newborns presenting with risk factors for developing MAS (Box 44-13). This requires a collaborative effort by the obstetric and neonatology teams. Because at-home delivery was associated with a threefold increased risk for MAS, mothers at risk, especially those who are postdate, should deliver in a facility where immediate medical intervention is available. Mothers at a gestational age of 41 weeks or greater with thick MSAF and nonreassuring fetal heart tracing require careful monitoring. Fetal scalp oximetry is a technique of fetal monitoring that might improve the accuracy of detecting newborns at risk. In fetuses with nonreassuring fetal heart rate patterns, fetal oxygen saturation below 30% had a high correlation with a scalp pH value of less than 7.2.[41] Infants born by emergency cesarean section, depressed neonates, and those with low 5-minute Apgar scores, are at very high risk for development of MAS and should be followed closely.

Amnioinfusion refers to the instillation of normal saline or lactated Ringer's solution into the uterus through a catheter for the purpose of replacing amniotic fluid in cases of oligohydramnios and MSAF. Amnioinfusion might decrease the incidence of MAS by two mechanisms: diluting meconium consistency and decreasing cord compression, thereby resolving asphyxia and gasping. A meta-analysis of 13 studies demonstrated that the use of prophylactic intrapartum amnioinfusion for moderate or thick MSAF shows two distinct patterns. When standard peripartum and expert neonatal care are available, amnioinfusion does not improve outcome. In contrast, where antenatal and neonatal care are limited, such as underserved African communities, 75% of MAS is prevented. Furthermore, amnioinfusion decreased the frequency of cesarean section rate (OR, 0.74), meconium below the vocal cords (OR, 0.18), and neonatal acidemia (OR, 0.42) with no increase in the rate of chorioamnionitis (OR, 0.47).[56] A large, multicenter, randomized trial involving 1998 women concluded that in clinical settings with standard peripartum surveillance, amnioinfusion in the presence of thick MSAF did not reduce the risk of perinatal death, moderate or severe MAS, or other serious neonatal disorders.[27] This led the American College of Obstetricians and Gynecologists to issue an opinion statement: "Based on current literature, routine prophylactic amnioinfusion for the dilution of meconium-stained amniotic fluid should be done only in the setting of additional clinical trials. However, amnioinfusion remains a reasonable approach in the treatment of repetitive variable decelerations, regardless of amniotic fluid meconium status."[5]

Suctioning of the oropharynx upon delivery of the head and before delivery of the shoulders is used commonly in obstetric practices to decrease the possibility of meconium aspiration with the first breath. A multicenter, randomized, prospective study concluded that antepartum suctioning is not warranted and does not decrease the incidence of MAS even in high-risk infants. On the contrary, it may lead to added complications including bradycardia, desaturations, and increased incidence of pneumothorax.[68] In 2000, Wiswell and colleagues documented in a multicenter, randomized, international study that intratracheal suctioning did not decrease the incidence of MAS in vigorous neonates born through MSAF.[70] The Neonatal Resuscitation Program (NRP) shortly afterward implemented the policy of reserving tracheal intubation for only depressed infants. Vigorous infants defined as those with strong cry, normal heart rate, and good tone should not be intubated for MSAF regardless of how thick it is. Following dissemination of this policy, Kabbur and colleagues documented a significant decrease in the rate of delivery room intubation in infants born through MSAF without a change in overall respiratory complications supporting the efficacy of NRP recommendations.[36]

In the Neonatal Intensive Care Unit

Management of patients with MAS consists mainly of supportive respiratory and cardiovascular care. Maintaining normal blood pressure, adequate perfusion, and preventing hypoxia are essential in decreasing complications. The use of antibiotics is indicated until infection is ruled out since MSAF could be the first sign of fetal sepsis or pneumonia, which may be indistinguishable from MAS on chest x-ray examination. Ventilatory support is indicated in the presence of respiratory failure or persistent hypoxemia nonresponsive to high fractional inspired oxygen. There is no clear evidence or consensus of an advantage of one ventilatory strategy. However, in the presence of air leak or failure of conventional ventilation, HFOV should be considered in units familiar with this ventilatory strategy. PaO_2 should be maintained at the high end of the recommended level (80 to 100 mm Hg) to minimize hypoxia-induced pulmonary vasoconstriction. Details of mechanical ventilation are discussed in Part 4.

Surfactant administration should be considered in severe cases of MAS. In a Cochrane review of available data, surfactant decreased the need for ECMO in patients with MAS (relative risk 0.64, 95% CI, 0.46, 0.91), and the number needed to treat to prevent one ECMO case was 6.[23] While surfactant administration in one study was associated with reduced hospital stay with a mean difference of 8 days, it did not affect mortality, days on ventilator or oxygen, BPD, pneumothorax, or pulmonary interstitial emphysema. The most effective method of delivering surfactant, bronchoalveolar lavage versus bolus administration, as well as which surfactant to use is controversial. In cases complicated by PPHN, iNO should be considered. ECMO can be life saving in patients with continued hypoxia despite aggressive treatment. In a recent review of the ECMO experience in the United Kingdom, MAS accounted for 48% of ECMO patients and was associated with 97% survival. Radhakrishnan and colleagues, in reviewing 4310 ECMO cases, noted a lower complication rate in MAS patients that required either venoarterial or venovenous ECMO than in non-MAS ECMO patients. They suggested that consideration should be made for more relaxed ECMO criteria in patients with MAS.[58]

Observational studies in infants with MAS showed some improvement of pulmonary function with the use of inhaled or systemic steroids. However, a Cochrane meta-analysis of data in 2003 concluded that there is insufficient evidence to assess the effects of steroid therapy in the management of MAS. Future directions for treatment of MAS aimed at reducing inflammation and cytokine production are promising. Multiple anti-inflammatory substances including aminophylline, Clara cell protein, monoclonal anti–mannose-binding lectin antibodies, caspase-3 inhibitor, and C1 complement inhibitor have shown some effect in animal models of MAS.

The ultimate prognosis depends not so much on the pulmonary disease as on the accompanying asphyxial insult and treatment required. No specific long-term deficits in pulmonary function have been attributed to this disorder, although BPD can result from prolonged assisted ventilation. Compromised infants born through MSAF have an increased incidence of acute otitis media, probably secondary to meconium contamination of the middle ear.

Other Aspiration Syndromes

Respiratory distress can develop in the newborn infant secondary to aspiration of other amniotic fluid material, including purulent amniotic fluid, vernix caseosa, and maternal blood. Small case reports have documented these entities. The clinical picture is that of respiratory distress as described above. X-ray findings can be indistinguishable from MAS, although lack of MSAF and other risk factors for MAS help in the diagnosis. Aspiration of maternal blood can be difficult to differentiate from pulmonary hemorrhage, especially if there is no history of antepartum hemorrhage. However, infants with pulmonary hemorrhage are usually sicker, with cardiovascular compromise including hypotension, poor perfusion, coagulopathy, and low platelets. Furthermore, the presence of swallowed blood in the stomach of affected infants suggests aspiration. Treatment with antibiotics is indicated if pneumonia is suspected secondary to aspiration of infected amniotic fluid.

Aspiration is most likely to be seen in preterm infants, those with disorders of swallowing, and infants with esophageal atresia and tracheoesophageal fistula. Small preterm infants are at greatest risk when fed excessive volumes per gavage or through misplaced orogastric tubes. These infants might initially present with cyanosis, desaturation, or apnea and subsequent respiratory distress, with pulmonary infiltrates visible on radiographs. The severity of disease varies; it can be indistinguishable from an inflammatory pneumonitis. Aspiration syndromes associated with disorders of swallowing may be suspected from the perinatal history (asphyxia), feeding history (cyanosis, excessive drooling, poor suck), and physical examination. The precise cause, however, might not be readily apparent, and these infants require extensive neurologic evaluation. Neonates with tracheostomies or gastrostomies are at risk for aspiration. Infants with recurrent aspiration, particularly those with disorders of the swallowing mechanism, present complex management problems.

Neonatal Pneumonia

Neonatal pneumonia continues to account for significant morbidity and mortality, especially in developing countries. Mortality has been found to be as high as 29 per 1000 live births in a rural area of India and as many as 800,000 neonatal deaths in developing countries have been attributed to acute respiratory infections according to World Health Organization estimates. However, in developed countries, the incidence varies between 1% in term neonates and 10% in ill infants with low birthweight. On the other hand, pneumonia was the cause of death in 50% of infants with extremely low birthweight in one series, and pneumonia was also diagnosed by the presence of inflammation in 15% to 38% of stillborn infants at autopsy.

ETIOLOGY

Neonatal pneumonia is classified as *early*, presenting before 3 days of life, and *late*, presenting after 3 days of life. Congenital pneumonia is one subset of early pneumonia that is acquired in utero and usually presents immediately after delivery. Congenital pneumonia is acquired through aspiration of infected amniotic fluid, ascending infection through intact or ruptured membranes, or hematogenous spread through the placenta. Early pneumonia can also be acquired during labor secondary to aspiration of infected amniotic fluid or bacteria colonizing the birth canal. Late neonatal pneumonia is usually a nosocomial infection and occurs most commonly in ventilated neonates, although infection through hematogenous spread can also occur.

Whereas bacterial, viral, and fungal agents can cause pneumonia, the etiologic agent is usually related to the timing of occurrence of pneumonia. Group B *Streptococcus* (GBS) is the most common cause of early pneumonia. However, the overall incidence of GBS sepsis has decreased dramatically since the introduction of universal screening and intrapartum antibiotic prophylaxis. The incidence of early GBS sepsis decreased by 33% between 2000 and 2003-2005 after the 2002 American Academy of Pediatrics (AAP) revised recommendations for universal screening for GBS colonization at 35 to 37 weeks. However, even though the overall incidence decreased to 0.33 per 1000 live births, the incidence increased in African American neonates from 0.52 to 0.89 per 1000 live births in the same time period. The etiology of this increase is not clearly understood. The contribution of African American race as an independent contributing factor persisted after correcting for socioeconomic differences.[14] The impact of the decreased incidence of GBS sepsis on the incidence of GBS pneumonia is not clear; however, the incidence of gram-negative sepsis, especially that caused by *Escherichia coli,* has increased following the implementation of the revised AAP guidelines.[12] Other bacterial causes of pneumonia include *Klebsiella, Enterobacter,* group A streptococci, *Staphylococcus,* and *Listeria monocytogenes.* Foul-smelling amniotic fluid is usually caused by anaerobes, but the contribution of these organisms to early-onset pneumonia is minimal. *Bacteroides* species occasionally is recovered.

Herpes simplex is the major cause of early viral pneumonia and is usually acquired during labor. Pneumonia is associated with 33% to 54% of disseminated herpes infection and is usually associated with high mortality rate. Other causes of early viral pneumonia include adenovirus, enterovirus, mumps, and rubella, whereas early pneumonia is an unusual presentation of congenital cytomegalovirus (CMV) infection. Other TORCH infections, including syphilis and toxoplasmosis, can also present with early-onset pneumonia. Up to

70% of disseminated candidal infections are associated with pneumonia, especially in premature infants.

Late-onset pneumonia is usually caused by organisms that colonize the newborn during the hospital stay. These include *Staphylococcus* species, including coagulase-negative staphylococci and *Staphylococcus aureus. Streptococcus pyogenes, Streptococcus pneumoniae, E. coli, Klebsiella, Serratia, Enterobacter cloacae, Pseudomonas, Bacillus cereus,* and *Citrobacter* can cause severe pneumonia especially in preterm infants. When *Chlamydia trachomatis* infection is acquired during labor, it usually manifests as pneumonia at 2 to 4 weeks of life because of its long incubation period. RSV is the most common viral agent causing late-onset pneumonia, although incidence and severity have decreased secondary to passive immunoprophylaxis. Other viral causes of late pneumonia include adenovirus, enteroviruses, parainfluenza, rhinoviruses, and influenza viruses and can result in severe disease. CMV pneumonia should always be considered in babies with congenital infection presenting with late respiratory decompensation. Prolonged courses of antibiotics and corticosteroids can increase the risk of candidal pneumonia, especially in colonized infants with extremely low birthweight.

CLINICAL PRESENTATION

Risk factors for early pneumonia are similar to those for neonatal sepsis and include prematurity, prolonged rupture of membranes, GBS colonization, chorioamnionitis, and intrapartum maternal fever. However, in one study, 22% of neonatal cases did not have risk factors, and in almost half, the only risk factor was early onset of labor. Therefore, risk factors should not determine whether to start antibiotics in neonates with respiratory distress, especially infants with extremely low birthweight. The presence and duration of mechanical ventilation and central venous lines were the main risk factors for development of late-onset pneumonia.[19] Other risk factors include abnormal neurologic conditions predisposing to aspiration pneumonia, poor nutrition, severe underlying disease, and prolonged hospitalization.

Clinical manifestations of early-onset pneumonia can be nonspecific; therefore a high index of suspicion should always be exercised. These symptoms include temperature instability, lethargy, apnea, tachycardia, metabolic acidosis, abdominal distention, poor feeding, and neurologic depression. Respiratory distress can present in the form of tachypnea and retractions in more than two thirds of affected neonates. Cough is an unusual symptom in neonatal pneumonia and was present in less than one third of neonates. Delay in diagnosis and treatment can lead to PPHN and septic shock.

Differential diagnosis for early neonatal pneumonia includes transient tachypnea of the newborn (TTN), RDS, MAS, and pulmonary congestion secondary to obstructed anomalous pulmonary venous return or other left heart obstructed lesions. Radiographic findings in pneumonia are nonspecific and thus do not help differentiate these disorders. Chest x-ray findings might include unilateral or bilateral streaky densities, confluent mottled opacified areas, or a diffusely granular appearance with air bronchograms. Differentiation from RDS is difficult in preterm infants, especially because preterm labor is a risk factor for pneumonia. Radiographic findings of TTN usually resolve by 48 hours and those of RDS are markedly improved after surfactant treatment, whereas radiologic changes of pneumonia may persist for weeks.

Late-onset pneumonia usually presents with nonspecific changes in the overall condition of the infant in the form of new-onset or increased apnea, abdominal distention or feeding intolerance, temperature instability, respiratory distress, hyperglycemia, or cardiovascular instability. Patients receiving ventilatory assistance usually present with an increased oxygen requirement or mechanical support.

The diagnosis of pneumonia requires a high index of suspicion in any infant with new onset of symptoms suggestive of sepsis. Sepsis workup, including blood culture, blood count, and differential should be obtained before starting antibiotics. The presence of elevated C-reactive protein, neutropenia, immature white blood cells, and thrombocytopenia is highly suggestive (although not diagnostic) of infection in newborn babies with risk factors. Tracheal Gram stain and culture should be considered in infants who require mechanical ventilation soon after intubation. A positive tracheal culture in the first 8 hours of life may correlate with a positive blood culture. After 8 hours, a positive tracheal culture might be secondary to colonization. Analysis and culture of pleural fluid, if present in adequate amount, can aid in the diagnosis in infants not responding to empirical therapy. Specific studies for viral or unusual bacterial infections should be obtained if suspected. Diagnosis of ventilator-associated pneumonia (VAP) can be troublesome, especially in preterm infants with underlying lung disease. Typically these infants' tracheas are colonized, discounting the validity of tracheal cultures. The Centers for Disease Control and Prevention has proposed stringent diagnostic criteria to diagnose VAP in infants younger than 1 year of age that relies on clinical symptoms of respiratory distress, hyperthermia, purulent tracheal secretions, increased requirement for ventilatory support, and new changes in chest radiograph that persist in at least two consecutive films.[26] However, the validity of these criteria in diagnosing VAP in preterm infants with underlying lung disease has not been substantiated. Further studies are clearly needed to better diagnose and treat pneumonia in ventilated infants with low birthweight.

MANAGEMENT

Successful treatment depends on identification of the causative organism, institution of early and adequate antibiotic therapy, and supportive care. Empirical antibiotic therapy is usually started before isolation of the organism. In early-onset pneumonia, ampicillin and gentamicin (dose based on gestational age and kidney function) are adequate initial therapy. However, with the increasing incidence of antibiotic-resistant gram-negative bacteria, this regimen may need to be altered based on specific institutional susceptibility data. Empirical therapy with vancomycin (for coagulase-negative staphylococci) and gentamicin is usually started for late-onset pneumonia. To decrease the possibility of developing vancomycin-resistant bacteria, an empirical regimen for late-onset sepsis/pneumonia may include nafcillin and gentamicin, and vancomycin is started once coagulase-negative *Staphylococcus* is identified or the clinical picture is deteriorating. In intubated infants, antibiotic coverage depends on the specific bacteria colonizing the trachea. Once the causative organism is isolated, specific therapy is started according to susceptibility profile. The

duration of therapy is dependent on the causative organism and response to treatment; however, in uncomplicated pneumonia, 10 to 14 days of therapy is usually adequate.

Whereas antibiotic therapy is the mainstay of treatment, supportive care is essential and has been shown to decrease the mortality and morbidity associated with pneumonia in developing countries. In the acute stage, circulatory support with fluids and inotropes might be needed, and mechanical ventilation and oxygen should be administered to correct hypoxemia. Special attention to correct acidosis, hypoglycemia, and other possible electrolyte imbalance is also warranted. Parenteral nutrition with amino acids, carbohydrates, and lipids can provide adequate nutrition and prevent protein catabolism as well as amino and fatty acid deficiency. Feeding should be started as soon as possible to supply adequate calories. In the absence of respiratory distress or abdominal pathology with concern for aspiration, gavage feedings can be started.

Transient Tachypnea of the Newborn

Transient tachypnea is a common physiologic disorder of the newborn resulting from pulmonary edema secondary to inadequate or delayed clearance of fetal alveolar fluid. The initial clinical picture is usually completely resolved by 48 to 72 hours, hence the term *transient*. However, TTN continues to represent a diagnostic dilemma secondary to the inability to differentiate its initial presentation from that of other causes of respiratory distress. The incidence has been estimated at 5.7 per 1000 births in term infants. Risk factors for development of TTN include premature or elective cesarean delivery without labor. The incidence of pulmonary pathology including TTN was found to be twofold to threefold higher in infants born after planned cesarean delivery compared with a planned vaginal delivery. TTN is also more common in infants of diabetic mothers and mothers with asthma, although the mechanism of the latter association is not clear.

Fetal alveolar fluid is continuously secreted during pregnancy through an epithelial chloride secretion mechanism and the rate of secretion decreases a few days before delivery. At birth, the balance of fluid movement in the alveolus switches from chloride secretion to sodium absorption, causing resorption of intra-alveolar fluid. Sodium (Na), and thereafter water, absorption occurs in two steps; initially Na moves passively from the alveolar lumen into the cell by passive movement through a concentration gradient maintained by the Na-K-ATPase pump. Next, sodium is actively transported into the interstitium by amiloride-sensitive epithelial sodium channels (ENaC). Thereafter, the sodium and fluid are cleared through the lymphatic and vascular systems. The mechanisms underlying failure or delay in clearance of intra-alveolar fluid in patients with TTN are not totally clear and have been studied mostly in animals. The mechanical force of birth canal squeeze, originally thought to be the major factor in lung fluid resorption, is now believed to be a minor contributor. Immaturity of ENaC has been shown, both in animals and newborn babies, to impair fluid resorption, and as ENaC expression is developmentally regulated, this is especially relevant in the late preterm infant. Hormonal changes associated with spontaneous labor, especially surge of catecholamines and endogenous steroid, seem to be important in increasing the expression and activity of ENaC, which partially accounts for the higher incidence of TTN in elective cesarean section cases not preceded by spontaneous labor.[33] The clinical picture of patients with TTN is secondary to the decrease in lung compliance associated with pulmonary edema. Collapse of airways might also occur in response to fluid accumulation in the interstitium and peribronchial lymphatics. The net result is variable degrees of hypoxemia and respiratory acidosis.

Patients with TTN usually present very early after birth with symptoms of respiratory distress. Tachypnea is the most consistent finding, although increased work of breathing with expiratory grunting, nasal flaring, and retractions may also be present. Hypoxemia necessitating modest oxygen requirement (usually less than 40%), together with hypercapnia, can occur, while respiratory failure requiring CPAP is unusual. The most characteristic feature of TTN is the transient nature of this disease. In most patients, rapid continuous improvement in the clinical condition occurs within 24 to 48 hours of life, although in some patients symptoms might persist beyond 72 hours of life. Characteristic radiographic findings consist of perihilar streaking that represents engorgement of the periarterial lymphatics and fluid-filled interlobar fissures. Both the horizontal and oblique fissures can be affected although the horizontal is affected more commonly. Fluid-filled alveoli can present as fluffy bilateral infiltrates. Atelectasis and pleural effusion can also be seen. Although these radiographic changes can readily be distinguished from classic changes of RDS, TTN can conceivably accompany RDS in preterm infants. Radiographic changes are essentially resolved by 48 hours. Recently, Copettia and Cattarossi described a characteristic ultrasound finding in patients with TTN that they designated "double lung point." This consisted of very compact comet-tail artifacts in the inferior fields of the lung that were rare in the superior fields.[17] This finding was not found in healthy newborns or those with other lung pathology. This finding, once substantiated, might help differentiate TTN from other disorders in equivocal cases. Differential diagnoses include RDS, pneumonia, MAS, and pulmonary edema of cardiac origin.

Treatment of TTN is supportive. However, because it is difficult to differentiate TTN from other disorders, most patients are usually started on antibiotics that can be discontinued after 48 hours if cultures are negative and the diagnosis is more clear. Lasix has no role in the treatment of TTN. Although not used in clinical practice to prevent TTN, antenatal steroids do enhance fluid resorption from alveolar spaces through increased transcription and activation of ENaC. Exogenous steroids or catecholamines do not seem to provide benefit after birth once the patient is symptomatic because recovery usually precedes the action of these agents. Delaying elective cesarean section until 39 to 40 weeks' gestation or until spontaneous labor starts will decrease the incidence of TTN. However, this should be weighed against possible complications of delaying a needed cesarean section.[29] Although TTN is considered a self-limited transient condition, there are increasing data to suggest that TTN increases a newborn's risk for developing a wheezing syndrome early in life.[47]

Pulmonary Hemorrhage

Pulmonary hemorrhage is a serious complication in neonates with RDS and has been associated with increasing risk for mortality and morbidity. Serious pulmonary hemorrhage has been defined as a gush of blood through an endotracheal tube in intubated neonates associated with a worsening clinical picture, requiring increased ventilatory support and blood product transfusion. The incidence of such severe hemorrhage is about 5% in very low birthweight infants and 10.2% in extremely low birthweight infants. Risk factors for development of pulmonary hemorrhage include extreme prematurity, surfactant administration, patent ductus arteriosus (PDA) with left to right shunting, multiple births, and male gender. Other risk factors include severe systemic illness, coagulopathy, and asphyxia. More than 80% of cases of serious pulmonary hemorrhage occur before 72 hours of life with a median of 40 hours; however, some babies might present after 1 week of life.[67]

The pathophysiology of pulmonary hemorrhage is believed to be secondary to sudden decrease in pulmonary vascular resistance, causing increased left-to-right shunting and pulmonary vascular engorgement, pulmonary edema, and ultimately rupture of pulmonary capillaries. This is especially true in patients with PDA after surfactant treatment. In post hoc analysis of patients enrolled in the trial for indomethacin prophylaxis in premature infants, a reduced risk for PDA accounted for 80% of the beneficial effect of prophylactic indomethacin on serious pulmonary bleeds.[6] However, pulmonary hemorrhage can also occur in patients who never received surfactant or had a PDA, highlighting the importance of other etiologies in the pathogenesis of pulmonary hemorrhage, including aggressive suctioning, especially using a closed circuit system.

Patients with pulmonary hemorrhage usually present with cyanosis, bradycardia, apnea, gasping, hypotension, increased work of breathing, hypoxia, and hypercapnia requiring increased ventilatory support. In almost one third of patients, serious pulmonary hemorrhage was preceded by prodromal episodes of suctioning frothy blood-tinged tracheal secretions. Chest radiographs demonstrate acute and varying degrees of worsening in underlying pulmonary disease, ranging from bilateral fluffy infiltrates to complete whiteout in severe cases.

Treatment of pulmonary hemorrhage is mostly supportive. Increased ventilatory support, especially positive end-expiratory pressure (PEEP), serves two purposes: It is needed for adequate ventilation and oxygenation, and it acts to tamponade and stop the bleeding. Suctioning should be limited during the acute hemorrhage. The efficacy of instillation of epinephrine, although used clinically, has not been proven in clinical trials. Transfusion of blood products and correction of underlying or secondary coagulopathy is essential. Pulmonary hemorrhage can cause deactivation of surfactant, and exogenous surfactant administration has been used successfully.[8] Prophylactic indomethacin decreased the incidence of pulmonary hemorrhage by 26% in infants with extremely low birthweight. Early recognition and treatment of PDA should be attempted in extremely premature neonates who are at the highest risk of mortality and morbidity associated with pulmonary hemorrhage. Pulmonary hemorrhage is associated with very high mortality approaching 50% in infants with extremely low birthweight. Whereas initial retrospective studies did not show worsening in neurodevelopmental outcome in survivors of pulmonary hemorrhage, a recent study showed increased incidence of cerebral palsy and cognitive delay (OR, 2.86 and 2.4, respectively).[6] Pulmonary hemorrhage was also associated with increased incidence of periventricular leukomalacia and seizures in survivors at 18 months of age.

Pulmonary Air Leak Syndromes

Air leak occurs more commonly in the newborn period than any other period of life. One percent to 2% of all live births were found to have pneumothorax on consecutive chest radiographs of term newborns in 1930. The incidence increases with decreasing gestational age. While the incidence was 6.3% in 1999 in very low birthweight infants in the Vermont-Oxford Network database, it approached 15% in those with a birthweight of 501 to 750 g.[32] Air leak syndromes include pneumothorax, pneumomediastinum, pulmonary interstitial emphysema, and pneumopericardium, and less commonly pneumoperitoneum and subcutaneous emphysema. Even though air leaks can occur spontaneously, they mostly occur in patients with lung pathology, including MAS, pneumonia, RDS, diaphragmatic hernia, and pulmonary hypoplasia, especially when positive pressure ventilation is required. The introduction of surfactant for treatment of RDS has caused a decrease in the incidence of air leaks. Conversely, the increasing practice of elective cesarean section before 39 completed weeks' gestation is associated with increased incidence of pneumothorax when compared with emergent cesarean section (OR, 4.2) or vaginal delivery (OR, 7.95).[72]

PATHOPHYSIOLOGY

Air leaks occur when overdistended alveoli rupture into the perivascular bundle, from where air tracks toward the hilum or pleura, causing pneumomediastinum or pneumothorax, respectively. In the preterm infant in whom the interstitium is more abundant and less dissectible, air can stay in the perivascular sheets causing pulmonary interstitial emphysema (PIE). Alveolar overdistention might occur in the presence of uneven alveolar ventilation or air trapping. Atelectasis in RDS and plugged small airways in MAS cause unequal distribution of the ventilated volume and transpulmonary pressure to the more distensible areas of the lung, increasing the risk of rupture and air leak. Partial obstruction during MAS causes air trapping when inspired air is not completely evacuated during exhalation. Further accumulation during subsequent breaths can rupture the alveolar space.

Different ventilatory strategies have been associated with the development of pneumothorax, including higher peak inspiratory pressure especially in the 24 hours preceding pneumothorax, long inspiratory time (greater than 0.5 seconds), and frequent suctioning in the 8 hours before pneumothorax. Elective initial use of high nasal CPAP (8 cm H_2O) in infants at 25 to 28 weeks' gestation was associated with increased incidence of air leak from 3% to 9% when compared with intubated infants who received surfactant therapy. However, there was no difference in the incidence of BPD or mortality rate between the two groups.[52] Recently, the use of CPAP (5 cm H_2O) in the delivery room in extremely low gestational age infants was associated with a decreased need

for intubation and postnatal corticosteroids for BPD, and fewer days of mechanical ventilation when compared to initial intubation and surfactant administration within 1 hour after birth without an increase in the incidence of pneumothorax.[65b] Factors possibly associated with decreased incidence of pneumothorax include positive pressure ventilation (rate greater than 60) and volume-targeted ventilation. The use of HFOV following pneumothorax was associated with a decreased incidence of secondary pneumothorax.[51]

CLINICAL PICTURE

Even though pneumothorax can be the presenting diagnosis, more commonly it complicates underlying lung pathology. Sudden worsening in respiratory distress should always raise the suspicion of development of pneumothorax. Tachypnea, grunting, flaring, and retractions occur most commonly. Hypoxemia with cyanosis and increased oxygen requirement occur early in the course of pneumothorax while hypercapnia follows. Hypoxemia develops secondary to hypoventilation and ventilation-perfusion mismatch as the affected lung collapses. Physical examination reveals distant breath sounds, overdistention of the chest wall, and bulging abdomen on the affected side secondary to downward displacement of the diaphragm in patients with unilateral pneumothorax. The cardiac apex is displaced away from the affected side, as is the trachea.

Larger volumes of leaked air can cause significant increase in intrathoracic pressure, which impairs venous blood return and compromises cardiac output, causing poor tissue perfusion and metabolic acidosis. Although bradycardia and hypotension were not seen in a piglet model of moderate pneumothorax (30 mL of air), they can develop with a severe tension pneumothorax. The decreased cardiac output may cause a compensatory increase in carotid bloodflow as the body tries to protect vital organs. The resultant increase in cerebral bloodflow together with impairment of cerebral venous return secondary to increased central venous pressure might explain the increased incidence of intraventricular hemorrhage (IVH) in patients with pneumothorax.

Pneumomediastinum is often asymptomatic if not associated with pneumothorax and is mostly found on radiographic evaluation of patients with respiratory distress or distant heart sounds. Dissection of air through the anterior mediastinum into the neck can cause subcutaneous emphysema that is most commonly felt as subcutaneous crepitus in the face, neck, or supraclavicular notch area.

Pneumopericardium is a rare and serious complication probably caused by dissection of leaked air through the vascular bundle of great vessels. Trapped air in the limited pericardial space can quickly cause cardiac tamponade, decreasing venous return and cardiac output. Pneumopericardium should be suspected in patients with an air leak and sudden cardiovascular compromise associated with a narrow pulse pressure. The clinical picture consists of worsening respiratory distress, hypotension, bradycardia, pallor, and/or cyanosis. Cardiac sounds are distant or muffled on cardiac auscultation and a pericardial rub might also be heard. Low voltage QRS complexes can also be seen.

Pneumoperitoneum occurs when an intrathoracic air leak decompresses into the abdomen. It is typically asymptomatic and usually diagnosed on radiographic evaluation. It should, however, be differentiated from free abdominal air secondary to ruptured viscus in which patients are usually symptomatic with signs and symptoms of peritonitis.

DIAGNOSIS

In unstable neonates with progressive deterioration of the clinical picture, transillumination of the chest might provide a quick bedside diagnostic tool and allow for immediate intervention before x-ray confirmation. The technique involves the use of a fiberoptic light probe that is placed on the infant's chest wall while the nursery is darkened. In the presence of a large Pneumothorax, the entire hemithorax on the affected side lights up and the opposite side shows diminished transillumination because of lung compression on that side. In such cases, decompression should be accomplished without awaiting radiographic confirmation. However, in stable neonates, radiographic confirmation should always be sought before intervention. Inconclusive results or inexperience with the use of transillumination should also be confirmed by x-ray before intervention. This allows for proper localization of the pneumothorax, as well as excluding other disorders that do not need evacuation, such as pneumomediastinum, congenital emphysema, or diaphragmatic hernia.

The diagnosis is clear on radiographic evaluation of patients with a large or tension pneumothorax. Air accumulates between the parietal and visceral pleura, separating the lung from the chest wall and collapsing the ipsilateral lung. This can be seen as a curvilinear line silhouetting the collapsed lung (Fig. 44-62). External artifacts can also appear as a curvilinear line on chest radiograph; however, artifact can be differentiated from a pneumothorax by its tendency to extend beyond the chest cavity in either direction. In tension pneumothorax, the mediastinal structures, including the heart, are shifted away from the affected side. Lung collapse might not be complete despite a severe pneumothorax in patients with RDS secondary to poor compliance of the affected lung. Smaller pneumothoraces might appear as a small sliver of free air lateral to the lung or above the diaphragm causing the edge of the diaphragm or costophrenic angle to appear crisp. An anterior pneumothorax causes the affected lung to look translucent compared with the contralateral side. Confirmation of a small pneumothorax can be obtained with a lateral decubitus chest radiograph, where the unaffected side is dependent. As the free air rises, the reflection of the parietal pleura is seen clearly as a curvilinear line beyond which no lung markings are seen. This might also identify any contralateral pneumothorax or pneumomediastinum.

Pneumomediastinum can be diagnosed on chest radiograph by elevation of the edge of the thymus from the pericardium by mediastinal free air in a characteristic crescent or spinnaker sail configuration. A large pneumomediastinum can be differentiated from a pneumothorax by lateral decubitus radiographs as described earlier.

Pneumopericardium appears on plain chest radiograph as free air completely surrounding the heart, but not extending beyond the aorta or pulmonary artery into the upper mediastinum. Although difficult to differentiate from a large pneumomediastinum, the presence of air between the heart and diaphragm is diagnostic of pneumopericardium (Fig. 44-63).

PIE is seen on chest radiograph as coarse, nonbranching radiolucencies that project toward the periphery of the lung in a disorganized fashion. This appearance must not be confused with an air bronchogram, a classic radiographic sign of respiratory distress syndrome. Air bronchograms show long, smooth, branching radiolucencies that follow normal anatomic distributions similar to the bronchial tree. Pathologically, PIE is seen in lung tissues as multiple irregular, air-filled cysts varying in diameter from 1 mm to 1 cm, localized to interlobular septa, and extending radially from the hilum. PIE can be localized to one lung or a lobe of a lung, or can be diffuse bilateral disease. There is usually hyperinflation on the affected side that persists even after weaning of ventilatory support.

MANAGEMENT

Treatment of a pneumothorax depends on the severity of clinical presentation and whether it occurs during mechanical ventilation. In asymptomatic patients without underlying

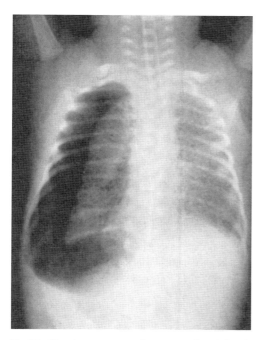

Figure 44–62. Tension pneumothorax on the right. An endotracheal tube is in place.

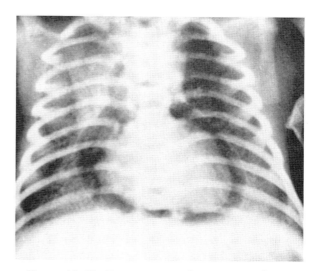

Figure 44–63. Pneumopericardium in a newborn.

pulmonary disease, no treatment is required; however, close observation for worsening pneumothorax and development of respiratory symptoms is clearly needed. The pneumothorax usually resolves spontaneously in 1 to 2 days. Follow-up radiographs can be obtained as mandated by the clinical picture. The association of symptomatic spontaneous pneumothorax with congenital renal malformations and the need for renal ultrasound evaluation in these patients is controversial. A review of 80 patients with spontaneous pneumothorax compared with normal controls showed no difference between the two groups in the rate of congenital renal malformations.[7]

Only supportive care is needed in the treatment of symptomatic patients with a mild pneumothorax without evidence of respiratory failure. While 100% oxygen given by a hood might lead to nitrogen washout and resolution or decrease in the size of the pneumothorax, this management strategy has not been adequately evaluated in infants. Oxygen is generally given only as needed to provide adequate oxgen saturations. Thoracocentesis is used for emergency evacuation of a large pneumothorax in unstable infants and might be the only treatment needed in nonventilated babies. However, recurrence of the pneumothorax should prompt the insertion of a chest tube. Thoracocentesis can also be used as a temporizing measure before chest tube insertion in ventilated infants.

In ventilated patients with a large or tension pneumothorax, the initial management is to wean PIP and PEEP to decrease further air leak while preparing for chest tube placement. Deciding on which brand of chest tube and which insertion technique to use depends most importantly on experience and comfort level. The tube should be inserted under complete aseptic technique and positioned anterior to the affected lung. This can be best achieved by starting in the anterior or middle axillary line. Position of the tube should be confirmed by anteroposterior and lateral chest radiographs. Once placed correctly, there is immediate improvement in oxygenation in affected patients, and the tube should be connected to an underwater seal with continuous suctioning at 10 to 20 cm H_2O. The chest tube should be secured once correct positioning is confirmed, with special attention given to prevent tension on the tube causing it to dislodge, particularly during radiologic examination. Chest tube insertion can be complicated by lung damage, which is usually diagnosed at autopsy, diaphragmatic paralysis secondary to

phrenic nerve damage, or bleeding (Fig. 44-64). The use of a trocar or other sharp instrument during insertion should be avoided to decrease the chance of these complications. Once air bubbling stops, the chest tube should be clamped overnight, and if the pneumothorax does not reaccumulate, the tube can be successfully removed. Isolated pneumomediastinum is usually self-limiting and does not need intervention. These patients should be closely observed, however, because they might develop a pneumothorax.

Management of PIE can present a challenge. Increased support may lead to enlargement of the more compliant PIE cysts, which in turn compresses the relatively normal adjacent alveoli, causing worsening hypoxia and hypercapnia. The treatment strategy instead should target decreasing mean airway pressure while accepting higher CO_2 levels and oxygen requirement to allow for collapse of the dilated interstitial cystic lesions and expansion of the normal alveoli. HFOV is an acceptable ventilatory strategy for PIE because of the lack of inflating volumes that tend to worsen the PIE. In the case of failure of conservative management and persistent PIE, different treatment strategies have been tried, especially in unilateral cases, with varying degrees of success. These include single lung ventilation, rupture of the PIE into a pneumothorax that can then be evacuated by a chest tube, and resection of the affected side. Rastogi and colleagues described successful management of 15 of 17 neonates with unilateral PIE who failed conservative management with single-lung ventilation.[59]

The occurrence of air leak is associated with increased incidence of mortality and morbidity. Together with the increased incidence of IVH mentioned earlier, very low birthweight infants who develop pneumothorax in the first 24 hours of life were 13 times more likely to die or develop bronchopulmonary dysplasia. Furthermore, extremely low birthweight infants with a pneumothorax who had a normal head ultrasound were more likely to develop cerebral palsy after controlling for other factors (OR, 2.3).[45] Therefore, management strategies directed at avoiding the development of a pneumothorax should always be sought, including using minimal effective inspiratory pressures, low inspiratory time, high-frequency positive pressure ventilation, volume-targeted ventilation, early administration of surfactant in eligible patients, and rapid weaning of mechanical ventilation.

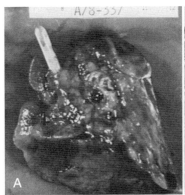 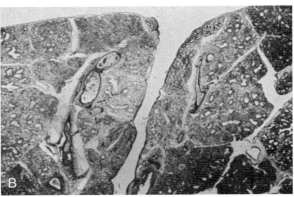

Figure 44-64. Perforation of the lung associated with insertion of chest tube by means of trocar and cannula. A, Gross appearance. B, Histologic features demonstrating tract into the lung.

RIB CAGE ABNORMALITIES

Thoracic cage and skeletal abnormalities are a rare group of conditions that can cause respiratory distress by restriction of thoracic volume. They include a number of entities incompatible with life. In this group of diseases are those with hypoplasia of the ribs and thorax, including asphyxiating thoracic dystrophy (Jeune syndrome), thanatophoric dwarfism, achondrogenesis, homozygous achondroplasia, osteogenesis imperfecta (severe form), Ellis–van Creveld syndrome (chondroectodermal dysplasia), hypophosphatasia, spondylothoracic dysplasia, and rib-gap syndrome.

Respiratory distress caused by structural abnormalities of the chest wall should be readily apparent. However, marked narrowing of the thorax can result in what appears to be a distended abdomen, and the respiratory problem can be erroneously attributed to an intra-abdominal pathologic condition. The presence of other associated anomalies, for example, short-limbed dwarfism, together with close observation of respiratory excursions, examination of the bony thorax, and measurement of the circumference of the chest, establishes the diagnosis even before a review is made of the thoracic and skeletal radiographs.

With structural abnormalities of the chest wall, asphyxia and respiratory distress are present from birth. The infants are cyanotic and tachypneic and demonstrate severe retractions and characteristically a virtually immobile chest. Diaphragmatic excursions are prominent; thus, respiration appears entirely abdominal. Pulmonary hypoplasia accompanies the thoracic dystrophy, and radiographically the lungs can appear airless.

Infants with asphyxiating thoracic dystrophy, thanatophoric dwarfism, achondrogenesis, homozygous achondroplasia, or Ellis–van Creveld syndrome have thoracic radiographs with a squared-off appearance, and the posterior rib arcs all appear to be the same length. The clavicles appear very high, and the diaphragms are low (Fig. 44-65). The transverse diameter of the thorax can appear diminished in comparison with the vertical diameter. On a lateral view, the ribs are very short and can appear clubbed anteriorly. The anteroposterior diameter of the thorax is decreased.

The lungs may be poorly aerated, infiltrates are often present, and the heart might appear enlarged. Differentiating among the various syndromes of thoracic cage and skeletal

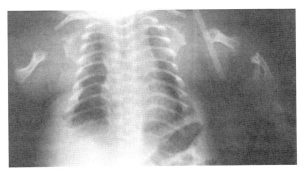

Figure 44–65. Radiographic appearance in thanatophoric dwarfism showing the narrow thorax, low diaphragm, and foreshortened humeri.

abnormalities usually is accomplished by means of a skeletal survey. Multiple fractures and bone demineralization are characteristic of osteogenesis imperfecta and hypophosphatasia.

Asphyxiating Thoracic Dystrophy

The hallmarks of asphyxiating thoracic dystrophy are extreme constriction and narrowing of the thorax, short ribs, and short-limbed dwarfism, with abnormalities of the bones of the pelvis and extremities. Associated anomalies include polydactyly and deformed teeth. Renal abnormalities may be present, and renal failure can occur later. The syndrome is inherited as an autosomal recessive trait. As mentioned previously, the chest appears narrow and the sternum is prominent. The thorax is relatively immobile, and the ribs are horizontally directed and short with bulbous ends. In addition to the thoracic abnormalities, the infants have trident iliac bones with a double-notch appearance of the acetabulum.

Thanatophoric Dwarfism

Thanatophoric dwarfism (see Chapter 29) was differentiated from achondroplasia in 1967. The disorder has been generally fatal in the perinatal period with rare exceptions and probably is the most common form of lethal neonatal dwarfism. Appearance at birth is characteristic and includes striking micromelia in association with a normal trunk, a large head, and a narrow thorax. The radiographic findings include severely flattened vertebral bodies with markedly widened intervertebral disc spaces, small iliac rings, and flaring of the metaphyses of the long bones. There is a high incidence of polyhydramnios, and the infants often present in the breech position. The condition is inherited as an autosomal recessive trait, occurring more frequently in the African American population.

Infants present at birth with severe pulmonary insufficiency, requiring mechanical ventilation and intensive neonatal care. Because there is no prognosis for mental and physical development, immediate and accurate diagnosis is important in guiding medical decisions about continuation of support.

PHRENIC NERVE INJURY PARALYSIS

Phrenic nerve injury with paralysis of the diaphragm is an unusual cause of respiratory distress. It is most commonly present on the right side following birth trauma; thus an associated brachial plexus injury or Horner syndrome can coexist in approximately 75% of the patients. However, injury can also occur after cardiovascular or thoracic surgeries or following invasive procedures. The injuries are observed in infants who are large for gestational age, especially following shoulder dystocia or difficult breech extractions. Fractures of the humerus or clavicle are often observed. The nerve roots of C3 to C5 are stretched, with lateral hyperextension and traction on the neck. Recovery depends on the degree of injury; avulsion results in permanent injury, and diaphragmatic eventration secondary to muscle atrophy ensues. Lesser injury or edema of the nerve roots results in a spectrum of respiratory symptoms, which can include cyanosis, weak cry, tachypnea, or apnea; decreased movement is noted on the affected side. On radiographic examination, the involved hemidiaphragm is elevated, and atelectasis usually is observed on that side. The heart and mediastinum are shifted away from the affected side (Fig. 44-66). Ultrasonographic or fluoroscopic evaluation should be diagnostic and reveal paradoxical movement of the diaphragm with elevation during inspiration and descent with expiration. Congenital eventration of the diaphragm also results in an elevated hemidiaphragm with paradoxical movement. Secondary pneumonia is the major source of morbidity and mortality. Treatment of phrenic nerve palsy initially is supportive and, in the absence of avulsion, spontaneous resolution is to be expected. Surgical plication of the diaphragm might be required for selected infants with avulsion.

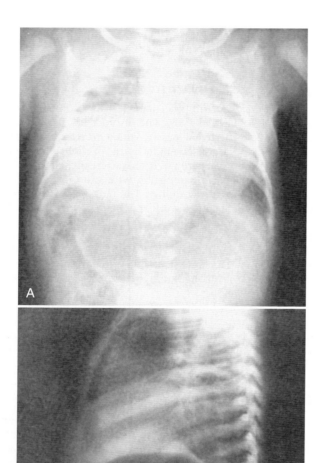

Figure 44–66. Phrenic nerve palsy. A, Note the elevated right dome of the diaphragm. B, Lateral view.

REFERENCES

1. Abu-Shaweesh JM, et al: Changes in respiratory timing induced by hypercapnia in maturing rats, *J Appl Physiol* 87:484, 1999.
2. Abu-Shaweesh JM: Maturation of respiratory reflex responses in the fetus and neonate, *Semin Neonatol* 9:169, 2004.
3. Abu-Shaweesh JM: Activation of central adenosine A$_{2A}$ receptors enhances superior laryngeal nerve stimulation-induced apnea in piglets via a GABAergic pathway, *J Appl Physiol* 103:1205, 2007.
4. Abu-Shaweesh JM, Martin RJ: Neonatal apnea: what's new? *Pediatr Pulmonol* 43:937, 2008.
5. ACOG Committee Opinion Number 346: Amnioinfusion does not prevent meconium aspiration syndrome, *Obstet Gynecol* 108:1053, 2006.
6. Alfaleh K, et al: Prevention and 18-month outcomes of serious pulmonary hemorrhage in extremely low birth weight infants: results from the trial of indomethacin prophylaxis in preterms, *Pediatrics* 121:e233, 2008.
7. Al Tawil K, et al: Symptomatic spontaneous pneumothorax in term newborn infants, *Pediatr Pulmonol* 37:443 2004.
8. Amizuka T, et al: Surfactant therapy in neonates with respiratory failure due to haemorrhagic pulmonary oedema, *Eur J Pediatr* 162:697, 2003.
9. Azizkhan RG, Crombleholme TM: Congenital cystic lung disease: contemporary antenatal and postnatal management, *Pediatr Surg Int* 24:643, 2008.
10. Back SA, et al: Protective effects of caffeine on chronic hypoxia-induced perinatal white matter injury, *Ann Neurol* 60:696, 2006.
11. Bellini C, et al: Congenital pulmonary lymphangiectasia, *Orphanet J Rare Dis* 1:43, 2006.
12. Bizzarro MJ, et al: Changing patterns in neonatal *Escherichia coli* sepsis and ampicillin resistance in the era of intrapartum antibiotic prophylaxis, *Pediatrics* 121:689, 2008.
13. Carroll JL, Kim I: Postnatal development of carotid body glomus cell O$_2$ sensitivity, *Respir Physiol Neurobiol* 149:201, 2005.
14. CDC: Perinatal group B streptococcal disease after universal screening recommendations–United States, 2003–2005. MMWR Morlo Mortal Wkly Rep. 56:701, 2007.
15. Collin P, et al: Pulmonary sequestration, *J Pediatr Surg* 22:750, 1987.
16. The Congenital Diaphragmatic Hernia Study Group: Defect size determines survival in infants with congenital diaphragmatic hernia, *Pediatrics* 120:e651, 2007.
17. Copettia R, Cattarossi L: The 'double lung point': an ultrasound sign diagnostic of transient tachypnea of the newborn, *Neonatology* 91:203, 2007.
18. Corbett HJ, Humphrey GM: Pulmonary sequestration, *Paediatr Respir Rev* 5:59, 2004.
19. Couto RC, et al: Risk factors for nosocomial infection in a neonatal intensive care unit, *Infect Control Hosp Epidemiol* 27:571, 2006.
20. Cunningham ML, Mann N: Pulmonary agenesis: a predictor of ipsilateral malformations, *Am J Med Genet* 70: 391, 1997.
21. Dargaville PA, et al: The epidemiology of meconium aspiration syndrome: incidence, risk factors, therapies, and outcome, *Pediatrics* 117:1712, 2006.
22. DiFiore JM, et al: Cardiorespiratory events in preterm infants referred for apnea monitoring studies, *Pediatrics* 108:1304, 2001.

23. El Shahed AI, et al: Surfactant for meconium aspiration syndrome in full term/near term infants, *Cochrane Database Syst Rev* 3:CD002054, 2007.

24. Everest NJ, et al: Outcomes following prolonged preterm premature rupture of the membranes, *Arch Dis Child Fetal Neonatal Ed* 93:F207, 2008.

25. Fleming P, Blair PS: Sudden infant death syndrome and parental smoking, *Early Hum Dev* 83:721, 2007.

26. Foglia E, et al: Ventilator-associated pneumonia in neonatal and pediatric intensive care unit patients, *Clin Microbiol Rev* 20:409, 2007.

27. Fraser, et al: Amnioinfusion for the prevention of the meconium aspiration syndrome, *N Engl J Med* 353:909, 2005.

28. Gozal D: Congenital central hypoventilation syndrome: an update, *Pediatr Pulmonol* 26:273, 1998.

29. Greene MF: Making small risks even smaller, *N Engl J Med* 360:183, 2009.

30. Hauck FR, et al: Do pacifiers reduce the risk of sudden infant death syndrome? A meta-analysis, *Pediatrics* 116:e716, 2005.

31. Hofstetter AO, et al: The induced prostaglandin E_2 pathway is a key regulator of the respiratory response to infection and hypoxia in neonates, *PNAS* 104:9894, 2007.

32. Horbar JD, et al: Trends in mortality and morbidity for very low birth weight infants 1991-1999, *Pediatrics* 110:143, 2002.

33. Jain L, Eaton DC: Physiology of fetal lung fluid clearance and the effect of labor, *Semin Perinatol* 30:34, 2006.

34. Jani JC, et al: Fetal lung-to-head ratio in the prediction of survival in severe left-sided diaphragmatic hernia treated by fetal endoscopic tracheal occlusion (FETO), *Am J Obstet Gynecol* 195:1646, 2006.

35. Janssen DJ, et al: Surfactant phosphatidylcholine metabolism in neonates with meconium aspiration syndrome, *J Pediatr* 149:634, 2006.

36. Kabbur PM, et al: Have the year 2000 Neonatal Resuscitation Program Guidelines changed the delivery room management or outcome of meconium-stained infants? *J Perinatol* 25:694, 2005.

37. Keller RL: Antenatal and postnatal lung and vascular anatomic and functional studies in congenital diaphragmatic hernia: implications for clinical management, *Am J Med Gen* 145C:184, 2007.

38. Kenny DP, et al: Antenatal diagnosis and postnatal treatment of intrapulmonary arteriovenous malformation, *Arch Dis Child Fetal Neonatal Ed* 92:F366, 2007.

39. Khan A, et al: Measurement of the CO_2 apneic threshold in newborn infants: possible relevance for periodic breathing and apnea, *J Appl Physiol* 98:1171, 2005.

40. Khazardoost S, et al: Risk factors for meconium aspiration in meconium stained amniotic fluid, *J Obstet Gynaecol* 27:577, 2007.

41. Kuhnert M, et al: Predictive agreement between the fetal arterial oxygen saturation and fetal scalp pH: results of the German multicenter study, *Am J Obstet Gynecol* 178:330, 1998.

42. Kumar AN: Perinatal management of common neonatal thoracic lesions, *Ind J Pediatr* 75:931, 2008.

43. Laje P, Liechty KW: Postnatal management and outcome of prenatally diagnosed lung lesions, *Prenat Diagn* 28:612, 2008.

44. Lakshmanan J, Ahanya SN, Rehan V, et al: Elevated plasma corticotrophin release factor levels and in utero meconium passage, *Pediatr Res* 61:176, 2007.

45. Laptook AR, et al: Adverse neurodevelopmental outcomes among extremely low birth weight infants with a normal head ultrasound: prevalence and antecedents, *Pediatrics* 115:673, 2005.

46. Lehtonen L, Martin RJ: Ontogeny of sleep and awake states in relation to breathing in preterm infants, *Semin Neonatol* 9:229, 2004.

47. Liem JJ, et al: Transient tachypnea of the newborn may be an early clinical manifestation of wheezing symptoms, *J Pediatr* 151:29, 2007.

48. Logan JW, et al: Congenital diaphragmatic hernia: a systematic review and summary of best-evidence practice, *J Perinatol* 27:535, 2007.

49. Malloy MH, Freeman DH Jr: Birth weight- and gestational age-specific sudden infant death syndrome mortality: United States, 1991 versus 1995, *Pediatrics* 105:1227, 2000.

50. Martin RJ, et al: Persistence of the biphasic ventilatory response to hypoxia in preterm infants, *J Pediatr* 132:960, 1998.

51. Miller JD, Carlo WA: Pulmonary complications of mechanical ventilation in neonates, *Clin Perinatol* 35:73, 2008.

52. Morley CJ: Nasal CPAP or intubation at birth for very preterm infants, *N Engl J Med* 58:700, 2008.

53. Nattie E: Central chemosensitivity, sleep, and wakefulness, *Respir Physiol* 129:257, 2001.

54. Nock ML, et al: Relationship of the ventilatory response to hypoxia with neonatal apnea in preterm infants, *J Pediatr* 144:291, 2004.

55. Peetsold MG, et al: The long-term follow-up of patients with a congenital diaphragmatic hernia: a broad spectrum of morbidity, *Pediatr Surg Int* 25:1, 2009.

56. Pierce J, et al: Intrapartum amnioinfusion for meconium stained fluid: meta-analysis of prospective clinical trials, *Obstet Gynecol* 95:1051, 2000.

57. Pillekamp F, et al: Factors influencing apnea and bradycardia of prematurity—implications for neurodevelopment, *Neonatology* 91:155, 2007.

58. Radhakrishnan RS, et al: ECMO for meconium aspiration syndrome: support for relaxed entry criteria, *ASAIO J* 53:489, 2007.

59. Rastogi S, et al: Treatment of giant pulmonary interstitial emphysema by ipsilateral bronchial occlusion with a Swan-Ganz catheter, *Pediatr Radiol* 37:1130, 2007.

60. Roehr CC, et al: Somatostatin or octreotide as treatment options for chylothorax in young children: a systematic review, *Intensive Care Med* 32:650, 2006.

61. Salvesen B, Nielsen EW, Harboe M, et al: Mechanisms of complement activation and effects of C1-inhibitor on the meconium-induced inflammatory reaction in human cord blood, *Mol Immunol* 46:688, 2009.

62. Schmidt B, et al: Long-term effects of caffeine therapy for apnea of prematurity, *N Engl J Med* 357:1893, 2007.

63. Singh SA, et al: Persistent pulmonary hypertension of newborn due to congenital capillary alveolar dysplasia, *Pediatr Pulmonol* 40:349, 2005.

64. Slocum C, et al: Infant apnea and gastroesophageal reflux: a critical review and framework for further investigation, *Curr Gastroenterol Rep* 9:219, 2007.

65. Stocker JT: The respiratory tract. In Stocker JT, Dehner LP, editors: *Pediatric pathology*, 2nd ed, vol 1, Philadelphia, 2001, Lippincott Williams & Wilkins.

65a. Supcun S, Kutz P, Pielemeier W, Roll C: Caffeine increases cerebral cortical activity in preterm infants, *J Pediatr* 156(3):490, 2010.

65b. SUPPORT Study Group of the Eunice Kennedy Shriver NICHD Neonatal Research Network, Finer NN, Carlo WA, Walsh MC, et al: Early CPAP versus surfactant in extremely preterm infants, *N Engl J Med* 362:1970, 2010.

66. Tamim H, et al: National Collaborative Perinatal Neonatal Network. Consanguinity and apnea of prematurity, *Am J Epidemiol* 158:942, 2003.

67. Tomaszewska M, et al: Pulmonary hemorrhage, clinical course and outcomes among very low-birth-weight infants, *Arch Pediatr Adolesc Med* 153:715, 1999.

68. Vain NE, et al: Oropharyngeal and nasopharyngeal suctioning of meconium-stained neonates before delivery of their shoulders: multicentre, randomized controlled trial, *Lancet* 364:597, 2004.

69. Wees-Mayer DE, et al: Sudden infant death syndrome: association with a promoter polymorphism of the serotonin transporter gene, *Am J Med Genet* 117A:268, 2003.

70. Wiswell TE, et al: Delivery room management of the apparently vigorous meconium-stained neonate: results of the multicenter, international collaborative trial, *Pediatrics* 105:1, 2000.

71. Young JK, et al: An astrocyte toxin influences the pattern of breathing and the ventilatory response to hypercapnia in neonatal rats, *Respir Physiol Neurobiol* 47:19, 2005.

72. Zanardo V, et al: The influence of timing of elective cesarean section on risk of neonatal pneumothorax, *J Pediatr* 150:252, 2007.

73. Zhang X, Kramer MS: Variations in mortality and morbidity by gestational age among infants born at term, *J Pediatr* 154:358, 2009.

PART 6

Upper Airway Lesions
Robert C. Sprecher and James E. Arnold

A spectrum of pathologic conditions can affect the neonatal upper airway, resulting in respiratory distress at birth or within the first few weeks of life. The clinical presentations of these disorders, however, are often quite similar. The most common symptom is stridor; other signs and symptoms include cyanosis, apnea, dyspnea, retractions, hypercapnia, difficulty feeding, abnormal cry, and cough. The physician's ability to arrive at a diagnosis and treatment plan in the neonate with respiratory distress requires an understanding of the unique anatomic and physiologic factors that affect neonatal upper airway physiology. Of primary importance in evaluating the neonatal airway is determining the degree of emergency and the need to establish an artificial airway (endotracheal intubation or tracheostomy).

The evaluation of an infant with a suspected airway problem should encompass the entire upper airway, from the anterior nasal vestibule to the tracheal bifurcation. Obstruction at any level can lead to respiratory distress. The duration and severity of the infant's symptoms and the progressive nature of the airway distress direct the examiner to either a congenital or acquired disorder. Division of the neonatal upper airway into four primary physiologic components—nasal, oral, laryngeal, and tracheal—allows orderly discussion of the pathologic conditions that could afflict the newborn infant's airway.

NASAL AND NASOPHARYNGEAL LESIONS
Pyriform Aperture Stenosis

Anterior nasal stenosis can occur as the result of bony overgrowth of the nasal process of the maxilla. The diagnosis can be confirmed with computed tomography (CT) scanning. In most patients, conservative therapy with judicious use of intranasal and systemic steroids to reduce mucosal edema provides symptomatic relief. In severe cases, the infants present with significant nasal obstruction similar to those with posterior choanal atresia. Rarely, surgical intervention involving drill-out of the bony pyriform aperture through a sublabial approach is necessary.[4]

Nasolacrimal Duct Cysts

Nasolacrimal duct cysts can occur either unilaterally or bilaterally. Children present with varying degrees of nasal obstruction. Often there is associated epiphora. Intranasal examination shows a smooth, mucosa-covered mass under the inferior turbinate. The diagnosis is confirmed with CT scanning (Fig. 44-67). Surgery is usually required to eliminate the nasal obstruction. Often, simply marsupializing the cyst results in complete resolution. This can be accomplished with a cup forceps or the CO_2 laser.

Choanal Atresia

Neonates are preferential nasal breathers for the first 4 to 6 weeks of life. The entire length of the neonate's tongue is in close proximity to the hard and soft palate, which creates a vacuum and resultant respiratory distress when nasal obstruction is present. Bilateral choanal atresia is the most common cause of complete nasal obstruction in the neonate,

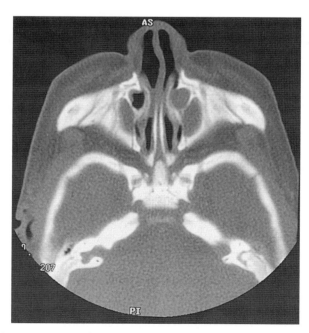

Figure 44–67. Bilateral nasolacrimal duct cysts causing complete anterior nasal obstruction.

occurring in approximately 1 in 7000 live births.[11] Associated anomalies occur in 20% to 50% of infants with choanal atresia.[29] The CHARGE syndrome includes coloboma or other ophthalmic anomalies, heart defect, atresia choanae, restriction of growth and developmental, genital hypoplasia, and ear anomalies with hearing loss.[8] Mutations in the *CHD7* gene (member of the chromodomain helicase DNA-binding protein family) located in chromosome 8q12 have been detected in more than two thirds of patients with CHARGE syndrome.[17,20] Recent data suggest overlap between CHARGE syndrome and 22q11.2 deletion syndrome in immunodeficiency states and hypocalcemia.[18] Children with CHARGE syndrome require intensive medical management as well as numerous surgical interventions. They also need multidisciplinary follow-up. A complete evaluation to rule out associated anomalies is therefore mandatory in all infants with bilateral choanal atresia.

Although bilateral obstruction always produces symptoms in the neonatal period, the degree of distress and cyanosis vary from severe asphyxia to cyanosis only with sucking. Typically, the infant has a history of distress when resting that is relieved with agitation and crying.

In a suspected case of choanal atresia, an attempt should be made to pass a 6-French catheter into the nasopharynx. Failure of the catheter to pass suggests choanal atresia. CT scan is required to differentiate between stenosis and atresia and to determine whether the atretic plate is bony or membranous.

Treatment of choanal atresia depends on the severity of the obstruction and the clinical presentation of the infant. Unilateral atresia rarely requires surgical intervention during infancy and is usually corrected before the child begins school (4 to 5 years of age). Bilateral atresia is usually repaired within the first few days of life. Historically, this was performed transpalatally, but today it is most commonly performed endoscopically through a transnasal route. Stenting of the repair has been associated with a higher rate of restenosis. As a result, single-stage repair is preferable.[36] Postoperatively, these patients do quite well, although repeated dilations may be necessary during the first year of life to maintain choanal patency. In CHARGE patients, tracheostomy may be preferable to immediate repair, depending on the severity of the associated anomalies.[1]

Intranasal Tumors

In addition to anomalous nasal development, nasal obstruction with airway distress can result from intranasal tumors such as dermoids, gliomas, encephaloceles, or teratomas. Any infant with an intranasal mass should be fully evaluated, including magnetic resonance imaging (MRI) to assess for skull base involvement and intracranial extension before intervention is undertaken. Biopsy of an unsuspected nasal encephalocele can lead to cerebrospinal fluid leak, meningitis, and death.

Gliomas and encephaloceles are rare lesions of neurogenic origin containing glial tissue. Gliomas are benign but locally aggressive tumors that are usually noticeable at birth or during early infancy. Approximately 15% of gliomas have a fibrous stalk with connection to the subarachnoid space.[14] Failure to recognize the fibrous stalk can lead to incomplete resection and tumor recurrence. Encephaloceles maintain their intracranial communication, with herniated brain tissue, dura, and cerebrospinal fluid constituting the tumor. Early surgical resection is generally recommended to alleviate the risk of meningitis that accompanies these tumors. In addition, progressive growth of the lesion can result in marked nasal deformity.

Teratomas are composed of multiple heterotopic tissues that are foreign to the site from which they arise. The etiology of these tumors is unknown, although they are believed to arise from rests of pluripotential cells sequestered during embryogenesis. The occurrence of nasopharyngeal teratomas is unusual, but when present they may be associated with significant airway distress.[5,7]

Generally, four classifications of teratomas are described. Dermoids are the most common subtype and are composed of epidermal and mesodermal elements. Teratoid tumors are composed of all three germ layers but are incompletely organized, whereas true teratomas are composed of all three germ layers with recognizable early organ differentiation. Epignathi are highly differentiated tumors and are rarely compatible with life.

Treatment of the nasopharyngeal teratoma involves airway stabilization and complete surgical resection. Prognosis is generally excellent with complete excision. Mortality in infants with teratomas is generally the result of airway obstruction.

Mucosal Obstruction

Generalized mucosal hypertrophy or edema can result in significant anterior nasal congestion and symptomatic obstruction in the neonate until oral breathing becomes reflexive. Treatment of these patients is generally conservative and includes humidification, saline drops, and judicious suctioning. Excessive attempts at suctioning can result in increased edema and exacerbation of the infant's symptoms. Gastroesophageal reflux may reach the level of the nasopharynx and can exacerbate nasal obstruction as well. Appropriate treatment of reflux may improve the nasal airway. Intranasal steroid drops might be helpful during periods of increased congestion such as that associated with viral rhinitis. Prolonged use of intranasal decongestants could lead to rhinitis medicamentosa (paradoxical mucosal swelling) and should be avoided.

Continuous Positive Airway Pressure Trauma

Care must be taken with the use of continuous positive airway pressure (CPAP) nasal prongs and masks in the neonate because nasal trauma can occur. Injuries such as excoriation of the nasal septum, necrosis of the columella, and lacerations of the nasal ala have been reported.[30] To prevent such injuries, nasal CPAP should be terminated as soon as possible. If injury is imminent and discontinuation of nasal CPAP is not possible, then changing to a different style of delivery may be useful.

ORAL AND OROPHARYNGEAL LESIONS

Normal oral cavity and oropharyngeal development is critical in establishing a patent upper airway. A variety of congenital anomalies have a known association with retrognathia, glossoptosis, and posterior tongue displacement and subsequent airway obstruction. Pierre Robin sequence,[11,34]

Treacher Collins syndrome, Goldenhar syndrome (oculoauriculovertebral dysplasia), Crouzon disease (Fig. 44-68), and Down syndrome are the most common congenital anomalies that have oropharyngeal airway obstruction as an important clinical feature (see Part 5 of this chapter and Chapter 29).

In most of these patients, normal growth and development results in an increase in oropharyngeal space and a decrease in obstructive symptoms. Any treatment plan for these patients must take into consideration the knowledge that normal growth alleviates much of the obstructive pathology. Often, placing the infant in a prone position with slight head elevation during sleep dramatically decreases the degree of symptomatic obstruction. A modified nipple (McGovern nipple) that maintains oral patency or the placement of a soft nasal trumpet may be sufficient to achieve adequate airway patency until growth of the mandible occurs. Nasal CPAP is a noninvasive means of establishing a patent upper airway in patients whose obstruction is primarily manifested as obstructive sleep apnea.[3]

In severe cases, surgical intervention may be necessary. Tracheostomy has been the mainstay of surgical management of patients with upper airway obstruction, but pediatric mandibular distraction osteogenesis has been successful in lengthening the mandible of patients with significant retrognathia. Bilateral internal microdistraction can avoid tracheostomy in selected infants, and it can facilitate decannulation in those with a preexistent tracheostomy.[16,28,31]

Lymphatic Malformations

Lesions of the floor of the mouth or base of the tongue that cause posterior tongue displacement also can be associated with secondary airway obstruction. Lymphatic malformations are known to infiltrate the soft tissue of the floor of the mouth and cause significant upper airway obstruction. Lymphatic abnormalities appear as persistent clusters of thin-walled vesicles, usually filled with clear, colorless fluid. Tissues affected by lymphatic anomalies are notorious for the speed at which infection can spread through them.[35] At the first signs of inflammation, aggressive antimicrobial therapy is mandatory. Such infections may be life threatening, especially if inflammation leads to increased airway obstruction.

Because of the infiltrative nature of these lesions in the oral cavity, extensive lymphatic anomalies are often not amenable to surgical excision. Serial resection is ineffective in most instances and could in fact exacerbate the degree of oropharyngeal obstruction. Spontaneous resolution is uncommon. For macrocystic cervicofacial lymphatic malformations, the immunostimulant OK-432 (Picibanil) has been shown to be effective.[33] Tracheostomy is the treatment of choice for patients with a large oral cavity and oropharyngeal lymphatic malformations and associated airway obstruction.

Tongue Cysts

Cysts of the base of the tongue are a rare but serious cause of airway obstruction in the newborn infant (Fig. 44-69). An acute airway crisis could appear shortly after birth or several months later. A 43% mortality rate has been reported in the literature, with most deaths attributed to delayed diagnosis and acute airway obstruction. In most patients, these cysts represent thyroglossal duct remnants that arise from the foramen cecum.[19]

Dermoid cysts have been reported in the literature as tongue lesions associated with airway obstruction in the young infant. In contrast with the infant with a thyroglossal duct cyst at the base of the tongue, oral dermoids have a more insidious onset of symptoms, with presentation after 6 months of age.[9] Airway obstruction is in part caused by the mass effect in the hypopharynx and inferoposterior displacement of the epiglottis, which causes supraglottic obstruction.

Surgical excision is the treatment of choice in these patients. Marsupialization may be an option for the large cyst that is not amenable to complete resection. Significant tongue

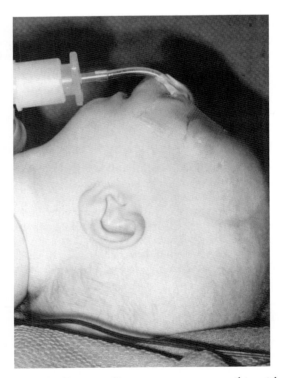

Figure 44–68. Crouzon disease: severe retrognathia with upper airway obstruction.

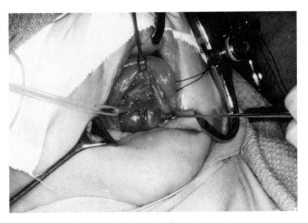

Figure 44–69. Oral cavity cyst.

swelling can develop postoperatively, and temporary intubation may be necessary to ensure a protected upper airway.

LARYNGEAL LESIONS

Embryologically, the larynx has three primary functions: airway protection, respiratory modulation, and voice production. The neonatal larynx has unique features, compared with that of an adult, that affect its ability to perform these three primary functions both in the normal and the diseased state.

Although the neonatal larynx is less than one-third the size of the adult larynx, the arytenoid cartilages are adult size at birth. This relationship between the supraglottic structures and the laryngeal inlet can contribute to the development of laryngomalacia in some infants. The subglottis is the smallest component of the pediatric larynx, whereas in the adult the glottic aperture is the size-limiting factor. The development of subglottic stenosis in the infant following endotracheal intubation is directly related to the small size of the subglottic opening.

In addition to differences in size, the infant larynx differs in its position in the neck relative to the cervical and facial skeleton. At birth the larynx may be found at approximately the level of the C4 vertebra. As the child grows, the larynx begins its inferior descent, ultimately resting at the level of C7. The high location of the larynx in the infant provides some protection against external trauma.

The cephalad location of the larynx also provides additional protection to the lower airway of the neonate, who has not yet fully developed the necessary protective reflexes to prevent aspiration during swallowing. In the young infant, the epiglottis rests on the nasopharyngeal surface of the soft palate. This position allows the infant to suckle without danger of aspiration and to breathe with the mouth closed.

Anatomically, the larynx may be subdivided into three components: supraglottis, glottis, and subglottis (Fig. 44-70). Disorders in one of these components produce a unique set of symptoms that allows the physician to begin narrowing the field of possible causes of airway distress in the infant. An attempt should be made to characterize stridor, when present, as inspiratory, expiratory, or biphasic.

Although not uniformly true, the level of obstruction is often reflected in the character of the stridor. Supraglottic lesions tend to produce a coarse, inspiratory stridor, whereas glottic and subglottic disorders are more "musical" in quality and often biphasic in nature. Pure tracheal lesions often manifest with a prolonged expiratory phase and expiratory stridor. Changes in the quality of the stridor with the level of activity and position of the infant are also a crucial aspect of the history. The quality of the child's cry (normal, weak, or aphonic) can direct one to a glottic lesion, although severe subglottic narrowing could produce an abnormal cry due to limited air movement.

The presence or absence of cough should be documented. A feeding history is critical. Symptoms of aspiration or cyanosis with feeds can signal a specific disorder. Failure to thrive or other signs of systemic illness could indicate a more chronic disorder. The infant's prenatal and perinatal history could reveal an unsuspected history of traumatic delivery or neonatal intubation.

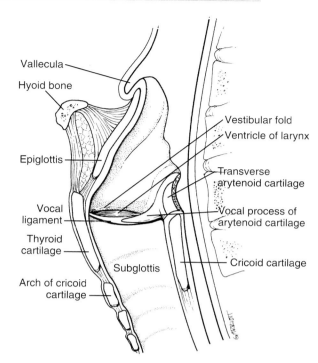

Figure 44–70. Parasagittal view of infant larynx demonstrating cartilaginous relationships.

If the infant is in extremis or there are signs to suggest significant airway compromise, extreme caution should be exercised. Manipulation of the infant should be minimized until the airway can be secured. The infant can be observed for tachypnea, tachycardia, retractions (supraclavicular, subcostal, intercostal), nasal flaring, cyanosis, drooling, cough, and level of consciousness (restless, agitated, stuporous) without increasing the level of the infant's anxiety.

Laryngeal examination should not be performed in the infant with an unstable airway unless the appropriate personnel and equipment are available for urgent airway access when necessary. Flexible fiberoptic nasolaryngoscopy is widely available and allows direct inspection of the larynx in the stable neonate.

Evaluation of the awake child has several distinct advantages. The larynx can be viewed in a dynamic fashion so that the degree of laryngeal collapse during active respiration is appreciated. In addition, vocal cord motion can be assessed. Flexible bronchoscopy allows further dynamic evaluation of the subglottic airway and lower tracheobronchial tree.

For more controlled laryngeal evaluation, direct laryngoscopy and rigid bronchoscopy under general anesthesia are necessary. If a deep inhalational anesthetic technique is used, dynamic laryngeal and tracheal function can be assessed using this method as well. Direct laryngoscopy with rigid bronchoscopy is the method of choice in evaluating an infant with air hunger, cyanosis, or any critical symptoms that may necessitate intubation.

Ancillary testing in the infant with a stable airway is useful in further identifying the site of the lesion before possible endoscopy and surgical intervention. Radiographic evaluation of the upper airway (usually with a CT scan with contrast) is useful in suspected subglottic stenosis (either congenital or iatrogenic), soft tissue laryngeal tumors (hemangiomas, papillomas), or congenital laryngeal or esophageal cysts. Less commonly, anteroposterior and lateral soft tissue radiographs of the neck can be obtained. Ballooning of the hypopharynx is often seen on the lateral neck radiograph in an infant with significant airway obstruction. Reversal of the cervical lordotic curvature is suggestive of a retropharyngeal process. Airway fluoroscopy allows a dynamic assessment of the airway and can be done in conjunction with a modified barium swallow to evaluate for vascular anomalies or tracheoesophageal fistula or to better define the contribution of a swallowing disorder to the airway symptoms. CT scan is also useful for evaluating the infant with a laryngeal tumor, for a severe laryngotracheal anomaly not fully delineated by endoscopy, or for the evaluation of laryngeal trauma. CT scanning is also useful for virtual bronchoscopy to map extensive tracheal or bronchial stenosis. MRI is useful for defining mediastinal anatomy in the infant with a suspected vascular anomaly.

Disorders of the neonatal larynx are best subdivided into congenital and acquired lesions. Severe congenital laryngeal anomalies are quite rare and in general manifest themselves within the first few minutes of life. These include complete atresia, severe stenosis, or near-total laryngeal webs. If these disorders are recognized, tracheostomy may be a life-saving procedure. Often these severe laryngeal anomalies are found in conjunction with other life-threatening neurologic, cardiac, gastrointestinal, and lower airway lesions. In the neonate, the acquired laryngeal injury is usually the result of endotracheal intubation (see Part 4). The overall prognosis for these neonates depends not only on the laryngeal problem but also on the infant's overall development and the impact of other concomitant lesions.

Laryngomalacia

Laryngomalacia (congenital flaccid larynx, congenital laryngeal stridor) is the most common cause of stridor in the infant and accounts for up to 60% of laryngeal problems in the pediatric population.[15] Clinically, the stridor develops between the second and fourth weeks of life, although it occasionally may be present at birth. The stridor is typically characterized as coarse inspiratory noise.

The infant is generally better in the prone position, because this serves to decrease the degree of supraglottic collapse on inspiration. Agitation tends to exacerbate the stridor, and stridor tends to disappear completely during rest. Feeding difficulties are unusual and cry is normal. However, the infant may present with failure to thrive. In these cases, surgical intervention is necessary. Severe airway obstruction is unusual and is generally seen in infants with underlying neuromuscular disorders.

The natural history of the disease is one of progression until 8 to 12 months of age, with complete resolution in most children by 2 years of age. The etiology of laryngomalacia remains elusive, although generalized neurologic immaturity of the infant's airway and digestive tract is believed to play a role. Gastroesophageal reflux is often present in these children and can affect the severity of the laryngeal symptoms.[20]

When the stridor is not associated with any severe cyanotic spells, fiberoptic office nasolaryngoscopy is useful in confirming the diagnosis of laryngomalacia. During inspiration, the supraglottic structures collapse into the laryngeal inlet, narrowing the air passage and creating the classic coarse stridor. Collapse of the arytenoids is often a key component in the development of clinically significant obstruction, rather than isolated epiglottic prolapse as initially hypothesized.

Airway fluoroscopy and modified barium swallow are useful adjuvants in the evaluation of these infants. Often, the skilled airway fluoroscopist can support the diagnosis of laryngomalacia. The subglottic airway may be indirectly evaluated using this technique, and a search can be made for possible vascular anomalies affecting the integrity of the airway.

Up to 20% of infants with laryngomalacia have a second airway lesion, most commonly congenital subglottic stenosis.[2] Direct laryngoscopy with rigid bronchoscopy is indicated in the atypical patient to confirm the suspected diagnosis of laryngomalacia and to evaluate for the possible existence of a secondary lesion below the level of the glottis.

In most cases, therapy for laryngomalacia is observation and reassurance. In more severe cases with feeding difficulties, endoscopic laser aryepiglottic fold incision (epiglottoplasty) can provide symptomatic relief without the need for tracheostomy (Fig. 44-71).[24,26] Tracheostomy is reserved for severe laryngomalacia that results in significant airway obstruction despite epiglottoplasty.

Bifid or Absent Epiglottis

Both the bifid epiglottis and the absent epiglottis are extremely rare (Fig. 44-72). Severe subglottic stenosis is usually seen with these unusual supraglottic anomalies. Tracheostomy is necessary because of the associated subglottic lesion. Aspiration is variable.

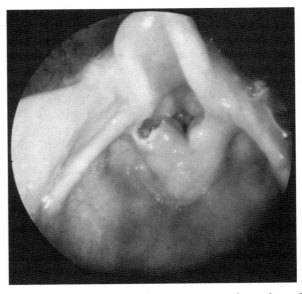

Figure 44–71. Infant supraglottis. Laser epiglottoplasty for laryngomalacia has been performed by cutting the left aryepiglottic fold.

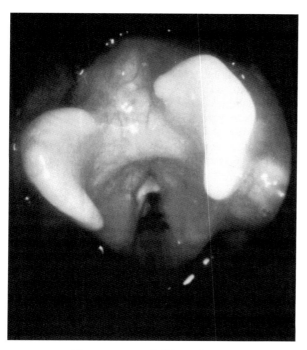

Figure 44–72. Bifid epiglottis.

Laryngeal Cysts

Most cysts of the larynx develop in the supraglottic location (aryepiglottic fold, epiglottis, vallecula) and gradually increase in size during the first few months of life (Fig. 44-73). Owing to the location of these lesions as well as their slowly progressive course, they may be indistinguishable clinically from laryngomalacia. These patients often have inspiratory stridor that worsens with agitation and when in the supine position. In older children, the voice can become muffled as the cyst

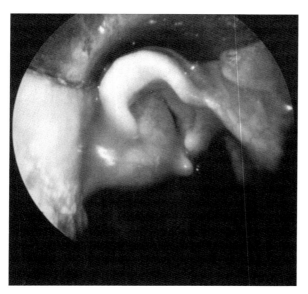

Figure 44–73. Infant supraglottis: left aryepiglottic fold cyst with glottic obstruction.

enlarges. Progressive dysphagia with aspiration is more commonly seen in these patients than in patients with classic laryngomalacia.[6]

If undetected and untreated, these cysts can become quite large and cause complete laryngeal obstruction. Fiberoptic evaluation confirms the presence of a supraglottic cyst and is the minimum requirement for all infants with new-onset, progressive inspiratory stridor. The treatment involves either endoscopic marsupialization or complete excision (either endoscopically or externally) of the cyst. Attempts to aspirate the cyst inevitably lead to cyst recurrence. Subglottic cysts can form just below the vocal cords and are caused by obstruction of mucosal glands related to intubation. Endoscopic marsupialization with the carbon dioxide laser is usually curative.

Vocal Cord Paralysis

Vocal cord paralysis is second only to laryngomalacia as a cause of stridor in the pediatric patient, accounting for 10% to 15% of new cases.[15] Although the paralysis might not be a true congenital lesion, it is often present at birth and is therefore grouped with other congenital anomalies of the larynx. Most of these lesions are unilateral.

Clinically, the infant is often symptomatic within the first week of life. In the case of unilateral injury, the infant might have a weak cry but develops stridor only when stressed (agitation, infection). The stridor is typically either inspiratory or biphasic in character. The child may have a history of choking, coughing, or brief cyanotic spells during feeds, which is indicative of aspiration.

Radiographic evaluation remains an important step in the management of these patients. Unilateral paralysis may be associated with cardiac atrial enlargement or anomalous great vessels, which can be detected on chest radiographs and barium swallow or echocardiogram. In the absence of a history of traumatic delivery or cardiothoracic surgery (e.g., ligation of patent ductus arteriosus [PDA], repair of tracheoesophageal fistula) that might have resulted in injury to the vagus or recurrent laryngeal nerve, the course of the vagus nerve should be investigated radiographically with a CT scan. Fiberoptic evaluation to confirm the diagnosis of vocal cord paralysis may be difficult if significant laryngomalacia is present, obscuring visualization of the laryngeal inlet during vocalization (crying). Ultrasonographic imaging is an alternative technique for assessing vocal cord function in the difficult patient.[10]

The treatment of unilateral vocal cord paralysis depends on the severity of the child's symptoms. Often the respiratory symptoms are minimal, and adjustments in the infant's diet could eliminate the problem with aspiration. Most cases of unilateral paralysis resolve spontaneously over 6 to 12 months. Direct surgical management of the paralyzed vocal cord is therefore generally not recommended. Tracheostomy is rarely necessary in unilateral vocal cord paralysis.

Bilateral paralysis creates more severe respiratory symptoms due to significant encroachment on the glottic aperture. Often, there are associated neurologic abnormalities, such as Chiari malformation and hydrocephalus, in infants with bilateral vocal cord paralysis. Evaluation of the infant with bilateral vocal cord paralysis should therefore include CT or

MRI imaging of the central nervous system and the base of the skull. Unlike unilateral paralysis, bilateral vocal cord paralysis often necessitates tracheostomy.

Laryngeal Web

A laryngeal web is the result of a failure to recanalize the laryngeal inlet at approximately 10 weeks' gestation. The web is a membrane of varying thickness and most frequently involves the glottis from the anterior commissure to the vocal process (Fig. 44-74). The infant might not be symptomatic at birth. As the level of activity increases, usually between 4 and 6 weeks of age, the infant develops biphasic stridor. The cry is often weak, and in severe cases the infant may be nearly aphonic. Feeding is not affected. Treatment of a laryngeal web depends on the thickness of the web itself and the degree of subglottic extension. Thin webs can often be treated endoscopically with the carbon dioxide laser. Thicker, more fibrotic webs might require tracheostomy and an external approach with stent or keel placement.

Congenital Subglottic Stenosis

The normal subglottis measures between 5 and 7 mm in the neonate. Congenital subglottic stenosis occurs when the subglottic diameter of a full-term infant is less than 4 mm at birth. Congenital stenosis often results from an abnormally shaped cricoid ring, elliptical rather than circular, or from excessive thickening of the subglottic tissue. Rarely, the first tracheal ring may be displaced superiorly and come to lie within the cricoid itself.

In mild forms, the stenosis can go undetected until the child is 2 to 3 years of age, at which point recurrent crouplike episodes prompt endoscopic evaluation. In more severe cases, biphasic stridor is present with a classic croupy cough in the absence of any systemic signs of a viral illness. The cry is usually normal, and feeding is only an issue in cases of significant shortness of breath due to airway compromise.

In general, congenital subglottic stenosis is concentric. Radiographic evaluation usually demonstrates symmetric subglottic narrowing.

Management of these lesions depends on the severity of the infant's symptoms and the age at presentation. Congenital subglottic stenosis is usually less severe than the iatrogenic form following endotracheal intubation. In select cases, an anterior cricoid split can prevent the need for tracheostomy in infants up to 18 months of age. In more severe cases of stenosis or in the older child, laryngotracheal reconstruction using rib for augmentation is the treatment of choice.

Subglottic Hemangioma

Subglottic hemangioma is the most common neoplasm of the infant airway and can lead to significant airway compromise if left untreated. A hemangioma is a vascular neoplasm characterized by proliferation of the capillary endothelium.[32] In the larynx, the lesion generally appears as a smooth, eccentric, compressible mass in the subglottis, most commonly located in the left, posterior subglottic space. Up to 50% of infants with a documented subglottic hemangioma have a cutaneous lesion as well.

The clinical presentation of a subglottic hemangioma is similar to that of subglottic stenosis. The infant typically has progressive biphasic stridor beginning at 4 to 6 weeks of age. Unlike with the static subglottic lesion, the symptoms associated with a hemangioma can fluctuate in severity from day to day. The fluctuating character of symptoms is strongly diagnostic of subglottic hemangioma. The stridor is worse with crying or agitation owing to vascular engorgement of the hemangioma. Feeding difficulties are unusual unless severe airway obstruction exists. The cry is generally normal. Radiographic evaluation (CT scan with contrast or anteroposterior soft tissue neck film) may show an asymmetric narrowing of the subglottis. The diagnosis of a subglottic hemangioma is confirmed at the time of direct laryngoscopy with rigid bronchoscopy (Fig. 44-75).

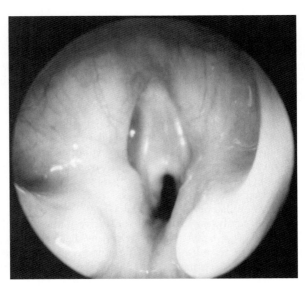

Figure 44-74. Glottic web.

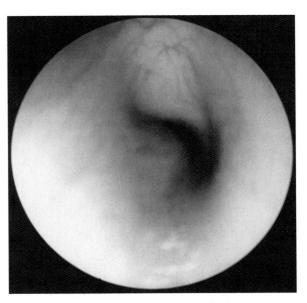

Figure 44-75. Subglottic hemangioma before treatment.

The treatment of subglottic hemangiomas must take into account the natural history of the neoplasm. Initially, the lesion undergoes rapid postnatal growth for 8 to 18 months (proliferative phase) followed by slow but inevitable regression for the next 5 to 8 years (involutive phase). Systemic steroids on a daily or every-other-day schedule may control the proliferative phase of the hemangioma in patients with minimal airway or feeding compromise and obviate the need for further surgical intervention. The CO_2 laser is a valuable tool in the treatment of larger lesions and those less responsive to systemic steroid therapy.[29] In cases of extensive airway involvement, a tracheostomy provides a secure airway until the tumor involutes. In patients with life-threatening or function-threatening hemangiomas who have failed or don't tolerate corticosteroid or other conservative management, other pharmacologic therapies (e.g., interferon, vincristine, or propanolol) may be considered.[21,25,27]

Laryngeal Cleft

Failure of fusion of the posterior cricoid lamina results in a posterior laryngeal cleft. This rare developmental anomaly usually manifests with respiratory distress precipitated by feeding. Other congenital anomalies are known to be associated with this lesion. If the cleft is mild, often dietary changes (thickened feeds) are sufficient to prevent aspiration. A gastrostomy is recommended if thickened feeds do not prevent aspiration, and open repair is advocated.

Congenital High Airway Obstruction Syndrome

Congenital high airway obstruction syndrome (CHAOS) was defined by Hedrick and colleagues[13] in 1994 as prenatally-diagnosed upper airway obstruction with concomitant findings of large echogenic lungs, dilated airways, flattened or inverted diaphragms with associated fetal ascites, or nonimmune hydrops. These hallmark findings are found consistently only when there is complete high upper airway obstruction with no tracheoesophageal connection. This leads to trapping of the fluid secreted by the fetal lung tissue. If the lung fields expand to the point of producing esophageal compression, then polyhydramnios may occur as a result of impaired swallowing of amniotic fluid. These findings necessitate a more detailed scan for other abnormalities because CHAOS may be one fetal presentation of Fraser syndrome characterized by variable expression of laryngeal atresia, cryptophthalmos, syndactyly, renal agenesis, and abnormalities of the ears and external genitalia.[22]

Possible airway anomalies include complete laryngeal atresia, severe congenital subglottic stenosis, and significant laryngeal web.[12] A laryngeal cyst that completely occludes the airway is less common.

This life-threatening condition was previously thought to be rare and uniformly fatal. Advances in prenatal imaging techniques have enabled this syndrome to be recognized more readily. Planning for the EXIT (ex utero intrapartum treatment) procedure can then be made to maximize survival.

If there is incomplete airway obstruction or a tracheoesophageal fistula, then the degree of fluid trapping is lessened and the diagnosis is less obvious on prenatal ultrasound imaging.

In these cases, with the diagnosis less obvious, survival depends on the degree of upper airway obstruction, the ability to tracheally intubate the child past the tracheoesophageal fistula or the ability to expeditiously perform a tracheostomy.

Intubation Trauma

The use of endotracheal intubation to secure the airway in the neonate for mechanical ventilation has become the standard of care for the critically ill newborn. Despite recent efforts to reduce the risk of iatrogenic injury, however, granuloma formation, arytenoid dislocation with true vocal cord fixation, and subglottic stenosis continue to occur.

Granuloma formation can follow endotracheal intubation. The infant is often hoarse following extubation, with progression rather than improvement of the symptoms with time. Evaluation of the larynx reveals a yellow-red pedunculated mass arising from the vocal process of the arytenoid. Subglottic cysts or mucoceles may develop when the opening of submucosal glands is interrupted by tissue reaction from an endotracheal tube. Microlaryngoscopy and removal of these lesions often result in resolution of the infant's symptoms. Repeat evaluation is recommended at 2 to 3 weeks to ensure that the granuloma has not reformed, which can be lessened by aggressive treatment of gastroesophageal reflux.

Several factors in the pediatric airway predispose the intubated neonate to subglottic stenosis (Fig. 44-76). The subglottic lumen is the narrowest aspect of the pediatric larynx. Premature infants and children with Down syndrome tend to have smaller cricoid rings than normal, thus increasing the overall risk of subglottic stenosis. Gastroesophageal reflux is an important factor in the pathogenesis of subglottic stenosis and is more frequently encountered in the premature infant and young child.[23] Difficulty in stabilizing the endotracheal tube in the neonate often results in repeated intubations and increased injury to the subglottis. Extreme immaturity

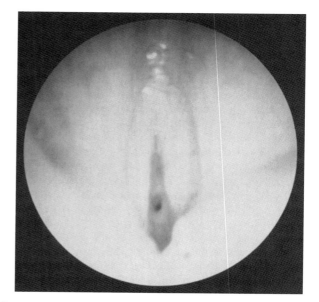

Figure 44–76. Iatrogenic subglottic stenosis following prolonged endotracheal intubation in a neonate.

requiring intubation periods of several months predisposes to subglottic injury. Hypoxia and sepsis are important variables in the development of subglottic tissue damage and are commonly seen in the neonatal intensive care setting. Injury to the subglottis may be reduced if the following steps are taken:

■ Use smaller endotracheal tubes.
■ Avoid cuffed endotracheal tubes in the infant and young child.
■ Aggressively treat systemic infection.
■ Minimize patient movement to prevent abrasions of the subglottic mucosa and resultant exposed cartilage as well as to prevent accidental extubation requiring further manipulation (sedation as necessary).
■ Consider tracheostomy if prolonged intubation is anticipated. Neonates tolerate intubation for much longer periods than the child or young adult.
■ Extubate under ideal conditions. In the difficult airway, high-dose systemic steroids for 24 to 48 hours before and after extubation may aid extubation. Use of inhaled epinephrine immediately following extubation can help reduce airway edema.

Treatment of iatrogenic subglottic stenosis depends on the severity of the stenosis, the age of the child, and concomitant medical problems. Tracheostomy remains the cornerstone of treatment, especially in the infant with multilevel airway involvement, multisystem failure, or significant pulmonary disease. The anterior cricoid split may be used in the neonate up to 18 months of age if mild stenosis exists. As in congenital subglottic stenosis, laryngotracheal reconstruction using rib cartilage is the method most commonly employed for treatment of significant pediatric subglottic stenosis. In selected patients, laryngotracheal reconstruction may be performed as a single-stage procedure, allowing immediate decannulation in the patient with a preexisting tracheostomy or avoidance of a tracheostomy altogether in the virgin trachea.

SUMMARY

Management of the neonate with upper airway obstruction requires that a rapid evaluation and diagnosis be made based on a complete understanding of the unique anatomic and physiologic characteristics of the neonatal airway. The airway should be assessed from nasal vestibule to tracheal bifurcation in a search for the etiology of acute or progressive respiratory distress. Treatment of the neonate with upper airway pathology is tailored to the specific abnormality as well as coexisting medical problems.

REFERENCES

1. Asher BF, et al: Airway complications in CHARGE association, *Arch Otolaryngol Head Neck Surg* 116:594, 1990.
2. Belmont JR, et al: Congenital laryngeal stridor (laryngomalacia): etiologic factors and associated disorders, *Ann Otol Rhinol Laryngol* 93:430, 1984.
3. Brooks LJ: Treatment of otherwise normal children with obstructive sleep apnea, *ENT J* 72:77, 1993.
4. Brown OE, et al: Congenital nasal pyriform aperture stenosis, *Laryngoscope* 99:86, 1989.
5. S, et al: Nasopharyngeal teratoma as a respiratory emergency in the neonate, *J Otolaryngol* 20:349, 1991.
6. Civantos FJ, et al: Laryngoceles and saccular cysts in infants and children, *Arch Otolaryngol Head Neck Surg* 118:296, 1992.
7. Cohen AF, et al: Nasopharyngeal teratoma in the neonate, *Int J Pediatr Otorhinolaryngol* 14:187, 1987.
8. Dobrowski JM, et al: Otorhinolaryngic manifestations of CHARGE association, *Otolaryngol Head Neck Surg* 93:798, 1985.
9. Flom GS, et al: Congenital dermoid cyst of the anterior tongue, *Otolaryngol Head Neck Surg* 100:602, 1989.
10. Friedman EM: Role of ultrasound in the assessment of vocal cord function in infants and children, *Ann Otol Rhinol Laryngol* 106:199, 1997.
11. Gunn TR, et al: Neonatal micrognathia is associated with small upper airways on radiographic measurement, *Acta Paediatr* 89:82, 2000.
12. Hartnick CJ, et al: Congenital high airway obstruction syndrome and airway reconstruction, *Arch Otolaryngol Head Neck Surg* 128:567, 2002.
13. Hedrick MH, et al: Congenital high airway obstruction syndrome (CHAOS): a potential for perinatal intervention, *J Pediatr Surg* 29:271,1994.
14. Hengerer AS, et al: Congenital malformations of the nose and paranasal sinuses. In Mackey T, editor: *Pediatric otolaryngology,* Philadelphia, 1990, Saunders.
15. Holinger LD: Etiology of stridor in the neonate, infant, and child, *Ann Otol Rhinol Laryngol* 89:397, 1980.
16. Izadi K, et al: Correction of upper airway obstruction in the newborn with internal mandibular distraction osteogenesis, *J Craniofac Surg* 14:493, 2003.
17. Jongmans M, et al: CHARGE syndrome: the phenotypic spectrum of mutation in the CHD7 gene, *J Med Genet* 43:306, 2005.
18. Jyonouchi S, et al: CHARGE (coloboma, heart defect, atresia choanae, retarded growth and development, genital hypoplasia, ear anomalies/deafness) syndrome and chromosome 22q11.2 deletion syndrome: a comparison of immunologic and nonimmunologic phenotypic features, *Pediatrics* 123:e871, 2009.
19. LaBagnara J Jr: Cysts of the base of the tongue in infants: an unusual cause of neonatal airway obstruction, *Otolaryngol Head Neck Surg* 101:108, 1989.
20. Lalani SR, et al: Spectrum of CHD7 mutations in 110 individuals with CHARGE syndrome and genotypic-phenotypic correlation, *Am J Hum Genet* 78:303, 2006.
21. Léauté-Labrèze C, et al: Propranolol for severe hemangiomas of infancy, *N Engl J Med* 358:24, 2008.
22. Lim FY, et al: Congenital high airway obstruction syndrome: natural history and management, *J Pediatr Surg* 38:940, 2003.
23. Little FB, et al: Effect of gastric acid on the pathogenesis of subglottic stenosis, *Ann Otol Rhinol Laryngol* 94:516, 1985.
24. McClurg FID, et al: Laser laryngoplasty for laryngomalacia, *Laryngoscope* 104:247, 1994.
25. Ohlms LA, et al: Interferon alfa-2A therapy for airway hemangiomas, *Ann Otol Rhinol Laryngol* 103:1, 1994.
26. Polonovski JM, et al: Aryepiglottic fold excision for the treatment of severe laryngomalacia, *Ann Otol Rhinol Laryngol* 99:625, 1990.

27. Rahbar R, et al: The biology and management of subglottic hemangioma: past, present, and future, *Laryngoscope* 114:1880, 2004.

28. Rhee ST, Buchman SR: Pediatric mandibular distraction osteogenesis: the present and the future, *J Craniofac Surg* 14:803, 2003.

29. Richardson MA, et al: Surgical management of choanal atresia, *Laryngoscope* 98:915, 1988.

30. Robertson NJ, et al: Nasal deformities resulting from flow driver continuous positive airway pressure, *Arch Dis Child* 75: 209, 1996.

31. Sidman JD, et al: Distraction osteogenesis of the mandible for airway obstruction in children, *Laryngoscope* 111:1137, 2001.

32. Sie KCY, et al: Subglottic hemangioma: ten years' experience with the carbon dioxide laser, *Ann Otol Rhinol Laryngol* 103:167, 1994.

33. Smith MC, et al: Efficacy and safety of OK-432 immunotherapy of lymphatic malformations, *Laryngoscope* 119:107, 2009.

34. Spier S, et al: Sleep in Pierre Robin syndrome, *Chest* 90:711, 1986.

35. AE, et al: Lymphatic malformations. In McAllister, editor: *Vascular birthmarks, hemangiomas, and malformations,* Philadelphia, 1988, Saunders.

36. Zuckerman JD, et al: Single-stage choanal atresia repair in the neonate, *Arch Otolaryngol Head Neck Surg* 134: 1090, 2008.

PART 7

Bronchopulmonary Dysplasia

Eduardo H. Bancalari and Michele C. Walsh

The introduction of mechanical ventilation for the management of premature infants with severe respiratory distress syndrome (RDS) in the 1960s changed the natural course of the disease, resulting in increased survival of smaller and sicker infants, many of whom had severe chronic lung damage. Northway and associates were the first to describe this condition in 1967 and introduced the term *bronchopulmonary dysplasia* (BPD).[43]

All infants in this original description were born prematurely, had severe respiratory failure, and received prolonged mechanical ventilation with high airway pressures and fraction of inspired oxygen (FiO_2). Their clinical and radiographic course ended with severe chronic lung changes characterized by persistent respiratory failure with hypoxemia and hypercapnia, frequent cor pulmonale, and a chest radiograph that revealed areas of increased density due to fibrosis and collapse surrounded by areas of marked hyperinflation.

Currently, this severe form of chronic lung disease (CLD) is less common and has been replaced by a milder form of chronic lung damage that occurs in many very small preterm infants who, with increasing frequency, are surviving after prolonged periods of mechanical ventilation. This milder form of lung damage often occurs in infants who initially have only mild pulmonary disease and do not require high airway pressures or FiO_2.[35,49] The terms *BPD* and *CLD* have

been used interchangeably but because the term *BPD* is more specific to the neonatal lung disease, this term is preferred here.

The incidence of BPD varies widely among different centers.[4] This is not only due to differences in patient susceptibility and in management but also to discrepancies in the way BPD is defined.[8] In 2001, a workshop conducted by the National Institutes of Health (NIH) proposed a definition that divides BPD into three categories based on the duration and level of oxygen therapy required (Table 44-7). Ehrenkranz and colleagues explored the validity of the NIH Consensus definition in the large NICHD Neonatal Research Network database.[24] Use of the consensus definition increases the number of infants diagnosed with BPD by adding the group who were on oxygen at 28 days of age, but in room air at 36 weeks to those defined as having BPD. The overall rate of BPD was increased from 46% to 77%. The assessment of severity of BPD adds richness to the outcome measure and identifies a spectrum of adverse pulmonary and neurodevelopmental outcomes. As the severity of BPD increases, the incidence of adverse events also increases. Also, the criteria for administering supplemental oxygen can greatly affect the reported incidence of BPD. A physiologic test to standardize the need for supplemental oxygen has been proposed as a way of reducing the variability in diagnostic criteria.[63]

With increasing survival of very small premature infants, the number of patients at risk of developing BPD increases. Available data suggest that surfactant therapy for RDS decreases mortality without independently affecting the incidence of BPD, but when both endpoints are combined the number of survivors without BPD is increased.[52]

The incidence of BPD in infants with RDS who receive intermittent positive-pressure ventilation (IPPV) is inversely related to the gestational age and birthweight, and although it can occur in full-term infants, it is uncommon in infants born after 32 weeks of gestation. Figure 44-77 shows the incidence of BPD in infants born in the United States between 1997 and 2002 and published in 2007.[25]

CLINICAL PRESENTATION

The diagnosis of BPD is based on the clinical and radiographic manifestations, but these are not specific. With rare exceptions, BPD follows the use of mechanical ventilation with IPPV during the first weeks of life. Mechanical ventilation is usually indicated for respiratory failure resulting from RDS, pneumonia, or poor respiratory effort. The development of BPD is often anticipated when mechanical ventilation and oxygen dependence extend beyond 10 to 14 days.

The major radiographic features of the more severe forms of BPD include hyperinflation and nonhomogeneity of pulmonary fields, with multiple fine or coarser densities extending to the periphery (Fig. 44-78). Only a radiographic picture showing chronic pulmonary involvement plus a clinical course that is compatible with BPD justifies this diagnosis with some degree of consistency. Once lung damage has occurred, these infants require mechanical ventilation and increased FiO_2 for several weeks or months.

Presently, most of these small infants have mild respiratory disease initially requiring ventilation with low pressures and oxygen concentration, but after a few days or weeks of

TABLE 44–7   Definition of Bronchopulmonary Dysplasia: Diagnostic Criteria

Gestational Age	<32 Weeks	≥32 Weeks
Time point of assessment	36 weeks' PMA or discharge to home, whichever comes first	>28 days but < 56 days' postnatal age or discharge to home, whichever comes first
	Treatment with > 21% Oxygen for at least 28 Days PLUS	
Mild BPD	Breathing room air 36 wk PMA or discharge, whichever comes first	Breathing room air by 56 days' postnatal age or discharge, whichever comes first
Moderate BPD	Need for < 30% oxygen at 36 wk PMA or discharge, whichever comes first	Need for < 30% oxygen at 56 days' postnatal age or discharge, whichever comes first
Severe BPD	Need for ≥ 30% oxygen and/or positive pressure (PPV or NCPAP) at 36 wk PMA or discharge, whichever comes first	Need for ≥ 30% oxygen and/or positive pressure (PPV or NCPAP) at 56 days' postnatal age or discharge, whichever comes first

BPD, bronchopulmonary dysplasia; NCPAP, nasal continuous positive airway pressure; PMA, postmenstrual age; PPV, positive pressure ventilation.
Adapted from Jobe AH, Bancalari E: Bronchopulmonary dysplasia, *Am J Respir Crit Care Med* 163:1723, 2001.

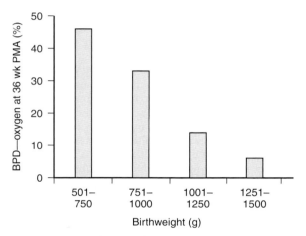

Figure 44–77. Incidence of bronchopulmonary dysplasia (BPD) defined as oxygen at 36 weeks' postmenstrual age (PMA) in the Neonatal Research Network. (*Data from Fanaroff AA, et al: Trends in neonatal morbidity and mortality for very low birthweight infants,* Am J Obstet Gynecol *196:147, 2007.*)

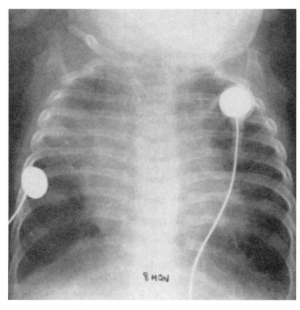

Figure 44–78. Chest radiograph shows hyperlucency in both bases with strands of radiodensity more prominent on the upper lung fields. This picture is characteristic of bronchopulmonary dysplasia stage IV. (*From Bancalari E, et al: Barotrauma to the lung. In Milunsky A, et al, editors:* Advances in perinatal medicine, *New York, 1982, Plenum, p 165, with kind permission of Springer Science and Business Media.*)

mechanical ventilation they show progressive deterioration in their lung function and BPD develops. This deterioration is often triggered by pulmonary or systemic infections or increased pulmonary bloodflow secondary to a patent ductus arteriosus (PDA).[27] In these cases the functional and radiographic changes are usually milder, revealing more diffuse haziness without the marked changes observed in the severe forms of BPD (Fig. 44-79). This entity has been termed *atypical BPD* or *new BPD*.[15,35]

Most survivors show a slow but steady improvement in their lung function and radiographic changes and, after variable periods, can be weaned from respiratory support and supplemental oxygen, but most infants persist with signs of respiratory compromise. In many infants, lobar or segmental atelectasis develops, resulting from retained secretions and airway obstruction.

Infants with more severe lung damage could die of progressive respiratory failure, cor pulmonale, or acute complications, especially intercurrent infections. In these infants, severe airway damage with bronchomalacia can lead to severe airway obstruction, especially during episodes of agitation and increased intrathoracic pressure.[40] Furthermore, anastomoses

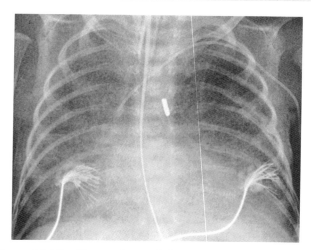

Figure 44–79. Chest radiograph from an infant with the new milder form of chronic lung disease showing diffuse haziness with no signs of hyperinflation.

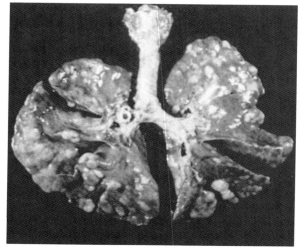

Figure 44–80. Macroscopic appearance of lungs with bronchopulmonary dysplasia showing uneven expansion. (*From Bancalari E, et al: Barotrauma to the lung. In Milunsky A, et al, editors:* Advances in perinatal medicine, *New York, 1982, Plenum, p 181, with kind permission of Springer Science and Business Media.*)

between the systemic and pulmonary circulations can aggravate their pulmonary hypertension.

Because of the respiratory failure, infants with BPD take oral feedings with difficulty and often require nasogastric or orogastric feeding. Weight gain is usually less than the expected normal even when they receive an amount of calories appropriate for their age. This lower weight gain can be due to chronic hypoxia and to the higher energy expenditure required by the increased work of breathing in these infants.

Signs of right heart failure may develop secondary to pulmonary hypertension, with cardiomegaly, hepatomegaly, and fluid retention. In these cases, the need for fluid restriction further limits the number of calories that can be provided. Right ventricular heart failure is seen less commonly than in the past, most likely because milder forms of BPD are seen today and because of the more aggressive maintenance of normal levels of oxygenation.

The diagnosis of BPD is based on the clinical and radiographic course described earlier, but these signs are not specific for any given etiology. For this reason, specific etiologies that could lead or contribute to the lung damage must be considered before concluding that the infant has BPD. Among these, one must rule out congenital heart disease, pulmonary lymphangiectasia, chemical pneumonitis resulting from recurrent aspiration, cystic fibrosis, or disorders of surfactant homeostasis.

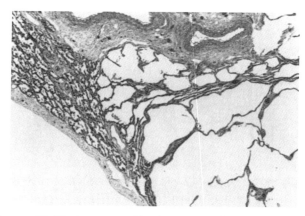

Figure 44–81. Low-magnification view showing areas of emphysema alternating with areas of partial collapse. (*From Bancalari E, et al: Barotrauma to the lung. In Milunsky A, et al, editors:* Advances in perinatal medicine, *New York, 1982, Plenum, p 181, with kind permission of Springer Science and Business Media.*)

PATHOLOGY

Macroscopically, the lungs of infants with severe BPD have a grossly abnormal appearance. They are firm and heavy and have a darker color than normal. The surface is irregular, often showing emphysematous areas alternating with areas of collapse (Fig. 44-80). On histologic examination the lungs are characterized by areas of emphysema, sometimes coalescing into larger cystic areas, surrounded by areas of atelectasis (Fig. 44-81). Widespread bronchial and bronchiolar mucosal

hyperplasia and metaplasia reduce the lumina in many of the small airways and can interfere with mucus transport (Fig. 44-82).

In some cases, excessive mucus persists throughout the course of the disease, but the involvement of the small airways is more prominent during the early stages, becoming less marked after the first months of evolution. In addition, there is interstitial edema and an increase in fibrous tissue with focal thickening of the basal membrane separating capillaries from alveolar spaces (Fig. 44-83). Lymphatics are usually dilated

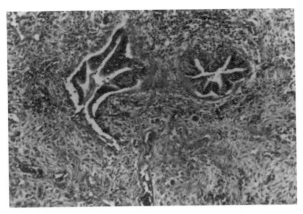

Figure 44–82. Small airways showing hyperplasia of the epithelium partially obstructing the lumen. Peribronchial muscle is hypertrophied, most alveoli are collapsed, and there is an increase in interstitial fibrous tissue. (*From Bancalari E, et al: Barotrauma to the lung. In Milunsky A, et al, editors: Advances in perinatal medicine, New York, 1982, Plenum, p 182, with kind permission of Springer Science and Business Media.*)

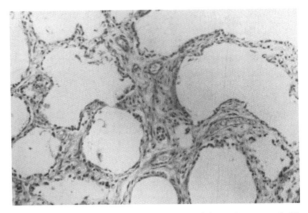

Figure 44–83. Alveolar septa thickened by edema and fibroblastic proliferation. (*From Bancalari E, et al: Barotrauma to the lung. In Milunsky A, et al, editors: Advances in perinatal medicine, New York, 1982, Plenum, p 182, with kind permission of Springer Science and Business Media.*)

and tortuous. Often there are vascular changes of pulmonary hypertension, such as medial muscle hypertrophy and elastic degeneration, and there is a reduction in the branching of the pulmonary vascular bed. There also may be evidence of right ventricular hypertrophy and, in many cases, left ventricular hypertrophy as well.

Infants who receive antenatal steroids and surfactant and have milder forms of BPD have a more diffuse injury with less emphysema and little or no fibrosis. A striking morphologic change in lungs with BPD is a marked reduction in the number of alveoli and capillaries and a reduction in the gas exchange surface area.[16,33,35] It is not known whether this alteration is reversible with increasing age, but it is the most striking and consistent change in the lungs of infants who die with BPD today.

PATHOGENESIS

BPD occurs almost exclusively in preterm infants who receive mechanical ventilation with positive pressure; therefore prematurity and mechanical overdistention have been considered the most important factors in the pathogenesis of BPD. Other factors that can contribute to the pathogenesis of BPD are oxygen toxicity, pulmonary or systemic infections, pulmonary vascular damage, and edema resulting from a PDA or excessive fluid administration.

Prematurity

The prevalence of BPD in mechanically ventilated infants is inversely related to gestational age and birthweight, strongly suggesting that incomplete development of the lungs plays an important role in the pathogenesis of BPD. As mentioned earlier, BPD is extremely uncommon in infants older than 32 to 34 weeks of gestation.

Mechanical Trauma

Although some forms of chronic lung damage have been described in infants who were not ventilated, most premature infants with BPD have received mechanical ventilation, although this may not be prolonged. This, plus the frequent association between pulmonary interstitial emphysema (PIE) and BPD, has led to the conclusion that lung overdistention secondary to positive pressure ventilation plays an important role in the pathogenesis of BPD. In fact, the lower incidence of BPD at some centers could be largely attributable to avoidance of mechanical ventilation in extremely premature infants.[58] The role of the endotracheal tube itself is difficult to separate from that of the mechanical ventilation, but the tube hinders the drainage of bronchial secretions and increases the risk of pulmonary infections.

Although peak inspiratory pressure is a major factor implicated as a cause of BPD, it is difficult to determine whether the high pressures have a causal effect on the chronic lung damage or whether these high settings are required after lung damage is already established. The damaging effect of high airway pressure and tidal volume on the surfactant-deficient lung has been demonstrated in preterm experimental animals. Lung compliance was decreased after only a few breaths with excessive tidal volumes given before surfactant replacement.[11] No significant differences in the incidence of BPD have been shown between infants ventilated with low pressures and prolonged inspiration and those ventilated with higher pressures and shorter inspiration, but experimental evidence strongly suggests that excessive tidal volumes can damage the lung, initiate an inflammatory cascade, and interfere with normal lung development. (See Part 4.)

Finally, the duration of assisted ventilation and duration of oxygen therapy could be important factors in the pathogenesis of BPD, but it is difficult to separate their role from the severity of the underlying disease. The smaller the infant and the more severe the disease, the higher the settings and the longer the time required for assisted ventilation.

Oxygen Toxicity

Clinical and experimental evidence suggest that pulmonary oxygen toxicity is a major factor in the pathogenesis of BPD. Although many tissues can be injured by high oxygen concentrations, the lung is exposed directly to the highest partial pressure of oxygen. The precise concentration of oxygen that is toxic to the immature lung probably depends on a large number of variables, including gestational age, nutritional and endocrine status, and duration of exposure to oxygen and other oxidants. Although a safe level of inspired oxygen has not been established, any concentration in excess of room air might increase the risk of lung damage when administered over a period of many days.

The pulmonary changes of oxygen toxicity are nonspecific and consist of atelectasis, edema, alveolar hemorrhage, inflammation, fibrin deposition, and thickening of alveolar membranes. There is early damage to capillary endothelium in animals, and plasma leaks into interstitial and alveolar spaces. Pulmonary surfactant can be inactivated, adding to the risk of atelectasis. Type I alveolar lining cells also are injured early, and bronchiolar and tracheal ciliated cells can also be damaged by oxygen. Total resolution after oxygen toxicity is possible if the initial exposure is not overwhelming. Cellular pathologic processes similar to those described in animals probably also occur in humans.

Continued exposure to high inspired oxygen levels is accompanied by influx of polymorphonuclear leukocytes containing proteolytic enzymes. In addition, the antiprotease defense system is significantly impaired in infants exposed to prolonged high inspired oxygen levels, favoring proteolytic damage of structural elements in alveolar walls. This could be an important pathogenic factor in oxygen toxicity and BPD. High inspired oxygen has also been shown to interfere with the process of alveolar and capillary formation.

Although the cellular basis for oxygen toxicity has not been completely elucidated, the principal mechanisms involve the univalent reduction of molecular oxygen and formation of free radical intermediates. The latter can react with intracellular constituents and membrane lipids, thus initiating chain reactions that can cause tissue destruction (Fig. 44-84).

To resist the detrimental effects of oxygen, the organism has evolved a number of antioxidant systems. Antioxidant enzymes such as superoxide dismutase, catalase, and glutathione peroxidase seem to play an important role in preventing the toxic effects of oxygen. Other elements, such as vitamin E, glutathione, and selenium are also part of the endogenous antioxidant mechanisms. The capacity for synthesizing these enzymes in some animal species follows a maturational trend similar to the production of surfactant; therefore animals born prematurely have lower concentrations of antioxidant enzymes than those born at full term.

Loss of mucociliary function may be an additional pathogenic factor in BPD because exposure to high oxygen concentrations results in a reduction of ciliary movements.

Infection and Inflammatory Reaction

Increasing evidence supports the role of antenatal and postnatal infections in the development of BPD. The role of infection appears to be especially important in very small infants

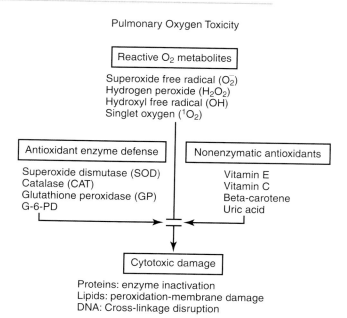

Pulmonary Oxygen Toxicity

Figure 44–84. Mechanisms of oxygen toxicity.

in whom the occurrence of nosocomial infections is associated with a marked increase in the risk for development of BPD.[49] This is even more striking when the infection occurs in an infant with a PDA.[27] Evidence suggests that perinatal adenovirus and cytomegalovirus infection might also increase the risk for BPD.

Several studies have suggested an association between *Ureaplasma urealyticum* tracheal colonization and the development of severe respiratory failure and BPD in infants with very low birthweight, but results have not been consistent.[17,31,44,64] There is also increasing evidence that maternal infections and specifically chorioamnionitis are associated with an increased risk of BPD in the infant.[65,71]

The role of inflammatory reaction in the development of BPD is receiving more attention. Inflammation could be triggered by factors such as oxygen, positive pressure ventilation, PDA, and prenatal or postnatal infections. Increased concentration of inflammatory mediators could contribute to the bronchoconstriction and vasoconstriction and the increased vascular permeability characteristic of these infants.[28] The inflammatory reaction might also be responsible for the decreased alveolarization characteristic of infants with BPD.[13,35,68]

Bronchoalveolar fluid examinations in infants with BPD reveal elevated neutrophil counts and increased elastase.[67] Increased desmosine excretion in the urine during the first week of life has been described in infants who subsequently develop BPD, indicating increased elastin degradation resulting from lung inflammation and injury. On the other hand, higher concentrations of fibronectin have been measured in tracheal lavage fluid from infants with BPD, which could foster the development of interstitial fibrosis in these patients.

Inflammatory mediators such as chemokines, interleukin, leukotrienes, and platelet activating factor also are found in high concentrations in lung lavage fluid of infants with BPD.[5,9,28] The potential role of inflammation is supported by the reported beneficial effects of steroids and possibly cromolyn sodium in some infants with BPD.[20]

Pulmonary Edema and Patent Ductus Arteriosus

There is an association between the presence of a PDA and the increased risk for BPD (Fig. 44-85).[27,49] Clinical evidence suggests that infants with RDS who receive greater fluid intake or do not show a diuretic phase during the first days of life have a higher incidence of BPD.[57] This may be because high fluid intake increases the incidence of a PDA. Increased pulmonary bloodflow because of PDA and the resulting increase in interstitial fluid cause a decrease in pulmonary compliance.[26] Combined with increased airway resistance, this can prolong the need for mechanical ventilation with higher ventilatory pressures and oxygen concentrations, increasing the risk for BPD. Moreover, the increased pulmonary bloodflow can also induce neutrophil margination and activation in the lung and contribute to the progression of the inflammatory cascade.[60]

Recent data from studies in preterm baboons showed decreased alveolarization in animals that remained for a longer time with an open ductus arteriosus, supporting the role of a persistent ductus arteriosus in the pathogenesis of BPD.[41]

For unknown reasons, infants with BPD have a predisposition to fluid accumulation in their lungs. Possible causes are functional alterations in pulmonary vascular resistance, plasma oncotic pressure, and increased capillary permeability that favor the extravascular accumulation of fluid. Pulmonary vascular pressure can be increased because of hypoxemia, hypercapnia, and a reduced pulmonary vascular bed. In some cases, fluid accumulation it is secondary to the left ventricular dysfunction that has been described in patients with chronic respiratory failure. Plasma oncotic pressure is often decreased because of decreased plasma protein concentration resulting from poor nutrition. Capillary permeability might be increased secondary to the effects of high FiO_2, mechanical trauma, increased flow due to a PDA, and infection on the capillary endothelium. During spontaneous breathing, the interstitial pressure in the lung is lower than normal because of the increased inspiratory effort necessary to overcome the low compliance and high pulmonary resistance. Finally, lymphatic drainage might be impaired because of compression of pulmonary lymphatics by interstitial fluid or gas and fibrous tissue, and because of the increased central venous pressure in cases of cor pulmonale.

Infants with BPD also have increased plasma levels of vasopressin and reduced urine output and free water clearance.[38] This is an additional alteration that can contribute to increased lung water in these patients. The abnormal accumulation of lung fluid in infants with BPD further compromises their lung function, perpetuating a cycle in which more aggressive respiratory assistance is required, which produces further lung damage.

Airway Damage

Increased airway resistance can alter the time constant of different regions of the lung and impair the distribution of the inspired gas, favoring uneven lung expansion. Airway obstruction can occur in these infants secondary to the bronchiolar epithelial hyperplasia and metaplasia and to mucosal edema secondary to trauma, oxygen toxicity, and infection. Pulmonary edema secondary to PDA or fluid overload also can increase airway resistance. These infants could also have bronchoconstriction resulting from smooth muscle hypertrophy. Inflammatory mediators such as leukotrienes and platelet-activating factor are present in high concentrations in the airways of infants with BPD, possibly contributing to the increased airway resistance that is characteristic in these infants. In some infants with severe BPD, tracheobronchomalacia develops, which is responsible for marked airway obstruction, especially during periods of agitation and increased intrathoracic pressure.

Other Factors

A decreased concentration of α_1-proteinase inhibitor could be another factor that predisposes the neonatal lung to damage produced by elastase and other proteolytic enzymes derived from neutrophils. This is especially important when pulmonary infection supervenes.

The possibility of a genetic predisposition to abnormal airway reactivity in infants with BPD has also been raised because of a stronger family history of asthma in infants with BPD. There is also evidence that vitamin A deficiency could increase the risk for BPD in preterm infants. Infants with BPD had lower vitamin A levels than did those who recovered without lung sequelae. This possible association is supported by the similarities between some of the airway epithelial changes observed in BPD and vitamin A deficiency. Early adrenal insufficiency has also been suggested as a contributing factor in the development of BPD in the smallest infants. Infants with lower cortisol levels in the first week of life have an increased incidence of PDA, more lung inflammation, and increased incidence of BPD.[66]

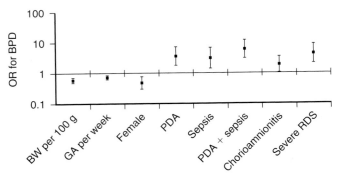

Figure 44–85. Perinatal and postnatal risk factors for bronchopulmonary dysplasia (BPD) defined as 28 days' duration of oxygen dependency during hospitalization. Obtained by logistic regression analysis from all extremely premature infants born at University of Miami Jackson Medical Center during the period 1995-2000. (N = 505 alive at 28 days; birthweight [BW], 500 to 1000 g; gestational age [GA], 23 to 32 weeks). OR, odds ratio; PDA, patent ductus arteriosus; RDS, respiratory distress syndrome. (*From Bancalari E, et al: Bronchopulmonary dysplasia: changes in pathogenesis, epidemiology and definition, Semin Neonatol 8:63, 2003.*)

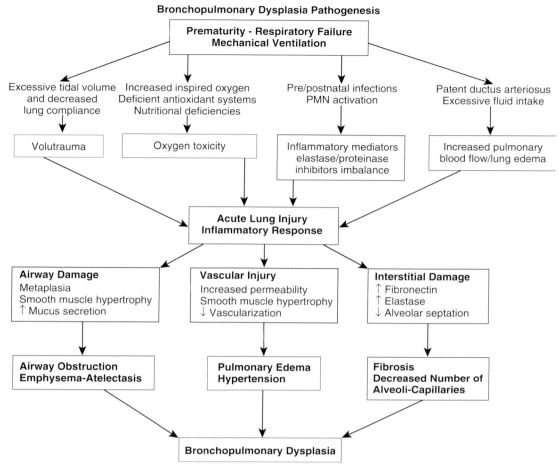

Figure 44-86. Algorithm for pathogenesis of bronchopulmonary dysplasia. PMN, polymorphonu-cleocytes.

Figure 44-86 summarizes some of the factors that have been implicated in the pathogenesis of BPD.

Prediction of Bronchopulmonary Dysplasia

A number of studies have been performed to develop scores that can predict the risk for BPD in ventilated preterm infants. Most of these scores include the state of maturation of the infant and factors that reflect the severity of the initial respiratory failure. These scores are helpful in identifying patients for clinical trials and could become more useful in the future if effective preventive therapies become available.

PULMONARY FUNCTION

The disruption of pulmonary function in BPD is explained by the severe structural alterations of these lungs. Minute ventilation is usually increased, but because of the lower lung compliance, this is accomplished with a smaller tidal volume and a higher respiratory rate than normal. Thus, there is an increase in dead space ventilation, partially accounting for the alveolar hypoventilation and CO_2 retention seen in these patients.

Infants with severe BPD characteristically have a marked increase in airway resistance and airway hyperreactivity.[48] This results in a decreased dynamic compliance, because with airway obstruction, dynamic compliance becomes frequency dependent; therefore, compliance decreases at higher respiratory rates. Lung compliance is also decreased because of fibrosis, overdistention, and collapse of lung parenchyma. It is also possible that some of these infants have a decreased concentration or inactivation of surfactant on their alveolar surface. The high resistance and decreased compliance result in a markedly increased work of breathing that contributes to the hypoventilation and hypercapnia.

Increased airway resistance is not specific for infants with BPD, and it is observed in many premature infants who survive after receiving IPPV, even when they do not have clinical or radiographic evidence of residual pulmonary disease. Airway resistance can be markedly increased, especially during active expiratory efforts associated with episodes of physical agitation. Airway obstruction can be severe in infants with tracheobronchomalacia.

Functional residual capacity is initially low or normal but could be increased later in cases of severe BPD. Infants with advanced BPD have abnormal distribution of ventilation, reflecting involvement of the small airways, but in infants with milder forms of BPD, the distribution of the inspired gas is usually normal as measured by nitrogen clearance delay.

Most infants with severe BPD have marked hypoxemia and hypercapnia and require supplemental oxygen to maintain acceptable oxygenation levels. The hypoxemia mainly results from a combination of ventilation-perfusion mismatch and alveolar hypoventilation. The oxygen requirement decreases gradually as the disease process improves, but it can increase during feedings, physical activity, or episodes of pulmonary infection or edema.

The increased $PaCO_2$ is also secondary to alveolar hypoventilation and to an increased alveolar-arterial CO_2 gradient produced by a ventilation-perfusion mismatch and increased alveolar dead space. The chronic hypercapnia often results in an increased serum bicarbonate concentration that tends to compensate for the respiratory acidosis. This increase in base is often exaggerated by the use of loop diuretics.

As discussed later, evaluation of pulmonary function in infants with BPD shows persistence of the abnormal airway function into adulthood in the more severe cases.

MANAGEMENT

Prevention of further lung damage is the cornerstone of management by avoiding, as much as possible, all factors that predispose to more injury.

Respiratory Support

See also Part 4.
When mechanical ventilation is used, the lowest peak airway pressure necessary to obtain adequate ventilation must be applied, using inspiratory times between 0.3 and 0.5 second. Shorter inspiratory times and higher flow rates can exaggerate the maldistribution of the inspired gas, but longer inspiratory times can increase the risk of alveolar rupture and cardiovascular side effects. An end-expiratory pressure between 4 and 6 cm H_2O is applied so that the minimum oxygen concentration necessary to keep the partial pressure of arterial oxygen (PaO_2) above 50 mm Hg is used. In infants with severe airway obstruction, especially those with bronchomalacia, the use of positive end-expiratory pressure levels of 5 to 8 cm H_2O can help reduce expiratory airway resistance and improve alveolar ventilation. The duration of mechanical ventilation must be limited as much as possible to reduce the risk of mechanical trauma and infection.

Weaning these patients from the ventilator is difficult and must be accomplished gradually. When the patient can maintain an acceptable PaO_2 and $PaCO_2$ with low peak pressures (lower than 15 to 18 cm H_2O) and an FiO_2 lower than 0.3 to 0.4, the ventilator rate is gradually reduced to allow the infant to perform an increasing proportion of the respiratory work. During the process of weaning, it may be necessary to increase the FiO_2. Concurrently, the $PaCO_2$ can rise, but as long as the pH is within acceptable limits, some degree of hypercapnia must be tolerated to wean the patient from the ventilator. In small infants, aminophylline or caffeine is used as a respiratory stimulant during the weaning phase. When the patient is able to maintain acceptable blood gas levels for several hours on low ventilator rates (10 to 15 breaths/minute), extubation should be attempted.

During the days after the extubation, it is important to provide chest physiotherapy to prevent airway obstruction and lung collapse caused by retained secretions. In smaller infants, the use of nasal continuous positive airway pressure (CPAP) after extubation can stabilize respiratory function and reduce the need to reinstitute mechanical ventilation.

Although it is necessary to reduce the FiO_2 as quickly as possible to prevent oxygen toxicity, it is important to maintain the PaO_2 at a level sufficient to ensure adequate tissue oxygenation and to prevent the pulmonary hypertension and cor pulmonale that can result from chronic hypoxemia. Furthermore, infants with BPD might respond with increased airway resistance to episodes of acute hypoxemia.

Because oxygen therapy does not produce respiratory depression in infants with BPD, the PaO_2 must be maintained above 50 to 55 mm Hg to prevent the effects of hypoxemia. Oxygen can be administered through a hood, tent, facemask, or nasal cannula. Because the oxygen consumption increases and the PaO_2 may decrease during feedings, it might be necessary to provide a higher FiO_2 to prevent hypoxemia.

Oxygen therapy could be required for several weeks or months. Some of these patients are discharged with oxygen therapy at home. This practice offers significant advantages, such as a better environment for the patient and cost savings, but it requires a supportive family and home environment to be accomplished safely and successfully.

Adequacy of gas exchange should be monitored continuously to avoid hypoxemia or hyperoxemia. Blood gas determinations obtained by arterial puncture are usually not reliable because the infant responds to pain with crying or apnea. Transcutaneous PO_2 electrodes are also inaccurate in these infants because they underestimate the true PaO_2. Pulse oximeters offer the most reliable estimate of arterial oxygenation and have the advantage of simplicity of use and the possibility of assessing oxygenation during feeding and crying.

Although there are no conclusive data in the literature on the optimal level of oxygenation for these infants, in general it is recommended to maintain their oxygen saturation in the range of high 80s to low or mid 90s. This range should minimize the risk of oxygen exposure and toxicity and prevent hypoxemia that can lead to pulmonary hypertension and poor weight gain.[2,54,55] Several international trials evaluating lower saturations ranges are underway.

Fluid Management

Infants with BPD tolerate excessive or even normal amounts of fluid intake poorly and, as mentioned earlier, have a marked tendency to accumulate excessive interstitial fluid in the lung. This excess can lead to a deterioration of their pulmonary function, with exaggeration of hypoxemia and hypercapnia and longer ventilator dependency.

To reduce lung fluid in infants with BPD, water and salt intake should be limited to the minimum required to provide the calories necessary for metabolic needs and growth. When increased lung water persists despite fluid restriction, diuretic therapy can be used successfully. The use of diuretics in infants with BPD is associated with an acute improvement in lung compliance and decrease in resistance, but blood gases do not always show improvement. Similar effects have been reported after the administration of furosemide by nebulization. The reduction in pulmonary capillary pressure observed after furosemide administration is not only due to the increased elimination of sodium and water but seems, in part, secondary to an increase in venous capacitance and reduced pulmonary bloodflow produced by this drug. Complications of chronic diuretic therapy include potential ototoxicity, hypokalemia, hyponatremia, metabolic alkalosis, hypercalciuria with nephrocalcinosis, and hypochloremia. Some of these side effects can be reduced by using an alternate-day schedule with furosemide.

Because increased metabolic demands in infants with BPD are associated in severe cases with low arterial oxygen tension, it is important to maintain a relatively normal blood hemoglobin concentration. This may be accomplished with blood transfusions or by the administration of recombinant erythropoietin.

Bronchodilator Therapy

Infants with severe BPD have airway smooth muscle hypertrophy and airway hyperreactivity. Because hypoxia can increase airway resistance in these patients, maintenance of adequate oxygenation is important for avoiding bronchoconstriction. Bronchodilators, most of them β-agonists, administered by inhalation have been shown to reduce airway resistance in infants with BPD. However, their safety and efficacy have never been evaluated in randomized clinical trials. Their effect is usually short-lived, and many of these drugs have cardiovascular side effects such as tachycardia, hypertension, and possible arrhythmias. Because of this, it is preferred to limit their use to the management of acute exacerbations of airway obstruction.

Methylxanthines (aminophylline and caffeine) also have been shown to reduce airway resistance in these infants. These drugs have other potential beneficial effects, such as respiratory stimulation and mild diuretic effect, and aminophylline can also improve respiratory muscle contractility.

Because of the increased concentration of leukotrienes in bronchial secretions of infants with BPD, cromolyn sodium has been suggested as a drug that might reduce airway resistance, but the experience is too limited to recommend its widespread use.

Nutrition

Infants with BPD frequently have impaired growth.[34] Adequate nutrition is a key aspect of care for these infants, who have an increase in resting oxygen consumption partially caused by the elevated work of breathing. Malnutrition can delay somatic growth and the development of new alveoli, making successful weaning from mechanical ventilation less likely. The malnourished patient is also more prone to infection and oxygen toxicity.

For these reasons, an aggressive approach should be taken toward supplying a parenteral or oral caloric intake that is adequate for growth. High-calorie formulas and supplements of protein, calcium, phosphorus, and zinc can be used to maximize the intake of calories while restricting fluid intake to prevent congestive heart failure and pulmonary edema. If for any reason enteral nutrition is precluded for more than 3

or 4 days, parenteral alimentation with glucose, amino acids, and fat should be substituted until the gastrointestinal tract again becomes functional.

Adequacy of nutrition should be closely monitored, and growth charts for weight, head circumference, and height must be kept. Other means of assessment include arm anthropometry to determine muscle mass and fat deposits and measurement of serum levels of albumin. Rib fractures noted on routine chest radiographs together with generalized bone demineralization are often observed in infants with BPD and are usually a manifestation of rickets. The cause could relate to dietary or parenteral deficiency of calcium or vitamin D or to the calciuria resulting from long-term diuretic therapy. Administration of extra calcium and vitamin D is necessary to prevent rickets in these infants.

In infants with established BPD, the use of a high-fat formula can increase the caloric intake and reduce carbon dioxide production. Infants who receive exclusively parenteral nutrition for prolonged periods are more susceptible to developing deficiency of specific nutrients, such as vitamins A and E, and trace elements such as iron, copper, zinc, and selenium, all of which play a role in antioxidant function, protection against infection, and lung repair.

Decreased caloric intake potentiates oxygen-induced lung damage and can interfere with cell multiplication and lung growth. Deficiency of sulfur-containing amino acids could also affect lung levels of glutathione, a potent antioxidant. Infants with severe BPD have been shown to have lower plasma levels of vitamin A, and a deficiency of this vitamin in experimental animals results in loss of ciliated epithelium and squamous metaplasia in the airways, changes similar to those observed in BPD. Clinical trials in preterm infants with severe RDS suggest that maintenance of normal plasma levels of vitamin A reduces the incidence and severity of BPD.[56]

Gastroesophageal reflux is often observed in infants with BPD, and when severe, may contribute to the chronic inflammatory process and lung damage. When severe reflux is documented, antireflux management might be indicated to alleviate the respiratory symptoms.

Control of Infection

See also Chapter 39.

Any infection can have serious consequences for the child with BPD, and bacterial, viral, or fungal infection generally results in profound setback. As a result, the child must be closely watched for early evidence of infection. Tracheal secretions are collected for culture and Gram stain or if a change in the quality and quantity of secretions indicates possible infection. A complete blood count, blood culture, and chest radiograph are obtained if pneumonia is suspected.

Although it is difficult to distinguish between colonization of the airway and true infection, this distinction is important because overtreatment with antibiotics could result in the emergence of resistant and more virulent organisms. Selection of antibiotics is based on the sensitivity of the implicated organism, and treatment is continued until the infection has been controlled. Measures to prevent pulmonary nosocomial infection are important. These include careful handwashing before handling the airway, maintenance of sterility of the respiratory equipment, and isolation from individuals with respiratory infections.

Corticosteroids

Because of the importance of inflammation in the pathogenesis of BPD, there has been interest in exogenous administration of corticosteroids during the early stages of the disease to reduce its progression. Several reports showed rapid improvement in lung function after the administration of steroids, facilitating weaning from the ventilator when compared with controls who received placebo.[3,19] The optimal age of treatment, dose schedule, and duration of therapy have not been established, and long-term respiratory outcome has not clearly improved in treated infants.[1,10,30,46]

Many mechanisms for the beneficial effect of steroids in BPD have been proposed. They include enhanced production of surfactant and antioxidant enzymes, decreased bronchospasm, decreased pulmonary and bronchial edema and fibrosis, improved vitamin A status, and decreased responses of inflammatory cells and mediators in the injured lung.

Potential complications of prolonged steroid therapy include masking the signs of infection, arterial hypertension, hyperglycemia, increased proteolysis, adrenocortical suppression, somatic and lung growth suppression, and hypertrophic cardiomyopathy. In addition, long-term follow-up studies suggest that infants who received postnatal steroid therapy have worse neurologic outcome than control infants.[45,70] Because of the seriousness of some of these complications, the American Academy of Pediatrics does not recommend the use of steroids except as part of a clinical trial or in the presence of life-threatening disease with parental consent. It remains to be seen whether treatment with shorter courses and lower doses beyond the first week of life offers significant advantage.

Controversy still exists regarding the possible beneficial effects of lower steroid doses and shorter durations of treatment. Doyle and colleagues studied low-dose dexamethasone after the first week of life and showed shorter duration of intubation among ventilator-dependent infants with extremely low birthweight (ELBW), without any obvious short-term complications, reopening the debate regarding the potential role of low-dose dexamethasone therapy specifically for infants at high risk for BPD.[22] Furthermore, a recent metaregression analysis reported a significant effect modification by risk for BPD. With a risk for BPD below 35%, corticosteroid treatment increased the chance of death or cerebral palsy, whereas when the risk for BPD exceeded 65%, corticosteroid treatment reduced this risk.[23] Wilson-Costello and colleagues examined the impact of dexamethasone dose, and timing in a large cohort of infants with ELBW.[69] Overall 16% of the cohort was exposed to dexamethasone. The authors confirmed the previous observation by Doyle and colleagues that the risk of the composite outcome of death or neurodevelopmental impairment was modified by the predicted risk of BPD[22]. Neonates at more than 50% predicted risk of BPD experienced less harm than those at lower risk (high-risk odds ratio [OR], 1.9; 95% confidence interval [CI], 1.4-2.6; low-risk OR, 2.9; 95% CI, 1.8-4.8). Infants at even higher predicted risk of BPD crossed a point where the risk of postnatal steroid treatment was offset by the risk of deteriorating

pulmonary status and its associated detrimental effects. Thus, the optimal corticosteroid type and the optimal dose are unknown, but it appears that the avoidance of steroids may in fact be detrimental to a class of infants at high risk for BPD.

In an attempt to induce the beneficial effects on the lung but minimize the systemic side effects, steroids have been administered by nebulization to a group of ventilator-dependent infants. This therapy resulted in a significant improvement in lung compliance and resistance only after 3 weeks of treatment. A subsequent study showed that inhaled steroids could reduce the need for systemic steroids, reducing the side effects associated with prolonged systemic therapy.[18] Data on topical steroids are not conclusive enough to recommend routine use of this therapy.

Pulmonary Vasodilators

Oxygen therapy to prevent hypoxemia is probably the most effective treatment to reduce pulmonary hypertension in these infants. Because pulmonary vascular resistance is extremely sensitive to changes in alveolar PO_2 in infants with BPD, it is important to ensure normal oxygenation not only when the infant is asleep but also when the infant is performing physical activity, such as feeding and crying.

In infants with severe pulmonary hypertension and cor pulmonale, the calcium channel blocker nifedipine decreases pulmonary vascular resistance. This drug is also a systemic vasodilator and can produce a depression of myocardial contractility. Its safety and long-term efficacy in these infants has not been established. Inhaled nitric oxide (iNO) is another alternative to reduce pulmonary vascular resistance in infants with severe pulmonary hypertension. Data are emerging on the potential role of iNO in the prevention of BPD. Trials that administered nitric oxide early in life for brief durations did not improve pulmonary outcomes at 2 years of age, although they did suggest some neuroprotection on imaging studies, and in the study by Mestan and coworkers.[37,39,51] In contrast, the NO CLD trial led by Ballard and coworkers found that treatment of ventilated preterm infants at a mean age of 16 days for 24 days significantly improved the likelihood of survival without BPD at 36 weeks of postmenstrual age.[6,7] Compared with infants who received placebo gas, infants who were treated with iNO were hospitalized for fewer days, needed supplemental oxygen for a shorter period, and had less severe disease. In addition, treated infants required fewer days of ventilatory support and hospitalization,[72] and were less likely to require treatment with pulmonary medications in the first year.[32] There was no evidence of adverse neurodevelopmental outcomes at 2 years of age.[61] Thus, while nitric oxide may prevent BPD, likely by modifying alveolarization and angiogenesis, its clinical role remains to be determined.

Infant Stimulation

The infant with severe BPD could be ventilator dependent for many months and thus deprived of normal parental stimulation. Developmental delays are common and are compounded if any gross neurologic disability exists. A well-organized program of infant stimulation can help the infant achieve maximum potential. Such a program instructs the caretakers in helping the infant with various social, language, cognitive, and motor skills (see also Chapter 43). As a child grows, speech therapy is useful in teaching communication skills, which are especially important for children with a tracheostomy. Beanbag chairs, strollers, and other adaptive tools are employed to mobilize the child and teach gross motor skills. Progress is monitored by periodic developmental evaluations, and emphasis is placed on areas in which delay is evident.

Parental Support

The parents of an infant with severe BPD lose considerable control of their child to the hospital staff, particularly in areas related to medical care. Parental participation is critical for the child's development and for establishment of normal relationships. Therefore, parents are encouraged to visit as frequently as possible and to participate in the day-to-day care of their child. They are educated about relevant medical equipment and procedures. In time many are able to assume complete responsibility for procedures such as chest physiotherapy and tracheal suctioning in addition to holding and playing with their child. During the prolonged hospitalization every effort must be made to assign a permanent physician and nursing team to oversee the child's care and be available for continuing parental support. Parental support groups may also be a valuable resource for these families.

OUTCOME

The outcome of infants with BPD has improved in part because of better management, but mainly because of the milder presentation of the disease.

The mortality rate for infants with BPD is low; when death occurs it is usually a result of respiratory failure, intercurrent infections, or intractable pulmonary hypertension and cor pulmonale. With adequate nutrition, somatic growth, and control of infection and heart failure, gradual improvement in pulmonary function may be accompanied by resolution of cor pulmonale and radiographic evidence of healing.

Lower respiratory tract infections are common during the first year of life in patients with BPD. Among survivors of BPD, hospitalizations for episodes of wheezing suggestive of bronchiolitis or asthma are common during the first 2 years of life, and infection with respiratory syncytial virus (RSV) can be life threatening. The American Academy of Pediatrics has recommended that all infants with BPD receive palivizumab during RSV season (see Chapter 39, Part 4). Acute radiographic evidence of hyperinflation can be difficult to appreciate in infants with severe BPD who generally are already in a state of pulmonary hyperinflation. Such episodes of bronchiolitis are often accompanied by focal, transient areas of atelectasis.

Pulmonary function studies of infants with a history of severe BPD indicate that pulmonary function may be impaired for many years even though the infants may be asymptomatic.[12,29,36,48] Northway and associates have reevaluated pulmonary function in their original cohort of infants with severe BPD reported in 1967.[42] At a mean age of 18 years, these adolescents and young adults still exhibited some evidence of pulmonary dysfunction, including airway obstruction and hyperactivity as well as hyperinflation. The ultimate clinical consequences of these findings remain to be determined, but most long-term studies suggest that with growth, pulmonary function tends to normalize.

Infants with severe BPD also have more neurodevelopmental sequelae when compared with similar control groups, and they exhibit transiently impaired growth curves. These neurodevelopmental and pulmonary impairments persist at 8 years of age, with 54% requiring special education classes compared with 37% of survivors born at very low birthweight without BPD.[21,53] Neurodevelopmental prognosis also depends on the severity of the BPD and on other associated risk factors that could be present in these infants. Infants with BPD also have been reported to have an increased risk for sudden infant death, but the evidence for this is not conclusive.

PREVENTION

The incidence of severe BPD has decreased, but there is a wide variation in incidence among different centers.[4,62] This variation suggests that certain steps in the management of preterm infants can influence the risk of BPD, although attempts to modify BPD have met with variable levels of success.[47] Because many factors play a role in the pathogenesis of BPD, it is important to focus on all of them and try to prevent as many as possible.

Prevention of BPD should start prenatally by attempting to prolong pregnancy as much as possible in cases of preterm labor. By postponing birth a few days or weeks, it is possible to substantially reduce the severity of RDS and the risk of BPD in the offspring. When birth is imminent, one effective means of reducing the risk of BPD in the infant is by administering antenatal steroids. Steroid administration reduces the incidence and severity of RDS, although the effect on the incidence of BPD has been less consistent.[59]

After birth, the effort should be initially directed to reduce as much as possible the infant's exposure to high airway pressures and FiO2. Although the use of early CPAP to reduce the use of mechanical ventilation has not been shown to reduce BPD, a conservative indication of mechanical ventilation and minimization of airway pressures and duration of IPPV are considered important steps to reduce lung damage and the incidence of BPD. The use of high-frequency ventilation has not been shown to be effective in reducing BPD in infants but data obtained in experimental animals suggest that high-frequency ventilation can reduce lung injury. Fluid restriction and early closure of a symptomatic PDA are important as is prevention of pulmonary and systemic infections. Proper nutrition and adequate supply of substrates that are important for the antioxidant mechanisms must be provided early in the course of the respiratory failure. The administration of caffeine to wean infants from mechanical ventilation has been associated with a significant reduction in the incidence of BPD.[50]

Exogenous administration of specific antioxidants, such as superoxide dismutase, metalloporphyrins, or inducers of the cytochrome P-450 system, is still experimental but could become an important part of BPD prevention in the future.[14] The possibility that exogenous surfactant administration to infants with RDS could reduce the incidence of BPD is still controversial. Large controlled trials have not shown a significant effect of exogenous surfactant administration on the incidence of BPD alone, but when combined with survival, infants who received surfactant had a significant advantage.

Although it can be expected that surfactant will reduce the incidence of BPD in infants who previously developed severe RDS, it is unlikely that it will have a significant effect on the BPD that occurs with increasing frequency in infants with extremely low birthweight who require prolonged IPPV because of poor respiratory effort rather than severe RDS. In these infants, a conservative use of mechanical ventilation, combined with an aggressive approach to close the PDA and efforts to reduce the risk of nosocomial infections, are probably the most effective ways to reduce the incidence and severity of BPD.

REFERENCES

1. Arias-Camison JM, et al: Meta-analysis of dexamethasone therapy started in the first 15 days of life for prevention of chronic lung disease in premature infants, *Pediatr Pulmonol* 28:167, 1999.
2. Askie LM, et al: Oxygen-saturation targets and outcomes in extremely preterm infants, *N Engl J Med* 349:10, 2003.
3. Avery GB, et al: Controlled trial of dexamethasone in respiratory-dependent infants with bronchopulmonary dysplasia, *Pediatrics* 75:106, 1985.
4. Avery ME, et al: Is chronic lung disease in low birth weight infants preventable? A survey of eight centers, *Pediatrics* 79:26, 1987.
5. Baier RJ, et al: CC Chemokine concentrations increase in respiratory distress syndrome and correlate with development of bronchopulmonary dysplasia, *Pediatr Pulmonol* 37:137, 2004.
6. Ballard RA, et al: Inhaled nitric oxide in preterm infants undergoing mechanical ventilation, *N Engl J Med* 355:343, 2006. Erratum in: *N Engl J Med* 357:1444, 2007.
7. Ballard RA: Inhaled nitric oxide in preterm infants — correction, *N Engl J Med* 357:1444, 2007.
8. Bancalari E, et al: Bronchopulmonary dysplasia: changes in pathogenesis, epidemiology and definition, *Semin Neonatol* 8:63, 2003.
9. Beresford MW, Shaw NJ: Detectable Il-8 and IL-10 in bronchoalveolar lavage fluid from preterm infants ventilated for respiratory distress syndrome, *Pediatr Res* 52:6, 2002.
10. Bhuta T, et al: Systematic review and meta-analysis of early postnatal dexamethasone for prevention of chronic lung disease, *Arch Dis Child Fetal Neonatal Ed* 79:F26, 1998.
11. Bjorklung LJ, et al: Manual ventilation with a few large breaths at birth compromises the therapeutic effect of subsequent surfactant replacement in immature lambs, *Pediatr Res* 42:348, 1997.
12. Blayney M, et al: Bronchopulmonary dysplasia: improvement in lung function between 7 and 10 years of age, *J Pediatr* 118:201, 1991.
13. Bry K, et al: Intraamniotic interleukin-1 accelerates surfactant protein synthesis in fetal rabbits and improves lung stability after premature birth, *J Clin Invest* 99:2992, 1997.
14. Chang LYL, et al: A catalytic antioxidant attenuates alveolar structural remodeling in bronchopulmonary dysplasia, *Am J Respir Crit Care Med* 167:57, 2003.
15. Charafeddine L, et al: Atypical chronic lung disease patterns in neonates, *Pediatrics* 103:759, 1999.
16. Coalson JJ, et al: Decreased alveolarization in baboon survivors with bronchopulmonary dysplasia, *Am J Respir Crit Care Med* 152:640, 1995.
17. Colayzy TT, et al: Detection of ureaplasma DNA in endotracheal samples is associated with bronchopulmonary dysplasia after adjustment for multiple risk factors, *Pediatr Res* 61:578, 2007.
18. Cole CH, et al: Early inhaled glucocorticoid therapy to prevent bronchopulmonary dysplasia, *N Engl J Med* 340:1005, 1999.
19. Collaborative Dexamethasone Trial Group: Dexamethasone therapy in neonatal chronic lung disease: an international placebo-controlled trial, *Pediatrics* 88:421, 1991.
20. Davis JM, et al: Drug therapy for bronchopulmonary dysplasia, *Pediatr Pulmonol* 8:117, 1990.
21. Doyle LW: Impact of perinatal lung injury in later life. In Bancalari E, Polin R, editors: *The newborn lung: neonatology questions and controversies*, Philadelphia, 2008, Saunders.
22. Doyle LW, DART Study Investigators, et al: Low dose dexamethasone facilitates extubation among critically ventilator-dependent infants: a multicenter, international, randomized, controlled trial, *Pediatrics* 117(1):75, 2006.
23. Doyle LW, et al: Impact of postnatal systemic corticosteroids on mortality and cerebral palsy in preterm infants: effect modification by risk for chronic lung disease, *Pediatrics* 115(3):655, 2005.
24. Ehrenkranz RA, et al: Validation of the National Institutes of Health consensus definition of bronchopulmonary dysplasia, *Pediatrics* 116:1353, 2005.
25. Fanaroff AA, Stoll BJ, Wright LL, et al: Trends in neonatal morbidity mortality for very low birthweight infants, *Am J Obstet Gynecol* 106:147, 2007.
26. Gerhardt T, et al: Lung compliance in newborns with patent ductus arteriosus before and after surgical ligation, *Biol Neonate* 38:96, 1980.
27. Gonzalez A, et al: Influence of infection on patent ductus arteriosus and chronic lung disease in premature infants weighting 1000 grams or less, *J Pediatr* 128:470, 1996.
28. Groneck P, et al: Association of pulmonary inflammation and increased microvascular permeability during the development of bronchopulmonary dysplasia: a sequential analysis of inflammatory mediators in respiratory fluids of high-risk preterm neonates, *Pediatrics* 93:712, 1994.
29. Gross SJ, et al: Effect of preterm birth on pulmonary function at school age: a prospective controlled study, *J Pediatr* 133:188, 1998.
30. Halliday HL, et al: Clinical trials of postnatal corticosteroids: inhaled and systemic, *Biol Neonate* 76:29, 1999.
31. Hannaford K, et al: Role of *Ureaplasma urealyticum* in lung disease of prematurity, *Arch Dis Child Fetal Neonatal Ed* 81:F162, 1999.
32. Hibbs AM, et al: One-year respiratory outcomes of preterm infants enrolled in the Nitric Oxide [to prevent] Chronic Lung Disease Trial, *J Pediatr* 153:525, 2008.
33. Husain AN, et al: Pathology of arrested acinar development in postsurfactant bronchopulmonary dysplasia, *Hum Pathol* 29:710, 1998.
34. Huysman WA, et al: Growth and body composition in preterm infants with bronchopulmonary dysplasia, *Arch Dis Child Fetal Neonatal Ed* 88:F46, 2003.
35. Jobe A: The new BPD: an arrest of lung development, *Pediatr Res* 46:6, 1999.

36. Kilbride HW, et al: Pulmonary function and exercise capacity for ELBW survivors in preadolescence: effect of neonatal chronic lung disease, *J Pediatr* 143:488, 2003.

37. Kinsella JP, et al: Early inhaled nitric oxide therapy in premature newborns with respiratory failure, *N Engl J Med* 355:354, 2006.

38. Kojima T, et al: Changes in vasopressin, arterial natriuretic factor, and water homeostasis in the early stage of bronchopulmonary dysplasia, *Pediatr Res* 27:260, 1990.

39. Mestan KK, et al: Neurodevelopmental outcomes of premature infants treated with inhaled nitric oxide, *N Engl J Med* 353:23, 2005.

40. McCoy KS, et al: Spirometric and endoscopic evaluation of airway collapse in infants with bronchopulmonary dysplasia, *Pediatr Pulmonol* 14:237, 1992.

41. McCurnin D, et al: Ibuprofen-induced patent ductus arteriosus closure: physiologic, histologic, and biochemical effects on the premature lung, *Pediatrics* 121:945, 2008

42. Northway WH, et al: Late pulmonary sequelae of bronchopulmonary dysplasia, *N Engl J Med* 323:1793, 1990.

43. Northway WH, et al: Pulmonary disease following respiratory therapy of hyaline membrane disease: bronchopulmonary dysplasia, *N Engl J Med* 276:357, 1967.

44. Ollikainen J, et al: *Ureaplasma urealyticum* infection associated with acute respiratory insufficiency and death in premature infants, *J Pediatr* 122:756, 1993.

45. O'Shea TM, et al: Randomized placebo-controlled trial of a 42-day tapering course of dexamethasone to reduce the duration of ventilator dependency in very low birth weight infants: outcome of study participants at 1-year adjusted age, *Pediatrics* 104:15, 1999.

46. O'Shea TM, et al: Follow-up of preterm infants treated with dexamethasone for chronic lung disease, *Am J Dis Child* 147:658, 1993.

47. Payne NR, Breathsavers Group, Vermont Oxford Network Neonatal Intensive Care Quality Improvement Collaborative, et al: Reduction of bronchopulmonary dysplasia after participation in the Breathsavers Group of the Vermont Oxford Network Neonatal Intensive Care Quality Improvement Collaborative, *Pediatrics* 118:S73, 2006.

48. Robin B, et al: Pulmonary function in bronchopulmonary dysplasia, *Pediatr Pulmonol* 37:236, 2004.

49. Rojas M, et al: Changing trends in the epidemiology and pathogenesis of neonatal chronic lung disease, *J Pediatr* 126:605, 1995.

50. Schmidt, et al: Caffeine therapy for apnea of prematurity, *N Engl J Med* 354:2112, 2006.

51. Schreiber MD, et al: Inhaled nitric oxide in premature infants with the respiratory distress syndrome, *N Engl J Med* 349:2099, 2003.

52. Schwartz RM, et al: Effect of surfactant on morbidity, mortality, and resource use in newborn infants weighing 500 to 1500 g, *N Engl J Med* 330:1476, 1994.

53. Short EJ, et al: Cognitive and academic consequences of bronchopulmonary dysplasia and very low birth weight: 8-year-old outcomes, *Pediatrics* 112:e359, 2003.

54. STOP-ROP Multicenter Study Group: Supplemental therapeutic oxygen for prethreshold retinopathy of prematurity (STOP-ROP), a randomized, controlled trial, *Pediatrics* 105:2, 2000.

55. Thibeault DW, et al: Acinar arterial changes with chronic lung disease of prematurity in the surfactant era, *Pediatr Pulmonol* 36:482, 2003.

56. Tyson JE, et al: Vitamin A supplementation for extremely-low-birth-weight infants, *N Engl J Med* 340:1968, 1999.

57. Van Marter LJ, et al: Hydration during the first days of life and the risk of bronchopulmonary dysplasia in low birth weight infants, *J Pediatr* 116:942, 1990.

58. Van Marter LJ, et al: Do clinical markers of barotraumas and oxygen toxicity explain interhospital variation in rates of chronic lung disease? *Pediatrics* 105:1194, 2000.

59. Van Marter LJ, et al: Antenatal glucocorticoid treatment does not reduce chronic lung disease among surviving preterm infants, *J Pediatr* 138:198, 2001.

60. Varsila E, et al: Closure of patent ductus arteriosus decreases pulmonary myeloperoxidase in premature infants with respiratory distress syndrome, *Biol Neonate* 67:167, 1995.

61. Walsh MC, et al, for the NO CLD Study Group: Two-year neurodevelopmental outcomes of ventilated preterm infants treated with inhaled nitric oxide (The NO-CLD Trial), *J Pediatr* 156:556, 2010.

62. Walsh MC, et al, for NICHD Neonatal Research Network: A cluster randomized trial of benchmarking and multi-modal quality improvement to improve rates of survival free of bronchopulmonary dysplasia for infants with birthweights of less than 1250 grams, *Pediatrics* 119:876, 2007.

63. Walsh MC, et al: Safety, reliability, and validity of a physiologic definition of bronchopulmonary dysplasia, *J Perinatol* 23:451, 2003.

64. Wang EEL, et al: Role of *Ureaplasma urealyticum* and other pathogens in the development of chronic lung disease of prematurity, *Pediatr Infect Dis* 7:547, 1988.

65. Watterberg KL, et al: Chorioamnionitis and early lung inflammation in infants in whom bronchopulmonary dysplasia develops, *Pediatrics* 97:210, 1999.

66. Watterberg KL, et al: Links between early adrenal function and respiratory outcome in preterm infants: airway inflammation and patent ductus arteriosus, *Pediatrics* 105:320, 2000.

67. Watterberg KL, et al: Secretory leukocyte protease inhibitor and lung inflammation in developing bronchopulmonary dysplasia, *J Pediatr* 125:264, 1994.

68. Willet KE, et al: Antenatal endotoxin and glucocorticoid effects on lung morphometry in preterm lambs, *Pediatr Res* 48:782, 2000.

69. Wilson-Costello D, et al, for the Eunice Kennedy Shriver Eunice Kennedy Shriver National Institute of Child Health and Human Development Neonatal Research Network: Impact of postnatal corticosteroid use on neurodevelopment at 18 to 22 months' adjusted age: effects of dose, timing, and risk of bronchopulmonary dysplasia in extremely low birth weight infants, *Pediatrics* 123:e430, 2009.

70. Yeh TF, et al: Outcomes at school age after postnatal dexamethasone therapy for lung disease of prematurity, *N Engl J Med* 350:13, 2004.

71. Yoon BH, et al: Amniotic fluid cytokines (interleukin-6, tumor necrosis factor-α, interleukin-1β, and interleukin-8) and the risk for the development of bronchopulmonary dysplasia, *Am J Obstet Gynecol* 177:825, 1997.

72. Zupancic J, et al, NO CLD Study Group: Economic evaluation of inhaled nitric oxide in ventilated preterm infants, *Pediatrics* 124:1325 2009.

PART 8

Therapy for Cardiorespiratory Failure

Eileen K. Stork

Assisted ventilation and oxygen therapy remain the standard of care for neonatal respiratory failure. A few term and preterm infants with a wide range of diagnoses develop intractable cardiorespiratory failure despite maximal ventilatory support. In these patients, severe pulmonary hypertension often contributes to persistent hypoxemia.

Two unique therapies for such patients are presented in this section: extracorporeal membrane oxygenation (ECMO), which is now well established as a rescue therapy for intractable respiratory failure in neonates, and inhaled nitric oxide (iNO), a noninvasive inhalational therapy that can elicit selective pulmonary vasodilation.

EXTRACORPOREAL MEMBRANE OXYGENATION

In ECMO, techniques of cardiopulmonary bypass, modified from those originally developed for open heart surgery, are used over a prolonged period to support heart and lung function. In newborns with hypoxic respiratory failure, this allows the lungs to rest and recover, and prevents the often damaging effects of aggressive artificial ventilation and 100% FiO_2.

ECMO offers support for term or near-term neonates with life-threatening cardiopulmonary disease. Because of serious inherent risks, such as systemic and intracranial hemorrhage, the procedure is currently reserved for neonates with reversible pulmonary disease in whom trials of conventional or high-frequency ventilation as well as inhaled nitric oxide have failed.

Several randomized trials have demonstrated improved survival in infants supported with ECMO. The most rigorous prospective, randomized trial was conducted in the United Kingdom, where 185 infants with severe respiratory failure were randomized to ECMO or conventional ventilatory management.[18] Survival in the ECMO-treated patients was 68% compared with 41% survival in the control arm ($P = .0005$), equivalent to one extra survivor for every three or four infants allocated to ECMO. Neurologic outcome was similar among survivors of either treatment arm, making it unlikely that ECMO contributed any added morbidity to this cohort of critically ill newborns.

Respiratory disease in the newborn is often complicated by persistent pulmonary hypertension of the neonate (PPHN), also called persistent fetal circulation. In this circumstance the pulmonary vascular resistance approaches or exceeds systemic vascular resistance, offering significant impedance to pulmonary bloodflow. Desaturated blood returning to the right heart is shunted to the systemic circulation (following the path of least resistance) across two persistent fetal channels, the patent ductus arteriosus (PDA), and the foramen ovale, resulting in marked cyanosis.

The clinical course of such infants is variable, depending on the severity of the underlying disease process and the degree to which PPHN contributes to the cyanosis. Diagnoses associated with severe hypoxic respiratory failure in neonates include meconium aspiration syndrome (MAS), respiratory distress syndrome (RDS), group B streptococcal sepsis and pneumonia, congenital diaphragmatic hernia (CDH), and asphyxia neonatorum. Idiopathic pulmonary hypertension is sometimes seen in patients who exhibit minimal or no lung disease and have clear chest radiographs. The International Extracorporeal Life Support Organization (ELSO) Registry reports the distribution of primary diagnoses and survival for patients undergoing bypass; data are shown in Figure 44-87.[17]

Traditional therapy for respiratory failure complicated by PPHN consists of the use of oxygen, mechanical ventilation, alkalosis, and pharmacologic vasodilators in an attempt to decrease pulmonary vascular resistance and increase bloodflow to the lungs. iNO is a selective pulmonary vasodilator that enhances pulmonary bloodflow and improves oxygenation in PPHN. For infants who do not respond to these measures, however, ECMO can be useful therapy.

Basic Techniques

The standard ECMO procedure used in most newborn intensive care units today is venoarterial (VA) bypass because it provides both pulmonary and cardiac support. The right atrium is cannulated via the right internal jugular vein with a Silastic or polyvinyl chloride catheter (10- to 14-French diameter); blood is siphoned to a level below the heart where a roller head or centrifugal pump circulates the blood through the artificial lung. These pumps are servoregulated to slow or shut down if venous return is not adequate to meet circuit flow demands. As the blood circulates through the artificial lung, gas exchange occurs against a filtered mixture of oxygen

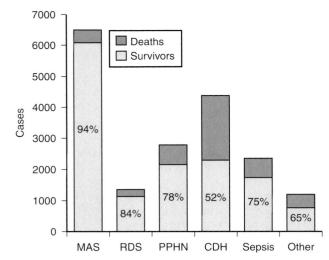

Figure 44–87. International ECMO experience (through January 2010). Data are derived from the Extracorporeal Life Support Organization Registry. MAS, meconium aspiration syndrome; RDS, respiratory distress syndrome; PPHN, persistent pulmonary hypertension of the neonate; CDH, congenital diaphragmatic hernia,

and CO_2. The most common artificial lung currently used in neonates is a 0.6 or 0.8 m^2, thin, gas-permeable silicone sheet membrane that serves as a blood-gas interface, similar to the alveolar capillary membrane. Countercurrent flow of blood and gas on opposite sides of the membrane allows for effective diffusion of gases between the blood and gas phases. The larger the patient, the larger the membrane lung must be to provide adequate gas exchange. In older children (more than 10 kg) and adults, a smaller, but more efficient, hollow fiber membrane lung (Quadrox D) has largely replaced the sheet membranes used for the past 25 years. Advantages of this newer artificial lung include a low priming volume and reduced blood/foreign surface area contact. This new generation of artificial lung also incorporates a heat exchanger to rewarm the oxygenated blood returning to the patient. Neonatal sized Quadrox membrane lungs for neonates and will be available in late 2010.

Oxygenation can be regulated by varying bloodflow through the ECMO circuit. The higher the volume of cardiac output diverted through the membrane lung, the better the oxygen delivery from the ECMO circuit. Oxygenated blood exiting the artificial lung is returned to the infant via an 8- to 12-French catheter positioned in the ascending aortic arch through a right common carotid artery cannulation.

Bloodflow through the ECMO circuit, at a rate of 90 to 120 mL/kg per minute, is usually adequate to provide excellent cardiac and respiratory support with maintenance of adequate blood pressure and oxygenation. Arterial wave dampening with narrowed pulse pressure is noticeable at flow rates approaching the infant's cardiac output because the ECMO circuit provides relatively nonpulsatile bloodflow. Pressor support, vasodilators, and paralytic agents can usually be stopped while the infant is on venoarterial (VA) ECMO support because perfusion pressure from the pump largely replaces cardiac output. Systemic anticoagulation therapy with unfractionated heparin is administered for the duration of the bypass procedure to prevent clotting in the circuit and possible thromboembolization. Activated clotting times are measured hourly and are maintained within a range of 180 to 240 seconds.

Once the infant is placed on ECMO, ventilator and oxygen support is reduced to a minimum to avoid any further barotrauma or oxygen toxicity to the lung. Infants can be maintained in room air with a peak inspiratory pressure (PIP) of 14 to 20 cm H_2O and a ventilator rate (IMV) of 12 to 20 for the duration of VA bypass. If volume ventilation is preferred, 3 to 6 mL/kg tidal volume is used to effect mild chest rise with each delivered breath. This helps maintain lung inflation and allows for continued pulmonary toilet. The respiratory status of the infant can be monitored with intermittent arterial blood gases obtained from the umbilical or peripheral arterial line. An oxygen saturation electrode inserted on the venous side of the circuit allows continuous monitoring of the mixed venous saturation at the level of the superior vena cava and right atrium. A mixed venous saturation of 70% or greater reflects adequate oxygen delivery.

As lung function improves or pulmonary hypertension abates, or both, the mixed venous saturation and partial pressure of arterial oxygen (PaO_2) rise above the baseline oxygenation provided through the artificial lung. Bloodflow through the artificial circuit can then be decreased in small increments (10 to 20 mL) while mixed venous and arterial oxygenation remain adequate. When ECMO flow has been reduced to 10 to 20 mL/kg per minute, the infant can be weaned from extracorporeal support.

Increased ventilator support is provided as the patient approaches decannulation. Bypass support may be required for 2 to 45 days with an average need for 8.9 days of support.[17] Continued ventilator support following ECMO can be quite variable (days to weeks) depending on the underlying cause of respiratory/cardiac failure, as well as the degree of barotrauma incurred before initiation of ECMO.

In most ECMO centers, the right carotid artery and internal jugular vein are permanently ligated at decannulation. This approach is technically easier and prevents any concern about acute embolic complications associated with vascular reconstruction. However, some surgeons reanastomose these vessels if the patient has been on bypass less than 10 days to prevent future ischemic risks to the developing newborn brain as well as during later adult life. Studies show no disadvantage to this approach. Magnetic resonance (MR) angiograms and Doppler flow studies confirm good antegrade flow through the reconstructed carotid artery postoperatively in the majority of these infants. However, long-term patency of the reconstructed carotid remains a question. Ultrasound vascular studies in children up to 5 years of age with reconstructed carotid arteries confirm good antegrade flow through the vessels in most cases, with no embolic sequelae reported.[16] Neurodevelopmental outcome and neuroimaging were equally favorable. Longer-term neurologic follow-up of these patients compared with ECMO survivors with carotid ligation is of interest to surgeons and neonatologists alike. Carotid artery ligation carries a small but definite risk for development of ischemic sequelae during VA bypass, whereas the risk for future ischemic stroke remains unknown.

Venovenous Extracorporeal Membrane Oxygenation

A growing experience supports the ability of venovenous ECMO to provide adequate oxygen delivery in patients with serious respiratory failure, but adequate heart function. In adults this technique usually involves draining desaturated blood from the right atrium and returning oxygenated blood through the femoral vein.

Venovenous (VV) bypass in infants has been greatly improved by the development of double-lumen catheters of varying sizes (12, 15, 18 French) that allow bypass support with cannulation of the right atrium alone. Desaturated blood is withdrawn from the right atrium through the outer fenestrated venous catheter wall. Oxygenated blood from the ECMO circuit is returned to the inner arterial catheter, which is angled to direct blood across the tricuspid valve. Higher flow rates are required to maintain adequate oxygen delivery with VV bypass because of recirculation of desaturated and oxygenated blood within the right atrial chamber.

Advantages of VV bypass include avoidance of carotid artery cannulation and maintenance of pulmonary bloodflow. The major disadvantage is that, unlike VA bypass, VV ECMO does not provide cardiac support. Oxygen delivery in VV bypass remains dependent on native cardiac output.

Survival data, complication rate, and length of bypass support compare favorably with those of VA bypass cases. The ELSO Registry reports that more than 6000 newborns have undergone VV bypass with only 11% requiring conversion to venoarterial support.[17] Because it avoids carotid ligation, VV bypass has enormous appeal and has become the treatment of choice in newborns with adequate cardiac function.

Personnel Needs

ECMO is the most labor-intensive procedure in the neonatal intensive care unit (NICU). Specialists trained in managing patients on ECMO must remain at the patient's bedside for the duration of bypass. In addition to monitoring the infant's respiratory status, specialists must regulate the rates of blood and gas flow through the extracorporeal circuit to meet the infant's respiratory demands. They must adjust anticoagulation by measuring the activated clotting time in the blood every 30 to 60 minutes and titrate the heparin infusion accordingly. Additionally, they must evaluate the patient for bleeding and replace losses appropriately. The specialists can be physicians, nurses, perfusionists, or respiratory therapists who have completed extensive training in perfusion support.

An ECMO physician trained in the clinical management of bypass patients must always be readily available for consultation, especially in case of mechanical failure or acute clinical decompensation. Additional support services required include 24-hour availability of personnel trained in radiology (ultrasonography), pediatric surgery, neurology, genetics, cardiology, and cardiothoracic surgery. The expertise and personnel needed to support these patients are extensive and costly.

Criteria for Patient Selection

The cumulative experience of many ECMO centers has resulted in the establishment of criteria that are currently used to decide whether ECMO support is appropriate.[62] These are described in Box 44-14.

GESTATIONAL AGE OF 34 WEEKS OR OLDER

Preterm newborns with respiratory failure carry a higher risk for intracranial hemorrhage (ICH) compared with term infants at baseline, and this risk is heightened with systemic

---

BOX 44-14	Patient Selection Criteria for Neonatal Extracorporeal Membrane Oxygenation [62]

Gestational age of 34 weeks or older
Normal cranial ultrasound (grade I intraventricular hemorrhage is a relative contraindication)
Absence of complex congenital heart disease
Less than 10 to 14 days of assisted ventilation
Reversible lung disease, including congenital diaphragmatic hernia
Failure of maximum medical therapy
No lethal congenital anomalies or evidence of irreversible brain damage

---

heparinization required during ECMO support. Furthermore, changes in cerebral bloodflow patterns associated with cardiopulmonary bypass can also place the immature brain at increased risk for bleeding.

In the early ECMO trials, premature infants less than 35 weeks' gestation had an 89% incidence of spontaneous ICH associated with heparinization.[6] Subsequent studies, (all retrospective) revisiting this issue, reported improvement in outcome, but confirmed increasing rates of ICH as gestational age decreases, with the incidence of ICH approaching 50% at gestational ages younger than 34 weeks.[62]

Technical refinements in bypass support have made ECMO possible for infants weighing as little as 1800 g. However, gestational age remains a strong predictor of ICH risk. In a recent study, postconceptional age (PCA) proved to be the highest predictor for ICH risk. In a retrospective study of 1524 neonates less than 37 weeks' gestation treated with ECMO between 1992 and 2000, ICH developed in 26% of patients younger than 32 weeks' PCA compared with 6% of patients with PCA of 38 weeks ($P = .004$).[26] Neurodevelopmental outcome in surviving preterm infants treated with ECMO in the first 2 weeks of life has not been well studied. This, together with the higher morbidity and mortality among ECMO-treated preterm infants, forms the basis of the recommendation that ECMO support be reserved for term and near-term infants.

NO MAJOR INTRACRANIAL HEMORRHAGE

The catastrophic extension of intracranial bleeds, along with the attendant neurologic sequelae, is the primary risk reported in the early series of Bartlett and associates.[6] Some centers have successfully managed infants with grade I or stable grade II intraventricular hemorrhage on bypass using a minimal heparin dosage to lessen bleeding complications and high ECMO flow rates to prevent clotting in the extracorporeal circuit. Uncontrolled bleeding from surgical wounds, chest tubes, or other sites also worsens with heparin therapy and is a contraindication to ECMO. The septic infant is of concern in this regard because of the commonly associated coagulopathy. Although these infants have a higher risk of bleeding complications on ECMO, meticulous correction of their coagulopathy and careful heparin management have allowed these infants to be successfully treated.[17]

ABSENCE OF COMPLEX CONGENITAL HEART DISEASE

Infants in severe respiratory failure must have an echocardiogram to rule out congenital heart disease as the underlying cause for refractory hypoxemia. In some instances, the degree of hypoxemia is not easily explained based on the heart lesion alone (e.g., in a newborn with an atrioventricular canal complicated by meconium aspiration or sepsis). ECMO can provide cardiovascular support to stabilize such a patient until the reversible component of the lung disease is no longer an issue, rendering the baby a more viable surgical candidate at some later date.

Similarly, an infant with suspected cyanotic congenital heart disease may present to an ECMO center with profound cyanosis and cardiogenic shock despite the use of prostaglandins and inotropes. Preoperative ECMO can stabilize such infants who are believed to have reparable cardiac defects, but who are deemed to be poor surgical candidates by virtue of their clinical instability. Both venovenous and venoarterial ECMO have been used preoperatively in infants with cyanotic congenital heart disease and cardiovascular instability.[31,34] Indications for ECMO include arterial saturations of 60% or less accompanied by hypotension and metabolic acidosis unresponsive to mechanical ventilation and pharmacologic support with inotropes and vasodilators. For most infants presenting with isolated cyanotic congenital heart disease, however, prompt surgical intervention, not ECMO, is the obvious treatment of choice.

LESS THAN 10 TO 14 DAYS OF ASSISTED VENTILATION

Although ECMO can support cardiovascular function for days to weeks, it does not reverse serious preexisting pulmonary damage. In early studies infants subjected to prolonged mechanical ventilation with high pressures and FiO_2 before ECMO suffered extensive barotrauma and did not recover despite prolonged support (more than 2 weeks) on bypass.[6] Severe bronchopulmonary dysplasia (BPD), or inability to wean from ECMO support, was the result. Infants who have recovered from BPD, however, are eligible for ECMO later in life. BPD survivors have been placed on ECMO in later infancy or toddlerhood for life-threatening bronchiolitis with good survival results: 59 of 76 (78%) patients in one study.[17] One center, however, reported severe pulmonary and neurodevelopmental sequelae among four of seven survivors with BPD who required ECMO beyond the neonatal period.[28]

Recent changes in ventilatory management wherein lower pressure and volume settings are used to avoid barotrauma (permissive hypercapnea or gentle ventilation) may protect the neonatal lung from irreversible damage for longer periods than earlier studies suggested. Use of surfactant and inhaled nitric oxide (iNO) may also blunt ventilator-induced lung injury. Nevertheless, the longer an infant is ventilated with high FiO_2 before initiating ECMO, the longer that infant will take to recover, owing to the barotrauma and oxygen toxicity superimposed upon the infant's underlying lung disease. Therefore, if a patient fails to respond favorably to respiratory measures available, ECMO support should be considered expeditiously.

REVERSIBLE LUNG DISEASE

Using reversible lung disease as a criterion to determine whether to use ECMO is intended to exclude infants with severe lung hypoplasia incompatible with life. Patients with marked renal dysplasia and prolonged oligohydramnios, large congenital diaphragmatic hernia (CDH) presenting in extremis at birth, and hydrops fetalis fall into this category. However, infants with respiratory failure in all these categories have survived with ECMO support, making the judgment of irreversible lung disease in the newborn extremely problematic.

The Dilemma of Congenital Diaphragmatic Hernia

CDH is defined as an anatomic defect in the diaphragm that permits abdominal contents to herniate into the thoracic cavity. In some cases the abdominal viscera are covered with a membranous sac. The incidence of CDH is 1 in 2500 live births. The type of hernia depends on the location of the diaphragmatic defect. The most common is the posterolateral hernia, also called the *Bochdalek hernia*, which accounts for 90% to 95% of CDH cases. The defect occurs more frequently on the left side of the diaphragm (78% to 84%) than on the right side (14% to 20%), whereas bilateral hernias occur rarely (0.9% to 2%).[23]

In CDH, the fetal lungs have a reduced number of arterioles and conducting airways. There are fewer alveoli, thickened alveolar walls, and increased interstitial tissue resulting in markedly diminished alveolar airspace and gas exchange surface area. Vascular development parallels that of the airways. There are a reduced number of vessels, adventitial thickening, medial muscle hyperplasia, and peripheral extension of the muscular layer into the smaller intra-acinary arterioles. Both lungs are affected, the ipsilateral one more than the contralateral one, and the hypoplasia is progressive beyond 30 weeks.[25] After delivery, these morphologic changes compromise effective gas exchange, resulting in respiratory failure and pulmonary hypertension. Survivors additionally suffer from variable degrees of pulmonary, gastrointestinal (gastroesophageal reflux and feeding problems), orthopedic (scoliosis, rib cage hypoplasia), and hearing and neurodevelopmental issues.

Infants with CDH who present with cyanosis and respiratory distress at delivery often suffer significant pulmonary hypoplasia, although the degree of lung restriction is difficult to assess radiographically because of the bowel contents in the chest. Volatile pulmonary hypertension in the first few days of life complicates the clinical course, even when adequate lung volume is available for gas exchange.

Infants in whom profound cyanosis develops, despite oxygen, mechanical ventilation, bowel decompression, and judicious volume and pressor support of blood pressure, make up the subset of patients with CDH for whom ECMO support is justified. As shown in Figure 44-87, CDH is the second most common diagnosis for which ECMO support is used in neonates. In the 2010 ELSO Registry (a national registry of ECMO cases), survival of newborns with CDH supported with ECMO (n = 5721) is 51%. This stands in marked contrast to the 94% survival achieved among infants with meconium aspiration treated with ECMO (n = 7438).[17]

Prenatal diagnosis of CDH is now common, but a substantial number of cases are still missed. In a prospective, population-based study of congenital anomalies in the United Kingdom, only 63 of 100 cases of CDH were diagnosed prenatally between 1997 and 2000 out of 125,380 live births. By comparison, during the same time period the prenatal diagnosis rate for hypoplastic left heart syndrome was 88% and the detection rate for gastroschisis was 94%. The prenatal diagnosis rate for all registered anomalies reported improved significantly over each 4-year epoch recorded from 1985 through 2000. Of note, termination of pregnancy for all fetal malformations rose from 23 to 47 per 10,000 registered births between 1985 and 2000.[56] In a retrospective study of 51 CDH cases recorded in the Auvergne Birth Defect Registry between 1992 and 2003, the prenatal detection rate of nonisolated CDH (detecting either the CDH or another major anomaly) was 73% while the detection rate of isolated CDH was only 45% (P = .03). Prenatal diagnosis in the presence of associated anomalies predicted poor outcome with survival of only 23%. Paradoxically, infants with isolated CDH who escaped prenatal detection had the highest survival rate (81%).[22,23]

The pathogenesis of CDH and the causes of pulmonary hypoplasia in this anomaly are slowly being unraveled. Nitrofen is a teratogenic herbicide (banned in the United States and United Kingdom since the 1980s) which produces CDH in rodents. When administered to pregnant dams between days 8 and 11 postconception, a high rate of CDH with associated pulmonary hypoplasia and pulmonary vascular anomalies occurs in the offspring, remarkably similar to the human malformation. A "dual hit hypothesis" has been proposed to explain the severe pulmonary hypoplasia often seen in this condition.[37] The first insult is caused by nitrofen and affects both lungs before diaphragm development is complete. The second insult affects the growth the ipsilateral lung due to compression of that lung by herniated viscera. The origin of the diaphragmatic defect lies in the disruption of the mesenchymal substrata of the pleuroperitoneal folds which form the scaffold for the eventual migration of muscular precursor cells into the nacent diaphragm. In human embryology this would point to a defect as early as 4 to 5 weeks' gestation, long before the formation of the "muscular" diaphragm.[12,50]

A defect in the retinoid signaling pathway, specifically, inhibition of retinal dehydrogenase-2 (Raldh2), has been proposed as the likely etiology of the embryonic disruption resulting in CDH.[23,24,32,50] Retinoids play a central role during embryogenesis and lung development in particular. During early lung morphogenesis, retinoic acid promotes mesodermal proliferation and induces fibroblast growth factor expression in the foregut. Retinoic acid is decreased in nitrofen-induced hypoplastic lungs in rodents. Furthermore, coadministration of large doses of vitamin A (25,000 units) and nitrofin to pregnant rodent dams reduces the incidence of CDH by 15% to 30% and attenuates lung hypoplasia, suggesting that the teratogenic effect of nitrofen on the embryonic lung and diaphragm is mediated through suppression of the retinoic pathway. Right-sided diaphragmatic hernias are also seen in offspring of dams fed a vitamin A–deficient diet. The incidence of herniation is decreased when vitamin A is introduced into the diet at midgestation.[24]

Human infants with CDH have a 40% to 60% risk for major nonpulmonary anomalies, including serious cardiac malformations.[58] Renal, central nervous system, and gastrointestinal anomalies are also reported. To date, a genetic role has not been described in isolated CDH. However, the 2% recurrence rate and association of chromosomal anomalies in 10% of nonisolated CDH cases (CDH+) suggests that there is a genetic component to this malformation. Some cases of CDH+ are associated with aneuploidy, including trisomies 13, 18, 21 and Turner syndrome (45 XO).[32,58] Structural chromosomal anomalies, including deletions, inversions, duplications, and translocations are also reported.[58] Genetic analysis has identified a CDH critical region on chromosome 15q26, which codes for four genes involved in diaphragmatic morphogenesis.[12] Microdeletions in this region have been described in several patients with nonisolated CDH and are associated with very high mortality. Other CDH "hot spots" include 1q41-q42, 3q22, 4p16, 8p23, 8q22, 11p13. Haploinsufficiency or decreased expression of one or more genes encoded in

these regions may cause or predispose to the development of CDH.[32,58]

In patients with CDH for whom a syndrome diagnosis can be provided, the most frequent is Fryns syndrome, which has an autosomal recessive inheritance pattern.[32] Other phenotypic variations of Fryns syndrome have also been linked to microdeletions in the chromosomal regions mentioned earlier.

For all the reasons discussed, amniocentesis for chromosomal analysis is recommended in all cases of CDH diagnosed antenatally. After birth, G-banded chromosomal analysis should be performed in all cases of CDH, including those who had amniocentesis. Furthermore, in nonisolated cases of CDH, array-based comparative genomic hybridization (aCGH) should also be considered because this technique is useful for identifying small chromosomal deletions and duplications below the resolution of G-band chromosomal analysis.[23,58]

Infants delivered at or near term with isolated CDH have the best prognoses, with 68% to 80% overall survival in tertiary care centers within the U.S. Among infants with isolated CDH identified in utero, liver herniation into the fetal chest and low lung area-to-head circumference ratio (LHR) < 1.4 in the contralateral lung reflect an especially high risk cohort.[25] Both findings predict a marked degree of lung hypoplasia and high mortality risk. Fetal surgery intervention has been actively studied in this unique group of CDH patients. Using a novel tracheal occlusion technique, this pioneering procedure has been shown in animal models of CDH to induce often dramatic growth of the hypoplastic left lung.[14]

However, in a prospective, randomized trial in human infants with isolated left CDH, fetal tracheal occlusion did not improve survival.[27] Infants enrolled in this study between 22 and 27 weeks' gestation all had liver herniation into the left chest and LHR less than 1.4 reflecting significant pulmonary hypoplasia. Eight of 11 (73%) infants treated with fetal surgery survived, compared with 10 of 13 (77%) infants receiving standard care at a tertiary care NICU with ECMO available. Moreover, preterm delivery (mean 31.8 weeks) was more common in the fetal intervention group, although rates of neonatal morbidity reportedly did not differ between the groups.

In addition to the fetal surgery centers in the United States, three European fetal surgical centers (Belgium, Spain, and the United Kingdom) continue to refine selection criteria and surgical technique in the performance of fetal tracheal occlusion (FETO).[14,15,60] Following epidural anesthesia in the mother, along with nifedipine tocolysis and fentanyl/pancuronium anesthesia in the fetus, investigators insert a single 3.3-mm cannula through the uterine wall and into the fetus' upper airway. An inflatable balloon is inserted between the vocal cords and carina to block the egress of lung fluid and thus distend the diminutive left lung. FETO is performed ideally between 26 and 28 weeks' gestation with reversal of the tracheal occlusion planned at 34 weeks unless preterm labor intervenes. The average gestation at delivery following this procedure is 33.5 weeks with 70% delivering beyond 32 weeks.[36,60] The European FETO centers offer prenatal intervention when the degree of pulmonary hypoplasia is severe, reflected by an LHR of less than 1.0 along with liver herniation in the chest. Survival in this cohort is reportedly only 15% with expected management. Following FETO, survival improved to 61.5% in 13 infants with fetal LHR of

0.6 to 0.7, and to 77.8% in 9 infants with LHR of 0.8 to 0.9.[36] A randomized, controlled trial by the European Consortium is under discussion.

The postnatal management of CDH has changed considerably in the past several years. For one thing, CDH is no longer treated as a surgical emergency. The timing of surgical repair is usually delayed until the patient's condition is stabilized with regard to oxygenation, blood pressure, and acid-base status, sometimes for a period of several days. Two prospective studies of delayed versus immediate repair failed to show any survival advantage. Conversely, these studies did not show any adverse outcomes associated with delayed surgery.[61] The CDH Study Group, a consortium of 62 international centers tracking the outcome of patients with CDH, reports that surgical repair is now accomplished at an average of 73 hours of life in newborns not requiring ECMO support.[10]

Surfactant treatment in CDH has been used in several tertiary care nurseries based on preliminary reports of surfactant deficiency in animal models of CDH and a few human case series, even at term gestation. However, a large retrospective study has failed to substantiate the efficacy of surfactant treatment in term and near term CDH infants. Using the CDH Study Group Registry, investigators identified 448 neonates with isolated CDH who were ≥35 weeks' gestation and who were treated with ECMO within the first 7 days of life. One hundred fourteen infants received surfactant treatment while 334 infants did not. Surfactant replacement did not provide significant benefit in the infants' clinical course with respect to survival, length of intubation, or subsequent need for supplemental oxygen.[13] In an autopsy study comparing ipsilateral lung samples from 16 preterm fetuses with CDH to age-matched controls who died of nonpulmonary disease, no differences were found in surfactant protein or phospholipid concentrations.[9]

The optimal timing for ECMO support in patients with CDH remains controversial. It has been used preoperatively in unstable patients or post-CDH repair if pulmonary hypertension supervenes. Repair of the hernia can be accomplished, while the patient is on bypass support if necessary, although in this circumstance bleeding complications are higher because the patient is anticoagulated.

Autopsy studies of CDH lungs confirm diminished lung volumes and show evidence of severe barotrauma often when ventilator exposure was relatively short. Wung and associates had previously established the efficacy of avoiding hyperventilation in infants with PPHN.[69] Based on this experience, investigators at Morgan Stanley Children's Hospital of New York Presbyterian first applied the technique of gentle ventilation to patients with CDH in the hope of avoiding barotrauma and preserving the integrity of the vulnerable hypoplastic lungs. Permissive hypercapnia, rather than hyperventilation, was the goal of this strategy, using low respiratory pressures (usually ≤25 cm H_2O) to achieve adequate chest rise rather than a target CO_2. Preductal saturations greater than 90% are the goals in oxygenation, but oxygen saturations between 80% and 89% are tolerated if the patient is otherwise stable. High-frequency oscillatory ventilation (HFOV) is used when the patient's preductal oxygen saturation is less than 80 or the P_{CO_2} persistently > 65 torr. Postductal saturations are often lower. ECMO is used to support infants with isolated CDH whose condition cannot be stabilized with gentle ventilation.

Using this approach, Boloker and colleagues reported 76% (91 of 120) survival in a cohort of 120 consecutive infants with CDH treated with delayed surgery and gentle ventilation.[8] Excluding 18 infants who were not offered surgery (lethal anomalies, overwhelming pulmonary hypoplasia, neurologic complications), 84% survived to discharge. ECMO was used in only 13.3% of infants.

Wilson and associates previously reported no significant improvement in CDH survival with the adoption of delayed surgery or ECMO at Boston Children's Hospital.[68] They subsequently adopted a treatment protocol emphasizing permissive hypercapnea, control of pulmonary hypertension, and judicious support of cardiac function. Using this strategy, 36 of 39 (93%) consecutive infants survived to discharge. Of particular interest was the survival in 8 of 10 (80%) infants with structural heart defects. Previously few infants with serious congenital heart lesions and CDH had survived at Boston Children's Hospital or elsewhere.

In fact, the true impact of ECMO on CDH survival remains unproved. Many small studies report improved survival with ECMO use, but these tend to use historical controls that tend to exaggerate treatment effect. The same is true for high-frequency ventilation studies in CDH. Of all therapeutic interventions used in the treatment of patients with CDH and hypoxic respiratory failure (HRF), only iNO has been studied in a prospective, randomized trial. Disappointingly, neither the mortality rate nor the need for ECMO was diminished in those infants receiving iNO in two studies involving 83 patients.[11,19]

FAILURE OF MAXIMAL MEDICAL THERAPY

Because ECMO is an invasive procedure, it is currently reserved for infants receiving optimal conventional therapy who meet criteria indicating a 60% to 80% or greater chance of dying. It is critical that these infants be identified quickly so that adjunctive therapies, such as surfactant, HFOV, and iNO can be used to stabilize, and hopefully reverse, respiratory failure short of ECMO. For infants whose respiratory status cannot be stabilized, however, ECMO should be initiated without delay, certainly before the infant is moribund.

The nature of maximal conventional therapy for respiratory failure in the newborn varies considerably among tertiary care units around the world and remains the source of much debate and controversy. No randomized trials have addressed the efficacy of several modalities employed in the treatment of neonatal respiratory failure complicated by PPHN.[67] These included muscle paralysis, hyperventilation to induce respiratory alkalosis, alkali therapy to promote metabolic alkalosis, and vasodilator therapy, including tolazoline (no longer commercially available), prostaglandins E and D, nitroprusside, and magnesium sulfate. The use of the aforementioned vasodilators has been limited by their unpredictable side effect of systemic hypotension.

Using high-frequency ventilation with the aim of decreasing ventilation-perfusion ($\dot{V}/\dot{Q}$) mismatch and improving oxygenation has been successful in some series.[10] Surfactant use has also been shown to decrease the need for ECMO in newborns with parenchymal disease (e.g., RDS, pneumonia, meconium aspiration) and respiratory failure.[45] Inhaled NO is a pulmonary vasodilator that selectively lowers pulmonary vascular resistance without adversely affecting systemic blood pressure. In prospective randomized trials of iNO in newborns with PPHN (including CDH), iNO improved oxygenation in most infants and decreased the need for ECMO by 40%.[20]

ECMO Referral

One of the hardest decisions faced by neonatologists in tertiary care is when to refer a newborn in respiratory failure to an ECMO center. Because of the volatile nature of PPHN, the risk of sudden cardiorespiratory decompensation and death remains high in any infant not responding favorably to conventional supportive measures. Likewise, transporting these unstable babies is problematic, with one series reporting a 25% mortality among ECMO transports.[7] In another study, the use of iNO during transport improved oxygenation in a cohort of 25 high-risk neonates with unstable cardiopulmonary disease. All 25 infants survived transport, many over long distances.[40]

It is essential that ECMO referrals be made as expeditiously as possible, certainly before the infant is moribund and preferably before the baby reaches ECMO-eligible respiratory criteria. Early and frequent telephone contact with an ECMO physician to discuss the details of each case can help establish transport criteria agreeable to both parties.

The parameters most often used to predict poor outcome in infants failing conventional or high-frequency ventilator support and regarded as entry criteria for ECMO are listed in Box 44-15. These criteria are applied when the infant has reached optimal ventilatory support on 100% oxygen.

One criterion is the oxygenation index (OI):

$$OI = \frac{\text{mean airway pressure} \times FiO_2 \times 100}{\text{Postductal } PaO_2}$$

This equation has a certain appeal in that it reflects the ventilator support being used to achieve any given PaO_2. The oxygenation index is the parameter used in most ECMO centers today to gauge the severity of respiratory insufficiency.

Another criterion is the alveolar-arterial oxygen gradient ($AaDO_2$):

$$AaDO_2 = FiO_2(P - 47) - PaO_2 - PaCO_2\left[FiO_2 + \frac{(1 - FiO_2)}{R}\right]$$

where P is the barometric pressure, 47 is the partial pressure of water vapor, R is the respiratory quotient (0.8), FiO_2 is the fractional inspired oxygen concentration, PaO_2 is the partial pressure of arterial oxygen, and $PaCO_2$ is the partial pressure of arterial carbon dioxide. When FiO_2 is 100% and assuming PaO_2 (partial pressure of alveolar oxygen) is equivalent to PaO_2, the equation reduces to

$$AaDO_2 = P - 47 - PaO_2 - PaCO_2$$

where P is 760 mm Hg at sea level.

An OI of ≥ 40 or an $AaDO_2$ gradient of ≥ 620 serve as baseline criteria for ECMO eligibility. Assessment of respiratory failure parameters begins after infants have received surfactant or iNO, or both, when clinically relevant. Supporting cardiac output with judicious use of volume

---

BOX 44–15 Formulas and Criteria for Neonatal Extracorporeal Membrane Oxygenation

OXYGENATION INDEX (OI)
$OI = (MAP \times FiO_2 \times 100)/PaO_2$
Usual criterion is OI of 35 to 60 for 0.5 to 6 hours.

ALVEOLAR-ARTERIAL OXYGEN ($AaDO_2$) GRADIENT
$AaDO_2 = FiO_2 (P - 47) - PaO_2 - PaCO_2 [FiO_2 + (1 - FiO_2)/R]$
Usual criterion is $AaDO_2 > 605\text{-}620$ mm Hg (at sea level) for 4 to 12 hours.

PARTIAL PRESSURE OF ARTERIAL OXYGEN
Usual criterion is $PaO_2 < 40$ mm Hg for 2 hours.

ACIDOSIS AND SHOCK
Usual criterion is pH < 7.25 for longer than 2 hours or with hypotension.

From Van Meurs KP, et al: ECMO for neonatal respiratory failure. In: Van Meurs L, et al, editors: *ECMO: extracorporeal cardiopulmonary support in critical care*, 3rd ed, Ann Arbor, MI, 2005, ELSO, pp 273-296.

---

loading and pressor infusion is key to maintaining adequate oxygen delivery in newborns with borderline blood pressure and respiratory insufficiency. In the ventilatory management of these infants equal attention must be paid to providing optimal ventilation without overdistending the lung, which compromises venous return and hence adversely affects cardiac output. Hyperventilation (to induce respiratory alkalosis) is no longer recommended in the ventilatory management of PPHN.

For the infant who remains severely hypoxic and hypotensive despite every supportive measure offered the choice for ECMO is easily made. However, for the infant whose blood gases and systemic blood pressure are marginally stable on maximal support including iNO, but who is unable to wean from these supports, the choice between invasive bypass support (ECMO) and the risk for extended volutrauma to the lungs remains difficult.

One large study in newborns with respiratory failure and PPHN confirmed that aggressive weaning of iNO over 96 hours can be accomplished without increasing the risk for ECMO.[11] Judicious but steady weaning of both FiO_2 and ventilator settings is recommended to avoid serious lung injury. If the infant's respiratory status fails to stabilize and improve over a number of days, then ECMO is an alternative.

ECMO Follow-up

More than 23,000 infants have been treated for respiratory failure in more than 100 ECMO centers worldwide for an overall survival of 76%.[17] The outcome of these children compares favorably with that of term and near-term infants surviving severe respiratory compromise and PPHN with conventional management.

A valid criticism of early ECMO follow-up studies was the lack of proper control data, that is, the outcome of infants with severe respiratory compromise who were managed during the ECMO era with conventional treatment alone. Such control data are essential for distinguishing morbid outcome caused by the underlying disease process and NICU management of respiratory failure, or both, from the morbidity that is secondary to the ECMO procedure itself.

To address this issue, Walsh-Sukys and associates were the first to report on the neurodevelopmental outcome of 74 consecutive neonates older than 34 weeks' gestation admitted to Rainbow Babies and Children's Hospital with severe respiratory failure.[66] Eighteen of 24 (75%) infants treated conventionally survived, whereas 43 of 48 (90%) treated with ECMO survived. Patients were evaluated at 8 and 20 months. Sixty-two of 72 (91%) survivors were seen in follow-up. Four of 17 (24%) conventionally treated survivors, and 10 of 38 (26%) ECMO-treated survivors had neurodevelopmental impairment defined as either Mental Developmental Index Score lower than 80 or neurosensory impairment. The conventionally treated group had significantly more chronic lung disease, longer duration of oxygen therapy, more chronic reactive airway disease, and more rehospitalizations than those treated with ECMO. Macrocephaly was noted in 24% of ECMO survivors, all treated with VA bypass, but in none of the conventional group. This study concluded that ECMO survivors did not suffer increased neurologic morbidity compared with similarly ill neonates managed conventionally and they may have fewer pulmonary sequelae.

Vaucher and colleagues prospectively assessed growth and neurodevelopmental outcome in a cohort of 190 infants surviving neonatal respiratory failure who met institutional criteria for the use of ECMO.[64] Fifty-two were managed with conventional or high-frequency ventilation, and 138 required ECMO. At 12 to 30 months of age the mean developmental scores of ECMO survivors were similar to those for infants who survived without ECMO. Neuroimaging abnormalities or diagnosis of bronchopulmonary dysplasia each independently predicted adverse neurodevelopmental outcome regardless of treatment strategies used in the NICU. This observation mirrors the same predictors of poor outcome described in another high-risk cohort familiar to neonatologists, namely, infants with very low birthweight (less than 1000 g).

In 2006, the UK Collaborative ECMO Trial Group published the 7-year follow-up of their surviving patients from the largest prospective randomized ECMO trial carried out so far.[47] In this study, a single psychologist assessed 90 of the 100 children available for follow-up without prior knowledge of treatment allocation (ECMO versus conventional management). At age 7 years, there was no difference in cognitive function between the 56 patients randomized to ECMO versus the 34 controls; 68 (76%) children recorded a cognitive level within the normal range. Learning problems were similar in the two groups. There were notable difficulties with spatial and processing tasks; the children also had particular difficulty completing tasks of reading comprehension with 35 (39%) scoring below the 10th percentile. There was no difference in laterality of neuromotor disability between the two groups. A higher respiratory morbidity and increased risk of behavioral problems among children treated conventionally (first reported in the 4-year follow-up) persisted. In the conventionally treated group, 11 (32%) of 30 children continued to have wheezing attacks and 14 (41%) of 32 regularly used an inhaler over the 12 months before study assessment. These compared with 6 (11%) of 43 ECMO children who

wheezed and 14 of 48 (25%) using an inhaler. In behavioral assessment, the total deviant score was higher in the conventionally treated group—38% versus 18% in ECMO survivors. The most commonly described difficulty reported by parents and teachers in both groups was hyperactivity; overall, 22 of 85 (26%) children had difficulty with hyperactivity.

The primary outcome of known death or severe disability occurred in 37% of the ECMO group compared with 59% in the conventional group (relative risk 0.64; $P = .004$) leading the authors to reaffirm that ECMO remains a beneficial treatment. These results, which have not changed from the 4-year follow-up, are equivalent to one additional child surviving without severe disability for every four to five children referred for ECMO.

Overall, 31 of 56 (55%) ECMO survivors and 17 of 34 (50%) conventionally treated survivors were assessed with no disability at 7 years. The authors concluded that the data collected at 1, 4, and now 7 years' follow-up of the UK ECMO Trial participants suggest that the underlying disease process (and associated physiologic instability) appears to be the major influence in long-term outcome. Their findings confirm significant long-term morbidity in many surviving children who had life-threatening respiratory failure soon after birth, regardless of their subsequent medical treatment. Furthermore, while both groups had problems, the beneficial influence of ECMO persists to 7 years. Clearly, newborns presenting with PPHN and severe respiratory failure require ongoing developmental assessment well beyond their NICU experience, and whether or not they required ECMO support.

Cost Analysis

ECMO saves lives, but it does cost more than conventional management of neonatal respiratory failure. A cost-effectiveness analysis of neonatal ECMO was published based on 7-year results from the UK Collaborative ECMO Trial.[55] Mean health service costs during the first 7 years of life were £30,270 in the ECMO group compared with o £10,229 in the conventional management group. Data for this analysis included air and ground transport costs, initial and all subsequent hospitalizations, outpatient hospital care, and community health care, as well as other health care services. These combined costs over 7 years translated into a cost of £13,385 per life-year gained. The incremental cost per disability-free life-year gained was estimated at £23,566. These incremental costs should decrease as the surviving children grow older. The authors concluded that ECMO was not only clinically effective, but also as cost-effective as other intensive care technologies in common use.

Alternative Uses for ECMO

ECMO support has been extended to a broader array of high-risk candidates. A small number (5%) of infants undergoing surgical repair of their heart defects cannot be successfully weaned from cardiopulmonary bypass (CPB) or they develop low cardiac output syndrome several hours after repair.[31] VA ECMO can provide circulatory support for these patients until their cardiac function improves. However, survival in postcardiotomy infants requiring ECMO is low (38%) compared with respiratory case survival (76%).[17]

In a single center retrospective study of 671 patients undergoing open heart surgery between January 2001 and October 2003, 36 (5.4%) infants received extracorporeal life support within one day after surgery (age younger than 30 days, n = 34). Overall, 28 patients (78%) were weaned from extracorporeal support successfully, and 24 (67%) survived to hospital discharge. These infants had a variety of disorders including single ventricle anatomy as well as failed hemodynamics postcardiotomy. The authors concluded that expanded use of extracorporeal support may improve outcome in some of the highest risk neonates, especially those with univentricular anatomy.[3] In another single center review from Vanderbilt University Medical Center, 84 children with congenital heart disease required postcardiotomy ECMO between January 2001 and September 2004. The median age of the patients was 128 days (1 day to 5 years), and median weight was 4.5 kg (2 to 18 kg). Fifty-two (61.9%) survived for more than 24 hours after decannulation, but only 31 (36.9%) survived to discharge. High arterial lactate levels at the time of ECMO initiation were strongly correlated with poor outcome. Inability to wean off ECMO by 6 days correlated with high mortality.[59]

ECMO has been used as a bridge to cardiac transplantation in infants with myocarditis or complex congenital heart disease, as well as support for early graft failure following heart transplantation in infancy. ECMO has also been used to stabilize infants with refractory supraventricular tachycardia until antiarrhythmic drugs could be maximized or radioablation of the aberrant pathway accomplished.[65] Tracheal reconstruction in infants with serious congenital defects of the upper airway has also been successfully accomplished while on ECMO.[30]

ECMO Present and Future

ECMO has become an established treatment for cases of hypoxic respiratory failure refractory to conventional management. Because of advances in neonatal respiratory care, the number of annual neonatal respiratory ECMO cases has declined from a peak of 1418 in 1992 to 800 infants in 2007.[17] Surfactant treatment, gentle ventilation, permissive hypercapnea, high-frequency ventilation, and inhaled nitric oxide have all contributed to the welcomed decline in the need for ECMO rescue in neonatal respiratory failure.

Research efforts continue to focus on PPHN treatment that could preclude the need for bypass altogether. Randomized, controlled trials over the past decade have proven the efficacy of iNO as the selective pulmonary vasodilator that decreases the need for ECMO (see later). Other drugs used extensively in the treatment of adult and pediatric idiopathic pulmonary hypertension have been reported, so far in small case series only, to hold promise in the treatment of PPHN. As the number of neonatal pulmonary cases declines, the use of ECMO support for cardiac low-output syndrome, as in myocarditis or postcardiotomy has increased. Time is needed to determine whether this use of extracorporeal support will translate into increased survival or improve neurodevelopmental outcome in this high-risk cohort.

NITRIC OXIDE THERAPY

PPHN is a serious and sometimes lethal cardiorespiratory complication of the transition to extrauterine life. The incidence ranges from 0.43 to 6.8 per 1000 live births.[67] It is well recognized that in the absence of congenital malformations of the lung, this condition improves if the patient can be supported through the period when pulmonary vascular resistance is most volatile, often exceeding systemic vascular resistance. Support is required for a matter of only days, usually less than 2 weeks.

Potent vasodilators such as tolazoline, nitroprusside, prostaglandin E_1 (PGE_1), and prostaglandin D (PGD) have been shown in small trials to reverse the severe pulmonary vasoconstriction that causes profound hypoxemia in PPHN. Although all these medications are efficacious in lowering pulmonary vascular resistance, their use is severely limited by a lack of pulmonary selectivity. Systemic vasodilation invariably occurs, leading to hypotension, compromised tissue perfusion, and inadequate oxygen delivery to vital organs.

In 1980, Furchgott and associates described an endogenous vasodilator called *endothelium-derived relaxing factor* (EDRF).[21] In 1987, NO was identified as the molecule responsible for the biologic activity of EDRF.[35] Previously recognized as a toxic component in cigarette smoke and atmospheric pollution, NO has proven to be an important endogenous mediator of multiple physiologic processes in the human body, including regulation of vascular tone. When delivered by inhalation, NO can decrease pulmonary vascular resistance and improve pulmonary bloodflow without compromising systemic blood pressure or worsening $\dot{V}/\dot{Q}$ mismatch. At present, NO is the most selective pulmonary vasodilator available for clinical use.

Physiology and Pharmacology

NO is a short-lived, highly reactive molecule, cleaved from its precursor, arginine, by the enzyme nitric oxide synthase (NOS). NOS has been classified into two forms. The constitutive enzyme is found in endothelium, neurons, platelets, the adrenal medulla, and the macula densa of the kidney. The inducible form is generated under pathologic conditions by macrophages, hepatocytes, and airway epithelial and smooth muscle cells. NOS converts arginine to citrulline, and NO, as follows:

$$\text{Arginine} \xrightarrow{\text{NOS}} \text{Citrulline} + \text{NO}$$

Pulmonary endothelial cells are an active site of NOS activity in both fetal and newborn lung. NO generated in the endothelium enters the adjacent vascular smooth muscle where it binds to soluble guanylate cyclase. This induces a conformational change and upregulation of this enzyme, promoting synthesis of cyclic guanosine monophosphate (cGMP) from guanosine triphosphate (GTP) (Fig. 44-88). Activation of a cascade of GMP-dependent protein kinases results in calcium efflux from the cells, resulting in smooth muscle relaxation and hence pulmonary vasodilation. Intracellular cGMP is therefore a key modulator of vascular smooth muscle tone. Its biologic half-life is short, however; a family of phosphodiesterases hydrolyze and inactivate cGMP and help regulate the concentration

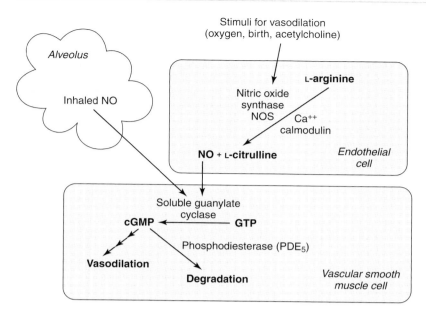

Figure 44–88. Nitric oxide (NO) is produced in the vascular endothelium during the conversion of L-arginine to L-citrulline by the enzyme NO synthase (NOS). Endogenous NO from the endothelium or exogenous NO inhaled into the alveolus diffuses to the vascular smooth muscle cell, stimulating soluble guanylate cyclase, which increases cyclic guanosine monophosphate (cGMP) production. Phosphodiesterase, specifically PDE5, hydrolyzes cGMP, reversing smooth muscle relaxation. GTP, guanosine triphosphate.

and duration of action of cGMP within the smooth muscle cell.

Lung endothelial NOS mRNA and protein are present in the early fetus and increase with advancing gestation in utero in the rat model. In the fetal lamb, intrapulmonary infusion of NOS inhibitors increases basal pulmonary vascular resistance by 35% as early as the second trimester.[1] Endogenous NO plays a pivotal role in the acute decrease in pulmonary vascular resistance at birth along with other vasodilators such as adenosine and prostacyclin. NOS expression is largely responsible for postnatal adaptation of the lung circulation following delivery. Nitrovasodilators, such as sodium nitroprusside, nitroglycerin, and the organic nitrates, donate NO through the NO cGMP pathway to promote vasodilation. When administered by inhalation NO rapidly diffuses across the alveolar membrane to relax the pulmonary vascular bed through upregulation of cGMP production. In contrast with intravenous vasodilators, inhaled NO has minimal effect on systemic vascular tone because of rapid binding and deactivation by reduced hemoglobin within the pulmonary vascular bed.

Nitric Oxide Toxicity

Clinicians should be aware of toxicity issues when using inhaled nitric oxide (iNO) in human subjects. Nitric oxide reacts with oxygen to form nitrogen dioxide (NO_2). Both NO and NO_2 are toxic, causing death in dogs at concentrations between 0.1% and 2% due to methemoglobinemia and pulmonary edema.[20] This concentration is much higher than the inhaled dose of NO used therapeutically in newborns (1 to 80 ppm) or the endogenous levels of NO produced in the endothelium (ppb). When NO reacts with superoxide in the lungs peroxynitrite is formed, which can result in membrane lipid peroxidation. Furthermore, at levels used in clinical trials, NO can inhibit platelet aggregation and adhesion. In one study, prolonged bleeding time was noted in healthy adults breathing 30 ppm iNO. However, no studies to date have reported issues of systemic bleeding with

iNO treatment. Occupational safety guidelines limit exposure to NO in the workplace to 8 hours a day at levels of 25 ppm, while 3 ppm is the upper limit for NO_2.[20] Patients treated with iNO must have methemoglobin levels monitored to ensure that levels do not exceed 5% to 7%. This is rarely a problem in neonates treated with 20 ppm or lower.

Neonatal Studies of Inhaled Nitric Oxide
TERM INFANTS

iNO has emerged as the best-studied pulmonary vasodilator in human neonates with hypoxic respiratory failure and PPHN. To date, 14 prospective, randomized trials have been published on the use of iNO in term or near-term infants with severe respiratory failure. The largest of these was the NINOS trial sponsored by the National Institute of Child Health and Human Development, in which 235 infants older than 34 weeks' gestation who had a diagnosis of hypoxic respiratory failure were randomized to iNO at 20 to 80 ppm in 91% to 96% FiO_2 versus standard ventilator management with 100% oxygen. The primary endpoint of this trial was death or ECMO. Although the mortality rate was no different in either treatment arm, there was a 40% reduction in need for ECMO among the babies treated with inhaled NO: 54% of infants required ECMO in the control arm, 39% required ECMO in the iNO treatment arm.[54] Follow-up of survivors at 2 years showed no difference in neurodevelopmental outcome between treated and control patients.[53]

In Kinsella and colleagues' study, 205 infants with PPHN were randomized to iNO and conventional ventilation or to HFOV alone.[39] Failure to respond to either treatment scheme led to crossover to the alternate study arm, and failing this, the infants received iNO plus HFOV. Treatment with HFOV and iNO proved more successful than either treatment alone in newborns with severe PPHN.

In another large multicenter trial of iNO in newborns, Clark and coworkers reported a 38% reduction in ECMO use and no difference in mortality among 248 infants with PPHN randomized to low-dose, short-duration (96 hours) iNO treatment versus control.[11] This study, unlike previous trials, showed a significant decrease in chronic lung disease in infants treated with iNO.

A meta-analysis of the results from 14 randomized trials (including the three studies detailed earlier) of iNO use in newborns with PPHN demonstrated that 50% of hypoxic near-term and term infants responded to iNO within 30 to 60 minutes.[20] The PaO_2 in the patients treated with iNO was 53 mm Hg higher (weighted mean difference) than in controls, and the OI was 15 units lower than in control patients. Mortality was not reduced in any study of iNO, perhaps because ECMO was used as a rescue therapy in nonresponders in whom severe hypoxic respiratory failure persisted.

As mentioned earlier in this section, iNO was found to be of no acute benefit in newborns with CDH. In a prospective, randomized trial of 52 infants with CDH, randomized separately in the NINOS trial, iNO neither reduced mortality nor decreased the need for ECMO. In fact, the need for ECMO was higher in the infants treated with iNO in this trial.[19] Most infants with CDH do have transient improvement in oxygenation when treated with iNO, but this response is not sustained. This observation exemplifies the importance of choosing clinically robust endpoints when testing a new drug for clinical efficacy rather than a target physiologic response (such as Po_2) which may not be sustained long enough to alter clinical outcome.

In contrast, Kinsella's group reported inhaled NO to be useful in treating a subset of older CDH patients, after surgical repair, whose pulmonary hypertension, by echocardiographic measurements, remained severe at the time of elective extubation (26 ± 3 days). Although their respiratory status was much improved (OI average 4 ± 1) after surgical repair, 10 of 47 CDH infants were found to have protracted pulmonary hypertension and were successfully treated with iNO administered through nasal cannulae until subsystemic pulmonary artery pressures were achieved. The infants received iNO in this fashion for a median of 17 days (range 5 to 60 days).[41]

The toxicity of NO and its metabolites in the newborn lung bears careful monitoring, particularly with regard to long-term exposure. The incidence of chronic lung disease is not higher in infants treated with iNO compared to untreated controls with similar disease severity. On the contrary, a prospective randomized study of low dose (5 ppm) iNO treatment in newborns greater than 34 week's gestation with PPHN reported a substantial reduction in the rate of BPD among survivors treated with iNO.[11] Despite its known antiplatelet activity, there have been no increased bleeding complications reported among preterm neonates treated with NO in randomized clinical trials.

On the evidence available, including the neurodevelopmental and general medical outcome information, near-term and term infants with hypoxic respiratory failure unresponsive to oxygen and ventilator support, excluding infants with CDH, should have a trial of iNO. This therapy significantly reduces the need for ECMO with the number needed to treat (NNT) of 5.3.[20] Therapy should be confined to infants who are severely ill with an OI greater than 25. Starting treatment earlier does not further reduce mortality or the need for ECMO.[43]

PREMATURE INFANTS

In preterm infants, survival and outcome are limited by respiratory distress syndrome (RDS) and its sequela, bronchopulmonary dysplasia (BPD). There are many potential short-term and long-term benefits of iNO in preterm newborns (Box 44-16). However, the use of iNO in this high-risk cohort was approached with trepidation because of the increased risk of intracranial hemorrhage and NO's known antiplatelet effect. Early pilot trials confirmed acute improvement in oxygenation in preterm (less than 1500 g) infants with severe hypoxic respiratory failure treated with iNO. However, survival was not improved, and the rate of intracranial bleeding was alarmingly high.

Several large randomized trials of iNO use in preterms have now been completed where the primary outcome focuses on survival without BPD. In a single center trial, Schreiber and colleagues randomized 207 infants with low birthweight (less than 1500 g) to treatment with a 7-day course of iNO or placebo starting on the first day of life. The authors reported a 24% reduction in the incidence of BPD and death in the iNO groups, largely accrued in the subset of infants with milder respiratory failure (OI <6.94). A 47% decrease in severe intracranial hemorrhage (ICH) and periventricular leukomalacia (PVL) was also noted.[57] At 2-year follow-up, 24% of the iNO-treated patients had abnormal neurodevelopment compared with 46% of the control group (NNT=5).[49]

Van Meurs and colleagues enrolled 420 newborns (401 to 1500 g birthweight) in a multicenter randomized, controlled trial through the NICHD.[63] Only responders (i.e., infants showing improved PaO_2) continued on inhaled NO; the average treatment duration was 76 hours. They found no difference in the incidence of death or BPD at 36 weeks' postmenstrual age between the iNO and control groups. Post hoc analysis revealed that NO reduced these rates in neonates weighing more than 1000 g, however. A higher rate of ICH and PVL noted in the infants weighing less than 1000 g (43% iNO versus 33% control) was concerning. An editorial accompanying this manuscript pointed out that Van Meurs and colleagues' patients were smaller, more immature, and had more severe respiratory

---

BOX 44–16 Potential Benefits of Inhaled Nitric Oxide in Preterm Infants

SHORT-TERM
Selective pulmonary vasodilation
Improvement in $\dot{V}/\dot{Q}$ matching
Decreased neutrophil accumulation and activation
Improvement in oxygenation and hypoxic respiratory failure

LONG-TERM
Reduced need for oxygen and decrease in oxidant stress
Improved surfactant function
Decreased airway resistance
Improved lung growth due to stimulation of angiogenesis and alveolarization

From Arul N, Konduri GG: Inhaled nitric oxide for preterm neonates, *Clin Perinatol* 36:43, 2009.

failure at study entry compared with Schreiber's study, making comparisons between the two trials problematic.

In 2006, two large prospective, randomized trials of iNO in preterm babies were published. Kinsella and colleagues randomized 793 newborns, less than 34 weeks' gestation, within 48 hours of birth, to 5 ppm iNO versus placebo gas for 21 days or until extubation. OI at study entry was 5.4 to 5.8. There was no difference in the incidence of death or BPD between groups. However, iNO reduced the incidence of BPD by 50% for infants with birthweights greater than 1000 g ($P = .001$, NNT 3). Low-dose iNO reduced the combined incidence of intracranial hemorrhage, PVL, and ventriculomegaly for the entire study population receiving iNO ($P = .032$, NNT 16).[42]

Ballard and colleagues, also in 2006, reported on the outcome of their prospective, randomized, controlled and masked trial of iNO treatment of preterm infants.[4] Five hundred eighty-two infants who required ventilatory support between 7 and 21 days of age were randomized (birthweight 500 to 1250 g). Infants were enrolled in the study with an estimated OI between 5 and 9; treatment with iNO versus study gas lasted a minimum of 24 days. The incidence of survival without BPD was increased in the iNO treatment group (43.9%) compared with controls (36.8%, $P = .04$, NNT 14). This effect was largely noted in those treated between 7 and 14 days of life, suggesting that early treatment is important to prevent BPD. One-year follow-up of study survivors was notable for decreased pulmonary sequelae reflected in decreased medication requirement in the iNO cohort.[29]

Recently, a large multicenter masked, placebo-controlled trial of inhaled nitric oxide (iNO) for the prevention of bronchopulmonary dysplasia (BPD) in preterm infants was published. Eight hundred infants between 24 and 28 6/7 weeks' gestation were randomized from 36 centers in 9 countries in the European Union. Infants were enrolled within 24 hours of birth and received either low-dose iNO (5 ppm) or placebo (nitrogen gas) for 7 to 21 days. In this industry-sponsored study, neither survival nor the incidence of BPD at 36 weeks' postmenstrual age was improved with iNO treatment.[48]

In summary, the available evidence from randomized trials detailed in this section suggests that low-dose iNO may be safe and effective in reducing the risk of death or BPD for the subset of preterm infants weighing more than 1000 g at birth. A neuroprotective effect was present in some, but not all, treated patients. This effect was larger in infants with lower disease severity at study entry. The apparent lack of efficacy in the tiniest, most immature preterm infants is disappointing, especially in light of animal data, which suggest that NO plays a key role in lung morphogenesis.[2]

Alternative Treatments and Avenues for Future Research

Future clinical trials of nitric oxide will better define the neonatal patient population for whom this inhalational treatment is efficacious. The optimum dose and duration of therapy require further refinement. For the 30% to 40% of near-term and term newborns with PPHN who fail to respond to iNO, or who do not sustain improvement in oxygenation, other drugs are available for study. Particularly in countries with limited medical resources, alternative treatment to costly iNO or ECMO would be most welcome.

A different, but related, approach to the treatment of PPHN would be to augment endogenous vasodilator therapy by inhibiting the rapid degradation of cyclic nucleotide second messengers, cGMP and cAMP, which play a central role in modulating smooth muscle relaxation in the pulmonary vascular bed. Phosphodiesterases (PDEs) have a wide distribution in normal mammalian tissues. They are divided into 11 distinct families based on substrate specificity and sensitivity. PDE5 inhibitors block the degradation of cyclic GMP (NO pathway) and PDE3 blocks the degradation of cyclic AMP (prostacycline pathway), both of which potentiate vasodilation.

Sildenafil is a specific PD5 inhibitor used primarily to treat erectile dysfunction. A number of small case studies have explored the therapeutic potential of sildenafil in treating PPHN because the lung is particularly rich in PDE5. In a double-blind, randomized, placebo-controlled study in 278 adults with primary pulmonary hypertension, sildenafil reduced mean pulmonary artery pressure and improved functional class of disease severity over 12 weeks of treatment. Sustained improvement over 1 year of treatment with sildenafil in adults with pulmonary arterial hypertension (PAH) was also confirmed, leading to Food and Drug Administration (FDA) approval for this drug in adults with PAH. However, safety and efficacy of sildenafil in the treatment of newborns with PPHN has not yet been established. In one small study, 13 patients were randomized to sildenafil treatment (n = 7) or placebo (n = 6). HFOV, iNO, and ECMO were not available in this center. The study was terminated early due to the deaths of six patients enrolled, five of whom were in the control arm.[5] Large randomized studies investigating the role of sildenafil as a single treatment agent, or in combination with iNO, for refractory PPHN have yet to be done.

A study on the kinetics of intravenous sildenafil in 36 infants with PPHN has been published.[52] Affected infants were treated within 72 hours of birth for a mean duration of 77 hours. Sildenafil clearance increased rapidly over the first 7 days of life, presumably due to increased hepatic clearance. Adverse side effects were mild to moderate in severity, and included hypotension (three subjects), labile blood pressure (one subject), and PDA (one subject). These data will pave the way for future clinical trials of this drug in newborns who are particularly sensitive to systemic vasodilation and $\dot{V}/\dot{Q}$ mismatch. The use of this potent vasodilating agent should be limited to prospective randomized trials until more information on the drug's safety and efficacy in the neonate becomes available.

Prostacyclin (Flolan; epoprestenol sodium), which affects pulmonary relaxation through upregulation of cyclic AMP levels, has emerged as one of the primary treatments of idiopathic pulmonary hypertension in adults and children where the drug is given by continuous intravenous infusion in nanogram doses.[33,46] Randomized trials of prostacyclin in PPHN have not been done. This drug has been used in small case series for the treatment of pulmonary hypertension in infants beyond the newborn period, however, with some success. Milrinone, a PD3 inhibitor, is widely used in intensive care as an inotrope and afterload-reducing agent. It has been described in case series to be useful in the treatment of pulmonary hypertension, particularly in the face of cardiac dysfunction. In the laboratory, milrinone enhances relaxation to prostacyclin and iloprost in pulmonary arteries isolated from a lamb model of PPHN.[44]

Iloprost, an aerosolized prostanoid, has been proven efficacious in adults with pulmonary hypertension, and has been successful in small case series in PPHN. Its drawback in adults is the requirement for aerosol treatments eight to 10 times per day. In the NICU, given the time frame of PPHN, this could be achievable. Blood pressure instability remains an issue with this as with any prostanoid; therefore, the use of iloprost should be confined to investigational pilot trials for the time being.[46]

Endothelin is a potent vasoconstrictor and a smooth muscle mitogen that may contribute to the development of PPHN. Increased endothelin levels have been measured in newborns with PPHN. Medications are available that block the endothelin receptors on vascular smooth muscle cells in the lung and ameliorate pulmonary vasoconstriction in adults with pulmonary hypertension. Bosentan is the most widely studied of these and is approved by the FDA for the treatment of pulmonary hypertension in adults. Bosentan improved cardiac index, and reduced mean PAP and PVR; functional class also improved in patients treated with bosentan. Liver toxicity, which appears to be dose dependent, is seen in 25% of bosentan-treated adults.[33,46] Whether this drug has any therapeutic efficacy in PPHN remains to be elucidated.

As with many new therapies, early reports of treatment response to NO were almost euphoric. Randomized, controlled trials have proven the efficacy of this inhaled vasodilator in PPHN, but they have also tempered our enthusiasm with the reality that up to 40% of term and near-term newborns with severe respiratory failure will not respond to iNO and still require ECMO support. For the preterm infant, the efficacy of iNO remains less certain. The lack of response in the more immature preterm infants (less than 1000 g birthweight) raises the question of whether these patients might require a longer course of iNO in order to enjoy the same benefits as their more mature counterparts with birthweights greater than 1000 g.

Lastly, the treatment of late-onset pulmonary hypertension in surviving infants with very low birthweight and BPD has emerged as a serious therapeutic challenge. Mortality in this cohort is high, and treatment with a variety of pulmonary vasodilators is being used with little evidence for which drug combinations are efficacious. A recent study of patients with BPD and pulmonary hypertension reported survival rates of 64% at 6 months and 52% at 2 years after the diagnosis of pulmonary hypertension.[38] Mourani and coworkers reported the effects of long-term sildenafil use for the treatment of pulmonary hypertension in infants younger than 2 years with chronic lung disease stemming from the neonatal period.[51] Eighteen of 25 were infants with low birthweight and BPD. The drug was judged to be well tolerated and effective in treated patients; median treatment duration was 241 days (range 28 to 950 days). However, 28% of treated patients also received other drugs for pulmonary vasodilation, including NO, calcium channel blockers, milrinone, and bosentan. Five of the 25 died during the 8-month follow-up period, emphasizing the vulnerability of this uniquely fragile cohort of NICU graduates.

Adjunctive therapies, as those discussed above, appear promising and may enhance the benefit of iNO, or replace this inhalational agent altogether. Within the relatively short period of neonatal intensive care, the discovery and use of one selective pulmonary vasodilator, such as iNO, represents a significant advance. Hopefully we can look forward to several treatment options for pulmonary hypertension once the therapeutic efficacy of these agents has been rigorously tested.

REFERENCES

1. Abman SH: Abnormal vasoreactivity in the pathophysiology of persistent pulmonary hypertension of the newborn, *Pediatr Rev* 20:e103, 1999.
2. Abman SH: Recent advances in the pathogenesis and treatment of persistent pulmonary hypertension of the newborn, *Neonatology* 91:283, 2007.
3. Alsoufi B, et al: Extracorporeal life support in neonates, infants, and children after repair of congenital heart disease: modern era results in a single institution, *Ann Thorac Surg* 80:15, 2005.
4. Ballard RA, et al: Inhaled nitric oxide in preterm infants undergoing mechanical ventilation, *N Engl J Med* 355: 343, 2006.
5. Baquero H, et al: Oral sildenafil in infants with persistent pulmonary hypertension of the newborn: a pilot randomized blinded study, *Pediatrics* 117:1077, 2006.
6. Bartlett RH, et al: Extracorporeal membrane oxygenation (ECMO) in neonatal respiratory failure. 100 cases, *Ann Surg* 204:236, 1986.
7. Boedy RF, et al: Hidden mortality rate associated with extracorporeal membrane oxygenation, *J Pediatr* 117:462, 1990.
8. Boloker J, et al: Congenital diaphragmatic hernia in 120 infants treated consecutively with permissive hypercapnea/spontaneous respiration/elective repair, *J Pediatr Surg* 37:357, 2002.
9. Boucherat O, et al: Surfactant maturation is not delayed in human fetuses with diaphragmatic hernia, *PLoS Med* 4:e237, 2007.
10. Clark RH, et al: Current surgical management of congenital diaphragmatic hernia: a report from the Congenital Diaphragmatic Hernia Study Group, *J Pediatr Surg* 33:1004, 1998.
11. Clark RH, et al: Low-dose nitric oxide therapy for persistent pulmonary hypertension of the newborn. Clinical Inhaled Nitric Oxide Research Group, *N Engl J Med* 342:469, 2000.
12. Clugston RD, et al: Gene expression in the developing diaphragm: significance for congenital diaphragmatic hernia, *Am J Physiol Lung Cell Mol Physiol* 294:L665, 2008.
13. Colby CE, et al: Surfactant replacement therapy on ECMO does not improve outcome in neonates with congenital diaphragmatic hernia, *J Pediatr Surg* 39:1632, 2004.
14. Deprest J, et al: Fetal intervention for congenital diaphragmatic hernia: the European experience, *Semin Perinatol* 29:94, 2005.
15. Deprest J, et al: Current consequences of prenatal diagnosis of congenital diaphragmatic hernia, *J Pediatr Surg* 41:423, 2006.
16. Desai SA, et al: Five-year follow-up of neonates with reconstructed right common carotid arteries after extracorporeal membrane oxygenation, *J Pediatr* 134:428, 1999.
17. Extracorporeal Life Support Organization: *ELSO Registry Report: International Summary.* 2010, Ann Arbor, MI
18. Field J: UK collaboration randomized trial of neonatal extracorporeal membrane oxygenation, *Lancet* 348:75, 1996.

19. Finer N: Inhaled nitric oxide and hypoxic respiratory failure in infants with CDH, *Pediatrics* 99:838, 1997.

20. Finer NN, Barrington KJ: Nitric oxide for respiratory failure in infants born at or near term, *Cochrane Database Syst Rev* CD000399, 2006.

21. Furchgott RF, Zawadzki JV: The obligatory role of endothelial cells in the relaxation of arterial smooth muscle by acetylcholine, *Nature* 288:373, 1980.

22. Gallot D, et al: Antenatal detection and impact on outcome of congenital diaphragmatic hernia: a 12-year experience in Auvergne, France, *Eur J Obstet Gynecol Reprod Biol* 125:202, 2006.

23. Gaxiola A, et al: Congenital diaphragmatic hernia: an overview of the etiology and current management, *Acta Paediatr* 98:621, 2009.

24. Greer JJ, et al: Etiology of congenital diaphragmatic hernia: the retinoid hypothesis, *Pediatr Res* 53:726, 2003.

25. Gucciardo L, et al: Prediction of outcome in isolated congenital diaphragmatic hernia and its consequences for fetal therapy, *Best Pract Res Clin Obstet Gynaecol* 22:123, 2008.

26. Hardart GE, et al: Intracranial hemorrhage in premature neonates treated with extracorporeal membrane oxygenation correlates with conceptional age, *J Pediatr* 145:184, 2004.

27. Harrison MR, et al: A randomized trial of fetal endoscopic tracheal occlusion for severe fetal congenital diaphragmatic hernia, *N Engl J Med* 349:1916, 2003.

28. Hibbs A, et al: Outcome of infants with bronchopulmonary dysplasia who receive extracorporeal membrane oxygenation therapy, *J Pediatr Surg* 36:1479, 2001.

29. Hibbs AM, et al: One-year respiratory outcomes of preterm infants enrolled in the Nitric Oxide (to prevent) Chronic Lung Disease trial, *J Pediatr* 153:525, 2008.

30. Hines MH, Hansell DR: Elective extracorporeal support for complex tracheal reconstruction in neonates, *Ann Thorac Surg* 76:175, 2003.

31. Hines MH: ECMO and congenital heart disease, *Semin Perinatol* 29:34, 2005.

32. Holder AM, et al: Genetic factors in congenital diaphragmatic hernia, *Am J Hum Genet* 80:825, 2007.

33. Humbert M, et al: Treatment of pulmonary arterial hypertension, *N Engl J Med* 351:1425, 2004.

34. Hunkeler NM, et al: Extracorporeal life support in cyanotic congenital heart disease before cardiovascular operation, *Am J Cardiol* 69:790, 1992.

35. Ignarro LJ, et al: Endothelium-derived relaxing factor produced and released from artery and vein is nitric oxide, *Proc Natl Acad Sci U S A* 84:9265, 1987.

36. Jani JC, et al: Fetal lung-to-head ratio in the prediction of survival in severe left-sided diaphragmatic hernia treated by fetal endoscopic tracheal occlusion (FETO), *Am J Obstet Gynecol* 195:1646, 2006.

37. Keijzer R, et al: Dual-hit hypothesis explains pulmonary hypoplasia in the nitrofen model of congenital diaphragmatic hernia, *Am J Pathol* 156:1299, 2000.

38. Khemani E, et al: Pulmonary artery hypertension in formerly premature infants with bronchopulmonary dysplasia: clinical features and outcomes in the surfactant era, *Pediatrics* 120:1260, 2007.

39. Kinsella JP, et al: Randomized, multicenter trial of inhaled nitric oxide and high-frequency oscillatory ventilation in severe, persistent pulmonary hypertension of the newborn, *J Pediatr* 131:55, 1997.

40. Kinsella JP, et al: Use of inhaled nitric oxide during interhospital transport of newborns with hypoxemic respiratory failure, *Pediatrics* 109:158, 2002.

41. Kinsella JP, et al: Noninvasive delivery of inhaled nitric oxide therapy for late pulmonary hypertension in newborn infants with congenital diaphragmatic hernia, *J Pediatr* 142:397, 2003.

42. Kinsella JP, et al: Early inhaled nitric oxide therapy in premature newborns with respiratory failure, *N Engl J Med* 355:354, 2006.

43. Konduri GG, et al: A randomized trial of early versus standard inhaled nitric oxide therapy in term and near-term newborn infants with hypoxic respiratory failure, *Pediatrics* 113:559, 2004.

44. Lakshminrusimha S, et al: Milrinone enhances relaxation to prostacyclin and iloprost in pulmonary arteries isolated from lambs with persistent pulmonary hypertension of the newborn, *Pediatr Crit Care Med* 10:106, 2009.

45. Lotze A, et al: Multicenter study of surfactant (beractant) use in the treatment of term infants with severe respiratory failure. Survanta in Term Infants Study Group, *J Pediatr* 132:40, 1998.

46. McLaughlin VV, et al: ACCF/AHA 2009 expert consensus document on pulmonary hypertension: a report of the American College of Cardiology Foundation Task Force on Expert Consensus Documents and the American Heart Association: developed in collaboration with the American College of Chest Physicians, American Thoracic Society, Inc., and the Pulmonary Hypertension Association, *Circulation* 119:2250, 2009.

47. McNally H, et al: United Kingdom collaborative randomized trial of neonatal extracorporeal membrane oxygenation: follow-up to age 7 years, *Pediatrics* 117:e845, 2006.

48. Mercier JC, Hummler H, Durrmeyer X, et al: from the EUNO Study Group: Inhaled nitric oxide for prevention of bronchopulmonary dysplasia in premature babies (EUNO): a randomized controlled trial, *Lancet* 376:346, 2010.

49. Mestan KK, et al: Neurodevelopmental outcomes of premature infants treated with inhaled nitric oxide, *N Engl J Med* 353:23, 2005.

50. Montedonico S, et al: Congenital diaphragmatic hernia and retinoids: searching for an etiology, *Pediatr Surg Int* 24:755, 2008.

51. Mourani PM, et al: Effects of long-term sildenafil treatment for pulmonary hypertension in infants with chronic lung disease, *J Pediatr* 154:379, 2008.

52. Mukherjee A, et al: Population pharmacokinetics of sildenafil in term neonates: evidence of rapid maturation of metabolic clearance in the early postnatal period, *Clin Pharmacol Ther* 85:56, 2009.

53. Neonatal Inhaled Nitric Oxide Study Group: Inhaled nitric oxide in term and near-term infants: neurodevelopmental follow-up of the neonatal inhaled nitric oxide study group (NINOS), *J Pediatr* 136:611, 2000.

54. Neonatal Inhaled Nitric Oxide Study Group [NINOS]: Inhaled nitric oxide in full term and nearly full term infants with hypoxic respiratory failure, *N Engl J Med* 336:597, 1997.

55. Petrou S, et al: Cost-effectiveness of neonatal extracorporeal membrane oxygenation based on 7-year results from the United Kingdom Collaborative ECMO Trial, *Pediatrics* 117:1640, 2006.

56. Richmond S, Atkins J: A population-based study of the prenatal diagnosis of congenital malformation over 16 years, *Br J Obstet Gynaecol* 112:1349, 2005.

57. Schreiber MD, et al: Inhaled nitric oxide in premature infants with the respiratory distress syndrome, *N Engl J Med* 349:2099, 2003.

58. Scott DA: Genetics of congenital diaphragmatic hernia, *Semin Pediatr Surg* 16:88, 2007.

59. Shah SA, et al: Clinical outcomes of 84 children with congenital heart disease managed with extracorporeal membrane oxygenation after cardiac surgery, *Asaio J* 51:504, 2005.

60. Sinha CK, et al: Congenital diaphragmatic hernia: prognostic indices in the fetal endoluminal tracheal occlusion era, *J Pediatr Surg* 44:312, 2009.

61. Skarsgard ED, Harrison MR: The surgeon's prospective, *Pediatr Rev Online* 20:e71, 1999.

62. Van Meurs KP, et al: ECMO for neonatal respiratory failure. In: Van Meurs L, et al, editors: *ECMO: extracorporeal cardiopulmonary support in critical care,* 3rd ed, Ann Arbor, MI, 2005, ELSO, pp 273-296.

63. Van Meurs KP, et al: Inhaled nitric oxide for premature infants with severe respiratory failure, *N Engl J Med* 353:13, 2005.

64. Vaucher YE, et al: Predictors of early childhood outcome in candidates for extracorporeal membrane oxygenation, *J Pediatr* 128:109, 1996.

65. Walker GM, et al: Extracorporeal life support as a treatment of supraventricular tachycardia in infants, *Pediatr Crit Care Med* 4:52, 2003.

66. Walsh-Sukys MC, et al: Severe respiratory failure in neonates: mortality and morbidity rates and neurodevelopmental outcomes, *J Pediatr* 125:104, 1994.

67. Walsh-Sukys MC, et al: Persistent pulmonary hypertension of the newborn in the era before nitric oxide: practice variation and outcomes, *Pediatrics* 105:14, 2000.

68. Wilson JM, et al: Congenital diaphragmatic hernia—a tale of two cities: the Boston experience, *J Pediatr Surg* 32:401, 1997.

69. Wung JT, et al: Congenital diaphragmatic hernia: survival treated with very delayed surgery, spontaneous respiration, and no chest tube, *J Pediatr Surg* 30:406, 1995.

CHAPTER **45**

The Cardiovascular System

The practice of the care of children with heart disease has increasingly become a neonatal specialty. Fetal diagnosis of congenital heart defects is now routine. Reparative cardiovascular surgery is commonplace in the first month of life and is now undertaken in utero. Defects once considered inoperable, most notably hypoplastic left heart syndrome, can be treated, with greatly improved long-term results. In parallel with these clinical advances, there has been exciting progress in understanding the cellular and molecular basis of normal and abnormal cardiogenesis and the relationship of heart defects to other congenital defects. The expansion in our understanding from combining clinical and basic science findings may lead to better predict the severity and consequences of congenital heart defects and also lead to strategies for alleviating the consequences to children and adults.

PART 1

Cardiac Embryology
Michiko Watanabe, Katherine S. Schaefer, Jamie Wikenheiser, Florence Rothenberg, and Ganga Karunamuni

The development of the heart has been a topic of study for hundreds of years. Nonetheless, many surprisingly basic questions have yet to be answered. For example, how does the cardiac pacemaking and conduction system develop, what factors allow the heart tube to bend in one direction and not the other, and how does the coronary vasculature develop in a stereotyped pattern? With the advent of new technologies and fields of study, these and other questions are being revisited, and answers are beginning to emerge. In combination with the traditional techniques, these new approaches have significantly advanced our understanding of normal and abnormal development.

Much of the current knowledge about cardiovascular development is based on studies of species other than humans, notably the chicken, quail, mouse, rabbit, fruit fly, and zebrafish. Remarkable similarities have been detected

in molecular and cellular developmental mechanisms among these diverse species. Research on the developmental genetics of the fruit fly, for example, has made an impact on our basic understanding of genes important for vertebrate systems, including humans. In the other direction, information from clinics has been analyzed in detail in more easily accessible and manipulable systems such as the fruit fly, zebrafish, chicken, or mouse. The distance between the bedside and the bench is getting shorter.

The mature heart is the product of gene expression driven by endogenous and exogenous influences. The developing heart manifests its morphologic and physiologic plasticity under stress. A detailed understanding of the effects of the factors that drive normal cardiogenesis is necessary for understanding the causes and consequences of abnormal development. Errors in cardiac morphogenesis involved with septation, valve formation, and proper patterning of the great vessels are responsible for most forms of congenital heart disease. Normal heart development requires precise timing for coordination of the complex three-dimensional contortions of tissues, but paradoxically, these tissues also have a remarkable capacity for regulation that compensates for mistakes. This compensation can allow abnormal heart structures and functions to be compatible with life up to and even after birth, but complicates identification of primary and secondary cardiac anomalies.

It is possible to investigate cardiovascular development at various levels using a variety of disciplines: molecular biology, biochemistry, biomedical engineering, cell and tissue biology, genetics, physiology, and epidemiology. Significant results have emerged when information was shared across disciplines. For example, the hemizygous deletion in the elastin gene has been shown to be responsible for Williams syndrome (or Williams-Beuren syndrome), the autosomal dominant form of supravalvular aortic stenosis.[35] Predictions about the clinical manifestations of this disease were elucidated after mutant elastin proteins were found in humans; existence of these mutant proteins was proposed based on knowledge about the protein structure provided by studies at the bench. In the reverse direction, analysis of the mutant human proteins in animal models, in tissue cultures, and in in vitro studies advanced understanding of the disease and of the biochemistry and role of elastin in vascular cell signaling. The passage of information across these investigative levels has resulted in a remarkably productive synergy.

OVERVIEW OF NORMAL HEART DEVELOPMENT

The following description of human heart development, especially the earlier events, is synthesized from information provided by studies of animal models and human embryonic and fetal tissues. A timetable of selected events in human heart development is presented in Table 45-1.[29,32,40] Figure 45-1 is a diagram depicting the major transitions in early mammalian heart development.[43]

The primordia of the heart are identified as bilaterally symmetric heart fields derived from the lateral plate mesoderm. These primordia migrate through the primitive streak between the ectoderm and endoderm layers to become symmetric mesoderm regions on either side of the primitive streak. These tissues fuse cranially to form a tubular structure comprising an inner layer of endocardium, a thick layer of extracellular matrix, and an outer layer of myocardium. This simple tube begins to contract rhythmically and grows differentially so that dilations (primordia of the heart chambers) and constrictions (primordia of the partitions between chambers) appear along its length. Later additions to the distal ends of the tubular heart form the outflow tract (OFT) and the sinus venosus. Dextral looping of the tube brings the venous caudal portion to a more dorsal position and to the left of the arterial cranial portion as septation of the tubular heart begins. The epicardium arises from tissue dorsal to the heart at the level of the atrioventricular (AV) junction and spreads over the outer surface of the myocardium as a layer of squamous epithelial cells and associated connective tissue during the early phase of septation.

The atrial chamber, arising from expansion of a caudal region, divides into two chambers by the growth of a crescentic ridge from the anterodorsal wall at the narrowest point of the atrial chamber. This ridge grows and fuses with the dorsal and ventral endocardial cushions, which are themselves growing and fusing with each other. Before the atrial septum completely closes the ostium primum, perforations appear and coalesce in the dorsal portion of the septum to form a single opening: the ostium secundum, later termed the *foramen ovale*. A second atrial septum subsequently grows to the right of the primary atrial septum; in conjunction with the primary atrial septum, it forms a one-way valve (right-to-left blood flow only) between the two atria in the fetus. This avenue of blood flow is permanently closed shortly after birth to complete atrial septation.

Ventricular septation begins after the primary atrial septum is formed. The ventricular septum results from the growth and remodeling of trabecular sheets, continues with expansion of the ventricular chambers, and ends with the fusion of several tissues, including endocardial cushions and the muscular septum, to form the membranous and muscular interventricular septum. The OFT septation is the result of growth and fusion of spiraling ridges that eventually divide the truncus into aortic and pulmonary tracts. The venous and arterial vessels (aortic arches) undergo degeneration, fusion, and growth to attain the mature structures.

The human heart has completed the major morphogenetic processes 8 weeks after fertilization. What follows is the completion of maturation of structures, growth, accumulation of cellular junctions at the intercalated discs, biochemical adjustments, and compensation for the changes in patterns of blood flow after birth, such as permanent closure of the foramen ovale of the atrial septum and closure and fibrosis of the ductus arteriosus.

SCIENTIFIC BASIS OF CARDIOGENESIS

Precardiac to Cardiac Tissues: Commitment and Formation of Primary Axes

The tissue regions giving rise to the heart have been mapped by the application of dyes, particles, and radiolabels to stages when the vertebrate embryo comprises two layers: the epiblast (or ectoderm) and the endoderm. The process of gastrulation, the movement of precardiac epiblast cells through the primitive streak, appears to be important in specification. These early determinative events have been elucidated largely by studying fruit fly genetics and by manipulating amphibian and avian embryos.

Transcription factors are proteins that bind as complexes to specific DNA sequences and influence the expression of genes (Fig. 45-2).[8,12] Such factors influence many aspects of cardiogenesis[12] and include members of the following families: the helix-loop-helix proteins (dHand and eHand), zinc finger proteins (GATAs), homeobox gene proteins (NKX2.5), and MADS box proteins related to serum response factor. Of the zinc finger proteins, GATA4, 5, and 6 are much studied members of the evolutionarily conserved transcription factor subfamily that recognizes a "GATA" DNA sequence motif. These have been implicated in the early specification of embryonic tissue destined to become heart.

An example from the homeobox gene family demonstrates how the study of fruit flies has advanced our understanding of human heart development. The dorsal vessel pumps hemolymph (insect blood) and is considered the insect heart. It is derived from mesoderm under the influence of homeobox genes. The mutation of one of these genes, *tinman*, results in absence of the dorsal vessel. Frog and mouse homologues of these homeobox genes were identified and localized in expression to the developing heart. Transgenic mice lacking a *tinman* homologue (NKX2.5) do not lack a heart but die at 9 days of development with a severely abnormal heart.[25] Humans in whom the *tinman* homologue NKX2.5 is mutated suffer atrial septal defects with associated AV conduction delay.[38] The fruit fly findings led to the study of a set of genes critically important in many aspects of human heart development.

The Tubular and Looping Heart

Tubular morphogenesis is initiated as two epithelia form a tube-within-a-tube structure from the migrating primordial heart tissue. Concurrent with this process, endocardial and myocardial cells—which form the layers of the developing heart—emerge from a common precursor.[23] This tissue progression requires cell differentiation, sorting, and polarization. Evidence supports both negative and positive influences from the surrounding neural tissue and endoderm on these processes.

During the tubular heart stages, the primordia of the peripheral cardiac structures continue to be added sequentially

TABLE 45–1   Developmental Landmarks in Cardiac Morphogenesis

Week	Days	Somites	Length (mm)*	Stage†	Developmental Events
3	15			VIII	(Primitive streak)
	16				
	17				
	18	1-3	1.5	IX	Blood islands in chorion, stalk, yolk sac
	19				
	20	1	1.5		Cardiogenic plate
	21	4			Tubes (2) connect with blood vessels
4	22	4-7	2	X	Tubes fuse
	23			X	Single median tube (first contractions), looping begins
	24	13-20	2.5-3	XI	
	25				
	26	21-29	3.5	XII	Cardiac loop
	27				Single atrium
	28	25	4-5	XIII	Bilobed atrium, primary AS begins growth
5	29		6-7	XIV	IVS appears
	30	28			Primary AS continues growth (placental circulation begins)
	31		7-8	XV	Ridges form inside outflow tract
	32				Primary AS begins perforation formation
	33		9-10	XVI	
	34			XVII	Secondary AS begins to grow; primary AS has foramen secundum
	35		11-14		AV cushions begin fusion (three-chambered heart)
6	36				Arterial (aortic arch) and venous morphogenesis begins
	37		14-16	XVIII	IVS growing
	38				
	39		17-20	XIX	
	40				Septation of bulbus and ventricle, valve formation
	41		21-23	XX	IVS maturation continues, AV canal splits into two
	42				
7	43		22-24	XXI	Beginning of separation of AV myocardial connection
	44		25-27	XXIII	(Fetal stages begin)
	45				
	46				
	47				
	48				
	49				Membranous and muscular IVS is complete, resulting in four-chambered heart
24-40			210-360		Birth and beginning of neonatal circulation

*Crown-to-rump measurements.
†Roman numerals refer to Streeter horizons.
AS, atrial septum; AV, atrioventricular; IVS, interventricular septum.
Data from Moore KL: *The developing human: clinically oriented embryology*, Philadelphia, 1982, Saunders; Pansky B: *Review of medical embryology*, New York, 1982, Macmillan; and Sissman NJ: Developmental landmarks in cardiac morphogenesis: comparative chronology, *Am J Cardiol* 25:141, 1970.

Figure 45–1. Major transitions in early mouse heart development. A, Cardiac crescent at mouse embryonic day 7.5 (human embryonic day 18); B, in cross section. C, Linear heart tube at mouse embryonic day 8.25 (human embryonic day 22); D, in cross section. E, Looping heart at mouse embryonic day 10.5 (human embryonic day 25); F, in cross section. G, Remodeling chambered heart at mouse embryonic day 12.5 (human embryonic day 35); H, in cross section. *Dark shading* represents myocardial tissue. AV, atrioventricular; E, embryonic day; LA, left atrium; LV, left ventricle; RA, right atrium; RV, right ventricle. (*Reprinted from Solloway MJ, Harvey RP: Molecular pathways in myocardial development: a stem cell perspective, Cardiovasc Res 58:264, 2003. Copyright 2003 with permission from The European Society of Cardiology.*)

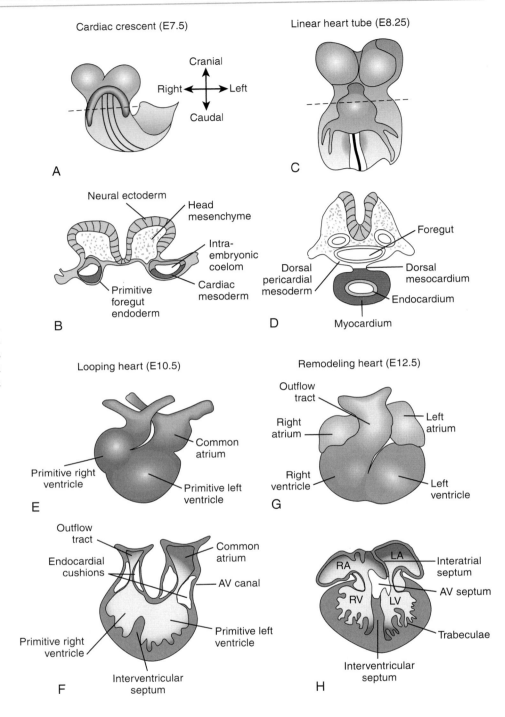

from the proximal to the distal at both the arterial and venous ends. The myocardial cells of the tubular heart begin very early to express cardiac-specific cytoskeletal components.

How is this program for cardiac muscle differentiation turned on and regulated? This question has been approached by studying the transcription factors that bind to promoter regions of the cardiac-specific cytoskeletal genes coding for molecules that appear in the early tubular heart. The discovery of myoD, a helix-loop-helix DNA-binding protein that controls skeletal muscle expression, led investigators to search for similar factors in cardiac muscle. To date, no such single factor has been defined. Current findings support the idea that both positive and negative regulators of cardiac genes exist and that they work in complexes that define the spatiotemporal pattern of expression of cardiac genes (see Fig. 45-2).

Closely related to the question of cardiac-specific gene regulation is the question of regional specification of the heart tube. Segmentation, although not as obvious in the vertebrate heart as it is in the insect body plan, is important in cardiogenesis. Chamber-specific expression of a number of endogenous genes and promoter-driven reporter genes suggests that the

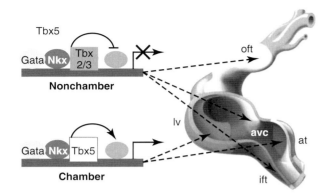

Figure 45–2. Model of transcription regulation of cardiac chamber and nonchamber genes. *NKX2.5, GATA4,* and *TBX5* are widely expressed in the developing heart and promote chamber-specific gene expression (chamber), whereas *TBX2* and *TBX3* are differentially expressed and inhibit chamber-specific gene expression by competing with *TBX5* binding (nonchamber). Chambers are the left ventricle (lv) and the atrium (at). Nonchamber regions include the outflow tract (oft), atrioventricular canal (avc), and inflow tract (ift). These proteins bind to DNA at specific sequences that are involved in controlling gene expression. The combinatorial effect of the binding of these proteins depresses or stimulates the transcription of cardiac-specific genes. (*Modified from Dunwoodie SL: Combinatorial signaling in the heart orchestrates cardiac induction, lineage specification and chamber formation,* Semin Cell Dev Biol *18:54, 2007; originally from Christoffels, et al: Architectural plan for the heart: early patterning and delineation of the chambers and the nodes,* Trends Cardiovasc Med *14:301, 2004.*)

outflow tract (OFT), the left and right ventricles, the atria, and the sinus venosus can in some cases be considered separate cardiac segments. However, many of the endogenous cardiac genes do not strictly follow chamber-specific expression but rather appear to be modularly controlled based on their position along the anteroposterior axis.[17]

An understanding of segment specification has been greatly advanced by the study of the homeobox genes in the fruit fly.[1] The identity and differentiation of segments are determined by interactions among homeobox and other genes. These interactions occur between the mesoderm, which gives rise to the heart tissues, and the tissues adjacent to the mesoderm.

The vertebrate heart tube normally loops to the right side of the embryo. Sidedness appears to be influenced by factors acting at a time when the heart is not recognizable as a distinct organ structure.[36] Transplantation studies using the early chicken embryo suggest that left and right sidedness are already determined in the precardiac mesoderm stages. Sidedness can also be regulated in part by retinoids. Retinoic acid–soaked bead implants in chicken embryos or application of all-*trans* retinoic acid in mouse embryos causes transposition of the great arteries.[20] Abnormalities in the direction of cardiac looping occur in humans.[5] These abnormalities are linked to an autosomal recessive gene defect that has been detected in the Amish population and another gene defect in

the X chromosome (Xq24-q27.1) in the general population.[6] Interestingly, abnormalities in genes associated with left-right asymmetry may also be responsible for apparently isolated cases of congenital heart defects. Mutations in the laterality *CFC1* gene have manifested as transposition of the great arteries in humans without other obvious laterality defects.

Two mouse mutants have abnormalities in sidedness. The iv/iv mutant mouse develops L-looping and dextrocardia 50% of the time.[18] A large percentage of these mice have a combination of cardiac defects, including persistent sinus venosus, atrial and ventricular septal defects, common AV canal, double-outlet right ventricle, tetralogy of Fallot, and transposition of the great arteries. This gene has been mapped to mouse chromosome 12, which is homologous to human chromosome 14. The inv/inv mutant mouse develops situs inversus close to 100% of the time.[46] Mutations screens using the zebrafish have uncovered a number of genes involved in laterality specification and indicate that there are organ-specific laterality regulators.[7] Identification of the genes involved in these human, mouse, and zebrafish mutations could provide valuable insight into the mechanisms of normal dextral looping of the heart.[3]

Septation

ENDOCARDIAL DEVELOPMENT: FORMATION OF CUSHION TISSUE

Septation of the heart begins with the swelling of the extracellular matrix between the endocardium and the myocardium at specific regions of the heart tube. These regions include the AV junction, the OFT, the leading edge of the primary atrial septum, and the ridge of the interventricular septum. A complex set of inductive events has been elucidated by studying cushion formation of the AV junction and the OFT.[33] These events include signaling between the specialized myocardium and a subset of competent activatable endocardial cells through growth factors (e.g., transforming growth factor-β, vascular endothelial growth factor) and extracellular matrix molecules. Various proteases and homeobox genes are also involved.

The subsequent cascade of events includes release and migration of cells from the endocardial epithelium (termed *epithelial-mesenchymal transition*) and proliferation and death of these endocardial mesenchyme cells within a complex matrix. In the OFT, the cushions are also populated by cardiac neural crest cells. The endocardial cushions of the AV junction are also invaded by cells originating from the embryonic epicardium. The cushions eventually give rise to—or at least greatly influence—the subsequent development of septa and valves of the heart. Because a number of factors, cell types, and tissues are involved in this process at multiple levels and at different stages, there are many sites where mistakes can occur. It is therefore not surprising that septation defects are so common. The differentiation of resilient valves requires remodeling of the extracellular matrix, an aspect that is poorly understood. However, it has been revealed recently that steps in cardiac valve differentiation and maturation share mechanisms with those of cartilage, tendon, and bone development.[24] The sharing of information across disciplines may therefore lead to rapid advances in understanding cardiac valve development and disease.

NEURAL CREST CONTRIBUTION TO CARDIOGENESIS

A subset of neural crest cells that originate and migrate from the dorsal region of the neural tube contributes significantly to the development of the heart and associated vessels (Fig. 45-3).[19,27] The role of the neural crest has been determined by the study of avian embryos using immunohistochemical neural crest markers, transplantation (quail-chicken chimeras), ablation, and genetic manipulation of mice. The neural crest cells from the cranial and trunk regions contribute to the walls of the aortic arch arteries, including the proximal aorta, the stems of the proximal coronary arteries, and the sympathetic and parasympathetic innervation of the heart (cardiac ganglia). A subset enters the heart within the endocardium and is involved in septation of the aortic and pulmonary trunk. A subset also appears to enter the heart and contributes in some way to the formation of the cardiac conduction system.[16]

Neural crest cells migrate from the cranial region of the neural folds through the pharyngeal arches and contribute to the aorticopulmonary septum and the tunica media of the great arteries that branch from the aorta. Removal of this subset of neural crest cells causes cardiac inflow anomalies, including double-inlet left ventricle, tricuspid atresia, and straddling tricuspid valve; cardiac outflow anomalies, including persistent truncus arteriosus; and abnormalities in the aortic arch arteries, including interruption of the aorta, double aortic arch, variable absence of the carotid arteries, and left aortic arch. In contrast, the systemic and pulmonary venous structures are not as affected by cardiac neural crest ablation.

A more global role for the cardiac neural crest is now recognized after the findings that removal or disturbance of cardiac neural crest cells can influence the function and proliferation of cardiomyocytes before neural crest cells migrate into the heart.[10] Recent findings point to a role for cardiac neural crest–derived cells in influencing the mesenchyme of the secondary or anterior heart–forming field that

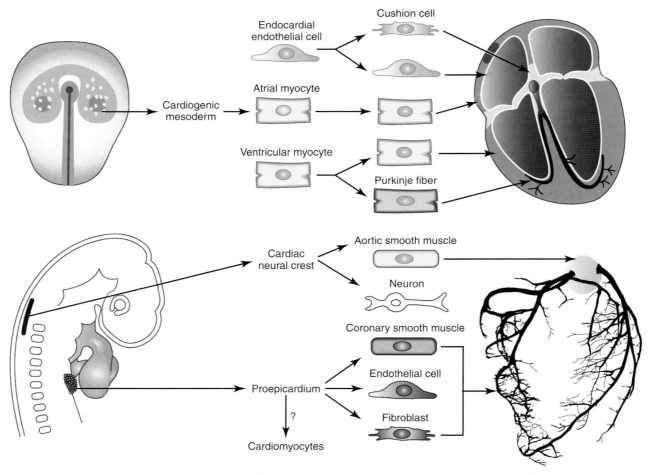

Figure 45–3. Lineage of cardiac cell types. Each cardiac cell type is established by lineage diversification of embryonic cells that arise from one of three distinct origins: cardiogenic mesoderm, neural crest, or proepicardium. This diagram illustrates the chronology and distribution for the development of cell lineages in the avian heart. Newly hypothesized is the epicardial source of a subset of cardiomyocytes. (*Modified from Mikawa T: Cardiac lineages. In Harvey RP, Rosenthal N, editors:* Heart development, *New York, 1999, Academic Press, p 19.*)

produces late-forming cardiac structures, including the out-flow tract.[42,47]

Because disturbances of neural crest development have the potential to cause cardiovascular anomalies, factors controlling normal neural crest cell development are receiving much attention. DiGeorge and related syndromes that include craniofacial and OFT abnormalities are believed to result from disruption of neural crest cell development.[13] These syndromes are associated with deletions in 22q11, a region of human chromosome 22 that is under close scrutiny.

The search for "the DiGeorge syndrome gene" has been confounded by the number of candidate genes in the DiGeorge critical region and by the differences between the phenotypes of mice and humans mutated in homologous genes. It is also puzzling that individuals without the deletion can closely resemble those with the DiGeorge region missing. *TBX1* and *CRKL* are currently described as the best candidate genes within the most common 22q11 deletion. However, researchers continue to propose that there is no single affected gene responsible for the defects associated with DiGeorge or the 22q11 deletion syndrome. Rather, a combination of affected genes within that region, as well as those outside that region, appear to regulate the same critical cellular processes. Recent data suggest that many of the mutations identified in individuals with a range of craniofacial and cardiac syndromes that include DiGeorge are in genes associated with the ERK pathway.[2,31] These genes include upstream genes such as *TBX1* and *CRKL* and downstream genes such as *SRF*. A broader hypothesis is emerging that anything that dysregulates the activity of the ERK pathway up or down in developing neural crest cells results in craniofacial and cardiac syndromes.

DEVELOPMENT OF THE CARDIAC CONDUCTION SYSTEM

Primordia of the pulse-generating system function early in the caudal region of the tubular heart and allow unidirectional blood flow, but subsequent events in the development of the cardiac conduction system (CCS) are not well understood. Investigations of CCS embryogenesis in a variety of species, including the mouse, chicken, and zebrafish, have contributed to this understanding.[21] Classic histologic analyses are limited in the information they provide because the early CCS cannot be readily distinguished histologically or even ultrastructurally from the surrounding myocardium. Biochemical markers have been detected that transiently stain portions of the CCS and have been used to follow these tissues during the three-dimensionally complex morphogenesis of the heart. The rabbit model is unique in that there is a marker for it, NF-150, an antibody to neurofilament proteins, that delineates its cardiac conduction system throughout its development and into the adult. These markers show that some of the tissues that give rise to the CCS can be distinguished from other cardiomyocytes as early as the tubular heart stages because they have a different pattern of gene expression and cell proliferation.

The role of the differentially expressed CCS markers is still not understood; nevertheless, the markers have clarified issues about normal and abnormal morphogenesis. Marking the early CCS by using the markers' specific properties has

allowed the CCS to be used as a point of reference to deduce which portion of the heart is growing and moving relative to others.[30]

Lineage tracing of myocardial cells provided clues to the origin of the CCS. The clonal relationship between CCS cells and working cardiomyocytes suggests that these specialized myocardia can be recruited from unspecialized myocardial cells. Evidence from avian systems supports the hypothesis that the vasculature can be the source of factors that initiate such recruitment, with endothelin-1 being a strong candidate for signaling.[14]

Less is known about the physiology of the developing CCS primarily because of technical barriers to resolution. This barrier is, however, being overcome by advances in biomedical engineering technologies such as optical mapping using voltage-sensitive fluorescent dyes and optical coherence tomography that allow the capture of images of the tiny beating heart at high spatiotemporal resolution. Different strategies are used by the embryo at different stages of cardiogenesis for coordinating the contraction of the heart. The tubular heart has a peristaltic-type contraction pattern resulting from a pulse-generating focus of cells and a slow distribution of action potentials radiating evenly from that region in all directions.[22] In the septating heart, alternating regions of relatively slow and fast conduction allow pumping of blood in one direction, with the endocardial cushions acting as primitive valves. Slow regions cause a delay of the impulse between the sinus venosus and atrial and ventricular chambers and through the OFT.[11] The ventricular conduction system achieves its mature morphology simultaneous with the appearance of the mature sequence of activation.[9] Subsequent differentiation allows for increasing speed of action potential conduction through the fascicular portion of this system and compensation for the growth of the heart. Maturation of the fibrous ring that separates the atrial from ventricular muscle and the connective tissue sheath around the conduction system also follows.

EPICARDIUM

The epicardium is a relatively late-forming cardiac tissue that does not appear until septation is underway. It provides the bulk of the noncardiomyocyte cellular components, including smooth muscle cells, fibroblasts, and endothelial cells. The progression of epicardial development has been studied in detail using avian and mouse models. The epicardium, the outer layer of the heart, forms by the growth of epithelial tissue from the dorsal mesothelium of the sinus venosus region. This single-cell layer spreads in a stereotyped pattern over the myocardium. The squamous epithelium of the primitive epicardium and the myocardium are initially juxtaposed, but a rapid accumulation and differentiation of connective tissue components between these layers ensues to thicken the epicardium. The cells of the epicardium invade the myocardium and the endocardium, giving rise to fibroblasts, smooth muscle cells, and all components of the coronary vasculature.[26] The epicardium is also the tissue in which cardiac ganglia develop, nerves travel, and fat cells accumulate. Recently, new evidence suggests that the embryonic epicardium may also include cells that can contribute a subset of cardiomyocytes.[4,48] This interesting tissue and its interaction with the myocardium are the focus of much current research.

LYMPHATICS

Although it is known that the adult vertebrate heart is incorporated with an extensive lymphatic network, the lymphatic vasculature of the embryonic heart has not been investigated in detail. The mature heart is thought to have two plexuses: (1) the deep plexus immediately under the endocardium, and (2) the superficial plexus subjacent to the visceral pericardium.[15,28] The deep plexus opens into the superficial plexus, whose efferent vessels will form right and left collecting trunks. The study of lymphatic development during cardiogenesis is now revived with the identification of lymphatic markers. This area of study is in its early stages. One of the many questions not yet answered in this field is, where do the lymphatic precursors come from? Lymphatic cells, whether or not they originate in the epicardium, do end up in the epicardium surrounding coronary vessels. An understanding of the mechanisms driving development of the lymphatic vasculature of the developing heart and of lymphangiogenesis in this region may help in treating edema or similar conditions in the future.

CELL DIVISION AND CELL DEATH

Differential control of cell division and cell death can in part account for the enormous differences in morphologic features of the various regions of the heart. For example, the cells of the thin-walled atria divide less than the cells of the thick-walled ventricle. The central structures of the fascicular CCS slow their proliferation rate early compared with surrounding myocardium.[39]

Apoptosis—programmed cell death—is a developmentally controlled strategy in the morphogenesis of many structures. It occurs during the pruning of the nervous system and the sculpting of digits, and it occurs at many sites throughout cardiogenesis.[34] Endocardial mesenchyme cells, which include cardiac neural crest cells, undergo a high level of apoptosis during septation. A high frequency of apoptosis of cardiomyocytes occurs coincident with OFT morphogenesis. Experimental manipulation to increase or decrease cell death at this stage results in conotruncal abnormalities.[37] Thus, regulated apoptosis of OFT cardiomyocytes is critical for the normal docking of the great arteries with the ventricles. Environmental and genetic factors that alter the level of apoptosis at these critical stages and sites in the developing heart may contribute to congenital heart defects.

HUMAN GENETICS

The entire human genome is sequenced, and efforts have been made to allow clinicians, basic scientists, industry scientists, and others to tap into the database and exchange information. Knowledge of the human genome helps in predicting potential problems, forming the basis for the growing field of genetic counseling. In addition, the study of human genetics allows identification of regions of the genome that might be adversely affected in patients with heart disease. Eventually, this information may be used in developing therapies for heart disease. Comparison of the human genome sequences with those of many other species has also provided important information. Sequences conserved across species often indicate regions of a gene that are critical for a particular function and are worth focused scrutiny. The field

of human genetics also provides information for the basic sciences, the "bedside to the bench" links. Genetic analysis of individuals with certain syndromes can pinpoint genes and proteins that can be studied in detail to identify critical functions.

Therapy

Strategies to repair heart tissue are relevant to both pediatric and adult cardiology and have been the focus of much effort. The problem is that human myocardial cells lose their ability to divide soon after birth. This terminal differentiation appears to be irreversible. It had been believed that, within adult heart tissue, no stem cells existed that could be activated to replace defective or damaged cardiomyocytes. Inspired by new information, investigators are seeking ways to initiate cell division in cardiomyocytes or to initiate myocardial differentiation in fibroblasts by turning on or off gene expression of various factors. Fibroblasts are being considered because they continue to divide, are abundant in the postnatal and adult myocardium, and have been successfully transdifferentiated into skeletal muscle by initiating expression of the transcription factor myoD. A proposed treatment of muscular dystrophy involves seeding healthy stem cells, embryonic or fetal cells, or genetically engineered cells into unhealthy tissues.

Heart tissue also appears amenable to such strategies. Myocardial cells (cell lines or embryonic myocytes) can integrate to some extent into the adult heart of animal models. Thus, they undergo some differentiation and integration in a foreign environment. Findings suggest that stem cells exist in the interstices of the adult heart and can be capable of differentiating into cardiomyocytes.[32] Endothelial cells, bone marrow cells, and umbilical cord cells are known to differentiate into cells with cardiac markers and are under study as potential candidates for use in cardiac tissue repair. Recent studies provide evidence that epicardial progenitor cells may have the capacity to contribute to the cardiomyocyte lineage in the developing heart.[4,48] Furthermore, investigators were able to induce the differentiation of adult epicardial cells into endothelial cells.[41] These findings suggest different strategies for therapy. The question remains whether any of these cells will be able to differentiate, integrate, and function appropriately in the adult heart as cardiomyocytes or endothelial cells without becoming malignant. The potential for causing cancer or arrhythmias is possible with some of these therapies.

A newly exploding area of research is the study of micro-RNAs and their potential therapeutic value.[44,45] Micro-RNAs are single-stranded RNAs, about 22 noncoding nucleotides in length, that are present endogenously. They act as specific regulators of gene expression in development and disease by interfering with translation of messenger RNAs or by enhancing the degradation of messenger RNAs. The ability of a particular micro-RNA to regulate RNAs from related sets of genes has raised the possibility that manipulating the levels of micro-RNAs may be a comprehensive strategy to prevent or reverse complex disease. Intriguing is the finding that sequences for micro-RNAs are found within the very genes that they control.

Gene therapy, in combination with intravascular stents, is being considered for treatment of coronary and peripheral vascular disease in adults. Exogenous genes can be introduced by a variety of means to the heart or vasculature. In vitro studies or those in animal models have also shown that physiologically significant genes (e.g., plasminogen activator) can be introduced and cause significant levels of protein expression for enough time to have therapeutic effects.

The most controversial approach for therapy involves manipulating the genome of the germ cells so that the entire embryo can go through development with the corrected gene. This approach requires that the manipulation result in little or no effect besides the desired effect. Introducing the gene into a genome can by itself cause inadvertent wide-ranging defects. Such methods also require a thorough understanding of the gene being manipulated so that all controlling elements, as well as the structural portion of the gene, are intact.

Another strategy in preventing congenital heart defects is to correct at a level farther along the pathway from the genome. This can be done by turning on alternative biochemical pathways or by boosting compensatory mechanisms. This approach requires a thorough understanding of the network of pathways and all of its interactions and feedback loops.

Finding the appropriate strategy for therapy is complicated because defects involve a combination of genes and environmental factors and include direct and indirect effects that are difficult to control with current knowledge and techniques. However, with the great and often serendipitous advances in our understanding of cardiovascular development, certain defects might be preventable or reversed in our lifetime.

REFERENCES

1. Akazawa H, Komuro I: Cardiac transcription factor Csx/Nkx2.5: its role in cardiac development and diseases, *Pharmacol Ther* 107:252, 2005.
2. Aoki Y, et al: The RAS/MAPK syndromes: novel roles of the RAS pathway in human genetic disorders, *Hum Mutat* 29:992, 2008.
3. Bisgrove BW, Morelli SH, Yost HJ: Genetics of human laterality: insights from vertebrate model systems, *Annu Rev Genomics Hum Genet* 4:1, 2003.
4. Cai CL, et al: A myocardial lineage derives from Tbx18 epicardial cells, *Nature* 454:104, 2008.
5. Carmi R, et al: Human situs determination is probably controlled by several different genes, *Am J Med Genet* 44:246, 1992.
6. Casey B, et al: Mapping a gene for familial situs abnormalities to human chromosome Xq24-q27.1, *Nat Genet* 5:403, 1993.
7. Chen JN, et al: Genetic steps to organ laterality in zebrafish, *Comp Funct Genomics* 2:60, 2001.
8. Christoffels, et al: Architectural plan for the heart: early patterning and delineation of the chambers and the nodes, *Trends Cardiovasc Med* 14:301, 2004.
9. Chuck ET, et al: Changing activation sequence in the embryonic chick heart: implications for the development of the His-Purkinje system, *Circ Res* 81:470, 1997.
10. Creazzo TL, et al: Role of cardiac neural crest cells in cardiovascular development, *Annu Rev Phys* 60:267, 1998.
11. de Jong F, et al: Persisting zones of slow impulse conduction in developing chicken hearts, *Circ Res* 71:240, 1992.
12. Dunwoodie SL: Combinatorial signaling in the heart orchestrates cardiac induction, lineage specification and chamber formation, *Semin Cell Dev Biol* 18:54, 2007.
13. Emanuel BS, et al: The genetic basis of conotruncal cardiac defects: The chromosome 22q11.2 deletion. In Harvey RP, Rosenthal N, editors: *Heart Development*, San Diego, 1999, Academic Press, p 463.
14. Gourdie RG, et al: Development of the cardiac pacemaking and conduction system, *Birth Defects Res Part C Embryo Today* 69:46, 2003.
15. Gray H: *Anatomy of the Human Body*, Philadelphia, 1918, Lea & Febiger.
16. Gurjarpadhye A, et al: Cardiac neural crest ablation inhibits compaction and electrical function of conduction system bundles, *Am J Physiol Heart Circ Physiol* 292:H1291, 2007.
17. Habets PEMH, et al: Regulatory modules in the developing heart, *Cardiovasc Res* 58:246, 2003.
18. Hummel KP, et al: Visceral inversion and associated anomalies in the mouse, *J Hered* 50:9, 1959.
19. Hutson MR, Kirby ML: Neural crest and cardiovascular development: a 20-year perspective, *Birth Defects Res Part C Embryo Today* 69:2, 2003.
20. Irie K, et al: All-trans-retinoic acid induced cardiovascular malformations. In Bockman DE, et al, editors: *Embryonic Origins of Defective Heart Development*, New York, New York, 1990, Academy of Science, p 387.
21. Jongbloed MR, et al: Development of the cardiac conduction system and the possible relation to predilection sites of arrhythmogenesis, *Sci World J* 8:239, 2008.
22. Kamino K: Optical approaches to ontogeny of electrical activity and related functional organization during early heart development, *Physiol Rev* 71:53, 1991.
23. Linask KK, Lash JW: Dynamics of endocardial cell sorting suggests a common origin with cardiomyocytes, *Dev Dyn* 195:62, 1993.
24. Lincoln J, Lange AW, Yutzey KE: Hearts and bones: shared regulatory mechanisms in heart valve, cartilage, tendon, and bone development, *Dev Biol* 294:292, 2008.
25. Lyons I, et al: Myogenic and morphogenetic defects in the heart tubes of murine embryos lacking the homeobox gene Nkx2-5, *Genes Dev* 9:1654, 1995.
26. Manner J, et al: The origin, formation and developmental significance of the epicardium: a review, *Cells Tissues Organs* 169:89, 2001.
27. Mikawa T: Cardiac lineages. In Harvey RP, Rosenthal N, editors: *Heart Development*, New York, 1999, Academic Press, p 19.
28. Milliard FP: *Applied Anatomy of the Lymphatics*, Kirksville, 1922, The Journal Printing Company.
29. Moore KL: *The Developing Human: Clinically Oriented Embryology*, Philadelphia, 1982, WB Saunders.
30. Moorman AF, et al: Cardiac septation revisited: The developing conduction system as a reference-structure, *J Perinat Med* 1:195, 1991.
31. Newbern J, et al: Mouse and human phenotypes indicate a critical conserved role for ERK2 signaling in neural crest development, *Proc Natl Acad Sci U S A* 105:17115, 2008.
32. Pansky B: *Review of Medical Embryology*, New York, 1982, Macmillan.
33. Person AD Klewer SE, Runyan RB: Cell biology of cardiac cushion development, *Int Rev Cytol* 243:287, 2005.

34. Pexieder T: Cell death in the morphogenesis and teratogenesis of the heart, *Adv Anat Embryol Cell Biol* 51:3, 1975.

35. Pober BR, Johnson M, Urban Z: Mechanisms and treatment of cardiovascular disease in Williams-Beuren syndrome, *J Clin Invest* 118:1606, 2008.

36. Ramsdell AF: Left-right asymmetry and congenital cardiac defects: getting to the heart of the matter in vertebrate left-right axis determination, *Dev Biol* 288:1, 2005.

37. Rothenberg F, et al: Sculpting the cardiac outflow tract, *Birth Defects Res Part C Embryo Today* 69:38, 2003.

38. Schott JJ, et al: Congenital heart disease caused by mutations in the transcription factor NKX2-5, *Science* 281:108, 1998.

39. Sedmera D, et al: Spatiotemporal pattern of commitment to slowed proliferation in the embryonic mouse heart indicates progressive differentiation of the cardiac conduction system, *Anat Rec* 274A:773, 2003.

40. Sissman NJ: Developmental landmarks in cardiac morphogenesis: Comparative chronology, *Am J Cardiol* 25:141, 1970.

41. Smart N, et al: Thymosin beta-4 is essential for coronary vessel development and promotes neovascularization via adult epicardium, *Ann N Y Acad Sci* 1112:171, 2007.

42. Snarr N, et al: Origin and fate of cardiac mesenchyme, *Dev Dyn* 237:2804, 2008.

43. Solloway MJ, Harvey RP: Molecular pathways in myocardial development: a stem cell perspective, *Cardiovasc Res* 58:264, 2003.

44. Thum T, Catlucci D, Bauersachs J: MicroRNAs novel regulators in cardiac development and disease, *Cardiovasc Res* 79:562, 2008.

45. van Rooj E, Marshall WS, Olson EN: Toward micro-RNA-based therapeutics for heart disease: the sense in antisense, *Circ Res* 103:919, 2008.

46. Yokoyama T, et al: Reversal of left-right asymmetry: a situs inversus mutation, *Science* 260:679, 1993.

47. Yutzey KE, Kirby ML: Wherefore heart thou? Embryonic origins of cardiogenic mesoderm, *Dev Dyn* 223:307, 2002.

48. Zhou B, et al: Epicardial progenitors contribute to the cardiomyocyte lineage in the developing heart, *Nature* 454:109, 2008.

PART 2

Pulmonary Vascular Development

Robin H. Steinhorn

Normal prenatal and postnatal development of pulmonary vascular structure and function is essential for the lung to perform its basic physiologic function of allowing gas exchange across a thin blood-gas interface. Survival of the newborn is therefore dependent on rapid adaptation of the fetal cardiopulmonary system to the demands of extrauterine life, and on sustained low pulmonary vascular resistance (PVR) as postnatal development continues.

FETAL PULMONARY VASCULAR DEVELOPMENT

Structural Development

Fetal lung development is classically described as occurring in five distinct but overlapping stages: embryonic, pseudoglandular, canalicular, saccular, and alveolar. Pulmonary vascular development begins during the embryonic phase of lung development. Endodermal lung buds arise from the ventral aspect of the foregut by the fifth week of gestation. The pulmonary trunk, derived from the truncus arteriosus, divides into the aorta and pulmonary trunks by 8 weeks of gestation by growth of the spiral aortopulmonary septum.[48] The pulmonary trunk connects to the pulmonary arch arteries, which are derived from the sixth branchial arch arteries. The mesenchyme surrounding the lung bud then develops into the vascular network.

As gestation progresses, there is close synchronization between the development of the pulmonary arterial tree and airway branching. In the human lung, the preacinar vascular branching pattern is present by the 20th week of fetal life.[23] In contrast, intra-acinar arteries form later in fetal life and after birth during the alveolar phase of lung development.[22] Airway and vascular development are highly interactive processes, and disrupted development of one system is likely to have important consequences on the development of the other, ultimately affecting lung structure and function. Development of the pulmonary veins parallels that of the arteries, but they arise separately from the loose mesenchyme of the lung septa and subsequently connect to the left atrium.[11]

Angiogenesis and vasculogenesis are two distinct morphogenetic processes that contribute to the development of the pulmonary vasculature. Vasculogenesis is the de novo organization of blood vessels by in situ differentiation of endothelial progenitor cells (angioblasts) from the mesoderm. These angioblasts migrate, adhere, and form vascular channels that become arteries, veins, or lymphatics depending on the local factors within the mesenchyme.[36] Endothelial precursor cells, after differentiation into the endothelium, either contribute to the expression of smooth muscle phenotype in the surrounding mesenchyme or recruit existing smooth muscle cells to the forming vessel.

Angiogenesis refers to the budding, sprouting, and branching of the existing vessels to form new ones. New evidence indicates that vasculogenesis and angiogenesis are not necessarily sequential processes, and that both may occur early in lung development, perhaps giving rise to heterogeneous cell populations in the vasculature.[49] In addition, a process of vascular fusion has been described that connects the angiogenic and vasculogenic vessels to allow for expansion of the vascular network.[11,48] Numerous local growth and transcription factors, such as vascular endothelial growth factor, transforming growth factor-β, fibroblast growth factors, platelet-derived growth factor, angiopoietin, and others, play an important role in vascular development and cell differentiation in the developing lung.[7,51] Growth factor function is also regulated through specific receptors, including the bone morphogenetic protein receptor-2 (BMPR2), a receptor for the transforming growth factor-β superfamily. Mutations of

BMPR2 are now known to be associated with familial and idiopathic pulmonary hypertension in adults and children.[32]

As gestation and fetal lung growth progress, the number of small pulmonary arteries increases, both in absolute terms and per unit volume of the lung.[30] In fetal lambs, lung weight increases 4-fold during the last trimester, whereas the number of small blood vessels in the lungs increases 40-fold. Thus, the number of small blood vessels within each lung increases 10-fold, preparing the lungs to accept the 10-fold increase in blood per unit of lung that occurs at birth. This increase in the capacity of the pulmonary arteries indicates that vascular constriction must play a key role in maintaining high pulmonary vascular tone during fetal life.

Mediators of Fetal Pulmonary Vascular Tone

Pulmonary hypertension is normal and necessary for the fetus. Because the placenta serves as the organ of gas exchange, most of the right ventricular output in the fetus bypasses the lung and crosses the ductus arteriosus to the aorta. Pulmonary pressures are equivalent to systemic pressures due to elevated PVR, and only about 10% of the combined ventricular output is directed to the pulmonary vascular bed.

Multiple mechanisms are in place to maintain low pulmonary blood flow in the fetus. The low oxygen environment of the fetus almost certainly plays a key role in maintaining high PVR. Normal fetal oxygen tension is about 25 mm Hg, a level that promotes normal growth and differentiation of pulmonary vascular cells and supports normal branching morphogenesis in the fetal lung.[18] Because oxygen regulates activity of enzymes such as nitric oxide synthase, the low oxygen environment of the fetus may maintain low production of vasoactive mediators such as nitric oxide and prostacyclin. For instance, a modest increase in PaO_2 (to levels of about 50 mm Hg) in the near-term fetal lamb activates nitric oxide synthase and increases pulmonary blood flow to levels comparable to postnatal lambs.[52] The fetal pulmonary circulation also exhibits a marked myogenic response as gestation progresses, meaning that the vasculature responds to vasodilatory stimuli with active vasoconstriction.[50]

Vasoactive mediators likely play an important role in maintaining the normal patterns of fetal circulation. Although it is assumed that vasoconstrictors help maintain high pulmonary vascular tone in utero, surprisingly little is known about their specific roles throughout gestation. Some of the proposed fetal pulmonary vasoconstrictors include endothelin-1, as well as vasoconstrictor products of arachidonic acid metabolism such as thromboxane and leukotrienes. It is also possible that low basal production of vasodilators such as nitric oxide or prostacyclin may maintain high PVR, although it is interesting to note that this low production occurs despite an increase in pulmonary expression of endothelial nitric oxide synthase and cyclooxygenase-1 during late gestation. Recent evidence points toward a critical role for the RhoA/Rho kinase signal transduction pathway,[39] a central downstream pathway that promotes vasoconstriction through inactivation of myosin light chain phosphatase, thus increasing calcium sensitivity of the smooth muscle cell.

PULMONARY VASCULAR TRANSITION

At birth, a rapid and dramatic decrease in PVR allows half of the combined ventricular output to be redirected from the placenta to the lung, leading to an 8- to 10-fold increase in pulmonary blood flow. Increased pulmonary blood flow increases pulmonary venous return and left atrial pressure, promoting functional closure of the one-way valve of the foramen ovale. Systemic vascular resistance increases at birth, at least in part because of removal of the low resistance vascular bed of the placenta.

The largest drop in PVR occurs shortly after birth, although resistance continues to drop over the first several months of life until it reaches the low levels normally found in the adult circulation. As PVR falls below systemic levels, blood flow through the patent ductus arteriosus reverses. Over the first several hours of life, the ductus arteriosus functionally closes, largely in response to the increased oxygen tension of the newborn. This effectively separates the pulmonary and systemic circulations and establishes the normal postnatal circulatory pattern.

The stimuli that appear to be most important in decreasing PVR are lung inflation with a gas and an increase in oxygen tension. Each of these stimuli by itself will decrease PVR and increase pulmonary blood flow, with the largest effects seen when the two events occur simultaneously. Mechanical distention of the lungs initiates the process of rapid structural adaptation of the pulmonary vessels. The external diameter of the nonmuscular arteries increases, and the prominent endothelial cells assume a flattened appearance (Fig. 45-4). There is an increase in cell length and surface-to-volume ratio as the cells spread within the vessel wall to increase lumen diameter and lower resistance.[4] This process is likely facilitated by the paucity of interstitial connective tissue, allowing for greater plasticity of the vessel. In postmortem arterial-injected specimens, the number of nonmuscular arteries that fill with injection

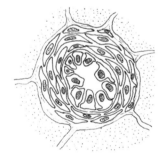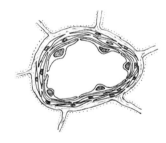

Figure 45–4. Changes in the small muscular pulmonary arteries during transition. Muscularized small pulmonary arteries from a near-term gestation fetus (*left*) demonstrate swollen endothelial cells and increased thickness of the muscular layer. Within 24 hours after birth (*right*), a considerable increase in luminal diameter is noted secondary to flattening of the endothelial cells, spreading of the smooth muscle cells, and an increase in external diameter due to relaxation of the smooth muscle. These events contribute to the drop in pulmonary vascular resistance after birth. (*From Lakshminrusimha S, et al: Pulmonary vascular biology during neonatal transition,* Clin Perinatal 26:601, 1999.)

material increases rapidly during the first 24 hours, suggesting that there is a rapid increase in the number of precapillary arteries recruited into the pulmonary circulation after birth.[21]

An increase in oxygen tension will reduce PVR independent of the effects of lung inflation. This oxygen response emerges at about 70% gestation in the fetal lamb and continues to develop as gestation progresses.[35] As noted earlier, the full vasodilatory effect of oxygen can be achieved with quite modest increases in arterial concentrations: PaO_2 levels of about 50 mm Hg in the near-term fetal lamb will decrease pulmonary vascular resistance and increase pulmonary blood flow to levels comparable to those in postnatal lambs.[52] Evidence indicates that in addition to facilitating vasodilation, oxygen may also promote the rapid endothelial spreading and remodeling described previously.[56]

Finally, the initial increase in pulmonary blood flow increases shear stress in the pulmonary vasculature, which further promotes rapid vasodilation in the pulmonary circulation of the newborn and late-gestation fetus.[1] The mechanisms of shear stress–mediated responses are complex but appear to involve stimulation of K^+ channels and activation of nitric oxide synthases.[6,53]

Vasoactive Mediators of the Pulmonary Vascular Transition

No single vasoactive agent has been identified as the primary mediator of transitional pulmonary vasodilation; rather, it is believed that numerous factors interact to facilitate the mechanical events described earlier. Increases in vasodilators appear to be more important than decreases in vasoconstrictors; of these, nitric oxide has emerged as one of the most important. Pulmonary expression of all three isoforms of nitric oxide synthase and its receptor molecule, soluble guanylate cyclase, increase late in gestation. Increased nitric oxide production serves to activate soluble guanylate cyclase and increase concentrations of the second messenger cyclic guanosine monophosphate (cGMP) in vascular smooth muscle cells. cGMP then initiates the cascade that decreases intracellular calcium and produces vasorelaxation. Acute or chronic inhibition of nitric oxide synthase in fetal lambs produces pulmonary hypertension after delivery, illustrating the critical importance of the nitric oxide–cGMP pathway in facilitating normal transition.[2,16] Data indicate that low fetal nitric oxide synthase activity may be maintained during fetal life in part through increased levels of asymmetric dimethyl arginine, a endogenous competitive inhibitor of nitric oxide synthase.[5,40] Expression of cGMP-specific phosphodiesterases also increases during late lung development, possibly serving to mediate tight regulation of intracellular cGMP concentrations and signal transduction at birth.[42]

Prostacyclin is a second central vasodilator that is upregulated in response to ventilation of the lung. Cyclooxygenase and prostacyclin synthase generate prostacyclin from arachidonic acid. Cyclooxygenase-1 in particular is upregulated during late gestation, leading to an increase in prostacyclin production in late gestation and early postnatal life.[8,29] Prostacyclin stimulates adenylate cyclase to increase intracellular cyclic adenosine monophosphate (cAMP) levels, which, as with cGMP, leads to vasorelaxation through a decrease in intracellular calcium concentrations.

ABNORMALITIES OF PULMONARY VASCULAR DEVELOPMENT

Persistent Pulmonary Hypertension of the Newborn (See also part 8)

Persistent pulmonary hypertension (PPHN) describes the failure of normal pulmonary vascular adaptation at birth. This syndrome complicates the course of about 10% of term and preterm infants with respiratory failure and remains a source of considerable mortality and morbidity. PPHN can be generally characterized as one of three types: (1) the abnormally constricted pulmonary vasculature due to lung parenchymal diseases, such as meconium aspiration syndrome, respiratory distress syndrome, or pneumonia; (2) the lung with normal parenchyma and remodeled pulmonary vasculature, also known as idiopathic PPHN; or (3) the hypoplastic vasculature as seen in congenital diaphragmatic hernia. Although idiopathic pulmonary hypertension is responsible for only 10% to 20% of all infants with PPHN, severe cases of PPHN associated with parenchymal disease are complicated by a significant degree of vascular remodeling.

Pulmonary vascular remodeling occurs antenatally in infants presenting with severe PPHN shortly after birth. Pathologic findings include significant remodeling of the pulmonary arteries, characterized by vessel wall thickening, and smooth muscle hyperplasia. An important feature includes extension of the smooth muscle to the level of the intra-acinar arteries (Fig. 45-5), which does not normally occur until much later in the postnatal period.[38] One cause of idiopathic PPHN is constriction of the fetal ductus arteriosus *in utero*, which can occur after exposure to nonsteroidal anti-inflammatory drugs during the third trimester.[3,31] Because it is difficult to gain sufficient mechanistic insights in the clinical setting, animal models have provided valuable insights into the antenatal and postnatal vascular abnormalities associated with PPHN. Ductal constriction or ligation can be surgically performed *in utero* in lambs and produces rapid antenatal remodeling of the pulmonary vasculature. Pathologic and physiologic findings in PPHN lambs are similar to those observed in human infants, including increased fetal pulmonary artery pressure, pulmonary vascular remodeling, and profound hypoxemia after birth.

New data suggest that maternal exposure to selective serotonin reuptake inhibitors during late gestation is associated with a sixfold increase in the prevalence of PPHN,[10] although it is not clear how many infants developed severe disease. Newborn rats exposed *in utero* to fluoxetine develop pulmonary vascular remodeling, abnormal oxygenation, and higher mortality when compared with vehicle-treated controls.[17] Because selective serotonin reuptake inhibitors have been reported to reduce pulmonary vascular remodeling in adult models of pulmonary hypertension, these findings also serve to highlight the unique vulnerability of fetal pulmonary vascular development.

Disruptions in the production or function of vasoactive mediators at birth will also lead to pulmonary vasoconstriction. Based on work from animal models and human infants, there is strong evidence that disruptions of the nitric oxide–cGMP,

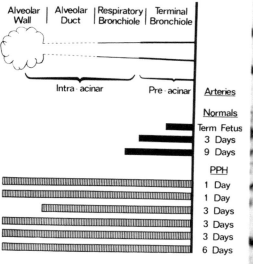

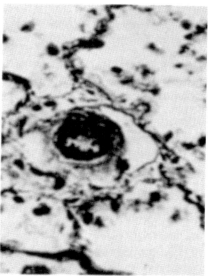

Figure 45–5. Vascular maldevelopment is a hallmark of persistent pulmonary hypertension (PPH). The pulmonary vessels show thickened walls with smooth muscle hyperplasia. Further, the smooth muscle extends to the level of the intra-acinar arteries, which does not normally occur until much later in the postnatal period. *(From Murphy JD, et al: The structural basis of persistent pulmonary hypertension of the newborn infant, J Pediatr 98:962, 1981.)*

prostacyclin-cAMP, and endothelin signaling pathways play an important role in the vascular abnormalities associated with PPHN. The nitric oxide–cGMP pathway has been a topic of particularly intense investigation over the past decade, at least in part because of the ability to deliver exogenous (inhaled) nitric oxide as a therapeutic agent. Decreased expression and activity of endothelial nitric oxide synthase have been documented in animal models,[45,54] and decreased endothelial nitric oxide synthase expression has been reported in umbilical venous endothelial cell cultures from human infants with meconium staining who develop PPHN.[12] There is also evidence that PPHN is associated with disruptions of endothelial nitric oxide synthase activity through "uncoupling" of the enzyme, which not only reduces synthesis of nitric oxide but also promotes production of reactive oxygen species, such as superoxide. Further, the vascular abnormalities appear to include downstream alterations in accumulation of the critical second messenger, cGMP. For instance, vessel studies from PPHN lambs suggest that soluble guanylate cyclase is less sensitive to nitric oxide, meaning that cGMP concentrations are reduced in the diseased vascular smooth musculature, even when exogenous nitric oxide is administered.[47] In addition to decreased cGMP production, increased activity of phosphodiesterase-5 has been reported in animal models, which would further decrease cGMP concentrations by increasing its inactivation.[20]

Although prostacyclin appears to be important in the normal pulmonary vascular transition, less is known about the role of abnormal prostacyclin-cAMP signaling in PPHN. Some data suggest abnormalities in prostacyclin synthesis and downstream adenylate cyclase responses exist, analogous to the abnormalities reported for nitric oxide–cGMP signaling.[28,44] In addition, production of the vasoconstrictor arachidonic acid metabolite, thromboxane, plays a role in pulmonary hypertension produced by chronic hypoxia.[14]

Circulating levels of the potent vasoconstrictor endothelin-1 are elevated in lambs and newborn infants with PPHN.[27,41] Endothelin-1 effects are mediated through two receptors, endothelin-A receptors on smooth muscle cells that mediate vasoconstriction and endothelin-B receptors on

endothelial cells that mediate vasodilation. There is evidence that the balance of endothelin receptors is shifted to the vasoconstrictor (endothelin-A) pathways.[24] In addition, endothelin may affect vascular tone by increasing production of reactive oxygen species such as superoxide and hydrogen peroxide, which also act as vasoconstrictors.[55] Therefore, the elevated endothelin levels in PPHN may increase vasoconstriction through preferential stimulation of endothelin-A receptors and through increased production of superoxide.

There is mounting evidence that oxidant stress plays an important role in the pathogenesis of PPHN. An increase in reactive oxygen species such as superoxide and hydrogen peroxide in the smooth muscle and adventitia of pulmonary arteries has been demonstrated in animal models of pulmonary hypertension.[9,15] Possible sources for elevated concentrations of reactive oxygen species include increased expression and activity of NADPH oxidase, uncoupled nitric oxide synthase activity, and a reduction in superoxide dismutase activity. Once present in the lung, elevated concentrations of reactive oxygen species promote vasoconstriction directly and by increasing production of other constrictors such as isoprostanes. Reactive oxygen species also increase vascular smooth muscle cell proliferation and blunt cGMP accumulation through increased activity of cGMP-specific phosphodiesterases.[13]

Congenital Diaphragmatic Hernia

(see also Chapter 44.)

Congenital diaphragmatic hernia (CDH) occurs in approximately 1 in 3000 births, and represents ~8% of all major congenital anomalies. CDH is an abnormality of diaphragm development, resulting in a defect that allows abdominal viscera to enter the chest and compress the lung. Herniation occurs most often in the posterolateral segments of the diaphragm, and 80% of the defects occur on the left side. While *in utero* compression of the lung is typically believed to produce lung hypoplasia, there is some evidence that the lung hypoplasia may be a primary event that occurs independently of the diaphragmatic defect. Severe CDH develops early in the course of lung development, and an arrest in the normal pattern of airway branching is noted in both lungs, associated with reduced lung volume and impaired alveolarization.

Because development of the pulmonary arterial system parallels development of the bronchial tree, a similar developmental arrest occurs in pulmonary arterial branching, resulting in a reduced cross-sectional area of the pulmonary vascular bed. Further, the media and adventitia of small arterioles are thickened, and abnormal medial muscular hypertrophy extends as far distally as the acinar arterioles.[34] Functionally, pulmonary blood flow is decreased because of the hypoplastic pulmonary vascular bed, as well as by abnormal pulmonary vasoconstriction. The mediators of altered pulmonary vascular reactivity in CDH are not well understood, although most evidence points to similar patterns of disruption of nitric oxide–cGMP and endothelin signaling as described previously for PPHN.

Abnormalities of cardiac development and function also play an important role in the pathophysiology of CDH. The left ventricle, left atrium, and intraventricular septum are hypoplastic in infants that die from CDH relative to age-matched controls,[46] perhaps owing to low fetal and postnatal pulmonary blood flow as well as compression by the hypertensive right ventricle. Left ventricular hypoplasia and dysfunction would be expected to increase left atrial and pulmonary venous pressure, and this unique feature of CDH may explain the relatively poor responses to inhaled nitric oxide during the first few days of life. Some infants may have exceptionally severe left ventricular dysfunction that leads to dependence on the right ventricle for systemic perfusion; this subset may benefit from clinical strategies that maintain patency of the ductus arteriosus.

Alveolar Capillary Dysplasia

Alveolar capillary dysplasia refers to a rare developmental abnormality of the lung that typically presents as severe idiopathic PPHN. It was first described by this name in 1981[25] and is believed to be a universally fatal condition. It is now recognized that the pulmonary phenotype is relatively consistent and includes a paucity of pulmonary capillaries, increased muscularization of pulmonary arterioles, simplification of the pulmonary architecture, and malposition of pulmonary veins adjacent to pulmonary arteries ("misaligned veins," Fig. 45-6). More than 50% of infants present with other anomalies, most commonly affecting the genitourinary, cardiovascular, and gastrointestinal systems. The diagnosis can only be made with certainty based on microscopic examination of the lung. Therefore, a complete postmortem evaluation should be recommended for all newborns who die as a result of unexplained pulmonary hypertension, and a lung biopsy should be considered in infants with prolonged, refractory PPHN. Although alveolar capillary dysplasia classically presents in the neonatal period, there is increasing recognition of late presentation at several months of life in some infants. About 10% of infants have a familial association, leading some to propose an autosomal recessive inheritance.[43] While the search for a candidate gene has proven difficult, a recent report showed an

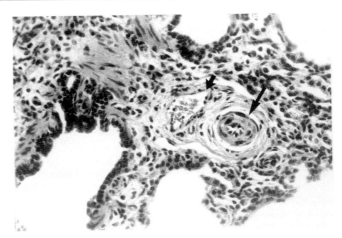

Figure 45–6. Vascular abnormalities associated with alveolar capillary dysplasia. The lung parenchyma shows airspace simplification and widened alveolar walls. A central membranous bronchiole is accompanied by adjacent thick-walled arteries (*long arrow*) with associated dilated veins (*short arrow*). The prominently muscularized arteries extend into adjacent alveolar walls, where they are also accompanied by dilated veins.

association with haploinsufficiency for the forkhead (FOX) transcription factor gene cluster and ACD/MPV associated with additional congenital heart defects and/or gastrointestinal anomalies.[46a]

Bronchopulmonary Dysplasia

(See also Chapter 44, Part 7.)
Extremely preterm infants (≤26 weeks' gestation) are born during the early saccular phase of lung development; in this setting, much of the saccular and all of the alveolar stages of lung development occur postnatally. Although recent advances in neonatal care have improved survival of this population, they have not reduced the incidence of bronchopulmonary dysplasia (BPD). However, the nature of BPD has changed during the past 2 decades from one defined primarily by lung injury and fibrotic changes to one consisting of abnormal and simplified patterns of alveolarization.

Abnormal vascularization of the lung is now recognized as a critically important component of BPD and is characterized by reductions in the size and number of intra-acinar pulmonary arteries, resulting in a reduced cross-sectional area of the pulmonary vascular bed. There is increasing recognition that abnormal vascular development may precede or promote abnormal lung growth.[19] The morphologic vascular alterations are accompanied by functional changes, characterized by increased pulmonary vascular tone and heightened vasoconstrictor responses to acute hypoxia.[37] Identifying pulmonary hypertension in this population requires a high index of suspicion and careful longitudinal evaluation with echocardiography and cardiac catheterization. Although the incidence and spectrum of pulmonary hypertension associated with BPD remains ill defined, the disease appears to be worst in infants with severe chronic lung disease and in those who are small for gestational age.[26] Further, the presence of severe pulmonary hypertension appears to be associated with exceptionally high mortality in infants with BPD.

Work during the past decade has begun to elucidate early abnormalities of vascular signaling in models of evolving BPD, and downregulation of nitric oxide production appears to be important.[33] Less is known about signaling abnormalities of the remodeled vessel in an infant with established pulmonary hypertension and BPD. Early clinical experience indicates that alterations in the nitric oxide-cGMP, prostacyclin-cAMP, and endothelin pathways will probably all play a role, and these data will be important in developing effective treatment strategies.

REFERENCES

1. Abman SH, et al: Acute effects of partial compression of ductus arteriosus on fetal pulmonary circulation, *Am J Physiol Heart Circ Physiol* 26:H626, 1989.
2. Abman SH, et al: Role of endothelium-derived relaxing factor during transition of pulmonary circulation at birth, *Am J Physiol* 259:H1921, 1990.
3. Alano MA, et al: Analysis of nonsteroidal antiinflammatory drugs in meconium and its relation to persistent pulmonary hypertension of the newborn, *Pediatrics* 107:519, 2001.
4. Allen K, et al: Human postnatal pulmonary arterial remodeling: ultrastructural studies of smooth muscle cell and connective tissue maturation, *Lab Invest* 59:702, 1988.
5. Arrigoni FI, et al: Metabolism of asymmetric dimethylarginines is regulated in the lung developmentally and with pulmonary hypertension induced by hypobaric hypoxia, *Circulation* 107:1195, 2003.
6. Ayajiki K, et al: Intracellular pH and tyrosine phosphorylation but not calcium determine shear stress-induced nitric oxide production in native endothelial cells, *Circ Res* 78:750, 1996.
7. Bourbon J, et al: Control mechanisms of lung alveolar development and their disorders in bronchopulmonary dysplasia, *Pediatr Res* 57:38R, 2005.
8. Brannon TS, et al: Prostacyclin synthesis in ovine pulmonary artery is developmentally regulated by changes in cyclooxygenase-1 gene expression, *J Clin Invest* 93:2230, 1994.
9. Brennan LA, et al: Increased superoxide generation is associated with pulmonary hypertension in fetal lambs: a role for NADPH oxidase, *Circ Res* 92:683, 2003.
10. Chambers CD, et al: Selective serotonin-reuptake inhibitors and risk of persistent pulmonary hypertension of the newborn, *N Engl J Med* 354:579, 2006.
11. deMello DE, et al: Embryonic and early fetal development of human lung vasculature and its functional implications, *Pediatr Dev Pathol* 3:439, 2000.
12. Esterlita M, et al: Decreased gene expression of endothelial nitric oxide synthase in newborns with persistent pulmonary hypertension, *Pediatr Res* 44:338, 1998.
13. Farrow KN, et al: Hyperoxia increases phosphodiesterase 5 expression and activity in ovine fetal pulmonary artery smooth muscle cells, *Circ Res* 102:226, 2008.
14. Fike CD, et al: Thromboxane inhibition reduces an early stage of chronic hypoxia-induced pulmonary hypertension in piglets, *J Appl Physiol* 31:31, 2005.
15. Fike CD, et al: Reactive oxygen species from NADPH oxidase contribute to altered pulmonary vascular responses in piglets

with chronic hypoxia-induced pulmonary hypertension, *Am J Physiol Lung Cell Mol Physiol* 295:L881, 2008.
16. Fineman JR, et al: Chronic nitric oxide inhibition in utero produces persistent pulmonary hypertension in newborn lambs, *J Clin Invest* 93:2675, 1994.
17. Fornaro E, et al: Prenatal exposure to fluoxetine induces fetal pulmonary hypertension in the rat, *Am J Respir Crit Care Med* 176:1035, 2007.
18. Gebb SA, et al: Hypoxia and lung branching morphogenesis, *Adv Exp Med Biol* 543:117, 2003.
19. Gien J, et al: Intrauterine pulmonary hypertension impairs angiogenesis in vitro: role of vascular endothelial growth factor nitric oxide signaling, *Am J Respir Crit Care Med* 176:1146, 2007.
20. Hanson KA, et al: Chronic pulmonary hypertension increases fetal lung cGMP phosphodiesterase activity, *Am J Physiol* 275:L931, 1998.
21. Haworth SG: Normal structural and functional adaptation of extrauterine life, *J Pediatr* 98:915, 1981.
22. Haworth SG: Development of the normal and hypertensive pulmonary vasculature, *Exp Physiol* 80:843, 1995.
23. Hislop A, et al: Intrapulmonary arterial development during fetal life: branching pattern and structure, *J Anat* 113:35, 1975.
24. Ivy DD, et al: Increased lung preproET-1 and decreased ETB-receptor gene expression in fetal pulmonary hypertension, *Am J Physiol* 274:L535, 1998.
25. Janney CG, et al: Congenital alveolar capillary dysplasia-an unusual cause of respiratory distress in the newborn, *Am J Clin Pathol* 76:722, 1981.
26. Khemani E, et al: Pulmonary artery hypertension in formerly premature infants with bronchopulmonary dysplasia: clinical features and outcomes in the surfactant era, *Pediatrics* 120:1260, 2007.
27. Kumar P, et al: Plasma immunoreactive endothelin-1 concentrations in infants with persistent pulmonary hypertension of the newborn, *Am J Perinatol* 13:335, 1996.
28. Lakshminrusimha S, et al: Milrinone enhances relaxation to prostacyclin and iloprost in pulmonary arteries isolated from lambs with persistent pulmonary hypertension of the newborn, *Pediatr Crit Care Med* 10:106, 2009.
29. Leffler CW, et al: The onset of breathing at birth stimulates pulmonary vascular prostacyclin synthesis, *Pediatr Res* 18:938, 1984.
30. Levin DL, et al: Morphological development of the pulmonary vascular bed in fetal lambs, *Circulation* 53:144, 1976.
31. Levin DL, et al: Constriction of the fetal ductus arteriosus after administration of indomethacin to the pregnant ewe, *J Pediatr* 94:647, 1979.
32. Machado RD, et al: BMPR2 haploinsufficiency as the inherited molecular mechanism for primary pulmonary hypertension, *Am J Hum Genet* 68:92, 2001.
33. McCurnin DC, et al: Inhaled NO improves early pulmonary function and modifies lung growth and elastin deposition in a baboon model of neonatal chronic lung disease, *Am J Physiol Lung Cell Mol Physiol* 288:L450, 2005.
34. Mohseni-Bod H, et al: Pulmonary hypertension in congenital diaphragmatic hernia, *Semin Pediatr Surg* 16:126, 2007.
35. Morin III FC, et al: Development of pulmonary vascular response to oxygen, *Am J Physiol Heart Circ Physiol* 254:H542, 1988.
36. Morin III FC, et al: Persistent pulmonary hypertension of the newborn, *Am J Respir Crit Care Med* 151:2010, 1995.
37. Mourani PM, et al: Pulmonary vascular effects of inhaled nitric oxide and oxygen tension in bronchopulmonary dysplasia, *Am J Respir Crit Care Med* 170:1006, 2004.

38. Murphy JD, et al: The structural basis of persistent pulmonary hypertension of the newborn infant, *J Pediatr* 98:962, 1981.

39. Parker TA, et al: Rho kinase activation maintains high pulmonary vascular resistance in the ovine fetal lung, *Am J Physiol Lung Cell Mol Physiol* 291:L976, 2006.

40. Pierce CM, et al: Asymmetric dimethyl arginine and symmetric dimethyl arginine levels in infants with persistent pulmonary hypertension of the newborn, *Pediatr Crit Care Med* 5:517, 2004.

41. Rosenberg AA, et al: Elevated immunoreactive endothelin-1 levels in newborn infants with persistent pulmonary hypertension, *J Pediatr* 123:109, 1993.

42. Sanchez LS, et al: Cyclic-GMP-binding, cyclic-GMP-specific phosphodiesterase gene expression is regulated during rat pulmonary development, *Pediatr Res* 43:163, 1998.

43. Sen P, et al: Expanding the phenotype of alveolar capillary dysplasia (ACD), *J Pediatr* 145:646, 2004.

44. Shaul PW, et al: Prostacyclin production and mediation of adenylate cyclase activity in the pulmonary artery: alterations after prolonged hypoxia in the rat, *J Clin Invest* 88:447, 1991.

45. Shaul PW, et al: Pulmonary endothelial NO synthase gene expression is decreased in fetal lambs with pulmonary hypertension, *Am J Physiol Lung Cell Mol Physiol* 272:L1005, 1997.

46. Siebert JR, et al: Left ventricular hypoplasia in congenital diaphragmatic hernia, *J Pediatr Surg* 19:567, 1984.

46a. Stankiewicz P, et al: Genomic and genic deletions of the FOX gene cluster on 16q24.1 and inactivating mutations of FOXF1 cause alveolar capillary dysplasia and other malformations, *Am J Hum Genet* 84:780, 2009.

47. Steinhorn RH, et al: Disruption of cyclic GMP production in pulmonary arteries isolated from fetal lambs with pulmonary hypertension, *Am J Physiol Heart Circ Physiol* 268:H1483, 1995.

48. Stenmark KP, et al: Lung vascular development: implications for the pathogenesis of bronchopulmonary dysplasia, *Annu Rev Physiol* 67:623, 2005.

49. Stevens T, et al: Lung vascular cell heterogeneity: endothelium, smooth muscle, and fibroblasts, *Proc Am Thorac Soc* 5:783, 2008.

50. Storme L, et al: In vivo evidence for a myogenic response in the fetal pulmonary circulation, *Pediatr Res* 45:425, 1999.

51. Thebaud B, et al: Bronchopulmonary dysplasia: where have all the vessels gone? Roles of angiogenic growth factors in chronic lung disease, *Am J Respir Crit Care Med* 175:978, 2007.

52. Tiktinsky MH, et al: Increasing oxygen tension dilates fetal pulmonary circulation via endothelium-derived relaxing factor, *Am J Physiol Heart Circ Physiol* 265:H376, 1993.

53. Uematsu M, et al: Regulation of endothelial cell nitric oxide synthase mRNA expression by shear stress, *Am J Physiol* 269:C1371, 1995.

54. Villamor E, et al: Chronic intrauterine pulmonary hypertension impairs endothelial nitric oxide synthase in the ovine fetus, *Am J Physiol Lung Cell Mol Physiol* 272:L1013, 1997.

55. Wedgwood S, et al: Role for endothelin-1-induced superoxide and peroxynitrite production in rebound pulmonary hypertension associated with inhaled nitric oxide therapy, *Circ Res* 89:357, 2001.

56. Wojciak-Stothard B, et al: Rac and Rho play opposing roles in the regulation of hypoxia/reoxygenation-induced permeability changes in pulmonary artery endothelial cells, *Am J Physiol Lung Cell Mol Physiol* 288:L749, 2005.

PART 3

Genetic and Environmental Contributions to Congenital Heart Disease

Kenneth G. Zahka

Insight into the causes of congenital heart disease can be gained from analysis of genetic and environmental factors[14,15,24,27] and consideration of associated noncardiac abnormalities. Animal models have provided an understanding of the role of a number of gene defects in a variety of transcription factors and signaling molecules that are associated with congenital heart defects. These include the transcription factors NKX2.5, TBX5, GATA4, and FOG2 and the signaling molecules PTPN11, JAG1, and CFC1.[15]

From population-based studies, principally the Baltimore-Washington Infant Study, it is known that more than 25% of infants with congenital heart disease have noncardiac abnormalities.[9] Chromosomal abnormalities and well-defined genetic syndromes constitute two thirds of these cases. The major chromosomal defects are summarized in Table 45-2, although there are many more recognized deletions with a known association with heart disease (see Chapter 29).

Infants with syndromes clearly related to excess or deleted chromosomal material have a pattern of anomalies that are pathogenetically related. Infants who have clusters of defects that appear in a nonrandom fashion and that do not correspond to either syndromes or particular developmental fields during cardiogenesis could have one of several recognized associations. The cause of these associations, including VACTERL (*v*ertebral abnormalities, *a*nal atresia, *c*ardiac abnormalities, *t*racheoesophageal fistula or *e*sophageal atresia, *r*enal agenesis and dysplasia, and *l*imb defects)[19,20] is not yet known, although midline defects might represent defects in blastogenesis. Mutations in the *CHD7* gene have been found in most patients with CHARGE association (*c*oloboma, *h*eart disease, choanal *a*tresia, *r*estricted *g*rowth and development or other central nervous system anomalies, genital hypoplasia, and *e*ar anomalies or deafness).[18,21]

CHROMOSOMAL DEFECTS

Molecular karyotyping yields an etiological diagnosis in at least 18% of patients with a syndromic CHD. Higher resolution evaluation results in an increasing number of variants of unknown significance.[3a]

The association of congenital heart disease with chromosomal defects, especially trisomies 13, 18, and 21, has been known for many years. Congenital heart defects are not present in all infants with trisomy 21 despite the apparent duplication of genetic material in each child. Equally intriguing is the narrow spectrum of heart defects observed in the 40% of infants with trisomy 21 and congenital heart disease (Table 45-3).[11] Sixty-five percent have endocardial cushion defects, a proportion many times that seen in children with heart defects and normal chromosomes.[30] Furthermore, many defects, including

TABLE 45–2 Major Chromosomal and Inherited Syndromes Associated with Heart Defects

Syndrome	Defects
Trisomy 8	Variable
Trisomy 13	ASD, PDA, VSD
Trisomy 18	ASD, ECD, PDA, TOF, VSD
Turner (XO)	AS, COA, HLHS[31]
Klinefelter (XXY)	MVP, TOF
Deletion 22q11	IAA, TOF, truncus
Marfan (AD, chromosome 15)	Aortic dilation, aortic dilation, TVP
DiGeorge (AD, chromosome 22)	IAA, TOF, truncus arteriosus
Williams (AD, chromosome 7)	Branch pulmonary artery stenosis, supravalvular aortic stenosis[7]
Holt-Oram (AD, chromosome 12)	ASD, COA, VSD[17]
Ellis-van Creveld (AR)	Common atrium
Meckel-Gruber (AR)	AS, ASD, COA, TGA, VSD
Radial aplasia-thrombocytopenia	ASD, TOF
Smith-Lemli-Opitz (AR)	TAPVC
Noonan (AD)	Cardiomyopathy, PS[32]
Kartagener (AR)	Dextrocardia
Neurofibromatosis (AD)	PS, aortic dilation, MVP, HCM[35]

AD, autosomal dominant; AR, autosomal recessive; AS, aortic stenosis; ASD, secundum atrial septal defect; COA, coarctation of the aorta; ECD, endocardial cushion defect; HCM, hypertrophic cardiomyopathy, HLHS, hypoplastic left heart syndrome; IAA, interrupted aortic arch; MVP, mitral valve prolapse; PDA, patent ductus arteriosus; PS, pulmonary valve stenosis; TAPVC, total anomalous pulmonary venous connection; TGA, transposition of the great arteries; TOF, tetralogy of Fallot; TVP, tricuspid valve prolapse; VSD, ventricular septal defect.

transposition of the great arteries and truncus arteriosus, which are common in infants with normal chromosomes, are rare or unreported in children with trisomy 21. The proportion of infants with trisomies 13 and 18 and heart disease is higher than that of infants with trisomy 21, yet the spectrum of defects is also narrower than in the general population.

The understanding of the mechanism of abnormal cardiogenesis is an area of intense interest in cardiovascular genetics. Collagen type VI has been studied for its role in the pathogenesis of heart defects in children with Down syndrome. Studies suggest that genetic variation in the *COL6A1* gene might be associated with an increased prevalence of heart defects.[6] The *SH3BGR* gene on chromosome 21 has been proposed as a critical candidate gene for cardiac defects and hypotonia.[34]

SINGLE GENE DEFECTS

Cardiovascular abnormalities are a feature of a number of syndromes that are clearly due to single gene defects. In Marfan syndrome, the defect has been linked to mutations in the fibrillin gene on chromosome 15.[8] Loeys-Dietz syndrome is a newly described connective tissue disorder due to mutations in the receptor for transforming growth factor-β, which can present in the neonatal period with aortic dilation and mitral valve prolapse.[23] Williams syndrome is associated with a defect in the elastin gene on chromosome 7.[36] Holt-Oram and other hand-heart syndromes have been found on chromosome 12. Holt-Oram syndrome is caused by mutations in the *TBX5* gene, which is believed to be critical for heart and limb development.[17]

Recognition that microdeletions of chromosome 22 are associated with the phenotype of velocardiofacial syndrome[13] and DiGeorge syndrome, both of which have a high prevalence of conotruncal heart defects, has increased the interest in abnormalities of this chromosome as a cause of other conotruncal defects. Goldmuntz and associates screened 250 consecutive children with conotruncal defects and found that 50% of children with interrupted aortic arch, 35% with truncus arteriosus, and 16% with tetralogy of Fallot had a microdeletion of chromosome 22.[12] Children with right aortic arch or aberrant subclavian artery were particularly likely to have a deletion.

Mutations in the *NKX2.5* gene are associated with heart defects and conduction abnormalities.[25] The cardiovascular abnormalities in Alagille syndrome are seen in children with *JAG1* mutation.[26]

TABLE 45–3 Cardiovascular Diagnoses in Infants with Down Syndrome and Isolated Cardiac Malformations

Diagnosis	No. of Patients	PERCENTAGE OF PATIENTS WITH DEFECT					
		CAVSD	PAVSD	VSD	ASD	TOF	PDA
Down syndrome	160	51	13	16	10	6	4
Isolated cardiac malformation	540	2	4	58	16	15	6

ASD, secundum atrial septal defect; CAVSD, complete atrioventricular septal defect; PAVSD, partial atrioventricular septal defect; PDA, patent ductus arteriosus; TOF, tetralogy of Fallot; VSD, perimembranous ventricular septal defect.
Adapted from Schneider DS, et al: Patterns of cardiac care in infants with Down syndrome, *Am J Dis Child* 143:363, 1989.

ENVIRONMENTAL TOXINS

Epidemiologic studies have occasionally linked exposure to drugs or environmental toxins to congenital heart defects (see Chapter 12). The timing of exposure during early cardiogenesis is critical, and in some cases, as in exposure to lithium,[2] the evidence remains controversial. Abuse of substances such as ethanol and probably cocaine increases the risk for congenital heart defects. Anticonvulsant therapy with phenytoin and valproic acid is associated with fetal congenital heart defects. Warfarin therapy is a major concern for mothers with congenital heart defects because the risk for congenital heart disease in offspring might be additive with any potential genetic risk.

Prostaglandin synthetase inhibitors, principally indomethacin, have been used in the third trimester to treat premature labor. Transient partial constriction of the fetal ductus arteriosus has been documented by fetal echocardiography and Doppler studies in up to 25% of fetuses during several days of maternal administration of indomethacin.[22] The narrowing resolves after discontinuation of the drug, although prolonged administration to animals can result in right ventricular dysfunction and tricuspid regurgitation as a result of right ventricular hypertension.

MATERNAL DISEASES

Mothers who have diabetes mellitus during cardiogenesis have a twofold to fourfold risk for having babies with congenital heart disease, most commonly ventricular septal defect, transposition of the great arteries, tetralogy of Fallot, and double-outlet right ventricle (see Chapter 16 and Chapter 49, Part 1).[1] The mechanism of this risk is unknown but is presumed to be metabolic abnormalities that occur during critical phases of development. Heart defects are less common in mothers with normal hemoglobin A_{1c} levels.[29] In late gestation, poor control of diabetes increases fetal insulin concentration in response to the increased transplacental glucose load. Insulin is a growth factor for fetal myocardium, and the infants could be born with hypertrophic cardiomyopathy. This myopathy is usually asymptomatic and resolves during the first weeks of life. A small number of infants have significant diastolic dysfunction or dynamic outflow tract obstruction, with tachypnea and signs of congestive heart failure or poor cardiac output at presentation. Treatment is usually supportive, with avoidance of inotropes, which could exacerbate the systolic obstruction.

Mothers with anti-Ro or anti-La antibodies because of lupus erythematosus have a small (about 5%) but important risk for fetal heart block (see Chapter 18).[4] There is transplacental passage of immunoglobulin G antibody, with antibody and complement deposition in the fetal myocardium. The risk is not related to the severity of the maternal disease, and the diagnosis of the maternal collagen vascular disease could be prompted by the observation of fetal conduction abnormalities. Fetal conduction defects worsen during gestation and in the early years of life.[4] In utero symptoms are rare; however, when they are present, such as hydrops fetalis, congestive heart failure could be related to both decreased heart rate and myocardial inflammation.

Maternal treatment with dexamethasone in an attempt to reduce potential inflammation in the fetal myocardium and conduction system does not appear to be effective in reversing established rhythm abnormalities.[5] Careful postnatal follow-up is important for assessing symptoms and the ventricular rate. Temporary or permanent pacing might be advantageous even in the neonatal period if the ventricular rate is slow (less than 60 beats per minute) or there is feeding intolerance, and many children require permanent pacemakers early in life.[4] Cardiomyopathy might be present in the newborn period or could develop over the first months of life in these babies.[33]

Neonatal diagnosis has improved the prognosis of phenylketonuria in children. Women who have benefited from dietary therapy are reaching childbearing age, and poor control of the maternal disease during cardiogenesis is associated with a high risk for congenital heart defects.[28]

INFLUENCE OF GENETICS, SEX, AND RACE

Multiple epidemiologic studies suggest a multifactorial cause of congenital heart disease with a relatively low (3% to 5%) risk for recurrence in siblings or offspring of parents with congenital heart defects.[3] In some families, left heart defects or conotruncal defects might be under much greater genetic control.[16] Genetic analysis of these families, especially those with several affected members, will provide insight into the pathogenesis of congenital heart disease. Aortic stenosis and transposition of the great arteries are more common (65%) in male patients. Racial differences in the prevalence or type of congenital heart defects are surprisingly few.[10] The exception is the large percentage of supracristal ventricular septal defects in Japanese people. A group of Amish infants have been described with a lethal form of neonatal hypertrophic cardiomyopathy and found to be homozygous for a mutation in the myosin binding protein C3 (*MYBPC3*) gene, which has been associated in its heterozygous form with adult-onset hypertrophic cardiomyopathy.[38]

MAJOR ASSOCIATED NONCARDIAC DEFECTS

Two major associations, VACTERL and CHARGE, highlight the spectrum of associated defects observed in neonates with congenital heart defects. Although neither VACTERL nor CHARGE is caused by a single pathogenetic mechanism, recognition of these associations is helpful in facilitating multidisciplinary care and diagnosing all components of the association.

The VACTERL association describes a coincidence of defects, including vertebral abnormalities, anal atresia, tracheoesophageal fistula, renal abnormalities, congenital heart disease, and limb abnormalities. Seventy percent of infants with VACTERL have three affected systems, 25% have four components, and 10% have five components. The variability of the individual components is great, and congenital heart disease is present in about three fourths of infants with the VACTERL association. Ventricular septal defect, tetralogy of Fallot, and coarctation of the aorta are the most common defects. Vertebral abnormalities include hemivertebrae, hypoplastic vertebrae, and extra vertebrae. The vertebral abnormalities are often associated with rib abnormalities. Renal abnormalities, including fistula and urethral obstruction, are particularly important in neonates who also have anal atresia. Limb defects might be unilateral or bilateral and could include displaced or absent thumbs and radial abnormalities.

CHARGE is the association of *colobomas*, *heart* defects, *choanal atresia*, *growth* and developmental *restriction*, *genital hypoplasia*, and *ear* abnormalities.[37] There is at least a 50% incidence of congenital heart defects in CHARGE association patients, with a preponderance of tetralogy of Fallot defects, including tetralogy of Fallot, tetralogy of Fallot with atrioventricular septal defect, tetralogy of Fallot with pulmonary atresia, and tetralogy of Fallot with Ebstein anomaly. Atrioventricular canal defects, double-outlet right ventricle, double-inlet left ventricle, and transposition of the great arteries have also been reported.

REFERENCES

1. Aberg A, et al: Congenital malformations among infants whose mothers had gestational diabetes or preexisting diabetes, *Early Hum Dev* 61:85, 2001.
2. Altshuler LL, et al: Pharmacologic management of psychiatric illness during pregnancy: dilemmas and guidelines, *Am J Psychiatry* 153:592, 1996.
3. Boughman J, et al: Familial risks of congenital heart disease assessed by a population-based epidemiologic study, *Am J Med Genet* 26:839, 1987.
3a. Breckpot J, Thienpont B, Peeters H, et al: Array comparative genomic hybridization as a diagnostic tool for syndromic heart defects, *J Pediatr* 156(5):810, 2010.
4. Buyon JP, et al: Autoimmune-associated congenital heart block: Demographics, mortality, morbidity and recurrence rates obtained from a national neonatal lupus registry, *J Am Coll Cardiol* 31:1658, 1998.
5. Buyon JP, et al. Autoimmune associated congenital heart block: integration of clinical and research clues in the management of the maternal/foetal dyad at risk, *J Intern Med* 265:653, 2009.
6. Davies GE, et al: Unusual genotypes in the COL6A1 gene in parents of children with trisomy 21 and major congenital heart defects, *Hum Genet* 93:443, 1994.
7. Eronen M, et al: Cardiovascular manifestations in 75 patients with Williams syndrome, *J Med Genet* 39:554, 2002.
8. Faivre L, et al: Clinical and molecular study of 320 children with Marfan syndrome and related type I fibrillinopathies in a series of 1009 probands with pathogenic FBN1 mutations, *Pediatrics* 123:391, 2009.
9. Ferencz C, et al: Congenital cardiovascular malformations: Questions on inheritance, *J Am Coll Cardiol* 14:756, 1989.
10. Fixler D, et al: Ethnicity and socioeconomic status: impact on the diagnosis of congenital heart disease, *J Am Coll Cardiol* 21:1722, 1993.
11. Freeman SB, et al: Population-based study of congenital heart defects in Down syndrome, *Am J Med Genet* 80:213, 1998.
12. Goldmuntz E, et al: Frequency of 22q11 deletions in patients with conotruncal defects, *J Am Coll Cardiol* 32:492, 1998.
13. Goldmuntz E, Emanuel BS: Genetic disorders of cardiac morphogenesis: the DiGeorge and velocardiofacial syndromes, *Circ Res* 80:437, 1997.
14. Harris JA, et al: The epidemiology of cardiovascular defects. Part 2: A study based on data from three large registries of congenital malformations, *Pediatr Cardiol* 24:222, 2003.
15. Hinton RB Jr, et al: Congenital heart disease: genetic causes and developmental insights, *Prog Pediatr Cardiol* 20:101, 2005.
16. Hinton RB, et al: Hypoplastic left heart syndrome links to chromosomes 10q and 6q and is genetically related to bicuspid aortic valve, *J Am Coll Cardiol* 53(12):1065, 2009.
17. Huang T: Current advances in Holt-Oram syndrome, *Curr Opin Pediatr* 14:691, 2002.
18. Jyonouchi S, et al: CHARGE (coloboma, heart defect, atresia choanae, retarded growth and development, genital hypoplasia, ear anomalies/deafness) syndrome and chromosome 22q11.2 deletion syndrome: a comparison of immunologic and nonimmunologic phenotypic features, *Pediatrics* 123:e871, 2009.
19. Källén K, et al: VATER non-random association of congenital malformations: study based on data from four malformation registers, *Am J Med Genet* 101:26, 2001.
20. Kim J, et al: The VACTERL association: lessons from the sonic hedgehog pathway, *Clin Genet* 59:306, 2001.
21. Lalani SR, et al: Spectrum of CHD7 mutations in 110 individuals with CHARGE syndrome and genotype-phenotype correlation, *Am J Hum Genet* 78:303, 2006.
22. Levy R, et al: Indomethacin and corticosteroids: an additive constrictive effect on the fetal ductus arteriosus, *Am J Perinatol* 16:379, 1999.
23. Loeys BL, et al: Aneurysm syndromes caused by mutations in the TGF-beta receptor, *N Engl J Med* 355:788, 2006.
24. Maron BJ, et al: Impact of laboratory molecular diagnosis on contemporary diagnostic criteria for genetically transmitted cardiovascular diseases: hypertrophic cardiomyopathy, long-QT syndrome, and Marfan syndrome. A statement for healthcare professionals from the Councils on Clinical Cardiology, Cardiovascular Disease in the Young, and Basic Science, American Heart Association, *Circulation* 98:1460, 1998.
25. McElhinney DB, et al: NKX2.5 mutations in patients with congenital heart disease, *J Am Coll Cardiol* 42:1650, 2003.
26. McElhinney DB, et al: Analysis of cardiovascular phenotype and genotype-phenotype correlation in individuals with a JAG1 mutation and/or Alagille syndrome, *Circulation* 106:2567, 2002.
27. Pradat P, et al: The epidemiology of cardiovascular defects, part I: A study based on data from three large registries of congenital malformations, *Pediatr Cardiol* 24:195, 2003.
28. Rouse B, et al: Maternal phenylketonuria syndrome: congenital heart defects, microcephaly, and developmental outcomes, *J Pediatr* 136:57, 2000.
29. Schaefer-Graf UM, et al: Patterns of congenital anomalies and relationship to initial maternal fasting glucose levels in pregnancies complicated by type 2 and gestational diabetes, *Am J Obstet Gynecol* 182:313, 2000.
30. Schneider DS, et al: Patterns of cardiac care in infants with Down syndrome, *Am J Dis Child* 143:363, 1989.
31. Sybert VP, McCauley E: Turner's syndrome, *N Engl J Med* 351:1227, 2004.
32. Sznajer Y, et al: The spectrum of cardiac anomalies in Noonan syndrome as a result of mutations in the PTPN11 gene, *Pediatrics* 119:e1325, 2007.
33. Taylor-Albert E, et al: Delayed dilated cardiomyopathy as a manifestation of neonatal lupus: case reports, autoantibody analysis, and management, *Pediatrics* 99:733, 1997.

34. Vidal-Taboada JM, et al: High-resolution physical map and identification of potentially regulatory sequences of the human SH3BGR located in the Down syndrome chromosomal region, *Biochem Biophys Res Commun* 241:321, 1997.
35. Williams VC, et al: Neurofibromatosis type 1 revisited, *Pediatrics* 123:124, 2009.
36. Wu YQ, et al: Delineation of the common critical region in Williams syndrome and clinical correlation of growth, heart defects, ethnicity, and parental origin, *Am J Med Genet* 78:82, 1998.
37. Wyse R, et al: Congenital heart disease in CHARGE association, *Pediatr Cardiol* 14:75, 1993.
38. Zahka K, Kalidas K, Simpson MA, et al: Homozygous mutation of MYBPC3 associated with severe infantile hypertrophic cardiomyopathy at high frequency among the Amish, *Heart* 94:1326, 2008.

PART 4

Fetal Cardiac Physiology and Fetal Cardiovascular Assessment

Francine Erenberg

PHYSIOLOGY

The physiology of congenital heart disease is best understood in the context of understanding fetal blood flow patterns and the subsequent transition to a postnatal circulation.[21] Most significant cardiac lesions diagnosed in the newborn period are compatible with a relatively normal intrauterine existence. It is the transition to extrauterine life that makes most cardiac lesions hemodynamically significant.

As described in more detail later, in the fetal circulation, very little blood flow is required to go to the lungs because the placenta provides fetal oxygenation, and both ventricles are responsible for perfusing the systemic circulation. Many critical newborn lesions involve severely diminished pulmonary blood flow (e.g., pulmonary atresia, tricuspid atresia) and, therefore, are well tolerated in utero when this is the norm, but they become clinically significant in the neonate. Similarly, defects involving a single ventricle or large ventricular septal defect with mixing of right and left ventricular blood are well tolerated during fetal life when both ventricles normally act as "systemic ventricles." Finally, because the right ventricle also contributes to the perfusion of the aorta and systemic circulatory system, even lesions of severe left heart obstruction (e.g., interrupted aortic arch, hypoplastic left heart syndrome) can be well tolerated in the fetus.

After birth, however, closure of the ductus arteriosus results in inadequate pulmonary or systemic blood flow, leading to rapid demise if no intervention is undertaken. In many such infants, early management has as its goal the return of the circulation to the in utero situation for a period long enough to reach a diagnosis and begin definitive therapy.

Fetal Circulation

Circulation in the normal fetus differs from that of the normal newborn because of the following in utero characteristics:

- There is high pulmonary vascular resistance and low systemic vascular resistance.
- Right and left ventricles contribute to systemic perfusion and circulation.
- Additional structures are present: foramen ovale, ductus arteriosus, and ductus venosus.
- The placenta is the site of gas exchange for the fetus.

As opposed to that found in the child or adult, vasoconstriction of the pulmonary arteriolar bed maintains high resistance in the pulmonary circuit; this directs most of the right ventricular blood across the ductus arteriosus and into the descending aorta rather than to the branch pulmonary arteries and lungs. The right ventricle therefore provides blood to the descending aorta and the placenta through the ductus arteriosus. The left ventricle supplies the ascending aorta and the upper portion of the body, including the brain, and sends a small amount down the descending aorta to mix with the right ventricular output. Therefore, the two ventricles are essentially pumping in parallel, not in series, and there is a functional, but not absolute, separation in the systemic circulation in the fetus. From this separation, the right ventricle supplies the lower portion of the body, and the placenta and the left ventricle supply the upper portion of the body.

Oxygenation occurs in the placenta, and blood of higher oxygen content passes from the placenta into the umbilical vein. Umbilical venous blood is distributed to both lobes of the liver, whereas portal venous blood is distributed almost completely to the right lobe of the liver. About half of the umbilical vein blood bypasses the ductus venosus and enters directly into the inferior vena cava. Thus, inferior vena cava blood in the fetus contains relatively more oxygen. In contrast, superior vena cava blood is highly deoxygenated because it is the venous return from the head and upper body, and it has no admixture of oxygen-rich blood from the placenta.

Although both superior and inferior caval blood arrive in the right atrium, patterns of streaming within the right atrium continue to separate the blood in terms of oxygen content. Blood from the superior vena cava, which is low in oxygen content, preferentially crosses the tricuspid valve and is sent by the right ventricle, through the ductus arteriosus, to the descending aorta and placenta (where it is oxygenated). Blood from the inferior vena cava, which is higher in oxygen content because of the contribution from the placenta, preferentially crosses the foramen ovale to fill the left atrium and left ventricle; from there, it is sent predominantly to the upper portion of the body, the brain, and the coronary circulation. Thus, blood in the ascending aorta has more oxygen than that in the descending aorta, resulting in the brain receiving blood with a higher oxygen content than does the lower body and placenta.

Transition to Extrauterine Circulation

With birth, a number of important events take place that result in important physiologic changes to the newborn infant circulation. These changes include the following:

- Increase in the systemic vascular resistance
- Decrease in the pulmonary vascular resistance
- Closure of the ductus arteriosus and ductus venosus
- Transition to left-to-right shunting through the foramen ovale
- Eventual closure of the foramen ovale

Occlusion of the umbilical cord removes the low-resistance capillary bed from the systemic circulation, thus increasing the systemic vascular resistance of the infant. Breathing is followed by a marked fall in pulmonary vascular resistance.

The fall in pulmonary vascular resistance results in increased pulmonary venous return to fill the left atrium. The increased left atrial filling then limits and eventually eliminates flow from the inferior vena cava through the foramen ovale into the left atrium. The increased filling and pressure in the left atrium direct blood left to right across the atrial septum, eventually functionally closing the foramen ovale flap. Because blood that returns from the lungs is more completely oxygenated than the blood that was provided by the placenta, arterial oxygen saturation in the left heart (and thus the body) then increases, and the baby becomes pink.

There is loss of endogenous prostaglandins produced by the placenta. The increase in arterial oxygen saturation of the blood primarily brings about closure of the ductus arteriosus and ductus venosus. Most of the transition from fetal to neonatal circulation takes place in the first several minutes of life and is due to changes in vascular resistance. Functional closure of the ductus arteriosus takes place within 10 to 15 hours after birth, but anatomic closure occurs only within days to 2 weeks. The foramen ovale typically remains patent, with little to no flow through it for weeks or months, and in fact could remain patent into adulthood.

Pulmonary Vascular Bed

The pulmonary vascular bed is a key component in the pathophysiology of congenital heart disease, affecting its presentation and management. Thus, special attention is paid to the pulmonary vascular bed during neonatal life. The first breath is accompanied by a sudden and dramatic fall in pulmonary vascular resistance, and a further decrease in resistance occurs within the first several days of life as pulmonary arterioles relax and subsequently mature. In normal infants, the pulmonary vascular bed resembles the adult pattern, both in resistance and in histologic appearance, by several weeks of age. In some infants, however, this maturation of the pulmonary vascular bed does not occur, or it occurs over a longer period.

Two factors could be responsible for this difference. First, alveolar hypoxemia can maintain pulmonary vasoconstriction after birth, as in infants born at high altitudes and those with lung disease.[45] Second, primary or secondary changes in the pulmonary vasculature can result in persistent or recurrent increase in arteriolar tension, resulting in pulmonary hypertension. Secondary pulmonary hypertension is much more common and could be a result of severe, persistent intrinsic lung disease or hypercarbia, as in a child with severe bronchopulmonary dysplasia, or it could be a result of congenital heart disease. An example of the latter is an infant with a large left-to-right shunt, such as a large ventricular septal defect. In this instance, the presence of the defect allows transmission of systemic left ventricular systolic pressure to the right ventricle and in turn to the pulmonary artery and pulmonary vascular bed.

This pulmonary hypertension interferes with the normal fall in pulmonary resistance described earlier, and the resistance could stay high until 1 or 2 months of age. In some patients with very large left-to-right shunts, often with the combination of excessive pulmonary blood flow, pulmonary resistance never falls, or after briefly falling, it becomes secondarily elevated again. Defects of this type, if not corrected surgically, eventually result in irreversible pulmonary vascular disease, or Eisenmenger syndrome.

CARDIOVASCULAR ASSESSMENT

Fetal cardiology is a field that requires the combined expertise of the pediatric cardiologist, the perinatal obstetrician, the geneticist, and the neonatologist. The main tool in fetal cardiac assessment is the fetal two-dimensional echocardiogram and Doppler examination, which is used in the diagnosis and follow-up of fetuses with structural congenital heart disease, arrhythmia, and myocardial disease or congestive heart failure. Fetal three- and four-dimensional echocardiography is also used to expand some of the diagnostic ability and precision of the two-dimensional scan.[39,56] Fetal electrocardiography, fetal magnetocardiography, and fetal cardiac magnetic resonance imaging are other techniques used, but these continue to have limitations and are generally used only in selected clinical scenarios or centers and not as screening or routine tools.

Fetal electrocardiography using maternal abdominal electrodes has been attempted, but with little success because of several limitations. These limitations include the insulating effect of the vernix caseosa after 27 weeks' gestation, the lack of consistent positioning of the fetus within the maternal abdomen, and the preferred conduction pathways between the fetal heart and maternal abdomen after about 27 weeks' gestation.[57] Fetal magnetocardiography has been used in attempts to increase the sensitivity of fetal heart rate tracings in the assessment of fetal well-being and in the diagnosis of arrhythmias. Its current role remains extremely limited because it is time consuming, expensive, and available only at a few centers.[47]

In addition to identifying specific lesions, fetal echocardiography can be used to aid our understanding of the physiology and natural history of conditions throughout pregnancy and for monitoring the heart during cardiac and noncardiac fetal interventions.

Indications for Fetal Cardiovascular Assessment

The incidence of congenital heart disease in the general population is about 1 per 125 live births.[2] The incidence in fetal life is actually higher because of fetal wastage from the heart defects, associated aneuploidy, or other congenital defects. A detailed fetal echocardiogram is both time intensive and labor intensive; for this reason, its use has been directed toward those pregnancies considered at increased risk for having a fetus with congenital heart disease. These include a family history of congenital heart disease in one of the parents or a previous sibling. Compared with the baseline risk, a family history raises the risk for fetal heart defects from 0.5 to 1 per 100 in the general population to 3 to 14 per 100.[41] Given this incremental risk, it is considered an important indication for fetal screening.

High-risk groups can further be divided into those with increased maternal risks and those with increased fetal risk factors.[10,44] These risk factors are listed in Box 45-1.

Certain extracardiac malformations have an especially high association with congenital heart disease. These include omphalocele (30%), diaphragmatic hernia, duodenal atresia, single umbilical artery, tracheoesophageal fistula, cystic hygroma, and increased nuchal translucency. Increased nuchal translucency is often seen in trisomy 21 or other chromosome abnormalities; in this context, the association with congenital heart defects is as high as 90%. Even in the absence of abnormal karyotype, increased nuchal translucency has a significant association with congenital heart disease, especially with increasing levels of edema.[24] Newer work suggests that increased nuchal translucency is not an appropriate screening test for congenital heart defects, but that the finding of increased nuchal translucency on screening ultrasound demands a formal fetal echocardiogram and more thorough evaluation for the presence of a structural heart defect.[35,55,63]

Box 45-2 lists indications for performing echocardiography in the fetus.

Finally, referrals sent secondary to suspected abnormality from a screening obstetric ultrasound have the highest yield; at least half of all mothers referred for detailed fetal cardiac studies on this basis are found to have fetuses with cardiac abnormalities.[1,8] The yield may be even higher depending on the skill level of the referring center. However, it should be noted that recent data from California indicate that overall

---

BOX 45–1 **Risk Factors for Congenital Heart Disease**

MATERNAL RISK FACTORS
Maternal metabolic disorders (diabetes, phenylketonuria)
Exposure to known teratogen (viral or drug), especially earlier than 8 weeks of gestation
Maternal autoantibodies (fetal heart block)
Maternal congenital heart disease: 5% to 10% recurrence risk, depending on lesion

FETAL RISK FACTORS
Suspicion of congenital heart disease on obstetric ultrasound
Extracardiac malformations or major anomalies of other organ systems
Aneuploidy or abnormal karyotype
Increased nuchal thickening, even in the absence of abnormal karyotype
Arrhythmia
Fetal hydrops, about 25% of which is cardiac

BOX 45–2 **Indications for Fetal Echocardiography**

Abnormal screening obstetric ultrasound
Fetal arrhythmia
Family history of congenital heart disease
Maternal diabetes
Maternal teratogen exposure (first trimester)
Extracardiac anomalies
Aneuploidy or abnormal karyotype
Hydrops fetalis
Increased nuchal translucency

---

prenatal detection of major congenital heart disease only occurs in less than 50% of cases.[20] In other series, the numbers range from 57% to 65%. To identify most lesions that can occur in the fetus, in addition to the traditional four-chamber view, it is necessary to include a view of the outflow tract using the most sophisticated equipment and have highly trained operators.[14]

Timing

The ideal timing of screening for fetal congenital heart defects is a compromise between obtaining adequate images for diagnosis in most routine patients and yet offering diagnosis as early as possible for parents to consider all options, including termination of pregnancy, if applicable.[38] Scanning must, therefore, occur sufficiently late to have adequate anatomic assessment and not miss late-developing lesions, and it must be early enough for all pregnancy outcomes to be considered. For the low-risk patient, this window is generally about 20 weeks of gestation. For those at high risk, such as fetuses with significant nuchal translucency or a family history, especially of left heart obstructive lesions, a preliminary examination at 11 to 15 weeks by transabdominal or transabdominal plus transvaginal echocardiogram should be considered and has been shown to have reasonable accuracy. Studies performed in the late first trimester are generally followed up with a more detailed study at 18 to 20 weeks' gestation.[3,25] In one series, 160 fetal echocardiograms were performed at a mean gestational age of 13.5 weeks in a population at high risk for anomalies. Twenty cardiac defects were found in this cohort, 14 of which were identified at the early echocardiogram, and 6 which were identified at the later study.[4]

Methods

Despite newer techniques, the two-dimensional and Doppler fetal echocardiogram remains the mainstay of fetal diagnosis, often supplemented with newer techniques targeted to provide additional anatomic or functional information. Studies are generally performed at 18 to 20 weeks' gestational age, although transabdominal, and certainly transvaginal, imaging can be performed as early as 11 weeks.

Adequate images can be obtained in nearly all pregnancies, although maternal obesity can limit the studies. The standard examination uses the approach known as *segmental anatomy*, the same method used in the pediatric echocardiogram, and consists of several views. The goal of the segmental anatomy approach is to scan from multiple standard views to assess the heart in terms of its segments, specifically the venous-atrial connections, the atrioventricular (AV) connections, and the ventriculoarterial connections, on both the right and left side of the heart. The basic anatomy is thus visualized by the two-dimensional component of the echocardiogram and is composed of a series of views aimed at assessing the various structures and their anatomic relationships.[3]

Fetal echocardiography is performed both by perinatologists and pediatric cardiologists, and sometimes jointly, as a collaborative effort. The ongoing assessment of the fetus is necessarily a collaborative effort between the two, with the perinatologist able to provide expertise during the antenatal period, and the pediatric cardiologist able to provide to the patient appropriate counseling and background regarding the congenital cardiac defect, the expected or possible postnatal courses, and the natural history of the abnormalities. As the field of antenatal cardiac imaging has developed, there has been interest in standardizing the tool. Recommendations have been made by several organizations to provide guidelines and consensus in this area.[31,49]

In addition to the two-dimensional imaging, pulsed and continuous-wave Doppler and color flow mapping permit evaluation of normal and abnormal flow patterns. These studies are useful for assessing for valvular stenoses, ventricular septal defects, and particularly left heart obstructive lesions, where the flow across the foramen ovale becomes left to right (due to the left heart obstruction), instead of the right-to-left flow seen in the normal fetus. Additional tools potentially useful in the fetal cardiac assessment are the three-dimensional fetal heart assessment and the three- and four-dimensional color Doppler using spatiotemporal image correlation. This is an automated procedure whereby a volume of data is acquired from the fetal heart, which includes both gray-scale three-dimensional images and color Doppler. The information is then presented in multiple planes, which can be evaluated without significant postprocessing. Limitations remain with this technique that are largely technical, including low discrimination of signal, especially early in gestation.[13] These newer techniques have been shown to add some level of detail but are probably only marginally additive to a thorough two-dimensional and Doppler echocardiogram performed by an expert.[26,62]

Cardiac size, growth, and ventricular function can also be assessed by the echocardiogram, and serial examinations can be used to compare interval change in size and function. In addition to the data typically obtained in an anatomic survey, various modalities exist to quantitatively assess the heart size and function in situations of fetal congestive heart failure. These include the comparisons of the cardiac to thoracic area or circumference, which are expressed as a ratio[48] (Fig. 45-7). Assessment of actual cardiac function can be undertaken in the fetus using techniques such as cardiac output or shortening fraction of both ventricles. Methods aimed at assessing overall cardiac performance include the Doppler-derived Tei index,[60] used in the fetus on both the right and left ventricles,[22] and a cardiovascular profile scoring system has been proposed that combines assessment of cardiac function with assessment for abnormality in venous and arterial Doppler pulsations, heart size, and evidence of hydrops.[17]

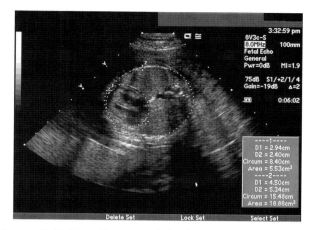

Figure 45–7. Two-dimensional fetal echocardiogram showing measurement of the fetal heart (1) and thorax (2) circumferences, used in calculating the cardiac-to-thoracic ratio.

Finally, fetal arrhythmias can be extensively investigated by comparing the timing of atrial and ventricular wall motion from M-mode recordings or from the Doppler flow patterns across the mitral and aortic valves.

Recognition of Fetal Cardiac Abnormalities
CONGENITAL HEART DEFECTS

Despite significant advances in fetal imaging, most congenital heart disease remains undetected until after birth. Well over one third of cases occur in pregnancies not otherwise identified as high risk.[15,59] For this reason, prenatal detection of congenital heart disease relies heavily on the screening fetal ultrasound. For many years, therefore, incorporation of a four-chamber view of the heart into formal guidelines for the screening fetal ultrasound has existed.

Most significant cardiac defects are excluded by a normal four-chamber view, but those not resulting in ventricular hypoplasia and those predominantly involving abnormalities of the outflow tracts will still be missed. Therefore, there has been interest in including outflow tract visualization in the standard screening fetal ultrasound. This appears to have an incremental value in the detection rate of congenital heart defects from 50% to as high as 85% to 90%.[11,28] Defects not detected with this screening tend toward those not requiring neonatal intervention. False-positive findings are also possible, and they often involve coarctation of the aorta or small ventricular septal defects.[8,42]

Defects associated with hypoplasia of the right or left ventricle are easily identified on the four-chamber view. Similarly, abnormal size of the aorta or pulmonary artery caused by semilunar valve stenosis or diminished arterial flow is readily seen. Milder degrees of aortic or pulmonary stenosis can be difficult to identify if they are not associated with abnormal arterial size or dramatic valve deformity. Large ventricular septal defects are easily identified, particularly when associated with tetralogy of Fallot or with AV septal defects. Greater difficulty is encountered in trying to identify small or medium-sized ventricular septal defects.[5] For this reason, there is a skew toward the fetal diagnosis of more complex forms of congenital heart disease compared with the general distribution of defects. This, coupled with fetal wastage due to the cardiac (or more often the associated noncardiac) genetic or somatic defects, results in a worsened natural history for congenital heart disease diagnosed prenatally compared with patients whose heart disease is diagnosed after birth.

Abnormalities of the superior vena cava or the inferior vena cava, such as an interrupted inferior vena cava with azygous continuation, are readily seen, and they are often noted because of their association with complex problems such as the heterotaxy syndromes. Color flow Doppler mapping has improved the ability to document pulmonary venous flow into the left atrium, improving the prenatal diagnosis of abnormalities of pulmonary venous connection. Pulsed Doppler recordings of the pulmonary veins are useful in assessing obstruction of the foramen ovale in fetuses with hypoplastic left heart syndrome.[6,27]

Structures that are normal in the fetus but abnormal in postnatal life cannot be diagnosed antenatally. Coarctation of the aorta can be challenging to identify because it might not become obstructive until the ductus arteriosus closes. More severe forms of coarctation are usually associated with varying degrees of transverse arch hypoplasia and are less likely to be overlooked.[27,51]

ARRHYTHMIAS

Intermittent premature atrial or ventricular contractions are often noted during fetal echocardiography.[58] They are rarely predictive of more complex arrhythmias, and they share the same benign prognosis as they do in the infant. Sustained fetal arrhythmias can be divided into tachyarrhythmias and bradyarrhythmias, as in the neonate or child.

Fetal tachyarrhythmias are much more common than bradyarrhythmias. Fetal AV reentry tachycardia, atrial tachycardia, or flutter[33] is usually easily differentiated from the rare fetal ventricular tachycardia[29] by the timing of atrial and ventricular wall motion on M-mode echocardiography (Fig. 45-8). Intermittent atrial tachycardia, or that at a relatively low rate

(<190 beats per minute) is usually well tolerated.[54] Sustained fetal tachycardia, however, especially when it occurs in midgestation, is poorly tolerated and often leads to fetal hydrops[40] (Fig. 45-9).

Fetal bradycardia is usually due to complete heart block or conduction abnormalities. This is most commonly associated with maternal autoantibodies (anti-SSA, anti-SSB) or with congenital heart disease, especially complex AV septal defects, heterotaxy syndrome, and ventricular inversion.[9] Isolated complete heart block is usually well tolerated in utero, as opposed to complete heart block associated with congenital heart disease, which has a grave prognosis for development of hydrops and fetal demise.[9]

FETAL CONGESTIVE HEART FAILURE AND MYOCARDIAL DISEASE

The cardiac physiology of the fetus allows adaptation to many of the cardiac defects that cause significant problems after birth. Specifically, postnatal congestive heart failure caused by significant left-to-right intracardiac shunting and pulmonary overcirculation is not expressed in the fetus. Congestive heart failure in the fetus, conversely, is generally caused either by myocardial dysfunction or severe regurgitation of the AV valves. Such lesions are poorly tolerated by the fetus, and this type of congestive heart failure often results in hydrops fetalis. Types of hydrops fetalis related to cardiovascular function are listed in Box 45-3.

Regurgitation from the AV valves of the right or left ventricle produces a significant fetal volume load that is not well tolerated. Lesions in which this is seen include Ebstein anomaly of the tricuspid valve,[45] pulmonary atresia with intact ventricular septum, AV septal defects with severe AV valve regurgitation,[53] and severe tricuspid insufficiency seen in the recipient twin in twin-to-twin transfusion syndrome.[46] In most fetuses with critical aortic stenosis, the left ventricle is simply bypassed, and the systemic circulation is perfused with the right ventricle through the ductus arteriosus, but severe left ventricular dilation and dysfunction, with mitral regurgitation, can develop.[52]

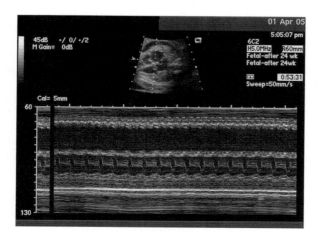

Figure 45–8. M-mode fetal scan through the atrial and ventricular walls, demonstrating atrial flutter. The atrial wall motion (*top of frame*) is twice that of the ventricular wall motion (*bottom of frame*).

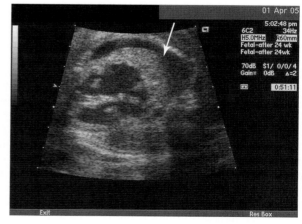

Figure 45–9. Two-dimensional fetal echocardiogram showing a four-chamber fetal heart with a large pleural effusion (*arrow*). The fetus had sustained tachycardia.

BOX 45–3   Nonimmune Hydrops Fetalis Related to Cardiovascular Function

ATRIOVENTRICULAR OR SEMILUNAR VALVE REGURGITATION
Atrioventricular canal defect
Ebstein anomaly or tricuspid valve dysplasia
Absent pulmonary valve syndrome

CRITICAL AORTIC STENOSIS

ARRHYTHMIAS
Supraventricular tachycardia
Atrial flutter
Complete atrioventricular block
Sinus or junctional bradycardia

MYOCARDIAL DISEASE
Myocarditis
Myocardial infarction
Cardiomyopathy

MISCELLANEOUS
Premature closure of the ductus arteriosus
Arteriovenous fistulas
Severe anemia

Conditions that affect myocardial function, such as viral myocarditis and intrauterine myocardial infarction, can severely compromise cardiac output and cause congestive heart failure in utero. Similarly, fetal cardiomyopathies are a rare and heterogeneous group of lesions that can even evolve throughout the pregnancy or beyond.[46] Premature closure of the ductus arteriosus can result in severe right ventricular pressure overload as the right ventricle becomes unable to unload its output to either the pulmonary or systemic circulations. Maternal indomethacin therapy, for example for preterm labor, is known to be associated with premature closure of the ductus arteriosus.[32] Women receiving this treatment during gestation are generally followed closely, with attention paid to the patency of the ductus arteriosus, development of tricuspid insufficiency, and development of fetal congestive heart failure.

Arrhythmias are also an important cause of fetal congestive heart failure. Bradyarrhythmias caused by complete heart block, especially when associated with structural lesions such as L-transposition of the great arteries, heterotaxia, or AV septal defects, can lead to fetal congestive heart failure. Fetal heart rates less than 55 beats per minute are usually poorly tolerated by the fetus. The fetus might also poorly tolerate tachyarrhythmias, such as persistent supraventricular tachycardia or atrial flutter. Finally, noncardiac causes of congestive heart failure in utero, such as arteriovenous fistulas, large sacrococcygeal teratomas, and severe anemia, should be considered.

Treatment

Most congenital heart disease can now be repaired safely in infancy with excellent surgical survival and good long-term prognosis. For these defects, therefore, there would be no need for fetal intervention. In utero intervention has been limited to those disease states that lead either to in utero demise (largely fetal arrhythmias) or to palliative procedures in defects that might be progressive during fetal life, and theoretically improved outcome could therefore be expected if intervention is undertaken earlier. The latter has largely been an experience with fetal intervention for aortic or pulmonary valve stenoses, with the ultimate goal of limiting progression to ventricular hypoplasia. Technical success for the procedure has been achieved at several centers worldwide.[30,37] The ultimate question of whether progression of ventricular hypoplasia can be halted remains guarded; recent analyses, however, have assessed technical aspects of the procedures, including patient selection and technique, with an eye toward increasing the success rate.[36] Large pericardial effusions have also been drained successfully in utero (see also Chapter 11).

As opposed to in utero intervention for structural congenital heart defects, antenatal management of fetal arrhythmias has the longest history and greatest success for fetal cardiovascular therapy. Tachyarrhythmias, particularly supraventricular tachycardia, have been successfully controlled by maternal administration of antiarrhythmic medications. Indications for treatment of fetal arrhythmias are still not clearly defined, but single ectopic beats and short, nonsustained runs of tachycardia do not appear to be associated with morbidity. Sustained tachycardia at rates greater than 200 beats per minute may lead to hydrops and ultimately to fetal demise and is a generally accepted indication for fetal therapy.

Digoxin remains a first-line drug at many institutions, although many drugs have been used, including flecainide,[23] verapamil, propranolol, sotalol,[43] and amiodarone.[54,58] Nonhydropic fetuses have a high success rate for transplacental treatment, although fetuses presenting with hydrops have a worse prognosis, with 27% mortality in one series.[54] In severe fetal hydrops, direct administration of drugs by umbilical vein puncture improves drug delivery but clearly has higher risk to the fetus. For fetal bradycardia, maternal steroids have been administered for treatment of fetal heart block caused by maternal lupus erythematosus.[50] Early treatment of an affected fetus can improve or prevent the loss of AV nodal conduction (complete heart block).

Outcome

With the exception of cases of large pericardial effusion with tamponade, balloon valvuloplasty of the aortic valve, and treatment of sustained arrhythmia, the prenatal diagnosis of congenital heart disease generally does not result in direct intervention to the fetus. This is not to say that the impact of a prenatal diagnosis of a congenital heart defect does not affect the pregnancy; it is likely to have an important role in terms of parental counseling, decisions regarding termination of pregnancy, perinatal planning, and fetal outcome.

Outcome studies regarding the impact of fetal echocardiography and fetal cardiac diagnosis have been performed. Many assess individual defects, including hypoplastic left heart syndrome,[7,34] truncus arteriosus,[16] AV septal defects,[19] and aortic stenosis. Initial reviews comparing the natural history for groups of fetuses with congenital heart defects diagnosed prenatally and those of children with defects diagnosed after birth show a worse outcome as a group for those with prenatal diagnosis.[18] These findings are attributable to the higher detection rate of complex defects (versus simple defects) before birth, the increasing severity of lesions detected prenatally compared with postnatally, and the higher association of prenatal heart defects with extracardiac anomalies that can add to their morbidity.

Direct comparisons of cohorts of infants with fetal versus postnatal diagnosis of complex congenital heart defects have shown improved outcome of children with defects diagnosed prenatally, however. Several series of infants with hypoplastic left heart syndrome, severe left heart obstructive lesions, and transposition of the great arteries have shown significantly less metabolic acidosis in infants with prenatal diagnosis as opposed to those with postnatal diagnosis.[12,61] A large, single-center study has already shown improved neurologic outcome and less metabolic acidosis in infants with prenatal diagnosis.[34] Future studies are needed to assess the relationship of improved perinatal management strategies on the ultimate outcome.

REFERENCES

1. Achiron R, et al: Extended fetal echocardiographic examination for detecting malformations in low risk pregnancies, *BMJ* 304:671, 1992.
2. Allan L, et al: Isolated major congenital heart disease, *Ultrasound Obstet Gynecol* 17:370, 2001.
3. Allan L: Technique of fetal echocardiography, *Pediatr Cardiol* 25:223, 2004.
4. Allan LD: Cardiac anatomy screening: what is the best time for screening in pregnancy? *Curr Opin Obstet Gynecol* 15:143, 2003.
5. Allan LD, et al: The accuracy of fetal echocardiography in the diagnosis of congenital heart disease, *Int J Cardiol* 25:279, 1989.
6. Better DJ, et al: Pattern of pulmonary venous blood flow in the hypoplastic left heart syndrome in the fetus, *Heart* 81:646, 1999.
7. Brackley KJ, et al: Outcome after prenatal diagnosis of hypoplastic left-heart syndrome: a case series, *Lancet* 356:1143, 2000.
8. Bromley B, et al: Fetal echocardiography: accuracy and limitations in a high and low risk for heart defects, *Am J Obstet Gynecol* 166:1473, 1992.
9. Buyon JP, et al: Autoimmune-associated congenital heart block: demographics, mortality, morbidity, and recurrence rates obtained from a national neonatal lupus registry, *J Am Coll Cardiol* 31:1658, 1998.
10. Callan NA, et al: Fetal echocardiography: indications for referral, prenatal diagnoses, and outcomes, *Am J Perinatol* 8:390, 1991.
11. Carvalho J, et al: Improving the effectiveness of routine prenatal screening for major congenital heart defects, *Heart* 88:387, 2002.
12. Chang AC, et al: Diagnosis, transport, and outcome in fetuses with left ventricular outflow tract obstruction, *J Thorac Cardiovasc Surg* 102:841, 1991.
13. Chaoui R, Heling KS: Three-dimensional (3D) and 4D color Doppler fetal echocardiography using spatio-temporal image correlation (STIC), *Ultrasound Obstet Gynecol* 23:535, 2004.
14. Chew C, et al: Population-based study of antenatal detection of congenital heart disease by ultrasound examination, *Ultrasound Obstet Gynecol* 29:619, 2007.
15. Cooper M, et al: Fetal echocardiography: retrospective review of clinical experience and an evaluation of indication, *Obstet Gynecol* 86:577, 1995.
16. Duke C, et al: Echocardiographic features and outcome of truncus arteriosus diagnosed during fetal life, *Am J Cardiol* 88:1379, 2001.
17. Falkensammer CV, et al: Fetal congestive heart failure: correlation of the Tei index and cardiovascular score, *J Perinat Med* 29:390, 2001.
18. Fesslova V, et al: Evolution of long term outcome in cases with fetal diagnosis of congenital heart disease: Italian multicentre study, *Heart* 82:594, 1999.
19. Fesslova V, et al: Spectrum and outcome of atrioventricular septal defect in fetal life, *Cardiol Young* 12:18, 2002.
20. Friedberg MK, et al: Prenatal detection of congenital heart disease, *J Pediatr* 155:26, 2009.
21. Friedman AH, Fahey JT: The transition from fetal to neonatal circulation: normal responses and implications for infants with heart disease, *Semin Perinatol* 17:106, 1993.
22. Freidman D, et al: Fetal cardiac function assessed by Doppler myocardial performance index (Tei Index), *Ultrasound Obstet Gynecol* 21:33, 2003.
23. Frohn-Mulder IM, et al: The efficacy of flecainide versus digoxin in the management of fetal supraventricular tachycardia, *Prenat Diagn* 15:1297, 1995.
24. Ghi T, et al: Incidence of major structural cardiac defects associated with increased nuchal translucency but normal karyotype, *Ultrasound Obstet Gynecol* 18:610, 2001.
25. Haak, MC, van Vugt JMG: Echocardiography in early pregnancy, *J Ultrasound Med* 22:271, 2003.
26. Hata T, et al: Real-time three-dimensional color Doppler fetal echocardiographic features of congenital heart disease, *J Obstet Gynaecol Res* 34:670, 2008.
27. Hornberger LK, et al: Antenatal diagnosis of coarctation of the aorta: a multicenter experience, *J Am Coll Cardiol* 23:417, 1994.
28. Kirk JS, et al: Prenatal screening for cardiac anomalies: the value of routine addition of the aortic root to the four-chamber view, *Obstet Gynecol* 84:427, 1994.
29. Kleinman CS, et al: In utero diagnosis of fetal supraventricular tachycardia, *Semin Perinatol* 9:113, 1989.
30. Kohl T, et al: World experience of percutaneous ultrasound-guided balloon valvuloplasty in human fetuses with severe aortic valve obstruction, *Am J Cardiol* 85:1230, 2000.
31. Lee W: ISUOG consensus statement: what constitutes a fetal echocardiogram, *Ultrasound Obstet Gynecol* 32:239, 2008.
32. Levy R, et al: Indomethacin and corticosteroids: an additive constrictive effect on the fetal ductus arteriosus, *Am J Perinatol* 16:379, 1999.
33. Lisowski LA, et al: Atrial flutter in the perinatal age group: diagnosis, management, and outcome, *J Am Coll Cardiol* 35:771, 2000.
34. Mahle WT, et al: Impact of prenatal diagnosis on survival and early neurologic morbidity in neonates with the hypoplastic left heart syndrome, *Pediatrics* 107:1277, 2001.
35. Maiz N, et al: Ductus venosus Doppler in fetuses with cardiac defects and increased nuchal translucency thickness, *Ultrasound Obstet Gynecol* 31:256, 2008.
36. Makikallio K, et al, Fetal aortic valve stenosis and the evolution of hypoplastic left heart syndrome: patient selection for fetal intervention, *Circulation* 113:1401, 2006.

37. Marshall A, et al: Aortic valvuloplasty in the fetus: technical characteristics of successful balloon dilatation, *J Pediatr* 147:535, 2005.

38. McAuliffe FM, et al: Early fetal echocardiography—a reliable prenatal diagnosis tool, *Am J Obstet Gynecol* 193:1253, 2005.

39. Meyer-Whitkopf M, et al: Three-dimensional (3-D) ultrasonography for obtaining the four and five-chamber view: comparison with cross-sectional (2-D) fetal sonographic screening, *Ultrasound Obstet Gynecol* 15:397, 2000.

40. Naheed ZJ, et al: Fetal tachycardia: mechanisms and predictors of hydrops fetalis, *J Am Coll Cardiol* 27:1736, 1996.

41. Nora JJ: Etiologic factors in congenital heart disease, *Pediatr Clin North Am* 18:1059, 1971.

42. Ott WJ: The accuracy of antenatal fetal echocardiography screening in high- and low-risk patients, *Am J Obstet Gynecol* 172:1741, 1995.

43. Oudijk MA, et al: Treatment of fetal tachycardia with sotalol: transplacental pharmacokinetics and pharmacodynamics, *J Am Coll Cardiol* 42:765, 2003.

44. Paladini D, et al: Prenatal diagnosis of congenital heart disease and fetal karyotyping, *Obstet Gynecol* 81:679, 1993.

45. Pavlova M, et al: Factors affecting the prognosis of Ebstein's anomaly during fetal life, *Am Heart J* 135:1081, 1998.

46. Pedra SRFF, et al: Fetal cardiomyopathies: pathogenic mechanisms, hemodynamic findings and clinical outcome, *Circulation* 106:585, 2002.

47. Quatero H, et al: Clinical implications of fetal magnetocardiography, *Ultrasound Obstet Gynecol* 20:142, 2002.

48. Respondek M, et al: 2D echocardiographic assessment of the fetal heart size in the 2nd and 3rd trimester of uncomplicated pregnancy, *Eur J Obstet Gynecol Reprod Biol* 44:185, 1992.

49. Rychik J, et al: American Society of Echocardiography Guidelines and Standards for Performance of the Fetal Echocardiogram, *J Am Soc Echocardiogr* 17:803, 2004.

50. Saleeb S, et al: Comparison of treatment with fluorinated glucocorticoids to the natural history of autoantibody-associated congenital heart block: retrospective review of the research registry for neonatal lupus, *Arthritis Rheum* 42:2335, 1999.

51. Sharland GK, et al: Coarctation of the aorta: difficulties in prenatal diagnosis, *Br Heart J* 71:70, 1994.

52. Sharland GK, et al: Left ventricular dysfunction in the fetus: relation to aortic valve anomalies and endocardial fibroelastosis, *Br Heart J* 66:419, 1991.

53. Silverman NH, Schmidt KG: Ventricular volume overload in the human fetus: observations from fetal echocardiography, *J Am Soc Echocardiogr* 3:20, 1990.

54. Simpson JM, Sharland GK: Fetal tachycardias: Management and outcome of 127 consecutive cases, *Heart* 79:576, 1998.

55. Simpson LL, et al: Nucahl translucency and the risk of congenital heart disease, *Obstet Gynecol* 109:376, 2005.

56. Sklansky M, et al: Usefulness of gated three-dimensional fetal echocardiography to reconstruct and display structures not visualized with two-dimensional imaging, *Am J Cardiol* 80:665, 1997.

57. Stinstra JG, Peters MJ: The influence of fetoabdominal tissues on fetal ECGs and MCGs, *Arch Physiol Biochem* 110:165, 2002.

58. Strasburger JF, et al: Amiodarone therapy for drug-refractory fetal tachycardia, *Circulation* 109:375,2004.

59. Stumpflen I, et al: Effect of detailed echocardiography as part of routine prenatal ultrasonographic screening on detection of congenital heart disease, *Lancet* 348:854, 1996.

60. Tei C, et al: Noninvasive Doppler-derived myocardial performance index: correlation with simultaneous measurements of cardiac catheterization measurements, *J Am Soc Echocardiogr* 10:169, 1997.

61. Verheijen PM, et al: Prenatal diagnosis of congenital heart disease affects preoperative acidosis in the newborn patient, *J Thorac Cardiovasc Surg* 121:798, 2001.

62. Wanitpongpan P, et al: Spatio-temporal image correlation (STIC) used by general obstetricians is marginally clinically effective compared to 2D fetal echocardiography scanning by experts, *Prenat Diagn* 28:923, 2008.

63. Westin M, et al: Is measurement of nuchal translucency thickness a useful screening tool for heart defects? A study of 16,383 fetuses, *Ultrasound Obstet Gynecol* 27:632, 2006.

PART 5

Principles of Neonatal Cardiovascular Hemodynamics
Kenneth G. Zahka

The following pathophysiologic principles provide the background needed for understanding the consequences of the transition from fetal to newborn life with normal and abnormal cardiac development. These principles are essential to an understanding of cardiac catheterization data and are integral to the clinical care of neonates with congenital heart disease.[7]

PRESSURE, FLOW, AND RESISTANCE

The pressure (P) in a chamber or vessel is related to the blood flow ($\dot{Q}$) and the resistance (R):

$$\Delta P = \dot{Q} \times R$$

or

$$\frac{\Delta P}{\dot{Q}} = R$$

Pressure is measured directly by catheterization or by sphygmomanometry. In neonates, flow is measured from oxygen data or thermodilution in the cardiac catheterization laboratory. It can also be estimated from noninvasive echocardiography and Doppler data. Resistance is always calculated from pressure and flow data.

The most basic application of this principle is the calculation of systemic and pulmonary vascular resistance. Resistance is directly related to the pressure drop across the vascular bed (ΔP, or the mean arterial pressure minus the mean atrial pressure) and inversely related to the blood flow. In the neonate, the normal postnatal fall in pulmonary artery pressure might be explained by a drop in left atrial pressure, a fall in pulmonary blood flow, or a decrease in the resistance to blood flow through the lungs. Clearly, on the basis of known data, the decrease in resistance is the only plausible factor.

In a neonate with high pulmonary artery pressure and a congenital heart defect, it is essential to know whether the high pulmonary artery pressure is due to high flow with low resistance or to normal flow with high resistance. Measurement of pressure and flow with calculation of resistance directs logical therapy in these infants. If the pressure is elevated because of increased flow with normal resistance, treatment to lower the resistance will likely only increase the flow and make the infant's condition worse.

This principle also explains the minimal pressure gradients across the aortic valve in critical aortic stenosis and left ventricular failure. If the resistance is high (in this case, the aortic valve) and the flow is low (poor cardiac output caused by left ventricular failure), the pressure drop across the valve will be small. Opening the valve (lowering the resistance) and improving left ventricular function (increasing flow) usually increase the pressure gradient (ΔP) in these infants.

MEASUREMENT OF BLOOD FLOW

Blood flow (systemic, $\dot{Q}s$; pulmonary, $\dot{Q}p$) can be estimated from the oxygen consumption and the arteriovenous oxygen difference with the Fick principle:

$$\dot{Q}s = \frac{\dot{V}_{O_2}}{[(Ao\ sat - SVC\ sat) \times 13.6 \times (g\ Hb/dL)]}$$

$$\dot{Q}p = \frac{\dot{V}_{O_2}}{[(PV\ sat - PA\ sat) \times 13.6 \times (g\ Hb/dL)]}$$

where oxygen consumption ($\dot{V}_{O_2}$) is in milliliters per minute; aortic (Ao), superior vena caval (SVC), pulmonary venous (PV), and pulmonary arterial (PA) oxygen saturations (sat) are expressed as decimals (e.g., 98% = 0.98); and oxygen capacity (in milliliters per liter) is 13.6 times the hemoglobin concentration in grams of hemoglobin per deciliter.

Oxygen saturation is measured by hemoximetry or is calculated from a blood gas measurement. If the infant is receiving supplemental oxygen, then dissolved oxygen might not be trivial ($P_{O_2} = 0.03$ mL/mm Hg) compared with bound oxygen, and it must be included in the calculation of oxygen content:

$$\text{Oxygen content} = sat \times 13.6 \times Hb\ \text{concentration} + 0.03\ mL \times P_{O_2}$$

where oxygen content is measured in milliliters per liter and hemoglobin concentration in grams per deciliter. In this case, systemic and pulmonary blood flow can be calculated as follows:

$$\dot{Q}s = \frac{\dot{V}_{O_2}}{(Ao\ content - SVC\ content)}$$

$$\dot{Q}p = \frac{\dot{V}_{O_2}}{(PV\ content - PA\ content)}$$

where Ao content, SVC content, PV content, and PA content are derived from the oxygen content equation. The Fick principle provides a convenient and reliable means of measuring blood flow in the cardiac catheterization laboratory or intensive care unit with appropriate vascular access to obtain the samples. It also gives excellent insight into the factors that have an impact on oxygen delivery and use.

Oxygen consumption varies with activity and metabolic state. In neonates, oxygen consumption can be measured by analysis of expired gas with a metabolic cart and use of the polarographic method. More typically, it is estimated from body surface area, 150 mL/m² per minute. Deviations from that assumed value because of activity or illness alter the calculated output, but it can also be seen that if oxygen consumption increases, the blood flow must increase, the arteriovenous difference must increase, or the oxygen content must increase. The neonate with adequate cardiovascular reserve increases blood flow. The infant with poor cardiac output must extract more oxygen, or an oxygen debt will develop in the tissues. The critical and therapeutic role of transfusion or oxygen therapy for the neonate with limited reserve can also be seen.

Thermodilution and dye dilution are techniques for measuring blood flow in older children but that require special adaptation for newborn infants. In both cases, a known amount of an indicator (cold or green dye) is injected into the circulation. Sampling (with a thermistor or photocell) is done distal to the injection site. The amount of dilution of the indicator is directly related to the blood flow between the injection and sampling sites. These techniques are most likely to be applicable to neonates with structurally normal hearts.

Estimation of flow by Doppler is integrated into all echocardiography machines:

$$\dot{Q} = VTI \times CSA$$

where VTI is the velocity time integral, or mean velocity, and CSA is the cross-sectional area of the vessel at that site calculated from the diameter. This calculation assumes laminar flow and is sensitive to accurate measurement of the diameter.

INTRACARDIAC SHUNTING

The location of a left-to-right or right-to-left shunt can be detected by an increase or decrease in the oxygen saturation at the atrial, ventricular, or arterial level. The magnitude of the shunt is indicated by a change in oxygen saturation.

This concept is an extension of principles outlined under "Measurement of Blood Flow," earlier. If there is no shunting, then pulmonary artery oxygen saturation must be the same as superior vena caval oxygen saturation. In practice, there is some variation in oxygen saturation throughout the right side of the heart because of differences in oxygen extraction by the head, liver, and other abdominal organs. Thus, it is useful to take multiple samples to identify the site of shunting and to avoid errors resulting from uneven mixing of venous flows. A change in saturation of 5% is likely to be significant.

The relative pulmonary and systemic blood flow can be estimated without measuring the $\dot{V}_{O_2}$ or calculating oxygen capacity ($13.6 \times g\ Hb/dL$):

$$\dot{Q}p/\dot{Q}s = (Ao\ sat - SVC\ sat)/(PV\ sat - PA\ sat)$$

This approach does not permit calculation of vascular resistance or flow, but it does give an estimate of relative pulmonary flow and systemic flow. For babies with a left-to-right shunt, $\dot{Q}p/\dot{Q}s$ of less than 1.5 is small, 1.5 to 2.5 is moderate, and greater than 2.5 is large. For newborn infants with a right-to-left shunt, $\dot{Q}p/\dot{Q}s$ of 0.9 to 1.0 is small, 0.7 to 0.9 is moderate, and less than 0.7 is large.

When two chambers or vessels are connected (e.g., ventricular septal defect), the flow through the connection is related to the size of the connection and the relative resistance to blood flow leaving the chamber or vessel (e.g., the aorta and the pulmonary artery). If the resistances are equal, no significant flow will cross the defect regardless of its size. If the defect is tiny, not much flow will cross the defect regardless of the relative systemic and pulmonary resistance.

This principle helps explain why a newborn infant with ventricular septal defect does not have a murmur in the delivery room when pulmonary vascular resistance is high. It also introduces the concept of a restrictive and a nonrestrictive defect. A nonrestrictive defect provides no resistance to flow and allows equalization of pressure between the two chambers. In contrast, small defects have resistance to flow and do not allow pressures to equalize.

CHAMBER AND VESSEL SIZE

Chamber and vessel size are proportional to the blood flow through them. Why do cardiac structures grow or dilate? Whether the consideration is the normal increase in cardiac output with growth or an increased flow resulting from congenital heart disease, the heart is sized relative to volume load. Important exceptions are if the wall is weak (e.g., the aorta in Marfan syndrome) or if the muscle is weak and the diastolic pressure is high (cardiomyopathy in the left ventricle, dilation of the left atrium because of mitral stenosis). If an echocardiogram or angiogram shows a dilated chamber, there must be an explanation based on this principle. The same is true for chambers that are smaller than normal.

WALL THICKNESS

Wall thickness (hypertrophy) develops in response to the factors that increase wall stress: the pressure in the chamber and the size of the chamber. Usually, hypertrophy occurs in an attempt to normalize wall stress. For this reason, with normal ventricular growth, the wall thickens in proportion to the chamber size. It is also the reason that left ventricular wall thickness is a good sign of the severity of aortic stenosis or systemic hypertension. Important exceptions are hypertrophic cardiomyopathy, in which the feedback to muscle mass is inappropriate, and infiltrative diseases.

ASSESSMENT AND DEVELOPMENTAL ASPECTS OF MYOCARDIAL PERFORMANCE

The characterization of ventricular function or myocardial performance has been the focus of decades of research, with the goal of defining myocardial contractility, afterload, and preload in the complex neurohumoral environment of the intact circulation. Superimposed on this challenge are the developmental changes in heart rate and the confounding factor of normal growth.[5]

Developmental Changes in Myocardial Structure

Myocyte number (hyperplasia) and size (hypertrophy) increase during maturation until shortly after birth, when only hypertrophy occurs.[9] Myofibrillar density and organization are lower in the immature myocardium. Only 30% of the fetal myocardial cell consists of myofibrils, in comparison with 60% in the adult myocardium. Ion channels and pumps, which regulate calcium, sodium, potassium, and hydrogen passage in the sarcolemma and T tubules, change from those in the fetus to those in the mature animal, although the impact on function is not clear. Mitochondrial size and complexity increase during development, and there is maturation of the energy-producing enzymes within the mitochondria. Fatty acid transport is deficient in the newborn infant's myocardium, and carbohydrate is the principal energy source.

Myofibrils are composed of a number of proteins, including myosins, actin, tropomyosins, and troponins. The isoforms of troponin T that are present in the fetal and neonatal myocardium appear to be less sensitive to calcium than those in the adult myocardium. Sarcoplasmic reticulum density and organization are decreased in the immature myocardium, which impairs calcium transport into the myofibrils. These developmental changes in myocardial structure, energy use, and ion transport likely have implications for the functional development of the myocardium from the fetus to the adult.[2]

Systolic Ventricular Function

PEAK DEVELOPED PRESSURE

The simplest measure of ventricular function is systolic blood pressure. Systolic pressure gradually increases in the fetus and during the first months of life, yet adult levels of blood pressure are not reached until late childhood (see Appendix B). Although blood pressure is useful because the clinician is able to integrate the imponderables of age, afterload, and preload, blood pressure as a measure of systolic function has limitations. A simple interpretation of that observation is that because the neonatal heart does not develop the same peak force as an adult heart, the immature myocardium is intrinsically functionally impaired compared with the mature myocardium. These observations do not account for the cross-sectional area of muscle mass, nor do they explain the ability to generate high pressures in response to obstruction.

STROKE VOLUME AND CARDIAC OUTPUT

The fetal circulation dictates a consideration of the combined ventricular output rather than separate right and left ventricular output.[12] Fetal cardiac output is sensitive to heart rate and is relatively insensitive to preload and afterload. After birth, there is a dramatic increase in left ventricular output[1] and a high level of endogenous β-adrenergic stimulation. This high level of β-adrenergic stimulation and the immaturity of myocardial calcium handling are in part responsible for the decreased contractile reserve of the neonate.

Cardiac output increases dramatically from the neonate to the adult. When the cardiac output is indexed for body surface area, which provides the cardiac index, normal neonatal left ventricular flow is between 4.0 and 6.5 L/m² per minute depending on the modality used to measure the output.

EJECTION FRACTION AND SHORTENING FRACTION

Ejection fraction (EF) and shortening fraction (SF) are measures of relative shortening of the myocardium during systole:

$$EF(\%) = 100 \times \frac{(EDV - ESV)}{EDV}$$

$$SF(\%) = 100 \times \frac{(EDD - ESD)}{EDD}$$

where EDV is end-diastolic volume, ESV is end-systolic volume, EDD is end-diastolic dimension, and ESD is end-systolic dimension. Each measurement is easily calculated from either angiography or echocardiography. Normal values (EF, 65% to 80%; SF, 28% to 40%) vary surprisingly little with age. Muscle shortening is afterload dependent, and acutely increasing the vascular resistance decreases the EF without necessarily changing intrinsic myocardial contractility.

VELOCITY OF CIRCUMFERENTIAL FIBER SHORTENING

Velocity of circumferential fiber shortening (VCF) is a measure of systolic function that indexes the SF by dividing the SF by the ventricular ejection time (VET):

$$VCF = \frac{SF}{VET}$$

The VCF value (normal, 1.25 + 0.15 circumferences per second) does change with heart rate and can be rate corrected. Corrected VCF (VCFc; normal, 1.01 + 0.11 circumferences per second) is calculated by dividing the VCF by the square root of the R-R interval:

$$VCFc = \frac{VCF}{\sqrt{R - R}}$$

WALL STRESS

Wall stress (WS), or force per unit area, has been assumed to be constant during one's lifetime and reflects the law of Laplace, which states:

$$WS = P \times \frac{D}{h}$$

where P is pressure, D is dimension, and h is wall thickness at any given time in the cardiac cycle. Peak systolic wall stress is about 225 g/cm². In the infant with aortic stenosis, increased cavity pressure typically increases wall thickness, and during growth, an increase in chamber size and pressure is accompanied by an increase in wall thickness. End-systolic wall stress (ESWS) is the best estimate of afterload. ESWS (in grams per square centimeter) can be estimated by the following equation, with measurements of end-systolic pressure (P_{es}) and dimension (D_{es}) (end-systolic pressure must be estimated from a carotid pulse tracing and aortic pressure):

$$ESWS = \frac{(1.35 \times D_{es} \times P_{es})}{4 \times h_{es} \times [1 + (h_{es}/D_{es})]}$$

The relationship between VCFc and wall stress has been used as a load-independent index of myocardial contractility.[4,8,11]

These data suggest that myocardial contractility does not change after the first 3 years of life. In contrast, premature infants, term neonates, and infants past the neonatal stage have higher mean VCFc and lower ESWS, with the observation most dramatic in the premature infant. This suggests a higher basal contractile state, which is not explained by afterload. Because the relationship between VCFc and ESWS is steeper in infants, they may be more sensitive to the effects of afterload.

REGIONAL WALL MOTION

The normal left ventricular end-systolic cross-sectional geometry is circular. With increased right ventricular pressure, the interventricular septum is flattened and the systolic left ventricle is D shaped. These changes are the result of altered septal motion, which regresses during the first week of life.

Diastolic Function

Ventricular compliance is the incremental change in ventricular volume for a change in pressure. The relationship between ventricular diastolic volume and pressure is nonlinear, and thus compliance decreases as preload increases. Compliance is affected by the intrinsic properties of the myofibrils, the connective tissue, and the pericardium. Comparison of right and left ventricular compliance in the fetus and the neonate reveals comparable right and left diastolic pressure-volume curves. In the adult, the left ventricular curve is shifted to the left, indicating that, at any given volume, left ventricular pressures are higher than right ventricular pressures. This observation is expected because hypertrophy is one of the determinants of diastolic function and because the fetal and neonatal right ventricular wall thickness is comparable to that of the left ventricle.

Analysis of the passive tension radius relationships in fetal, neonatal, and adult left ventricular myocardium suggests that the fetal ventricle is stiffer than the neonatal or adult ventricle. In the beating heart, diastolic compliance is affected by myocardial relaxation. Relaxation is an active process that requires transport of calcium from troponin C into the sarcoplasmic reticulum. Neonatal myocardium has a limited ability to sequester calcium, and this can impair relaxation.

The clinical assessment of diastolic function has relied on several echocardiographic and Doppler indexes. All have shortcomings, and unfortunately a clear understanding of diastolic function is even more elusive than that of systolic function. Echocardiographically determined rates of left ventricular posterior wall thinning increase dramatically during the first month of life, suggesting improved compliance or relaxation.[6] A similar index, the maximum velocity of lengthening of the left ventricular cavity, suggests that diastolic function is further impaired in premature infants.[3]

Doppler studies of atrioventricular valve and venous flow patterns have led to a number of parameters that are affected by diastolic ventricular function. In the fetus and the neonate, the proportion of blood that enters the ventricles during atrial systole (A wave) is higher than the flow during early diastole (E wave). This relationship can be expressed either as peak E and A velocities or areas or as the ratio of E to A velocities or areas. The isovolumic relaxation time can be measured from the end of aortic flow to the beginning of mitral valve flow. Retrograde flow into the hepatic veins during atrial systole occurs in normal infants and is usually attenuated by inspiration. If there is qualitatively more retrograde flow, or if the retrograde flow persists during inspiration, right ventricular compliance is probably reduced.

The interaction of ventricular relaxation, ventricular compliance, and preload make interpretation of these data difficult and prone to error. In clinical practice, infants who have persistent dominance of atrioventricular flow during atrial systole probably have some degree of diastolic dysfunction. Serial studies in individual infants might also be useful if there are no changes in preload.

Heart Rate

The embryonic heart rate gradually increases during cardiogenesis and then stabilizes in the second trimester. After birth, heart rate generally falls throughout childhood to adult levels. Heart rate is related to intrinsic properties of the pacemaker cells and endogenous catecholamines and hormones. These factors do not explain the remarkable relationship between heart rate and body size, ranging from more than 500 beats per minute in small rodents to less than 20 beats per minute in large mammals.

The major factor is likely the importance of ventricular-arterial coupling.[10] Blood flow occurs in a pulsatile fashion, and the total ventricular afterload is best described by vascular impedance, which includes the role of arterial diameter, distensibility, and length and wave reflections, as well as peripheral vascular resistance. Moreover, analysis of impedance permits the calculation of the energy required to move blood in a pulsatile fashion. Matching stroke volume and heart rate to arterial mechanics suggests that energy is minimized by high heart rates in a small aorta and low heart rates in a large aorta. In the embryo, developmental changes in aortic impedance resulting from changes in distensibility might favor lower heart rates despite the small size of the aorta.[13]

REFERENCES

1. Agata Y, et al: Changes in left ventricular output from fetal to early neonatal life. *J Pediatr* 119:441, 1991.
2. Anderson PA: Maturation and cardiac contractility, *Cardiol Clin* 7:209, 1989.
3. Appleton RS, et al: Altered early left ventricular diastolic cardiac function in the premature infant, *Am J Cardiol* 59:1391, 1987.
4. Colan SD, et al: Developmental modulation of myocardial mechanics: age- and growth-related alterations in afterload and contractility, *J Am Coll Cardiol* 19:619, 1992.
5. Dewey FE, et al: Does size matter? Clinical applications of scaling cardiac size and function for body size, *Circulation* 117:2279, 2008.
6. Fouron JC, et al: Left ventricular diastolic function during the first month of life, *Biol Neonate* 53:1, 1988.
7. Griftka RG: Cardiac catheterization and angiography, In Allen HD, et al, editors: *Heart Disease in Infants, Children, and Adolescents*, 7th ed., Baltimore, 2008 ,Williams & Wilkins, p 208.
8. Lee LA, et al: Left ventricular mechanics in the preterm infant and their effect on the measurement of cardiac performance, *J Pediatr* 120:114, 1992.
9. Mahoney L: Development of myocardial structure and function, In Allen HD, et al, editors: *Heart Disease in Infants, Children, and Adolescents*, 6th ed., Baltimore, 2008, Williams & Wilkins, p 573.
10. Milnor W: Aortic wavelength as a determinant of the relation between heart rate and body size in mammals, *Am J Physiol* 237:R3, 1979.
11. Rowland DG, Gutgesell HP: Noninvasive assessment of myocardial contractility, preload, afterload in healthy newborn infants, *Am J Cardiol* 75:818, 1995.
12. Teitel D, Rudolph AM: Perinatal oxygen delivery and cardiac function, *Adv Pediatr* 32:321, 1985.
13. Zahka KG, et al: Aortic impedance and hydraulic power in the chick embryo from stages 18 to 29, *Circ Res* 64:1091, 1989.

PART 6
Approach to the Neonate with Cardiovascular Disease
Kenneth G. Zahka

PRESENTATION OF CONGENITAL HEART DISEASE

Most patients with serious (life-threatening) congenital heart disease initially are seen by the physician in the neonatal period, many in the first several days of life. At this time, urgent intervention, either medical, surgical, or both, is often necessary. The mode of presentation depends on the cardiac lesion or combination of lesions, as well as on the timing of ductus arteriosus closure, fall in pulmonary vascular resistance, or ductus venosus closure. The superimposition of other disease processes in patients with serious structural cardiac disease can make the initial recognition and classification of such infants difficult and confusing. The most important examples of these superimposed disease processes are bacterial sepsis, pulmonary disease, and severe anemia. Such patients are at high risk; heart disease might not be recognized in a patient with clear bacterial sepsis, or perhaps worse, sepsis might go undiagnosed in a patient with obvious heart disease. The clinician must keep an open mind to all the diagnostic possibilities.

DIAGNOSTIC TECHNIQUES
Physical Examination

Cyanosis is one of the most important findings in recognizing congenital heart disease in an infant (Box 45-4).[17] Central cyanosis is the outward manifestation of reduced arterial oxygen saturation. The estimation of oxygen saturation based on the intensity of cyanosis can be inaccurate, however. The intensity of cyanosis is determined by the concentration of desaturated hemoglobin rather than by the actual oxygen saturation. Therefore, infants with marked polycythemia might appear

---

BOX 45-4 Distinctive Physical Signs

TO-AND-FRO SYSTOLIC AND DIASTOLIC MURMURS
Aortic stenosis and regurgitation
Truncal stenosis and regurgitation
Absent pulmonary valve syndromes: pulmonary stenosis
  and regurgitation
Left ventricular-to-aortic tunnel

DIFFERENTIAL CYANOSIS

Upper Normal and Lower Hypoxic
- Coarctation of the aorta, patent ductus arteriosus,
  ventricular septal defect
- Aortic arch interruption, patent ductus arteriosus,
  ventricular septal defect
- Mitral stenosis, patent ductus arteriosus
- Persistence of the transitional circulation with ductal
  right-to-left shunting and minimal atrial right-to-left
  shunting

Upper Hypoxic and Lower Normal
Transposition of the great arteries, coarctation of the aorta

---

cyanotic despite relatively minor arterial desaturation, because of the high absolute concentration of desaturated hemoglobin. On the other hand, infants with significant anemia appear relatively pink despite significant arterial desaturation. The latter situation is most common at 1 to 2 months of age, when normal physiologic anemia can occur. Infants who are somewhat cold, especially in the delivery room, can manifest impressive peripheral cyanosis, which does not reflect central arterial desaturation. Arterial desaturation can be a sign of right-to-left shunting of blood (as in a variety of congenital heart lesions and in persistent fetal circulation), transposition of the great arteries with delivery of systemic venous blood directly to the aorta, pulmonary venous desaturation caused by alveolar hypoxia (as in pulmonary edema, pneumonia, or atelectasis with perfusion of unventilated alveoli), or a combination of these factors.

The degree of respiratory distress should be noted because it is a clue to the cause of the problem. In general, cardiac lesions with reduction in pulmonary blood flow do not result in significant respiratory distress unless cyanosis is profound. Lesions with poor systemic output and acidosis, as well as those with increased pulmonary blood flow, cause respiratory distress. Infants with primarily pulmonary disease and those with superimposed pulmonary disease have respiratory distress (see Chapter 44).

Palpation of the cardiac impulse is helpful in assessing the anatomy and physiology of the lesion. Clear cardiac malpositions such as mirror-image dextrocardia might be obvious with palpation of the apex well to the right. A dramatically increased right or left ventricular impulse indicates increased ventricular pressure or, much more commonly, increased ventricular volume. An example would be an infant with total anomalous pulmonary venous return, in which both pulmonary and systemic venous returns enter the right side of the heart. Such an infant has a dramatically increased right ventricular impulse. In contrast, an infant with tetralogy of Fallot is likely to have no

increase in cardiac impulse because pulmonary blood flow is reduced.

Auscultation of the heart sounds is valuable but rarely diagnostic. The second heart sound is of the greatest importance in evaluating congenital heart disease, but accurate assessment can be difficult and is a skill that takes a great deal of practice to acquire. The second heart sound is single in lesions associated with significant pulmonary hypertension, as well as in transposition, pulmonary atresia, and certain other conditions. Surprisingly, it is occasionally split in truncus arteriosus despite the presence of only one semilunar valve in this condition. The auscultation of cardiac murmurs in newborn infants rarely provides diagnostic or even specific information, with several exceptions. A to-and-fro systolic-diastolic murmur is characteristic of absent pulmonary valve syndrome, truncus arteriosus with truncal stenosis, and regurgitation. The loudest murmurs often occur in children with relatively benign lesions, such as small ventricular septal defects, whereas children with severe heart disease might have little or no murmur. Transient murmurs can be caused by tricuspid regurgitation or a patent ductus arteriosus.

Detection of hepatomegaly is helpful but also nonspecific. It indicates high systemic venous pressure, which can result from congestive heart failure of any cause or from conditions such as total anomalous pulmonary venous return or systemic arteriovenous fistula in which right ventricular volume is increased.

A careful assessment of the pulses and peripheral perfusion is critical in the infant with suspected heart disease. The femoral pulses are compared with an upper extremity pulse, usually the radial or brachial pulse, in assessing the possibility of aortic coarctation. Many experienced clinicians believe that such a careful comparison by palpation is more reliable than the determination of four-limb blood pressures (see discussion later). Conditions that cause a decreased pulse in all sites include any condition with decreased systemic blood flow and especially lesions that are dependent on the patency of the ductus arteriosus for systemic flow, such as hypoplastic left ventricle.

Blood Pressure Measurement

See also Chapter 31.
Blood pressure measurement is more helpful for following changes in hemodynamic condition than for diagnosing particular defects. This is true both for standard cuff pressures and for those obtained automatically by machine. The reason is that the act of inflating a cuff in a conscious infant is often associated with agitation and straining on the part of the infant. Nonsimultaneous measurements, therefore, are from somewhat different hemodynamic states, making comparisons of upper and lower extremity pressures unreliable. One approach to making such comparisons somewhat more reliable is to use two automatic machines simultaneously on the upper and lower extremities and then to switch the machines and repeat the procedure, taking the average difference between the two readings to correct for intermachine variation. There can be as much as a 15-mm Hg difference in the arm and leg blood pressure in normal newborns.[2]

Pulse Oximetry

See also Chapter 31 and Chapter 44, Part 3.

The pulse oximetry technique provides an excellent method of assessing arterial oxygen saturation noninvasively, using a probe attached to the palm or foot in the infant. Although the measurement of arterial blood gas tension is always useful, pulse oximetry avoids a painful needle stick, which can cause agitation, struggling, and underventilation, making such direct measurements somewhat unreliable.

Measurements should always be made from the right hand and from a foot to provide information about ductus arteriosus flow patterns. For example, patients with severe aortic coarctation or interruption and a patent ductus arteriosus providing flow from the pulmonary artery to the descending aorta have a much lower saturation in the feet than in the hands. On the other hand, patients with transposition and aortic coarctation can have a much higher saturation in the feet than in the hands because pulmonary arterial blood is highly saturated and passes from the pulmonary artery into the ductus arteriosus and descending aorta.

To prevent problems created by intermachine variability, one should use two machines simultaneously and then switch the leads, taking the average difference between the upper and lower extremity readings. Numerous studies have suggested that routine screening of all newborns can identify a greater percentage of infants with cyanotic congenital heart defects than clinical assessment alone, although screening in the first hours of life has a high false-positive rate.[4] Infants with left heart defects may be missed by this strategy, and careful clinical assessment remains important; in one study it was as effective as pulse oximetry for screening for critical heart defects.[15]

Hyperoxic Test

See also Chapter 44, Part 2.

For the hyperoxic test, the infant is allowed to breathe 100% oxygen, and an arterial blood gas measurement is obtained and compared with one obtained before the use of oxygen.[17] It can be performed either with arterial blood or with a transcutaneous monitor or pulse oximeter to estimate Po_2 or oxygen saturation. Patients with pulmonary disease alone generally have a rise in Po_2 of greater than 20 to 30 mm Hg or a rise in saturation of greater than 10%. Those with a fixed right-to-left shunt might have a small rise in oxygenation but generally less than these amounts. A fixed right-to-left shunt is a lesion in which no increase is possible either in pulmonary blood flow or in mixing of systemic and pulmonary venous return. Therefore, in such patients, pulmonary venous blood is already nearly completely oxygenated, and little additional oxygenation is possible. A good example is in tetralogy of Fallot, in which there is both a high resistance to pulmonary flow because of pulmonary stenosis and a right-to-left shunt through a ventricular septal defect.

Despite a common misconception, the hyperoxic test is not used to rule out congenital heart disease. Indeed, patients with large left-to-right shunts and systemic hypoxemia might have large increases in oxygenation because added inspired oxygen normalizes pulmonary venous saturation, which may be low as a result of pulmonary edema and the accompanying oxygen diffusion gradient. Patients with mixing of pulmonary and systemic venous return and no obstruction to pulmonary flow could also have a large rise in O_2 saturation because additional inspired oxygen can cause pulmonary arteriolar vasodilation, raising pulmonary flow and increasing the quantity of pulmonary venous blood available for admixture. The best example of this phenomenon is total anomalous pulmonary venous return without obstruction, in which there is a large amount of pulmonary flow, but cyanosis is caused by mixing that occurs in the right atrium.

Supplemental inspired oxygen can increase arterial saturation somewhat because of additional increases in pulmonary flow. The same effect can be seen with the use of pulmonary vasodilators such as prostaglandin E_1. If supplemental oxygen is continued, however, this increase in an already high pulmonary flow could be detrimental, leading to pulmonary edema, congestive heart failure, and eventually acidosis.

Radiography

See also Chapter 37.

The chest radiograph can provide subtle information concerning possible types of heart disease, but the most common use is for assessing heart size and determining pulmonary blood flow (Box 45-5 and Figs. 45-10 and 45-11). For the determination of heart size, the width of the cardiothymic silhouette is measured and compared with the width of the chest at its largest dimension. The ratio should be 0.65 or less. Because true posteroanterior projections are unusual in infants, the measurement is made with an anteroposterior chest film; the most reliable measurements are from a film on which a good inspiration was obtained, with the diaphragm seen at the posterior margin of the 9th or 10th rib. The heart can appear falsely enlarged if the film is taken on expiration. One could be seeing heart, thymus, and pericardial fluid as part of the cardiothymic silhouette. The degree of pulmonary vascularity should be noted as normal, increased, or decreased, and the presence or absence of interstitial fluid, which is seen in pulmonary edema, must also be noted. Perhaps with the exception of the position of the aortic arch, which is ascertained by the deviation of the trachea or massive cardiomegaly, the chest

---

BOX 45–5   Distinctive Radiographic Signs

NEONATAL PULMONARY EDEMA (see Fig. 45-10)
Obstructed total anomalous pulmonary venous drainage
Cor triatriatum
Supravalvular mitral ring
Hypoplastic left heart syndrome with restrictive atrial
    septal defect
Mitral stenosis with restrictive atrial septal defect
Critical aortic stenosis with left ventricular dysfunction

RIGHT AORTIC ARCH
Tetralogy of Fallot
Truncus arteriosus
Transposition of the great arteries with ventricular septal
    defect and pulmonary stenosis

MASSIVE CARDIOMEGALY (see Fig. 45-11)
Ebstein anomaly

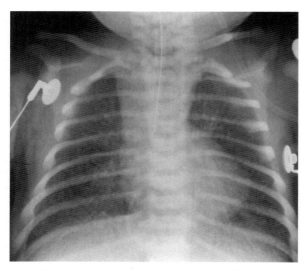

Figure 45–10. Chest radiograph of a newborn with an obstructed total anomalous pulmonary venous connection to innominate vein through the vertical vein. Bilateral pulmonary edema is due to pulmonary venous congestion.

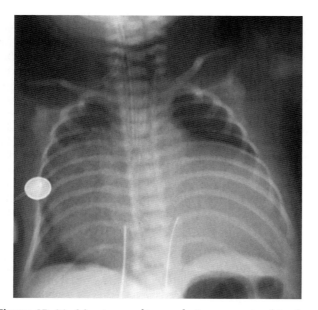

Figure 45–11. Massive cardiomegaly is present in this chest radiograph of a 1-day-old infant with severe Ebstein malformation of the tricuspid valve. The entire right cardiac silhouette is from right atrial enlargement. Diminished pulmonary vascularity is due to associated pulmonary atresia.

radiograph is relatively insensitive for specific cardiac diagnoses. It should not be used to exclude important heart defects when there is clinical suspicion of heart disease.[5]

Electrocardiography

Use of the electrocardiogram in the diagnosis of congenital heart disease is largely applicable to ventricular hypertrophy. Normal newborn infants have a relative predominance of the

right ventricle over the left ventricle. This predominance shifts to left ventricular predominance in the first year of life because of the fall in pulmonary artery pressure and the consequent fall in right ventricular systolic pressure. All electrocardiographic interpretations in children must be made relative to the normal right or left ventricular predominance existing at that particular age.

Electrocardiographic diagnosis of hypertrophy can be determined by recognizing that the right ventricle is oriented to the right, superior, and anterior, whereas the left ventricle is oriented to the left, inferior, and posterior. Leads that represent these orthogonal directions are V_5 and V_6 (right-left), aVF (superior-inferior), and V_1 and V_2 (anterior-posterior). One can then compare the forces present in these leads with normal standards for age to arrive at a judgment of relative ventricular predominance.

The T-wave main vector is an additional aid for diagnosing right ventricular hypertrophy. In normal neonates, the T wave is upright in leads V_1, $_RV_3$, and $_RV_4$ and inverts by 1 week of age, remaining inverted until about age 5 to 8 years. If it is upright between the ages of several days and 5 years, right ventricular hypertrophy is likely.

Except for the diagnosis of arrhythmias, the electrocardiogram is rarely diagnostic in the evaluation of the newborn with cardiac disease (Box 45-6). However, although one might suppose that a lesion obstructing the left ventricle, such as aortic coarctation, would produce left ventricular hypertrophy, in fact such lesions are seen more often with right ventricular hypertrophy, probably because, in the intrauterine circulation, the right ventricle is responsible for more of the combined ventricular output when the left ventricle is obstructed. The same is often true of lesions obstructing the right ventricle, which are often seen with left ventricular hypertrophy.

The electrocardiographic picture varies greatly within each of the diagnostic groups, and the electrocardiogram of infants with serious disease such as transposition is often completely normal. In practice, the clinician uses the electrocardiogram to confirm the impression that there is heart disease when the electrocardiogram fits the suspected diagnosis.

Echocardiography

Cardiac ultrasonography is the definitive diagnostic method for evaluating suspected cardiac disease in infants. It is noninvasive and safe, can be done at the bedside of sick neonates, and can be used successfully in premature infants of all sizes. The resolution is sufficient to make complete anatomic diagnoses in even the smallest hearts. Doppler echocardiography and color flow Doppler mapping have added the ability to study intracardiac and extracardiac flow patterns for assessing valve function and sites of obstruction.

BOX 45–6   Distinctive Electrocardiographic Signs
Left axis deviation
Endocardial cushion defect
Tricuspid atresia
Noonan syndrome
Left ventricular hypertrophy

The quality of the diagnostic information is such that many infants who would previously have undergone cardiac catheterization are now referred for cardiac surgery on the basis of the echocardiogram alone. Patients should be recommended for echocardiography on the basis of a cardiac evaluation, including physical examination, oxygen saturation measurement, electrocardiography, and other modalities. Echocardiography must be directed with knowledge of the infant's presenting signs and the results of the evaluation to date. Otherwise, important and often subtle findings might be missed.

CARDIAC IMAGING

Echocardiography relies on the reflection of ultrasound from interfaces in cardiac tissue such as those between arterial walls and the blood. Because the velocity of ultrasound in tissue is known, the time between the generation of the ultrasound and its reflection back to the transducer is proportional to distance. The strength of the reflections is a function of the tissue qualities. When arrays of different ultrasound crystals are coordinated simultaneously, two-dimensional images can be assembled. These are obtained from many standard precordial, subcostal, and suprasternal views. Evaluation of multiple planes from these sites results in a complete picture of cardiac structure (Box 45-7). Three-dimensional echocardiography can provide improved understanding of valve or spacial anatomy in selected neonates.

Technically, excellent transthoracic studies are the rule in neonates except in the postoperative period and obviously in the operating room after cardiopulmonary bypass. These limitations have been addressed by the development of pediatric transesophageal transducers, and intraoperative transesophageal echocardiography to assess the results of surgery has become routine.[3] Because of the relative size of the transducer and the proximity to the airway, postoperative neonates who need transesophageal echocardiography are intubated and sedated.

A quantitative approach to echocardiography is essential even in the neonate. Measurement of ventricular diastolic and systolic dimensions can be made either from two-dimensional images or from M-mode recordings. In M-mode recordings, a cursor is directed through the two-dimensional image across the structure to be measured (e.g., the left ventricle), and a continuous recording of dimensions along that cursor is made with time. Quantitative measurement of ventricular volume is done by planimetry of two-dimensional images. This quantitative approach often suggests physiologic abnormalities, such as left ventricular hypertrophy caused by increased left ventricular pressure.

DOPPLER ECHOCARDIOGRAPHY

Doppler echocardiography measures blood flow velocity and direction. Pulsed Doppler selects a specific site in the heart (e.g., the aortic valve) and measures velocity and direction with time. The maximum velocity that pulsed Doppler can detect is limited and is affected by the distance from the transducer and the frequency of the ultrasound transducer. The advantage of pulsed Doppler is that the velocities being measured are range-gated; that is, the velocities measured are from a specific structure within the heart.

Continuous-wave Doppler overcomes the problem of aliasing but sacrifices the range-gating. Velocities measured by continuous-wave Doppler could come from any structure along the cursor through the two-dimensional image. Continuous-wave Doppler is useful for measuring high-velocity flow such as occurs with stenotic or regurgitant valves.

Pulsed Doppler and continuous-wave Doppler provide highly quantitative velocity data from limited areas of the heart displayed as a function of time. Color flow mapping provides velocity information at many simultaneous sites encoded by color directly on the two-dimensional image. Blood flow toward the transducer is coded in shades of yellow or red, and flow away from the transducer is coded in shades of blue. The higher the velocity, the brighter the color that codes the flow. These color maps are updated up to 30 times per second and give a remarkable picture of the direction of blood flow through the heart. Color flow mapping dramatically enhances the identification of intracardiac shunts and disturbed blood flow at valves and along blood vessels.

The application of the Bernoulli principle to cardiac Doppler imaging has facilitated the quantitative assessment of physiologic changes caused by congenital heart defects. The Bernoulli principle in its simple form states that the change in pressure (ΔP) across an obstruction of flow is proportional to a constant times the square of velocity distal to the obstruction.[7,9,11]

MEASUREMENT OF CARDIAC FUNCTION

Table 45-4 and Box 45-8 summarize the data available from two-dimensional imaging and Doppler studies to define cardiac systolic and diastolic function.[14] The use of two-dimensional echocardiographic and Doppler parameters to define pulmonary artery pressure is outlined in Table 45-5.[8,12,16]

Computed Tomography and Magnetic Resonance Imaging

See also Chapter 37.
Computed tomography and magnetic resonance imaging are important tools for evaluating cardiac structure and function in the child and adult. Newer techniques for rapid acquisition

---

BOX 45-7   Echocardiographic Definition of Cardiac Structure

Cardiac position
Abdominal and atrial situs
Systemic and pulmonary venous connections
Mitral and tricuspid valve anatomy
Atrioventricular connections
Ventricular morphologic features, size, and wall thickness
Ventriculoarterial connections
Semilunar valve anatomy
Aortic arch anatomy
Pulmonary artery anatomy
Thymus

TABLE 45–4 Two-Dimensional and Doppler Assessment of Systolic Cardiac Function

Parameter	Formula	Modality
Wall Motion		
Shortening fraction (SF,%)	$100 \times (LVD - LVS)/LVD$	M-mode
Ejection fraction (EF,%)	$100 \times (LVD^3 - LVS^3)/LVD^3$	M-mode
	$100 \times (LVD - LVS)/LVD$	Two dimensional
VCF (circ/sec)	SF/VET	M-mode
VCF wall stress		M-mode, pressure
Regional wall motion analysis		Two dimensional
Blood Flow		
Systemic blood flow (L/min)	$(EDV - ESV) \times HR$	Two dimensional
	Ao VTI $\times$ Ao CSA $\times$ HR	Doppler, two dimensional
Pulmonary blood flow (L/min)	PA VTI $\times$ PA CSA $\times$ HR	Doppler, two dimensional

Ao, aortic; circ/sec, circumferences per second; CSA, cross-sectional area (πr^2); EDV, left ventricular end-diastolic volume; ESV, left ventricular end-systolic volume; HR, heart rate; LVD, left ventricular diastolic dimension; LVS, left ventricular systolic dimension; PA, pulmonary artery; VTI, velocity time integral; VCF, velocity of circumferential fiber shortening; VET, ventricular ejection time.

BOX 45–8 Two-Dimensional and Doppler Assessment of Diastolic Cardiac Function

TWO-DIMENSIONAL ASSESSMENT
Velocity of posterior wall thinning

DOPPLER ASSESSMENT

Right Ventricle
Tricuspid early diastole and atrial systole peak velocities
Tricuspid early diastole and atrial systole time integrals
Retrograde hepatic vein flow during atrial systole

Left Ventricle
Mitral early diastole and atrial systole peak velocities
Mitral early diastole and atrial systole time integrals
Retrograde pulmonary vein flow during atrial systole
Isovolumic relaxation time
Myocardial tissue Doppler indexes[10]

TABLE 45–5 Two-Dimensional and Doppler Assessment of Pulmonary Hypertension: Interpretation of Normal Values

Variables	Values
Two-Dimensional Assessment	
RV hypertrophy	Normal < 3 mm
Mid-systolic pulmonary valve closure	Normal: none
Systolic septal flattening: circularity index	Normal > 93%
Systolic time interval: RV pre-ejection period and RV ejection time	Normal < 0.3 indicates normal PA diastolic pressure
Doppler Assessment	
Systolic time interval: RV pre-ejection period and RV ejection time	Normal < 0.3 indicates normal PA diastolic pressure
RVOT acceleration time/ejection time	Normal > 0.36 indicates normal mean PA pressure
Tricuspid regurgitation velocity	Low velocity indicates low RV systolic pressure
Pulmonary regurgitation velocity	Low velocity indicates low PA diastolic pressure
Ductal velocity	High velocity indicates low PA diastolic pressure
Ventricular septal defect velocity	High velocity indicates low RV systolic pressure

PA, pulmonary artery; RV, right ventricular; RVOT, right ventricular outflow tract.

---

of images has made these modalities available to the neonate. Magnetic resonance and computed tomography imaging in the neonate are particularly strong in delineating the anatomy of the aortic arch, pulmonary artery, pulmonary veins, and ventricular volumes.[6,13]

Computed tomography clearly demonstrates the relationship of the bronchi and the cardiac structures, which is invaluable in assessing respiratory distress in neonates with vascular rings and tracheal compromise resulting from enlarged pulmonary arteries. Software enhancements and cardiac gating have also helped define ventricular anatomy and function. Flow studies are possible and permit calculations similar to those of Doppler echocardiography for pressure gradients.

The principal disadvantage of these modalities for the sick neonate is the inability to come to the bedside for the study. However, ventilators and monitors are available that make these studies possible.

Cardiac Catheterization

Although routine neonatal diagnostic cardiac catheterization is rare, there remains a role for diagnostic catheterization and angiography, especially when decisions must be made regarding neonatal repair or palliation of complex defects. Pressure data can usually be inferred from echocardiography but directly measured only by catheterization. Neonatal repair of many defects can be undertaken without precise hemodynamic measurement of pressure and blood flow and calculation of vascular resistance. Elective catheterization is usually more useful after neonatal palliation with shunts or pulmonary artery bands to assess pulmonary artery hemodynamics. An understanding of the principles of hemodynamic catheterization is, however, essential for postoperative care, when atrial and arterial monitoring catheters are available for oxygen sampling and pressure measurement.

DIAGNOSTIC GROUPS OF CONGENITAL HEART DISEASE

The spectrum of congenital heart disease includes scores of particular lesions with variable presentations within each diagnosis. These variations often determine the type and timing of corrective cardiac surgery, but they do not preclude a general grouping of defects. Grouping of defects by symptoms enhances the recognition of which infants require echocardiography, transfer to a specialized center, and, most important, prostaglandin E_1 to maintain or restore ductal patency.

The reduction in neonatal cardiovascular morbidity and mortality rates since the introduction of prostaglandin E_1 in the late 1970s cannot be underestimated, and the timely identification of infants with ductal-dependent heart defects is essential. These defects include those with restricted pulmonary blood flow (e.g., pulmonary atresia), restricted systemic blood flow (critical aortic stenosis or coarctation), and separate circulations with poor mixing (transposition of the great arteries). Preliminary diagnosis identifies which infants have excessive pulmonary flow and limited systemic blood flow, for whom supplemental oxygen will be detrimental, such as infants with hypoplastic left heart syndrome.

A summary of defects by diagnostic category is given in Box 45-9. Varieties of several defects appear in more than one category if there is a spectrum of common clinical presentations.

Cyanosis

Varying degrees of cyanosis might be present in many neonates with congenital heart disease at presentation. Cyanosis is the most prominent feature, as opposed to respiratory distress, congestive heart failure, or poor systemic flow, in infants with restricted pulmonary blood flow and those with separate circulations and poor mixing. A lesser degree of hypoxia is seen with mixing lesions, pulmonary disease, or pulmonary edema.

BOX 45–9 Classification of Congenital Heart Disease

SEVERE CYANOSIS CAUSED BY SEPARATE CIRCULATIONS AND POOR MIXING
D-Transposition of the great arteries
D-Transposition of the great arteries and ventricular septal defect
Double-outlet right ventricle with subpulmonary ventricular septal defect (Taussig-Bing)

SEVERE CYANOSIS CAUSED BY RESTRICTED PULMONARY BLOOD FLOW
Tetralogy of Fallot
Double-outlet right ventricle with subaortic ventricular septal defect and pulmonary stenosis
Tricuspid atresia
Pulmonary atresia with intact interventricular septum
Critical pulmonary stenosis
Ebstein anomaly
Single ventricle with pulmonary stenosis
Persistent pulmonary hypertension

MILD CYANOSIS CAUSED BY COMPLETE MIXING WITH NORMAL OR INCREASED PULMONARY BLOOD FLOW
Total anomalous pulmonary venous connection
Truncus arteriosus
Single ventricle without pulmonary stenosis
Double-outlet right ventricle with subaortic ventricular septal defect

SYSTEMIC HYPOPERFUSION AND CONGESTIVE HEART FAILURE WITH MILD OR NO CYANOSIS
Aortic stenosis*
Coarctation of the aorta and aortic arch interruption
Hypoplastic left heart syndrome
Multiple left heart defects
Single ventricle with subaortic stenosis or coarctation of the aorta
Myocardial diseases: cardiomyopathy and myocarditis*
Cardiac tumor*
Arteriovenous malformation*
Hypertension*

ACYANOSIS WITH NO OR MILD RESPIRATORY DISTRESS
Normal murmurs
Pulmonary stenosis
Ventricular septal defect†
Atrial septal defect
Endocardial cushion defect†
Patent ductus arteriosus†
Aortopulmonary window†
L-Transposition of the great arteries
Arteriovenous malformation
Hypertension

---

*No symptoms with mild forms of disease.
†Congestive heart failure can develop as left-to-right shunt increases with decrease in pulmonary vascular resistance.

SEVERE CYANOSIS CAUSED BY SEPARATE CIRCULATIONS AND POOR MIXING

Severe cyanosis caused by separate circulations and poor mixing is a diagnostic group that includes lesions in which there is prominent cyanosis but a normal or increased pulmonary blood flow. The neonates have transposition of the great arteries with a small atrial or ventricular septal communication or a related lesion with similar blood flow patterns (double-outlet right ventricle with subpulmonary ventricular septal defect). In such cases, the cyanosis is due to inadequate mixing between the systemic and pulmonary venous returns, so that the systemic venous return is delivered to the aorta through the right ventricle, with little admixture of oxygenated blood. Patients with this group of defects could benefit from a patent ductus arteriosus because the ductal flow enhances atrial mixing.

SEVERE CYANOSIS CAUSED BY RESTRICTED PULMONARY BLOOD FLOW

In the lesions of severe cyanosis caused by restricted pulmonary blood flow, there is an anatomic obstruction to pulmonary blood flow, including obstruction of the pulmonic valve or tricuspid valve. Because neonates with these lesions are dependent on patency of the ductus arteriosus, a prostaglandin E_1 infusion should be started immediately. A dramatic improvement in saturation resulting from prostaglandin E_1 infusion confirms that a particular lesion is in this group.

Within this group with decreased pulmonary flow, several lesions have characteristic findings that allow one to be more confident of the actual diagnosis. For example, a cyanotic infant with decreased pulmonary flow and a huge cardiac silhouette most likely has Ebstein anomaly of the tricuspid valve. A small heart and a harsh ejection murmur but decreased pulmonary flow most likely indicate tetralogy of Fallot. The murmur is due to a stenotic, but not atretic, pulmonic valve.

MILD CYANOSIS CAUSED BY COMPLETE MIXING WITH NORMAL OR INCREASED PULMONARY BLOOD FLOW

Most patients with lesions in the diagnostic group of mild cyanosis caused by complete mixing with normal or increased pulmonary blood flow have evidence of pulmonary overcirculation, as seen on the chest radiograph, and their most prominent presenting sign is usually respiratory distress. In the mixing lesions, arterial desaturation is due to mixing of systemic and pulmonary venous blood before ejection into the aorta. Because pulmonary flow is increased or normal, cyanosis is not profound.

Because pulmonary flow is capable of increasing under the influence of inhaled oxygen, the arterial saturation often rises dramatically with the hyperoxic test. Arterial saturation does not become normal, however, because some admixture of systemic and pulmonary venous blood is always present. This decreased response to oxygen helps differentiate these infants from those with primarily left-to-right shunts and mild cyanosis caused by pulmonary overcirculation and resultant pulmonary edema. Similarly, infants with pulmonary edema caused by left ventricular dysfunction and high pulmonary venous pressures have a normal response to oxygen.

Examples of a mixing lesion with increased pulmonary flow are total anomalous pulmonary venous connection, truncus arteriosus, and single ventricle without pulmonary stenosis. Infants with these defects do not require prostaglandin E_1 unless there are associated defects. A patent ductus arteriosus is unlikely to be deleterious if prostaglandin E_1 is started empirically. In contrast, supplemental oxygen or hyperventilation can dramatically increase pulmonary blood flow and decrease systemic blood flow and should be avoided in this group of babies.

Systemic Hypoperfusion and Congestive Heart Failure with Mild or No Cyanosis

Some degree of hypoperfusion might be present in infants with cyanosis, especially with the injudicious use of oxygen. However, infants with systemic hypoperfusion and congestive heart failure with mild or no cyanosis have poor systemic perfusion as the most prominent feature.[1] The classic example of this group of lesions is hypoplastic left heart syndrome. The babies with these lesions are ductal dependent for systemic flow because all or a large portion of systemic flow must traverse the ductus arteriosus from the pulmonary artery. Also in this group of lesions are critical aortic stenosis, critical coarctation of the aorta, and aortic arch interruption. In these lesions, the mild cyanosis might be limited to the lower portion of the body because the ductus arteriosus perfuses the descending aorta with a variable degree of retrograde ascending aortic flow.

The differential diagnosis for this group includes a number of cardiac conditions that are not dependent on the ductus arteriosus for systemic flow, as well as several noncardiac conditions. Cardiac conditions that do not depend on a patent ductus arteriosus and that include systemic hypoperfusion at presentation include cardiomyopathies and arrhythmias. Noncardiac conditions that could have systemic hypoperfusion at presentation, mimicking forms of congenital heart disease, include neonatal sepsis and metabolic disease.

Acyanosis with No or Mild Respiratory Distress

In the neonatal period, most infants with uncomplicated left-to-right shunts, including ventricular septal defect and patent ductus arteriosus, are in the group of acyanosis with no or mild respiratory distress. Prostaglandin E_1 is not necessary; however, unlike the infants with a single ventricle, these infants, when given supplemental oxygen, rarely have difficulty with impaired systemic flow because of excessive pulmonary flow. Respiratory distress or poor perfusion should suggest an associated obstruction of the left side of the heart.

REFERENCES

1. Abu-Harb M, et al: Presentation of obstructive left heart malformations in infancy, *Arch Dis Child Fetal Neonatal Ed* 71:F179, 1994.
2. Crossland DS, et al: Variability of four limb blood pressure in normal neonates, *Arch Dis Child Fetal Neonatal Ed* 89:F325, 2004.
3. Drinker LR, et al: Use of the monoplane intracardiac imaging probe in high-risk infants during congenital heart surgery, *Echocardiography* 25:999, 2008.

4. de-Wahl Granelli A, et al: Impact of pulse oximetry screening on the detection of duct dependent congenital heart disease: a Swedish prospective screening study in 39,821 newborns, *BMJ* 338:3037, 2009.

5. Fonseca B, et al: Chest radiography and the evaluation of the neonate for congenital heart disease, *Pediatr Cardiol* 26:367, 2005.

6. Hirsch R, et al: Computed tomography angiography with three-dimensional reconstruction for pulmonary venous definition in high-risk infants with congenital heart disease, *Congenit Heart Dis* 1:104, 2006.

7. Houston AB, et al: Doppler flow characteristics in the assessment of pulmonary pressure in ductus arteriosus, *Br Heart J* 62:284, 1989.

8. Hsieh KS, et al: Right ventricular systolic time intervals: comparison of echocardiographic and Doppler-derived values, *Am Heart J* 112:103, 1986.

9. Marx GR, et al: Doppler echocardiographic estimation of pulmonary artery pressure in patients with aortic-pulmonary shunts, *J Am Coll Cardiol* 7:880, 1986.

10. Mori K, et al: Pulsed wave Doppler tissue echocardiography assessment of the long axis function of the right and left ventricles during the early neonatal period, *Heart* 90:175, 2004.

11. Murphy DJ Jr, et al: Continuous-wave Doppler in children with ventricular septal defect: noninvasive estimation of interventricular pressure gradient, *Am J Cardiol* 57:428, 1986.

12. Portman MA, et al: Left ventricular systolic circular index: an echocardiographic measure of transseptal pressure ratio, *Am Heart J* 114:1178, 1987.

13. Prakash A, et al: Usefulness of magnetic resonance angiography in the evaluation of complex congenital heart disease in newborns and infants, *Am J Cardiol* 100:715, 2007.

14. Riggs TW, et al: Doppler echocardiographic evaluation of right and left diastolic ventricular function in normal neonates, *J Am Coll Cardiol* 13:700, 1989.

15. Sendelbach DM, et al: Pulse oximetry screening at 4 hours of age to detect critical congenital heart defects, *Pediatrics* 122:e815, 2008.

16. Stevenson JG: Comparison of several noninvasive methods for estimation of pulmonary artery pressure, *J Am Soc Echocardiogr* 2:157, 1989.

17. Yabek SM: Neonatal cyanosis: reappraisal of response to 100% oxygen breathing, *Am J Dis Child* 138:880, 1984.

PART 7

Congenital Defects

Kenneth G. Zahka and Francine Erenberg

CYANOTIC HEART DEFECTS: POOR MIXING

D-Transposition of the Great Arteries

ANATOMY AND PATHOPHYSIOLOGY

In D-transposition of the great arteries, the aorta connects to the right ventricle, and the pulmonary artery connects to the left ventricle. The aorta is anterior and slightly to the right, and the pulmonary artery is posterior and to the left.

In contrast to the blood flow pattern in the normal heart, in which the pulmonary and systemic circulations are in series, in transposition of the great arteries, the pulmonary and systemic circulations are in parallel. Thus, the venous blood returning to the right atrium flows through the tricuspid valve into the right ventricle and is ejected into the aorta, supplying the body with poorly oxygenated blood, which then returns to the right atrium to repeat the cycle. Fully oxygenated blood from the lungs enters the left atrium, flows through the mitral valve into the left ventricle, and is ejected into the pulmonary artery to perfuse the lungs and return to the left atrium without delivering oxygen to the body. In the absence of shunting across connections between the systemic and pulmonary circulations, this results in profound, lethal systemic hypoxia.

The persistence of two fetal connections, the foramen ovale and the ductus arteriosus, provides sites for intracardiac shunting during the first hours and days of life. After spontaneous closure of the ductus arteriosus, bidirectional shunting at the atrial level is essential for survival.

Right ventricular pressure is high because of high vascular resistance in the aorta and systemic vasculature. The high right ventricular pressure and systemic resistance maintain the right ventricular muscle mass. With the fall in pulmonary vascular resistance, left ventricular and pulmonary artery pressures fall, which results in regression of the normal neonatal left ventricular hypertrophy.

ASSOCIATED DEFECTS

Associated defects have a dramatic effect on the presentation and pathophysiology of newborn infants with transposition of the great arteries. At a minimum, an atrial septal defect with balanced bidirectional shunting is essential for survival.[92] This shunting occurs in a phasic manner over the cardiac cycle, with shunting from the left to right atrium favored during ventricular systole. The addition of a patent ductus arteriosus permits nearly exclusive shunting from the aorta to the pulmonary artery at the arterial level, with an equal volume of left-to-right atrial shunting at the atrial level. This combination provides excellent palliation of the systemic hypoxia.

A ventricular septal defect occurs in about 25% of infants with transposition of the great arteries. Because of the relative aortic and pulmonary artery resistance, flow at a ventricular septal defect is from the right ventricle to the left ventricle and pulmonary artery in systole. This right-to-left shunt is usually balanced by a left-to-right shunt at the atrial level or the ventricular level in diastole.

Arch obstruction, either coarctation of the aorta or aortic arch interruption, occurs in association with transposition of the great arteries and ventricular septal defect.[82] Flow to the descending aorta comes from the pulmonary artery and has a high saturation. Valvular and subvalvular pulmonary stenosis limits pulmonary blood flow and shunting from the left to the right atrium and from the right ventricle to the pulmonary artery.

CLINICAL PRESENTATION

Transposition of the great arteries is the most common cyanotic heart defect identified in the first week of life, and the diagnosis should be considered in any cyanotic neonate. Fetal diagnosis is common but not uniform; however, even with prenatal diagnosis, profound hypoxia due to a highly restrictive patent foramen ovale can lead to rapid deterioration and death in the first hours of life.[50,98] Respiratory symptoms are absent or limited to hyperpnea or tachypnea without dyspnea. The second heart sound is persistently single in transposition of the great arteries because of the anterior position of the aorta and the posterior position of the pulmonary artery. A holosystolic murmur suggests an associated ventricular septal defect; a systolic ejection murmur is heard with pulmonary stenosis. In the absence of these associated defects, murmurs are typically not heard. The peripheral pulses are normal unless coarctation of the aorta is present. Persistent ductal patency or high pulmonary vascular resistance will affect the clinical findings of an associated ventricular septal defect or coarctation of the aorta.

LABORATORY EVALUATION

The electrocardiogram is normal, although right ventricular hypertrophy might be evident after the first week of life. Similarly, the classic egg-shaped heart with increased pulmonary vascularity on the chest radiograph might not be seen in the newborn period. Echocardiography defines the associated defects and coronary artery anatomy.[79] Preoperative identification of anatomic coronary variations, including an intramural course of the coronary arteries, is central to surgical planning for the arterial switch operation.[61] Cardiac catheterization is usually reserved for neonates requiring balloon atrial septostomy, but it is occasionally useful for clarifying coronary or other anatomic details (Fig. 45-12).

MANAGEMENT AND PROGNOSIS

Establishing patency of the ductus arteriosus with prostaglandin E_1 in newborn infants who have transposition of the great arteries often improves arterial oxygenation by increasing shunting from the aorta into the pulmonary artery. This in turn increases the pulmonary venous return, distending the left atrium and facilitating shunting from the left to the right atrium of fully saturated blood across the foramen ovale.

If prostaglandin E_1 treatment does not result in adequate systemic oxygenation, a balloon atrial septostomy is performed. At cardiac catheterization or at the bedside with echocardiographic guidance, a balloon-tipped catheter is advanced from the inferior vena cava into the right atrium and through the foramen ovale to the left atrium. The balloon is inflated with dilute radiographic contrast medium. The catheter is then sharply tugged, resulting in rapid withdrawal of the inflated balloon from the left atrium to the junction of the right atrium and inferior vena cava. The atrial septum tears, enlarging the foramen ovale into an atrial septal defect and allowing improved mixing of the systemic and pulmonary venous return at the atrial level.

History

Surgical management of transposition of the great arteries has changed dramatically since the 1960s and, in particular, since the 1980s. Surgical creation of an atrial septal defect with the technique described by Blalock and Hanlon in 1950 was eventually replaced by the atrial baffling operations described by Senning in 1959 and Mustard in 1964. In these operations, the arterial and ventricular connections remained transposed, and the venous inflow into the atria was redirected. The superior and inferior vena caval blood was tunneled across the atrium to the mitral valve, and the pulmonary veins were directed to the tricuspid valve.

This physiologic repair resulted in fully oxygenated blood in the right ventricle and aorta and in poorly oxygenated blood in the left ventricle and pulmonary artery; however, the anatomic ventriculoarterial relationships of the heart remained

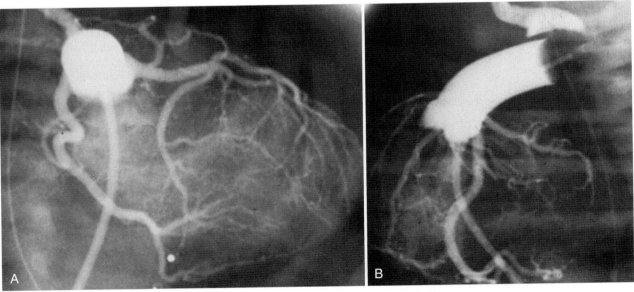

Figure 45-12. **A,** Anterior "laid back" view in balloon occlusion aortogram demonstrating the most common coronary arterial anatomy found in transposition of great arteries. Great arteries are front to back, and the right coronary artery arises from the right posterior-facing sinus, whereas the left coronary artery arises from the left posterior-facing sinus and gives rise to the left anterior descending and circumflex arteries. **B,** Lateral view of the same, showing ideal balloon position and occlusion of the aorta at the time of injection.

abnormal. Long-term postoperative problems included atrial arrhythmias, pulmonary and systemic venous obstruction, and right ventricular enlargement and dysfunction.[3,42]

Arterial Switch Operation

Jatene and later Yacoub pioneered the anatomic repair of transposition of the great arteries, using the arterial switch operation. This operation requires transection of the aorta and pulmonary artery to move the pulmonary artery anteriorly to the right ventricle and the aorta posteriorly to the left ventricle. The coronary arteries are moved from their original position on the aorta to the newly created aorta, and atrial and ventricular septal defects are repaired.

The arterial switch operation in infants with transposition of the great arteries and with an intact ventricular septum is optimally performed in the first 2 weeks of life. During this time, the left ventricle has sufficient hypertrophy to support systemic blood pressure. After 2 weeks, unless there is a large ventricular septal defect, left ventricular pressure is low, and the left ventricular muscle mass has regressed in a similar fashion to that of the right ventricle in children with normally related great arteries.

The follow-up to date for the arterial switch operation is favorable.[63,98,107] Risk factors for early mortality include prematurity and right ventricular hypoplasia.[16] Coronary anatomy (especially intramural coronary arteries), a risk factor in the earlier experience, can now be managed effectively, although with a higher hospital morbidity.[16,61] Long-term follow-up studies demonstrate excellent ventricular function, normal rhythm, and a low incidence of obstruction at the aortic and coronary suture lines.[23,88] Narrowing in the supravalvular pulmonary area could require subsequent surgery or catheter interventions.[5,31,74,98] Dilation of the neoaortic root and aortic regurgitation are found in some children but rarely require intervention.[62,98] Neurodevelopmental outcome is, in general, good in infants who do not require intraoperative circulatory arrest. Motor deficits, rather than impaired intelligence quotient scores, are seen in infants with transposition of the great arteries who had circulatory arrest.[15]

CYANOTIC DEFECTS: RESTRICTED PULMONARY BLOOD FLOW

Tetralogy of Fallot

ANATOMY AND PATHOPHYSIOLOGY

In 1888, Fallot described the association of infundibular (subvalvular) and valvular pulmonary stenosis, a large ventricular septal defect, a large aorta overriding the ventricular septum, and right ventricular hypertrophy.

A variable degree of pulmonary artery hypoplasia, an atrial septal defect or foramen ovale, patent ductus arteriosus, or systemic-to-pulmonary collateral vessels are often present. In the most severe form of tetralogy of Fallot, atresia of the pulmonary valve or of the entire right ventricular outflow tract (OFT) and main pulmonary artery occurs.

Obstruction of the right ventricular OFT reduces pulmonary blood flow and produces systemic arterial desaturation by diverting poorly oxygenated right ventricular blood across the ventricular septal defect into the ascending aorta. The extent of right-to-left shunting is determined by the relative resistance to systemic and pulmonary blood flow. Whereas systemic resistance is determined by peripheral arteriolar resistance, total resistance to pulmonary blood flow is the combination of pulmonary infundibular, valvular, and arteriolar resistance. Acutely increasing the pulmonary infundibular obstruction, such as probably occurs with the release of endogenous catecholamine, exacerbates the shunting.

ASSOCIATED DEFECTS

Right aortic arch is seen in about 25% of neonates with tetralogy of Fallot. Surgically important variants include origin of the anterior descending coronary artery from the right coronary artery. This branch crosses the right ventricular OFT at the level of the site of the infundibular incision and could limit the possibility of excising the subpulmonary obstruction. The branch pulmonary arteries might be discontinuous and supplied by one or more collateral vessels from the aorta. Tetralogy of Fallot with absent pulmonary valve includes hypoplasia of the pulmonary valve annulus and rudimentary cusps. Infants with this defect also have marked poststenotic dilation of the branch pulmonary arteries and compression of the bronchi.

CLINICAL PRESENTATION

The spectrum of the clinical presentation of tetralogy of Fallot is directly related to the severity of the pulmonary stenosis. The intensely cyanotic newborn infant generally has severe pulmonary stenosis or atresia and markedly diminished pulmonary blood flow. The minimally cyanotic or even acyanotic newborn infant being examined for a systolic murmur has just enough pulmonary stenosis to prevent a left-to-right shunt through the ventricular septal defect without producing a right-to-left shunt.

There is usually a palpable right ventricular impulse, reflecting the right ventricular hypertension, and a single second heart sound with an absent pulmonary component because of the anterior location of the aorta and the marked abnormality of the pulmonary artery OFT. The systolic ejection murmur heard in neonates with tetralogy of Fallot is produced by turbulent blood flow across the pulmonary stenosis; therefore, the intensity of the murmur is directly related to the amount of pulmonary blood flow and inversely related to the severity of the pulmonary obstruction.

The absence of a systolic ejection murmur in children with tetralogy of Fallot implies atresia of the right ventricular OFT. In this case, a continuous murmur indicates blood flow through a patent ductus arteriosus or through systemic-to-pulmonary collateral vessels as the sole source of pulmonary blood flow.

LABORATORY EVALUATION

The electrocardiogram of the neonate is normal. Electrocardiographic criteria for right ventricular hypertrophy develop during the first month of life. The echocardiogram demonstrates the ventricular septal defect and aortic override (Fig. 45-13). Of particular echocardiographic importance is documentation of the sites of pulmonary obstruction, with determination of the size of the main and branch pulmonary arteries and the presence of a patent ductus arteriosus or collateral vessels.

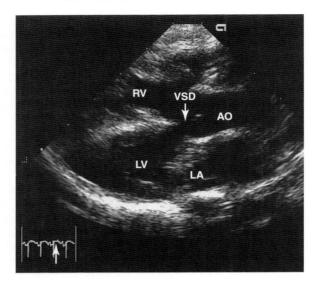

Figure 45–13. Echocardiogram showing parasternal long-axis view in a newborn infant with tetralogy of Fallot. The right ventricle (RV) is anterior, and left ventricle (LV) is posterior, with a large ventricular septal defect (VSD) and overriding aorta (AO). LA, left atrium.

Coronary artery anatomy can usually be defined. In newborn infants, the chest radiograph does not show the typical "boot-shaped" heart, although decreased vascularity or a right aortic arch might be evident. Cardiac catheterization is now only indicated before surgery if the pulmonary artery anatomy and sources of pulmonary blood flow cannot be defined noninvasively by echocardiogram, computed tomography, or magnetic resonance imaging.

MANAGEMENT AND PROGNOSIS

Neonates with severe cyanosis are stabilized by an infusion of prostaglandin E_1 to dilate the ductus arteriosus and increase pulmonary blood flow. These infants often have severely hypoplastic pulmonary arteries and must have a palliative procedure to establish a source of pulmonary blood flow. This includes a systemic-to-pulmonary shunt, with either a direct connection of the subclavian artery to the pulmonary artery (Blalock-Taussig shunt) or a synthetic tubular graft (Gore-Tex) between the aorta or one of its branches and the pulmonary artery. Balloon dilation or stenting of the stenotic pulmonary valve has been favored in a few centers as an alternative to shunts.[27] In babies with marked pulmonary artery hypoplasia, the right ventricular OFT can be widened surgically without closing the ventricular septal defect. Rehabilitation of branch pulmonary artery stenosis by surgery or interventional catheterization is important either at the time of primary repair or as part of a staged approach.[57]

Neonatal repair of tetralogy of Fallot is feasible for babies with appropriate pulmonary artery anatomy. Surgical repair of tetralogy of Fallot consists of closure of the ventricular septal defect, excision of the pulmonary stenosis, and enlargement of the right ventricular OFT with a patch. In the absence of marked pulmonary artery hypoplasia or unfavorable coronary artery anatomy, surgery can be undertaken at virtually any age.[86]

Tricuspid Atresia
ANATOMY AND PATHOPHYSIOLOGY

Tricuspid atresia usually results in complete absence of the components of the tricuspid valve, with a smooth floor of the right atrium at the usual location of the tricuspid valve. In rare instances, tricuspid valve tissue and chordae are present, but the valve is imperforate. Associated right ventricular hypoplasia and pulmonary artery hypoplasia are proportional to the size of the ventricular septal defect and the degree of subpulmonary and pulmonary valve stenosis.

Systemic venous return from the inferior and superior venae cavae enters the right atrium and crosses the atrial septum, with resultant complete mixing of the systemic and pulmonary venous return in the left atrium. Pulmonary blood flow is supplied by left-to-right shunting through either the ductus arteriosus or the ventricular septal defect. The degree of systemic hypoxia is proportional to the relative systemic and pulmonary blood flow. Neonates with tricuspid atresia, small ventricular septal defect, and severe pulmonary stenosis have severely limited pulmonary blood flow and are ductal dependent. Those with large ventricular septal defects and no pulmonary stenosis have high pulmonary artery pressure and flow. When pulmonary artery resistance falls in these babies, pulmonary flow dramatically increases, and hypoxia is minimal. The babies are, in contrast, at risk for congestive heart failure as a result of excessive pulmonary blood flow and left ventricular volume loading.

ASSOCIATED DEFECTS

An atrial septal defect is essential for postnatal survival in all neonates with tricuspid atresia. Associated lesions have been reported with tricuspid atresia, including transposition of the great arteries, truncus arteriosus, and atrioventricular (AV) septal defect. The size of the ventricular septal defect is extremely important in neonates with the combination of tricuspid atresia and transposition of the great arteries. Those with restrictive ventricular septal defects have limited systemic blood flow and a high prevalence of associated coarctation of the aorta.

CLINICAL PRESENTATION

The typical neonatal presentation is cyanosis at the time of ductal closure and a murmur. Precordial activity is normal, and the second heart sound is single. There is a systolic ejection murmur arising from the subpulmonary and pulmonary valve stenosis. Absence of a harsh systolic murmur in a baby with tricuspid atresia suggests associated pulmonary atresia. A continuous murmur of ductal flow can be heard. If the ventricular septal defect is large, tachypnea, a left ventricular impulse, and a third heart sound develop during the first few days of life as the pulmonary vascular resistance falls. Hepatic enlargement is an important sign of a restrictive atrial septal defect and elevated right atrial pressures.

LABORATORY EVALUATION

The electrocardiogram is usually diagnostic in neonates with tricuspid atresia. The left anterior bundle conducts abnormally, and there is an abnormal superior and leftward frontal plane vector or axis. The right ventricular hypoplasia leads to diminished right ventricular forces and to an electrocardiographic diagnosis of left ventricular hypertrophy. The chest radiograph is nonspecific, although severely cyanotic neonates show decreased pulmonary vascularity. The echocardiogram (Fig. 45-14) defines the anatomy of the right ventricular OFT and the pulmonary artery, the presence of a ductus arteriosus, and a nonrestrictive atrial septal defect. Catheterization is rarely needed to assess pulmonary artery anatomy before surgery.

MANAGEMENT AND PROGNOSIS

Antegrade pulmonary flow across the ventricular septal defect may be adequate in the first months of life. It is usually possible to predict by echocardiogram when babies require a patent ductus arteriosus to maintain adequate arterial saturations. Balloon atrial septostomy is rarely necessary unless there is significant restriction at the atrial septal defect.

If the baby is ductal dependent or if hypoxia increases in the first month of life, a systemic-to-pulmonary shunt is necessary for providing adequate pulmonary blood flow and oxygenation. The long-term effect of left ventricular volume loading caused by systemic-to-pulmonary shunts and the risk for distortion of the pulmonary arteries must be considered; conversion to a bidirectional Glenn anastomosis is usually considered when an infant is between 3 and 6 months of age.[53] Some babies with well-balanced systemic and pulmonary flows can proceed directly to an early bidirectional Glenn operation[85] or to a Fontan operation at about 1 year of age. Among children who undergo the Fontan type of operation, those with tricuspid atresia have the best long-term prognosis, with a low prevalence of ventricular dysfunction, mitral regurgitation, arrhythmias, and systemic venous congestion (see Table 45-12 in Part 10).[96]

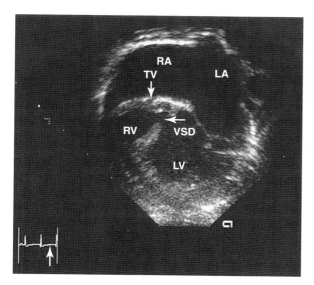

Figure 45–14. Apical four-chamber view of neonate with tricuspid atresia. Shown are a fibromuscular floor of the right atrium (TV), small ventricular septal defect (VSD), and hypoplastic right ventricle (RV). A large atrial septal defect permits free flow from the right atrium (RA) to the left atrium (LA) and into the left ventricle (LV).

Pulmonary Atresia with Intact Ventricular Septum and Critical Pulmonary Stenosis

ANATOMY AND PATHOPHYSIOLOGY

Neonatal critical pulmonary stenosis and pulmonary atresia share several important anatomic and pathophysiologic issues. The extent of right ventricular obstruction is profound, and the degree of right ventricular hypertrophy and dysfunction is high. Neonates with atresia of the pulmonary valve have a spectrum of disease from a thick membrane with hypoplastic annulus to well-developed sinuses with complete fusion of the cusps. Critical pulmonary stenosis lies at the latter end of the spectrum with a small amount of anterograde flow. There is an additional component of tricuspid valve and right ventricular inflow hypoplasia with hypoplasia of the trabecular portion of the body of the right ventricle. Despite the right ventricular hypoplasia and limited anterograde flow, the pulmonary arteries are usually well developed because of in utero ductal flow.

Systemic venous return largely crosses the atrial septum and mixes completely with the pulmonary venous return in the left atrium. Anterograde flow that does cross the tricuspid valve is ejected back into the atrium with minimal or no net anterograde flow. Right ventricular pressure exceeds left ventricular pressure. Flow to the pulmonary arteries is primarily by the ductus arteriosus.

ASSOCIATED DEFECTS

Fistulas between the right ventricle and the coronary arteries are the most critical associated lesions in this defect. They decompress the right ventricle by carrying desaturated systemic venous blood back to the aorta. They can also supply the coronary arteries, and in some cases they are the sole source of coronary flow with atresia of the coronary arteries at the aorta. The associated atrial septal defect is rarely restrictive in the neonatal period. Occasional neonates with pulmonary atresia have an associated mild degree of aortic stenosis or a bicuspid aortic valve.

CLINICAL PRESENTATION

Neonates with pulmonary atresia and an intact ventricular septum have severe hypoxia at the time the ductus arteriosus closes. A right ventricular impulse and a single second heart sound are present. A high-pitched holosystolic murmur of tricuspid regurgitation might be audible, or a murmur with systolic and diastolic components from flow in the coronary fistulas can be heard. The liver is enlarged because of the tricuspid regurgitation and right ventricular diastolic dysfunction. Fetal diagnosis frequently can identify the risk factors for subsequent interventional and surgical management, including tricuspid valve hypoplasia and coronary artery fistulas.[33]

LABORATORY EVALUATION

The electrocardiogram might be normal or might show a variable degree of right ventricular hypertrophy. Unlike neonates with tricuspid atresia, the neonates with pulmonary atresia might have a relatively normal right ventricular muscle mass despite a component of ventricular hypoplasia. The chest radiograph shows cardiomegaly caused by right atrial enlargement. The echocardiogram defines the degree of tricuspid valve and right ventricular hypoplasia. Color flow mapping can detect patency of the valve, and the right ventricular pressure can be estimated by the tricuspid regurgitation velocity. Flow in coronary fistulas may be seen on the epicardium and within the myocardium by color flow mapping. Fistulas must also be suspected if there is anterograde tricuspid valve flow and no tricuspid regurgitation. Cardiac catheterization is usually indicated to assess coronary flow and consider balloon dilation of the pulmonary valve.

MANAGEMENT AND PROGNOSIS

Prostaglandin E_1 therapy is essential in maintaining ductal patency. Careful assessment of the individual baby's anatomy and physiology provides a framework for interventional and surgical management.[6] Balloon pulmonary valvuloplasty is feasible in all babies with even a tiny orifice in the pulmonary valve, and novel techniques, including radiofrequency ablation to open the valve in the catheterization laboratory, can be considered (see "Neonatal Interventional Catheterization" in Part 10).[4]

If interventional catheterization is unsuccessful, surgical valvotomy is indicated unless there is clear dependence of the coronary flow on the right ventricle. In that circumstance, decompression of the right ventricle could result in coronary hypoperfusion, so that a systemic-to-pulmonary shunt is a better option.

In babies with successful surgical or interventional valvotomies, right ventricular growth is possible, and biventricular circulation can be expected.[41,46]

Severe tricuspid hypoplasia or right ventricle-dependent coronary circulation is an indication for a long-term Glenn and Fontan approach to separate the systemic and pulmonary circulations.[38] Babies who have right ventricular hypoplasia might also be candidates for a bidirectional Glenn operation combined with closure of the atrial septal defect. This procedure directs the inferior vena caval blood across the hypoplastic tricuspid valve and uses the right ventricle (see Table 45-12 in Part 10).

Ebstein Anomaly

ANATOMY AND PATHOPHYSIOLOGY

The tricuspid valve annulus is displaced downward into the right ventricle and the tricuspid valve leaflets are tethered to the wall in Ebstein anomaly. The area of the right ventricle between the true and functional annulus is thin walled, or "atrialized." The extent of displacement is variable; however, in severe forms, the displacement of the valve could also obstruct the right ventricular OFT.

The valve could have both impaired filling and regurgitation, leading to elevated right atrial pressures and right-to-left shunt at the atrial level. The degree of atrial-level shunting usually parallels the severity of the malformation of the valve. Right ventricular pressure is low, and the functional volume of the right ventricle is diminished.

ASSOCIATED DEFECTS

Ebstein anomaly usually occurs as an isolated defect or in association with an atrial septal defect or patent foramen ovale. Occasional patients with coarctation of the aorta are

described. Wolff-Parkinson-White syndrome or concealed bypass tracts are found in about 20% of patients. If there is associated L-transposition of the great arteries, the Ebstein malformation still occurs in the anatomic right ventricle. In these babies, AV valve regurgitation and ventricular dysfunction may be severe.

CLINICAL PRESENTATION

At presentation, neonates with severe Ebstein malformation have severe cyanosis caused by atrial-level right-to-left shunting. They have a diffusely active precordium, multiple systolic clicks, and a low-frequency holosystolic murmur of tricuspid regurgitation. If the malformation is mild, the diagnosis could be suggested by a click or during evaluation for neonatal supraventricular tachycardia.

LABORATORY EVALUATION

The electrocardiogram of babies with severe Ebstein malformation shows an RSR'S' pattern across the right side of the chest, suggesting right ventricular dilation. The chest radiograph shows marked cardiomegaly caused by right atrial dilation. The area of the right atrium and of the atrialized right ventricle has been a useful sign of severity and outcome.[108]

MANAGEMENT AND PROGNOSIS

Mild forms of Ebstein anomaly require no specific treatment, and the infants generally do well.[95a] The severely affected neonate might be ductal dependent and might have no anterograde flow through the right ventricle.[108] Maintaining patency of the ductus arteriosus with prostaglandin E_1 can be useful in the short term; however, ductal flow into the pulmonary artery can make anterograde flow more difficult, and the right ventricle can fill by pulmonary regurgitation. In severe Ebstein anomaly, measures to lower the pulmonary vascular resistance, including nitric oxide and several attempts to wean the infant from prostaglandin E_1, might be necessary before anterograde flow becomes established.[9] Brief support with extracorporeal membrane oxygenation to facilitate this transition has been successful in a few babies. Surgical repair or replacement of the valve is feasible in older children who have symptomatic disease but has not been useful in neonates. Either surgical exclusion of the right ventricle, with plans for a long-term Fontan repair, or transplantation might be the only alternative for the neonate with severe, persistent cyanosis.[56]

CYANOTIC DEFECTS: COMPLETE MIXING
Total Anomalous Pulmonary Venous Connection
ANATOMY AND PATHOPHYSIOLOGY

Total anomalous pulmonary venous connection comprises a group of defects in which the pulmonary veins enter the right side of the heart rather than the left atrium. The common sites of anomalous connection to the pulmonary veins are to the superior vena cava through the innominate vein, to the right atrium or coronary sinus, and to the inferior vena cava through the portal venous system. The veins connecting the pulmonary venous confluence to the right atrium are nearly always obstructed as they pass through the liver. In a smaller fraction of newborn infants, the vertical vein connecting the pulmonary venous confluence to the innominate vein is compressed as it passes between the left pulmonary artery and the left bronchus. If the pulmonary veins do not share a common confluence, the pulmonary venous connection could be mixed with veins from different lung segments draining through connections above and below the diaphragm.

Pulmonary venous return mixes completely with systemic venous return in the right atrium. Blood flow to the left side of the heart is entirely by shunting from the right atrium to the left atrium through the foramen ovale. In the absence of pulmonary venous obstruction, pulmonary blood flow is increased and hypoxia is mild. In contrast, if the pulmonary venous connection is obstructed as it passes through the mediastinum or liver, there is pulmonary venous hypertension with pulmonary edema and diminished pulmonary blood flow. The combination of decreased pulmonary blood flow and impaired pulmonary function caused by edema results in profound systemic hypoxia.

ASSOCIATED DEFECTS

An atrial septal defect is essential for postnatal survival and is rarely obstructed in the neonatal period. At the time of presentation, neonates often have a patent ductus arteriosus. Left heart defects, transposition of the great arteries, and tetralogy of Fallot have been reported with total anomalous pulmonary venous connection. The most common association is in neonates with asplenia syndrome and complex single ventricular anatomy. Total anomalous pulmonary venous connection occurs in a large portion of these babies, including those with pulmonary atresia.

CLINICAL PRESENTATION

The clinical presentation of the newborn infant with total anomalous pulmonary venous connection is variable. Cyanosis and respiratory distress are usually limited to babies with obstructed pulmonary venous connections. These babies have a right ventricular impulse, a single second heart sound, and no murmur. In most neonates without pulmonary venous obstruction, tachypnea and right ventricular heave gradually develop because of the increased right ventricular and pulmonary blood flow. Pulmonary artery pressure is not necessarily elevated, and the second heart sound could be split. A systolic ejection murmur at the upper left sternal border with radiation to the lungs is usually present because of the increased flow, but it is not necessarily harsh and obviously pathologic.

LABORATORY EVALUATION

The electrocardiogram in the neonatal period is normal. Pulmonary edema seen on the chest radiograph is highly suggestive of pulmonary venous obstruction. Dilated mediastinal veins can give an appearance of fullness (snowman sign) to the superior mediastinum, although in neonates, this is usually masked by the thymus. The echocardiogram (Fig. 45-15) should demonstrate the entry of each pulmonary vein into the confluence and define the course of the drainage of the confluence. Sites of venous obstruction are seen by imaging and turbulent flow by color flow mapping and Doppler imaging.

The size of the individual pulmonary veins and of the confluence should be measured because pulmonary venous

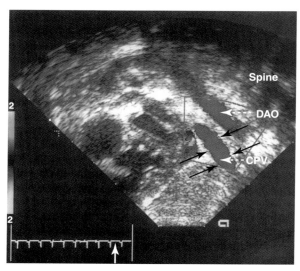

Figure 45–15. Subcostal Doppler echocardiogram illustrates anatomy and blood flow of a neonate with a total anomalous pulmonary venous connection below the diaphragm. In this study, the spine is on the *right*. Superior mediastinal structures are at the *top*, and the liver is at the *bottom* of the frame. Structures shown, from posterior to anterior (*left* of frame), are descending aorta (DAO), common pulmonary vein and descending vertical vein (CPV), small left ventricle, and dilated right ventricle. Blood flow is from superior to inferior in these views. Blood flow (outlined by *black arrows*) in the dilated CPV is going below the diaphragm, where it enters the liver and returns to the inferior vena cava.

diameters less than 2 mm are associated with a poor prognosis.[49] Evidence of restriction of the atrial septal defect is important to recognize. Cardiac catheterization is helpful in further delineating the venous anatomy if it is uncertain by echocardiography, especially in newborn infants with possible mixed pulmonary venous connection patterns.

MANAGEMENT AND PROGNOSIS

Unobstructed total anomalous pulmonary venous connection requires little specific medical management. Neonates with evidence of restrictive atrial septal defects should be started on a regimen of prostaglandin E_1 therapy to maintain patency of the ductus arteriosus and ensure systemic blood flow. Neonates with pulmonary venous obstruction are profoundly hypoxic and require significant respiratory and metabolic support. Extracorporeal membrane oxygenation has been used as a bridge to total repair (see Chapter 44, Part 8).

Elective repair—anastomosis of the common pulmonary venous confluence to the left atrium—in the first month of life is appropriate for neonates with unobstructed flow. Urgent surgery is essential for those with pulmonary venous obstruction. Postoperative pulmonary artery hypertension and pulmonary vascular reactivity is most troublesome in neonates with preoperative pulmonary venous obstruction. The long-term prognosis is excellent except in those neonates with hypoplastic pulmonary veins[49] or single ventricle anatomy.[40] Recurrent or persistent pulmonary venous obstruction at the anastomosis or within the veins is difficult to treat either by surgery or interventional catheterization.[59] Arrhythmias and a poor chronotropic response to exercise have been reported in some patients after surgery.[101]

Truncus Arteriosus
ANATOMY AND PATHOPHYSIOLOGY

In truncus arteriosus, there is a common origin of aorta and pulmonary artery from a single semilunar valve. The relationship of the origin of the pulmonary arteries from the truncus is variable. In type 1 truncus, the pulmonary arteries arise from the left lateral aspect of the truncus, with a short main pulmonary artery. In type 2 truncus, there is no main pulmonary artery, and the origin of the right and left pulmonary arteries is directly from the posterior or lateral aspect of the truncus arteriosus. In type 3 truncus, either the right or left pulmonary artery is absent, or it arises from the ductus arteriosus, and a large subarterial ventricular septal defect with deficiency of the conal portion of the septum produces overriding of the truncus over the ventricular septum.

The pulmonary artery pressure is comparable to aortic pressure, and diastolic pressure is decreased in the aorta because of the nonrestrictive connection with the low-impedance pulmonary vascular bed. The systemic and pulmonary venous returns completely mix in the truncus. Partitioning of the flow to the pulmonary artery and the aorta is determined by the relative systemic and pulmonary vascular resistance. In the first days of life, as the pulmonary vascular resistance falls, there is a relative increase in pulmonary blood flow. The pulmonary blood flow increases with a relatively constant systemic blood flow, and the arterial oxygen saturation in the truncus increases. The hemodynamic consequences are increased pulmonary arterial and left ventricular flow with resultant pulmonary venous hypertension and left atrial and left ventricular dilation.

ASSOCIATED DEFECTS

Truncal valve stenosis or regurgitation is present in about 20% of neonates. The truncal valve can have two, three, or four cusps, with a variable degree of thickening or abnormal coaptation. Truncal stenosis places an additional pressure load on both the right and left ventricles. Truncal regurgitation often increases left ventricular stroke volume, although truncal regurgitation into the right ventricle can occur. Unilateral or bilateral branch pulmonary artery stenosis occurs in 10% of children, reducing both the pulmonary artery pressure and the flow to the affected lung. Atresia of the origin of a branch pulmonary artery usually causes the vascular supply of the lung to be from aortic to pulmonary collateral vessels. Coronary artery stenosis and malposition are rare but surgically important variations.[1] These include origin of the left coronary artery in the proximal pulmonary artery. A right aortic arch is found in 15% to 25% of neonates with truncus. A small number of neonates have truncus arteriosus and aortic arch interruption, with a small ascending aorta branching into the innominate artery and the left carotid artery. The left subclavian artery and the descending aorta come from the truncus through a large patent ductus arteriosus.

CLINICAL PRESENTATION

The neonatal presentation of uncomplicated truncus arteriosus can be subtle. Mild tachypnea or cyanosis might be the only symptom. The left ventricular impulse increases as the pulmonary vascular resistance falls. Neonates with abnormal truncal valves have a systolic ejection click. The second heart sound is single, and there may be an apical third heart sound. The pulses are bounding, and the pulse pressure is wide with decreased diastolic pressure. A vibratory systolic ejection murmur from increased truncal valve flow and a mid-diastolic murmur from increased mitral valve flow could also be present. A harsh systolic ejection murmur and a blowing early diastolic murmur suggest associated truncal valve stenosis and regurgitation. Early signs of congestive heart failure suggest in utero pressure and volume loading resulting from truncal valve stenosis and regurgitation. Poor perfusion and decreased leg pulses indicate ductal narrowing if there is associated arch interruption.

LABORATORY EVALUATION

The electrocardiogram is usually normal in the neonatal period. ST-T segment changes suggest poor coronary perfusion caused by low diastolic pressures. Left ventricular hypertrophy can be seen in neonates with in utero truncal stenosis and regurgitation. The chest radiograph identifies the side of the aortic arch.

After the initial diagnosis, echocardiography must be directed to the definition of associated defects, including those of the truncal valve, branch pulmonary arteries, arch anatomy, and coronary arteries. The size of the thymus must also be defined. Cardiac catheterization is reserved only for neonates in whom the presence of associated defects is uncertain.

Pulse oximetry and arterial oxygen saturation are usually about 85%. Lower saturations are seen before the pulmonary vascular resistance falls or if either branch pulmonary artery stenosis or pulmonary dysfunction caused by edema is present. Acidosis suggests decreased systemic blood flow and is most commonly seen in neonates with associated truncal stenosis and regurgitation or arch interruption. The serum calcium concentration can fall in neonates with associated DiGeorge anomaly. All neonates with truncus arteriosus should be examined for microdeletion of chromosome 22.

MANAGEMENT AND PROGNOSIS

Supplemental oxygen can decrease pulmonary vascular resistance and should be avoided unless severe hypoxia and pulmonary edema are present. Tachypnea caused by increased pulmonary flow often responds to digoxin and furosemide. Medical management of neonates with significant truncal stenosis or regurgitation is usually unsuccessful, and their hemodynamic difficulties can be further complicated by tracheal compression caused by truncal dilation. Hypocalcemia resulting from hypoparathyroidism should be corrected.

Truncus arteriosus is routinely repaired in the first month of life and often in the neonatal period. The ventricular septal defect is closed, and a connection is made from the right ventricle to the pulmonary artery, usually with a homograft. Postoperative pulmonary hypertensive crises are minimized by repair in the first month of life. Associated defects, including truncal valve stenosis, arch interruption, coronary abnormalities, and branch pulmonary artery atresia, increase risk but do not preclude repair.[102] If truncal stenosis and regurgitation are severe, homograft truncal valve replacement is necessary to provide a competent neoaortic valve.[17]

The long-term prognosis is excellent for children with truncus arteriosus. Homograft replacement is required by age 5 years in about 20% of patients.[43] Neoaortic valve stenosis and regurgitation gradually worsen and can require repair or replacement of the valve in 25% of patients.[44] Ventricular dysfunction and arrhythmias are not expected.

CYANOTIC DEFECTS: VARIABLE PHYSIOLOGY

Single Ventricle

The anatomic variability of neonates with a single ventricle is broad. Two forms of single ventricle—tricuspid atresia and hypoplastic left heart syndrome—are discussed in separate sections.

A methodical segmental approach to venous, atrial, ventricular, and arterial size and connections does permit accurate anatomic diagnosis. Connections between the atria and the ventricles can be concordant or discordant. Similarly, the ventricular-arterial relationship may be normal, or D-transposition or L-transposition might be present. The hypoplastic ventricle can be either the anatomic right or anatomic left ventricle. Several pathophysiologic principles unite the defects and are the foundation of effective neonatal management.

Complete mixing of the systemic and pulmonary venous blood flow occurs in all forms of single ventricle. The cause can be anomalous pulmonary venous return, atresia of one of the AV valves with atrial-level shunting, or double inlet of the mitral and tricuspid valves into a single ventricle. Regardless of the site of mixing, the oxygen saturation in the ventricle and the aorta is determined by the relative systemic and pulmonary blood flow. Babies with defects involving pulmonary stenosis and restricted blood flow have low arterial oxygen saturation, and those with unrestricted pulmonary flow have relatively higher oxygen saturation.

It is particularly important to recognize babies in this latter group because they are sensitive to oxygen as a pulmonary vasodilator, and supplemental oxygen can therefore markedly increase pulmonary blood flow and reduce systemic blood flow.

The origin of one of the great arteries is usually from a hypoplastic outlet chamber. Especially in babies with L-transposition of the great arteries, hypoplastic right ventricle, and double-inlet left ventricle, the bulboventricular foramen (ventricular septal defect) could be restrictive.[68] The result, subaortic obstruction in utero and postnatally, is often associated with coarctation of the aorta. It is particularly important to recognize this defect before placing a pulmonary artery band to reduce pulmonary flow and pressures. Banding can hasten the natural progression of the subaortic obstruction or cause ventricular dysfunction because of the combined afterload of the band and the subaortic narrowing. A Damus-Kaye-Stansel operation or a

modification of the Norwood operation anastomoses the main pulmonary artery to the ascending aorta and could be needed in the first month of life to bypass the subaortic obstruction.[21,26,71] Pulmonary blood flow is provided by a systemic-to-pulmonary shunt in a fashion similar to the Norwood procedure. Other babies could have an arterial switch operation to relieve the obstruction (see Table 45-12 in Part 10).[58]

Babies with hypoxia caused by pulmonary stenosis and single ventricle are managed with a shunt in the neonatal period. Although a neonatal bidirectional Glenn procedure would be ideal, high pulmonary vascular resistance makes a venous-to-pulmonary artery connection prone to high systemic venous pressures. For babies with excessive pulmonary flow, a pulmonary artery band might be needed for several months before the bidirectional Glenn procedure can be performed.

The most challenging group of babies with single ventricle are those with pulmonary atresia, discontinuous pulmonary arteries, collateral supply of pulmonary blood flow, and pulmonary venous obstruction. These babies often have asplenia syndrome, and because of their unfavorable pulmonary artery architecture and venous obstruction, they are poor long-term candidates for the Fontan approach to single ventricle (see Table 45-12 in Part 10).

Long-term surgical planning for babies with single ventricle must begin in the neonatal period. Because they eventually must have a Fontan procedure, careful attention to the preservation of pulmonary arterial anatomy and low resistance is essential. Shunts from the systemic to the pulmonary circulation must not distort the pulmonary arteries or excessively volume-load the ventricle. Conversion of the shunt to a bidirectional Glenn procedure at as early as 3 months of age improves ventricular volume loading and ensures low pulmonary artery pressures.[2,85] Relief of subaortic obstruction improves systemic blood flow and ventricular diastolic function.[21,26,71] Any degree of pulmonary venous obstruction caused either by left AV valve stenosis or anomalous pulmonary venous return must be repaired before the Glenn procedure, and repair might be needed when there is a shunt from the systemic to the pulmonary artery circulation.

Double-Outlet Right Ventricle

ANATOMY AND PATHOPHYSIOLOGY

In double-outlet right ventricle, the aorta and the pulmonary artery arise side by side from the right ventricle. The pulmonary valve is to the left, the aortic valve is to the right, and the semilunar valves are at the same level. This defect is caused by a bilateral subarterial conus, which also distorts the normal aorta to mitral valve fibrous continuity. The location of the ventricular septal defect defines the type of double-outlet right ventricle. Babies with a subaortic ventricular septal defect have streaming from the left ventricle to the aorta, and the pathophysiology is similar to that in babies with a large ventricular septal defect. Those with subpulmonary ventricular septal defect, Taussig-Bing malformation, have streaming from the left ventricle into the pulmonary artery and have a circulation similar to transposition of the great arteries with ventricular septal defect.[89] Less commonly, the ventricular septal defect could be doubly committed below both arteries or remote in the muscular septum.

ASSOCIATED DEFECTS

The most important associated defect is pulmonary and sub-pulmonary stenosis. The additional obstruction to pulmonary blood flow in double-outlet right ventricle with subaortic ventricular septal defect causes a malformation similar to tetralogy of Fallot. Similarly, babies with a subpulmonary ventricular septal defect and pulmonary stenosis have the combination of transposition flow patterns with diminished pulmonary flow and pressure. The ventricular septal defect could be restrictive, leading to suprasystemic right ventricular pressures.

CLINICAL PRESENTATION

At presentation, double-outlet right ventricle usually is manifested by neonatal cyanosis or murmurs. If there is a subaortic ventricular septal defect and no pulmonary stenosis, the initial examination could reveal only a mildly hyperactive precordium and a single second heart sound; however, congestive heart failure develops in the first few weeks of life.

LABORATORY EVALUATION

The electrocardiogram and chest radiograph are nonspecific. The most important echocardiographic goal is to define the size and location of the ventricular septal defect relative to the great arteries.

MANAGEMENT AND PROGNOSIS

Neonatal repair of double-outlet right ventricle with a sub-pulmonary ventricular septal defect uses the arterial switch approach to move the aorta closer to the ventricular septal defect and permit an intraventricular baffle from the left ventricle to the neoaorta.[18,89] If there is a subpulmonary ventricular septal defect and pulmonary stenosis or atresia, the left ventricular outflow is baffled to the aorta. The pulmonary artery is removed from the heart and connected to the body of the right ventricle with a conduit. Babies with subaortic ventricular septal defect are managed similarly to those with tetralogy of Fallot or uncomplicated ventricular septal defect.[18]

SYSTEMIC HYPOPERFUSION WITH CONGESTIVE HEART FAILURE

Aortic Stenosis

ANATOMY AND PATHOPHYSIOLOGY

Aortic valve disease is a spectrum of malformations from an isolated bicuspid aortic valve to critical aortic valve stenosis with poorly differentiated valve cusps. Aortic stenosis has an in utero hemodynamic impact, and neonates have left ventricular hypertrophy, which generates the increased left ventricular pressure to overcome the obstruction. Mild to moderate obstruction is well tolerated in utero and postnatally with maintenance of good left ventricular systolic function. However, with severe obstruction, the left ventricle can develop significant dilation and dysfunction. It is the group

of neonates with this latter defect who might be dependent on the ductus arteriosus at birth. In these neonates, a significant portion of the systemic blood flow is supplied by shunting across the ductus arteriosus from the pulmonary artery to the aorta. In a steady state, this blood flow comes from atrial-level left-to-right shunting, which is enhanced because of high left ventricular diastolic pressures. The physiology in these babies is similar to that in babies with hypoplastic left heart syndrome.

ASSOCIATED DEFECTS

See also "Multiple Left Heart Defects," later.

Mild aortic stenosis accompanied by a large patent ductus arteriosus might present a challenging problem in an assessment of the aortic valve disease. Because the flow past the aortic valve is increased by the left-to-right shunt at the ductus, the pressure gradient across the aortic valve is exaggerated. Reassessment after spontaneous, surgical, or temporary balloon ductal closure might be needed to determine the true severity of the aortic valve obstruction.

Aortic regurgitation is rare in neonates with aortic valve stenosis. The presence of a diastolic decrescendo murmur of aortic regurgitation should raise the possibility of a tunnel from the left ventricle to the aorta.[67] This defect is just outside the aortic annulus, which is an additional pathway for ejection during systole and a site of regurgitation in diastole. The aortic valve might also be abnormal. Careful evaluation of the site of regurgitation by color flow mapping usually identifies this defect.

Aortic root dilation is found even with mild aortic stenosis. There may be a component of supravalvular aortic stenosis just distal to the aortic sinuses in these babies. Babies with Williams syndrome have more diffuse supravalvular aortic stenosis beyond the sinotubular junction.[55] Diffuse aortic root hypoplasia usually is a sign of associated coarctation of the aorta or left heart hypoplasia with severe aortic valve stenosis.

CLINICAL PRESENTATION

A bicuspid aortic valve can cause a systolic ejection click but no murmur in a neonate with no symptoms. Commonly, the defect is not detected until several years of age. Mild or moderate aortic stenosis causes a systolic ejection click and a harsh systolic ejection murmur that is audible shortly after birth. In the neonate, the murmur can be difficult to differentiate from a murmur caused by pulmonary stenosis, although radiation to the neck instead of the back should suggest aortic stenosis. The pulses and precordial activity are normal in these babies. With increasing severity of aortic stenosis, the murmur becomes louder, but the pulse volume can decrease.

Critical aortic stenosis has a clinical presentation similar to that of hypoplastic left heart syndrome. Poor feeding and respiratory distress caused by decreased cardiac output and pulmonary edema are frequent symptoms. There is a right ventricular heave, no click, and a soft systolic ejection murmur. If the ductus arteriosus is patent, the pulses are palpable, but with ductal narrowing, the pulses diminish. Right ventricular volume and pressure overload cause elevated right atrial pressures and hepatomegaly. Shock, acidosis, and multisystem failure occur with ductal closure.

LABORATORY EVALUATION

Because the severity of neonatal aortic stenosis is difficult to assess clinically, careful noninvasive assessment is essential. The electrocardiogram is usually normal, although occasional neonates with severe stenosis and in utero left ventricular dilation and hypertrophy have left ventricular hypertrophy on the electrocardiogram. The chest radiograph is most useful in detecting pulmonary edema. The echocardiogram (Fig. 45-16A) must be used to assess the anatomy to the aortic valve, the pressure gradient estimated by Doppler imaging (see Fig. 45-16B), and the presence of associated defects of the left side of the heart. Any indication of right-to-left shunting at the ductal level must be assumed to indicate either severe stenosis or associated coarctation of the aorta or mitral stenosis. Pulse oximetry or

arterial blood gas determination in the right arm and the umbilical artery or leg also suggests right-to-left ductal shunting. Arterial blood gas or electrolyte measurements can be followed as an indication of tissue perfusion and renal function.

MANAGEMENT AND PROGNOSIS

Neonatal bicuspid aortic valve or mild aortic stenosis without associated defects is well tolerated and requires no specific medical treatment except prophylaxis for bacterial endocarditis. Moderate and severe aortic stenosis can progress during the first few months of life, and careful follow-up is essential. Any indication of congestive heart failure or ventricular dysfunction in an infant with severe aortic stenosis is an indication for balloon or surgical valvotomy. Critical aortic stenosis is a neonatal emergency and continues to result in morbidity and death.

Success rates with neonatal balloon aortic valvuloplasty have been good, although residual or recurrent stenosis and aortic regurgitation are common (see "Neonatal Interventional Catheterization" in Part 10).[39,70] Valvotomy or transventricular dilation remains an alternative as a primary procedure or if balloon valvuloplasty is unsuccessful.[72] Either approach has limitations in neonates with marked annular hypoplasia, unicuspid aortic valve, associated subaortic obstruction, and ventricular hypoplasia or dysfunction. For these neonates, a Norwood approach to bypass the left ventricle or an aortic root enlargement and pulmonary autograft replacement[77] might be a more suitable long-term solution (see Table 45-12 in Part 10). The selection of babies with borderline criteria for a two-ventricle approach remains challenging.[22,25]

Coarctation of the Aorta and Aortic Arch Interruption

ANATOMY AND PATHOPHYSIOLOGY

Aortic arch obstruction occurs at several predictable levels distal to the aortic root. Coarctation of the aorta is the most common and consists of narrowing in the juxtaductal region distal to the left subclavian artery. It can be associated with transverse aortic and isthmic hypoplasia. Aortic arch interruption can occur at the same site (type A), but in aortic arch interruption, there is complete discontinuity of the aorta between the left subclavian artery and the insertion of the ductus arteriosus into the descending aorta. Type B aortic arch interruption is between the left carotid artery and the left subclavian artery. The origin of the right subclavian artery from the aorta distal to the ductus arteriosus can be found with either coarctation of the aorta or aortic arch interruption.

Coarctation of the aorta presents an increased afterload to the left ventricle, resulting in left ventricular hypertrophy and hypertension. Dilated collateral vessels develop between the branches of the ascending aorta and the descending aorta distal to the coarctation to carry flow to the distal aorta. In some neonates with coarctation of the aorta and in all neonates with aortic arch interruption, the severity of the obstruction results in either left ventricular failure or inadequate lower body perfusion at the time of ductal closure. The ductus arteriosus is critical to survival in these babies because it can perfuse the descending aorta from the pulmonary artery. The

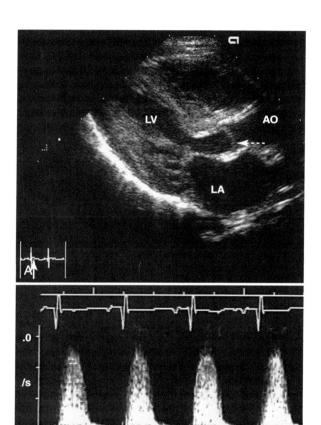

Figure 45–16. A, This 1-week-old infant was referred for evaluation of a systolic murmur. The echocardiogram, in long-axis view, shows thickened, domed aortic valve (*arrow*) and dilated ascending aorta (AO). There is left ventricular (LV) hypertrophy and hyperdynamic systolic function. LA, left atrium. B, Continuous-wave Doppler from the suprasternal notch shows left ventricular outflow tract velocity of 4.6 m/sec (85 mm Hg peak systolic gradient). Each mark on the scale on the left of frame is a velocity of 2 m/sec. Full scale is 6 m/sec. Mean velocity predicted gradient of 58 mm Hg, which is comparable to the systolic gradient measured before successful aortic balloon valvuloplasty.

right-to-left ductal-level shunting is balanced by an equal volume of atrial- or ventricular-level left-to-right shunting. This left-to-right shunt increases the oxygen saturation in the main pulmonary artery and the descending aorta. In some babies with juxtaductal coarctation of the aorta, right-to-left shunting is not significant; however, closure of the ductus arteriosus can further narrow the site of coarctation and cause poor distal perfusion.

ASSOCIATED DEFECTS

Coarctation of the aorta is a frequent component of diffuse left-heart disease (multiple left-heart defects). Bicuspid aortic valve and ventricular septal defect are common isolated associated defects. Aortic arch interruption is invariably associated with ventricular septal defect, aortic pulmonary window, truncus arteriosus, or transposition of the great arteries. The ventricular septal defect can be malaligned and can cause subaortic obstruction. Partial or complete DiGeorge syndrome or microdeletion of chromosome 22 is found in association with aortic arch interruption and occasionally in association with coarctation of the aorta.

CLINICAL PRESENTATION

Symptom-free newborn infants who have diminished leg pulses on a routine discharge examination have mild coarctation of the aorta and usually no associated aortic valve stenosis or septal defects. Early signs and symptoms of congestive heart failure should raise concern about associated defects. Careful palpation of all pulses, including the neck (Table 45-6), can provide valuable anatomic data. The pulse discrepancy should be confirmed by blood pressure measurement in both arms and both legs. Precordial hyperactivity, a single second heart sound, a gallop rhythm, and hepatomegaly indicate significant obstruction or associated defects. Holosystolic murmurs suggest either a ventricular septal defect or mitral regurgitation. The typical systolic murmur, well localized to the back, which is heard in older children with coarctation of the aorta, is not usually heard in neonates.

LABORATORY EVALUATION

The electrocardiogram and chest radiograph of a neonate with coarctation of the aorta or aortic arch interruption are usually normal. Significant cardiomegaly suggests associated lesions or ventricular dilation or dysfunction after the ductus arteriosus closes. Echocardiography (Fig. 45-17) can define the arch with considerable accuracy, although predicting the severity of the coarctation with the ductus arteriosus open is occasionally difficult. Right-to-left ductal shunting is an important sign of significant obstruction. Transverse arch hypoplasia, especially with a long segment between the left carotid and left subclavian arteries, suggests a significant coarctation of the aorta. Pulse oximetry and arterial blood gas measurements in the upper and lower extremities can confirm ductal shunting and perfusion.

MANAGEMENT AND PROGNOSIS

Uncomplicated coarctation of the aorta can be repaired electively in early childhood. Indications for repair in early infancy are significant hypertension or any sign of ventricular dysfunction. Surgical repair with end-to-end anastomosis remains the primary approach in many centers. Balloon angioplasty of native coarctation of the aorta can also be considered (see "Neonatal Interventional Catheterization" in Part 10).

Neonates with congestive heart failure or signs of poor perfusion must be treated with prostaglandin E_1 to maintain or restore ductal patency. All neonates with aortic arch interruption must have primary surgical repair of both the aortic arch abnormality and associated defects. Long-term results with interrupted aortic arch and aortopulmonary window or ventricular septal defect are good; however, recurrent arch obstruction and subaortic stenosis are frequent problems.[69] Mortality and morbidity in newborns with interrupted aortic arch and truncus arteriosus remain significant. Similarly, neonates with coarctation of the aorta and a large ventricular septal defect undergo primary repair.[51,83] Those with significant arch hypoplasia might require mobilization of the descending aorta to provide enough tissue to relieve the obstruction.[24]

Severe coarctation of the aorta without hemodynamically important associated defects is repaired through the left side of the chest. Balloon angioplasty of native coarctation of the aorta is usually reserved for older children but might be useful in the treatment of selected neonates.[78,90a] Postoperative systemic hypertension, the hallmark of coarctation in older children, is rare in neonates. Long-term growth of the repair might be an issue in up to 30% of babies, with premature infants having a higher risk.[52] Balloon angioplasty has been effective in the treatment of recurrent coarctation.

TABLE 45–6 Pulses or Blood Pressure				
Site	Coarctation or Interruption Distal to Left Subclavian Artery	Interruption Distal to Left Carotid Artery	Coarctation with Aberrant Right Subclavian Artery	Interruption Distal to Left Carotid Artery with Aberrant Right Subclavian Artery	Aortic Stenosis, Aortic Atresia, and Cardiomyopathy
Right arm	+	+	−	−	−
Neck	+	+	+	+	−
Left arm	+	−	+	−	−
Legs	−	−	−	−	−

+, normal; −, diminished.

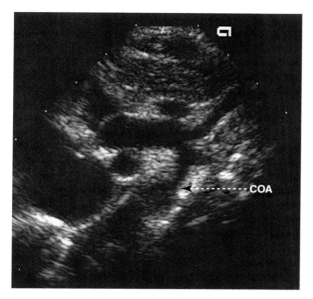

Figure 45-17. Echocardiogram from the suprasternal notch, demonstrating coarctation of the aorta (COA) just distal to the left subclavian artery. Mild hypoplasia of the transverse arch and poststenotic dilation of descending aorta are seen. Doppler study of this 1-week-old infant showed continuous high-velocity flow at the coarctation site and no evidence of patent ductus arteriosus.

Hypoplastic Left Heart Syndrome

Before 1980, no effective palliation was available for hypoplastic left heart syndrome. The Norwood operation[75] and the application of cardiac transplantation to the neonate[14] with hypoplastic left heart syndrome have afforded new hope to the families of newborn infants with this lethal heart defect. The advances in both of these approaches have brought us much closer to the reality of an acceptable quality and duration of life.

ANATOMY AND PATHOPHYSIOLOGY

Hypoplastic left heart syndrome includes aortic valve atresia, mitral valve atresia, and severe left ventricular and proximal aortic hypoplasia. Aortic coarctation is often associated.[64] Left ventricular endocardial fibroelastosis or infarction can develop because of in utero subendocardial ischemia. Coronary artery abnormalities have been recognized but have uncertain impact on long-term myocardial function.[11] Variations on this classic anatomy include degrees of aortic and mitral valve stenosis and left ventricular and aortic hypoplasia.

In hypoplastic left heart syndrome, the entire systemic circulation is supplied by blood from the main pulmonary artery that crosses the ductus arteriosus and enters the aorta. Flow from the ductus arteriosus goes retrograde to the ascending aorta and anterograde to the descending aorta. In utero, with high pulmonary vascular resistance, this circulation provides excellent organ perfusion, and the growth of the fetus is often normal. After birth, even when pulmonary vascular resistance falls and pulmonary blood flow increases, right ventricular output is usually adequate to supply both the systemic and the pulmonary circulations. However, closure of

the ductus arteriosus dramatically alters this balance and results in profound systemic hypoperfusion with acidosis and multisystem organ failure.

ASSOCIATED DEFECTS

The most important associated defects are anomalies of pulmonary venous return[95] or of the right aortic arch. Occasional neonates with aortic atresia have a normal mitral valve and normal left ventricular size because of an associated ventricular septal defect. The absence of an atrial septal defect creates severe in utero pulmonary venous hypertension and limits pulmonary blood flow after birth.[35] Central nervous system anomalies, including absent corpus callosum, might be more common in babies with hypoplastic left heart syndrome.[36]

CLINICAL PRESENTATION

In utero diagnosis has dramatically changed the presentation of neonates with hypoplastic left heart syndrome. For families who have early prenatal diagnosis and choose to continue the pregnancy, the place and time of delivery can be tailored to the intended surgical management.

Babies with hypoplastic left heart syndrome have tachypnea and mild cyanosis. There is a moderate right ventricular impulse, a single second heart sound, and a third heart sound. Murmurs, if present, are caused by increased pulmonary flow or tricuspid valve regurgitation. If the ductus arteriosus is patent, the pulses can be nearly normal; however, as the ductus arteriosus closes, it is difficult to palpate the pulses, and the perfusion is poor.

A restrictive atrial septal defect is initially beneficial because it tends to limit the pulmonary blood flow and promote systemic blood flow. However, if the atrial septal defect is highly restrictive, total pulmonary resistance is very high, and pulmonary blood flow is markedly diminished. Left atrial and pulmonary venous pressures are high, and pulmonary edema is present. The combination of pulmonary edema and restricted pulmonary blood flow produces profound hypoxia.[10,35]

LABORATORY EVALUATION

The electrocardiogram shows dominant right ventricular forces, often with a QR pattern in the right chest leads. Pulse oximetry averages 70% to 90%, depending on the pulmonary blood flow and the degree of pulmonary edema. The chest radiograph shows cardiomegaly and increased pulmonary blood flow with some degree of pulmonary venous congestion. The echocardiogram (Fig. 45-18) defines right ventricular function, tricuspid regurgitation, venous anatomy, and the atrial septal defect, all possible risk factors for surgery.

MANAGEMENT AND PROGNOSIS

The ability to sustain the life of a baby with hypoplastic left heart syndrome by maintaining ductal patency and systemic blood flow with prostaglandin E_1 and the advances in neonatal cardiopulmonary care have made both the Norwood operation and cardiac transplantation (see also Part 10) important therapies for these neonates. The choice of the Norwood operation or cardiac transplantation[13] is guided by several factors, including donor availability and the evolving experience and results with both approaches. The improved

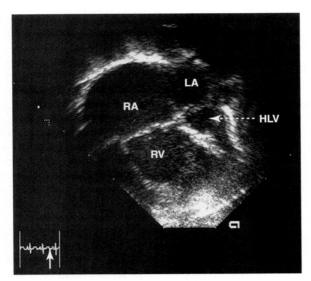

Figure 45–18. Neonate with diminished pulses and poor perfusion. Echocardiogram showed left-sided hypoplasia with a 3-mm aortic valve and a 4-mm mitral valve. Apical four-chamber view demonstrates marked size discrepancy between right ventricle (RV) and hypoplastic left ventricle (HLV). RA, right atrium; LA, left atrium.

results of the staged Norwood palliation since the mid-1990s have favored this approach over transplantation in many centers, except in babies with poor ventricular function.[48] Careful preoperative assessment and management for preventing the complications of excessive pulmonary blood flow are essential for good long-term results.

The goal of the Norwood stepwise approach to the surgical management of hypoplastic left heart syndrome is first to ensure systemic blood flow and protect the lungs from excessive pulmonary flow and pulmonary hypertension. Subsequently, the systemic venous drainage and the pulmonary venous drainage are separated, providing normal arterial oxygen saturation and ventricular stroke volume. The surgical management has evolved during the past decade in the effort to solve problems recognized during the early experience with the operation.

The first-stage operation, done in the newborn period with the use of cardiopulmonary bypass, fundamentally changes the defect from aortic atresia to pulmonary atresia. The branch pulmonary arteries are separated from the main pulmonary artery. The ascending aorta is opened along its length from at least the transverse aorta to distal to the ductus arteriosus. The main pulmonary artery is anastomosed to the aorta, and the anastomosis is augmented, when necessary, with homograft tissue to minimize the distortion of the arch and relieve any area of coarctation. The pulmonary blood flow is established by a shunt between the systemic and the pulmonary circulation. An alternative to the aortic-to-pulmonary shunt is a right ventricle-to-pulmonary shunt (*Sano modification*).[19] The atrial septum is excised to prevent any pulmonary venous obstruction.

A second alternative strategy has developed with the advent of a hybrid, interventional catheterization and surgery,

approach to hypoplastic left heart syndrome. The first-stage palliation is replaced with stenting of the patent ductus arteriosus and banding of the branch pulmonary arteries. The actual arch reconstruction is done at a second stage at the time of a bidirectional Glenn procedure.[32] The potential advantage of this approach is that it can avoid circulatory arrest in the newborn and shifts the major surgical procedure to an older age.

The postoperative management of the infant after the first stage of the Norwood operation follows principles similar to those for the preoperative care; however, the restriction of pulmonary blood flow by the systemic-to-pulmonary or right ventricle-to-pulmonary shunt permits a greater flexibility in modulating the systemic vascular resistance with afterload reduction and increased carbon dioxide. This, coupled with inotropic support, has improved systemic oxygen delivery without excessive pulmonary blood flow. Even in the era of improved surgical and intensive care techniques, a proportion of newborns after first-stage palliation require extracorporeal membrane oxygenation support for 24 to 48 hours to achieve stability.[84]

The second stage of the Norwood operation exchanges the shunt between the systemic and the pulmonary circulation for a bidirectional Glenn anastomosis or a hemi-Fontan operation.[28] This operation, done between 2 and 6 months of age, directs the superior vena caval blood flow to both right and left pulmonary arteries. The previous shunt is ligated, and the systemic venous return from the upper half of the body becomes the sole source of pulmonary flow. The typical result is an arterial saturation of 70% to 75%. The volume load on the ventricle is reduced, and the possibility of ventricular systolic or diastolic dysfunction is minimized.

The final surgical step, done between 12 months and 3 years of age, is to completely separate the systemic and the pulmonary venous return by a modification of the Fontan operation. The superior aspect of the right atrium is anastomosed to the underside of the pulmonary artery, and the atrium is partitioned with a baffle to direct the inferior vena caval flow into the pulmonary artery. Alternatively, an extracardiac conduit can be placed between the inferior vena cava and the right pulmonary artery. Although this technique is usually used in older children, it offers the advantage that it can be done without cardiopulmonary bypass and requires fewer suture lines in the atrium.[80] Limiting the atrial suture lines can reduce the long-term risk for arrhythmias.

The cumulative mortality and morbidity rates during the development of the Norwood operation were high. The early experience with first-stage palliation resulted in a 1-year survival rate of less than 50%. The most recent experience has improved these first-stage results, and the staged approach through the Glenn to the Fontan operation shows considerable early promise for improved quality of life and survival.[7,26,48] Most series comparing the traditional systemic-to-pulmonary shunt with the Sano modification or the hybrid have failed to demonstrate a significant difference in outcome.[30,34,45] A multicenter prospective clinical trial is underway comparing Blalock-Taussig and right ventricle-to-pulmonary artery shunts in the Norwood procedure.[76]

Risk factors for poor first-stage survival are low birthweight, a highly restrictive atrial septal defect, ventricular dysfunction, and tricuspid regurgitation.[10,26,48,91,105] Long-term morbidity includes recurrent coarctation,[60] AV valve regurgitation, sinus node dysfunction, and ventricular dysfunction. The improved mortality rate provides an opportunity to assess the impact of multiple surgeries and underlying central nervous system defects on neurodevelopmental outcome. Early data suggest that babies with hypoplastic left heart syndrome are at a higher risk for neurodevelopmental delay.[8,37,54,66]

Multiple Left Heart Defects

Associated left heart defects are common and can be multiple. Mitral valve abnormalities can be subtle, with mild hypoplasia and minimal distortion of the chordal and papillary muscle geometry. Shortening and fusion of the chordae tendineae or alterations in papillary muscle spacing increase the obstruction of the mitral valve. A single mitral valve papillary muscle (parachute deformity) causes significant stenosis.[47,93,103] Mild subaortic obstruction is seen with an isolated thin membrane just below the aortic valve. As the narrowing becomes more diffuse, it tends to be more severe and is associated with more severe forms of aortic valve disease. Coarctation of the aorta with varying degrees of aortic arch hypoplasia is an important component of multiple defects of the left side of the heart. The consequence of abnormal left ventricular inflow, because of either mitral valve disease or abnormal left ventricular diastolic function, is the additional component of left ventricular hypoplasia.

Atrial septal defects in neonates with left heart defects usually consist of stretching and incompetence of the foramen ovale as a result of left atrial hypertension rather than true defects of tissue. Associated ventricular septal defects can significantly alter the presentation and pathophysiology of neonates with left heart defects. Even a ventricle of small to moderate size can allow significant left-to-right shunting in a neonate with aortic stenosis or coarctation of the aorta. If there is mitral stenosis or left ventricular hypoplasia, filling of the aorta will occur through the ventricular septal defect. If the defect is large, the aortic valve and arch can be normal, and systemic blood flow will be preserved. A smaller defect might be inadequate to support systemic flow at birth or in the first weeks of life.

ACYANOTIC DEFECTS WITH NO OR MILD RESPIRATORY DISTRESS

Normal Murmurs

Normal murmurs are generated by laminar blood flow across normal valves into normal blood vessels. The vibratory systolic ejection murmur heard in newborn infants radiates uniformly over the chest. The vibratory systolic ejection murmurs from the pulmonary artery that are localized to the upper left sternal border and are heard from the aorta from the lower left sternal boarder radiating to the neck, which are heard in older children, are unusual in neonates. The precordial activity, second heart sound, and pulses are normal.

The murmur is best heard with the baby breathing quietly and is obliterated by crying or straining. Clearly pulmonary in origin by its radiation to the lungs, it is similar to but less harsh than the murmur heard in babies with branch pulmonary artery stenosis. Thus, despite the absence of true stenosis, it

has been labeled *peripheral pulmonary artery stenosis*. Perhaps the addition of the word *physiologic* would help clarify its normalcy.

Echocardiographic studies suggest that this murmur arises from the abrupt increase in velocity as the flow in the main pulmonary arteries turns into relatively small branch pulmonary arteries.[90] This size difference is due to the fetal circulation, which largely bypasses the lungs across the ductus arteriosus. An increase in velocity from 1.4 to 2.5 m per second is typical as the 8-mm main pulmonary artery branches into 3-mm left and right pulmonary arteries.

The murmur of physiologic peripheral pulmonary artery stenosis is accentuated by increased pulmonary flow caused by an atrial septal defect or a patent foramen ovale. If the murmur has harsh components and is best heard at the upper left sternal border, mild pulmonary stenosis should be considered. With growth during the first year, the size discrepancy between the main and the branch pulmonary arteries resolves, and the acceleration of flow into the lungs is considerably lower. Laboratory studies are rarely needed to diagnose this condition and are needed only if the murmur persists beyond infancy.

Pulmonary Stenosis

ANATOMY AND PATHOPHYSIOLOGY

Neonatal valvular pulmonary stenosis is differentiated from critical pulmonary stenosis or atresia by the presence of a normal tricuspid valve and normal right ventricular size. The pulmonary annulus is normal, and the valve leaflets are thickened and fused. Poststenotic dilation of the main and proximal branch pulmonary arteries is present. A thickened, immobile, dysplastic valve might not have any enlargement of the pulmonary arteries. Right ventricular systolic and diastolic function is normal, and atrial-level right-to-left shunting is unusual. Right ventricular pressure and hypertrophy are in proportion to the degree of obstruction. Right ventricular pressure is less than left ventricular pressure.

ASSOCIATED DEFECTS

Babies with severe stenosis usually have a component of dynamic subpulmonary stenosis. Branch pulmonary artery stenosis is atypical in association with valvular pulmonary stenosis. Atrial-level left-to-right shunting is common, and the increased flow across the pulmonary valve can exaggerate the estimate of severity by pressure gradient.

CLINICAL PRESENTATION

Neonates with pulmonary stenosis are free of symptoms and are identified by auscultation of an early systolic ejection click or a harsh systolic ejection murmur that radiates to the lungs. The intensity of the murmur correlates with the severity of obstruction. In moderate or severe stenosis, the right ventricular impulse persists, and the pulmonary component of the second heart sound is diminished and delayed. The peripheral pulses and liver are normal.

LABORATORY EVALUATION

Examination of all neonates with the clinical diagnosis of pulmonary stenosis is warranted. The differentiation from tetralogy of Fallot on clinical examination alone can be unreliable.

The electrocardiogram of neonates with pulmonary stenosis is normal. The chest radiograph might show dilation of the pulmonary artery segment, although it is often obscured by the thymus. Echocardiography is diagnostic, especially with moderate or severe stenosis. Because the entire cardiac output crosses the valve, the gradient estimated by Doppler study is an accurate measure of severity. The normal neonatal pulmonary valve is somewhat echogenic, and occasionally newborn infants who have very mild pulmonary valve stenosis on newborn echocardiograms are found to be normal on later follow-up.

MANAGEMENT AND PROGNOSIS

The natural history of isolated valvular pulmonary stenosis is excellent. Neonates with moderate or severe stenosis should be followed closely because progression during the first few months of life does occur. Pulmonary balloon valvuloplasty (see "Neonatal Interventional Catheterization" in Part 10) is indicated for infants with severe stenosis. Despite significant pressure loading of the right ventricle, these infants rarely have symptoms, and the timing of the procedure is determined by the gradient and the severity of right ventricular hypertrophy. Balloon valvuloplasty for children with moderate stenosis is undertaken between 1 and 3 years of age. Surgical pulmonary valvotomy is now reserved for infants with dysplastic pulmonary valves who do not respond to balloon valvuloplasty or for children with associated atrial septal defects.

Ventricular Septal Defect

ANATOMY AND PATHOPHYSIOLOGY

Defects in the ventricular septum occur in the inlet septum, muscular septum, perimembranous septum, and supracristal portion of the septum. The defects could be any size from less than 1 mm to the size of the aorta and can occur in combination. High pulmonary vascular resistance at the time of birth effectively limits shunt through the defect. With the fall in the pulmonary vascular resistance during the first few days of life, flow increases across the defect. Primarily, this flow is throughout systole from the left ventricle to the right ventricle, although diastolic flow can occur. The extent of flow across the defect is determined by the size of the defect and the relative systemic and pulmonary vascular resistance. Small defects, even with low pulmonary vascular resistance, do not allow significant shunting. Large defects allow equalization of pressures in the right and left ventricles, and the flow across the defect is limited only by the relative systemic and pulmonary vascular resistance.

ASSOCIATED DEFECTS

Ventricular septal defects are commonly seen in association with many other cardiovascular defects. Left-heart defects, especially aortic stenosis and coarctation of the aorta, can dramatically change the natural history of either defect in isolation.

CLINICAL PRESENTATION

Small perimembranous ventricular septal defects are routinely identified by their characteristic holosystolic murmur at the time of the discharge physical examination. Similarly, small muscular ventricular septal defects have a harsh early systolic murmur. The abbreviated nature of the murmur is likely due to a change in the size of the defect during systole. Even at 1 or 2 days of age, the pulmonary vascular resistance has fallen enough to establish turbulent flow across the defect. The babies have no symptoms, and the remainder of the examination findings are normal, including the precordial activity, second heart sound, and pulses.

Larger defects can be more challenging to identify before discharge because the large defect offers no resistance to flow and generates no turbulence, despite the early changes in the pulmonary vascular resistance. A persistent right ventricular impulse or narrow splitting of the second heart sound, or a low-frequency systolic murmur, can be a clue to the underlying defect. However, most children with isolated ventricular septal defect are discharged from the hospital with no symptoms, and many ventricular septal defects are not diagnosed until the first well-child check at several weeks of age.

LABORATORY EVALUATION

Small ventricular septal defects are easily diagnosed on a clinical examination. The electrocardiogram and chest radiograph are normal and, although reassuring, are not diagnostic. Echocardiographic diagnosis of ventricular septal defects by imaging and color flow mapping is accurate and provides reassurance that associated defects are not present. If the typical murmur persists or if there is any question about the diagnosis, echocardiography is indicated. If a large defect is suspected on clinical examination, even in the symptom-free baby who is ready for discharge, an echocardiogram is essential to exclude more complex disease.

MANAGEMENT AND PROGNOSIS

Spontaneous closure of small and some large ventricular septal defects is common. Small defects do not cause symptoms even when they stay patent. Larger defects can cause congestive heart failure in the first months of life and present a long-term risk for pulmonary vascular disease. If there is no evidence of spontaneous closure except a finding of persistent congestive heart failure or pulmonary hypertension, surgical repair is indicated in infancy.

Atrial Septal Defect

An isolated ostium secundum atrial septal defect in a neonate is nearly always an incidental finding on an echocardiogram obtained to evaluate a murmur. Many apparent defects in neonates represent stretching or incomplete closure of the foramen ovale and resolve by 1 year of age. This is especially true of babies with associated patent ductus arteriosus or ventricular septal defect in whom increased left atrial pressure stretches the atrial septum and permits shunting across the foramen ovale. Clinical signs of an atrial septal defect on routine follow-up during childhood indicate the need for further cardiovascular evaluation at that time.

Endocardial Cushion Defects

ANATOMY AND PATHOPHYSIOLOGY

Endocardial cushion defects are a spectrum of malformations resulting from failure of the endocardial cushions to fuse completely. The most severe malformation is a complete AV septal defect with a common AV valve, a large inlet ventricular septal defect, and a large ostium primum atrial septal defect. Intermediate forms have a small ventricular component, together with some separation of the tricuspid and mitral components of the AV valves. Ostium primum atrial septal defect and cleft mitral valve are milder forms of endocardial cushion defects.

The pathophysiology of endocardial cushion defects is similar to that of perimembranous ventricular septal defect and ostium secundum atrial septal defects. A high degree of pulmonary vascular resistance in the newborn period effectively limits the flow across the defects, and neonatal problems are unusual.

ASSOCIATED DEFECTS

A small degree of AV valve regurgitation is common; however, significant regurgitation causes early congestive heart failure. Common atrium is a form of endocardial cushion defect and is associated with anomalies of the systemic and pulmonary veins, including left superior vena cava to the roof of the left atrium. Unbalanced ventricular development with right or left ventricular hypoplasia can be associated with hypoplasia of the mitral or tricuspid component or with obstruction of the aortic or pulmonary outflow.

CLINICAL PRESENTATION

Endocardial cushion defects are common in babies with Down syndrome, and a large number of these defects are diagnosed as part of the evaluation for Down syndrome in the nursery (see Chapter 29). The high-pitched holosystolic murmur of mitral regurgitation can be heard in the nursery. However, the septal defects present the same limitations that preclude routine neonatal diagnosis of ostium secundum atrial septal defects and ventricular septal defects. Cyanosis caused by atrial right-to-left shunting is present in some neonates with large AV septal defects, especially if there is tricuspid regurgitation.

LABORATORY EVALUATION

The electrocardiogram of babies with endocardial cushion defects is helpful because the maldevelopment of the endocardial cushion produces abnormal activation of the left anterior bundle. These babies have an abnormal superior frontal plane vector (left axis deviation). They are easily differentiated from the baby with tricuspid atresia because they have normal right ventricular forces.

MANAGEMENT AND PROGNOSIS

Elective repair of complete AV septal defects is done in the first several months of life with a high degree of success.[99,100] Long-term issues are primarily AV valve function. Infants with less extensive defects, no pulmonary hypertension, or failure to thrive undergo repair in the first year of life.

Patent Ductus Arteriosus

ANATOMY AND PATHOPHYSIOLOGY

The ductus arteriosus, connecting the pulmonary artery and the aorta, is an essential structure during fetal life. Because fetal pulmonary vascular resistance is high, nearly 90% of the blood ejected by the fetal right ventricle flows through the ductus arteriosus to the descending aorta. The ductus arteriosus closes in the first few days after birth, and the entire right ventricular output is ejected into the pulmonary arterial bed.

If the ductus arteriosus remains patent postnatally and pulmonary vascular resistance falls, blood flow through the ductus arteriosus is from the aorta to the pulmonary artery. Furthermore, because the connection is open during both systole and diastole and pulmonary artery pressure is lower than the respective aortic pressure, blood flows across the patent ductus arteriosus continuously throughout the cardiac cycle. The volume overload and enlargement of the pulmonary artery, pulmonary veins, left atrium, left ventricle, and aorta are directly related to the volume of blood through the patent ductus arteriosus, which in turn is determined by the size of the ductus arteriosus and the relative systemic and pulmonary vascular resistances.

An important exception to this pattern of left atrial and left ventricular volume loading occurs in newborn infants with persistent transitional circulation. In these infants, the pulmonary vascular resistance is comparable to or higher than the systemic vascular resistance. Blood flow during systole is from the pulmonary artery to the aorta and from the aorta to the pulmonary artery in diastole. If the pulmonary vascular resistance is significantly higher than systemic resistance, flow across the ductus arteriosus is from pulmonary artery to aorta in both systole and diastole.

The mechanisms responsible for constriction of the ductus arteriosus at birth are not fully understood. The ductus arteriosus is highly sensitive to changes in oxygen tension; the increase in arterial oxygen tension that normally occurs after birth probably serves as the stimulus for closure of the ductus arteriosus. How this response is mediated is less certain; it is likely attributable to a complex interaction between autonomic chemical mediators, nerves, prostaglandin, and the ductal musculature. The ductus arteriosus functionally closes in most full-term infants during the first day of life, but anatomic obliteration of the ductus arteriosus does not occur until after the first week of life. A persistently patent ductus arteriosus is uncommon in otherwise normal children. In contrast, 30% of infants who weighed less than 1.5 kg at birth have a patent ductus arteriosus, possibly as a result of hypoxia and immaturity of the ductal closure mechanisms.[87] Spontaneous permanent PDA closure only occurred by 4 postnatal days in approximately one third of infants <1000 g birth weight.[56a] Therefore, a majority of such infants are potential candidates for pharmacologic or surgical intervention, although the merits of active therapy for PDA closure are controversial.

ASSOCIATED DEFECTS

A patent ductus arteriosus is present at birth in all but a few congenital heart defects. Although the presenting features of the associated defects are usually clear, occasionally the ductus arteriosus is the most easily recognized component clinically and by echocardiogram. Coarctation of the aorta is clearly more difficult to diagnose in the presence of a large ductus arteriosus.

The absence of the ductus arteriosus is notable in some neonates with tetralogy of Fallot and pulmonary atresia. In these babies, the central pulmonary arteries are markedly hypoplastic where the ductus would insert, and there are aortic-to-pulmonary collateral vessels from other sites. The ductus arteriosus is also often absent in neonates with the absent pulmonary valve syndrome, in which the failure of ductal formation or closure at a critical time in cardiogenesis can play a role in the pathogenesis of the pulmonary valve and arterial abnormality.

CLINICAL PRESENTATION

The clinical presentation of the neonate with a patent ductus arteriosus is unlike that of the infant or child in whom a continuous murmur is the classic feature. In newborn infants, especially premature ones, the diastolic flow through the ductus arteriosus is difficult to hear. A systolic murmur with uneven intensity throughout systole is best heard at the upper left sternal border. Even in the absence of a murmur, the hemodynamic consequences of a patent ductus arteriosus could be clinically evident. Increased pulmonary blood flow causes an oxygen requirement and difficulty in weaning the infant from ventilatory support. The left ventricular volume load produces an increased left ventricular impulse or a third heart sound. The diastolic flow into the pulmonary artery lowers aortic diastolic pressures, causing bounding pulses. These clinical signs can lag behind echocardiographic signs of a significant patent ductus arteriosus.[97]

LABORATORY EVALUATION

In babies with symptoms, the clinical suspicion of a patent ductus arteriosus should be confirmed by echocardiography. Similar physical findings are present in infants with aortic-pulmonary collateral vessels, an aortic-pulmonary window, origin of the right pulmonary artery from the ascending aorta (hemitruncus), fistula between the coronary artery and the right ventricle, and a ruptured sinus-of-Valsalva aneurysm. Echocardiography (Fig. 45-19) permits an accurate diagnosis—with assessment of both the hemodynamic impact of the shunt, as reflected by the extent of left atrial and ventricular enlargement, and the estimated pulmonary artery pressure by Doppler imaging—and excludes other associated defects. Electrocardiography is of limited value in the assessment. Chest radiographs offer an estimate of heart size but are not diagnostic. B-type natriuretic peptide (BNP)

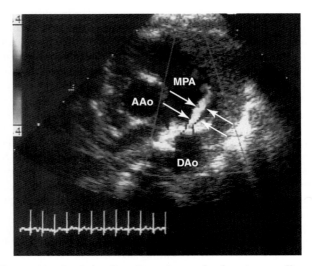

Figure 45–19. Color flow Doppler study showing small patent ductus arteriosus with flow outlined by *arrows* from descending aorta (DAo) to main pulmonary artery (MPA) in parasternal short-axis view. AAo, ascending aorta.

is produced in response to increased myocyte stretch and may be a useful bedside screening tool for the presence of a PDA or response to therapy in premature infants.[38a, 46a]

MANAGEMENT AND PROGNOSIS

Full-term neonates with the clinical diagnosis of a small patent ductus arteriosus can be followed clinically. Careful assessment of the precordial activity and pulses and documentation of normal pulse oximetry usually is adequate to exclude clinically important associated heart defects in a symptom-free baby. An electrocardiogram and a chest radiograph can be reassuring but are of limited value beyond the clinical examination. If there is uncertainty about the diagnosis or if symptoms develop, the diagnosis should be confirmed by echocardiography.

Spontaneous closure of a patent ductus arteriosus can occur in the first months of life. Persistent ductal patency does have an important long-term risk for bacterial endocarditis, and closure is usually recommended after age 6 months. Conventional surgical closure or video-assisted thoracoscopic surgery[20] is appropriate for infants with a moderate to large patent ductus arteriosus. Interventional catheterization closure with coils is useful for smaller defects (see "Neonatal Interventional Catheterization" in Part 10).

In the premature infant, spontaneous closure is common; however, persistent or recurrent congestive heart failure and respiratory distress can require therapy to close the ductus arteriosus. A rapid or progressive increase in ventilator settings and inspired oxygen can be manifestations of congestive heart failure caused by a patent ductus arteriosus in such patients. Medical management with fluid restriction and diuretics is occasionally effective.

Indomethacin, a prostaglandin synthetase inhibitor, has been shown to close the ductus arteriosus in a large fraction of premature infants up to 14 days of age and occasionally as late as 1 month of age. A common dosing regimen is 0.1 to 0.2 mg/kg per dose given intravenously, administered at 12- to 24-hour intervals for up to three doses. Contraindications to indomethacin therapy are renal failure (creatinine concentration level higher than 1.2 to 1.5 mg/dL), active bleeding, or significant thrombocytopenia. Failure of indomethacin therapy has been related to extreme immaturity and to greater postnatal age at initiation of therapy.[106] Longer treatment courses can be used (0.1 to 0.2 mg/kg per day) for 5 days. However, there appears to be no clear advantage to prolonged low-dose indomethacin regimes for patent ductus arteriosus closure[100] (see Appendix A).

Prophylactic indomethacin improves the rate of permanent ductus closure by increasing the degree of initial constriction. Narayanan and associates[73] showed that prophylactic indomethacin neither affected the remodeling process nor altered the inverse relationship between infant maturity and subsequent reopening. Even when managed with prophylactic indomethacin, the rate of ductus arteriosus reopening remained unacceptably high in the most immature infants. Prophylactic indomethacin has its advocates, and an additional benefit of this approach could be to decrease the incidence of intraventricular hemorrhage (see Chapter 40, Part 3). However, a large prospective study that documented a decrease in the incidence of patent ductus arteriosus from 50% to 25% failed to alter the incidence of intraventricular or periventricular hemorrhage or to improve neurodevelopmental outcome at 18 months of corrected age.[94] Using echocardiography to direct the duration of indomethacin therapy appears to achieve similar closure rates while limiting drug exposure and its attendant risks.[20a]

Ibuprofen has been shown to be equally effective for ductal closure with fewer renal side effects.[81] Surgical ligation of the ductus arteriosus has been associated with increased morbidity and adverse neurodevelopmental outcome.[65] A relatively high incidence of left vocal cord paralysis has been reported postoperatively in extremely low birth weight infants.[15a] Surgery is indicated if the ductus arteriosus remains hemodynamically significant by clinical or echocardiographic criteria after indomethacin or ibuprofen therapy, or if pharmacotherapy is contraindicated.

Aortopulmonary Window

ANATOMY AND PATHOPHYSIOLOGY

An aortopulmonary window is typically a large defect between the ascending aorta and the main pulmonary artery. Smaller, restrictive defects do occur but are the exception. The pathophysiology mimics a patent ductus arteriosus with pulmonary hypertension and a left-to-right shunt that increases as the pulmonary vascular resistance falls.

ASSOCIATED DEFECTS

An aortopulmonary window can be seen in conjunction with aortic arch interruption or tetralogy of Fallot.

CLINICAL PRESENTATION

Clinical signs of congestive heart failure can occur in the first week of life. Precordial hyperactivity, a single second heart sound, a low-frequency systolic murmur of increased pulmonary blood flow, and bounding pulses might be evident even before tachypnea and poor feeding become problems.

LABORATORY EVALUATION

The electrocardiogram is normal in the neonatal period and shows combined ventricular hypertrophy as the pulmonary vascular resistance falls and pulmonary blood flow increases. The chest radiograph demonstrates cardiomegaly and increased pulmonary vascular markings. Echocardiography shows the defect; however, specific attention must be directed to excluding an associated patent ductus arteriosus or aortic arch interruption.

MANAGEMENT AND PROGNOSIS

Surgical closure of an aortopulmonary window is usually done shortly after diagnosis, with excellent short- and long-term results.[12]

L-Transposition of the Great Arteries

ANATOMY AND PATHOPHYSIOLOGY

L-Transposition of the great arteries, or ventricular inversion, is the connection of the right atrium to the left ventricle and of the left ventricle to the pulmonary artery, and the connection of the left atrium to the right ventricle and of the right ventricle to the aorta. The ventricles are usually side by side, with the ventricular septum directed from the anterior to the posterior portion. The anatomic right ventricle is to the left, and the anatomic left ventricle is to the right. The aorta is anterior and to the left, and the pulmonary artery is posterior and to the right. Because the aorta arises from the right ventricle, a subaortic infundibulum is present, and the aortic valve is superior to the pulmonary valve.

Unless associated lesions are present, there is no shunting, but normal pressures and saturations are found in the aorta and pulmonary artery. Because the systemic ventricle is the anatomic right ventricle in this condition, right ventricular systolic pressure is comparable to aortic pressure. Similarly, the pulmonary ventricle is the anatomic left ventricle and has low systolic pressure.

ASSOCIATED DEFECTS

Associated defects are nearly always found in babies with L-transposition of the great arteries. Ventricular septal defect, pulmonary stenosis, and Ebstein malformation of the tricuspid valve are frequent. L-Transposition of the great arteries with hypoplastic subaortic left ventricle, restrictive ventricular septal defect, and coarctation of the aorta is a well-recognized form of single ventricle. Acquired complete AV block occurs in children with L-transposition of the great arteries and might be present at birth.

CLINICAL PRESENTATION

Uncomplicated L-transposition of the great arteries is rare and is unlikely to be detected in the newborn period. Associated defects are diagnosed because of cyanosis or murmurs.

LABORATORY EVALUATION

The electrocardiogram might be abnormal in the newborn period because of abnormal septal activation with Q waves in the right chest leads. On the chest radiograph, the ascending aorta forms a straight left heart border that angles medially to the superior mediastinum. A methodical echocardiogram is necessary for identifying the spatial and anatomic connections.

MANAGEMENT AND PROGNOSIS

Management and prognosis are driven by the associated lesions. The prognosis in uncomplicated L-transposition of the great arteries can be excellent with good long-term systemic right ventricular function. Severe Ebstein malformation of the tricuspid valve is a cause of severe neonatal congestive heart failure. Repair or replacement of the systemic AV valve has limitations.[104] For infants and children with systemic right ventricular failure, a combined atrial and arterial switch operation might offer improved survival.[29]

REFERENCES

1. Adachi I, et al: Relationship between orifices of pulmonary and coronary arteries in common arterial trunk, *Eur J Cardiothorac Surg* 35:594, 2009.
2. Alejos JC, et al: Factors influencing survival in patients undergoing the bidirectional Glenn anastomosis, *Am J Cardiol* 75:1048, 1995.
3. Alonso de Begona J, et al: The Mustard procedure for correction of simple transposition of the great arteries before 1 month of age, *J Thorac Cardiovasc Surg* 104:1218, 1992.
4. Alwi M, et al: Pulmonary atresia with intact ventricular septum percutaneous radiofrequency-assisted valvotomy and balloon dilation versus surgical valvotomy and Blalock Taussig shunt, *J Am Coll Cardiol* 35:468, 2000.

5. Angeli E, et al: Late reoperations after neonatal arterial switch operation for transposition of the great arteries, *Eur J Cardiothorac Surg* 34:32, 2008.

6. Ashburn DA, et al: Determinants of mortality and type of repair in neonates with pulmonary atresia and intact ventricular septum, *J Thorac Cardiovasc Surg* 127:1000, 2004.

7. Ashburn DA, et al: Outcomes after the Norwood operation in neonates with critical aortic stenosis or aortic valve atresia, *J Thorac Cardiovasc Surg* 125:1070, 2003.

8. Atallah J, et al for the Western Canadian Complex Pediatric Therapies Follow-Up Group: Two-year survival and mental and psychomotor outcomes after the Norwood procedure: an analysis of the modified Blalock-Taussig shunt and right ventricle-to-pulmonary artery shunt surgical eras, *Circulation* 118:1410, 2008.

9. Atz AM, et al: Diagnostic and therapeutic uses of inhaled nitric oxide in neonatal Ebstein's anomaly, *Am J Cardiol* 91:906, 2003.

10. Atz AM, et al: Preoperative management of pulmonary venous hypertension in hypoplastic left heart syndrome with restrictive atrial septal defect, *Am J Cardiol* 83:1224, 1999.

11. Baffa J, et al: Coronary artery abnormalities and right ventricular histology in hypoplastic left heart syndrome, *J Am Coll Cardiol* 20:350, 1992.

12. Bagtharia R, et al: Outcomes for patients with an aortopulmonary window, and the impact of associated cardiovascular lesions, *Cardiol Young* 14:473, 2004.

13. Bailey LL: Transplantation is the best treatment for hypoplastic left heart syndrome, *Cardiol Young* 14(Suppl 1):109, 2004.

14. Bailey LL, et al, for the Loma Linda University Pediatric Heart Transplant Group: Bless the babies: one hundred fifteen late survivors of heart transplantation during the first year of life, *J Thorac Cardiovasc Surg* 105:805, 1993.

15. Bellinger DC, et al: Neurodevelopmental status at eight years in children with dextro-transposition of the great arteries: The Boston Circulatory Arrest Trial, *J Thorac Cardiovasc Surg* 126:1385, 2003.

15a. Benjamin JR, Smith PB, Cotten CM, et al: Long-term morbidities associated with vocal cord paralysis after surgical closure of a patent ductus arteriosus in extremely low birth weight infants, *J Perinatol* 30:408, 2010.

16. Blume ED, et al: Evolution of risk factors influencing early mortality of the arterial switch operation, *J Am Coll Cardiol* 33:1702, 1999.

17. Bove EL, et al: Results of a policy of primary repair of truncus arteriosus in the neonate, *J Thorac Cardiovasc Surg* 105:1057, 1993.

18. Bradley TJ, Karamlou T, Kulik A, et al: Determinants of repair type, reintervention, and mortality in 393 children with double-outlet right ventricle, *J Thorac Cardiovasc Surg* 134:967, 2007.

19. Bradley SM, et al: Hemodynamic status after the Norwood procedure: a comparison of right ventricle-to-pulmonary artery connection versus modified Blalock-Taussig shunt, *Ann Thorac Surg* 78:933, 2004.

20. Burke RP, et al: Video-assisted thoracoscopic surgery for patent ductus arteriosus in low birth weight neonates and infants, *Pediatrics* 104:227, 1999.

20a. Carmo KB, Evans N, Paradisis M: Duration of indomethacin treatment of the preterm patent ductus arteriosus as directed by echocardiography, *J Pediatr* 155:819, 2009.

21. Clarke AJ, et al: Mid-term results for double inlet left ventricle and similar morphologies: timing of Damus-Kaye-Stansel, *Ann Thorac Surg* 78:650, 2004.

22. Colan SD, et al: Validation and re-evaluation of a discriminant model predicting anatomic suitability for biventricular repair in neonates with aortic stenosis, *J Am Coll Cardiol* 47:1858, 2006.

23. Colan SD, et al: Status of the left ventricle after the arterial switch operation for transposition of the great arteries: Hemodynamic and echocardiographic evaluation, *J Thorac Cardiovasc Surg* 109:311, 1995.

24. Conte S, et al: Surgical management of neonatal coarctation, *J Thorac Cardiovasc Surg* 109:663, 1995.

25. Corno AF: Borderline left ventricle, *Eur J Cardiothorac Surg* 27:67, 2005.

26. Daebritz SH, et al: Results of Norwood stage I operation: comparison of hypoplastic left heart syndrome with other malformations, *J Thorac Cardiovasc Surg* 119:358, 2000.

27. Dohlen G, et al: Stenting of the right ventricular outflow tract in the symptomatic infant with tetralogy of Fallot, *Heart* 95:142, 2009.

28. Douglas WI, et al: Hemi-Fontan procedure for hypoplastic left heart syndrome: outcome and suitability for Fontan, *Ann Thorac Surg* 68:1361, 1999.

29. Duncan BW, et al: Results of the double switch operation for congenitally corrected transposition of the great arteries, *Eur J Cardiothorac Surg* 24:11, 2003.

30. Edwards L, et al: Norwood procedure for hypoplastic left heart syndrome: BT shunt or RV-PA conduit? *Arch Dis Child Fetal Neonatal Ed* 92:F210, 2007.

31. Formigari R, et al: Treatment of pulmonary artery stenosis after arterial switch operation: stent implantation vs. balloon angioplasty, *Catheter Cardiovasc Interv* 50:207, 2000.

32. Galantowicz M, et al: Hybrid approach for hypoplastic left heart syndrome: intermediate results after the learning curve, *Ann Thorac Surg* 85:2063, 2008.

33. Gardiner HM, et al: Morphologic and functional predictors of eventual circulation in the fetus with pulmonary atresia or critical pulmonary stenosis with intact septum, *J Am Coll Cardiol* 51:1299, 2008.

34. Ghanayem NS, et al: Right ventricle-to-pulmonary artery conduit versus Blalock-Taussig shunt: a hemodynamic comparison, *Ann Thorac Surg* 82:1603, 2006.

35. Glatz JA, et al: Hypoplastic left heart syndrome with atrial level restriction in the era of prenatal diagnosis, *Ann Thorac Surg* 84:1633, 2007.

36. Glauser TA, et al: Congenital brain anomalies associated with the hypoplastic left heart syndrome, *Pediatrics* 85:984, 1990.

37. Goldberg CS, et al: Neurodevelopmental outcome of patients after the Fontan operation: a comparison between children with hypoplastic left heart syndrome and other functional single ventricle lesions, *J Pediatr* 137:646, 2000.

38. Guleserian KJ, et al: Natural history of pulmonary atresia with intact ventricular septum and right-ventricle-dependent coronary circulation managed by the single-ventricle approach, *Ann Thorac Surg* 81:2250, 2006.

38a. Hammerman C, Shchors I, Schimmel MS, et al: N-terminal-pro-B-type natriuretic peptide in premature patent ductus arteriosus: a physiologic biomarker, but is it a clinical tool? *Pediatr Cardiol* 31(1):62, 2010.

39. Han RK, et al: Outcome and growth potential of left heart structures after neonatal intervention for aortic valve stenosis, *J Am Coll Cardiol* 50:2406, 2007.

40. Hancock Friesen CL, et al: Total anomalous pulmonary venous connection: an analysis of current management strategies in a single institution, *Ann Thorac Surg* 79:596, 2005.

41. Hannan RL, et al: Midterm results for collaborative treatment of pulmonary atresia with intact ventricular septum, *Ann Thorac Surg* 87:1227, 2009.

42. Hayes C, Gersony W: Arrhythmias after the Mustard operation for transposition of the great arteries: a long-term study, *J Am Coll Cardiol* 7:133, 1986.

43. Heinemann MK, et al: Fate of small homograft conduits after early repair of truncus arteriosus, *Ann Thorac Surg* 55:1409, 1993.

44. Henaine R, et al: Fate of the truncal valve in truncus arteriosus, *Ann Thorac Surg* 85:172, 2008.

45. Honjo O, et al: Clinical outcomes, program evolution, and pulmonary artery growth in single ventricle palliation using hybrid and Norwood palliative strategies, *Ann Thorac Surg* 87:1885, 2009.

46. Hirata Y, et al: Pulmonary atresia with intact ventricular septum: limitations of catheter-based intervention, *Ann Thorac Surg* 84:574, 2007.

46a. Hsu J, Yang S, Chen H, et al: B-type natriuretic peptide predicts responses to indomethacin in premature neonates with patent ductus arteriosus, *J Pediatr* 157:79, 2010.

47. Ikemba CM, et al: Mitral valve morphology and morbidity/mortality in Shone's complex, *Am J Cardiol* 95:541, 2005.

48. Jacobs ML, et al, for the Congenital Heart Surgeons Society: Intermediate survival in neonates with aortic atresia: a multiinstitutional study, *J Thorac Cardiovasc Surg* 116:417, 1998.

49. Jenkins KJ, et al: Individual pulmonary vein size and survival in infants with anomalous pulmonary venous connection, *J Am Coll Cardiol* 22:201, 1993.

50. Jouannic JM, et al: Sensitivity and specificity of prenatal features of physiological shunts to predict neonatal clinical status in transposition of the great arteries, *Circulation* 110:1743, 2004.

51. Kanter KR, et al: What is the optimal management of infants with coarctation and ventricular septal defect? *Ann Thorac Surg* 84:612, 2007.

52. Karamlou T, et al: Factors associated with arch reintervention and growth of the aortic arch after coarctation repair in neonates weighing less than 2.5 kg, *J Thorac Cardiovasc Surg* 137:1163, 2009.

53. Karamlou T, et al, for the Members of the Congenital Heart Surgeons' Society: Matching procedure to morphology improves outcomes in neonates with tricuspid atresia, *J Thorac Cardiovasc Surg* 130:1503, 2005.

54. Kern JH, et al: Early developmental outcome after the Norwood procedure for hypoplastic left heart syndrome, *Pediatrics* 102:1148, 1998.

55. Kim YM, et al: Natural course of supravalvar aortic stenosis and peripheral pulmonary arterial stenosis in Williams' syndrome, *Cardiol Young* 9:37, 1999.

56. Knott-Craig CJ, et al: Repair of neonates and young infants with Ebstein's anomaly and related disorders, *Ann Thorac Surg* 84:587, 2007.

56a. Koch J, Hensley G, Roy L, et al: Prevalence of spontaneous closure of the ductus arteriosus in neonates at a birth weight of 1000 grams or less, *Pediatrics* 117;1113, 2006.

57. Kreutzer J, et al: Tetralogy of Fallot with diminutive pulmonary arteries: preoperative pulmonary valve dilation and transcatheter rehabilitation of pulmonary arteries, *J Am Coll Cardiol* 27:1741, 1996.

58. Lacour-Gayet F, et al: Early palliation of univentricular hearts with subaortic stenosis and ventriculoarterial discordance: the arterial switch option, *J Thorac Cardiovasc Surg* 104:1238, 1992.

59. Lacour-Gayet F, et al: Surgical management of progressive pulmonary venous obstruction after repair of total anomalous pulmonary venous connection, *J Thorac Cardiovasc Surg* 117:679, 1999.

60. Larrazabal LA, et al: Ventricular function deteriorates with recurrent coarctation in hypoplastic left heart syndrome, *Ann Thorac Surg* 86 :869, 2008.

61. Li J, et al: Coronary arterial origins in transposition of the great arteries: factors that affect outcome. A morphological and clinical study, *Heart* 83:320, 2000.

62. Losay J, et al: Aortic valve regurgitation after arterial switch operation for transposition of the great arteries: incidence, risk factors, and outcome, *J Am Coll Cardiol* 47:2057, 2006.

63. Losay J, et al: Late outcome after arterial switch operation for transposition of the great arteries, *Circulation* 104:I1121, 2001.

64. Machii M Becker AE: Nature of coarctation in hypoplastic left heart syndrome, *Ann Thorac Surg* 59:1491, 1995.

65. Madan JC, et al, for the National Institute of Child Health and Human Development Neonatal Research Network: Patent ductus arteriosus therapy: impact on neonatal and 18-month outcome, *Pediatrics* 123:674, 2009.

66. Mahle WT, et al: Neurodevelopmental outcome and lifestyle assessment in school-aged and adolescent children with hypoplastic left heart syndrome, *Pediatrics* 105:1082, 2000.

67. Martins JD, et al: Aortico-left ventricular tunnel: 35-year experience, *J Am Coll Cardiol* 44:446, 2004.

68. Matitiau A, et al: Bulboventricular foramen size in infants with double-inlet left ventricle or tricuspid atresia with transposed great arteries: influence on initial palliative operation and rate of growth, *J Am Coll Cardiol* 19:142, 1992.

69. McCrindle BW, et al for the Congenital Heart Surgeons Society: Risk factors associated with mortality and interventions in 472 neonates with interrupted aortic arch: A Congenital Heart Surgeons Society study, *J Thorac Cardiovasc Surg* 129:343, 2005.

70. McElhinney DB, et al: Left heart growth, function, and reintervention after balloon aortic valvuloplasty for neonatal aortic stenosis, *Circulation* 111:451, 2005.

71. Miura T, et al: Management of univentricular heart with systemic ventricular outflow obstruction by pulmonary artery banding and Damus-Kaye-Stansel operation, *Ann Thorac Surg* 77:23, 2004.

72. Mosca RS, et al: Critical aortic stenosis in the neonate: a comparison of balloon valvuloplasty and transventricular dilation, *J Thorac Cardiovasc Surg* 109:147, 1995.

73. Narayanan M, et al: Prophylactic indomethacin: factors determining permanent ductus arteriosus closure, *J Pediatr* 136:330, 2000.

74. Nogi S, et al: Fate of the neopulmonary valve after the arterial switch operation in neonates, *J Thorac Cardiovasc Surg* 115:557, 1998.

75. Norwood WI, et al: Physiologic repair of aortic atresia-hypoplastic left heart syndrome, *N Engl J Med* 308:23, 1983.

76. Ohye RG, et al, for the Pediatric Heart Network Investigators. Design and rationale of a randomized trial comparing the Blalock-Taussig and right ventricle-pulmonary artery shunts in the Norwood procedure, *J Thorac Cardiovasc Surg* 136:968, 2008.

77. Ohye RG, et al: The Ross/Konno procedure in neonates and infants: Intermediate-term survival and autograft function, *Ann Thorac Surg* 72:823, 2001.

78. Park Y, et al: Balloon angioplasty of native aortic coarctation in infants 3 months of age and younger, *Am Heart J* 134:917, 1997.

79. Pasquini L, et al: Coronary echocardiography in 406 patients with D-loop of the great arteries, *J Am Coll Cardiol* 24:763, 1994.

80. Petrossian E, Reddy VM, Collins KK, et al: The extracardiac conduit Fontan operation using minimal approach extracorporeal circulation: early and midterm outcomes, *J Thorac Cardiovasc Surg* 132:1054, 2006.

81. Pezzati M, et al: Effects of indomethacin and ibuprofen on mesenteric and renal blood flow in preterm infants with patent ductus arteriosus, *J Pediatr* 135:733, 1999.

82. Pocar M, et al: Long-term results after primary one-stage repair of transposition of the great arteries and aortic arch obstruction, *J Am Coll Cardiol* 46:1331, 2005.

83. Quaegebeur JM, et al: Outcomes in seriously ill neonates with coarctation of the aorta: a multi-institutional study, *J Thorac Cardiovasc Surg* 108:841, 1994.

84. Ravishankar C, et al: Extracorporeal membrane oxygenation after stage I reconstruction for hypoplastic left heart syndrome, *Pediatr Crit Care Med* 7:319, 2006.

85. Reddy VM, et al: Primary bidirectional superior cavopulmonary shunt in infants between 1 and 4 months of age, *Ann Thorac Surg* 59:1120, 1995.

86. Reddy VM, et al: Routine primary repair of tetralogy of Fallot in neonates and infants less than three months of age, *Ann Thorac Surg* 60:S592, 1995.

87. Reller MD, et al: Review of studies evaluating ductal patency in the premature, *J Pediatr* 122:S59, 1993.

88. Rhodes LA, et al: Arrhythmias and intracardiac conduction after the arterial switch operation, *J Thorac Cardiovasc Surg* 109:303, 1995.

89. Rodefeld MD, Ruzmetov M, Vijay P, et al: Surgical results of arterial switch operation for Taussig-Bing anomaly: is position of the great arteries a risk factor? *Ann Thorac Surg* 83:1451, 2007.

90. Rodriguez RJ, Riggs TW: Physiologic peripheral pulmonary stenosis in infancy, *Am J Cardiol* 66:1478, 1990.

90a. Rothman A, Galindo A, Evans WN, et al: Effectiveness and safety of balloon dilation of native aortic coarctation in premature neonates weighing ≤2,500 grams, *Am J Cardiol* 105(8):1176, 2010.

91. Sano S, et al: Risk factors for mortality after the Norwood procedure using right ventricle to pulmonary artery shunt, *Ann Thorac Surg* 87:178, 2009.

92. Satomi G, et al: Blood flow pattern of the interatrial communication in patients with complete transposition of the great arteries: a pulsed Doppler echocardiographic study, *Circulation* 73:95, 1986.

93. Schaverien MV, et al: Independent factors associated with outcomes of parachute mitral valve in 84 patients, *Circulation* 109:2309, 2004.

94. Schmidt B, et al: Long-term effects of indomethacin prophylaxis in extremely-low-birth-weight infants, *N Engl J Med* 344:1966, 2001.

95. Seliem MA, et al: Patterns of anomalous pulmonary venous connection/drainage in hypoplastic left heart syndrome: diagnostic role of Doppler flow mapping and surgical implications, *J Am Coll Cardiol* 19:135, 1992.

95a. Shinkawa T, Polimenakos AC, Gomez-Fifer CA, et al: Management and long-term outcome of neonatal Ebstein anomaly, *J Thorac Cardiovasc Surg* 139(2):354, 2010.

96. Sittiwangkul R, et al: Outcomes of tricuspid atresia in the Fontan era, *Ann Thorac Surg* 77:889, 2004.

97. Skelton R, et al: A blinded comparison of clinical and echocardiographic evaluation of the preterm infant for patent ductus arteriosus, *J Paediatr Child Health* 30:406, 1994.

98. Skinner J, et al: Transposition of the great arteries: from fetus to adult, *Heart* 94:1227, 2008.

99. Suzuki T, et al: Results of definitive repair of complete atrioventricular septal defect in neonates and infants, *Ann Thorac Surg* 86:596, 2008.

100. Tammela O, et al: Short versus prolonged indomethacin therapy for patent ductus arteriosus in preterm infants, *J Pediatr* 134:552, 1999.

101. Tanel RE, et al: Long-term noninvasive arrhythmia assessment after total anomalous pulmonary venous connection repair, *Am Heart J* 153:267, 2007.

102. Thompson LD, McElhinney DB, Reddy M, et al: Neonatal repair of truncus arteriosus: continuing improvement in outcomes, *Ann Thorac Surg* 72:391, 2001.

103. Uva M, et al: Surgery for congenital mitral valve disease in the first year of life, *J Thorac Cardiovasc Surg* 109:164, 1995.

104. van Son JA, et al: Late results of systemic atrioventricular valve replacement in corrected transposition, *J Thorac Cardiovasc Surg* 109:642, 1995.

105. Vlahos AP, et al: Hypoplastic left heart syndrome with intact or highly restrictive atrial septum: outcome after neonatal transcatheter atrial septostomy, *Circulation* 109:2326, 2004.

106. Weiss H, et al: Factors determining reopening of the ductus arteriosus after successful clinical closure with indomethacin, *J Pediatr* 127:466, 1995.

107. Williams WG, et al: Outcomes of 829 neonates with complete transposition of the great arteries 12-17 years after repair, *Eur J Cardiothorac Surg* 24:1, 2003.

108. Yetman AT, et al: Outcome in cyanotic neonates with Ebstein's anomaly, *Am J Cardiol* 81:749, 1998.

PART 8

Cardiovascular Problems of the Neonate

Kenneth G. Zahka

CARDIAC MALPOSITION AND ABNORMALITIES OF ABDOMINAL SITUS

The normal cardiac position is the ventricular apex pointed to the left with the left atrium and stomach on the left and the right atrium and liver on the right. The morphologic three-lobed lung is on the right, and there is early branching of the right bronchus with an epiarterial bronchus. The morphologic two-lobed lung is on the left, with a long segment of left main bronchus before the bronchus branches.[31] The assessment of normal cardiac position can be made by physical examination and by routine chest radiography and echocardiography. Abdominal situs is ascertained by palpation of the liver; an abdominal radiograph for the stomach bubble; and ultrasonography to define the stomach, liver, and spleen. A liver-spleen scan might be helpful in finding the spleen if it is not seen on ultrasonography. Howell-Jolly bodies are seen on a blood smear in patients who do not have normal splenic function.

Dextrocardia is present when the heart is in the right side of the chest. If the heart is in the midline, mesocardia is present. Situs solitus is the normal location of the atria and abdominal organs. Situs inversus is present when the right atrium is on the left, the left atrium is on the right, and the liver and stomach are similarly reversed. In situs inversus, the morphologic right lung is on the left, and the morphologic left lung is on the right. Situs ambiguous, with the liver and stomach in the midline, is seen in neonates with bilateral right-sidedness or bilateral left-sidedness. Babies with bilateral right-sidedness have asplenia, and their atrial and pulmonary morphologic features are characteristic of bilateral right atria and lungs. Babies with bilateral left-sidedness have polysplenia and bilateral morphologic left atria and lungs.

Associated Lesions

The importance of these cardiac and situs abnormalities lies in the associated lesions. Dextrocardia with situs inversus is a mirror image of normal anatomy and often has no associated cardiac lesions. It could, however, be associated with Kartagener, or immotile cilia, syndrome. In contrast, babies with dextrocardia with situs solitus often have associated congenital heart defects, including uncomplicated septal defects and L-transposition of the great arteries. Neonates with situs inversus with levocardia always have associated heart defects. Intestinal obstruction can cause intestinal malrotation in these babies.[8]

Asplenia syndrome should be suspected whenever complex heart defects are associated with total anomalous pulmonary venous connection.[50] Because there is no morphologic left atrium, pulmonary venous drainage is rarely directly to the atrium. Similarly, the coronary sinus, which lies posterior to the normal left atrium, is usually absent. Systemic venous drainage is also abnormal, with bilateral superior venae cavae. The left superior vena cava might enter directly into the roof of the left-sided morphologic right atrium, whereas the right superior vena cava enters the right atrium in a normal fashion. The right inferior vena cava is present, and there might be an additional left inferior vena cava. Dextrocardia, with a common atrium and a single atrioventricular valve, and either a common ventricle or a large ventricular septal defect, is common. Severe pulmonary stenosis or atresia is common.[12] In addition to the liability of complex congenital heart disease, these babies are immunologically compromised because of their asplenia.[52] Daily administration of a prophylactic antibiotic to reduce the risk for bacterial sepsis is important.

Absent hepatic segment of the inferior vena cava, so-called interrupted inferior vena cava, is an excellent clue to the presence of polysplenia in a neonate with ambiguous abdominal situs.[60] Because there is no right atrium, the course of the inferior vena cava is not normal. Drainage of the inferior vena cava is to the azygos or hemiazygos veins and into the superior vena cava. With bilateral left atria, the pulmonary veins also usually enter in a bilateral fashion. Polysplenia is often associated with levocardia, normally related great arteries, a common atrium, and two ventricles with a ventricular septal defect. The pulmonary valve is usually normal. Although there are multiple small spleens, splenic function is typically normal, although the

presence of Howell-Jolly bodies on blood smear may indicate hyposplenism in some patients.[45]

COR PULMONALE

See also Chapter 44, Part 7.

Cor pulmonale is heart disease caused by chronic lung disease or upper airway obstruction. It is the result of abnormal cardiovascular systolic and diastolic loading, at least in its early phases, related to increased right ventricular afterload caused by hypoxic pulmonary vasoconstriction. Other factors, including loss or underdevelopment of pulmonary parenchyma and its associated vascular bed, can also be important in infants with bronchopulmonary dysplasia[23] or diaphragmatic hernia. If the normal fall in pulmonary vascular resistance does not occur because of lung disease, right ventricular hypertrophy will persist. Right ventricular dilation and dysfunction are usually present in proportion to the severity of the underlying lung disease.

Diagnosis

Clinical recognition of cor pulmonale can be hampered by respiratory distress and lung sounds from the underlying respiratory disease. A right ventricular impulse and narrow splitting of the second heart sound with an accentuated pulmonary closure sound should be present in infants with cor pulmonale but can be difficult to recognize. Hepatomegaly resulting from right ventricular diastolic dysfunction could be assumed to be due to hyperinflation.

Electrocardiographic evidence of right ventricular hypertrophy is usually associated with significant cor pulmonale. Echocardiography has a greater role in the screening and follow-up of cor pulmonale, especially in at-risk babies with difficult cardiac examinations. Initial and longitudinal echocardiographic evaluation provides the opportunity to demonstrate the earliest indications of this complication and to determine the degree of correlation between echocardiographic signs of cor pulmonale and the clinical severity of pulmonary dysfunction. With recognition of the importance of ventricular interdependence, echocardiographic parameters of ventricular function should be applied not only to the right ventricle but also to the left ventricle. Because in some babies the degree of hypoxia and respiratory distress can vary during the course of the day or during a period of several weeks, the echocardiographic signs of cor pulmonale can reflect in an integrated fashion the status of lung function averaged across time.

Changes in right ventricular diastolic size and geometry and increased right ventricular wall thickness are the early indicators of chronic cor pulmonale. The severity of these abnormalities often, but not always, correlates with the degree of clinical chronic pulmonary dysfunction. Infants with exacerbations of their disease can demonstrate acute changes in right ventricular physiology, expressed by increased pulmonary and tricuspid regurgitation velocities and by acceleration time, without dramatic changes in their chronic right ventricular hypertrophy and chamber dilation. Right ventricular diastolic dysfunction assessed by retrograde flow in the hepatic veins during atrial systole and changes in early and late diastolic filling patterns can also be useful in assessing babies with cor pulmonale.

Serum B-type natriuretic peptide can be elevated in patients with pulmonary hypertension and evidence of congestive heart failure. Serial measurements may also complement clinical and echocardiographic assessment of the response to therapy.

Cardiac catheterization has not been needed as part of the assessment of cor pulmonale because two-dimensional and Doppler echocardiography are normally used. Cardiac catheterization is essential, however, if there is any question about structural heart disease, including pulmonary venous obstruction as a cause of pulmonary hypertension, or if there is any uncertainty about the elevation (per kg) of pulmonary vascular resistance before starting pulmonary vasodilator medications. Aortic-to-pulmonary collateral vessels develop in babies with chronic lung disease and can be recognized by color flow mapping.[2] If the collaterals appear large, coil embolization at the time of cardiac catheterization can be helpful.

Treatment

Treatment of the lung disease and airway obstruction and relief of hypoxia are the foundation of therapy for cor pulmonale. Diuretics have been used to decrease pulmonary interstitial edema and fluid retention caused by right ventricular dysfunction. The value of digoxin therapy in babies with cor pulmonale remains controversial, although with careful monitoring, the risk for digoxin use should be minimal.

Initial studies using calcium channel blockers to decrease pulmonary vascular resistance did not demonstrate benefit and raised concerns that perfusion of vascular beds that are poorly ventilated would exacerbate hypoxia.[7] Inhaled nitric oxide has become the standard treatment for persistent pulmonary hypertension of the newborn and may be used for rescue treatment for acute exacerbations of pulmonary hypertension associated with chronic lung disease. The introduction of oral phosphodiesterase type 5 inhibitors, including sildenafil, into the treatment of pulmonary hypertension in children and adults has opened their use for the treatment of cor pulmonale associated with pulmonary hypertension.[54]

Coil embolization of collateral vessels or of a small ductus arteriosus (see "Neonatal Interventional Catheterization" in Part 10) can be performed and decreases pulmonary blood flow and left ventricular volume loading. The improvement in pulmonary function is modest, and other collateral vessels can develop.

Surgical closure of a larger patent ductus arteriosus should be considered early in the course of the disease to decrease the risk for surgical morbidity, which is higher in the setting of severe lung disease. Surgical closure of a small foramen ovale is also not advisable because left-to-right shunting is mild, and right-to-left shunting usually indicates significant right ventricular diastolic dysfunction.

Prognosis

The long-term prognosis for a baby with cor pulmonale is usually determined by the lung disease. Babies receiving long-term ventilatory therapy or in respiratory failure with severe right ventricular dilation have significant morbidity and mortality rates. Mild to moderate right ventricular dilation is often reversible as the lung disease improves and is not a factor in long-term quality of life. Significant pulmonary hypertension in the setting of chronic lung disease remains an important marker for mortality.[32]

ARTERIOVENOUS MALFORMATIONS
Diagnosis

Cerebral arteriovenous malformations manifest in the neonatal period with signs of congestive heart failure, including a hyperdynamic precordium and hepatomegaly. Most defects identified in the neonatal period are vein of Galen malformations, although neonates with large pial malformations and congestive heart failure have been described. Intracranial hemorrhage could be an additional presenting feature in the neonate with a pial arteriovenous malformation. A cranial bruit and a systolic ejection murmur of increased aortic and pulmonary artery flow are present. The chest radiograph shows cardiomegaly, and the echocardiogram demonstrates enlargement of all chambers and the ascending aorta and carotid arteries. Doppler study of the aorta usually indicates significant diastolic runoff in the carotid arteries. Color flow mapping is particularly useful in identifying the multiple flow channels into the vein of Galen.

Treatment

Medical therapy with inotropes and diuretics in neonates with congestive heart failure caused by cerebral arteriovenous malformations improves symptoms before surgical intervention. The use of digoxin is controversial in this group of neonates because of concern about poor renal perfusion and toxicity.[21] Surgical management of cerebral arteriovenous malformations is difficult because of their size and location and because of the multiple feeder vessels. Embolization, with catheter-delivered metal coils or cyanoacrylate, of the arterial and venous channels before surgery has improved the results; however, complete cure of the defect is still unusual. Mortality and morbidity rates have improved dramatically in the past decade, but neurologic function after a combined interventional and surgical approach can be abnormal in up to 50% of survivors.[35]

HYPERTENSION

See also Chapter 51.

Measurement of blood pressure in newborn and intensive care nurseries has become routine since the introduction of oscillometric methods (see Chapter 31). The principles of accurate blood pressure measurement that have been developed for children and adults apply to neonates. Proper cuff size is essential, and the variety of disposable cuffs available in nurseries should permit the use of a cuff that fits the upper arm or thigh with the bladder nearly encircling the extremity. When the neonate rests quietly, the correlation with arterial blood pressure has been good even in small premature babies, and normal values for systolic and diastolic blood pressures are well established (see Appendix B).

Healthy neonates might have blood pressure measured once during their hospital course, although the standard of care is not well defined. Babies in intensive care units have multiple measurements, and those with arterial catheters have continuous monitoring of blood pressure.

Diagnosis

In addition to routine blood pressure screening, nonspecific clinical clues or maternal factors, including neonatal irritability and lethargy, should prompt additional measurements. Guidelines established by the Second Task Force on Blood Pressure Control in Children indicate that for full-term babies in the first week of life, significant hypertension is a systolic blood pressure greater than 96 mm Hg, and severe hypertension is greater than 106 mm Hg. In the first month, the guidelines are 104 mm Hg for significant and 110 mm Hg for severe hypertension. For newborn premature babies, the upper limits of normal blood pressure range from 58/38 mm Hg at 1 kg to 65/42 mm Hg at 2 kg (see Appendix B).

The mechanisms of blood pressure regulation in the neonate are similar to those in the child and adult; however, the fundamental disease processes that trigger those pathways are less diverse in the neonate. The differential diagnosis of neonatal hypertension[24,72] is summarized in Box 45-10. The aortic arch obstructions can be readily diagnosed by palpation of brachial and femoral pulses and measurement of arm and leg blood pressure. In contrast with the older child, significant hypertension is not a consistent feature of neonates with coarctation of the aorta. Marked elevation of the blood pressure in neonates with vascular catheters should always suggest renovascular complications and may lead to hypertensive cardiomyopathy.[49] Aortic mural thrombi or catheter-related emboli can occur at any point, including during unsuccessful attempts, in the course of umbilical arterial catheterization. Ultrasound and Doppler flow studies of the aortic arch, renal vessels, and renal parenchyma usually clarify these etiologic factors.

Moderate hypertension, especially if it develops gradually, is well tolerated, and there is compensatory left ventricular hypertrophy to match the increased afterload. In some neonates with acutely increased blood pressure caused by renovascular

---

BOX 45–10   Differential Diagnosis of Neonatal Hypertension

AORTIC ARCH OBSTRUCTION
Coarctation of the aorta
Aortic arch interruption
Descending aorta thrombosis

RENAL AND RENOVASCULAR PROBLEMS
Renal artery thrombosis or embolus
Renal artery stenosis
Renal vein thrombosis (late)
Cystic renal disease
Obstructive uropathy

PHARMACOLOGIC ADVERSE EFFECTS
Catecholamines
Cocaine
Dexamethasone
Theophylline

OTHER CAUSES
Exogenous fluid administration
Environmental cold or noise stress
Seizures
Chronic lung disease

---

complications, left ventricular dysfunction and diminished cardiac output develop. Therapy is indicated if the infant is symptomatic or if the hypertension is sustained above a mean of 70 mm Hg (see Appendix B). Afterload reduction with intravenous administration of sodium nitroprusside is necessary until renal and cardiac function improves.

Treatment

If urine output is poor because of renal dysfunction, fluid restriction is necessary. Orally administered angiotensin-converting enzyme inhibitors such as captopril are excellent antihypertensive agents; however, they are contraindicated in the treatment of babies with coarctation of the aorta, unilateral renal artery disease, and hyperkalemia. They also must be used with care in babies with chronic hypertension because an abrupt drop in blood pressure, even when the pressure is not outside the normal range, can cause neurologic and renal side effects.[24]

Thrombectomy is rarely needed in babies with hypertension caused by catheter complications unless complete thrombosis of the aorta occurs. Gradual recovery with a good long-term prognosis is typical.[20]

PERSISTENT PULMONARY HYPERTENSION (PERSISTENT FETAL CIRCULATION)

See also part 2 of this chapter and Chapter 44, Part 8.
The normal transition to the extrauterine circulation is multifaceted; however, central to the process is a dramatic decrease in pulmonary vascular resistance. The mediators of neonatal pulmonary vasodilation include mechanical factors relating to stretching of the lung, oxygen factors, and vascular endothelial factors.

Endothelin type 1 is a potent vasoconstrictor produced by the fetal vascular endothelium. The effect of endothelin type 1 is mediated through receptors in the endothelium and vascular smooth muscle. Constriction of vascular smooth muscle is probably mediated by inhibition of nitric oxide production by vasoactive peptides such as endothelin type 1. Nitric oxide is recognized as a potent vasodilator that likely has an important role in the fall in neonatal pulmonary vascular resistance, although a host of other mediators have the potential to mediate pulmonary vascular resistance.[33]

Etiology

Delayed relaxation of the pulmonary vascular bed is a feature of many neonatal pulmonary problems, including lung hypoplasia (e.g., congenital diaphragmatic hernia), meconium aspiration syndrome, perinatal asphyxia, bacterial pneumonia, and sepsis. It can also occur in the absence of obvious triggering diseases, presumably because of abnormal muscularization of pulmonary arterioles or transient defects in endothelial function.

High pulmonary vascular resistance causes pulmonary and right ventricular hypertension. The neonatal right ventricle is well adapted to this increased afterload because of the high in utero right ventricular pressures and rarely has difficulty in meeting the challenge of generating high pressures. Intracardiac shunting at the ductus arteriosus and foramen ovale produce the hallmark of the disease, namely hypoxemia out of proportion to abnormalities on the chest radiograph.

Two factors promote right-to-left atrial shunting through the foramen ovale. The fetal right ventricle is less compliant than the left ventricle, and high postnatal right ventricular pressures can compound this diastolic dysfunction. Blood returning to the right atrium crosses the atrial septum at the foramen ovale if right ventricular diastolic pressure is elevated. Perinatal asphyxia could be associated with dysfunction of the tricuspid papillary muscle, which causes tricuspid regurgitation. The tricuspid regurgitation increases right atrial pressures and causes right-to-left shunting during ventricular systole. In some babies, color flow mapping can demonstrate a jet of tricuspid regurgitation directed into the fossa ovalis. Atrial-level right-to-left shunting causes left atrial, left ventricular, and systemic arterial desaturation. In this way, the disease mimics right heart defects such as critical pulmonary stenosis with impaired right ventricular filling.

Right-to-left ductal-level shunting in neonates with persistent pulmonary hypertension of the newborn (PPHN) occurs primarily during ventricular systole (Fig. 45-20). During diastole, there is left-to-right shunting. However, when the pulmonary vascular resistance is very high, shunting from the pulmonary artery to the aorta can occur during diastole. If right-to-left shunting is limited to the ductus, systemic arterial desaturation is limited to the descending aorta. Saturations in the ascending aorta, right arm, and cerebral circulation are normal.

The atrial and arterial connections are, in a sense, protective for the neonate with PPHN. If the pulmonary vascular resistance is significantly higher than systemic resistance, the right ventricle might not be able to generate the pressure required to overcome the high resistance. Without atrial or arterial connections, the output through the right side of the heart falls, and there is inadequate pulmonary blood flow, pulmonary venous return, and left ventricular filling. The result is high systemic venous (right atrial) pressure and low left atrial, left ventricular, and systemic arterial pressures. Arterial hypotension is avoided when the left atrium is filled across the foramen ovale or the aorta from the pulmonary artery. Although the result of this shunting is systemic arterial hypoxemia, the shunt does provide normal blood pressure and flow. Organ perfusion is maintained, and oxygen delivery can be nearly normal by increasing tissue extraction.

Diagnosis

The recognition of risk factors for PPHN has been one of the major diagnostic tools to differentiate babies with PPHN from those with structural heart disease. The physical examination might be of limited value. A modest right ventricular impulse and single second heart sound are features of many cyanotic heart defects. The presence or absence of a murmur is not helpful. Neonates with transposition of the great arteries do not have murmurs, and those with PPHN might have the murmur of high-velocity tricuspid regurgitation. Significant precordial hyperactivity is unusual in PPHN and suggests structural heart disease, most often total anomalous pulmonary venous return. The chest radiograph might document the parenchymal disease, which could be the triggering factor for PPHN. Evidence of pulmonary edema should suggest structural heart disease.

Preductal and postductal blood gas measurements have been used to differentiate PPHN from structural heart disease. Babies with PPHN might have nearly normal right arm oxygen tension (PaO_2) and oxygen saturations (SaO_2), but the ductal-level right-to-left shunt causes lower PaO_2 and saturation measured from an umbilical artery sample. This approach has clear limitations. If atrial-level right-to-left shunting is a prominent feature of PPHN, both the right arm and the right leg saturations will be low. Conversely, babies with patent ductus arteriosus and coarctation of the aorta might have differential cyanosis without a significant blood pressure difference. The clinical course and response to treatment are often the most valuable signs.

Because PPHN is a labile disease, documentation of normal arterial PaO_2 at some point during the course does help exclude congenital heart disease. Echocardiography can usually provide a definitive structural diagnosis. Of equal importance is the physiologic data available from Doppler studies of atrial and ductal flow. Measurement of ductal and tricuspid regurgitation velocities with simultaneous blood pressure measurement provides an accurate indication of right-sided pressures and physiology.

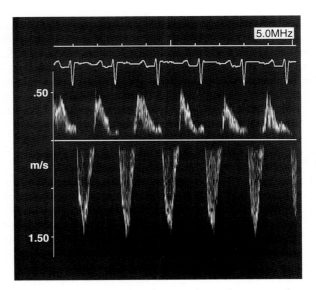

Figure 45–20. Doppler recording made in the patent ductus arteriosus of a neonate with severe persistent pulmonary hypertension of the newborn. It documents pulmonary artery to aorta (right-to-left) shunting during systole and left-to-right (above baseline) flow in diastole.

Treatment

The primary goal of therapy is to lower the pulmonary vascular resistance selectively. Years of experimental and empirical therapy have identified a number of effective strategies for neonates with PPHN (Table 45-7). Management of PPHN typically requires integration of therapeutic strategies simultaneously directed toward the pulmonary hypertension and, if present, the underlying lung disease. In cases of congenital diaphragmatic hernia, a small cross-sectional area of the pulmonary vessels results in high pulmonary vascular resistance.

TABLE 45–7 Proposed Treatment Strategies for Persistent Pulmonary Hypertension

Type	Proven Therapies*	Potentially Beneficial Therapies	Unproven Therapies
Pulmonary treatments	Oxygen Surfactant for RDS and meconium aspiration syndrome	High-frequency ventilation	Marked respiratory alkalosis
Pharmacologic treatments	Inhaled nitric oxide	—	Alkali infusion Other intravenous vasodilators
Cardiac support	Support of cardiac output with dopamine, fluid Normalization of ionized calcium	—	—
Environmental strategies	—	Avoidance of noise Reduced light	Paralysis
Rescue treatments	Inhaled nitric oxide Extracorporeal membrane oxygenation	—	—

*Efficacious in well-designed randomized trials.
RDS, respiratory distress syndrome.

Attempts to relieve pulmonary hypertension must be coordinated with optimal timing for surgery (see Chapter 44, Parts 5 and 8). Fetal surgical therapy for diaphragmatic hernia is addressed in Chapter 11.

Appropriate management of any underlying parenchymal lung disease must be aggressively pursued in patients with PPHN. Surfactant deficiency (or inactivation) can contribute to respiratory failure in term infants with PPHN who have nonspecific lung disease (which could be a variant of respiratory distress syndrome), meconium aspiration syndrome, or neonatal pneumonia. Exogenous surfactant therapy may improve lung function and outcome in some patients. High-frequency ventilation can optimize lung volume and enhance alveolar ventilation (see Chapter 44, Part 4). Modest respiratory alkalosis can prove useful in inducing pulmonary vasodilation.

Data from animal studies suggested that alkalosis, whether respiratory or metabolic, could lower pulmonary vascular resistance. Neonatologists quickly embraced alkali infusion as a treatment of PPHN on the assumption that hyperventilation and alkali infusion were equivalent. However, no randomized, controlled trials of either hyperventilation or alkali infusion are available. A review of a cohort of 385 newborns with PPHN indicated that a modest hyperventilation strategy might be associated less often with the need for extracorporeal membrane oxygenation or long-term oxygen than alkali administration.[70] These data, together with work on metabolic alkalosis in critically ill adults, have led many to question the role of alkali infusion.[71] A common compromise in management of PPHN is to maintain pH in the 7.4 to 7.45 range by modest hyperventilation, avoiding more severe alkalosis which can have detrimental neurodevelopmental consequences.

Pharmacologic management aims to normalize systemic pressures (e.g., dopamine) while relieving pulmonary hypertension and thus to minimize the risk for right-to-left shunting. Many vasodilators (e.g., nitroprusside, prostaglandin, isoproterenol) have been used; however, none appears to cause selective pulmonary vasodilation. Calcium channel blockers are of no benefit. Nonrandomized studies have demonstrated an improvement in PPHN in a small number of babies receiving magnesium sulfate infusion.[65] Available animal data suggest that magnesium sulfate does not have a selective pulmonary vasodilator effect.[56] The use of magnesium sulfate cannot be encouraged.

The discovery of nitric oxide's role in inducing endothelium-derived relaxation has delivered a selective modulator of pulmonary vascular resistance. Studies with low doses of inhaled nitric oxide (<20 ppm) have suggested that the number of babies requiring extracorporeal membrane oxygenation to survive PPHN is reduced by 40% (see Chapter 44, Part 8). A randomized, controlled trial of high-frequency ventilation and inhaled nitric oxide suggested that the combination was more effective than either treatment individually.[33] The apparent toxicity of nitric oxide appears to be low. Concerns about downregulation of endogenous nitric oxide synthesis, effects on bleeding time, and pulmonary immune function have been raised in early experimental studies but have been significant in clinical use.

Preliminary experience with intravenous sildenafil (inhibitor of cGMP-specific phosphodiesterase) has demonstrated improved oxygenation in neonates with PPHN, many of whom were already receiving inhaled nitric oxide. The most commonly reported adverse event was hypotension. A randomized clinical trial will be needed to determine if there is a therapeutic role for this therapy.[62a]

There has been a broad and favorable experience with continuous intravenous infusion of prostacyclin for treating pulmonary hypertension in children and adults.[4,5] The experience in neonates is limited but encouraging, and it can emerge as a treatment in selected neonates with chronic pulmonary hypertension.[17] The dose of prostacyclin used in the Eronen and associates study,[17] a mean dose of 60 ng/kg per minute, was higher than that typically used for older children, and unlike studies in older children, it was used for only a few days. The experience with the oral prostacyclin analogue in children is limited; however, studies in adults with primary pulmonary hypertension suggest a long-term benefit of this drug.[27,44]

MYOCARDIAL DISEASES: CARDIOMYOPATHY AND MYOCARDITIS

Cardiomyopathy refers to a diverse group of myocardial diseases with multiple causes. Definition and classification of cardiomyopathy are hampered by this diversity and uncertain pathogenesis. Because cardiomyopathy could be familial, these diseases have been the focus of intense metabolic and, most recently, genetic research to uncover the molecular basis of cardiomyopathy. Myocarditis, an inflammatory, usually infectious, process affecting the myocardium, can cause a cardiomyopathy (see Chapter 50).

Congestive or dilated cardiomyopathies are diseases in which there is both ventricular dilation and systolic dysfunction. The myocardial dysfunction in dilated cardiomyopathy could be due to primary disorders of the myocardium or to abnormalities of coronary perfusion (coronary embolism), afterload (hypertension, aortic stenosis), or arrhythmia (persistent supraventricular tachycardia). Fetal or neonatal congestive heart failure usually occurs when there is significant myocardial impairment. Poor perfusion and pulses with respiratory distress are present shortly after birth. Babies are initially well, but during the first weeks of life have either a sudden insult such as a coronary embolism or previously unrecognized and compensated myocardial dysfunction, which is worsened by an intercurrent infection or stress. Clinical clues to milder forms of cardiomyopathy include loud third heart sounds and the murmur of mitral regurgitation. Myocarditis causing cardiomyopathy should be suspected when there is a history of maternal infection, in babies with ST-T segment changes on the electrocardiogram, or in those with pancarditis (pericardial effusion, atrioventricular valve regurgitation, and myocardial dysfunction) by echocardiography.

Hypertrophic cardiomyopathies are structural abnormalities of the myocardium in which ventricular mass is out of proportion to the afterload of the ventricle. The process usually involves the left ventricular walls and is either asymmetric or concentric. Either asymmetric or concentric hypertrophic cardiomyopathies can be obstructive and nonobstructive. The left ventricular cavity could be either normal in size or small. The primary physiologic abnormality is ventricular diastolic dysfunction. Babies with obstructive hypertrophic cardiomyopathy have the additional problem of systolic obstruction to left ventricular ejection. In babies with primary disorders of the myocardium, hypertrophy and myofibrillar disarray could be the result of mutations of the proteins of the cardiac sarcomere.[38,42] Severe hypertrophic cardiomyopathies with impaired systolic function should suggest the possibility of inherited genetic abnormalities from both parents.[73] Babies with storage diseases could have features similar to hypertrophic cardiomyopathy with thickening of the myocardium because of infiltration of the muscle. They might not have the normal or hyperdynamic systolic function that is present with primary hypertrophic cardiomyopathy. The myopathy seen in infants of diabetic mothers is the most common form of hypertrophic

cardiomyopathy seen in the neonatal period (see Chapter 16 and Chapter 49, Part 1).

Restrictive cardiomyopathy is characterized by impairment of diastolic filling, usually with normal systolic function. The result is atrial dilation and normal ventricular size. Isolated restrictive cardiomyopathy is rare in the neonate. However, babies with the contracted form of endocardial fibroelastosis have a significant restrictive cardiomyopathy caused by the scarring of the endocardium. This disease is manifested in the first few months of life with congestive heart failure caused by the diastolic dysfunction. Systolic function is usually near normal.

Diagnosis

The approach to neonates with suspected cardiomyopathy or myocarditis must include a methodical approach to the diagnosis (Boxes 45-11 to 45-13)* and a level of support appropriate for their clinical symptoms. The inclusion of a myocardial, skin, or skeletal muscle biopsy as part of the examination of the baby with cardiomyopathy should be guided by the clinical course and the results of the initial blood and urine tests. The myocardial biopsy can guide therapy or help in defining the prognosis by identifying pathologic features by light and electron microscopy, by searching for viral ribonucleic acid, or by using new techniques for assessing mitochondrial function.[55] Evidence of active inflammation or immune suppression can be treated with intravenously administered immune globulin, although its role in the treatment of myocarditis remains to be fully validated.[16,26] The prognosis is often good if the baby can be managed through an episode of myocarditis. In contrast, if a biopsy shows endocardial fibroelastosis or the echocardiogram shows endocardial thickening, the likelihood of recovery of myocardial function is small.

Treatment

Babies with dilated cardiomyopathy and minimal symptoms can be successfully managed with digoxin, diuretics, and captopril. Those with poor cardiac output are initially supported with mechanical ventilation, intravenous inotropes, and afterload reduction, and then the transition to oral agents is made. Ventricular and atrial arrhythmias are poorly tolerated in babies with severe myocardial dysfunction and must be effectively treated (see the discussion of arrhythmias in Part 9). Shock with acidosis and organ dysfunction is an indication for extracorporeal membrane oxygenation, especially if the cause is reversible or if transplantation is being considered.

CARDIAC TUMORS

Cardiac tumors can be identified on fetal echocardiography or on evaluation of murmurs or arrhythmias. The most common neonatal tumors are rhabdomyomas, and some babies have tuberous sclerosis.[29] Rhabdomyomas arise on the ventricular endocardial surface, and if they are large enough, they can interfere with ventricular filling or emptying. When they are located near the atrioventricular valves, the tissue can serve as a bypass tract and mimic the features of Wolff-Parkinson-White syndrome.[41] Confirmation by myocardial biopsy in a

---

*References 13-15,46,57,58,62,66-69.

BOX 45–11   Causes of Dilated Cardiomyopathy in Infants

MYOCARDITIS
Viral: Coxsackie virus group B, parvovirus, adenovirus
Bacterial: group B streptococcal sepsis

ENDOCARDIAL FIBROELASTOSIS
Primary: in utero myocarditis or infarction
Secondary: critical aortic stenosis

NEONATAL AND INFANT MYOCARDIAL INFARCTION
Amniotic fluid embolus, air embolus, clot
Protein C, protein S deficiency
Homocystinuria
Origin of left coronary artery from pulmonary artery

ARRHYTHMIAS
Incessant atrial or ventricular tachycardia

STORAGE DISORDERS
Glycogenesis type IIa (Pompe disease, acid maltase deficiency)*
Infantile glycogenesis type IV (debrancher deficiency with phosphorylase deficiency)
Cardiac glycogenesis (cardiac phosphorylase kinase deficiency)
$G_{M2}L$: gangliosidosis with ascites (β-galactosidase deficiency)
G_{M2}: gangliosidosis (hexosaminidase deficiency)

CARNITINE DEFICIENCY*
Renal tubular and gastrointestinal wasting of carnitine[28]
Neonatal transient carnitine deficiency

MITOCHONDRIAL DISEASES
NADH dehydrogenase (cytochrome complex I) defect
Cytochrome c oxidase (cytochrome complex IV) defect
Coenzyme Q cytochrome c reductase (cytochrome complex III) defect

X-LINKED MITOCHONDRIAL DISORDERS
Barth syndrome[9,22]
Type II X-linked 3-methylglutaconic aciduria[47]
Thiamine-responsive defects in oxidative phosphorylation

MYOSIN MUTATIONS
Mutation of mtDNA in the tRNA (Leu[UUR]) gene[61]

MISCELLANEOUS
Congenital adrenal hyperplasia*
Selenium deficiency

*Could have features of hypertrophic myopathy.
mtDNA, mitochondrial DNA; NADH, nicotinamide adenine dinucleotide, reduced; tRNA, transfer ribonucleic acid.

BOX 45–12   Hypertrophic Cardiomyopathy

Infant of a diabetic mother
B cell adenoma[25]
Beckwith-Wiedemann syndrome
Noonan syndrome[59]
Dexamethasone or ACTH therapy[30]
Familial: chromosomes 1, 14, and 15[64]
Mitochondrial disorders
Carbohydrate-deficient glycoprotein syndrome[11]
Congenital cataracts and hypertrophic cardiomyopathy
Barth syndrome[51]

ACTH, adrenocorticotropic hormone.

BOX 45–13   Laboratory Studies to Be Considered in Infantile Cardiomyopathy of Suspected Metabolic Origin

BLOOD
Carnitine
Amino acids
Blood gases
Lactate, pyruvate
Leukocyte preparations for enzyme assays
Genetic testing for mutations of the cardiac sarcomere

URINE
Amino acids
Organic acids
Oligosaccharides

ELECTROMYOGRAPHY

SKIN BIOPSY
Morphologic studies for storage disorders
Fibroblast cultures for specific enzymatic studies

MUSCLE BIOPSY
Morphologic studies for skeletal myopathy
Biochemical studies for carnitine deficiency and mitochondrial disorders

MYOCARDIAL BIOPSY
Light and electron microscopy
Viral ribonucleic acid
Mitochondrial function

symptom-free neonate is not necessary, especially if the skin and central nervous system features of tuberous sclerosis are present. Rhabdomyomas typically regress,[39] and surgical excision is not needed unless the tumor is obstructing flow and is discrete or pedunculated enough to allow excision. Radiofrequency ablation of the tumors has been successfully performed for medically resistant arrhythmias.

Other rare tumors that can occur in the neonate include myocardial hemangioma,[6] hamartoma,[37] fibroma, and pericardial teratomas. Myocardial hemangiomas are tumors with dense capillary beds which can have connections to the coronary arteries. They are on the epicardial surface with intrusion into the myocardium. Hemangiomas can cause subpulmonary stenosis if they are located in the right ventricular outflow tract. Small hamartomas cause histiocytoid or oncocytic cardiomyopathy, which is associated with severe and persistent ventricular arrhythmias. Myocardial fibroma can be located in the myocardium or on the atrial wall or can involve the mitral valve and cause obstruction (Fig. 45-21). Intrapericardial teratoma is a benign tumor attached to the base of the aorta. It is associated with mediastinal compression and pericardial effusion in the fetus, neonate, or young infant. Successful excision of intrapericardial teratoma has been reported, although large tumors can

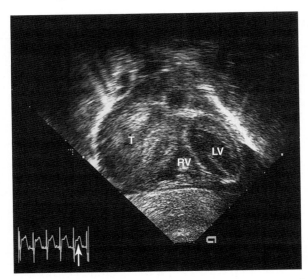

Figure 45–21. Subcostal echocardiogram of symptom-free 2-week-old infant with murmur. A large tumor (T) nearly completely filled the right ventricle (RV). The tumor was successfully excised and histologic study showed fibroma. LV, left ventricle.

cause fetal death. Atrial myxomas are not reported in the neonatal period.

A redundant eustachian valve or Chiari network in the right atrium might be mistaken for an atrial tumor. Atrial masses in neonates with a history of central venous catheters probably represent thrombi. Bacterial or fungal infection of these thrombi is a frequent concern, although excision of the masses is unusual. Thrombi beginning in the superior or inferior vena cava can be difficult to extract successfully once they have begun to organize. Thrombolysis carries risk for bleeding and seldom dissolves a clot that has been present for more than a few days. Similarly, anticoagulation has uncertain benefit, unless there is a documented increase in the thrombus size. Embolization of a right atrial thrombus rarely occurs, even when it appears to be highly mobile and pedunculated.

VASCULAR RINGS

In the first month of life, respiratory distress caused by vascular rings usually indicates severe obstruction. Severe obstruction is caused by either a double aortic arch or a pulmonary artery sling. Neither left aortic arch with aberrant right subclavian artery nor right aortic arch with aberrant left subclavian artery and right ductus arteriosus causes a ring or obstruction. Right aortic arch with aberrant left subclavian artery and left ductus arteriosus does form a ring, but symptoms in the neonatal period are unusual. Diagnosis of these arch abnormalities can be made on the basis of a combination of echocardiography, barium swallow radiography, computed tomography, and magnetic resonance imaging (see Chapter 44, Part 5).

Several variants of double aortic arch should be considered as part of the presurgical assessment. The dominant arch should be preserved and the smaller or atretic side divided. Both a right and a left ductus might be present, and coarctation of the aorta has been reported with double aortic arch. Any of these variants produces the bilateral and posterior indentation

on the esophagus seen by barium swallow radiography. Echocardiography and magnetic resonance imaging do not identify any atretic segments. The atretic side is inferred by the origin of the arch vessels on the atretic side (usually the left) from an anterior and a posterior aortic diverticulum. Coarctation of the aorta must be identified by imaging because the Doppler or magnetic resonance flow disturbances are not present until the arch is divided. Careful color flow Doppler mapping should permit identification of the location of either a right or left patent ductus arteriosus. There is considerable experience with surgical division of the vascular rings[1,3,10] and with video-assisted thoracoscopic surgery in older children.[34]

Pulmonary artery sling is caused by the origin of all or part of the left pulmonary artery from the right pulmonary artery. The aberrant pulmonary artery courses posteriorly between the trachea and esophagus and along the left main bronchus. Diagnosis is suggested by the echocardiogram and the distinctive anterior impression on the esophagus on a barium swallow radiograph. Pulmonary artery sling occurs as an isolated defect or in association with ventricular septal defect. Mobilization and reimplantation of the left pulmonary artery help relieve the obstruction; however, tracheomalacia or tracheal rings can cause persistent respiratory distress.

PERICARDIAL EFFUSION

Pericardial effusion is seen in neonates who have had fetal congestive heart failure caused by anemia or myocarditis. Small effusions may be associated with neonatal pneumonia. Effusions can also occur after open heart surgery and as a complication of hyperalimentation with central venous catheters as a result of local irritation of the atrial or superior vena caval wall by fluids with high osmolality. Pneumopericardium is a complication of mechanical ventilation and can have hemodynamic effects similar to those of fluid. If the pericardial fluid accumulated gradually, intrapericardial pressure remains low and symptoms are few until the effusion is large. Rapid accumulation of fluid, either blood or intravenous fluid, can cause pericardial tamponade with much smaller volumes.

The diagnosis of pericardial tamponade should be suspected in any baby with early signs of poor cardiac output, including tachycardia and poor perfusion. Pulsus paradoxus, an exaggerated fall in blood pressure with inspiration, is easiest to observe in neonates with arterial lines for continuous blood pressure monitoring. A dramatic increase in heart size on a chest radiograph supports the clinical diagnosis. Intrapericardial air is usually obvious on the radiograph and can be differentiated from mediastinal air because it encircles the heart. Echocardiography is the best way to confirm the diagnosis and assess the physiologic impact of the effusion. Diastolic collapse of the right atrium and right ventricle suggests a significant effusion. Pericardiocentesis by the subxiphoid approach can drain enough fluid or air to relieve symptoms. If the fluid or air returns, a small catheter can be placed percutaneously or surgically.

NEONATAL MARFAN SYNDROME

In the absence of a known familial genotype, the clinical diagnosis of Marfan syndrome in the neonate who has an affected parent requires a careful multisystem evaluation, including echocardiography to assess aortic root dimension. The diagnosis is usually difficult to establish in neonates referred for evaluation solely on the basis of their family history. Aortic root dimensions are usually within the normal range, and mitral valve prolapse is absent. This is in contrast to the neonates with dramatic multisystem involvement, who nearly always represent new mutations.[19,43] Skeletal features are recognizable, and clinical signs of congestive heart failure caused by mitral or tricuspid regurgitation could be evident in the first days of life. Aortic root dimensions are often increased, and aortic regurgitation can be seen by color flow mapping. Genetic testing to exclude Loeys-Dietz syndrome may also be indicated in the neonate presenting with physical findings of connective tissue abnormalities.[36]

Medical management of the mitral regurgitation might improve symptoms, but early mitral valve repair is often needed. Aortic root dilation must be carefully followed and elective aortic root replacement performed if aortic dilation becomes severe.[18] Multicenter studies are underway to evaluate the relative benefit of beta blockade or angiotensin receptor blockade to slow the progression of the aortic root enlargement and permit surgery at a later time.[48]

THE PREMATURE BABY WITH CONGENITAL HEART DISEASE

Patent ductus arteriosus is obviously the most prevalent heart defect in the premature baby. The clinical recognition, echocardiographic assessment, medical management, and when needed, surgical management, are well established and are effective even in the baby weighing 500 g. A population-based study suggests that cardiovascular defects, in general, may be more prevalent in preterm babies despite the assumption that most defects are well tolerated in utero.[63] Many defects in preterm babies are not hemodynamically important and do not require specific management. For preterm babies with cyanotic heart defects, large ventricular septal defects, or left heart obstruction, the nutritional and respiratory needs of the premature baby can dramatically add to the challenge of a congenital heart defect. The initial pulmonary vascular resistance in a premature baby may be lower because of less well developed muscular arterioles, which can lead to early signs of congestive heart failure in babies with defects causing excessive pulmonary blood flow.

Case reports of successful surgical or interventional catheterization of a number of defects in premature babies weighing between 1 and 2 kg certainly indicate that these babies can be helped. Reddy and colleagues reviewed their experience with heart surgery in 102 newborns weighing between 700 and 2500 g (including 16 weighing less than 1500 g).[53] The overall mortality was 18%, but many babies were successfully treated. Long-term infusion of prostaglandin E$_1$ in babies with cyanotic or left heart defects does permit a period for maturation of the lungs and nutrition and, for many premature babies, is preferable to open heart surgery in those weighing less than 1800 g. The risk that pulmonary vascular disease will develop within several months, even in a baby with truncus arteriosus or transposition of the great arteries, is small. The most important risk of conservative management is the occurrence of necrotizing enterocolitis. If heart failure or hypoxia is unmanageable,

palliation or correction can be undertaken. Defects with atrioventricular valve regurgitation, severe aortic stenosis, and defects with pulmonary venous obstruction are difficult to manage medically and are probably more likely to have a good outcome with aggressive surgical or catheter therapy. Associated bronchopulmonary dysplasia also increases the risk associated with surgical treatment.[40]

REFERENCES

1. Alsenaidi K, et al: Management and outcomes of double aortic arch in 81 patients, *Pediatrics* 118:e1336, 2006.
2. Ascher DP, et al: Systemic to pulmonary collaterals mimicking patent ductus arteriosus in neonates with prolonged ventilatory courses, *J Pediatr* 107:282, 1985.
3. Backer CL, et al: Trends in vascular ring surgery, *J Thorac Cardiovasc Surg* 129:1339, 2005.
4. Barst RJ: Recent advances in the treatment of pediatric pulmonary artery hypertension, *Pediatr Clin North Am* 46:331, 1999.
5. Barst RJ, et al: Vasodilator therapy for primary pulmonary hypertension in children, *Circulation* 99:1197, 1999.
6. Brizard C, et al: Cardiac hemangiomas, *Ann Thorac Surg* 56:390, 1993.
7. Brownlee JR, et al: Acute hemodynamic effects of nifedipine in infants with bronchopulmonary dysplasia and pulmonary hypertension, *Pediatr Res* 24:186, 1988.
8. Choi M, et al: Heterotaxia syndrome: the role of screening for intestinal rotation abnormalities, *Arch Dis Child* 90:813, 2005.
9. Christodoulou J, et al: Barth syndrome: clinical observations and genetic linkage studies, *Am J Med Genet* 50:255, 1994.
10. Chun K, et al: Diagnosis and management of congenital vascular rings: a 22-year experience, *Ann Thorac Surg* 53:597, 1992.
11. Clayton PT, et al: Hypertrophic obstructive cardiomyopathy in a neonate with the carbohydrate-deficient glycoprotein syndrome, *J Inherit Metab Dis* 15:857, 1992.
12. Cohen MS, et al: Controversies, genetics, diagnostic assessment, and outcomes relating to the heterotaxy syndrome, *Cardiol Young* 17(Suppl 2):29, 2007.
13. Cohen N, Muntoni F: Multiple pathogenetic mechanisms in X linked dilated cardiomyopathy, *Heart* 90:835, 2004.
14. Daubeney PE, et al, for the National Australian Childhood Cardiomyopathy Study: Clinical features and outcomes of childhood dilated cardiomyopathy: results from a national population-based study, *Circulation* 114:2671, 2006.
15. Debray FG, et al: Disorders of mitochondrial function, *Curr Opin Pediatr* 20:471, 2008.
16. Drucker NA, et al: Gamma-globulin treatment of acute myocarditis in the pediatric population, *Circulation* 89:252, 1994.
17. Eronen M, et al: Prostacyclin treatment for persistent pulmonary hypertension of the newborn, *Pediatr Cardiol* 18:3, 1997.
18. Everitt MD, et al: Cardiovascular surgery in children with Marfan syndrome or Loeys-Dietz syndrome, *J Thorac Cardiovasc Surg* 137:1327, 2009; discussion 1332-3.
19. Faivre L, et al: Clinical and molecular study of 320 children with Marfan syndrome and related type I fibrillinopathies in a series of 1009 probands with pathogenic FBN1 mutations, *Pediatrics* 123:391, 2009.
20. Flynn JT: Neonatal hypertension: diagnosis and management, *Pediatr Nephrol* 14:332, 2000.
21. Friedman DM, et al: Recent improvement in outcome using transcatheter techniques for neonatal aneurysmal malformations of the vein Galen, *Pediatrics* 91:583, 1993.

22. Gedeon AK, et al: X-linked fatal infantile cardiomyopathy maps to Xq28 and is possibly allelic to Barth syndrome, *J Med Genet* 32:383, 1995.

23. Gorenflo M, et al: Pulmonary vascular changes in bronchopulmonary dysplasia: a clinicopathologic correlation in short- and long-term, *Pediatr Pathol* 11:851, 1991.

24. Guignard JP, et al: Arterial hypertension in the newborn infant, *Biol Neonate* 55:77, 1989.

25. Harris JP, et al: Reversible hypertrophic cardiomyopathy associated with nesidioblastosis, *J Pediatr* 120:272, 1992.

26. Hia CP, et al: Immunosuppressive therapy in acute myocarditis: an 18 year systematic review, *Arch Dis Child* 89:580, 2004.

27. Ichida F, et al: Acute effect of oral prostacyclin and inhaled nitric oxide on pulmonary hypertension in children, *J Cardiol* 29:217, 1997.

28. Ino T, et al: Cardiac manifestations in disorders of fat and carnitine metabolism in infancy, *J Am Coll Cardiol* 11:1301, 1988.

29. Isaacs H Jr: Fetal and neonatal cardiac tumors, *Pediatr Cardiol* 25:252, 2004.

30. Israel BA, et al: Hypertrophic cardiomyopathy associated with dexamethasone therapy for chronic lung disease in preterm infants, *Am J Perinatol* 10:307, 1993.

31. Jacobs JP, et al: The nomenclature, definition and classification of cardiac structures in the setting of heterotaxy, *Cardiol Young* Suppl 2:1, 2007.

32. Khemani E, et al: Pulmonary artery hypertension in formerly premature infants with bronchopulmonary dysplasia: clinical features and outcomes in the surfactant era, *Pediatrics* 120:1260, 2007.

33. Kinsella JP, et al: Randomized, multicenter trial of inhaled nitric oxide and high-frequency oscillatory ventilation in severe, persistent pulmonary hypertension of the newborn, *J Pediatr* 131:55, 1997.

34. Kogon BE, et al: Video-assisted thoracoscopic surgery: is it a superior technique for the division of vascular rings in children? *Congenit Heart Dis* 2:130 2007.

35. Lasjaunias PL, et al: The management of vein of Galen aneurysmal malformations, *Neurosurgery* 59(Suppl 3):S184, 2006; discussion S3-13.

36. Loeys BL, et al: Aneurysm syndromes caused by mutations in the TGF-beta receptor, *N Engl J Med* 355:788, 2006.

37. Marian AJ, Roberts R: Molecular genetics of hypertrophic cardiomyopathy, *Annu Rev Med* 46:213, 1995.

38. Maron BJ, et al: Impact of laboratory molecular diagnosis on contemporary diagnostic criteria for genetically transmitted cardiovascular diseases: hypertrophic cardiomyopathy, long-QT syndrome, and Marfan syndrome. A statement for healthcare professionals from the Councils on Clinical Cardiology, Cardiovascular Disease in the Young, and Basic Science, American Heart Association, *Circulation* 98:1460, 1998.

39. Matsuoka Y, et al: Disappearance of a cardiac rhabdomyoma complicating mitral regurgitation as observed by serial two-dimensional echocardiography, *Pediatr Cardiol* 11:98, 1990.

40. McMahon CJ, et al: Preterm infants with congenital heart disease and bronchopulmonary dysplasia: postoperative course and outcome after cardiac surgery, *Pediatrics* 116:423, 2005.

41. Mehta A: Rhabdomyoma and ventricular preexcitation syndrome: a report cases and review of literature, *Am J Dis Child* 147:669, 1993.

42. Morita H, et al: Shared genetic causes of cardiac hypertrophy in children and adults, *N Engl J Med* 358:1899, 2008.

43. Morse R, et al: Diagnosis and management of infantile Marfan syndrome, *Pediatrics* 86:888, 1990.

44. Nagaya N, et al: Effect of orally active prostacyclin analogue on survival of outpatients with primary pulmonary hypertension, *J Am Coll Cardiol* 34:1188, 1999.

45. Nagel BH, et al: Splenic state in surviving patients with visceral heterotaxy, *Cardiol Young* 15:469, 2005.

46. Nugent AW, et al; National Australian Childhood Cardiomyopathy Study: Clinical features and outcomes of childhood hypertrophic cardiomyopathy: results from a national population-based study, *Circulation* 112:1332, 2005.

47. Ostman-Smith I, et al: Dilated cardiomyopathy due to type II X-linked aciduria: successful treatment with pantothenic acid, *Br Heart J* 72:349, 1994.

48. Pearson GD, et al, for the National Heart, Lung, and Blood Institute and National Marfan Foundation Working Group: Report of the National Heart, Lung, and Blood Institute and National Marfan Foundation Working Group on research in Marfan syndrome and related disorders, *Circulation* 118:785, 2008.

49. Peterson AL, et al: Presentation and echocardiographic markers of neonatal hypertensive cardiomyopathy, *Pediatrics* 118:e782, 2006.

50. Phoon CK, Neill CA: Asplenia syndrome: insight into embryology through an analysis of cardiac and extracardiac anomalies, *Am J Cardiol* 73:581, 1994.

51. Pignatelli RH, et al: Clinical characterization of left ventricular noncompaction in children: a relatively common form of cardiomyopathy, *Circulation* 108:2672, 2003.

52. Price VE, et al: The prevention and management of infections in children with asplenia or hyposplenia, *Infect Dis Clin North Am* 21:697, viii-ix, 2007.

53. Reddy VM, et al: Results of 102 cases of complete repair of congenital heart defects in patients weighing 700 to 2500 grams, *J Thorac Cardiovasc Surg* 117:324, 1999.

54. Rosenzweig EB, Barst RJ: Pulmonary arterial hypertension in children: a medical update, *Curr Opin Pediatr* 20:288, 2008.

55. Rustin P, et al: Endomyocardial biopsies for early detection of mitochondrial disorders in hypertrophic cardiomyopathies, *J Pediatr* 124:224, 1994.

56. Ryan CA, et al: Effects of magnesium sulfate and nitric oxide in pulmonary hypertension induced by hypoxia in newborn piglets, *Arch Dis Child* 71:F151, 1994.

57. Saudubray JM, et al: Recognition and management of fatty acid oxidation defects: a series of 107 patients, *J Inherit Metab Dis* 22:488, 1999.

58. Schwartz ML, et al: Clinical approach to genetic cardiomyopathy in children, *Circulation* 94:2021, 1996.

59. Sharland M, et al: A clinical study of Noonan syndrome, *Arch Dis Child* 67:178, 1992.

60. Sheley RC, et al: Azygous continuation of the interrupted inferior vena cava: A clue to prenatal diagnosis of the cardiosplenic syndromes, *J Ultrasound Med* 14:381, 1995.

61. Silvestri G, et al: a new mtDNA mutation in the tRNA (Leu[UUR]) gene associated maternally inherited cardiomyopathy, *Hum Mutat* 3:37, 1994.

62. Spencer CT, Bryant RM, Day J, et al: Cardiac and clinical phenotype in Barth syndrome, *Pediatrics* 118:e337, 2006.

62a. Steinhorn RH, Kinsella JP, Pierce C, et al: Intravenous sildenafil. In the treatment of neonates with persistent pulmonary hypertension, *J Pediatr* 155:841, 2009.

63. Tanner K, Sabrine N, Wren C: Cardiovascular malformations among preterm infants, *Pediatrics* 116:e833, 2005.
64. Thierfelder L, et al: A familial hypertrophic cardiomyopathy locus maps to chromosome 15q2, *Proc Natl Acad Sci U S A* 90:6270, 1993.
65. Tolsa JF, et al: Magnesium sulfate as an alternative and safe treatment for severe persistent pulmonary hypertension of the newborn, *Arch Dis Child Fetal Neonatal Ed* 72:F184, 1995.
66. Towbin JA, Lipshultz SE: Genetics of neonatal cardiomyopathy, *Curr Opin Cardiol* 14:250, 1999.
67. Towbin JA, et al: Incidence, causes, and outcomes of dilated cardiomyopathy in children, *JAMA* 296:1867, 2006.
68. Tsirka AE, et al: Improved outcomes of pediatric dilated cardiomyopathy with utilization of heart transplantation, *J Am Coll Cardiol* 44:391, 2004.
69. van der Ploeg AT, Reuser AJ: Pompe's disease, *Lancet* 372:1342, 2008.
70. Walsh-Sukys MC, et al: Persistent pulmonary hypertension of the newborn in the era before nitric oxide: practice variation and outcomes, *Pediatrics* 105:14, 2000.
71. Webster NR, Kulkarni V: Metabolic acidosis in the critically ill, *Crit Rev Clin Lab Sci* 36:497, 1999.
72. Wilson D, et al: Infantile hypertension caused by unilateral renal arterial disease, *Arch Dis Child* 65:881, 1990.
73. Zahka K, et al: Homozygous mutation of MYBPC3 associated with severe infantile hypertrophic cardiomyopathy at high frequency among the Amish, *Heart* 94:1326, 2008.

PART 9
Neonatal Arrhythmias
George F. Van Hare

The diagnosis and treatment of cardiac arrhythmias in neonates can be challenging and often different from diagnosis and treatment of the same arrhythmias in older children. For example, infants can sustain very fast sinus rates, and so sinus tachycardia may masquerade as paroxysmal supraventricular tachycardia. The neonatal normal range of electrocardiographic values must be considered when one is interpreting electrocardiograms. Also, the natural history of arrhythmias occurring in the neonatal period is often dramatically different from those occurring later in life.

METHODS OF DIAGNOSIS
Heart Rate

The observation of an abnormal heart rate can be the first sign of an arrhythmia, yet determining the exact heart rate is often difficult. The pulse might be too fast to count by palpation or auscultation. Bedside cardiac monitors that automatically display the heart rate as a digital read-out might oversense or undersense the QRS complex, yielding incorrect values. Pulse oximeters count only the beats that produce an appreciable pulse and so may underestimate actual heart rate, and they are prone to artifact. The most accurate method is to determine the rate from an electrocardiogram. All QRS

complexes are counted for a period of 6 seconds, and the rate per minute is obtained by multiplying by 10. The only pitfall of this method is machine malfunction causing paper drag, which results in a slower paper speed and a more rapid apparent heart rate.

Electrocardiogram

Although some arrhythmias can be diagnosed directly from the cardiac monitor, analysis of a paper record of the electrocardiogram is the standard for accurately diagnosing arrhythmias. Small variations in the PR or R-R interval are detectable only with the paper record. The manner of initiation and termination of tachycardias, the morphology and duration of the QRS complex, and the P wave configuration determined from the electrocardiogram are important diagnostic features of arrhythmias. All electrocardiograms of interest should be preserved for later analysis and consultation because future treatment decisions are often made on the basis of these recordings.

Similarly, cardiac monitors employing three or four chest electrodes provide a great deal of information, but details such as P wave axis, QRS complex duration, and ST segment morphologic features are best evaluated by the pediatric standard 15-lead electrocardiogram (the standard 12 leads plus V_{3R}, V_{4R}, and V_7). Therefore, when time and hemodynamic condition allow, it is important to obtain a complete 15-lead electrocardiogram.

Ambulatory Monitoring and Telemetry

Conventional neonatal monitors and electrocardiograms offer brief opportunities to record the heart rhythm. For the neonate with a sustained arrhythmia, these technologies are usually adequate and may be diagnostic. For the neonate with intermittent symptoms or rhythm disorders, continuous recording of the rhythm with the ability to analyze the range of heart rates and the onset and cessation of arrhythmias is invaluable for diagnosis and management. Continuous monitoring is available either in inpatient full-disclosure telemetry units or with portable ambulatory electrocardiography (Holter monitoring).

Esophageal Electrocardiogram

The atrial electrogram can be recorded by passing a flexible bipolar electrode down the esophagus and positioning it behind the left atrium. These leads are connected to a filtering box and recorded with simultaneous limb and chest leads. The amplitude of the transesophageal atrial electrogram is larger than the surface P wave. The atrial electrogram can be compared with the QRS complex on the simultaneous surface electrocardiogram or with ventricular electrograms from the transesophageal lead. The atrium can also be paced by this electrode, and transesophageal pacing can be used to terminate various types of reentrant tachycardias.

Electrophysiologic Testing

Formal transvenous electrophysiologic studies to elucidate the mechanisms of arrhythmias or to guide treatment of arrhythmias are rarely necessary in the neonatal period. Limited but often diagnostic studies can be performed with the temporary atrial and ventricular epicardial pacing wires placed at the time of open heart surgery. These wires are used for recording the atrial and ventricular electrograms and for pacing to assess the conduction system and to terminate atrial tachycardias.

Blood Pressure

Automatic blood pressure monitors are convenient and provide accurate blood pressure determinations in most neonates with arrhythmias. Some devices function poorly in babies with tachycardia, particularly at rates seen in the neonate.

Intra-arterial blood pressure monitoring is the most accurate technique for measuring blood pressure in the neonate who has poor cardiac output and an arrhythmia.

MECHANISMS OF TACHYCARDIA
General Mechanisms

The two general mechanisms for tachyarrhythmias seen in clinical practice (Tables 45-8 and 45-9) are reentry and increased automaticity. Reentry is the circular movement of electrical impulses within the atrium, atrioventricular (AV)

TABLE 45–8 Mechanisms of Tachycardia with Normal QRS Duration

Diagnosis	Findings on Electrocardiogram
Reentrant Tachycardias	
Atrial and sinoatrial reentry	P waves present, precede next QRS complex Terminates with QRS rather than P wave Variable AV conduction possible; AV block does not terminate atrial rhythm P wave axis superior or inferior, depending on origin
Atrial flutter	Sawtooth flutter waves AV block does not terminate atrial rhythm Atrial rate up to 500 beats/min in neonates Variable AV conduction is common
Tachycardia mediated by accessory pathway (WPW syndrome and concealed accessory pathway)	P waves follow QRS, typically on upstroke of T wave Superior or rightward P wave axis AV block always terminates tachycardia Typically terminates with P wave After termination, those with WPW syndrome have pre-excitation
Permanent form of junctional reciprocating tachycardia	Incessant P waves precede QRS complex Inverted P waves in leads II, III, aVF AV block always terminates tachycardia May terminate with QRS complex or with P wave No pre-excitation after termination
Atrioventricular node reentry	P waves usually not visible; superimposed on QRS complex AV block usually terminates tachycardia
Atrial fibrillation (probably reentrant)	Irregularly irregular; no two R-R intervals exactly the same P waves difficult to see or bizarre and chaotic
Increased Automaticity Tachycardias	
Sinus tachycardia	Normal P wave axis P waves precede QRS Causes: extrinsic factor such as heart failure, fever, anemia, catecholamine, or theophylline infusion Continue in presence of AV block
Atrial ectopic tachycardia	Incessant Abnormal P wave axis that predicts location of focus P waves precede QRS Continues in presence of AV block
Junctional ectopic tachycardia	Incessant Usually with atrioventricular dissociation and slower atrial than ventricular rate Capture beats with no fusion

AV, atrioventricular; WPW, Wolff-Parkinson-White.

TABLE 45–9   Mechanisms of Tachycardia with Prolonged QRS Duration

Diagnosis	Findings on Electrocardiogram
Ventricular tachycardia	Often with AV dissociation Capture beats with narrower QRS complex than on other beats Fusion beats
Supraventricular tachycardia with preexisting bundle branch block	QRS morphologic features similar to those of sinus rhythm QRS morphologic features are those of right or left bundle branch block
Supraventricular tachycardia with rate-dependent bundle branch block	QRS morphologic features usually similar to those of right or left bundle branch block Rare in small children Difficult to distinguish from ventricular tachycardia in children
Antidromic supraventricular tachycardia in WPW syndrome	QRS morphologic features similar to those of pre-excited sinus rhythm but wider, never with AV dissociation
Atrial fibrillation with WPW syndrome	Irregularly irregular wide QRS tachycardia

AV, atrioventricular; WPW, Wolff-Parkinson-White.

node, or ventricles. Reentrant tachycardias include sinoatrial and intra-atrial reentry, AV node reentry, AV reciprocating tachycardia involving an accessory pathway, atrial flutter, the permanent form of junctional reciprocating tachycardia (PJRT), and the reentrant form of ventricular tachycardia. Increased automaticity is the abnormal state in which cardiac cells display autonomous repetitive depolarization at a rate faster than normal. Automatic tachycardias include sinus tachycardia, atrial ectopic tachycardia (AET), junctional ectopic tachycardia (JET), and the automatic focus form of ventricular tachycardia.

Three conditions are needed o support reentrant tachycardias. First, an anatomically distinct reentrant circuit must be present, allowing for the circular movement of excitation. Second, unidirectional conduction block must occur, allowing subsequent reversed conduction in that segment. Third, there must be an area of conduction delay in the reentry circuit sufficient to allow recovery of all components of the circuit before the arrival of the next wave of activation.

The definitive example of a reentrant supraventricular tachyarrhythmia is the reciprocating AV reentrant tachycardia in babies with Wolff-Parkinson-White syndrome. Typically, a premature atrial contraction blocks in the accessory pathway but is conducted with a significant delay down the AV node and His-Purkinje system. Impulses arriving in the ventricle are then conducted retrograde in the accessory pathway back to the atrium. The conduction delay in the AV node allows the accessory pathway and atrium sufficient time to recover and thus allows establishment of the tachycardia. Orthodromic tachycardias use the AV node for anterograde conduction, and antidromic tachycardias use the AV node for retrograde conduction.

A major characteristic of the reentrant tachycardias that helps differentiate them from the automatic tachycardias is their tendency to start and stop suddenly. Premature atrial and ventricular contractions can initiate or terminate these rhythms. Direct-current cardioversion is usually successful in terminating reentrant tachycardias but not automatic focus tachycardias.

Specific Mechanisms

SINUS TACHYCARDIA

Sinus tachycardia can masquerade as a paroxysmal supraventricular tachycardia in neonates. Sinus tachycardia is nearly always secondary to some other problem. Identification and treatment of that problem can facilitate the diagnosis of sinus tachycardia. For example, gradual slowing of a narrow QRS tachycardia after an intravenous fluid bolus in a hypovolemic neonate provides strong evidence for sinus tachycardia and against other forms of paroxysmal supraventricular tachycardia. Other causes of sinus tachycardia include heart failure, high fever, pain, hypoxia, exogenous chronotropic agents such as isoproterenol or dobutamine, xanthine therapy, undersedation in paralyzed infants supported by mechanical ventilation, or rarely, hyperthyroidism.

The criteria for sinus tachycardia are normal P wave axis, gradual onset and termination, and rates less than 250 beats per minute. Narrow-complex tachycardias with rates between 180 and 250 beats per minute can be either sinus tachycardia or some form of abnormal tachycardia.

The correct diagnosis must be established, if possible, before antiarrhythmic therapy is instituted. This can be difficult because in infants, the P wave often is partially superimposed on the preceding T wave. Several leads should be carefully analyzed for deformation of the T wave by a P wave.

Vagal maneuvers and other methods of converting supraventricular tachycardia will not terminate sinus tachycardia. Vagal maneuvers can briefly slow the rhythm, but because the underlying cause of sinus tachycardia is unaffected by such maneuvers, the rhythm resumes immediately. Therapy should be directed to the likely underlying causes of the sinus tachycardia. The response to such measures could well be diagnostic.

ACCESSORY PATHWAY REENTRANT TACHYCARDIA

Wolff-Parkinson-White syndrome is seen in neonates with structurally normal hearts and those with heart defects. The most common defect is Ebstein malformation of the tricuspid valve; as many as 25% of these patients have an accessory pathway.[12]

Wolff-Parkinson-White syndrome is caused by an accessory pathway electrically connecting the atrial tissue and the ventricular tissue. Neonates with manifest Wolff-Parkinson-White syndrome have a delta wave or other evidence of pre-excitation on a baseline electrocardiogram in sinus rhythm. Neonates with concealed accessory pathways do not have manifest pre-excitation, and anterograde conduction is absent in the accessory pathway. In both cases, orthodromic tachycardia typically is elicited by a premature atrial or ventricular contraction, proceeds with conduction down the AV node and His-Purkinje system, and continues up the accessory pathway to the atria to complete the reentrant circuit. In rare neonates with antidromic tachycardia, the accessory pathway is used for anterograde conduction, and the AV node or a second accessory pathway is used for retrograde conduction.

During orthodromic tachycardia, there is no delta wave. The tachycardia rate is typically 250 to 300 beats per minute in infants. Because of brisk AV conduction, the P waves can fall halfway between the QRS complexes or can be difficult to discern on the T wave (Fig. 45-22). There is little or no variation in the R-R interval, and because the AV node is part of the reentry circuit, AV block always terminates the tachycardia, for at least several beats, although immediate reonset is often seen. If bundle branch block develops during the tachycardia in the same ventricle as the accessory pathway, the ventriculoatrial time lengthens, and the tachycardia rate often slows. In antidromic tachycardia, the ventricle is activated entirely from the accessory pathway so that QRS complexes are wide. P waves can be seen just before the wide QRS complexes.

Differentiation of antidromic tachycardia with bundle branch block from ventricular tachycardia can be clarified by analyzing the relationship between atrial and ventricular activation.

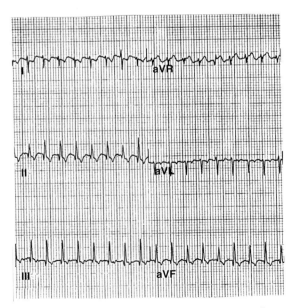

Figure 45–22. Six-lead electrocardiogram in an infant with accessory pathway tachycardia. Note suggestion of P waves superimposed on upstroke of T waves, best seen in lead II.

AV dissociation excludes reentrant tachycardia depending on an accessory pathway in either direction and suggests ventricular or junctional tachycardia.

PERMANENT FORM OF JUNCTIONAL RECIPROCATING TACHYCARDIA

A related form of accessory pathway tachycardia is PJRT. The rhythm is due to a concealed slow-conducting accessory pathway, usually in the posterior-septal region. The slow retrograde accessory pathway conduction makes consistent AV node conduction possible by the time the impulse reaches the atrium through the accessory pathway. Therefore, the tachycardia in PJRT is relatively incessant, or "permanent." Left ventricular dysfunction and even congestive heart failure, believed to be due to chronic tachycardia, have developed in infants with PJRT and persistently high ventricular rates.[9]

In PJRT, the slow retrograde accessory pathway conduction causes the P wave to be located nearer the subsequent QRS complex than the previous one. Spontaneous terminations can occur with block in either the pathway or the AV node; thus, these rhythms can end with either a P wave or a QRS complex. Because of the incessant nature of these rhythms and the location of the P wave, a misdiagnosis of incessant atrial tachycardia or even sinus tachycardia is often made. The P wave axis, however, should be superior (i.e., negative P waves in leads II, III, aVF) rather than inferior, as it would be in sinus tachycardia.

ATRIOVENTRICULAR NODE REENTRANT TACHYCARDIA

AV node reentrant tachycardia (AVNRT) is due to reentry involving dual pathways in the AV node: one fast pathway, generally with a long effective refractory period (ERP), and one slow pathway with a shorter ERP. During normal sinus rhythm, both pathways simultaneously conduct, and the impulse from the fast pathway arrives first in the bundle of His. Tachycardia is initiated when a premature atrial contraction is blocked in the fast, long ERP pathway. It is conducted through the slow pathway, and if the conduction delay is long enough, it allows enough time for the fast pathway to recover and permit retrograde conduction. This establishes the reentrant circuit and tachycardia. In neonates, AVNRT could also be initiated by sudden sinus slowing followed by a junctional escape beat or by a premature ventricular beat.

In the usual form of AVNRT, the reentrant circuit is made up of conduction down the slow pathway and up the fast pathway. Because transit from the distal node up the fast pathway to the atria takes about as long as transit from the distal node to the ventricles, the P waves are superimposed on the QRS complex and are usually not easily discernible on the surface electrocardiogram. In some children, the P wave might be visible slightly before the QRS complex. The reason is that in children, the fast AV node pathway is fast enough so that it is traversed retrograde more rapidly than the distal conduction system is traversed anterograde. In the typical form of AVNRT, the P wave originates in the low atrial septum at the site of the AV node, and the retrograde conduction produces a superior P wave axis. There is little or no variability in R-R intervals. The tachycardia starts and terminates suddenly. AV block, occurring spontaneously or induced by vagal maneuvers or medication, should with rare exception terminate the tachycardia. The rhythm could terminate with a P wave or QRS complex, depending on the site of block.

In the unusual form of AVNRT, conduction is up the slow pathway and down the fast pathway. Because conduction up the slow pathway to the atria takes longer than conduction to the ventricles, the P waves are discernible, usually closer to the subsequent QRS complex than to the previous QRS complex.

In general, AVNRT is thought to be quite rare in neonates, but accessory pathway tachycardia is much more common.

ATRIAL FLUTTER

Atrial flutter results from reentry involving a circuit in a large part of atrial muscle. Atrial flutter rates are as high as 400 to 500 beats per minute in newborn infants, in contrast with older children and adults, who normally have atrial rates of about 300 beats per minute. Atrial flutter can be seen in neonates without associated heart defects and in those with atrial dilation caused by AV valve stenosis or regurgitation.

The neonatal AV node cannot conduct atrial rates of 400 to 500 beats per minute in a 1:1 relationship, and so there is some degree of AV block. If every other atrial beat is conducted, there is 2:1 AV conduction; if every third beat is conducted, there is 3:1 conduction. The degree of AV block can vary, or there could be variable Wenckebach conduction leading to changes in the atrial and ventricular conduction intervals. In neonates with 2:1 conduction, the characteristic sawtooth appearance of flutter waves can be difficult to recognize because of superimposition on the QRS complex and the T waves. Examining multiple leads, especially leads II, III, and aVF, can facilitate the diagnosis. Episodes of increased AV block (spontaneously occurring or induced by vagal maneuvers or medication) do not usually terminate atrial reentrant tachycardias because the AV node is not part of the reentrant circuit. However, such episodes are helpful in making the diagnosis (Fig. 45-23).

The variable R-R intervals resulting from variable AV conduction can mimic the irregular R-R intervals seen in atrial fibrillation and may also cause bundle branch aberration, with some QRS complexes wider than others. Differentiation of atrial flutter from atrial fibrillation can be aided by analysis of the atrial electrocardiogram recorded from an esophageal lead or from atrial temporary pacing wires. Atrial flutter starts suddenly, stops suddenly, and ends with a QRS complex rather than a P wave, because AV block is not necessary for termination.

ATRIAL ECTOPIC TACHYCARDIA

The mechanism of AET likely involves a site with abnormal automaticity somewhere in the right or left atrium. Atrial rates range from slightly faster than normal sinus rates up to 300 beats per minute. Although neonates with AET occasionally have symptoms, this rhythm is more often incessant and causes symptoms only after weeks or months of accelerated ventricular rates. Congestive heart failure develops because of dilated cardiomyopathy. This constellation is termed *tachycardia-induced cardiomyopathy*, and it is believed that the sustained ventricular rates are directly responsible for the myocardial damage. Neonates with symptomatic AET might have had fetal tachycardia, and AET is one mechanism for nonimmune hydrops fetalis.

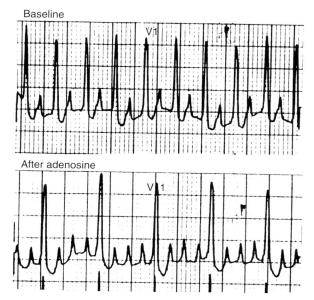

Figure 45-23. Atrial flutter in newborn infant. *Top,* P waves are not clearly discernible. *Bottom,* After administration of adenosine intravenously, flutter waves with rate of 400 beats/min are easily seen.

The most important characteristics of AET are an abnormal P wave axis and morphologic features together with an accelerated rate. Often the PR interval is prolonged, and episodes of Wenckebach conduction can occur. The continuation of the tachycardia despite AV block strongly suggests that the mechanism does not involve the AV node. In an infant with dilated cardiomyopathy and any degree of tachycardia, the P waves must be carefully examined to determine whether they are sinus or ectopic waves. This can be a difficult task, particularly when rapid rates cause superimposition of P waves on T waves. In this case, waiting for a spontaneous Wenckebach cycle or administering adenosine to produce transient AV block allows examination of a nonsuperimposed P wave. The location of the atrial focus can then be predicted on the basis of the P wave axis. For example, P waves that are inverted in leads I and aVL would predict a left atrial location.

JUNCTIONAL ECTOPIC TACHYCARDIA

The mechanism of JET is believed to involve a small focus within the AV node or bundle of His exhibiting abnormal automaticity. As with AET, these rhythms are often incessant, and although they might be well tolerated hemodynamically in the short term, they can lead to cardiomyopathy if not well controlled. They can also manifest in the newborn infant as nonimmune hydrops fetalis. The congenital form of JET had a high mortality rate in the era before the availability of catheter ablation.[7,19,20]

The classic electrocardiographic appearance of JET is a narrow QRS tachycardia with AV dissociation and capture beats (Fig. 45-24). The ventricular rate is faster than the atrial rate, often as fast as 300 beats per minute. AV dissociation is due to lack of retrograde conduction from the junctional focus back to the atrium. Capture beats are caused by

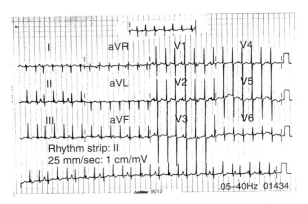

Figure 45–24. Twelve-lead electrocardiogram of infant with congenital junctional ectopic tachycardia. Note easily seen atrioventricular dissociation. *(From Van Hare GF, et al: Successful transcatheter ablation of congenital junctional ectopic tachycardia in a ten-month-old infant using radiofrequency energy, Pacing Clin Electrophysiol 13:730, 1990.)*

dissociated sinus beats that periodically occur at a time when anterograde AV nodal conduction is possible. The R-R interval shortens suddenly, and the QRS complex of the capture beat is no narrower than the QRS complex during tachycardia.

Occasionally, JET can be seen in which retrograde conduction is intact. In such patients, there are no AV dissociation or capture beats, which makes the diagnosis more challenging. Burst esophageal pacing or adenosine infusion can be used to produce brief episodes of AV block, facilitating the diagnosis.

VENTRICULAR TACHYCARDIA

Neonates with idiopathic incessant or paroxysmal ventricular tachycardia typically have structurally normal hearts. Infants with incessant tachycardia and rapid rates have signs of congestive heart failure at presentation. The paroxysmal form of ventricular tachycardia seen in neonates is usually better described as ventricular accelerated rhythm because the rates are only slightly faster than sinus rhythm. This rhythm usually resolves spontaneously within several

months or years.[18] Infants with the long QT syndrome occasionally have episodes of torsades de pointes in the newborn period (Fig. 45-25).

Ventricular tachycardia is recognized from wide QRS complexes, AV dissociation, and capture beats (Fig. 45-26). Unlike JET, in which the capture beats are no narrower than the tachycardia beats, in ventricular tachycardia the capture beats should be narrower than the tachycardia beats, often with a normal QRS duration and morphologic picture. The reason is that the capture beat is a random sinus beat that finds the AV conducting system no longer refractory. It conducts down the conducting system normally, narrowing the QRS. In infants, however, AV dissociation might not be seen because ventriculoatrial conduction is often present. Moreover, because sustained bundle branch aberration is rarely seen in infants with supraventricular tachycardia, many or most wide QRS tachycardias that one encounters in this age group are due to ventricular tachycardia.

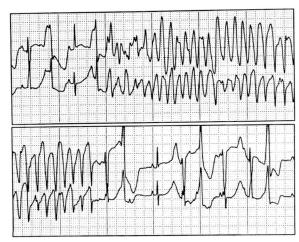

Figure 45–25. Torsades de pointes in infant with long QT syndrome who had an irregular heart rate in the delivery room. *(From Van Hare GF, et al: Successful transcatheter ablation of congenital junctional ectopic tachycardia in a ten-month-old infant using radiofrequency energy, Pacing Clin Electrophysiol 13:730, 1990.)*

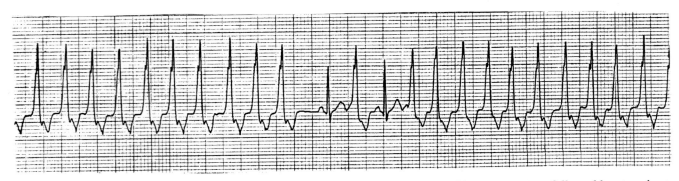

Figure 45–26. Ventricular tachycardia at rate of 230 beats/min in an infant. Note sudden termination, followed by sinus beat, followed by immediate reinitiation.

MECHANISMS OF BRADYCARDIA
Specific Mechanisms
SINUS BRADYCARDIA

Newborn infants are thought to have incomplete sympathetic cardiac innervation and are predominantly vagally innervated. As a result of this autonomic imbalance, episodic sinus bradycardia is fairly common. Sinus bradycardia is recognized as a regular slow atrial rate with normal P waves and 1:1 conduction. Pathologic causes of sinus bradycardia include hypoxia, acidosis, increased intracranial pressure, abdominal distention, and hypoglycemia. Drugs such as digoxin and propranolol can also cause significant sinus bradycardia. Episodic bradycardia often accompanies apnea of prematurity (see also Chapter 44).

SECOND-DEGREE ATRIOVENTRICULAR BLOCK

Second-degree AV block is classified as either Mobitz type 1 (Wenckebach) or Mobitz type 2. Wenckebach conduction is characterized by progressive prolongation of the PR interval, which eventually results in a single blocked atrial beat. Wenckebach conduction is caused by block in the AV node, and it can usually be reversed with catecholamines or with vagolytic agents. Type 2 block lacks the characteristic progressive PR prolongation with shortening after the blocked beat seen in Wenckebach conduction. It is usually not reversible with medication. Type 1 second-degree AV block generally has a better prognosis than type 2. One specific form of second-degree block requires immediate attention: the form of 2:1 conduction seen in infants with markedly prolonged QR intervals. Two-to-one conduction in such infants is an important risk factor for the development of torsades de pointes and sudden death.

COMPLETE ATRIOVENTRICULAR BLOCK

Complete AV block can be congenital, surgically induced, or acquired, for example, after myocarditis. It is due to complete block of conduction either in the AV node or in the distal (His-Purkinje) system. It is recognized as AV dissociation with regular R-R intervals and regular P-P intervals. The atrial rate is usually greater than the ventricular rate, and P waves that occur well after the T wave have no effect on the R-R interval. Congenital AV block can be associated with maternal lupus (see Part 2 of this chapter and Chapter 18), ventricular inversion, and mutations in the NKX2.5 gene.[5]

Miscellaneous Causes

Other causes of bradycardia are sinus exit block, in which sinus P waves intermittently disappear because impulses leaving the region of the node are blocked, and frequent premature atrial contractions, which occur too early to be conducted to the ventricles and therefore slow the resulting ventricular rate.

CAUSES OF PREMATURE BEATS

The new onset of frequent premature beats often is the clue to underlying conditions such as toxic effects of digoxin or other drugs, myocarditis, hypoxia, hypokalemia, hypercapnia, or acidosis.

Supraventricular Premature Contractions

Supraventricular premature contractions are caused by a focus in the right atrium, left atrium, or proximal AV node that depolarizes before the sinus node. Those that originate in the atrium produce a premature P wave that is superimposed on and deforms the previous T wave. This sign can be subtle, however, and requires examination of multiple leads. The premature P wave is followed by a premature narrow QRS beat. Supraventricular premature contractions can also have wide QRS complexes because of a bundle branch aberration. In these babies, the observation of a preceding premature P wave is essential for differentiating an aberrant beat from a ventricular premature contraction. Premature atrial contractions are fairly common in newborn infants and are benign in the absence of structural cardiac disease or other illnesses.

Ventricular Premature Contractions

Ventricular premature contractions occur from a ventricular focus that depolarizes before the atrial beat is conducted through the AV node. They are wide premature beats without a preceding early P wave. Differentiating between ventricular contractions and aberrantly conducted supraventricular contractions is sometimes difficult or impossible from the surface electrocardiogram. Although, traditionally, premature ventricular beats can be differentiated from supraventricular beats by the presence of a full compensatory pause, this sign is somewhat unreliable in children. Fusion beats, in which a sinus beat occurs simultaneously with a premature beat, thus creating an intermediate morphologic picture, help to establish the premature beat as ventricular in origin. When premature ventricular beats are identified in a newborn infant, a careful search for structural or functional cardiac disease is required, together with an evaluation to rule out electrolyte disorders.

INITIAL MANAGEMENT OF TACHYCARDIA
Severity Assessment

When an infant is first found to have a cardiac arrhythmia, the physician should immediately make an assessment of the hemodynamic condition. Some arrhythmias require emergency therapy (electrical cardioversion, pacing), whereas others are less urgent and allow more time for evaluation and electrocardiographic analysis before therapy is instituted. Infants can be free of symptoms, can have mild symptoms, or can be seriously ill or critically ill at first identification.

SYMPTOM-FREE OR MILDLY AFFECTED INFANTS

It is not unusual for infants with moderate or short episodes of tachycardia to be completely free of symptoms during the arrhythmia. These cases are detected on routine examination or are noticed by nurses or parents. The decision to treat the child depends on the presence of structural heart disease, Wolff-Parkinson-White syndrome, and other factors. Some symptom-free neonates do not require short- or long-term treatment. In other cases, episodes are notable by a change in activity on the part of the infant when no respiratory distress or other signs of compromise are present. In these cases or when there is an increased risk for prolonged arrhythmia, long-term treatment is necessary (Tables 45-10 and 45-11).

SERIOUSLY ILL INFANTS

When major symptoms develop in a neonate, emergency treatment is required. The time required to develop congestive heart failure varies according to age, heart rate, and the presence or absence of structural heart disease. Newborn infants can tolerate rates of 300 beats per minute and higher for many hours before signs of congestive heart failure develop. In children with structural heart disease, particularly with significant cyanosis, chronic congestive heart failure, or significant valvular obstruction, tachycardia is usually poorly tolerated.

The seriously ill infant might be fretful and irritable, sweaty, pale, and tachypneic and could be feeding poorly. The liver might be enlarged, with a prominent left lobe. Infants rarely manifest pulmonary edema with rales on auscultation of the chest but might have wheezing and appear to be having primarily a pulmonary problem. Cardiac auscultation might reveal an abnormally fast heart rate, often with a gallop rhythm.

Further evaluation should include questioning of the parents for a history of heart disease, arrhythmias, antiarrhythmic or other medications, and allergies to medications. A chest radiograph might reveal cardiomegaly, and pulmonary venous congestion.

CRITICALLY ILL INFANTS

Heart rates sufficiently fast or slow can result in critically low blood pressure, nonpalpable pulses, altered sensorium, complete loss of consciousness. Although seriously ill patients are generally stable enough to tolerate a small delay of therapy for gathering information, placing intravenous lines, measuring arterial blood gas tensions, obtaining a complete electrocardiogram, and attempting nonpharmacologic maneuvers, critically ill patients require definitive treatment within 2 or 3 minutes of the onset of the arrhythmia. If there will be any delay before electrical cardioversion or the institution of pacing, cardiopulmonary resuscitation or mechanical support required to support the circulation.

Rapid Classification of Abnormal Tachycardia

After assessing the hemodynamic status of the neonate with tachycardia, the rhythm is classified as either a wide or narrow QRS tachycardia. A narrow QRS tachycardia has a QRS duration similar to that during normal sinus rhythm or is in the normal range for age. The QRS duration in wide-complex tachycardia is significantly longer than the duration in normal sinus rhythm, or longer than the 95th percentile for age. Nearly all narrow QRS tachycardias in infants are supraventricular in origin, and most wide QRS tachycardias are ventricular in origin.

Any form of narrow QRS tachycardia could manifest *aberration*, defined as widening of the QRS complex. Aberration is usually due to rate-dependent bundle branch block. The onset of aberration can be progressive, and once established, aberration can persist until termination. Because widening of the QRS complex results from rate-dependent bundle branch block, it usually resembles a right or left pattern of bundle branch block.

Aberration with supraventricular tachycardia often occurs at the onset of the tachycardia in the absence of preexisting bundle branch block, but sustained bundle branch aberration

TABLE 45–10 Intravenous Antiarrhythmic Agents

Agent	Dosage	Comments
Esmolol	50-500 micrograms/kg/min	Monitor pulse, blood pressure Contraindicated in congestive heart failure Do not give with verapamil
Procainamide	10-15 mg/kg IV over 30-45 min	Can cause hypotension Continuous blood pressure monitoring is essential
Digoxin	10 micrograms/kg IV as initial load; second dose in 6 hr and third at 24 hr	Do not use in hypokalemia or if toxic reaction to digoxin is suspected
Lidocaine	1-2 mg/kg IV over 15 min; continuous infusion of 30-50 micrograms/kg/min	
Phenylephrine	20 micrograms/kg IV slowly	Used for raising blood pressure and eliciting a baroreceptor vagal reflex
Adenosine	Start IV dose of 100 micrograms/kg; double dose repeatedly until effect is seen, to maximum of 400 micrograms/kg	Contraindicated in preexisting second- and third-degree AV block without pacemaker Use with caution in severe asthma; half-life is 10 sec in serum Occasionally induces atrial fibrillation
Amiodarone	5 mg/kg IV over 15-30 min or as 5 separate 1 mg/kg aliquots	Given by central line diluted in D_5W Can cause gasping syndrome in infants due to benzyl alcohol Continuous infusion probably should not be used in infants

IV, intravenously.

TABLE 45–11   Oral Antiarrhythmic Agents

Agent	Dosage	Comments
Propranolol	0.25-1 mg/kg PO every 6 hr	Observe for wheezing and symptoms of hypoglycemia
Atenolol	0.5-2 mg/kg/day PO divided every 12 hr	
Procainamide	50-100 mg/kg/day PO divided every 8 hr	Monitor both procainamide and NAPA levels
Quinidine sulfate	30-60 mg/kg/day PO divided every 6 hr	
Flecainide	50-200 mg/m²/day PO divided every 12 hr or 6.7-9.5 mg/kg/day divided every 8 hr	Flecainide levels >1.0 micrograms/mL correlate with toxic effects
Mexiletine	1.4-5.1 mg/kg PO every 8 hr	
Digoxin	10 micrograms/kg PO as initial load. Second dose in 6 hr, third in 24 hr; reduce dosage in premature infants	Do not use in hypokalemia or if digoxin toxic reaction is suspected
Amiodarone	5 mg/kg PO bid × 2 wk, then 2.5 mg/kg PO bid	Monitor thyroid and pulmonary function
Sotalol	2-8 mg/kg/day PO divided every 8 hr	Torsades de pointes is likely with hypokalemia

bid, twice a day; NAPA, N-acetylprocainamide; PO, orally.

with supraventricular tachycardia is rare in infants. Therefore, most wide QRS tachycardias in infants are due to ventricular tachycardia.

Therapeutic Options

The therapeutic options are listed in Box 45-14.

General Acute Therapeutic Approach
NARROW QRS TACHYCARDIA

For critically ill infants with any form of narrow QRS tachycardia, synchronized electrical cardioversion is indicated. For seriously ill infants, in whom there can be signs of congestive heart failure but who have a measurable blood pressure and are conscious, the clinician must judge the stability of the patient's hemodynamic status. If the status is unstable, the patient should have electrical cardioversion after placement of an intravenous line. More stable patients are managed by means of vagal maneuvers followed by adenosine, with electrical cardioversion as an option if these measures fail (Box 45-15).

WIDE QRS TACHYCARDIA

Most infants with wide QRS tachycardia have ventricular tachycardia rather than supraventricular tachycardia with an aberration. Because it may be nearly impossible to differentiate these possibilities in neonates with only a surface electrocardiogram, patients with wide QRS tachycardia are treated as if they have ventricular tachycardia. In practice, this means that electrical cardioversion is indicated in most cases.

In patients who are not seriously or critically ill, one can defer cardioversion while pharmacologic agents are administered. In this situation, procainamide would be a good choice because it is effective both for ventricular and supraventricular arrhythmias. Lidocaine can be used if the diagnosis of ventricular tachycardia is certain.

For infants with few or no symptoms, beta blockers such as propranolol are often effective. Propranolol should be used with great care; however, if tachycardia is not controlled by propranolol, the hypotension and poor cardiac contractility that can be produced by propranolol will be poorly tolerated in the presence of continuing tachycardia.

Infants in whom the long QT syndrome with polymorphous ventricular tachycardia (torsades de pointes) is suspected should not receive procainamide or lidocaine. They should instead receive propranolol, possibly intravenously, with the possible addition of temporary ventricular pacing, particularly if they also manifest episodes of second-degree AV block.

Therapy for Specific Tachyarrhythmias
ATRIAL FLUTTER

Therapy can be directed toward converting the tachycardia to sinus rhythm or toward limiting the ventricular response. Vagal maneuvers can be successful in converting the rhythm but can also be useful diagnostically by causing a short episode of AV block without terminating the tachycardia and revealing the underlying flutter waves. Digoxin, propranolol, or esmolol can be used to slow the ventricular response and can also assist in converting the tachycardia.

Procainamide can be effective in converting the tachycardia, but there is a chance of slowing the atrial rate without converting the rhythm. If the faster atrial rate was associated with variable AV conduction, the slower rate can allow 1:1 AV conduction, paradoxically increasing the ventricular rate. For this reason, procainamide should be used only after a drug that limits AV conduction, such as digoxin, is given.

If tachycardia conversion is necessary immediately, the first choice is esophageal atrial overdrive pacing. This method is effective, particularly in small children, and does not require anesthesia. In postoperative cardiac surgery patients,

BOX 45–14   Therapeutic Options for Tachycardia

VAGAL MANEUVERS

Use with IV line in place; do not continue for more than 5 minutes in seriously ill infants before trying other modalities.

Elicit gag with nasogastric tube.

Elicit diving reflex by placing a bag filled with ice over the face and ears for 15 seconds.

Do not perform carotid massage or apply orbital pressure.

ADENOSINE

Used for supraventricular tachycardias that involve the AV node as part of reentrant circuit.[14]

Give by rapid IV injection; onset of effect seen in 7 or 8 seconds, half-life in blood is less than 10 seconds; AV blockade is brief. Do not give by umbilical artery.

If conversion is successful, provides evidence against other forms of tachycardia.

Transient AV block can reveal flutter waves in atrial flutter, so diagnosis can be made.

Caution: Adenosine is a negative inotrope, but this factor is rarely a problem.

DIGOXIN

Effective for most neonatal narrow QRS tachycardias.

Disadvantage is a relatively long period needed to achieve therapeutic drug levels safely.

Do not give if baby has hypokalemia or if toxic reaction to digoxin is suspected.

Give with care if renal failure is suspected (excretion of digoxin entirely renal); acts by slowing sinus node, lengthening PR interval.

Only antiarrhythmic drug that improves contractility.

CLASS I AGENTS (SODIUM CHANNEL BLOCKERS)

Procainamide

Effective in atrial arrhythmias and in some AV reciprocating tachycardias or AV node reentrant tachycardias.

Give IV or PO; hypotension is common with loading dose.

Drug levels correlate with efficacy.

Measure both procainamide and *N*-acetylprocainamide.

Can cause negative inotropic effects and lupus-like syndrome.

Quinidine

Similar electrophysiologic effect to procainamide, less effect on contractility.

Do not give intravenously; diarrhea is most common side effect in infants.

Quinidine and Procainamide

In atrial flutter, fibrillation, or atrial ectopic tachycardia, both agents slow atrial rate but shorten AV node refractory period, increasing ventricular rate by decreasing block at AV node.

Best to give digoxin or propranolol before procainamide or quinidine therapy in such patients.

Both prolong QT interval and should not be given to infants with long QT syndrome.

Effect is additive with several drugs, including erythromycin.

Other signs of toxic effects with both are prolongation of PR interval and QRS duration.

Mexiletine and Lidocaine

Both drugs shorten QT interval but have no effect on sinus rates and conduction.

Mexiletine is given PO and lidocaine is given IV.

Flecainide

Limited use in children because adult trials showed excessive mortality rate when used for ventricular arrhythmias.

Not considered arrhythmogenic in children with structurally normal hearts; has been used to treat atrial arrhythmias.[10]

Drug is a negative inotrope; slows sinus node and prolongs PR interval.

Propafenone

Used for junctional ectopic tachycardia and other refractory atrial tachycardias.[13]

Shares similar hemodynamic and electrophysiologic characteristics with other type I agents but tends to slow sinus rate.

CLASS II AGENTS (BETA BLOCKERS)

Propranolol

Limited side effects; decreased contractility, hypoglycemia, asthma, and fatigue seen in older children.

Atenolol

Little experience in very young children. Might have fewer central nervous system side effects than propranolol.

Half-life longer than propranolol in adults, shorter in young children; twice-daily dosing could be required.

Both Agents

Negative inotropes; slow sinus node and prolonged PR interval.

CLASS III AGENTS (POTASSIUM CHANNEL BLOCKERS)

Sotalol

Has both class III and beta-blocking properties.

Given orally.

Effective in atrial arrhythmias in children.[3,16]

Amiodarone

Long used in Europe.[6]

Used in refractory atrial arrhythmias.

IV loading followed by oral administration overcomes long time required for oral loading.

If used IV, has additional beta-blocking and calcium channel blocking properties.

Sotalol and Amiodarone

Increase PR interval and QRS duration and slow sinus node.

CLASS IV AGENTS (CALCIUM CHANNEL BLOCKERS)

Verapamil

IV form never given to infants (causes hypotension and asystolic cardiac arrests in those <6 months of age).

Oral form is used in atrial flutter.

Has negative inotropic effects, slows sinus nodes, and prolongs PR interval.

ESOPHAGEAL AND TRANSVENOUS ATRIAL PACING

Works well in neonatal period.[4]

Brief atrial overdrive pacing at rate higher than tachycardia might allow termination of atrial tachycardias, including atrial flutter.

BOX 45-14 Therapeutic Options for Tachycardia—cont'd

Transvenous
Place sheath in large vein (femoral, internal jugular, or subclavian) and direct bipolar pacing catheter to right atrium or right ventricle.

Esophageal
Position esophageal lead behind left atrium for pacing; use pulse generators that generate long pulse widths (at lest 10 msec) because outputs required for capture at conventional pulse widths (>2 msec) are very uncomfortable for the infant.

Using Fluoroscopy
With pacing leads connected to external pulse generator, select rate, turn on generator, and increase output until capture is achieved.

ELECTRICAL CARDIOVERSION
Used rarely in newborn infants.
Cardioverter-defibrillator must deliver very low amplitude shocks and have small paddles (those used for direct delivery to epicardial surface of heart in older patients intraoperatively are appropriate).
Initial dose is 0.5-1.0 J/kg.
Converts narrow QRS tachycardias in synchronous mode to avoid delivery on T wave.

Perform defibrillation for ventricular fibrillation in asynchronous mode.
With wide QRS tachycardias in synchronous mode to avoid delivery on T wave.
Perform defibrillation for ventricular fibrillation in asynchronous mode.
With wide QRS tachycardias, initially use synchronous mode; some forms of ventricular tachycardia appear almost sinusoidal, and cardioverter-defibrillator might not sense R wave well. Therefore, use of asynchronous mode might be needed.
No specific precautions are needed with therapeutic doses of digoxin, but with high levels of toxic reaction to digoxin, give initial bolus of lidocaine, 1 mg/kg IV, before cardioversion.

TRANSCATHETER ABLATION
Treatment of choice for many atrial tachycardias in children and adults with symptoms.
In very young children, concerns involve depth of scar, growth of scar over time, and risk for injury to adjacent structures (see discussion of accessory pathway reentrant tachycardia).

BOX 45-15 Treatment of Supraventricular Tachycardia

ACUTE CONDITIONS
Critically Ill Infants
Synchronized cardioversion, 0.5 J/kg

All Others
Electrocardiographic monitoring and IV access
Vagal maneuvers
Nasogastric stimulation
Ice to face for 30 sec
Adenosine, 100 micrograms/kg, given by rapid IV infusion (not in umbilical artery)
Repeat 200 micrograms/kg and then give 400 micrograms/kg if no effect
Esophageal pacing, atrial pacing, or cardioversion

CHRONIC CONDITION
For infants with Wolff-Parkinson-White syndrome or if status is unknown: propranolol, 0.5 mg/kg PO every 6 hr
For infants with no documented accessory pathway: digoxin, 5 micrograms/kg PO every 12 hr after initial load

IV, intravenous; PO, orally.

include flecainide, given two or three times a day,[10] or propafenone, given three times a day.[13]

When atrial flutter occurs in the newborn period, it often disappears within the first 6 months of life.[4] Although traditionally such infants have been treated for 1 year with digoxin, there is evidence that they can be successfully followed without medication after initial conversion.

ATRIOVENTRICULAR NODE REENTRANT TACHYCARDIA

Short-term treatment of AVNRT is directed at achieving a brief episode of AV block. Neonates might respond to vagal maneuvers or rectal stimulation. If vagal measures fail, our first choice of medication is intravenously administered adenosine. Intravenous administration of esmolol or digoxin might also be effective. Esophageal or intracardiac atrial overdrive pacing is effective. Neonates with refractory AVNRT also respond to electrical synchronous cardioversion.

Long-term management is directed at changing conduction through the slow AV nodal pathway. Oral digoxin or propranolol might be effective. AV node modification with radiofrequency energy or by cryoablation is possible but is rarely employed in the neonate.

The natural history of this condition in infants is unknown, but the condition may well disappear with time. Therefore, it is reasonable to treat such infants with antiarrhythmic medications for several years with the hope of avoiding transcatheter ablation.

ACCESSORY PATHWAY REENTRANT TACHYCARDIA

As in AVNRT, acute treatment can be directed at either the antegrade AV node conduction or the retrograde accessory pathway conduction. Vagal maneuvers or drugs such

temporary atrial pacing wires can be used. If this method fails or is not available, electrical cardioversion with deep sedation or anesthesia will be effective.

For long-term treatment, the first choice is digoxin or propranolol orally. If therapy with one of these drugs fails, one can add sotalol, given three times a day.[3,16] Other choices as adenosine,[14] digoxin, or propranolol can be used to affect the antegrade limb of the reentrant circuit. The retrograde accessory pathway conduction can be affected by procainamide or flecainide.[10] Esophageal pacing is effective in terminating an episode, either by atrial overdrive or extrastimulation, and is the second choice when available and when vagal maneuvers fail. Electrical cardioversion is also effective.

Long-term management depends on the severity of the problem and the frequency of the attacks. For infants with rare, mildly symptomatic attacks of supraventricular tachycardia that are easily terminated, we advise no treatment at all. Infants with more frequent or symptomatic attacks are treated initially with beta blockers. Digoxin is used only if there is no evidence of pre-excitation in sinus rhythm. About one third of adults with pre-excitation treated with digoxin have a shortening of the anterograde ERP of the accessory pathway, which could be dangerous if atrial fibrillation develops. Although atrial fibrillation is uncommon in infants and digoxin has been used for years in the treatment of children with pre-excitation, with few if any documented problems, some reports suggest the possibility of sudden death in infants treated with digoxin.[8]

Transcatheter ablation of the accessory pathway is increasingly being used as first-line therapy in children, but its use in infants is still limited.[11] The reason is the concern of complications such as perforation, AV block, and damage or occlusion of major coronary arteries. In addition, the natural history of accessory pathway tachycardia in infancy is favorable: 75% to 90% of such infants have spontaneous resolution of tachycardia by 12 months of age.[15] Ablation is reserved for life-threatening, medically refractory cases.[1] Often, the patients have PJRT and dramatically compromised left ventricular function.

PERMANENT FORM OF JUNCTIONAL RECIPROCATING TACHYCARDIA

Treatment of children with PJRT is often challenging. In addition to the techniques and drugs used for infants with Wolff-Parkinson-White syndrome, amiodarone is often effective, and spontaneous resolution is occasionally observed.[17]

ATRIAL ECTOPIC TACHYCARDIA

Treatment of AET is difficult, and rate control might be the only achievable therapy. The atrial focus could be slowed by beta blockers, flecainide, or propafenone or by class III agents such as sotalol and amiodarone. The goal of treatment is to protect the patient from the subsequent development of tachycardia-induced cardiomyopathy. Definitive intervention for cure of tachycardia, either by radiofrequency ablation or cryoablation or by surgical cryoablation, should be done at the earliest signs of poor cardiac function shown by echocardiography.[21]

JUNCTIONAL ECTOPIC TACHYCARDIA

The pharmacologic approach to AET can also be effective in the treatment of JET. Although no agent is reliably effective in treating this arrhythmia, amiodarone is often effective. In selected patients, transcatheter ablation has been employed to eliminate the junctional focus. In very small infants, because of the proximity of the JET focus to the AV node, there is a risk for causing complete AV block at the time of the ablation, although this risk is likely to be lower with cryoablation. The potential for permanent pacemaker implantation limits the applicability of this technique to the sickest infants who have not responded to all classes of antiarrhythmic agents.[7,19]

Postoperative JET is usually seen in babies with low cardiac output. In this situation, JET could be caused by the poor cardiac output or could be contributing to the hemodynamic compromise. Intravenous amiodarone is widely used in this setting.[6] Surface cooling can slow the junctional rate and allow effective AV sequential pacing. This restores AV synchrony, which often improves the cardiac output.[2] Unlike congenital JET, postoperative JET is transient and resolves as the myocardium recovers.[22]

VENTRICULAR TACHYCARDIA

Pharmacologic suppression of ventricular tachycardia, when it is dependent on catechol stimulation for induction, usually includes the use of moderate to high doses of beta-blocking medications. When the use of esmolol, propranolol, or atenolol is not successful, or when the rhythm is not dependent on catecholamines, class I agents such as mexiletine and flecainide can be used. Class III agents such as sotalol and amiodarone might also be effective. Infants with ventricular accelerated rhythm, however, probably do not require any treatment because the tachycardia rate is not fast enough to produce hemodynamic compromise and because these rhythms usually resolve by several months of age.[18]

TREATMENT OF BRADYARRHYTHMIAS

The hemodynamic effect of a slow heart rate depends on the actual rate and the degree of difference from the baby's usual heart rate. Sudden decreases in rate can be poorly compensated by increases in stroke volume, particularly in neonates with preexisting poor cardiac function. Bradycardia caused by sinus slowing can be induced by hypoxia, vagal stimulation during nasogastric tube placement, or gastroesophageal reflux. Blocked premature atrial beats, when they occur in a bigeminal pattern, cause sustained bradycardia.

Despite episodic rates of 70 beats per minute, this rhythm rarely requires treatment in otherwise normal babies. Congenital complete AV block could require treatment if there is coexisting heart disease or particularly slow ventricular escape rates. Postoperative complete AV block is treated in the acute stage by temporary pacing and, if it persists, by permanent pacing.

If treatment is indicated, initial treatment with atropine, followed by continuous isoproterenol infusion, increases sinus rates, improves AV conduction, and can increase the rate of subsidiary pacemakers. After initial stabilization with medications, temporary transvenous pacing should be instituted, particularly in cases with very low ventricular rates (less than 45 beats per minute in the neonate) and those with hemodynamic compromise. Subsequently, implantation of a permanent pacemaker might be necessary if bradycardia does not improve.

TREATMENT OF PREMATURE BEATS

In the absence of tachycardia, neonates only rarely need treatment for premature beats of any kind. Supraventricular premature contractions virtually never require treatment. Ventricular premature contractions could require treatment in the following situations:

- When they are multiform
- When they occur in couplets or short runs of ventricular tachycardia
- When they are seen in association with a recently converted ventricular tachycardia
- When they exhibit the "R on T" phenomenon (i.e., they fall repeatedly on the early part of the T wave of the preceding beat)

Decisions concerning treatment of premature beats are difficult and should be made in consultation with a cardiologist. As usual, possible inciting factors such as hypoxia and acidosis should be corrected. If ventricular premature contractions require emergency treatment, the agents of choice are lidocaine or amiodarone, given as a bolus followed by a continuous intravenous infusion.

REFERENCES

1. Aiyagari R, et al: Radiofrequency ablation for supraventricular tachycardia in children ≤15 kg is safe and effective, *Pediatr Cardiol* 26:622, 2005.
2. Bash SE, et al: Hypothermia for the treatment of postsurgical greatly accelerated junctional ectopic tachycardia, *J Am Coll Cardiol* 10:1095, 1987.
3. Beaufort-Krol GC, Bink-Boelkens MT: Sotalol for atrial tachycardias after surgery for congenital heart disease, *Pacing Clin Electrophysiol* 20:2125, 1997.
4. Benson DW, et al: Transesophageal cardiac pacing: history, application, technique, *Clin Prog Pacing Electrophys* 2:360, 1984.
5. Benson DW, et al: Mutations in the cardiac transcription factor NKX2.5 affect diverse cardiac developmental pathways, *J Clin Invest* 104:1567, 1999.
6. Bucknall CA, et al: Intravenous and oral amiodarone for arrhythmias in children, *Br Heart J* 56:278, 1986.
7. Collins KK, et al: Pediatric nonpost-operative junctional ectopic tachycardia medical management and interventional therapies, *J Am Coll Cardiol* 53:690, 2009.
8. Deal BJ, et al: Wolff-Parkinson-White syndrome and supraventricular tachycardia during infancy: Management and follow-up, *J Am Coll Cardiol* 5:130, 1985.
9. Dorostkar PC, et al: Clinical course of persistent junctional reciprocating tachycardia, *J Am Coll Cardiol* 33:366, 1999.
10. Fish, FA, et al, for the Pediatric Electrophysiology Group: Proarrhythmia, cardiac arrest, and death in young patients receiving encainide and flecainide, *J Am Coll Cardiol* 18:356, 1991.
11. Kugler JD, et al, for the Pediatric EP Society, Radiofrequency Catheter Ablation Registry: Radiofrequency catheter ablation for paroxysmal supraventricular tachycardia in children and adolescents without structural heart disease, *Am J Cardiol* 80:1438, 1997.
12. Lev M, et al: Ebstein's disease with Wolff-Parkinson-White syndrome, *Am Heart J* 49:724, 1955.
13. Musto B, et al: Electrophysiologic effects and clinical efficacy of propafenone in children with recurrent paroxysmal supraventricular tachycardia, *Circulation* 78:863, 1988.
14. Overholt ED, et al: Usefulness of adenosine for arrhythmias in infants and children, *Am J Cardiol* 61:336, 1988.
15. Perry JC, Garson A: Supraventricular tachycardia due to Wolff-Parkinson-White syndrome in children: early disappearance and late recurrence, *J Am Coll Cardiol* 16:1215, 1990.
16. Tipple M, Sandor G: Efficacy and safety of oral sotalol in early infancy, *Pacing Clin Electrophysiol* 14:2062, 1991.
17. Vaksmann G, et al: Permanent junctional reciprocating tachycardia in children: a multicentre study on clinical profile and outcome, *Heart* 92:101, 2006.
18. Van Hare GF, Stanger P: Ventricular tachycardia and accelerated ventricular rhythm presenting in the first month of life, *Am J Cardiol* 67:42, 1991.
19. Van Hare GF, et al: Successful transcatheter ablation of congenital junctional ectopic tachycardia in a ten-month-old infant using radiofrequency energy, *Pacing Clin Electrophysiol* 13:730, 1990.
20. Villain E, et al: Evolving concepts in the management of congenital junctional ectopic tachycardia: a multicenter study, *Circulation* 81:1544, 1990.
21. Walsh EP, et al: Transcatheter ablation of ectopic atrial tachycardia in young patients using radiofrequency current, *Circulation* 86:1138, 1992.
22. Walsh EP, et al: Evaluation of a staged treatment protocol for rapid automatic junctional tachycardia after operation for congenital heart disease, *J Am Coll Cardiol* 29:1046, 1997.

PART 10

Principles of Medical and Surgical Management

Kenneth G. Zahka and Ernest S. Siwik

GENERAL PRINCIPLES

General principles that apply to the care of critically ill neonates are the basis of medical care of the baby with congenital heart disease. Thermal regulation, nutritional and metabolic derangements, identification and treatment of infections, and the techniques of ventilatory support are discussed in other chapters in detail.

For the baby with congenital heart disease, it is essential that the clinician understand the anatomy, pathophysiology, and natural history of the defect. This guides the decision to start medical or surgical therapy. One goal of therapy may be to modify the anatomy with prostaglandin E_1, interventional catheterization, or surgery. Another goal may be to alter the physiology through changes in heart rate, preload, afterload, or contractility.[3]

After neonatal surgery, a precise knowledge of the type of surgery and the expected changes in the circulation can help predict the baby's needs. Careful serial physical examination and review of available physiologic data make management of the postoperative patient not only safer and effective but also more gratifying. Anticipating problems by evaluating trends in systemic and pulmonary arterial blood pressure, atrial pressures, heart rate, and systemic venous oxygen saturation[60] and thus initiating therapy can improve outcomes. Intraoperative and postoperative echocardiography has greatly added to our ability to assess residual defects and ventricular function. If these data do not answer the question of why a baby is struggling after surgery, cardiac catheterization must be performed with the goal of identifying residual defects or problems that might be amenable to medical therapy or surgery.

Oxygen and Ventilation

Experience with the preoperative and postoperative management of infants with hypoplastic left heart syndrome has raised the awareness of the unique pathophysiology of the child with potentially limited systemic blood flow and exuberant pulmonary blood flow.[66] Preoperatively, the ductus arteriosus is large, and balancing the systemic and pulmonary blood flow requires attention to both the systemic vascular and pulmonary vascular resistance.[5] Therapies that decrease total pulmonary resistance or increase systemic resistance direct an excessive amount of flow to the lungs and steal flow from the systemic circulation. This results in poor systemic perfusion despite a widely patent ductus arteriosus. This is especially deleterious in babies with impaired ventricular function or tricuspid regurgitation. Conversely, pulmonary vasoconstriction or systemic vasodilation limits pulmonary blood flow and increases systemic blood flow. This results in lower systemic arterial oxygen saturation, which, if severe, can compromise tissue oxygen delivery despite good blood flow. In this setting, a highly restrictive atrial septal defect further reduces pulmonary blood flow and limits systemic oxygen delivery.

Babies at risk for excessive pulmonary flow or decreased systemic flow can usually breathe room air unless severe pulmonary edema causes pulmonary venous desaturation. Similarly, hyperventilation with the resultant hypocapnia and alkalosis lowers the pulmonary vascular resistance. Unless there is poor respiratory effort or concern about apneic episodes related to prostaglandin E_1, spontaneous breathing offers the advantage of allowing the infant to achieve normal ventilation. If the infant has undergone intubation and is sedated, the minute ventilation should be adjusted to achieve normal arterial carbon dioxide tension ($PaCO_2$) and pH. In babies with hypoplastic left heart syndrome, atrial septostomy is usually avoided unless the atrial opening is critically small. A modest degree of left atrial hypertension adds to the total pulmonary resistance and limits pulmonary blood flow. There are babies with hypoplastic left heart syndrome for whom this conservative approach is inadequate, and they develop signs of systemic hypoperfusion. In these babies, hypoventilation using mechanical ventilation and muscle relaxants and subambient oxygen levels[66] are important techniques for avoiding hemodynamic instability.

Babies with restricted pulmonary blood flow can be treated with supplemental oxygen without risk but with the recognition that there might be little increment in the arterial oxygen saturation. If there is clinical or echocardiographic evidence that pulmonary hypertension with high pulmonary vascular resistance is causing the reduced pulmonary flow and hypoxia, supplemental oxygen is essential. Further approaches to modulating the pulmonary vascular resistance are discussed in Part 8 under "Persistent Pulmonary Hypertension (Persistent Fetal Circulation)."

Postoperatively, the restriction to pulmonary blood flow provided by a systemic-pulmonary shunt or right ventricle-to-pulmonary artery conduit permits a greater focus on optimizing systemic oxygen delivery through reduction of systemic vascular resistance.[42] Systemic vascular resistance can be modulated by the addition of milrinone or a specific systemic vasodilator such as nitroprusside or phenoxybenzamine. Increasing arterial CO_2 either through permissive hypoventilation or the addition of carbon dioxide to the ventilator circuit drops cerebral vascular resistance and improves oxygen delivery, as evidenced by increased systemic venous saturation, and simultaneously reduces oxygen consumption.[42] Splanchnic blood flow, however, is reduced by this strategy, raising concern that in some neonates there is an increased risk for intestinal ischemia.

Blood

Oxygen delivery to the tissues is dependent on adequate hemoglobin concentration. Anemia causes a higher cardiac output to maintain oxygen delivery. If the infant is unable to produce an increased cardiac output, increased oxygen extraction leads to lower systemic venous oxygen saturation. For the neonate with a normal arterial oxygen saturation and adequate cardiac output, mild anemia is well tolerated. For the baby with severe hypoxia or poor cardiac output, anemia impairs oxygen delivery because increased extraction might not be possible or because it taxes the fragile cardiovascular reserve.

With recognition of the risks of blood transfusion, it is prudent to use all means to minimize blood loss and maximize erythropoiesis. Transfusion to maintain a hematocrit of at least 40% for babies with significant cyanosis or with impaired cardiac output should be considered when clinical symptoms are evident. The clinician might need to take special precautions to avoid volume overload in babies with congestive heart failure, prolonging either the transfusion or giving concomitant diuretics. Radiation of the blood is essential for any baby in whom the DiGeorge syndrome is suspected.

Prostaglandin E_1

Neonates who are expected to fit one of the categories in which ductal dependence is likely or who are known from fetal studies to be ductal dependent should begin prostaglandin E_1 therapy immediately.[23] In general, the more severe the cyanosis or the systemic hypoperfusion, the more urgent the administration of prostaglandin E_1. If there is some doubt about the proper category and the infant is ill with respiratory distress, it is reasonable to begin treatment with prostaglandin E_1 while further evaluation is undertaken.

The response of the ductus arteriosus to prostaglandin E_1 is related to the time since spontaneous closure. Cyanosis in newborn infants is usually recognized shortly after ductal closure; therefore, the infants respond well to prostaglandin E_1. Babies with cyanosis beginning at several weeks of age should not be assumed to be unresponsive to prostaglandin E_1. It is possible that the ductus arteriosus had recently closed, and thus it may well respond to prostaglandin E_1.

Babies with coarctation of the aorta might be able to survive for several days with marginal blood flow through the obstruction before they are recognized to be in trouble. Although they might respond to prostaglandin E_1, they have the highest likelihood of not responding and of needing urgent surgery.

Prostaglandin E_1 is administered intravenously through a peripheral vein or central venous catheter. The initial studies also include umbilical artery administration with no apparent adverse effects.[23] The initial dose is 0.05 μg/kg per minute, and this can be decreased to 0.03 μg/kg per minute once an effect is seen. The principal side effect of short-term administration of prostaglandin E_1 is apnea, which is most frequent in premature infants and at the higher doses but can occur in full-term infants. Apnea can occur several hours after the start of prostaglandin E_1 administration. Doses as low as 0.01 μg/kg per minute can be effective and tend to decrease the risk of apnea.[38] Depending on the type of transport, elective intubation before transport might be advisable. Other dose-dependent, short-term side effects include skin flushing and fever.

Long-term administration of prostaglandin E_1 could be required for the neonate with other medical problems or for the premature baby. Oral administration of prostaglandin E_2 has been used with some success; however, intravenous administration of prostaglandin E_1 is the more reliable treatment. Long-term side effects include periosteal thickening,[75] which can cause painful swelling of the hands and feet and can be seen in the ribs on chest radiographs. There are also reports of a higher prevalence of pyloric stenosis in babies who have received long-term treatment with prostaglandin E_1.[55]

Heart Rate

The importance of heart rate and rhythm as a determinant of myocardial performance must be decided clinically. The neonate with congenital complete atrioventricular (AV) block might be well, and the postoperative neonate with a comparable rate and rhythm might need pacing. Similarly, supraventricular tachycardia that is tolerated by the normal neonate for at least 24 hours causes low output and low blood pressure in a postoperative baby. Details of the evaluation and treatment of arrhythmias, including those seen after cardiac surgery, are discussed in Part 9.

Preload

The clinical assessment of preload is indirect and includes serial measurement of body weight, liver size, and tissue fluid. Unfortunately, these parameters might not reflect the quantity of intravascular fluid. Atrial and ventricular end-diastolic pressures are more quantitative but are also affected by ventricular diastolic function and AV and semilunar valve function. Because

the goal is to produce an adequate cardiac output and blood pressure, the preload that is needed is also determined by ventricular contractility and afterload. In clinical practice, if the baby is well perfused and has good blood pressure and urine output, preload is adequate. If the lungs are clear and there is no evidence of pleural fluid or ascites, fluid overload is not present.

Several specific fluid issues apply to the postoperative neonate. After cardiopulmonary bypass, even with the current techniques of ultrafiltration when bypass is being terminated, total body fluid is increased. Routine daily fluid administration should be less than calculated maintenance. This could require concentration of medications or hyperalimentation or, in the days after surgery, enteral feedings. Blood losses should be replaced to maintain the hematocrit, and coagulopathies should be corrected with fresh frozen plasma or platelets as indicated. If perfusion, blood pressure, or urine output is reduced, the role of hypovolemia should be assessed by analysis of fluid balance and atrial pressures. Low atrial pressures or atrial pressures that have been falling are the best sign that intravascular volume is depleted. Fluid administration helps improve the cardiac output in a baby with impaired contractility; however, it usually is at the cost of increased body fluid and does not address the fundamental physiologic problem.

Diuretics are commonly used to improve fluid balance in the preoperative and postoperative neonate. Tachypnea, hepatomegaly, inappropriate weight gain, or pulmonary edema on a chest radiograph are typical signs of fluid overload requiring treatment with oral or intravenous diuretics. Depending on the degree of physiologic impairment, furosemide and bumetanide, each used alone or in combination with chlorothiazide, are the most commonly used diuretics. Oral metolazone has been used to manage chronic fluid retention. The addition of spironolactone, a potassium-sparing diuretic, or potassium chloride supplements is important in treating the inevitable hypokalemic, hypochloremic alkalosis that results from long-term diuretic therapy.

Afterload

Systemic arterial afterload reduction has become an important short- and long-term treatment for ventricular dysfunction or AV valve regurgitation.[3,27] The clearest indication for afterload reduction is the combination of normal blood pressure, normal filling pressures, and poor peripheral perfusion in the postoperative baby. Selective intravenously administered vasodilators, such as nitroprusside, have the advantage of very short duration of action and dosing titrated to effect. Dobutamine has both short-acting inotropic and vasodilator properties. Amrinone and milrinone have excellent and longer-acting inotropic and vasodilator effects. Of all the orally administered agents, captopril is still the most commonly used in neonates. Renal function and potassium levels must be monitored, especially in babies with poor renal perfusion. Pulmonary vasodilators are discussed in Part 8 under "Persistent Pulmonary Hypertension (Persistent Fetal Circulation)." In the postoperative baby, recognition and management of pulmonary hypertension is often facilitated by pulmonary artery monitoring lines, which permit assessment of the response to therapy.

Systemic afterload augmentation is rarely needed in the neonate. Treatment of cyanotic spells before surgery or decreased arterial saturation after a systemic-to-pulmonary shunt can include increasing the systemic vascular resistance with phenylephrine. By changing the relative systemic and pulmonary resistance, more flow is directed through the shunt or pulmonary valve. Similarly, increasing the pulmonary vascular resistance by decreasing the inspired oxygen, while avoiding hyperventilation or bleeding carbon dioxide into the ventilator circuit, might be needed for the baby with excessive pulmonary blood flow. This is most important in babies with single-ventricle physiology who have limited ventricular functional reserve.

Contractility

Orally administered digoxin has been used for decades to treat congestive heart failure. Its safety in older children is well established, and with dose modifications, it may be used in the neonate.[28] Toxic effects are rare but can be treated with digoxin-specific Fab fragments.[76] There remains considerable skepticism about the efficacy of digoxin in babies with left ventricular volume overloading, and in some centers, digoxin is reserved for treating arrhythmias and overt ventricular dysfunction. When other oral inotropic agents are unavailable, and with appropriate care in dosing, digoxin can have a role in the treatment of these and other babies with congestive heart failure.

There is also considerable experience with intravenous administration of β-adrenergic blocking agents in preoperative and postoperative management of ventricular dysfunction with low cardiac output or low blood pressure. Contractility is the physiologic problem when there is low cardiac output and adequate atrial pressures for the clinical situation. Decreased wall motion, as shown by postoperative echocardiography, especially if systemic vascular resistance and blood pressure are not high, also suggests impaired contractility.

Dopamine and dobutamine[8] have a similar inotropic effect.[10] Dobutamine causes somewhat more tachycardia and can be associated with hypotension as a result of systemic vasodilation. Premature babies usually have a greater blood pressure response to dopamine.[26,35] Epinephrine in low doses is a potent inotrope with acceptable chronotropic and peripheral vasoconstriction, which can be a problem at high doses. Isoproterenol has inotropic, chronotropic, and some systemic and pulmonary vasodilatory effects. Tachycardia often limits its usefulness. Amrinone is a longer-acting intravenously administered inotrope that acts by increasing cyclic adenosine monophosphate by inhibiting phosphodiesterase. It has excellent inotropic and peripheral vasodilator effects.[40] Its principal side effect is thrombocytopenia. Milrinone improves cardiac index and lowers systemic resistance after cardiac surgery in neonates.[31] Milrinone should be used with caution in neonates with renal failure.

Long-term intravenous administration of inotropes increases the risk for development of diastolic dysfunction and receptor downregulation. Every effort should be made to wean the baby from these medications on the basis of clinical and invasive monitoring.

Treatment of Cyanotic Spells

Although cyanotic spells are most common at several months of age, they can occur in the first month of life. If the initial spell is atypical and is not preceded by crying or occurs without the hyperpnea, the possibility must be considered that a previously unrecognized patent ductus arteriosus has closed. Prompt recognition and treatment of spells can prevent the neurologic and metabolic sequelae of severe, prolonged hypoxia (Box 45-16). Some of the therapy is based on clinical observations dating back to the early experience with the Blalock-Taussig operation; newer therapies have been based on further thoughts about the pathophysiology of spells.

Supplemental oxygen, in theory, should not have much effect in babies with markedly diminished pulmonary blood flow, but it continues to be used. Morphine, and more recently fentanyl, might work by decreasing endogenous catecholamines and reducing dynamic subpulmonary obstruction. Similarly, propranolol blocks the effect of endogenous catecholamines. This cannot be the only effect because these drugs appear also to help babies with pulmonary atresia and spells who cannot have increased dynamic infundibular obstruction. Increasing systemic resistance with phenylephrine drives more blood into the lungs if there is no change in pulmonary vascular resistance.

Fluid administration probably helps either by increasing end-systolic volume and reducing dynamic infundibular obstruction or by increasing arterial blood pressure. The prolonged hypoxia causes metabolic acidosis, which should be treated with sodium bicarbonate.

Some babies with refractory spells respond to intubation and hyperventilation, which suggests that there is a component of pulmonary vascular reactivity. Anesthetic doses of fentanyl can be added once the airway and ventilation are secure. Finally, urgent repair or a shunt might be considered on the basis of the underlying anatomy.

Prevention of Bacterial Endocarditis

Bacterial endocarditis is an exceedingly rare and isolated problem in early infancy. Occasional babies have endocarditis or endovascular infections after cardiac surgery or as a complication of prolonged vascular access.[51] The once well-established recommendations for antibiotic prophylaxis were dramatically modified in 2007 and are now limited to individuals with unrepaired cyanotic heart defects, prosthetic valves, and heart transplantation or who have had prosthetic material placed within the last 6 months either by surgery or cardiac catheterization.[74]

BOX 45–16 Treatment of Cyanotic Spells

Oxygen
Intubation and hyperventilation
Morphine, 0.1-0.2 mg/kg IV or SC
Fentanyl, 1-4 μg/kg
Ketamine, 1 mg/kg IV
Fluid (5% albumin, blood if anemic), 5-20 mL/kg
Sodium bicarbonate, 1 mEq/kg IV
Propranolol, 0.05-0.15 mg/kg slow IV
Phenylephrine, 0.01 mg/kg IV, 0.1 mg/kg SC or IM; 1-20 μg/kg/min IV

IM, intramuscularly; IV, intravenously; SC, subcutaneously.

Although many neonates will fit into these categories, the procedures which result in bacteremia are either uncommon or not performed in neonates, and thus prophylactic antibiotics are often used empirically rather than based on evidence of need or efficacy. Furthermore, many babies who have gastrointestinal, genitourinary, or tracheal surgery are often receiving antibiotics for other reasons.

Two situations arise that might not warrant prophylactic antibiotics. Transesophageal echocardiography has a low incidence of bacteremia and no documented relationship to endocarditis in adults. Circumcision has been performed for centuries on babies with congenital heart disease, without endocarditis as a known complication. There are no recommendations from the American Heart Association or the American Dental Association, and local or individual preference dictates whether to administer one dose of amoxicillin orally before and one after neonatal circumcision to babies with heart defects.

Surgery

The ingenuity of neonatal cardiovascular surgery has dramatically improved the prognosis for babies with heart disease. Many surgical procedures have been named after the innovative surgeon who first reported the advance (Table 45-12). Specific surgical management is discussed under the individual lesions. The general principles of surgery—accurate preoperative diagnosis and careful correction of defects with preservation of myocardial and, when possible, valvular function—pertain to all surgeries. Residual defects, obstruction, and valve incompetence are less likely to be tolerated in the neonate. Moderate hypoxia is usually preferable to excessive volume loading for large systemic-to-pulmonary shunts in babies with pulmonary atresia (including hypoplastic left heart syndrome) after neonatal palliation. The mortality rate for neonatal heart surgery for many defects is low, and attention has been focused on strategies to reduce morbidity. The deleterious effects of circulatory

TABLE 45–12   Named Operations

Procedure	Operation
Systemic-to-Pulmonary Shunts	
Blalock-Taussig	Anastomosis of subclavian artery to pulmonary artery
Waterston	Anastomosis of ascending aorta to right pulmonary artery
Potts	Anastomosis of descending aorta to left pulmonary artery
Gore-Tex*	Vascular graft of expanded polytetrafluoroethylene
Closed Heart Procedures	
Brock	Closed pulmonary valvotomy
Blalock-Hanlon	Closed surgical atrial septectomy
Waldhausen	Subclavian flap angioplasty for coarctation of the aorta
Glenn	End-to-end anastomosis of SVC to RPA
Open Heart Procedures	
Jatene	Arterial switch for D-transposition of the great arteries
Mustard	Intra-atrial pericardial baffle for D-transposition of the great arteries
Senning	Intra-atrial baffle using mostly the atrial septum and walls for D-transposition of the great arteries
Rastelli	Extracardiac conduit for treatment of pulmonary atresia
Bidirectional Glenn	End-to-side anastomosis of SVC to RPA; often done as a "hemi-Fontan" procedure with anastomosis of proximal SVC to underside of RPA, but patching over of this opening until completion of modified Fontan
Modified Fontan	Anastomosis of right atrium (proximal SVC) to pulmonary artery, with intra-atrial baffling of IVC to proximal SVC; done at same time as or after bidirectional Glenn
Damus-Kaye-Stansel	Anastomosis of main pulmonary artery to ascending aorta, to bypass subaortic obstruction in single ventricle
Norwood	First stage: anastomosis of proximal pulmonary artery to hypoplastic ascending aorta, systemic-to-pulmonary shunt, atrial septectomy Second stage: bidirectional Glenn Third stage: modified Fontan
Sano	Right ventricle to pulmonary artery conduit as part of Norwood palliation.

*Named after the founders of the company that developed the polytetrafluoroethylene (Gore-Tex) graft.
IVC, inferior vena cava; RPA, right pulmonary artery; SVC, superior vena cava.

arrest have been carefully documented in babies with transposition of the great arteries, which favors, when possible, low-flow cardiopulmonary bypass over circulatory arrest for neonates.[7]

Neonatal Heart Transplantation

Neonatal heart transplantation initially focused on the baby with hypoplastic left heart syndrome and was driven by the disappointing early results with the Norwood operation and by the improved survival rate after adult cardiac transplantation with the introduction of cyclosporine as an immunosuppressive agent. Bailey,[4] at Loma Linda University, performed a xenotropic heart transplantation (on Baby Faye) in 1983, and this was followed by the first orthotropic heart transplantation for hypoplastic left heart syndrome in 1985. Although the results with surgical palliation of hypoplastic left heart syndrome have improved, there remains an interest in and an acceptance of transplantation for hypoplastic left heart syndrome and severe neonatal myopathies.

Clinical experience and experimental studies suggest that the newborn period might be a particularly favorable time for transplantation because of the immaturity of the immune system and low levels of antibody. This tolerance is further demonstrated by the transplantation of ABO-incompatible hearts in infants.[73]

Preoperative assessment and careful hemodynamic management are important because limited donor availability dictates careful recipient selection and waiting times of up to several months. Anatomic variants of hypoplastic left heart are not impediments to transplantation, although precise definition of pulmonary venous drainage is important. Pretransplantation evaluation by the transplant team maximizes the family's understanding of the long-term commitment needed for transplantation.

In view of the high incidence of genetic and neurologic malformations, screening studies including chromosome analysis and cranial and renal ultrasonography are performed on all babies. During the waiting period, medical management based on an understanding of single-ventricle physiology can minimize pulmonary blood flow and favor systemic blood flow. Pulmonary venous hypertension caused by a restrictive atrial septal defect and poor ventricular function are major limitations to successful medical management. Careful monitoring for infection, strict adherence to central venous line technique, and early nutrition are as important as therapy with prostaglandin E_1 to the survival of infants awaiting a transplant. Blood transfusion, when necessary, is with irradiated, cytomegalovirus-negative, leukocyte-filtered blood. There has been interest in the successful use of erythropoietin to minimize blood transfusions in neonates awaiting transplant surgery.[62]

The surgical technique for neonatal heart transplantation for hypoplastic left heart syndrome is now well developed.[58] Particular attention to the distal aortic anastomosis and wide excision of the ductus arteriosus minimize the subsequent development of coarctation of the aorta. Impaired ventricular function in the immediate postoperative period is managed with conventional inotropic drugs or with extracorporeal membrane oxygenation if profound dysfunction threatens survival. Postoperative pulmonary hypertension can occur, particularly in neonates who have had highly restrictive atrial septal defects and pulmonary venous hypertension. Death

before transplantation and prolonged average waiting times remains a challenge.[17] ABO-incompatible donors[72] and transplantation after donor cardiocirculatory death[14] have been used in newborns to help overcome this problem.

Prevention, assessment, and treatment of rejection are a significant long-term challenge. Immunosuppression protocols generally start with tacrolimus, prednisone, and mycophenolate mofetil.[2] Most neonates can be successfully weaned from steroids during the first few months after transplantation.[16] Rejection surveillance is by clinical, electrocardiographic, echocardiographic, and myocardial biopsy criteria.[41] Clinical criteria for rejection include fever and irritability. Unfortunately, these symptoms are common in young infants and can be nonspecific. Close follow-up is essential in identifying subtle signs that can suggest rejection rather than intercurrent illness. Electrocardiographic and echocardiographic changes, including voltage, wall thickness, and systolic and diastolic ventricular function, can supplement the clinical assessment; however, they are not generally reliable.[49] Dobutamine stress testing has been used to identify transplant patients at risk for cardiac events.[20]

Mild rejection can cause a decreased rate of posterior wall thinning. Increased left ventricular mass, especially if associated with changing systolic function, suggests severe rejection. Myocardial biopsy is possible but technically more challenging in neonates.[77] In neonates, biopsies rarely identify rejection when it is not suspected clinically, and biopsy specimens show negative results about 50% of the time when rejection is clinically evident. In the Loma Linda neonatal experience, the median number of rejection episodes is one, which usually occurs in the first 3 months.

Side effects of immunosuppression have improved with newer protocols. Growth and bone strength are rarely a problem in neonates rapidly weaned from steroids. Cyclosporine-associated renal dysfunction and hypertension occur in more than half of the babies. These side effects are dose related, and lower doses after the first year are stabilized or improve the effect. Both problems are much less prevalent with the use of tacrolimus. Hirsutism and gingival hyperplasia, although not medically harmful, are of cosmetic concern for the children and their families. Lymphoproliferative diseases have been reported with older children and adults and can be anticipated with infants after transplantation.

Opportunistic infections remain a constant threat to immunocompromised patients, and prophylactic antibiotic and antiviral agents are occasionally used, especially in the immediate post-transplantation period.[13] Cytomegalovirus-related pneumonia and gastrointestinal and blood infections are the most common. In children, they usually are caused by preexisting infection or the use of infected donors. Routine blood cell counts and electrolyte measurements are essential in following up the impact of the immunosuppressive agents on bone marrow and renal function. Immunization with killed vaccines is appropriate.

The 5-year survival rate is 72%; however, most deaths occur within the first month.[17] For babies with hypoplastic left heart syndrome, survival rate at 5 years must also include the proportion of babies who die awaiting transplantation. When this pretransplantation mortality rate is considered, the 5-year survival rate falls to 54%.[17]

Graft survival is not ensured, and dramatically premature atherosclerosis could require retransplantation or lead to sudden death. Graft atherosclerosis occurs in about 7% of children an average of 2 years after transplantation.[52] It does appear to be more prevalent in children with multiple episodes of rejection. The only effective treatment in young children at present is retransplantation, although newer immunosuppressive drugs, including rapamycin, hold promise to both prevent and treat graft vasculopathy.[45] Cholesterol-lowering drugs appear to reduce the risk for graft vascular disease.[71]

Pediatric follow-up data from the 2008 report of the Registry for International Society for Heart Transplantation indicate that for babies undergoing transplantation in the first year of life, the survival over the next 4 years is 88% for those who survive the first year after the transplantation.[34] Hypertension, renal dysfunction, hyperlipidemia, graft atherosclerosis, and malignancies remain important long-term issues.[17,34,69] Neurodevelopmental follow-up of infant heart transplant recipients demonstrates low-normal functional status.[6]

NEONATAL INTERVENTIONAL CATHETERIZATION

Catheter-directed therapies for congenital and acquired heart disease were described more than 40 years ago. However, balloon atrial septostomy, which was introduced in 1966, was the first to be widely and successfully used in pediatrics.[57] Since the mid-1980s, the variety of interventions has increased dramatically and now includes blade septostomy; balloon septal angioplasty; balloon dilation of stenotic valves, arteries, and veins including native or postoperative coarctation of the aorta and stenotic central or branch pulmonary arteries; occlusion of various types of congenital and acquired vascular lesions; cutting balloon dilations for resistant lesions; radiofrequency wire perforation of atretic valves or imperforate atrial septum; and endovascular stent implantation including for neonatal indications. Many procedures, such as balloon dilation of valvular pulmonary stenosis, are now considered first-line therapy, and with increased clinical experience and the evolution of less traumatic and smaller catheter and delivery systems, most of these procedures are now successfully and safely performed in the newborn infant.

Creation of Atrial Septal Defects

INDICATIONS

The initial therapy for transposition of the great arteries in neonates is balloon atrial septostomy, even when primary repair is to be performed in the newborn period. In addition, septostomy is indicated when an unrestrictive atrial shunt is mandatory, as in absent right or left AV connection or valve atresias, pulmonary atresia with intact ventricular septum, or total anomalous pulmonary venous connection balloon. Despite surgical advancements facilitating early surgical repair for many complex lesions, balloon septostomy remains a vital treatment modality in infants with lesions including absent AV connection, in whom primary repair is not feasible in the neonatal period.

TECHNIQUES

Balloon Atrial Septostomy

The basic technique for balloon atrial septostomy has remained essentially unaltered since originally described by Rashkind and Miller in 1966.[57] Modifications in catheters have made the procedure simpler and more effective. Percutaneous femoral or umbilical access has essentially eliminated the need for venous cutdown, and the use of a larger balloon that accommodates 4 mL of fluid has resulted in a larger effective dilating diameter (Fig. 45-27). The procedure traditionally has been performed in the cardiac catheterization laboratory; however, it has been increasingly performed at the bedside under ultrasound guidance, which can expedite correction of hypoxia in the very fragile infant.

The tear occurs in the valve of the foramen ovale. Success can be assessed by an increase in arterial oxygen saturation, by equalization of atrial pressures, and by two-dimensional echocardiographic imaging and Doppler flow studies across the defect created.

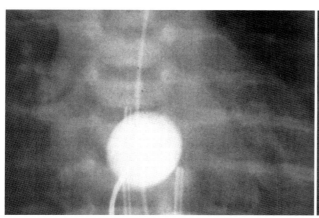 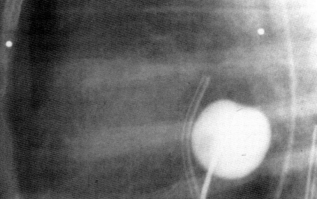

Figure 45–27. Anterior (*left*) and lateral (*right*) projections of inflated 4-mL septostomy balloon in the left atrium of a neonate with transposition of the great arteries before withdrawal into the right atrium across the atrial septum.

There are no absolute contraindications to balloon septostomy; however, the procedure cannot be performed in the absence of the hepatic portion of the inferior vena cava (azygos continuation) and is difficult when the left atrium is hypoplastic (i.e., hypoplastic left heart syndrome) or there is left juxtaposition of the right atrial appendage. In the latter two conditions, fluoroscopic guidance may be useful in addition to echocardiographic imaging in facilitating proper catheter position.

Serious complications are rare but can include perforation and tearing of the atrial wall or pulmonary veins or rupture of the tricuspid valve. Such complications require prompt recognition but may not be fatal. Atrial dysrhythmias are usually transient. Cerebral complications caused by an embolus or subarachnoid hemorrhage and pneumopericardium have also been reported but are similarly rare and can be virtually eliminated by careful catheterization and imaging techniques.

Blade Atrial Septostomy

Beyond the first weeks of life, balloon atrial septostomy is rarely successful because of thickening of the atrial septum. Through experimental studies, a blade atrial septostomy catheter was developed for such clinical situations, and its feasibility, efficacy, and safety were established.[53] This technique was previously employed primarily in patients with transposition of the great arteries and poor atrial mixing; however, with implementation of primary atrial or arterial repairs in the newborn period, this population no longer exists. In neonates, other techniques have supplanted its usefulness in addressing problematic atrial septal restriction.

The main indication remains in older infants and children with an absent left or right AV connection, who require an unrestrictive atrial communication and in whom the atrial defect has become progressively smaller with age. It has also been used in children receiving extracorporeal membrane oxygenation for acute myocarditis to decompress the left atrium, although atrial septal angioplasty with or without stent placement is becoming a more accepted approach to this problem.[61]

Balloon Septal Angioplasty and Stent Placement

Some infants who require an atrial septal defect to relieve left atrial hypertension have an extremely small left atrium, either because of associated left heart hypoplasia or because of leftward deviation of the attachments of the septum primum. The atrial septum in these infants is usually thick but also might be intact with decompression of the pulmonary veins through other routes. In these infants, the risk for atrial laceration with either balloon or blade septostomy is high, and adequate palliation might be technically impossible with either technique. In this circumstance, the successful creation of an adequate atrial septal defect has been achieved by performing atrial septal puncture, followed by balloon dilation, with or without stent placement. The creation of multiple holes in the atrial septum might be required. This procedure is particularly useful in the patient with hypoplastic left heart syndrome and a severely restrictive atrial septal defect, before either first-stage surgical palliation or cardiac transplantation. Radiofrequency perforation wires currently play an important role in facilitating transseptal

puncture in the setting of an imperforate or thick atrial septum, and are technically better suited to neonatal interventions than traditional transseptal needles (Brockenbrough needles).

Valvuloplasty

PULMONARY VALVE STENOSIS

Extensive experience in children and adults has convincingly demonstrated that percutaneous balloon dilation of the pulmonary valve can effectively reduce the transvalvular gradient to a degree equivalent to that of a surgical valvotomy, thus avoiding the need for open heart surgery.[33] The cyanotic newborn infant with critical pulmonary stenosis and an intact ventricular septum requires emergent treatment. Surgical valvotomy with or without a pulmonary-to-systemic shunt had been the traditional approach. With experience in percutaneous balloon valvotomy in the older child, the technique was successfully adapted to the neonate.

Pulmonary valve dilation in the neonate with critical pulmonary stenosis is a technically somewhat more challenging procedure than in older children; the most difficult aspect is crossing the pinpoint orifice of the pulmonary valve (Fig. 45-28). Gradient relief, however, is reported to be comparable to that achieved by balloon dilation in older children and by surgery in neonates.

The immediate postprocedure gradient might not accurately reflect relief of obstruction in infants who have a patent ductus arteriosus; however, subsequent noninvasive imaging usually confirms adequate and often persistent relief of obstruction. Less ideal candidates for the procedure might have associated right ventricular or tricuspid valve hypoplasia or a poorly expanded subpulmonary infundibulum. Although complications (annular or venous tears, cardiac perforation) in neonates

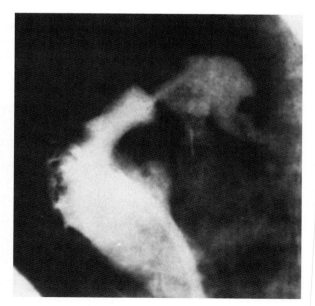

Figure 45–28. Lateral projection of right ventriculogram of a neonate with critical pulmonary stenosis. Note pinpoint central jet with poor filling of main pulmonary artery.

had been reported at significantly higher rates than in older children, with contemporary equipment and approaches, the incidence of serious complications is certain to be much lower.[15] Even infants with complete membranous atresia of the pulmonary valve can be effectively decompressed by wire-guided perforation of the valve followed by balloon dilation.[70]

BALLOON DILATION OF THE PULMONARY VALVE IN COMPLEX CONGENITAL HEART DISEASE

Balloon dilation of a stenotic pulmonary valve in cyanotic heart defects, including single ventricle with pulmonary stenosis and tetralogy of Fallot, can eliminate the immediate need for a systemic-to-pulmonary shunt, which has risks that include pulmonary artery distortion. The balance between the severity of the obstruction at the valvular level and severity at the subvalvular level reflects the success of the procedure.

Despite a number of reports,[30,47] its role remained controversial. Sreeram and coworkers[65] reported 82 successful procedures in patients with tetralogy of Fallot, with arterial oxygen saturation increasing from an average of 74% to 90.5%. Of 67 patients, 11 required an aortopulmonary shunt within 1 month of dilation. Serious complications occurred in 4 patients and included transient pulmonary edema (1 patient), sepsis (1 patient), and cardiac tamponade requiring emergency surgical repair (2 patients). More encouraging results were demonstrated recently after right ventricular outflow tract stent placement in symptomatic infants with tetralogy of Fallot. In these 9 patients, median arterial saturation increased from 73% to 94%, with most infants going on to complete repair at a later age. In these patients, the pulmonary valve and annulus were thought to be inadequate to avoid ultimate transannular patching, and this strategy was employed to allow definitive, complete repair to take place at a more favorable age and size.[21]

PULMONARY VALVE ATRESIA

The traditional surgical approach to pulmonary valve atresia in neonates consists of creating a systemic-to-pulmonary artery shunt, together with an open pulmonary valvotomy or right ventricular outflow patch at the same or a later procedure. Currently, percutaneous transcatheter techniques can help avoid neonatal surgery. Typically, this involves perforation of the atretic valve with radiofrequency wires, followed by balloon dilation.

The long-term efficacy of these techniques is encouraging, with results comparable to surgery in selected patients.[1] Moreover, infants with a problematic degree of right-to-left atrial shunting due to associated tricuspid and right ventricular hypoplasia, stenting of the ductus arteriosus can be performed concomitantly to augment pulmonary blood flow in lieu of a surgical aortopulmonary shunt, allowing time for beneficial right heart remodeling and growth. Use of this strategy in appropriate patients can allow for establishing biventricular circulation, without surgery, in most patients.[46]

AORTIC VALVE STENOSIS

Balloon dilation of congenital aortic valve stenosis in children was initially reported by Lababidi in 1983.[39] Application of this technique to neonates with critical aortic stenosis followed shortly thereafter. As in the case of pulmonic stenosis,

the technical considerations and risks of the procedure differ for neonates from those for infants and children. Balloon dilation remains an important treatment for neonates with critical aortic stenosis. The mortality rate among neonates with this lesion was initially high, whether treated surgically or by interventional catheterization. The neonatal mortality rate for critical aortic stenosis was 18% versus 0.5% in children beyond the neonatal period, with serious morbidity in 36% of neonates versus 0.2% of children in the older group.[59] Careful selection of patients and improved techniques have resulted in good results even in ductal-dependent neonates with aortic stenosis.[22]

For neonates judged to have favorable anatomy for balloon valvuloplasty, the valve is often approached retrograde through the femoral or umbilical arteries, although the valve can also be successfully crossed antegrade from the left ventricle after the crossing the atrial septum. Alternatively, accessing the right carotid artery through a surgical cutdown provides a technically straightforward approach to the valve and appears to be well tolerated.[12]

Given the disorganized nature of the valve and its eccentric opening, crossing the valve with a guide wire can, at times, be difficult. Inadvertent wire perforation of the valve leaflet and subsequent dilation, or avulsion of the leaflet from the aortic ring, has been described and can result in severe aortic regurgitation. Although there has been a dramatic reduction in catheter and sheath size, femoral artery trauma or thrombosis can still occur in neonates but often favorably responds to medical therapy with heparin or thrombolytics, or both.

MITRAL VALVE STENOSIS

Percutaneous balloon dilation of rheumatic mitral stenosis was first described in 1984 and in children the following year; application of the technique to congenital mitral stenosis was reported in 1986. In patients with congenital mitral stenosis, results are variable. Among nine patients reported by Moore and associates,[48] seven had a significant immediate increase in valve area and decrease in mean gradient, although two of those had evidence of restenosis within 2 months of the procedure. Experience with neonates is extremely limited.

Angioplasty

NATIVE COARCTATION OF THE AORTA

Coarctation of the aorta traditionally has been treated by surgery. Although a variety of surgical techniques have been employed, there has been a low mortality rate, especially in those infants without additional congenital heart defects and managed with preoperative prostaglandin E_1 to maintain peripheral perfusion. However, the recurrence rates range between 10% and 30%, which has prompted alternative strategies for management. Balloon angioplasty of recurrent aortic coarctation in a critically ill infant was first reported by Singer and colleagues[64] in 1982. Experimental work in excised segments of human coarctation and in animal models demonstrated that successful balloon dilation required relatively high pressures and was associated with tears of the intima and media; the adventitia remained intact.[43] This finding generated concern about late aneurysm formation and has led to considerable controversy over the issue of whether native coarctation of the aorta should undergo angioplasty. Aneurysm formation has been reported in a small number of children, although long-term follow-up, of large numbers of patients, is incomplete.

Successful gradient relief has been reported, although primarily it has been accomplished in the older infant and child. Experience suggests that in the newborn period, however, gradient relief can be transient and obstruction recurs, requiring further intervention.[54,56] As in any arterial intervention in the neonate, femoral arterial complications are more frequent. To prevent these complications, successful coarctation angioplasty can be performed from the venous anterograde approach. The current role of angioplasty in native coarctation, in most centers, is as a selective palliative technique that allows for hemodynamic and clinical stabilization in neonates deemed high-risk surgical candidates.

RECURRENT COARCTATION OF THE AORTA

Surgery for recurrent coarctation is not uniformly successful and can be technically difficult because of surgical scarring. Balloon angioplasty for recurrent coarctation has been very effective in this setting.[29] The type of initial repair does not appear to influence the outcome of balloon angioplasty. Angioplasty typically is not performed until 6 to 8 weeks after the initial operation in order to prevent inadvertent rupture of the suture line. Under these circumstances, the surgical scar, which is the major component of the recurrent obstruction, limits the extent of the tear. As in any arterial intervention, femoral artery complications are a possible complication. The incidence of late aneurysm formation is unknown. The procedure has become the initial management approach in this patient group. Coarctation restenosis has been recognized as a common complication of the first stage of the Norwood procedure and appears to respond to balloon dilation.[67]

PERIPHERAL PULMONARY ARTERY STENOSIS

Pulmonary artery stenosis beyond the hilum and diffuse hypoplasia of the pulmonary arteries are difficult or impossible to treat surgically. Rehabilitation of branch pulmonary artery stenosis by balloon dilation and endovascular stents has been useful in infants and children with challenging pulmonary artery anatomy.[39,78] When the outcome after surgical repair of associated lesions is heavily dependent on correction of peripheral pulmonary artery stenoses, as in some children with tetralogy of Fallot and in those with single ventricle physiology who will eventually undergo a Fontan repair, it seems advantageous to be able to assess and palliate important pulmonary stenoses preoperatively. Early balloon dilation of branch pulmonary artery stenoses can afford maximal growth potential coincident with somatic growth. The use of endovascular stents in infants currently is limited by the largest stent diameter that can be reached through sequential dilations with somatic growth. Although many stents can be delivered even in the neonatal setting, they might not suffice from the standpoint of ultimate adult vessel diameter and require surgical revision or removal. Ongoing research is focusing on the development of stents that are either biodegradable or can be disarticulated in situ by balloon dilation, thus freeing the vessel to be further dilated if needed. Cutting balloons, angioplasty balloons with an array

of longitudinal microtomes, have provided a useful tool in addressing severe peripheral arterial stenoses, especially in the setting of genetic arteriopathies, such as seen in Williams syndrome.[9] Their use in neonates, however, is limited.

PULMONARY VEIN STENOSIS

The results of surgical treatment of pulmonary vein stenosis are poor, and even when improvement occurs, early recurrence is common. Early reports of balloon angioplasty, as well as of the use of balloon-expandable endovascular stents, have indicated that, like surgery, dilation is short lived, and recurrent obstruction dominates the clinical picture.[50]

DILATION OF SURGICALLY CREATED SHUNT BETWEEN THE SYSTEMIC ARTERIAL AND THE PULMONARY ARTERIAL CIRCULATION

Neonates requiring a shunt between the systemic arterial and the pulmonary arterial circulations might have progressive cyanosis postoperatively because of kinking or stenosis at the shunt site. On the basis of limited early experience, it appears that this type of narrowing can be amenable to balloon dilation or, more reliably, stent placement using low-profile coronary or other premounted stents. Obviously, if profound cyanosis is present, emergent surgical shunt revision is warranted.

Stents to Maintain Patency of the Ductus Arteriosus

In infants who have ductus-dependent heart defects, long-term prostaglandin E_1 infusion has multiple side effects. Several investigators have attempted to maintain ductal patency through stent implantation, which could replace surgical creation of a shunt from the systemic to the pulmonary circulation.[18] Previous experience focused on infants who had hypoplastic left heart syndrome and were awaiting heart transplantation. Recently, however, the evolution of a "hybrid approach" to the treatment of these patients has made stent placement in the ductus arteriosus commonplace at centers that have adopted this approach. Typically, this is done by a sternotomy through a small pursestring incision in the main pulmonary artery under fluoroscopic guidance and using both surgical and medical expertise.[24] Neonates with ductal dependent pulmonary blood flow, similarly, can be candidates for maintaining ductal patency through endovascular stenting in lieu of a surgical aortopulmonary shunt.[25] These infants typically undergo placement of premounted coronary stents to achieve an appropriate ductal diameter.

Vessel Occlusion

Embolization or occlusion of abnormal vascular communications is possible with a variety of materials, including coils, tissue adhesives, detachable balloons, foam, and umbrella devices. Vessels and defects successfully treated by transcatheter therapy include aortopulmonary collateral vessels; systemic circulation pulmonary artery shunts; patent ductus arteriosus; atrial and ventricular septal defects; and a variety of arteriovenous malformations involving the hepatic, pulmonary, coronary, or cerebral circulations. The effectiveness of occluding aortopulmonary collateral vessels, which develop in infants with bronchopulmonary dysplasia, has not been established; the emergence of a new collateral supply is likely.

The usefulness of these techniques in the treatment of neonates is determined by the size of the device or delivery systems. Coils that can be delivered through 4-Fr systems are most applicable to the neonate. Coil occlusion of patent ductus arteriosus has become the treatment of choice for infants and children with persistent ductal patency.[32] Neonates in this group, most of whom are infants with low birthweight, largely remain treated by surgery because of the technical limitations of interventional procedures. Newer generation, nitinol-based occluders are available for atrial septal defects and patent ductus arteriosus, and, although the indications in neonates are uncommon, these occluders could be delivered through a percutaneous approach in certain situations. A range of devices for ventricular septal defects are available but would probably have limited utility in the neonatal population, unless delivered by periventricular approach in the operating room.

Line Placements: Transhepatic Catheterization

In some children with congenital heart disease, as well as in chronically ill neonates, conventional venous access (femoral, subclavian, or internal jugular veins) might become unavailable. The technique of percutaneous transhepatic venous access for cardiac catheterization or with subsequent Broviac insertion for long-term administration of parenteral nutrition or antibiotics has been used and in short-term follow-up provides an effective and safe alternative in children.[63] As more experience with the technique evolves, this could prove to be a preferred route for percutaneous venous access in certain children.

Endomyocardial Biopsy

Endomyocardial biopsy has proved to be a safe and effective means of diagnosing a wide variety of myocardial diseases in the older child and adult. Although the indications are rare (myocarditis, cardiomyopathies, after neonatal heart transplantation, metabolic disease), it can be safely performed in neonates and infants. No significant complications have been reported, although using a soft size 3-Fr bioptome, often with echocardiographic and fluoroscopic guidance, is recommended to minimize the risk for cardiac perforation.

Catheter Retrieval of Foreign Bodies

The first catheter retrieval of a foreign body from a child's heart was reported by Rashkind and Miller in 1966.[57] An international review of experience with this procedure reported 90% success with no complications in 180 retrievals.[11] Embolization of sheared catheter fragments or lost guide wires is a ubiquitous (albeit preventable) event. Even in very small infants, such fragments can be safely retrieved from the heart or vasculature percutaneously with the use of a snare, forceps, or basket.

Procedural Complications

Complications during interventional studies are more common in the neonate because of hemodynamic and biochemical instability. As with diagnostic procedures, diligent patient monitoring is performed, with particular attention paid to the neonate's vital signs, blood volume, hemoglobin concentration, temperature, ventilatory status, and electrolyte and glucose balance; the duration of the procedures is kept to a minimum. The risk for diagnostic catheterization is less than 0.5%.[19] Fortunately, more serious complications such as chamber or vessel perforation, valve disruption, and embolization related to any invasive procedure are relatively rare, even as the repertoire of neonatal interventional procedures has expanded.

Vascular complications dominate the problems associated with therapeutic procedures in the neonate. The preferred method of vascular access is by the umbilical vein or artery (depending on the lesion) and by percutaneous entry of the femoral vessels, the latter being associated with occlusion of the iliac vein or distal vena cava in 5% to 15% of infants.[68] Arterial trauma is a more pervasive problem in the neonate.

For diagnostic studies, femoral arterial entry is not usually required because the umbilical artery, a ventricular septal defect, or a patent foramen ovale or patent ductus arteriosus allows transcatheter arterial access. However, interventional manipulations are often difficult through these circuitous routes, and direct femoral arterial cannulations might be required. The introduction of small French catheters and low-profile balloons for many of the procedures has reduced the incidence of thrombosis. Vessel recannulation has been demonstrated with the use of heparin and, if necessary, fibrinolytic therapy.[37]

Fetal Interventional Catheterization

See also Chapter 11.

The practice of pediatric cardiology and cardiovascular surgery has advanced significantly with respect to the ability to perform neonatal catheterization interventions and surgical repairs. An extension of this progress is to perform these techniques during fetal life.[36] Establishing normal blood-flow patterns in the fetus who has critical valve stenosis or atresia can allow for more normal growth of vessels and ventricles with the potential for longer postnatal survival and better quality of life. To date, this has primarily focused on the fetuses at risk for ultimate evolution of hypoplastic left heart syndrome and relief of severe semilunar valve stenosis or restrictive atrial septum.[44]

Any form of fetal intervention for cardiovascular disease requires extensive understanding of the fetal pathophysiologic responses to intervention. Research is ongoing to attempt to perform direct surgical corrective and palliative procedures, fetal cardiac bypass, and catheterization interventions. The advancement of technical aspects of such interventions is promising; however, moral and ethical issues and the allocation of medical resources remain key determinants of further progress in the management of the fetus with congenital heart disease.

REFERENCES

1. Alwi M, et al: Pulmonary atresia with intact ventricular septum percutaneous radiofrequency-assisted valvotomy and balloon dilation versus surgical valvotomy and Blalock Taussig shunt, *J Am Coll Cardiol* 35:468, 2000.
2. Amerduri A, et al: Current practice in immunosuppression in pediatric heart transplantation, *Prog Ped Cardiol* 26:31, 2009.
3. Auslender M, Artman M: Overview of the management of pediatric heart failure, *Prog Ped Cardiol* 11:231, 2000.
4. Bailey LL: Role of cardiac replacement in the neonate, *J Heart Transplant* 4:506, 1985.
5. Barnea O, et al: Balancing the circulation: theoretic optimization of pulmonary/systemic flow ratio in hypoplastic left heart syndrome, *J Am Coll Cardiol* 24:1376, 1994.
6. Baum M, et al: Neuropsychological outcome of infant heart transplant recipients, *J Pediatr* 145:365, 2004.
7. Bellinger DC, et al: Neurodevelopmental status at eight years in children with dextro-transposition of the great arteries: The Boston Circulatory Arrest Trial, *J Thorac Cardiovasc Surg* 126:1385, 2003.
8. Berg RA, et al: Dobutamine infusions in stable, critically ill children: pharmacokinetics and hemodynamic actions, *Crit Care Med* 21:678, 1993.
9. Bergersen L, et al: Follow-up results of cutting balloon angioplasty used to relieve stenoses in small pulmonary arteries, *Cardiol Young* 15:605, 2005.
10. Bhatt-Mehta V, Nahata MC: Dopamine and dobutamine in pediatric therapy, *Pharmacotherapy* 9:303, 1989.
11. Bloomfield DA: The nonsurgical retrieval of intracardiac foreign bodies—an international survey, *Cathet Cardiovasc Diagn* 4:1, 1978.
12. Borghi A, et al: Surgical cutdown of the right carotid artery for aortic balloon valvuloplasty in infancy: midterm follow-up, *Pediatr Cardiol* 22:194, 2001.
13. Bork J, et al: Infectious complications in infant heart transplantation, *J Heart Lung Transplant* 12:S199, 1993.
14. Boucek MM, et al: Denver Children's Pediatric Heart Transplant Team. Pediatric heart transplantation after declaration of cardiocirculatory death, *N Engl J Med* 359:709, 2008.
15. Boucek MM, et al: Balloon pulmonary valvotomy: palliation for cyanotic heart disease, *Am Heart J* 115:318, 1988.
16. Canter CE, et al: Steroid withdrawal in the pediatric heart transplant initially treated with triple immunosuppression, *J Heart Lung Transplant* 13:74, 1994.
17. Chrisant MR, et al, for the Pediatric Heart Transplant Study Group: Fate of infants with hypoplastic left heart syndrome listed for cardiac transplantation: a multicenter study, *J Heart Lung Transplant* 24:576, 2005.
18. Coe JY, Olley PM: A novel method to maintain ductus arteriosus patency, *J Am Coll Cardiol* 18:837, 1991.
19. Cohn HE, et al: Complications and mortality associated with cardiac catheterization in infants under one year: a prospective study, *Pediatr Cardiol* 6:123, 1985.
20. Di Filippo S, et al: Non-invasive detection of coronary artery disease by dobutamine-stress echocardiography in children after heart transplant, *J Heart Lung Transplant* 22:876, 2003.
21. Dohlen G, et al: Stenting of the right ventricular outflow tract in the symptomatic infant with tetralogy of Fallot, *Heart* 95:142, 2009.
22. Egito ES, et al: Transvascular balloon dilation for neonatal critical aortic stenosis: early and midterm results, *J Am Coll Cardiol* 29:442, 1997.
23. Freed MD, et al: Prostaglandin E_1 infants with ductus arteriosus-dependent congenital heart disease, *Circulation* 64:899, 1981.
24. Galantowicz M, et al: Hybrid approach for hypoplastic left heart syndrome: intermediate results after the learning curve, *Ann Thorac Surg* 85:2063, 2008; discussion 2070-1.
25. Gewillig M, et al: Stenting the neonatal arterial duct in duct-dependent pulmonary circulation: new techniques, better results, *J Am Coll Cardiol* 43:107, 2004.
26. Greenough A, Emery EF: Randomized trial comparing dopamine and dobutamine in preterm infants, *Eur J Pediatr* 152:925, 1993.
27. Grenier MA, et al: Angiotensin-converting enzyme inhibitor therapy for ventricular dysfunction in infants, children and adolescents: a review, *Prog Ped Cardiol* 11:91, 2000.
28. Hastreiter AR, et al: Maintenance digoxin dosage and steady-state plasma concentration in infants and children, *J Pediatr* 107:140, 1985.
29. Hellenbrand WE, et al: Balloon angioplasty for aortic recoarctation: Results of Valvuloplasty and Angioplasty of Congenital Anomalies Registry, *Am J Cardiol* 65:793, 1990.
30. Heusch A, et al: Balloon valvoplasty in infants with tetralogy of Fallot: Effects on oxygen saturation and growth of the pulmonary arteries, *Cardiol Young* 9:17, 1999.
31. Hoffman TM, et al: Efficacy and safety of milrinone in preventing low cardiac output syndrome in infants and children after corrective surgery for congenital heart disease, *Circulation* 107:996, 2003.
32. Ing FF, Sommer RJ: The snare-assisted technique for transcatheter coil occlusion of moderate to large patent ductus arteriosus: Immediate and intermediate results, *J Am Coll Cardiol* 33:1710, 1999.
33. Kan JS, et al: Percutaneous transluminal balloon valvuloplasty for pulmonary valve stenosis, *Circulation* 69:554, 1984.
34. Kirk R, et al: Registry of the International Society for Heart and Lung Transplantation: eleventh official pediatric heart transplantation report, *J Heart Lung Transplant* 27:970, 2008.
35. Klarr JM, et al: Randomized, blind trial of dopamine versus dobutamine for treatment of hypotension in preterm infants with respiratory distress syndrome, *J Pediatr* 125:117, 1994.
36. Kohl T, et al: World experience of percutaneous ultrasound-guided balloon valvuloplasty in human fetuses with severe aortic valve obstruction, *Am J Cardiol* 85:1230, 2000.
37. Kothari SS, et al: Thrombolytic therapy in infants and children, *Am Heart J* 127:651, 1994.
38. Kramer HH, et al. Evaluation of low-dose prostaglandin E1 treatment for ductus-dependent congenital heart disease, *Eur J Pediatr* 154:700, 1995.
39. Lababidi Z: Aortic balloon valvuloplasty, *Am Heart J* 106:751, 1983.
40. Laitinen P, et al: Amrinone versus dopamine and nitroglycerin in neonates after arterial switch operation for transposition of the great arteries, *J Cardiothorac Vasc Anesth* 13:186, 1999.
41. Levi DS, et al: The yield of surveillance endomyocardial biopsies as a screen for cellular rejection in pediatric heart transplant patients, *Pediatr Transplant* 8:22, 2004.
42. Li J, et al: Carbon dioxide—a complex gas in a complex circulation: its effects on systemic hemodynamics and oxygen

transport, cerebral, and splanchnic circulation in neonates after the Norwood procedure, *J Thorac Cardiovasc Surg* 136:1207, 2008.

43. Lock J, et al: *Diagnostic and Interventional Catheterization in Congenital Heart Disease,* Boston, 1987, Martinus-Nijhoff.

44. Mäkikallio K, et al: Fetal aortic valve stenosis and the evolution of hypoplastic left heart syndrome: patient selection for fetal intervention, *Circulation* 113:1401, 2006.

45. Mancini D, et al: Use of rapamycin slows progression of cardiac transplantation vasculopathy, *Circulation* 108:48, 2003.

46. Marasini M, et al: Long term results of catheter based treatment of pulmonary atresia and intact ventricular septum, *Heart* 95:1473-1474, 2009.

47. Massoud I, et al: Palliative balloon valvoplasty of the pulmonary valve in tetralogy of Fallot, *Cardiol Young* 9:24, 1999.

48. Moore P, et al: Severe congenital mitral stenosis in infants, *Circulation* 89:2099, 1994.

49. Neuberger S, et al: Comparison of quantitative echocardiography with endomyocardial biopsy to define myocardial rejection in pediatric patients after cardiac transplantation, *Am J Cardiol* 79:447, 1997.

50. O'Laughlin M, et al: Use of endovascular stents in congenital heart disease, *Circulation* 83:1923, 1991.

51. Opie GF, et al: Bacterial endocarditis in neonatal intensive care, *J Paediatr Child Health* 35:545, 1999.

52. Pahl E, et al: Posttransplant coronary artery disease in children: a national survey, *Circulation* 90:II-56, 1994.

53. Park SC, et al: Blade atrial septostomy: collaborative study, *Circulation* 66:258, 1982.

54. Park Y, et al: Balloon angioplasty of native aortic coarctation in infants three months of age and younger, *Am Heart J* 134:917, 1997.

55. Peled N, et al: Gastric outlet obstruction induced by prostaglandin therapy in neonates, *N Engl J Med* 327:505, 1992.

56. Rao PS, et al: Five- to nine-year follow-up results of balloon angioplasty of native aortic coarctation in infants and children, *J Am Coll Cardiol* 27:462, 1996.

57. Rashkind WJ, Miller WW: Creation of an atrial septal defect without thoracotomy: a palliative approach to complete transposition of the great arteries, *JAMA* 196:991, 1966.

58. Razzouk AJ, et al: Transplantation as a primary treatment for hypoplastic left heart syndrome: intermediate-term results, *Ann Thorac Surg* 62:1, 1996.

59. Rocchini AP, et al: Balloon aortic valvuloplasty: Results of the Valvuloplasty and Angioplasty of Congenital Anomalies Registry, *Am J Cardiol* 65:784, 1990.

60. Rossi AF, et al: Usefulness of intermittent monitoring of mixed venous oxygen saturation after stage I palliation for hypoplastic left heart syndrome, *Am J Cardiol* 73:1118, 1994.

61. Seib PM, et al: Blade and balloon atrial septostomy for left heart decompression in patients with severe ventricular dysfunction on extracorporeal membrane oxygenation, *Catheter Cardiovasc Interv* 46:179, 1999.

62. Shaddy RE, et al: Epoetin alfa therapy in infants awaiting heart transplantation, *Arch Pediatr Adolesc Med* 149:322, 1995.

63. Shim D, et al: Transhepatic therapeutic cardiac catheterization: a new option for the pediatric interventionalist, *Catheter Cardiovasc Interv* 47:41, 1999.

64. Singer MI, et al: Transluminal aortic balloon angioplasty for coarctation of the aorta in the newborn, *Am Heart J* 103:131, 1982.

65. Sreeram N, et al: Results of balloon pulmonary valvuloplasty as a palliative procedure in tetralogy of Fallot, *J Am Coll Cardiol* 18:159, 1991.

66. Theilen U, Shekerdemian L: The intensive care of infants with hypoplastic left heart syndrome, *Arch Dis Child Fetal Neonatal Ed* 90:F97, 2005.

67. Tworetzky W, et al: Balloon arterioplasty of recurrent coarctation after the modified Norwood procedure in infants, *Catheter Cardiovasc Interv* 50:54, 2000.

68. Vitiello R, et al: Complications associated with pediatric cardiac catheterization, *J Am Coll Cardiol* 32:1433, 1998.

69. Webber SA, et al, for the Pediatric Heart Transplant Study: Lymphoproliferative disorders after paediatric heart transplantation: a multi-institutional study, *Lancet* 367:233, 2006.

70. Weber HS: Initial and late results after catheter intervention for neonatal critical pulmonary valve stenosis and atresia with intact ventricular septum: a technique in continual evolution, *Catheter Cardiovasc Interv* 56:394, 2002.

71. Wenke K, et al: Simvastatin initiated early after heart transplantation: 8-year prospective experience, *Circulation* 107:93, 2003.

72. West LJ, et al: Impact on outcomes after listing and transplantation, of a strategy to accept ABO blood group-incompatible donor hearts for neonates and infants, *J Thorac Cardiovasc Surg* 131:455, 2006.

73. West LJ, et al: ABO-incompatible heart transplantation in infants, *N Engl J Med* 344:793, 2001.

74. Wilson W, et al, for the American Heart Association Rheumatic Fever, Endocarditis, and Kawasaki Disease Committee; American Heart Association Council on Cardiovascular Disease in the Young; American Heart Association Council on Clinical Cardiology; American Heart Association Council on Cardiovascular Surgery and Anesthesia; Quality of Care and Outcomes Research Interdisciplinary Working Group: Prevention of infective endocarditis: guidelines from the American Heart Association. A guideline from the American Heart Association Rheumatic Fever, Endocarditis, and Kawasaki Disease Committee, Council on Cardiovascular Disease in the Young, and the Council on Clinical Cardiology, Council on Cardiovascular Surgery and Anesthesia, and the Quality of Care and Outcomes Research Interdisciplinary Working Group, *Circulation* 116:1736, 2007.

75. Woo K, et al: Cortical hyperostosis: a complication of prolonged prostaglandin infusion in infants awaiting cardiac transplantation, *Pediatrics* 93:417, 1994.

76. Woolf AD, et al: The use of digoxin-specific Fab fragments for severe digitalis intoxication in children, *N Engl J Med* 326:1739, 1992.

77. Zales VR, et al: Role of endomyocardial biopsy in rejection surveillance after transplantation in neonates and children, *J Am Coll Cardiol* 23:766, 1994.

78. Zeevi B, et al: Midterm clinical impact versus procedural success of balloon angioplasty for pulmonary artery stenosis, *Pediatr Cardiol* 18:101, 1997.

CHAPTER 46

The Blood and Hematopoietic System

PART 1

Hematologic Problems in the Fetus and Neonate

Lori Luchtman-Jones and David B. Wilson

HEMATOPOIETIC DEVELOPMENT

Hematopoietic Stem Cells

All blood cells are derived from hematopoietic stem cells that originate in differentiating mesoderm.[63] These stem cells are found both in hematopoietic organs (yolk sac, liver, and bone marrow) and in the circulating blood of the embryo, fetus, and infant. Hematopoietic stem cells are pluripotential; each of these cells can give rise to different types of committed progenitors (Fig. 46-1). Like other stem cells of the body, hematopoietic stem cells are capable of self-renewal. At any given time, most hematopoietic stem cells are not cycling but rather are in a resting state. This property, together with a knowledge of surface markers found on these cells (e.g., CD34), has been exploited to isolate highly purified populations of human stem cells. Proliferation and differentiation of stem cells require the proper microenvironment, including supporting adventitial cells and humoral factors. The anatomic sites of hematopoiesis, the nature of the supporting cells, and the growth factors that influence stem cell differentiation change during development.[63]

ANATOMIC AND FUNCTIONAL SHIFTS IN HEMATOPOIESIS

As in other vertebrates, hematopoiesis in the human embryo begins in the yolk sac. Embryonic red blood cells (RBCs) are visible in the yolk sac as early as 2 weeks' gestation.[63] Before the chorioallantoic placenta forms, the yolk sac is solely responsible for uptake and delivery of nutrients and oxygen to the growing embryo; thus, it is not surprising that this organ is the first site of hematopoiesis in the embryo.

Hematopoiesis in the yolk sac is restricted to production of RBCs and macrophages. Other types of blood cells (e.g., neutrophils, platelets, and lymphocytes) are not generated in the yolk sac, implying that these latter cell types are not essential for early development. The red blood cells produced by the yolk sac are extremely large (mean corpuscular volume [MCV] = 200) and remain nucleated throughout their brief life span. These cells express embryonic hemoglobins and distinctive surface markers. The metabolic characteristics of yolk sac erythroblasts also differ from those of erythrocytes produced later in development. Studies on chicken and mouse embryos suggest that yolk sac endoderm cells support hematopoietic stem cell differentiation during embryonic development. The humoral or cell-associated factors that regulate yolk sac hematopoiesis are unknown but probably differ from those that control later stages of hematopoiesis, such as erythropoietin or stem cell factor.[42]

At 6 weeks' gestation, the liver becomes the major site of hematopoiesis.[63] Most cells produced during the hepatic stage of hematopoiesis are erythroid, although platelets, neutrophils, and other blood cells also are generated. Between the third and fifth month of life, as many as 50% of the cells within the liver are erythroid precursors. The RBCs produced during this stage of hematopoiesis do not remain nucleated and are smaller than those produced by the yolk sac. During liver hematopoiesis, fetal hemoglobins are the predominant hemoglobins synthesized. The metabolic parameters and surface antigens of these cells differ from yolk sac erythroblasts. Hepatocytes appear to function as support cells for stem cell differentiation during this stage of hematopoiesis. Erythropoietin, possibly derived from extrarenal sources, and other growth factors appear to be required for this stage of hematopoiesis.[42]

By 24 weeks' gestation and after birth, the bone marrow is the principal site of blood cell production.[1] All types of blood cells are generated during marrow hematopoiesis. Beginning in late gestation and continuing through the first year of life, a gradual shift occurs from production of fetal hemoglobins to the so-called adult hemoglobins (see later). Over this period, the MCV of the RBCs continues to decline. Bone marrow stromal cells function as essential support cells during the marrow

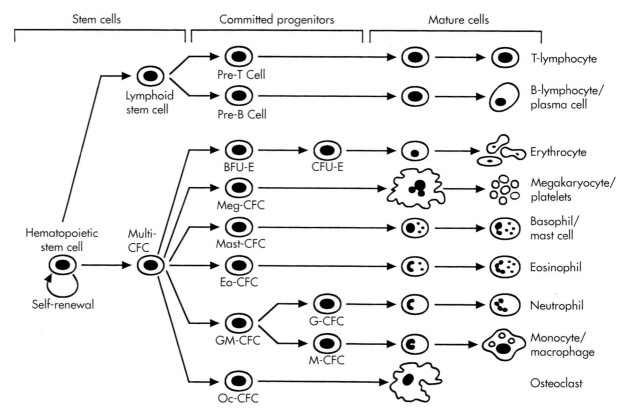

Figure 46–1. Hematopoietic stem cell differentiation. BFU-Ee, burst-forming units, erythroid; CFC, colony-forming cells; CFU-E, colony-forming unit, erythroid; Eo-CFC, eosinophil colony-forming cells; G-CFC, granulocyte colony-forming cells; GM-CFC, granulocyte-macrophage colony-forming cells; M-CFC, macrophage colony-forming cells; Meg-CFC, megakaryocyte colony-forming cells; Oc-CFC, osteoclast colony-forming cells.

phase of hematopoietic development. Bone marrow hematopoiesis depends on a number of growth factors, including erythropoietin and stem cell factor. Erythropoietin levels rise with gestational age, and by birth they exceed adult levels.[42]

Hematopoietic Growth Factors

Growth factors regulate the proliferation, differentiation, and survival of hematopoietic stem cells and committed progenitor cells.[42] In some instances, these factors also influence the survival and function of fully differentiated cells, including nonhematopoietic cells such as endothelial cells. Some hematopoietic growth factors are synthesized by support cells in the vicinity of hematopoietic progenitors, whereas other growth factors are synthesized at more distant sites. The past decade has witnessed a dramatic increase in our understanding of hematopoietic growth factors. Table 46-1 lists the currently known hematopoietic growth factors and their functions. To date, only a few of the glycoprotein growth factors are widely used clinically, although this number is likely to increase in the coming years.

The nomenclature associated with growth factors is complex. Many of these proteins have several names, reflecting the diversity of effects elicited by these factors in vitro and in vivo. For example, stem cell factor (SCF) is also known as kit ligand (KL), mast cell growth factor (M-CGF), and steel factor (SF). Some of the first hematopoietic growth factors identified were called colony-stimulating factors (CSFs), based on in vitro observations that these factors stimulate progenitor cells to form colonies of recognizable maturing cells. In the CSF nomenclature system, prefixes denote the cell types seen in the maturing colonies (e.g., GM-CSF, granulocyte-macrophage CSF). Another group of factors, the interleukins (ILs), were named for their cellular source or action on leukocytes. Still other factors derived their names from the cell surface receptor to which they bind because the receptor was identified before the ligand was characterized (e.g., kit ligand). Some hematopoietic growth factors, such as IL-3 and GM-CSF, support proliferation, differentiation, and survival of a broad range of precursors, including stem cells. Other growth factors, such as erythropoietin and granulocyte CSF (G-CSF), are lineage restricted. Clinical uses for the various hematopoietic growth factors are discussed later in the context of specific hematologic conditions.

RED BLOOD CELLS
Hemoglobins and Oxygen-Carrying Capacity

The function of RBCs is to transport oxygen (O_2) to tissues to meet metabolic demands. Hemoglobin (Hb), the most abundant protein in erythrocytes, facilitates oxygen delivery

TABLE 46-1   Hematopoietic Growth Factors

Factor	Source	Receptor	Target Cells	Effects
Erythropoietin (EPO)	Kidney, hepatocytes	EPO-R	E, Meg	Stimulates growth and differentiation of erythroid precursors
Stem cell factor (SCF) (also known as steel factor [SF], KIT ligand [KL], and mast cell growth factor [MCGF])	Ubiquitous	KIT	E, mast cells, melanocytes, germ cells	Stimulates growth and differentiation of erythroid and myeloid precursors; enhances growth of mast cells
Granulocyte colony-stimulating factor (G-CSF)	Stromal cells, macrophages	G-CSF-R	N	Stimulates growth and differentiation of neutrophil precursors; activates phagocytic function of mature neutrophils
Granulocyte-macrophage colony-stimulating factor (GM-CSF)	Stromal cells	GM-CSF-R (α and β chains)	M, N, Eo, Endo	Stimulates growth and differentiation of neutrophils, eosinophils, and monocytes; activates endothelial cells; induces cytokine expression by monocytes
Macrophage colony-stimulating factor (M-CSF)	Mesenchymal cells	FMS	M	Stimulates growth and differentiation of monocytes; induces phagocytic function in monocytes and macrophages; is involved in bone remodeling
Interleukin 1 (IL-1)	Ubiquitous	IL-1RI, IL-1RII	T, E, B, M, S	Induces production of cytokines and prostaglandins by stromal cells, T cells, and many other cell types; induces fever
Interleukin 2 (IL-2)	T cells	P55, P75	B, T, NK	Induces proliferation and activation of T, B, and NK cells; induces IL-1 expression by monocytes
Interleukin 3 (IL-3)	T cells	IL-3Rα, GM-CSF-Rβ	M, N, Eo, Meg	Stimulates growth and differentiation of myeloid and erythroid precursors, induces cytokines
Interleukin 4 (IL-4)	T cells, mast cells, basophils	IL-4R	M, Ba, B, T	Induces proliferation and activation of B and T cells
Interleukin 6 (IL-6)	Ubiquitous	IL-6R/GP130	B, N	Induces activation of neutrophils; induces B cell maturation, synergistic with IL-3
Interleukin 7 (IL-7)	Stromal cells	IL-2R	B, T, meg	Stimulates T cells; induces monocytes
Interleukin 8 (IL-8)	Stromal cells, macrophages, T cells	IL-8R	T, N	Induces neutrophils and chemotaxis
Interleukin 10 (IL-10)	T cells, macrophages	IL-10R	Meg, E	Induces B and mast cells; inhibits T cells
Interleukin 11 (IL-11)	Stromal cells	IL-11R, GP130	Meg	Stimulates megakaryocytes
Interleukin 12 (IL-12)	Neutrophils, monocytes	IL-12R	T, NK	Induces differentiation of cytotoxic T cells
Thrombopoietin (TPO)	Unknown	MPL	Meg	Stimulates megakaryocytes

B, B cells; Ba, basophil; E, erythroid precursors; Endo, endothelial cell; Eo, eosinophil; Meg, megakaryocyte; M, monocyte; N, neutrophil; NK, natural killer cell; S, stroma cell; T, T cell.

Adapted from Bagby CC: Hematopoiesis. In Stamatoyannopoulos G, et al, editors: *The molecular basis of blood diseases,* vol. 2, Philadelphia, 1994, Saunders, p 76.

TABLE 46–2   Human Hemoglobins Expressed During Development

Hemoglobin (Hb)	Globin Chain Composition	Stage of Expression	Primary Site of Production
Hb Gower 1	$\zeta_2\epsilon_2$	Embryonic	Yolk sac
Hb Gower 2	$\alpha_2\epsilon_2$	Embryonic	Yolk sac
Hb Portland	$\zeta_2\gamma_2$	Embryonic	Yolk sac
Hb F	$\alpha_2{}^{A}\gamma_2$ or $\alpha_2{}^{G}\gamma_2$	Fetal	Liver
Hb A_2	$\alpha_2\delta_2$	Adult	Bone marrow
Hb A	$\alpha_2\beta_2$	Adult	Bone marrow

by reversibly binding O_2 molecules. Individual molecules of hemoglobin are composed of four globin chains, each of which is covalently bound to a heme prosthetic group. Different globin chains are expressed in the course of normal development (Table 46-2) and in certain pathologic states. The physiologic hemoglobins are tetramers consisting of two α-type globins (α-globin or ζ-globin) and two β-type globins (β-globin, ε-globin, $^{A}\gamma$-globin, $^{G}\gamma$-globin, or δ-globin). For example, the major adult hemoglobin, Hb A, is composed of two α-globin chains and two β-globin chains ($\alpha_2\beta_2$). In states of globin synthetic imbalance (e.g., the thalassemias), Hb molecules composed of four identical chains can be formed, such as Hb Barts (γ_4) or Hb H (β_4). The binding of oxygen to hemoglobin tetramers is cooperative, resulting in the familiar sigmoidal oxygen dissociation curve (Fig. 46-2). The affinity of Hb molecules for oxygen is influenced by a variety of factors, including temperature, pH, carbon dioxide pressure (P_{CO_2}), and the concentration of red cell organic phosphates (e.g., 2,3-diphosphoglycerate [2,3-DPG]). In the case of Hb A, oxygen affinity for the molecule varies directly with pH and inversely with temperature and the concentration of 2,3-DPG. A high content of fetal hemoglobin (Hb F) is associated with high oxygen affinity, as is explained later (see also Chapter 44).

In the transition from yolk sac to liver to marrow hematopoiesis, different globin genes are sequentially expressed in RBC precursors, a process known as *hemoglobin switching* (Fig. 46-3). The two α-type globin genes, α-globin and ζ-globin, are adjacent on chromosome 16 and are arranged with the ζ gene 5′ to a pair of duplicated α-globin genes. The β-type genes are located on chromosome 11 and are oriented 5′ to 3′ as ε-, $^{A}\gamma$-, $^{G}\gamma$-, δ-, and β-globin genes. The protein products of the $^{A}\gamma$- and $^{G}\gamma$-globin genes differ only at a single amino acid residue and are functionally indistinguishable. During development, α-type and β-type globin gene clusters are activated sequentially from the 5′ (embryonic) end to the 3′ (adult) end. The mechanisms that control globin switching are complex. Temporal and cell-specific expression of specific globin genes is influenced by cis-elements within individual globin gene promoters, a distant 5′-enhancer called the *locus control region*, and a host of positively acting transcription factors, such as GATA1, GATA2, NFE2, MYB, EKLF, RBTN2, and SCL. Other mechanisms that also regulate globin switching are silencers, DNA conformational changes, and DNA methylation.[63]

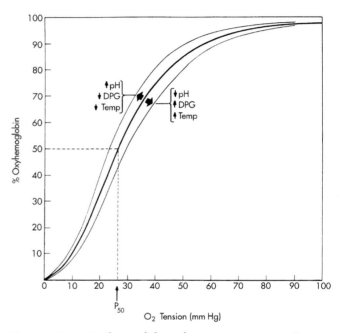

Figure 46–2. Oxyhemoglobin dissociation curve. Factors that influence the position of the curve are indicated. DPG, diphosphoglycerate. (*Adapted from Bunn HF, et al: Hemoglobin: molecular, genetic, and clinical aspects, Philadelphia, 1969, Saunders.*)

During yolk sac hematopoiesis, RBCs produce the embryonic hemoglobins (Hb Gower 1 [$\zeta_2\epsilon_2$]; Hb Gower 2 [$\alpha_2\epsilon_2$]; and Hb Portland [$\zeta_2\gamma_2$]). Hb F ($\alpha_2\gamma_2$), the predominant hemoglobin of the fetus and newborn, contains two α chains and two γ chains ($^{A}\gamma$ or $^{G}\gamma$, or both). Production of the major adult hemoglobin (Hb A) increases significantly between birth and 6 months of age, commensurate with a decline in the synthesis of Hb F. Synthesis of Hb A_2, a minor adult globin, also increases gradually over the first months of life. In anyone older than 6 months of age, Hb F usually constitutes less than 1% of the total hemoglobin and is unevenly distributed among red blood cells. Normally, only 0.1% to 7% of RBCs contain detectable Hb F. In the cells that express Hb F (F cells), Hb F constitutes about 20% of the cell's total hemoglobin.

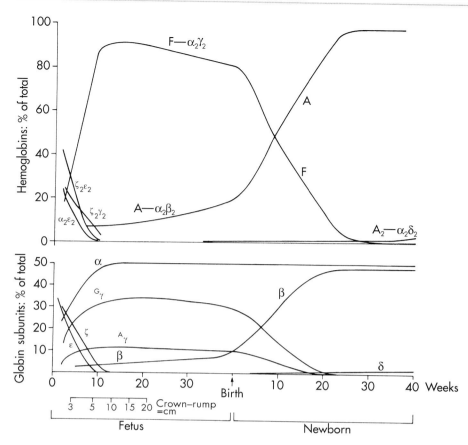

Figure 46–3. Changes in expression of hemoglobin tetramers (*upper panel*) and individual globin chains (*lower panel*) during development. (*Adapted from Bunn HF, et al: Hemoglobin: molecular, genetic, and clinical aspects, Philadelphia, 1969, Saunders.*)

The process of hemoglobin switching has been conserved through vertebrate evolution, suggesting that embryonic, fetal, and adult globins serve essential roles in development. Each of these different types of globin exhibits distinctive functional properties. Fetal erythrocytes, which are rich in Hb F, have a considerably higher oxygen affinity than adult red cells. This property is thought to facilitate the transport of oxygen from Hb A-bearing erythrocytes in the maternal circulation across the placenta to fetal red blood cells. The increased O_2 affinity of fetal hemoglobin has been ascribed to the diminished interactions of Hb F with red blood cell organic phosphates. Embryonic erythrocytes also display a greater affinity for oxygen than adult cells.

Erythropoietin Levels and Erythropoiesis

Fetal erythropoiesis is primarily under the control of the fetus. Erythropoietin (EPO) is a glycoprotein produced primarily in the fetal liver as well as in the cortical interstitial cells of the kidney. EPO regulates RBC production in response to tissue oxygen delivery and the oxygen saturation of hemoglobin. Adult erythropoiesis is controlled by the kidney. Levels of EPO in cord blood are higher than in adult blood samples (Table 46-3), but there is a dramatic decrease after birth in response to higher levels of tissue oxygenation. By 1 month of age, serum levels in healthy term infants reach their nadir. This is followed by a rise to maximal levels at 2 months of age, and then a slow drift down to adult values.[27] The postnatal changes in tissue oxygenation and erythropoietin

production result in a physiologic anemia of infancy with mean minimal hemoglobin concentrations in healthy term infants of about 11 g/dL at 6 to 9 weeks of life (Fig. 46-4; and see Table 46-5, later). Because of the shorter red blood cell life span in preterm infants, this physiologic anemia of infancy is noted earlier and may be more severe. Other causes of blood loss and suppression of erythropoiesis in the ill neonate can contribute to more severe and earlier anemia. Although preterm infants will respond to hypoxia with a rise in EPO levels, the increase is lower than that expected for term infants. The suboptimal EPO response may be due to developmental changes in transcription factors or to the site of fetal EPO production. The use of recombinant EPO in premature and sick newborn infants is discussed later.

Red Blood Cell Indices during Prenatal and Postnatal Development

The RBC count, Hb concentration, and hematocrit (Hct) increase throughout gestation, as shown in Table 46-4. In term infants, the mean capillary hemoglobin at birth is 19.3 g/dL (Table 46-5). The Hct has a mean of 61 g/dL. Premature infants have lower Hct levels than do full-term infants (see Table 46-4). In addition to gestational age, Hb and Hct levels are influenced by a variety of factors that must be kept in mind when analyzing the neonate with anemia or polycythemia. One important determinant of blood Hct is the site of sampling: capillary hematocrit values are higher than peripheral venous samples, and umbilical venous Hct results are the

TABLE 46–3 Serum Erythropoietin Levels During Infancy

Postnatal Age (days)	Serum Erythropoietin Level (mU/mL)	Sample Size
0-6	33.0 ± 31.4	11
7-50	11.7 ± 3.6	7
51-100	21.1 ± 5.5	13
101-150	15.1 ± 3.9	5
151-200	17.8 ± 6.3	6
>200	23.1 ± 9.7	10

From Yamashita H, et al: Serum erythropoietin levels in term and preterm infants during the first year of life, *Am J Pediatr Hematol Oncol* 16:213, 1994.

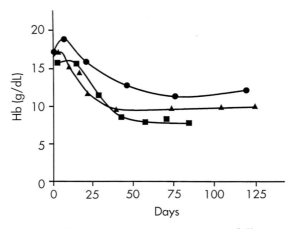

Figure 46–4. Hemoglobin concentrations in full-term and premature infants. (●) Full-term infants; (▲) premature infants, birthweight 1200 to 2350 g; (■) premature infants, birthweight less than 1200 g. (*Adapted from Oski F: The erythrocyte and its disorders. In Nathan D, et al, editors:* Hematology of infancy and childhood, *4th ed, Philadelphia, 1993, Saunders, p 18.*)

lowest. The interval between delivery and clamping of the umbilical cord also can significantly affect a newborn's blood volume and total RBC mass. The placenta contains about 100 mL of blood, and the mean blood volume of a full-term infant is about 85 mL/kg. Early or delayed clamping of the umbilical cord alters this mean blood volume by about 10% lower or higher, respectively. The average Hct at birth is relatively unchanged; however, 48 hours later, after redistribution of plasma volume, Hct values will reflect the lower or higher red cell mass. Racial differences also occur: one study reported significantly higher Hb, Hct, and MCV in white infants compared with black infants of similar gestational ages.[3] Reticulocyte counts in the cord blood of infants average 4% to 5%, and nucleated RBCs are evident in most cord blood samples (40,000/μL). These findings are presumed to reflect high EPO production secondary to low oxygen retention in utero. Infants who experience placental insufficiency and intrauterine growth restriction have higher than normal

EPO production and an even greater degree of erythrocytosis. The mean MCV of RBCs in the newborn is increased. The RBCs of the neonate have an increased Hb content, but the mean corpuscular hemoglobin concentration is comparable to that of adults.

Red Blood Cell Survival

The normal life span of adult RBCs is about 120 days. The life span of RBCs in newborns at term is about 60 to 80 days, and it is even more truncated in preterm infants. When the RBC life span is less than 2 standard deviations below the mean for age, hemolysis is occurring. In general, red blood cell survival is affected by changes related to aging (senescence) and by random hemolysis of red blood cells, or portions of red blood cells, in the spleen and the rest of the reticuloendothelial system. Aging erythrocytes with declining RBC enzyme activity become progressively less tolerant of oxidative challenges during the transportation of oxygen molecules and exposure to circulating oxidants. Any additional deficiencies in the enzymatic pathways of the RBC may affect the ability of the erythrocyte to tolerate oxidative challenges and further shrink red blood cell survival. With transit through the kidneys and lungs, the RBCs experience cycles of osmotic swelling and shrinkage. Shear forces in high-pressure areas of the circulation buffet the erythrocytes. Each passage through the cords of Billroth within the spleen requires the RBCs to deform and squeeze through tiny slits in the walls of the cords or face destruction if they cannot. Congenital or acquired defects in membrane stability or decreases in the ratio of surface area to red blood cell volume will also decrease erythrocyte survival. Alterations in the deformability of neonatal erythrocytes and relative intolerance to oxidative challenges result in shorter survival for neonatal red blood cells. Random hemolysis can be increased with splenic enlargement or activation of the phagocytic system. Infants with hemolysis may have exaggerated anemia because of decreased erythropoiesis, enhanced splenic filtration, and activation of phagocytes.

RED BLOOD CELL DISORDERS
Anemia
DEFINITION

Anemia is defined by a hemoglobin or hematocrit value that is more than 2 standard deviations below the mean for age. In the neonate, the causes of anemia can be divided into two broad categories: anemia resulting from accelerated loss or destruction of red blood cells and anemia caused by a defect at some stage of red blood cell production (Box 46-1). The defects may be congenital or acquired, and the abnormality may be intrinsic to the RBCs or extrinsic. Anemias also may be categorized on a morphologic basis. Using the normal range of the MCV for age and gestation, the anemia may be characterized as microcytic, normocytic, or macrocytic (Box 46-2). Hypochromicity, abnormal RBC shapes (poikilocytes), polychromasia, and cell inclusions (e.g., basophilic stippling or Howell-Jolly bodies) also provide clues to the etiology of the anemia (Table 46-6).

TABLE 46–4   Red Blood Cell Values (Arterial Samples) on First Postnatal Day at Different Gestational Ages*

Variables	Group 1	Group 2	Group 3
	23-25 wk (n = 40)	*26-28 wk (n = 60)*	*29-31 wk (n = 88)*
Hematocrit (%)	43.5 ± 4.2[†]	45.0 ± 4.5[‡]	48.0 ± 5.0[‡†]
	(36.0, 43.8, 51.0)	(37.5, 45.0, 54.3)	(39.4, 47.6, 56.0)
Hemoglobin (g/dL)	14.5 ± 1.6є	15.1 ± 1.6[‡]	16.2 ± 1.7[‡†]
	(12.0, 14.7, 17.4)	(12.5, 15.0, 18.3)	(13.2, 16.1, 18.8)
Mean corpuscular hemoglobin (pg)	38.6 ± 2.2[†]	38.3 ± 2.9	37.3 ± 2.5[†]
	(35.0, 38.6, 43.0)	(33.4, 38.4, 43.2)	(32.0, 37.5, 40.6)
Mean corpuscular volume (fL)	115.6 ± 5.6[†]	114.0 ± 7.6[‡]	110.4 ± 6.6[‡†]
	(107.0, 114.5, 125.7)	(98.4, 114.0, 126.6)	(97.3, 111.2, 120.0)
Mean corpuscular hemoglobin concentration (g/dL)	33.4 ± .9	33.6 ± .6	33.7 ± .7
	(32.3, 33.3, 34.6)	(32.3, 33.6, 34.6)	(32.5, 33.6, 34.9)
Red cell distribution width	15.9 ± 1.4	16.5 ± 1.9	16.4 ± 1.5
	(14.2, 15.6, 18.5)	(14.5, 16.0, 21.0)	(14.6, 16.0, 19.4)

*Values are reported as mean ± standard deviation and 5th, 50th, and 95th percentiles in parentheses.
[†] *P* value of <.01 between groups 1 and 3.
[‡] *P* value of <.01 between groups 2 and 3.
Modified from Alur P, et al: Impact of race and gestational age on red blood cell indices in very low birth weight infants, *Pediatrics* 106:306, 2000.

TABLE 46–5   Red Cell Values (Capillary Samples) for Term Infants During the First 12 Weeks of Life

Age	Hemoglobin (g/dL) ± SD	Red Blood Cells (× 10¹²/L) ± SD	Hematocrit (%) ± SD	Mean Corpuscular Volume (fL) ± SD	Mean Corpuscular Hemoglobin Concentration (g/dL) ± SD	Reticulocytes (%) ± SD
Days						
1	19.3 ± 2.2	5.14 ± 0.7	61 ± 7.4	119 ± 9.4	31.6 ± 1.9	3.2 ± 1.4
2	19.0 ± 1.9	5.15 ± 0.8	60 ± 6.4	115 ± 7.0	31.6 ± 1.4	3.2 ± 1.3
3	18.8 ± 2.0	5.11 ± 0.7	62 ± 9.3	116 ± 5.3	31.1 ± 2.8	2.8 ± 1.7
4	18.6 ± 2.1	5.00 ± 0.6	57 ± 8.1	114 ± 7.5	32.6 ± 1.5	1.8 ± 1.1
5	17.6 ± 1.1	4.97 ± 0.4	57 ± 7.3	114 ± 8.9	30.9 ± 2.2	1.2 ± 0.2
6	17.4 ± 2.2	5.00 ± 0.7	54 ± 7.2	113 ± 10.0	32.2 ± 1.6	0.6 ± 0.2
7	17.9 ± 2.5	4.86 ± 0.6	56 ± 9.4	118 ± 11.2	32.0 ± 1.6	0.5 ± 0.4
Weeks						
1-2	17.3 ± 2.3	4.80 ± 0.8	54 ± 8.3	112 ± 19.0	32.1 ± 2.9	0.5 ± 0.3
2-3	15.6 ± 2.6	4.20 ± 0.6	46 ± 7.3	111 ± 8.2	33.9 ± 1.9	0.8 ± 0.6
3-4	14.2 ± 2.1	4.00 ± 0.6	43 ± 5.7	105 ± 7.5	33.5 ± 1.6	0.6 ± 0.3
4-5	12.7 ± 1.6	3.60 ± 0.4	36 ± 4.8	101 ± 8.1	34.9 ± 1.6	0.9 ± 0.8
5-6	11.9 ± 1.5	3.55 ± 0.4	36 ± 6.2	102 ± 10.2	34.1 ± 2.9	1.0 ± 0.7
6-7	12.0 ± 1.5	3.40 ± 0.4	36 ± 4.8	105 ± 12.0	33.8 ± 2.3	1.2 ± 0.7
7-8	11.1 ± 1.1	3.40 ± 0.4	33 ± 3.7	100 ± 13.0	33.7 ± 2.6	1.5 ± 0.7
8-9	10.7 ± 0.9	3.40 ± 0.5	31 ± 2.5	93 ± 12.0	34.1 ± 2.2	1.8 ± 1.0
9-10	11.2 ± 0.9	3.60 ± 0.3	32 ± 2.7	91 ± 9.3	34.3 ± 2.9	1.2 ± 0.6
10-11	11.4 ± 0.9	3.70 ± 0.4	34 ± 2.1	91 ± 7.7	33.2 ± 2.4	1.2 ± 0.7
11-12	11.3 ± 0.9	3.70 ± 0.3	33 ± 3.3	88 ± 7.9	34.8 ± 2.2	0.7 ± 0.3

Adapted from Matoth Y, et al: Postnatal changes in some red cell parameters, *Acta Paediatr Scand* 60:317, 1971.

BOX 46–1 Anemias by Etiology

ACCELERATED LOSS
Hemorrhage
- Fetal
- Placental
- Traumatic delivery
- Coagulation defect
Early umbilical cord clamping
Twin-twin transfusion
Fetal-maternal transfusion

ACCELERATED DESTRUCTION
Hemolytic anemia
- Immune
    Alloimmune: Rh, ABO, minor blood group
    Autoimmune
- Nonimmune
    Hemoglobinopathy
    Thalassemias
    Unstable hemoglobin
    Red blood cell enzymatic defect
    Structural defect of red blood cell membrane
    Mechanical destruction
    Microangiopathic hemolytic anemia
    Infection
    Vitamin E deficiency

DIMINISHED RED BLOOD CELL PRODUCTION
Congenital
- Diamond-Blackfan anemia
- Fanconi anemia
- Anemia of prematurity
- Congenital dyserythropoietic anemia
Acquired
- Parvovirus B19
- Transient erythroblastopenia of childhood
- Human immunodeficiency virus infection
- Syphilis
- Iron deficiency
- Lead toxicity
- Excess phlebotomy losses

BOX 46–2 Classification of the Anemias According to Mean Corpuscular Volume

MACROCYTIC ANEMIA
Reticulocytosis
Folic acid deficiency*
Vitamin B_{12} deficiency*
Organic aciduria, acidemia (orotic aciduria, or MMA)
Diamond-Blackfan anemia
Fanconi anemia
Acquired aplastic anemia
Drugs

MICROCYTIC ANEMIA
Iron deficiency
Lead poisoning
Thalassemia
Chronic infection

NORMOCYTIC ANEMIA
Low reticulocyte count
- Infection
- Parvovirus B19
- Transient erythroblastopenia of childhood
- Chronic disease
- Immune HA
- Mechanical HA
- Drugs
- Leukemia
- Hemoglobinopathy
- Unstable hemoglobin

Normal or high reticulocyte count
- Blood loss
- Sequestration
- Red blood cell enzyme defects

*Macro-ovalocytes.
HA, hemolytic anemia; MMA, methylmalonic aciduria.

EVALUATION

The clinician begins the evaluation of anemia by taking a thorough history. Appropriate data vary with the patient's age but often include the medical and dietary history of the pregnancy, the estimated gestational age at birth, the chronologic age, the infant's diet, and details of any previous anemia, blood loss, transfusions, medications, and illnesses, as well as the family history of anemia. The physical examination should evaluate the infant's general health, growth, and development. Identification of any dysmorphic features, abnormal masses, or skin lesions can aid the diagnosis (Table 46-7). The patient also should be assessed for jaundice, hepatosplenomegaly, cardiovascular function, and lymphadenopathy.

The initial laboratory evaluation includes a complete blood count (CBC) with RBC indexes, a reticulocyte count, and evaluation of the peripheral blood smear (Fig. 46-5). The results of the preliminary laboratory testing, combined with information from the history and physical examination, should dictate the need for further tests, such as hemoglobin analysis of the infant or parents, CBCs and blood smears of the parents, analysis of hepatic or renal function, direct or indirect antiglobulin (Coombs) testing, cultures or titers to identify infectious agents, a bone marrow aspirate or biopsy, osmotic fragility tests, and quantitative or qualitative testing for glucose-6-phosphate dehydrogenase (G6PD) deficiency.

The neonatal patient presents the diagnostician with a number of unique challenges. Because of the small total blood volume of the infant, who already is anemic, testing must be limited. Major pediatric medical centers can perform many of the necessary tests on very small quantities of blood, especially if the tests are appropriately batched when they are submitted. Because of the many morphologic and biochemical differences in fetal and infant RBCs, some diagnoses are best made by testing the parents for evidence of disease or carrier states. At times, a definitive diagnosis can be made only with repeat testing later in infancy, when the infant would be expected to have a much higher percentage of

TABLE 46–6	Morphologic Findings on Peripheral Blood Smears
Morphologic Finding	**Etiologies**
Hypochromia	Iron deficiency, thalassemia, lead poisoning
Target cells	HB C, S, or E; thalassemia; liver disease; abetalipoproteinemia
Sickle cells	Hb S disease and variants
Basophilic stippling	Iron deficiency; lead poisoning; hemolytic anemia; thalassemia
Heinz bodies	Normal in newborn; hemolytic anemias—enzymatic defects
Howell-Jolly bodies	Splenic hypofunction or postsplenectomy
Spherocytes	Immune HA ABO more common than Rh; G6PD deficiency; structural defects of red blood cell membrane cytoskeleton
Elliptocytes	Structural defects of red cell membrane cytoskeleton
Schistocytes	Microangiopathic hemolytic anemia
Nucleated red blood cells	Normal in newborn; hemolytic anemia; semi-acute blood loss
Polychromasia	Normal in newborn; proliferative response to anemia

G6PD, glucose-6-phosphate dehydrogenase; HA, hemolytic anemia.

TABLE 46–7	Physical Findings in Neonatal Anemia
Physical Finding	**Etiologies**
Short stature	Fanconi anemia; Diamond-Blackfan anemia
Microcephaly	Congenital infection
Dysmorphic features	Fanconi anemia; Diamond-Blackfan anemia
Jaundice	Hemolytic anemia
"Blueberry muffin" spots	Congenital infection
Petechiae	Bone marrow infiltration/failure; disseminated intravascular coagulation; sepsis
Congestive heart failure	Chronic anemia causing decompensation
Cardiac disease	"Waring blender" syndrome
Giant hemangioma	Kasabach-Merritt syndrome

adult-type RBCs or when the infant has recovered from an acute hemolytic crisis that might have destroyed the older, more biochemically or morphologically abnormal cells.

RATIONALE FOR TRANSFUSION THERAPY

See also Chapter 46, Part 2.

Because the primary function of the RBC is to transport oxygen from the pulmonary bed to other tissues for release, anemia diminishes oxygen-carrying capacity and can compromise tissue oxygenation. Tissue oxygenation is a complex concept involving not only the Hb concentration but also the oxygen affinity of the hemoglobin in the patient's red blood cells and the patient's cardiorespiratory status. The only absolute indications for rapidly correcting anemia by RBC transfusion are to restore tissue oxygenation and to expand blood volume after severe, acute loss. In most pediatric centers, the sicker patients, especially those with cardiopulmonary dysfunction, receive transfusions to maintain the Hb and Hct values closer to normal for that age. Neonatal exchange transfusions are also performed with the goal of replacing "doomed" infant RBCs with healthy adult RBCs, which have superior oxygen-transporting ability. This has the triple benefit of limiting hyperbilirubinemia from RBC breakdown, reducing the body load of maternal antibodies, and supplementing with cells that contain Hb A.

ANEMIA CAUSED BY BLOOD LOSS

Blood loss can occur in the fetus, at birth, or in the postnatal period. The bleeding can be acute or chronic. Anemia caused by chronic blood loss generally is better tolerated because the neonate will at least partly compensate for a gradual reduction in RBC mass. Chronic blood loss can be diagnosed by identifying signs of compensation. Doppler assessment of the fetal middle cerebral artery peak systolic velocity is a noninvasive method for determination of fetal anemia, independent of the etiology. The infant may be pale and might exhibit signs and symptoms of congestive heart failure. Anemia will be present, often with reticulocytosis, hypochromia, and microcytosis.

An infant with acute blood loss may not be anemic if blood sampling is done soon enough after the acute event that hemodilution has not yet occurred. Anemia usually develops within 3 to 4 hours after blood loss; repeat testing 6 to 12 hours after the event should reveal the true extent of the loss. In acute blood loss, the infant might exhibit signs and symptoms of hypovolemia and hypoxemia (e.g., tachycardia, tachypnea, and hypotension). The RBCs should be morphologically normal. With either kind of hemorrhage, infants tend to have fewer problems with hyperbilirubinemia because they have a reduced RBC mass.

Either maternal or fetal factors can cause prenatal blood loss. In a study of 259 patients in a neonatal intensive care unit, Faxelius and colleagues[30] correlated reduced RBC mass with a maternal history of vaginal bleeding, placenta previa, abruptio placentae, nonelective cesarean delivery, and cord compression. Infants with 1-minute Apgar scores of 6 or lower also had a lower RBC volume at birth or shortly thereafter. Hemorrhage from the umbilical cord may be the result of intrinsic vascular abnormalities, inflammation of the cord, velamentous insertion of the cord, or an unusually short cord. A normal cord can rupture during a precipitous or assisted delivery or if it becomes tangled around the infant. Placental abnormalities such as abruptio placentae or placenta

Figure 46–5. Algorithm for diagnosis of anemia in the neonate. MCV, mean corpuscular volume.

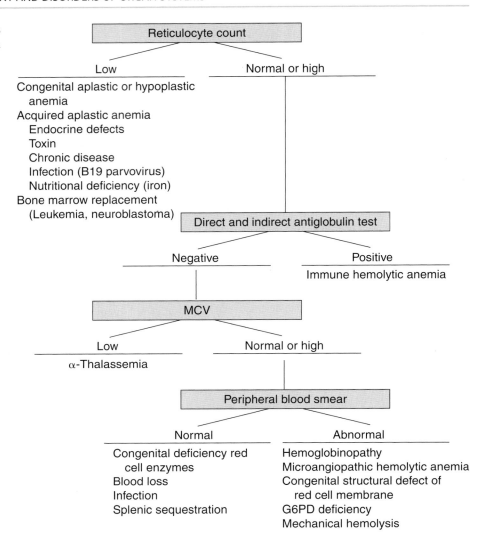

previa can cause hemorrhage. Accidental incision of the placenta during delivery also can result in bleeding.

The acid elution technique, or Kleihauer-Betke test, can be used to look for fetal RBCs in vaginal or peripheral blood samples from women with vaginal bleeding late in pregnancy. This method exploits the stability of Hb F-containing RBCs in acid solution relative to cells containing Hb A. False-positive test results are seen in women with any condition, including many of the hemoglobinopathies, that elevates their own Hb F level. Some centers now offer immunofluorescence flow cytometry testing, which can sort RBCs by whether they are Rh negative or positive. This is useful for evaluating the amount of Rh positive fetal blood that is present in a blood sample from an Rh negative mother.[33]

Fetal-Maternal Hemorrhage

Fetal cells may be found in the maternal circulation in about half of all pregnancies. In about 8% of pregnancies, the transfer of blood is estimated to be between 0.5 and 40 mL; in about 1% of pregnancies, the volume of blood transferred exceeds 40 mL.[33] Fetal-maternal hemorrhage is more common after procedures such as an external cephalic version before delivery or a

traumatic amniocentesis. The diagnosis is made by demonstrating fetal RBCs in a maternal blood sample; therefore, the analysis must be done before the fetal cells are cleared from the maternal circulation. The test usually is performed within the first few hours after delivery; in cases of ABO blood group incompatibility, the red cells may be cleared faster than this, and the test may be falsely negative. The most commonly performed test is the Kleihauer-Betke test, although flow cytometry is available in many major centers. If the maternal Hb F level is above normal, another type of test that is based on differential agglutination should be used.

TWIN-TWIN TRANSFUSION

In monozygotic multiple births with monochorial placentas, blood can be exchanged between the fetuses through vascular anomalies (see Chapters 19 and 24). The incidence of twin-twin transfusions has been estimated at 9% to 15% of monochorionic pregnancies and can be associated with a high risk for fetal and neonatal morbidity and mortality. Transfusion can be problematic for the hypovolemic donor who develops oligohydramnios, but the recipient often experiences greater difficulties with hyperbilirubinemia, hypervolemia, and hyperviscosity that arise from the increased RBC mass. Cardiac, neurologic, and developmental disorders have been associated with twin-twin transfusion syndrome.[66]

HEMORRHAGE

Internal bleeding can occur if the fetus has anatomic abnormalities or defects in the hemostatic system, or with a history of interventional obstetric procedures. Often the first signs of internal hemorrhage in the newborn are those of hypovolemic shock and hypoxemia. Jaundice occurs later when the entrapped RBCs break down. A surprisingly large amount of blood can be lost within a cephalohematoma (see Chapter 28), and even greater bleeding can occur in the subaponeurotic area of the scalp (subgaleal hemorrhage), where bleeding is not limited by periosteal attachments. Traumatic or assisted deliveries and vitamin K deficiency are commonly associated with such bleeding. Full-term infants might have intracranial bleeding, which usually occurs in the subarachnoid or subdural regions (see Chapter 40). Although the cause might not be found, full-term infants with intracranial hemorrhage should be evaluated for hemostasis abnormalities because this type of bleeding is associated with qualitative and quantitative platelet defects and with abnormalities of several of the coagulation proteins. Hemorrhage into the adrenals, kidneys, liver, spleen, or retroperitoneum also can occur after difficult or breech deliveries. Splenic or hepatic rupture can occur after trauma, especially if the organs are enlarged as a result of extramedullary hematopoiesis. Occult or superficial vascular tumors can bleed and sequester large volumes of red blood cells and platelets.

HEMOLYTIC ANEMIA: ACCELERATED DESTRUCTION OF RED BLOOD CELLS

See also "Red Blood Cell Survival."
Accelerated destruction of RBCs is the endpoint of a number of intrinsic, extrinsic, congenital, and acquired RBC abnormalities. Because the RBCs of premature infants and newborns

have a shorter life span, *hemolysis* is defined as a process that shortens the survival of the RBCs relative to the life span expected for the infant's gestational and postnatal age. In contrast to anemia caused by blood loss, most infants with hemolysis have some evidence of indirect hyperbilirubinemia and elevated lactate dehydrogenase for age. Reticulocytosis should accompany the hemolysis, although in conditions complicated by bone marrow suppression (e.g., congenital infections, chronic illness, or nutritional deficiency) or decreased EPO production, the reticulocyte count may be inappropriately low for the degree of anemia present. With maximal bone marrow response, RBC survival of 20 to 30 days can be compensated for without anemia. The bone marrow may show hyperplasia and a reversal of the usual myeloid-to-erythroid ratio of 3:1. Because optimal conditions for bone marrow response are not present in the newborn, hemolysis with anemia and hyperbilirubinemia may be evident in the neonate. In chronic hemolytic states, compensatory hypertrophy of the bone marrow may result in bony changes over time, especially of the skull and hands.

Intrinsic hemolytic anemias are caused by inherited abnormalities of the RBC membrane, hemoglobin, or RBC intracellular enzymes. Extrinsic factors cause hemolytic anemia by damaging the RBC chemically, physically, or immunologically. Some intrinsic hemolytic anemias also result in extrinsic damage to RBCs. Extrinsic hemolysis can be divided into immune and nonimmune etiologies (Table 46-8); the most common causes of immune hemolytic disease are discussed first.

ALLOIMMUNE HEMOLYTIC ANEMIA

See Chapter 21.
Alloimmune hemolytic disease of the newborn (HDN) is caused by the destruction of fetal or neonatal RBCs by maternal immunoglobulin G (IgG) antibodies. Alloimmune HDN involves the major blood group antigens of the Rhesus (Rh),

TABLE 46–8   Acute Hemolytic Anemia: Causative Mechanisms and Representative Infectious Agents

Mechanism	Infectious Agent
Release of hemolysin	*Clostridium perfringens*
Direct invasion of red blood cell	Malaria
Alteration of red blood cell surface	
By adherence of organism	*Bartonella* organisms
By alteration of antigenic phenotype by neuramidase	Influenza virus
By cold agglutinin	Epstein-Barr virus
By absorption of capsular polysaccharide	*Haemophilus influenzae*
Microangiopathy	Any agent causing disseminated intravascular coagulation or hemolytic-uremic syndrome
Enhanced oxidative damage in patients with enzyme deficiency	*Campylobacter jejuni* enteritis in neonates with a diminished cytochrome-b_5 reductase system

From Ritchey AK, et al: Hematologic manifestations of childhood illness. In Hoffman R, et al, editors: *Hematology: basic principles and practice,* 2nd ed, New York, 1995, Churchill Livingstone, p 1722.

A, B, AB, and O systems, but minor blood group incompatibilities (Kell, Duffy, MNS, and P systems) can also be associated with clinically significant disease. Particularly for Rh (D), anti-c, anti-E, and anti-K (Kell) antibodies, intrauterine or direct fetal transfusion may be indicated prenatally, and exchange transfusion may be necessary postnatally. Maternal IgG antibodies can cross the placenta, enter the fetal circulation, and cause hemolysis, anemia, hyperbilirubinemia, and hydrops fetalis. In utero, the process is called *erythroblastosis fetalis*, while postnatally it is called hemolytic disease of the newborn (HDN). Maternal sensitization occurs through a prior transfusion of incompatible RBCs, after fetal-maternal hemorrhage of incompatible fetal RBCs, or from production of a preexisting antibody developed against antigens from bacteria, viruses, or food. Transfer of antibodies across the placenta depends on the F_c component of the IgG molecule. Because both IgM and IgA antibodies lack this component, only IgG antibodies cause hemolytic disease of the newborn. IgG1 antibodies cross the placenta earlier and are responsible for more prenatal hemolysis. IgG3 antibodies cross the placenta later in gestation and are responsible for more severe hemolysis postnatally.

Rh Hemolytic Disease

The original description of HDN was due to Rh (D) incompatibility, and it remains the most severe cause. The spectrum of clinical problems caused by Rh HDN ranges from mild, self-limited hemolytic anemia to hydrops fetalis. With the widespread use of antenatal and postpartum Rh immunoglobulin administration, Rh(D) sensitization is less common in pregnancies in which prenatal care is received. Failure to administer Rh immunoglobulin when indicated, nonrecognition of a large fetal bleed, and chronic transplacental hemorrhage account for most of the cases currently seen.

The Rh antigens are inherited as a linked group of two genes, *RHD* and *RHCE*, located on chromosome 1. People are typed as Rh negative or positive based on the expression of the major D antigen on the RBC, and their RBCs will also express C or c and E or e antigens. Rarely, Rh deletions of D, C/c, and E/e loci can occur. Anti-c and anti-E are emerging as the most frequent causes of isoimmune HDN as the incidence of Rh(D) disease decreases. The incidence of Rh disease depends on the prevalence of Rh-negative antigens in the population studied (Table 46-9). Even in white populations, only a small percentage of pregnancies are affected because not all women who are Rh negative develop antibodies, Rh immunization of the mother does not usually occur during the first pregnancy, and some of the second infants will be Rh negative.

The interaction of the anti-D IgG with a D-positive RBC does not usually involve complement. Hemolysis generally is extravascular. Hyperbilirubinemia and jaundice can occur in the first day of life because the placenta no longer is available to clear bilirubin from hemolyzed RBCs. The peripheral blood smear might show anemia, reticulocytosis, and macrocytosis. Microspherocytes are usually not seen in Rh disease. A direct antiglobulin (Coombs) test should demonstrate anti-D IgG. Partial or total exchange transfusions may be necessary to reduce the load of antibody and remove the antibody-coated cells. Management of hyperbilirubinemia is discussed in Chapter 48. In a series of 101 babies born to Rh(D)-negative mothers who received one or two doses of anti-D

TABLE 46–9	**Prevalence of Rh-Negative Genotype (CDE/CDE) by Population**
Population Group	**Percent Affected**
European whites	11-21
U.S. whites	14.4
Indians (India)	8
U.S. African Americans	5.5
Native Americans	0
Chinese	0
Japanese	0

Adapted from Prokop O, et al: *Human blood and serum groups,* Barking, UK, 1969, Elsevier.

immunoglobulin, no signs of hemolysis were noted in the Rh(D)-positive or Rh(D)-negative infants. Twenty percent of Rh-positive babies whose mothers received two doses of anti-D immunoglobulin had a positive direct Coombs test, compared with 2.4% of those whose mothers received only one dose.[49]

ABO Hemolytic Disease

Although the incidence of blood group O mothers delivering babies of blood group A or B is about 15%, ABO hemolytic disease is estimated to occur in only 3% of pregnancies and requires treatment with exchange transfusion in less than 0.1% of pregnancies. In contrast to Rh hemolytic disease, ABO hemolytic disease tends to be less severe (i.e., less frequently requires exchange transfusion), and the severity does not depend on birth order. Maternal anti-A or anti-B IgG antibodies, which might have been raised against A or B substances occurring in food or on bacteria, can cross the placenta and react with the sparsely distributed A or B antigens on the neonatal RBCs. ABO HDN occurs in infants with type A or B blood. African-American infants with type B blood can have more severe hemolysis, presumably because the B antigen is more developed in this group of neonates.

Hemolysis is primarily extravascular. Infants may develop anemia, reticulocytosis, and hyperbilirubinemia within the first 24 hours of life. The hallmark of ABO hemolytic disease (in contrast to Rh disease) is the presence of microspherocytes on the peripheral blood smear. The direct antiglobulin test should be at least weakly positive for anti-A or anti-B; however, because of the sparse distribution of antigenic sites on a newborn's RBCs, ABO hemolytic disease may be present even without a positive result on the direct antiglobulin test. The maternal serum should have high titers of IgG directed against A or B (positive indirect antiglobulin test). In the absence of clinical hemolytic disease, laboratory evidence of erythrocyte sensitization should not be considered HDN.

Minor Blood Group Hemolytic Diseases

The incidence of HDN for minor blood group antigens is related to the antigenicity of the particular blood group antigen and the expression of that antigen on fetal RBCs. Maternal antibodies against minor blood group antigens develop after exposure from a transfusion or prior pregnancy, or from contact with bacteria or viruses that express the antigen. HDN has been associated with the minor group antigens Kell, Duffy, MNS system, and P system. Most clinically significant HDN not attributed to ABO or Rh incompatibility is due to anti-Kell, anti-E, and anti-c. Kell HDN may require intrauterine intervention. The severity of anti-Kell HDN is due both to hemolysis and to suppression of erythropoiesis in progenitor cells. Screening for minor group antibodies is recommended for all women in the 34th week of pregnancy: routine screening with cells containing only high-frequency antigens would not detect antibodies to low-frequency antigens. The diagnosis and treatment of hemolytic disease are identical to those for Rh hemolytic disease (see Chapters 21 and 48). Identification of low-frequency antibodies associated with HDN is especially important for mothers who plan additional pregnancies.

Natural History of Hemolytic Diseases of the Newborn
Hydrops fetalis is the most severe consequence of hemolysis, but anemia generally is less problematic than hyperbilirubinemia in the acute phase of illness. Hyperbilirubinemia may be evident within the first 24 hours of life. Anemia can occur in the first few weeks in both those who received exchange transfusions and those who required only phototherapy for management of hyperbilirubinemia. Many causes for the anemia have been postulated, including ongoing destruction of native cells by anti-blood group IgG, hypersplenism, inadequate replacement by transfused red blood cells, and shortened survival of transfused red blood cells. Because the half-life of IgG molecules is about 28 days, hemolysis should resolve within the first 3 or 4 months. Resolution often occurs sooner if the antibodies are cleared by adhering to RBCs or by exchange transfusion. Thrombocytopenia and bleeding can complicate hemolytic disease. Usually thrombocytopenia, without other laboratory evidence of disseminated intravascular coagulation (DIC), is noted, but DIC can be triggered by massive hemolysis or shock and acidosis.

Other Immune Hemolytic Anemias
The other immune hemolytic diseases of early childhood are relatively rare. Autoimmune hemolytic anemia occurs, as do anemias associated with infections, drugs, and immunodeficiency syndromes. IgG antibodies, with or without complement, are often directed against one of the Rh erythrocyte antigens. These antibodies are most active at 37°C and often are called *warm autoantibodies*. The IgG-coated cells, with or without the assistance of complement, are cleared by the spleen and, to a lesser extent, by the liver. Congenital infections (syphilis, cytomegalovirus [CMV], rubella, toxoplasmosis, herpes), bacterial infections, and viral infections, such as infection with the human immunodeficiency virus (HIV) and hepatitis, can cause hemolytic anemia and bone marrow suppression with reticulocytopenia (see Chapter 39). IgM autoantibodies can cause disease and usually are referred to as *cold agglutinins* because they are most active at between 0° and 30°C. These antibodies, with complement, coat RBCs and are usually cleared in the liver. Intravascular hemolysis is less common. The best known causes of cold hemagglutinin disease are *Mycoplasma pneumoniae* and Epstein-Barr virus. IgA-mediated hemolysis is quite rare but is remarkable for its severity.

The natural history of autoimmune hemolytic disease in infancy is that of a rapid onset of anemia with hyperbilirubinemia, splenomegaly or hepatomegaly, and hemoglobinuria. Initially, reticulocytopenia may be noted, especially if antibodies are directed against RBC progenitors in the bone marrow, but a brisk reticulocytosis usually follows. Resolution within 3 to 6 months is common. Anemia with reticulocytosis and spherocytosis may be seen on the peripheral blood smear, but the diagnosis depends on demonstration of antibody-coated cells, with or without complement, in the direct and indirect antiglobulin tests. Therapy includes treatment of underlying infection, removal of the offending drug, and supportive measures to limit hyperbilirubinemia. Response to corticosteroids is common, as is complete recovery. Steroids are less effective in IgM-mediated disease. A subset of patients younger than 2 years and with a slower onset of disease at presentation develop chronic hemolytic anemia. Difficulties with identifying compatible blood during a hemolytic crisis, as well as the usually self-limited nature of the disease, restrict blood transfusions to cases in which severe anemia impairs tissue oxygenation.

NONIMMUNE HEMOLYTIC ANEMIA
Erythrocyte Structural Defects
During its lifetime, a normal RBC traverses the circulation thousands of times, enduring tremendous mechanical and metabolic stress with each passage. The smallest capillaries have an internal diameter that is smaller than the diameter of the RBC; thus the blood cells must deform to squeeze through the capillaries and then return to their normal shape as they enter distal venules. During their rapid transit, the RBCs must endure tremendous fluctuations in pH, Po_2, and osmotic pressure. The lipid bilayer that forms the cell membrane is the site of numerous biologic functions mediated by integral proteins. It also is the attachment site for the proteins of the cytoskeleton, which confer the shape and stability necessary for proper membrane function. Some abnormalities in the membrane-cytoskeleton unit result in morphologic defects of RBCs (Fig. 46-6).[34] Because abnormally shaped RBCs are removed from the circulation by the reticuloendothelial system, many of these defects cause some degree of hemolytic anemia. Analysis of these defects has led to an understanding of the erythrocyte membrane and cytoskeleton.

The more common erythrocyte cytoskeletal defects originally were described by morphologic, genetic, and clinical criteria. As knowledge of the cytoskeleton at a molecular level accumulated, it became clear that various mutations in genes coding for a few structural proteins were responsible for a family of inherited hemolytic anemias with overlapping morphologic, clinical, and genetic features. Mutations in the genes encoding α-spectrin, β-spectrin, ankyrin, protein 4.1, glycophorin C, protein 4.2, and band 3 all have been reported in patients with hereditary spherocytosis, hereditary elliptocytosis, hereditary ovalocytosis, and hereditary pyropoikilocytosis.[34]

The following discussion of the most common disorders uses the classic morphologic criteria. These defects commonly manifest during childhood and occasionally cause hepatosplenomegaly, hyperbilirubinemia, and hemolytic

Figure 46–6. Molecular origins of hereditary spherocytosis (HS) and hereditary elliptocytosis-pyropoikilocytosis (HE/HPP) based on the hypothesis of vertical and horizontal defects. Vertical interactions are those needed to stabilize the attachment of the spectrin lattice to the lipid bilayer. Abnormalities in this attachment result in destabilization of the lipid bilayer, membrane loss during splenic conditioning, and HS. Horizontal interactions reversibly hold spectrin dimers and tetramers together, allowing stretching and distortion of the red blood cell membrane during circulation. Weakening of these interactions results in loss of elasticity. GP, glycoproteins. (*Adapted from Palek J: Red cell membrane disorders. In Hoffman R, et al, editor:* Hematology: basic principles and practice, *New York, 1991, Churchill Livingstone, p 472.*)

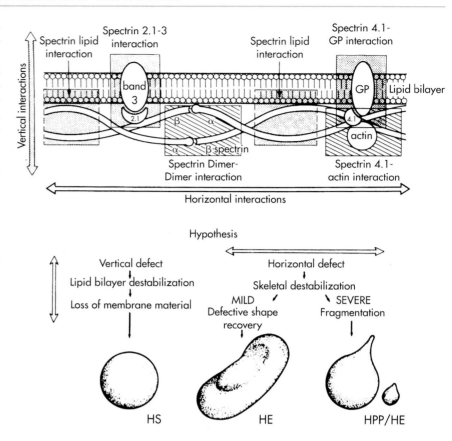

anemia in the neonate. Often the specific diagnosis depends on evaluation of family members and serial examinations of the infant's blood smear over time. Aplastic crisis, attributed to drugs or an infectious agent such as parvovirus B19, or splenic sequestration might cause life-threatening anemia in patients with hemolytic anemia. The more severe cases of hemolytic anemia can require splenectomy, although surgery generally is delayed beyond the first few years of life.

HEREDITARY SPHEROCYTOSIS

Hereditary spherocytosis is characterized by the appearance of spherocytes on the peripheral blood smear, accompanied by a hemolytic anemia of varying severity and by splenomegaly. Hereditary spherocytosis is noted predominantly in those of Northern European ancestry. Inheritance usually is autosomal dominant, but autosomal recessive inheritance and autosomal dominant inheritance with reduced penetrance also have been reported.[11] The defects studied alter the stability of the cytoskeleton attachment to the lipid bilayer, so that pieces of membrane are removed in the spleen. Defect or deficiency in spectrin are the most common, with some accompanying defects in ankyrin, band 3, and protein 4.2.[34] Nondeformable spherocytes with a decrease in the surface area are more susceptible to lysis on exposure to the metabolic and deformation stresses of the splenic sinuses or with incubation in hypo-osmolar solutions. The osmotic fragility test exposes the suspected cells and normal control cells to progressively more hypotonic solutions and compares their ability to resist lysis.

HEREDITARY ELLIPTOCYTOSIS AND HEREDITARY PYROPOIKILOCYTOSIS

The findings on the peripheral blood smears in hereditary elliptocytosis and hereditary pyropoikilocytosis are distinct (Fig. 46-7). Hereditary elliptocytosis is an autosomal dominant condition characterized by elliptical RBCs. In hereditary pyropoikilocytosis, the RBC morphology is bizarre, marked by fragments, elliptocytes, and spiculated cells. The disorders are caused by defects in various proteins; the defects weaken the structural interactions necessary for cellular stability and reversible deformability.[11] The RBCs tend to retain deformed shapes and are cleared by the reticuloendothelial system. Hemolysis in hereditary elliptocytosis generally is milder than in hereditary spherocytosis, although patients with hereditary elliptocytosis can exhibit hemolysis and hyperbilirubinemia in the neonatal period. Persons with hereditary pyropoikilocytosis have inherited genes encoding abnormal structural proteins (e.g., hereditary elliptocytosis alleles) from each parent. Hereditary pyropoikilocytosis is associated with more severe hemolysis and hyperbilirubinemia, often requiring exchange transfusion or phototherapy in the neonatal period.[23] Examination of blood smears from each parent is helpful in making this diagnosis.

Membrane Lipid Defects

Membrane lipid abnormalities can be inherited but most often are acquired. Their presence, detected by morphologic abnormalities on the peripheral blood smear, usually is most important as the signal of an underlying disease. Target cells form when the surface-to-volume ratio of the red blood cell

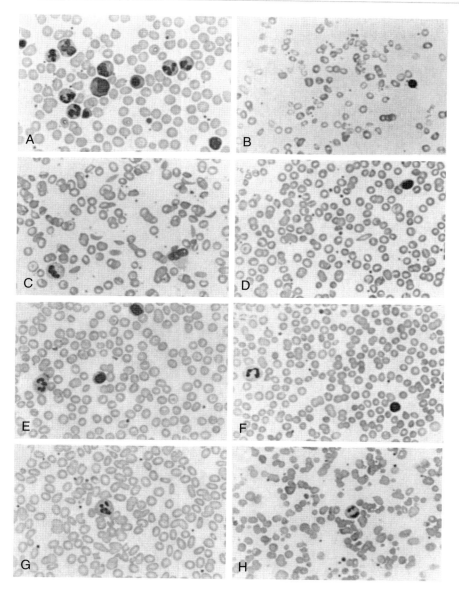

Figure 46–7. Peripheral blood smears. **A**, Premature newborn of 26 weeks' gestation. **B**, Iron deficiency. **C**, Hemoglobin SS. **D**, Hemoglobin SC. **E**, Hemoglobin CC. **F**, Hereditary spherocytosis. **G**, Hereditary elliptocytosis. **H**, Hereditary pyropoikilocytosis.

increases, either because of poorly hemoglobinated cells (iron deficiency, thalassemias, Hb C) or because lipids are added to the RBC membrane (liver disease with intrahepatic cholestasis, lecithin-cholesterol acyltransferase deficiency). Acanthocytes form when the membrane lipid composition is altered between the inner and outer leaflets of the bilayer, as in liver disease and abetalipoproteinemia.[34]

Inherited Enzymatic Defects

The mature RBC, lacking a nucleus, polyribosomes, and mitochondria with which to perform protein synthesis, must circulate through extremes of pH, Po_2, and osmotic gradients while maintaining deformability and integrity. It also must metabolize glucose through the Embden-Meyerhof pathway and hexose monophosphate shunt to provide energy for maintaining ionic pumps, to achieve reduction of methemoglobin to hemoglobin, and to synthesize small molecules such as adenine, guanine, pyrimidine nucleotides, glutathione, and lipids. Defects in the enzymatic machinery of the

erythrocyte have been studied since the 1940s. The most commonly affected enzyme, G6PD, has been extensively evaluated at the clinical, biochemical, and molecular level.[17] Many other enzymatic defects have been reported, but the rarity of the disorders has hindered investigation. Enzymatic defects of the RBC known to be associated with hemolytic anemia are listed in Box 46-3. A few of the enzyme deficiencies cause abnormalities in other tissues. The end result of these defects is hemolytic anemia of varying severity, sometimes called *hereditary nonspherocytic anemia.* The RBCs are generally morphologically normal and usually produce normal results on osmotic fragility testing, but they have a shorter life span. The milder cases cause little difficulty in the neonatal period. Occasionally, the hemolysis is severe, requiring chronic transfusion therapy and encouraging investigators to evaluate the possibilities of gene transfer therapy.

G6PD deficiency is the only common defect of RBC enzymes, and its prevalence among some ethnic groups initiated studies that suggested a selective advantage for

---

BOX 46–3 Red Blood Cell Enzymatic Defects Associated with Hemolysis

GLYCOLYTIC PATHWAY
Pyruvate kinase
Hexokinase
Glucose phosphate isomerase
Phosphofructokinase
Aldolase
Triose phosphate isomerase
Glyceraldehyde-3-phosphate dehydrogenase
Phosphoglycerate kinase
2,3-Diphosphoglycerate mutase
Enolase
Acquired disorders
- Hyperphosphatemia, uremia
- Hypophosphatemia
- Magnesium deficiency (?)
- Iron deficiency
- Hypothyroidism (?)

HEXOSE MONOPHOSPHATE PATHWAY
Glutathione synthetase
γ-Glutamyl cysteine synthetase
Glutathione reductase
Glutathione S-transferase
Glutathione peroxidase

ERYTHROCYTE NUCLEOTIDE METABOLISM
Elevated adenosine deaminase levels
Pyrimidine 5'-nucleotidase
Adenylate kinase

---

deficiency in areas where *Plasmodium falciparum* malaria occurred. As an enzyme in the pentose phosphate pathway, G6PD supplies NADPH and reduced glutathione to the RBC. Deficiency limits the cell's ability to recover from oxidative stress. The gene is X-linked recessive in inheritance; males are affected most commonly, but females may also be affected in cases in which X-inactivation is unbalanced. Eleven variants have been described among various ethnic groups. In the United States, African-American males are the most commonly affected, with an estimated prevalence of 11% to 14%.[17] The A-minus variant, common in the African population, shows a mild reduction in both catalytic activity and stability. The variant common among Mediterranean, some Asian, and Ashkenazi Jewish populations involves a severe reduction of enzyme activity, resulting in chronic moderate to severe hemolytic anemia that could prove fatal in the face of severe oxidant challenge. In affected patients, the oldest RBCs are most deficient, resulting in a normal or minimally shortened erythrocyte life span, but exposure to oxidant drugs and toxins or a febrile episode can precipitate severe hemolysis. Hemolysis occurs within 24 to 48 hours of exposure and is accompanied by abdominal pain, vomiting, diarrhea, low-grade fever, jaundice, splenomegaly, hemoglobinuria, and anemia.

Neonates may present with hemolytic anemia and hyperbilirubinemia within 24 hours of life and are susceptible to developing methemoglobinemia (see later). Management

involves avoidance of precipitating agents, hydration, phototherapy, and, if needed, transfusion (partial volume exchange or simple). Common drugs to be avoided or used with caution in this disorder include antimalarials, sulfonamides and sulfones, nitrofurans, anthelminthics, ciprofloxacin, methylene blue, acetaminophen, aspirin, and vitamin K analogues. Enzyme levels are highest in younger cells, and evaluation immediately after a hemolytic episode could be inconclusive because the older, more biochemically abnormal cells have been destroyed. Repeat quantitative testing at a later time, as well as evaluation of maternal enzyme levels, can be useful. Genetic testing of the common variants is available. Some states and countries include G6PD deficiency screening as part of their newborn screening program.

Vitamin E Deficiency

Vitamin E (α-tocopherol) is a fat-soluble antioxidant that reduces the peroxidation of polyunsaturated fatty acids by reactive oxygen species during oxidative enzyme activity. Preterm infants and infants with low birthweight have low serum and tissue levels of this vitamin. Patients who have cystic fibrosis or other causes of chronic fat malabsorption are the most likely to develop symptomatic vitamin E deficiency. A deficiency state in preterm infants and those with very low birthweight has been described, characterized by hemolytic anemia, reticulocytosis, thrombocytosis, chronic lung disease, intracranial hemorrhage, and retinopathy of prematurity. In a 2003 Cochrane review[11] of 26 randomized controlled clinical trials, vitamin E supplementation in preterm infants was found to lower the risk for intracranial hemorrhage but increase the risk for sepsis. Similarly, it was associated with reduction of severe retinopathy of prematurity and blindness in infants with very low birthweight but increased the risk for sepsis. There was a small increase in hemoglobin level. Evidence does not support supplementation with intravenous or high-dose vitamin E.

The Thalassemias

The thalassemias are a group of hereditary anemias that arise from defects in the synthesis of globin chains. In their milder forms, thalassemias are among the most common heritable disorders. The α-thalassemias are most common in the Chinese subcontinent, Malaysia, Indochina, and Africa. β-Thalassemia is common in Mediterranean and African populations but also has a higher incidence in China, Pakistan, India, and the Middle East. The four α-thalassemia syndromes (silent carrier, α-thalassemia trait, Hb H disease, and hydrops fetalis) are caused by diminished production of α-globin protein due to defects in one, two, three, or four of the α-globin genes, respectively. There is considerable heterogeneity within these four categories because the clinical outcome is affected by whether the genetic defects result in diminished or absent expression of each of the affected genes. Although only two genes for β-globin production are inherited, there also are four clinical classifications for β-thalassemia: silent carrier, β-thalassemia trait, thalassemia intermedia, and thalassemia major. The clinical outcome in this disease is a result of complex interactions involving the type of genetic defect, the degree of β-globin production, and the ratio of α-globin chains produced relative to the number of β-globin chains. Coinheritance of α-globin and β-globin defects may result in a less severe thalassemia because the ratio of α-globin to β-globin chains is rebalanced.

Prenatal diagnosis strategies are available for both α- and β-thalassemia. If evaluation of the parents' RBCs produces evidence of thalassemia, molecular detection strategies can be undertaken. After 18 to 20 weeks' gestation, fetal reticulocytes may be tested for globin chain biosynthetic ratios. Fetal tissue from chorionic villus sampling or amniocentesis can be analyzed by a number of DNA-based methodologies (see Chapter 8).

α-THALASSEMIA

Because the production of α-globin chains predominates from mid-gestation onward, defects in α-globin synthesis can be detected at birth. Before the debut of molecular analysis, the various α-thalassemia syndromes were assigned according to clinical criteria. Hydrops fetalis, the most severe and rarest form of α-thalassemia, occurs when an infant inherits deletions of both α-globin genes from each of the parents (see Chapter 21). Such an infant produces small quantities of Hb Portland to maintain in utero viability. The excess γ and β chains form tetramers with themselves, resulting in functionally useless Hb Barts (γ_4) present in the newborn and Hb H (β_4) present in the older infant. The tetramers accumulate in the bone marrow and reticuloendothelial system, resulting in ineffective erythropoiesis. These mutant hemoglobins can precipitate to form inclusion bodies that adhere to cell membranes, promote oxidative damage to the membrane, diminish cell deformability, and shorten RBC survival. The blood smear shows hypochromic microcytes, target cells, and nucleated RBCs. Bizarre RBC shapes and fragments are also common. The fetus with four α-globin gene defects experiences congestive heart failure in utero secondary to severe anemia and, in the absence of fetal transfusion, becomes grossly hydropic (hydrops fetalis). There is evidence of extensive extramedullary hematopoiesis and placental hypertrophy. Most are stillborn at 30 to 40 weeks' gestation or die shortly after delivery. Infants with hepatosplenomegaly, jaundice, and a moderate hypochromic, microcytic hemolytic anemia should be evaluated for deletion of three α-globin genes, Hb H disease. At birth, large amounts of Hb Barts may be seen as well as Hb H. Incubation of the RBCs with brilliant cresyl blue reveals many small inclusions. Treatment is supportive and includes supplementation with folic acid, avoidance of oxidant drugs, transfusion of RBCs, and recognition and treatment of the patients as having compromised splenic function. Hypersplenism, characterized by leukopenia, thrombocytopenia, and worsening anemia, might necessitate splenectomy, although this usually is deferred beyond the first few years of life. Iron overload from chronic transfusions is a significant cause of morbidity and mortality.[37]

α-Thalassemia trait is characterized by a mild anemia with microcytosis, hypochromia, and erythrocytosis. Hb Barts is mildly elevated, 4% to 6% at birth. After the neonatal period, there is no simple laboratory evaluation that is diagnostic for α-thalassemia trait, although β- to α-biosynthetic ratio of reticulocytes or restriction endonuclease mapping can be performed. The diagnosis usually is made in an iron-replete patient with a normal hemoglobin electrophoresis and appropriate family history for α-thalassemia. As the name

implies, silent carriers of α-thalassemia could have slightly microcytic RBCs but usually are asymptomatic. Several states now use molecular testing for *HBA1* and *HBA2*, the genes coding for α_1-globin and α_2-globin, respectively.[37]

β-THALASSEMIA

β-Thalassemia is not usually diagnosed at birth unless blood loss or RBC destruction has created an unusually high demand for replacement of RBCs. The disease generally manifests after 6 months of age, when a microcytic anemia persists beyond the time course for physiologic anemia. The more severe manifestations of the disease traditionally were called *Cooley anemia*, but these have been separated into *thalassemia major* and *thalassemia intermedia*. Affected patients exhibit splenomegaly, poor growth, microcytic hemolytic anemia with ineffective erythropoiesis, target cells on the peripheral blood smear, and extramedullary expansion of erythropoiesis. An abnormal hemoglobin analysis reveals elevations of Hb F and Hb A_2 and a decrease in Hb A.[37]

Patients are categorized as having thalassemia intermedia if they are able to maintain a hemoglobin level greater than 7 g/dL without routine transfusion. Thalassemia major patients require regular transfusions and iron chelation therapy to maintain a hemoglobin value adequate for growth and development. Iron overload is a significant cause of morbidity and mortality starting in the second decade of life. Evidence of hypersplenism might necessitate splenectomy in either type of patient. Bony deformities from expansion of extramedullary hematopoiesis occur in incompletely transfused patients.

β-Thalassemia trait is characterized by abnormalities on the blood smear: microcytosis, hypochromia, erythrocytosis, and the appearance of elliptocytes and target cells. Occasionally, a patient has hepatosplenomegaly. Hemoglobin analysis generally is helpful because of a mild elevation of Hb A_2 and Hb F, although this is not true if the genetic mutation also interferes with production of δ-globin or γ-globin or if Hb A_2 and Hb F production are depressed because of coexistent iron deficiency anemia. The silent carrier state of β-thalassemia is associated with normal findings on the peripheral blood smear and hemoglobin electrophoresis and usually is identified by family studies of patients with a more severe β-thalassemia syndrome.

Hemoglobin Variants

In the fetus, switching from one type of globin chain expression to another occurs several times (see earlier), and over the first few months of the postnatal period, the final switch to the adult-type hemoglobin ($\alpha_2\beta_2$) occurs. Some hereditary defects in fetal globin gene products can produce a hemolytic anemia that resolves as β-globin gene expression predominates. Similarly, a neonate who is asymptomatic at birth can develop a hemolytic anemia over the subsequent months as production of β-globin–containing hemoglobin assumes major importance. Because α chains are produced from the fetal period onward, defects in α-globin are present at birth. If the combination of the mutant α-globin and the γ-globin is more unstable than that of α- and β-globin or α- and δ-globin, the infant experiences a transient hemolytic anemia that resolves as Hb A predominates.

More than 500 structurally different hemoglobin variants have been reported.[47] Several of the important variants are summarized in Box 46-4. Most involve a single amino acid substitution in one of the globin polypeptide chains due to a single nucleotide change in DNA. Other variants are the result of gene deletions or fusions due to uneven crossover. Some of the more commonly important hemoglobin mutations are discussed later.

HEMOGLOBIN S AND SICKLE CELL ANEMIA

Sickle cell (Hb SS) disease is a common medical problem in the United States, where 1 in 400 newborns is affected. By definition, *sickle cell anemia* refers to the doubly heterozygous inheritance of abnormal genes that code for the substitution of valine in place of glutamic acid at position 6 in the β chain of hemoglobin. There are a number of other sickle hemoglobinopathies in which one gene coding for Hb S is inherited along with a second abnormal β-globin gene coding for other hemoglobins, such as Hb C or β-thalassemia. The clinical courses of affected patients may be indistinguishable from, or milder than, those of Hb SS disease. As with the thalassemias, prenatal diagnostic techniques are available. Newborn screening programs have been instituted (Fig. 46-8) in many parts of the world, including much of the United States. Samples of cord or capillary blood are subjected to testing, usually hemoglobin electrophoresis or isoelectric focusing. Infants with electrophoretic patterns demonstrating Hb S and Hb F but not Hb A are presumed to have sickle cell anemia and are referred for confirmatory testing and disease counseling. This screening method also identifies patients with Hb SC disease.

Heterozygotes for Hb S (sickle cell trait) were thought to be clinically unaffected but there are reports of hematuria, decreased urinary concentrating ability, and occasional reports of sudden death related to high altitude and extreme exercise. Associations have been made between sickle cell trait and venous thrombosis, renal medullary carcinoma, and a more severe course of diabetes mellitus.

The clinical hallmark of Hb SS disease is hemolytic anemia with reticulocytosis and the appearance of irreversibly sickled cells on the peripheral blood smear. The onset of signs and symptoms correlates with the decrease in Hb F and increasing expression of the mutant β-globin gene products during the first year of life. Neonates generally are asymptomatic, although older infants are at risk for several disease-related complications. Problems reported in neonates include fever, hepatosplenomegaly, and hyperbilirubinemia. Because of splenic dysfunction, bacterial infections are a major cause of mortality and morbidity in infants and young children. A suddenly pale, listless infant may be experiencing life-threatening anemia caused by hepatic or splenic sequestration. Aplastic crisis, triggered by infection or drugs, also may occur. Vaso-occlusive pain crises most commonly occur in infants' hands and feet. Hand-foot syndrome (dactylitis) manifests with pain, warmth, and swelling of the hands and feet.

Identification of affected newborns through newborn screening programs and enhancements in parent education and supportive care such as penicillin prophylaxis until the sixth year of life, immunization against *Streptococcus pneumoniae* and *Haemophilus influenzae*, and early identification of hepatic or splenic sequestration have decreased the death rate for infants and children. The natural history of sickle cell anemia includes stroke, pulmonary hypertension, overwhelming sepsis from splenic dysfunction, avascular necrosis of joints, retinopathy, acute and chronic lung disease, and transfusion-related iron overload.

Treatment of the sickle hemoglobinopathies has been largely supportive. Penicillin prophylaxis is recommended for all infants with sickle cell anemia. Blood transfusions may be needed to restore tissue oxygenation or to reverse a vaso-occlusive episode in a critical organ. Oral or intravenous chelation therapy decreases iron overload in chronically transfused patients. Extended RBC phenotyping and crossmatching decrease the incidence of transfusion-associated alloimmunization. Hydration, narcotics, and nonsteroidal antiinflammatory drugs are useful during painful crises. Hydroxyurea decreases the number and severity of vaso-occlusive events in many people with sickle cell anemia: its use in young children has been favorably reported. The Baby HUG study, looking at the effects of hydroxyurea therapy in infants as young as 9 months of age, is currently ongoing. Bone marrow transplantation, the only established cure for sickle cell anemia, has been limited by the availability of suitable donors and the uncertainty in predicting which children will express a more severe phenotype. Ongoing studies of less toxic preparative regimens for bone marrow transplantation and more inclusive donor options, as well as risk stratification of sickle cell patients, may allow larger number of patients to undergo bone marrow transplantation in the future.

BOX 46–4   **Clinically Important Hemoglobin Variants**

SICKLE CELL SYNDROMES
Hb SS
Hb SC
Hb S-β^Thal

STRUCTURAL VARIANTS THAT RESULT IN A THALASSEMIC PHENOTYPE
β-Thalassemic phenotypes
- Hb-E syndromes
  Hb AE (mild microcytic anemia)
  Hb EE (moderate microcytic anemia)
  Hb E-β^Thal (moderate to severe anemia)
- Hb Lepore (an δβ fusion globin caused by nonhomologous crossover of adjacent genes)

α-Thalassemic phenotypes
- Hb Constant Spring (an α-chain termination mutation)
- Hb H disease (three dysfunctional α genes)
- Hydrops fetalis (four dysfunctional α genes)

UNSTABLE HEMOGLOBINS (congenital heinz body hemolytic anemias)

Hb WITH ABNORMAL OXYGEN AFFINITY
High affinity—erythrocytosis
Low affinity—cyanosis
Hb M (a cause of congenital methemoglobinemia)

Hb, hemoglobin.

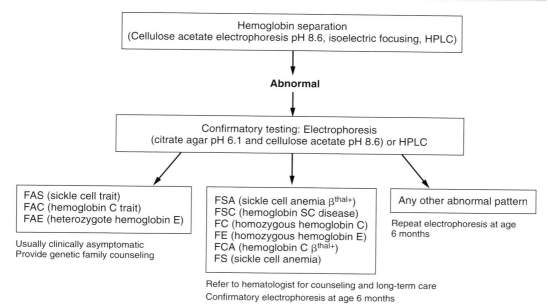

Figure 46–8. Algorithm for investigating abnormal results on hemoglobinopathy screening tests in newborns. FAC, FAE, FAS, FC, FCA, FE, FS, FSA, FSC, sickle-cell traits; HPLC, high-performance liquid chromatography.

HEMOGLOBIN E

Hemoglobin E is one of the most common hemoglobinopathies in the world. This mutant hemoglobin is particularly abundant among people of Southeast Asian ancestry, especially individuals from Laos, Cambodia, and Thailand. Hb E is caused by a single nucleotide substitution in the coding region of the β-globin gene. The resultant β-globin chain contains a Glu26Lys substitution, but it associates normally with α-globin to form a functional hemoglobin tetramer with essentially normal stability and oxygen-dissociation characteristics. Persons with Hb E are anemic because the mutation creates a cryptic splice site in the β-globin message. During RNA processing, a portion of the β-globin message is spliced into an abnormal, unstable transcript. Consequently, the total level of β-globin messenger RNA is reduced, resulting in a thalassemic phenotype. Those who are heterozygous or homozygous for Hb E have chronic, mild to moderate, microcytic anemia but are otherwise well. However, patients who inherit an Hb E allele from one parent and a β-thalassemia allele from the other have a moderate to severe anemia that can be transfusion dependent. Hb levels in these patients range from 2 to 7 g/dL, and children with this condition can develop hepatosplenomegaly and growth failure. Hb E-β thalassemia disease now is the most common form of transfusion-dependent thalassemia in the United States and other parts of the world. Hb E coinherited with sickle cell trait also results in a more severe sickle phenotype.

UNSTABLE HEMOGLOBINS

Most of these mutations affect β-globin and involve amino acid substitutions in hydrophobic residues around the heme pocket. These amino acid replacements alter the hydrophobic interior of the molecule, predisposing these molecules to instability and precipitation in the form of Heinz bodies. Because the amino acid substitutions often involve replacing one neutral amino acid with another, the hemoglobin electrophoretic mobility might not change. Patients usually develop anemia and jaundice in late infancy or early childhood as β-globin synthesis increases. Mutations in fetal or embryonic globins can cause symptoms at birth but not later in life. The diagnosis is confirmed by staining for Heinz bodies, which are usually present, and testing for hemoglobin stability.[47]

Anemia Caused by Inefficient Production of Red Blood Cells

IRON-DEFICIENCY ANEMIA

Although the prevalence of iron deficiency anemia is decreasing in the United States, it remains the leading cause of anemia in infancy and childhood. Factors associated with the declining rates of iron deficiency anemia include the increasing number of infants receiving breast milk, the extensive use of iron-supplemented infant formulas and baby cereals during the first year of life, and delaying introduction of cow's milk into the infant diet until after 1 year of age.

Iron is an essential nutrient. Most iron is bound to the heme proteins, hemoglobin, and myoglobin. The storage proteins, ferritin and hemosiderin, contain most of the rest, though a small percentage is bound in enzyme systems such as cytochromes and catalase. In healthy adults, most of the body's iron is recycled from the breakdown of RBCs; little iron needs to be absorbed from the intestines, and little is lost through fecal or urinary excretion. Because neonates must rapidly expand muscle mass and blood volume, they require a much higher percentage of dietary iron intake. The amount of iron stored in the neonate's body is proportionate to birthweight. For a full-term infant, this should be sufficient for the first 4 to 6 months of life. Preterm infants and those born small for gestational age weigh less at birth, have a much faster rate of postnatal growth, and are at risk for iron deficiency within the first 3 months of life (Table 46-10). Infants born anemic and those who have accelerated iron losses from repeated laboratory testing, trauma, surgery, or anatomic abnormalities may also become deficient. Babies born to mothers with iron deficiency anemia are at increased risk for developing iron deficiency anemia during the first year of life.

Although both breast milk and cow's milk contain iron, the bioavailability of the iron in breast milk is much superior. Full-term infants who are breast-fed should not require iron supplementation until 4 to 6 months of age. Two daily servings of an iron-fortified cereal will meet this requirement. Infants who are premature, ill, or have low birthweight and who are breast-fed will require supplementation as early as 2 months of age (Table 46-11). Formula-fed infants should be given an iron-supplemented formula. Infant cereal fortified with iron should be one of the earliest solid foods introduced. After 6 months of age, one daily serving of a vitamin C–rich food should be introduced. Because the protein in cow's milk can cause occult

gastrointestinal bleeding in the neonate and because of the poor bioavailability of iron in cow's milk, it is recommended that babies avoid cow's milk until after 1 year of age.

Iron deficiency in infancy has been associated with impairment of psychomotor development and may negatively affect social and emotional behavior. Whether these deficits are fully resolved by subsequent iron supplementation is unclear. Although severe iron deficiency is fairly simple to diagnose, milder deficiency may not yet have caused anemia or may be difficult to distinguish from other causes of microcytic anemia, especially in patients with chronic or acute illness. The American Academy of Pediatrics recommends that testing for anemia should include Hb or Hct values between ages 9 and 12 months. Given emerging information about the early effects of iron deficiency and identification of at-risk populations of infants, the American Academy of Pediatrics also recommends a risk assessment as early as 4 months of age for healthy infants. A careful dietary history should be taken, and consideration should be given to special circumstances such as ongoing blood loss, malabsorption, and birth history.

In early iron deficiency, the bone marrow stores are depleted, and the RBC distribution width increases. Subsequently, the iron transport levels fall, resulting in lower serum levels of iron, ferritin, and transferrin. Finally, erythrocyte production is affected. A hypochromic, microcytic anemia becomes apparent. Screening test results such as serum iron, total iron-binding capacity, ferritin, and transferrin saturation may be inconclusive because of acute or chronic illness. A therapeutic trial of iron for presumptive iron deficiency anemia is a cost-effective strategy. Ferrous sulfate, in a dose of 2 to 6 mg/kg per day of elemental iron, may be given for 1 month. If the hemoglobin rises by at least 1 g/dL (in the absence of ongoing blood loss), the diagnosis of iron deficiency is made, and the iron supplementation should be continued for 2 or 3 more months or until 1 or 2 months after the Hb and Hct values are in the normal range. Screening for lead exposure should be done as part of routine well-baby care and particularly considered if a hypochromic, microcytic anemia is detected.

ANEMIA OF PREMATURITY

Anemia of prematurity is characterized by a low reticulocyte count and an inadequate response to erythropoietin (EPO). Infants with extremely low birthweight often undergo transfusion because they are critically ill, need artificial ventilation, and have the highest blood sampling loss in relation to their weight. More centers are using restrictive transfusion guidelines and have been able to decrease the number of transfusions and donor exposures. Although appreciable levels of EPO are present in the serum of most premature infants, the neonate produces an insufficient amount of this growth factor and is amenable to pharmacologic supplementation with recombinant EPO.

Multiple placebo-controlled trials have established that EPO therapy effectively increases reticulocyte counts and hematocrit.[62] Unfortunately, in most studies, although the total volume of blood transfused was reduced, donor exposures were not reduced. Thus, EPO alone does not appear to be an effective strategy to reduce transfusion

TABLE 46–10 Risk Factors for Iron Deficiency Anemia in the First 6 Months of Life

Prematurity
Small for gestational age
Anemia at birth
Fetal-maternal hemorrhage
Twin-twin transfusion syndrome
Perinatal hemorrhage
Erythropoietin use
Maternal iron deficiency anemia
Iatrogenic or other ongoing blood loss
Insufficient dietary intake or malabsorption
Early introduction of whole cow's milk

TABLE 46–11 Guidelines for Iron Supplementation for Breast-Fed Infants in the First Year of Life

Status at Birth	Minimum Daily Requirement (maximum 15 mg)	Begin By
Full-term	1 mg/kg	4 mo
Premature	2 mg/kg	2 mo
Very low birth-weight (<1500 g)	3-4 mg/kg	2 mo

Adapted from American Academy of Pediatrics. Recommendations for preventive pediatric health care (periodicity schedule). http.//practice.aap.org/content.aspx?aid=1599.

needs. It remains to be seen if blood conservation, combined with EPO replacement, will be effective in reducing transfusions.

TRANSIENT ERYTHROBLASTOPENIA OF CHILDHOOD

Transient erythroblastopenia of childhood is an acquired, transient, normocytic, hypoplastic anemia affecting children. The etiology of transient erythroblastopenia is unknown but is postulated to be the result of viral injury to erythroid precursors. Familial cases have been reported. This syndrome is exceedingly rare in neonates; most cases of the condition cluster at 2 to 3 years of age. The degree of anemia can range from moderate to severe. Occasionally, hemoglobin levels as low as 3 g/dL are seen. Transient erythroblastopenia is a diagnosis of retrospect. Treatment consists of supportive measures, including RBC transfusion if needed, until bone marrow recovery. Most patients recover in 1 to 2 months. The condition may be confused with Diamond-Blackfan anemia and parvovirus-induced anemias.

PARVOVIRUS-INDUCED ANEMIA

Parvovirus B19, which proliferates in human erythroid precursors, causes several diseases. In normal children or adults, the virus produces fifth disease. Thirty to 60% of adults in the United States have antibody to the virus.[29] The rash and joint symptoms associated with this generally minor illness are due to vascular deposition of antibody complexes generated in response to the infection. In patients with underlying hemolytic anemias (e.g., sickle cell anemia or hereditary spherocytosis), parvovirus infection can cause a transient, severe aplastic crisis. The virus also can cause chronic anemia by means of a persistent infection in erythroblasts in immunocompromised hosts. Chronic parvovirus anemia responds to administration of intravenous γ-globulin that contains antiparvovirus antibody.

The virus binds to blood group P-antigen on the surface of erythroid precursors, is internalized, and then replicates, disrupting normal erythroid differentiation. P-antigen is also expressed on cells not known to be permissive for parvovirus replication. Endothelial cell P-antigen is postulated to participate in placental transmission of the virus. This antigen is also found on fetal cardiomyocytes, a finding consistent with the fact that the fetus infected with parvovirus can develop myocarditis. Infection rate during pregnancy is estimated to be in the 3% range. Parvovirus infection during pregnancy can result in anemia, hydrops fetalis (see Chapter 22), fetal loss, or congenital infection. The rate of transplacental transmission of the virus has been estimated at 33%. Initial reports of more than 30% rates of stillbirth and fetal loss have been reduced, and it is recognized that most of the mortality occurs during the first 20 weeks of gestation. Fetal loss associated with the infection is 11% before 20 weeks and less than 1% after this point in gestation. Hydrops is reported in 3.9% of infections diagnosed before 32 weeks of gestation, compared with 0.8% after this time.[29] Severe thrombocytopenia occurs in more than one third of cases and can complicate intrauterine transfusion. Parvovirus-induced hydrops can be detected by ultrasound, and treatment of suspected hydropic infants includes intrauterine RBC transfusion.

Parvovirus infection of the fetus may persist after birth as a cause of congenital RBC aplasia.

DIAMOND-BLACKFAN ANEMIA

Diamond-Blackfan anemia is a rare syndrome of congenital macrocytic anemia with reticulocytopenia.[7] The median hemoglobin at birth for these patients is 7 g/dL, and the reticulocyte count usually is 0% to 1%. Bone marrow examination reveals decreased numbers of erythroid precursors and abnormal erythroid maturation. Serum EPO levels are elevated as a compensatory response to inefficient RBC production by the marrow. RBC adenosine deaminase levels also are elevated in this syndrome. Patients with Diamond-Blackfan anemia often have one or more physical anomalies, such as low birthweight, short stature, abnormal facies, skeletal abnormalities (including abnormal thumbs), and visceral anomalies. The median age of diagnosis is 2 months. Although the phenotypes of Diamond-Blackfan anemia and Fanconi anemia overlap, several features distinguish these syndromes. Patients with Diamond-Blackfan anemia are anemic from birth, whereas those with Fanconi anemia generally develop reticulocytopenia later in life. Finally, laboratory evaluation reveals increased chromosome fragility in Fanconi cells but not in Diamond-Blackfan anemia cells.

Erythroid precursors from patients with Diamond-Blackfan anemia display abnormal maturation in vitro, and the syndrome can be corrected by allogeneic bone marrow transplantation, indicating that it is caused by a defect in stem cell differentiation. Family studies have documented autosomal dominant and autosomal recessive patterns of inheritance. Several genes have been identified whose mutations together account for about 45% of patients with Diamond-Blackfan anemia. All mutations identified affect proteins of the small (RPS) or large (RPL) ribosomal subunit, suggesting that this is a disorder of ribosome biogenesis.[7] Heterozygous mutations in RPS19 are evident in 25% of cases.

About two thirds of patients with Diamond-Blackfan anemia respond to glucocorticoid therapy with an increase in Hb concentration and the reticulocyte count. Prednisone therapy usually is initiated at a dose of 2 mg/kg per day, and an increase in the reticulocyte count generally is noted in 1 to 2 weeks. For glucocorticoid responders, the prednisone dose is slowly tapered until the patient is on an alternate-day dose that maintains a reasonable Hb level. Many patients remain on small alternate-day doses of steroids for years. Steroid nonresponders are managed with chronic RBC transfusion therapy, with the long-term complication of iron overload. Chelation therapy is indicated when transfusion-dependent patients develop significantly increased iron stores, as documented by an elevated serum ferritin value greater than 1000 ng/mL or increased urinary excretion of iron after a desferrioxamine challenge. Bone marrow transplantation from an HLA-matched unaffected sibling is a consideration for transfusion-dependent patients.

Despite advances in medical therapy, patients with Diamond-Blackfan anemia have a shortened expected life span. As is true for other congenital bone marrow failure syndromes, Diamond-Blackfan anemia is associated with an increased risk for aplastic anemia, myelodysplastic syndrome, and acute leukemia later in life.

FANCONI ANEMIA

Although Fanconi anemia is not a cause of pure anemia in the neonate, this congenital bone marrow failure syndrome is discussed here in the context of other congenital hematologic diseases. Originally characterized as familial aplastic anemia with birth defects, the condition has been extended to include patients with characteristic chromosome fragility findings, with or without aplastic anemia, and with or without birth anomalies.[7] Hematologic abnormalities other than macrocytosis usually are not evident in infants with Fanconi anemia. The condition often is not recognized until the onset of aplastic anemia, at a mean age of 8 years.

The physical anomalies associated with Fanconi anemia are listed in Table 46-12. Only a minority of Fanconi patients have thumb anomalies, the birth defect traditionally associated with this condition.

Cells from patients with Fanconi anemia exhibit increased chromosome breakage in response to certain alkylating agents, and this now is the basis of diagnostic testing for this condition. Patient lymphocytes are cultured and exposed to the alkylating agent diepoxybutane, and then metaphase smears of the chromosomes are examined for breaks. Complementation studies using somatic cell hybrids have shown that mutations in at least seven genes can produce the Fanconi anemia phenotype.

The proteins encoded by the *FANC-A*, *-C*, *-E*, *-F*, *-G*, *-L*, and *-M* genes assemble into a multisubunit nuclear complex. DNA damage caused by alkylating agents activates this protein complex, leading to monoubiquitination of *FANC-D2*, which interacts with the tumor suppressor *BRCA1* to effect DNA repair. The product of the "*FANC-D1* gene" is *BRCA2*, another tumor suppressor that physically interacts with *BRCA1*. Researchers postulate that disruption of the Fanconi

anemia complex and impaired monoubiquitination of *FANC-D2* result in the cellular and clinical phenotypes common to most of the complementation groups.[7]

Hematopoietic progenitor cells from patients with Fanconi anemia display a distinct hypersensitivity to interferon-γ, which causes apoptosis of these progenitor cells. Interferon-γ hypersensitivity might account for the development of progressive bone marrow failure in these patients.

CONGENITAL DYSERYTHROPOIETIC ANEMIAS

Patients with these rare disorders have congenital anemia with ineffective, morphologically abnormal erythroid production. The degree of anemia can range from moderate to severe and can be macrocytic, normocytic, or microcytic. Type II is the most common of the three described types. The bone marrow shows multinucleated RBC precursors and asynchrony in the maturation of erythroid nuclei and cytoplasm. Defects in glycosylation of erythroid precursor surface glycoproteins and glycolipids have been associated with some cases. The disease often remains undiagnosed in the neonatal period, although many patients are noted to have anemia and jaundice early on. Dysmorphic features can be associated with the anemia.[74] Management includes transfusion and chelation of iron excess. Bone marrow transplantation has been attempted in severe cases.

SIDEROBLASTIC ANEMIAS

The sideroblastic anemias are congenital hypochromic, microcytic, or normocytic anemias that are unresponsive to iron therapy. Both X-linked and autosomal varieties exist. Acquired sideroblastic anemia occurs later in life. These anemias are caused by abnormalities in the mitochondrial enzymes of the heme biosynthetic pathway. Adequate iron stores are available, but iron is not incorporated into heme. The iron accumulates in the mitochondria of the nucleated erythrocyte and forms a ring around the nucleus. Prussian blue staining of the marrow reveals erythroid hyperplasia and large numbers of these ringed sideroblasts. Some respond to pharmacologic doses of pyridoxine because some of the heme biosynthetic enzymes (e.g., aminolevulinic acid synthetase) use this vitamin as a cofactor. Bone marrow transplantation has been suggested as a treatment for severe disorders.

Pearson syndrome is a refractory sideroblastic anemia characterized by vacuolization of bone marrow precursors due to deletion of mitochondrial DNA. The disease is frequently associated with exocrine pancreatic insufficiency, hepatic failure, and renal tubular dysfunction. The disorder becomes evident during early infancy, and most patients die before the age of 3 years.

Other Erythrocyte Disorders

METHEMOGLOBINEMIA

Methemoglobinemia results when methemoglobin production is increased or when the ability to reduce methemoglobin is decreased. For hemoglobin to reversibly bind oxygen, the heme iron must be in the ferrous (Fe^{2+}) state. As the RBC circulates and is exposed to various oxidants, the oxyhemoglobin is slowly oxidized to methemoglobin in the ferric

TABLE 46–12	**Physical Anomalies Associated with Fanconi Anemia**
Anomaly	**Percentage**
Skin hyperpigmentation or café-au-lait spots	76
Microsomy	65
Low birthweight	47
Thumb anomalies	40
Hypogenitalia	33
Renal anomalies	32
Skeletal anomalies (except thumbs)	28
Strabismus	23
Microphthalmia	19
Mental retardation	18
Ear anomalies or deafness	12
Congenital heart disease	7

Adapted from Alter BP, et al: Long-term outcome in Fanconi's anemia: description of 26 cases and a review of the literature. In German J, editor: *Chromosome mutation and neoplasia*, New York, 1983, Alan R Liss.

(Fe^{3+}) state. Partial oxidation of hemoglobin markedly increases the oxygen affinity of the other hemes in the tetramer and decreases oxygen delivery to tissues. Reduction of methemoglobin in the RBC depends largely on two electron carriers, cytochrome-b_5 and NADH, as well as the enzyme cytochrome-b_5 reductase. An alternate pathway using G6PD to generate NADPH in the hexose monophosphate shunt can be driven by the addition of electron carriers such as methylene blue. It is estimated that methemoglobin accumulates in adults at a rate of 2% to 3% a day, but RBCs with an intact cytochrome-b_5 reductase system contain less than 0.6% methemoglobin.[53] Neonates and premature infants have a transient enzymatic deficiency and lower cytochrome-b_5 levels for the first few months of life. Ingestion of nitrates, usually from contaminated well water, and their subsequent conversion to oxidizing nitrites by gut bacteria, are the leading cause of acquired methemoglobinemia in infants. Although the cause is unclear, there is an association between diarrheal illness in infants and methemoglobinemia even when toxin exposure has not been detected. Xylocaine and its derivatives and dapsone are the most common drugs precipitating methemoglobinemia.

Cyanosis occurs when relatively high levels of deoxyhemoglobin are present (generally, >5 g/dL) or when a nonphysiologic hemoglobin (e.g., methemoglobin) is present (>1.5 g/dL). The differential diagnosis of cyanosis is addressed in Chapters 44 and 45. Congenital methemoglobinemia is due either to a defect in the cytochrome-b_5 reductase system or to inheritance of one of the M hemoglobins (Hb M), which have an alteration in either the α or β chain, resulting in preferential binding of ferric iron. Acquired methemoglobinemia is caused by metabolic acidosis and exposure to certain drugs and chemicals with oxidant potential, such as nitrites. Neonates are at higher risk for developing toxic methemoglobinemia from environmental toxins and pharmacologic agents. The onset of symptoms in patients with one of the M hemoglobins corresponds with expression of the affected globin chains. Patients with cytochrome-b_5 reductase deficiency type I are asymptomatic other than cyanosis; the more rare type II disease presents with cyanosis, failure to thrive, and a severe neurologic phenotype. Many with type II disease die in infancy.

Patients have cyanosis that is unresponsive to oxygen therapy. Their blood is a characteristic chocolate brown. A fresh sample of blood is analyzed by co-oximetry to detect absorbance in the 630-nm range. False-positive tests results may be due to the presence of other pigments that absorb near the same wavelength, such as sulfhemoglobin and methylene blue.[53] Confirmatory testing of positive results is performed by the Evelyn-Mally method, in which the addition of cyanide abolishes absorbance methemoglobin at 630 nm. Hb analysis identifies abnormal hemoglobin in patients with M hemoglobins. Both quantitative and qualitative tests are available for evaluating defects in the cytochrome-b_5 reductase system.

Inheritance of the Hb M variants is autosomal dominant, whereas defects in the cytochrome-b_5 reductase system are inherited in an autosomal-recessive fashion. Homozygotes and compound heterozygotes usually are affected, but heterozygotes can become symptomatic after exposure to oxidant drugs or toxins. Patients with congenital methemoglobinemia may be cyanotic but otherwise asymptomatic. Similarly, patients with chronic methemoglobinemia, with methemoglobin levels of up to 40% or 50%, may be physiologically well compensated and exhibit minimal symptoms. Acute methemoglobinemia with levels above 20% produces the signs and symptoms of hypoxia. Levels greater than 70% can result in coma and death, although there are reports of neonates who survived levels as high as 85%.[53]

Therapy is initiated for symptomatic patients with cytochrome-b_5 reductase deficiency and those with methemoglobin levels above 40%. The usual treatment is oral methylene blue, given in a dose of 1 to 2 mg/kg. If the patient does not show a good response within 1 hour, the treatment may be repeated, although consideration should be given that the patient could have G6PD deficiency. Patients with G6PD deficiency should not be treated with methylene blue because it is often not beneficial and it also causes oxidant stress and hemolysis. Alternative therapy with ascorbic acid, 200 to 500 mg/kg per day, may be used with caution because of concerns about calcium kidney stone formation. High-dose ascorbic acid also has oxidant potential and can trigger hemolysis in G6PD-deficient patients. No treatment exists for those with Hb M variants. All patients with congenital methemoglobinemia and known heterozygotes for cytochrome-b_5 reductase deficiency should avoid aniline derivatives and nitrates.

POLYCYTHEMIA

Polycythemia is defined as an increase in RBC mass more than 2 standard deviations above mean for age and gestation. For a term infant, polycythemia occurs when a peripheral venous blood sample has an Hb greater than 22 g/dL or a hematocrit greater than 65%. Capillary blood samples are generally higher than those drawn from peripheral blood, and central venous values are lower still. The real issue is viscosity, which has a linear relationship to the hematocrit up to about 60%. Blood viscosity increases more rapidly above 60% hemacrit, but less predictably.[69] Laboratory testing for hyperviscosity is not generally available, so decisions are made using the hematocrit or hemoglobin and clinical symptoms. Symptoms include listlessness, irritability, plethora, acrocyanosis, poor feeding, hypoglycemia, respiratory distress, and systemic thromboses. Persistent pulmonary hypertension of the newborn can be caused by increased pulmonary vascular resistance. The increased load of RBCs also contributes to hyperbilirubinemia. Symptoms often appear at or after 2 hours of life, when the hematocrit is highest due to fluid shifts. Some patients with excessive extracellular fluid losses may become symptomatic on day 2 or 3 of life.

Conditions that result in transfusion to the fetus, such as twin-twin or maternal-fetal transfusion or delayed clamping of the umbilical cord, can cause polycythemia. Exacerbations in the degree of intrauterine hypoxia, such as may be seen with placental insufficiency, maternal toxemia, and postmaturity, trigger increased production of EPO, which causes an increase in RBC mass. Maternal smoking has been associated with symptomatic polycythemia in infants. Several endocrine conditions are associated with increased RBC production and polycythemia, including maternal diabetes, hyperthyroidism or hypothyroidism, and congenital adrenal hyperplasia. Excessive EPO production and polycythemia also are seen in infants with Down syndrome and some other trisomies and

Beckwith-Wiedemann syndrome. Less commonly, an alteration in hemoglobin can greatly increase the affinity of the hemoglobin for oxygen, but most of the cases described have involved β-chain defects that would be expected to manifest later in infancy. Hereditary defects in the EPO receptor associated with polycythemia also have been reported.

Management remains controversial for most infants because exchange transfusion is associated with the usual transfusion risks as well as increased risk for necrotizing enterocolitis. Asymptomatic infants with a hematocrit of 60% to 70% should be monitored closely with adequate hydration and glucose levels. Symptomatic patients and those with a central hematocrit greater than 70% more often undergo partial volume exchange transfusion with normal saline to reduce the RBC mass (see Part 2 of this chapter), but some are still managed with supportive care.

PHAGOCYTES

Normal Physiology of Phagocytes

FUNCTION OF PHAGOCYTES

Leukocytes serve as major effector cells for host defense against invading organisms. Neutrophils circulate in the blood until they encounter specific chemotactic signals that promote adhesion to the vascular endothelium and migration through (diapedesis) and movement to the sites of microbial invasion (chemotaxis). Mononuclear phagocytes (monocytes, macrophages) function primarily as cells resident within certain tissues such as the spleen, lungs, and peritoneum, where they interact closely with lymphocytes to generate a local immune response. Both neutrophils and mononuclear phagocytes take up opsonized targets (internalization, phagocytosis), which are then destroyed within intracellular vacuoles by the release of hydrolytic enzymes and reactive oxygen intermediates (respiratory burst activity).

NUMBER OF PHAGOCYTES

Changes in the number of circulating leukocytes could represent either disordered leukocyte production or disordered leukocyte consumption, or both. *Neutropenia* is defined as a neutrophil blood count of less than 1500/μL. Although this definition is generally used for all ages and races, in the newborn the absolute neutrophil count (ANC) is elevated for the first few days of life. The ANC is the product of the total white blood cell (WBC) count and the percentage of mature neutrophils plus percentage of bands:

$$ANC = WBC \times (\% \text{ neutrophils} + \% \text{ bands}) \times 0.01$$

Neutrophilia is an elevation of the blood neutrophil count greater than 2 standard deviations above the mean.

Human myelopoiesis begins in the embryo (about 8 weeks). By 20 weeks of gestation, neutrophils demonstrate partial functional activity. However, even neutrophils from the normal newborn display limited functional activity. Neutrophil counts vary considerably during the neonatal period (Table 46-13), with a mean of 11,000/μL and a range of 6000 to 26,000/μL. Total WBC counts may be as high as 38,000/μL within 12 hours of age. However, after the first 12 hours of life, neutrophil counts fall, reaching a mean of about 5000/μL (1000 to

TABLE 46–13 Polymorphonuclear Leukocyte and Band Counts in the Newborn During the First 2 Days of Life*

Age (hr)	Absolute Neutrophil Count (per μL)	Absolute Band Count (per μL)	Band-to-Neutrophil Ratio
Birth	3500-6000	1300	0.14
12	8000-15000	1300	0.14
24	7000-13000	1300	0.14
36	5000-9000	700	0.11
48	3500-5200	700	0.11

*Normal values were obtained from the assessment of 3100 separate white blood cell counts obtained from 965 infants; 513 counts were from infants considered to be completely normal at the time the count was obtained and for the preceding and subsequent 48 hours. There was no difference in the normal ranges when infants were compared by either birthweight (whether more or less than 2500 g) or gestational age.

Modified from Manroe BL, et al: The differential leukocyte count in the assessment and outcome of early-onset neonatal group B streptococcal disease, *J Pediatr* 91:632, 1977.

10,000) in the first week of life. The WBC differential during this period resembles that of adults, with a majority of neutrophils. However, during the next 5 years, lymphocytes predominate in the peripheral blood differential. There is substantially greater variability in the changes from birth onward for the first several weeks of life in a premature infant.

KINETICS OF PHAGOCYTES

The circulating blood neutrophil pool reflects a dynamic equilibrium among several compartments: within the bone marrow are the dividing (or mitotic) pool, the differentiation (or maturation) pool, and the storage pool; outside the bone marrow are the circulating pool, the vascular marginated pool, and the peripheral tissue pool. Neutrophils transit the circulating pool only during the brief 3- to 6-hour period from bone marrow to tissue. Thus, changes in the WBC count or differential could reflect rapid changes in a relatively small yet highly fluctuant pool.

Estimates suggest that the peripheral blood neutrophil count represents less than 5% of the total neutrophil pool size. Neutrophil distribution studies demonstrate about 1 billion neutrophils per kilogram of body weight, of which about 20% are in the marrow neutrophil precursor pool, 75% are in the marrow storage pool, 3% are in the marginated vascular pool, and 2% are in the circulating blood (Table 46-14). About 1.5 billion neutrophils per kilogram of body weight are produced each day, with a residence time of 9 days in marrow, 3 to 6 hours in blood, and 1 to 4 days in peripheral tissues (see Table 46-14).

Neutrophils are derived from a common stem cell progenitor, which also gives rise to mature erythrocytes, megakaryocytes (and ultimately platelets), eosinophils, basophils, and monocytes (see Fig. 46-1). A variety of recently identified growth factors and cytokines regulate proliferation and differentiation along neutrophilic lineage (see Table 46-1).

TABLE 46-14   Adult Blood Neutrophil Pools and Kinetics

Pool	Definition/Calculation	Mean Pool Size ($\times 10^7$/kg)	95% Limits
Total blood neutrophil pool (TBNP)	All neutrophils in the circulation	70	14-160
Circulating neutrophil pool (CNP)	Blood neutrophil concentration multiplied by blood volume	31	11-46
Marginal neutrophil pool (MNP)	Total blood neutrophil pool less circulating pool (MNP = TBNP − CNP)	39	0-85

Kinetics	Definition/Calculation	Mean Value	95% Limits
$t_{1/2}$ (blood clearance half-time)	Disappearance time of half of the labeled neutrophils from circulation $$\frac{0.693 \times TBNP}{t_{1/2}}$$	6.7 hr	4-10 hr
Neutrophil turnover rate (NTR)		163×10^7/kg/day	$50\text{-}340 \times 10^7$/kg/day

Adapted from Beutler E, et al: *Williams' hematology*, 5th ed, New York, 1995, McGraw-Hill.

Phagocyte Abnormalities

NEUTROPENIA

Neutropenia (<1500/µL) can result from a decline in neutrophil production or from accelerated destruction, as well as from changes in the relative distribution of neutrophils between the circulating pool and the marrow and peripheral tissue pools. Most cases are due to acquired defects, many of which are transient.

Extrinsic Defects of Phagocyte Function
SEPSIS AND POSTINFECTIOUS NEUTROPENIA
Infection is the most common cause of neutropenia in the neonate. Neutropenia is a risk factor for infection and sepsis, but it can also occur as a result of overwhelming sepsis. Neonates are particularly at risk for this complication because their neutrophil storage pools are smaller. Neutrophil counts are sometimes unmeasurable in the peripheral blood if the bone marrow neutrophil pool is exhausted. Both increased vascular neutrophil margination and vascular-to-tissue neutrophil movement are associated with circulating neutropenia during sepsis.

Among hospitalized infants, neonatal sepsis continues to be a major cause of morbidity and mortality. Neonates with very low birthweight (500 to 1000 g) are most vulnerable and are prone to early- and late-onset sepsis. Cytokines such as G-CSF have been used without clear benefit in preventing or treating sepsis in neonates, but they are used more commonly in neutropenic neonates with infection or sepsis. Infusions of intravenous immunoglobulin (see Chapter 39) may also augment IgG levels.[14] Granulocyte transfusions are discussed in Part 2 of this chapter.

NEONATAL ALLOIMMUNE NEUTROPENIA
Neonatal alloimmune neutropenia is estimated to occur in 1 of 2000 live births and is analogous to Rh hemolytic disease of the newborn. The severe neonatal neutropenia is caused by maternal sensitization to paternally inherited human neutrophil antigens, resulting in maternal IgG that crosses the placenta, coats the infant's neutrophils, and causes their destruction by opsonization. Affected newborns often develop fever in the first few days of life with associated cutaneous infections, including umbilical stump infections. Upper and lower respiratory tract infections, otitis media, necrotizing enterocolitis, and sepsis are less common. The onset of symptoms coincides with the severe neutropenia.

Isolated neutropenia (<1000/uL) with normal maternal neutrophil count should trigger suspicion, but nonimmune causes of the neutropenia should be considered as well. Special testing using paternal granulocytes and maternal granulocytes and serum are used to detect maternal antibody to paternal or test panel granulocytes. If there is antibody to a paternal antigen present, the father is then tested serologically and genotypically to determine whether his antigen is homozygous or heterozygous. If the father is homozygous, the risk for future alloimmune neutropenia is 100%. As expected for the half-life of maternal IgG, infant neutrophil counts generally return to normal within the first 1 to 2 months of life. Antibodies to several neutrophil-specific antigens have been detected. Treatment of isoimmune neonatal neutropenia consists of appropriate antibiotics, and sometimes G-CSF or IgG.[22]

AUTOIMMUNE NEUTROPENIA OF INFANCY
Antineutrophil antibodies have been detected in the serum of infants in the first months of life. The incidence of autoimmune neutropenia is estimated at 1 per 100,000 infants. It is most commonly seen between the ages of 5 and 15 months. In primary autoimmune neutropenia (not associated with an underlying disorder), despite neutropenia in the 500 to 1000/µL range, infection is seen in only 12% of patients. A peripheral monocytosis may be present. Autoimmune neutropenia is self-limited, with resolution in the first 2 to 3 years of life. Secondary autoimmune neutropenia is more common in older

children and adults and tends to be associated with autoimmune disorders, infections, and drugs. If bone marrow analysis is done, there may be a paucity of neutrophils and myeloid progenitor cells, depending on the specificity of the antibody for mature or progenitor cell antigens. The overall bone marrow cellularity may be normal or hypercellular.

The autoantibodies are directed against human neutrophil antigens, which are usually glycosylated isoforms of FcγRIIIb (or CD 16b). Less commonly, the antibodies are directed against adhesion glycoproteins of the CD 11/Cd 18 (HNA-4a, HNA-4b) complex. Qualitative and quantitative defects in neutrophils have been noted. Qualitative defects may explain why a subset of patients with autoimmune neutropenia do develop serious infections.

A variety of assays (e.g., opsonization and immunochemical and direct antibody binding) have been used to detect circulating and bound neutrophil-specific antibodies. The degree of neutropenia is related to the specificity of the antibody as well as its titer and affinity.

Therapy for autoimmune neutropenia depends on the severity of the neutropenia-associated symptoms (e.g., fever and infection). Often no treatment is needed. Antibiotics, with or without the addition of G-CSF or intravenous γ-globulin, are sometimes necessary. Corticosteroid use is reported in the older literature, but this treatment is less frequent now that less toxic therapies are available.[16]

DRUG-INDUCED NEUTROPENIA

An enormous number of agents have been implicated as causes of neutropenia (Box 46-5). The mechanisms could involve direct bone marrow suppression or immune-mediated destruction (see "Autoimmune Neutropenia of Infancy," previously). Anti-inflammatory drugs, semisynthetic penicillins, antiseizure medications, and a host of others are commonly seen in the newborn nursery. Recovery from marrow toxic effects generally begins within several days after the offending agent is discontinued. As with recovery from chemotherapy-induced neutropenia, recovery of peripheral neutrophil counts is ushered in by a rise in circulating monocytes and immature neutrophils in the peripheral blood.

IDIOPATHIC NEUTROPENIA OF INFANTS WITH VERY LOW BIRTHWEIGHT

In 1998, Juul's group reported their evaluation of four infants with very low birthweight who had neutropenia from, or shortly following, delivery and lasting for 1 to 9 weeks.[41] Maternal antineutrophil antibody studies were negative. All patients responded to a 3-day trial of G-CSF by transiently normalizing blood neutrophil counts, and all four infants experienced complete resolution of neutropenia by week 9.

THERAPEUTIC USES OF G-CSF AND GM-CSF

The cytokines G-CSF and GM-CSF are members of a family of hematopoietic growth factors that stimulate production of mature WBCs in the bone marrow. These two cytokines also enhance neutrophil and monocyte functions, such as neutrophil oxidative metabolism, chemotaxis, and phagocytosis. Both are normally present at low concentrations in serum. G-CSF levels are about threefold higher in the cord blood of

premature infants than in term infants in the first 3 days of life.[13] G-CSF levels peak at 7 hours of life, followed by a rise in the neutrophil count at about 13 hours of life.

When normal adults are exposed to an infectious challenge, G-CSF levels rise, and peripheral neutrophilia follows. GM-CSF levels, on the other hand, remain steady. Whether preterm and full-term infants are capable of mounting an appropriate cytokine response to infection or sepsis and whether neonatal cells respond adequately to cytokines are still controversial issues. Although neonatal neutrophil GM-CSF and G-CSF receptors are quantitatively similar and share comparable binding affinities with those on adult cells, in vitro studies of adult and neonatal mononuclear cells demonstrated an eightfold lower cytokine response to mitogen stimulation by the neonatal cells. Regardless, some recent studies have documented an increase in serum G-CSF levels in full-term and preterm infants with bacterial infection compared with healthy term infants.

Some clinical trials using pharmacologic doses of G-CSF and GM-CSF have shown benefit in patients with acquired and congenital neutropenia by reducing infectious morbidity and mortality and improving quality of life. The utility of these growth factors in the treatment and prevention of sepsis in non-neutropenic infants, on the other hand, has not been clearly demonstrated.[6]

Inherited Disorders Associated with Neutropenia
SEVERE CONGENITAL NEUTROPENIA

Severe congenital neutropenia is a heterogeneous group of disorders first described in a large, consanguineous family by Swedish physician Rolf Kostmann. In the first several months of life, infants manifest recurrent severe infections (e.g., omphalitis, skin abscesses, respiratory tract infections, and otitis media) and a marked reduction or absence of circulating neutrophils. Bone marrow examination reveals a paucity of myeloid cells and an arrest at the promyelocyte or myelocyte stage. Staphylococcal and streptococcal infections are common, whereas yeast, fungal, and parasitic infections are rare.[83] According to the Severe Chronic Neutropenia International Registry data, mortality from sepsis is 0.4% per year in those who respond to G-CSF and 1.4% per year in those whose G-CSF response is less optimum.[83] Patients who survive through early childhood develop myelodysplastic syndrome and acute myelogenous leukemia at 10 years.[71]

Severe congenital neutropenia exhibits multiple patterns of inheritance, including autosomal dominant, autosomal recessive, X-linked, and sporadic. Most cases are caused by heterozygous missense mutations in the gene encoding neutrophil elastase (*ELA2*), a serine protease present in neutrophil and monocyte granules.[80] Emerging evidence suggests that these mutations trigger the unfolded protein response, leading to increased apoptosis of granulocyte progenitors.[80] Homozygous mutations of *HAX1* are associated with the autosomal recessive variant of severe congenital neutropenia. *HAX1* is a member of the antiapoptotic *BCL2* gene family, suggesting that increased apoptosis is the mechanism underlying this form of severe congenital neutropenia. There are three case reports of patients with severe congenital neutropenia who have germline heterozygous mutations in the G-CSF receptor gene (*CSFR3*).[7] Heterozygous germline mutations of *GFI1*,

BOX 46–5   Widely Used Drugs Associated with Idiosyncratic Neutropenia

ANALGESICS AND ANTI-INFLAMMATORY AGENTS
Gold salts
Indomethacin*
Pentazocine
Para-aminophenol derivatives*
- Acetaminophen
- Phenacetin
Pyrazolone derivatives*
- Aminopyrine
- Dipyrone
- Oxyphenbutazone
- Phenylbutazone

ANTIBIOTICS
Cephalosporins
Chloramphenicol*
Clindamycin
Gentamicin
Isoniazid
Para-aminosalicylic acid
Penicillins and semisynthetic penicillins*
Rifampin
Streptomycin
Sulfonamides*
Tetracyclines
Trimethoprim-sulfamethoxazole
Vancomycin

ANTICONVULSANTS
Carbamazepine
Mephenytoin
Phenytoin
Valproate

ANTIDEPRESSANTS
Amitriptyline
Amoxapine
Desipramine
Doxepin
Imipramine

ANTIHISTAMINES (H$_2$ BLOCKERS)
Cimetidine
Penicillamine
Ranitidine

ANTIMALARIALS
Amodiaquine
Chloroquine
Dapsone
Pyrimethamine
Quinine

ANTITHYROID AGENTS
Carbimazole
Methimazole
Propylthiouracil

CARDIOVASCULAR DRUGS
Captopril
Disopyramide
Hydralazine
Methyldopa
Procainamide
Propranolol
Quinidine
Tocainide

DIURETICS
Acetazolamide
Chlorothiazide
Chlorthalidone
Ethacrynic acid
Hydrochlorothiazide

HYPOGLYCEMIC AGENTS
Chlorpropamide
Tolbutamide

HYPNOTICS AND SEDATIVES
Chlordiazepoxide and other benzodiazepines
Meprobamate

PHENOTHIAZINES*
Chlorpromazine
Other phenothiazines

OTHER DRUGS
Allopurinol
Clozaril
Lemavisole
Ticlopidine

*More often reported to cause neutropenia in epidemiologic studies.
Adapted from Beutler E, et al: *Williams' hematology,* 5th ed, New York, 1995, McGraw-Hill.

which encodes a transcriptional repressor, have been reported in families with persistent neutropenia and lymphopenia.[7] An X-linked form of severe congenital neutropenia has been linked to gain-of-function mutations in *WAS*, the gene mutated in Wiscott-Aldrich syndrome and X-linked thrombocytopenia (see later).

Treatment with human recombinant G-CSF markedly reduces the number and degree of serious infections and corrects circulating neutrophil levels to normal in many patients. Some patients require high doses for response. A subset of patients with underlying defects in neutrophil function

remain at risk for sepsis even when the ANC is increased. Hematopoietic stem cell transplantation from an HLA-matched, unaffected sibling should be considered for patients with severe congenital neutropenia, especially those who respond poorly to G-CSF.

SHWACHMAN-DIAMOND SYNDROME
See also Chapter 47.
This rare syndrome of neutropenia (<500/μL) associated with pancreatic insufficiency and metaphyseal dysplasia is inherited in an autosomal recessive pattern. A variety of

physical abnormalities, including short stature, are common. Neutrophil counts generally are less than 500/μL, and moderate thrombocytopenia and anemia are common. Many patients have qualitative neutrophil defects. Defects in B, T, and NK lymphocytes have also been described. Severe, recurrent infections with *Staphylococcus* species, *Haemophilus* species, and gram-negative rods, as well as steatorrhea, are seen within the first 10 years of life. Transformation to acute leukemia occurs at a high rate. Serum trypsinogen is abnormal; sweat chloride testing is normal. The disease has been linked to homozygous mutations in the *SBDS* gene on chromosome 7q11. The function of this gene is unknown, but it might participate in RNA metabolism. The gene defect in most cases of Shwachman-Diamond syndrome is a conversion mutation from a pseudogene.[8] The etiology of the neutropenia is not understood, although it often responds to administration of G-CSF. Hematopoietic stem cell transplantation has been reported to have an increased incidence of transplant-related complications.

MYELOKATHEXIS

Another rare disorder with severe congenital neutropenia, severe and recurrent infections, and dysmorphic myeloid elements in the bone marrow, myelokathexis is more common in females and may have autosomal dominant inheritance. It may be part of the WHIM syndrome (warts, hypogammaglobulinemia, infections, myelokathexis).[51]

CONGENITAL DYSGRANULOPOIETIC NEUTROPENIA

This disease with severe congenital neutropenia, severe infections, and defects in primary and secondary myeloid granules is an autosomal recessive disorder.[44]

P14 DEFICIENCY

This disorder of congenital neutropenia, recurrent respiratory infections, reduced cytotoxic T-cell function, low IgM, short stature, partial albinism, and coarse facial features is responsive to G-CSF. P14, involved in MAP kinase signaling, is deficient in these patients.[9]

CYCLIC NEUTROPENIA

Children with cyclic neutropenia often display recurrent fevers and bacterial infections (e.g., stomatitis and pharyngitis), with cyclical patterns at intervals of 2 to 5 weeks. The cyclic nature of the neutropenia correlates precisely with the presence and severity of the infections. Individual patients maintain constant cycle times. Diagnosis is based on frequent CBCs (two to three times weekly) over a 6-week period demonstrating a cyclic rise and fall of the ANC. Platelet count and monocytes often rise and fall paradoxically with the ANC. Bone marrow examination reveals hypocellularity of the myeloid lineage with myelocyte arrest during times of peripheral neutropenia. Based on studies in humans and in the gray collie dog (an animal model), a regulatory defect at the level of the stem cell has been hypothesized.

This disorder, like severe congenital neutropenia, has been linked to single-base substitutions in the gene encoding neutrophil elastase.[40] It is unclear why these mutations affect the clocklike timing of hematopoiesis. Therapy consists of administering prophylactic antibiotics and G-CSF.

CARTILAGE-HAIR HYPOPLASIA

Cartilage-hair hypoplasia is a rare autosomal recessive disorder characterized by short-limbed dwarfism, fine hair, hyperextensible digits, increased susceptibility to infection, lymphopenia, and chronic neutropenia. Cellular immunity is abnormal. Cartilage-hair hypoplasia is an autosomal recessive disease caused by mutations in *RMRP*, a noncoding RNA gene involved in mitochondrial DNA replication, ribosome biogenesis, and ribosomal RNA processing.[7] The cellular defects have been treated with hematopoietic stem cell transplantation.

DYSKERATOSIS CONGENITA

Dyskeratosis congenita is characterized by neutropenia (and other cytopenias), abnormal skin pigmentation, nail dystrophy, and mucosal leukoplakia. Other features include immunodeficiency, fragile bones, tooth decay, short stature, alopecia or premature graying, gonadal hypoplasia, urethral abnormalities, pulmonary fibrosis, liver cirrhosis, esophageal strictures, mental retardation, and a predisposition to cancers of the skin, gastrointestinal tract, and other sites.

Impaired telomere maintenance has been implicated in the pathogenesis of dyskeratosis congenita. It is hypothesized that the clinical manifestations of dyskeratosis congenita, which develop at a variable rate during childhood, are caused by excessive telomere shortening in stem cells within rapidly dividing tissues (e.g., skin or bone marrow). Autosomal dominant dyskeratosis congenita has been linked to mutations in either the telomerase RNA (*TERC*) gene or telomerase catalytic subunit (*TERT*) gene, and the X-linked form of the disease is caused by mutations in *DKC1*, which encodes a protein implicated in telomerase RNA processing or stabilization. Mutations in *DKC1* have also been identified in Hoyeraal-Hreidarsson syndrome, a condition marked by prenatal growth restriction, pancytopenia, cerebellar atrophy, abnormal myelination of cerebral white matter, and hypoplasia of the corpus callosum. Hoyeraal-Hreidarsson syndrome is considered a severe variant of X-linked dyskeratosis congenita. Other telomere maintenance genes mutated in some cases of dyskeratosis congenita include *NOP10*, *TINF2*, and *NHP2*.[7]

Hematopoietic stem cell transplantation is the only cure for patients who develop severe bone marrow complications of dyskeratosis congenita. However, patients with dyskeratosis congenita who undergo conventional transplantation do poorly because of a high incidence of early and late transplant-related complications, including severe mucositis, sepsis, hepatic veno-occlusive disease, microangiopathic hemolytic anemia, and pulmonary fibrosis. Recent studies suggest that nonmyeloablative transplant conditioning regimens afford better outcomes in these patients.

RETICULAR DYSGENESIS

This is a rare syndrome of lymphoid hypoplasia, thymic aplasia, and agranulocytosis with normal bone marrow megakaryocyte and erythroid precursors. Patients have low serum IgM and IgA levels and die in infancy without hematopoietic stem cell transplantation. There is a maturation arrest in the myeloid lineage and also a global impairment of lymphoid maturation leading to severe reduction in both B- and T-cell numbers. The mitochondrial energy metabolism enzyme adenylate kinase 2 (AK2) is mutated in individuals with reticular dysgenesis.[65] Hematopoietic stem cell transplantation is the only curative treatment.

Congenital Neutropenia with Inborn Errors of Metabolism
GLYCOGEN STORAGE DISEASE TYPE 1 (VON GIERKE DISEASE)
Patients with type 1b have neutropenia, but those with type 1c also have a qualitative neutrophil defect that is associated with an increased susceptibility to infections. G-CSF has successfully decreased infection rates in patients with type 1b.[48]

COBALAMIN AND FOLATE DEFICIENCIES
Whether nutritional or due to an inherited disorder affecting vitamin B_{12} or folate metabolism, mild neutropenia is associated with the megaloblastic anemia of cobalamin and folate deficiencies.

Neutropenia Associated with Agammaglobulinemia
In this primary immunodeficiency disorder, severe immunodeficiency is accompanied by neutropenia. Hematopoietic stem cell transplantation can be life-saving.

NEUTROPHILIA

Neutrophilia is the specific elevation of the ANC more than 2 standard deviations above the mean (Box 46-6).

Intrinsic Defects that Cause Neutrophilia
LEUKEMOID REACTION
Newborns sometimes mount an exaggerated response to infection. As in older children, the circulating neutrophil count increases, and a left shift occurs (band forms, myelocytes, and metamyelocytes increase in the peripheral circulation). A significant increase in early neutrophil precursors in the peripheral blood, as well as an increase in the white blood cell count (generally exceeding 50,000/μL), is considered a leukemoid reaction. A normal newborn in the first 2 days of life displays a neutrophil-to-band ratio greater than 7:1 (see Table 46-13). A leukemoid reaction associated with severe infection in the newborn often is accompanied by cytoplasmic vacuoles within the neutrophil and by the appearance of toxic granulations. Infants with Down syndrome can have a type of leukemoid reaction (see "Down Syndrome," later). A rare, autosomal dominant hereditary neutrophilia has been described.[39]

A prospective study of all patients admitted to the neonatal intensive care unit at the University of Florida during a 12-month period identified 9 of 707 patients (1.3%) with a transient leukemoid reaction.[15] Of these 9 patients, 7 were identified in the first 4 days of life, and 1 presented on day 9 and 1 at day 25 of life. One infant had Down syndrome. Maternal betamethasone treatment was associated in 4 cases. Hyperviscosity and congenital infection were excluded in all 9. The duration of the reaction ranged from 5 to 32 days, the longest being in the infant with trisomy 21.

DOWN SYNDROME
About 10% of infants who have Down syndrome develop transient myeloproliferative disorder. This process also sometimes occurs in a phenotypically normal child with trisomy 21 mosaicism, including an isolated clone of trisomy 21 bone marrow cells. Transient myeloproliferative disorder is characterized by the presence of megakaryoblasts in the peripheral blood, variable thrombocytopenia, and hepatosplenomegaly. Abnormalities of all three hematopoietic cell lineages have been described. Additional cytogenetic abnormalities might be present in the blasts. In most cases, the reaction is transient and resolves within the first 3 months of life, although it can be life-threatening or fatal.[25] Occasionally, it reappears.

By some estimates, up to 30% of infants with Down syndrome and transient myeloproliferative disorder develop acute megakaryoblastic leukemia (AMKL) in the first 4 years of life, suggesting that transient myeloproliferative disorder is a preleukemic state. Somatic mutations in *GATA1* have been reported in nearly all cases of transient myeloproliferative disorder and Down syndrome AMKL but not in other forms of leukemia. In addition, several groups of investigators have found identical *GATA1* mutations in the transient myeloproliferative disorder and AMKL blasts of patients for whom sequential samples were available. Together, these findings demonstrate that the development of a *GATA1* mutation is an early event in Down syndrome myeloid leukemogenesis.[35]

Management of affected infants is controversial. Most pediatric oncologists adopt a wait-and-see approach in managing these leukemoid reactions, regardless of chromosomal abnormalities. Infants with organ infiltration or a severe course are more likely to receive treatment with chemotherapy.

Disorders of Phagocyte Function
ADHESION DISORDERS

Leukocyte Adhesion Deficiency
Leukocyte adhesion deficiency is a rare group of autosomal recessive disorders characterized by persistent leukocytosis, delayed separation of the umbilical cord, and recurrent infections.[21] Leukocyte adhesion deficiency type I is characterized by the impairment of respiratory burst generation of complement-opsonized microorganisms and associated with defects in neutrophil adhesion and chemotaxis (Fig. 46-9). The clinical picture varies depending on the relative deficiency of CD18. CD18 is the β_2-subunit of cell surface leukocyte integrins. These molecules are involved in adherence, chemotaxis, C3bi-mediated ingestion, degranulation, and neutrophil respiratory burst activation. Leukocyte adhesion deficiency should be suspected in any infant who has unusually severe bacterial infections accompanied by normal to increased blood leukocyte counts. There is a striking absence of pus at the site of infection because neutrophils do

---

BOX 46–6   **Intrinsic and Extrinsic Defects that Cause Neutrophilia In the Neonate**

INTRINSIC DEFECTS
Down syndrome
Leukocyte adhesion deficiency
Hereditary neutrophilia

EXTRINSIC DEFECTS
Infection
Stress
Rh disease and other hemolytic anemias
Drugs (glucocorticoids and beta-adrenergic agonists)
Asplenia

Figure 46–9. Attachment and spread of leukocyte adhesion deficiency (LAD) (**A**) and control (**B**) neutrophils through cell surface integrins, as visualized through scanning electron microscopy. Orientation and movement of LAD (**C**) and control (**D**) neutrophils to a chemotactic gradient (from the right), as visualized by means of scanning microscopy. (*Adapted from Anderson D, et al: Abnormalities of polymorphonuclear leukocyte function associated with a heritable deficiency of high-molecular-weight surface glycoproteins (GP 138): common relationship to diminished cell adherence, J Clin Invest 74:536, 1985.*)

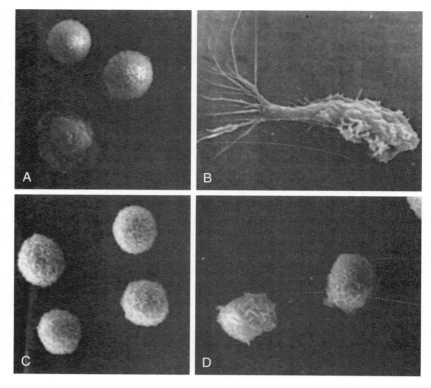

not migrate from the vasculature to sites of inflammation within tissues.

Diagnosis of leukocyte adhesion deficiency type I is made, generally by flow cytometric analysis, by demonstrating a severe deficiency of the β_2-subunit of neutrophil integrins (usually 0% to 10%). Carriers can be identified by the expression of an about 50% normal β_2-integrin level on circulating neutrophils. Therapy for patients with leukocyte adhesion deficiency type I depends on the clinical severity. Patients with a moderately severe clinical phenotype can be aggressively managed with antibiotics. However, patients with a severe phenotype often succumb to overwhelming infection in the first or second year of life. Hematopoietic stem cell transplantation is indicated for patients with severe leukocyte adhesion deficiency type I.[21]

Leukocyte Adhesion Deficiency Type II (Rombam-Hasharon Syndrome)

In addition to persistent leukocytosis and recurrent bacterial infections, this autosomal recessive clinical syndrome has been described in a few patients in Israel to include short stature, severe mental retardation, and the hh (Bombay) RBC phenotype.[21] Neutrophils from these patients exhibited markedly diminished chemotaxis in vitro, although the neutrophils displayed normal levels of CD18 and were able to phagocytose serum-opsonized particles. The molecular defect in these patients is a defect of fucosyl transferase, the enzyme responsible for carbohydrate linkages associated with the AB blood groups, specifically the sialyl-Lewis X structure. This has importance for neutrophil function because the sialyl-Lewis X structure is necessary for the formation of the neutrophil cell surface ligand recognized by the endothelial cell surface E-selectin and P-selectin receptors.

Neutrophil Actin Dysfunction

Neutrophil actin dysfunction is an autosomal recessive disorder with markedly diminished chemotaxis in vitro and a diminished ability to ingest opsonized particles.[21] The neutrophils exhibit dysfunctional actin polymerization in vitro. The patient first described with this disorder died, and subsequently the neutrophils of his parents and sister were shown to have half the actin polymerizability in vitro with normal in vivo function.[75]

CHEMOTAXIS DISORDERS

Newborns, particularly premature infants, are at increased risk for severe bacterial infections. Neonates' neutrophils have a variety of disorders associated with immune surveillance and neutrophil-mediated immune function, but the particular defects and mechanistic bases thereof are not clear. For example, neonatal neutrophils display reduced chemotaxis in vitro compared with adult neutrophils. This could result from diminished augmentation of β_2-integrin (i.e., Mac-1) upregulation after exposure to chemotactic stimuli. That is, neutrophils from fetuses and from preterm and term infants display about 50% levels of Mac-1 compared with neutrophils from adults. After exposure to chemotactic mediators (e.g., bacterial extracts), the intracellular membrane-bound pool of Mac-1 is inappropriately mobilized in these neutrophils compared with neutrophils from adults.[76]

INGESTION AND DEGRANULATION DISORDERS

Chédiak-Higashi Syndrome

Chédiak-Higashi syndrome is a rare autosomal recessive disorder characterized by oculocutaneous albinism, progressive neuropathy, platelet dysfunction, frequent neutropenia, and progression to an accelerated phase and lymphoma-like syndrome (see also Chapter 52). The responsible gene has been cloned, and its product functions as a vacuolar sorting protein. Giant cytoplasmic granules and giant organelles are seen in many cells throughout the body because trafficking of granular proteins and organelles is defective. The syndrome affects neutrophil, platelet, and lymphocyte function. Neutrophils from affected patients demonstrate abnormal adherence and chemotaxis, delayed granulation, and diminished killing of ingested microorganisms. Patients with this disorder are unduly susceptible to bacterial infections. Most patients also undergo an accelerated phase, marked by lymphohistiocytic infiltration of multiple organs. This lymphoproliferative syndrome appears to result principally from a lack of natural killer cell function. Death often occurs in the first decade from infection, bleeding, or development of the accelerated phase. Hematopoietic stem cell transplantation can be used to treat the hematologic complications of Chédiak-Higashi syndrome.

OXIDATIVE KILLING DISORDERS

Chronic Granulomatous Disease

Chronic granulomatous disease is a rare (about 1 in 200,000), genetically heterogeneous disorder characterized by inherited defects in the neutrophil respiratory burst generated by the reduced NADPH oxidase enzyme.[76] Affected patients develop severe recurrent bacterial and fungal infections, often caused by organisms not ordinarily considered pathogens (e.g., *Aspergillus* species). Most patients manifest symptoms within the first year of life (Box 46-7). Inadequate neutrophil killing or ingestion is associated with a chronic inflammatory response that culminates in the formation of macrophage-containing granulomas throughout the gastrointestinal and urinary tracts. Chronic granulomatous disease manifests as a clinically heterogeneous disorder in which a minority of patients have a milder clinical course.[76]

This disorder, first described in 1957, is associated with absent or markedly reduced respiratory burst oxidase (phagocyte NADPH oxidase, or PHOX) activity in neutrophils, monocytes, and macrophages.[76] Because four distinct gene products are required for functional NADPH oxidase activity, defects in any one of these components can lead to this disorder. Chronic granulomatous disease is usually X-linked in inheritance, associated with the gp91 protein, gp91-PHOX, but autosomal recessive forms are associated with defects in CYBA, NCFI, and other PHOX proteins (as shown in Table 46-15). Diagnosis of chronic granulomatous disease was classically made using the nitroblue-tetrazolium test, in which reduction of nitroblue-tetrazolium by superoxide free radical formation does not occur in patients. Currently dihydrorhodamine-stained neutrophils from a whole blood sample are incubated and stimulated to produce superoxide radicals (or not) to reduce dihydrorhodamine. A cytochrome C reduction assay can estimate the amount of superoxide free radical a patient can produce. Genetic analysis of affected patients can identify the specific genetic defect.[56] Therapy involves prophylactic antibiotics and antifungal agents. Recombinant interferon-γ-1b prophylaxis has also been effective in reducing the incidence of infections. γ-Retroviral gene therapy has been reported in some patients with chronic granulomatous disease and has been associated with benefit in a minority but also some severe toxicities, including death. Hematopoietic stem cell

---

BOX 46-7   Clinical Presentation of Chronic Granulomatous Disease*

CHRONIC CONDITIONS
Lymphadenopathy
Hepatomegaly
Splenomegaly
Anemia of chronic disease
Dermatitis
Aphthous stomatitis
Restrictive lung disease
Gingivitis
Hydronephrosis
Persistent diarrhea
Gastric antral narrowing (infants and children)

INFECTIONS
Pneumonia
Lymphadenitis
Cutaneous abscess and impetigo
Perirectal abscess
Hepatic abscess
Osteomyelitis
Sepsis
Conjunctivitis

Sinusitis
Pyelonephritis (often due to obstruction)
Rare but Important
- Pericarditis
- Brain abscess
- Meningitis

INFECTING ORGANISMS
Staphylococcus aureus
Klebsiella species
Serratia marcescens
Escherichia coli
Aspergillus species
Pseudomonas cepacia
Candida albicans
Salmonella species
Other enteric bacteria
Rare but Important
- *Nocardia* species
- Mycobacteria
- *Pneumocystis carinii*

*Each list is arranged in approximate order of frequency based on 35 patients followed at the Scripps Research Institute and on a review of the literature by Forrest and colleagues.[109]
Modified from Curnutte JT: Disorders of phagocyte function. In Hoffman R, et al, editors: *Hematology: basic principles and practice*, New York, 1991, Churchill Livingstone, p 575.

TABLE 46–15 Simplified Classification of Chronic Granulomatous Disease

Component Affected	Inheritance	NBT Score (% Positive)	Frequency (% of Cases)	IMMUNOBLOT LEVELS*			
				gp91	p22	p47	p67
gp91-PHOX†	X	0	50	0	0	N	N
		0	3	N	N	N	N
p22-PHOX‡	A	0	5	0	0	N	N
p47-PHOX	A	0	33	N	N	0	N
p67-PHOX	A	0	5	N	N	N	0

*Defined by immunoblotting with component-specific antibodies.
† A variant exists with low but detectable NBT activity, gp91/p22 at 3% frequency.
‡ A variant exists with no NBT activity, but detectable p22 immunoblot activity at 1% frequency.
A, autosomal recessive inheritance; N, normal level of protein; NBT, nitroblue tetrazolium; X, X-linked inheritance; 0, undetectable level of protein activity.
Modified from Curnutte JT: Molecular basis of the autosomal recessive forms of chronic granulomatous disease, *Immunodefic Rev* 3:149, 1992.

transplantation could also correct the defect in chronic granulomatous disease.

Myeloperoxidase Deficiency

Myeloperoxidase deficiency is the most common inherited disorder of neutrophils, with complete deficiency found in about 1 in 4000 persons and partial deficiency observed in 1 in 2000. However, most affected persons are notable for lack of any symptoms. The classic presentation in the subset of patients is immunodeficiency and infection with *Candida albicans*. It can mimic chronic granulomatous disease in certain screening tests.

HEMOSTASIS

Tissue injury triggers a number of immediate host responses whose goal is to maintain blood vessel integrity while more permanent repair processes are underway. Participants in the human hemostatic mechanism include the blood vessels, platelets, procoagulant and anticoagulant proteins, and fibrinolytic system. An abnormality in any component can disrupt the critical balance and result in excessive thrombosis or bleeding. Although much remains to be discovered, many alterations in the hemostatic mechanism have been described in the healthy fetus and newborn, and because the normal fetus and newborn do not suffer from excessive bleeding or thrombosis, these differences must be considered physiologic.

The first half of this section provides an overview of hemostasis, including a discussion of the known physiologic differences in hemostasis in the fetus and newborn. The second half examines the hemorrhagic and thrombotic disorders that commonly and sometimes almost exclusively occur in the neonate.

Components of Hemostasis

BLOOD VESSELS

The endothelial cell lining of blood vessels provides a structural interface between the blood and the subendothelial matrix. In its uninjured, inactive state, it presents an antithrombotic surface to which platelets do not adhere. Endothelial cell products with antithrombogenic properties include prostacyclin (PGI_2), the lipoxygenase pathway product 13-hydroxyoctadecadienoic acid, and heparan sulfate proteoglycans. Nitric oxide is produced by the intact endothelium and has vascular relaxation activity and contributes to inhibition of platelet adhesion and aggregation.

After injury, the smooth muscle layer of involved arterioles or venules contracts, resulting in localized vascular constriction and reduced blood loss from the injured site. When the endothelial surface is disrupted, thrombotic subendothelial substances are exposed to blood. Alternatively, exposure of the endothelium to various inflammatory or immune mediators as a result of systemic illness, infection, or tissue injury substantially alters the endothelium to an activated state. The vascular endothelium then becomes a contact point for adhesion and aggregation of activated platelets and leukocytes and for deposition of the coagulation proteins. Tissue factor can form a complex with circulating coagulation factor VIIa to initiate the fluid phase of coagulation.

The circulating procoagulant molecule thrombin also participates in anticoagulant processes by its association with thrombomodulin on the endothelial cell surface to promote activation of protein C (see "Physiologic Anticoagulation Strategies and Proteins," later). Fibrinolytic activities of cultured endothelial cells include production of urokinase and tissue plasminogen activator (t-PA). There are binding sites for plasminogen and t-PA on the cell surface.

Genetic and environmental factors influence alterations in the human vascular endothelium, which occur over a lifetime. Many of these changes enhance the thrombotic potential of the vasculature. Little is known about the functional differences between newborn and adult endothelium.

PLATELETS, ENDOTHELIUM, AND VON WILLEBRAND FACTOR

Platelets participate in the first phase of hemostasis, during which a platelet plug forms at the site of blood vessel injury. Platelets limit loss at the site of endothelial disruption within injured blood vessels, and they also provide a framework to facilitate fibrin clot formation by components of the plasma phase of coagulation. Platelets circulate as smooth discs, but on exposure to agonists released in response to vascular injury or endothelial activation, they become activated, adhere to the site of disrupted endothelium, aggregate, release their granule contents, and promote the generation of thrombin. The most active physiologic platelet activators are thrombin and collagen. Adenosine diphosphate and epinephrine are weaker agonists. Thrombin can cleave protease-activated receptors PAR-1 and PAR-4, members of the G-protein protease-activated receptor family of transmembrane signaling proteases. This appears to be the major physiologic activation process for platelets. Platelets also become activated through the collagen receptor glyoprotein (GP) IV and adhere to the subendothelium via collagen receptor GP Ia/IIa.

Activated platelets undergo shape change to extend adhesive pseudopods. Platelets adhere to von Willebrand factor (vWF) in the subendothelium through their GP Ib/IX/V surface glycoprotein receptor. Platelet activation also allows a conformational change in, and surface expression of, the glycoprotein receptor GP IIb/IIIa, which binds fibrinogen (as well as some vWF) and results in platelet aggregation. Additionally, the cytosolic part of GP IIb/IIIa in activated platelets binds to their cytoskeleton and participates in platelet shape changes and clot retraction. The resultant platelet plug functions not only as a physical barrier at the site of a break in the endothelium but also as an initiator for thrombin production and rapid formation of a localized fibrin clot. Activated platelets degranulate and secrete many substances that promote vasoconstriction, endothelial adhesion, platelet activation and recruitment, platelet aggregation, and thrombin formation. The exposure of surface prothrombotic phospholipids such as phosphatidylserine promotes the localized surface formation of procoagulant enzyme complexes. Coagulation factor V and fibrinogen are released by activated platelets, and the phospholipid of the platelet membrane assists in the formation of complexes of coagulation factors and calcium, so that fibrin clot formation proceeds rapidly and efficiently. Platelet function, physiologic alterations in the newborn, and qualitative and quantitative abnormalities of platelet function are discussed later.

vWF is a multimeric glycoprotein synthesized by megakaryocytes and endothelial cells that functions in platelet adhesion (through GP Ib/IX/V) and aggregation (through GP IIb/IIIa) (Fig. 46-10). It is secreted by activated platelets, is found in the subendothelial matrix, and also circulates in plasma as a carrier for coagulation factor VIII. vWF is a highly multimeric glycoprotein. The largest multimers are the most functional in platelet adhesion and aggregation activities. Platelet-vWF-fibrinogen interactions are measured most commonly by the platelet function screening tests such as the PFA-100 (Dade-Behring, Deerfield, IL). Bleeding time testing is generally not done in neonates (see "Laboratory Testing of the Neonatal Hemostatic System," later).

COAGULATION FACTORS

Coagulation proceeds through the sequential activation of zymogens (inactive proenzymes) to enzymes and the assembly of complexes of enzymes in association with cofactors, calcium, and phospholipids that produce a robust amount of thrombin and a strong fibrin clot. Effective localization of blood clot formation is necessary so that hemostasis is achieved and yet systemic thrombosis is avoided. The cellular participants in hemostasis, as well as most of the circulating procoagulant proteins, normally exist in their inactive states. The plasma concentrations of the zymogens are low enough that spontaneous activation is rare. The efficiency of the activation reactions improves enormously when the proteins are brought into close approximation with their activating enzymes and cofactors through the formation of calcium-containing complexes on a cellular phospholipid membrane.

In 1964, the coagulation cascade-waterfall hypothesis was introduced (Fig. 46-11). This theory proposed two pathways leading to activation of factor X, which then combined with cofactor Va to cleave prothrombin to thrombin. Thrombin cleaved fibrinogen to fibrin, leading to eventual fibrin clot formation. According to this theory, coagulation could be initiated either by the intrinsic pathway, so named because all the necessary components existed in plasma, or by the extrinsic pathway, which required addition of tissue factor. The extrinsic

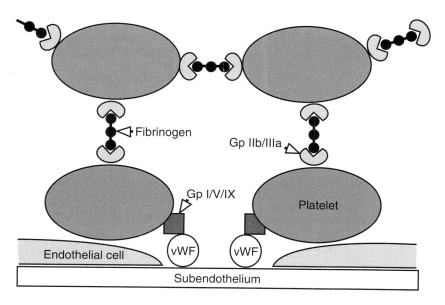

Figure 46–10. Schematic representation of the interaction of platelets with the subendothelium (see text for details). Gp, glycoprotein; vWF, von Willebrand factor.

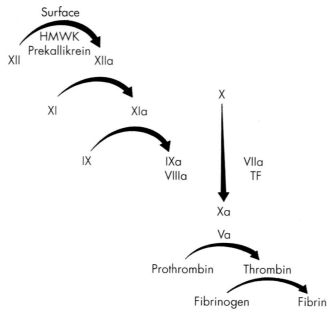

Figure 46–11. The cascade-waterfall hypothesis of blood coagulation. In this scheme, coagulation may be initiated by the extrinsic or intrinsic pathway, either of which can lead to thrombin-mediated formation of a fibrin clot via a common pathway involving factor Xa, factor Va, and phospholipids. HMWK, high-molecular-weight kallikrein; TF, tissue factor.

and intrinsic pathways could be tested separately by the prothrombin time (PT) and partial thromboplastin time (PTT) assays, respectively. The PT and activated partial thromboplastin time (aPTT) tests have proved invaluable for evaluation of coagulation factor deficiencies; however, a number of clinical and laboratory observations could not be explained by the cascade-waterfall hypothesis. A physiologic activator of the intrinsic pathway's contact activators has not been found, and people who are deficient in these contact activation factors, factor XI, prekallikrein, or high-molecular-weight kininogen,

have prolonged aPTT assay results but do not bleed abnormally. Patients with severe hemophilia A (factor VIII deficiency) or hemophilia B (factor IX deficiency) have serious clinical bleeding abnormalities. In contrast, those with deficiency of another intrinsic pathway member, factor XI, have a milder clinical course. Severe factor VII deficiency (extrinsic pathway) results in hemorrhagic abnormalities.

In 1991, Gailani and associates[33a] proposed the revised hypothesis of coagulation (Fig. 46-12). Clotting is initiated when subendothelial tissue factor is exposed to circulating factor VII or VIIa. The factor VIIa-tissue factor complex associates with calcium on a phospholipid surface to form the *extrinsic tenase complex*, which activates factor X and factor IX. Some of the factor Xa complexes with cofactor Va, calcium, and phospholipid (the *prothrombinase complex*) and cleaves prothrombin to thrombin. This initial thrombin activates platelets. Factor IXa, in combination with cofactor VIIIa, calcium, and a phospholipid membrane, forms the *intrinsic tenase complex*, activates additional factor X, and produces more thrombin. This thrombin activates factor XI, which activates factor IX and then promotes robust thrombin production through the intrinsic tenase complex, followed by the prothrombinase complex. Thrombin can cleave fibrinogen to fibrin, leading to production of a fibrin clot. Fibrin monomers spontaneously polymerize into strands, but covalent bonding of the strands into a stable clot is accomplished by the transglutaminase, factor XIII. Factor XIII is activated by thrombin. In addition, premature breakdown of the clot is prevented by the thrombin-activated fibrinolysis inhibitor. When coagulation factors or cofactors are defective or deficient, less thrombin is generated. This affects the quality as well as the quantity of fibrin clot formation.

Interestingly, thrombin also promotes anticoagulant and antifibrinolytic processes.

PHYSIOLOGIC ANTICOAGULANT STRATEGIES AND PROTEINS

Balancing the efficient, localized formation of clot at a site of injury are the anticoagulant complexes, which bind to endothelial cells and efficiently inactivate clotting factors to prevent

Figure 46–12. Revised hypothesis of blood coagulation, in which coagulation is initiated by factor VIIa- and tissue factor (TF)-mediated activation of factors IX and X, sustained through the participation of factors VIIIa and IXa, and consolidated by factor XIa. Tissue factor pathway inhibitor (TFPI) inhibits factor Xa, and in a factor Xa-dependent fashion, feeds back and inhibits the factor VIIa-tissue factor complex.

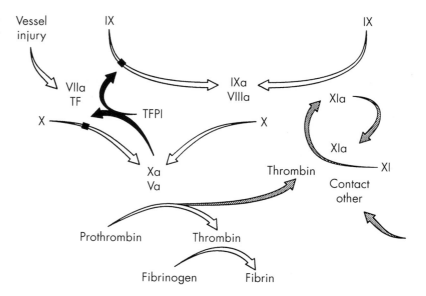

excessive coagulation and systemic thrombosis. In pathologic states, diffuse and unregulated activation of the hemostasis can occur, resulting in systemic thrombosis. Normally, some activated coagulant factors drift away from the coagulation complexes and are diluted in the bloodstream. Clotting factors are proteolytically degraded. In addition to nonspecific limitations of clot formation, anticoagulant systems also prevent excessive clot formation. Thrombin is a necessary component of clot formation, but it also serves to localize and limit the process by complexing with anticoagulant proteins and the fibrinolytic system to localize and enhance the efficiency of the anticoagulation and fibrinolytic reactions.

One inhibitor of coagulation, tissue factor pathway inhibitor, is present at low concentration in the plasma and is stored in the endothelium. Factor Xa can combine with tissue factor pathway inhibitor and become inhibited. Additionally, the tissue factor pathway inhibitor–factor Xa complex produces feedback inhibition of the factor VIIa–tissue factor complex. Tissue factor pathway inhibitor is produced in the microvascular endothelium and its release into plasma is enhanced by heparin.

A second coagulation inhibitor is antithrombin, formerly referred to as antithrombin III. Antithrombin inactivates a number of coagulation proteases, the most important of which is factor IIa (thrombin), as well as factors XIa, Xa, and IXa. The anticoagulant drug heparin and naturally occurring endothelial cell surface heparan sulfate greatly accelerate the activity of antithrombin. The anticoagulant effect of heparin is largely due to enhancement of inhibition of thrombin and factor Xa through interactions with a critical pentasaccharide region.

Thrombin also binds thrombomodulin on the endothelial surface, promoting protein C activation. Activated protein C, with its cofactor protein S, in the presence of calcium and phospholipids, proteolytically inactivates factors Va and VIIIa. Qualitative or quantitative defects in the anticoagulant proteins or in their ability to inactivate factor V by cleavage shift the balance toward excessive thrombus formation.

FIBRINOLYTIC SYSTEM

When repair of injured tissues is complete, the fibrin clot is dissolved by the enzyme plasmin. The fibrinolytic system is composed of the zymogen plasminogen and its thrombin-activated counterpart plasmin; the plasminogen activators (PAs) urokinase type (u-PA) and tissue type (t-PA); and their inhibitors, plasminogen-activator inhibitors PAI-1 and PAI-2 and α_2-antiplasmin (Fig. 46-13). Plasmin cleaves fibrinogen as well as fibrin. Cleavage of the cross-linked fibrin clot produces fibrin degradation products. D-Dimer is fibrin degradation products produced from the cleavage of two cross-linked fibrin monomers, releasing a fragment with two cross-linked D domains. Inhibition of the action of plasmin can occur by the activator inhibitors PAI-1 or PAI-2 or by inhibition of the enzyme itself with α_2-antiplasmin. u-PA is active in the extravascular compartment, whereas t-PA functions to activate plasminogen within the vasculature. Antithrombin also inhibits plasminogen activation. Defects in the fibrinolytic system have been associated with excessive thrombosis or bleeding. Recombinant t-PA is used to lyse pathologic thrombi.

PHYSIOLOGIC ALTERATIONS OF COAGULATION AND FIBRINOLYSIS IN THE NEONATE

Many differences in the neonatal coagulation system have been described. Understanding of the newborn hemostatic system has been hampered by difficulties in obtaining adequate control groups of healthy newborns and because the values of many coagulation factors change rapidly as gestational age and postnatal age progress. Coagulation and fibrinolytic factors do not cross the placenta and are reported to begin to appear in the fetal circulation by 10 weeks' gestational age. Normal ranges for most components of the coagulation, anticoagulation, and fibrinolytic systems are available for full-term infants and for infants born as prematurely as 30 weeks' gestation (Tables 46-16 to 46-18) (see "Laboratory Testing of the Neonatal Hemostatic System," below). The proposed etiologies for the differences in the newborn hemostatic system relative to the adult system include decreased synthesis of factors in the immature liver; decreased post-translational modification of some factors to active forms due to low vitamin K levels; enhanced clearance; general activation of the coagulation system at birth, with resultant consumption of factors; and synthesis of less-active fetal

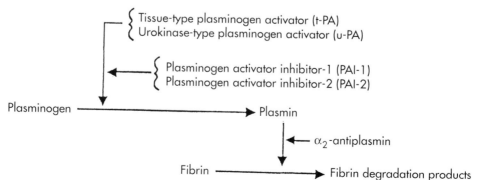

Figure 46–13. Plasminogen activation cascade. The proenzyme plasminogen is activated to the enzyme plasmin by tissue-type plasminogen activator (t-PA) or urinary-type plasminogen activator (u-PA). These two enzymes are inactivated after reaction with plasminogen activator inhibitor-1 (PAI-1) or plasminogen activator inhibitor-2 (PAI-2). Plasmin is capable of degrading fibrin clots to low-molecular-weight fibrin degradation products. Plasmin may be inactivated by α_2-antiplasmin.

TABLE 46–16 Reference Values for Coagulation Tests in the Healthy Full-Term Infant During the First 6 Months of Life

Tests	Day 1 (N)	Day 5 (N)	Day 30 (N)	Day 90 (N)	Day 180 (N)	Adult (N)
PT (sec)	13.0 ± 1.43 (61)	12.4 ± 1.46 (77)	11.8 ± 1.25 (67)	11.9 ± 1.15 (62)	12.3 ± 0.79 (47)	12.4 ± 0.78 (29)
aPTT (sec)	42.9 ± 5.80 (61)	42.6 ± 8.62 (76)	40.4 ± 7.42 (67)	37.1 ± 6.52 (62)	35.5 ± 3.71 (47)	33.5 ± 3.44 (29)
TCT (sec)	23.5 ± 2.38 (58)	23.1 ± 3.07 (64)	24.3 ± 2.44 (53)	25.1 ± 2.32 (52)	25.5 ± 2.86 (41)	25.0 ± 2.66 (19)
Fibrinogen (g/mL)	2.83 ± 0.58 (61)	3.12 ± 0.75 (77)	2.70 ± 0.54 (67)	2.43 ± 0.68 (60)	2.51 ± 0.68 (47)	2.78 ± 0.61 (29)
Factor II (U/mL)	0.48 ± 0.11 (61)	0.63 ± 0.15 (76)	0.68 ± 0.17 (67)	0.75 ± 0.15 (62)	0.88 ± 0.14 (47)	1.08 ± 0.19 (29)
Factor V (U/mL)	0.72 ± 0.18 (61)	0.95 ± 0.25 (76)	0.98 ± 0.18 (67)	0.90 ± 0.21 (62)	0.91 ± 0.18 (47)	1.06 ± 0.22 (29)
Factor VII (U/mL)	0.66 ± 0.19 (60)	0.89 ± 0.27 (75)	0.90 ± 0.24 (67)	0.91 ± 0.26 (62)	0.87 ± 0.20 (47)	1.05 ± 0.19 (29)
Factor VIII (U/mL)	1.00 ± 0.39 (60)	0.88 ± 0.33 (75)	0.91 ± 0.33 (67)	0.79 ± 0.23 (62)	0.73 ± 0.18 (47)	0.99 ± 0.25 (29)
vWF (U/mL)	1.53 ± 0.67 (40)	1.40 ± 0.57 (43)	1.28 ± 0.69 (40)	1.18 ± 0.44 (40)	1.07 ± 0.45 (46)	0.92 ± 0.33 (29)
Factor IX (U/mL)	0.53 ± 0.19 (59)	0.53 ± 0.19 (75)	0.51 ± 0.15 (67)	0.67 ± 0.23 (62)	0.86 ± 0.25 (47)	1.09 ± 0.27 (29)
Factor X (U/mL)	0.40 ± 0.14 (60)	0.49 ± 0.15 (76)	0.59 ± 0.14 (67)	0.71 ± 0.18 (62)	0.78 ± 0.20 (47)	1.06 ± 0.23 (29)
Factor XI (U/mL)	0.38 ± 0.14 (60)	0.55 ± 0.16 (74)	0.63 ± 0.13 (67)	0.69 ± 0.14 (62)	0.86 ± 0.24 (47)	0.97 ± 0.15 (29)
Factor XII (U/mL)	0.53 ± 0.29 (60)	0.47 ± 0.18 (75)	0.49 ± 0.16 (67)	0.67 ± 0.21 (62)	0.77 ± 0.19 (47)	108 ± 0.27 (29)
Prekallikrein (U/mL)	0.37 ± 0.16 (45)	0.48 ± 0.14 (51)	0.57 ± 0.17 (48)	0.73 ± 0.16 (46)	0.86 ± 0.15 (43)	1.12 ± 0.25 (29)
HMW-K (U/mL)	0.54 ± 0.24 (47)	0.74 ± 0.28 (63)	0.77 ± 0.22 (50)	0.82 ± 0.32 (46)	0.82 ± 0.23 (48)	0.92 ± 0.22 (29)
Factor XIIIa (U/mL)	0.79 ± 0.26 (44)	0.94 ± 0.25 (49)	0.93 ± 0.27 (44)	1.04 ± 0.34 (44)	1.04 ± 0.29 (41)	1.05 ± 0.25 (29)
Factor XIIIb (U/mL)	0.76 ± 0.23 (44)	1.06 ± 0.37 (47)	1.11 ± 0.36 (45)	1.16 ± 0.34 (44)	1.10 ± 0.30 (41)	0.97 ± 0.20 (29)
Plasminogen (U/mL)	1.95 ± 0.35 (44)	2.17 ± 0.38 (60)	1.98 ± 0.36 (52)	2.48 ± 0.37 (44)	3.01 ± 0.40 (47)	3.36 ± 0.44 (29)

All factors except fibrinogen and plasminogen are expressed as units per milliliter where pooled plasma contains 1 U/mL.
Plasminogen units are those recommended by the American Society of Hematology Committee on Thrombolytic Agents (CTA). All values are expressed as mean ± 1 SD.
aPTT, activated partial thromboplastin time; HMWK, high-molecular-weight kininogen; PT, prothrombin time; TCT, thrombin clotting time; vWF, von Willebrand factor.
From Andrew M, et al: The development of the human coagulation system in the full-term infant, *Blood* 70:165, 1987.

forms of some proteins. Most factors have reached adult levels by 6 months of life if not sooner. Factors VIII, V, fibrinogen, and XIII levels are normal at birth. Protein C levels remain low until later in childhood.

Several differences in the fibrinolytic system exist in the newborn: plasminogen and α_2-antiplasmin levels are low, whereas t-PA and PAI levels are twice the normal level for adults. α_2-Macroglobulin, an inhibitor of many proteolytic enzymes, including thrombin and plasmin, has been reported in infants at levels 2½ times the normal values for adults.

The cumulative result of these alterations is that plasmin activity is diminished in the newborn.

Defects in the Hemostatic System

In addition to physiologic changes, acquired and congenital defects in the hemostatic system can occur in the neonate, placing the infant at risk for bleeding or thrombosis. Evaluation of the hemostatic system must distinguish alterations that are considered physiologic for gestational and postnatal

TABLE 46–17   Reference Values for Coagulation Tests in Healthy Premature Infants (30 to 36 Weeks' Gestation) During First 6 Months of Life

Tests	DAY 1		DAY 5		DAY 30		DAY 90		DAY 180		ADULT	
	Mean	Range	Mean	Range	Mean	Range	Mean	Range	Mean	Range	Mean	Range
PT (sec)	13.0	(10.6-16.2)	12.5	(10.0-15.3)	11.8	(10.0-13.6)	12.3	(10.0-14.6)	12.5	(10.0-15.0)	12.4	(10.8-13.9)
aPTT (sec)	53.6	(27.5-79.4)	50.5	(26.9-74.1)	44.7	(26.9-62.5)	39.5	(28.3-50.7)	37.5	(21.7-53.3)	33.5	(26.6-40.3)
TCT (sec)	24.8	(19.2-30.4)	24.1	(18.8-24.4)	24.4	(18.8-29.9)	25.1	(19.4-30.8)	25.2	(18.9-31.5)	25.0	(19.7-30.3)
Fibrinogen (g/L)	2.43	(1.50-3.73)	2.80	(1.60-4.18)	2.54	(1.50-4.14)	2.46	(1.50-3.52)	2.28	(1.50-3.60)	2.78	(1.56-4.00)
Factor II (U/mL)	0.45	(0.20-0.77)	0.57	(0.29-0.85)	0.57	(0.36-0.95)	0.68	(0.30-1.06)	0.87	(0.51-1.23)	1.08	(0.70-1.46)
Factor V (U/mL)	0.88	(0.41-1.44)	1.00	(0.46-1.54)	1.02	(0.48-1.56)	0.99	(0.59-1.39)	1.02	(0.58-1.46)	1.06	(0.62-1.50)
Factor VII (U/mL)	0.67	(0.21-1.13)	0.84	(0.30-1.38)	0.83	(0.21-1.45)	0.87	(0.31-1.43)	0.99	(0.47-1.51)	1.05	(0.57-1.43)
Factor VIII (U/mL)	1.11	(0.50-2.13)	1.15	(0.53-2.05)	1.11	(0.50-1.99)	1.06	(0.58-1.88)	0.99	(0.50-1.87)	0.99	(0.50-1.49)
vWF (U/mL)	1.36	(0.78-2.10)	1.33	(0.72-2.19)	1.36	(0.66-2.16)	1.12	(0.75-1.84)	0.98	(0.54-1.58)	0.92	(0.50-1.58)
Factor IX (U/mL)	0.35	(0.19-0.65)	0.42	(0.14-0.74)	0.44	(0.13-0.80)	0.59	(0.25-0.93)	0.81	(0.50-1.20)	1.09	(0.55-1.63)
Factor X (U/mL)	0.41	(0.11-0.71)	0.51	(0.19-0.83)	0.56	(0.20-0.92)	0.67	(0.35-0.99)	0.77	(0.35-1.19)	1.06	(0.70-1.52)
Factor XI (U/mL)	0.30	(0.08-0.52)	0.41	(0.13-0.69)	0.43	(0.15-0.71)	0.59	(0.25-0.93)	0.78	(0.46-1.10)	0.97	(0.67-1.27)
Factor XII (U/mL)	0.38	(0.10-0.66)	0.39	(0.09-0.69)	0.43	(0.11-0.75)	0.61	(0.15-1.07)	0.82	(0.22-1.42)	1.08	(0.52-1.64)
Prekallikrein (U/mL)	0.33	(0.09-0.57)	0.45	(0.26-0.75)	0.59	(0.31-0.87)	0.79	(0.37-1.21)	0.78	(0.40-1.16)	1.12	(0.62-1.62)
HMWK (U/mL)	0.49	(0.09-0.89)	0.62	(0.24-1.00)	0.64	(0.16-1.12)	0.78	(0.32-1.24)	0.83	(0.41-1.25)	0.92	(0.50-1.36)
Factor XIIIa (U/mL)	0.70	(0.32-1.08)	1.01	(0.57-1.45)	0.99	(0.51-1.47)	1.13	(0.71-1.55)	1.13	(0.65-1.61)	1.05	(0.55-1.55)
Factor XIIIb (U/mL)	0.81	(0.35-1.27)	1.10	(0.68-1.58)	1.07	(0.57-1.57)	1.21	(0.75-1.67)	1.15	(0.67-1.63)	0.97	(0.57-1.37)
Plasminogen (U/mL)	1.70	(1.12-2.48)	1.91	(1.21-2.61)	1.81	(1.09-2.53)	2.38	(1.58-3.18)	2.75	(1.91-3.59)	3.36	(2.48-4.24)

All factors except fibrinogen and plasminogen are expressed as units per milliliters where pooled plasma contains 1 U/mL. Plasminogen units are those recommended by the Committee on Thrombolytic Agents (CTA).
All values are given as a mean and lower and upper boundary encompassing 95% of the population. Between 40 and 96 samples were assayed for each value for newborns.
aPTT, activated partial thromboplastin time; HMWK, high-molecular-weight kininogen; PT, prothrombin time; TCT, thrombin clotting time; vWF, von Willebrand factor.
From Andrew M, et al: Development of the human coagulation system in the healthy premature infant, *Blood* 72:1651, 1988.

TABLE 46–18 Reference Values for Inhibitors of Coagulation in Healthy Infants During First 6 Months of Life

Tests	DAY 1		DAY 5		DAY 30		DAY 90	
	Mean	Range	Mean	Range	Mean	Range	Mean	Range
AT III (U/mL)	0.38	(0.14-0.62)	0.56	(0.30-0.82)	0.59	(0.37-0.81)	0.83	(0.45-1.21)
α_2-M (U/mL)	1.10	(0.56-1.82)	1.25	(0.71-1.77)	1.38	(0.72-2.04)	1.80	(1.20-2.66)
α_2-AP (U/mL)	0.78	(0.40-1.16)	0.81	(0.49-1.13)	0.89	(0.55-1.23)	1.06	(0.64-1.48)
C_1-INH (U/mL)	0.65	(0.31-0.99)	0.83	(0.45-1.21)	0.74	(0.40-1.24)	1.14	(0.60-1.68)
α_2-AT (U/mL)	0.90	(0.36-1.44)	0.94	(0.42-1.46)	0.76	(0.38-1.12)	0.81	(0.49-1.13)
HC II (U/mL)	0.32	(0.00-0.60)	0.34	(0.00-0.69)	0.43	(0.15-0.71)	0.61	(0.20-1.11)
Protein C (U/mL)	0.28	(0.12-0.44)	0.31	(0.11-0.51)	0.37	(0.15-0.59)	0.45	(0.23-0.67)
Protein S (U/mL)	0.26	(0.14-0.38)	0.37	(0.13-0.61)	0.56	(0.22-0.90)	0.76	(0.40-1.12)

Tests	DAY 180		ADULT	
	Mean	Range	Mean	Range
AT III (U/mL)	0.90	(0.52-1.28)	1.05	(0.79-1.31)
α_2-M (U/mL)	2.09	(1.10-3.21)	0.86	(0.52-1.20)
α_2-AP (U/mL)	1.15	(0.77-1.53)	1.02	(0.68-1.36)
C_1-INH (U/mL)	1.40	(0.96-2.04)	1.01	(0.71-1.31)
α_2-AT (U/mL)	0.82	(0.48-1.16)	0.93	(0.55-1.31)
HC II (U/mL)	0.89	(0.45-1.40)	0.96	(0.66-1.26)
Protein C (U/mL)	0.57	(0.31-0.83)	0.96	(0.64-1.28)
Protein S (U/mL)	0.82	(0.44-1.20)	0.92	(0.60-1.24)

All values are expressed in units per milliliter, where pooled plasma contains 1.0 U/mL. All values are given as a mean followed by lower and upper boundary encompassing 95% of the population. Between 0 and 75 samples were assayed for each value for the newborn.
AP, antiplasmin; AT, antithrombin; C_1-INH, C_1 esterase inhibitor; HC, heparin cofactor; M, macroglobulin.
From Andrew M, et al: Development of the human coagulation system in the healthy premature infant, *Blood* 72:1651, 1988.

age from those that are abnormal. Consideration is then given to the patient's clinical status.

Although acquired defects are much more common, an otherwise healthy infant with excessive bleeding or thrombosis is more likely to have a congenital defect than is a sick infant with similar symptoms. Many patients with congenital abnormalities of hemostasis have symptoms and signs in infancy, and some of the presentations are unique to the neonatal period. Excessive bleeding can appear as an expanding cephalohematoma, prolonged bleeding after circumcision, oozing from venipuncture and line placement sites, or bleeding from the umbilicus. The ill infant can bleed from the bladder, gastrointestinal tract, or mucous membranes. Joint bleeding is distinctly uncommon in early infancy. Intracranial hemorrhage, especially in an otherwise healthy term infant, is an unusual but important presentation of a hemostatic defect.

LABORATORY TESTING OF THE NEONATAL HEMOSTATIC SYSTEM

Laboratory evaluation of a bleeding infant is especially challenging because the patient's small blood volume, often coupled with the poor regenerative potential of an ill infant, limits the total volume of blood available for testing. Because heparin adheres tightly to the walls of the tubing connected to intravenous catheters, most measures of coagulation are reliably performed only on free-flowing blood specimens obtained from an atraumatic venipuncture. Some centers place blood-drawing intravenous lines that are flushed or maintained with saline. Although sometimes successful, small clots can form within the catheter or at the tip, resulting in consumption of clotting factors and falsely abnormal results on coagulation testing. Cord blood may be used for coagulation factor assays and other testing if the specimen is immediately obtained by venipuncture from a double-clamped segment of the cord. Fetal blood specimens can be obtained, by ultrasound guidance, in fetuses as young as 20 weeks' gestation (see Chapter 8).

The higher hematocrit and resultant smaller volume of plasma per milliliter of whole blood in the newborn can alter the plasma-to-anticoagulant ratio, resulting in over-anticoagulation and falsely prolonged endpoints in some coagulation assays. Special sample tubes should be prepared for coagulation testing in infants with a hematocrit above 55%, so that the amount of anticoagulant added maintains the correct anticoagulation. If a patient is very anemic, excessive plasma per milliliter of whole blood will be sampled, and the plasma will be inadequately anticoagulated if standard sample tubes are used. To avoid falsely low results in some coagulation tests, special sample tubes should be prepared for patients whose hematocrit is below 25%.

Normal ranges for most components of the coagulation, anticoagulation, and fibrinolytic systems are available for full-term infants and for infants born as prematurely as 30 weeks' gestation (see Tables 46-16 to 46-18). In 2006, Monagle's group reevaluated the validity of these reference ranges and showed that the normal ranges are somewhat dependent on reagents and instruments used for testing.[59] Validation of reference ranges in the local laboratory is essential. Factors I, V, VIII, XIII, and vWF approximate adult ranges in the term newborn. Because the physiologic concentrations of some coagulation and fibrinolytic proteins is quite low in the neonatal period, definitive diagnosis can require repeat testing at a time when the expected normal range for age of the factor in question can be distinguished from a deficiency state (Fig. 46-14). The aPTT commonly is used as a screening coagulation test in older infants, children, and adults, but because most of the factors tested are normally low in the newborn, results are difficult to interpret. Results of the PT assay are only slightly prolonged in infants of more than 32 weeks' gestation. A small volume, whole blood, point-of-care assay for the activated clotting time (ACT) is discussed later in the "Extracorporeal Membrane Oxygenation" section.

Measurement of the non–γ-carboxyl glutamated clotting proteins induced by vitamin K absence (PIVKA) (Table 46-19) can be helpful in distinguishing vitamin K deficiency from factor deficiency. Des-γ-carboxy prothrombin (PIVKA II) is ordered for this indication. If gastrointestinal bleeding in an infant must be distinguished from swallowed maternal blood, a gastric aspirate, vomitus, or fecal material with gross blood present may be tested by the Apt test. Addition of 1% sodium hydroxide to a solution containing fetal hemoglobin retains the pink color of the mix. Adult hemoglobin turns yellowish brown if subjected to similar treatment.

Historically, bleeding time tests were used as a gross measurement of the interaction of platelets with the vascular endothelium and vWF in older children and adults. Bleeding time normal ranges for infants up to about 6 months of age are shorter than for adults. This has been attributed to the elevated levels of vWF, as well as the increase of the more functional high-molecular-weight multimers found in the newborn. The higher hematocrit and relative macrocytosis of the neonatal RBCs also may contribute. Bleeding time testing of the newborn is complicated by a lack of standardization and difficulties in reproducibility and has been largely replaced by platelet function screening tests such as the PFA-100 (Dade-Behring, Deerfield, IL), which measure platelet-vWF-fibrinogen interactions. Closure times in neonates tend to be shorter or within the lower limit of normal for older children and adults, presumably due to the presence of higher-molecular-weight multimers of vWF in neonates.

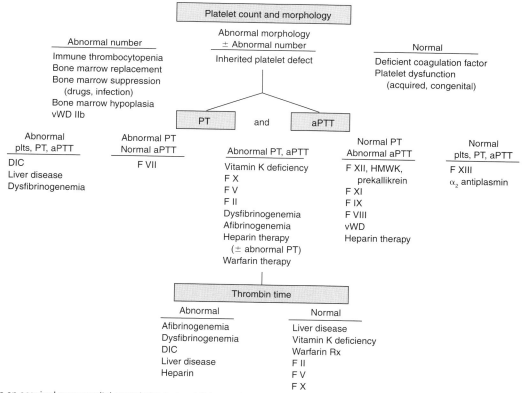

In an acquired or congenital coagulation factor deficiency state, a 50:50 mixture of patient plasma with pooled human plasma should yield normal results in a PT or aPTT assay. If these results are abnormal, investigation for a specific or nonspecific inhibitor of coagulation should be done.

Figure 46–14. Diagnostic algorithm for a bleeding neonate. aPTT, activated partial thromboplastin time; DIC, disseminated intravascular coagulation; F, factor; plts, platelets; HMWK, high-molecular-weight kallikrein; PT, prothrombin time; RX, treatment; vWD, von Willebrand disease.

TABLE 46–19   Laboratory Findings in Selected Coagulation Defects

Factor	Bleeding Time	PT	aPTT	Thrombin Time	Comments
I (Afibrinogenemia)	A	A	A	A	Low fibrinogen level
Dysfibrinogenemia	N	A	±A	A	Fibrinogen activity lower than antigen levels
Heparin therapy	±N	N	A	A	Check factor level; PT, aPTT normalize with 50:50 mix
VII	N	A	N	N	Check factor level; PT corrects with 50:50 mix
IX	N	N	A	N	Check factor level; aPTT corrects with 50:50 mix
X	N	A	A	N	Check factor level; aPTT corrects with 50:50 mix
XI	N	N	A	N	Check factor level; aPTT corrects with 50:50 mix
XII, prekallikrein, HMW kininogen	N	N	A	N	Check factor levels; deficiencies do not cause clinical bleeding
XIII	N	N	N	N	Check factor level; check clot solubility
vWD	±A	N	±A	N	Check vWF antigen, factor VIII activity, RIPA r (ristocetin-induced platelet aggregation), ristocetin cofactor, multimeric analysis
Inhibitor	N	±A	±A	N	Abnormality does not correct with 50:50 mix; check for lupus anticoagulant

A, abnormal; aPTT, activated partial thromboplastin time; HMW, high molecular weight; N, normal; PT, prothrombin time; vWD, von Willebrand disease; vWF, von Willebrand factor.

CONGENITAL DEFECTS IN HEMOSTASIS

Hemophilia A and B (factors VIII and IX deficiency, respectively) and von Willebrand Disease account for 95% to 98% of congenital bleeding disorders. Factors VIII and IX deficiencies are X-linked in inheritance, whereas von Willebrand disease can be inherited in an autosomal dominant or recessive fashion. The other congenital defects are recessively inherited coagulation disorders. All bleeding disorder patients should be managed with the help of hematologists expert in their care. In addition, genetic counseling about recurrence risks, family testing, and prenatal diagnosis is essential. Most defects with no detectable factor present are caused by deletions of a large portion of a gene (null mutation). Missense mutations can result in mild to severe disease. Rarely, combined deficiencies are due to defective genes coding for intracellular transport or involved in vitamin K metabolism or vitamin K-dependent post-translational modification. A North American Registry for rare congenital bleeding disorders tracks patients with deficiencies or defects in factors I, II, V, VII, X, and XIII.[1]

Hemophilias

A bleeding male infant, especially if otherwise clinically well, whose screening platelet count, PT, thrombin time, and fibrinogen concentration are within the normal range for age, is statistically most likely to have hemophilia. Because of the X-linked inheritance of both hemophilia A (factor VIII deficiency) and hemophilia B (factor IX deficiency), usually only males are affected, and more than half have a family history of the disorder. Factor VIII deficiency is five times as common as factor IX deficiency.[52]

Bleeding is less common in the newborn period than in later months, but for those who do bleed in the neonatal period, iatrogenic causes are most likely (circumcision, venipuncture, heel sticks). Less commonly, umbilical bleeding or intracranial hemorrhage may occur. Intracranial hemorrhage is often subdural rather than intraventricular. The incidence of intracranial hemorrhage in newborns with hemophilia has been estimated at about 3%. Hemorrhage into joints and deep muscle bleeding are the hallmarks of hemophilia. The clinical severity of the disease correlates with the patient's baseline factor level. Hemophilia is classified into three categories, based on the assumption that on average, a normal plasma factor activity level is 100%, and 1 mL of normal plasma has 1 unit of factor activity. Patients with severe, moderate, and mild disease have factor levels below 1%, between 1% and 5%, and above 5%, respectively. Patients with severe hemophilia bleed with little, or seemingly no, provocation (i.e., spontaneous hemorrhage). Both hemophilia A and hemophilia B are characterized by prolonged aPTT results with a normal PT test. Unfortunately, the physiologic prolongation of the neonatal aPTT makes diagnosis more difficult. Because factor VIII levels in the neonatal period approach adult levels, hemophilia A is reliably diagnosed, especially in those who are moderately or severely affected. An infant with evidence of factor VIII deficiency must at some point be evaluated for von Willebrand disease because this protein serves as the carrier for factor VIII, and an abnormality in the carrier protein can result in a low plasma factor VIII level. Because vWF levels are higher in the perinatal period, only severely affected patients (type 3 and some type 2 disease) might be expected to show bleeding problems. Factor IX levels are low at birth and do not reach adult values until 2 to 6 months postnatally. Severe factor IX deficiency can be diagnosed at birth, but mild and moderate hemophilia B often require subsequent confirmatory testing as the infant ages.

Therapeutic options include purified factor preparations and recombinant factors VIII or IX. Desmopressin (DDAVP) has been used for mild hemophilia A and for von Willebrand disease type 1 and some type 2 patients to increase release of factor VIII and vWF from endothelial stores. The antifibrinolytic agents ε-aminocaproic acid (Amicar) and tranexamic acid can be used in mucocutaneous bleeding to stabilize the fibrin clot and retard fibrinolysis. These agents are contraindicated in bladder or ureteral bleeding because of concerns about obstruction of urine flow by thrombi. Recombinant factor VIIa and prothrombin complex concentrates have been used in patients with coagulation factor inhibitors. Patients with hemophilia require specialty care by physicians expert in the disease management.

Von Willebrand Disease

Because vWF levels are higher at birth, and because there is an abundance of the most functional, highest-molecular-weight multimers during this period, the incidence of bleeding from von Willebrand disease in newborns is very low. Diagnosis usually requires repeat testing later in infancy. Because vWF serves as a carrier for factor VIII, those who are symptomatic in early infancy often have signs and symptoms associated with low factor VIII levels. The disorder can be classified into three types and many subtypes, and inheritance can be autosomal dominant or recessive. Type 1 disease is caused by a quantitative defect in vWF. vWF levels vary with blood type, with the lowest levels seen in patients with type O blood. Hematologists debate on whether type 1 should be called a disease because many affected patients and family members are not symptomatic. Those affected have mucosal type bleeding. Type 2 includes a large number of subtypes, all of which result from qualitative defects in vWF. These patients are more likely to have significant mucocutaneous bleeding symptoms. Patients with type 3 disease are either homozygotes or compound heterozygotes for qualitative and quantitative defects. These patients have a clinical presentation that is similar to hemophilia, including joint bleeding and intracranial hemorrhage. Laboratory tests include aPTT, platelet function screen, blood type, factor VIII coagulant activity, vWF antigen, vWF (ristocetin cofactor) activity, and multimeric analysis. Treatment is not needed for all patients. Mild cases (type 1 and some type 2 patients) can be managed with DDAVP and Amicar or tranexamic acid. Moderate or severe bleeding requires supplementation with one of the two currently available recombinant factor VIII concentrates that are copurified with vWF.

Factor XI Deficiency

Factor XI deficiency (hemophilia C) is inherited in an autosomal recessive manner and is not usually diagnosed in the neonatal period. It is most commonly reported in Ashkenazi Jews. Some patients may be diagnosed because an aPTT is prolonged. Unlike hemophilia A or hemophilia B, there is incomplete correlation between the degree of factor deficiency and hemorrhagic symptoms; some patients with very low levels have no bleeding history. Excessive bleeding typically occurs in the post-traumatic or postoperative setting. Certain anatomic locations, such as the genitourinary tract, are associated with an increased incidence of bleeding. These areas might have a high fibrinolytic rate that, according to the revised hypothesis of coagulation, would demand additional generation of factor Xa through the action of factor XIa.

Bleeding after circumcision has been reported. Because factor XI levels normally are low in the neonatal period, the diagnosis must be confirmed by repeat levels in the older infant. Treatment involves fresh-frozen plasma (FFP). Factor XI deficiency has been described as a common finding in Noonan syndrome.

Other Congenital Factor Deficiencies
FACTOR XIII DEFICIENCY
More than 80% of patients with homozygous factor XIII deficiency have delayed hemorrhage of the umbilical cord stump.[26] Up to one third of these infants have intracranial hemorrhage at some time. Later in life, patients experience delayed hemorrhages, wound dehiscence, hemarthroses, and repeated spontaneous abortions. Because of the autosomal recessive type of inheritance, the family history most commonly is unhelpful. Factor XIII activity is not measured by the PT, aPTT, or any other routine screening test. Laboratory testing is based on an abnormally low quantitative factor XIII level (more sensitive). The functional test looking at instability of a patient's blood clot in a 5M urea solution can be normal in some symptomatic patients.

FACTOR I DEFICIENCY AND DEFECTS
Deficiency of factor I (fibrinogen) can be characterized as afibrinogenemia, hypofibrinogenemia, or dysfibrinogenemia. Deficiencies and dysfunction can be associated with bleeding as well as thrombotic episodes. Both the aPTT and the PT will be prolonged. Replacement is generally achieved by using cryoprecipitate, although low levels of fibrinogen are present in FFP as well.

FACTOR II DEFICIENCY OR FACTOR X DEFICIENCY
Life-threatening bleeding may present early on and can include intracranial hemorrhage, hemarthroses, umbilical cord bleeding, and hematomas. The aPTT and PT will be prolonged. Replacement at low levels is done with FFP, but in general, higher levels are needed for management of bleeding. Prothrombin complex concentrates are used for higher replacement levels.

FACTOR V DEFICIENCY
Patients experience mucocutaneous bleeding and bleeding after trauma or surgery. The PT and aPTT are prolonged. Treatment is with FFP.

COMBINED DEFICIENCY OF FACTORS V AND VIII
Most commonly, a defect in the gene coding for a lectin mannose-binding protein (LMAN1) affects the intracellular transport of these factors to the surface of the platelet after activation. Another gene, MCFD2, which is a cofactor of LMAN1, is defective in a minority of patients. These patients have hemarthroses, mucocutaneous bleeding, and posttraumatic bleeding. The PT and aPTT are affected. Replacement with FFP is usual for bleeding patients. DDAVP can be used to raise the factor VIII level.[54]

FACTOR VII DEFICIENCY
As with factor XI deficiency, there is poor correlation between activity level and clinical course in patients with factor VII deficiency. Some infants present with intracranial hemorrhage,

whereas others with undetectable levels are asymptomatic. Mucocutaneous and deep tissue and joint bleeding can also be seen. Increased risk for thrombosis has been reported. The PT will be prolonged, whereas the aPTT should be normal for age. Treatment with a recombinant VIIa product is approved by the U.S. Food and Drug Administration for deficiency.

CONGENITAL MULTIPLE VITAMIN K-DEPENDENT FACTOR DEFICIENCY

This rare disorder is due to a defect in vitamin K epoxide reductase or in the γ-glutamyl carboxylase gene that adds glutamic acid as a post-translational modification to factors II, VII, IX, X, and proteins C and S. Umbilical cord bleeding, intracranial hemorrhage, mucocutaneous hemorrhage, and deep tissue bleeding can present early or later in life. Both the PT and aPTT will be prolonged.[10] Des-γ-carboxy prothrombin level will be normal, whereas prothrombin activity will be low. Treatment is with high-dose vitamin K and FFP.

ACQUIRED DEFECTS IN HEMOSTASIS

Hemorrhagic Disease of the Newborn

In 1894, Townsend described a series of 50 infants with self-limited bleeding that occurred mostly between the first and fifth day of life and that differed from classic hemophilia. Later investigators proposed decreased prothrombin levels as the cause of the bleeding tendency, and early feeding of infants with establishment of intestinal flora was shown to reduce the incidence of hemorrhage. Hemorrhagic disease of the newborn was formally defined and associated with a deficiency of vitamin K by the American Academy of Pediatrics Committee on Nutrition in 1961.

Vitamin K is a fat-soluble vitamin that is required for modifying coagulation proteins II (prothrombin), VII, IX, and X and anticoagulant proteins C and S. The post-translational γ-carboxylation of amino-terminal glutamic acid residues allows these factors to form complexes with other hemostatic proteins, through calcium, on a phospholipid surface. Localization of enzymes with their substrates and cofactors promotes very efficient reactions, and for the coagulation proteins, localization results in rapid, localized blood clot formation. Three forms of vitamin K have been identified: vitamin K_1 (phytonadione), which is present in green, leafy vegetables; vitamin K_2, which is synthesized by gastrointestinal flora; and vitamin K_3 (menadione), a synthetic, water-soluble form seldom used in neonates because of its association with hemolytic anemia. Placental transfer of the vitamin is poor, and vitamin K levels are low in newborn plasma and liver. Breast milk is a poor source of vitamin K relative to cow's milk or infant formulas supplemented with vitamin K. The gastrointestinal tract is sterile at birth, and its population with vitamin K-producing flora occurs after feedings are instituted. Because lactation requires several days to become established, infants who are exclusively breast-fed and those who are not fed orally are at risk for vitamin K deficiency. Broad-spectrum antibiotic therapy can be associated with vitamin K deficiency if the intestinal flora are eliminated. Because factors II, VII, IX, and X and proteins C and S are already low at birth, and deficiency of vitamin K results in production of dysfunctional coagulation proteins, infants with vitamin K deficiency are at

risk for serious bleeding problems. Although proteins C and S are involved with control of coagulation, the clinical presentation of vitamin K deficiency is that of bleeding and not thrombosis.

Hemolytic disease of the newborn can be temporally divided into three types. Early disease occurs in the first 24 hours of life and generally is seen in infants born to mothers taking oral anticoagulant or anticonvulsant drugs. These infants often have serious bleeding, including intracranial hemorrhage. Classic disease occurs from days 1 to 7 and usually is characterized by cutaneous, gastrointestinal, or circumcision bleeding in infants who did not receive vitamin K prophylaxis at birth. Late-onset disease occurs in infants beyond 1 week of age and sometimes is associated with exclusively breast-fed infants. It is more commonly associated with chronic diseases that impair absorption of the fat-soluble vitamins or that obliterate intestinal flora, such as α_1-antitrypsin deficiency, abetalipoproteinemia, biliary atresia, hepatitis, cystic fibrosis, celiac disease, chronic diarrhea, and antibiotic therapy. Affected infants may develop cutaneous, gastrointestinal, or intracranial hemorrhages (30% to 60%).

An infant with hemorrhagic tendencies and a prolonged PT, with normal fibrinogen level and platelet count, from a statistical consideration almost certainly has HDN. Administration of vitamin K should be followed by cessation of bleeding symptoms and improvement of the PT within 24 hours. Specific factor assays, assays for the decarboxylated forms of the vitamin K-dependent coagulation proteins produced in the absence of vitamin K (PIVKA) or the des-γ-carboxyl prothrombin (PIVKA II), and direct measurement of the vitamin K level are usually not necessary.

The American Academy of Pediatrics recommends that all newborns receive prophylaxis with vitamin K_1. This usually is given as 0.5 to 1 mg of intramuscular vitamin K_1, but if injections are contraindicated, 2 mg of oral vitamin K_1 may be substituted with the first feeding, and repeated at weeks 1, 4, and 8. There were initial concerns about absorption of the oral form of the vitamin and about ensuring that the entire dose delivered is received. Oral administration is equally effective in preventing classic disease, but intramuscular administration is more protective against late-onset disease.[4] Infants who are treated with total parenteral nutrition or prolonged antibiotic therapy and those with acute or chronic malabsorption should be treated with vitamin K routinely. Identification of early warning signs and prompt treatment of HDN will decrease the incidence of serious bleeding, particularly intracranial hemorrhage. Serious bleeding may be treated with 10 to 20 mL/kg of FFP. In the setting of life-threatening hemorrhage, a prothrombin complex concentrate, or recombinant factor VIIa may be used.

Hepatic Disease

Many coagulation factors are synthesized in the liver, including factor V and the vitamin K-dependent factors II, VII, IX, and X. Hepatic damage can result in lower levels of these proteins. Because of its physiologic level of about 60% in newborns and because of its short half-life, the factor VII level often is used as an indicator of hepatic dysfunction. Measurement of factor V, a non–vitamin K-dependent, hepatically synthesized clotting factor that has a short half-life and that is present in similar amounts in the newborn and adult, can distinguish vitamin K deficiency from hepatic dysfunction.

Because vitamin K is metabolized back to its active form by liver microsomes, liver disease also can herald the rise of incompletely γ-carboxylated glutamic acid residues of the vitamin K-dependent factors. Cholestasis can interfere with vitamin K absorption, resulting in lower levels of active vitamin K-dependent factors. Factor VIII levels are elevated in hepatitis, whereas in DIC, general consumption of factors would be expected. Factor VIII and vWF levels are usually elevated in chronic liver disease. Altered hepatic clearance of fibrin degradation products can cause an elevation of these in plasma. Hypofibrinogenemia can occur in chronic liver disease with cirrhosis, although the more common laboratory findings are normal fibrinogen concentration with abnormal sialic acid residues on the molecules and resultant dysfibrinogenemia. If ascites develops, a general coagulopathy due to loss of clotting factors occurs. Finally, hepatic dysfunction may be associated with development of DIC, making interpretation of laboratory test results difficult. Coagulopathy can be managed with vitamin K supplementation, FFP, and cryoprecipitate. There are reports of the use of recombinant factor VIIa in pediatric patients with hepatic dysfunction.

Disseminated Intravascular Coagulation

DIC occurs as a result of activation and dysregulation of the hemostatic system and is characterized by generation of activated platelets and coagulation proteases, fibrin clot formation, and accelerated fibrinolysis. Depending on the patient's compensatory capacity to inactivate and clear the products of hemostasis and fibrinolysis and to regenerate components of the hemostatic system, the patient could experience bleeding or thrombosis, or both, or might only show laboratory evidence of DIC.

DIC in the neonate is most commonly due to infection, hypoxia, or tissue damage and necrosis. Neonatal viral infections, including rubella virus, herpesvirus, cytomegalovirus, and enterovirus; toxoplasmosis; systemic candidiasis; and bacterial infections, especially with gram-negative organisms, are common causes. Vascular malformations may be associated with DIC. The Kasabach-Merritt syndrome of kaposiform hemangioendothelioma with thrombocytopenia and hypofibrinogenemia is associated with DIC and often includes a microangiopathic hemolytic anemia.[36] The lesion might not be obvious, and identification could require radiographic imaging of the most common locations (i.e., brain, liver, spleen, and gastrointestinal tract). The placenta might have chorioangiomatous malformations associated with development of DIC, which is terminated by delivery of the infant and clamping of the umbilical cord. Finally, massive hemolysis, such as is sometimes seen in Rh incompatibility, can trigger DIC.

Diagnosis of DIC depends on clinical findings and laboratory tests. Typical laboratory results include thrombocytopenia; microangiopathic hemolytic anemia; prolongation of the PT; low levels of factors I (fibrinogen), V, and VIII, as well as AT III, protein C, and heparin cofactor II; elevation of fibrin and fibrinogen split products; and general depletion of coagulation factors. The D-dimer test signals degradation of cross-linked fibrin. This test commonly is positive in premature infants without DIC. The diagnosis of DIC relies on clinical information supplemented by confirmatory laboratory testing.

The most important therapeutic intervention is to treat the underlying cause of the DIC. Infants with bleeding or thrombosis also should be treated to control their hemostatic problem. Infants without clinical evidence of DIC might not require therapy. Treatment options include FFP and cryoprecipitate for factor replacement, exchange transfusion to remove fibrin and fibrinogen split products, and platelet transfusion. Anticoagulant therapy is not generally used because the benefit has not proved to outweigh the added risk for hemorrhage. Many institutions use transfusions to maintain the platelet count above 50×10^9/L, the fibrinogen above 100 mg/dL, and the PT within the normal range for age.

Respiratory Distress Syndrome

Respiratory distress syndrome is associated with increased pulmonary surface tension due to surfactant deficiency (see Chapter 44). At autopsy, some preterm infants with respiratory distress syndrome have fibrin deposition not only in the lungs but also in the liver, kidneys, and other organs. Because of the abnormal systemic fibrin deposition, various coagulation and fibrinolytic parameters have been evaluated in these infants, and antithrombotic or thrombolytic therapies proposed without clear benefit.

Extracorporeal Membrane Oxygenation

See Chapter 44.

Extracorporeal membrane oxygenation (ECMO) has been used in the treatment of many life-threatening, potentially reversible disorders. Intracranial hemorrhage, other hemorrhagic complications, infection, and thrombosis are significant complications of ECMO. Severe thrombocytopenia and low birthweight are associated with increased risk of hemorrhage. Probable causes of intracranial hemorrhage include thrombocytopenia, alterations in vascular flow, and heparin therapy.

Systemic anticoagulation with heparin traditionally continues for the duration of ECMO support to minimize the potential for clotting within the circuit and subsequent embolization. Because heparin is associated with bleeding complications and because the patient response to dosage is variable, close monitoring is essential. Traditionally, heparin therapy in ECMO patients has been monitored by the ACT, a rapid, whole blood, point-of-care test that requires a small volume sample. Patients are usually maintained close to a target time of 200 seconds; adjustments to the heparin drip depend on the ACT results as well as clinical perceptions of excessive hemorrhagic or thrombotic events in the patient or artificial circuit. Testing is performed every 30 to 60 minutes. PT, fibrinogen, platelet count, and hemoglobin are also monitored. Patients receive FFP, cryoprecipitate, platelets, and packed RBC transfusions to keep these values within target ranges identified by institutional protocols.

Current areas of investigation include using the direct thrombin inhibitor bivalirudin in place of heparin because of the likelihood of less bleeding and thrombosis as well as more predictable pharmacokinetics. Performing brief periods of ECMO without systemic anticoagulation is also being tested.

Thrombotic Disorders

STROKE

Stroke is defined as an acute neurologic syndrome caused by injury of the cerebral vasculature. Perinatal stroke occurs in the time period between 20 weeks of gestation and 28 days of postnatal life. Strokes can be due to arterial occlusion (acute ischemic stroke or AIS), cerebral venous thrombosis (CVT), or intracerebral hemorrhage (ICH). Although rare throughout childhood, AIS is relatively common in the neonatal period. Infants present with seizures, sensorimotor deficits, irritability, lethargy, or jitteriness. AIS of the neonate is an important cause of chronic neurologic disability.[19]

The diagnosis of AIS could be delayed until later in infancy when focal neurologic deficits become apparent. Thromboembolism from the fetal-placental circulation is believed to be the most common etiology, followed by poor or absent arterial blood flow or venous outflow obstruction. Congenital heart disease, anatomic defects, infection, perinatal asphyxia, and, arguably, thrombophilia track with AIS. Diagnostic imaging with magnetic resonance imaging, particularly if augmented with magnetic resonance angiography, diffusion weighted images, or magnetic resonance venography, is more sensitive than computed tomography (CT) scan. Management of neonatal stroke is supportive with seizure control, correction of metabolic abnormalities, adequate oxygenation and ventilation, and antibiotic therapy if appropriate. Cardioembolic stroke is treated with anticoagulation unless the size of the stroke is large or there is a hemorrhagic component, so that the risk for bleeding precludes anticoagulation. Aspirin or anticoagulation may be indicated in patients at risk for recurrent stroke. In general, risk for recurrence of AIS is low and is most likely in patients with underlying anatomic abnormalities and thrombophilia. Long-term outcomes in neonates tend to be superior to those of older children and adults, presumably because of the adaptive capabilities of the immature brain. CVT and sinovenous thrombosis (SVT) may cause venous obstruction to blood flow and resultant hemorrhagic or AIS. Trauma to cerebral sinuses or impaired blood flow during delivery may result in SVT. It is associated with perinatal complications, dehydration, trauma, or anatomic abnormalities of the head and neck, ECMO, and possibly with thrombophilia. Nonhemorrhagic lesions are often treated with anticoagulation.[31,64,68]

NEONATAL THROMBOSIS

Thrombotic complications occur more often in neonates than in any other age group in pediatrics. There is an unusually high predilection for thrombosis of major vessels, especially the inferior vena cava, renal vein and artery, aorta, portal vein, femoral arteries, and cerebral arteries and veins. Most are associated with catheter placement. Renal vein thrombosis is the most common type of thrombosis not related to presence of an indwelling catheter. The predisposing factors for thrombosis include vascular injury, alteration in the dynamics of blood flow, activation of the vascular endothelium, and the physiologic alterations of neonatal hemostasis. In the neonatal period, vessel wall damage from the catheter or from substances infused through it can promote thrombus formation. Hyperviscosity and turbulent blood flow from congenital heart disease or catheter placement can also contribute. In contrast to adult patients, it is estimated that more than 95% of the children who present with venous thrombosis have a serious underlying disease or condition. The most frequently associated diagnoses are congenital heart disease, cancer, trauma, major surgery, and systemic lupus erythematosus.

Dehydration, polycythemia, hypoxia, impaired perfusion, maternal diabetes, intrauterine growth restriction, and congenital deficiency of anticoagulant proteins are associated with increased risk for clot formation.

Despite the common practice of infusing heparin-containing solutions into indwelling catheters, the incidence of line-associated clots is high. Presenting signs and symptoms include loss of catheter patency, thrombocytopenia, and swelling of the area of the body associated with the blood vessel. Chylothorax can be seen with severe superior vena cava thrombosis. Asymptomatic catheter-related thrombi might occur in 10% to 90% of patients, depending on the method used to diagnose the thrombi. The true incidence of catheter-related venous thrombosis is unknown because the published studies are small and generally use suboptimal imaging techniques. Clots in the upper venous system are notoriously difficult to image, yet increasing numbers of infants and children are using venous catheters in the upper system. Immediate sequelae of thrombi can include pain, renal hypertension, organ failure, intestinal necrosis, and gangrene. Portal vein thrombosis secondary to umbilical venous catheter placement, particularly in a site with low venous flow such as intrahepatic, can manifest with signs and symptoms of an acute abdomen. More commonly, portal vein thrombosis remains silent until symptoms of chronic obstruction (splenomegaly, gastrointestinal bleeding) occur. Any clot can break off, or embolize, to the lungs. Pulmonary embolism is associated with significant morbidity and mortality. Right atrial thrombi can be seen in association with central venous catheters. In addition to catheter dysfunction, presenting symptoms can include cardiac murmur, heart failure, or persistent bacteremia. Arterial thromboses are most often associated with arterial catheter placement. Impaired blood flow beyond the clot can present as pain, poor perfusion, or organ dysfunction.

Renal vein thrombosis (RVT) accounts for up to 10% of venous thrombosis in infants and newborns and occurs primarily at this age. The most common cause of non–catheter-associated thrombosis in this age group, it occurs in association with dehydration, acidosis, sepsis, hypoxia or asphyxia, polycythemia, and maternal diabetes. Presenting signs and symptoms include flank mass, hematuria, proteinuria, and thrombocytopenia. Unilateral and left-sided renal vein thrombosis are the most common. Findings on ultrasound include enlargement of the involved kidneys, thrombus, and altered intrarenal and renal vein blood flow. Hypertension and renal damage are the most common serious sequelae.

Infants with congenital heart disease are at increased risk for venous thrombosis, pulmonary embolus, right atrial thrombus, and stroke. Appropriate prophylactic anticoagulation and treatment of thromboembolic disease reduces morbidity and mortality.[58]

Congenital and Acquired Laboratory Risk Factors for Thrombosis

The episodic nature of thrombosis indicates that acquired or environmental risk factors combine with genetic defects. It is estimated that 70% of families with thrombophilia have at least one identifiable genetic risk factor, yet within these kindreds, there are asymptomatic members who carry the identical genetic defects (Table 46-20). Some single point mutations (e.g., factor V Leiden and prothrombin 20210A allele; see later) are common in the general population. Laboratory tests for risk factors for thrombosis can be divided into two categories: genetic factors and abnormal laboratory phenotypes. Genetic risk factors include all known mutations that, through a gain or loss of function, tip the balance toward thrombus formation. Such loss-of-function mutations include deficiencies of anticoagulants AT, protein C, and protein S. Proteins are either abnormal in function or are present at reduced levels. Gain-of-function mutations, such as factor V Leiden and the prothrombin 20210A allele, are common. Abnormal laboratory phenotypes that are associated with increased risk for thrombosis include activated protein C resistance, lupus anticoagulant, hyperhomocysteinemia, and elevated factor VIII levels. At present, all molecular risk factors for venous thromboembolism are found within the anticoagulant and procoagulant pathways. Within the fibrinolytic and antifibrinolytic pathways, both genetic defects (dysfibrinogenemia, hypoplasminogenemia, dysplasminogenemia) and abnormal phenotypes (high PAI-1 levels, low t-PA levels) have been reported. There is very limited information about most molecular risk factors and the incidence of thrombosis in the neonatal period.

The anticoagulant proteins, protein C, protein S, and AT, are all inherited in an autosomal dominant manner. The medical literature reports many studies associating heterozygous deficiency states with an increased incidence of thrombosis, although these events are rare in the neonatal period. It is not entirely clear whether heterozygous deficiency of one of the coagulation inhibitors is sufficient to increase the risk for thrombosis because not all who are heterozygous for deficiency of one of these anticoagulant proteins have excessive thrombosis (see Table 46-20). Heterozygotes are not treated unless they have had an episode of thrombosis. Older children and adults who are considered to be in a period of high risk for thrombosis, such as during and immediately after surgery or childbirth, may receive prophylactic anticoagulation.

Homozygous protein C or protein S deficiency causes serious thrombotic events in the postnatal period. In the first few hours or days of life, affected patients manifest purpura fulminans, severe DIC, and life-threatening thromboses. Diagnosis is aided by laboratory tests, which yield results consistent with DIC and show no measurable protein by functional or immunologic assay. If instituted early in the course of the purpura fulminans, treatment can dramatically alter the clinical outcome. Initial therapy for protein C or S deficiency usually involves FFP. A protein C concentrate is available on a compassionate-use basis in the United States. Primary therapy should not be discontinued until the patient is placed on lifelong warfarin and has a therapeutic international normalized ratio of 3.0 to 4.0. Liver transplantation has also been attempted.

FACTOR V LEIDEN

Families with venous thromboembolism whose plasma was poorly responsive to the addition of activated protein C in an aPTT assay have been described. Eventually, the defect was traced to mutations in coagulation factor V that render it resistant to cleavage by activated protein C, and resistance to activated protein C is now the most common laboratory abnormality identified in patients with excessive venous thrombosis. These defects are inherited in an autosomal dominant fashion, and the homozygous state has been identified with an even higher thrombosis risk. Interactions with protein C, protein S, and prothrombin 20210A alleles causing enhanced risk for thrombosis have been reported.

PROTHROMBIN 20210A ALLELE

A mutation in the 3'-untranslated region of the prothrombin gene at nucleotide 20210 is associated with elevated prothrombin levels. Prothrombin levels greater than 115% of normal values are linked to a 2.1-fold increased risk for thrombosis. The molecular basis of the enhanced risk is not known.[67] Heterozygous carriers have a 2.8-fold increased risk for venous clot. The mutation interacts with factor V Leiden and protein S deficiency.

ELEVATED FACTOR VIII LEVELS

In the Leiden thrombophilia study, blood group (non-O), elevated vWF (>150%), and high factor VIII levels (>150%) were all associated with increased incidence of venous thrombosis.

TABLE 46–20   Molecular Defects and Risk for Venous Thrombosis in Adults

Deficient Protein	Increased Risk for Thrombosis	Incidence in Healthy Individuals (%)	Incidence in DVT Patients (%)	Incidence in Families with Thrombophilia (%)
AT III heterozygous	5×	0.05-1	1	4
Protein C heterozygous	7×	0.3	3	6
Protein S heterozygous	6-10×	?	1-2	6
Factor V Leiden heterozygous	7×	2-16	18	40
Factor V Leiden homozygous	80×	—	—	—

AT III, antithrombin III; DVT, deep vein thrombosis.
From Bertina RM: Molecular risk factors for thrombosis, *Thromb Haemost* 82:601, 1999.

Factor VIII levels higher than 150% stood out as an independent risk factor.[45]

DYSFIBRINOGENEMIA

The dysfibrinogenemias can manifest with bleeding or venous or arterial thrombosis, or they can be clinically silent. This diverse and rare group of defects is inherited in an autosomal dominant manner. Laboratory testing includes functional and antigenic assays of fibrinogen, which should show higher antigenic than functional results. The PT and aPTT also are usually prolonged. Thrombin time is abnormally prolonged.

INHERITED ABNORMALITIES OF FIBRINOLYSIS

Cases of dysplasminogenemia and hypoplasminogenemia associated with excessive thrombosis have been reported rarely, although the same defects have been identified in other family members who did not experience thrombosis. Differences between immunochemical and functional levels of plasminogen, and its activators and inhibitors have been used to diagnose these rare abnormalities.

TREATMENT OF THROMBOSIS

Treatment of thromboses is controversial because of the absence of randomized, controlled clinical trials in the neonatal population. Therapeutic options include supportive care, nonspecific measures (e.g., warming the involved or contralateral limb), anticoagulants, fibrinolytic agents, and (rarely) surgical removal. Most infants with a catheter-related thrombus are clinically asymptomatic. In these cases, the thromboses are underdiagnosed, and those patients who are diagnosed are treated supportively, with good response. Line removal is recommended in all catheter-related clots if possible. Patients who develop limb or organ compromise secondary to thrombosis must be treated more aggressively.

Numerous attempts have been made to develop pharmacologic agents that successfully restore physiologic balance to the coagulation system and prevent excessive thrombosis. The goal of anticoagulation is to prevent clot extension while augmenting the naturally occurring anticoagulation processes, and without causing bleeding. Unfractionated heparin and low-molecular-weight heparin (LMWH) are the most commonly used anticoagulants in infants. Long-term oral anticoagulation with warfarin is rare in neonates and usually is used for patients with recurrent thrombosis, mechanical heart valves, or thrombosis with a significant, ongoing, predisposing factor (homozygous protein C, protein S, or AT deficiency). Baseline laboratory testing in thrombosis includes platelet count, Hb, aPTT, PT, and fibrinogen. The impact of D-dimers and factor VIII activity are unclear. Thrombophilia testing is also controversial but commonly includes risk factors discussed previously such as protein C, protein S, AT, factor V Leiden, and prothrombin gene mutation. General guidelines for management are to maintain platelet count above 50,000 and fibrinogen level above 1 g/L and to correct any severe bleeding tendencies. Baseline assessment should be done for intracranial hemorrhage with CT scan or, if not practical, at least ultrasound. In adults, there are relative contraindications for initiation of anticoagulation, which include recent surgery or active bleeding. In the absence of validated criteria for the newborn, the risks and benefits of treatment compared with supportive care are carefully weighed. Consultation with an experienced pediatric hematologist is recommended. Monagle and colleagues have authored the eighth edition of evidence-based guidelines for the management of neonatal and pediatric thrombosis. Recommendations for management of specific types of thromboses are given.[58]

Unfractionated Heparin

Unfractionated heparin is an indirect thrombin inhibitor that binds antithrombin through a unique pentasaccharide to enhance inhibition of thrombin and factor Xa primarily, as well as factors XIa and IXa. A ternary complex of unfractionated heparin with AT and thrombin facilitates thrombin inhibition and requires both the pentasaccharide and a critical length of the unfractionated heparin, which is not present in LMWH. Unfractionated heparin is inexpensive, widely available, and rapidly reversible. Unfortunately, it must be given as a continuous infusion. Unpredictable pharmacokinetics require frequent monitoring of aPTT or heparin levels. Heparin therapy in the neonate cannot be directly based on the adult experience. Heparin clearance in the newborn is accelerated because of the larger volume of distribution and enhanced hepatic metabolism. Lower AT levels may affect the response to heparin both in terms of aPTT prolongation and by suboptimal clinical response. AT supplementation with FFP is sometimes suggested. Adverse effects include bleeding, unintended heparin overdose, heparin-induced thrombocytopenia, and osteoporosis. If bleeding occurs, heparin should be stopped. Protamine sulfate will inactivate unfractionated heparin at a ratio of 1 mg per 100 units. The dose will depend on the amount of unfractionated heparin given as well as the half-life of heparin, which is estimated at 1 hour in the neonate. Box 46-8 provides suggested guidelines for initiation of heparin therapy.

Laboratory testing is most useful in ensuring that a newborn is not overly anticoagulated and placed at excessive risk for hemorrhage. Because of the lower AT levels, newborn plasma tested by the aPTT overestimates the amount of unfractionated heparin in the plasma, whereas plasma tested in assays based on AT inhibition of exogenous thrombin or factor Xa yields results that underestimate the amount of unfractionated heparin in the plasma. The whole blood clotting time or activated clotting time (ACT) is sometimes used to monitor heparin therapy because the results can be obtained quickly. The test evaluates the ability of whole blood to clot, and the result can be prolonged by any abnormality in the cellular or fluid phase of the hemostatic system.

Low-Molecular-Weight Heparin

Because of the difficulties in obtaining venous access for continuous infusion of unfractionated heparin and the need for frequent laboratory monitoring associated with unfractionated heparin therapy, LMWHs are widely used for treatment or prophylaxis of thrombosis in adults. Less is known about their use in children and infants, but they are often used. LMWHs contain the critical pentasaccharide to inhibit factor Xa through AT, but they cannot form the ternary complex with AT and thrombin. LMWH therapy results in selective inhibition of factor Xa and theoretically puts the patient less at risk for hemorrhage. LMWHs do not prolong the aPTT. The longer half-life allows for daily or twice-daily

BOX 46–8   **Recommendations for Unfractionated Heparin Therapy in Neonates**

Pretreatment laboratory testing: CBC with platelets, aPTT, PT, serum creatinine, ALT
Loading dose: 75 U/kg IV over 10 minutes
Maintenance dose: 28 U/kg/hr continuous infusion
Laboratory monitoring:
   aPTT 4 hr after heparin loading dose given (use table to adjust dosing), then daily, *or*
   Daily anti-Xa level, unfractionated heparin— target range 0.35-0.6 anti-Xa units, *or*
   Daily anti-factor IIa level—target range 0.2-0.4 U/mL
   Daily CBC with platelets

Unfractionated Heparin Dosing Adjustments Based on aPTT Results

aPTT (sec)	Bolus (U/kg)	Hold Infusion (min)	Percent Change In Infusion Rate	Repeat aPTT (hr)
<50	50	0	↑20	4
50-59	0	0	↑10	4
60-85	0	0	0	24
86-95	0	0	↓10	4
96-120	0	30	↓10	4
>120	0	60	↓15	4

Duration of therapy (see text):
   10-14 days, *or*
   5-7 days; add warfarin or LMWH day 1 or 2 (extensive clot or PE: start warfarin on day 5 and treat with heparin for 14 days)
Precautions:
   If platelet count drops <150,000/μL, consider heparin-induced thrombocytopenia
   Avoid IM injections and arterial punctures

Unfractionated Heparin Antidote: Protamine Sulfate 10 mg/ml at a Rate not to Exceed 5 mg/min, Maximum Dose 50 mg

Time Elapsed since Last Heparin Dose (min)	Protamine Sulfate Dose (mg/100 U Heparin Received)— Maximum 50 Mg	aPTT after Protamine (min)
<30	1	15
30-60	0.5-0.75	15
61-120	0.375-0.5	15
>120	0.25-0.375	15

ALT, alanine aminotransferase; aPTT, activated partial thromboplastin time; CBC, complete blood count; IM, intramuscular; IV, intravenous; LMWH, low-molecular-weight heparin; PE, pulmonary embolus; PT, prothrombin time.
Adapted from the Protocol for Heparin Therapy, Hospital for Sick Children, Toronto, Canada, 1995.

BOX 46–9   **Recommendations for Low-Molecular-Weight Heparin Therapy in Neonates**

Pretreatment laboratory testing
   CBC with platelets, aPTT, PT with international normalized ratio
   ALT, AST, bilirubin total and direct, serum creatinine
Recommended therapeutic target range: 0.5-1.0 antifactor Xa U/mL
Therapeutic dosing
   Enoxaparin
      <2 mo of age: 1.5 mg/kg SC q 12 hr
      >2 mo of age: 1.0 mg/kg SC q 12 hr
   Reviparin
      <2 mo of age: 150 U/kg SC q 12 hr
      >2 mo of age: 100 U/kg SC q 12 hr

Anti-Xa U/mL	Percent of Prior Dose	Repeat Anti-Xa
<0.35	125	4 hr after next dose
0.35-0.49	110	4 hr after next dose
0.5-1.0	Same dose (100)	Next day
1.1-1.5	80	4 hr after dose
1.6-2.0	70	4 hr after dose
>2.0	Hold until anti-Xa <0.5 U/mL, then 40	4 hr after dose

Laboratory monitoring
   Draw anti-Xa level 4 hr after dose given
   When anti-Xa level is 0.5-1.0 U/mL, repeat next day, then 1 week later and monthly after

ALT, alanine aminotransferase; aPTT, activated partial thromboplastin time; AST, aspartate aminotransferase; CBC, complete blood count; SC, subcutaneous.
Adapted from Lilleyman J, et al, editors: *Thromboembolic complications in pediatric hematology,* 2nd ed, New York, 1999m Churchill Livingstone.

Clinical studies in adults have shown that LMWH is as effective as crude heparin in preventing thrombosis but is associated with equal or fewer bleeding complications. Although the studies in pediatric patients are small, safety and efficacy have been reported for enoxaparin and dalteparin.[50,57] Pediatric dosing is age dependent and weight dependent (Box 46-9). Infants younger than 2 months require higher doses than older children to maintain therapeutic anti-Xa levels of 0.5 to 1.0 international units/mL. If bleeding occurs, the LMWH should be stopped. Protamine sulfate, given within 4 hours of LMWH dose at a ratio of 1 mg per 100 units of LMWH, will partially reverse the LMWH effect.

Oral Anticoagulation with Warfarin (Coumadin)

Oral therapy with warfarin (Coumadin) in neonates is often complicated by hepatic dysfunction, drug interactions, diet fluctuations, vitamin K supplementation in infant formulas, and poor venous access for laboratory monitoring. It is difficult to achieve and sustain therapeutic levels of drug. Efficacy and safety are related to time in the therapeutic range. Warfarin therapy should be supervised by an experienced pediatric hematologist or cardiologist. The action of warfarin is based

dosing subcutaneously in adults. More predictable pharmacokinetics allow less laboratory monitoring using the anti-Xa assay. This assay is less widely and rapidly available than the aPTT used to monitor unfractionated heparin therapy. Heparin-induced thrombocytopenia and osteoporosis risks are less.

on interruption of the vitamin K–dependent γ-carboxylation of factors II, VII, IX, and X and proteins C and S. The PT or international normalized ratio is used to monitor adequacy of anticoagulation (Box 46-10).

New Anticoagulation Agents in Infants

There is limited information on the use of the indirect thrombin inhibitor fondaparinux in children. This synthetic pentasaccharide is given subcutaneously and has been used in the treatment of patients with heparin-induced thrombocytopenia.[55] The direct thrombin inhibitor bivalirudin is of interest because its efficacy does not depend on AT levels in plasma and because this small molecule can become incorporated into the fibrin clot to inhibit both bound and circulating thrombin. Early reports of rapid clot resolution with less bleeding are intriguing and may suggest an alternative to fibrinolytic therapy or for anticoagulation in heparin-induced thrombocytopenia. The drug is administered by continuous infusion and is monitored by the aPTT.[81] Bivalirudin has also been used in patients with heparin-induced thrombocytopenia as an alternative anticoagulant.

Fibrinolytic Therapy

The goal of thrombolytic therapy is to degrade fibrin and dissolve the fibrin clot. Recombinant t-PA is the most commonly used agent (Box 46-11). It facilitates conversion of plasminogen to plasmin, enhancing degradation of fibrin, fibrinogen, and coagulation factors V and VIII. Bleeding complications have been a major concern in thrombolytic therapy in neonates, in addition to embolization or rethrombosis. Attention in older patients has focused on localizing therapy so that plasminogen associated with the thrombus is preferentially activated and systemic bleeding complications are minimized, but directed fibrinolysis is generally impractical in the small blood vessels of the neonate. In vitro and in vivo studies of thrombolytic therapies in the newborn have demonstrated different responses compared with adults, probably because of the physiologic differences in the fibrinolytic system. The neonate is resistant to t-PA and may require higher doses than those used in adults. Supplementation with heparin and FFP is sometimes appropriate. Consultation with an experienced pediatric hematologist is strongly encouraged for treatment and monitoring recommendations.

BOX 46-10 Recommendations for Warfarin Therapy in Neonates

Pretreatment laboratory testing
   CBC with platelets, aPTT, PT with international normalized ratio (INR)
   ALT, AST, bilirubin total and direct
Recommended target ranges for INR
   2.0-3.0, usual range
   2.5-3.5, mechanical heart valves
Loading period
   Lasts 3-5 days, or until a stable, therapeutic drug level is achieved
   Begins 1-2 days after initiation of heparin therapy (for extensive DVT or pulmonary embolus, begin at day 5 of heparin therapy)
   Dose on day 1: 0.2 mg/kg PO single daily dose, maximum 10 mg
   Fontan procedure patients: 0.1 mg/kg, maximum 5 mg
   Reduce loading dose if hepatic or renal dysfunction present or baseline INR >1.2
   Monitor closely if potential for drug interactions exists
   Consider amount of vitamin K in diet and supplements

Warfarin Dose Adjustments During Loading Period*

INR	Percent of Loading Dose to Be Given
1.1-1.3	100
1.4-3.0	50
3.1-4.0	25
>4.0	Hold until INR <4.5, then restart at 50

*Daily PO dose based on INR results.
Discontinue heparin 5 days after initiation of warfarin and when INR >2.0 daily × 2.

Warfarin Dose Adjustments During Maintenance Period*

INR	Percent of Previous Dose to Be Given
1.1-1.4	120
1.5-1.9	110
2.0-3.0	100
3.1-4.0	90
4.1-4.5	80
>4.5	Hold until INR <4.5, then restart at 80

*Daily PO dose based on INR results.
Discontinue heparin 5 days after initiation of warfarin and when INR >2.0 daily × 2.

Laboratory monitoring
   Daily INR until therapeutic level reached on 2 consecutive days
   INR weekly if stable; may require more frequent testing
Warfarin antidote
   No bleeding: vitamin K_1
      Rapid reversal and anticipate warfarin treatment in future: 0.5-1 mg SC
      Rapid reversal and no future need for warfarin: 2 mg SC
   Clinically significant bleeding: 2-5 mg vitamin K_1 IV over 10-20 min and fresh-frozen plasma (20 U/kg) or factor IX concentrate containing other vitamin K–dependent factors (50 U/kg).

DVT, deep vein thrombosis; IV, intravenous; SC, subcutaneous.
Adapted from the Protocol for Coumadin Therapy, Hospital for Sick Children, Toronto, Canada, 1995.

BOX 46–11 | Institutional Protocol* for t-PA Use in Blocked Catheters

Instill t-PA (2 mg/mL) into catheter; volume of t-PA should be based on catheter type.
 Infant Broviac: 0.5 mL
 Single-lumen Broviac: 1 mL
 Double-lumen Broviac: 1.5 mL each lumen
 Port-a-Cath: 2 mL
Allow the drug to dwell for 2 hours. At the end of 2 hours, the drug should be withdrawn.
This process may be repeated one additional time if needed.

*Protocol for St. Louis Children's Hospital, 2007.
t-PA, tissue plasminogen activator.

In the face of life- or limb-threatening thrombosis, thrombolytic therapy is considered. Dose, duration of thrombolysis, and concurrent or subsequent use of heparin are controversial (Table 46-21).[58]

Regulation of Platelet Production

Megakaryocytopoiesis is regulated in vivo mainly by thrombopoietin (TPO). In adults, the liver and, to a lesser extent, the kidney and bone marrow have been identified as sites of TPO production. Preterm infants have lower TPO levels than term infants, and TPO levels in infants are lower than those of adults, regardless of platelet count. Fetal and neonatal cells demonstrate a dose-response effect when exposed to TPO. The thrombocytopenia present in some neonates may be due to ineffective TPO production. In adults and children, serum TPO concentrations are inversely related to the mass of megakaryocytes and circulating platelets. The regulation of TPO levels appears to be mediated by the MPL receptor found on platelets and megakaryocytes, and on other hematopoietic progenitors in lesser concentrations. These cells bind, internalize, and degrade the constitutively produced growth factor. The therapeutic role of recombinant TPO in the neonatal period is not established.

The normal circulating platelet count for all ages ranges from 150,000 to 400,000/μL. Average platelet counts are slightly lower in preterm infants and increase with gestational age. Two thirds of total body platelets circulate; the other third are located within the spleen. The average platelet life span is 7 to 10 days, although survival of transfused platelets in a thrombocytopenic recipient is reduced proportionately to the severity of the thrombocytopenia.

Most patients with thrombocytopenia are asymptomatic. When it does occur, bleeding is usually mucocutaneous. Severe thrombocytopenia can manifest with petechiae. Larger purpuric lesions, ecchymoses, may appear at sites of injury. Epistaxis, hematuria, and prolonged bleeding at incision or venipuncture sites can occur.

Treatment decisions are difficult, because of the lack of direct correlation between platelet count and bleeding risk. The risk for hemorrhage is affected by other factors such as coexisting coagulation defects, trauma, surgery, and poorly understood patient characteristics. In older children and adults, serious spontaneous bleeding does not occur until the platelet count is less than 20,000/μL. Many physicians use 10,000 to 20,000/μL as the threshold for intervention. This is based on data from a study of children with leukemia in whom the risk for serious bleeding increased below this range. Because of the increased risk for intracranial hemorrhage in neonates, a threshold of 20,000 to 50,000/μL is often used for the first 96 hours of life, when the risk is highest (see Part 2 of this chapter). Consideration is given to the etiology of the thrombocytopenia. Patients with a production defect are more likely to have serious bleeding than those with a destructive platelet problem, because in the latter cases, the platelets tend to be larger and more functional. If bone marrow transplantation or frequent transfusions are anticipated, the transfusion threshold is generally lowered in an attempt to minimize the risk for alloimmunization or graft failure.

Platelet Function

Platelets adhere to subendothelial components at the site of endothelial injury through glycoprotein receptors GP Ib/IX/V, Ia/IIa, and IIb/IIIa. Receptor-ligand binding results in platelet activation with shape changes and degranulation from α-granules (vWF, platelet factor 4, thrombospondin, fibrinogen, fibronectin, factors V and VIII, platelet-derived growth factor) and dense granules (adenosine diphosphate, adenosine triphosphate, calcium, serotonin, epinephrine). Platelet aggregation is mediated through GP IIb/IIIa and fibrinogen to link platelets together. Platelets also host the formation of a fibrin clot on their phospholipid membrane surface in the presence of calcium and coagulation factors.

Quantitative defects of platelets, or thrombocytopenia, result in excessive bleeding and bruising when platelet counts drop below 100,000/μL. Spontaneous, serious hemorrhage from isolated thrombocytopenia is unusual when platelet counts are more than 20,000/μL. Thrombocytopenia can be accompanied by qualitative platelet disorders. Qualitative disorders in older children and adults are most commonly acquired and associated with drugs or uremia, but in the otherwise healthy newborn with mucocutaneous bleeding, consideration must be given to congenital defects in platelet function. Some of the defects are associated with decreased production or increased platelet clearance. A few are characterized by changes in platelet size or by associated defects in white blood cells. Congenital qualitative defects include abnormalities in glycoprotein receptors and defective or deficient granules or secretion of the granules.

Platelet counts are determined most commonly in an automated cell counter in the laboratory. Abnormally sized platelets require manual counting. Review of the peripheral blood smear for platelet morphology, color (rule out gray platelet syndrome), white blood cell inclusions, and evidence of schistocytes (DIC) is helpful. A common platelet function screening instrument, the PFA-100, can test the interaction of platelets with fibrinogen and vWF, assuming the platelet count is at least 100,000/μL. The gold standard test for platelet function, platelet aggregometry, is rarely done in the newborn period because it requires a large volume of blood. Testing for platelet glycoprotein receptor

TABLE 46–21	**Thrombolytic Therapy**					
Anticoagulation	Loading Dose	Continuous Infusion	Pretreatment Duration	Monitoring Tests	Reversal Tests	Agents
Urokinase	4400 U/kg	4400 U/kg/h	Up to 48 h or until clot lysis	CBC, plts, PT, PTT, fibrinogen, FDP, cranial ultrasound	Fibrinogen, FDP, clot imaging*†	Fresh-frozen plasma, cryoprecipitate
Recombinant t-PA	0.5 mg/kg	0.04-0.5 mg/kg/h	48-72 h or until clot lysis	CBC, plts, PT, PTT, fibrinogen, FDP, cranial ultrasound	Fibrinogen, FDP, clot imaging‡	Fresh-frozen plasma, cryoprecipitate
			If no response, consider concurrent plasminogen therapy			

*Schmidt B, Andrew M: Report of Scientific and Standardization Subcommittee on Neonatal Hemostasis Diagnosis and Treatment of Neonatal Thrombosis, *Thromb Haemost* 67:381, 1992.
†Local treatment: Corrigan JJ: Neonatal thrombosis and the thrombolytic system: pathophysiology and therapy, *Am J Pediatr Hematol Oncol* 10:83, 1988.
‡Dillon PW, et al: Recombinant tissue plasminogen activator for neonatal and pediatric vascular thrombolytic therapy, *J Pediatr Surg* 28:1264, 1993.
CBC, complete blood count; FDP, fibrin degradation product; plts, platelets; PT, prothrombin time; PTT, partial thromboplastin time; t-PA, tissue plasminogen activator.

components and markers of activation by flow cytometry is available in specialized laboratories. Unfortunately, specialized platelet studies must be performed rapidly on fresh platelets and so generally require travel by the patient to the reference laboratory.

Thrombocytopenia

Etiologies for thrombocytopenia can be divided into decreased production or increased destruction. Often, both are present in the neonate. Infection, liver disease, and drug effects can be associated with decreased production and increased destruction of platelets. Congenital cytomegalovirus and rubella often are complicated by thrombocytopenia secondary to both underproduction and increased destruction. HIV infection also can be associated with thrombocytopenia (see Chapter 39). Certain trisomies are also associated with thrombocytopenia, including trisomy 13 and trisomy 18. DIC, necrotizing enterocolitis, hypoxia, immune destruction, maternal history of preeclampsia, and thrombosis are examples where increased consumption of platelets can reduce counts. Cardiopulmonary bypass and ECMO are associated with activation of platelets and the coagulation system as well as hemodilution. In hypersplenism, a larger proportion of platelets remain in the spleen, so peripheral counts can be lower. Heparin-induced thrombocytopenia, triggered by immune response to anticoagulation, is a rare cause of thrombocytopenia in the neonate. Renal failure is associated with qualitative defects in platelet function and variable thrombocytopenia. Congenital qualitative and quantitative defects are rare causes of decreased platelet production. Infiltration of the bone marrow by malignant cells (leukemia, neuroblastoma) or by histiocytes in hemophagocytic lymphohistiocytosis (see "Hemophagocytic Lymphohistiocytosis Syndrome," later) is rare in the neonatal period.

Thrombocytopenia is rare in the healthy term infant (<1%) but commonly seen in the neonatal intensive care unit. One study estimated that 22% of the neonatal intensive care unit patients had low platelets.[18] Prematurity is one factor. In a retrospective study of 284 infants with extremely low birthweight, thrombocytopenia was reported in 73% of infants with birthweight of less than 1000 g. In infants weighing less than 800 g at birth, low platelets were seen in 85%. Counts were less than 50,000/μL and less than 100,000/μL for 28% and 56%, respectively.[20]

THROMBOCYTOPENIA RESULTING FROM INCREASED PLATELET DESTRUCTION

Neonatal Alloimmune Thrombocytopenia
See Chapter 18.

Neonatal alloimmune thrombocytopenia (NAIT) results from placental transfer of maternal alloantibodies directed against paternally inherited antigens that are present on the fetal platelets but absent from maternal platelets. In general, these are IgG antibodies, which recognize protein antigens rather than oligosaccharide determinants. This condition is analogous to Rh hemolytic disease of the newborn, but in contrast, NAIT can develop in the first pregnancy. The platelet antigens form early in gestation, and maternal antibody crosses the placenta and into the fetal circulation as early as midtrimester. Severe thrombocytopenia can result, with intracranial hemorrhage estimated to occur in 10% to 20% of affected infants. Many of the intracranial hemorrhages (25% to 50%) occur in utero.[12]

In white populations, the most frequently implicated alloantigen in NAIT is HPA-1a, which accounts for 78% of serologically confirmed cases. Incompatibility for the HPA-5b alloantigen is the next most common cause, followed by HPA-15b. About 98% of whites express the HPA-1a antigen on their platelets; most of the remaining 2% are homozygous for an alternative allele that encodes the HPA-1b antigen. The incidence of NAIT is about 1 in 2000 births, which is much lower than the predicted incidence based on the distribution of the HPA-1a and HPA-1b alleles in the population. Other immune response genes appear to regulate HPA-1a alloantibody formation. Women with the HLA-DR3 antigen have about a 20-fold relative risk for forming HPA-1a alloantibodies. In the Asian population, incompatibility of the HPA-4 (Pem) system is the most common cause of NAIT (80%), followed by HPA-3.[77]

NAIT should be suspected in an otherwise healthy infant with isolated thrombocytopenia at the time of birth. The degree of thrombocytopenia can be severe, with platelet counts often lower than $10,000/\mu L$ in the first day of life. The maternal platelet count is normal, an important laboratory value for distinguishing this condition from neonatal thrombocytopenia secondary to maternal idiopathic thrombocytopenic purpura (ITP) (discussed later). Mucocutaneous bleeding is common in patients with NAIT. These patients are at increased risk for intracranial hemorrhage, both prenatally and postnatally. The pronounced bleeding diathesis associated with anti-HPA-1a NAIT probably reflects the combination of severe thrombocytopenia and antibody-mediated interference with the function of the GP IIb-IIIa complex on the few remaining platelets.

The diagnosis of NAIT is confirmed by serologic testing of maternal serum for antiplatelet antibodies and immunophenotyping of maternal and paternal platelets. Genotyping of maternal and paternal blood to establish platelet antigen genotypes is preferable when available. Because delays may be associated with serologic and platelet antigen testing, therapy should be initiated as soon as the diagnosis is suspected. The treatment of choice for severe isoimmune thrombocytopenia is transfusion of washed irradiated maternal platelets. Term infants tend to receive platelet transfusion for bleeding and less than $30,000/\mu L$, whereas preterm infants and ill infants may have a transfusion threshold of less than $50,000/\mu L$. Suspected infants should have a head CT scan if possible, or alternatively, a cranial ultrasound to look for intracranial hemorrhage. Because the risk for intracranial hemorrhage drops after 3 to 4 days, the otherwise healthy term infant can be managed with lower platelet counts. When maternal platelets are not available, irradiated, randomdonor platelet infusions can be used; however, a modest and short-lived increase in the platelet count might be observed. Intravenous γ-globulin (1 g/kg daily for 2 days) or corticosteroids (methylprednisolone, 2 mg/kg per day), or both, also can be used as temporary measures. Platelets produced by neonates with NAIT often exhibit accelerated clearance until antiplatelet antibody is removed from the circulation. Consequently, it is not unusual for additional transfusions of maternal platelets to be required after the first few weeks of life.

The likelihood is high that subsequent infants born to these mothers will be affected. Because the severity of intracranial hemorrhage tends to increase in later pregnancies, detailed counseling about the risk for recurrence should be provided to the family at the time that the first infant's thrombocytopenia is diagnosed. Although the thrombocytopenia may have resolved before completion of the full diagnostic laboratory evaluation, it is important that the diagnosis and presumed antigen incompatibility be confirmed by formal serologic and genotypic testing in order to guide the management of future pregnancies. Antibody titers begin to decline after delivery, so the evaluation should be initiated in the postpartum period. Because the likelihood of thrombocytopenia in subsequent infants depends on whether the father is HPA-1a homozygous or HPA-1a or HPA-1b heterozygous, it is desirable to perform DNA-based genotyping.

Neonatal Thrombocytopenia Resulting from Maternal Immune Thrombocytopenia

Neonatal thrombocytopenia can occur in infants of mothers with ITP, lupus erythematosus, or other autoimmune disorders (see Chapter 18).[79] This diagnosis should be considered when both the neonate and the mother have evidence of thrombocytopenia. The diagnosis should be suspected in infants of mothers with a previous history of ITP because neonatal thrombocytopenia has been observed in infants of mothers rendered asymptomatic of chronic ITP by splenectomy. Maternal ITP must be distinguished from the mild decrease in platelets that often accompanies pregnancy at term, presumably due to plasma volume expansion.

The thrombocytopenia associated with maternal ITP is generally milder than in NAIT, and bleeding is less common. A large study of these patients revealed that the incidence of cord platelet counts of less than $50,000/\mu L$ is only about 3%. Affected infants should undergo evaluation for intracranial hemorrhage by head CT or cranial ultrasound. The babies should be followed closely until counts are clearly rising because platelet counts often fall in the first few days after birth. As described in the discussion on NAIT, prophylactic platelet transfusion is considered, especially in the first 96 hours of life and in ill or premature infants. Intravenous γ-globulin (1 g/kg daily for 2 days) elevates the platelet count in most patients. Corticosteroids (methylprednisolone, 2 mg/kg per day) may be used in addition to or instead of intravenous γ-globulin therapy.

The perinatal management of mothers with immune thrombocytopenia is controversial. Because the cord platelet count rarely is less than $50,000/\mu L$, perinatal intracranial hemorrhage is rare and not necessarily related to delivery. There are no reliable predictors of severe thrombocytopenia in the newborn except for direct determination of the fetal platelet count by percutaneous umbilical venous sampling, but this procedure is rarely justified in this condition. The degree of maternal thrombocytopenia is a poor predictor of the degree of neonatal thrombocytopenia. Measuring maternal platelet-associated IgG and maternal serum antiplatelet IgG has been proposed as a possible predictor, but has not proved generally useful.

Other Conditions Associated with Increased Platelet Destruction

Kasabach-Merritt syndrome associated with kaposiform hemangioendothelioma should be considered in cases of neonatal thrombocytopenia with DIC. Infection can trigger DIC, hepatosplenomegaly, and bone marrow suppression of platelet production. The relatively rare type 2b von Willebrand disease can manifest as isolated thrombocytopenia in the newborn period. Immune thrombocytopenia can accompany some cases of hemolytic disease of the newborn. For example, blood group O-B incompatibility can result in both hemolysis and thrombocytopenia because the B antigen is expressed on platelets. Maternal treatment with some drugs (penicillins, digoxin, and some anticonvulsants) may trigger an IgG response, which can cross into the fetal circulation and cause low platelets. Necrotizing enterocolitis is often associated with thrombocytopenia and bleeding. Thrombosis, particularly renal vein thrombosis, can be associated with consumption of platelets and low counts.

Another recently recognized cause of immune thrombocytopenia is autoimmune lymphoproliferative syndrome (ALPS).[70] This syndrome manifests early in childhood in persons who inherit mutations in genes critical for lymphocyte apoptosis. In autoimmune lymphoproliferative syndrome, defective lymphocyte apoptosis results in the survival of normally uncommon "double-negative" CD3[+], CD4[−], CD8[−] T cells and the development of autoimmune disease. Most cases of autoimmune lymphoproliferative syndrome involve mutations in the lymphocyte surface protein Fas or signaling molecules downstream of Fas. In addition to immune thrombocytopenia, children with ALPS can exhibit autoimmune hemolytic anemia, neutropenia, lymphadenopathy, and splenomegaly.

CONGENITAL THROMBOCYTOPENIA DUE TO UNDERPRODUCTION OF PLATELETS

Wiskott-Aldrich Syndrome

This X-linked syndrome is characterized by immunodeficiency, eczema, and thrombocytopenia secondary to decreased production.[60] Often only the thrombocytopenia is recognizable at birth. The platelets of patients with Wiskott-Aldrich syndrome are abnormally small (average diameter, 1.8 μm versus 2.2 μm). Cell-mediated immunity progressively declines with age. The number and phenotype of blood lymphocytes are normal. Serum immunoglobulins are abnormal: IgM is diminished, whereas IgA and IgE are elevated. The immune response to polysaccharide antigen is abnormal. The Wiskott-Aldrich gene *WAS* has been identified through positional cloning.[24] It encodes a cytoskeletal protein (WASP) that is expressed in hematopoietic progenitor cells. Symptomatic bleeding secondary to thrombocytopenia can be managed with irradiated single-donor platelet transfusions, although this rarely is necessary. The definitive treatment for Wiskott-Aldrich syndrome is allogeneic bone marrow transplantation.

Congenital Amegakaryocytic Thrombocytopenia

Amegakaryocytic thrombocytopenia is an autosomal recessive, rare cause of congenital thrombocytopenia. The degree of thrombocytopenia can be profound, with a count often less than 20,000/μL.[7] Bone marrow aspiration reveals a markedly reduced number of megakaryocytes, which may be dysplastic. Infants have severe mucocutaneous bleeding and can have intracranial hemorrhage in the perinatal period. As with other congenital bone marrow failure syndromes, this condition may evolve into progressive bone marrow failure or leukemia. Mutations in the *MPL* gene, which encodes the TPO receptor, are responsible for disease.[7]

Patients generally are dependent on platelet transfusions and have a short life span; the mean age of death is 5 years. Factors that contribute to this poor prognosis include the risk for hemorrhage, complications of chronic

platelet transfusion (i.e., sensitization), and the risk for evolution into bone marrow failure or leukemia. In addition to transfusion support with single-donor, irradiated platelets, trials of growth factors (e.g., IL-11, TPO) have been attempted, with mixed success. Allogeneic bone marrow transplantation should be considered if a healthy HLA-matched sibling is available.

Thrombocytopenia with Absent Radii Syndrome

Thrombocytopenia with absent radii (TAR) syndrome is another rare autosomal recessive cause of severe neonatal thrombocytopenia. Patients with this condition have no radii but can have normal or hypoplastic thumbs (Fig. 46-15).[7] Other skeletal anomalies can accompany the absent radii, including ulnar shortening, thumb hypoplasia, and scapular changes. Platelet counts in neonates are usually less than 50,000/μL. Bone marrow aspiration reveals a decrease in megakaryocytes, although this test is not required to make the diagnosis. Patients have mucocutaneous bleeding, especially in the first year of life, when the thrombocytopenia is most pronounced. As infants, these patients often require transfusions of single-donor, irradiated platelets to maintain a platelet count greater than 10,000/μL. After the first year of life, platelet-transfusion dependence usually diminishes. This condition has a much better prognosis than amegakaryocytic thrombocytopenia; the survival curve for TAR plateaus above 70% by 4 years of age.

The molecular pathogenesis of TAR is unknown. Levels of TPO are elevated in patients with TAR, yet TAR platelets fail to respond to recombinant TPO. Defective signal transduction through the *MPL* pathway has been suggested.[7] Comparative genomic hybridization studies have identified a 200-kb deletion on chromosome 1q21.1 in 30 of 30 affected individuals and in 32% of unaffected family members, suggesting that microdeletion on 1q21.1 is necessary but not

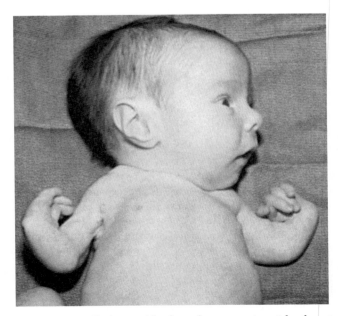

Figure 46–15. Patient with thrombocytopenia with absent radii syndrome.

sufficient to cause the disease.[43] Inheritance of an additional modifier is required to cause the phenotype, although the nature of this modifier is unknown.

Radial abnormalities are a sine qua non in TAR. In a patient with TAR, thumbs may be present in the absence of radii, whereas in Fanconi anemia, absence of the radius always is accompanied by thumb abnormalities. Despite these differences in clinical presentation, it is prudent to test patients who have a clinical picture of TAR for increased chromosome fragility to formally rule out Fanconi anemia.

Fanconi Anemia
See earlier discussion.

Although the phenotypes of TAR and Fanconi anemia overlap somewhat, several features distinguish these conditions. Cytopenias in the autosomal recessive disorder Fanconi anemia rarely present in the neonatal period, but the associated dysmorphic features such as hypopigmented skin lesions, café-au-lait spots, thumb abnormalities, short stature, microcephaly, and genitourinary abnormalities may be evident. Only about 30% of patients with Fanconi anemia have radial anomalies, whereas absent radius is always present in TAR. Fanconi patients develop progressive bone marrow failure as children or adults. Fanconi anemia patients have a cancer predisposition that is not affected by hematopoietic stem cell transplantation and correction of bone marrow failure.

X-Linked Thrombocytopenia with Dyserythropoiesis and Cryptorchidism
Boys with X-linked thrombocytopenia with dyserythropoiesis and cryptorchidism have a point mutation in the gene encoding GATA1, a transcription factor expressed in megakaryocytes, erythroid precursors, and Sertoli cells.[32] This mutation disrupts the interaction of GATA1 with the nuclear coactivator FOG1. The bone marrow from these patients is hypercellular and contains numerous small, dysplastic megakaryocytes.

CONGENITAL QUALITATIVE DEFECTS IN PLATELET FUNCTION

Glanzmann Thrombasthenia
Glanzmann thrombasthenia is an autosomal recessive condition caused by a deficiency in the platelet fibrinogen receptor GP IIb-IIIa.[61] This protein complex, a member of the integrin family of adhesion proteins, is also referred to as α-IIIb-β-III integrin. This complex is abundantly expressed on the surface of platelets. Each of the two subunits of the platelet fibrinogen receptor is encoded by a separate gene, and these genes are closely linked on chromosome 17. Patients with Glanzmann thrombasthenia exhibit decreased expression of functional GP IIb-IIIa on the platelet surface secondary to mutations in either the GP IIb or GP IIIa gene. These patients have mucocutaneous bleeding in the neonatal period and remain predisposed to bleeding throughout their lives.

Platelet counts and morphology are normal. The bleeding time is prolonged, although this test is notoriously difficult to perform and interpret in neonates. Clot retraction, which depends on platelet-platelet interactions, is abnormal in Glanzmann thrombasthenia and is a useful laboratory screening test, even in neonates. Abnormal platelet aggregation is seen in response to a variety of agonists, including collagen, adenosine diphosphate, epinephrine, arachidonic acid, and thrombin. GP IIb-IIIa levels on platelets of suspected patients can be measured by flow cytometry.

Bleeding in patients with Glanzmann thrombasthenia can be managed with platelet transfusions. However, platelet transfusions should be reserved for severe episodes of hemorrhage because high-titer alloantibodies that recognize GP IIb-IIIa can develop in these patients, making subsequent platelet transfusions less efficacious. Patients with Glanzmann thrombasthenia generally survive into adulthood.

Paris-Trousseau Syndrome
Paris-Trousseau syndrome is characterized by congenital thrombocytopenia, giant platelet α-granules, and a deletion at chromosome 11q23.[46] The thrombocytopenia reflects defective megakaryocyte maturation. Numerous micromegakaryocytes can be seen in the bone marrow. Congenital malformations, including facial dysmorphism and cardiac anomalies, can accompany the hematopoietic defects.

OTHER QUALITATIVE DEFECTS IN PLATELET FUNCTION

Patients with the autosomal recessive conditions Hermansky-Putlak and Chédiak-Higashi syndromes have albinism and a mild bleeding tendency secondary to abnormalities in platelet granules.

THE CONGENITAL MACROTHROMBOCYTOPENIA SYNDROMES

Bernard-Soulier Syndrome
Patients with Bernard-Soulier syndrome have a deficiency in the platelet vWF receptor, a complex structure that contains four proteins designated GP Ib-α, GP Ib-β, GP IX, and GP V. Mutations in the genes encoding GP Ib-α, GP Ib-β, and GP IX have been associated with the syndrome. The GP Ib-α-Ib-β-IX-V complex mediates adhesion of platelets to vWF deposited on vascular subendothelium (see Fig. 46-10).

The platelets in Bernard-Soulier syndrome patients are unusually large, approaching the size of mature lymphocytes. It is not clear why Ib-α-Ib-β-IX-V deficiency results in increased platelet size.

Bernard-Soulier syndrome is inherited as an autosomal recessive trait, and patients can have moderate to severe bleeding. The diagnosis is confirmed by failure of platelets to agglutinate in the presence of ristocetin, which induces binding of vWF to the glycoprotein complex. Agglutination in response to other agonists is normal.

May-Hegglin Anomaly
This autosomal dominant defect is known for giant platelets and moderate thrombocytopenia (macrothrombocytopenia) and leukocyte inclusions.

Alport Syndrome (Hereditary Nephritis) and Epstein Syndrome
Familial hematuria, progressive renal failure, deafness, and ocular abnormalities characterize the classic presentation of this syndrome. Some families with Epstein syndrome have a moderate macrothrombocytopenia with leukocyte inclusions.

NEOPLASMS IN THE NEONATE

The peak incidence of cancer in childhood (<15 years of age) occurs during the first year of life. The annual incidence rate for all cancers of infancy is 233 per million infants, according to the National Cancer Institute's statistics for the years 1976 to 1984 and 1986 to 1994. This represents 10% of all childhood malignancies. Figure 46-16 provides a graphic summary of cancer incidence by common types. In adults, cancer is thought to occur after a long interplay between environmental triggers and genetic predisposition. In infancy, especially in the neonatal period, cancer includes a rare spectrum of diseases in which the normal, genetically programmed protections against unregulated growth of cells fail very early. Researchers studying infant cancers may provide the clearest information about oncogenesis. The first year of life is the only time in childhood when the incidence of cancers is not higher in males than females, but is instead equal. Overall, the prognosis for infants compared with older children with the same histologic diagnoses is worse, despite the fact that infant neuroblastoma has a much superior survival rate. Many entities (e.g., retinoblastoma [see also Chapter 53], Wilms tumor [see also Chapter 51], and brain tumors [see also Chapter 40]) are discussed elsewhere.

Neuroblastoma

About half of infant neuroblastomas are diagnosed within the first 4 months of life. These tumors of neural crest origin can arise anywhere along the sympathetic chain. In infants, the most common sites of presentation are cervical and thoracic. Involvement of the adrenal gland, which presents as an abdominal mass, is most common in older children. Neuroblastomas can be detected by prenatal ultrasound. Many of these tumors secrete catecholamines, so urine homovanillic acid and vanillylmandelic acid levels are commonly used diagnostic tests. Mass infant screening programs using these urine tests in Japan, Quebec, and Europe have increased the detection of good-prognosis tumors, but have failed to change the mortality rate from high-risk neuroblastoma.

The most important variables for prognosis for infant neuroblastoma are the patient age at diagnosis, the stage of the tumor, DNA index, and *MYCN* amplification. Tumor hyperdiploidy (DNA index >1) is a favorable prognostic indicator, whereas *MYCN* amplification is associated with more aggressive disease. Infants (<1 year of age) with neuroblastoma have a better prognosis than older children, with an overall 5-year survival of about 80% (versus 45% for those >1 year at diagnosis). Children younger than 1 year of age with localized tumors have a 5-year survival rate of 95%. A significant proportion of infants with metastatic disease are in the prognostically favorable stage IV-S category. These infants have liver, skin, and bone marrow involvement in addition to a seemingly localized primary tumor (<1 year), but do not have evidence of bone metastases. Despite metastatic disease, this subgroup of infants has the unique, poorly understood characteristic of spontaneous tumor regression. Surgery, chemotherapy, high-dose chemotherapy with peripheral blood stem cell rescue, and radiation therapy are treatment options, depending on risk group. Infants with low-risk disease may be candidates for observation with close monitoring for resolution.

Infant Leukemia

Infant leukemias tend to present toward the second half of the first year of life. A number of clinical features that have been associated with a poorer prognosis are common in neonates and infants with acute lymphocytic leukemia (ALL): a large tumor cell burden (hyperleukocytosis), massive hepatosplenomegaly, involvement of the central nervous system, and hypogammaglobulinemia. The leukemic blasts in infant ALL often are CD10 negative, and cytogenetic abnormalities involving the *MLL* (mixed lineage leukemia) gene at chromosome 11q23 are common. Although neonates experience significant toxicities both from chemotherapy and central nervous system irradiation, the especially poor prognosis for infant ALL is due to the high incidence of bone marrow and extramedullary relapse. Progressively more intensive chemotherapeutic regimens and bone marrow transplantation have been used in these patients, but the event-free survival rate at 5 years is only in the 30% range.

In contrast to ALL, infants with acute myelogenous leukemia (AML) have similarly poor remission and disease-free survival rates indistinguishable from those for older children. Distinctive features of AML in the infant include very high incidences of cutaneous involvement (leukemia cutis) and central nervous system disease, hyperleukocytosis, and an unusually high number of cases with blasts of the monoblastic or myelomonocytic type. Cytogenetic abnormalities in the blasts are exceptionally common. Infants with Down syndrome who are diagnosed with AML have a superior survival rate compared with others with AML because they tend to

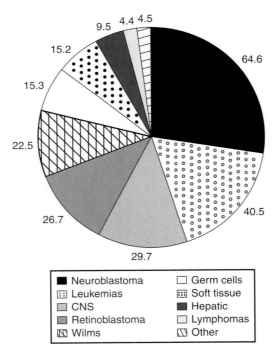

Figure 46–16. Average annual incidence per 1 million infants of cancers by type, SEER data, 1976-1984 and 1986-1994. *(Adapted from Gurney JG, et al: Cancer among infants. Available at: www.SEER.cancer.gov/publications.childhood/infant.pdf. 1999.)*

develop the acute megakaryocytic leukemia subset of AML (AMKL) and have a very high response rate to therapy.

Juvenile myelomonocytic leukemia (JMML; formerly juvenile chronic myelogenous leukemia), is a myeloproliferative disorder that accounts for about 1% of pediatric leukemias. Ten percent of cases are diagnosed before 3 months of age. Clinical manifestations include splenomegaly, rash, lymphadenopathy, failure to thrive, leukoerythroblastosis, monocytosis, thrombocytopenia, and elevated fetal hemoglobin. The abnormal growth of JMML cells has been linked to a dysregulated transduction signal through the pathway that involves GM-CSF, the GM-CSF receptor neurofibromin, and Ras. When cultured in vitro, JMML cells exhibit a hypersensitivity to GM-CSF. PTEN protein deficiency has been noted in a large number of patient leukemia cells tested and may explain the lack of negative growth signals that should counteract hyperactive Ras signaling.

About 15% to 20% of children with JMML have neurofibromatosis type I. *RAS* family oncogene mutations occur in the leukemia cells in 25% of sporadic JMML cases. Patients with Noonan syndrome, a disorder associated with gain-of-function mutations in *PTPN11*, the gene encoding the protein tyrosine phosphatase SHP-2, are at increased risk for developing JMML. Mutations in *PTPN11* are present in the leukemia cells of one third of spontaneous JMML cases. Patients diagnosed before 2 years of age and those with Noonan syndrome have a better prognosis. Although a variety of therapies have been employed to treat JMML, allogeneic bone marrow transplantation is the only curative treatment.[28]

Congenital Leukemia

Although rare (<5 cases per 1 million live births), leukemia can manifest in the newborn period. Associations between congenital defects or chromosomal abnormalities and congenital leukemia have been made. Eighty percent of congenital leukemias are nonlymphocytic. The infant may be symptomatic at the time of birth or may be diagnosed later in the neonatal period. It is often difficult to distinguish leukemia from a leukemoid reaction (see earlier) secondary to infection or associated with Down syndrome. Infiltration of nonhematopoietic organs by hematopoietic blasts and cytogenetic abnormalities (other than trisomy 21) in the blasts differentiates leukemia from the more benign processes. With the exception of Down syndrome patients with AMKL, congenital leukemia carries a grave prognosis.

Transient Myeloproliferative Disorder

See "Down Syndrome," earlier.

Teratomas and Other Germ Cell Tumors

Most infant germ cell tumors are diagnosed before the age of 2 months. Germ cell tumors originate early in life from preinvasive precursors that transform into overt tumors during infancy, adolescence, or young adulthood.[38] Whereas 90% of germ cell tumors diagnosed during adult life are gonadal, two thirds of childhood germ cell tumors are extragonadal. Most neonatal germ cell tumors, irrespective of location, are benign.

Teratomas are the most common neonatal germ cell tumors.[38] The term *teratoma* describes both benign and malignant tumors

composed of haphazardly intermixed tissues that originate from pluripotent stem cells and are foreign to the anatomic site in which they arise. Traditionally, tissue components from all three embryonic germ layers—endoderm, mesoderm, and ectoderm—should be represented in a teratoma. However, it is now generally accepted that tumors that are foreign to the site where they arise and consist of more than one embryonic layer can be classified as teratomas.

Sacrococcygeal teratomas are frequently detected at birth as a mass in the region of the sacrum or buttocks, sometimes accompanied by obstruction of the rectum or urinary tract. These tumors are most often postsacral but occasionally presacral. Vertebral anomalies can be seen in patients with sacrococcygeal teratomas.

The mainstay of therapy for germ cell tumors is surgical resection. Typically, teratomas have an excellent outcome. Immature teratomas have a prognosis comparable to mature teratomas, provided the tumor can be totally excised. In the case of sacrococcygeal teratomas, prematurity, perioperative hemorrhage, and other postoperative events result in a 10% to 20% risk for mortality. Endodermal sinus tumors of the infant testis have a better prognosis than those at later ages and other locations, including the ovary. See Table 46-22 for age-adjusted α-fetoprotein values.

TABLE 46–22	Postnatal Serum Concentrations of α-Fetoprotein in Preterm and Term Infants		
	AFP CONCENTRATION (μg/L)*		
Age	*10th percentile*	*Median*	*90th percentile*
Preterm Infants (27-35 Weeks' Gestational Age)			
Birth	149,700	252,125	335,375
1 wk	43,825	96,510	234,500
1 mo	21,825	41,975	66,460
2 mo	3,100	16,000	36,900
3 mo	560	1,250	10,140
4 mo	75	162	621
6 mo	22	67	170
9 mo	6	20	54
12 mo	5	10	28
Term Infants (38-42 Weeks' Gestational Age)			
Birth	17,200	30,875	44,350
2 mo	88	206	412
4 mo	16	77	127
6 mo	11	30	67
9 mo	5	12	27
12 mo	4	7	17

*1 μg/L AFP = 1.09 IU/mL.

Modified from Lahdenne P, et al: Biphasic reduction and concanavalin A binding properties of serum alpha-fetoprotein in preterm and term infants, *J Pediatr* 118:272, 1991.

Infantile Myofibromatosis

Infantile myofibromatosis generally occurs in the newborn period and is the most common fibrous tumor of infancy.[73] The disease can manifest as a solitary lesion or multiple lesions in the skin, subcutaneous tissue, skeletal muscle, bone, or viscera such as the lung. Histopathology reveals a spindle cell neoplasm with myofibroblastic proliferation. A unique feature of the neoplasm is its ability to spontaneously regress. The multifocal form of the disease may be associated with a high morbidity and mortality if visceral involvement is evident. Autosomal dominant inheritance has been reported in some cases.[2] Treatment depends on the location of the tumors, with surgery or chemotherapy reserved for rapidly progressive or symptomatic disease.[73]

Congenital Fibrosarcoma

Congenital fibrosarcoma is a spindle cell tumor of the soft tissues. It usually presents before the age of 2 years. Surgery is the mainstay of therapy. Although these malignancies can recur locally, they have a generally favorable prognosis and only rarely metastasize. A novel chromosomal translocation, t(12;15)(p13;q25), which gives rise to an ETV6-NTRK3 gene fusion, is present in these tumors. Polymerase chain reaction–based assays for this fusion protein are helpful in making this diagnosis and in differentiating this tumor from composite infantile myofibromatosis.[2]

Rhabdomyosarcoma

Rhabdomyosarcoma is a tumor of striated muscle cell origin that rarely occurs in the neonate. Neonatal rhabdomyosarcoma usually occurs in the abdomen or pelvis, rather than appearing as masses in the head and neck region, as is common in older patients. The prognosis depends on both the histologic type (embryonal, alveolar, botryoid, and pleomorphic in best to worst order of prognosis) and the extent of tumor resection. Both radiation therapy and chemotherapy are important adjuvants to surgical resection.[72]

Langerhans Cell Histiocytosis

Langerhans cell histiocytosis is a rare disorder, primarily of childhood, characterized by the infiltration of tissues with histiocytes. Histiocytosis can be present at birth, although the peak age of incidence is between 1 and 3 years of age. Langerhans cell histiocytosis includes localized and disseminated forms of disease. An isolated bone lesion (most commonly skull) is an example of low-risk disease that requires only observation. The disseminated form, formerly termed Letterer-Siwe disease, is often seen in infants and children younger than 2 years of age and manifests with rash, lymphadenopathy, fever, and wasting. Involvement of at-risk organs (lungs, liver, spleen, and bone marrow) portends a poor prognosis. High-risk disease is treated with chemotherapy. Multifocal bone lesions and those occurring in the so-called special sites, such as intraspinal or parameningeal, also require chemotherapy.[78]

Hemophagocytic Lymphohistiocytosis Syndrome

Hemophagocytic lymphohistiocytosis is a rare disease, generally affecting infants and children, which causes persistent T-cell activation and histiocytic infiltration of tissues. It is estimated to occur in 1.2 per 1 million children. A primary form, also known as familial hematophagocytic lymphohistiocytosis, is an autosomal recessive disease associated with mutations in the perforin genes (PRF1 and UNC13D), a gene involved in T-cell cytotoxicity (MUNC13-4), and the syntaxin 11 gene (STX11). The secondary form of the disease occurs in response to viral, bacterial, parasitic, or fungal infections, as well as cancers and rheumatologic disorders. Immune dysregulation, characterized by reduced or absent natural killer cell function, is present in most cases. Usually, infection will trigger an inflammatory process that abates with control of the infection. In hemophagocytic lymphohistiocytosis, immune dysregulation results in persistence of the inflammatory response. Common clinical features include persistent fever, thrombocytopenia, hepatosplenomegaly, a cutaneous maculopapular eruption, and central nervous system involvement. Laboratory findings include thrombocytopenia, very elevated ferritin level, anemia, hypofibrinogenemia, neutropenia, and cerebrospinal fluid pleocytosis. Biopsy of tissue, commonly bone marrow, will show phagocytosis of blood cells. Specialized tests for NK-cell function, perforin expression in lymphocytes, and genetic testing for the known mutations aid the diagnosis. The management of familial hemophagocytic lymphohistiocytosis should include genetic testing and counseling of family members. Without treatment, the familial syndrome is rapidly fatal. Chemotherapy can be used as a temporizing measure, but cure requires allogeneic bone marrow transplantation.[5]

REFERENCES

1. Acharya SS, et al: Rare bleeding disorder registry: deficiencies of factors II,V,VII, X, XIII, fibrinogen and dysfibrinogenemias, J Thromb Haemost 2:248, 2004.
2. Alaggio R, et al: Morphologic overlap between infantile myofibromatosis and infantile fibrosarcoma: a pitfall in diagnosis, Pediatr Dev Pathol 11:355, 2008.
3. Alur P, et al: Impact of race and gestational age on red blood cell indices in very low birth weight infants, Pediatrics 106:306, 2000.
4. American Academy of Pediatrics Committee on Fetus and Newborn: Controversies concerning vitamin K and the newborn, Pediatrics 112:191, 2003.
5. Arceci RJ: When T cells and macrophages do not talk: the hemophagocytic syndromes, Curr Opin Hematol 15:359, 2008.
6. Bell SG: Immunomodulation, part II: granulocyte colony-stimulating factors, Neonatal Netw 25:65, 2006.
7. Bessler M, et al: Inherited Bone Marrow Failure Syndromes. In Orkin SH, et al, editors: Nathan and Oski's Hematology of Infancy and Childhood, 7th ed., Philadelphia, 2008, Elsevier.
8. Boocock GR, et al: Mutations in SBDS are associated with Shwachman-Diamond syndrome, Nat Genet 33:97, 2003.
9. Bohn G, et al: A novel human primary immunodeficiency syndrome caused by deficiency of the endosomal adaptor protein p14, Nat Med 13:38, 2007.

10. Brenner B: Hereditary deficiency of all vitamin K-dependent coagulation factors, *Thromb Haemost* 84:935, 2000.

11. Brion LP, et al: Vitamin E supplementation for prevention of morbidity and mortality in preterm infants, *Cochrane Database Syst Rev* CD003665, 2003.

12. Bussel JB, et al: Fetal alloimmune thrombocytopenia, *N Engl J Med* 337:22, 1997.

13. Cairo MS, et al: Circulating steel factor (SLF) and G-CSF levels in preterm and term newborn and adult peripheral blood, *Am J Pediatr Hematol Oncol* 15:311, 1993.

14. Cairo MS, et al: Randomized trial of granulocyte transfusions versus intravenous immune globulin therapy for neonatal neutropenia and sepsis, *J Pediatr* 120:28, 1992.

15. Calhoun DA, et al: Incidence, significance, and kinetic mechanism responsible for leukemoid reactions in patients in the neonatal intensive care unit: a prospective evaluation, *J Pediatr* 129:403, 1996.

16. Capsoni F, et al: Primary and secondary autoimmune neutropenia, *Arthritis Res Ther* 7:208, 2005.

17. Cappellini MD, Fiorelli G: Glucose-6-phosphate dehydrogenase deficiency, *Lancet* 371:64, 2008.

18. Castle V, et al: Frequency and mechanism of neonatal thrombocytopenia, *J Pediatr* 108:749, 1986.

19. Chalmers EA: Perinatal stroke—risk factors and management, *Br J Haematol* 130:333, 2005.

20. Christensen RD, et al: Thrombocytopenia among extremely low birth weight neonates: data from a multihospital healthcare system, *J Perinatol* 26:348, 2006.

21. Curneutte JT, Dinauer MC: Genetic disorders of phagocyte killing. In Stammatoyannopoulous G, et al, editors: *The Molecular Basis of Blood Diseases*, 3rd ed., Philadelphia, 2001, Saunders Co.

22. Curtis BR, et al: Neonatal alloimmune neutropenia attributed to maternal immunoglobulin G antibodies against the neutrophil alloantigen HNA-1c (SH): a report of five cases, *Transfusion* 45:1308, 2005.

22a. Dahlback B, et al: Familial thrombophilia due to a previously unrecognized mechanism characterized by poor anticoagulant response to activated protein C: prediction of a cofactor to activated protein C, *Proc Natl Acad Sci USA* 90:1004, 1993.

23. DePalma L, Luban NL: Hereditary pyropoikilocytosis: clinical and laboratory analysis in eight infants and young children, *Am J Dis Child* 147:93, 1993.

24. Derry JM, et al: Isolation of a novel gene mutated in Wiskott-Aldrich syndrome, *Cell* 78:635, 1994.

25. Dixon H, et al: Clinical manifestations of hematologic and oncologic disorders in patients with Down Syndrome, *Am J Med Genet, part C, Semin Med Genet* 142C:149, 2006.

26. Duckert F, et al: A hitherto undescribed congenital haemorrhagic diathesis probably due to fibrin stabilizing factor deficiency, *Thromb Diath Haemorrh* 5:179, 1960.

27. Eckardt KU: The ontogeny of the biological role and production of erythropoietin, *J Perinat Med* 23:19, 1995.

28. Emanuel PD: Juvenile myelomonocytic leukemia, *Curr Hematol Rep* 3:203, 2004.

29. Enders M, et al: Fetal morbidity and mortality after the acute human parvovirus B19 infection in pregnancy: prospective evaluation of 1018 cases, *Prenat Diagn* 24:513, 2004.

30. Faxelius G, et al: Red cell volume measurements and acute blood loss in high-risk newborn infants, *J Pediatr* 90:273, 1977.

31. Fitzgerald KC, et al: Cerebral sinovenous thrombosis in the neonate, *Arch Neurol* 63:405, 2006.

32. Freson K, et al: Different substitutions at residue D218 of the X-linked transcription factor GATA1 lead to altered clinical severity of macrothrombocytopenia and anemia and are associated with variable skewed X inactivation, *Hum Mol Genet* 11:147, 2002.

33. Fung KAFK, et al: Clinical usefulness of flow cytometry in detection and quantification of fetomaternal hemorrhage, *J Matern Fetal Investig* 8:121, 1998.

33a. Gailani D, Broze GJ Jr: Factor XI activation in a revised model of blood coagulation, *Science*, 253: 909, 1991.

34. Gallagher PG, Benz EJ: The erythrocyte membrane and cytoskeleton: structure, function, and disorders. In Stammatoyannopoulous G, et al, editors: *The Molecular Basis of Blood Diseases*, 3rd ed., Philadelphia, 2004, Saunders Co.

35. Gurbuxani S, et al: Recent insights into the mechanisms of myeloid leukemogenesis in Down syndrome, *Blood* 103:399, 2004.

36. Hall GW: Kasabach-Merritt syndrome: pathogenesis and management, *Br J Haematol* 112:851, 2001.

37. Hartwell SK, et al: Review on screening and analysis techniques for hemoglobin variants and thalassemia, *Talanta* 65:1149, 2005.

38. Heikinheimo M, Wilson DB: Germ cell tumors. In Rudolph CD, et al, editors: *Rudolph's Pediatrics*, 21st ed., Philadelphia, 2002, Mosby-Year Book.

39. Herring WB, et al: Hereditary neutrophilia: *Am J Med* 56:729, 1974.

40. Horwitz M, et al: Mutations in ELA2, encoding neutrophil elastase, define a 21-day biological clock in cyclic haematopoiesis, *Nat Genet* 23:433, 1999.

41. Juul SE, et al: "Idiopathic neutropenia" in very low birthweight infants, *Acta Paediatr* 87:963, 1998.

42. Kaushansky K: Hematopoietic growth factors and receptors. In Stammatoyannopoulous G, et al, editors: *The Molecular Basis of Blood Diseases*, 3rd ed., Philadelphia, 2001, Saunders Co.

43. Klopocki E, et al: Complex inheritance pattern resembling autosomal recessive inheritance involving a microdeletion in thrombocytopenia-absent radius syndrome, *Am J Hum Genet* 80:232, 2007.

44. Koren A, et al: Congenital dysgranulopoietic neutropenia in two siblings: clinical, ultrastructural, and in vitro bone marrow culture studies, *Pediatr Hematol Oncol* 6:293, 1989.

45. Koster T, et al: Role of clotting factor VIII in effect of von Willebrand factor on occurrence of deep-vein thrombosis, *Lancet* 345:152, 1995.

46. Krishnamurti L, et al: Paris-Trousseau syndrome platelets in a child with Jacobsen's syndrome, *Am J Hematol* 66:295, 2001.

47. Kutlar F: Diagnostic approach to hemoglobinopathies, *Hemoglobin* 31:243, 2007.

48. Leuzzi R, et al: Inhibition of microsomal glucose-6-phosphate transport in human neutrophils results in apoptosis: a potential explanation for neutrophil dysfunction in glycogen storage disease type 1b, *Blood* 101:2381, 2003.

49. Maayan-Metzger A, et al: Maternal anti-D prophylaxis during pregnancy does not cause neonatal haemolysis, *Arch Dis Child Fetal Neonatal Ed* 84:F60, 2001.

50. Malowany JI, et al: Enoxaparin use in the neonatal intensive care unit: experience over 8 years, *Pharmacotherapy* 27:1263, 2007.

51. Mamlok RJ, et al: Neutropenia and defective chemotaxis associated with binuclear, tetraploid myeloid-monocytic leukocytes, *J Pediatr* 111:555, 1987.

52. Mannucci PM, Tuddenham EG: The hemophilias-from royal genes to gene therapy, *N Engl J Med* 344:1773, 2001.

53. Mansouri A, Lurie AA: Concise review: methemoglobinemia, *Am J Hematol* 42:7, 1993.

54. Mansouritorgabeh H, et al: Hemorrhagic symptoms in patients with combined factors V and VIII deficiency in north-eastern Iran, *Haemophilia* 10:271, 2004.

55. Mason AR, et al: Successful use of fondaparinux as an alternative anticoagulant in a 2-month-old infant, *Pediatr Blood Cancer* 50:1084, 2008.

56. Mauch L, et al: Chronic granulomatous disease (CGD) and complete myeloperoxidase deficiency both yield strongly reduced dihydrorhodamine 123 test signals but can be easily discerned in routine testing for CGD, *Clin Chem* 53:890, 2007.

57. Michaels LA, et al: Low molecular weight heparin in the treatment of venous and arterial thromboses in the premature infant, *Pediatrics* 114:703, 2004.

58. Monagle P, et al, for the American College of Chest Physicians: Antithrombotic therapy in neonates and children: American College of Chest Physicians evidence-based clinical practice guidelines (8th edition), *Chest* 133(6 Suppl):887S, 2008.

59. Monagle P, et al: Developmental haemostasis. Impact for clinical haemostasis laboratories, *Thromb Haemost* 95:362, 2006.

60. Notarangelo LD, et al: Wiskott-Aldrich syndrome, *Curr Opin Hematol* 15:30, 2008.

61. Nurden AT: Glanzmann thrombasthenia, *Orphanet J Rare Dis* 1:10, 2006.

62. Ohls RK: Human recombinant erythropoietin in the prevention and treatment of anemia of prematurity, *Paediatr Drugs* 4:111, 2002.

63. Orkin SH: Transcription factors that regulate lineage decisions. In Stammatoyannopoulous G, et al, editors: *The Molecular Basis of Blood Diseases*, 3rd ed., Philadelphia, 2001, Saunders.

64. Orkin SH, Zon LI: Hematopoiesis: an evolving paradigm for stem cell biology, *Cell* 132:631, 2008.

65. Pannicke U, et al: Reticular dysgenesis (aleukocytosis) is caused by mutations in the gene encoding mitochondrial adenylate kinase 2, *Nat Genet* 41:101, 2009.

66. Pochedly C, Musiker S: Twin-to-twin transfusion syndrome, *Postgrad Med* 47:172, 1970.

67. Poort SR, et al: A common genetic variation in the 3'-untranslated region of the prothrombin gene is associated with elevated plasma prothrombin levels and an increase in venous thrombosis, *Blood* 88:3698, 1996.

68. Raju TN, et al: Ischemic perinatal stroke: summary of a workshop sponsored by the National Institute of Child Health and Human Development and the National Institute of Neurological Disorders and Stroke, *Pediatrics* 120:609, 2007.

69. Ramamurthy RS, Brans YW: Neonatal polycythemia: I. Criteria for diagnosis and treatment, *Pediatrics* 68:168, 1981.

70. Rao VK, Straus SE: Causes and consequences of the autoimmune lymphoproliferative syndrome, *Hematology* 11:15, 2006.

71. Rosenberg PS, et al: The incidence of leukemia and mortality from sepsis in patients with severe congenital neutropenia receiving long-term G-CSF therapy, *Blood* 107:4628, 2006.

72. Ruymann FB, Grovas AC: Progress in the diagnosis and treatment of rhabdomyosarcoma and related soft tissue sarcomas, *Cancer Invest* 18:223, 2000.

73. Schurr P, Moulsdale W: Infantile myofibroma: a case report and review of the literature, *Adv Neonatal Care* 8:13, 2008.

74. Shalev H, et al: Neonatal manifestations of congenital dyserythropoietic anemia type I, *J Pediatr* 131:95, 1997.

75. Southwick FS, et al: Neutrophil actin dysfunction is a genetic disorder associated with partial impairment of neutrophil actin assembly in three family members, *J Clin Invest* 82:1525, 1988.

76. Stasia MJ, Li XJ: Genetics and immunopathology of chronic granulomatous disease, *Semin Immunopathol* 30:209, 2008.

77. Urwijitaroon Y, et al: Frequency of human platelet antigens among blood donors in northeastern Thailand, *Transfusion* 35:868, 1995.

78. Weitzman S, Egeler RM: Langerhans cell histiocytosis: update for the pediatrician, *Curr Opin Pediatr* 20:23, 2008.

79. Wilson DB: Acquired platelet defects In Nathan DG, et al, editors: *Hematology of Infancy and Childhood*, 6th ed., Philadelphia, 2003, Harcourt.

80. Xia J, Link DC: Severe congenital neutropenia and the unfolded protein response, *Curr Opin Hematol* 15:1, 2008.

81. Young G, et al: Pilot dose-finding and safety study of bivalirudin in infants <6 months of age with thrombosis, *J Thromb Haemost* 5:1654, 2007.

82. Zeidler C, et al: Congenital neutropenias, *Rev Clin Exp Hematol* 7:72, 2003.

PART 2

Blood Component Therapy for the Neonate

Ross Fasano and Naomi L. C. Luban

SPECIAL CONSIDERATIONS FOR TRANSFUSION THERAPY IN THE NEONATE

Neonates constitute one of the most heavily transfused patient groups in the hospital. Neonatal transfusion practices differ substantially from adult and pediatric transfusion practices owing to unique differences in neonatal physiology. Neonates have small blood volumes compared with older children and adults but high blood volume per body weight. Their immature organ system function predisposes them to metabolic derangements from blood products and additive solutions and to the infectious and immunomodulatory hazards of transfusion, such as transfusion-transmitted cytomegalovirus (TT-CMV) infection and transfusion-associated graft versus host disease (TA-GVHD). Neonates undergo rapid growth but have a limited capacity to expand their blood volume. In addition, passive transfer of maternal antibodies to the immunologically naive newborn creates unique compatibility scenarios not commonly seen in children or adults. Their responses to stresses, including hypothermia, hypovolemia, hypoxia, and acidosis, are dependent on gestational age, birthweight, and comorbidities. These considerations necessitate special approaches to transfusion therapy in the neonate.[24,35]

RISKS OF TRANSFUSION THERAPY

Advances in donor recruitment and blood screening and processing have decreased the risks associated with blood transfusion. Current transfusion considerations and guidelines focus on reducing both transfusion number and donor exposures. Nevertheless, hematologic, immunologic, infectious, cardiovascular, and metabolic complications can occur. Many of these risks exist for transfusion recipients of any age, whereas others pose a greater threat to the neonatal recipient. These potential risks affect the choice and processing of blood products. Parents must be advised of the risks, benefits, and alternatives to transfusion, and informed consent should be documented in the medical record along with the indications for and results of the prescribed transfusion.

Metabolic Complications

Neonates, especially extremely premature infants, are more susceptible to metabolic alterations because of the immaturity of many of their organ systems. Glucose imbalances, hyperkalemia, and hypocalcemia are the most common metabolic derangements related to transfusion resulting from the inability of the infant to efficiently metabolize or excrete many compounds within the blood components such as anticoagulants, preservatives, and other solutes.

HYPOGLYCEMIA

See also Chapter 49, Part 1.
Hypoglycemia can result from the combination of decreased glucose infusion rates during transfusion and impaired glycogenolysis and gluconeogenesis within the liver of the preterm neonate. Continuous glucose infusion rates of more than 3 to 4 mg/kg per minute are often required in preterm infants; if maintenance fluids are suspended during transfusion, glucose infusion rates can decrease to about 0.2 mg/kg per minute for citrate-phosphate-dextrose-adenine preserved (CPDA-1) red blood cells (RBCs) and to 0.5 mg/kg per minute for Adsol preserved (AS-1) RBCs. In a previous report of 31 fresh (<5 days old) small-volume RBC transfusions in 16 preterm infants (mean birthweight and gestational age, 863 g and 26 weeks, respectively), 15% of infants receiving AS-1 preserved RBCs and 64% of infants receiving CPDA-1 preserved RBCs required supplemental dextrose infusions during the transfusion because of hypoglycemia (blood glucose <35-40 mg/dL or symptoms of hypoglycemia).[21] Subsequent analysis has shown similar frequency of transfusion-associated hypoglycemia when older (5 to 21 days old) AS-1 preserved units were used. Furthermore, reported incidences of hypoglycemia in neonates either during or after exchange transfusions range from 1.4% to 3.6% with no difference in incidence when group O whole blood or reconstituted whole blood was used. Hypoglycemia occurring after exchange transfusion is believed to be due to intraprocedural hyperglycemia, which causes rebound hypoglycemia from insulin secretion.[45] Preventive measures for transfusion-associated hypoglycemia include recognizing those infants at risk for developing glucose homeostatic imbalances, continuing the infusion of maintenance fluids rich in dextrose (albeit at a slower rate) in order to maintain an adequate glucose infusion rate during simple transfusions, and close monitoring of blood glucose during both small and large volume transfusions.

HYPERKALEMIA

As stored RBCs age, potassium leaks out into the plasma and raises the extracellular potassium level within the component. RBC units in extended-storage media (AS-1, AS-3,

AS-5) have a hematocrit (Hct) of about 60%, and RBCs stored in CPDA have an Hct of about 70%. Furthermore, some pediatric transfusion centers centrifuge RBC aliquots before transfusions for neonates to further reduce the plasma component to 20% (i.e., RBC unit: Hct >80%). After 42 days of storage, K^+ levels in the plasma of an AS-1 preserved RBC unit approximates 0.05 mEq/mL. Therefore, infusing 15 mL/kg would yield a potassium dose of 0.3 mEq/kg (i.e., 1 kg infant receiving 15 mL RBC, 6 mL plasma). Conversely, after 35 days of storage of CPDA-1 preserved RBCs, potassium levels in the plasma approximate 0.07 to 0.08 mEq/mL. Transfusing 15 mL/kg of the CPDA-1 stored product would yield a potassium dose of 0.3 to 0.4 mEq/kg (i.e., 1 kg infant receiving 15 mL RBC, 4.5 mL plasma).[56] Given that the daily potassium requirement is about 2 to 3 mEq/kg, simple RBCs transfused slowly over 2 to 4 hours should pose no theoretical risk. It has been shown in multiple studies that transfusing dedicated RBC units to their expiration dates does not cause hyperkalemia even in extremely preterm infants.[23,30,34,45,57] Therefore, the routine practice of washing older RBCs is unnecessary for most small-volume RBC transfusions in infants, including those with birthweight less than 1.5 kg.[30]

This rationale may not apply to large-volume transfusions (>25 mL/kg) or rapid small-volume transfusions. There have been reports of hyperkalemia-induced electrocardiac abnormalities and cardiac arrest when RBC transfusions (fresh and old) have been administered through rapid infusion (10 to 20 mL/kg over 10 to 15 minutes) to neonates with concurrent low cardiac output states, when irradiated more than 24 hours before infusion, and when given by central line directly into the inferior vena cava. In cases of large-volume transfusions (i.e., exchange transfusion, cardiopulmonary bypass, and massive transfusion of neonates), fresh reconstituted whole blood (<7 days old) is often used because of concern for high potassium concentrations in older RBC units. In most cases, these RBCs are administered rapidly and in large amounts, thereby exposing the neonate to potentially toxic potassium concentrations.[34] In circumstances in which fresh reconstituted whole blood is unavailable for large-volume transfusions, saline-washed RBCs can be used.[24,34,50] Special considerations should be taken when RBCs need to be transfused rapidly, and this should be coordinated with the transfusion center so that proper preparation can be performed to avoid hyperkalemia.

HYPOCALCEMIA

See also Chapter 49, Part 2.
Infants, especially premature infants, are particularly susceptible to hypocalcemia within the first week of life owing to multiple factors. Because of the immaturity in neonatal liver and kidney function and the low amount of skeletal muscle mass, transfusion of citrate enriched blood can result in hypocalcemia from citrate toxicity. The amount of citrate infused into a neonate during a small-volume transfusion (10 to 15 mL/kg) is unlikely to cause hypocalcemia; however, the citrate load during an exchange transfusion can reach very high levels and lead to symptomatic hypocalcemia. In a retrospective review of 106 infants undergoing 140 exchange transfusions, symptomatic hypocalcemia was one of the most common serious side effects. Eighty-one infants were

classified as "healthy" if indication for exchange was solely asymptomatic hyperbilirubinemia; 25 infants were classified as "ill" if comorbid conditions existed. Incidences of asymptomatic and symptomatic hypocalcemia (defined as irritability, jitteriness, or electrocardiographic changes) were 34.6% and 5%, respectively, in the "healthy" infant population, and 40% and 8%, respectively, in the "ill" infant population.[22] Because clinical manifestations of hypocalcemia are often subtle or variable in premature infants, many recommend monitoring ionized calcium levels and QT intervals throughout exchange transfusion procedures, in addition to minimizing potentiating factors such as hypomagnesemia, hyperkalemia, alkalosis, and hypothermia in high-risk (ill) patients.[45]

TRANSFUSION-ASSOCIATED GRAFT-VERSUS-HOST DISEASE

TA-GVHD occurs when an immunosuppressed or immunodeficient patient receives cellular blood products, which possess immunologically competent lymphocytes.[31] The transfused donor lymphocytes are able to proliferate and engraft within the immunologic incompetent recipient because the recipient is unable to detect and reject foreign cells. The degree of similarity between HLA antigens of donor and recipient also increases the likelihood of developing TA-GVHD. As an example, in the setting of directed donation from a first-degree relative, donor lymphocyte homozygosity for an HLA haplotype for which the recipient is haploidentical predisposes to recipient tolerance, donor lymphocyte engraftment, and alloreaction leading to TA-GVHD.[35]

The clinical signs and symptoms of TA-GVHD include fever; generalized, erythematous rash that may progress to desquamation; watery diarrhea; mild hepatitis to fulminant liver failure; respiratory distress; and pancytopenia, which is usually severe because hematopoietic progenitor cells are preferentially affected. Onset is 3 to 30 days after transfusion of lymphocyte-replete cellular blood components. Neonates at "high risk" for TA-GVHD include those with impaired cellular immunity, such as severe combined immunodeficiency disease or Wiskott-Aldrich syndrome, those receiving intrauterine transfusions or neonatal exchange transfusion, and those receiving cellular blood components from family members or those who are genetically similar to the recipient. Extremely premature neonates are also considered by many to be at significant risk for TA-GVHD.[22,56]

No effective therapy is available for TA-GVHD, and owing to bone marrow hypoplasia, the mortality rate is 90% in the pediatric population. Fortunately, this complication can be prevented by pretransfusion gamma irradiation of cellular blood components at a dose of 2.5 Gy, which effectively abolishes lymphocyte proliferation.[31] The shelf life of irradiated RBCs is 28 days; however, no data currently exist on the safety in the neonatal population of gamma-irradiated RBCs that are stored for this amount of time. Because potassium and free hemoglobin increase after irradiation and storage of RBCs, it is preferable to irradiate cellular blood products close to administration time for neonates, who may not be able to tolerate high potassium loads.[17] There exists no "standard of care" regarding irradiation of blood products for otherwise not high-risk infants. Many transfusion centers irradiate all cellular blood products given to preterm infants

born weighing 1.0 to 1.2 kg or less, whereas some neonatal centers irradiate all cellular blood products for infants younger than 4 months, citing the lack of clinical studies on the incidence of TA-GVHD in the neonatal population and the concern for failing to recognize an infant with an undiagnosed congenital immunodeficiency. When an infant requires irradiated blood components, all cellular blood components for that infant should be irradiated; however, it is not necessary to irradiate acellular blood components, such as fresh frozen plasma (FFP). The known and presumed indications for irradiation of blood components for neonates are listed in Box 46-12.

Transfusion-Associated Infections

Many infectious agents can be transmitted by blood or blood component transfusion (Table 46-23). These include viruses, bacteria, protozoa, and other pathogens. Current transfusion-transmitted disease testing for allogeneic blood donation include hepatitis B surface antigen (HBsAg), hepatitis B core antibody (anti-HBc), anti-hepatitis C antibody (anti-HCV), antibody to HIV-1 and HIV-2 (anti-HIV-1/2), antibody to HTLV-I and HTLV-II, serology for syphilis and *Trypanosoma cruzi*, and nucleic acid testing (NAT) for HIV-1, HIV-2, HCV, and West Nile virus (WNV).[46]

CYTOMEGALOVIRUS

The prevalence of human CMV is 30% to 70% in blood donors and varies based on demographic differences within areas of the United States. This DNA virus remains latent within the leukocytes of immune persons and can be transmitted by transfusion of cellular blood components into seronegative recipients. Primary CMV infection occurs in a seronegative recipient from a blood component from a donor who has either active or latent infection. There is wide variation in clinical sequelae from transfusion-transmitted CMV (TT-CMV), ranging from asymptomatic serologic conversion to significant morbidity and mortality from CMV-related pneumonia, cytopenias, and hepatic dysfunction. Premature

---

BOX 46-12 Indications for Administering Irradiated Blood Components to Neonates

- Transfusion to a premature infant with birthweight <1200 g
- Intrauterine transfusion
- Known or suspected congenital cellular immunodeficiency
- Significant immunosuppression related to chemotherapy or radiation treatment
- Transfusion of a cellular blood component obtained from a blood relative
- Transfusion of an HLA-matched or platelet crossmatched product

Modified from Josephson CD: Neonatal and pediatric transfusion practice. In Roback JD, editor: *Technical manual of the American Association of Blood Banks*, 16th ed, Bethesda, MD, 2008, American Association of Blood Banks, pp 639-663; and Roseff SD, et al: Guidelines for assessing appropriateness of pediatric transfusion, *Transfusion*, 42:1398, 2002.

TABLE 46-23   Transfusion-Transmitted Infections

Infectious Agent	Infectious Risk
Bacterial contamination	(*Yersinia enterocolitica*, *Escherichia coli*, *Brucella* species)
Platelets	1 in 5000
Red blood cells	1 in 5 million
Hepatitis A	1 in 10 million
Hepatitis B	1 in 250,000 to 350,000
Hepatitis C	1 in 1.8 million
Human immunodeficiency virus	1 in 2.3 million
Cytomegalovirus	Unknown
Human T-cell lymphotrophic virus	1 in 641,000 to 921,000
West Nile virus	Extremely low
Chagas disease (*Trypanosoma cruzi*)	Extremely low*
Syphilis	Virtually nonexistent
Malaria	1 in 4 million
Babesiosis (*Babesia microti*)	Extremely low[†]
Creutzfeldt-Jakob disease	No cases reported in United States

*Although about 1 in 25,000 to 50,000 U.S. donors are seropositive, only 7 cases of transfusion-transmitted *T. cruzi* have been reported in the United States and Canada.
[†]May be as high as 1 in 1800 in highly endemic areas (Northeast United States).
Data from references 5, 18, and 35.

seronegative neonates weighting less than 1250 g, fetuses receiving intrauterine transfusions, severely immunocompromised individuals, and recipients of hematopoietic stem cell and solid-organ transplants are recipient groups at increased risk for post-transfusion CMV-related morbidity and mortality.[35] Infants born to seropositive mothers apparently have decreased risk for acquiring TT-CMV, but perinatal infection with a different strain of CMV has been reported infrequently.

Because the prevalence of CMV seropositivity among blood donors limits the availability of seronegative components, supplementary strategies can be used to minimize the risk for TT-CMV infection in high-risk infants. Use of third-generation leukoreduction filters at the time of collection of cellular products has been recommended for recipients at risk for TT-CMV. The American Association of Blood Banks states that leukoreduced blood products must contain fewer than 5×10^6 total WBCs per unit. Current third-generation leukocyte reduction filters consistently provide WBC reduction in accordance with these standards, with some filters yielding less than 1×10^6 per product. European standards maintain a more stringent definition of leukoreduced as less than 1×10^6 total WBCs per unit.[35]

Leukocyte reduction has been shown to be effective in preventing CMV infection in neonates, among other groups; however, whether leukocyte reduction is as efficacious as the use of CMV-seronegative blood has been disputed widely. In one study, equivalent rates of post-transfusion CMV infection in allogeneic hematopoietic stem cell transplant recipients were found for CMV-seronegative units and leukoreduced units (1.4% versus 2.4%, respectively).[12] A subsequent study

demonstrated similar rates of TT-CMV for leukoreduced and CMV-seronegative platelet products, but not for RBC products.[42] No formal consensus on the debate of equivalency has been developed, leading many to advise against the elimination of "dual inventories" of blood products for CMV-seronegative and seropositive units. Nonetheless, variable strategies for preventing TT-CMV currently exist depending on the number of high-risk patients treated at a given center, the regional donor demographics, and product availability.

HEPATITIS A VIRUS

Post-transfusion hepatitis A infection is an infrequent complication of transfusion because of the short period of viremia and the lack of an asymptomatic carrier state associated with the hepatitis A virus.[19] The risk for hepatitis A transmission increases when the transfused product is derived from a pool of products, such as cryoprecipitate and plasma-derived clotting factors. Purification processes used to treat derivatives of human plasma are ineffective against nonenveloped viruses such as hepatitis A.

HEPATITIS B VIRUS

Acute infection with hepatitis B virus (HBV) is symptomatic in about 50% of adults, and 5% to 10% of those infected become chronic carriers.[19] In contrast, HBV infection acquired in infancy and early childhood is often asymptomatic, yet 70% of those infected become chronic carriers. Elimination of paid blood donors, uniform screening of blood donations for HBV surface antigen (HBsAg), and routine immunization for hepatitis B have reduced the estimated incidence of transfusion-transmitted HBV (TT-HBV) to 1 in 150,000 to 300,000 units transfused. The residual risk for TT-HBV is attributed to infection from units of donors who donated within the HBsAg-negative window of early infection, donors who are chronic carriers with a level of HBsAg below the level of detection, and donors infected with a mutant strain of HBV that is not detected by current testing.[18]

HEPATITIS C VIRUS

Hepatitis C virus (HCV) is a well-known cause of transfusion-associated hepatitis. Acute HCV infection is often asymptomatic and anicteric, but the likelihood of developing chronic hepatitis exceeds 60%. About 20%-30% of those with untreated chronic hepatitis develop hepatic fibrosis and cirrhosis within two decades; those with cirrhosis have a 1% to 5% risk for hepatocellular carcinoma 20 years after cirrhosis is diagnosed.[35] Long-term outcome is dependent on the route of transmission, age when infected, sex, and coexisting morbidities. A retrospective study of 31 adults with transfusion-associated HCV acquired at birth (35 years earlier) described a milder disease with slower progression to hepatic fibrosis in perinatally acquired HCV compared with those who acquire HCV in early adulthood.[15,33] In a recent lookback study involving previously transfused infants and children, 88% of those with silent infection (positive anti-HCV enzyme immunoassay) had persistent HCV viremia 10 years after transfusion. This is in contrast to previously reported pediatric HCV clearance rates of 45% and 42% 19.5 and 35 years after transfusion, respectively, which indicated that children, unlike adults, may clear HCV over time.[33] Pediatric clinical trials are underway to determine the implications of early identification of those with silent HCV infection and the impact antiviral therapy may have on viral clearance and prevention of the long-term effects of HCV infection.

Since the advent of nucleic acid testing (NAT) for HCV in the late 1990s, the incidence of TT-HCV has decreased to 1 in 1.8 to1.9 million within the United States. This is due to shorter window periods from time of acute infection to laboratory markers of infection (16 to 32 days) within the donor population.[18,35]

HUMAN IMMUNODEFICIENCY VIRUS TYPES 1 AND 2

The retroviruses HIV-1 and HIV-2 are the agents responsible for AIDS. In the United States, most AIDS cases are related to HIV-1. About 1.9% of all reported cases of AIDS have been attributed to HIV-1 transmission by blood components, excluding factor concentrates.[18,35] Factor concentrates were responsible for an additional 0.75% of the more than 339,000 reported transfusion-transmitted AIDS cases. Virtually all these transfusion-transmitted infections occurred before 1985, when serologic screening for HIV was initiated, and numerous effective methods of viral inactivation for plasma-derived clotting factor concentrates subsequently became available. Today, the risk for HIV transmission from blood transfusion is less than 1 in 2.1 million owing to improved donor history screening and the advent of NAT testing in the late 1990s, which decreased the estimated window period to 12 to 13 days.[1]

EMERGING PATHOGENS

West Nile virus (WNV), a mosquito-borne, single-stranded RNA virus of the Flaviviridae family, has become a major public health concern since its first detection in the United States in 1999. The first cases of transfusion-transmitted WNV occurred in 2002, with growing numbers of cases through 2004. Infection results in neuroinvasive disease (meningoencephalitis, spastic paralysis) in roughly 20% of individuals, with more severe sequelae in elderly and immunocompromised patients. WNV NAT testing was implemented in 2003, and since being implemented through 2004, more than 1000 blood components from 519 WNV-positive donors have been identified, preventing release.[55] There have been 9 WNV transfusion transmissions since WNV NAT implementation, representing window period donations.[5]

Continuous attention is being paid to emerging infections such as WNV, *T. cruzi*, babesiosis, variant Creutzfeldt-Jakob disease, and malaria, among others. Despite extensive donor screening and laboratory testing, infections can still be transmitted through blood products. Pathogen inactivation offers the advantage of eliminating the risk for infection with any nucleic acid–containing agent, which includes viruses, bacteria, protozoa, and fungi (prions excluded). However, current pathogen inactivation techniques using nucleic acid–inactivating agents are still under investigation because no single technique has proved effective for all blood components.[4,5]

Transfusion Reactions

Transfusion reactions are less common in neonates than in older children or adults. When an acute transfusion reaction occurs, it is crucial to discontinue the transfusion immediately, maintain intravenous access, and verify that the correct unit was transfused while treating the patient's symptoms. Notifying the transfusion service for further laboratory evaluation of the reaction is essential to properly classify the reaction so that the patient can be managed appropriately.

FEBRILE NONHEMOLYTIC TRANSFUSION REACTIONS

Febrile nonhemolytic transfusion reactions (FNHTRs) are characterized by fever, chills, and diaphoresis. These reactions are believed to result from the release of pyrogenic cytokines by leukocytes within the plasma during storage. The incidence of FNHTRs has been decreased dramatically since the implementation of prestorage leukoreduction of RBCs and platelet products in 1999. Whereas FNHTRs occurred in about 10% of transfusions in the past, the incidence for all products since the introduction of leukoreduction is now 0.1% to 3% (about 0.2% for prestorage leukoreduction).[27,43] When FNHTR is suspected, the transfusion should be stopped and more serious reactions ruled out. A sample of blood from the patient may be sent to the laboratory for direct antibody testing (DAT), plasma hemoglobin quantification, serum lactate dehydrogenase level, and bilirubin level to ensure that the patient is not experiencing a hemolytic transfusion reaction. Bacterial contamination should be assessed by cultures of the transfused product and the patient's blood; empirical antibiotic therapy may be warranted. Most FNHTRs respond to antipyretics, and meperidine may be used for rigors.

The utility of premedication with antipyretics to prevent FNHTRs is controversial. Although a retrospective analysis of 385 pediatric patients receiving 7900 transfusions demonstrated no difference in the incidence of FNHTRs in those who received premedication with acetaminophen and dyphenhydramine,[54] a recent prospective, double-blind, placebo-controlled study of 315 adult oncology patients receiving

4199 transfusions revealed a marginal benefit with premedication in terms of reducing FNHTRs (0.34% for premedicated versus 0.64% for placebo; $P = 0.08$).[25]

ALLERGIC TRANSFUSION REACTIONS

Allergic transfusion reactions (ATRs) are marked by urticaria and itching but can include flushing, bronchospasm, and anaphylaxis in severe cases. For mild or localized cases, transfusion can be continued once symptoms have subsided; however, severe allergic reactions (anaphylactoid or anaphylactic reactions) may require treatment with corticosteroids or epinephrine, or both. The same blood unit should never be restarted in severe cases, even after symptoms have abated. Leukoreduction does not decrease the incidence of ATRs, as it has for FNHTRs.[43] Premedication with antihistamines with or without steroids is recommended for ATRs. Because these reactions are caused by an antibody response in a sensitized recipient to soluble plasma proteins within the blood product, washed RBCs and platelets may be used for severe or recurrent ATRs nonresponsive to medication. Severe ATRs leading to anaphylaxis can often be due to the development of anti-immunoglobulin A (anti-IgA) antibodies in recipients who are IgA deficient. In these instances, IgA-deficient plasma products may be obtained, but they require the use of rare donor registries.[59]

HEMOLYTIC TRANSFUSION REACTIONS

Acute hemolytic transfusion reactions occur when RBCs are transfused to a recipient with preformed antibodies to antigens on the transfused RBCs. Almost all acute hemolytic transfusion reaction fatalities are the result of transfusion of ABO-incompatible blood due to clerical errors and misidentification; however, nonimmune causes of acute hemolysis may also occur. These include hemolysis from shear or heat stress, or both, imposed on erythrocytes by extracorporeal circuits, infusion devices, filters, blood warmers, or phototherapy light exposure. These reactions are characterized by fever, chills, diaphoresis, abdominal pain, hypotension, and hemoglobinuria with potential progression to disseminated intravascular coagulopathy and acute renal failure. When a hemolytic transfusion reaction is suspected, the transfusion should be immediately stopped, blood cultures (from patient and blood components) should be obtained, and the blood bank should be notified. A clerical check, blood component inspection, post-transfusion hemolysis check, and DAT should be completed by the blood bank. The patient's hemoglobin, hematocrit, serum bilirubin, lactate dehydrogenase, and urobilinogen should be monitored, and intravenous fluids should be administered to offset hypotension and ensure adequate urine output. Mannitol may be administered to force diuresis, but osmotic diuresis in neonates is controversial because of concerns about alterations in cerebral microcirculation and risk for intraventricular hemorrhage. Although infants younger than 4 months have an absence of A and B hemagglutinins and other RBC alloantibodies, maternal IgG antibodies can cross the placenta, causing hemolysis of transfused RBCs, and, therefore, should be considered when transfusing infants.[16]

Delayed hemolytic transfusion reactions occur 3 to 10 days after RBC transfusion and manifest as unexplained anemia, hyperbilirubinemia, and abdominal pain. As with acute hemolytic reactions, the diagnosis is confirmed by a positive DAT, hyperbilirubinemia, and a reduction in hemoglobin. Delayed hemolytic transfusion reactions are extremely rare in neonates because of the immaturity of the immune system. Even though there have been case reports of anti-E and anti-Kell formation in infants as young as 18 days of life, most reports have supported the infrequency of RBC alloimmunization and delayed hemolytic transfusion reactions in infants younger than 4 months.[35,58]

TRANSFUSION-RELATED ACUTE LUNG INJURY

Transfusion-related acute lung injury (TRALI) is an uncommon, potentially fatal acute immune-related transfusion reaction, which typically occurs within 4 hours of transfusion and presents with respiratory distress due to noncardiogenic pulmonary edema (normal central venous pressure and pulmonary capillary wedge pressure), hypotension, fever, and severe hypoxemia. Differentiation from transfusion-associated circulatory overload, an acute, nonimmune transfusion reaction that presents with respiratory distress, cardiogenic pulmonary edema, and hypertension due to volume overload, is important because treatments differ. Furthermore, transient leukopenia, which is commonly seen with TRALI but is absent in transfusion-associated circulatory overload, can aid in differentiation of these reactions. Symptoms of TRALI usually improve within 48 to 96 hours; however, three fourths of patients require aggressive respiratory support. Treatment is mainly supportive, including fluid or vasopressor support in the face of hypotension. Although aggressive diuresis is often required in transfusion-associated circulatory overload, this should be avoided in TRALI.[29]

Although the exact mechanism of TRALI remains uncertain, it is generally believed to be caused by the passive transmission of HLA or neutrophil antibodies directed against recipient leukocytes. These antibodies activate and sequester recipient neutrophils within the endothelium of the lungs, ultimately leading to the production of vasoactive mediators and capillary leak. Plasma products (FFP, apheresis platelets) account for most severe TRALI cases, and multiparous women are the most commonly implicated donors.[29,52] Because of these findings, various preventative measures have been adopted in the United States and elsewhere. These include the use of male-only high-volume plasma products (FFP, platelets), or the selection of donor products from donors who have a low likelihood of being alloimmunized by pregnancy or prior transfusions. Although there have been no definitive cases of TRALI documented in the neonatal population, TRALI has been well documented in children. A case has been reported of a 4-month-old girl who experienced respiratory distress, hypoxemia, hypotension, and fever within 2 hours of completion of an RBC transfusion from her mother. HLA antibodies were identified in the mother's serum, demonstrating the possible role of HLA antibodies in the pathogenesis of TRALI in the setting of a designated blood transfusion between mother and infant.[52,61]

DONOR-SPECIFIC UNITS
Autologous Red Blood Cell Transfusions

Collection of autologous umbilical cord blood was first reported in 1992. Depending on the gestational age of the infant, the umbilical cord contains 75 to 120 mL of blood.

Although the procedure has been associated with bacterial contamination rates as high as 8.6% and the smallest volumes of RBCs are collected from the most premature infants, interest in autologous collection remains.[13,32] Additional large, randomized, controlled clinical trials are needed to validate the safety and efficacy of this process. Delayed clamping of the umbilical cord of premature infants has been reported as a successful variation of autologous transfusion. Meta-analysis of 454 preterm infants showed that delayed cord clamping (>30 seconds) is safe and is associated with higher circulating blood volumes during the first 24 hours of life, decreased immediate need of blood transfusions, and a decreased incidence of intraventricular hemorrhage.[47]

Parental Blood Donation

Concern about transfusion-associated infections has encouraged directed donor blood programs, including those that allow biologic parents to serve as directed donors for their neonates. No data exist to support the contention that directed donor programs increase safety, and parental blood products are a poor choice in neonates with immune-mediated hemolysis, hemolytic disease of the newborn, or neonatal alloimmune thrombocytopenia. In these cases, transfused paternal cells express the antigens to which the mother has been sensitized and are passively transferred through the placenta to the neonate. Maternal plasma may contain alloantibodies directed against paternal RBC, leukocyte, platelet, and HLA antigens. Antileukocyte and antiplatelet antibodies have been found in 16% and 12% of mothers, respectively.[20] Transfusion of any maternal blood component containing plasma exposes the infant to these antibodies, with the potential to cause significant hemolytic, thrombocytopenic, or pulmonary reactions. Given these concerns, when parental directed donation is considered for an infant, the following recommendations should be reviewed with families and the provider[10,11]:

- All parental cellular blood components must be irradiated before transfusion to the neonate to prevent TA-GVHD.
- If maternal RBCs or platelets are transfused, they should be given as washed cells or should be plasma reduced, and irradiated.
- Fathers are not recommended as RBC donors for their newborns.
- Fathers should not donate granulocytes or platelets to their infants unless maternal serum is shown to lack lymphocytotoxic antibodies.

BLOOD PRODUCTS
Red Blood Cell Transfusion

INDICATIONS

In the first few days of life, term infants have an elevated hemoglobin concentration (14 to 20 g/dL); however, because of physiologic decreases in erythropoietin (EPO) levels, hemoglobin concentration decreases to a nadir of 10 to 12 g/dL about 2 to 3 months before beginning to rise. This is referred to as the *physiologic anemia of infancy*. In preterm infants, this anemia is more significant with mean nadirs of 8 g/dL in

infants with very low birthweight (1.0 to 1.5 kg), and 7 g/dL in infants with extremely low birthweight (<1 kg). This is the result of lower hemoglobin concentrations at birth, frequent blood sampling, low total blood volume-to-sampling ratio, increased risk for other comorbidities, and diminished capacity of the premature infant to increase EPO.[11] Normal ranges of hemoglobin and hematocrit have been established for term and premature infants; however, guidelines for RBC transfusion therapy remain controversial because there are few randomized controlled studies that address appropriate neonatal transfusion triggers. Current guidelines for replacement transfusion therapy in neonates are given in Box 46-13. Infants with significant cardiac or respiratory disease generally receive more aggressive RBC transfusion therapy.[51,60] Two recent studies attempted to address high versus low threshold transfusion guidelines based on level of respiratory support in infants with very low or extremely low birthweight. Although very different in design and outcome, neither study clearly established an appropriate hemoglobin target. Although the multi-institutional Canadian Premature Infants in Need of Transfusion study[28] demonstrated no advantage for liberal transfusion practices, the Bell and colleagues' study[9] suggested that restrictive transfusion was associated with more apneic episodes, intraparenchymal brain hemorrhage, and periventricular leukomalacia. The question of long-term neurodevelopmental outcome is how being addressed in both infant study groups.[60]

Most RBC transfusions in newborns are administered to either replace blood loss or treat anemia of prematurity. Blood loss can result from hemorrhage or phlebotomy. Iatrogenic losses from phlebotomy can be considerable but can be minimized by judicious testing strategies, sampling from indwelling catheters, using microtainers for laboratory assays, and implementing point-of-care testing.

The use of recombinant human EPO has been proposed to decrease neonatal transfusion burden, donor exposure, anemia of prematurity, and other comorbidities. Meta-analysis of late (>8 days of life) EPO use involving 1302 preterm infants showed no clear benefit in terms of significantly decreasing

---

BOX 46–13 Guidelines for Red Blood Cell Replacement

IN HIGH-RISK NEONATES
- For severe cardiopulmonary disease*
  Maintain hematocrit >40%-45%
- For moderate cardiopulmonary disease:
  Maintain hematocrit >30%-35%
- For major surgery:
  Maintain hematocrit >30%-35%
- For infants with stable anemia†:
  Maintain hematocrit >20%

*Severe cardiopulmonary disease defined as: requiring mechanical ventilation with >0.35 FiO₂.
†Especially if unexplained breathing disorders, tachycardia, or poor growth.
Modified from Strauss RG: How I transfuse red blood cells and platelets to infants with anemia and thrombocytopenia of prematurity, *Transfusion*, 48:209, 2008; and Widness JA: Treatment and prevention of neonatal anemia, *NeoReviews*, 9:e526, 2008.

donor exposures, nor was there any effect on incidence of comorbidities. Although late administration of EPO reduced the number of RBC transfusions per infant and the total transfused volume of RBCs per infant, the clinical impact of these results is trivial (<1 transfusion per infant and 7 mL/kg of RBCs). Avoiding the use of RBC transfusions was not demonstrated because many infants had received one or more transfusion prior to receiving EPO at study entry.[2] A subsequent meta-analysis designed to assess the effectiveness and safety of early initiation of EPO (<8 days of life) in 1825 premature infants also showed no evidence of any substantial benefits with regard to donor blood exposure; however, a statistically significant increased risk for retinopathy of prematurity (higher than stage 3) was noted in neonates who received early EPO therapy. Again, RBC transfusion was not avoided when RBC transfusion before study entry was considered.[36,41] Therefore, no conclusive evidence currently exists that either early or late EPO use offers any clear benefit in regard to donor exposure or improvement of morbidity or mortality in preterm infants, and that early EPO use may increase risk for retinopathy of prematurity in the neonatal population with very low birthweight. The use of EPO as a neuroprotectant is under investigation.

PRETRANSFUSION TESTING

Before RBC transfusion, a blood sample is obtained for ABO and Rh determination (blood group and type) and to screen for antibodies against blood group antigens.[46] Because antibodies identified in the neonate's blood are most often of maternal origin, maternal blood can often serve as the source of serum and plasma for the antibody screen. A newborn's ABO group is assigned solely on the testing of the patient's RBCs for the A and B antigens (forward typing) because the isohemagglutinins anti-A and anti-B are not present in the serum at birth. The use of cord blood specimens for infant blood type determination is discouraged because of possible contamination with Wharton's jelly and because of concerns about proper identification of the specimen.

If the newborn's antibody screen is negative, ABO- and Rh-specific RBCs may be transfused, and the antibody screen does not need to be repeated during the infant's hospitalization during the first 4 months of life. If the screening identifies passively acquired maternal blood group antibodies, as in Rh hemolytic disease of the newborn, O-negative RBCs should be transfused until repeat testing is negative for antibodies reacting against the ABO- or Rh-specific units. When antibodies to other RBC antigens other than D are detected, blood should be selected that is ABO and Rh specific but negative for the identified antibody. In cases in which reconstituted whole blood is needed for large-volume transfusion procedures (i.e., exchange transfusions, cardiopulmonary bypass, extracorporeal membrane oxygenation [ECMO]), the neonate may be given plasma that is ABO compatible with the neonate's RBCs, but receive RBCs that are compatible with maternal serum. This may mean that the ABO group of the RBC and FFP units are different. An alternative used by some transfusion centers entails the use of low isohemagglutinin titer, group-O whole blood, if available.[11] Infants whose Rh-negative mothers were treated with Rh immune globulin (RhIG) during pregnancy often have a positive DAT, owing to circulating anti-D antibody from the RhIG. The clinician

must distinguish this situation from Rh hemolytic disease of the newborn.

In infants older than 4 months, repeat testing for blood group, Rh type, and antibody screening is performed within 72 hours of each RBC transfusion if the patient has received a transfusion during the past 3 months, or if the history is uncertain or unavailable.[46] Reverse ABO blood group testing, which detects anti-A and anti-B antibodies, is frequently deferred for the first 6 months of life because this testing is often weak or nonreactive in babies less than 1 year of age.

RED BLOOD CELL PREPARATIONS

RBC viability and functional activity require that RBCs be preserved in additive solutions that support their metabolic demands. All anticoagulant-preservative (AP) solutions contain citrate, phosphate, and dextrose (CPD), which function as an anticoagulant, a buffer, and a source of RBC metabolic energy, respectively. The addition of mannitol and adenine to existing additive solutions has increased the shelf life of RBCs from 21 days (CPD) to 35 days (CPDA-1) and to 42 days for newer AP solutions (Adsol, Optisol, Nutricell) by stabilizing the RBC membrane and maintaining 2.3-diphosphoglycenate and adenosine triphosphate within erythrocytes. Studies have shown that extended-storage preservative solutions are safe and as efficacious as CPDA-1 RBCs in increasing the hematocrit for neonates receiving small-volume (10 to 15 mL/kg) RBC transfusions.[23,57] However, no clinical studies have confirmed or refuted the effect of an AP on metabolic abnormalities in massive transfusion for the neonate. Therefore, many experts recommend avoiding RBCs stored in extended-storage media (Adsol, Optisol, Nutricell) for large-volume transfusions until such data have been published.

The highest relative blood volumes (in mL/kg) are found in neonates. Adult blood volumes on a per kilogram basis are achieved by 3 months of age (Table 46-24). A typical replacement transfusion is 10 to 15 mL of RBCs per kilogram. Because infants are so small, many pediatric transfusion centers dispense small aliquots from one RBC unit (300 to 350 mL) to one or several neonates who require multiple transfusions in order to decrease donor exposure and to conserve RBC inventory. This practice requires sterile connecting devices to ensure that the original RBC unit remains a closed system, and transfer packs or syringe sets that permit multiple aliquots to be removed. Studies have shown that CPDA-1 and AS-3 preserved split RBC packs effectively limit donor exposures and are safe for use in neonatal small-volume transfusions after 35 days of storage.[37]

TABLE 46-24 Estimated Blood Volumes

Age	Blood Volume (mL/kg)
Premature infant	90-105
Term newborn	82-86
1-7 days	78-86
1-12 months	72-78

From Price DC, et al: In Handmaker H, et al, editors: *Nuclear medicine in clinical pediatrics*, New York, 1975, Society of Nuclear Medicine, p 279.

Because RBC units are stored at 4° to 6°C, hypothermia can develop after massive transfusion unless the blood products are first warmed to body temperature. Inline blood warmers should be used for all RBC exchange transfusions, and radiant heaters should be avoided because they can result in hemolysis of the RBC component. When phototherapy is in progress, the blood component and tubing should be positioned to minimize exposure to phototherapy light, which may also cause hemolysis.[24]

Platelet Transfusion

INDICATIONS

As with older children and adults, platelet transfusions are administered to neonates therapeutically or prophylactically to prevent the hemorrhagic complications of thrombocytopenia. Neonates have different risks for bleeding given the same degree of thrombocytopenia. For example, thrombocytopenic neonates with neonatal alloimmune thrombocytopenia have a high risk for major bleeding, whereas those with sepsis or necrotizing enterocolitis and those with intrauterine growth restriction have an intermediate and low risk for major hemorrhage, respectively. Differences in platelet function or concurrent coagulopathy are likely causes for these discrepancies. The only randomized, controlled trial addressing whether platelet transfusions reduce major bleeding in neonates found no benefit of maintaining a normal platelet count (platelets >150,000/μL) in preterm neonates compared with those maintained at >50,000/μL. However, this study did not address bleeding risk or transfusion benefit for neonates with platelet counts below 50,000/μL.[7]

A number of platelet transfusion guidelines for the newborn have been proposed; however, given the lack of clinical trials addressing absolute bleeding risk in thrombocytopenia caused by different etiologies, they are based on expert panel recommendations garnered from clinical experience. Furthermore, because of the concern for intraventricular hemorrhage in the sick neonate, many physicians have traditionally adopted a fairly aggressive platelet threshold for transfusion. Murray and colleagues retrospectively studied 53 neonates (44 preterm) with severe thrombocytopenia and concluded that a threshold of 30,000/μL without other risk factors, or previous intraventricular hemorrhage, is safe for most neonates.[39] Thus, a generally accepted transfusion trigger for a platelet count of less than 30,000/μL has been endorsed for neonates without other risk factors, whereas some experts propose a higher trigger (<50,000/μL) for neonates with extremely low birthweight within the first week of life, clinically unstable neonates, and neonates with neonatal alloimmune thrombocytopenia (using HPA-compatible platelet products).[24a,49] Platelet transfusions are also indicated to treat hemorrhage associated with acquired (i.e., ECMO, cardiopulmonary bypass, uremia) or congenital qualitative platelet abnormalities (i.e., Glanzmann thrombasthenia, Bernard-Soulier syndrome), even if the platelet count is within the normal range.

PRETRANSFUSION TESTING

Platelets express intrinsic ABO antigens, but not Rh antigens. They should be ABO-group specific whenever possible, owing to reports of intravascular hemolysis following transfusion of ABO-incompatible platelets in infants and children.[8] Platelets do not routinely require crossmatching. If ABO-incompatible platelets must be used, plasma removal through volume reduction or washing or by selecting low isohemagglutinin (anti-A, anti-B) titer units are options. Routine volume reduction methods for all neonates should be avoided because about 20% of platelets are lost in the final product, which is resuspended in either saline or compatible plasma. Although Rh matching does not affect post-transfusion platelet survival, RBCs are present in small amounts of whole blood-derived platelet concentrate and can cause Rh sensitization in an Rh-negative recipient. A unit of whole blood derived platelets contains approximately 0.2-0.3 mL RBCs. Administration of RhIG should be strongly considered for any Rh-negative neonate, especially girls, within 72 hours of exposure to Rh-positive RBCs through a platelet transfusion. The recommended dose is 120 IU RhIG per 1 mL of RBCs transfused, administered intramuscularly (90 IU RhIG per 1 mL of RBCs intravenously).[26] When aliquots of apheresis platelets, which are relatively RBC free, are used, there should be limited to no concern for Rh sensitization.

COMPONENT DEFINITION

A standard unit of platelets, prepared from a single donation of whole blood, contains at least 5.5×10^{10} platelets in 50 to 70 mL of plasma. Apheresis platelets, often called single-donor platelets, contain a minimum of 3×10^{11} platelets in about 250 mL (range, 200 to 400 mL) of plasma, the equivalent of an estimated 6 units of whole blood-derived platelets. Single-donor platelets are split for neonatal use and offer the advantage of avoiding multiple donor exposures. Platelets are optimally stored at 20° to 24°C under constant agitation and have a shelf life of 5 days after collection. Transfusion of 10 to 15 mL/kg of platelets for neonates, or 0.1 to 0.2 unit/kg for children over 10 kg, should yield a platelet increment of 50,000/μL to 100,000/μL if no predisposing risk factors for refractoriness exist. It is important to account for device-related dead space (10 to 30 mL) when issuing the product because this can be considerable in relation to the overall platelet dose. The expected rise in the platelet count after transfusion may not be met because of destructive thrombocytopenia such as occurs with splenomegaly, fever, sepsis, disseminated intravascular coagulation, bleeding, or antibiotic therapy. Immune-mediated causes of platelet refractoriness, such as alloantibodies to platelet specific antigens (i.e. HPA-1a, 5b) in neonatal autoimmune thrombocytopenia, and autoantibodies to common platelet antigens in idiopathic thrombocytopenic purpura, require consideration in this population, so that appropriate management can be initiated.[11]

Granulocyte Transfusion

Neonates, particularly those with very low birthweight, are susceptible to overwhelming bacterial infection. Many factors contribute to this risk, including disruption of mucosal barriers, hypogammaglobulinemia, and qualitative neutrophil defects. Furthermore, preterm neonates may become neutropenic during sepsis, owing to a reduced capacity to increase myeloid progenitor cell proliferation with infections. Transfusion of granulocytes has been employed in the treatment of neonatal sepsis; however, the efficacy of such transfusions is controversial. Meta-analysis of the safety and efficacy of granulocyte infusion adjunctive to antimicrobial therapy in the treatment of septic neutropenic neonates failed to show that granulocyte infusions reduce morbidity or mortality.[38] However, granulocyte transfusion may be considered in neonates with qualitative neutrophil defects with severe (or progressive) bacterial or fungal infection, who have not responded to appropriate aggressive antimicrobial treatment.[51]

Granulocyte concentrates for neonatal transfusion are prepared by automated leukapheresis of healthy stimulated (dexamethasone with or without granulocyte colony-stimulating factor) donors and contain 1 to 2×10^9 neutrophils per kilogram in a volume of 10 to 15 mL/kg. Treatment should be continued daily until clinical improvement or neutrophil count recovery (absolute neutrophil count >3000/μL in first week of life; >1500/μL thereafter). All granulocytes should be gamma-irradiated and CMV negative because leukodepletion is contraindicated. Because granulocyte concentrates have a significant amount of RBCs (Hct, 15% to 20%), the component must be ABO, Rh, and crossmatch compatible with the intended neonatal recipient. Because granulocytes must be transfused within 24 hours of collection, U.S. Food and Drug Administration–mandated testing for blood products will not be completed before the product is released for administration, and therefore the risks and benefits of transfusing an untested blood product must be weighed by the medical team and the parents of the infant.[11]

There are unique risks to granulocyte transfusion. They include varying degrees of pulmonary reactions, from mild transient respiratory distress to severe pulmonary edema, hypoxia, and acute respiratory distress syndrome, and a high incidence of febrile transfusion reactions. Pulmonary complications have been reported in 4% of transfused infants,[38] and severe pulmonary reactions resembling TRALI have been reported.[40] Mild to moderate reactions occur in 25% to 50% and severe reactions in about 1% of all granulocyte transfusions. Administration of amphotericin B treatment should be not given within 6 hours of granulocytes owing to suspected increased risk for severe pulmonary reactions.

Although granulocyte colony-stimulating factor and granulocyte-macrophage colony-stimulating factor have been used successfully to stimulate neutrophil numbers, and intravenous immune globulin has been attempted to augment traditional antimicrobial therapy to support septic neonates, data on efficacy are inconclusive.[14,53] Because of the lack of clear consensus on their impact on improving host defense mechanisms and improving outcomes, these adjuncts to standard antimicrobial and antifungal therapy need further investigation.

Fresh-Frozen Plasma Transfusion

Plasma can be prepared by either whole blood separation or by apheresis. When the plasma product is frozen to −18°C or colder within 8 hours of collection, it is labeled as FFP (about 250 to 300 mL) and can be stored at this temperature for up to 1 year.[11] To conserve plasma inventory and limit donor exposures for infants who receive only fractions of an FFP unit, plasma can be separated into a system of multiple satellite bags and frozen as aliquots. Once thawed, FFP can be further subdivided into aliquots for multiple neonates by sterile connecting devices, stored at 1° to 6°C for up to 5 days and transfused as *thawed plasma*.[24] Although thawed plasma has about 40% factor V and VIII (heat labile factors) activity, effective hemostasis is maintained at this level, making thawed plasma clinically similar to FFP.

FFP is used primarily to treat acquired coagulation factor deficiencies as a result of disseminated intravascular coagulation, liver failure, vitamin K deficiency from malabsorption, biliary disease or warfarin therapy, or dilutional coagulopathy from massive transfusion. It can also be used for specific factor replacement in congenital factor deficiencies (e.g., factor X, factor XI, protein C, protein S, antithrombin) when specific factor concentrates or recombinant products are not manufactured or unavailable.[11,24,46] FFP is not indicated for volume expansion, for enhancement of wound healing, or as first-line treatment for congenital factor deficiencies when either a virally inactivated plasma-derived factor concentrate or recombinant factor is available.

Plasma transfusions should be ABO compatible with the neonate's RBCs to avoid passive transfer of isohemagglutinins from ABO-incompatible plasma resulting in hemolysis.[24] Because the freezing process renders the frozen-thawed plasma component free of viable leukocytes, FFP is not screened for CMV antibody, nor are leukoreduction and irradiation necessary for the prevention of CMV reactivation and TA-GVHD, respectively. However, passive administration of antibody to CMV in FFP may cause CMV IgG testing to become positive in the transfused neonate. This does not represent CMV infection, and the antibody disappears in a time course consistent with the 21-day half-life of γ-globulin.[50]

FFP is typically dosed at 10 to 15 mL/kg. Assuming that 1 mL of FFP generally equates to 1 mL of factor activity, one can predict the amount of replacement of most factors after plasma transfusion. For example, for a *preterm* infant, the calculations are as follows:

1. 1 mL of factor activity = 1 mL FFP
2. Total blood volume (TBV) = Weight (kg) × 100 mL/kg
3. Total plasma volume (TPV) = TBV × (1 − Hct)
4. Unit of factor needed = TPV × (desired factor [%] − initial factor [%])

Example: 1 kg preterm infant, with Hct: 55%; the desired increment in a given factor of 30%:

$$TBV = 100 \text{ mL, and } TPV = 45 \text{ mL}$$
$$\text{Units of Factor needed} = 45 \times (0.30) = 15 \text{ mL}$$
$$\text{Amount of FFP needed} = 15 \text{ mL (or 15 mL/kg)}$$

Using these calculations for a *preterm* infant, it is evident that 10 to 15 mL/kg of FFP will replace about 10% to 30% of most factors immediately after transfusion. It is important for the clinician to know the half-lives of the factors because factor half-lives vary. Furthermore, vitamin K-dependent factors are lower in neonates, thereby prolonging both the prothrombin time and activated partial thromboplastin time. Correlation of laboratory values to clinical status of the individual is therefore important when devising an FFP dosing schedule for a coagulopathic infant. It is critical that appropriately collected specimens for evaluation of coagulation factors be obtained in advance of FFP transfusion.

Cryoprecipitate Transfusion

Cryoprecipitate is the cold-insoluble precipitate prepared from FFP that has been thawed slowly at 1° to 6°C, the supernatant removed, and refrozen at −18°C. Each unit (bag) of cryoprecipitate is derived from a single whole blood donation and has a shelf life of up to 1 year. A unit (10 to 15 mL) of cryoprecipitate contains a minimum of 80 U of factor VIII activity and 150 mg of fibrinogen. There are no standards for the quantity of the other factors; however, there is about the same amount of von Willebrand factor and factor XIII in one unit as 10 to 15 mL/kg of FFP.[46] Therefore, it is a useful product in infants who require higher concentrations of factors VIII, XIII, von Willebrand factor, or fibrinogen levels, and who are volume restricted. Cryoprecipitate is indicated in the treatment of bleeding episodes associated with von Willebrand disease or hemophilia A only when U.S. Food and Drug Administration–licensed recombinant factor concentrates and viral inactivated pooled plasma-derived factor concentrates are not available. Cryoprecipitate is the treatment of choice for factor XIII deficiency, congenital afibrinogenemia, dysfibrinogenemia, and severe hypofibrinogenemia (<150 mg/dL) associated with bleeding.[11,50] In general, an infant should receive 1 unit of cryoprecipitate per 5 kg, which increases the total fibrinogen by about 100 mg/dL.

SPECIAL TOPICS IN NEONATAL TRANSFUSION

Exchange Transfusion

Exchange transfusion is the replacement of most or all of the recipient's RBC mass and plasma with appropriately compatible RBCs and plasma from one or more donors. The amount of blood exchanged generally is expressed in relation to the recipient's blood volume (e.g., as a single- or double-volume exchange, or a partial exchange).

INDICATIONS

Neonatal exchange transfusions are most commonly used in infants with hemolytic disease of the newborn. Double-volume exchange transfusions also are frequently used in newborns with severe jaundice from other causes to prevent kernicterus and other toxicity related to hyperbilirubinemia.[24] Bilirubin levels warranting exchange transfusion are discussed in Chapter 48. Meta-analysis has shown that intravenous immune globulin administration (0.5 to 1 g/kg) can result in significant reduction in the incidence of exchange transfusion for term infants with hemolytic disease of the newborn. Therefore, intravenous immune globulin should be considered early when serum bilirubin levels continue to rise despite aggressive phototherapy or when the bilirubin level is within 2 to 3 mg/dL of the exchange level.[3,6] Exchange transfusions can also be used, albeit infrequently, to remove exogenous (drugs) or endogenous (metabolic) toxins.

The efficiency of exchange transfusion diminishes exponentially as the procedure continues. The kinetics of exchange are very similar, regardless of whether a continuous technique (simultaneous withdrawal and replacement) or discontinuous technique (alternating withdrawal and replacement) is used.

The effectiveness of exchange transfusion varies with the component being removed. The efficiency is highest for RBC exchange. A double-volume exchange transfusion results in removal of about 85% of the neonate's RBCs; however, the amount of bilirubin or maternal alloantibody removed by exchange transfusion is significantly less (25% to 45%) because of an equilibrium between the intravascular pool and the extravascular tissues for bilirubin, antibody, and similar substances.

The optimal volume for an exchange transfusion is twice the infant's blood volume.[48] Little is gained by exceeding two blood volumes. When anticipating the volume needed for double-volume exchange, the total volume required depends on the whether the infant is preterm. For example, using $2 \times$ total blood volume (TBV):

- 2-volume exchange volume (preterm) = 100 mL/kg $\times$ 2, or 200 mL/kg
- 2-volume exchange volume (term) = 85 mL/kg $\times$ 2, or 170 mL/kg

To perform the exchange transfusion, aliquots of the reconstituted whole blood product are administered while equal amounts of the infant's blood are withdrawn, with careful attention not to exceed 5 mL/kg or 5% of TBV at a time (over 2 to 10 minutes).

CHOICE OF BLOOD COMPONENTS

Either stored whole blood if available or reconstituted whole blood (i.e., RBCs plus FFP) can be used for neonatal exchange transfusions. The RBC component should be group-O negative or ABO and Rh compatible to maternal serum for Rh hemolytic disease of the newborn. Fresh (<5 to 7 days) CPDA units should be used because the safety of extended storage media has not been amply studied for neonatal large volume transfusions. If only older CPDA units or extended storage units are available, the RBC units can be washed or the supernatant removed. The RBCs are reconstituted with AB or compatible plasma to a final hematocrit of 40% to 50%. Furthermore, components should be CMV risk reduced (leukodepletion), gamma-irradiated, and sickle negative. Both whole blood and reconstituted whole blood are deficient in platelets. Platelets are not added to reconstituted blood during an exchange because this could lead to increased microaggregate formation. Infants who are significantly thrombocytopenic (platelet count <30,000/μL) after an exchange transfusion or who are bleeding should receive platelet transfusion. For infants with hemolytic disease of the newborn caused by other RBC antibodies, the RBC product should be specifically selected to be negative for the offending antibodies.

Potential complications of exchange transfusion include hypocalcemia, hyperglycemia (with subsequent rebound hypoglycemia), dilutional thrombocytopenia, neutropenia, umbilical vein and arterial thrombosis, necrotizing enterocolitis, intracranial pressure fluctuations resulting in intraventricular hemorrhage, air embolization, and infection.[48] In a retrospective review of 55 neonates undergoing 66 exchange transfusions, most adverse events associated with exchange transfusions were asymptomatic laboratory abnormalities, with thrombocytopenia (44%), hypocalcemia (29%), and metabolic acidosis (24%), the most common abnormalities needing treatment. Adverse events were more frequent in exchanges done on preterm infants born before 32 weeks, in infants with other significant comorbidities, and when umbilical catheters were used compared with other methods of central venous access.[44]

Partial Exchange Transfusion

About 5% of all neonates are born with or develop polycythemia. Infants of diabetic mothers and neonates who are small for gestational age are at higher risk. Neonatal polycythemia is defined as a venous hematocrit greater than 65% within the first week of life. Partial exchange transfusion effectively lowers the hematocrit and reduces whole blood viscosity in polycythemic neonates who have hyperviscosity. Partial exchange transfusion is also useful for correcting severe anemia without the risk for fluid overload and heart failure.

The long-term benefit of early partial exchange transfusion in polycythemic neonates is controversial, at least partly because the prognosis for such infants depends greatly on the etiology. An hematocrit greater than 65% is generally used as the stimulus for exchange transfusion because as the hematocrit rises over this level, blood viscosity significantly increases, and oxygen transport diminishes.

A partial exchange is used to normalize the hematocrit to below 60% by removing infant whole blood and replacing with equal volume of isotonic crystalloid solution. Crystalloid solutions are preferable to plasma to decrease exposure to plasma and because necrotizing enterocolitis has been associated with the use of plasma as replacement solution. The volume of exchange required can be calculated with the following formula:

Volume of exchange (mL)

$$= \text{total blood volume (mL)}$$
$$\times \left[\frac{\text{observed Hct} - \text{desired Hct}}{\text{observed Hct}} \right]$$

Example: 1-kg preterm infant with Hct 68%, desired post-partial exchange Hct 55%

Volume of exchange (mL)

$$= 100 \text{ mL} \times \left[68 - \frac{55}{68} \right]$$
$$= \text{about 20 mL of crystalloid}$$
$$\text{exchanged with whole blood}$$

To correct severe anemia, packed RBCs are used as the replacement fluid for the whole blood withdrawn. The formula used to calculate the volume required for exchange is similar to the one above; however, the hematocrit of the RBC product used must be taken into account. RBCs in CPDA-1 usually have a hematocrit of approximately 70%; thus the formula is:

Volume of exchange (mL)

$$= \text{TBV (mL)} \times \left[\frac{\text{Desired Hct} - \text{Observed Hct}}{\text{Hct of unit} - \text{Observed Hct}} \right]$$

Example: 1-kg preterm infant with Hct 21%, desired post-partial exchange Hct 45%

Volume of exchange (mL)

$$= 100 \text{ mL} \times \left[\frac{45 - 21}{70 - 21} \right]$$
$$= 49 \text{ mL of CPDA RBCs}$$
$$\text{exchanged with whole blood}$$

If RBCs preserved in other solutions are used, the equation must be altered to take into account the average hematocrit of the product. The technique of partial exchange transfusion is similar to that used in larger-volume exchange. A discontinuous methodology is most often used; aliquots of 5 mL/kg or less should be used for each withdrawal and infusion.

Extracorporeal Membrane Oxygenation

See also Chapter 44, Part 8.

Because of the large volume of transfused RBCs used for ECMO, RBCs used in the bypass circuit should be less than 7 to 14 days old to avoid high potassium levels in older blood.[34] In the infant with presumed or suspected cellular immunodeficiency, the blood products should undergo CMV risk reduction (CMV seronegative *or* leukoreduced) and gamma irradiation. Although there is mounting anecdotal evidence that RBCs preserved in extended storage media (AS-1, AS-3) are safe for ECMO, most ECMO centers use RBC products stored in CPD or CPDA preservatives or reduce the additive before use.[24] Hemolysis from mechanical damage and phlebotomy contributes to ongoing RBC transfusion requirements. Thrombocytopenia occurs in all patients undergoing ECMO as a result of accelerated platelet destruction. This, coupled with the need for systemic anticoagulation with heparin to prevent clotting within the extracorporeal circuit (see Part 1 of this chapter), places infants on ECMO at significant risk for hemorrhage. Platelets should be maintained at greater than 50,000 to 150,000/μL or higher in infants undergoing major surgery like diaphragmatic hernia repair while on ECMO. Activated clotting times are used to measure coagulation parameters, and FFP and cryoprecipitate are often needed to maintain normal clotting factors.

REFERENCES

1. Adverse effects of blood transfusion. In: Gottschall J, editor: *Blood Transfusion Therapy: A physician's handbook*, 8th edition, Bethesda, MD, 2005, American Association of Blood Banks, pp 141–50.
2. Aher S, Ohlsson A: Late erythropoietin for preventing red blood cell transfusion in preterm and/or low birth weight infants, *Cochrane Database of Systematic Reviews* 2006, Issue 3. Art. No.: CD004868. DOI: 10.1002/14651858.CD004868.pub2
3. Alcock GS, Liley H: Immunoglobulin infusion for isoimmune haemolytic jaundice in neonates, *Cochrane Database Syst Rev* 3: CD003313, 2002.
4. Alter HJ: Pathogen reduction: a precautionary principle paradigm, *Transfus Med Rev* 22:97, 2008.

5. Alter HJ, et al. Emerging infectious diseases that threaten the blood supply, *Semin Hematol* 44:32, 2007.

6. American Academy of Pediatrics Subcommittee on Hyperbilirubinemia: Management of hyperbilirubinemia in the newborn infant 35 or more weeks of gestation, *Pediatrics* 114:297, 2004.

7. Andrew M, et al: A randomized, controlled trial of platelet transfusions in thrombocytopenic premature infants, *J Pediatr* 123:285, 1993.

8. Angiolillo A, Luban NL: Hemolysis following an out-of-group platelet transfusion in an 8-month-old with Langerhans cell histiocytosis, *J Pediatr Hematol Oncol* 26:267, 2004.

9. Bell EF, et al: Randomized trial of liberal versus restrictive guidelines for red blood cell transfusion in preterm infants, *J Pediatr* 115:1685, 2005.

10. Blanchette VS, et al: Platelet transfusion therapy in newborn infants, *Transfus Med Rev* 9:215, 1995.

11. Blood components. In: Roseff SD, editor: *Pediatric Transfusion: A physician's handbook*, 2nd edition, Bethesda MD, 2006, American Association of Blood Banks, pp 1–52.

12. Bowden RA, et al: A comparison of filtered leukocyte-reduced and cytomegalovirus (CMV) seronegative blood products for the prevention of transfusion-associated CMV infection after marrow transplant, *Blood* 86:3598, 2003.

13. Brune T, et al: Efficacy, recovery, and safety of RBCs from autologous placental blood: clinical experience in 52 newborns, *Transfusion* 43:1210, 2003.

14. Carr R, et al: G-CSF and GM-CSF for treating or preventing neonatal infections, *Cochrane Database Syst Rev* 3:CD003066, 2003.

15. Casiraghi MA, et al: Long-term outcome (35 years) of hepatitis C after acquisition of infection through mini transfusions of blood given at birth, *Hepatology* 39:90, 2004.

16. Davenport RD: Hemolytic transfusion reactions. In: Popovsky MA editor: *Transfusion Reactions*, 3rd ed Bethesda, MD, 2007, AABB Press, pp 1–56.

17. Davey RJ, et al: The effect of prestorage irradiation on postransfusion red cell survival, *Transfusion* 32:525, 1992.

18. Dodd RY: Current risk for transfusion transmitted infections, *Curr Opin Hematol* 14:671, 2007.

19. Dodd RY: Transfusion-transmitted hepatitis virus infection, *Hematol Oncol Clin North Am* 9:137, 1995.

20. Elbert C, et al: Biological mothers may be dangerous blood donors for their neonates, *Acta Haematol* 85:189, 1991.

21. Goodstein MH, et al: Comparison of two preservation solutions for erythrocyte transfusions in newborn infants, *J Pediatr* 123:783, 1993.

22. Jackson JC: Adverse events associated with exchange transfusion in healthy and ill newborns, *Pediatrics* 99:E7, 1997.

23. Jain R, Jarosz C: Safety and efficacy of AS-1 red blood cell use in neonates, *Transfus Apher Sci* 24:111, 2001.

24. Josephson CD: Neonatal and pediatric transfusion practice. In Roback JD, editor: *Technical manual of the American Association of Blood Banks*, 16th ed, Bethesda, MD, 2008, American Association of Blood Banks, pp 639–663.

24a. Josephson CD, Su LL, Christenson RD, et al: Platelet transfusion practices among neonatologists in the United States and Canada: results of a survey, *Pediatrics* 123(1):278, 2009.

25. Kennedy LD, et al: A prospective, randomized, double-blind controlled trial of acetaminophen and diphenhydramine pretransfusion medication versus placebo for the prevention of transfusion reactions, *Transfusion* 48:2285–2291, 2008.

26. Kennedy MS: Perinatal issues in transfusion practice. In Roback JD editor: *Technical Manual of the American Association of Blood Banks*, 16th ed, Bethesda MD, 2008, American Association of Blood Banks, pp 625–37.

27. King TE, et al: Universal leukoreduction decreases the incidence of febrile nonhemolytic transfusion reactions to red cells, *Transfusion* 44:25, 2004.

28. Kirpalani H, et al: The premature infant in need of transfusion (PINT) study: a randomized, controlled trial of a restrictive (low) versus liberal (high) transfusion threshold for extremely low birth weight infants, *J Pediatr* 149:301, 2006.

29. Kopko PM, Popovsky MA: Transfusion related acute lung injury. *In: Popovsky MA editor: Transfusion Reactions*, 3rd ed, Bethesda, MD, 2007, AABB Press, pp 207–28.

30. Lee DA, et al: Reducing blood donor exposures in low birth weight infants by the use of older, unwashed packed red blood cells, *J Pediatr* 126:280, 1995.

31. Linden JV, Pisciotto PT: Transfusion-associated graft-versus-host disease and blood irradiation, *Transfus Med Rev* 6:116, 1992.

32. Luban NL: Management of anemia in the newborn, *Early Hum Dev* 84:493, 2008.

33. Luban NL, et al: The epidemiology of transfusion-associated hepatitis C in a children's hospital, *Transfusion* 47:615, 2007.

34. Luban NL, et al: Commentary on the safety of red cells preserved in extended storage media for neonatal transfusions, *Transfusion* 31:229, 1991.

35. Luban NL, Wong EC: Hazards of transfusion. In: Arceci RJ, Hann IM, Smith OP, editors: *Pediatric Hematology*, 3rd ed, New York, 2006, Wiley Blackwell, pp 724–44.

36. Mainie P: Is there a role for erythropoietin in neonatal medicine? *Early Hum Dev* 84:525, 2008.

37. Mangel J, et al: Reduction of donor exposures in premature infants by the use of designated adenine-saline preserved split red blood cell packs, *J Perinatol* 6:363, 2001.

38. Mohan P, Brocklehurst P: Granulocyte transfusions for neonates with confirmed or suspected sepsis and neutropenia, *Cochrane Database Syst Rev* 4:CD003956, 2003

39. Murray NA, et al: Platelet transfusion in the management of severe thrombocytopenia in neonatal intensive care unit patients, *Transfus Med* 12:35, 2002.

40. O'Connor JC, et al: A near-fatal reaction during granulocyte transfusion of a neonate, *Transfusion* 28:173, 1988.

41. Ohlsson A, Aher SM: Early erythropoietin for preventing red blood cell transfusion in preterm and/or low birth weight infants, *Cochrane Database of Systematic Reviews* 2006, 3:CD004863.

42. Nichols WG, et al: Transfusion-transmitted cytomegalovirus infection after receipt of leukoreduced blood products, *Blood* 101:4195, 2003.

43. Paglino JC, et al: Reduction of febrile but not allergic reactions to red cells and platelets following conversion to universal prestorage leukoreduction, *Transfusion* 44:16, 2004.

44. Patra K, et al: Adverse events associated with neonatal exchange transfusion in the 1990s, *J Pediatr* 144:626, 2004.

45. Pisciotto PT, Luban NL: Complications of neonatal transfusion. In: Popovsky MA, editor: *Transfusion Reactions*, 3rd ed, Bethesda, MD, 2007, AABB Press, pp 459–499.

46. Price TH, editor: *Standards for Blood Banks and Transfusion Services*, 25th ed, Bethesda MD, 2008, American Association of Blood Banks, pp 41–7.

47. Rabe H, et al: Systematic review and meta-analysis of a brief delay in clamping the umbilical cord of preterm infants, *Neonatology* 93:138, 2008.

48. Ramasethu J, Luban NL: Alloimmune hemolytic disease of the newborn. In: Lichtman M, et al, editors: *Williams Textbook of Hematology*, 8th ed, New York, 2010, McGraw Hill.

49. Roberts I, Murray NA: Neonatal thrombocytopenia, *Semin Fetal Neonatal Med* 13:256, 2008.

50. Robitaille N, Hume HA: Blood components and fractionated plasma products: preparations, indications, and administration. In: Arceci RJ, et al, editors: *Pediatric Hematology*, 3rd ed, New York, 2006, Wiley Blackwell, pp 693–706.

51. Roseff SD, et al: Guidelines for assessing appropriateness of pediatric transfusion, *Transfusion*, 42:1398, 2002.

52. Sanchez R, Toy P: Transfusion related acute lung injury: a pediatric perspective, *Pediatr Blood Cancer* 45:248, 2005.

53. Sandberg K, et al: Preterm infants with low immunoglobin G have increased risk of neonatal sepsis but do not benefit from prophylactic immunoglobin G, *J Pediatr* 137:623, 2000.

54. Sanders RP, et al: Premedication with acetaminophen or diphenhydramine for transfusion with leucoreduced blood products in children, *Br J Haematol* 130:781, 2005.

55. Stramer SL, et al: West Nile virus among blood donors in the United States, 2003 and 2004, *N Engl J Med* 353:451, 2005.

56. Strauss RG: Data-driven blood banking practices for neonatal RBC transfusions, *Transfusion* 40:1528, 2000.

57. Strauss RG, et al: Feasibility and safety of AS-3 red blood cells for neonatal transfusions, *J Pediatr* 136:215, 2000.

58. Strauss RG, et al: Comparing alloimmunization in preterm infants after transfusion of fresh unmodified versus stored leukocyte-reduced red blood cells, *J Pediatr Hematol Oncol* 21:224, 1999.

59. Vamvakas EC: Allergic and anaphylactic reactions. In: Popovsky MA, editor: *Transfusion Reactions*, 3rd ed, Bethesda, MD, 2007, AABB Press, pp 105–156.

60. Widness JA: Treatment and prevention of neonatal anemia, *NeoReviews* 9:e526, 2008.

61. Yang X, et al: Transfusion-related acute lung injury resulting from designated blood transfusion between mother and child: a report of two cases, *Am J Clin Pathol* 121:590, 2004.

CHAPTER 47

The Gastrointestinal Tract

PART 1

Development and Basic Physiology of the Neonatal Gastrointestinal Tract

David K. Magnuson, Robert L. Parry, and Walter J. Chwals

The human gastrointestinal (GI) tract is a complex combination of organs whose primary function is to digest and absorb nutrients. Many important secondary functions are also performed, such as the endocrine function of the pancreas. In fact, what was once considered a simple system of digestion and absorption is now recognized as something much more complex and dynamic. Furthermore, as with the respiratory system, in order to perform its duties, the GI tract must be in continuity with the environment. This places the additional demand of having mechanisms in place to protect the host from toxins and pathogens. It is remarkable that this tube, open to the outside world at both ends and colonized by bacteria for a significant portion of its length, is tolerated so well and has relatively few complications associated with it. But troubles do occur, and in the neonate, most can be traced to developmental anomalies.

THE BEGINNING

During gestation, the alimentary canal can be simply considered as the folding of endoderm and splanchnic mesoderm into a tube at the end of week 3 and the beginning of week 4.[6] As the head fold forms, the cranial part of the yolk sac becomes enclosed within the embryo and becomes the foregut. Shortly thereafter, the caudal portion of the yolk sac becomes enclosed and forms the hindgut. The midgut resides between the foregut and the hindgut, near the yolk sac, which remains outside the embryo. The midgut remains in communication with the yolk sac until the yolk stalk closes during the 10th week of gestation. Initially, the digestive tube ends blindly—cranially at the oropharyngeal membrane and caudally at the cloacal membrane. These membranes, made up of endoderm and ectoderm, break down, with the oropharyngeal going first at the start of week 4 followed by the cloacal at the start of week 6.

ESOPHAGUS

The esophagus is the only portion of the GI tract that has neither digestive nor absorptive function. Rather, it serves as a conduit between mouth and stomach and, at the gastroesophageal junction, functions to avoid reflux of stomach contents back up the esophagus. Although this task sounds simple, the esophagus performs its roles so well that no esophageal replacement has been found that does anywhere near as good a job. All efforts are made to keep a native esophagus, even a severely compromised one, rather than go with any replacement.

The fully developed esophagus extends from the pharynx and cricopharyngeal sphincter in the neck to the lower esophageal sphincter and gastroesophageal junction in the abdomen. The blood supply to the esophagus is segmental. The upper esophagus is supplied by branches descending from the inferior thyroid artery. The middle and lower thirds of the esophagus are supplied by branches arising directly from the bronchial vessels or the descending thoracic aorta. The abdominal and lower esophagus also receive blood supply from the left gastric and inferior phrenic arteries. The esophagus varies in length from 13 to 25 cm depending on the age and height of the patient. There are four areas of natural anatomic constriction of the esophagus: (1) at the level of the cricopharyngeal sphincter, (2) as the aortic arch crosses anteriorly, (3) as the left main stem bronchus crosses anteriorly, and (4) at the level of the lower esophageal sphincter. Foreign bodies in the esophagus tend to lodge at one of these areas of constriction, and burns from caustic ingestion tend to be more severe in these regions.

The esophagus is differentiated from the primitive foregut during the 4th week of gestation.[7,9] A tracheoesophageal septum is evident at this time initiating the division of the trachea anteriorly from the foregut posteriorly. The septum remains at about the same level in the fetus while the body grows cranially. This leads to elongation of the esophagus, primarily from "ascent" of the pharynx rather than "descent" of the stomach. It reaches its full length, relative to the size of the developing fetus, during the 7th week of gestation. Aberrations during this phase of development result in esophageal atresia and tracheoesophageal fistulas.

The lumen of the esophagus is nearly obliterated during the 7th and 8th weeks of gestation, secondary to rapid proliferation of mucosal epithelial cells. Temporary obliteration of the lumen (as in the duodenum) is thought not to occur.

A single lumen is clearly present by the 10th week, with growth of the muscular wall.

The muscular wall of the esophagus is similar to that of the rest of the GI tract, with an outer longitudinal layer and a circular inner layer. The more highly developed longitudinal layer forms during the 9th week of gestation, whereas the circular layer forms during the 6th week. There is no serosa on the esophagus except in the short abdominal portion.

The epithelial lining of the esophagus is derived from the primitive endoderm. At the 10th week of gestation, this is ciliated, but a stratified, nonkeratinizing, squamous epithelium begins replacing the ciliated epithelium at about the 4th month of gestation. Some ciliated epithelium along the length of the esophagus may persist until birth. The striated muscle of the upper third arises from mesoderm of the branchial arches, whereas the smooth muscle of the distal two thirds is derived from splanchnic mesenchyme. Therefore, diseases of smooth muscle tend to affect the lower esophagus only.

Small glands of mucus- and bicarbonate-secreting cells with ducts opening onto the surface of the epithelium are scattered throughout the length of the esophagus, particularly in the lower third.

By 8 weeks' gestation, immature neurons are identifiable within the wall of the esophagus. These nerves are derived from both parasympathetic and sympathetic fibers. The cervical sympathetic trunks send fibers along the inferior thyroid artery to the upper third of the esophagus, whereas the middle and lower thirds are supplied by branches from the greater splanchnic nerves. The thoracic esophagus is supplied by branches of the esophageal vagal plexus, arising directly from the vagus trunks in the chest.

The act of swallowing is initiated by impulses from the swallowing center, an area in the reticular formation of the rostral medulla where the nuclei of cranial nerves IX and X are located. The initial event in esophageal peristalsis is stimulation of the longitudinal muscle layer, which is followed by the segmental activation of the circular muscle and relaxation of the lower esophageal sphincter. The peristaltic wave begins in the pharynx and continues through to the gastroesophageal junction without interruption. Whereas primary waves are initiated from the swallowing center, secondary peristalsis is mediated by local intramural pathways to return refluxed material in the lower esophagus to the stomach.

The upper esophageal sphincter corresponds to the cricopharyngeal muscle. There is no morphologic distinction in the muscular wall of the lower esophagus that would identify this sphincter, although clearly one functionally exists. The primary role of this sphincter is to prevent the reflux of gastric contents back into the lower esophagus. The lower esophageal sphincter relaxes as the primary peristaltic wave traverses the esophageal body, and it remains open until the peristaltic wave enters the sphincter and closes it. Disordered lower esophageal sphincter function is thought to be the primary mechanism for gastroesophageal reflux.

STOMACH

The stomach first appears as a fusiform dilation of the caudal part of the foregut at the end of the 4th week of gestation.[5] At this time, the stomach is suspended between the posterior and anterior body walls by a ventral and dorsal mesentery. During weeks 6 through 10, the stomach undergoes rotation in two planes, as well as growth differentials that lead to the appropriate size and orientation of the organ as seen at birth. One rotation is 90 degrees counterclockwise (viewed from below upward) along the longitudinal axis of the stomach. This brings the dorsal aspect of the stomach toward the fetus' left side, and the ventral aspect now points to the right. The two mesenteries follow this rotation, with the ventral mesentery finally extending horizontally from the stomach to the liver as the lesser omentum. The cranial portion of the dorsal mesentery runs horizontally to the spleen laterally as the gastrosplenic ligament, and it contains the short gastric vessels. A second, lesser rotation, in conjunction with a growth differential favoring greater growth on the dorsal (now left lateral) side of the stomach, leads to the organ's final position. This rotation is clockwise around the body's anterior-posterior axis when viewed from the front and brings part of the now left lateral (formerly dorsal) side of the stomach to point caudally. This part of the stomach still has the caudal portion of the stomach's dorsal mesentery attached, which now grows quite quickly caudally forming a two-layer fat pad that covers the bowel and extends to the pelvis. The two fat layers fuse to each other and to the colon and become the greater omentum. The space now created behind the stomach is called the lesser sac. It has one entrance, the epiploic foramen (foramen of Winslow), located beneath the free edge of the ventral mesentery that now extends from the area of the gastroduodenal junction to the liver.

The final shape of the stomach along with the various epithelial cell types that constitute its mucosal lining create distinct areas: the cardia around the gastroesophageal (GE) junction; the fundus, which projects cephalad from the gastroesophageal junction, the body, which is the vast majority of the gastric reservoir; and the antrum, the portion of the stomach immediately before the pylorus. There are three muscle layers of the stomach: the outer longitudinal, the intermediate circular, and the inner oblique. The three layers permit complex mixing and churning movements that help begin the process of digestion.

The blood supply to the stomach is extremely rich and is derived principally from the celiac axis. Four major vessels are felt to provide the stomach with blood: the right and left gastric and the right and left gastroepiploic. Also important are the short gastric arteries off the splenic artery. Venous drainage is via the portal system, with the exception of the gastroesophageal junction which can drain to the systemic system via esophageal veins (critical to the development of esophageal varices). The blood supply to the stomach is so redundant that the organ can survive if three of the four major arteries are divided.

The gastric epithelium is made up of a diverse cell population distributed in a regionally specific manner. The early gastric mucosa is initially a stratified or pseudostratified columnar epithelium that later becomes cuboidal. This mucus-secreting cuboidal epithelium then becomes peppered with gastric pits that are first observed between gestational weeks 6 and 9. By 20 weeks, the mucosa of the stomach is mature in appearance. At the base of the gastric pits are the gastric glands, which contain the effector and regulator cells of gastric secretion.

The different cell populations of the gastric glands in various regions of the stomach allow the stomach to be histologically and functionally compartmentalized. Parietal cells are found predominantly in the gastric fundus and body and less often in the proximal antrum and can be identified in gastric glands as early as week 10. They produce both hydrochloric acid and intrinsic factor under complicated regulatory control. Chief cells are found principally in the gastric fundus and body; first appearing in gestational week 12. They are located exclusively at the base of the gastric glands, where they synthesize, store, and secrete pepsinogen. Pepsinogen is hydrolyzed to the active proteolytic enzyme pepsin in the acid environment of the stomach.

Enteroendocrine cells are present throughout the stomach, duodenum, and distal intestine. Because of their ability to produce biologically active amines and peptides and to internalize certain precursor molecules, they are referred to as *amine precursor uptake and decarboxylation* (APUD) cells. There are many distinct types of enteroendocrine and neuroendocrine cells found in the gastric mucosa. These cells are among the first to populate the gastric glands, appearing at 8 to 9 weeks. The most common and well-characterized are the G cells, which produce gastrin, and the D cells, which produce somatostatin and amylin. These cells predominate in the gastric antrum. Other enteroendocrine cells are ubiquitous both within the gastric glands and within the duodenal wall. They are responsible for producing such diverse amines and peptides as histamine (from the enterochromaffin-like cells), serotonin, dopamine, vasoactive intestinal peptide (VIP), glucagon, gastric-releasing peptide (GRP), motilin, and ghrelin. Interestingly, the A cells, which produce glucagon, are present only in fetal and neonatal glands. Considered along with the trophic effect of many GI hormones, this suggests a growth and differentiation role for these substances, along with the digestive and regulatory roles they are currently known to have.

All three components of the autonomic nervous system—sympathetic, parasympathetic, and enteric—innervate the stomach. The parasympathetic and enteric predominate. Sympathetic innervation is predominantly inhibitory to GI function and primarily uses the postganglionic neurotransmitter norepinephrine.[3] The parasympathetic pathways mediated by acetylcholine are generally stimulatory. The enteric nervous system (ENS), on the other hand, uses a variety of neurotransmitters including dopamine, somatostatin, VIP, GRP, ghrelin, and cholecystokinin. The ENS is the largest and most complex compartment of the autonomic nervous system and comprises more than 10^8 resident neurons within the wall of the GI tract. The ENS is anatomically separate from the CNS (i.e., the sympathetic and parasympathetic systems).

Sympathetic innervation originates from cell bodies within the thoracic spinal cord and extends through presynaptic fibers in the greater splanchnic nerve to postsynaptic neurons in the celiac ganglion, whose axonal fibers follow blood vessels into the gastroduodenal wall. Parasympathetic presynaptic nerves originate in the brainstem and follow the vagus nerves to the stomach. ENS precursors differentiate from neuroblasts located in the vagal area of the neural crest and migrate with the vagus nerves to the developing GI tract. These ENS neurons then further differentiate, proliferate, and establish connections to each other, to other autonomic pathways, and to developing gastric secretory and muscle cells. There is significantly more ENS than CNS activity within the GI tract, suggesting a more powerful role for intrinsic (ENS) control than for extrinsic (CNS) control.

The stomach has two distinct functional zones based on motor activity differences. The proximal zone, which includes the fundus and the proximal third of the body of the stomach, serves as a reservoir in which an ingested meal is stored. Its ability to distend without increasing intraluminal pressure is important during bolus feeding. The proximal stomach generates slow, sustained tonic contractions under CNS control via the vagus. This action creates a constant pressure gradient that controls the passage of material through the stomach. Vagotomy significantly impairs this function, causing rapid emptying of fluids.

Motor activity in the stomach distal to the proximal third of the body of the stomach is characterized by spontaneous depolarizations that result in phasic, directional contractions. This gives this portion of the stomach the ability to mix and grind solid food and to empty mixed food particles into the duodenum in a controlled fashion. During the fasting state, gastric activity follows a 90- to 120-minute repetitive pattern called the interdigestive migrating motor complex. This four-phase complex runs from mechanically silent to coordinated contractions that empty the gastric lumen of all indigestible materials. The fed state occurs when the migrating motor complex is interrupted by the arrival of ingested food. Now, the stomach begins forceful, nonpropagated contractions in the distal stomach coupled with coordinated contractions of the pyloric sphincter that churn food into small particles. A gastric pacemaker located along the greater curvature at the proximal boundary of the distal zone triggers these contractions at a rate of three to four cycles per minute. When the average particle size reaches 1 mm, chyme is allowed to empty into the duodenum. Complex CNS and ENS coordination permits adequate breakdown of the food and ensures that the rate of gastric emptying is adjusted to provide an isocaloric flow of nutrients into the duodenum over time.

Gastric secretory function evolves early in development. By 10 weeks' gestation, parietal and enteroendocrine cells have begun to differentiate, and by 12 to 13 weeks, gastrin, hydrochloric acid, pepsin, and intrinsic factor (IF) can all be detected. Mucus and bicarbonate secretion commences later, at about the 16th week. The gastric luminal pH of full-term newborns is neutral, but it is as low as 3.5 within a few hours. By 48 hours, the pH is between 1.0 and 3.0. Premature infants have a prolonged period of alkalinity, often many days, that is related to the degree of prematurity.

The production and secretion of hydrochloric acid by gastric parietal cells is governed by complex neurocrine, endocrine, and paracrine pathways, with little evidence for a final common pathway. The parietal cell can receive input and respond to a large variety of inputs, making its regulation by medical and surgical treatments difficult. Gastric acid has many functions. One is to facilitate protein digestion, but the lack of malabsorption problems in patients with achlorhydria indicates that this role may not be critical. Normal acid secretion does, however, play an integral role in initiating the digestive process. Gastric acid also creates a barrier to the entrance of bacteria into the GI tract. This not only protects the upper aerodigestive tract but also insulates the bacteria downstream from constant challenges from above. This is consistent with recent data that acid suppression therapy for gastroesophageal reflux may be associated with a higher incidence of lower respiratory tract infections.[8]

DUODENUM, PANCREAS, AND BILIARY SYSTEM

The duodenum is the short retroperitoneal portion of the GI tract that connects the foregut to the midgut. At its proximal end, it connects to the outlet of the stomach, the pylorus, and it ends a short distance later at the ligament of Treitz, where the GI tract becomes an intraperitoneal organ once again and becomes the jejunum. Like the stomach, the duodenum undergoes a rotational process that brings it to its final C-loop configuration (Fig. 47-1). This 270-degree counterclockwise rotation swings the duodenum under the superior mesenteric artery. During this rotation, the duodenum's dorsal mesentery shortens, which allows the duodenum to become fixed in the retroperitoneal position across the upper abdomen from the

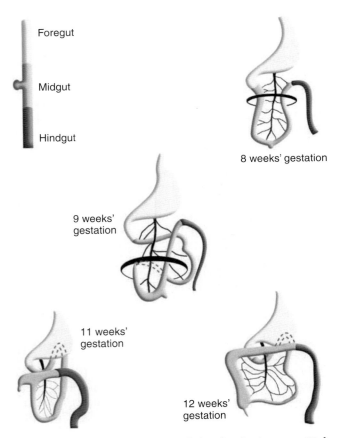

Figure 47–1. Normal rotation of the developing gut. Eight weeks' gestation: elongation of the midgut and superior mesenteric artery, herniating into the umbilical stalk. Nine and 11 weeks' gestation: 270-degree counterclockwise rotation of duodenal-jejunal segment and 270-degree counterclockwise rotation of ileo-colic segment. Twelve weeks' gestation: final orientation of the normally rotated gut.

pylorus (to the right of midline) to the ligament of Treitz (to the left of midline). This fixation is absolutely critical, because, from the ligament of Treitz to the cecum (the next retroperitoneal portion of the GI tract located in the right lower quadrant), the bowel is on a mesentery and free to float about the peritoneal cavity. The bowel thus becomes fixed within the peritoneal cavity at the two most widely separated points available—the ligament of Treitz in the left upper quadrant and the cecum in the right lower quadrant. Because the mesenteric base is therefore so broad, it is impossible for the floating, intraperitoneal bowel to twist on its mesentery, thus compromising its own blood supply. However, any failure of proper rotation and fixation of the bowel can lead to the twisting of the bowel on its mesentery (i.e., volvulus) and the subsequent catastrophe of interruption of the flow of blood to the bowel.

The rotation of the bowel occurs during the 6th to 10th weeks of gestation. Concurrently, there is a rapid epithelial proliferation (along with the rectum and esophagus) that obliterates the hollow lumen and converts the duodenum to a solid, cordlike structure. Vacuoles then appear and gradual recanalization occurs. The distal duodenum does not appear to pass through a solid phase. Defects in this proliferation and recanalization process are believed to lead to the problems of duodenal atresia, web, and stenosis.

The duodenum is divided into four portions corresponding to the curvatures of the C loop. The blood supply is derived from the celiac axis through the superior pancreaticoduodenal branches of the gastroduodenal artery, and the superior mesenteric artery through the inferior pancreaticoduodenal branches. Consistent with the location of the original liver bud, this transition from celiac to superior mesenteric blood supply defines the transition from foregut to midgut. A consistent landmark in the medial portion of the duodenum, near the end of the foregut, is the ampulla of Vater, which represents the confluence of common bile duct and pancreatic ducts and their entry into the duodenum.

The liver and biliary system develop within a bud along the free edge of the ventral mesentery, with stomach and bowel rotation bringing them to their final location in the right upper quadrant.[1] Also within this bud is the primordial ventral pancreas. Opposite this ventral pancreatic bud (including liver and biliary primordium) is the dorsal pancreatic bud. During rotation, the ventral pancreatic bud fuses to the dorsal bud and becomes one organ. Failure of this rotation leads to the problem of annular pancreas. The biliary and pancreatic drainage systems also fuse during rotation, so that the common bile duct descends in the remnant free edge of ventral mesentery, along with the portal vein and hepatic artery, then passes behind the duodenum to join with the main pancreatic duct at the ampulla of Vater. This main pancreatic duct is formed from the confluence of the original ventral pancreatic duct with the distal dorsal pancreatic duct. The proximal dorsal pancreatic duct remains as the accessory pancreatic duct. The biliary and pancreatic ductal systems are complete by the 10th to 12th gestational week. With so many rotation and fusion requirements to produce the "classic" biliary-pancreatic ductal anatomy, it is no wonder that one sees the "classic" form less than 50% of the time. Blood supply to the gallbladder arises from the celiac artery. The pancreas is supplied by numerous branches of the celiac and superior mesenteric arteries.

The layers of the duodenum are the muscularis, the submucosa, and the mucosa. The muscularis is made up of smooth muscle cells, which are divided distinctly into two separate layers: an outer, longitudinal layer and an inner, circular layer. The submucosa is a band of dense connective tissue lying just under the mucosa. The mucosa is the innermost layer and is composed of three distinct layers: the muscularis mucosa, the lamina propria, and the epithelial cell lining. The most striking feature is the villi, 1.5 mm tall in the duodenum and decreasing in size through to the ileum. Crypts of Lieberkühn surround the base of each villus and average one-third to one-fourth the height of the villi.

Like the rest of the small bowel, the duodenal mucosa is made up mainly of enterocytes, tall columnar epithelial cells that are responsible for absorption (see Small Intestine later). The duodenum is also richly populated with enteroendocrine cells, along with goblet cells, Paneth cells, and lymphoid aggregates of Peyer patches. The enteroendocrine cells are stimulated by nutritional substrates delivered from the stomach, and they secrete mediators that regulate a variety of digestive processes. Secretin is produced by the duodenal S cells in response to luminal acid, stimulating bicarbonate secretion from the pancreas, liver, and duodenal Brunner glands and mucosal cells. Cholecystokinin, produced by duodenal I cells in response to certain fatty acids and amino acids, stimulates gallbladder contraction and pancreatic exocrine secretion.

The pancreas is a central metabolic organ with key roles in both exocrine and endocrine function.[4] It is the primary source of digestive enzymes: more than 20 different enzymes are synthesized and stored in the secretory acini. The proteolytic enzymes such as trypsin, chymotrypsin, and carboxypeptidase are secreted as inactive proenzymes. They are converted to active enzymes by enterokinase, an intestinal brush border enzyme, when they reach the duodenal lumen. These enzymes, in turn, can activate other proenzymes. Pancreatic amylase and lipase are secreted in their active form. The secretory acinar cells are under complex CNS, ENS, and hormonal regulation. The ducts that drain the acini are lined by cells that secrete water and bicarbonate. Secretin stimulates this fluid and bicarbonate secretion, which raises intestinal pH and thereby facilitates pancreatic enzyme activity.

The pancreas also has an essential role in the hormonal regulation of metabolism and glucose homeostasis. These endocrine functions are provided by the islets of Langerhans, which make up about 1% to 2% of the pancreatic mass. These 1 to 2 million islets are more plentiful on the pancreatic tail and are also under complex CNS, ENS, and hormonal control. There are four distinct cell types within the islets: alpha cells for glucagon production, beta cells for insulin, gamma cells for somatostatin, and PP cells for pancreatic polypeptide.

SMALL INTESTINE

The small intestine is the major digestive and absorptive portion of the GI tract. The gut initially herniates out of the fetus's abdominal domain and lengthens rapidly during the 6th to 12th weeks of gestation.[11] As described earlier (see Duodenum,

Pancreas, and Biliary System), on reentry into the abdominal cavity, the small bowel undergoes a 270-degree twist around the superior mesenteric artery axis to bring it into its final anatomic position. This positioning is complete by the 20th week. The "small" of small intestine clearly relates only to the circumference of the structure, as its length is anything but small. The small intestine typically measures between 200 and 300 cm at birth in the full-term neonate after doubling its length between 26 and 38 weeks of gestation. After birth, the small intestine continues to grow, finally reaching its maximum length of 600 to 800 cm after 4 years of age.[10] During this time, and continuing through puberty, there are also increases in intestinal diameter, along with development of the plicae circulares, villi, and microvilli that enlarge the absorptive surface area of the small intestine from about 950 cm^2 at birth to 7500 cm^2 in the adult. The blood supply of the small intestine is provided solely by branches of the superior mesenteric artery running in the mesentery of the small intestine.

The circular muscles of the small intestine appear at 6 weeks of gestation and the longitudinal muscles at 8 weeks. Neuroblasts appear at 7 weeks of gestation, and the myenteric and submucosal plexuses are noted to appear between the 9th and 13th weeks. Although there is some peristalsis noted as soon as the plexuses appear, it is poorly coordinated. The appearance of myenteric muscle contractions at 32 to 34 weeks leads to more coordinated contractions, but intestinal transit time at this gestation time is as long as 9 hours—nearly twice as long as in the term infant. It is not until about 38 weeks' gestation that the myenteric muscle contractions are fully present and fasting motor activity is mature. Even so, limited feedings can be accomplished in infants as young as 25 weeks, as they appear to stimulate contractions, albeit immature.

Villi appear during weeks 8 to 11 and acquire their final, finger-like shape by week 14. However, the villi remain shorter in the ileum than in the jejunum, leading to a fourfold greater absorptive area in the jejunum. Microvilli appear and the enterocytes are morphologically mature and display a well-organized brush border by 14 weeks of gestation. Endocrine cells appear at 9 weeks and continue to proliferate, with all the various gut peptide hormones and neurotransmitters present by 20 weeks' gestation. These include enteroglucagon, neurotensin, gastrin, pancreatic polypeptide, motilin, and VIP. Although all are present at birth, many of them show remarkable increases in basal levels during the first 2 weeks of life in the fed infant. Interestingly, when feedings are withheld in infants, intestinal growth and functional maturation are delayed and basal levels of the intestinal peptides remain low, suggesting some form of cause-and-effect relationship.

It is generally held that the enteric ganglion cells are derived from vagal neural crest cells. As mentioned previously, neural crest-derived neuroblasts first appear in the developing esophagus at 5 weeks. They then begin a migration down to the anal canal in a craniocaudal direction during the 5th to 12th weeks of gestation. The neural crest cells first form the myenteric plexuses just outside the circular muscle layer. The mesenchymally derived longitudinal muscle layer then forms, sandwiching the myenteric plexus after it has been formed in the 12th week of gestation. Finally, the submucous plexus is formed by neuroblasts, which migrate from the myenteric plexus across the circular muscle layer and into the submucosa and the mucosa. This also progresses in a craniocaudal direction, but it occurs during the 12th to 16th weeks of gestation.

COLON, RECTUM, AND ANUS

The colon is a continuation of the intestine with two basic functions: (1) the absorption of water and electrolytes and (2) the storage and elimination of feces. Its absorptive function is significant, in that the colon absorbs more than 80% of the water left after passage through the small intestine. The rectum and anus are critical in the complex act of controlled defecation.

The colon is divided into six areas: the cecum, the appendix, and the ascending, transverse, descending, and sigmoid colon. Like the duodenum, the colon also undergoes a 270-degree counterclockwise rotation during the 10th to 12th weeks of gestation to bring it into the proper position.[2] Although this is nearly concurrent with the duodenal rotation, the two are not completely codependent. Either one, or both, can go astray, so it is possible to have a nonrotated colon with a properly rotated duodenum, and vice versa. If properly rotated, the cecum lies in the right lower quadrant, the ascending colon along the right gutter, the transverse colon from the hepatic flexure to the splenic flexure, and the descending colon along the left gutter; the sigmoid colon connects the descending colon to the rectum approximately at the level of the third sacral vertebrae. The ascending colon and the descending colon are retroperitoneal structures with peritoneum covering only their anterior and lateral surfaces. The cecum is variably fixed—sometimes completely retroperitoneal (along with the appendix) and sometimes on a short mesentery. The transverse and sigmoid colon are on a mesentery. The posterior border of the greater omentum is also attached to the transverse colon.

The blood supply of the colon is supplied by both the superior and inferior mesenteric arteries. The watershed area between the distribution of the two vessels is typically located around the mid transverse colon to the splenic flexure. This also marks the boundary of the midgut and hindgut. The rectum is supplied by the inferior mesenteric artery as well as branches off the iliac arteries.

Although it is developmentally similar to the small intestine in general structure, the colon has unique elements. Most obvious is the concentration of the longitudinal muscle coat into three bands—the teniae coli. The teniae create sacculations, called *haustra*, that permit radiographic differentiation of the small from the large intestine after infancy. The mucosa of the colon is characterized by crypts of Lieberkühn, which are lined with absorptive, goblet, and endocrine cells.

The development of the anorectum requires unique attention, because problems result in a wide variety of anorectal malformations. As mentioned previously, during the 3rd week of gestation, the bilaminar germ disc transforms into a trilaminar disc of ectoderm, mesoderm, and endoderm. At either end of the embryo, the endoderm and ectoderm fuse, excluding the mesoderm from these areas and giving rise to the oropharyngeal and cloacal membranes. The former breaks down in the 4th week to give rise to the mouth, whereas the cloacal membrane does not open until the 8th week. Between weeks 4 and 6, it is widely held that the primitive gut tube at the level of the cloacal membrane gets canalized and partitioned into an anterior urogenital sinus and a posterior anorectum by the cranial caudal growth of a mesodermally derived partition called the urorectal septum. Eventually, the urorectal septum fuses with the cloacal membrane, and the fusion site is called the *perineal body*. The newly formed anorectal canal remains closed by the posterior aspect of the cloacal membrane, which is now called the *anal membrane*. The ectoderm in this region then goes on to form the anal pit or proctodeum, so the distal third of the anal canal is eventually made up of ectoderm, the proximal two thirds is made up of mesoderm, and the two cell types are divided by the anal membrane. The membrane breaks down during week 8, and the two cell populations fuse at what is called the *pectinate* or *dentate line*.

Aside from the previously described migration of neural crest cells to form enteric ganglion cells, the anorectum has an important neurologic milestone during the 4th week of gestation. At this time, spinal nerves from sacral levels 2, 3, and 4, which contribute to the peripheral parasympathetic nervous system, form. In contrast to the motility problems noted with failure of migration and thus the absence of ganglion cells, problems related to the proper development of these spinal nerves during week 4 may lead to the proprioceptive and motility problems associated with anorectal malformations.

REFERENCES

1. Flake AW: Disorders of the gallbladder and biliary tract. In Oldham KT, et al, editors: *Surgery of infants in children: scientific principles and practice,* Philadelphia, 1997, Lippincott-Raven, p 1405.
2. Katz AL: Colon. In Oldham KT, et al, editors: *Surgery of infants in children: scientific principles and practice,* Philadelphia, 1997, Lippincott-Raven, p 1313.
3. Kutchai HC: Gastrointestinal motility. In Berne RM, Levy MN, editors: *Physiology,* 3rd ed, St Louis, 1993, Mosby Year Book, p 138.
4. Lillehei C: Pancreas. In Oldham KT, et al, editors: *Surgery of infants in children: scientific principles and practice,* Philadelphia, 1997, Lippincott-Raven, p 1415.
5. Magnuson DK, Schwartz MZ: Stomach and duodenum. In Oldham KT, et al, editors: *Surgery of infants in children: scientific principles and practice,* Philadelphia, 1997, Lippincott-Raven, p 1133.
6. Moore KL: The digestive system. *In The developing human,* 2nd ed, Philadelphia, 1977, Saunders, p 197.
7. O'Rahilly R, Muller F: The digestive system. *In Human embryology and teratology,* 2nd ed, New York, 1996, Wiley-Liss, p 225.
8. Orenstein SR, et al: Multicenter, double-blind, randomized, placebo-controlled trial assessing the efficacy and safety of proton pump inhibitor lansoprazole in infants with symptoms of gastroesophageal reflux disease, *J Pediatr* 154:514, 2009.
9. Rodgers BM, McGahren ED: Esophagus. In Oldham KT, et al, editors: *Surgery of infants in children: scientific principles and practice,* Philadelphia, 1997, Lippincott-Raven, p 1005.
10. Shorter NA: Tumors of the small bowel. In Oldham KT, et al, editors: *Surgery of infants in children: scientific principles and practice,* Philadelphia, 1997, Lippincott-Raven, p 1249.
11. Treen WR: Small intestine. In Oldham KT, et al, editors: *Surgery of infants in children: scientific principles and practice,* Philadelphia, 1997, Lippincott-Raven, p 1163.

PART 2

Disorders of Digestion

*Shaista Safder, Sundeep Arora, and
Gisela Chelimsky*

Neonates can present with a variety of problems pertaining to the digestive tract. The major focus of this chapter is to discuss the disorders that will affect neonates and infants in the achievement of good weight gain. This review is an overview of the evaluation and management of the newborn who presents with symptoms of poor weight gain, diarrhea, or malabsorption.

The main clinical expression of malabsorption is diarrhea. Diarrhea, when chronic, results in malnutrition and failure to thrive. Chronic diarrhea starting in the hours and days following birth is usually extremely severe, leading in a few weeks to life-threatening malnutrition. Malabsorption syndromes are characterized by the association of chronic diarrhea, abdominal distention, and failure to thrive.

INFANTILE DIARRHEA

In 1968, Avery and colleagues coined the term *intractable diarrhea of infancy* to define an entity characterized by the appearance of diarrhea in an infant younger than 3 months, lasting more than 2 weeks, with three or more negative stool cultures, and requiring long-term parenteral nutrition and possibly intestinal transplant for survival.[9] Little has changed in this definition since then. Intractable diarrhea of infancy should be contrasted with protracted diarrhea of infancy, which resolves despite its initial severity.[160]

Evaluation of the Infant with Chronic Diarrhea

The evaluation of the infant with chronic diarrhea should include a careful prenatal history, past medical history, feeding history, family history, a detailed physical examination, and then evaluation. For example, infants who are not breast fed are at increased risk to develop persistent diarrhea whereas breast feeding is a protective factor.[72] Table 47-1 summarizes the key points to be considered in the evaluation of infants and children with chronic diarrhea. Table 47-2 summarizes many of the causes of chronic diarrhea. In the evaluation of chronic diarrhea, it is important to differentiate between secretory and osmotic diarrhea. On many occasions, the diarrhea can be a result of a combination of both mechanisms, for example, in tufting enteropathy, phenotypic diarrhea, and diarrhea due to immunodeficiencies. The classification of secretory and osmotic diarrhea is based on the persistence of diarrhea in the absence of feeds and on the fecal osmolar gap. *Secretory diarrhea* is described as large volumes of watery stools that persist in the absence of enteral feeds, whereas osmotic diarrhea is dependent on enteral feeds and stool volumes are not as massive as in secretory diarrheas.

Secretory diarrheas are characterized by increased electrolytes and water fluxes toward the lumen secondary to either a block in intestinal absorption of NaCl or increase in chloride

TABLE 47–1   Approach to Infant with Diarrhea and Poor Weight Gain

Prenatal history	Polyhydramnios consistent with congenital sodium and chloride diarrhea
Past medical history	Surgeries, history of necrotizing enterocolitis, chronic liver disease
Physical examination	Emphasis on skin manifestations such as those with acrodermatitis enteropathica, facial features, and woolly hair of phenotypic diarrhea Evaluation of nutritional status and intervention for nutritional support
Family history	Important in elucidating a genetic cause for congenital diarrheas. A family history of immune or atopic disease would point to allergy or autoimmunity, or family history of cystic fibrosis.
Infectious workup (regardless of risk factors)	Stool cultures, stool parasites, and enteric viruses
Biochemical markers	Albumin, prealbumin, iron, micronutrient assessment
Test for etiology based on pathophysiology of diarrhea (secretory versus osmotic)	Measure osmotic gap, stool electrolytes for sodium and chloride, stool pH
Test for intestinal function	Stool α_1-antitrypsin, fecal elastase, stool-reducing substance, stool fat, stool for occult blood, stool for fecal leukocytes, fecal calprotectin
Structural evaluation	Endoscopy and histology Electron microscopy indicated in all forms of intractable diarrheas of unknown etiology to evaluate ultrastructural abnormalities
Immunohistochemistry	Evaluate mucosal immune activation,[27] study smooth muscle cells, neuronal cells, enterocytes, and components of basal membrane
Abdominal imaging	Evaluate anatomy

TABLE 47–2   Classification of Diarrheas and Malabsorption Syndromes

Pancreatic insufficiency	Cystic fibrosis, Shwachman-Diamond syndrome, Johanson-Blizzard syndrome, Donlan syndrome, Pearson syndrome, Jeune syndrome
Carbohydrate malabsorption	Disaccharides deficiency, congenital lactase deficiency, glucose-galactose malabsorption, maltase-glucoamylase deficiency
Protein malabsorption	Primary intestinal enteropeptidase deficiency, primary trypsinogen deficiency, lysinuric protein intolerance, primary intestinal lymphangiectasia
Fat malabsorption	Hypobetalipoproteinemia, abetalipoproteinemia, chylomicron retention disease Bile acid malabsorption
Electrolyte transport defects	Congenital chloride diarrhea, congenital sodium diarrhea
Villous architectural defects	Microvillous inclusion disease, tufting enteropathy, autoimmune enteropathy (IPEX), infectious enteropathy
Infantile intractable diarrhea	Syndromic or phenotypic diarrhea
Miscellaneous conditions	Acrodermatitis enteropathica, hormone-mediated secretory diarrhea, short gut syndrome
Motility disorders, usually associated with small intestinal bacterial overgrowth	Intestinal aganglionosis (long segment Hirschsprung disease) or chronic intestinal pseudo-obstruction syndrome
Immune mediated	Allergic enteropathy

secretion by secretory crypt cells. Examples of this kind of diarrhea are congenital Na and Cl diarrhea, microvillus inclusion disease, and autoimmune enteropathy.

Osmotic diarrheas generally occur when digestion and/or absorption is impaired. They are caused by nonabsorbed nutrients in the gastrointestinal tract and are generally associated with intestinal damage. The osmotic force driving water into the lumen is derived from nonabsorbable solutes from food or injured mucosa. Absence or reduction in pancreatic enzymes and bile acid disorders cause impaired digestion of carbohydrate, protein, and fat, contributing to this kind of diarrhea (Table 47-3). Infectious agents can cause diarrhea either by a secretory or osmotic mechanism.

The kind of diarrhea can also be differentiated by measuring the stool osmolality and the fecal osmolar gap. The normal fecal osmolality is similar to the plasma osmolality (i.e., 290 mOsm/kg).[35,36] The fecal osmolar gap is calculated by subtracting twice the sum of fecal sodium and potassium

(to account for anions) from the fecal osmolality. It is important that the fecal electrolytes be measured on a freshly collected specimen.

$$\text{Fecal osmolar gap} = 290 \text{ mOsm/kg} - [2\,(Na^+ + K^+)]$$

	Secretory diarrhea	Osmotic diarrhea
Osmotic gap	<50 mOsm/kg	>135 mOsm/kg
pH	>6	<5
Na concentration	>70 mEq/L	<70 mEq/L
Cl concentration	>40 mEq/L	<35 mEq/L

In secretory diarrhea, the fecal osmolar gap is usually less than 50, whereas in osmotic diarrhea, it is greater than 50.[15] It is important in the evaluation of the child with diarrhea to quantify stool output, even if this entails placing a urinary catheter to separate urine from stools. Another way to collect stools is to have the child wear one diaper inside out, surrounded by a second diaper in the usual fashion to absorb any stool that runs out.

Diarrhea can also be categorized based on the location of the disorder, either as a luminal or epithelial disorder. Among the luminal causes, alteration in intestinal transit times and surgical removal of absorptive surface of bowel contributes to diarrhea and malabsorption such as that seen in short gut syndrome.

Management of Intestinal Failure

Intestinal failure is a condition in which there is insufficient functional bowel to allow for adequate nutrient and fluid absorption to sustain adequate growth in children, necessitating parenteral nutrition. There can be medical and surgical causes for intestinal failure. Surgical causes include patients with necrotizing enterocolitis, intestinal atresias, and midgut volvulus, among others. Many of these conditions do not intrinsically cause intestinal failure, but their natural histories

TABLE 47–3   Components Required for Digestion of Macronutrients

Carbohydrates	Pancreatic amylase, glucoamylase, intestinal disaccharidases (maltase, sucrase, lactase), glucose transporters, colonic bacteria
Protein	Gastric pH, pepsin (stimulated by gastrin), chymotrypsin and trypsin (activated by enterokinase), dipeptidase, amino acid transporters
Fat	Bile acids, pancreatic lipase, chylomicron formation in enterocytes

often mandate surgical resection of bowel leading to short bowel syndrome and its complications. Medical causes of intestinal failure include infants with dysmotility disorders[29] or patients with severe intractable diarrheas. Children with surgical causes of intestinal failure have greater potential for bowel adaptation than children with medical causes of intestinal failure.[29] Patients with intestinal failure need intestinal rehabilitation which can be seen as a three-pronged strategy merging nutrition, pharmacologic, and surgical approaches to achieve the ultimate goal of enteral nutrition in these children. Intestinal transplantation is indicated in patients in whom long-term parenteral nutrition cannot be performed safely. Common reasons for intestinal transplantation include short bowel syndrome, congenital mucosal diseases, and motility disorders.[131] In children with intestinal failure, transplantation must be discussed early, and should evolve from being a rescue procedure to becoming a true therapeutic option.[131]

DISORDERS OF PANCREATIC INSUFFICIENCY

Cystic Fibrosis

Cystic fibrosis (CF) is one of the most common fatal genetic disorders.[28] It is an inherited disease of epithelial cell ion transport, and it is the most common cause of exocrine pancreatic insufficiency and severe progressive lung disease in childhood.[48] This disease was considered uniformly fatal, but with advances in management, the median survival today is estimated at 40 years.[137]

INCIDENCE

Cystic fibrosis is estimated to affect between 1 in 1900 and 1 in 3700 live births in the white population,[137] with a much lower frequency among African Americans (1 in 17,000)[137] and even lower in Asian populations (1 in 90,000).[28] Other geographic areas with higher incidences are Northern Ireland (1 in 1700) and Sweden (1 in 7700). As a result of inbreeding, certain areas have a higher than average incidence, such as 1 in 377 in Britain and 1 in 640 among the American Amish.[137] Nevertheless, CF is always considered in the differential for any child with the constellation of poor weight gain and chronic lung disease, irrespective of the race or the geographic origin of the patient.[122]

GENETICS

Cystic fibrosis is transmitted in an autosomal recessive manner.[48] In the white population, approximately 1 in 20 individuals carries the recessive form of the allele.[38] Thus, if both parents are CF carriers, there is a 25% chance of having an affected child, a 50% chance of having a carrier, and a 25% chance of having an unaffected child.[28]

MOLECULAR PATHOGENESIS

Kerem and colleagues[75] were successful in cloning the gene responsible for CF in 1989. This gene was mapped to chromosome 7 and was found to encode for a large, single-chain protein that forms a chloride channel with its associated regulatory regions, named the cystic fibrosis transmembrane regulator.[48] More than 800 different mutations have been described, of which the most important is the delta F508 mutation.

CLINICAL FEATURES

Affected newborns present with intestinal obstruction resulting from thick meconium plugs obstructing the ileum, also known as *meconium ileus*.[137] Abdominal radiography demonstrates dilated small bowel loops associated with bubbles of gas and meconium in the absence of air-fluid levels, also described as a ground-glass appearance (Neuhauser sign).[122] Other findings include a small-caliber colon (microcolon).[160] Half of the affected infants present with complications such as peritonitis, volvulus, atresia, and necrosis, which may be noted as calcifications on a plain abdominal radiograph.[122] Meconium plug syndrome, a transient distal colonic obstruction that is relieved by the passage of a meconium plug, signifies the possibility of CF.[122]

Extrahepatic biliary duct obstruction resulting from thick inspissated bile plugs or long-term parenteral nutrition support can result in prolonged conjugated hyperbilirubinemia.[122] Thus, sweat chloride is part of the workup of any neonate with prolonged conjugated hyperbilirubinemia.[137] A small percent of children (2% to 5%) present with symptomatic portal hypertension.[73] Poor weight gain is almost universal in patients with CF who have pancreatic insufficiency.[122] Respiratory symptoms include cough, wheezing, retractions, and tachypnea, with a variable degree of atelectasis on chest radiograph that typically presents later.[73]

DIAGNOSIS

The diagnosis is usually established by a supportive history along with laboratory investigations. Sweat chloride in excess of 60 mEq/L is diagnostic.[137] Ninety-nine percent of patients with CF have elevated sweat chloride concentrations.[137] However, conditions such as hypothyroidism, Addison disease, ectodermal dysplasia, glycogen storage disease, and technical errors such as evaporation and contamination may falsely elevate sweat chloride values. Likewise, edema, malnutrition, and sampling errors may give falsely negative values.[28,137] Thus it is important to carry out this test at a center certified by the Cystic Fibrosis Foundation.[28] Genotyping with commercially available tests can identify 80 common mutations in the cystic fibrosis transmembrane regulator, including delta F508, and can also be used when adequate sweat is difficult to obtain.[140]

Another measure of pancreatic insufficiency that is easily performed, inexpensive, and reproducible with a high sensitivity and specificity, is the measurement of fecal elastase 1 (E1).[146] Nissler and coworkers[101] established reference ranges after measuring E1 from the stool samples of 148 children. For an infant older than 2 weeks, E1 above 200 μg/g of feces is adequate, and less than 100 μg/g of stool is a measure of insufficiency.[101] Figure 47-2 describes the currently suggested evaluation in children with concerns for cystic fibrosis.

PRENATAL DIAGNOSIS

On the basis of the CF carrier status of the parents, a prenatal diagnosis can be established by mutational analysis of fetal cells obtained by chorionic villus sampling at 10 weeks of gestation or by amniocentesis at 15 to 18 weeks of gestation. If the pregnancy is carried to term, the neonate should be tested by sweat chloride analysis for confirmation.[122] Other radiologic signs that may be suggestive of CF include a

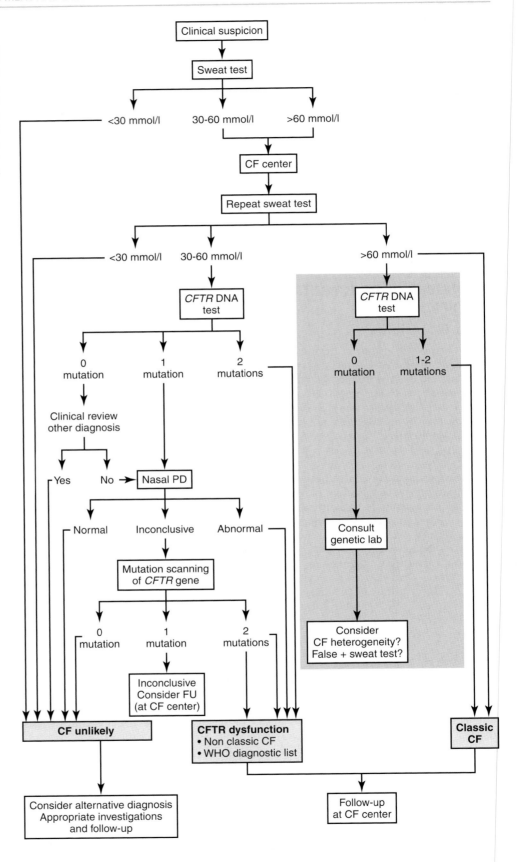

Figure 47–2. Cystic fibrosis (CF) diagnostic algorithm. FU, ; PD, potential difference; WHO, World Health Organization. (*Redrawn from De Boeck K, Wilschanski M, Castellani C, et al, on behalf of the Diagnostic Working Group: Cystic fibrosis: terminology and diagnostic algorithms. Thorax 61(7):627-635, 2006. Copyright © 2006, BMJ Publishing Group Ltd. and British Thoracic Society.*)

hyperechoic fetal bowel pattern, meconium peritonitis, and abdominal calcifications.[137]

MANAGEMENT

Management of the patient with CF is a multidisciplinary team effort involving the participation of a gastroenterologist, a pulmonologist, a nutritionist, and a social worker.[160] Attention must be focused on supplying adequate calories, replacing fat-soluble vitamins, and providing supportive care.[122] Pancreatic enzyme replacements have long been used and are generally well tolerated. However, the dosage should not exceed 50,000 U lipase per kilogram because of concerns of fibrosing colonopathy.[132]

Pulmonary disease is the main cause for late morbidity and mortality associated with CF. Clinical trials are underway to evaluate the potential for gene therapy as being the definitive treatment for CF pulmonary disease.

Shwachman-Diamond Syndrome

The Shwachman-Diamond syndrome complex,[31] characterized by exocrine pancreatic insufficiency, bone marrow failure, and skeletal changes, was originally described independently by Nezelof and Watchi (1961),[97] Bodian and colleagues in the United Kingdom (1964),[17] Burke and coworkers in Australia (1967),[20] and Shwachman in the United States (1964).[141] It is a very rare disorder of pancreatic insufficiency, but its importance is that it is the second most common cause of bone marrow failure after cystic fibrosis; the third most common cause is Fanconi, followed by Diamond-Blackfan anemia.[32]

INCIDENCE

The estimated incidence in the North American population is about 1 in 50,000. Recent reports have noted the existence of Shwachman-Diamond syndrome in European, Asian, and African population cohorts.[160]

GENETICS

An autosomal recessive mode of inheritance has been proposed by observation of different family pedigrees. In 2002, researchers from Toronto identified the gene that is altered in Shwachman-Diamond syndrome and the locus has been mapped to chromosome 7.[33] Unlike Fanconi anemia, which may result from mutations in more than five different genes, and Diamond-Blackfan anemia (25% of families have mutations in the RPS19 gene), more than 90% of the Shwachman-Diamond syndrome patients had alterations in one single gene on chromosome 7. The SBDS gene (named after Shwachman-Bodian-Diamond), located on 7q11, is predicted to code for a 250 amino acid protein of (currently) unknown function. The transcript of the normal gene is widely expressed in the pancreas, bone marrow, and leukocytes and assumed to be necessary for the normal development of these tissues.[51]

CLINICAL FEATURES

The disease is highlighted by failure to thrive in infancy associated with exocrine pancreatic insufficiency and varying degrees of bone marrow failure.[123] Pancreatic insufficiency results in malabsorption and steatorrhea, which in turn results in poor weight gain.[160] Neutropenia with defective neutrophil chemotaxis is the most common hematologic abnormality which

results in frequent bacterial infections such as otitis media and pneumonia.[31] Neutropenia is characteristically intermittent, with cycles of low to normal values.[32] Anemia and thrombocytopenia have also been described in patients with Shwachman-Diamond syndrome.[160] Bone marrow is hypocellular and is replaced with fatty infiltration.[33] When a case of Shwachman-Diamond syndrome is suspected, the diagnostic criteria listed in Table 47-4 should help establish the diagnosis. The presence of skeletal abnormalities, short stature, and hepatic impairment would support the diagnosis.

MANAGEMENT

The following recommendations for managing Shwachman-Diamond syndrome were outlined at the 3rd International Congress on Shwachman-Diamond syndrome in June 2005, Cambridge, UK.[51]

Gastrointestinal

As in cystic fibrosis, the pancreatic insufficiency is treated with pancreatic enzyme supplements, fat-soluble vitamins, and a high caloric diet. The enzyme dose should be regulated according to symptoms, such as steatorrhea, abdominal pain, and growth parameters.

Hematologic

Febrile neutropenia or overt infection is treated with broad-spectrum antibiotics. Granulocyte colony-stimulating factor (G-CSF) can be used, but is usually reserved for cases of severe life-threatening sepsis and rarely as prophylaxis. Blood and platelet transfusions are given as required for anemia and thrombocytopenia.

Johanson-Blizzard Syndrome

Johanson-Blizzard syndrome (JBS) is a rare autosomal recessive disorder that was first described in 1971 by Johanson and Blizzard.[69] Only about 30 cases have been described in

TABLE 47-4	Diagnostic Criteria for Shwachman-Diamond Syndrome[31]
Exocrine pancreatic insufficiency (at least one of the following)	Abnormal quantitative pancreatic stimulation test Serum cationic trypsinogen below normal range Abnormal 72-hour fecal fat Evidence of pancreatic lipomatosis by computed tomography or ultrasound
AND	
Hematologic abnormalities (at least one of the following)	Chronic single lineage or multi-lineage cytopenia Neutrophil less than 1.5×10^9/L Hemoglobin less than 2 standard deviations below mean Thrombocytopenia less than 150×10^9/L Myelodysplastic syndrome

the literature.[32] This disorder is characterized by multisystem involvement.[39] More than a dozen subjects have positional cloning identified loss-of-function mutations in the *UBRI* gene on the long arm of chromosome 15.[167] In patients with Johanson-Blizzard syndrome, the absence of *UBRI* results in early prenatal destruction of the exocrine pancreas that involves impaired apoptosis, induced necrosis, and prominent inflammation.

Affected infants have characteristic phenotypic features, including aplastic alae nasi (which gives the appearance of a beaklike nose with large nostrils),[8] extension of the hairline to the forehead with upswept frontal hair,[50] low-set ears, large anterior fontanelle, micrognathia, thin lips, microcephaly,[39] aplasia cutis (patchy distribution of hair with areas of alopecia), dental anomalies, postnatal growth restriction and pancreatic exocrine aplasia, and anorectal anomalies (predominantly, imperforate anus).[8,151] Other features include mental retardation, deafness, genitourinary abnormalities, hypothyroidism, and cardiac malformations.[8] These infants have significant intrauterine growth restriction because of the lack of insulin resulting from pancreatic insufficiency,[50] and they grow up to exhibit dwarfism. Takahashi and colleagues described a neonate with a diagnosis of Johanson-Blizzard syndrome whose poor growth was determined to be caused by growth hormone deficiency.[151] This patient also demonstrated poor glucagon secretion in response to hypoglycemia. Al-Dosari reported a case of an infant with classic Johanson-Blizzard syndrome who also had unusually severe neonatal cholestatic liver disease that progressed to liver fibrosis and portal hypertension.[3]

As a result of exocrine pancreatic insufficiency, affected patients present with severe malabsorption, which leads to poor weight gain, failure to thrive, hypoalbuminemia, edema, and anemia.[8] Prenatally, diagnosis has been suggested by ultrasonographic findings of beaklike nose and of dilation of sigmoid colon as a result of imperforate anus.[8] Affected individuals have a normal karyotype[8] as well as normal sweat chloride. The presence of anatomic dysmorphisms, exocrine pancreatic insufficiency, and normal sweat chloride distinguishes this condition from cystic fibrosis.

Miscellaneous Causes of Pancreatic Insufficiency

Many other syndromes and diagnoses can be associated with pancreatic insufficiency. Donlan syndrome is similar to JBS, with the notable exception of the presence of normal alae nasi and cleft palate.[50] Pearson syndrome is characterized by features of pancreatic insufficiency, sideroblastic anemia,[50] variable neutropenia, thrombocytopenia, and vacuolization of bone marrow precursors.[160] Jeune syndrome is a rare autosomal recessive disorder of pancreatic insufficiency and asphyxiating thoracic dystrophy.[160] Isolated deficiencies of amylase, lipase, colipase, and trypsinogen have also been described. Familial pancreatitis with mutations in the trypsinogen gene can cause chronic pancreatitis, pancreatic insufficiency, and chronic diarrhea.

DISORDERS OF CARBOHYDRATE ABSORPTION

The enterocytes lining the small intestine have, at their apical surface brush border, various enzymes responsible for digestion of carbohydrates.[160] These carbohydrate hydrolases convert disaccharides and oligosaccharides into simple monosaccharides that are absorbed easily via transport proteins that exist on the intestinal surface.[98] Examples include maltase-glucoamylase, sucrase-isomaltase (SI), and lactase-phlorhizin hydrolase.[99] The clinical symptoms of carbohydrate malabsorption occur either because of the deficiency of a particular enzyme (e.g., congenital sucrase-isomaltase deficiency) or because of an abnormality in a transport protein involved with the absorption of digestion product (e.g., glucose-galactose malabsorption). There is often a correlation between the age a disorder appears and the age at which a particular food is introduced into the baby's diet (Table 47-5).

Patients with carbohydrate malabsorption disorders, regardless of the cause, present with severe watery diarrhea, which results from osmotic action exerted by the malabsorbed oligosaccharide,[160] that is, lactose, sucrose, or glucose, in the intestinal lumen. An important aspect is the regression of diarrhea when oral feeds are discontinued. The malabsorbed sugars are in turn acted on by colonic bacteria, generating a mixture of gases (e.g., hydrogen, methane, and carbon dioxide),[160] along with short-chain fatty acids. The gases form the basis of carbohydrate-specific breath hydrogen testing, which is often used in diagnosis.[121] The short-chain fatty acids are absorbed via the colonic epithelium, and they not only provide energy but also help decrease the colonic osmolality. In the presence of a large carbohydrate load, these protective mechanisms become overwhelmed, leading to worsening of the diarrhea.[160] The increased volume, coupled with low pH, stimulates gut motility and decreases intestinal transit time.[74]

Disaccharidase Deficiencies

CONGENITAL SUCRASE-ISOMALTASE DEFICIENCY

Congenital sucrase-isomaltase deficiency is the most common congenital disorder of carbohydrate malabsorption.[90] It is characterized by decreased activity of the enzyme responsible for hydrolysis of dietary sucrose[11] in the brush border epithelium of the small intestine. It is transmitted in an autosomal

TABLE 47-5	Age of Onset of Different Malabsorption Syndromes
Age of Onset	*Disorder*
Immediate neonatal period	Glucose-galactose malabsorption Congenital lactase deficiency
Weaning age	Glucoamylase deficiency Congenital sucrase-isomaltase deficiency

recessive form[119] and has been mapped to chromosome 3.[90] A higher prevalence has been noted among congenital sucrase-isomaltase deficiency populations of Canadian, native Alaskan, and Greenlander descent (3% to 10%)[90] compared with native North Americans (0.2%).[160]

Etiology
Congenital sucrase-isomaltase deficiency is caused by reduced activity of the brush border enzyme sucrase-isomaltase.[119] Several theories have been proposed for the pathogenesis of this enzyme deficiency. A point mutation in the *SI* gene,[105] resulting in substitution of glutamine by arginine at position 117,[147] interferes with its transport out of the endoplasmic reticulum and the Golgi bodies, resulting in intracellular accumulation and degradation. The sucrase-isomaltase (SI) gene from 11 patients of Hungarian origin with congenital sucrase-isomaltase deficiency was examined by Sander and colleagues.[130] Analyses revealed 43 *SI* variants in total, 15 within exons and one at a splice site. Eight of the exonic mutations lead to amino acid exchanges, causing null alleles. One new variation affects a splice site, which is also predicted to result in a null allele. All potential pathologic alterations were present on one allele only. In 6 of the 11 patients, the phenotype of congenital sucrase-isomaltase deficiency was accounted for by compound heterozygosity.[130]

Clinical Features
The patient presents with diarrhea, usually noticed around the age of 3 to 6 months when the infant is weaned from breast milk to baby foods that contain sucrose. If the baby has been switched to a sucrose-containing formula (e.g., Isomil), diarrhea is noted earlier. Affected infants present with severe, chronic or intermittent watery diarrhea, abdominal distention, cramping,[153] and failure to thrive.[11] The stool pH is noted to be less than 7 as a result of fermentation by colonic bacteria, but because sucrose is a nonreducing sugar, Clinitest or a test for stool reducing substances is negative.[90]

Diagnosis and Treatment
The history from the caregiver should describe feedings, formula changes, age at weaning, and age of onset of diarrhea. Patients present with severe watery diarrhea, metabolic acidosis, and poor weight gain.[11] Stools are acidotic but test negative for reducing substances. Stool osmolality reveals an elevated osmolar gap (greater than 50 mOsm), indicating the presence of malabsorbed sugars. Sucrose hydrogen breath testing[52] offers a noninvasive assessment, but the results must be interpreted in the light of other clinical findings, as secondary disaccharidase deficiency is a known consequence of mucosal injury from any cause.[90] Endoscopy, with analysis of duodenal biopsies for actual enzyme levels, is the gold standard for diagnosis. The treatment of congenital sucrase-isomaltase deficiency is highlighted by strict lifelong avoidance of sucrose-containing fruits and beverages.[90]

CONGENITAL LACTASE DEFICIENCY
Congenital lactase deficiency is an exceedingly rare autosomal recessive disorder. Patients present with watery diarrhea, vomiting, poor weight gain, lactosuria, aminoaciduria, and nervous system changes in the days after birth.[65,85] A majority of the patients described in the literature are from Finland, where more than 42 cases[65] have been described since the first diagnosis in 1959.[61]

Congenital lactase deficiency is caused by the deficiency of lactase, a disaccharidase in the small intestine that has been linked to 2q21.[65] Villous architecture of the intestinal mucosa is preserved, as noted on biopsy specimens of the small intestine.[160] However, congenital lactase deficiency is different from adult-type hypolactasia, which is caused by decreased activity of the lactase-phlorhizin hydrolase enzyme, which resides more than 2 Mb away from the congenital lactase deficiency locus.[65] Usually, congenital lactase deficiency is an isolated deficiency, but as reported by Nichols and colleagues, it may be associated with deficiencies of other disaccharidases such as maltase-glucoamylase.[98]

The appearance of the watery diarrhea coincides with the introduction of lactose-containing milk (either in breast milk or in lactose-based commercial formulas) into the baby's diet, and it is usually noticed within the first 10 days.[65] The stool pH is less than 7 as a result of fermentation of the malabsorbed lactose by colonic bacteria. The diarrhea resolves after switching to a lactose-free formula,[160] which clinches the diagnosis. Apart from diarrhea, these babies are lively and have a good appetite; they exhibit poor weight gain but no vomiting.[128] Saarela and colleagues described 11 infants with congenital lactase deficiency who were found to have hypercalcemia and nephrocalcinosis.[128] The hypercalcemia probably resulted from either metabolic acidosis or enhanced calcium absorption in the ileum, as facilitated by nonabsorbed lactose. Interestingly, the hypercalcemia was corrected after a lactose-free diet was instituted.[128] As a result of metabolic acidosis, a decreased urinary excretion of citrate is noted.[106] Thus hypercalcemia in the presence of hypocitruria sets the stage for nephrocalcinosis.

Congenital lactase deficiency can be diagnosed by its classic presentation, and it can be objectively demonstrated by the lack of a rise of blood reducing sugars after an oral load of lactose.[85] Patients have flat lactose tolerance curves with a normal elevation of blood sugar after the administration of individual monosaccharides and other disaccharides.[85] The diagnostic gold standard is quantification of the enzyme levels from duodenal biopsy specimens,[160] but this may not be possible in all cases.[85]

Treatment consists of avoidance of lactose-containing formula for the neonate. Patients with congenital lactase deficiency have good catch-up growth with normal psychomotor development when maintained on a lactose-free diet.

MALTASE-GLUCOAMYLASE DEFICIENCY
Maltase-glucoamylase is a brush border hydrolase[98] that serves as an alternate pathway for starch digestion. It compensates partially for the lack of sucrase-isomaltase.[160] Congenital maltase-glucoamylase deficiency, first described in 1994, is very rare,[99] with an estimated incidence of 1.8% among children who are investigated for congenital diarrhea. Maltase-glucoamylase bears a striking similarity to SI (59% homology), and it has two catalytic sites that are identical to those of SI.[98] Thus it is not uncommon to see maltase-glucoamylase deficiency in patients with congenital sucrase-isomaltase deficiency.

Clinical Features

Patients present with diarrhea, abdominal distention, and bloating. Symptoms usually coincide with the introduction of starch into the infant's diet at the time of weaning.[160]

Diagnosis and Treatment

Diagnosis is usually established by demonstrating decreased levels of the enzyme on intestinal biopsies. Affected infants should be fed lactose-free formulas. Starch elimination is helpful beyond the neonatal period.[160]

Transport Defects

GLUCOSE-GALACTOSE MALABSORPTION

Glucose-galactose malabsorption is a rare disorder. Patients present with severe watery diarrhea in the neonatal period, which can lead to rapid dehydration and death.[160] It is clinically indistinguishable from congenital lactase deficiency.[106] It was reported in 1962 by Lindquist and Meeuwisse in Sweden.[86] It is transmitted in an autosomal recessive manner.[152]

Incidence

Glucose-galactose malabsorption is rare, and its highest prevalence occurs among populations with a high rate of consanguineous marriages. Approximately 300 cases have been described in the literature worldwide.[160]

Molecular Pathophysiology

Glucose-galactose malabsorption stems from a defect in the intestinal glucose-galactose transport protein, SGLT1.[160] SGLT1 transports glucose and galactose, intracellularly coupled with Na^+, using an electrical gradient to transport against the concentration gradient.[106] It has been mapped to chromosome 22, and mutation analysis is possible. Kianifar and colleagues reported D28G mutations in family members of a patient with glucose-galactose malabsorption using the polymerase chain reaction restriction fragment length polymorphism method.[76]

Clinical Features

Affected infants present with severe watery diarrhea, urine-like in appearance, and coinciding with the start of breast-feeding or ingestion of glucose-containing formula.[160] The predominant sugar of breast milk is lactose, which is hydrolyzed to glucose and galactose prior to being absorbed. The diarrhea can lead to rapid dehydration and electrolyte imbalance.[152] The malabsorbed sugar behaves like an osmotic agent, resulting in diarrhea, which is acidic because of fermentation by colonic bacteria.[160] If prompt attention is not paid to the correction of fluid and electrolyte imbalances, glucose-galactose malabsorption can be rapidly fatal. Stools test positive for reducing substances, indicating malabsorption of reducing sugars.[106] The results of an oral glucose tolerance test demonstrate a flat glucose tolerance curve with the presence of glucose in stools. Endoscopy and colonoscopy show normal colonic and small bowel histology. The onset of diarrhea after the introduction of glucose, the presence of glucose in stools, hypoglycemia, hypernatremic dehydration, and normal intestinal morphology clinch the diagnosis. Because SGLT1 is also expressed in renal tubular cells,

patients may also have glucosuria.[106] Case reports of nephrocalcinosis and urinary calculus formation in patients with glucose-galactose malabsorption have been described in the literature.[106,152] The mechanisms responsible for renal stone formation, as explained earlier for congenital lactase deficiency, may exist in glucose-galactose malabsorption. As with congenital lactase deficiency, hypercalcemia resolved after a glucose-free diet was instituted and diarrhea was controlled.[106]

Diagnosis and Treatment

Diarrhea that improves on elimination of glucose, galactose, and lactose from the diet, coupled with a positive glucose breath hydrogen test and a normal intestinal biopsy, establishes the diagnosis.[160] Infants with glucose-galactose malabsorption can be safely treated with fructose-containing formula, because fructose is absorbed via a different carrier, GLUT5, which is unaffected.[106]

DISORDERS OF PROTEIN ABSORPTION

Primary Intestinal Enteropeptidase Deficiency

Enteropeptidase, formerly known as *enterokinase*, resides in the proximal small intestine and belongs to the group of serine proteases.[62] This enzyme plays a key role in the initiation of protein digestion in the small intestine by bringing about the conversion of trypsinogen to active trypsin, which in turn activates other pancreatic zymogens.[45] It was initially described in 1969 and very few cases are known worldwide. Affected infants present with diarrhea, failure to thrive, and protein-losing enteropathy.[11] When the edema that resulted from hypoproteinemia gets remarkably better after the baby is switched from an intact-protein-based formula to a protein-hydrolysate formula, the diagnosis is confirmed.[160]

Congenital enteropeptidase deficiency is a rare recessively inherited disorder. The genomic structure of the proenteropeptidase gene (25 exons, total gene size 88 kb) was characterized in order to perform DNA sequencing in three clinically and biochemically proved patients with congenital enteropeptidase deficiency who were from two families. Holzinger and associates found compound heterozygosity for nonsense mutations (S712X/R857X) in two affected siblings and found compound heterozygosity for a nonsense mutation (Q261X) and a frameshift mutation (FsQ902) in the third patient. In accordance with the biochemical findings, all four defective alleles identified were predicted null alleles leading to a gene product not containing the active site of the enzyme.[62] These data provide first evidence that proenteropeptidase-gene mutations are the primary cause of congenital enteropeptidase deficiency.[62]

LABORATORY INVESTIGATIONS

Affected infants present with watery diarrhea with normal osmolality and absent osmolar gap, suggesting transport defects. The serum hypoalbuminemia and hypoproteinemia are striking. Enteropeptidase deficiency can be demonstrated either by quantification of the enzyme levels on small intestinal biopsies or by assaying enzyme levels in the duodenal fluid.[45]

TREATMENT

Once the diagnosis has been established, the infant should be switched to protein-hydrolysate formula.[160]

Primary Trypsinogen Deficiency

Primary trypsinogen deficiency results in clinical symptoms very similar to those of primary enteropeptidase deficiency. It is usually described in children with cystic fibrosis who have pancreatic exocrine deficiency.[160]

Lysinuric Protein Intolerance

Lysinuric protein intolerance, also known as *hyperdibasic aminoaciduria type 2* or *familial protein intolerance*,[107] is a disorder of amino acid transport that is characterized by subnormal plasma levels of dibasic amino acids, such as ornithine, arginine, and lysine, and their enhanced urinary excretion. This disorder is transmitted in an autosomal recessive manner and is found at a higher prevalence in three main geographic areas: Finland, Italy, and Japan.[107] Affected patients usually present around the time of weaning, when they are switched from breast feeding to high-protein foods.[107] Citrulline supplementation (200 mg/kg per day) and a protein-restricted diet (1.5 g/kg per day) are the mainstays of therapy.[160]

Primary Intestinal Lymphangiectasia or Waldmann Disease

In 1961, Waldmann and coworkers described the first 18 cases of idiopathic hypercatabolic hypoproteinemia.[159] These patients had edema associated with hypoproteinemia and low serum albumin and gammaglobulin levels. Microscope examination of the small intestine biopsies showed variable degrees of dilation of the lymph vessels in the mucosa and submucosa. The authors also proposed the term *intestinal lymphangiectasia*.[159]

Primary intestinal lymphangiectasia is a rare disorder characterized by dilated intestinal lacteals resulting in lymph leakage into the small bowel lumen and responsible for protein-losing enteropathy leading to lymphopenia, hypoalbuminemia, and hypogammaglobulinemia. Primary intestinal lymphangiectasia is generally diagnosed before 3 years of age but may be diagnosed in older patients. Prevalence is unknown.

Primary intestinal lymphangiectasia may be suspected at birth or during pregnancy based on ultrasonography images, which can detect fetal ascites or lower limb lymphedema.[133]

ETIOLOGY

To date, primary intestinal lymphangiectasia etiology is unknown. Intestinal lymphangiectasia is responsible for lymph leakage into the bowel lumen, which leads to hypoalbuminemia and lymphopenia. Edema is the consequence of hypoproteinemia with decreased oncotic pressure. Several genes, such as *VEGFR3* (vascular endothelial growth factor receptor 3), prospero-related homeobox-transcriptional factor *PROX1*, forkhead transcriptional factor *FOXC2*, and *SOX18* are implicated in the development of the lymphatic system. In a recent paper, Hokari and colleagues reported inconsistently changed expressions of regulatory molecules for lymphangiogenesis in the duodenal mucosa of patients with primary intestinal lymphangiectasia.[59]

CLINICAL FINDINGS

The main symptom is peripheral edema of variable degree, usually symmetric, from moderate (lower limb edema) to severe, including the face and external genitalia.[82] Edema may be moderate to severe with anasarca and includes pleural effusion, pericarditis, and chylous ascites. Fatigue, abdominal pain, weight loss, inability to gain weight, moderate diarrhea, and fat-soluble vitamin deficiencies due to malabsorption may also be present. In some patients, limb lymphedema is associated with primary intestinal lymphangiectasia and is difficult to distinguish lymphedema from edema. Moderate diarrhea is the main digestive symptom.[83]

Five syndromes are associated with intestinal lymphangiectasia: von Recklinghausen, Turner (X0), Noonan, Klippel-Trenaunay, and Hennekam.[55]

DIAGNOSIS

Primary intestinal lymphangiectasia diagnosis is confirmed by the presence of intestinal lymphangiectasia based on endoscopic findings with the corresponding histology of intestinal biopsy specimens.[158] Protein-losing enteropathy is confirmed by the elevated 24-hour stool alpha-1 antitrypsin clearance.

MANAGEMENT

Low-fat diet associated with supplementary medium-chain triglycerides is the cornerstone of primary intestinal lymphangiectasia medical management.[66] It is likely that the absence of fat in the diet prevents engorgement of the intestinal lymphatics with chyle, thereby preventing their rupture with its ensuing protein and T-cell loss. Medium-chain triglycerides are directly absorbed into the portal venous circulation and thus provide nutrient fat avoiding lacteal engorgement. Other inconsistently effective treatments have been proposed for primary intestinal lymphangiectasia patients, such as antiplasmin, octreotide, and corticosteroids. Surgical small bowel resection is useful in the rare cases with segmental and localized intestinal lymphangiectasia.[158]

Other Causes of Protein-Losing Enteropathy

Congenital disorders of glycosylation and Fontan surgery to correct univentricular hearts can also cause protein-losing enteropathy. Bode and coworkers hypothesized that protein-losing enteropathy develops when genetic insufficiencies collide with simultaneous or sequential environmental insults; they found the loss of heparan sulfate proteoglycans specifically from the basolateral surface of intestinal epithelial cells of subjects with protein-losing enteropathy, suggesting a direct link to protein leakage.[16] Heparan sulfate is a glycosaminoglycan. Congenital heparan sulfate deficiency is an extremely rare disorder with severe albumin loss from the gastrointestinal tract presenting within the first week of life.

Congenital disorders of glycosylation are caused by defects in protein N-glycosylation. Congenital disorders of glycosylation are usually associated with mental and psychomotor retardation, but some forms cause coagulopathy, hypoglycemia, and liver fibrosis without neurologic involvement.[64] Westphal reported protein-losing enteropathy in a patient with a congenital disorder of glycosylation who showed reduced heparan sulfate accumulation in the enterocytes.[162]

DISORDERS OF FAT ABSORPTION

Hypobetalipoproteinemia and Abetalipoproteinemia

Hypobetalipoproteinemia is an autosomal dominant disorder characterized by decreased or absent plasma concentrations of apolipoprotein (apo)-B-containing lipoproteins and low-density lipoprotein (LDL) cholesterol.[134] In heterozygous individuals, the disorder is usually clinically silent, because the concentrations of apo-B and LDL cholesterol are 25% to 50% of normal, whereas homozygous individuals have extremely low levels.

In patients with the severe form of homozygous hypobetalipoproteinemia, there is complete absence of beta-lipoproteins, so they present clinically with fat malabsorption, acanthocytosis, retinitis pigmentosa, and neuromuscular degeneration.[87] Homozygous patients are clinically indistinguishable from patients with abetalipoproteinemia, which is an autosomal recessive condition of the apo-B deficiency state.[87] Abetalipoproteinemia (ABL) is a rare autosomal recessive disorder characterized by fat malabsorption, acanthocytosis, and hypocholesterolemia in infancy. Later in life, deficiency of fat-soluble vitamins is associated with development of atypical retinitis pigmentosa, coagulopathy, posterior column neuropathy, and myopathy. ABL results from mutations in the gene encoding the large subunit of microsomal triglyceride transfer protein (MTP). To date at least 33 MTP mutations have been identified in 43 patients with ABL.[166] Management strategies include a low-fat diet and fat-soluble vitamin supplementation.[160]

Chylomicron Retention Disease

Chylomicron retention disease, also known as *Anderson disease*,[160] is an autosomal recessive disorder of lipoprotein assembly[13] that is characterized by hypocholesterolemia, fat malabsorption, and failure to thrive. As a result of mutations in the large polypeptide subunit of microsomal triglyceride transfer protein,[13] enterocytes fail to secrete chylomicrons across the basolateral membrane.[160] It is not unusual to diagnose chylomicron retention disease in neonates who present with diarrhea, but case reports have cited delayed diagnosis in adolescents who present with vitamin E deficiency. Clinically, the presentation is similar to that of hypobetalipoproteinemia and abetalipoproteinemia, but retinitis pigmentosa and neuromuscular manifestations are less severe.[160] Vacuolated enterocytes that stain strongly with oil red[13] indicate the presence of fat within the enterocytes. On electron microscopy, lipid-laden enterocytes are seen.[13] Treatment centers on a low-fat diet and fat-soluble vitamin supplementation.[160]

Primary Bile Acid Malabsorption

Alterations in bile acid metabolism and in the enterohepatic circulation are often associated with chronic diarrhea and should be considered when more common causes of chronic diarrhea have been excluded. Bile acid diarrhea most often occurs in disease or resection of the terminal ileum, in which there is increased exposure of the colonic mucosa to bile salts with consequent activation of fluid and electrolyte secretion. Congenital or acquired defects in the enterohepatic circulation of bile acids also may lead to diarrhea.[120]

Enterohepatic circulation of bile is the primary mechanism by which the body reabsorbs 98% of the bile[94] that is reused as bile salts, and a disruption in this pathway leads to diarrhea, steatorrhea, and decreased blood cholesterol levels.[104] Primary bile acid malabsorption is an idiopathic disorder that has been linked to a missense mutation in the sodium-bile acid cotransporter gene, SCL10A2.[95,104] The diarrhea is exacerbated with the addition of dietary fats, and a remarkable improvement is noted on a trial of cholestyramine and a low-fat diet. Bile acid absorption by the ileum may be measured by using the bile acid analogue 75 Se-homocholic acid taurine test.

Akobeng and associates[2] reported an inborn error in bile acid synthesis presenting as malabsorption leading to rickets. Deficiency of 3β-hydroxy-Δ^5-C_{27}-steroid dehydrogenase (3β-HSDH), the enzyme that catalyses the second reaction in the principal pathway for the synthesis of bile acids, has been reported to present with prolonged neonatal jaundice with the biopsy features of neonatal hepatitis. It has also been shown to present between the ages of 4 and 46 months with jaundice, hepatosplenomegaly, and steatorrhea (a clinical picture resembling progressive familial intrahepatic cholestasis).[2]

DISORDERS OF ELECTROLYTE ABSORPTION

Congenital Chloride Diarrhea

Congenital chloride diarrhea[160] is the most common cause of congenital secretory diarrhea with intact mucosal histopathology.[57] It is transmitted in an autosomal recessive manner,[58] and it is characterized by the passage of severe voluminous watery diarrhea that is rich in chloride. It is being recognized with increasing frequency. After an initial report on 45 cases by Hartikainen-Sorri in 1980,[53] more than 250 cases have been reported in the literature, of which greater than 50% have been reported from Finland alone. This disease is uniformly fatal without treatment. Although long-term prognosis is uncertain, survival is possible with adequate treatment.[53]

INCIDENCE

Congenital chloride diarrhea is estimated to occur at a higher frequency in Finland (1 in 20,000), Poland, and the Arab lands (1 in 32,000).[57,160]

MOLECULAR PATHOPHYSIOLOGY

Congenital chloride diarrhea is due to mutations in the intestinal Cl^- $HCO3^-$ exchange (SLC26A3) which results in sodium chloride and fluid depletion leading to hypochloremic and hypokalemic metabolic alkalosis. Chloride is absorbed predominantly along the entire length of the colon and terminal ileum.[160] SLC26A3 is the transport carrier that functions to absorb chloride in exchange for $HCO3^-$. The chloride ion is absorbed as NaCl, coupled with the sodium ion provided by the Na^+/H^+ exchanger (NHE) (Fig. 47-3),

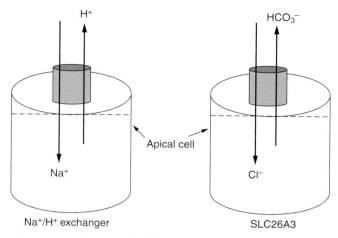

Figure 47–3. Sodium (Na^+) and chloride (Cl^-) absorption across a normal enterocyte. Sodium absorption is via a sodium hydrogen (Na^+H^+) exchanger, and chloride absorption is through the solute carrier (SLC26A3).

which is deficient in patients with congenital sodium diarrhea (see later). However, the amount of chloride secreted into the bowel is not different from the amount secreted in normal individuals; rather, the absorption is faulty at the level of the colon and ileum.[1]

CLINICAL FEATURES

Congenital chloride diarrhea is characterized by profuse watery diarrhea beginning in the immediate neonatal period. The stool has a high chloride concentration, which persists despite fasting.[1] Absence of the passage of meconium is noted, which could be explained by severe intrauterine diarrhea.[58] Wedenoja and colleagues reported a high incidence of mild chronic kidney disease in 35 other patients with congenital chloride diarrhea.[161] The main feature of the renal injury was nephrocalcinosis, without hypercalciuria or nephrolithiasis with small sized kidneys and commensurately reduced glomerular filtration rates. This suggests that diarrhea-related sodium chloride and volume depletion, the first signs of nonoptimal salt substitution, promote urine supersaturation and crystal precipitation.[161]

LABORATORY INVESTIGATION

Affected infants have watery bowel movements with high fecal chloride concentration (greater than 90 mmol/L).[57] Patients are hypokalemic, with low fecal bicarbonate concentrations.[160]

PRENATAL DIAGNOSIS

There is at present no definitive prenatal diagnosis for this condition, but a high index of suspicion must be maintained if there is a positive family history. Polyhydramnios is noted on the prenatal ultrasound,[47,77,88,109,114] and these pregnancies usually result in premature delivery. Poor visualization of the gastrointestinal canal by amniofetography, elevated amniotic fluid bilirubin levels in the absence of Rh immunization, and high amniotic fluid α-fetoprotein levels have

been suggested as being indicative of congenital chloride diarrhea, but should be interpreted in the context of the clinical findings.[53,88,138]

TREATMENT

Treatment centers around oral potassium supplementation to maintain eukalemia.[160] Proton pump inhibitors have recently been shown to be beneficial by decreasing the chloride load to the gut.[1] Oral butyrate in treatment of congenital chloride diarrhea was reported.[23] The short-chain fatty acid butyrate stimulates intestinal water and ion absorption through a variety of mechanisms, including the activation of a parallel Cl^-/butyrate and Na^+/H^+ exchanger.

Congenital Sodium Diarrhea

Congenital sodium diarrhea, first described by Holmberg and Perheentupa,[60] is characterized by voluminous secretory diarrhea noted to start soon after birth, with supranormal fecal sodium content (in stark contrast to congenital chloride diarrhea, as described earlier). It is an exceedingly rare disease and only a few cases have been reported in the literature worldwide.[92] The age of onset is quite variable. The youngest patient described in the literature is a 31-week premature infant, suggesting that the disease manifests in utero.[60]

GENETICS

Congenital sodium diarrhea is transmitted in an autosomal recessive manner.[92] Parental consanguinity and common ancestral inheritance were noted by Muller and coworkers in a kindred of five children with congenital sodium diarrhea from Austria when traced back five generations.[92]

MOLECULAR PATHOPHYSIOLOGY

Congenital sodium diarrhea is related to a defect in the sodium-hydrogen exchanger in the jejunal brush border,[18] which is responsible for the absorption of Na^+ in exchange for H^+. Muller and colleagues studied five related infants with secretory diarrhea in Austria to understand the sodium-hydrogen transporter (NHE) defect in congenital sodium diarrhea. Using the techniques of multipoint linkage analysis and homozygosity mapping, they were able to rule out the known transporters, NHE1 to NHE5, as the culprits. NHE3-knockout mice were found to have a sodium secretory state that bore a close resemblance to congenital sodium diarrhea; however, the diarrhea was mild.[92] Further research to identify the specific transport defect is ongoing. Intractable secretory diarrhea in a Japanese boy with mitochondrial respiratory chain complex I deficiency was reported by Murayama and colleagues.[93]

CLINICAL FEATURES

Congenital sodium diarrhea appears very early in life with severe secretory urine-like diarrhea, which is rich in sodium and has a pH of greater than 7. Sodium losses in excess of 100 to 150 mmol/L have been described, leading to profound and rapid hyponatremia, dehydration, and metabolic acidosis.[92] Affected children may require in excess of 300 mL/kg per day of fluids and 50 mmol/kg per day of sodium to maintain electrolyte balance.[4] It is of paramount importance to closely monitor urine output in these children, even if it entails placement of an indwelling catheter. Profound volume loss via stools can lead to acute renal failure, and the caregiver can be easily misled by wet diapers, thinking them an indication of a good urine output with minimal stools.[18] Urine sodium concentrations are low normal.[92]

Affected babies can also present with abdominal distention and failure to pass meconium within 24 hours after birth, mimicking bowel obstruction or Hirschsprung disease,[4] which can lead to unnecessary surgical interventions. Thus a correct diagnosis is very important.

The results of biopsies of the small intestine are normal in patients with congenital sodium diarrhea.[160] However, Muller and colleagues did report cryptic hyperplasia with jejunal villous atrophy on light microscopy in three patients, which on transmission electron microscopy had vacuolation of the surface epithelium.[92]

LABORATORY INVESTIGATION

An infant who presents with severe watery diarrhea should have fecal electrolytes, stool osmolality, and pH checked. Stool osmolality of less than 50 mOsm, high fecal sodium losses, and alkaline stool pH are characteristic of congenital sodium diarrhea.[160] Serum hyponatremia, metabolic acidosis, and hypokalemia are noted, which is in contrast to patients with congenital chloride diarrhea (Table 47-6). However, because of the rarity of the condition, it is not often entertained in the differential diagnosis, and affected infants may be diagnosed very late in the course of the disorder.[4]

TABLE 47-6   Characteristics of Congenital Chloride Diarrhea and Congenital Sodium Diarrhea

	Congenital Chloride Diarrhea	Congenital Sodium Diarrhea
Inheritance	Autosomal recessive	Autosomal recessive
Incidence	Common in Finnish, Polish, Middle-Eastern populations	Very rare; only six known cases in literature
Serum pH	Metabolic alkalosis	Metabolic acidosis
Serum chloride	Low	Normal to high
Serum potassium	Low	High
Serum sodium	Low	Low or normal
Stool bicarbonate	Low	High
Stool pH	Acidic	Alkaline
Stool sodium	—	High

PRENATAL DIAGNOSIS

Polyhydramnios may be noted antenatally, which suggests the intrauterine manifestation of the disease.[4] Failure to pass meconium postnatally may be explained by the severe secretory diarrhea experienced by the baby in utero.[92]

TREATMENT

Aggressive fluid and electrolyte replacement, either orally or parenterally, is necessary for survival.

DISORDERED VILLOUS ARCHITECTURE
Microvillus Inclusion Disease

Microvillus inclusion disease (MVI), also known as *microvillus atrophy*, was initially described as a clinical entity more than 3 decades ago. It is an important cause of neonatal diarrhea, occurring in both a congenital form (which presents in the first few days after birth) and a late-onset form (which has a better prognosis).[110] It is a congenital defect of the intestinal epithelial brush border that leads to severe intractable diarrhea requiring long-term parenteral nutrition.[26] Early small bowel transplantation alone or small bowel-plus-liver transplantation offers the only hope for long-term survival.[124] A multicenter survey of 23 patients by Phillips and Schmitz revealed a poor prognosis for the condition, with a 75% death rate among affected infants younger than age 9 months.[110] Metabolic complications, sepsis, and liver failure were responsible for a majority of the deaths associated with microvillus inclusion disease.[126] It is transmitted in an autosomal recessive fashion, but it has not been able to be linked to a particular gene.[125] Different series report either male[79] or female[115] dominance. Several reports of microvillus inclusion disease in members of the same family and in children delivered to consanguineously married couples have suggested a genetic association. Pohl and colleagues[115] noted a higher incidence in the Navajo population in northern Arizona, with a 1:12,000 prevalence in surviving infants.[49] In contrast to other causes of neonatal diarrhea (e.g., congenital sodium diarrhea and congenital chloride diarrhea), a history of polyhydramnios during pregnancy is absent.[139]

CLINICAL FEATURES

Microvillus inclusion disease presents with severe secretory diarrhea in the first few days after birth. Intestinal failure secondary to diarrhea is definitive. Diarrhea is watery (urine-like or cholera-like)[111] with an electrolyte concentration that is very similar to that of fluid derived from small intestine.[160] Diarrhea is profuse, and the affected infant could pass up to 500 mL/kg of body weight per day.[110] This persists even when the patient is not fed. Mucus is noted to be abundant in the diarrheal fluid, but blood is absent. Stool cultures are negative for the common pathogens, and the pH is neutral.[111] Reducing substances, if tested, are notably absent unless the baby is fed orally.[110] Massive losses of water lead to dehydration, electrolyte imbalance, and acidosis, which are the major causes of mortality unless the baby is treated with total parenteral nutrition and intravenous fluids.

Phillips and colleagues reported patients with late-onset microvillus inclusion disease, which usually presents beyond the neonatal period and carries a better prognosis.[111] They noted some atypical features (e.g., megaloblastosis with low vitamin B_{12} levels, muscular atrophy, metabolic acidosis, seizures, and cholestatic jaundice) in a few patients. These patients may also present with a picture of intestinal pseudo-obstruction in the neonatal period, and with abdominal distention that may be a diagnostic challenge.[160]

Gathunga and associates reported the association of microvillus inclusion disease with coarctation of the aorta and bicuspid aortic valve, cardiac malformations within the spectrum of left ventricular outlet tract obstruction.[40]

HISTOLOGIC APPEARANCE

When biopsy specimens from these patients are analyzed under light microscopy, villus atrophy without crypt lengthening is noticed.[42] Ultrastructural analyses reveal (1) a partial to total atrophy of microvilli on mature enterocytes with apical accumulation of numerous secretory granules in immature enterocytes and (2) the highly characteristic inclusion bodies containing rudimentary or fully differentiated microvilli in mature enterocytes.[126] Light microscopy shows accumulation of PAS-positive granules at the apical pole of immature enterocytes, together with atrophic band indicating microvillus atrophy and, in parallel, an intracellular PAS or CD10-positive line (marking the microvillous inclusion bodies seen on electron microscopy).[46] Recently, CD10 staining has become a valuable tool in identifying patients with microvillus inclusion disease. CD10 is a leukemia antigen that is normally associated with brush border epithelium in normal small bowel.

PATHOPHYSIOLOGY

The pathogenesis of the disease is unknown.[155] It has been suggested that there is a failure of migration of vesicles from the normal-appearing Golgi apparatus[111] to the surface of the enterocytes,[5] and that it is this migration that is responsible for the transportation of the microvilli.[94]

TREATMENT

Affected infants require lifelong parenteral nutrition. Isolated small bowel transplantation[19,155] or small bowel-plus-liver transplantation[56] is the definitive cure.

Tufting Enteropathy

Tufting enteropathy, also known as *intestinal epithelial dysplasia*, was first described by Reifen and colleagues in 1994 in three children who presented with severe watery diarrhea and weight loss, and whose symptoms did not meet the diagnostic criteria for other well-defined clinical entities.[117] Tufting enteropathy presents in the first few weeks of life with severe life-threatening urine-like diarrhea, weight loss, and persistence despite formula changes.[160] This diarrhea persists despite bowel rest and parenteral nutrition. Affected infants are usually of Middle Eastern or North African descent, and a history of consanguinity is not unusual.[94] To date, no epidemiologic data are available; however, the prevalence can be estimated at around 1 in 50,000 to 1 in 100,000 live births in Western Europe.[42] Histologically, epithelial shedding is noted, which proceeds in an irregular fashion, and associated changes of cryptic hyperplasia and increased mitosis in the crypts are noted.[9,117] The so-called tufts[9] refer to the closely packed surface enterocytes that are seen toward the villus tip and may affect up to 70% of the villi.[160] Various degrees of villous atrophy with low or without mononuclear cell infiltration of the lamina propria are seen. Several associated specific features, including abnormal deposition of laminin and heparan sulfate proteoglycan in the basement membrane, increased expression of desmoglein and ultrastructural changes in the desmosomes, and abnormal distribution of $\alpha_2\beta_1$ integrin adhesion molecules were reported.[42] Sivagnanam and coworkers identified epithelial cell adhesion molecule (EpCAM) as the gene for congenital tufting enteropathy[143] in a family with two children affected with tufting enteropathy.

Affected children require lifelong parenteral nutrition, and intestinal transplantation offers the hope for long-term survival.[108] Some infants are reported to have associated choanal, rectal, or esophageal atresia. Nonspecific punctuated keratitis was reported in more than 60% of patients.[42]

Autoimmune Enteropathy

Autoimmune enteropathy is characterized by severe intractable watery diarrhea with persistent villus atrophy, requiring lifelong total parenteral nutrition.[160] Murch and colleagues[95] were among the first to coin the term *autoimmune enteropathy* for a syndrome that was characterized by severe watery diarrhea that occurred in immunocompetent individuals and that was associated with other autoimmune conditions. Key features of this diarrhea are that it persists even after stopping oral feeding and that it is usually noticed within the first few weeks of life.[124]

IPEX syndrome, the best-characterized form of autoimmune enteropathy,[12,124] is a rare disorder with very few known cases.[160] The acronym is intended to suggest that it is a disorder of *immune dysfunction, polyendocrinopathy*, and *enteropathy*, and that it is transmitted in an *X*-linked fashion[12] (males are affected). It is caused by a mutation in the DNA-binding protein FOXP3, also known as *scurfin*,[163] which is responsible for the development of regulatory T cells.[100] The gene has been mapped to chromosome X, very close to the locus of the Wiskott-Aldrich syndrome gene.[12]

CLINICAL FEATURES

The initial presenting features of patients with IPEX syndrome include diarrhea,[163] type I diabetes mellitus,[84] eczema or atopic dermatitis,[100] poor feeding,[84] anemia,[84] thrombocytopenia,[163] hypothyroidism,[84] lymphadenopathy,[163] respiratory distress,[163] and bruising.[84] The first signs of the disease are usually noticed in the immediate neonatal period.[163] Affected infants come to attention because of severe watery diarrhea, which persists despite bowel rest, and hyperglycemia, which becomes a challenge to manage despite aggressive insulin therapy.[163] Diabetes mellitus is caused by the inflammatory destruction of the islet cells, and as the disease progresses, other autoimmune diseases become apparent.[84]

Autoimmune enteropathy must be differentiated from other causes of primary or secondary immunodeficiencies that can present in a similar manner.[160] Wiskott-Aldrich syndrome is characterized by eczema, thrombocytopenia, diarrhea, and enteropathy with low CD8[+] counts,[160] which are normal in IPEX.

The treatment of autoimmune enteropathy focuses primarily on immunosuppression and bone marrow transplantation.[124] Yong and associates reported their success with the use of sirolimus in children with IPEX.[165] Children with autoimmune enteropathy are predominantly dependent on parenteral nutrition for their survival.[124]

Syndromic or Phenotypic Diarrhea

Syndromic diarrhea, also known as *phenotypic diarrhea* or *tricho-hepato-enteric syndrome*, is a congenital enteropathy presenting with early-onset severe intractable diarrhea in infants born small for gestational age and associated with nonspecific villous atrophy with low or no mononuclear cell infiltration of the lamina propria or specific histologic abnormalities involving the epithelium. The diarrhea is associated with facial dysmorphism, immune disorders, and in some patients, early onset of severe liver cirrhosis,[43] hypertelorism, and woolly, easily removable hair with trichorhexis nodosa. Jejunal biopsy specimens showed total or subtotal villous atrophy with crypt necrosis and inconstant T-cell activation in some cases. Colon biopsy specimens showed moderate nonspecific colitis. All the patients had defective antibody responses despite normal serum immunoglobulin levels, and defective antigen-specific skin tests despite positive proliferative responses in vitro.[41] Two cases have been reported by Stankler and coworkers as unexplained diarrhea and failure to thrive in two siblings with unusual facies and abnormal scalp hair shafts.[148] Some cases reported by Girault and colleagues.[41] in 1994 presented with an early-onset severe cholestatic disease that rapidly progressed to cirrhosis and death. A recent report (including two cases with severe liver disease) and the review of the published cases suggested that these patients had the same heterogeneous disease (inappropriately separated into different entities), suggesting that syndromic diarrhea and tricho-hepato-enteric syndrome are two sides of a now well recognized disease of unclear origin.[37]

Clinical findings comprise intrauterine growth restriction, severe protracted diarrhea of infancy, abnormal facies, abnormal hair with tricorrhexis nodosa,[81] immune deficiency,[41] long-term growth failure, and, commonly, mental retardation. Liver disease is associated in about half of the patients and is variable in severity.[43,156]

To date, no epidemiologic data are available. The estimated prevalence is approximately 1 in 300,000 to 1 in 400,000 live births in western Europe.[44] Ethnic origin does not appear to be associated with syndromic diarrhea. Infants are born small for gestational age and present with facial dysmorphism including prominent forehead and cheeks, broad nasal root, and hypertelorism. Hair is woolly, easily removed, and poorly pigmented.[43] Severe and persistent diarrhea starts within the first 6 months of life (1 month or earlier in most cases) and is accompanied by severe malabsorption leading to early and relentless protein energy malnutrition with failure to thrive. Liver disease affects about half of patients with extensive fibrosis or cirrhosis. There is currently no specific biochemical profile, although a functional T-cell immune deficiency with defective antibody production

was reported.[156] Microscopic analysis of the hair shows twisted hair (pili torti), anisotrichosis, poilkilotrichosis, and trichorrhexis nodosa.[81] Histopathologic analysis of small intestine biopsy shows nonspecific villous atrophy with low or no mononuclear cell infiltration of the lamina propria, and no specific histologic abnormalities involving the epithelium. The etiology remains unknown. The frequent association of the disorder with parental consanguinity or affected siblings suggests a genetic origin with an autosomal recessive mode of transmission. Early management consists of total parenteral nutrition. Some infants have a milder phenotype with partial parenteral nutrition dependency, or require only enteral feeding. Prognosis of this syndrome is poor, but most patients survive, and about half of the patients may be weaned from parenteral nutrition at adolescence, although they experience failure to thrive and final short stature.[44,156]

OTHER CAUSES OF DIARRHEA
Infectious Enteropathy

Diarrhea can be caused by any number of viral and bacterial agents and can be prolonged.[74] Stool studies for bacterial cultures and viral antigen detection should be a part of the workup for infantile diarrhea (see also Chapter 39). Gastrointestinal infections are worldwide the most frequent cause of enteropathy by increasing mucosal permeability, local expression of costimulatory molecules allowing antigen penetration in the mucosa, and T-cell activation leading sometimes to disruption of oral tolerance.[129] Concomitant malnutrition impairs not only the immunologic response but also the recovery of damaged mucosa with secondary intestinal and pancreatic enzymatic reductions manifesting as lactose intolerance.

Allergic Enteropathy

Food protein-induced allergic colitis very commonly affects infants in the first few months of life.[105] Offending antigens are usually derived from commercially prepared infant formulas[80] or via breast milk in breast-fed infants.[103] Affected infants present with hematochezia, with or without diarrhea, with prompt resolution of symptoms after elimination of the antigen from the diet.[103] The usual age of presentation is around 66 days,[103] but Kumar and colleagues[80] reported three neonates in whom symptoms were noted at as early as 2 days of life, which suggests in utero sensitization. The most commonly implicated antigens are cow's milk protein and soy protein, which form the basis for the majority of the proprietary formulas.[80] Furthermore, infants diagnosed with cow's milk protein allergy have a 30% to 40% chance of being allergic to soy protein.[103] The dietary approach to allergic disease is currently evolving from passive allergen avoidance to active modulation of the immune system to establish or reestablish tolerance. The gastrointestinal flora provides maturational signals for the lymphoid tissue, improves balance of inflammatory cytokines, reduces bacterial invasiveness and dietary antigen load, and normalizes gut permeability. Major attention has recently focused on the immune effects of dietary lipids in terms of possible prevention of allergic sensitization by downregulating the inflammatory response and protecting the epithelial barrier and host-microbe interactions modifying the adherence of microbes to the mucosa.[129]

Motility Disorders and Small Intestinal Bacterial Overgrowth

Severe and extensive motility disorders such as total or subtotal intestinal aganglionosis (long-segment Hirschsprung disease) or chronic intestinal pseudo-obstruction syndrome may also cause permanent intestinal failure. Small intestinal bacterial overgrowth is a common problem in motility disorders and contributes to diarrhea and malabsorption. Children undergoing bowel surgery in the neonatal period and those having more than one procedure are at greater risk of developing small intestinal bacterial overgrowth postoperatively.

Small intestinal bacterial overgrowth is characterized by nutrient malabsorption associated with an excessive number of bacteria in the proximal small intestine. The pathology of this condition involves competition between bacteria and the human host for ingested nutrients. This competition leads to intraluminal bacterial catabolism of nutrients, often with production of toxic metabolites and injury to the enterocytes. The excess bacteria classically produce diarrhea and malabsorption by deconjugating bile acids, rendering them inadequate for micellar formation and fat digestion Therefore villous atrophy may not be present.[112] Small intestinal bacterial overgrowth is characterized by diarrhea, bloating, flatulence, nausea, abdominal pain, and weight loss.[30,149] Subjects with small intestinal bacterial overgrowth may have protein, carbohydrate, and fat malabsorption. Vitamin B_{12} deficiency produces megaloblastic anemia. Steatorrhea due to fat malabsorption is also a common finding. Small intestinal bacterial overgrowth leads to carbohydrate malabsorption by reducing brush border disaccharidase levels.[139] Lactose intolerance is common and contributes to the diarrhea that typifies small intestinal bacterial overgrowth. Bacterial fermentation of carbohydrates contributes to abdominal discomfort and bloating in small intestinal bacterial overgrowth. The carbohydrate malabsorption is the basis for various breath tests used to diagnose this problem. Protein malabsorption in small intestinal bacterial overgrowth is caused by a number of factors, such as decreased absorption of amino acids and peptides, leading to mucosal damage,[71] low level of enterokinase, which may impair the activation of pancreatic proteases,[127] and protein-losing enteropathy.[78] Small intestinal histologic findings are generally normal in patients with small intestinal bacterial overgrowth, but transient abnormalities of the small intestinal mucosa may be present in some patients.[118]

The most common underlying factors are dysmotility, small intestinal obstruction, and blind or afferent loops. Small intestinal bacterial overgrowth can be diagnosed by jejunal aspirate culture for bacterial counts and hydrogen breath testing using glucose or lactulose.[116] Treatment usually consists of the eradication of bacterial overgrowth with repeated course of antimicrobials, correction of associated nutritional deficiencies, and when possible, correction of the underlying predisposing conditions. Interestingly, loss of the ileocecal valve does not seem to be associated with an increased risk of bacterial overgrowth.[89]

Acrodermatitis Enteropathica

Acrodermatitis enteropathica is a rare autosomal recessive disorder resulting from zinc deficiency. Patients present with poor weight gain, diarrhea, and dermatitis, most noticeably in the perirectal and perioral areas (see also Chapter 52).[160] The SLC39A (solute carrier 39A)[7] gene family consists of 14 members, which are thought to control zinc uptake into the cytoplasm. Among these, zinc-iron transporter protein (ZIP4) is known to be particularly important for zinc homoeostasis. Mutations in this gene cause acrodermatitis enteropathica.[7]

Hormonally Mediated Secretory Diarrhea

In 1958, Verner and Morrison[157] described a syndrome of watery diarrhea and hypokalemia associated with pancreatic tumors in the adult population.[142,154] Vasoactive intestinal polypeptide (VIP) was subsequently isolated in 1975[145] and found to be responsible for causing chronic high-volume watery diarrhea with hypokalemia and acidosis syndrome.[74] Affected children usually present between the ages of 1 and 3 years[74] with severe watery diarrhea that persists despite gut rest.[96] Stool sodium and potassium concentrations are elevated, and fecal osmolar gap is less than 50.[96] The serum VIP concentration, which must be measured if the diagnosis is suspected, is elevated.[74] The most common VIP-secreting tumors (VIPomas) in children originate from neural crest and are usually ganglioneuromas or ganglioneuroblastomas.[96] These tumors are most often localized to the adrenal medulla or the sympathetic chain.[74]

Steroids have been reported to afford transient improvement, but the VIPomas must be aggressively located via either computed tomography or selective arteriography from different parts of the body, because removal of these tumors is curative.[145]

Short Bowel Syndrome

Short bowel syndrome (SBS) is characterized by a complex of symptoms, including malabsorption, diarrhea, and failure to thrive that occur in neonates who underwent small bowel resection. Congenital short bowel in a neonate born with only 50 cm of small bowel has been reported by Hasosah and associates.[54] Most neonates with SBS may have suffered bowel loss as a result of congenital anomalies, such as omphalocele, gastroschisis, or intestinal atresia, or they may have acquired intestinal ischemia from volvulus or necrotizing enterocolitis.[144] Malabsorption in neonates with SBS may ultimately resolve because of the ability of the remaining bowel to grow and to adapt functionally. The small intestine of neonates is 250 cm long and grows to 750 cm by adulthood. In addition, proximal small bowel can differentiate to assume absorptive functions. When the intestine adapts to SBS, the symptoms of malabsorption may improve. In the meantime, nutritional needs must be met parenterally. Factors associated with a reduced likelihood of recovery of bowel function include a remaining small bowel with a length of less than 40 cm, together with either colonic resection or absent ileocecal valve. The health of the remaining bowel and its ability to adapt are important but largely unpredictable factors. Cole and colleagues reported small intestinal bacterial overgrowth to be a negative factor in gut adaptation in patients with short gut.[25] Patients with SBS are predisposed to intestinal mucosal barrier breakdown, bowel dilation, and bacterial overgrowth, all of which may increase the risk of food allergies.

Treatment of neonates with SBS involves a combination of aggressive parenteral nutrition and prompt but cautious enteral feedings. It is important to deliver enteral nutrition, even though absorption is of limited nutritional consequence, to promote intestinal adaptation. Joly and associates report that in patients with SBS, continuous tube feeding (exclusively or in conjunction with oral feeding) following the postoperative period significantly increases the absorption of nutrients compared with oral feeding.[70] Glucagon-like peptide 2 (GLP-2) has generated recent attention as a potential agent in the management of patients with intestinal failure. Several studies have described the various gastrointestinal properties of GLP-2, such as enhanced epithelial and mucosal proliferation,[34,135] improved gastric motility,[164] and decreased gastric secretion.[164] The initial studies using GLP-2, or its protease-resistant analogue teduglutide, have demonstrated improvements in intestinal absorption and decreases in fecal volumes.[67,68] Anecdotally, growth hormone alone or in combination with glutamine has been used in the treatment of SBS; to date, there is insufficient evidence to support the use of growth hormone, glutamine, or a combination of the two as standard therapy in SBS patients.[21,22,136]

Morbidity from SBS is related primarily to nutritional deficiencies, cholestatic liver disease, central line-associated sepsis, and critical limitation of venous access. Pharmaceutical care of the patient with SBS is complex and always changing as intestinal function improves or complications develop. Pharmacologic therapy is directed at controlling gut motility, enhancing intestinal adaptation, minimizing small bowel overgrowth, and preventing nutrient deficiencies and hepatic complications. Rapid intestinal transit may be treated pharmaceutically. Gastric acid hypersecretion may occur in proportion to the degree of bowel resection and is treated with histamine blockers or proton pump inhibitors. Cholestyramine may be used to bind bile salts in patients with choleretic diarrhea. Cholestatic liver disease may be treated with phenobarbital and ursodeoxycholic acid to enhance bile flow. It is helpful to follow stool-reducing substances to document intestinal carbohydrate malabsorption, and to limit feeding advances in the face of malabsorption. Because most absorption of carbohydrate, fat, protein, and micronutrients occurs in the proximal small intestine, losses in this region are associated with micronutrient deficiencies. Careful monitoring of serum levels of fat-soluble vitamins, vitamin B[12], zinc, and copper is recommended when long-term total parenteral nutrition is required. The management of SBS includes also as a key component bowel conservation (especially small intestine) and the prompt reestablishment of bowel continuity.[6]

Surgical procedures, such as longitudinal intestinal lengthening and tapering (LILT) or serial transverse enteroplasty (STEP), can increase mucosal surface area and may enhance intestinal adaptation. Survival after longitudinal intestinal lengthening and tapering ranges from 30% to 100%.[14,63] Survivors that were successfully weaned off parenteral nutrition ranged from 28% to 100%.[14,63]

In the serial transverse enteroplasty procedure a stapler is applied across the dilated bowel in an alternating fashion,

leaving a zigzag-shaped bowel. This approach accomplishes two results, to lengthen and to taper the dilated bowel without damaging the mesenteric blood supply or diminishing mucosal surface area. The serial transverse enteroplasty procedure is simple to perform. Because of the adaptation process, there can be redilation of the bowel after a longitudinal intestinal lengthening and tapering operation. Multiple serial transverse enteroplasty procedures are possible by repeating the operation after the process of adaptation and dilation has occurred.[91,113] Data show a substantial increase in intestinal length and improvement of enteral tolerance, nutrition parameters and ability to wean off parenteral nutrition.[24,102]

Many children with SBS require transplantation. The most common indications for transplantation include failure to wean off parenteral nutrition, parenteral nutrition-associated liver disease, recurrent central catheter sepsis, and loss of vascular access to provide parenteral nutrition.[10] Similar to the longitudinal intestinal lengthening and tapering and serial transverse enteroplasty procedures, intestinal transplantation should be viewed as an adjunct to intestinal rehabilitation. Historically, intestinal transplantation was complicated by significant morbidity and mortality. With recent advances in immunosuppression, specifically the use of tacrolimus, outcomes such as mortality, cost-effectiveness, and quality of life have improved over the last decade.[150] Currently, patients undergoing intestinal transplants experience 1-year graft survivals of 80% and survival of 80% per the Intestinal Transplant Registry. Three different types of transplants can be offered to patients depending on the nature and extent of their intestinal failure: isolated intestinal, liver-intestinal, and multivisceral (e.g., stomach, duodenum, pancreas, intestine, and liver). Recent data show that of pediatric intestinal transplantations, 50% are liver-intestinal, 37% are isolated, and 13% are multivisceral per the Intestinal Transplant Registry (www.intestinaltransplant.org). The decision regarding the type of transplantation should be based on each patient's specific disease and condition.

CONCLUSIONS

Malabsorption syndromes are characterized by the association of chronic diarrhea, abdominal distention, and failure to thrive. There are many causes of malabsorption and chronic diarrhea in the newborn ranging from insufficiency of key elements required in the digestion of carbohydrates, protein, and fat, to electrolyte transport defects, disorders of villous architecture, motility disorders, and congenital causes leading to bowel resection and short bowel syndrome. Any of these disorders can lead to intestinal insufficiency or intestinal failure. Bowel rehabilitation is a key element in the survival of these children, and often requires a multidisciplinary approach for the diagnosis and management of these neonates with the help of a team comprising neonatologist, pediatric gastroenterologist, pediatric surgeon, pediatric pathologist, and nutritionist.

REFERENCES

1. Aichbichler BW, et al: Proton-pump inhibition of gastric chloride secretion in congenital chloridorrhea, *N Engl J Med* 336:106, 1997.

2. Akobeng AK, et al: An inborn error of bile acid synthesis (3beta-hydroxy-delta5-C27-steroid dehydrogenase deficiency) presenting as malabsorption leading to rickets, *Arch Dis Child* 80:463, 1999.

3. Al-Dosari MS, et al: Johanson-Blizzard syndrome: report of a novel mutation and severe liver involvement, *Am J Med Genet A* 146A:1875, 2008.

4. Al Makadma AS, et al: Congenital sodium diarrhea in a neonate presenting as acute renal failure, *Pediatr Nephrol* 19:905, 2004.

5. Ameen NA, Salas PJ: Microvillus inclusion disease: a genetic defect affecting apical membrane protein traffic in intestinal epithelium, *Traffic* 1:76, 2000.

6. Andorsky DJ, et al: Nutritional and other postoperative management of neonates with short bowel syndrome correlates with clinical outcomes, *J Pediatr* 139:27, 2001.

7. Andrews GK: Regulation and function of Zip4, the acrodermatitis enteropathica gene, *Biochem Soc Trans* 36:1242, 2008.

8. Auslander R, et al: Johanson-Blizzard syndrome: a prenatal ultrasonographic diagnosis, *Ultrasound Obstet Gynecol* 13:450, 1999.

9. Avery GB, et al: Intractable diarrhea in early infancy, *Pediatrics* 41:712, 1968.

10. Barksdale EM, Stanford A: The surgical management of short bowel syndrome, *Curr Gastroenterol Rep* 4:229, 2002.

11. Belmont JW, et al: Congenital sucrase-isomaltase deficiency presenting with failure to thrive, hypercalcemia, and nephrocalcinosis, *BMC Pediatr* 2:4, 2002.

12. Bennett CL, Ochs HD: IPEX is a unique X-linked syndrome characterized by immune dysfunction, polyendocrinopathy, enteropathy, and a variety of autoimmune phenomena, *Curr Opin Pediatr* 13:533, 2001.

13. Berriot-Varoqueaux N, et al: Apolipoprotein B48 glycosylation in abetalipoproteinemia and Anderson's disease, *Gastroenterology* 121:1101, 2001.

14. Bianchi A: From the cradle to enteral autonomy: the role of autologous gastrointestinal reconstruction, *Gastroenterology* 130:S138, 2006.

15. Binder HJ: The gastroenterologist's osmotic gap: fact or fiction? *Gastroenterology* 103:702, 1992.

16. Bode L, et al: Heparan sulfate plays a central role in a dynamic in vitro model of protein-losing enteropathy, *J Biol Chem* 281:7809, 2006.

17. Bodian M, et al: Congenital hypoplasia of the exocrine pancreas, *Acta Paediatr* 53:282, 1964.

18. Booth IW, et al: Defective jejunal brush-border Na^+/H^+ exchange: a cause of congenital secretory diarrhoea, *Lancet* 1:1066, 1985.

19. Bunn SK, et al: Treatment of microvillus inclusion disease by intestinal transplantation, *J Pediatr Gastroenterol Nutr* 31:176, 2000.

20. Burke V, et al: Association of pancreatic insufficiency and chronic neutropenia in childhood, *Arch Dis Child* 42:147, 1967.

21. Byrne TA, et al: Growth hormone, glutamine, and a modified diet enhance nutrient absorption in patients with severe short bowel syndrome, *JPEN J Parenter Enteral Nutr* 19:296, 1995.

22. Byrne TA, et al: Growth hormone, glutamine, and an optimal diet reduces parenteral nutrition in patients with short bowel syndrome: a prospective, randomized, placebo-controlled, double-blind clinical trial, *Ann Surg* 242:655, 2005.

23. Canani RB, et al: Butyrate as an effective treatment of congenital chloride diarrhea, *Gastroenterology* 127:630, 2004.

24. Chang RW, et al: Serial transverse enteroplasty enhances intestinal function in a model of short bowel syndrome, *Ann Surg* 243:223-228, 2006.

25. Cole CR, Ziegler TR: Small bowel bacterial overgrowth: a negative factor in gut adaptation in pediatric SBS, *Curr Gastroenterol Rep* 9:456, 2007.

26. Croft NM, et al: Microvillous inclusion disease: an evolving condition, *J Pediatr Gastroenterol Nutr* 31:185, 2000.

27. Cuenod B, et al: Classification of intractable diarrhea in infancy using clinical and immunohistological criteria, *Gastroenterology* 99:1037, 1990.

28. Davis PB (2001) Cystic fibrosis, *Pediatr Rev* 22:257, 1990.

29. Diamanti A, et al: Irreversible intestinal failure: prevalence and prognostic factors, *J Pediatr Gastroenterol Nutr* 47:450, 2008.

30. Dibaise JK, et al: Enteric microbial flora, bacterial overgrowth, and short-bowel syndrome, *Clin Gastroenterol Hepatol* 4:11, 2006.

31. Dror Y: Shwachman-Diamond syndrome, *Pediatr Blood Cancer* 45:892, 2005.

32. Dror Y, Freedman MH: Shwachman-diamond syndrome, *Br J Haematol* 118:70, 2002.

33. Dror Y, et al: Immune function in patients with Shwachman-Diamond syndrome, *Br J Haematol* 114:712, 2001.

34. Drucker DJ, et al: Induction of intestinal epithelial proliferation by glucagon-like peptide 2, *Proc Natl Acad Sci U S A* 93:7911, 1996.

35. Duncan A, et al: The fecal osmotic gap: technical aspects regarding its calculation, *J Lab Clin Med* 119:359, 1992.

36. Eherer AJ, Fordtran JS: Fecal osmotic gap and pH in experimental diarrhea of various causes, *Gastroenterology* 103:545, 1992.

37. Fabre A, et al: Intractable diarrhea with "phenotypic anomalies" and tricho-hepato-enteric syndrome: two names for the same disorder, *Am J Med Genet A* 143:584, 2007.

38. Farrell MH, Farrell PM: Newborn screening for cystic fibrosis: ensuring more good than harm, *J Pediatr* 143:707, 2003.

39. Fichter CR, et al: Perioperative care of the child with the Johanson-Blizzard syndrome, *Paediatr Anaesth* 13:72, 2003.

40. Gathungu GN, et al: Microvillus inclusion disease associated with coarctation of the aorta and bicuspid aortic valve, *J Clin Gastroenterol* 42:400, 2008.

41. Girault D, et al: Intractable infant diarrhea associated with phenotypic abnormalities and immunodeficiency, *J Pediatr* 125:36, 1994.

42. Goulet O, et al: Intestinal epithelial dysplasia (tufting enteropathy), *Orphanet J Rare Dis* 2:20, 2007.

43. Goulet O, et al: Syndromic (phenotypic) diarrhea in early infancy, *Orphanet J Rare Dis* 3:6, 2008.

44. Goulet OJ, et al: Syndrome of intractable diarrhoea with persistent villous atrophy in early childhood: a clinicopathological survey of 47 cases, *J Pediatr Gastroenterol Nutr* 26:151, 1998.

45. Green JR, et al: Primary intestinal enteropeptidase deficiency, *J Pediatr Gastroenterol Nutr* 3:630, 1984.

46. Groisman GM, et al: CD10: a valuable tool for the light microscopic diagnosis of microvillous inclusion disease (familial microvillous atrophy), *Am J Surg Pathol* 26:902, 2002.

47. Groli C, et al: Congenital chloridorrhea: antenatal ultrasonographic appearance, *J Clin Ultrasound* 14:293, 1986.

48. Grosse SD, et al: Newborn screening for cystic fibrosis: evaluation of benefits and risks and recommendations for state newborn screening programs, *MMWR Recomm Rep* 53:1, 2004.

49. Guandalini S: Congenital microvillus atrophy. *eMed Journal* 3, 2002.

50. Guzman C, Carranza A: Two siblings with exocrine pancreatic hypoplasia and orofacial malformations (Donlan syndrome and Johanson-Blizzard syndrome), *J Pediatr Gastroenterol Nutr* 25:350, 1997.

51. Hall GW, et al: Shwachman-Diamond syndrome: UK perspective, *Arch Dis Child* 91:521, 2006.

52. Harms HK, et al: Enzyme-substitution therapy with the yeast *Saccharomyces cerevisiae* in congenital sucrase-isomaltase deficiency, *N Engl J Med* 316:1306, 1987.

53. Hartikainen-Sorri AL, et al: Congenital chloride diarrhea: possibility for prenatal diagnosis, *Acta Paediatr Scand* 69:807, 1980.

54. Hasosah M, et al: Congenital short bowel syndrome: a case report and review of the literature, *Can J Gastroenterol* 22:71, 2008.

55. Hennekam RC, et al: Autosomal recessive intestinal lymphangiectasia and lymphedema, with facial anomalies and mental retardation, *Am J Med Genet* 34:593, 1989.

56. Herzog D, et al: Combined bowel-liver transplantation in an infant with microvillous inclusion disease, *J Pediatr Gastroenterol Nutr* 22:405, 1996.

57. Hoglund P, et al: Genetic background of congenital chloride diarrhea in high-incidence populations: Finland, Poland, and Saudi Arabia and Kuwait, *Am J Hum Genet* 63:760, 1998.

58. Hoglund P, et al: Distinct outcomes of chloride diarrhoea in two siblings with identical genetic background of the disease: implications for early diagnosis and treatment, *Gut* 48:724, 2001.

59. Hokari R, et al: Changes in regulatory molecules for lymphangiogenesis in intestinal lymphangiectasia with enteric protein loss, *J Gastroenterol Hepatol* 23:e88, 2008.

60. Holmberg C, Perheentupa J: Congenital Na$^+$ diarrhea: a new type of secretory diarrhea, *J Pediatr* 106:56, 1985.

61. Holzel A, et al: Defective lactose absorption causing malnutrition in infancy, *Lancet* 1:1126, 1959.

62. Holzinger A, et al: Mutations in the proenteropeptidase gene are the molecular cause of congenital enteropeptidase deficiency, *Am J Hum Genet* 70:20, 2002.

63. Hosie S, et al: Experience of 49 longitudinal intestinal lengthening procedures for short bowel syndrome, *Eur J Pediatr Surg* 16:171, 2006.

64. Jaeken J, et al: The carbohydrate-deficient glycoprotein syndrome. A new inherited multisystemic disease with severe nervous system involvement, *Acta Paediatr Scand Suppl* 375:1, 1991.

65. Jarvela I, et al: Assignment of the locus for congenital lactase deficiency to 2q21, in the vicinity of but separate from the lactase-phlorhizin hydrolase gene, *Am J Hum Genet* 63:1078, 1998.

66. Jeffries GH, et al: Low-fat diet in intestinal lymphangiectasia. Its effect on albumin metabolism, *N Engl J Med* 270:761, 1964.

67. Jeppesen PB, et al: Glucagon-like peptide 2 improves nutrient absorption and nutritional status in short-bowel patients with no colon, *Gastroenterology* 120:806, 2001.

68. Jeppesen PB, Sanguinetti EL, Buchman A, et al: Teduglutide (ALX-0600), a dipeptidyl peptidase IV resistant glucagon-like peptide 2 analogue, improves intestinal function in short bowel syndrome patients, *Gut* 54:1224, 2005.

69. Johanson A, Blizzard R: A syndrome of congenital aplasia of the alae nasi, deafness, hypothyroidism, dwarfism, absent permanent teeth, and malabsorption, *J Pediatr* 79:982, 1971.

70. Joly F, Dray X, Corcos O, et al: tube feeding improves intestinal absorption in short bowel syndrome patients, *Gastroenterology* 136:824, 2009.

71. Jones EA, et al: Protein metabolism in the intestinal stagnant loop syndrome, *Gut* 9:466, 1968.

72. Karim AS, et al: Risk factors of persistent diarrhea in children below five years of age, *Ind J Gastroenterol* 20:59, 2001.

73. Katkin J: Overview of gastrointestinal disease in children with cystic fibrosis, *UpToDate online*, 16.3, 2008.

74. Keating JP: Chronic diarrhea, *Pediatr Rev* 26:5, 2005.

75. Kerem B, et al: Identification of the cystic fibrosis gene: genetic analysis, *Science* 245:1073, 1989.

76. Kianifar HR, et al: D28G mutation in congenital glucose-galactose malabsorption, *Arch Iran Med* 10:514, 2007.

77. Kim SH: Congenital chloride diarrhea: antenatal ultrasonographic findings in siblings, *J Ultrasound Med* 20:1133, 2001.

78. King CE, Toskes PP: Protein-losing enteropathy in the human and experimental rat blind-loop syndrome, *Gastroenterology* 80:504, 1981.

79. Kucinskiene R, et al: Microvillous inclusion disease, *Medicina (Kaunas)* 40:864, 2004.

80. Kumar D, et al: Allergic colitis presenting in the first day of life: report of three cases, *J Pediatr Gastroenterol Nutr* 31:195, 2000.

81. Landers MC, Schroeder TL: Intractable diarrhea of infancy with facial dysmorphism, trichorrhexis nodosa, and cirrhosis, *Pediatr Dermatol* 20:432, 2003.

82. Le Bougeant P, et al: Familial Waldmann's disease, *Ann Med Interne (Paris)* 151:511, 2000.

83. Lee WS, Boey CC: Chronic diarrhoea in infants and young children: causes, clinical features and outcome, *J Paediatr Child Health* 35:260, 1999.

84. Levy-Lahad E, Wildin RS: Neonatal diabetes mellitus, enteropathy, thrombocytopenia, and endocrinopathy: further evidence for an X-linked lethal syndrome, *J Pediatr* 138:577, 2001.

85. Lifshitz F: Congenital lactase deficiency, *J Pediatr* 69:229, 1966.

86. Lindquist B, Meeuwisse GW: Chronic diarrhoea caused by monosaccharide malabsorption, *Acta Paediatr* 51:674, 1962.

87. Linton MF, et al: Familial hypobetalipoproteinemia, *J Lipid Res* 34:521, 1993.

88. Lundkvist K, et al: Congenital chloride diarrhoea: a prenatal differential diagnosis of small bowel atresia, *Acta Paediatr* 85:295, 1996.

89. Maestri L, et al: Small bowel overgrowth: a frequent complication after abdominal surgery in newborns, *Pediatr Med Chir* 24:374, 2002.

90. Mahant S, Friedman J: Index of suspicion. Case 3. Congenital sucrase-isomaltase deficiency, *Pediatr Rev* 21(1):24, 2000.

91. Modi BP, et al: First report of the international serial transverse enteroplasty data registry: indications, efficacy, and complications, *J Am Coll Surg* 204:365, 2007.

92. Muller T, et al: Congenital sodium diarrhea is an autosomal recessive disorder of sodium/proton exchange but unrelated to known candidate genes, *Gastroenterology* 119:1506, 2000.

93. Murayama K, et al: Intractable secretory diarrhea in a Japanese boy with mitochondrial respiratory chain complex I deficiency, *Eur J Pediatr* 168:297, 2008.

94. Murch SH: The molecular basis of intractable diarrhoea of infancy, *Baillieres Clin Gastroenterol* 11:413, 1997.

95. Murch SH, et al: Autoimmune enteropathy with distinct mucosal features in T-cell activation deficiency: the contribution of T cells to the mucosal lesion, *J Pediatr Gastroenterol Nutr* 28:393, 1999.

96. Murphy MS, et al: Persistent diarrhoea and occult VIPomas in children, *BMJ* 320:1524, 2000.

97. Nezelof C, Watchi M: Lipomatous congenital hypoplasia of the exocrine pancreas in children (2 cases and review of the literature), *Arch Fr Pediatr* 18:1135, 1961.

98. Nichols BL, et al: Congenital maltase-glucoamylase deficiency associated with lactase and sucrase deficiencies, *J Pediatr Gastroenterol Nutr* 35:573, 2002.

99. Nichols BL, et al: Human small intestinal maltase-glucoamylase cDNA cloning. Homology to sucrase-isomaltase, *J Biol Chem* 273:3076, 1998.

100. Nieves DS, et al: Dermatologic and immunologic findings in the immune dysregulation, polyendocrinopathy, enteropathy, X-linked syndrome, *Arch Dermatol* 140:466, 2004.

101. Nissler K, et al: Pancreatic elastase 1 in feces of preterm and term infants, *J Pediatr Gastroenterol Nutr* 33:28, 2001.

102. O'Keefe SJ, et al: Short bowel syndrome and intestinal failure: consensus definitions and overview, *Clin Gastroenterol Hepatol* 4:6, 2006.

103. Odze RD, et al: Allergic colitis in infants, *J Pediatr* 126:163, 1995.

104. Oelkers P, et al: Primary bile acid malabsorption caused by mutations in the ileal sodium-dependent bile acid transporter gene (SLC10A2), *J Clin Invest* 99:1880, 1997.

105. Ouwendijk J, et al: Congenital sucrase-isomaltase deficiency. Identification of a glutamine to proline substitution that leads to a transport block of sucrase-isomaltase in a pre-Golgi compartment, *J Clin Invest* 97:633, 1996.

106. Pahari A: Neonatal nephrocalcinosis in association with glucose-galactose malabsorption, *Pediatr Nephrol* 18:700, 2003.

107. Palacin M, et al: Lysinuric protein intolerance: mechanisms of pathophysiology, *Mol Genet Metab* 81 Suppl 1:S27, 2004.

108. Paramesh AS, et al: Isolated small bowel transplantation for tufting enteropathy, *J Pediatr Gastroenterol Nutr* 36:138, 2003.

109. Patel PJ, et al: Antenatal sonographic findings of congenital chloride diarrhea, *J Clin Ultrasound* 17:115, 1989.

110. Phillips AD, Schmitz J: Familial microvillous atrophy: a clinicopathological survey of 23 cases, *J Pediatr Gastroenterol Nutr* 14:380, 1992.

111. Phillips AD, et al: Periodic acid-Schiff staining abnormality in microvillous atrophy: photometric and ultrastructural studies, *J Pediatr Gastroenterol Nutr* 30:34, 2000.

112. Pimentel M, et al: Eradication of small intestinal bacterial overgrowth reduces symptoms of irritable bowel syndrome, *Am J Gastroenterol* 95:3503, 2000.

113. Piper H, et al: The second STEP: the feasibility of repeat serial transverse enteroplasty, *J Pediatr Surg* 41:1951, 2006.

114. Poggiani C, et al: Darrow-Gamble disease: ultrasonographic and radiographic findings, *Pediatr Radiol* 23:65, 1993.

115. Pohl JF, et al: A cluster of microvillous inclusion disease in the Navajo population, *J Pediatr* 134:103, 1999.

116. Rana SV, Bhardwaj SB: Small intestinal bacterial overgrowth, *Scand J Gastroenterol* 43:1030, 2008.

117. Reifen RM, et al: Tufting enteropathy: a newly recognized clinicopathological entity associated with refractory diarrhea in infants, *J Pediatr Gastroenterol Nutr* 18:379, 1994.

118. Riordan SM, et al: Small intestinal mucosal immunity and morphometry in luminal overgrowth of indigenous gut flora, *Am J Gastroenterol* 96:494, 2001.

119. Ritz V, et al: Congenital sucrase-isomaltase deficiency because of an accumulation of the mutant enzyme in the endoplasmic reticulum, *Gastroenterology* 125:1678, 2003.

120. Robb BW, Matthews JB: Bile salt diarrhea, *Curr Gastroenterol Rep* 7:379, 2005.

121. Romagnuolo J, et al: Using breath tests wisely in a gastroenterology practice: an evidence-based review of indications and pitfalls in interpretation, *Am J Gastroenterol* 97:1113, 2002.

122. Rosenstein BJ: What is a cystic fibrosis diagnosis? *Clin Chest Med* 19:423, 1998.

123. Rothbaum R, et al: Shwachman-Diamond syndrome: report from an international conference, *J Pediatr* 141:266, 2002.

124. Ruemmele FM, et al: Autoimmune enteropathy: molecular concepts, *Curr Opin Gastroenterol* 20:587, 2004.

125. Ruemmele FM, et al: New perspectives for children with microvillous inclusion disease: early small bowel transplantation, *Transplantation* 77:1024, 2004.

126. Ruemmele FM, et al: Microvillous inclusion disease (microvillous atrophy), *Orphanet J Rare Dis* 1:22, 2006.

127. Rutgeerts L, et al: Enterokinase in contaminated small-bowel syndrome, *Digestion* 10:249, 1974.

128. Saarela T, et al: Hypercalcemia and nephrocalcinosis in patients with congenital lactase deficiency, *J Pediatr* 127:920, 1995.

129. Salvatore S, et al: Chronic enteropathy and feeding in children: an update, *Nutrition* 24:1205, 2008.

130. Sander P, et al: Novel mutations in the human sucrase-isomaltase gene (SI) that cause congenital carbohydrate malabsorption, *Hum Mutat* 27:119, 2006.

131. Sauvat F, et al: Is intestinal transplantation the future of children with definitive intestinal insufficiency? *Eur J Pediatr Surg* 18:368, 2008.

132. Schibli S, et al: Proper usage of pancreatic enzymes, *Curr Opin Pulmonol Med* 8:542, 2002.

133. Schmider A, et al: Isolated fetal ascites caused by primary lymphangiectasia: a case report, *Am J Obstet Gynecol* 184:227, 2001.

134. Schonfeld G: Familial hypobetalipoproteinemia: a review, *J Lipid Res* 44:878, 2003.

135. Scott RB, et al: GLP-2 augments the adaptive response to massive intestinal resection in rat, *Am J Physiol* 275:G911, 1998.

136. Seguy D, et al: Low-dose growth hormone in adult home parenteral nutrition-dependent short bowel syndrome patients: a positive study, *Gastroenterology* 124:293, 2003.

137. Shalon LB, Adelson JW: Cystic fibrosis. Gastrointestinal complications and gene therapy, *Pediatr Clin North Am* 43:157, 1996.

138. Shanthala CC, et al: Congenital chloride diarrhoea, *Indian J Pediatr* 63:254, 1996.

139. Sherman PM, et al: Neonatal enteropathies: defining the causes of protracted diarrhea of infancy, *J Pediatr Gastroenterol Nutr* 38:16, 2004.

140. Shulman LP, Elias S: Cystic fibrosis, *Clin Perinatol* 28:383, 2001.

141. Shwachman H, et al: The syndrome of pancreatic insufficiency and bone marrow dysfunction, *J Pediatr* 65:645, 1964.

142. Sitaraman S: The VIPoma syndrome, *Gastroenterol Hepatol* 12, 2004.

143. Sivagnanam M, et al: Identification of EpCAM as the gene for congenital tufting enteropathy, *UpToDate online* 17.1, 2009.

144. Snyder CL, et al: Survival after necrotizing enterocolitis in infants weighing less than 1,000 g: 25 years' experience at a single institution, *J Pediatr Surg* 32:434, 1997.

145. Socha J, et al: Chronic diarrhea due to VIPoma in two children, *J Pediatr Gastroenterol Nutr* 3:143, 1984.

146. Soldan W, et al: Sensitivity and specificity of quantitative determination of pancreatic elastase 1 in feces of children, *J Pediatr Gastroenterol Nutr* 24:53, 1997.

147. Spodsberg N, Jacob R, Alfalah M, et al: Molecular basis of aberrant apical protein transport in an intestinal enzyme disorder, *J Biol Chem* 276:23506, 2001.

148. Stankler L, et al: Unexplained diarrhoea and failure to thrive in 2 siblings with unusual facies and abnormal scalp hair shafts: a new syndrome, *Arch Dis Child* 57:212, 1982.

149. Stein JM, Schneider AR: Bacterial overgrowth syndrome, *Z Gastroenterol* 45:620, 2007.

150. Sudan D: Cost and quality of life after intestinal transplantation, *Gastroenterology* 130:S158, 2006.

151. Takahashi T, et al: Johanson-blizzard syndrome: loss of glucagon secretion response to insulin-induced hypoglycemia, *J Pediatr Endocrinol Metab* 17:1141, 2004.

152. Tasic V, et al: Nephrolithiasis in a child with glucose-galactose malabsorption, *Pediatr Nephrol* 19:244, 2004.

153. Treem WR, et al: Sacrosidase therapy for congenital sucrase-isomaltase deficiency, *J Pediatr Gastroenterol Nutr* 28:137, 1999.

154. Udall JN, et al: Watery diarrhea and hypokalemia associated with increased plasma vasoactive intestinal peptide in a child, *J Pediatr* 88:819, 1976.

155. Ukarapol N, et al: Microvillus inclusion disease as a cause of severe protracted diarrhea in infants, *J Med Assoc Thai* 84:1356, 2001.

156. Verloes A, et al: Tricho-hepato-enteric syndrome: further delineation of a distinct syndrome with neonatal hemochromatosis phenotype, intractable diarrhea, and hair anomalies, *Am J Med Genet* 68:391, 1997.

157. Verner JV, Morrison AB: Islet cell tumor and a syndrome of refractory watery diarrhea and hypokalemia, *Am J Med* 25:374, 1958.

158. Vignes S, Bellanger J: Primary intestinal lymphangiectasia (Waldmann's disease). *Orphanet J Rare Dis* 3:5, 2008.

159. Waldmann TA, et al: The role of the gastrointestinal system in "idiopathic hypoproteinemia", *Gastroenterology* 41:197, 1961.

160. Walker W: *Pediatric Gastrointestinal Disease*, Philadelphia, 2004, BC Decker.

161. Wedenoja S, et al: The impact of sodium chloride and volume depletion in the chronic kidney disease of congenital chloride diarrhea, *Kidney Int* 74:1085, 2008.

162. Westphal V, et al: Reduced heparan sulfate accumulation in enterocytes contributes to protein-losing enteropathy in a congenital disorder of glycosylation, *Am J Pathol* 157:1917, 2000.

163. Wildin RS, et al: Clinical and molecular features of the immunodysregulation, polyendocrinopathy, enteropathy, X linked (IPEX) syndrome, *J Med Genet* 39:537, 2002.

164. Wojdemann M, et al: Inhibition of sham feeding-stimulated human gastric acid secretion by glucagon-like peptide-2, *J Clin Endocrinol Metab* 84:2513, 1999.

165. Yong PL, et al: Use of sirolimus in IPEX and IPEX-like children, *J Clin Immunol* 28:581, 2008.

166. Zamel R, et al: Abetalipoproteinemia: two case reports and literature review, *Orphanet J Rare Dis* 3:19, 2008.

167. Zenker M, et al: Genetic basis and pancreatic biology of Johanson-Blizzard syndrome, *Endocrinol Metab Clin North Am* 35:243, 2006.

PART 3

Selected Gastrointestinal Anomalies

Edward M. Barksdale, Jr., Walter J. Chwals, David K. Magnuson, and Robert L. Parry

THORACIC ANOMALIES

Esophageal Atresia and Tracheoesophageal Fistula

Combined anomalies of the esophagus and trachea are regular occurrences in most tertiary neonatal units caring for high-risk infants. The spectrum of recognized deformities comprises a variety of combinations involving esophageal atresia (EA) and tracheoesophageal fistula (TEF). These malformations are well-recognized entities, yet they continue to stimulate a great deal of interest for a variety of reasons, and almost all are lethal unless surgically corrected. Many have concurrent pulmonary complications and most are associated with other congenital anomalies that require careful coordination of interdisciplinary care. The majority can expect a satisfactory outcome if all these considerations are properly addressed. There are few conditions, if any, that require a greater degree of cooperation between neonatologist and surgeon.

The reported incidence of EA/TEF is roughly 1 to 2 per 5000 live births.[48,103] The incidence of EA/TEF is higher in white populations than in nonwhite. There is also a slight preponderance of males and a disproportionate rate of twinning among affected infants. Although the majority of cases are sporadic, there are numerous well-recognized genetic associations. Approximately 7% of affected infants have a chromosomal abnormality such as trisomy 13, 18, or 21. Additionally, EA/TEF has been reported in infants with the Pierre-Robin, DiGeorge, Fanconi, and polysplenia syndromes.

Although usually sporadic, most cases of EA/TEF are not isolated. Most affected infants, up to 70% in some series, have at least one other anomaly.[34] The likelihood of coexisting anomalies is considered to be greatest with pure EA and least with pure TEF. The most widely recognized relationship between EA/TEF and other congenital anomalies is within the constellation of defects referred to as the VACTERL association—abnormalities involving vertebral, anorectal, cardiac, tracheal, esophageal, renal/genitourinary, and limb structures. There is a lesser association with CHARGE syndrome (coloboma, heart defects, atresia choanae, retarded development, genital hypoplasia, ear defects/deafness). Gastrointestinal anomalies (other than anorectal defects) associated with EA/TEF include duodenal atresia, annular pancreas, jejunoileal atresia, and intestinal malrotation. Neurologic defects, especially hydrocephalus, may be associated with EA/TEF, as may diaphragmatic hernia and abdominal wall defects. In order of approximate frequency, the affected organ systems most commonly associated with EA/TEF are cardiovascular (35% to 45%), gastrointestinal (25%), genitourinary (25%), skeletal (15%), and neurologic (10%).

The anatomy of EA/TEF includes five well-recognized variants. A number of anatomic classifications have been devised but have been largely discarded in favor of simple descriptive nomenclature. The most common variant is the combination of a proximal esophageal atresia and a distal tracheoesophageal fistula. The proximal atresia/distal fistula variant occurs in about 85% of affected patients. It manifests classically as a dilated, blind-ending proximal pouch that extends to the lower neck or upper mediastinum, and a distal esophageal segment that originates from the posterior membranous wall of the trachea, carina, or main stem bronchus and connects to the stomach in a normal fashion. The next two most common variants are isolated EA and isolated TEF, both of which occur in approximately 5% to 10% of patients. An isolated TEF is often referred to as an H-type fistula; the fistula itself is usually angled downward, with the esophageal end inferior to the tracheal end. The rarest variants include the proximal fistula/distal atresia, and the double fistula, both occurring in no more than 1% or 2% of patients.

Theories regarding the pathogenesis of EA/TEF are currently undergoing reappraisal. Normal development of the esophagus and trachea includes the formation of a primordial lung bud as a diverticulum of the ventral foregut during the 4th week of gestation. The appearance of this diverticulum is associated with a pair of lateral infoldings of the foregut—the laryngotracheal folds—which begin at the caudal end of the lung bud and fuse to form the tracheoesophageal septum. This process of lateral invagination and fusion was historically believed to proceed cranially, displacing the orifice of the lung bud in a cephalad direction and separating the developing trachea from the esophagus as the tracheal bifurcation moved caudally in a relative sense. Therefore, in the traditional model for the cause of tracheoesophageal malformations, the esophagus and trachea shared a common foregut precursor over a significant distance, becoming separated by the cephalad movement of the tracheoesophageal septum. Perturbations of this process would account for the observed variety of abnormal connections between these two adjacent structures. This theory of cephalad migration of a tracheoesophageal septum is now controversial. Evidence suggests that the position of the laryngeal orifice remains constant relative to the developing notochord, and that the tracheal bifurcation descends simply as a result of linear tracheal growth without any cephalad movement of a tracheoesophageal septum.[69]

Given this alternative scheme of tracheoesophageal development, a different etiologic theory is required to explain tracheoesophageal anomalies. One such theory has arisen from observations in the Adriamycin-treated rat model of VACTERL deformities. In this model, pregnant rats are exposed to Adriamycin during early gestation and give birth to offspring that express VACTERL phenotypes, including EA/TEF. Investigations have demonstrated that the distal "esophageal" segment in EA/TEF arises from a respiratory precursor, descends from the carina along with the two main stem bronchi, and elongates caudally to merge with the stomach. A respiratory origin for this third structure is supported by the finding of pseudostratified respiratory epithelium and respiratory-specific thyroid transcription factor-1 (TTF-1) in distal fistulas from Adriamycin-treated rat model sources, and of TTF-1 expression in distal fistula specimens from human sources.[14,15,94] This structure does not branch as the developing bronchi do, because of abnormal epithelial-mesenchymal interactions caused by deficiencies of mesenchymal fibroblast growth factor (FGF-1) and epithelial FGF receptors.[16] In support of this hypothesis, findings document a brief stage in the Adriamycin-treated rat model during which the stomach is anatomically disconnected from the rest of the developing foregut.[93]

If current proposals of a respiratory-derived distal fistula are accurate, the proximal atresia must therefore have a separate etiology. One proposed explanation is an abnormal concentration gradient of the early embryonic morphogen known as *sonic hedgehog* (Shh), which is elaborated by the developing notochord and is believed to participate in early foregut differentiation. Notochord abnormalities have been documented in the Adriamycin-treated rat model, and in specimens of human distal fistulas that been shown to be specifically deficient in Shh.[27,95] A unifying theory that links these newer models and provides a comprehensive explanation for tracheoesophageal maldevelopment is still lacking.

The clinical presentation of infants with EA/TEF depends on the specific anatomic variant encountered. Most cases of EA/TEF are not diagnosed prenatally, but current prenatal imaging techniques may raise a suspicion of EA/TEF in a significant number of infants. The combination of maternal polyhydramnios and a small or absent stomach has both sensitivity and a positive predictive value for EA/TEF of approximately 40% to 60% in most series.[39,91] The finding of a dilated upper pouch in the neck by high-resolution ultrasonography or magnetic resonance imaging can increase the diagnostic accuracy in this selected group of patients to nearly 100%.[49,85]

In most affected infants, the diagnosis is made in the immediate postnatal period. The infant cannot swallow secretions and appears to drool excessively. As the upper pouch fills, tracheal compression and antegrade aspiration may occur, leading to significant coughing, respiratory distress, and cyanosis. In patients with a distal fistula, the stomach may dilate with air, leading to the reflux of gastric secretions back into the lungs, resulting in significant and progressive respiratory distress due to reactive bronchoconstriction and chemical pneumonitis.

Attempted passage of a gastric tube is usually diagnostic. The tube fails to pass distally and extrudes back through the mouth. A simple chest radiograph usually establishes the diagnosis by demonstrating the radiopaque catheter curled in the upper pouch (Fig. 47-4). If the diagnosis is still in question,

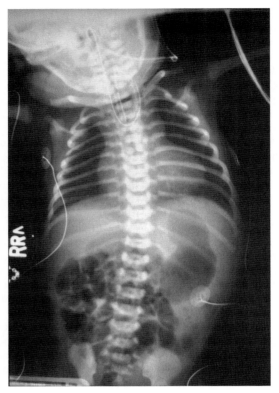

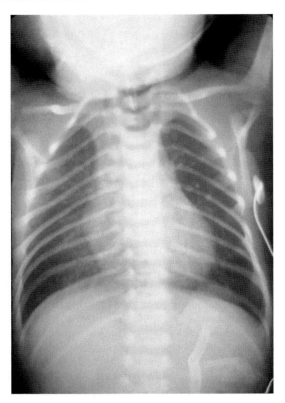

Figure 47–4. Typical chest radiograph of a patient with a tracheoesophageal fistula, with proximal atresia and a distal fistula.

Figure 47–5. Chest radiograph of patient with pure esophageal atresia.

the upper pouch should not be studied with barium or water-soluble contrast agents, as aspiration of these can cause parenchymal lung injury. Air itself makes an excellent contrast agent, and the catheter can be pulled back under fluoroscopic guidance until the tip is positioned in the proximal esophagus, and then 5 to 10 mL of air is injected slowly. A radiolucent dilated pouch is then easily documented. If there is no luminal gas below the diaphragm, the anomaly can be further defined as a pure or distal atresia (Fig. 47-5). The clinical presentation of an H-type TEF is typically much more subtle and delayed. It usually includes a history of coughing during feedings and occasionally the development of pneumonia due to aspiration through the fistula. An H-type TEF may be very difficult to confirm radiographically. Contrast must be injected through a tube positioned in the thoracic esophagus, with the patient prone and in the Trendelenburg position, allowing the contrast to flow back up the angled fistula. Often, an H-type fistula is documented only on rigid bronchoscopy during evaluation for respiratory distress.

Once the diagnosis is established, efforts are made to prevent aspiration-induced lung injury, to provide respiratory support if necessary, and to define associated anomalies while preparing the patient for surgical correction. Gastric acid blockade is immediately instituted while the infant is maintained in a slightly head-up position to reduce reflux of gastric secretions into the airway. A small-caliber sump tube is kept in the upper pouch and suctioned intermittently. The use of preoperative broad-spectrum antibiotics during the first several days is advisable. Spontaneous ventilation is preferred to

minimize the introduction of air into the stomach, as gastric decompression is possible only by percutaneous needle aspiration. This is particularly important in the presence of distal intestinal obstruction. The use of continuous positive airway pressure is contraindicated. If parenchymal lung disease mandates the use of positive-pressure ventilation, mean airway pressures are minimized to avoid shunting of tidal volume through the fistula. This may be difficult in patients with lung disease and poor compliance. Under these circumstances, the use of high-frequency oscillatory ventilation (HFOV) may allow adequate gas exchange to occur at lower peak airway pressures, preventing the loss of ventilation through the fistula. The failure or unavailability of HFOV in a patient requiring aggressive ventilatory support may be an indication for urgent surgical intervention to ligate the fistula, ligate the gastroesophageal junction, or occlude the fistula with a balloon catheter.

A thorough evaluation for other VACTERL-associated defects is mandatory. A preoperative radiograph provides much information regarding cardiopulmonary status, diaphragmatic integrity, and the presence of vertebral abnormalities. The only other studies necessary before surgical management of the EA/TEF are an echocardiogram in all patients and a renal ultrasound in patients with inadequate urine output. Echocardiography not only identifies significant intracardiac anomalies that may influence anesthetic management but also establishes the presence of aortic arch anomalies that may alter the surgical approach.

The nature and timing of surgical intervention depend on the specific anatomic variant being treated. Surgical strategies include immediate primary repair, delayed primary repair, staged repair, and esophageal replacement. Immediate primary repair is appropriate for the majority of infants with EA/TEF. Rigid bronchoscopy immediately before surgical repair is often a useful adjunct to confirm the diagnosis before thoracotomy and to obtain useful information: The location of the fistula can be determined, the presence of a second upper pouch fistula can be detected, and the structural status of the trachea can be assessed (Fig. 47-6). The repair is approached through a right extrapleural thoracotomy, or through the left side if preoperative echocardiography documents a right-sided aortic arch. An extrapleural approach is preferred to avoid a pleural empyema if an anastomotic leak subsequently develops. The fistula is divided and the tracheal side closed transversely to prevent narrowing of the trachea. A primary anastomosis between the proximal esophageal pouch and the distal esophageal segment is then performed. Single-layer end-to-end anastomotic technique is now universal as it results in less tension than two layers and does not substantially increase the likelihood of an anastomotic leak. A closed suction drain is placed and the thoracotomy closed.

In most patients, a gap of some degree exists between the proximal and distal esophagus, requiring mobilization of both ends, and still resulting in some degree of tension at the anastomosis. Anastomotic ischemia caused by overaggressive mobilization or excessive tension leads to fibrosis and stricture formation. The blood supply to the cervical esophagus originates proximally and extends distally through the submucosal plexus, allowing extensive mobilization of the upper pouch without causing ischemia at the distal tip. The blood supply to the normal thoracic esophagus derives from the intercostal vessels and is therefore more segmental. Whether or not this limits the ability to mobilize the distal fistula without causing ischemia is debated. If careful mobilization does

not sufficiently reduce tension at the anastomosis, two options are available. The first option is to lengthen the upper pouch by performing a circular or spiral myotomy. Dividing only the muscle layers allows the redundant mucosa/submucosa to be stretched farther to gain significant additional length. Myotomies may result in the later development of pseudodiverticula and must be performed judiciously. A second option is to perform a staged lengthening of both the upper and lower pouches before performing the anastomosis. This technique, pioneered by Dr. John Foker of the University of Minnesota, is described in more detail later.

The postoperative care of patients with primary esophageal repairs must be meticulous and conservative. Removal of the endotracheal tube should occur only after respiratory mechanics have been optimized, as failure of extubation may lead to aggressive bag-mask ventilation and reintubation—events that place the tracheal repair at risk for disruption. Extubation should occur only when the operating surgeon or other experienced clinician is available to perform reintubation. If a sump tube has been left proximal to the anastomosis, as some surgeons prefer, the tube should not be advanced or reinserted if it is pulled back inadvertently. Some surgeons leave a soft, silicone transanastomotic feeding tube to initiate early enteral feedings. In all cases, the head of the bed is elevated and gastric acidity neutralized to minimize reflux injury to the healing anastomosis. After 5 to 7 days, if the patient is clinically stable without signs of sepsis, a contrast esophagram is carefully performed with a water-soluble agent followed by barium. If no leak is demonstrated, oral feedings are initiated and the chest tube is removed. Small, asymptomatic leaks that are adequately controlled by the existing extrapleural chest tube may be managed nonoperatively and repeat studies performed until healing is documented. Large leaks and intrapleural leaks mandate exploration for repair or diversion.

In many clinical situations, the described primary approach is neither feasible nor appropriate. In the premature infant with very low birthweight, or in any infant with a significant cardiac defect, respiratory compromise, or sepsis, primary anastomosis should be postponed until the patient is a better surgical candidate. If the anticipated surgical delay is brief, careful upper pouch suctioning and parenteral nutrition may be used until the delayed primary repair can be carried out. If a lengthy or indeterminate delay is expected, a staged approach may be required. This strategy provides temporizing measures that allow later esophageal repair to be undertaken electively. Typically, a gastrostomy tube is placed for decompression and feeding, and the fistula is divided via an extrapleural approach to protect the lungs from further injury. Later, a transpleural approach may be taken to restore esophageal continuity.

The list of postoperative complications that occur in this complex group of patients is long and varied. Beyond the immediate postsurgical period, when anastomotic leak is the most feared problem, anastomotic strictures represent the most common complications of surgical treatment, occurring in up to 40% of patients in some series.[42] Strictures result from fibrosis during healing, which in turn results from ischemia, excessive tension, leakage, or acid-peptic injury. An anastomotic stricture should be suspected whenever dysphagia or respiratory symptoms occur in a patient

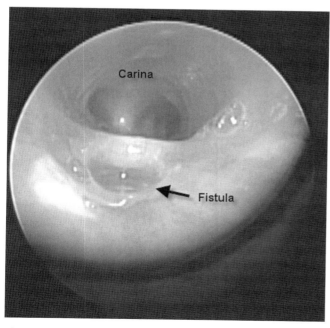

Figure 47–6. Bronchoscopic view of tracheoesophageal fistula.

who had previously tolerated oral feedings. A contrast esophagram reliably demonstrates the stricture and often demonstrates distention of the upper pouch with posterior compression of the trachea—the so-called upper pouch syndrome (Fig. 47-7). Strictures are best treated by tangential dilation under fluoroscopic guidance and control of acid reflux. Near-occlusive strictures require placement of an indwelling transanastomotic guide line that can be used to pull sequential dilators safely through the stricture on a frequent basis. If pharmacologic suppression of gastric acid secretion fails to prevent recurrent strictures, an antireflux procedure may be required. Finally, a stricture refractory to aggressive management may require segmental resection.

Recurrent fistulas occur in 5% to 10% of cases and usually present with respiratory distress during feeding or with recurrent aspiration pneumonia.[22] Diagnosis is made with a dilute barium esophagram in the prone position. Most recurrent fistulas result from small, contained anastomotic leaks that cause chronic inflammatory changes and gradually erode back through the tracheal repair. Surgical options range from primary closure to segmental esophageal resection, and they must include interposition of healthy, well-vascularized soft tissue such as a pleural or strap muscle rotation flap. Some repairs can be approached from a cervical incision, which limits the complications associated with secondary leaks.

Functional disturbances of the esophagus are nearly universal after repair of EA/TEF. Occasionally, dysphagia is associated with severe esophageal dysmotility in the absence of a stricture. Solid-phase esophagography demonstrates that solid foods have great difficulty traversing the anastomosis and lower esophagus because of a lack of peristaltic force. In these situations, dietary modification and adjustment of feeding behavior may be all that can be offered. Gastroesophageal reflux (GER) disease is present to some degree in most of these patients and may be clinically significant in up to 50% of patients with tracheoesophageal malformations.[104] Deficient autonomic and enteric innervation, intrinsic developmental abnormalities of the lower esophageal muscle, shortening of the intra-abdominal esophagus, and distortion of the angle of His may all contribute to lower esophageal sphincter (LES) dysfunction in varying degrees. LES incompetence is exacerbated by esophageal dysmotility, reducing clearance of gastric acid from the esophagus. The major consequence of uncontrolled reflux is anastomotic stricture. Some degree of tracheomalacia is also expected in all patients with EA/TEF. Most patients exhibit the typical raspy cough caused by vibration of the weak and flattened tracheal wall, and they outgrow these minor symptoms with age.

In patients with isolated EA, a long gap is anticipated, and primary repair, immediate or delayed, is not feasible. Historically, long-gap EA had been an absolute indication for esophageal substitution without attempts at staged primary repair. Over the past two decades, however, the proportion of patients with pure atresia who eventually undergo successful esophageal repair has increased dramatically, obviating esophageal substitution in a large number of children.[10,24] There is no universal agreement regarding the maximal gap that will permit esophageal repair.[74,96] However, a fluoroscopically measured gap of greater than four vertebral bodies with the segments in neutral position, or greater than two vertebral bodies (Fig. 47-8) with the segments stretched toward each other, portends a low likelihood of successful primary anastomosis. Elongating the upper and lower

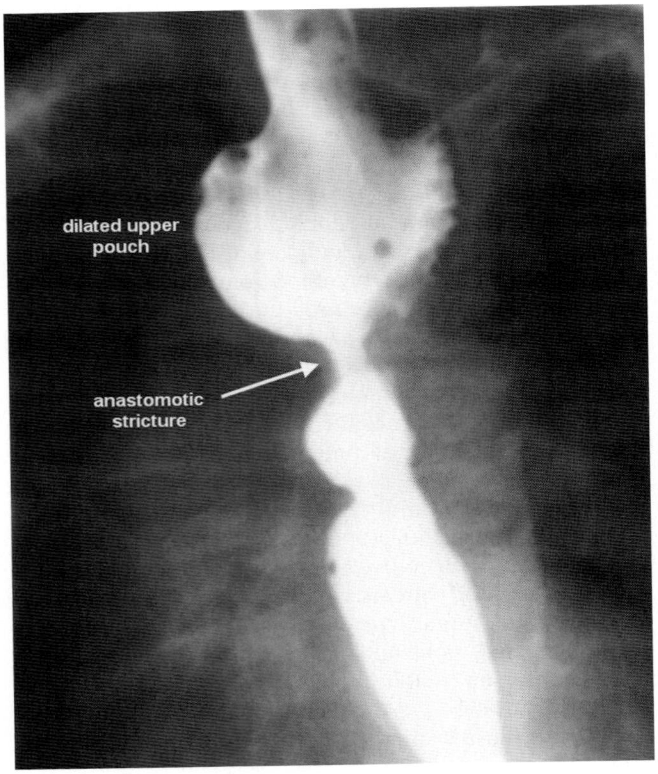

Figure 47–7. Barium esophagram demonstrating anastomotic stricture and upper pouch dilation.

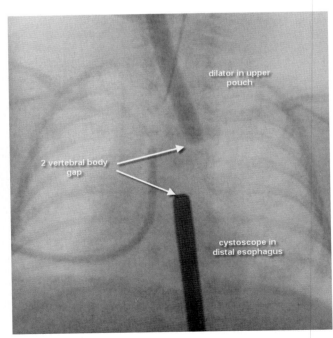

Figure 47–8. Measuring gap length in pure esophageal atresia.

pouches over a 1- to 3-week period, followed by primary anastomosis, has been very successful at keeping the native esophagus and avoiding esophageal replacement. Foker has performed no interpositions since 1983 while treating more than 70 patients with long-gap esophageal atresia.[24] Figures 47-9 and 47-10 show preoperative and postoperative contrast images of a patient with a long-gap atresia of nearly seven vertebral bodies treated by elongation and primary repair. Reflux requiring fundoplication is common in these patients as are dilations to relieve strictures. However, when compared with the multiple, significant complications associated with esophageal replacement using either small or large bowel, the Foker procedure requires strong consideration in all patients with long-gap esophageal atresia. Esophageal replacement is reserved for those cases of long-gap atresia unsuitable for immediate or delayed primary repair, and when attempted primary repair has failed irretrievably due to leakage or stricture.

Long-term outcomes for all variants of EA/TEF have improved steadily over the last three to four decades. Waterston and colleagues were the first to stratify patients on the basis of risk factors shown to affect prognosis, and to recommend treatment strategy based on this stratification.[111] In this analysis, prognosis was dependent on birthweight, associated anomalies, and the presence of pneumonia. Many stratification schemes subsequently evolved, and Spitz and associates refined this prognostic model to include only birthweight and presence of significant congenital heart disease (Table 47-7).[97] In the current era, most infants born with tracheoesophageal anomalies ultimately experience a positive outcome owing equally to refinements in surgical technique and to neonatal support over the past several decades.

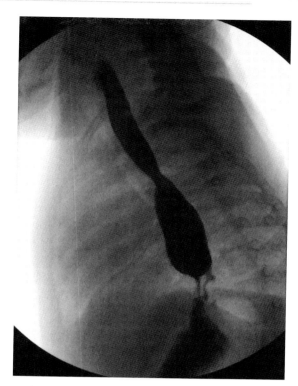

Figure 47–10. Same patient as in Figure 47-9 after Foker repair and Nissen fundoplication. Patient is able to eat all foods without difficulty.

TABLE 47–7   Determinants of Survival in Cases of Tracheoesophageal Malformation

Group	Characteristics	Survival
I	Birthweight >1500 g without CHD	97%
II	Birthweight <1500 g or CHD	59%
III	Birthweight <1500 g and CHD	22%

CHD, major congenital heart disease.

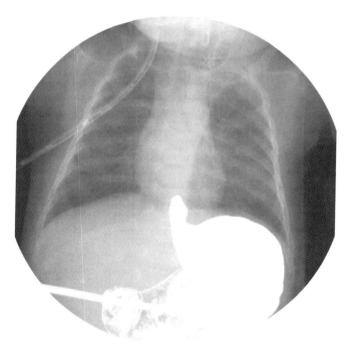

Figure 47–9. Long-gap esophageal atresia. Note proximal air-filled upper pouch and small distal esophagus. Gap is approximately seven vertebral bodies in length.

ESOPHAGEAL DUPLICATIONS

Esophageal duplication cysts are uncommon causes of esophageal obstruction during infancy. These structures result either from abnormalities in the vacuolization process that reestablishes the esophageal lumen after obliterative epithelial proliferation during early embryonic development, or from the "budding" and separation of a portion of the developing foregut. These structures are usually cystic, but they may be tubular and may be located within the muscular wall of the esophagus or exist separately in the posterior mediastinum. They contain an epithelial lining derived from any foregut structure: squamous, columnar, or pseudostratified ciliated respiratory epithelium. They may also contain gastric epithelium and pancreatic or adrenal rests.

Infants with esophageal duplication cysts are usually asymptomatic, and the diagnosis is made when chest radiography unexpectedly demonstrates a mediastinal mass. Some

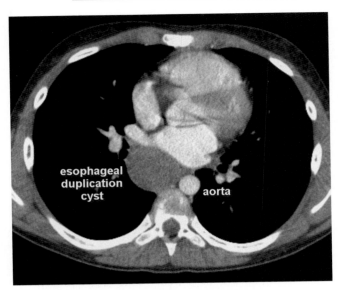

Figure 47–11. Esophageal duplication cyst demonstrated by computed tomography.

infants, however, experience feeding difficulties or respiratory compromise if the cystic structure compresses the adjacent esophagus or trachea. Cysts containing gastric mucosa may present with complications of acid-induced injury: upper gastrointestinal hemorrhage, ulceration, perforation, or erosion into the bronchial tree.

Although the diagnosis may be suggested by a plain chest radiograph or by contrast esophagram, computed tomography is definitive and helpful in planning the operative approach (Fig. 47-11). Magnetic resonance imaging provides additional information about the status of the spinal cord, which may be abnormal, and should be obtained in all patients with a vertebral abnormality or a cystic structure in close proximity to the spine. Esophagoscopy is unnecessary and potentially harmful.

Surgical treatment involves resection of the cyst and repair of any esophageal defect. This may require a thoracotomy, but many lesions lend themselves to thoracoscopic resection. Cysts complicated by infection with abscess formation or by internal hemorrhage may expand rapidly and may require urgent drainage before resection. Duplications that are deemed unresectable because of their extensive nature, which may include extension into the abdomen, should be treated by stripping the mucosa from the duplication and leaving the muscular remnant to heal to the existing esophageal wall. Excellent results can be expected in most patients.

CONGENITAL DIAPHRAGMATIC HERNIA

See also Chapters 11 and 44.

Congenital diaphragmatic hernia (CDH) is a condition in which the defective development of one or more diaphragmatic precursors results in an abnormal communication between the thorax and abdomen, leading to herniation of abdominal contents into the chest. This complex malformation is discussed more thoroughly in Chapter 44, as the principal causes of morbidity and mortality actually relate to

secondary pulmonary hypoplasia, pulmonary hypertension, and cardiac maldevelopment. However, a number of gastrointestinal issues related to CDH merit separate discussion.

Most instances of CDH involve a posterolateral defect, the foramen of Bochdalek, resulting from a failure of the embryonic pleuroperitoneal canal to close. The majority of these, approximately 85%, occur on the left side, although the number of right-sided hernias is probably under-reported, as the liver may block smaller defects and render them asymptomatic. Bilateral hernias are rare and usually fatal. Less commonly, defective development of the central septum transversum leads to an anteromedial defect, the foramen of Morgagni. Morgagni hernias are usually diagnosed before the onset of symptoms when imaging studies are obtained for unrelated reasons. The overall incidence of all types of CDH is approximately 2 to 5 per 10,000 live births.[20] The true incidence may be higher, as a number of affected fetuses experience in utero demise as a result of associated defects, and a number expire in the immediate postnatal period before transfer to a tertiary neonatal center can be arranged, and thus may not be included in statistical surveys.

Current treatment of CDH includes preoperative stabilization, delayed repair, frequent use of prosthetic material to reconstruct the diaphragm, and a variety of management strategies to deal with varying degrees of pulmonary hypoplasia and hypertension. These include permissive hypercapnia, early use of HFOV, inhaled nitric oxide, and extracorporeal membrane oxygenation (ECMO). Advancements in the perioperative physiologic stabilization of these patients have led to an increase in survival rates from less than 50% to approximately 80%.[20] Accurate assessment of the impact of these modalities on survival has proved challenging, however, because of difficulties in applying these technologies in a prospective randomized fashion, and it is unlikely that precise outcome statistics will ever be ascertained.

The most common gastrointestinal complication of CDH is the development of GER, which occurs in approximately 15% to 60%, depending on study criteria and sample pool characteristics.[78,106] GER can be particularly damaging when it results in aspiration pneumonitis in a child with pre-existing pulmonary hypoplasia. Esophageal dysmotility and ectasia are also increased in CDH, potentially exacerbating the peptic complications of GER such as esophageal stricture. Careful surveillance for GER and aggressive medical therapy are therefore mandatory in all survivors of CDH. Surgical treatment of GER may be compromised by dysphagia because of the effects of increased resistance on a dyskinetic esophagus. Therefore, in some circumstances, an incomplete fundoplication may be preferable to a fully competent fundoplication. The proportion of infants with CDH who require fundoplication has been as high as one third in some series.[42]

Although intestinal malrotation is nearly universal in infants with posterolateral CDH, midgut volvulus is uncommon in this population. Retrospective data suggest an incidence of midgut volvulus in survivors of CDH of 3% to 9%.[54,79] This relatively low incidence may result from the extensive intra-abdominal adhesions that form after CDH repair, especially if significant postoperative bleeding occurs as a result of anticoagulation for ECMO. There are no universally accepted recommendations regarding the advisability of performing a Ladd procedure and appendectomy for malrotation at the time of CDH repair. Certainly, the extensive dissection required for a Ladd procedure is contraindicated if the operation is undertaken after the patient has received anticoagulant therapy for ECMO, and appendectomy is ill-advised when placing a prosthetic patch for diaphragm repair because of the potential infectious complications. It may be wise to repair the CDH only, allowing adhesion formation to stabilize the intestinal tract against volvulus.

GASTROESOPHAGEAL REFLUX

Any discussion of GER in neonates must begin with the disclaimer that GER is a normal condition in this age group. Therefore, distinguishing pathologic from physiologic GER is often an exercise in semantics. The proper diagnosis and treatment of GER in neonates requires an understanding of the normal development of physiologic antireflux mechanisms and the natural history and complications of untreated GER. Only then can the somewhat fluid definition of GER be applied meaningfully to individual newborn patients.

Under normal circumstances, gastric contents are prevented from retrograde flow back into the esophagus by the actions of the lower esophageal sphincter. In spite of its accepted name, the LES does not actually consist of a simple circumferential muscle but instead represents the cumulative effects of several discrete physiologic and anatomic components. These include (1) the intra-abdominal esophagus, (2) the angle of His, (3) the gastroesophageal (GE) junction, and (4) the diaphragmatic crura. The intra-abdominal esophageal segment functions in the simple fashion of a Starling resistor—an external positive pressure produces a compressive force against the compliant esophageal wall as it emerges from the negative pressure environment of the thorax. The *angle of His* refers to the oblique angle at which the esophagus connects to the stomach. This obliquity transmits intraluminal pressure in the gastric fundus to the GE junction in an orientation that increases resistance through the GE junction. The circumferential muscle layer of the esophagus at the GE junction also functions somewhat independently, demonstrating anatomic thickening and manometrically detectable muscular tone. The diaphragmatic crura exert a caudad and rightward displacement on the intra-abdominal esophagus during inspiration, resulting in a pinch-cock effect when intrathoracic pressure is most negative. These individual components compose a functional antireflux sphincter that can be quantified in terms of pressure and length.

The LES may be approximately defined in any patient as a high pressure zone by esophageal manometry. The LES resting pressure is approximately 2 to 3 mm Hg at birth and increases linearly to adult levels of 10 to 15 mm Hg by the end of the 2nd month of life on average, and by 6 months of age at the latest.[9] The maturation of the LES by several months of life is seen in both full-term and premature neonates. Significant GER during the first months of life may, therefore, be physiologic and usually resolve without adverse clinical consequences.

The diagnosis of GER in neonates may be made on clinical grounds or bedside assessment via esophageal pH monitoring or the technique of multiple intraluminal impedance. The former is a measure of esophageal acidity, while the latter can quantify retrograde peristaltic waves in the esophagus via specially designed esophageal catheters.[87] When the diagnosis is unclear, a contrast esophagram may be helpful. Esophagography has a low sensitivity in neonates, but it is quite accurate when it does demonstrate reflux. Contrast esophagography is indicated in all neonates with pathologic reflux, to exclude anatomic reasons for excessive vomiting such as malrotation and intrinsic duodenal anomalies. Radionuclide scans are purported to achieve higher sensitivity and specificity than esophagography, but their utility is compromised by a significant false positive rate. They are more useful for assessing delayed gastric emptying, which may contribute significantly to GER and may require specific medical or surgical treatment.

Significant GER in high-risk neonates and infants who do not demonstrate improvement by 6 months of age may be considered an indication for medical therapy. Head-up positioning may be effective, as is the thickening of formula feedings with small amounts of cereal. Prokinetic agents to accelerate gastric emptying may have a beneficial effect. Because these agents increase mean intragastric pressure, they may also exacerbate GER in some patients and must be assessed for efficacy on an individual basis. The hallmark of medical therapy is neutralization of gastric acidity, which does not reduce GER events but does protect the esophagus from peptic injury secondary to prolonged exposure to gastric acid. This may be accomplished with either antacids or antisecretory agents, such as histamine blocking agents and proton pump inhibitors, although increased risk of infection is a potential side effect.[70]

Surgical treatment for GER is reserved for high-risk infants who have complications of GER and for those who are refractory to medical therapy. Complications of GER include failure to thrive, aspiration pneumonia, reactive airway disease, and esophagitis with bleeding, stricture, ulceration, or Barrett metaplasia. Antireflux surgery may also be performed electively in the older child who prefers surgery to a lifetime of medication. Finally, surgical intervention is often necessary in certain select groups—infants with coexisting tracheoesophageal malformations, congenital diaphragmatic hernia, hiatal hernia, and severe neurodegenerative conditions.

There are many surgical options for the treatment of GER, a reflection of the fact that no antireflux surgery is completely effective or without a significant incidence of complications. The Nissen fundoplication, which includes a complete, circumferential wrap of the gastric fundus, has emerged as the most effective option in most clinical settings. In this procedure, a high pressure zone is created just above the GE junction by the fundic wrap, which has been mobilized by dividing its normal attachments to the spleen and diaphragm. Crucial elements of this procedure include creation of a loose wrap 1 to 2 cm in length, provision of an adequate length of intra-abdominal esophagus, and secure closure and reinforcement of the diaphragmatic crural fibers behind the esophagus to prevent postoperative hiatal hernia. This procedure can be performed with similar results using either traditional open or minimally invasive techniques.

There is little controversy that Nissen fundoplication provides excellent control of GER in children, as assessed by symptom relief or quantitative pH measurement. The rate of complications, however, is more difficult to ascertain. Most postoperative complications are associated with symptoms of recurrent reflux or excessive resistance. The most common serious complication of fundoplication is hiatal herniation of the wrap, the incidence of which ranges between 3% and 10% in unselected studies to between 10% and 20% in neurologically impaired children.[57,88] Hiatal hernias occur when increased intra-abdominal pressure is transmitted to the wrap, which pushes up through the crural repair. Patients with hypertonia, spasticity, seizure disorders, constipation, and reactive airway disease may all be at risk for this complication. The wrap may also be pulled up into the chest by negative intrathoracic pressure, a congenitally short esophagus, and an intrinsically weak crural mechanism. These conditions exist in neonates with congenital hiatal hernia, esophageal atresia, and diaphragmatic hernia. The rate of wrap dehiscence is negligible in virtually every contemporary series. When recurrent GER occurs after antireflux surgery, hiatal hernia of the wrap is the most likely underlying problem.

The other main complication of fundoplication is dysphagia and gas-bloat syndrome, in which the patient is unable to relieve gastric distention by vomiting or belching. These occur when an over-tight wrap generates excessive resistance to flow in either direction. This complication should be minimal when a loose, "floppy" wrap is constructed. The goal of surgery is not to prevent all reflux but to reduce reflux to near-physiologic levels.

A major contributing factor to wrap herniation, wrap failure, and gas-bloat syndrome after fundoplication is delayed gastric emptying, which results in a distended stomach under increased pressure. Delayed gastric emptying results from dysfunction of the autonomic and enteric nervous systems, and it occurs frequently in patients with profound neurologic compromise and those with diffuse metabolic disorders. Diagnosis can be best made by radionuclide imaging, and treatment includes pyloroplasty at the time of fundoplication.[3]

In certain patients, a circumferential, fully competent fundoplication can be predicted to cause dysphagia and gas-bloat syndrome. Patients shown to have severe esophageal dysmotility may achieve a better clinical result with a partial fundoplication. The Toupet fundoplication, which includes a posterior partial wrap, and the Thal fundoplication, which includes an anterior imbrication of the fundus over the GE junction, are both less effective than the Nissen fundoplication at reducing reflux but produce less resistance and dysphagia. Careful preoperative patient selection should determine the most appropriate surgical option on an individualized basis.

ABDOMINAL ANOMALIES
Abdominal Wall Defects

The most common abdominal wall defects seen in neonates are omphalocele and gastroschisis, occurring in approximately 4 per 10,000 live births. These conditions result from different developmental miscues and manifest as distinct clinical entities. In the case of omphalocele, a central abdominal wall defect of variable size is covered by a domelike mesenchymal membrane composed of amnion. The umbilical cord connects to the central portion of this membrane (Fig. 47-12). The underlying abdominal organs are protected

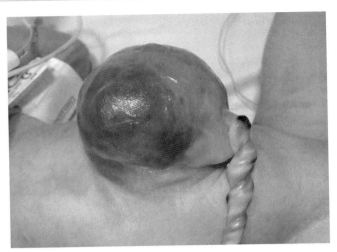

Figure 47–12. Typical medium-size omphalocele.

from exposure to amniotic fluid. In gastroschisis, the defect is usually smaller and located to the right of the umbilical attachment. There is no protective membranous covering. The abdominal contents, therefore, are eviscerated and suspended in amniotic fluid during gestation (Fig. 47-13).

Omphalocele results from a failure in the folding mechanism that converts the flat trilaminar germ disc into a complex "tubular" structure starting at about 5 weeks' gestation. The lateral body folds and craniocaudal folds converge at the umbilical ring, which contracts, closing the ventral abdominal wall. In patients with omphalocele, this ring fails to contract and leaves a round defect of variable size and a corresponding sac composed of amnion. The liver and small intestine usually occupy a portion of the sac, along with a variable amount of other abdominal contents. The underlying failure of umbilical ring closure may be related to aberrant development and migration of abdominal wall muscular components, or to failure of the developing midgut to return to the abdominal cavity after a period of herniation into the umbilical stalk. Rarely, the defect is cephalad to the umbilicus, producing a complex deformity referred to as the

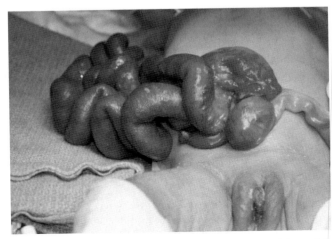

Figure 47–13. Typical gastroschisis defect with mild "peel."

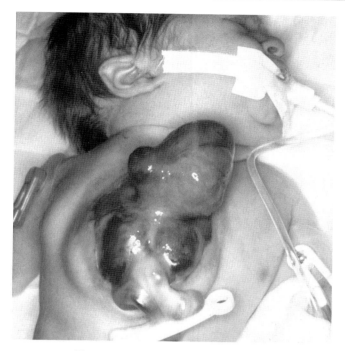

Figure 47–14. Pentalogy of Cantrell.

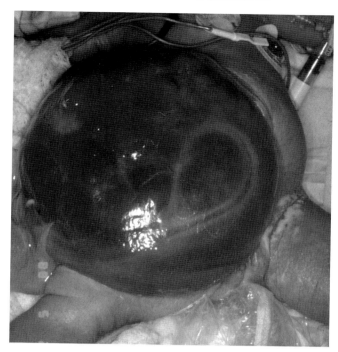

Figure 47–15. Giant omphalocele with predominate liver component.

pentalogy of Cantrell: sternal, diaphragmatic, and pericardial defects, upper abdominal omphalocele, and ectopia cordis (Fig. 47-14). When centered below the umbilicus, bladder or cloacal exstrophy may occur. The cause of gastroschisis is equally unclear, but it may involve a rupture of the umbilical stalk during the period of midgut herniation. Competing theories involving thromboembolic infarction of the developing abdominal wall or a failure of mesenchymal migration are less convincing.

The factors influencing morbidity and survival in these two distinct conditions are very different. Omphalocele, with a stable incidence of about 2 to 2.5 per 10,000 live births, is associated with other structural or genetic defects in 50% to 75% of affected infants.[13] These associated anomalies, which may involve the cardiovascular, gastrointestinal, genitourinary, or central nervous systems, account for most of the morbidity in these patients. Because the abdominal contents are protected throughout gestation, little morbidity accrues from injury to the intestinal tract. The discrepancy between the volume of eviscerated abdominal organs and the size of the abdominal cavity— the "loss of domain"—accounts for the other major source of morbidity in these patients. In a giant omphalocele, eventual closure of the abdominal wall by any means may be challenging, leading to a variety of problems related to structural integrity of the torso, chronic ventral hernias, and posture and gait development (Fig. 47-15). Additionally, infants with giant omphaloceles may have a high incidence of pulmonary hypoplasia, resulting in respiratory compromise and pulmonary hypertension.[5]

The syndromes most often associated with omphalocele include the VACTERL association, Beckwith-Wiedemann syndrome (macrosomia, macroglossia, visceromegaly, hemihypertrophy, hypoglycemia, renal pathology), EEC syndrome (ectodermal dysplasia, ectrodactyly, cleft palate), and OEIS

complex (omphalocele, exstrophy, imperforate anus, spinal defects). An oft-reported association of omphalocele with cryptorchidism is unsubstantiated. Chromosomal abnormalities, including trisomies 13, 18, and 21, occur in 25% to 50% of affected patients. The presence of a small sac, the absence of liver in the sac, and the presence of other malformations strongly predict an abnormal karyotype.[18,26]

Gastroschisis, in contrast, is sporadic in the vast majority of cases. The incidence of gastroschisis is approximately 1.5 per 10,000 live births and increasing. Risk factors for gastroschisis include young maternal age, lower socioeconomic status, and exposure to external agents such as vasoconstricting decongestants, nonsteroidal anti-inflammatory agents, cocaine, and possibly pesticides/herbicides.[29,102] The 5% to 20% incidence of associated defects is lower than for omphalocele, and it represents mostly intestinal atresias directly associated with ischemic or mechanical injury to the eviscerated bowel during gestation. Abnormalities not directly related to the abdominal wall defect are uncommon.

Morbidity in infants with gastroschisis, as opposed to those with omphalocele, is almost entirely related to intestinal dysfunction caused by in utero injury to the eviscerated bowel. The spectrum of injury displayed by the eviscerated bowel in gastroschisis ranges from mild to catastrophic. Morphologically, the bowel appears edematous, matted, and foreshortened. Often, the mass appears to be contained within an inflammatory rind—the "peel" of gastroschisis (Fig. 47-16). Histologically, the intestine is characterized by villous atrophy and blunting, submucosal fibrosis, muscular hypertrophy and hyperplasia, and serosal inflammation.[51,98] The cause of injury is unclear, but it is probably related to a combination of two separate insults. Exposure to amniotic fluid appears to be a major contributing

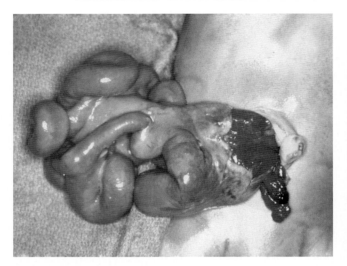

Figure 47–16. Gastroschisis with moderately severe peel.

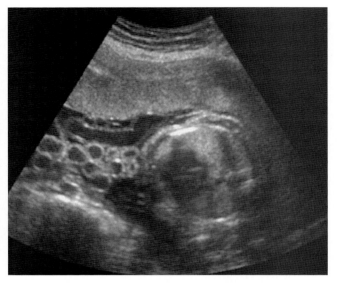

Figure 47–17. Ultrasound of fetus with gastroschisis.

factor, as amniotic fluid exchange can prevent peel formation.[2] The second cause of injury may be the partial closure of the defect around the base of the eviscerated intestinal mass. This causes progressive constriction around the intestinal mesentery, resulting in the obstruction of luminal, lymphatic, and venous outflow.

The functional consequences of these structural changes include impaired absorption, reduced brush border enzyme synthesis, and a prolonged motility disorder related to rigidity of the bowel wall and possible derangements in the production of enteric neurotransmitters such as nitric oxide.[6] These changes concur with the clinical observation that infants with a dense peel suffer prolonged gastrointestinal dysfunction that requires precise nutritional management. This nutritional failure and the complications arising from prolonged enteral and parenteral nutritional therapy constitute a significant proportion of the adverse clinical outcomes in these patients.

The prenatal diagnosis of abdominal wall defects by fetal ultrasonography is well established (Fig. 47-17). Any uncertainty in distinguishing omphalocele from gastroschisis may be eliminated by measuring amniotic fluid α-fetoprotein levels, which should be elevated in gastroschisis only. A prenatal diagnosis of omphalocele should prompt a thorough sonographic survey of the entire fetus to evaluate for associated anomalies. Chromosomal analysis may also be helpful in determining postnatal management and prognosis.

The obstetric decisions related to timing and route of delivery continue to engender considerable debate. In the case of omphalocele, if the membrane is intact, the pregnancy should be carried to term if possible, as early delivery has no theoretical benefit for the fetus. Cesarean delivery has historically been recommended to prevent rupture of the omphalocele membrane, which would necessitate emergent surgical intervention without the benefit of preoperative evaluation and stabilization. Studies, however, have suggested that the route of delivery has no effect on morbidity or prognosis in abdominal wall defects in general.[4,37,84] Recommendations regarding the route of delivery for a fetus

with a giant omphalocele or associated anomalies should be individualized.

In gastroschisis, the belief that prolonged exposure of the eviscerated intestine to amniotic fluid and progressive mechanical constriction causes intestinal injury has led to the proposal that early delivery and repair might improve intestinal function and reduce morbidity. Early delivery after lung maturation has been enthusiastically endorsed by some, but definitive evidence that this strategy confers any statistically verifiable benefit is lacking. A more selective approach in which early delivery is undertaken when sonographic surveillance suggests progressive bowel injury, as defined by bowel dilation and wall thickening, has yielded numerous conflicting reports.[38,62] Until the efficacy of selective early delivery for gastroschisis has been studied in a prospective, randomized fashion, support for this intuitively appealing strategy will remain anecdotal. Serial amniotic fluid exchange in gastroschisis with oligohydramnios has been reported to reduce bowel injury, but this has not been subjected to a large scale randomized study.[19] Regardless of the timing of delivery, almost all infants with gastroschisis may be delivered vaginally without increased injury to the bowel.

The surgical goal of establishing complete fascial and skin closure without causing further injury to the underlying bowel is common to patients with both omphalocele and those with gastroschisis. The surgical strategies applied to these two conditions are, however, quite different. In patients with gastroschisis, emergent closure or coverage of the defect is of the highest priority to limit intestinal injury and reduce morbidity. The eviscerated intestine should be completely covered in the delivery room to prevent water and heat loss through evaporation, conduction, and convection. Temporary coverage can be provided by wrapping the torso with transparent plastic film or by placing the baby in a transparent surgical "bowel bag" and cinching the drawstring closed gently under the axillae. This arrangement effectively limits heat and water loss, and it allows the intestine to be visualized at all times so that inadvertent volvulus and ischemia can be detected and reversed. A lateral decubitus position is often better tolerated than supine. A gastric decompression tube is placed immediately to prevent intestinal dilation.

Many infants with gastroschisis are born prematurely, and aggressive respiratory care including supplemental oxygen, endotracheal intubation, and intratracheal surfactant may be necessary. Intravenous access is established for fluid resuscitation and administration of broad-spectrum antibiotics. As soon as the baby is physiologically stable, transport to the operating room for surgical management is advisable. Unnecessary delay only compounds the problems of further bowel swelling and possible ischemia.

Gastroschisis can be managed by either primary or staged closure, depending on the size discrepancy and the infant's physiologic status. Although 60% to 70% of gastroschisis cases can be closed primarily, the decision to do so is individualized in each circumstance. As the intestine is returned to the abdominal cavity and the abdominal fascia approximated, increased abdominal pressure may prevent safe, complete closure. In infants with preexisting pulmonary compromise, the restriction of diaphragmatic excursion may decrease extrinsic compliance and cause ventilatory pressures to rise to unacceptable levels. Increased abdominal pressures may also impair mesenteric, hepatic, and renal perfusion. Intraoperative monitoring of abdominal pressure by connecting a bladder catheter to a pressure transducer can provide useful information.

When respiratory problems or abdominal pressures prevent safe primary closure, placement of a temporary prosthetic "silo" allows for more gradual reduction of the eviscerated intestine into the abdominal cavity and delayed primary closure at a later time (Fig. 47-18). Previous retrospective studies had documented improved survival with primary closure, prompting an era marked by an aggressive approach to immediate closure. Appreciation of the fact that this survival advantage simply represented a selection bias, along with recognition of the deleterious effects of high intra-abdominal

pressures, has led to a more liberal use of temporary silo coverage. Usually, the fascial opening is extended to produce a broad-based defect, and a cylinder of reinforced silicone or other nonporous material is sutured to the fascial rim. Many surgeons have abandoned the use of traditional handmade silos in favor of prefabricated silos that consist of an elongated prosthetic bag with an elastic, springlike base. These silos can be installed without sutures and may be placed in the delivery room, obviating an emergent trip to the operating room.

When a silo has been constructed, the intestinal contents are squeezed back into the abdominal cavity in daily increments. Abdominal wall cellulitis related to the open wound and presence of the prosthetic material limits the use of a silo to a period of approximately 2 weeks. When reduction of the silo contents is complete, the patient is returned to the operating room for final closure (Fig. 47-19). Broad-spectrum antibiotics are given until the silo is removed. Placement of a silo does not preclude postoperative extubation, and spontaneous ventilation during staged closure is preferable to positive-pressure ventilation. Infants should be maintained on a ventilator to allow for neuromuscular paralysis in only the most severe cases of abdominoviscerial disproportion requiring aggressive closure. When postoperative mechanical ventilation is required, increased levels of positive end-expiratory pressure are necessary to maintain functional residual capacity and optimize compliance.

During staged closure, parenteral nutrition is administered through a peripherally inserted central venous catheter, or one placed at the time of silo placement. Complete bowel rest and gastric decompression are maintained during reduction of the silo. After abdominal wall closure, whether primary or delayed, enteral feedings should be initiated only after clinical resolution of the ileus is apparent—cessation of bilious gastric aspirates, presence of bowel sounds, and passage of meconium. Advancement of enteral feedings should be conservative, as infants with gastroschisis, especially those with a dense peel requiring silo closure, are extremely sensitive to changes in nutritional substrate load. Delayed enteral feedings and prolonged parenteral infusions are a principal

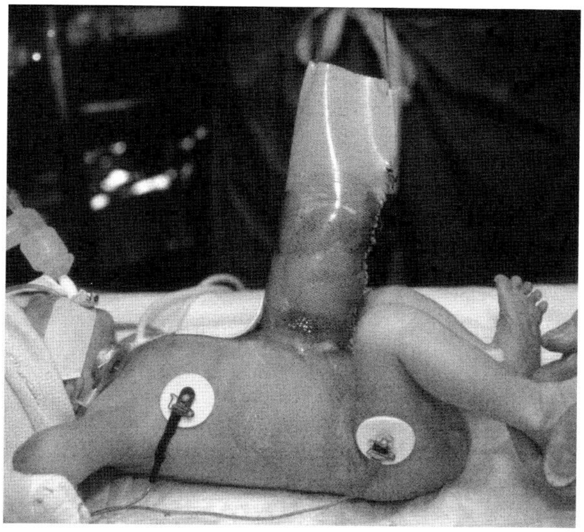

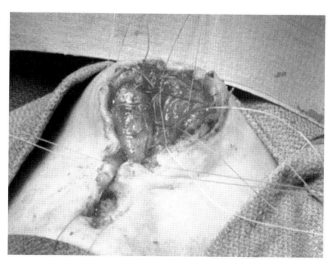

Figure 47–18. Silastic "silo" for delayed primary closure of abdominal wall defects.

Figure 47–19. Final reduction and closure of abdominal wall defect after silo reduction.

source of morbidity in this group. Development of cholestatic jaundice is common, and hepatic dysfunction and fibrosis may occur in a small number of refractory patients. Early administration of partial enteral mini-feedings, meticulous avoidance of infection, and reduction of copper and manganese have all been advocated to reduce the incidence of cholestatic liver disease.[59]

The coexistence of intestinal atresias with gastroschisis deserves special mention. Intestinal atresias occur in 5% to 25% of patients with gastroschisis, and they are one of several independent variables that have a negative impact on prognosis in gastroschisis. They are commonly felt to be related to vascular compromise caused by in utero constriction on the intestinal mesentery, although this relationship has been cited by some as supportive evidence for a thromboembolic etiology for both conditions.[112] When atresias are recognized at the time of surgery, options include primary anastomosis if no peel exists and a straightforward abdominal closure is anticipated, or simple internalization of the uncorrected atresia if a peel exists or staged closure is necessary.[89] This is then followed by later reexploration and repair after the peel resolves in several weeks. Construction of an enterostomy in the presence of a silo is associated with an increased incidence of abdominal wall infectious complications.[30] In a patient who fails to exhibit intestinal patency within 2 weeks of abdominal wall closure, a water-soluble lower gastrointestinal contrast study should be obtained to exclude the presence of an unrecognized atresia.

The surgical options for abdominal wall closure for omphalocele are similar to those for gastroschisis. The main difference relates to the preoperative management of these patients. A careful assessment of physiologic status and a thorough search for syndromic and chromosomal anomalies is imperative to guide anesthetic management and to identify prognostic factors. The presence of a protective membrane allows a careful and unhurried preoperative evaluation. Small rents in the membrane may be sutured at bedside to maintain this elective posture. In some cases, neither primary nor staged closure is appropriate. These include cases associated with lethal anomalies, patients with profound cardiac compromise, those with severe pulmonary hypoplasia or pulmonary hypertension, and those with giant omphaloceles with no hope for autogenous tissue closure. In these circumstances, nonoperative management may be used. The membrane is preserved and treated by topical application of an antimicrobial agent such as silver sulfadiazine, allowing slow epithelialization of the amnion. This results in durable coverage and a chronic ventral hernia. If the patient survives the short-term medical challenges, removal of the amnion and placement of a prosthetic patch with overlying skin closure allows for gradual stepwise reduction of the patch and eventual abdominal wall closure later in childhood.

As defined previously, the factors affecting prognosis for gastroschisis and omphalocele are quite distinct. Prematurity, degree of peel formation, and associated atresias account for most of the morbidity in gastroschisis, which has an overall survival rate of 90% to 95%.[33,66] Most of the deaths attributed to gastroschisis are related to perioperative complications, such as sepsis, necrotizing enterocolitis, and abdominal visceral ischemia, or to late hepatic failure caused by parenteral nutrition-related cholestatic disease. Surprisingly, midgut

volvulus related to obligatory intestinal malrotation in these patients is virtually nonexistent, possibly because of the development of peritoneal adhesions that limit mobility of the intestine. The reported survival rate for infants with omphalocele ranges from 30% to 80%.[65,113] When mortality caused by associated malformations is excluded, the survival rates approach those for gastroschisis. Long-term tolerance of enteral feedings, as well as physical growth and development, are usually normal after 1 or 2 years, even in severe cases. With thoughtful management and attention to the prevention of parenteral nutrition-related hepatic complications, most infants born with abdominal wall defects should survive with an acceptable quality of life.

GASTRIC VOLVULUS

Congenital deficiencies of mesenteric fixation of the stomach to the surrounding structures predispose to gastric volvulus and can take two distinct forms. Absence or laxity of the gastrohepatic and gastrosplenic ligaments allows the stomach to rotate around its longitudinal axis, producing an organoaxial volvulus. Similar abnormalities of the gastrophrenic ligament and duodenal attachments allow rotation around the stomach's transverse axis, referred to as a *mesentericoaxial volvulus*. Organoaxial volvulus is the more common of the two types in infants and children. A strong association has been found between gastric volvulus and malrotation, asplenia, and congenital abnormalities of the diaphragm.[58] Gastric volvulus may also be associated with conditions that result in gastric distention, such as aerophagia and hypertrophic pyloric stenosis. Because these entities all result in absence or stretching of stabilizing attachments, a causative role is assumed.

Although gastric volvulus can occur as either an acute or a chronic problem, the acute form is more common in children. The classic presentation of sudden epigastric pain, retching without emesis, and inability to advance a nasogastric tube into the stomach is rarely encountered in the actual clinical setting. Children may experience emesis, which can be bilious or nonbilious, and may not have abdominal distention. Intermittent gastric volvulus may be considered in the workup of infants presenting with apparent life-threatening events.[68] Any combination of symptoms suggesting a partial or complete proximal mechanical obstruction may be present. Profound physiologic decompensation, hemodynamic instability, or unrelenting metabolic acidosis suggests strangulation, ischemic necrosis, and possibly perforation.

Radiologic assessment can reveal several characteristic findings. On plain abdominal radiographs, massive gastric dilation can usually be seen, often with a distinct incisura pointing toward the right upper quadrant. The spleen and small intestine may be displaced inferiorly. If a contrast study has been attempted, the contrast column may be confined to the esophagus, with a long, gradual tapering at the bottom. Occasionally, a paraesophageal hiatal hernia is detected. Classic findings on barium upper gastrointestinal study include transverse lie of the stomach and inversion of the greater curvature and pylorus (Fig. 47-20). Operative treatment of acute gastric volvulus includes gastric decompression by nasogastric suction or needle aspiration and reduction of the volvulus. Perforations are closed primarily or, depending on

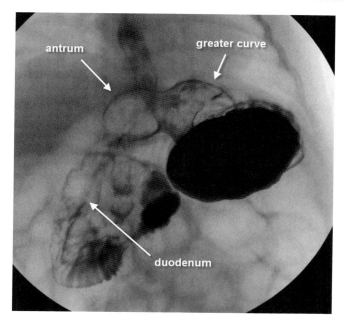

Figure 47–20. Upper gastrointestinal contrast study demonstrating gastric volvulus with rotation of the greater curve and antrum of the stomach above the duodenal bulb.

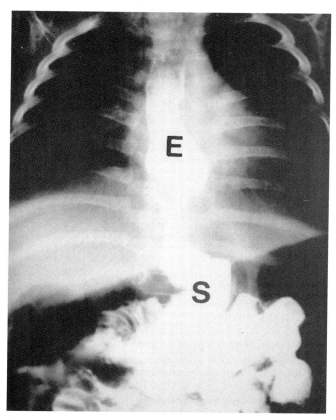

Figure 47–21. Upper gastrointestinal contrast study of patient with microgastria (S) and megaesophagus (E).

their location, around a Malecot tube; more extensive necrosis requires resection. Coexisting anomalies, such as malrotation and diaphragmatic defects, should be corrected. Recurrent volvulus is prevented by performing an anterior gastropexy. Historically, a Stamm-type gastrostomy has been used to increase stability of the gastropexy by creating a fibrotic scar that traverses all layers of the abdominal and gastric walls, although there are no data that suggest this is mandatory. Both laparoscopic and open approaches are effective. Recurrence is rare.

MICROGASTRIA

Congenital microgastria is a rare anomaly in which the stomach is characterized by very small volume, a tubular shape, and abnormal fixation. Gastric volume does not undergo complete compensatory growth and remains relatively small as the child ages.[8] Associated abnormalities include megaesophagus, GER, intrinsic duodenal obstruction, malrotation, biliary anomalies, situs inversus, asplenia, and skeletal defects.

Microgastria presents with vomiting and failure to thrive in the infant, often associated with persistent diarrhea. Vomiting may be due to gastric insufficiency, GER, or duodenal obstruction. Diarrhea is presumed to be due to rapid gastric transit and dumping. The diagnosis is established by contrast upper gastrointestinal tract study, which reveals a small stomach with a transverse lie and frequently a large, patulous esophagus (Fig. 47-21). Particular attention should be given to the anatomy of the duodenum and the ligament of Treitz.

The initial management of microgastria includes continuous drip enteral feeding and supplemental parenteral nutrition. When continuous feedings can be maintained for several

weeks, the stomach may undergo some enlargement, allowing for a gradual transition to bolus and ad libitum feedings. Antireflux precautions, including small frequent meals, may be required indefinitely. Although case reports of successful management by gastrojejunostomy exist, the favored surgical approach involves gastric augmentation with a Roux-en-Y jejunal reservoir.[108]

GASTRIC PERFORATION

The causes of gastric perforation in neonates can be categorized as traumatic, ischemic, or spontaneous.

In addition, the use of postnatal steroids for bronchopulmonary dysplasia (possibly in combination with cyclooxygenase inhibitors for ductal closure) has been implicated (see Chapter 44). Traumatic perforations are generally caused by puncture of the stomach during placement of a gastric tube, or by gastric distention from bag-mask ventilation or positive-pressure ventilation in an infant with a tracheoesophageal fistula. Usually, these appear as short lacerations or discrete puncture wounds. Ischemic perforations occur in the setting of severe physiologic stress, such as extreme prematurity, perinatal asphyxia, or necrotizing enterocolitis. The pathophysiology of these lesions is presumed to be associated with a reduction in submucosal blood flow resulting in impaired mucosal defense and/or focal infarction of the gastric wall. It is possible that some of these lesions represent perforated stress ulcers. Rarely, a healthy neonate presents with a spontaneous gastric perforation of unknown cause. The most common location is high on the greater curvature near the gastroesophageal junction.

The most constant diagnostic feature of gastric perforation in the neonate is massive pneumoperitoneum, unless the perforation is posterior and contained within the lesser sac. Surgical management is individualized to either simple débridement and closure, or closure around a temporary gastrostomy tube. Extensive gastric resections have not been necessary. Outcomes depend on the cause of the perforation and any associated disease, such as respiratory failure and complex congenital malformations. Reported mortality rates of 50% to 60% have changed little over the last two decades.[40,71]

LACTOBEZOARS

Lactobezoars are compact aggregations of undigested milk constituents that develop within the gastric lumen in infants. Little is known about their underlying cause, although a single etiology is unlikely. Historically, they were believed to result from commercial formulas of high caloric density, particularly those rich in casein protein, which precipitated in the stomachs of premature neonates. Lactobezoars, however, have been reported in term neonates and older infants on diets of human milk and homogenized cow milk.[86,105]

The majority of infants with lactobezoars present with abdominal distention, nonbilious emesis, and diarrhea. A palpable mass may be detectable on physical examination. Plain radiographs often display a frothy appearance in the gastric lumen. An upper gastrointestinal tract contrast series is diagnostic. Ultrasonography, which can detect a hyperechoic intraluminal gastric mass, may also be used to establish the diagnosis.[63] Treatment is nonsurgical in the great majority of patients who do not present with perforation. Simple withholding of enteral feedings and administration of parenteral nutrition usually results in spontaneous resolution of the bezoar; gastric lavage may hasten this process.[21] After follow-up imaging studies document resolution, enteral feedings can be reinstituted using the same formula. Recurrence has not been reported.

PYLORIC ATRESIA

Congenital partial or complete gastric outlet obstructions are rare causes of feeding intolerance in infants. The obstruction may involve either the antrum or the pylorus and may take the form of a segmental defect (gap), which is sometimes bridged by a fibrous cord, or a membrane (web), which can have one or more apertures through which gastric contents pass. Histologically, such membranes consist of mucosa and submucosa without a muscularis. Prepyloric membranes become redundant after exposure to antegrade propulsive pressures, creating a "windsock" web that can prolapse through the pyloric channel. Pyloric webs account for two thirds of these obstructions, pyloric atresia accounts for about a quarter, and most of the remainder are antral webs and atresias. Another, rare cause for the obstruction is the presence of ectopic pancreatic tissue within the submucosa of the pyloric channel that bulges into the lumen and causes a partial obstruction.

The etiology of antral and pyloric atresia is not understood. An in utero vascular accident, such as results in jejunoileal atresias, is unlikely because of the stomach's redundant blood supply. As the stomach (unlike the duodenum) does not undergo a solid embryonic phase, failure of recanalization cannot account for these anomalies. Instead, some form of foregut segmentation mechanism is proposed but unproved. A genetic cause has been identified for some cases of pyloric atresia that occur in association with epidermolysis bullosa lethalis (Herlitz and Carmi syndromes), which is inherited in an autosomal recessive manner. A hemidesmosome defect has been identified in the gastric mucosal epithelium in this syndrome, and genetic studies have documented a variety of mutations in the genes coding for cell-surface beta 4 integrins.[64] This condition is marked by extreme mucocutaneous fragility and is usually lethal in the first year of life.

Complete membranes or atresias appear in the first few days of life as acute gastric outlet obstruction with nonbilious vomiting. There is often a history of maternal polyhydramnios. Gastric distention leading to respiratory compromise can occur, and frank gastric perforation has been reported as early as 12 hours of life. Incomplete gastric outlet obstruction due to perforated membranes or heterotopic pancreatic tissue can present early in the neonatal period or later in childhood. Radiologic evaluation reveals a large gastric air bubble, with little or no gas in the distal intestine (Fig. 47-22). Because neonatal gastric hypotonia can reproduce these radiographic

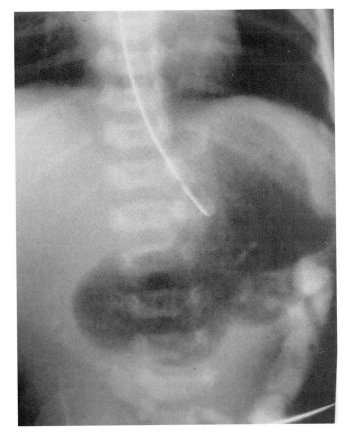

Figure 47–22. Plain radiograph of gastric bubble in patient with pyloric atresia.

findings, upper gastrointestinal tract contrast studies are mandatory. These studies either show nonfilling of the duodenum or delineate the membrane when viewed laterally. Ectopic pancreatic tissue can cause an eccentric protrusion into the pyloric channel.

Preoperative resuscitation and gastric decompression are necessary in infants with complete gastric outlet obstruction. A chloride-responsive contraction alkalosis is often seen and requires specific measures to restore fluid volume and correct chloride and potassium deficits. Prolonged vomiting in the neonate can also lead to profound hypoglycemia, which must be anticipated and corrected. In general, webs can be excised and closed transversely to avoid stenosis. Complete atresias with anatomic disconnection can usually be corrected by primary anastomosis, such as gastroduodenostomy. Gastrojejunostomy is poorly tolerated in the neonate and should be avoided whenever possible. Recognition of windsock deformities and distal atresias by passage of a balloon catheter proximally and distally can be helpful in defining the exact anatomy and in detecting additional distal obstructions. Ectopic pancreatic tissue in the pylorus requires excision of the mass and reconstruction of the pylorus.

HYPERTROPHIC PYLORIC STENOSIS

Hypertrophic pyloric stenosis (HPS) is an acquired condition in which the circumferential muscle layer of the pyloric sphincter becomes thickened, resulting in narrowing and elongation of the pyloric channel. This produces a high-grade gastric outlet obstruction with compensatory dilation, hypertrophy, and hyperperistalsis of the stomach. The incidence of HPS ranges between 0.1% and 1% in the general population and appears to be rising. A longitudinal study using ultrasound in 1400 randomly selected term neonates documented that all nine infants (0.65%) in whom HPS later developed had normal pyloric dimensions at birth.[83] There is a significant male predominance of about 4:1, although the long-held belief that HPS primarily afflicts first-born males is unproven. The incidence in whites exceeds that in blacks by severalfold; the incidence in Asian infants is low. The transmission of HPS appears to involve multifactorial threshold inheritance or the effects of multiple interacting loci. Transmission from mothers is more common than from fathers: HPS develops in 19% of boys and 7% of girls whose mothers had HPS as infants, and in 5% of boys and 2.5% of girls whose fathers were previously affected.[61]

The cause of HPS remains unknown. One hypothesis is that dyscoordination between gastric peristalsis and pyloric relaxation results in simultaneous gastric and pyloric contraction and work hypertrophy of the pyloric muscle.[41] This initiates a cycle of escalating pyloric resistance and gastric hyperperistalsis. Although functional disturbances in gastric emptying in the first weeks of life have not been proven to occur in neonates in whom HPS later develops, a report of in utero gastric dilation in a neonate who later developed HPS suggests a possible role for prenatal gastric emptying dysfunction. An association between maternal and infant exposure to erythromycin and the development of HPS has been identified, and a causal link has been postulated.[28,56,76,90] Erythromycin stimulates phase III migrating myoelectric complex activity and may expose the immature pylorus to markedly elevated gastric pressures.

The pathophysiology underlying pyloric dysfunction in HPS is undetermined. Observations of decreased ganglion cell density and elevated levels of prostaglandins E_2 and F_2 have not been causally linked to the development of HPS. Gastric outlet obstruction due to pylorospasm has been reported in neonates receiving prostaglandin infusions, but pyloric dysfunction in these infants does not lead to muscular hypertrophy.[60]

Perhaps a more promising hypothesis for the pathophysiology of HPS is a primary abnormality of the enteric nervous system (ENS). Axonal degeneration in both the myenteric plexus and the intramuscular nerves has been observed in patients with HPS. Studies have documented decreased and disordered innervation of the circumferential muscle layer in specimens of pyloric muscle taken at the time of pyloromyotomy.[45,50] Furthermore, the muscle layer in HPS appears to be nearly devoid of neurotrophins—peptides that govern differentiation and survival of ENS neurons.[32] Circumstantial evidence exists to suggest that such neural immaturity is transient, consistent with the observation that HPS does not recur after reconstitution of the pyloric sphincter after pyloromyotomy.[46] Immunohistochemical staining for neuropeptides has revealed a marked reduction in a variety of neuropeptides, such as gastrin-releasing peptide, vasoactive intestinal peptide, somatostatin, and substance P, in patients with HPS.[1] Nitric oxide synthase, which can be identified in significant concentrations in the circular and longitudinal pyloric muscle layers and the myenteric plexus in normal controls, has been shown to be selectively absent in the circular muscle layer in patients with HPS.[107] This has also been documented for nitric oxide synthase mRNA.[47] A deficiency of nitric oxide, a ubiquitous paracrine and neurocrine mediator of smooth muscle relaxation, might be a final common pathway in the dysregulation of pyloric function in HPS.

The typical patient is a term male infant between 3 and 6 weeks of age who has progressive, nonbilious, projectile vomiting. Many infants with HPS are significantly dehydrated at the time of presentation, and chemistry analyses may reflect a hypochloremic, hypokalemic, contraction metabolic alkalosis with paradoxical aciduria. Significant hypoglycemia can also be present and may precipitate seizures. Unconjugated hyperbilirubinemia is common and correlates with a decrease in hepatic glucuronyltransferase activity. This jaundice is transient and resolves as soon as the gastric outlet obstruction is corrected, making it attractive to speculate that the hepatic defect is secondary to abnormal enteroendocrine feedback between the stomach and the hepatocyte.

The hallmark of the diagnosis is the finding of a small, mobile, ovoid mass in the epigastrium. The process of detecting this mass, the "olive," on examination may be quite difficult. A positive examination is very accurate, with a selectivity value of more than 97%.[28] If the pylorus is unequivocally felt, the diagnosis is established, and no further diagnostic maneuvers are necessary.

If the pylorus is not detected and the clinical presentation is sufficiently suggestive to warrant further evaluation, radiologic evaluation can be definitive. Real-time ultrasonography has supplanted barium upper gastrointestinal tract study as the procedure of choice. The hypertrophied pylorus appears to have a characteristic appearance on B-mode ultrasound, and measurement of pyloric dimensions accurately establishes the diagnosis of HPS. Parameters measured include overall diameter, single wall thickness, and pyloric channel length, with the latter two being the most commonly used (Fig. 47-23). Measurements found to have greater than 90% positive predictive value include overall diameter of 17 mm or more, muscular wall thickness of 4 mm or greater, and channel length of 17 mm or greater. In infants 30 days of age or younger, it has been suggested that diagnostic criteria for wall thickness be reduced to 3 mm. When parameters are equivocal, an upper gastrointestinal tract study can be diagnostic by demonstrating an elongated and narrowed pyloric channel, with the characteristic shoulders of the hypertrophied pylorus bulging into the gastric lumen. Although an accurate diagnosis based on physical examination should be possible in most cases, and should be attempted in all, it is evident that an increasing reliance on ultrasonography will continue to erode the skills of examiners. A review comparing diagnostic accuracy between two eras in a single pediatric institution found that the sensitivity of physical examination declined by half during a period of increasing reliance on ultrasound.[55]

Preoperative preparation is critical once the diagnosis is made. HPS is not a surgical emergency, so careful correction of fluid and electrolyte losses should be accomplished before operative intervention. The infant who presents early in the course of the disease with no clinical dehydration, normal serum electrolytes and glucose, and a normal urine output can be operated on at the earliest convenience. Many patients, however, present with dehydration, hypoglycemia, or a contraction alkalosis of sufficient severity to require preoperative resuscitation for 24 to 48 hours. Once volume status and urine output have improved, serum chloride, potassium, and bicarbonate have normalized, and paradoxical aciduria has resolved, surgery can be conducted safely.

The treatment of HPS is pyloromyotomy. Historically, the operation is performed through a transverse right upper quadrant incision. Over the past decade, the minimally invasive approach has gained widespread popularity (Fig. 47-24). The time to full feedings and discharge may be slightly shorter when the operation is done laparoscopically, and cosmesis is better.[25] Both approaches to pyloromyotomy are acceptable, and the choice of one or the other depends on individual factors and operator preference. In both approaches, the most common operative complication is inadvertent extension of the pyloromyotomy incision through the duodenal or gastric mucosa, resulting in a perforation. The reported rates of perforation range from 3% to 30%, although rates above 10% are unusual. If recognized at the time of surgery, the defect may be repaired primarily and the ramifications limited to a short delay in the resumption of feedings. A feeding regimen is begun 4 to 8 hours after operation with a small volume of sugar water, advancing volume and osmolarity every 2 to 3 hours until the infant is taking formula or breast milk ad libitum. It is common for occasional emesis to occur after pyloromyotomy; this should not delay the progression of the feeding schedule in most cases. In general, most infants so managed can be discharged within 24 to 48 hours of surgery.

Persistent postoperative vomiting beyond 48 hours is uncommon. In this circumstance, the possibilities of an incomplete myotomy or unrecognized perforation should be considered. Radiologic studies are of little value in evaluating the completeness of the myotomy because the fluoroscopic and sonographic appearances of the hypertrophied pylorus before and after myotomy are similar. A contrast study should be obtained to exclude a mucosal leak, which may produce a fluid collection that compresses the gastric outlet. In the absence of a leak or complete obstruction, an interval of at least 2 weeks is allowed to pass before the presumptive diagnosis of incomplete myotomy prompts reexploration.

Most children treated for HPS can expect excellent short- and long-term outcomes. With appropriate resuscitation, expert anesthesia, and a standard surgical approach, mortality

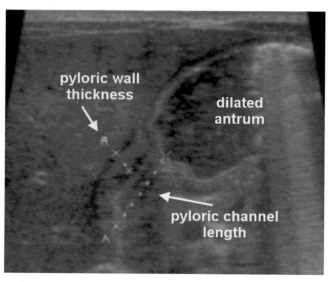

Figure 47-23. Abdominal ultrasound of patient with hypertrophic pyloric stenosis.

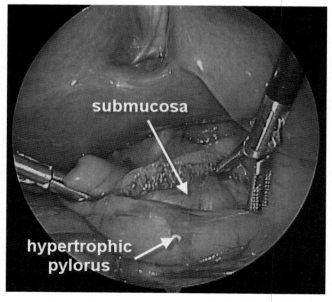

Figure 47-24. Laparoscopic pyloromyotomy.

has been virtually eliminated. Wound infection and dehiscence, significant problems in previous eras, are relatively uncommon today. Postoperative ultrasound studies have documented a return to normal muscle thickness within 4 weeks, associated with healing of the pyloric muscle and return of function. A study addressing gastric emptying and abdominal symptoms after pyloromyotomy found no differences between treatment and control groups several decades after surgery.[53]

DUODENAL ATRESIA AND STENOSIS

Congenital duodenal obstruction may be complete or partial, intrinsic or extrinsic. Intrinsic atresias or stenoses have an incidence of about 1 in 7000 live births and account for about half of all small intestinal atresias. Extrinsic obstruction has many causes, including malrotation with Ladd bands, pre-duodenal portal vein, gastroduodenal duplications, cysts or pseudocysts of the pancreas and biliary tree, and annular pancreas. Annular pancreas is commonly associated with an intrinsic cause of duodenal obstruction.

Intrinsic duodenal obstructions and annular pancreas result from events that occur during early development of the foregut. Duodenal atresia and stenosis are believed to result from a failure of recanalization of the embryonic duodenum, which becomes solid as a result of early epithelial proliferation. Annular pancreas occurs when the ventral pancreatic bud fails to rotate behind the duodenum, leaving a nondistensible ring of pancreatic tissue fully encircling the second portion of the duodenum.[100] Annular pancreas frequently coexists with intrinsic duodenal anomalies and anomalies of the pancreaticobiliary ductal system, suggesting closely linked mechanisms of pancreatic, duodenal, and biliary development during this stage.

Atresias of the duodenum have several basic morphologies. Type I atresias constitute luminal webs or membranes, some of which contain a central defect or fenestration of variable size, and result in a marked size discrepancy with mural continuity (Fig. 47-25). Type II atresias have dilated proximal

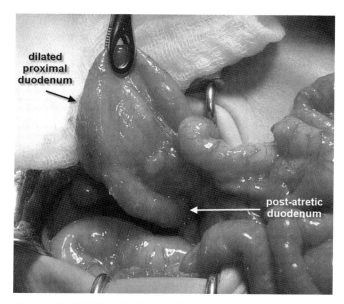

Figure 47–25. Type I duodenal atresia with continuity of muscular wall.

and diminutive distal segments connected by a fibrous cord. Type III atresias are characterized by a complete discontinuity between the segments. The relationship between the point of obstruction and the ampulla of Vater is important. Most series document a predominance of postampullary obstructions, although some have described a preampullary predominance. Obstructions caused by type I membranes are frequently associated with anomalies of the common bile duct in which the common bile duct may terminate within the membrane itself.

Congenital duodenal obstructions are often associated with other congenital anomalies, which account for most of the morbidity and mortality in these patients. Various reports put the incidence of associated conditions between 50% and 80%. Congenital heart disease and trisomy 21 are the most common associated conditions, each occurring in about 30% of cases.[31] Not infrequently, all three conditions coexist in the same patient.[23] Among patients with trisomy 21 who underwent prenatal ultrasonography, about 4% were found to have prenatal evidence of duodenal atresia.[67] Other associated anomalies include intestinal malrotation (20%), esophageal atresia, or imperforate anus (10% to 20%), thoracoabdominal heterotaxia, and gallbladder agenesis. The outcome for patients with duodenal atresia depends more on the severity of these associated anomalies and the ease with which they can be corrected than on the surgical management of the obstruction itself.

Many patients with duodenal atresia have the diagnosis suggested by prenatal ultrasonography. A maternal history of polyhydramnios is common in congenital duodenal obstruction, approaching 75% in one series.[92] Prenatal sonographic evaluation of the fetus at 22 to 23 weeks of gestation can reliably detect two dilated fluid-filled structures consistent with a double bubble. The unavailability of a sonographic diagnosis until relatively late in gestation frequently results in an ethical dilemma for prospective parents, who may consider elective termination based on the association of duodenal atresia with trisomy 21. Reliable data regarding the rate of false-positive examinations for duodenal obstruction in the fetus are unavailable.

The clinical presentation of the infant with congenital duodenal obstruction depends on the presence or absence of a membranous aperture, its size, and the location of the obstruction relative to the ampulla. The classic presentation of a complete postampullary obstruction includes bilious vomiting within 24 hours of birth in an otherwise stable infant with a nondistended abdomen. Plain radiographs of the abdomen typically show the classic double-bubble sign—two distinct gas collections or air-fluid levels in the upper abdomen resulting from the markedly dilated stomach and proximal duodenal bulb (Fig. 47-26). If the infant's stomach has been decompressed by vomiting or previous nasogastric aspiration, 30 to 60 mL of air may be injected carefully through the nasogastric tube and the double-bubble sign reproduced. Air makes an excellent contrast agent, obviating a barium or water-soluble contrast study in routine cases. The distal intestinal tract may be gasless or may contain a small amount of intraluminal air due to a membranous aperture or perforation, or an anomalous bile duct with openings on both sides of the obstructing diaphragm.[73]

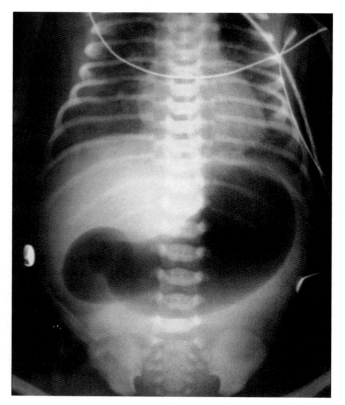

Figure 47–26. Plain abdominal radiograph in patient with duodenal atresia.

The importance of differentiating intrinsic duodenal obstruction from intestinal malrotation with a midgut volvulus in the infant who presents with bilious vomiting cannot be overstated. A clue may be derived from the appearance of the duodenum on the plain radiograph. In the classic double-bubble sign, the duodenum appears distended and round because of chronic intrauterine obstruction. When a distended stomach is associated with a normal-caliber duodenum, the diagnosis of malrotation with duodenal obstruction secondary to Ladd bands or volvulus must be entertained. In an unstable patient, echocardiography and contrast studies may be required to distinguish hemodynamic compromise caused by volvulus from that caused by cardiac disease. Even when the diagnosis of duodenal atresia is established in the stable patient, cardiac anatomy and function should be evaluated before surgical correction.

Preoperative preparation includes nasogastric decompression, fluid and electrolyte replacement, and a thorough evaluation for associated anomalies. If malrotation is ruled out, surgical correction of duodenal atresia can be temporarily postponed, and more urgent conditions evaluated and treated. Prophylactic perioperative antibiotics are begun preoperatively.

The surgical management of an intrinsic duodenal web is usually limited to excision of a portion of the web and an enteroplasty to widen the duodenal lumen at that point. As the membrane occasionally contains the terminal common bile duct, great caution must be taken in excising or incising the membrane to avoid biliary injury and stricture formation. The most widely accepted surgical management of both true

atresia and annular pancreas involves constructing an anastomosis between the dilated proximal duodenum and the diminutive distal duodenum. The diamond duodenoduodenostomy has yielded consistently good results and remains the procedure of choice.[43] The diamond anastomosis is fashioned in such a way as to approximate the ends of one incision to the midpoints of the other incision. The tension resulting from this orientation tends to hold the anastomosis open in a self-stenting manner.

A feeding gastrostomy should not be necessary for postoperative management of an uncomplicated duodenal repair. Gastroduodenal function usually returns within 5 to 7 days, at which time enteral feeding can be initiated with small boluses and the volume progressively advanced as tolerated. One of the most problematic issues following repair of duodenal atresia is delayed transit, usually associated with a persistently dilated and dyskinetic proximal duodenum. Even with the preferred diamond anastomosis, a persistent megaduodenum with symptomatic partial obstruction and stasis can occur. This complication may be managed either by tapering duodenoplasty or by lateral seromuscular resection.[44] A significant number of infants with corrected duodenal atresia also experience GER, which may be exacerbated by an impairment in gastric emptying. Survival rates of 95% are reported in those who are deemed satisfactory surgical candidates. As mentioned earlier, morbidity and mortality are usually related to associated anomalies.

GASTROINTESTINAL DUPLICATIONS

The stomach and duodenum are the least common regions of the gastrointestinal tract in which duplications occur. For most congenital lesions of the stomach and duodenum included in this category, the term *duplication* may be a misnomer. The actual embryologic cause of these lesions is unknown, but the designation of *enterogenous cyst* or *congenital diverticulum* may be more accurate. Nevertheless, it is important to recognize that gastric and duodenal duplications are occasionally associated with other gastrointestinal duplications or with vertebral anomalies. Communications with or attachments to an abnormal vertebral column suggest they may be caused by aberrant splitting of the primitive notochord during early embryonic development.

Classically, four pathologic criteria are considered necessary to establish the diagnosis of gastric duplication: (1) contiguity with the stomach, (2) an outer smooth muscle layer, (3) a shared blood supply with the stomach, and (4) a gastric epithelial lining (which may also contain pancreatic tissue). Most gastric duplications are cystic, do not communicate with the gastric lumen, and are located along the greater curvature of the stomach. When a luminal communication is present, it may result from peptic ulceration of the common wall between the two structures. Tubular duplications are less common, frequently communicate with the gastric lumen, and are also most commonly found on the greater curvature (Fig. 47-27). Extragastric cystic structures lined by gastric epithelium and exhibiting a muscular wall, however, are usually referred to as gastric duplications regardless of their proximity to the stomach.

In the neonatal period, duplications often present with symptoms and signs of proximal gastrointestinal obstruction.

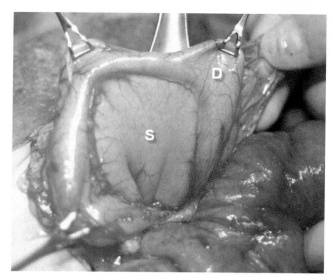

Figure 47–27. Gastric duplication of greater curvature. D, duplication; S, stomach.

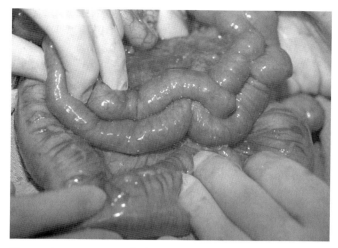

Figure 47–28. Long tubular duplication on mesenteric side of small intestine.

Vomiting is common and can be bilious or nonbilious, depending on the location of the extrinsic compression relative to the ampulla of Vater. Case reports of gastric duplications, both adjacent to the stomach and in the retroperitoneum, have described connections to the pancreatic ductal system and have resulted in chronic pancreatitis and pseudocyst formation. Connections to the biliary system and to extrapulmonary sequestrations have also been reported. Duodenal duplications most commonly occur in the first or second portion, usually on the posterior surface, and may be lined with gastric mucosa. These may also cause pancreatitis by compression of the pancreatic duct within the duodenal wall. Gastroduodenal hemorrhage or perforation secondary to peptic ulceration is the usual emergency indication for surgery. Gastrointestinal hemorrhage secondary to ulcer penetration from a noncommunicating duplication cyst into an adherent loop of intestine or colon has been reported.

Gastroduodenal duplications are being detected by antenatal ultrasound with increasing frequency and should be considered along with choledochal cysts and omental cysts in the differential diagnosis of a fetal right upper quadrant cystic mass. Postnatally, an upper gastrointestinal tract contrast study may demonstrate an extrinsic compression of the stomach or duodenum, but ultrasound and computed tomography can definitively reveal the mass itself. Technetium-99m scans may identify duplications distant from the stomach if they contain ectopic gastric mucosa but are not specific for duplications per se.

Resection of the entire duplication, either by enucleation or by limited gastric resection, is the treatment of choice. Successful laparoscopic resection has been reported and may be advisable for smaller, uncomplicated lesions. Extensive duplications, however, require removal of the entire mucosal cyst lining to avoid potential malignant degeneration. Adenocarcinoma arising from the gastric epithelium has been described in later life. Partial excision of the duplication with stripping of the residual mucosa is acceptable for lesions around the pylorus and duodenum for which en bloc resection of the contiguous gastroduodenal wall would necessitate sacrificing important structures (e.g., the common bile duct). Internal drainage into the adjacent duodenum or a Roux-en-Y jejunal limb is reserved for the rare circumstance in which resection or mucosal stripping is not feasible. Partial resection of a contiguous aberrant pancreatic lobe or internal drainage of an associated pseudocyst may also be required. Marsupialization should be avoided.

Duplications of the small or large intestine are more common than those of the stomach and duodenum. They are usually cystic but may be tubular and extend for a variable distance (Fig. 47-28). Cystic duplications may cause obstruction or volvulus, and they may present with a palpable mass. Either type may present with hemorrhage. Simple cystic duplications of the small or large intestine are most easily managed by resection and primary anastomosis. Long tubular duplications may be managed by mucosal stripping to prevent future peptic complications and to remove potentially dysplastic epithelium. Long colonic duplications may result in anal duplication. If the second anus is within the muscular sphincter, division of the septum to establish a common lumen may be sufficient. Cystic rectal duplications must be distinguished from sacrococcygeal teratomas and meningoceles before trans-sacral or posterior sagittal resection is undertaken.

MALROTATION AND MIDGUT VOLVULUS

As described in the development section, the bowel undergoes two independent 270-degree counterclockwise rotations during the 6th to 12th weeks of gestation. One involves the duodenojejunal junction around the axis of the superior mesenteric artery, and the other involves the ileocolic junction around the same axis. Although this is difficult to grasp spatially, the concept is simple. When the bowel rotates appropriately during development, it fixes itself in the abdomen in such a way that it absolutely cannot twist and obstruct itself or, as occurs in volvulus, compromise its own blood supply. This is remarkable, considering the length of bowel involved. However, if the bowel does not rotate and fix itself in the abdomen properly, the stage is set for later obstruction or volvulus. Yet malrotation, more comprehensively described as an anomaly of intestinal fixation and rotation, is not a problem in itself. It is estimated that nearly 1 in 100 people have some form of improper rotation or fixation, yet 1% of the population do not have the related clinical symptoms. Rather, 1 in 6000 live births leads to a clinical discovery.[12,110] So, anomalies of intestinal fixation and rotation are only potential time bombs, some much worse than others, that may, or may never, go off.

Because so many variations of malrotation can exist, there are many possible clinical presentations. Any case of unexplained abdominal pain or emesis should have malrotation somewhere in the differential diagnosis. However, the main symptom complexes can be grouped together as those related to acute volvulus, to duodenal obstruction, to evidence of intermittent or chronic abdominal pain, or as an incidental finding in an otherwise asymptomatic patient. More than half of patients present in the first month of life, with half of the rest in the first year. However, 25% can still present at any other time in life.[99] Bilious emesis in any child younger than 1 year of age should be assumed to be due to malrotation until proven otherwise.

The preoperative evaluation of the malrotation or midgut volvulus is the radiologic determination of the position of the ligament of Treitz, and secondarily, its distance and relation to the ileocecal junction.[109] The initial film is typically a plain radiograph. Although alone it is not sufficient for a diagnosis, obvious obstruction of the stomach with little or no distal air in an acutely ill newborn or infant can be enough to warrant taking the child immediately to the operating room. Midgut volvulus is one of the few pediatric emergencies in which operating takes precedence over resuscitation. More typically, plain radiographs are nonspecific and further urgent evaluation is warranted.

The upper gastrointestinal series is the gold standard for making the diagnosis of malrotation. The procedure must be performed in the radiology suite by a trained radiologist using fluoroscopy. In cases of volvulus, the site of obstruction is in the second or third portion of the duodenum and has the appearance of a bird's beak. If the duodenum is partially obstructed, a spiral or corkscrew configuration may be seen (Fig. 47-29). In diagnosing malrotation alone, the position of the duodenojejunal junction must be documented. Normally, it is to the left of midline, rising to approximately the level of the pylorus and fixed well posteriorly. In a patient with malrotation, it is anterior, low, and often midline or to the right of midline (Fig. 47-30). The diagnosis requires judgment and, therefore, an experienced and confident radiologist.

Barium enema was historically the procedure of choice, but it has several limitations. Most importantly, the cecum can be in the proper position in the patient with duodenojejunal malrotation, and the latter can therefore be missed. As the risk for midgut volvulus is related to duodenojejunal malrotation and not jejunoileal, the barium enema cannot be depended on. A contrast enema can, however, help determine the potential width of the mesenteric base, and therefore the risk of volvulus, in a child when the location of the duodenojejunal junction on upper gastrointestinal investigation is unclear.

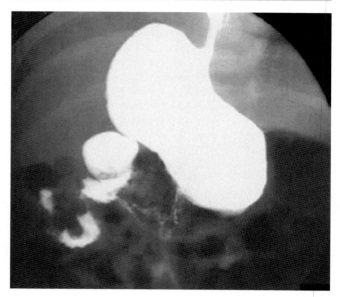

Figure 47–29. Upper gastrointestinal contrast study in patient with malrotation and midgut volvulus.

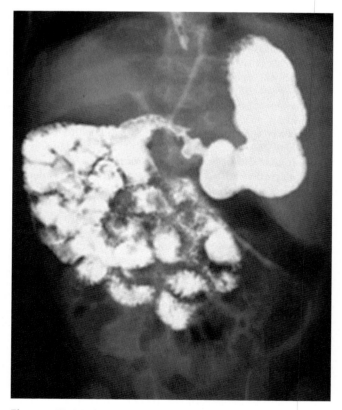

Figure 47–30. Upper gastrointestinal contrast study in patient with malrotation without volvulus. Note location of duodenal-jejunal junction and small intestine to right of midline.

Ultrasonography can be used to determine the orientation of the superior mesenteric vessels and thus may be helpful in the diagnosis of malrotation. Normally, the superior mesenteric vein lies to the right of the superior mesenteric artery. If the superior mesenteric vein lies either anterior or to the left of the superior mesenteric artery, malrotation may be present. However, this is inconsistent and does not lead to a definitive diagnosis.

An acutely ill child with the presumed diagnosis of volvulus requires urgent operative intervention even at the expense of full resuscitation. As the operation gets underway, intravenous fluids continue, bladder and stomach catheters can be placed, blood is drawn for type and crossmatch, and broad-spectrum antibiotics are administered. Time is critical. In patients with malrotation without volvulus or obstruction, urgency is somewhat less. As long as all caregivers are vigilant for the development of volvulus, early operation (within a day or two of diagnosis) would appear to be justified. Older individuals with intermittent symptoms can be treated more electively.

The surgical treatment of these patients involves seven aspects: evisceration of the bowel, detorsion of a volvulus, division of Ladd bands, widening the mesenteric base, relieving duodenal obstruction, incidental appendectomy, and nonrotational return of the bowel to the abdomen. Ladd bands extend from the ascending colon (on the medial aspect of the duodenum in patients with malrotation) across the duodenum and attach to the posterior aspect of the right upper quadrant. They presumably represent the attempt of the ascending colon to become retroperitoneal, as it is in the normally rotated individual. They must be completely divided. Techniques to widen the mesenteric base and relieve duodenal obstruction are then used. Incidental appendectomy and nonrotational return of the bowel to the abdomen may seem unusual. It would seem logical to try to rotate the bowel properly or to try to fix it in place. However, this does not work in practice. Experience has shown that returning the bowel with the small bowel on the right and the large bowel on the left (total nonrotation) is effective. Unfortunately, this typically leaves the appendix in the left upper quadrant, so it is removed to avoid possibly confusing clinical presentations of appendicitis in the future.

Mortality for the operative correction of malrotation ranges from 3% to 9% and is increased in patients with volvulus, intestinal necrosis, prematurity, and other abnormalities. Recurrent volvulus is relatively infrequent (less than 10%) but must always be considered. Gastrointestinal motility disturbances are not uncommon after operative correction of malrotation. Other complications can occur as a result of compromised bowel from ischemia caused by volvulus, such as reperfusion injury with hemodynamic instability and delayed stricture formation. Adhesive bowel obstruction is possible in any patient after abdominal exploration. Finally, midgut volvulus accounts for nearly 20% of the cases of short gut syndrome in the pediatric population.

MECONIUM SYNDROMES

Meconium syndromes are associated with intestinal obstruction resulting from thick, inspissated meconium. These syndromes are broadly characterized by several patterns of clinical presentation, including meconium ileus, meconium plug syndrome, meconium peritonitis, and meconium ileus equivalent. In meconium ileus, which is almost always associated with cystic fibrosis, the inspissated meconium typically obstructs the small bowel, usually at the level of the distal jejunum or the proximal ileum. Meconium plug syndrome is observed more frequently in preterm infants and involves obstruction at the level of the colon. It is thought to occur as a result of poor intestinal motility, but it can be associated with cystic fibrosis in a minority of infants. Meconium peritonitis results from bowel perforation, usually intrauterine, which is secondary to meconium-related obstruction. Meconium ileus equivalent is a condition associated with stool-related bowel obstruction in older children with cystic fibrosis.

Meconium Ileus

Meconium ileus occurs in approximately 10% to 20% of newborns with cystic fibrosis. Cystic fibrosis is caused by mutations in the gene that codes for a protein called *cystic fibrosis transmembrane conductance regulator* (CFTR), which regulates chloride transport across epithelia.[17,82] Luminal epithelial cells of patients with cystic fibrosis either lack or have defective CFTR, and are relatively impermeable to chloride and excessively reabsorb sodium. This leads to dehydration and hyperviscosity of secretions with secondary obstruction of the lumina that these cells line, including the mucus-secreting glands of the bowel wall and the ductal cells of the exocrine pancreas.

The hyperviscosity of mucosal cell secretion leads to the formation of thick, tarlike meconium, which becomes increasingly inspissated farther along the small bowel lumen, eventually resulting distally in the formation of small, dense meconium pellets and a microcolon. Resultant small bowel obstruction is usually present at birth and can even be diagnosed antenatally on ultrasonic examination of the maternal abdomen. Postnatal clinical signs of bowel obstruction usually evolve within 24 to 48 hours, including increased abdominal distention associated with failure to defecate and eventual bilious vomiting. Bowel loops, which have a pliant, doughlike quality, can often be palpated on abdominal examination. Abdominal radiographs may have a granular, soap-bubble appearance as a result of air bubbles in the meconium. This clinical picture is classically used to characterize *simple meconium ileus*. However, luminal bowel obstruction of this sort can progress to volvulus, necrosis, and perforation, and these clinical situations constitute *complicated meconium ileus*. If bowel necrosis and perforation have occurred in utero, a pseudocyst may form and present as a palpable mass on abdominal examination at birth. Volvulus can also present as a palpable abdominal mass. In addition to the classic features of intestinal obstruction (i.e., multiple distended bowel loops), abdominal radiography may reveal a large mass containing calcified material (pseudocyst) or calcifications distributed throughout the peritoneal cavity (meconium peritonitis) in association with this process. Ascites, free air, or a granular, soap-bubble appearance caused by air bubbles in the meconium may also be present. The absence of any or all of these radiographic findings does not necessarily rule out meconium ileus. However, a contrast enema almost always demonstrates a microcolon, usually associated with small, "rabbit-pellet" meconium concretions seen proximally. The differential diagnosis includes meconium plug syndrome, small bowel and proximal colonic atresia, total colonic Hirschsprung disease, and congenital hypothyroidism.

Management options to treat meconium ileus depend on the type of presentation. General management principles always include prompt rehydration with adequate fluid and electrolyte support, gastric decompression with a dual-lumen sump nasogastric tube, and appropriate antibiotic coverage.

Simple meconium ileus can be treated either nonoperatively or operatively. Nonoperative intervention requires that other causes of distal bowel obstruction be ruled out and that complicated meconium ileus (volvulus, necrosis, perforation, pseudocyst, or peritonitis) does not exist. A hyperosmolar solution (typically Gastrografin) is administered as an enema and allowed to reflux into the ileum. The hypertonic solution (1900 mOsm/L) establishes a concentration gradient across the bowel wall that draws fluid into the lumen and promotes passage of the meconium. It is extremely important that the infant receive adequate intravenous fluid therapy before and during this procedure to compensate for the rapid fluid shift out of the plasma compartment as a result of the intestinal osmotic load. This procedure should be performed by an appropriately trained and experienced pediatric radiologist, with a pediatric surgeon available. Although the technique is successful a little over 50% of the time, there is also an 11% perforation rate.[80] Furthermore, necrotizing enterocolitis can result from the exposure of the bowel to the hyperosmolar solution. Surgical treatment involves evacuation of the meconium from the intestine. This can be accomplished by creating an enterotomy and irrigating the bowel with 2% to 4% N-acetyl-L-cysteine, which helps to partially dissolve the inspissated meconium, making it easier to flush through the lumen. In addition, the bowel can be partially diverted using a variety of techniques (Bishop-Koop, Santulli-Blanc, or Mikulicz procedures), which allow for evacuation of the meconium over a longer term with gradual resumption of distal bowel utilization.

Complicated meconium ileus requires an exploratory laparotomy. Volvulus can be relieved by untwisting the bowel. Bowel resection is usually required to treat atresia, necrotic and perforated bowel, and in some instances, remarkably dilated bowel. Partial or complete temporary intestinal diversion is usually required along with the irrigation techniques previously mentioned. Initial postoperative care involves adequate fluid and electrolyte support, continued nasogastric sump tube decompression of the stomach, and appropriate antibiotic therapy. Careful ostomy irrigation by the pediatric surgeon can be continued postoperatively to facilitate further meconium evacuation if needed. Bowel function usually returns within 3 to 5 days, at which time oral nutritional support can be initiated, first with elemental formulations if the inflammation encountered at exploration was extensive or if surgery was complicated by intra-abdominal infection. Pancreatic enzyme supplementation should also be considered. If bowel function does not return within this period, parenteral nutritional support should be initiated. Early postoperative recovery is usually good. Proper ostomy care is essential and surgical closure is usually carried out 4 to 6 weeks after the initial surgery. Because long-term mortality in patients with cystic fibrosis is most frequently associated with respiratory complications, aggressive pulmonary toilet during the initial postoperative period is mandatory.

Meconium Peritonitis

Intestinal obstruction from a variety of causes, including, but not limited to, meconium ileus, volvulus, atresia, peritoneal bands, and internal hernia, can result in bowel necrosis and perforation during the fetal period. Meconium escaping into the peritoneal cavity combined with intestinal necrosis can cause an inflammatory reaction, leading to calcification and extensive scarring (fibroadhesive peritonitis), which seals the perforation; cystic meconium peritonitis (if a seal does not form and meconium continues to leak into the peritoneal cavity); or meconium pseudocyst (when loops of bowel and necrotic tissue are encased in scar tissue and surround the extramural meconium). Meconium ascites presents as a large amount of liquid meconium, presumably resulting from a recent perforation just before birth, which fills the peritoneal cavity.

Asymptomatic patients with radiographic evidence of intraperitoneal calcification can be managed conservatively; however, babies with meconium peritonitis who present with bowel obstruction usually require surgical intervention. Surgical management is based on the findings at laparotomy and may include resection of necrotic bowel or temporary intestinal diversion, or both. Every attempt should be made to preserve as much bowel length as possible to decrease the risk of developing short gut syndrome. The principles of postoperative care are similar to those for meconium ileus.

Meconium Plug Syndrome

Meconium plug syndrome is believed to relate to colonic hypomotility. It is more frequently observed in preterm infants and in infants of diabetic mothers, and it has been alternatively termed *functional inertia of prematurity* or *neonatal small left colon syndrome* (see also Chapter 49, Part 1). Several factors known to affect bowel motility have been implicated. These include hypermagnesemia and hypoglycemia. A hypermagnesemia-associated decrease in the release of acetylcholine can result in myoneural depression. This mechanism has been used to explain meconium plug syndrome observed in preterm neonates whose mothers received magnesium to treat eclampsia. Furthermore, immature development of the myenteric plexus of preterm infants may impair intestinal motility, accounting for the increased observation of meconium plug syndrome in this patient population. Hypoglycemia, frequently observed in infants of diabetic mothers, is thought to induce increased glucagon secretion, and may be associated with intestinal hypomotility.

Meconium ileus is seen in preterm infants who present with abdominal distention associated with minimal passage of meconium. Multiple dilated bowel loops are present on abdominal radiography. Although a digital rectal examination can sometimes result in the passage of the obstructing meconium, a water-soluble contrast enema is valuable both for diagnostic purposes (usually demonstrating a microcolon distal to the obstruction) and for therapy (to induce passage of the obstructing meconium plug). Surgical therapy is infrequently required to relieve the blockage. Because of the association of meconium plug syndrome with cystic fibrosis and Hirschsprung disease, patients with this disorder may need to be evaluated for cystic fibrosis and undergo a rectal biopsy.

JEJUNOILEAL ATRESIA AND STENOSIS

The potential pathogenesis of small bowel atresia is varied and includes events during the second and third trimester of intrauterine life such as intussusception, internal herniation of bowel, volvulus, bowel perforation, vascular constriction in association with gastroschisis (and, less frequently, omphalocele), mesenteric thrombosis, and possibly excessive resorption of the intestinal attachment of the omphalomesenteric remnant. The suggestion of in utero vascular compromise as an etiologic factor was first demonstrated in beagle puppies by Christian Barnard and colleagues, who observed that the late-gestational ligation of mesenteric vessels resulted in a classic V-shaped mesenteric defect in association with a noncontiguous gap atresia (most likely caused by resorption of the ischemic bowel supplied by the ligated vessels).[52]

These observations have subsequently been confirmed in a number of different animal models. The notion that the etiologic events occur after the 12th week of embryonic life is supported by the frequent clinical finding of bile pigments and lanugo hairs in the postatretic bowel segment, because secretion of bile into the bowel lumen and fetal swallowing of amniotic fluid begin during the 11th to 12th week of gestation. Another potential etiologic factor is linked to the concept of epithelial plugging. From the 5th to 8th week of gestation, the intestine undergoes a period of epithelial growth so rapid that it can completely obliterate the intestinal lumen (solid-cord stage). After the 8th week, the intestinal lumen is reestablished through a process termed *revacuolization*. Lack of complete revacuolization has been postulated to account for the development of intestinal stenoses and webs (membranous atresias).

The classification of jejunoileal atresia is as follows. Operative management of intestinal atresia and stenosis is based on pathologic findings.

Type I: Mucosal (membranous) web
Type II: Blind ends connected by a fibrous cord
Type IIIa: Blind ends separated by a V-shaped mesenteric defect
Type IIIb: Apple-peel or Christmas-tree deformity (blind ends; distal small bowel segment forms corkscrew around ileocecal artery terminus)
Type IV: Multiple atresias (string of sausages)

The anatomic distribution is approximately 50% in the jejunum (proximal 30%, distal 20%) and 50% in the ileum (proximal 15%, distal 35%). Approximately 90% of all small bowel atresias are single. Type IV atresias more often involve the proximal jejunum.

The initial diagnosis is often entertained when pregnant mothers present with polyhydramnios resulting from the inability of the fetus to absorb amniotic fluid via the obstructed bowel. Prenatal ultrasonography shows distended loops of fetal bowel consistent with obstruction. Newborn infants typically present with the abdominal distention and bilious vomiting often associated with failure to pass meconium. A more proximal (higher) location of the obstruction is characterized by an earlier onset of bilious vomiting and less abdominal distention in comparison with a more distal (lower) obstruction. On plain abdominal radiography, distended air-filled bowel loops are usually observed. The lower the obstruction, the greater is the number of distended loops and air-fluid levels. Often, a markedly distended loop (relative to other bowel loops) is visualized, which may help to identify the location of the blind end of the obstructed bowel. A contrast enema typically reveals a microcolon, which results from the fact that little or no succus has passed distal to the obstruction.

The differential diagnosis includes malrotation (with or without volvulus), meconium syndromes, duodenal or colonic atresia, internal hernia, intestinal duplication, and total colonic Hirschsprung disease. The particular distinguishing features of these conditions are discussed elsewhere in this chapter; however, jejunoileal atresia may coexist with malrotation (10% to 18%), meconium peritonitis (12%), meconium ileus (10%), and, less frequently, with other comorbid obstructive conditions. Intestinal ileus secondary to sepsis can also present with abdominal distention and bilious vomiting. When the level and pattern of obstruction suggest the possibility of malrotation, a limited upper gastrointestinal contrast study should be performed to demonstrate a normally positioned ligament of Treitz (located to the left of the vertebral column at the level of the pylorus).

Initial treatment should include prompt adequate intravenous hydration and orogastric decompression of the stomach with a sump tube placed at intermittent suction with frequent regular irrigation of the tube to ensure patency. The operative management of the child should not be undertaken until the fluid and electrolyte status is within normal range. Bilious drainage from the stomach should be replaced with equal amounts of intravenous lactated Ringer's solution every 4 hours. Fluid management should be administered to maintain a urine output of 3 to 4 mL/kg per hour.

Operative intervention is based on the type of atresia, the presence of associated surgical comorbidities, and the condition of the bowel at the time of surgical exploration. Abdominal exploration is usually carried out through a transverse incision above the level of the umbilicus. In considering the most appropriate operation, a general strategy is to preserve as much viable bowel as possible. Although dilation of the bowel proximal to the obstructing blind end is always present, a marked and relatively abrupt increase in the caliber of dilation is often found at the terminus itself, creating a large, bulbous pouch (Fig. 47-31). Because peristalsis of massively dilated bowel is thought to be ineffective, a primary anastomosis between such a pouch and the small-caliber, unused distal bowel should not be attempted. Instead, the pouch should be surgically tapered (or resected, if the involved segment is appropriately limited to avoid creating short gut syndrome) to allow for better postoperative peristalsis and to facilitate a more appropriately proportioned end-to-oblique end anastomosis. Side-to-side anastomoses are not generally used because of the association with blind-loop syndrome.

Before creation of the anastomosis, the distal lumen of the bowel is gently irrigated (inflated) to ensure that no further

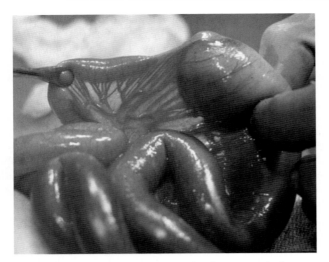

Figure 47–31. Operative photograph of a type II ileal atresia.

atretic segments or webs are present. Multiple atresias can be managed either by multiple resections and anastomoses or by intramural stenting.[11] This latter method may help to preserve intestinal length. Particular care is required in handling the distal bowel involved in the fragile apple-peel deformity, as the entire length of the segment is based on a delicate, easily injured ileocecal artery terminus. If the bowel is compromised by inflammation or ischemia, a primary anastomosis is postponed and the bowel is diverted.

Postoperative care involves adequate nutritional support, often administered parenterally until adequate bowel function is present. Elemental formulas may be useful to transition over to a full regular-formula diet. The most serious postoperative complications usually involve anastomotic leakage and sepsis. Over the longer term, anastomotic stricture can be problematic.

HIRSCHSPRUNG DISEASE

Congenital intestinal aganglionosis (Hirschsprung disease) is the result of arrested fetal development of the myenteric nervous system (see Small Intestine in Part 1). Hirschsprung disease is the most common cause of intestinal obstruction in the neonate. It occurs in about 1 in 5000 live births with a male-to-female ratio of 3.4:1. Total-colon Hirschsprung disease, noted in up to 8% of cases, favors females at a ratio of 1.6:1. More than 75% of the time, the transition zone from normal to involved colon is located in the rectosigmoid region. Down syndrome is the most commonly associated anomaly, occurring in 8% to 16% of patients. Approximately 5% of patients with Down syndrome have Hirschsprung disease. Family history is important because the risk of a sibling having Hirschsprung disease is 1% to 5% for short-segment disease and 9% to 33% with long-segment disease. Familial Hirschsprung disease occurs in 4% to 8% of patients.[36,77,81,101] Hirschsprung disease or tumors of neural crest origin (neuroblastoma, ganglioneuroblastoma, and ganglioneuroma) occur in association with congenital central hypoventilation syndrome in approximately 20% and 6% of cases, respectively.[7]

Approximately 80% to 90% of patients present in the neonatal period with complete intestinal obstruction characterized by abdominal distention, emesis, and failure to pass meconium. Approximately 95% of normal full-term infants pass meconium in the first 24 hours, whereas an equal number of patients with Hirschsprung disease do not. Physical examination shows a distended, soft abdomen, but rectal examination can produce an explosive stool. A contrast examination can be diagnostic in 80% of newborns. Findings may include a rectum with a smaller diameter than the sigmoid colon, a transition zone, normal caliber in the majority of the colon, and failure to completely evacuate on a 24-hour delayed film. Contrast enemas in all age groups are performed on unprepared bowel if the diagnosis of Hirschsprung disease is being considered. The definitive diagnosis of Hirschsprung disease, however, rests on demonstration of aganglionosis and hypertrophy of the nerve trunks on biopsy. In newborns, adequate biopsy specimens can often be obtained by the suction technique in the nursery.

Hirschsprung-associated enterocolitis occurs in 10% of patients overall and is more common beyond the neonatal period. This can be fatal and can happen even after treatment for Hirschsprung disease has been completed. All practitioners should be aware of this complication and treat for it whenever it is suspected. Enterocolitis is associated with abdominal distention, fever, emesis, and spontaneous diarrhea or an explosive diarrheal stool with gas during and after rectal examination. Enterocolitis is treated with decompression of the rectum with a large catheter and with warm saline irrigations using 20 mL/kg three or four times per day, volume resuscitation, and administration of broad-spectrum antibiotics.

The initial goal of treatment is decompression. Traditionally, this was performed with a leveling ostomy. Leveling here refers to the intraoperative determination of where on the bowel the ganglion cells make an appearance. This is done by taking seromuscular biopsies and having the pathologist review the frozen sections. The ostomy is then placed proximal to this to ensure its adequate function. Primary pull-through procedures are being performed with much greater frequency. Here, instead of the traditional three stages (ostomy, definitive repair, ostomy takedown), the operation is done in one stage, and without a protective stoma. Occasionally, a primary repair with a protective ostomy is performed—a two-stage operation, in that ostomy takedown is still required.

If a primary procedure is to be performed, the bowel must be decompressed and not too dilated. In the newborn, this is easily accomplished with rectal irrigations of saline at a volume of 20 mL/kg three times daily via a large catheter located high in the rectum or sigmoid colon. These irrigations can be performed by competent caregivers for a few days to a few weeks before the definitive pull-through procedure. Perioperative broad-spectrum antibiotics are recommended.

The three traditional surgical methods used to treat Hirschsprung disease are (1) Swenson, (2) Soave, and (3) Duhamel. No statistically significant difference has been shown between the outcomes of any of these procedures if they are performed properly. In the Swenson procedure, the aganglionic bowel is removed completely and the ganglionic bowel is anastomosed full-thickness to full-thickness rectum just above the dentate line. In the

Soave, only the distal mucosa of the bowel is removed, from just above the dentate line to about the level of the peritoneal reflection. The remaining aganglionic bowel is removed. The ganglionic bowel is then brought down into the sleeve of bowel left behind and anastomosed full-thickness to partial-thickness rectum just above the dentate line. The Duhamel leaves the last segment of aganglionic distal bowel in place and brings the ganglionic segment down behind it. The two segments are then stapled and sewn together to create a common channel above the dentate line, with aganglionic bowel anteriorly and ganglionic bowel posteriorly. Most laparoscopic procedures done today are slight variants based on the Soave technique. Total colonic Hirschsprung disease requires much more involved and less successful procedures. Many variants have been proposed and are performed, with the goal of all surgical procedures being to bring ganglionated bowel down the anorectal junction, with or without the formation of a reservoir.

Regardless of the procedure performed, these patients must be followed for years postoperatively. Postoperative care and long-term issues are similar to those for patients with anorectal malformations. Mandatory dilations are not necessary in Hirschsprung disease, as a neorectum is not created. However, strictures are not uncommon, and these patients need to be diligently followed during the first year. If any narrowing is noted, a full dilation program is started. As there appears to be no detriment to dilations, some surgeons start a dilator program in all patients. Also, enterocolitis is not typically seen in patients with anorectal malformations but can absolutely occur after repair in a patient with Hirschsprung disease. All patients with Hirschsprung disease, at any time in their lives, should have enterocolitis included in their differential diagnosis whenever they have abdominal pain, distention, or diarrhea. Also unique to patients with Hirschsprung disease is the possibility of a retained aganglionic segment contributing to ongoing, postoperative constipation. This occurs when poorly vascularized, poorly ganglionated, or frankly aganglionic bowel is brought down in the pull-through. Repeat biopsy is necessary. Anal sphincter achalasia can also occur, and injection with botulinum toxin can help make this diagnosis. If suspected, an anal myomectomy can provide a permanent solution. All the potential complications, however, must be balanced by the long-term results, which indicate that approximately 90% of these patients ultimately achieve normal or near-normal bowel function.

ANORECTAL ANOMALIES

Anorectal malformations, or imperforate anus, are a class of congenital malformations that covers a wide spectrum of defects.[35,72,75] They can be quite minor in appearance—for example, a mildly anteriorly displaced anus—or quite severe. Overall, most patients do reasonably well, with more than 75% attaining a good degree of bowel control when they have adequate treatment.[76] The most severe forms of pelvic malformations, such as cloacal exstrophy, are not discussed here; this discussion is limited to malformations of the anus and rectum alone.

Imperforate anus occurs in 1 of every 4000 to 5000 newborns. The estimated risk for a couple having a second child with an anorectal malformation is approximately 1%. The frequency of this defect is slightly higher in male than in female patients.

Traditionally, the terms *high, intermediate,* and *low* were used to describe various degrees of imperforate anus. However, terminology should relate to the location of the rectal fistula for both prognostic and therapeutic implications.

More than 80% of male patients with imperforate anus have a fistulous connection between the rectum and the urinary tract. This can go from the rectum to the bladder (rectovesical), to the prostatic urethra (rectoprostatic), and to the bulbar urethra (rectobulbar). When the rectal fistula opens onto the perineal skin, it is called a *perineal fistula.* An unusual form of imperforate anus occurs when the rectum ends blindly in the pelvis. More than 50% of these patients have Down syndrome and almost all patients with Down syndrome and imperforate anus have this variant.

In female patients, there are three main types of malformations: perineal fistulas, vestibular fistulas, and complex malformations called *cloacae.* In the perineal fistula, the rectum opens on the perineal skin anterior to the anal dimple. A vestibular fistula opens in the posterior aspect of the introitus but outside the hymen. A cloaca is a malformation in which the rectum, vagina, and urethra all open into a common channel of variable length, which then opens onto the perineum. A rectovaginal fistula is extremely uncommon; these are usually rectovestibular fistulas.

Anorectal malformations may be associated with malformations of the sacrum and spine. One missing vertebra does not appear to have prognostic significance; however, two or more missing sacral vertebrae is a poor prognostic sign in terms of bowel continence and, sometimes, urinary control. Hemivertebrae in the thoracic and lumbar spine are also associated with imperforate anus.

Tethered cord is a defect frequently associated with imperforate anus, seen in up to 25% of cases. The actual repercussions of tethered cord are more difficult to determine. It usually coincides with very high anal defects, a very abnormal sacrum, or spina bifida. Cause and effect is unclear, as is the benefit of surgical treatment of the tethered cord, but the current standard of care is to look for tethered cord in all patients with imperforate anus and surgically treat if discovered.

The frequency of associated genitourinary defects varies from 20% to 50%. The width of the range is most likely related to how diligently the defects are sought. The higher the malformation, the more frequent are the associated urologic abnormalities. Patients with a persistent cloaca or rectovesical fistula have a 90% chance of an associated genitourinary abnormality. Conversely, children with perineal fistulas have less than a 10% chance of an associated urologic defect. Hydronephrosis, urosepsis, and metabolic acidosis from poor renal function are the main sources of mortality and morbidity in newborns with anorectal malformation. In fact, a thorough urologic evaluation should take precedence over the colostomy itself in patients with high lesions. In patients with lower lesions such as perineal fistulas, the urologic evaluation can be performed on an elective basis. This evaluation must include an ultrasonographic study of the kidneys and the entire abdomen to rule out the presence of hydronephrosis or any other obstructive process.

Approximately 5% of patients with imperforate anus have associated esophageal atresia, and up to 10% have significant cardiac malformations such as tetralogy of Fallot, ventricular septal defect, or patent ductus arteriosus.

The initial diagnosis of imperforate anus is almost always made during the first newborn physical examination. Occasionally, a mild perineal fistula is missed. Two important questions need to be answered within the first 24 hours. The first is whether a colostomy will be needed, deferring definitive repair until later in life, or whether to proceed with definitive repair. The second is to determine whether associated defects, such as urologic abnormalities, require more urgent treatment. It should be stressed that imperforate anus is not a surgical emergency and rarely needs to be operated on within the first 24 hours of life. This time should be used to complete the workup and discuss options with the family. On the other hand, some associated abnormalities can carry morbidity and mortality risks in the first 24 hours, and these must be addressed. Intravenous fluids, antibiotic coverage, an abdominal ultrasound, a radiograph of the spine, anteroposterior and lateral radiographs of the sacrum, a cardiac evaluation, and a nasogastric tube are indicated.

The decision to perform a colostomy or to proceed with the definitive repair can be answered within the first 24 hours by physical examination alone in more than 80% of male patients and 95% of female patients (Figs. 47-32 and 47-33). In the male, the presence of a well-developed midline groove between the buttocks, a prominent anal dimple, and meconium exiting through a small orifice located anterior to the sphincter in the midline of the perineum are evidence of a perineal fistula. Occasionally, there is a prominent skin bridge that an instrument can be passed beneath (known as a "bucket handle") or a midline raphe "black ribbon" of subepithelial meconium. These malformations can be repaired via a perineal approach during the newborn period without a colostomy. On the other hand, flat buttocks with no evidence of a perineal opening and the presence of meconium in the urine are indications of a rectourethral fistula. A small gauze pad over the tip of the penis can be helpful in spotting meconium in the urine. Most surgeons place a colostomy in these patients.

It can take up to 24 hours for enough pressure to build up in the colon to push meconium out a perineal fistula. So, unless meconium is definitely seen in the urine, waiting is appropriate. If the diagnosis is still in doubt after 24 hours, a cross-table lateral radiograph of the abdomen and pelvis with the infant in the prone position is indicated. By identifying the anal dimple with a lead marker, the distance between the

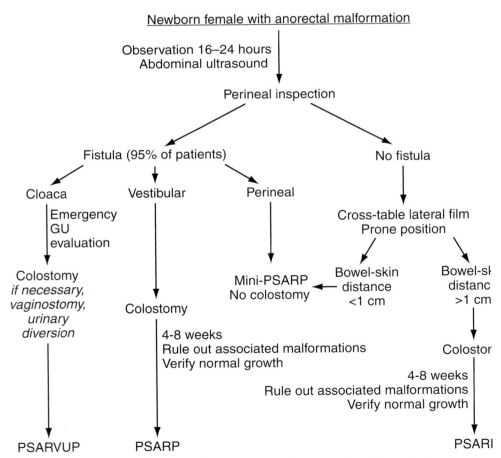

Figure 47–32. Algorithm for neonatal management of anorectal malformation in female patients. GU, genitourinary; PSARP, posterior sagittal anorectoplasty; PSARVUP, posterior sagittal anorectal vaginourethroplasty.

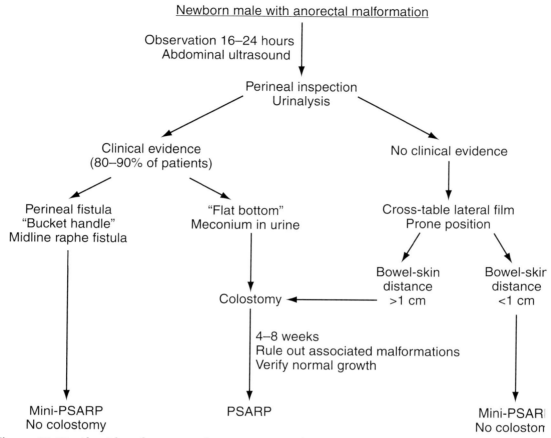

Figure 47–33. Algorithm for neonatal management of anorectal malformation in male patients. GU, genitourinary; PSARP, posterior sagittal anorectoplasty.

end of the dilated bowel and the skin can be estimated. If this distance is less than 1 cm, a primary repair can be attempted. It is important to wait 24 hours before obtaining this radiograph, because pressure within the colon is necessary for its prognostic value. Fewer than 20% of male patients need this radiograph.

In the female patient, physical examination alone can lead to the proper initial surgical treatment in more than 95% of cases. If a single perineal opening is observed where the urethra is normally located, the diagnosis of cloaca is established and a colostomy is indicated. A girl with a normal urethra and an opening within the vestibule of the female genitalia but outside of the hymen confirms the diagnosis of rectovestibular fistula. Initial treatment of this defect is the most variable. Pediatric surgeons experienced in its repair often either temporarily dilate the fistula and perform a definitive repair in a few weeks or proceed directly to definitive repair. The most conservative option is to place a colostomy and perform the repair at a later date. This is by far the most common defect seen in girls.

A fistula tract located anterior to the center of the sphincter but posterior to the vestibule of the genitalia establishes the diagnosis of perineal fistula. These babies undergo primary anoplasty without a protective colostomy. In the absence of any fistulous tract in the female patient, imperforate anus without fistula is the diagnosis, particularly in patients with

Down syndrome. The cross-table film is needed for fewer than 5% of female patients.

The surgical care of patients with anorectal malformations often involves a complex interplay between clinical judgment and technical expertise. Surgical strategies include the creation of a temporizing or palliative colostomy and various types of corrective repairs. Some of the principles that influence surgical decisionmaking follow.

Colostomy

The main purpose of a colostomy is to provide immediate relief of bowel obstruction related to imperforate anus. It also allows the medical and surgical team time to plan the definitive repair, and it permits other medical and surgical issues, some of which may be more pressing, to be properly addressed. A colostomy is nearly always a temporary measure, as patients with imperforate anus very rarely require permanent diversion.

Most colostomies are placed at the junction of the descending and sigmoid colon in the patient's left lower quadrant. This limits the amount of prolapse that can occur and leaves adequate colon to perform the pull-through in the future. A divided colostomy is required, as loop colostomies can provide incomplete diversion. Overflow of stool into the distal limb exposes the patient to fecal contamination of the genitourinary tract and can lead to massive distention of the distal colon, compromising the ability to perform a successful pull-through. The stoma appliance should not include both stomas to avoid this same problem. A technical point is that the distal colon should be irrigated of all meconium at the time of the colostomy. An exception to the descending/sigmoid colostomy placement is that in the female patient with a persistent cloaca, a divided transverse colon colostomy is performed, despite its greater risk of prolapse, because more distal colon may be needed to perform a vaginal reconstruction.

It is extremely important that the surgeon know the exact location of the fistula before undertaking the definitive repair. A distal colostogram must be obtained for all male patients who undergo a colostomy and all female patients with a cloaca. This study accurately shows the location of the fistula between the rectum and the genitourinary tract, the length of available colon from the colostomy to the fistula site, the distance from the rectum to the anal dimple, its relationship with the sacrum, the characteristics of the urethra in the male patient, the characteristics of the vagina in a female patient, and the presence or absence of vesicoureteral reflux. It is important that the radiologist apply some pressure to the contrast material to get full benefit from the examination.

Definitive Repair

The goal of the definitive repair is to place a neoanus in the appropriate location allowing control by the patient. The vast majority of patients with imperforate anus can be approached via the posterior sagittal route by a posterior sagittal anorectoplasty. Male patients with a bladder neck fistula and female patients with a long common channel (greater than 2.5 cm) require combined abdominal and posterior sagittal approaches. In the posterior sagittal approach, the patient is placed in the prone position with the pelvis elevated. An incision is made from above the coccyx to below the anal dimple. Fine-tip cautery is used, and an electrical stimulator is critical to determine the location of the sphincter mechanism. Dissection proceeds exactly on midline until the rectum is found. In male patients, fistulas to the urethra must be isolated and divided, and the rectum freed. Perineal fistulas in both sexes and vestibular fistulas in female patients are tracked directly to the rectum, which must still be freed from the common wall it may have with other genitourinary structures. The now mobilized rectum is then brought down to the perineum into the proper location within the sphincter mechanism as determined by electrical stimulation. The rectum occasionally needs to be tapered at this time. The surrounding muscle and soft tissue is then appropriately closed in layers. In the male patient, a Foley catheter must be placed at the start of the operation and left in place for 4 to 7 days postoperatively.

Postoperative Care

After colostomy, broad-spectrum antibiotics are continued for 2 to 3 days. A stoma appliance is fitted, and the mucous fistula is typically left exposed. Once the colostomy is productive, feedings are begun. Recovery after posterior sagittal anorectoplasty is typically quite rapid—patients can often eat on the day of surgery. Broad-spectrum antibiotics are continued for 2 days.

Patients can often go home after 2 days, but male patients should have their Foley catheters left in until postoperative day 4 to 7. If the catheter accidentally comes out, it should not be replaced until the patient is given ample opportunity to void spontaneously, because replacing the Foley can cause significant injury.

Two to 3 weeks after surgery, dilations are begun using Hegar dilators. That this procedure is critical for success must be impressed on the patient's caregivers. Dilations continue for 6 to 12 months postoperatively. If this process is interrupted, there is a high likelihood that a stricture will develop. If a colostomy is present, it can be closed once the desired anal size is reached, typically a 14 Hegar dilator in a 6-month-old child. The importance of dilation cannot be overstated.

After colostomy closure or primary definitive repair, the usual multiple bowel movements frequently produce severe perianal excoriations. These may take time to heal and caregivers should be forewarned. Every attempt to prevent prolonged contact of stool and skin should be made. Barrier products are frequently used, but it is most helpful to avoid using a diaper on the patient as much as possible.

Special Considerations for Cloaca Patients

In patients with a cloaca, certain characteristics of the common channel determine the various operative approaches. As noted earlier, a cloaca is a common opening in the perineum, seen in female patients only, into which the bladder, vagina, and rectum typically enter. It is not to be confused with cloacal exstrophy, a defect seen in both sexes in which the incomplete hindgut, genitals, and bladder are exposed in conjunction with a deformed pelvis. Cloacal exstrophy is not discussed in this chapter. In cloacal malformations, the major treatment determinant is the length of the common channel. A *common channel* is defined as the distance from the introitus to the first fistula tract, that is, bladder, bowel, or vagina. Most pediatric surgeons believe that a common channel of more than 3.5 cm changes the technical aspects of the repair from performing a urogenital mobilization from below to requiring a combined abdominoperineal approach that may include an interposition graft of bowel to create a neovagina. In a urogenital mobilization, the rectal fistula is divided from the cloaca and placed appropriately in the muscle complex, as is done for all anorectal malformations described earlier. The common bladder and vagina complex is then extensively mobilized and brought down to the introitus. By not dividing the urethra and vagina, many complications can be avoided. With a long common channel, both an abdominal and perineal approach is required. Frequently in these cases, inadequate vaginal tissue is available and a neovagina of colon or small bowel is required. Despite the complexity of these reconstructions, with meticulous surgical care and careful operative planning, these patients can do very well and a number have gone on to have children of their own. All should achieve some level of social continence and be able to be sexually active.

Long-term Follow-up

These patients need life-long follow-up. Constipation is the most common sequela in patients with anorectal malformations, and it can be most severe in the benign group of malformations.

The more complex malformations have a poorer prognosis in terms of bowel control but less chance for constipation. Constipation must be treated aggressively, and prolonged use of laxatives in this population is indicated.

Twenty-five percent of patients with anorectal malformations suffer from some level of fecal incontinence and require some form of bowel management.[72,75,76] Urinary incontinence is not common in boys—99% enjoy control. In females with cloacae, 50% to 60% have control, 20% require a continent diversion, and the rest remain dry with intermittent catheterization.

REFERENCES

1. Abel RM, et al: A quantitative study of the morphological and histochemical changes within the nerves and muscle in infantile hypertrophic pyloric stenosis, *J Pediatr Surg* 3 3:682, 1998.
2. Aktug T, et al: Amnio-allantoic fluid exchange for the prevention of intestinal damage in gastroschisis: an experimental study on chick embryos, *J Pediatr Surg* 30:384, 1995.
3. Alexander F, et al: Delayed gastric emptying affects outcome of Nissen fundoplication in neurologically impaired children, *Surgery* 122:690, 1997.
4. Anteby EY, Yagel S: Route of delivery of fetuses with structural anomalies, *Eur J Obstet Gynecol Reprod Biol* 106:5, 2003.
5. Argyle JC: Pulmonary hypoplasia in infants with giant abdominal wall defects, *Pediatr Pathol* 9:43, 1989.
6. Bealer JF, et al: Gastroschisis increases small bowel nitric oxide synthase activity, *J Pediatr Surg* 31:1043, 1996.
7. Berry-Kravis EM, Zhou L, Rand CM, et al: Congenital central hypoventilation syndrome; *PHOX2B* mutations and phenotype, *Am J Respir Crit Care Med* 174:1139, 2006.
8. Blank E, Chisholm AJ: Congenital microgastria: a case with a 26-year followup. *Pediatrics* 51:1037, 1973.
9. Boix-Ochoa J, Canals J: Maturation of the lower esophagus, *J Pediatr Surg* 11:749, 1976.
10. Boyle EM Jr, et al: Primary repair of ultra-long-gap esophageal atresia: results without a lengthening procedure, *Ann Thorac Surg* 57:576, 1994.
11. Chaet MS, et al: Management of multiple jejunoileal atresias with an intraluminal Silastic stent, *J Pediatr Surg* 29:1604, 1994.
12. Clark LA, Oldham KT: Malrotation, In Ashcraft KW, editor: *Pediatric surgery*, 3rd ed, Philadelphia, 2000, Saunders, p 425.
13. Colozari E, et al: Omphalocele and gastroschisis in Europe: a survey of 3 million births 1980-1990. EUROCAT Working Group, *Am J Med Genet* 58:187, 1995.
14. Crisera CA, et al: Esophageal atresia with tracheoesophageal fistula: suggested mechanism in faulty organogenesis, *J Pediatr Surg* 34:204, 1999.
15. Crisera CA, et al: TTF-1 and HNF-3beta in the developing tracheoesophageal fistula: further evidence for the respiratory origin of the distal esophagus, *J Pediatr Surg* 34:1322, 1999.
16. Crisera CA, et al: Defective fibroblast growth factor signaling allows for nonbranching growth of the respiratory-derived fistula tract in esophageal atresia with tracheoesophageal fistula, *J Pediatr Surg* 35:1421, 2000.
17. Davis PB, Drumm M, Konstan MW: Cystic fibrosis: state of the art, *Am J Respir Crit Care Med* 154:1229, 1996.
18. DeVeciana M, et al: Prediction of an abnormal karyotype in fetuses with omphalocele, *Prenat Diagn* 14:487, 1994.
19. Dommergues M, et al: Serial transabdominal amniotransfusion in the management of gastroschisis with severe oligohydramnios, *J Pediatr Surg* 31:1297, 1996.
20. Doyle NM, Lally KP: The CDH Study Group and advances in the clinical care of the patient with congenital diaphragmatic hernia, *Semin Perinatal* 28:174, 2004.
21. DuBose TM 5th, et al: Lactobezoars: a patient series and literature review, *Clin Pediatr* 40:603, 2001.
22. Engum SA, et al: Analysis of morbidity and mortality in 227 cases of esophageal atresia and/or tracheoesophageal fistula over two decades, *Arch Surg* 130:502, 1995.
23. Fogel M, et al: Congenital heart disease and fetal thoracoabdominal anomalies: associations in utero and the importance of cytogenetic analysis, *Am J Perinatol* 8:411, 1991.
24. Foker JE, et al: Development of a true primary repair for the full spectrum of esophageal atresia, *Ann Surg* 226:533, 1997.
25. Fujimoto T, et al: Laparoscopic extramucosal pyloromyotomy versus open pyloromyotomy for infantile hypertrophic pyloric stenosis: which is better? *J Pediatr Surg* 34:370, 1999.
26. Gilbert WM, Nicolaides KH: Fetal omphalocele: associated malformations and chromosomal defects, *Obstet Gynecol* 70:633, 1987.
27. Gillick J, et al: Notochord anomalies in the Adriamycin rat model: morphologic and molecular basis for the VACTERL association, *J Pediatr Surg* 38:469, 2003.
28. Godbole P, et al: Ultrasound compared with clinical examination in infantile hypertrophic pyloric stenosis, *Arch Dis Child* 75:335, 1996.
29. Goldblum G, et al: Risk factors for gastroschisis, *Teratology* 42:397, 1990.
30. Gornall P: Management of intestinal atresia complicating gastroschisis, *J Pediatr Surg* 24:522, 1989.
31. Grosfeld JL, Rescorla FJ: Duodenal atresia and stenosis: reassessment of treatment and outcome based on antenatal diagnosis, pathologic variance, and long-term follow-up, *World J Surg* 17:301, 1993.
32. Guarino N, et al: Selective neurotrophin deficiency in infantile hypertrophic pyloric stenosis, *J Pediatr Surg* 36:1280, 2001.
33. Haddock G, et al: Gastroschisis in the decade of prenatal diagnosis: 1983-1993, *Eur J Pediatr Surg* 6:18, 1996.
34. Harmon CM, Coran AG: Congenital anomalies of the esophagus. In O'Neill JA Jr, et al, editors: *Pediatric surgery*, 5th ed, St Louis, 1998, Mosby, p 945.
35. Hirschl RB, Coran AG: Anorectal disorders and imperforate anus. In O'Neill JA, et al, editors: *Principles of pediatric surgery*, 2nd ed, St Louis, 2004, Mosby, p 587.
36. Holschneider A, Ure BM: Hirschsprung's disease. In Ashcraft KW, editor: *Pediatric surgery*, 3rd ed, Philadelphia, 2000, Saunders, p 453.
37. How HY, et al: Is vaginal delivery preferable to elective cesarean delivery in fetuses with a known ventral wall defect? *Am J Obstet Gynecol* 182:1527, 2000.
38. Huang J, et al: Benefits of term delivery in infants with antenatally diagnosed gastroschisis, *Obstet Gynecol* 100:695, 2002.
39. Kalish RB, et al: Esophageal atresia and tracheoesophageal fistula: the impact of prenatal suspicion on neonatal outcome in a tertiary care center, *J Perinat Med* 31:111, 2003.
40. Kara CS, et al: Neonatal gastric perforation: review of 23 years' experience, *Surg Today* 34:243, 2004.

41. Kawahara H, et al: Motor abnormality in the gastroduodenal junction in patients with infantile hypertrophic pyloric stenosis, *J Pediatr Surg* 36:1641, 2001.

42. Kieffer J, et al: Gastroesophageal reflux after repair for congenital diaphragmatic hernia, *J Pediatr Surg* 30:1330, 1996.

43. Kimura K, et al: Diamond-shaped anastomosis for duodenal atresia: an experience with 44 patients over 15 years, *J Pediatr Surg* 25:977, 1990.

44. Kimura K, et al: Elliptical seromuscular resection for tapering the proximal dilated bowel in duodenal or jejunal atresia, *J Pediatr Surg* 31:1405, 1996.

45. Kobayashi H, et al: Pyloric stenosis: new histopathologic perspective using confocal laser scanning, *J Pediatr Surg* 36:1277, 2001.

46. Kobayashi H, et al: Age-related changes in innervation in hypertrophic pyloric stenosis, *J Pediatr Surg* 32:1704, 1997.

47. Kusafuka T, Puri P: Altered messenger RNA expression of the neuronal nitric oxide synthase gene in infantile hypertrophic pyloric stenosis, *Pediatr Surg Int* 12:576, 1997.

48. Kyyronen P, Hemminki K: Gastro-intestinal atresias in Finland in 1970-79, indicating time-place clustering, *J Epidemiol Commun Health* 42:257, 1988.

49. Langer JC, et al: Prenatal diagnosis of esophageal atresia using sonography and magnetic resonance imaging, *J Pediatr Surg* 36:804, 2001.

50. Langer JC, et al: Hypertrophic pyloric stenosis: ultrastructural abnormalities of enteric nerves and the interstitial cells of Cajal, *J Pediatr Surg* 30:1535, 1995.

51. Langer JC, et al: Etiology of intestinal damage in gastroschisis. I: Effects of amniotic fluid exposure and bowel constriction in a fetal lamb model, *J Pediatr Surg* 24:992, 1989.

52. Louw JH, Barnard CN: Congenital intestinal atresia: observations on its origin, *Lancet* 269:1065, 1955.

53. Ludtke FE, et al: Gastric emptying 16 to 26 years after treatment of infantile hypertrophic pyloric stenosis, *J Pediatr Surg* 29:52, 1994.

54. Lund DP, et al: Congenital diaphragmatic hernia: the hidden morbidity, *J Pediatr Surg* 29:258, 1994.

55. Macdessi J, Oates RK: Clinical diagnosis of pyloric stenosis: a declining art, *Br Med J* 306:553, 1993.

56. Mahon BE, et al: Maternal and infant use of erythromycin and other macrolide antibiotics as risk factors for infantile hypertrophic pyloric stenosis, *J Pediatr* 139:380, 2001.

57. Martinez DA, et al: Sequelae of antireflux surgery in profoundly disabled children, *J Pediatr Surg* 27:267, 1992.

58. McIntyre RC Jr, et al: The pediatric diaphragm in acute gastric volvulus, *J Am Coll Surg* 178:234, 1994.

59. Meehan JJ, Georgeson KE: Prevention of liver failure in parenteral nutrition-dependent children with short bowel syndrome, *J Pediatr Surg* 32:473, 1997.

60. Mercado-Deane MG, et al: Prostaglandin-induced foveolar hyperplasia simulating pyloric stenosis in an infant with cyanotic heart disease, *Pediatr Radiol* 24:45, 1988.

61. Mitchell LE, Risch N: The genetics of infantile hypertrophic pyloric stenosis: a reanalysis, *Am J Dis Child* 147:1203, 1993.

62. Moir CR, et al: A prospective trial of elective preterm delivery for fetal gastroschisis, *Am J Perinatol* 21:289, 2004.

63. Naik DR, et al: Demonstration of lactobezoar by ultrasound, *Br J Radiol* 60:506, 1987.

64. Nakano A, et al: Epidermolysis bullosa with congenital pyloric atresia: novel mutations in the beta 4 integrin gene ITGB4 and genotype/phenotype correlations, *Pediatr Res* 49:618, 2001.

65. Nicolaides KH, et al: Fetal gastrointestinal and abdominal wall defects: associated malformations and chromosomal abnormalities, *Fetal Diagn Ther* 7:107, 1992.

66. Novotny A, et al: Gastroschisis: an 18-year review, *J Pediatr Surg* 28:650, 1993.

67. Nyberg DA, et al: Prenatal sonographic findings of Down syndrome: review of 94 cases, *Obstet Gynecol* 76:370, 1990.

68. Okada K, et al: Discharge diagnoses in infants with apparent life-threatening event, *Pediatr Int* 45:560, 2003.

69. O'Rahilly R, Muller F: Respiratory and alimentary relations in staged human embryos: new embryological data and congenital anomalies, *Ann Otol Rhinol Laryngol* 93:421, 1984.

70. Orenstein SR, Hassall E, Furmaga-Jablonska W, et al: Multicenter, double-blind, randomized, placebo-controlled trial assessing the efficacy and safety of proton pump inhibitor lansoprazole in infants with symptoms of gastroesophageal reflux disease, *J Pediatr* 154:514, 2009.

71. Ozturk H, et al: Gastric perforation in neonates: analysis of five cases, *Acta Gastroenterol Belg* 66:271, 2003.

72. Paidas CN, Pena A: Rectum and anus. In Oldham KT, et al, editors: *Surgery of infants and children: scientific principles and practice,* Philadelphia, 1997, Lippincott-Raven, 1997, p 1323.

73. Panuel M, et al: Duodenal atresia with bifid termination of the common bile duct, *Arch Fr Pediatr* 49:365, 1992.

74. Pederson JC, et al: Gastric tube as the primary procedure for pure esophageal atresia, *J Pediatr Surg* 31:1233, 1996.

75. Pena A: Imperforate anus and cloacal malformations. In Ashcraft KW, editor: *Pediatric surgery,* 3rd ed, Philadelphia, 2000, Saunders, p 473.

76. Pena A, Hong AR: Anorectal malformations. In Mattei P, editor: *Surgical directives: pediatric surgery,* Philadelphia, Lippincott Williams & Williams, 2002, p 413.

77. Puri P: Hirschsprung's disease. In Oldham KT, et al, editors: *Surgery of infants and children: scientific principles and practice,* Philadelphia, 1997, Lippincott-Raven, p 1277.

78. Rais-Bahrami K, et al: Congenital diaphragmatic hernia: outcome of preoperative extracorporeal membrane oxygenation, *Clin Pediatr* 34:471, 1995.

79. Rescorla FJ, et al: Anomalies of intestinal rotation in childhood: analysis of 447 cases, *Surgery* 108:710, 1990.

80. Rescorla FJ, Grosfeld JL: Contemporary management of meconium ileus, *World J Surg* 17:318, 1993.

81. Ricketts RR: Hirschsprung's disease. In Mattei P, editor: *Surgical directives: pediatric Surgery,* Philadelphia, 2002, Lippincott Williams & Williams, p 371.

82. Riordan JR: Therapeutic strategies for treatment of CF based on knowledge of CFTR, *Pediatr Pulmonol Suppl* 18:83, 1999.

83. Rollins MD, et al: Pyloric stenosis: congenital or acquired? *Arch Dis Child* 64:138, 1989.

84. Segel SY, et al: Fetal abdominal wall defects and mode of delivery: a systematic review, *Obstet Gynecol* 98:867, 2001.

85. Shulman A, et al: Prenatal identification of esophageal atresia: the role of ultrasonography for evaluation of functional anatomy, *Prenat Diagn* 22:669, 2002.

86. Singer JI: Lactobezoar causing an abdominal triad of colicky pain, emesis and a mass, *Pediatr Emerg Care* 4:194, 1988.

87. Slocum C, Arko M, DiFiore J, et al: Apnea, bradycardia, and desaturation in preterm infants before and after feeding, *J Perinatol* 29:209, 2009.

88. Smith CD, et al: Nissen fundoplication in children with profound neurologic disability: high risks and unmet goals, *Ann Surg* 215:654, 1992.

89. Snyder CL, et al: Management of intestinal atresia in patients with gastroschisis, *J Pediatr Surg* 36:1542, 2001.

90. Sorensen HT, Skriver MV, Pedersen L, et al: Risk of infantile hypertrophic pyloric stenosis after maternal postnatal use of macrolides, *Scand J Infect Dis* 35:104, 2003.

91. Sparey C, et al: Esophageal atresia in the Northern Region Congenital Anomaly Survey, 1985-1997: prenatal diagnosis and outcome, *Am J Obstet Gynecol* 182:427, 2000.

92. Spigland N, Yazbeck S: Complications associated with surgical treatment of congenital intrinsic duodenal obstruction, *J Pediatr Surg* 25:1127, 1990.

93. Spilde TL, et al: Complete discontinuity of the distal fistula tract from the developing gut: direct histologic evidence for the mechanism of tracheoesophageal fistula formation, *Anat Rec* 267:220, 2002.

94. Spilde TL, et al: Thyroid transcription factor-1 expression in the human neonatal tracheoesophageal fistula, *J Pediatr Surg* 37:1065, 2002.

95. Spilde TL, et al: A role for sonic hedgehog signaling in the pathogenesis of human tracheoesophageal fistula, *J Pediatr Surg* 38:465, 2003.

96. Spitz L, et al: Gastric transposition for esophageal substitution in children, *Ann Surg* 206:69, 1987.

97. Spitz LO, et al: Oesophageal atresia: at-risk groups for the 1990s, *J Pediatr Surg* 29:723, 1994.

98. Srinathan SK, et al: Etiology of intestinal damage in gastroschisis. III: Morphometric analysis of smooth muscle and submucosa, *J Pediatr Surg* 30:379, 1995.

99. Stolar CJ: Rotational anomalies and volvulus. In O'Neill JA, et al, editors: *Principles of pediatric surgery*, 2nd ed, St Louis, 2004, Mosby, p 477.

100. Suda K: Immunohistochemical and gross dissection studies of annular pancreas, *Acta Pathol Jpn* 40:505, 1990.

101. Teitelbaum DH: Hirschsprung's disease. In O'Neill JA, et al, editors: *Principles of pediatric surgery*, 2nd ed, St Louis, 2004, Mosby, p 573.

102. Torfs CP, et al: Maternal medications and environmental exposures as risk factors for gastroschisis, *Teratology* 54:84, 1996.

103. Torfs CP, et al: Population-based study of tracheoesophageal fistula and esophageal atresia, *Teratology* 52:220, 1995.

104. Tovar JA: Ambulatory 24-hour manometric and pH metric evidence of permanent impairment of clearance capacity in patients with esophageal atresia, *J Pediatr Surg* 30:1224, 1995.

105. Usmanni SS, Levenbrown J: Lactobezoar in a full-term breast-fed infant, *Am J Gastroenterol* 84:647, 1988.

106. Vanamo K, et al: Long-term gastrointestinal morbidity in patients with congenital diaphragmatic defects, *J Pediatr Surg* 31:551, 1996.

107. Vanderwinden JM, et al: Nitric oxide synthase activity in infantile hypertrophic pyloric stenosis, *N Engl J Med* 327:511, 1992.

108. Velasco AL, et al: Management of congenital microgastria, *J Pediatr Surg* 25:192, 1990.

109. Warner BW: Malrotation. In Mattei P, editor: *Surgical directives: pediatric surgery*, Philadelphia, 2002, Lippincott Williams & Williams.

110. Warner BW: Malrotation. In Oldham KT, et al, editors: *Surgery of infants and children: scientific principles and practice*, Philadelphia, 1997, Lippincott-Raven, p 1229.

111. Waterston DJ, et al: Oesophageal atresia: tracheo-esophageal fistula—a study of survival in 218 infants, *Lancet* 1:819, 1962.

112. Werler MM, et al: Association of vasoconstrictive exposures with risks of gastroschisis and small intestinal atresia, *Epidemiology* 14:349, 2003.

113. Yazbeck S, et al: Omphalocele: a 25-year experience, *J Pediatr Surg* 21:761, 1986.

PART 4

Neonatal Necrotizing Enterocolitis: Clinical Observations, Pathophysiology, and Prevention

Michael S. Caplan

Neonatal necrotizing enterocolitis (NEC) is a common and devastating gastrointestinal emergency that primarily afflicts premature infants in neonatal intensive care units (NICUs) worldwide. Despite advances in neonatal care and significant clinical and basic science investigation, the etiology remains incompletely understood, specific treatment strategies are lacking, and morbidity and mortality from this disease remain high. This section reviews the epidemiology and classic clinical features of NEC, describes the current understanding of the pathophysiology, and relates new, exciting approaches to prevention.

EPIDEMIOLOGY

The incidence of NEC varies among US centers and across continents, but ranges between 3% and 28% with an average of approximately 6% to 10% in infants born weighing less than 1500 g.[126] There is an inverse correlation between gestational age/birthweight and incidence of NEC; the incidence increases dramatically in the smallest and most premature infants, and intrauterine growth restriction confers a higher risk of disease than that of a normally grown preterm infant. Whereas there appears to be a slightly increased prevalence in boys, some data suggest higher NEC rates in African Americans compared with whites or Hispanic neonates.[106] Most (90% to 95%) preterm infants in whom NEC develops are previously fed, although the onset of disease may be several weeks after enteral nutrition begins. Although most neonates in whom NEC develops are preterm, 5% to 10% of cases occur in babies born greater than or equal to 37 weeks' gestation.[136] In this population, NEC is almost always associated with a specific risk factor such as asphyxia, intrauterine growth restriction (IUGR), polycythemia/hyperviscosity, exchange transfusion, umbilical catheters, gastroschisis, congenital heart disease, or myelomeningocele. In these situations, overt intestinal ischemia is often suspected, and therefore the pathophysiology may differ from that in the preterm neonate with NEC (see Pathophysiology). Despite significant advances in neonatal care, the mortality resulting from NEC has not improved over the last three decades, with reports of NEC mortality ranging between 10% and 30%.[49]

CLINICAL FEATURES

Presentation

NEC can present with a variety of symptoms and signs; preterm neonates may demonstrate symptoms of hematochezia, emesis or increased gastric residuals, abdominal distention, lethargy, apnea, and bradycardia, as well as signs of neutropenia, thrombocytopenia, metabolic acidosis, tachycardia, abdominal tenderness, abdominal discoloration, respiratory failure, and, if severe, shock.[134] Guaiac-positive stools are quite common in nasogastric tube-fed preterm neonates (60% to 75%) and therefore are not a useful indicator of NEC. Feeding intolerance occurs frequently in this population of preterm neonates, but studies indicate that intolerance is not a reliable marker for the development of intestinal injury.

Diagnosis

The diagnosis is typically made by the identification of pneumatosis intestinalis (air in the bowel wall) or portal venous gas on abdominal radiograph, although in some cases of NEC, commonly in unfed patients, pneumatosis is not appreciated (Fig. 47-34). In these situations, NEC may be diagnosed surgically or pathologically, or in some instances by ultrasound appreciation of portal venous air. Bell and colleagues suggested a classification scheme that differentiates suspected NEC (stage I) from proven NEC (stage II) and advanced NEC (stage III with peritonitis or perforation) (Table 47-8).[6] In this scheme, stage I NEC includes mild systemic signs, abdominal distention with changes of feeding intolerance, but no confirmatory radiographic evidence. Stage II or proven NEC has similar symptoms or signs with pneumatosis and/or portal venous gas, and stage III demonstrates significant systemic signs with radiographic evidence of intestinal perforation (pneumoperitoneum). This classification scheme is useful in occasional circumstances, especially when one analyzes studies that evaluate NEC; readers should be wary of interventions that appear to influence stage I suspected disease without altering definitive NEC.

Treatment

No specific treatment approaches have influenced the outcome of NEC; therefore interventions are supportive and include fluid resuscitation, withholding feedings with gastric decompression; antibiotics to cover likely enteric pathogens; correction of acidosis, anemia, and thrombocytopenia; and blood pressure support. Whereas blood cultures are positive in approximately 30% of NEC cases and are thought to reflect a breakdown in the mucosal barrier leading to bacterial translocation, intraluminal enteric bacterial pathogens are thought to contribute to the pathophysiology (see later).[66] Antibiotic

coverage in this condition typically includes ampicillin and an aminoglycoside or third-generation cephalosporin, although only occasionally. Staphylococcal species are heavy colonizers of the intestinal tract, and nafcillin or vancomycin should be considered. In situations with suspected or proven intestinal perforation, aggressive anaerobic coverage with clindamycin is often added. Although routine treatment with NPO and antibiotics in uncomplicated medical NEC usually proceeds for 7 to10 days, length of treatment has not been carefully studied, and a recent report has suggested earlier refeeding after ultrasonographic evidence of portal venous air has resolved.[16]

Surgical intervention for NEC is required in 30% to 50% of cases reported, although the approach and timing of these procedures remain controversial. Most physicians agree that intestinal perforation in a patient with NEC requires surgery, but based on three recent clinical trials, patients treated with a peritoneal drain had similar rates of death and short-term intestinal function as those undergoing definitive laparotomy.[15,80,101] In surgical trials for NEC treatment, almost 50% of cases treated with a drain never required a second procedure.[37] In patients without perforation but with worsening disease as manifested by abdominal discoloration and distention, persistent thrombocytopenia and acidosis, and respiratory failure, exploratory laparotomy is often undertaken to remove a discrete segment of necrotic bowel, or to confirm the viability of enough remaining intestine to sustain life. Nonetheless, the timing and utility of these procedures in these complex cases has not been adequately studied.

Outcome

Approximately 30% of patients with radiologic evidence of pneumatosis intestinalis have mild disease and require a period of bowel rest but no surgical intervention. Another 30% of patients eventually die of the disease, with most presenting acutely with rapid deterioration and death. Survivors of NEC have a significant risk for intestinal stricture; in some reports, partial bowel obstruction will develop in as many as 25% in weeks or months following the initial presentation. Short bowel syndrome from NEC develops in some patients; postsurgical patients have an incidence of short bowel syndrome as high as 11%, and these patients are an extremely difficult group to care for. Novel medical and surgical interventions have made only modest improvements in the morbidity and mortality rates associated with this dreaded complication. Of concern, accumulating data suggest that the neurodevelopmental outcome of NEC patients is significantly worse than their gestational age/birthweight-matched controls with similar respiratory disease.[129] The morbidity includes mental retardation as well as an increased incidence of cerebral palsy, hypothetically related to white matter injury from cytokine mediators involved in the systemic inflammatory cascade.[130] Further studies are needed to confirm this association and to clarify the significance of these important results. Nonetheless, NEC is a major financial burden nationwide, with increased initial hospital costs (due primarily to longer length of stay) of $60,000 for a case of medical NEC and up to $200,000 per patient for surgical disease.[14] Based on the current epidemiology, this projects an annual cost burden of $1 billion to the US health care industry without taking into account the long-term care issues associated with impaired survivors.

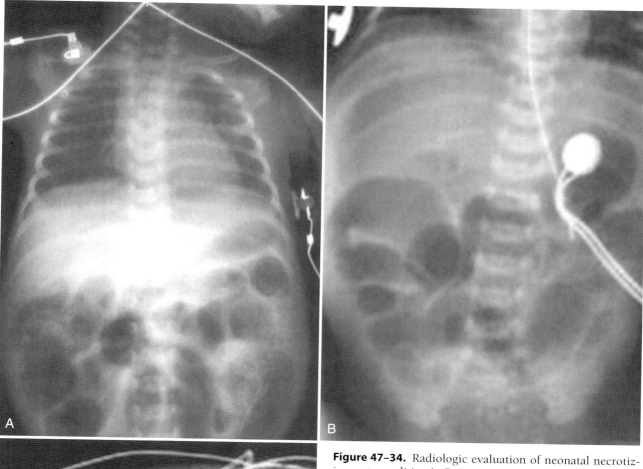

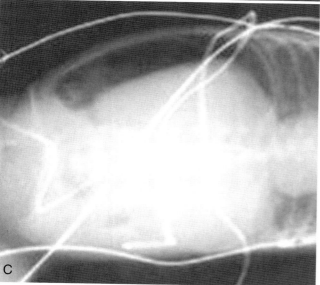

Figure 47–34. Radiologic evaluation of neonatal necrotizing enterocolitis. **A**, Pneumatosis intestinalis. **B**, Perforation with free air seen on supine film. **C**, Free air seen on cross-table lateral radiograph.

Pathology

Clues to the etiology are suggested by the pathologic changes observed in surgical specimens and autopsy material, including coagulation necrosis (suggesting some component of ischemic injury), inflammation (acute and/or chronic), and less commonly, ulceration, hemorrhage, reparative change, bacterial overgrowth, edema, and pneumatosis intestinalis.[5]

PATHOPHYSIOLOGY

Although the specific etiology of NEC is still controversial, epidemiologic analyses of this disease have identified key risk factors of prematurity, enteral feeding, intestinal ischemia/asphyxia, and bacterial colonization. Studies have begun to delineate the mechanisms that link these risk factors to the final common pathway of bowel necrosis. It has been

TABLE 47–8 Modified Bell Staging Criteria for Necrotizing Enterocolitis

Stage	Classification	Clinical Signs	Radiologic Signs
I	Suspected NEC	Abdominal distention Bloody stools Emesis/gastric residuals Apnea/lethargy	Ileus/dilation
II	Proven NEC	As in stage I, plus: Abdominal tenderness ±Metabolic acidosis Thrombocytopenia	Pneumatosis intestinalis and/or portal venous gas
III	Advanced NEC	As in stage II, plus: Hypotension Significant acidosis Thrombocytopenia/disseminated intravascular coagulation Neutropenia	As in stage II, with pneumoperitoneum

Modified from Walsh MC, Kliegman RM: Necrotizing enterocolitis: treatment based on staging criteria, *Pediatr Clin North Am* 33:179, 1986.

suggested that mucosal injury associated with impaired host defense leads to the activation of the inflammatory cascade with subsequent intestinal injury, occasionally associated with the systemic inflammatory response syndrome.

Prematurity

Greater than 90% of NEC cases occur in premature infants; there is consistently a higher risk with lower gestational age and birthweight,[77,106,126] and prematurity is the most consistent and important risk factor. Even though there are many known differences between preterm and full-term neonates, the specific underlying mechanisms responsible for this predilection of NEC in the premature condition remain incompletely elucidated. Studies in humans and animals have identified alterations in multiple components of intestinal host defense,[11,46,131] motility,[8,17] bacterial colonization,[20,25,34,38,39] bloodflow regulation,[87] and inflammatory response[19,41,84] that may contribute to the development of intestinal injury in this unique population.

Enteral Feeding

Because most cases of NEC occur after feedings have been introduced (>90%), enteral alimentation is a significant risk factor for disease in premature infants. Historical reports identified the onset of NEC several days following the first feeding, but in studies of infants with extremely low birthweight, NEC may be diagnosed several weeks after initiating enteral supplementation.[126] This change may reflect current neonatal practice, which typically uses early trophic or hypocaloric feedings, characterized by small volumes and slow rates of increase, without a significant impact on the development of NEC.[40,124] While the precise relationship between enteral feedings and NEC

remains poorly understood, studies have identified the importance of breast milk (versus formula), volume and rate of feeding advancement, osmolality, and substrate fermentation as important factors.[36,65,125]

Breast milk feeding appears to reduce the incidence of NEC in human studies and in carefully controlled animal models.[20,53,77] Breast milk contains multiple bioactive factors that influence host immunity, inflammation, and mucosal protection, including secretory IgA, leukocytes, lactoferrin, lysozyme, mucin, cytokines, growth factors, enzymes, oligosaccharides, and polyunsaturated fatty acids, many of which are absent in neonatal formula preparations (Table 47-9). Specific intestinal host defense factors acquired from breast milk such as epidermal growth factor (EGF), polyunsaturated fatty acid, platelet-activating factor (PAF)-acetylhydrolase, IgA, and macrophages are effective in reducing the incidence of disease in animals,[23,26,41,98] and some have been effective in limited human trials.[43] Nonetheless, breast milk is not completely protective against NEC in premature infants; the largest prospective trial identified a reduction by 50% in most birthweight-specific groups, although there was not a statistically significant reduction in disease observed in a randomized subset from this cohort.[67,77] Due to ethical considerations, it seems unlikely that such an investigation will be accomplished, although there is renewed interest in evaluating donor milk samples and alternative human milk preparations in this context.[110] Because most premature infants receive breast milk via the nasogastric route after artificial collection by mothers and subsequent freezing, it has been suggested that the lack of the normal maternal-infant physical interaction during feeding interferes with specific milk immunity, thereby reducing the protection against the neonate's unique microbial flora. The particular microbial profile in the neonate's intestinal environment may contribute to initiation of NEC (see later).

TABLE 47–9 Factors in Breast Milk That May Influence Pathophysiology of Necrotizing Enterocolitis

Molecule	Effective in Animal Model	Effective in Human Trial
IgA, IgG	+	±
Leukocytes	+	NA
Oligosaccharides	NA	NA
Polyunsaturated fatty acids	+	±
Lactoferrin	NA	±
Glutamine	+	-
Arginine	+	±
Platelet-activating factor-acetylhydrolase	+	NA
Epidermal growth factor	+	NA
Interleukin-10	+	NA
Erythropoietin	±	NA

NA = not applicable

Specific components of milk feedings have been implicated to cause mucosal injury in the high-risk neonate and to subsequently stimulate the development of NEC. Studies have shown that hyperosmolar formulas resulted in disease and that addition of medication to feedings can markedly increase osmolality.[135] Animal studies have shown that short chain fatty acids such as propionic or butyric acid can cause damage to developing intestine, and that colonic fermentation leading to production of these acids by the host microflora may occur in situations of carbohydrate malabsorption.[18,30,75]

This pathway may be especially problematic in the premature infant who is partially deficient in lactase activity and other brush border enzymes. Finally, an intriguing new hypothesis suggests that bile acid accumulation may lead to mucosal injury in the unique environment of the preterm neonate.[54]

Different approaches to feeding have been associated with the initiation of NEC. Early studies suggested that rapid volume increases with full-strength formula increased the incidence of disease, and protocols were designed to limit feeding advancement. Several studies have shown that early hypocaloric or trophic feedings are safe and improve gastrointestinal function in infants with very low birthweight.[40,111,124] Feeding advancement has been evaluated, and the results suggest that judicious volume increase may be safer.[9,65] It has been postulated that overdistention of the stomach with aggressive volumes may compromise splanchnic circulation, leading to intestinal ischemia. Nonetheless, there remains little clarity on the safety of differing feeding practices on the

incidence of NEC, and additional trials are needed to answer this challenging question.

Intestinal Ischemia/Asphyxia

Early observations on the pathophysiology of NEC suggested that profound intestinal ischemia led to intestinal necrosis in unusual clinical situations.[3,122] Similar to the "diving reflex" observed in aquatic mammals, it was hypothesized that in periods of stress, bloodflow was diverted away from the splanchnic circulation resulting in bowel injury. While early epidemiologic observations identified asphyxia as an important risk factor, subsequent studies have shown that the majority of NEC cases are not associated with profound impairment in intestinal perfusion.[134] In animal models, studies have shown that the reperfusion following intestinal ischemia is required in the initiation of bowel necrosis[112]; occlusion of the mesenteric artery for a prolonged period of time results in only mild histologic changes atypical for full-blown NEC.

Neonatal animals have been shown to have differences in the intestinal circulation that may predispose them to NEC. The basal intestinal vascular resistance is elevated in the fetus, and soon following birth decreases significantly, allowing for rapid increase in intestinal bloodflow that is necessary for robust intestinal and somatic growth. It has been shown that this change in the resting vascular resistance is dependent on *the balance between* the dilator (nitric oxide), constrictor (endothelin) molecules, and the myogenic response,[82] and altered levels of these vasoactive mediators have been identified in human NEC samples.[88,89] Perhaps more relevant than basal vascular tone, studies have shown that the newborn has alterations in response to circulatory stress, resulting in compromised intestinal flow and/or vascular resistance. In response to hypotension, newborn animals (3-day-old but not 30-day-old swine) appear to have defective pressure-flow autoregulation, resulting in compromised intestinal oxygen delivery and tissue oxygenation.[87] In addition, in the face of arterial hypoxemia, the newborn intestinal circulatory response differs from that in older animals. Even though intestinal vasodilation and increased intestinal perfusion occur following modest hypoxemia, severe hypoxemia causes vasoconstriction and intestinal ischemia or hypoxia, mediated in part by loss of nitric oxide production. There are multiple chemical mediators (nitric oxide, endothelin, substance P, norepinephrine, and angiotensin) that impact on intestinal vasomotor tone, and in the stressed newborn, abnormal regulation of these may result in compromised circulatory autoregulation, leading to perpetuation of intestinal ischemia and tissue necrosis.[83,90]

Bacterial Colonization

Although reports have documented isolated epidemics of NEC associated with specific bacteria (e.g., *Clostridium* sp., *Escherichia coli*, *Klebsiella* sp., *Staphylococcus epidermidis*), most cases occur endemically and demonstrate a variety of bacterial isolates from stool cultures that are similar to the flora isolated from patients without intestinal symptoms.[39,97] Blood cultures are positive in only 20% to 30% of affected cases, and this likely occurs from mucosal damage and subsequent bacterial translocation. At birth, the intestine is a sterile environment, and no cases of NEC have been described in utero, supporting the importance of bacterial colonization in the pathophysiology. Healthy breast-fed infants develop colonization with several organisms by 1 week of age, including a predominance of anaerobic species of *Bifidobacterium* and *Lactobacillus*, while the hospitalized, extremely premature infant intestine has less species diversity and fewer or absent anaerobes.[47,105,121,137] This imbalance may allow for pathologic proliferation, binding, and invasiveness of otherwise nonpathogenic intestinal bacteria, and a reduction in anti-inflammatory effects and mucosal defense that has been attributed to probiotic organisms.[132] Evidence suggests that contamination or colonization of nasogastric feeding tubes in formula-fed premature infants predisposes some infants to develop NEC.[79] The specific mechanisms by which bacteria initiate NEC remain unclear; mounting evidence suggests that bacterial cell wall products (e.g., endotoxin and lipoteichoic acids) activate specific toll-like receptors on intestinal epithelium and activate the inflammatory cascade leading to the final common pathway of intestinal injury.[13,34,35,138] Nonetheless, certain bacteria such as adherent *E. coli* produce disease in a rabbit model of NEC, whereas nonpathogenic strains of gram-positive organisms prevent disease.[95] Furthermore, accumulating evidence suggests that early colonization by probiotics (facultative anaerobes, e.g., bifidobacteria and lactobacilli) reduces the risk of NEC in animal and human studies, which is discussed further in a subsequent section.[25,56] In summary, bacterial colonization is an important factor in the initiation of intestinal injury, but the specific events in the pathophysiology are not well delineated.

FINAL COMMON PATHWAY: IMBALANCE BETWEEN MUCOSAL INJURY AND HOST DEFENSE/REPAIR WITH ACTIVATION OF THE PROINFLAMMATORY CASCADE

It has been suggested that mild or moderate stress or injury to intestinal epithelium (e.g., from feeding, intestinal ischemia, or bacterial products) without adequate host defense and repair can activate the inflammatory response leading to intestinal injury and NEC.

Host Defense

Gastrointestinal host defense is markedly impaired in the preterm infant, and this imbalance further increases the risk for injury in this population. This intricate system includes (1) physical barriers such as skin, mucous membranes, intestinal epithelia and microvilli, epithelial cell tight junctions, and mucin, (2) immune cells such as polymorphonuclear leukocytes, macrophages, eosinophils, and lymphocytes, and (3) multiple biochemical factors.* Intestinal permeability to macromolecules including immunoglobulins, proteins, and carbohydrates is known to be greater in the neonate than in older children and adults, and in premature infants this permeability may be more pronounced. Intestinal mucus, a

complex gel consisting of water, electrolytes, mucins, glycoprotein, immunoglobulins, and glycolipids, protects against bacterial and toxin invasion, and is abnormal in developing animals and perhaps premature infants.[68,114] Additionally, key bacteriostatic proteins are secreted from epithelium that bind to or inactivate the function of invading organisms. Intestinal trefoil factor is one such molecule that appears to be developmentally regulated and, therefore, deficient in the premature neonate.[74,109,119] Human defensins (or cryptidins) are bacteriostatic proteins synthesized and secreted from paneth cells that protect against bacterial translocation and are altered in premature infants and those with NEC.[92,107]

Immunologic host defense is abnormal in developing animals.[50,96,102] It is known that intestinal intraepithelial lymphocytes (IEL) are decreased in neonates (B and T cells), and do not approach adult levels until 3 to 4 weeks of life. Newborns have markedly reduced secretory IgA in salivary samples, reflecting the decreased activity presumed in intestine.[43,104] Breast milk feeding provides significant supplementation; formula fed neonates have impaired intestinal humoral immunity, and this deficiency may predispose to the increased incidence of infectious diseases and NEC noted in this population.[128,137]

Several biochemical factors that are present in the intestinal milieu play an important role in the maintenance of gut health and integrity. Substances such as lactoferrin,[71] glutamine,[85] growth factors such as EGF,[41] HB-EGF,[44] TGF,[86] insulin-like growth factor (IGF),[103] and erythropoietin,[62,70] gastric acid, oligosaccharides,[32] polyunsaturated fatty acids,[26] and nucleotides,[120] among others, affect mucosal barrier function, intestinal inflammation, and the viability of intraluminal bacteria. Many of these factors are deficient or absent in the preterm neonate, especially in those patients not receiving breast milk feedings.

Based on a growing body of evidence, mucosal stress coupled with inadequate host defense and repair can result in a final common pathway of intestinal injury involving the activation of the inflammatory cascade.[22,24,57] This cascade involves a complex balance of pro- and anti-inflammatory endogenous mediators, receptors, signaling pathways, second messengers, and a variety of downstream effects that ultimately results in end-organ damage in certain clinical circumstances. *Inflammation can be* initiated by a variety of factors, the prototype most commonly described by exposure to the bacterial cell wall product, endotoxin. It has now been clearly shown that bacterial pathogens initiate downstream events following the binding of specific pathogen-associated molecular patterns to a series of human toll-like receptors (TLRs) that are expressed on most cells in the body.[1,2] For example, endotoxin or lipopolysaccharide, the cell wall product of gram-negative bacteria, binds to and activates TLR4, which is normally downregulated on the surface of intestinal epithelium but which has been shown to be abundantly expressed in stressed animals and human neonates.[61,69] Additional work has shown that TLR4 dysfunction reduces the risk of experimental NEC in neonatal mice. Following TLR4 activation, a series of signaling events occurs, allowing for activation of nuclear factor kappa B (NFκB) and translocation into the nucleus with subsequent production of a variety of cytokines including PAF, tumor necrosis factor (TNF), IL-1, and IL-8.[7,78,84,91,100,123] In intestine, subsequent events lead to

---

*References 52, 57, 63, 68, 93, 94, 127, 131.

chemotaxis, transmigration, and activation of leukocytes, as well as synthesis and release of many products from epithelial and inflammatory cells such as IL-6, IL-8, IL-10, IL-18, arachidonic acid metabolites, thromboxanes, leukotrienes, prostaglandins, nitric oxide, endothelin-1, and oxygen free radicals.* If counter-regulatory responses are insufficient (e.g., with decreased or absent IL-1 receptor antagonist, IL-11, IL-12, PAF-acetylhydrolase, IκB leading to increased NFκB), pathologic changes to gut mucosa occur and may include accentuated apoptosis of epithelial cells, perturbation of tight junctional proteins and complexes, increased mucosal permeability, bacterial translocation, alterations of vascular tone and microcirculation, and additional neutrophil infiltration and accumulation (Fig. 47-35). This process may then be perpetuated by the activation of the secondary inflammatory response, and the final common pathway will result in intestinal necrosis. While these events remain localized in some cases, in others this activation results in the systemic inflammatory response syndrome, in which patients develop capillary leak, hypotension, metabolic acidosis, thrombocytopenia, renal failure, respiratory failure, and often, death.[117] In summary, proinflammatory signaling follows TLR4 activation on the intestinal epithelium and leads to a cascade culminating in intestinal necrosis in neonatal animals, similar to that in humans, neonatal NEC.

Although endotoxin is a well-characterized activator of inflammation, additional factors may play a role in stimulating

the NEC cascade in premature infants. Asphyxia or ischemia-reperfusion activate the early mediators of inflammation in many tissues including intestine. Neonatal animal studies have shown that the stress of formula feeding stimulates phospholipase A_2 gene expression, intestinal PAF production, and stimulation of apoptosis and the inflammatory response with resulting NEC.[21,22] Therefore many of the purported risk factors for NEC may activate the inflammatory response, which results in the final common pathway described earlier.

The evidence suggests that the premature neonate may have an abnormal balance between proinflammatory and anti-inflammatory mediator regulation, thereby increasing the predisposition for diseases such as NEC. PAF is a potent phospholipid inflammatory mediator that is associated with NEC in several experimental models and human analyses.[28,29,48,58,99] PAF infusion causes intestinal necrosis in animals, and PAF receptor antagonists prevent injury following hypoxia, endotoxin challenge, TNF infusion, and ischemia-reperfusion.[27,81,116] It has been shown that neonates are markedly deficient in their ability to degrade PAF due to decreased activity of the PAF-specific enzyme PAF-acetylhydrolase.[19] PAF-acetylhydrolase is present in breast milk but absent in commercial formula, which may in part account for the beneficial effects of breast milk feeding. IL-10 is an anti-inflammatory cytokine thought to be important in reducing intestinal inflammation and possibly NEC in animals and humans.[42,76] In neonatal rats, maternal milk feedings increased IL-10 and reduced the incidence of NEC, while in human milk specimens, a significant percentage of NEC patient-pairs were deficient in this

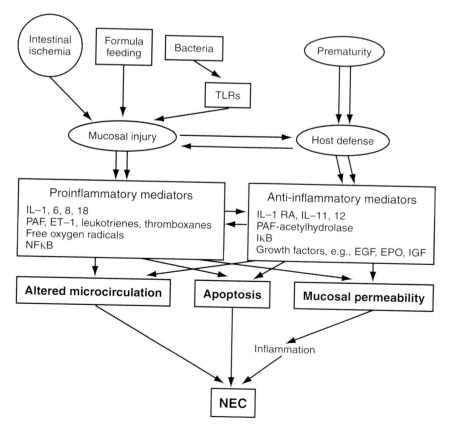

Figure 47–35. Hypothetical events in the pathophysiology of neonatal necrotizing enterocolitis (NEC). EGF, epidermal growth factor; EPO, erythropoietin; ET, endothelin; IGF, insulin-like growth factor; IL, interleukin; PAF, platelet activating factor; TLR, toll-like receptors.

important cytokine. Studies have compared proinflammatory response to endotoxin and/or IL-1 in different cell lines and have found that IL-8 response is significantly higher in fetal intestinal epithelium compared with mature, adult intestine.[84] These results suggest that the neonatal balance of the inflammatory response may be weighted toward the proinflammatory side and may be more likely to result in the pathologic outcome of NEC.

PREVENTION OF NEONATAL NECROTIZING ENTEROCOLITIS

Based on the unique epidemiologic features and understanding of the pathophysiology, there have been multiple approaches attempted to prevent NEC in animal and human studies. Human prevention trials with sufficient power to demonstrate a reduction in NEC incidence from 10% to 5% (e.g., in babies born weighing less than 1500 g) would require a large number of patients, approximating 350 patients per treatment group. Reduction of disease in animal models has been shown with breast milk feeding, IgA supplementation, antibiotic prophylaxis, steroids, probiotics, polyunsaturated fatty acids, PAF antagonists, PAF-acetylhydrolase, EGF, trefoil factor, leukocyte depletion, and oxygen radical scavengers. In human studies, there remains no standard effective alternative for NEC prevention, although careful enteral feeding with breast milk is the best approach that neonatologists have to offer. Prevention trials with IgA/IgG,[43] steroids,[51] polyunsaturated fatty acids, arginine,[4] and antibiotics[113] have been conducted with limited success, but because of various problems including poor study design, risks of intervention, lack of reproducibility, and weak statistical power, these approaches have yet to become routine strategies in the neonatal intensive care unit for preterm infants.

Probiotic supplementation is a promising approach for the prevention of NEC in infants with very low birthweight. There have now been several international prospective randomized trials that demonstrate efficacy for probiotic prophylaxis for this indication, and additional trials in the United States are planned to confirm these findings (Table 47-10).* As described earlier, probiotic colonization in infants with very low birthweight appears inadequate, and studies have

*References 12, 33, 56, 72, 73, 108.

defined multiple plausible mechanisms whereby probiotics could improve gastrointestinal health and prevent proinflammatory signaling and disease. As seen in Table 47-10, five of the six recent studies showed a reduction in NEC, and although the specific probiotic species and dosing varied somewhat, the cumulative results identified a reduction in NEC from 142 in 2143 controls (6.6%) to 53 in 2093 treated (2.5%, $P < .01$). Of additional importance, probiotics reduced the incidence of death in this vulnerable population ($P < .05$), and there were no reported cases of probiotic sepsis in any of these cohorts.

Although there is much excitement and appropriate optimism regarding this promising strategy, there are several important reasons why additional studies are warranted before clear standard-of-care can be recommended. First, different probiotic species have differing effects, and the optimal probiotic combination and optimal dosing strategy are not clearly elucidated. Second, probiotic preparations have not been rigorously regulated, and because some studies have shown inaccuracies in the reported organism species and content, appropriate quality control measures are warranted. Finally, although probiotic sepsis has not been observed in this unique population, additional safety concerns have been raised with recent reports demonstrating increased death in an adult population of patients in intensive care units, and increased wheezing and asthma in pediatric patients treated in the newborn period.[10,64] Nonetheless, after a large, multicenter trial with similar efficacy and safety in infants with very low birthweight has been reported as in other countries, it is likely that in the United States this approach will soon become routine in neonatal intensive care units.

SUMMARY

In conclusion, NEC is an increasing clinical burden to patients, families, and the neonatology health care team. Although the diagnosis is straightforward, the morbidity and mortality associated with the disease are not improving. Risk factors of prematurity, formula feeding, intestinal ischemia/hypoxia, and bacterial colonization accentuate the imbalance toward mucosal stress with impaired host defense, in some cases leading to uncontrolled intestinal inflammation and necrosis. The premature infant differs from term infants and older patients in multiple ways, including enteral feeding characteristics, bacterial colonization patterns, autoregulation of splanchnic bloodflow, host defense, and the regulation of the inflammatory cascade.

TABLE 47–10	Randomized Trials for Probiotic Prophylaxis					
	Hoyos 1999	Dani 2002	Lin 2005	Bin-Nun 2005	Lin 2008	Samanta 2008
Probiotic Species	*Lactobacillus acidophilus Bifidobacterium infantis*	*Lactobacillus strain GG*	*L. acidophilus B. infantis*	ABC Dophilus *Streptococcus thermophilus Bifidobacterium bifidum, Bifidobacterium infantis*	*L. acidophilus Bifidobacterium bifidum*	*B. infantis B. bifidum Bifidobacterium longum L. acidophilus*
Effect	Decreased NEC vs. historic controls	1.4% vs 2.7%, NS	1.1% vs 5.3%, $P < .05$	1% vs. 14%, $P < .05$	1.8% vs 6.5%, $P = .02$	5.5% vs 15.8%, $P = .04$

NEC, neonatal necrotizing enterocolitis; NS, not significant.

Although several strategies to prevent NEC have been tested in humans and animals, most have had limited success. Recent results from studies using probiotic supplementation have been exciting, and following additional investigation, this novel approach may significantly impact the incidence, morbidity, and mortality associated with neonatal NEC.

REFERENCES

1. Akira S: Toll-like receptor signaling, *J Biol Chem* 278:38105, 2003.
2. Akira S, Hemmi H: Recognition of pathogen-associated molecular patterns by TLR family, *Immunol Lett* 85:85, 2003.
3. Alward CT, Hook JB, Helmrath TA, et al: Effects of asphyxia on cardiac output and organ blood flow in the newborn piglet, *Pediatr Res* 12:824, 1978.
4. Amin HJ, Zamora SA, McMillan DD, et al: Arginine supplementation prevents necrotizing enterocolitis in the premature infant, *J Pediatr* 140:425, 2002.
5. Ballance WA, Dahms BB, Shenker N, et al: Pathology of neonatal necrotizing enterocolitis: a ten-year experience, *J Pediatr* 117:S6, 1990.
6. Bell MJ, Ternberg JL, Feigin RD, et al: Neonatal necrotizing enterocolitis. Therapeutic decisions based upon clinical staging, *Ann Surg* 187:1, 1978.
7. Benveniste J: PAF-acether, an ether phospholipid with biological activity, *Progress Clin Biol Res* 282:73, 1988.
8. Berseth CL: Neonatal small intestinal motility: motor responses to feeding in term and preterm infants, *J Pediatr* 117:777, 1990.
9. Berseth CL, Bisquera JA, Paje VU: Prolonging small feeding volumes early in life decreases the incidence of necrotizing enterocolitis in very low birth weight infants, *Pediatrics* 111:529, 2003.
10. Besselink MG, van Santvoort HC, Buskens E, et al: Probiotic prophylaxis in predicted severe acute pancreatitis: a randomised, double-blind, placebo-controlled trial, *Lancet* 371:651, 2008.
11. Bines JE, Walker WA: Growth factors and the development of neonatal host defense, *Adv Exp Med Biol* 310:31, 1991.
12. Bin-Nun A, Bromiker R, Wilschanski M, et al: Oral probiotics prevent necrotizing enterocolitis in very low birth weight neonates, *J Pediatr* 147:192, 2005.
13. Birchler T, Seibl R, Buchner K, et al: Human Toll-like receptor 2 mediates induction of the antimicrobial peptide human beta-defensin 2 in response to bacterial lipoprotein, *Eur J Immunol* 31:3131, 2001.
14. Bisquera JA, Cooper TR, Berseth CL: Impact of necrotizing enterocolitis on length of stay and hospital charges in very low birth weight infants, *Pediatrics* 109:423, 2002.
15. Blakely ML, Lally KP, McDonald S, et al: Postoperative outcomes of extremely low birth-weight infants with necrotizing enterocolitis or isolated intestinal perforation: a prospective cohort study by the NICHD Neonatal Research Network, *Ann Surg* 241:984, 2005.
16. Bohnhorst B, Muller S, Dordelmann M, et al: Early feeding after necrotizing enterocolitis in preterm infants, *J Pediatr* 143:484, 2003.
17. Bueno L, Ruckebusch Y: Perinatal development of intestinal myoelectrical activity in dogs and sheep, *Am J Physiol* 237:E61, 1979.
18. Butel MJ, Roland N, Hibert A, et al: Clostridial pathogenicity in experimental necrotising enterocolitis in gnotobiotic quails and protective role of bifidobacteria, *J Med Microbiol* 47:391, 1998.
19. Caplan M, Hsueh W, Kelly A, et al: Serum PAF acetylhydrolase increases during neonatal maturation, *Prostaglandins* 39:705, 1990.
20. Caplan MS, Hedlund E, Adler L, et al: Role of asphyxia and feeding in a neonatal rat model of necrotizing enterocolitis, *Pediatr Pathol* 14:1017, 1994.
21. Caplan MS, Hedlund E, Adler L, et al: The platelet-activating factor receptor antagonist WEB 2170 prevents neonatal necrotizing enterocolitis in rats, *J Pediatr Gastroenterol Nutr* 24:296, 1997.
22. Caplan MS, Jilling T: New concepts in necrotizing enterocolitis, *Curr Opin Pediatr* 13:111, 2001.
23. Caplan MS, Lickerman M, Adler L, et al: The role of recombinant platelet-activating factor acetylhydrolase in a neonatal rat model of necrotizing enterocolitis, *Pediatr Res* 42:779, 1997.
24. Caplan MS, MacKendrick W: Inflammatory mediators and intestinal injury, *Clin Perinatol* 21:235, 1994.
25. Caplan MS, Miller-Catchpole R, Kaup S, et al: Bifidobacterial supplementation reduces the incidence of necrotizing enterocolitis in a neonatal rat model, *Gastroenterology* 117:577, 1999.
26. Caplan MS, Russell T, Xiao Y, et al: Effect of polyunsaturated fatty acid (PUFA) supplementation on intestinal inflammation and necrotizing enterocolitis (NEC) in a neonatal rat model, *Pediatr Res* 49:647, 2001.
27. Caplan MS, Sun XM, Hsueh W: Hypoxia causes ischemic bowel necrosis in rats: the role of platelet-activating factor (PAF-acether), *Gastroenterology* 99:979, 1990.
28. Caplan MS, Sun XM, Hsueh W: Hypoxia, PAF, and necrotizing enterocolitis, *Lipids* 26:1340, 1991.
29. Caplan MS, Sun XM, Hseuh W, et al: Role of platelet activating factor and tumor necrosis factor-alpha in neonatal necrotizing enterocolitis, *J Pediatr* 116:960, 1990.
30. Clark DA, Thompson JE, Weiner LB, et al: Necrotizing enterocolitis: intraluminal biochemistry in human neonates and a rabbit model, *Pediatr Res* 19:919, 1985.
31. Cueva JP, Hsueh W: Role of oxygen derived free radicals in platelet activating factor induced bowel necrosis, *Gut* 29:1207, 1988.
32. Dai D, Nanthkumar NN, Newburg DS, et al: Role of oligosaccharides and glycoconjugates in intestinal host defense, *J Pediatr Gastroenterol Nutr* 30:S23, 2000.
33. Dani C, Biadaioli R, Bertini G, et al: Probiotics feeding in prevention of urinary tract infection, bacterial sepsis and necrotizing enterocolitis in preterm Infants. a prospective double-blind study, *Biol Neonate* 82:103, 2002.
34. Deitch EA: Role of bacterial translocation in necrotizing enterocolitis. *Acta Paediatrica (suppl)* 396:33, 1994.
35. Deitch EA, Specian RD, Berg RD: Endotoxin-induced bacterial translocation and mucosal permeability: role of xanthine oxidase, complement activation, and macrophage products, *Crit Care Med* 19:785, 1991.
36. Di Lorenzo M, Bass J, Krantis A: An intraluminal model of necrotizing enterocolitis in the developing neonatal piglet, *J Pediatr Surg* 30:1138, 1995.
37. Dimmitt RA, Meier AH, Skarsgard ED, et al: Salvage laparotomy for failure of peritoneal drainage in necrotizing enterocolitis in infants with extremely low birth weight, *J Pediatr Surg* 35:856, 2000.

38. Duffy LC, Zielezny MA, Carrion V, et al: Bacterial toxins and enteral feeding of premature infants at risk for necrotizing enterocolitis, *Adv Exp Med Biol* 501:519, 2001.

39. Duffy LC, Zielezny MA, Carrion V, et al: Concordance of bacterial cultures with endotoxin and interleukin-6 in necrotizing enterocolitis, *Dig Dis Sci* 42:359, 1997.

40. Dunn L, Hulman S, Weiner J, et al: Beneficial effects of early hypocaloric enteral feeding on neonatal gastrointestinal function: preliminary report of a randomized trial, *J Pediatr* 112:622, 1988.

41. Dvorak B, Halpern MD, Holubec H, et al: Epidermal growth factor reduces the development of necrotizing enterocolitis in a neonatal rat model, *Am J Physiol Gastrointest Liver Physiol* 282:G156, 2002.

42. Edelson MB, Bagwell CE, Rozycki HJ: Circulating pro- and counterinflammatory cytokine levels and severity in necrotizing enterocolitis, *Pediatrics* 103:766, 1999.

43. Eibl MM, Wolf HM, Furnkranz H, et al: Prevention of necrotizing enterocolitis in low-birth-weight infants by IgA-IgG feeding, *N Engl J Med* 319:1, 1988.

44. Feng J, El-Assal ON, Besner GE: Heparin-binding epidermal growth factor-like growth factor decreases the incidence of necrotizing enterocolitis in neonatal rats, *J Pediatr Surg* 41:144, 2006.

45. Ford H, Watkins S, Reblock K, et al: The role of inflammatory cytokines and nitric oxide in the pathogenesis of necrotizing enterocolitis, *J Pediatr Surg* 32:275, 1997.

46. Furlano RI, Walker WA: Immaturity of gastrointestinal host defense in newborns and gastrointestinal disease states, *Adv Pediatr* 45:201, 1998.

47. Gewolb IH, Schwalbe RS, Taciak VL, et al: Stool microflora in extremely low birthweight infants, *Arch Dis Child Fetal Neonatal Ed* 80:F167, 1999.

48. Gonzalez-Crussi F, Hsueh W: Experimental model of ischemic bowel necrosis. The role of platelet-activating factor and endotoxin, *Am J Pathol* 112:127, 1983.

49. Grosfeld JL, Chaet M, Molinari F, et al: Increased risk of necrotizing enterocolitis in premature infants with patent ductus arteriosus treated with indomethacin, *Ann Surg* 224:350, 1996.

50. Guy-Grand D, Griscelli C, Vassalli P: The mouse gut T lymphocyte, a novel type of T cell. Nature, origin, and traffic in mice in normal and graft-versus-host conditions, *J Exp Med* 148:1661, 1978.

51. Halac E, Halac J, Begue EF, et al: Prenatal and postnatal corticosteroid therapy to prevent neonatal necrotizing enterocolitis: a controlled trial, *J Pediatr* 117:132, 1990.

52. Haller D, Bode C, Hammes WP, et al: Non-pathogenic bacteria elicit a differential cytokine response by intestinal epithelial cell/leucocyte co-cultures, *Gut* 47:79, 2000.

53. Halpern MD, Holubec H, Dominguez JA, et al: Upregulation of IL-8 and IL-12 in thr ileum of neonatal rats with necrotizing enterocolitis, *Pediatr Res* 51:733, 2002.

54. Halpern MD, Holubec H, Saunders TA, et al: Bile acids induce ileal damage during experimental necrotizing enterocolitis, *Gastroenterology* 130:359, 2006.

55. Hammerman C, Goldschmidt D, Caplan MS, et al: Amelioration of ischemia-reperfusion injury in rat intestine by pentoxifylline-mediated inhibition of xanthine oxidase, *J Pediatr Gastroenterol Nutr* 29:69, 1999.

56. Hoyos AB: Reduced incidence of necrotizing enterocolitis associated with enteral administration of *Lactobacillus acidophilus* and *Bifidobacterium infantis* to neonates in an intensive care unit, *Int J Infect Dis* 3:197, 1999.

57. Hsueh W, Caplan MS, Sun X, et al: Platelet-activating factor, tumor necrosis factor, hypoxia and necrotizing enterocolitis, *Acta Paediatrica (suppl)* 396:11, 1994.

58. Hsueh W, Gonzalez-Crussi F, Arroyave JL: Platelet-activating factor-induced ischemic bowel necrosis. An investigation of secondary mediators in its pathogenesis, *Am J Pathol* 122:231, 1986.

59. Hsueh W, Gonzalez-Crussi F, Arroyave JL: Release of leukotriene C4 by isolated, perfused rat small intestine in response to platelet-activating factor, *J Clin Investigation* 78:108, 1986.

60. Hsueh W, Gonzalez-Crussi F, Arroyave JL: Sequential release of leukotrienes and norepinephrine in rat bowel after platelet-activating factor. A mechanistic study of platelet-activating factor-induced bowel necrosis, *Gastroenterology* 94:1412, 1988.

61. Jilling T, Simon D, Lu J, et al: The roles of bacteria and TLR4 in rat and murine models of necrotizing enterocolitis, *J Immunol* 177:3273, 2006.

62. Juul SE, Joyce AE, Zhao Y, et al: Why is erythropoietin present in human milk? Studies of erythropoietin receptors on enterocytes of human and rat neonates, *Pediatr Res* 46:263, 1999.

63. Kagnoff MF: Immunology of the intestinal tract. *Gastroenterology* 105:1275, 1993.

64. Kalliomaki M, Salminen S, Poussa T, et al: Probiotics during the first 7 years of life: a cumulative risk reduction of eczema in a randomized, placebo-controlled trial, *J Allergy Clin Immunol* 119:1019, 2007.

65. Kamitsuka MD, Horton MK, Williams MA: The incidence of necrotizing enterocolitis after introducing standardized feeding schedules for infants between 1250 and 2500 grams and less than 35 weeks of gestation, *Pediatrics* 105:379, 2000.

66. Kliegman RM, Fanaroff AA: Necrotizing enterocolitis. *N Eng J Med* 310:1093, 1984.

67. Kliegman RM, Pittard WB, Fanaroff AA: Necrotizing enterocolitis in neonates fed human milk, *J Pediatr* 95:450, 1979.

68. Laboisse CL: Structure of gastrointestinal mucins: searching for the Rosetta stone, *Biochimie* 68:611, 1986.

69. Leaphart CL, Cavallo J, Gribar SC, et al: A critical role for TLR4 in the pathogenesis of necrotizing enterocolitis by modulating intestinal injury and repair, *J Immunol* 179:4808, 2007.

70. Ledbetter DJ, Juul SE: Erythropoietin and the incidence of necrotizing enterocolitis in infants with very low birth weight, *J Pediatr Surg* 35:178, 2000.

71. Lee WJ, Farmer JL, Hilty M, et al: The protective effects of lactoferrin feeding against endotoxin lethal shock in germfree piglets, *Infect Immun* 66:1421, 1998.

72. Lin HC, Hsu CH, Chen HL, et al: Oral probiotics prevent necrotizing enterocolitis in very low birth weight preterm infants: a multicenter, randomized, controlled trial, *Pediatrics* 122:693, 2008.

73. Lin HC, Su BH, Chen AC, et al: Oral probiotics reduce the incidence and severity of necrotizing enterocolitis in very low birth weight infants, *Pediatrics* 115:1, 2005.

74. Lin J, Holzman IR, Jiang P, et al: Expression of intestinal trefoil factor in developing rat intestine, *Biol Neonate* 76:92, 1999.

75. Lin J, Nafday SM, Chauvin SN, et al: Variable effects of short chain fatty acids and lactic acid in inducing intestinal mucosal injury in newborn rats, *J Pediatr Gastroenterol Nutr* 35:545, 2002.

76. Lindsay JO, Ciesielski CJ, Scheinin T, et al: The prevention and treatment of murine colitis using gene therapy with adenoviral vectors encoding IL-10, *J Immunol* 166:7625, 2001.
77. Lucas A, Cole TJ: Breast milk and neonatal necrotising enterocolitis, *Lancet* 336:1519, 1990.
78. Medzhitov R: Toll-like receptors and innate immunity, *Nature Rev Immunol* 1:135, 2001.
79. Mehall JR, Kite CA, Saltzman DA, et al: Prospective study of the incidence and complications of bacterial contamination of enteral feeding in neonates, *J Pediatr Surg* 37:1177, 2002.
80. Moss RL, Dimmitt RA, Barnhart DC, et al: Laparotomy versus peritoneal drainage for necrotizing enterocolitis and perforation, *N Engl J Med* 354:2225, 2006.
81. Mozes T, Braquet P, Filep J: Platelet-activating factor: an endogenous mediator of mesenteric ischemia-reperfusion-induced shock, *A J Physiol* 257, 1989.
82. Nankervis CA, Nowicki PT: Role of endothelin-1 in regulation of the postnatal intestinal circulation, *Am J Physiol Gastrointest Liver Physiol* 278:G367, 2000.
83. Nankervis CA, Reber KM, Nowicki PT: Age-dependent changes in the postnatal intestinal microcirculation, *Microcirculation* 8:377, 2001.
84. Nanthakumar NN, Fusunyan RD, Sanderson I, et al: Inflammation in the developing human intestine: A possible pathophysiologic contribution to necrotizing enterocolitis, *Proc Natl Acad Sci U S A* 97:6043, 2000.
85. Neu J, Roig JC, Meetze WH, et al: Enteral glutamine supplementation for very low birth weight infants decreases morbidity, *J Pediatr* 131:691, 1997.
86. Neurath MF, Fuss I, Kelsall BL, et al: Experimental granulomatous colitis in mice is abrogated by induction of TGF-beta-mediated oral tolerance, *J Experimental Med* 183:2605, 1996.
87. Nowicki PT: Effects of sustained flow reduction on postnatal intestinal circulation, *Am J Physiol* 275:G758, 1998.
88. Nowicki PT, Caniano DA, Hammond S, et al: Endothelial nitric oxide synthase in human intestine resected for necrotizing enterocolitis, *J Pediatr* 150:40, 2007.
89. Nowicki PT, Dunaway DJ, Nankervis CA, et al: Endothelin-1 in human intestine resected for necrotizing enterocolitis, *J Pediatr* 146:805, 2005.
90. Nowicki PT, Minnich LA: Effects of systemic hypotension on postnatal intestinal circulation: role of angiotensin, *Am J Physiol* 276:G341, 1999.
91. O'Neill LA: The interleukin-1 receptor/Toll-like receptor superfamily: signal transduction during inflammation and host defense, *Sci STKE* 2000:RE1, 2000.
92. Ouellette AJ: Paneth cells and innate immunity in the crypt microenvironment, *Gastroenterology* 113:1779, 1997.
93. Pang KY, Bresson JL, Walker WA: Development of the gastrointestinal mucosal barrier. Evidence for structural differences in microvillus membranes from newborn and adult rabbits, *Biochim Biophys Acta* 727:201, 1983.
94. Pang KY, Newman AP, Udall JN, et al: Development of gastrointestinal mucosal barrier. VII. In utero maturation of microvillus surface by cortisone, *Am J Physiol* 249:G85, 1985.
95. Panigrahi P, Gupta S, Gewolb IH, et al: Occurrence of necrotizing enterocolitis may be dependent on patterns of bacterial adherence and intestinal colonization: studies in Caco-2 tissue culture and weanling rabbit models, *Pediatr Res* 36:115, 1994.

96. Perkkio M, Savilahti E: Time of appearance of immunoglobulin-containing cells in the mucosa of the neonatal intestine, *Pediatr Res* 14:953, 1980.
97. Peter CS, Feuerhahn M, Bohnhorst B, et al: Necrotising enterocolitis: is there a relationship to specific pathogens? *Eur J Pediatr* 158:67, 1999.
98. Pitt J, Barlow B, Heird WC: Protection against experimental necrotizing enterocolitis by maternal milk. I. Role of milk leukocytes, *Pediatr Res* 11:906, 1977.
99. Rabinowitz SS, Dzakpasu P, Piecuch S, et al: Platelet-activating factor in infants at risk for necrotizing enterocolitis, *J Pediatr* 138:81, 2001.
100. Read RC, Wyllie DH: Toll receptors and sepsis, *Curr Opin Crit Care* 7:371, 2001.
101. Rees CM, Eaton S, Kiely EM, et al: Peritoneal drainage or laparotomy for neonatal bowel perforation? A randomized controlled trial. *Ann Surg* 248:44, 2008.
102. Rieger CH, Rothberg RM: Development of the capacity to produce specific antibody to an ingested food antigen in the premature infant, *J Pediatr* 87:515, 1975.
103. Riegler M, Sedivy R, Sogukoglu T, et al: Effect of growth factors on epithelial restitution of human colonic mucosa in vitro, *Scandinavian J Gastroenterol* 32:925, 1997.
104. Roberts SA, Freed DL: Neonatal IgA secretion enhanced by breast feeding, *Lancet* 2:1131, 1977.
105. Rubaltelli FF, Biadaioli R, Pecile P, et al: Intestinal flora in breast- and bottle-fed infants, *J Perinat Med* 26:186, 1998.
106. Ryder RW, Shelton JD, Guinan ME: Necrotizing enterocolitis: a prospective multicenter investigation, *Am J Epidemiol* 112:113, 1980.
107. Salzman NH, Polin RA, Harris MC, et al: Enteric defensin expression in necrotizing enterocolitis, *Pediatr Res* 44:20, 1998.
108. Samanta M, Sarkar M, Ghosh P, et al: Prophylactic Probiotics for Prevention of Necrotizing Enterocolitis in Very Low Birth Weight Newborns, *J Trop Pediatr* 55:128, 2009.
109. Sands BE, Podolsky DK: The trefoil peptide family, *Annu Rev Physiol* 58:253, 1996.
110. Schanler RJ, Lau C, Hurst NM, et al: Randomized trial of donor human milk versus preterm formula as substitutes for mothers' own milk in the feeding of extremely premature infants, *Pediatrics* 116:400, 2005.
111. Schanler RJ, Shulman RJ, Lau C, et al: Feeding strategies for premature infants: randomized trial of gastrointestinal priming and tube-feeding method [see comments]. *Pediatrics* 103:434, 1999.
112. Schoenberg MH, Beger HG: Reperfusion injury after intestinal ischemia, *Crit Care Med* 21:1376, 1993.
113. Siu YK, Ng PC, Fung SC, et al: Double blind, randomised, placebo controlled study of oral vancomycin in prevention of necrotising enterocolitis in preterm, very low birthweight infants, *Arch Dis Child Fetal Neonatal Ed* 79:F105, 1998.
114. Snyder JD, Walker WA: Structure and function of intestinal mucin: developmental aspects, *Int Arch Allergy Appl Immunol* 82:351, 1987.
115. Sun X, Rozenfeld RA, Qu X, et al: P-selectin-deficient mice are protected from PAF-induced shock, intestinal injury, and lethality, *Am J Physiol* 273, 1997.
116. Sun XM, Hsueh W: Bowel necrosis induced by tumor necrosis factor in rats is mediated by platelet-activating factor, *J Clin Investigation* 81:1328, 1988.

117. Takakuwa T, Endo S, Inada K, et al: Assessment of inflammatory cytokines, nitrate/nitrite, type II phospholipase A2, and soluble adhesion molecules in systemic inflammatory response syndrome, *Res Commun Mol Pathol Pharmacol* 98:43, 1997.

118. Tan X, Sun X, Gonzalez-Crussi FX, et al: PAF and TNF increase the precursor of NF-kappa B p50 mRNA in mouse intestine: quantitative analysis by competitive PCR, *Biochimica et Biophysica Acta* 1215:157, 1994.

119. Tan XD, Hsueh W, Chang H, et al: Characterization of a putative receptor for intestinal trefoil factor in rat small intestine: identification by in situ binding and ligand blotting, *Biochem Biophys Res Communications* 237:673, 1997.

120. Tanaka M, Lee K, Martinez-Augustin O, et al: Exogenous nucleotides alter the proliferation, differentiation and apoptosis of human small intestinal epithelium, *J Nutr* 126:424, 1996.

121. Tomkins AM, Bradley AK, Oswald S, et al: Diet and the faecal microflora of infants, children and adults in rural Nigeria and urban U.K, *J Hyg (Lond)* 86:285, 1981.

122. Touloukian RJ, Posch JN, Spencer R: The pathogenesis of ischemic gastroenterocolitis of the neonate: selective gut mucosal ischemia in asphyxiated neonatal piglets, *J Pediatr Surg* 7:194, 1972.

123. Tracey KJ, Beutler B, Lowry SF, et al: Shock and tissue injury induced by recombinant human cachectin, *Science* 234:470, 1986.

124. Troche B, Harvey-Wilkes K, Engle WD, et al: Early minimal feedings promote growth in critically ill premature infants, *Biol Neonate* 67:172, 1995.

125. Tyson JE, Kennedy KA: Minimal enteral nutrition for promoting feeding tolerance and preventing morbidity in parenterally fed infants, *Cochrane Database Syst Rev* 2, 2000.

126. Uauy RD, Fanaroff AA, Korones SB, et al: Necrotizing enterocolitis in very low birth weight infants: biodemographic and clinical correlates. National Institute of Child Health and Human Development Neonatal Research Network, *J Pediatr* 119:630, 1991.

127. Udall JN Jr: Gastrointestinal host defense and necrotizing enterocolitis, *J Pediatr* 117:S33, 1990.

128. Villalpando S, Hamosh M: Early and late effects of breast-feeding: does breast-feeding really matter? *Biol Neonate* 74:177, 1998.

129. Vohr BR, Wright LL, Dusick AM, et al: Neurodevelopmental and functional outcomes of extremely low birth weight infants in the National Institute of Child Health and Human Development Neonatal Research Network, 1993-1994, *Pediatrics* 105:1216, 2000.

130. Volpe JJ: Postnatal sepsis, necrotizing enterocolitis, and the critical role of systemic inflammation in white matter injury in premature infants, *J Pediatr* 153:160, 2008.

131. Walker WA: Role of nutrients and bacterial colonization in the development of intestinal host defense, *J Pediatr Gastroenterol Nutr* 30:S2, 2000.

132. Walker WA: Mechanisms of action of probiotics, *Clin Infect Dis* 46 Suppl 2:S87, 2008.

133. Wallace JL, Cirino G, McKnight GW, et al: Reduction of gastrointestinal injury in acute endotoxic shock by flurbiprofen nitroxybutylester, *Eur J Pharmacol* 280:63, 1995.

134. Walsh MC, Kliegman RM: Necrotizing enterocolitis: treatment based on staging criteria, *Pediatr Clin North Am* 33:179, 1986.

135. Willis DM, Chabot J, Radde IC, et al: Unsuspected hyperosmolality of oral solutions contributing to necrotizing enterocolitis in very-low-birth-weight infants, *Pediatrics* 60:535, 1977.

136. Wiswell TE, Robertson CF, Jones TA, et al: Necrotizing enterocolitis in full-term infants. A case-control study, *Am J Dis Child* 142:532, 1988.

137. Wold AE, Adlerberth I: Breast feeding and the intestinal microflora of the infant—implications for protection against infectious diseases, *Adv Exp Med Biol* 478:77, 2000.

138. Yoshimura A, Lien E, Ingalls RR, et al: Cutting edge: recognition of gram-positive bacterial cell wall components by the innate immune system occurs via Toll-like receptor 2, *J Immunol* 163:1, 1999.

CHAPTER 48

Neonatal Jaundice and Liver Disease

Michael Kaplan, Ronald J. Wong, Eric Sibley, and David K. Stevenson

Bilirubin is one of the biologically active end products of heme catabolism. Its clinical significance in the neonate relates to its propensity for deposition in the skin and mucous membranes, producing easily identifiable jaundice (French *jaune*, yellow) or icterus (Greek *ikteros*). The yellow color, or the serum (or plasma) total bilirubin (TB) concentration at any point in time, represents the combined processes of bilirubin production minus bilirubin elimination from the body, the latter primarily due to bilirubin conjugation. As long as these processes remain in balance, a moderate degree of jaundice should develop, which should not endanger an otherwise healthy, nonhemolyzing infant. An imbalance between bilirubin production and its elimination may result in increasing jaundice or hyperbilirubinemia. In rare cases, the degree of bilirubin production relative to bilirubin elimination may be so great that bilirubin may deposit in the brain, where it may cause transient dysfunction (acute bilirubin encephalopathy, or ABE) and, occasionally, chronic bilirubin encephalopathy with resultant permanent neuronal damage known as kernicterus. Because as many as 60% of otherwise healthy, term newborns develop some degree of elevated TB levels, whereas, in contrast, severe hyperbilirubinemia with its potentially devastating sequelae is rare, it is important to distinguish between normal processes of bilirubin physiology from pathologic conditions. All those caring for newborns should possess a thorough understanding of normal bilirubin physiology, on the one hand, and a healthy respect for the potential complications of severe hyperbilirubinemia, on the other.

BILIRUBIN METABOLISM
Bilirubin Biochemistry

Throughout life, there is a continuum of bilirubin production and elimination from the body. Ongoing lysis of red blood cells (RBCs) or hemolysis, whether physiologic or at increased rates, releases iron protoporphyrin (heme), the oxygen-carrying component of hemoglobin. Catalyzed by heme oxygenase (HO), heme is then converted to biliverdin from which bilirubin is derived. This unconjugated bilirubin is transported to the liver bound to albumin (Fig. 48-1). In the hepatocyte, bilirubin is conjugated to glucuronic acid by the enzyme uridine diphosphoglucuronate (UDP)-glucuronosyltransferase 1A1 (UGT1A1). This water-soluble conjugated bilirubin can be now excreted into the bile, from which it reaches the bowel and is eliminated from the body.[182] This simplified overview of bilirubin biochemistry will be reviewed in greater detail in the pages to come.

Heme oxygenase-1 (HO-1), the inducible isoform of HO, a membrane-bound enzyme found in cells of the liver and other organs, catalyzes the first step in the pathway by which heme is converted to biliverdin through oxidation of the former molecule's α-methene bridge carbon (Fig. 48-2). This rate-limiting step produces free iron (which can be reutilized for hemoglobin synthesis) and carbon monoxide (CO) (which is excreted in the lungs) in equimolar amounts. Biliverdin is a blue-green water-soluble pigment that can be readily excreted by the liver and kidneys. In amphibians, reptiles, and certain avian species, the major pigmented end product of heme catabolism is biliverdin. In mammals, however, biliverdin is converted to bilirubin by biliverdin reductase in the cytosol.

The degradation of 1 g of hemoglobin forms 34 mg of bilirubin. The isomeric form of bilirubin formed by this two-step process is IX-α (the Z,Z isomer), defining the relative positions of the four pyrrole rings and the hydrogen molecules on the two linking lateral carbons. This form of bilirubin is insoluble owing to tertiary structural changes that internalize the keto and carboxy groups that would otherwise interact with water molecules. Intramolecular hydrogen bonding maintains this folded bilirubin structure.

Because bilirubin is a weak acid and is neither water soluble nor readily excreted at pH 7.4, it must be conjugated to

Figure 48–1. Metabolic pathway of the degradation of heme and the formation of bilirubin. Heme released from the hemoglobin of red blood cells or from other hemoproteins is degraded by heme oxygenase (HO), the first and rate-limiting enzyme in a two-step reaction requiring nicotinamide adenine dinucleotide phosphate (NADPH) and oxygen, and resulting in the release of iron and the formation of carbon monoxide (CO) and biliverdin. Metalloporphyrins, synthetic heme analogues, can competitively inhibit HO activity (indicated by the *X*). Biliverdin is further reduced to bilirubin by the enzyme biliverdin reductase. CO can activate soluble guanylyl cyclase (sGC) and lead to the formation of cyclic guanosine monophosphate (cGMP). It can also displace oxygen from oxyhemoglobin or be exhaled. The bilirubin that is formed is taken up by the liver and conjugated with glucuronides to form bilirubin monoglucuronide or diglucuronide (BMG and BDG, respectively), in reactions catalyzed by uridine diphosphoglucuronate glucuronosyltransferase (UGT). The bilirubin glucuronides are then excreted into the intestinal lumen but can be deconjugated by bacteria so that the bilirubin is reabsorbed into the circulation, as shown. (*Modified from Vreman HJ, et al: Carbon monoxide in breath, blood, and other tissues. In: Penney DG, editor. Carbon monoxide toxicity, Boca Raton, FL, 2000, CRC Press, pp 22-30.*)

Figure 48–2. Catabolism of heme to bilirubin by microsomal heme oxygenase and biliverdin reductase. (*From Tenhunen R, et al: The enzymatic conversion of hemoglobin to bilirubin, Trans Assoc Am Physicians 82:363, 1969.*)

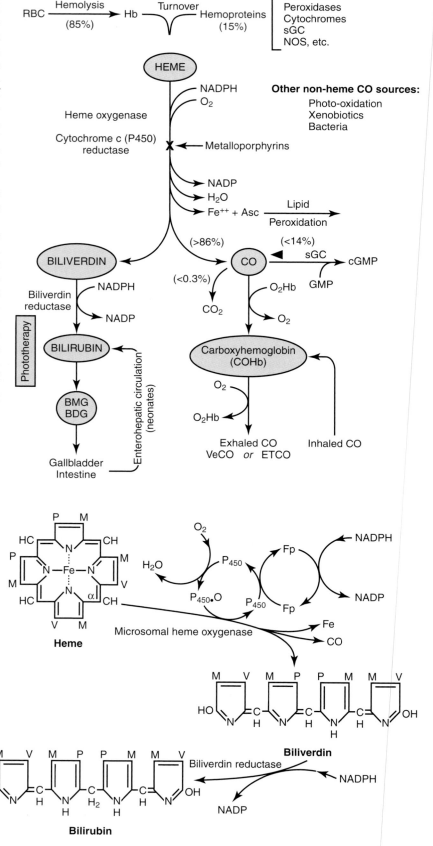

glucuronic acid before excretion by the specific hepatic enzyme isozyme (UGT1A1).[112] What evolutionary advantage is derived by mammalian species in the development of such an intricate energy-dependent system that first produces bilirubin from a water-soluble precursor and then converts it back to a water-soluble form for excretion is presently uncertain. The mammalian placenta is capable of removing unconjugated bilirubin, but not biliverdin. Biliverdin accumulation in the mammalian fetus would presumably result in the accumulation of large amounts of potentially toxic heme metabolites. Evidence has shown that bilirubin and even CO may be biologically useful molecules.[144,205] The inducibility of HO-1 would appear to indicate that bilirubin production is helpful to cells when they are stressed.[69] Bilirubin is an antioxidant that readily binds to membrane lipids and is capable of limiting membrane damage by preventing their peroxidation. Biologic evidence of potentially beneficial effects of bilirubin, on the one hand, is tempered by the association of high levels of unconjugated bilirubin with neuronal dysfunction and necrosis, on the other. Although cells may be potential beneficiaries of small amounts of bilirubin, in greater circulating quantities the same bilirubin molecule may be a causative factor of severe neuronal damage. The dilemma that faces the clinician is determining the desirable or "safe" level of bilirubin appropriate for any particular neonate.

The CO formed by heme degradation binds to hemoglobin to form carboxyhemoglobin (COHb) and is then transported in the circulation to the lung. Here, the CO separates from hemoglobin and is excreted in exhaled breath. Although there are other potential endogenous and exogenous sources of CO, such as lipid peroxidation and photo-oxidation,[236] the main source of endogenous CO is derived from heme catabolism. Therefore, quantitative estimation of its synthesis or excretion (in infants without significant lung disease or oxygen exposure) offers a reasonably accurate assessment of the rate of heme degradation from which the rate of bilirubin synthesis can be derived. It is believed that other hemoproteins undergo the same degradative process.

Bilirubin Production

The pathway of bilirubin synthesis, transport, and metabolism is summarized in Figure 48-3. In the normal adult, bilirubin is derived primarily from the degradation of heme, which is released from senescing RBCs, in the reticuloendothelial cells. Normally, about 20% of the bilirubin excreted into bile is derived from erythrocyte precursors and other hemoproteins (mainly cytochromes, catalase). Carbon monoxide excretion in humans and more direct measurements in animals have demonstrated that, on the first day of life, bilirubin production is increased two to three times the rate of adults, to an estimated average of 8 to 10 mg/kg of body weight per day.[204,232] Bilirubin production decreases rapidly during the first 2 postnatal days.[114] Several factors may explain this increased production in the newborn. The circulating RBC life span is shortened to 70 to 90 days compared with 120 days in the adult. Increased heme degradation arises from the very large pool of hematopoietic tissue, essential to intrauterine well-being, but which ceases to function shortly after birth. An additional factor may possibly include an increased turnover of cytochromes. Another major addition to the bilirubin pool in the neonate, in addition to increased synthesis, is an increase

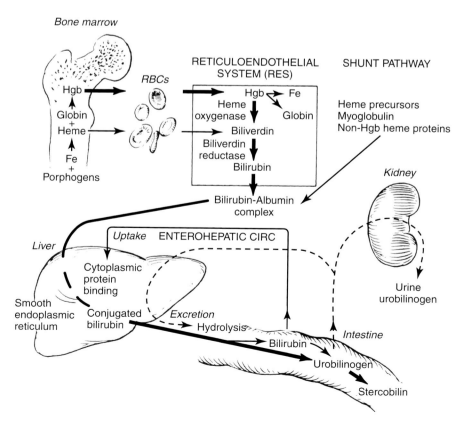

Figure 48–3. The pathways of bilirubin synthesis, transport, and metabolism. Hgb, hemoglobin; RBCs, red blood cells. *(From Assali NS: Pathophysiology of gestation, New York, Academic Press, 1972.)*

in bilirubin absorbed from the bowel as part of the enterohepatic circulation. This mechanism results from both reformation of unconjugated bilirubin from conjugated bilirubin in the bowel and enhanced absorption of unconjugated bilirubin by the intestinal mucosa (see "Enterohepatic Absorption of Bilirubin," later).

Transport of Bilirubin in Plasma

Unconjugated bilirubin is almost insoluble in water at pH 7.4, with a solubility of less than 0.01 mg/dL, and when released into the circulation by the reticuloendothelial cells, it is rapidly bound to albumin. Each molecule of adult albumin is capable of binding at least two molecules of bilirubin; the first molecule is more tightly bound than the second. Additional binding sites with weaker affinities may also exist but are probably of little clinical importance. On average, 7 to 8 mg/dL of unconjugated bilirubin can be bound to each gram of albumin. Physiologically, newborns have a lower plasma-binding capacity for bilirubin compared with adults or older children. This occurs because of reduced neonatal serum albumin concentrations and reduced molar binding capacities. Binding of unconjugated bilirubin by albumin is believed to be of some importance in determining bilirubin toxicity to the brain and neural tissue (acute bilirubin encephalopathy or kernicterus and auditory neuropathy). The unbound bilirubin concentration is thought to be a more sensitive predictor of bilirubin neurotoxicity than the clinically used TB.[249] However, there is currently no reliable and clinically available measurement to make determination of unbound concentrations a useful clinical tool in evaluating the risk to the newborn for developing bilirubin toxicity.

Bilirubin exists in four different forms in circulation: (1) unconjugated bilirubin reversibly bound to albumin, which makes up the major portion; (2) a relatively minute fraction of unconjugated bilirubin not bound to albumin (known as free or unbound bilirubin); (3) conjugated bilirubin, comprising mainly monoglucuronides and diglucuronides, which have effluxed from the hepatocyte to the circulation and which are readily excretable through the renal or biliary systems; and (4) conjugated bilirubin covalently bound to albumin, known as δ-bilirubin. The latter has a plasma disappearance rate similar to that of serum albumin (Fig. 48-4).[33] Conjugated bilirubin, but not δ-bilirubin, gives a "direct" reaction with standard diazo reagents, whereas bound or unbound unconjugated bilirubin yields an "indirect" reaction. The terms indirect and direct bilirubin tend to be used interchangeably with unconjugated and conjugated bilirubin, respectively. δ-Bilirubin can be measured only with newer techniques. It is found in detectable amounts in normal older neonates and children, and in significantly increased concentrations in those with prolonged conjugated hyperbilirubinemia resulting from various liver disorders.[34] However, it is virtually absent from the serum during the first 2 weeks of life.[129]

Hepatic Uptake of Bilirubin

Bilirubin dissociates from circulating albumin before entering the liver cell. The latter process occurs partly by a passive process of carrier-mediated diffusion, and partly by

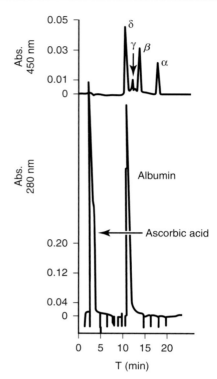

Figure 48–4. Separation of serum bilirubin fractions by high-performance liquid chromatography, showing bilirubin profiles at 450 nm (*upper trace*) and 280 nm (*lower trace*). α, Unconjugated bilirubin; β, monoconjugated bilirubin; δ, delta fraction bilirubin; γ, diconjugated bilirubin; Abs, absorption. (*From Wu TW: Bilirubin analysis: the state of the art and future prospects,* Clin Biochem 17:221, 1984.)

mediation by organic anion transporter proteins (OATP). In the liver cell cytoplasm, the unconjugated bilirubin is bound to glutathione-S-transferase A, also known as ligandin, or with B-ligandin (Y protein). These are major intracellular transport proteins, and their bilirubin binding ability helps keep the potentially toxic unbound portion low. Z protein, another hepatic cytoplasmic carrier, also binds bilirubin but with a lower affinity. The equilibrium between the rates of bilirubin entry into the circulation, from de novo synthesis, enterohepatic recirculation and tissue shifts, on the one hand, and hepatic cell bilirubin uptake, conjugation of bilirubin and conjugated bilirubin excretion, on the other, determines the TB concentrations under both normal and abnormal circumstances.

A reduced capacity of net hepatic uptake of unconjugated bilirubin has been implicated in the development of physiologic jaundice. In the newborn monkey, deficiency of B-ligandin and reduced clearance of sulfobromophthalein were demonstrated in the first 3 days of life, the period during which this animal frequently has physiologic jaundice. Studies in the human indicate that deficiency of bilirubin uptake is probably of less importance in the pathogenesis of unconjugated hyperbilirubinemia than immaturity of the bilirubin conjugation system during the first 3 or 4 days of life. However, the relative contribution of uptake deficiency may be greater during the second week of life when the rate of bilirubin conjugation increases and approaches that of normal adults.[199]

Conjugation of Bilirubin

In order for bilirubin to be excreted into the bile, the non-polar, water-insoluble unconjugated bilirubin must be converted to a more polar, water-soluble substance. The aim of this process is to alter the bilirubin molecule by solubilizing bilirubin IX-α. Bilirubin is presumed to be transported by hepatic ligandin from the liver cell plasma membrane to the endoplasmic reticulum, at which site the conjugating enzyme, UGT1A1, is situated. The conjugation process comprises a two-step enzymatic process, in which each molecule of bilirubin is conjugated with two molecules of glucuronic acid. Glucuronic acid derives from activated uridine diphosphoglucuronic acid (UDPGA), itself synthesized by the soluble cytoplasmic enzyme uridine diphosphoglucose dehydrogenase from uridine diphosphoglucose, which, in turn, is synthesized from free glucose. The UGT1A1 enzyme first catalyzes the transfer of one glucuronic acid molecule from one of the two propionic acid side groups on one of the central pyrrole rings of bilirubin, in an ester linkage, to form bilirubin monoglucuronide. A reduction in enzyme activity to less than 1% of normal may result in unconjugated hyperbilirubinemia.

Although bilirubin monoglucuronide is water soluble and capable of being excreted into bile without further alteration, about two thirds of the total bilirubin excreted into bile in the adult human is in the form of a diglucuronide. The second step of the enzymatic conjugation process involves the esterification of a second glucuronide molecule to the now monoconjugate. This process is catalyzed primarily by the same UGT1A1 enzyme on the endoplasmic reticulum, although a second enzyme, located in the canalicular portion of the hepatocyte plasma cell membrane, UDP-glucuronate glucuronosyltransferase (transglucuronidase), may also play a role. The substrate for the canalicular transglucuronidation is believed to be bilirubin monoglucuronide. The enzyme transfers one molecule of glucuronic acid from one molecule of bilirubin monoglucuronide to another, resulting in the formation of one molecule of bilirubin diglucuronide. The latter molecule is excreted into the bile canaliculus, whereas the remaining molecule of now unconjugated bilirubin is returned to the endoplasmic reticulum for subsequent reconjugation. In circumstances such as severe chronic hemolysis, increased loads of bilirubin are delivered to the liver, which results in retention of conjugated bilirubin in the form of bilirubin monoglucuronide.

The result of the esterification is to disrupt the intramolecular hydrogen bonds, thereby opening the molecule and rendering the conjugated bilirubin water soluble. The water-soluble form of bilirubin is excretable in the bowel. Water solubility also decreases the amount of bilirubin reabsorbed from the bowel because hydrophilic agents do not pass through the intestinal wall easily.[72]

In the normal adult, glucuronide conjugation accounts for the disposal of about 90% of all bilirubin. The remaining portion is converted to water-soluble substances by conjugation with substances other than glucuronic acid, or by oxidation,

hydroxylation, or reduction. In humans, bilirubin forms a conjugate with glucose, xylose, possibly other carbohydrates, sulfates, and taurine. These nonglucuronide conjugates account for no more than 10% of the total bilirubin conjugates excreted in the bile.

A number of in vitro studies have demonstrated the existence of deficiencies in hepatic UGT activity in newborns of many species, including the human. In newborn rhesus monkeys, hepatic bilirubin conjugating capacity is extremely low during the first hours of life, and functions at about 5% of adult capacity (Fig. 48-5). However, by 24 hours of age, UGT activity increases sufficiently to process the bilirubin load presented to the liver, and the TB concentration begins to fall. In 1-day-old rats, the proportion of both xylose and glucose conjugates of bilirubin equals that of glucuronide conjugates. Total conjugating capacity increases to the adult level by the fourth day of life, when a mature pattern of glycoside distribution is present, with 75% of all conjugates being glucuronides. In human newborns, the monoglucuronide conjugate is the predominant bile pigment conjugate. UGT activity in term infants is about 1% of that of healthy adults, and increases at an exponential rate until 3 months of age, when adult levels are reached.[172] Nonglucuronide conjugates are insignificant in this period.[124]

Excretion of Bilirubin

Excretion of the now polar, water-soluble bilirubin appears to be an energy-dependent concentrative process. The bilirubin conjugates are incorporated into mixed micelles along with bile acids, phospholipids, and cholesterol.[72] The conjugates are excreted against a concentration gradient, and as a result, bile bilirubin concentration is about 100-fold that of the hepatocyte cytoplasm. Although the capacity for bilirubin excretion into bile is limited in newborn rhesus monkeys (Fig. 48-6), excretory deficiency is not a rate-limiting factor in the overall hepatic elimination of bilirubin in the human newborn. In newborn babies, bilirubin uptake into the hepatocyte and the enzyme-mediated conjugation processes are the more restrictive steps and may result in a "bottleneck" effect. By contrast, in older humans and in the mature rhesus

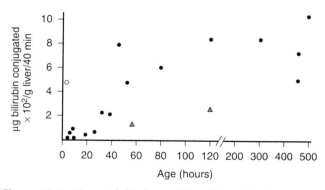

Figure 48–5. Hepatic bilirubin uridine diphosphoglucuronate glucuronosyltransferase (UGT) activity in term (*filled circles*), premature (*triangles*), and postmature (*open circle*) newborn rhesus monkeys. (*From Gartner LM, et al: Development of bilirubin transport and metabolism in the newborn rhesus monkey,* J Pediatr *90:513, 1977.*)

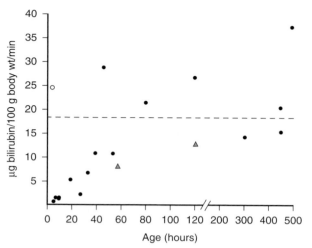

Figure 48–6. Maximal hepatic bile bilirubin excretion in term (*filled circles*), premature (*triangles*), and postmature (*open circle*) newborn rhesus monkeys. The *horizontal dashed line* represents mean normal hepatic bile bilirubin excretion for nine adult rhesus monkeys (18.2 $\pm$ 1.0 SEM). (*From Gartner LM, et al: Development of bilirubin transport and metabolism in the newborn rhesus monkey,* J Pediatr 90:513, 1977.)

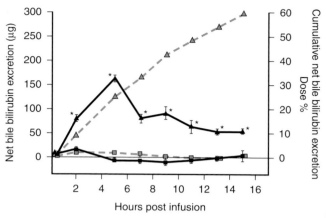

Figure 48–7. Net rate of bilirubin excretion in adult rat bile over 15 hours after intraduodenal administration of 1000 mg unconjugated bilirubin in normal human milk at pH 8.6 (*filled squares,* mean $\pm$ SEM; $n = 5$) and human milk from mothers of infants with breast milk jaundice syndrome, pH 8.6 (*filled triangles,* mean $\pm$ SEM; $n = 5$). Cumulative net bilirubin excretion in bile for the same experiments expressed as a percentage of administered dose (*gray squares,* bilirubin in normal human milk; *gray triangles,* bilirubin in human milk from mothers of infants with breast milk jaundice syndrome). *Asterisks* indicate $P < .01$ for bilirubin in normal human milk versus bilirubin in human milk from mothers of infants with breast milk jaundice syndrome. (*From Gartner LM, et al: Development of bilirubin transport and metabolism in the newborn rhesus monkey,* J Pediatr 90:513, 1977.)

monkey and other mammals beyond the newborn period, hepatic excretion of conjugated bilirubin into bile predominates as the rate-limiting step in the presence of a large bilirubin load. At any age, in the presence of hepatic cell injury and biliary obstruction, hepatic excretory transport is the step most severely restricted, resulting in efflux of conjugated bilirubin from the hepatocyte to the serum with resultant conjugated hyperbilirubinemia. Thus, the hepatic excretory step may have the least reserve capacity of all the processes contributing to bilirubin elimination.

Enterohepatic Absorption of Bilirubin

Conjugated bilirubin is not absorbed from the intestine. However, the monoglucuronides and diglucuronides of bilirubin are relatively unstable conjugates that are readily hydrolyzed to unconjugated bilirubin. Having reverted to this form, unconjugated bilirubin may now be readily absorbed across the intestinal mucosa, contributing, through the enterohepatic circulation, to the circulating unconjugated bilirubin pool, and again being presented to the liver for conjugation. Of importance in the mechanism of the enterohepatic circulation is the enteric mucosal enzyme β-glucuronidase, which is present in both term and premature neonates in high concentrations. Mild alkaline conditions present in the duodenum and jejunum contribute to the deconjugation process.

A study in adult rats demonstrates that enteric absorption of unconjugated bilirubin occurs predominantly in the duodenum and colon.[79] The extent of absorption varies widely, depending on diet and caloric intake (Fig. 48-7). Although quantitative estimates of the disposal of bilirubin have been performed only for adult humans, these data do

indicate that about 25% of the TB excreted into the intestine is reabsorbed as unconjugated bilirubin. About 10% of the total is excreted in stool as unaltered bilirubin. The remaining pigment is converted to urobilinoids, most of which are excreted in stool, with a small portion being reabsorbed in the colon for subsequent excretion by both the liver and kidney.

Neonates have relatively high concentrations of unconjugated bilirubin in the intestine that contribute to the enterohepatic circulation. Intestinal bilirubin is derived from increased bilirubin production, exaggerated hydrolysis of bilirubin glucuronide, and high concentrations of bilirubin found in meconium. The relative lack of bacterial flora in the newborn bowel to reduce bilirubin to urobilinogen further increases the intestinal bilirubin pool in comparison with that of the older child and adult. The increased hydrolysis of bilirubin conjugates in the newborn is enhanced by high mucosal β-glucuronidase activity and the excretion of predominantly monoglucuronide conjugates (in the newborn) rather than diglucuronides (in the adult). Oral administration of nonabsorbable bilirubin-binding substances, such as agar, activated charcoal, or a lipase inhibitor (e.g., Orlistat),[92,166] may retain bilirubin in the bowel, thereby further increasing stool bilirubin content and reducing bilirubin reabsorption, in this way decreasing TB. Studies of intestinal bilirubin binding contribute to our understanding of the contribution of the enterohepatic circulation to unconjugated hyperbilirubine-mia of the newborn.[58]

GENETIC CONTROL OF BILIRUBIN ELIMINATION

Genetic Control of Uptake of Bilirubin into the Hepatocyte

This process by which unconjugated bilirubin is taken up from the hepatic sinusoids and crosses the hepatocyte membrane to enter into that cell is facilitated by a carrier molecule, organic anion-transporting polypeptide-2 (OATP2, gene *SLC21A6*). Human OATP2 may play an important role in the metabolism of bilirubin and in the prevention of hyperbilirubinemia by facilitating the entry of bilirubin into hepatocytes.[57] A mutation in the *SLC21A6* gene leading to an impaired maturation of the protein with reduced membrane localization and abolished transport function has been described,[151] and a number of single-nucleotide polymorphisms have been identified, some of which are associated with an altered in vitro transport capability.[213]

Genetics of Diminished Bilirubin Conjugation

Perhaps one of the most important advances in our understanding of the genomics of bilirubin metabolism is the elucidation of the *UGT* gene encoding the bilirubin conjugating enzyme, UGT1A1. Next we provide a short overview to allow the reader to comprehend mutations of this gene and interactions of these mutations with genetic or environmental factors in the mechanism of jaundice.[31,40,50,125,134,189,215]

The *UGT* Gene

The *UGT* gene is a superfamily of genes whose function is to encode a biochemical reaction leading to the conjugation of glucuronic acid to certain target substrates in order to facilitate their elimination from the body. The *UGT2* genes are located on chromosomes 4q13 and 4q28. The enzymes encoded by this family preferentially conjugate endobiotic substances, such as steroids and bile acids, and although of physiologic and pharmacologic importance, they are of little relevance to bilirubin metabolism. In contrast, the UGT1A1 gene isoform, which belongs to the UGT1 gene family, is of major importance to the conjugation, and therefore elimination, of bilirubin. This gene isoform has been mapped to chromosome 2q37.[225] *UGT1A1* was cloned by Ritter and associates in 1991.[181] The gene encodes isoform 1A1 of the UGT enzyme, which is of paramount importance in the conjugation of bilirubin. The gene consists of four common exons (exons 2, 3, 4, and 5) and 13 variable exons, of which only variable exon A1 is of any importance regarding bilirubin conjugation; the remaining exons play a role in the detoxification of a diverse range of chemical substances (Fig. 48-8). The variable exon A1 functions in conjunction with common exons 2 to 5: in response to a specific signal, transcription processing splices messenger RNA from the variable exon to the common exons. This process provides a template for the synthesis of an individual enzyme isoform. Upstream of each variable exon is a regulatory noncoding promoter that contains a TATAA box sequence of nucleic

Most frequently encountered promoter (TATAA box) genotypes

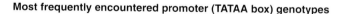
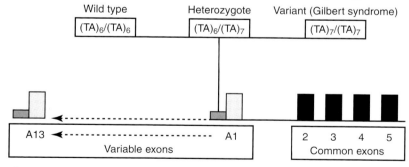

Figure 48–8. The human *UGT1* gene locus. Schematic representation of the genomic structure of the *UGT1* gene complex. Variable exon 1A1 and common exons 2 to 5 of the gene complex have been identified as those sites encoding the bilirubin conjugating enzyme, UDP-glucuronosyltransferase. Variable exons 1A2 to 1A13 do not participate in bilirubin metabolism. Genetic mutations associated with absent or decreased enzyme activity, which cause deficiencies of bilirubin conjugation, have been localized to this variable exon 1A1 (light gray box), its promoter (dark gray box), or the common exons 2 to 5 (black boxes). The *upper section* of the diagram demonstrates the common exon 1A1 promoter TATAA box genotypes. (*Redrawn from Kaplan M, Hammerman C: Bilirubin and the genome: the hereditary basis of unconjugated neonatal hyperbilirubinemia,* Curr Pharmacogenom *3:30, 2005.*)

acids. Mutations of variable exon A1, its promoter, or the common exons 2 to 5, may result in deficiencies of bilirubin conjugation. Polymorphisms of the noncoding promoter area affect bilirubin conjugation by diminishing expression of a normally structured enzyme, whereas mutations of the gene coding area may affect enzyme function by altering the structure of the enzyme molecule. Further information is supplied in the section on "Conjugated Hyperbilirubinemia," later.

NONPATHOLOGIC UNCONJUGATED HYPERBILIRUBINEMIA

In contrast with the older pediatric and adult patient, elevations in unconjugated bilirubin occur ubiquitously in the human neonatal population. In a sense, this "normal" increase in TB levels is not true hyperbilirubinemia when compared with a reference group of all newborns. A more appropriate term that would add to our understanding of the phenomenon and distinguish the normal or physiologic state with the pathologic entity implied in the term *hyperbilirubinemia* may be *physiologic bilirubinemia*.[136] A study of the hour-of-life specific bilirubin nomogram (Fig. 48-9) will reflect the natural increase in TB during the first days of life, reaching a peak at about 5 days.

Unconjugated hyperbilirubinemia in the human, regardless of age, is defined as an indirect-reacting bilirubin concentration of 2.0 mg/dL (34 μmol/L) or greater, depending on the standard used in calibration of the reaction. Nearly all adults and older children normally have indirect-reacting bilirubin concentrations in circulation of less than 0.8 mg/dL (14 μmol/L) and δ-bilirubin of 0.2 to 0.3 mg/dL (3 to 5 μmol/L). Conjugated hyperbilirubinemia is defined as an elevation of the direct-reacting fraction in the van den Bergh diazo reaction of greater than 1.5 mg/dL (26 μmol/L) provided it comprises more than 10% of the TB concentration. The latter portion of the definition is added to guard against overinterpretation of direct reactions in newborns with markedly elevated indirect-reacting bilirubin concentrations because up to 10% of the unconjugated pigment behaves as direct-reacting pigment in the van den Bergh-type methods.

Clinical situations in which the direct-reacting bilirubin concentration is equal to or close to the TB concentration are extremely rare, especially in the newborn period. In the neonate with conjugated hyperbilirubinemia, the hyperbilirubinemia is usually "mixed," the elevated direct-reacting fraction accounting for 20% to 70% of the total pigment. Thus, a neonate with mixed hyperbilirubinemia should be considered primarily to have *conjugated* hyperbilirubinemia, and pathology resulting from interference with hepatic cell excretion and bile transport, rather than from abnormalities of increased bilirubin production or deficient hepatic bilirubin uptake or conjugation, should be sought.

Fetal Bilirubin

During the last stages of human gestation, the normal degradation of erythrocytes formed earlier in fetal life results in about a 150% increase in bilirubin production per unit of body weight compared with adults. The mammalian fetus of all species appears to be capable of degrading heme without limitation, through the two enzymatic steps responsible for the formation of unconjugated bilirubin IX-α, HO and biliverdin (see Fig. 48-2). However, notable species differences exist in the pattern of development of hepatic bilirubin conjugation. Marked deficiency in the conjugating enzyme (UGT) activity is noted in rat, rabbit, guinea pig, sheep, dog, monkey, and human fetuses. At term, UGT activity in the rhesus monkey is only 1% to 5% of that in the adult. In the human fetus, UGT activity is extremely low before 30 weeks of gestation at about 0.1% of adult activity, and gradually increases to about 1% at term.

Diminished UGT activity is the central rate-limiting step that, in conjunction with additional processes including increased bilirubin production, enhanced enterohepatic circulation, and diminished uptake into the hepatocyte, manifests as physiologic jaundice in monkeys and humans.

Significant hyperbilirubinemia is unusual in the human fetus because the placenta transports unconjugated bilirubin from the fetus to the mother. Administration of radioactive unconjugated bilirubin into the fetal circulation of a dog,

Figure 48–9. Zones of risk for pathologic hyperbilirubinemia based on hour-specific serum bilirubin levels. (*From Bhutani VK, et al: Predictive ability of a predischarge hour-specific serum bilirubin for subsequent significant hyperbilirubinemia in healthy term and near-term newborns, Pediatrics 103:6, 1999.*)

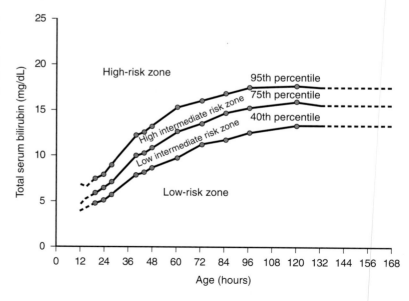

guinea pig, or monkey shows a rapid disappearance from the fetal side and recovery in the maternal bile. Even in states of severe intrauterine hemolysis from conditions such as Rh isoimmunization, the degree of anemia by far exceeds the level of hyperbilirubinemia, and clinical jaundice is usually mild at birth.[29] After delivery and separation of the placenta from the infant, rapid increases in TB may be expected. By contrast, the placenta is barely permeable to conjugated bilirubin. Thus, in the absence of evidence of hemolytic disease, if clinical jaundice is present at birth, a conjugated hyperbilirubinemia, caused by intrauterine hepatic pathology, should be suspected.

A large amount of bilirubin is found in meconium, indicating appreciable activity of fetal hepatic bilirubin conjugation. A significant level of β-glucuronidase activity is found in meconium, suggesting that conjugated bilirubin in the fetal intestine can be hydrolyzed back to unconjugated bilirubin and then absorbed from the bowel into the portal circulation. This absorbed bilirubin may reenter the hepatocyte for subsequent reconjugation and re-excretion, or may be transferred through the placenta into the maternal circulation. The efficiency of this process is protective to the fetus against severe hyperbilirubinemia, even when hemolysis is severe.

Conjugated hyperbilirubinemia in the mother, which may occur in hepatitis or recurrent jaundice of pregnancy, is not reflected in the cord blood. Severe hemolytic disease in the fetus results in small, but significant, increases in amniotic fluid bilirubin concentrations. How bilirubin enters the amniotic fluid pool is not known, but suggestions have ranged from direct transfer across the placenta from the maternal circulation, to transudation of pigment across the amniotic membranes or cord vessels, to secretion of bilirubin in the pulmonary fluids flowing from the fetal lung into the fetal pharynx and oral cavity and then into the amniotic fluid. Although to a great extent replaced by noninvasive measurement of anterior cerebral artery flow as an index of fetal anemia, in recent decades, measurement of amniotic fluid bilirubin concentrations by spectrophotometry, combined with percutaneous umbilical blood sampling allowing for serial hematocrit determinations and fetal intravascular transfusions, resulted in markedly improved outcome for the now rare fetus and infant with Rh erythroblastosis (see Chapter 21).

Neonatal Hyperbilirubinemia

TERM NEONATE

In the full-term newborn, physiologic jaundice is characterized by a progressive rise in TB concentration from about 2 mg/dL (34 μmol/L) in cord blood to a mean peak of 5 to 6 mg/dL (86 to 103 μmol/L) between 48 and 120 hours of age in white and African-American babies, with most infants peaking at 72 to 96 hours of age, and 10 to 14 mg/dL (171 to 239 μmol/L) between 72 and 120 hours of age in Asian-American babies. This is followed by a rapid decline to about 3 mg/dL (51 μmol/L) by the 5th day of life (Fig. 48-10) in white and African-American neonates and by the 7th to 10th day in Asian-American neonates. This early period of physiologic jaundice has been designated as *phase 1* physiologic jaundice. During the period from the 5th to 10th day of life in white and African-American infants, TB concentrations

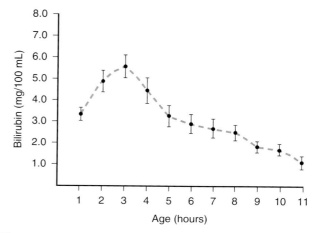

Figure 48–10. Mean total bilirubin (TB) concentrations in 22 full-term normal white and African-American infants during the first 11 days of life. *Vertical bars* represent standard error of the mean. (*From Gartner LM, et al: Development of bilirubin transport and metabolism in the newborn rhesus monkey,* J Pediatr 90:513, 1977.)

decline slowly, reaching the normal adult value of less than 2 mg/dL (34 μmol/L) by the end of that period. This late neonatal period of minimal, slowly declining hyperbilirubinemia has been designated as *phase 2* physiologic jaundice. The epidemiology is dependent, in part, on the prevalence of breast feeding in a population because lower peak TB values will be found among predominantly formula-fed infants.

Studies in the newborn rhesus monkey, an animal with a pattern of physiologic jaundice of the newborn that is similar to that in humans, show that phase 1 results from the combination of a sixfold postnatal increase in the load of bilirubin presented to the liver combined with a markedly diminished UGT activity. The presence of either of these factors alone would result in retention of unconjugated bilirubin to a lesser extent than when in combination. Hepatic uptake and excretion of bilirubin are also decreased during this period, although their function as rate-limiting steps in the transport of bilirubin from plasma into bile is dwarfed by the combination of increased bilirubin load to the liver and diminished conjugative capacity. The very large increase in bilirubin load appears to result from both increased de novo bilirubin synthesis and enteric reabsorption of unconjugated bilirubin. In the newborn monkey, the markedly increased load persists for 3 to 6 weeks, primarily because of enhanced intestinal bilirubin absorption. Similar data are not yet available for the human neonate.

In the human, UGT activity is extremely low in the fetal period. After birth, UGT activity increases at an exponential rate, reaching the adult level by 6 to 12 weeks of age (Fig. 48-11). The early deficiency in enzyme activity may result from insufficient enzyme synthesis, inhibition of enzymatic activity by naturally occurring substances, deficient synthesis of the glucuronide donor UDPGA, or a combination of these factors. Phase 2 physiologic jaundice appears to result from an imbalance in which hepatic uptake of bilirubin remains diminished while the increased bilirubin load presented to the liver persists. Developmental deficiency of B-ligandin may contribute to deficient uptake of bilirubin.

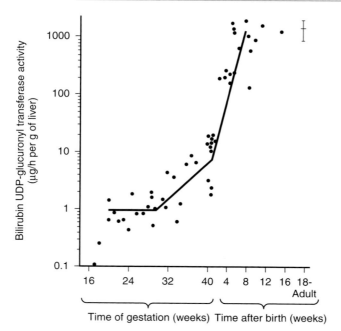

Figure 48–11. Developmental pattern of hepatic bilirubin uridine diphosphoglucuronate (UDP)-glucuronosyltransferase activity in humans. *(From Kawade N, Onishi S: The prenatal and postnatal development of UDP-glucuronyltransferase activity towards bilirubin and the effect of premature birth on this activity in the human liver,* Biochem J *196:257, 1981. Reprinted by permission of the Biochemical Society, London.)*

Despite the development of physiologic jaundice of some degree in nearly every newborn, only half of all white and African-American term newborns become visibly jaundiced during the first 3 days of life. Cutaneous icterus in the newborn will not become evident until TB concentrations exceed 5 to 6 mg/dL (86 to 103 μmol/L). This situation contrasts with that of the older child and adult, in whom jaundice may be noticeable in the sclerae and skin at TB concentrations as low as 2 mg/dL (34 μmol/L). Variations in duration of hyperbilirubinemia, in skin color, and in perfusion may account for these differences. As the intensity of jaundice increases, clinical icterus progresses in a caudal direction. At lower levels of TB, only the head and sclerae may be affected, with the chest, abdomen, legs, and feet becoming jaundiced in parallel to increasing TB concentrations. Because routine daily TB determinations are not usually performed on full-term or even premature newborns, careful scrutiny of the nursery population several times a day by experienced personnel is essential to detect infants who are becoming jaundiced. Some of these may subsequently develop significant hyperbilirubinemia and require further TB testing. Visual assessment of jaundice, however, is largely subjective, inaccurate, and dependent on observer experience. Development of transcutaneous devices intended to measure the skin color objectively and noninvasively may improve on the reliability of visual estimation and facilitate daily bilirubin determinations (see section on "Transcutaneous Bilirubinometry" later in this chapter). This is especially important in predischarge assessment of newborns, especially those discharged before 72 hours of age.

PRETERM NEONATE

Physiologic jaundice in premature neonates is more severe than in term neonates, with mean peak TB concentrations reaching 10 to 12 mg/dL (171 to 205 μmol/L) by the fifth day of life. This delay in reaching the maximal concentration compared with term neonates primarily reflects the delay in maturation of hepatic UGT activity. Because mean peak unconjugated bilirubin concentrations as low as 10 to 12 mg/dL (171 to 205 μmol/L) may be associated with acute bilirubin encephalopathy or kernicterus in certain high-risk, low-birthweight neonates, all degrees of visible jaundice in premature neonates should be monitored closely and investigated fully.[44]

Despite lower UGT activity in premature neonates than in term neonates at birth, UGT activity increases rapidly, far exceeding the expected maturational rate noted in utero (Fig. 48-12). This observation indicates that there are two components in the maturational process of hepatic UGT: (1) chronologic maturation and (2) accelerated maturation related to birth. Nevertheless, normal TB concentrations in

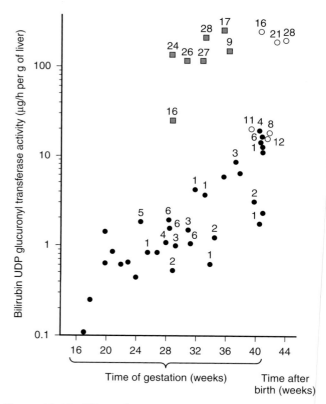

Figure 48–12. Effect of premature birth on development of hepatic bilirubin uridine diphosphoglucuronate (UDP) glucuronosyltransferase (UGT) activity in humans. Numbers beside symbols represent age (days) at which activities were measured. Symbols represent enzyme activities for premature *(squares)* and full-term *(open circles)* infants who lived more than 8 days after birth, and for fetuses and premature and full-term infants who died within 7 days of delivery *(filled circles).* *(From Kawade N, Onishi S: The prenatal and postnatal development of UGT activity towards bilirubin and the effect of premature birth on this activity in the human liver,* Biochem J *196:257, 1981. Reprinted by permission of the Biochemical Society, London.)*

premature neonates may not be reached in many cases until the end of the first month of life.[124]

LATE PRETERM NEONATE

Late preterm gestation (newborns born between 34 and 36 completed weeks) is an important risk factor for the development of severe neonatal hyperbilirubinemia and kernicterus. At this point of gestation, hepatic conjugative capacity is still immature and may contribute to the greater prevalence, severity, and duration of neonatal jaundice in these infants. Many of these infants will be feeding with human breast milk. Additional factors that may increase the incidence of severe hyperbilirubinemia include large for gestational age status, male sex, and glucose-6-phosphate dehydrogenase (G6PD) deficiency. Scrupulous attention to screening for jaundice in the newborn nursery, adequate lactation support, parental education, and appropriate postdischarge follow-up should facilitate institution of treatment when clinically indicated.[245]

POST-TERM NEONATE

Nearly all postmature neonates and about half of all term neonates who are small for gestational age (SGA) may be expected to have little or no physiologic jaundice, with peak TB concentrations of less than 2.5 mg/dL (43 μmol/L). The mechanism for this acceleration of hepatic maturation is unknown. Similarly, neonates of mothers treated with phenobarbital, a drug known to stimulate hepatic UGT activity and the concentration of ligandin,[171] and neonates of heroin users have less than the anticipated severity of physiologic jaundice. Other drugs, less well investigated, also may have similar "maturing" effects.[220,243]

GENETIC, ETHNIC, AND CULTURAL EFFECTS

The severity of physiologic jaundice varies significantly among different ethnic populations. Mean maximal TB concentrations in Chinese, Japanese, Korean, American-Indian, and other Asian term newborns are between 10 and 14 mg/dL (171 to 239 μmol/L), about double those of the white and African-American populations. The incidence of bilirubin toxicity as defined by autopsy-proven kernicterus is also increased significantly in Asian newborns. There is no clinical evidence for increased hemolysis in Asian newborns to account for these dramatic differences,[74,130] although some studies of CO production have suggested that bilirubin synthesis may be slightly increased compared with that in white or African-American neonates. A mutation (Gly71Arg) in the gene for UGT frequently found in Japanese, Koreans, and Chinese, but rare in whites, is associated with Gilbert syndrome in Asian populations has been shown to be associated with an increased incidence of neonatal hyperbilirubinemia in these groups.[8] In contrast, variation in the number of thymidine-adenine (TA) repeats in the promoter for *UGT1A1* gene are commonly encountered in whites and are associated with Gilbert syndrome in that population group (see section on "Genetic Control of Bilirubin Conjugation," earlier). The promoter polymorphism is rare in Asian communities.[24] Thus, there is mounting evidence that the phenotypic variability in neonatal TB levels seen in different populations results in part from genotypic heterogeneity.

Certain geographically distinct populations may demonstrate a markedly increased incidence of neonatal unconjugated hyperbilirubinemia without associated hemolysis. The most dramatic of these are from certain Greek islands, especially the islands of Lesbos and Rhodes. Although the incidence of G6PD deficiency in these populations is markedly increased compared with the remainder of the Greek population and the world incidence, the incidence of hyperbilirubinemia was not directly correlated with the frequency of G6PD deficiency, suggesting interaction of additional icterogenic factors.[219] Unless aggressively treated with phenobarbital prophylaxis, phototherapy, and exchange transfusion, the incidence of kernicterus was also much greater in the newborns from these Greek islands than in those of the mainland population.[220]

It has been speculated that the increased incidence of neonatal unconjugated hyperbilirubinemia in Asian and geographically identifiable populations may result either from environmental influences, such as the maternal ingestion of certain ethnically characteristic herbal medications or foods, or from a genetic predisposition to slower maturation of bilirubin metabolism and transport. Asian-origin infants born in the United States, and Greek newborns born in Australia, appear to be at similar risk for neonatal jaundice as natives of Asia and Greece, respectively, suggesting that geographic factors alone are not determinant. Differentiating the influence of drugs, foods, or traditional practices from that of genetic factors requires further investigation. Severe hyperbilirubinemia can result from hemolysis associated with sepsis or, if genetically vulnerable (e.g., in G6PD deficiency), exposure to chemicals (such as naphtha in mothballs) or pharmaceutical agents (such as antimalarials, sulfonamides, sulfones, antipyretics, and analgesics). In some societies with a high incidence of G6PD deficiency, application of henna to the skin or use of menthol-containing umbilical potions may precipitate severe hyperbilirubinemia and potentiate bilirubin encephalopathy. Even though some of these agents and stressors have received public attention, others represent generally unsuspected dangers, such as the intramuscular (IM) injection of vitamin K_3 (menadione) or the inhalation of paradichlorobenzene, which is used in moth repellents, air fresheners, and bathroom deodorizers.[197,221] In addition, newborn exposure to a hemolytic agent, especially in the presence of G6PD deficiency, can occur transplacentally or through breast milk, through both of these as in the case of maternal ingestion of fava beans, or directly by inhalation, ingestion, or injection.

PATHOLOGIC UNCONJUGATED HYPERBILIRUBINEMIA

Elevated concentrations of unconjugated bilirubin are of concern because of the danger of bilirubin encephalopathy or neuropathy associated with this fraction of bilirubin. Although there have been some reports of bilirubin encephalopathy associated with elevated levels of conjugated bilirubin, the role of conjugated hyperbilirubinemia in the mechanism of bilirubin encephalopathy is not clear. Most studies of kernicterus have related to the TB concentration, of which the conjugated fraction usually comprises a small fraction. Elevated levels of conjugated bilirubin frequently indicate disease processes of hepatic origin. The following discussion therefore relates primarily to unconjugated, or indirect, hyperbilirubinemia, and is followed by a section on conjugated hyperbilirubinemia.

The TB level at any point in time reflects a multiplicity of forces in delicate balance. Processes including bilirubin production, transport, uptake, conjugation, excretion, and reabsorption are not only interdependent but are also influenced by tremendous physiologic flux present in this complex system in the first few days of the neonatal period. Examples of such changes include differences in the rate of heme catabolism and progressive maturation of the bilirubin conjugation system. Physiologically, the net result is an increase in TB up to about the fifth day of life, after which point it levels off and then gradually decreases. Superimposed on these physiologic alterations of bilirubin metabolism may be specific disorders that may further exaggerate or prolong the normal pattern of elevated TB. These conditions may affect the entire spectrum of bilirubin metabolism and include disorders of bilirubin production as well as bilirubin conjugation and elimination.

Causes of Unconjugated Hyperbilirubinemia

DISORDERS OF PRODUCTION

Although increased bilirubin production could result from pathologic states in which degradation of nonhemoglobin heme (i.e., hemoproteins such as cytochromes, catalase) and erythrocyte hemoglobin precursor heme are increased, such disorders in fact have not been identified in the newborn period. The most common pathologic causes of unconjugated hyperbilirubinemia in the newborn include isoimmune hemolytic disease caused by blood group incompatibility between mother and fetus, and G6PD deficiency. Disorders associated with increased erythrocyte destruction are listed in Box 48-1 (see Chapter 21).

BOX 48-1 Conditions Associated with Increased Erythrocyte Destruction

ISOIMMUNIZATION
Rh incompatibility
ABO incompatibility
Other blood group incompatibilities
ERYTHROCYTE BIOCHEMICAL DEFECTS
Glucose-6-phosphate dehydrogenase deficiency
Pyruvate kinase deficiency
Hexokinase deficiency
Congenital erythropoietic porphyria
Other biochemical defects
STRUCTURAL ABNORMALITIES OF ERYTHROCYTES
Hereditary spherocytosis
Hereditary elliptocytosis
Infantile pyknocytosis
Other
INFECTION
Bacterial
Viral
Protozoal
SEQUESTERED BLOOD
Subdural hematoma and cephalohematoma
Ecchymoses
Hemangiomas

Neonates who are acutely hemolyzing appear to be at a higher risk for developing bilirubin-induced brain damage compared with those without hemolysis. Indeed, the first association to be recognized between increasing bilirubin levels and the risk for kernicterus was made in newborns with Rh isoimmunization.[99] Subsequently, some reports suggested that kernicterus in hyperbilirubinemic newborns with hemolytic disease may occur more frequently than that in counterparts without evidence of hemolytic disease, as reviewed by Newman and Maisels.[163] Surveying the literature up to 1983, Watchko and Oski[248] reinforced the concept that hyperbilirubinemia among neonates without hemolytic disease was less dangerous with regard to the development of kernicterus than in cases in which hemolysis was present. A similar stand was taken by Newman and Maisels[164] several years later. However, there are few data to substantiate this view. A study shedding some light on this question was performed by Ozmert and colleagues.[174] In 102 children aged 8 to 13 years, indirect hyperbilirubinemia ranging from 17 to 48 mg/dL (291 to 821 µmol/L) associated with a positive direct Coombs test, presumed to reflect ongoing hemolysis, was associated with lower intelligence quotient (IQ) scores and a higher incidence of neurologic abnormalities. In these same children, the incidence of detected neurologic abnormalities increased as the time of exposure to high bilirubin levels became more prolonged. Similarly, in Norway, Nilsen and coworkers[165] found that of males born in the early 1960s who developed neonatal hyperbilirubinemia, those with a positive Coombs test and hyperbilirubinemia for greater than 5 days had significantly lower IQ scores than average for that country.

Although there is to date no hard evidence demonstrating higher levels of unbound bilirubin in hemolyzing neonates, many believe hemolysis to be a potential factor increasing the risk for bilirubin-related brain damage. Although a TB concentration of 20 to 24 mg/dL (342 to 410 µmol/L) may be associated with kernicterus in a neonate with Rh isoimmunization, a healthy, term infant without an obvious hemolytic condition will rarely be endangered by TB concentrations in this range. Conditions associated with hemolysis, including direct Coombs-positive Rh and ABO immunization or other isoimmunizations and G6PD deficiency, may pose an increased threat to an otherwise healthy newborn. The Subcommittee on Hyperbilirubinemia of the American Academy of Pediatrics (AAP) includes jaundice developing within the first 24 hours, blood group incompatibility with a positive direct antiglobulin test (DAT) (also known as the Coombs test), and other known conditions including G6PD deficiency, all associated with increased hemolysis, as major risk factors for the development of severe hyperbilirubinemia.[13] The AAP recommends initiating phototherapy or performing exchange transfusions at lower levels of TB in neonates with hemolytic conditions than in apparently nonhemolyzing counterparts. However, we do not propose that a hyperbilirubinemic newborn, but without an obvious hemolytic condition will be unaffected by bilirubin encephalopathy. Patients with kernicterus have been reported in whom no evidence of hemolysis was evident.[140] Crigler-Najjar syndrome, a condition not associated with increased hemolysis, is frequently complicated by bilirubin-induced neurologic dysfunction.

Hemolytic conditions in the newborn are generally divided into two major etiologic groups: immune and nonimmune.

Isoimmunization

The hallmark of isoimmunization is a positive DAT, also known as the Coombs test. This is indicative of maternally produced antibody that has traversed the placenta and is now found within the fetus. The test is termed *direct* if the antiglobulin is adhered to the RBCs. An *indirect* test refers to the antibody being detected in the serum.

Rh DISEASE

In past decades, Rh hemolytic disease was the most common cause of severe hemolytic hyperbilirubinemia and a frequent cause of kernicterus. However, maternal prophylaxis with high-titer anti-D immunoglobulin G (RhoGAM), combined with aggressive fetal surveillance and intrauterine blood transfusions, has greatly reduced the incidence and severity of this disease. Mothers sensitized before the development of immune serum prophylaxis are no longer commonly encountered. Those without access to preventive treatment, immigrants from countries in which prophylaxis was not widely available, or those who did not receive prophylaxis following abortion or invasive procedures may continue to deliver affected infants.

The Rh blood group proteins are a highly antigenic group of proteins capable of causing severe isoimmunization with a high risk for fetal hydrops and death. Although several systems of nomenclature exist, the CDE system is most commonly used. These three loci each contain two major alleles (C,c; D,d; E,e) and several minor alleles. The D antigen may produce maternal sensitization with a fetomaternal hemorrhage as small as 0.1 mL. Whereas C and E alleles are relatively uncommon causes of isoimmunization, they can, on occasion, lead to severe hemolysis and hyperbilirubinemia. Rh disease in pregnancy is highly associated with both intrauterine hemolysis and severe hemolytic disease following delivery. Untreated, the condition can lead to intrauterine anemia and severe *hydrops fetalis*, with rapid postnatal evolvement of hyperbilirubinemia with the potential of kernicterus.

The immunization process may begin if an Rh-negative woman, usually D negative, is exposed to a D antigen. This usually occurs by antepartum or intrapartum transplacental fetomaternal transfusion of fetal RBCs containing a D antigen, or by transfusion of Rh-positive RBCs during abortion, blood administration, or procedures including amniocentesis, chorionic villus sampling, or fetal blood sampling. Following exposure to the D antigen on the fetal RBCs, the mother's immune system responds by forming anti-D immunoglobulin G (IgG) antibodies. The IgG then crosses the placenta and adheres to fetal RBCs containing the D antigen. The subsequent antigen-antibody interaction leads to hemolysis and anemia. The immune response may become more severe and more rapid with progressive pregnancies. Resultant anemia causes bone marrow stimulation, with increased numbers of immature RBCs appearing in the circulation (*erythroblastosis*) and extramedullary hematopoiesis. *Fetal hydrops*, a condition characterized by generalized tissue edema and pleural, pericardial, and peritoneal effusions, may result from a combination of hypoproteinemia, tissue

hypoxia, and capillary leak. Anemia with resultant poor myocardial function may further exacerbate the hydrops by causing congestive cardiac failure and venous congestion.[154]

Elevated COHb levels, detected in blood obtained by cordocentesis in affected fetuses of nonsmoking isoimmunized mothers, demonstrate that destruction of erythrocytes begins in utero.[254] However, the primary manifestation of the in utero hemolysis is that of anemia. Although large amounts of bilirubin are produced concomitantly, erythroblastotic infants are not severely icteric at birth. TB concentrations are usually kept below 5 mg/dL (86 μmol/L) by transfer of unconjugated bilirubin across the placenta. Jaundice may appear, however, within 30 minutes after delivery. Classically, the serum bilirubin is all indirect reacting, although small amounts of conjugated bilirubin have been noted. After some days of excessive bilirubin load, the excretory system may become overwhelmed with efflux of conjugated bilirubin into the serum, and an increasing conjugated bilirubin fraction is not uncommonly seen. Hepatic conjugation may mature more rapidly than excretory function as a result of stimulation by chronic exposure to high concentrations of bilirubin in utero. Furthermore, hepatic excretory function may also be adversely affected by development of hepatic congestion secondary to heart failure and swelling caused by extramedullary hepatic hematopoiesis, anemia, and poor hepatic perfusion.

ABO HETEROSPECIFICITY

With the reduction of the incidence of Rh isoimmunization by immune prophylaxis, DAT-positive ABO incompatibility is now the single most prominent cause of immune hemolytic disease in the neonate. The clinical picture is usually milder than that of Rh disease, although infrequently severe hemolysis with hyperbilirubinemia may occur.

By ABO blood group heterospecificity, we refer to the situation in which a blood group A or B baby is born to a group O mother, a setup occurring in about 12% of pregnancies. In some instances, women with blood group O have a high titer of naturally occurring anti-A or anti-B antibodies. High titers of anti-A or anti-B antibodies can sometimes be found in blood group O women even before their first pregnancy. This contrasts to Rh isoimmunization, in which immune sensitization occurs progressively with subsequent pregnancies.[90] In contradistinction to blood group A or B individuals, in whom their respective anti-B or anti-A antibodies are IgM molecules with limited ability to cross the placenta, the respective antibodies of blood group O individuals are predominantly smaller IgG molecules and may cross the placenta. Attachment to corresponding fetal RBCs may follow, provided these cells have the A or B antigen. Extravascular hemolysis of the IgG-coated RBCs is thought to be mediated within the reticuloendothelial system by Fc-receptor–bearing cells. As with Rh isoimmunization, the immune process may commence in utero. However, unlike the Rh situation, there is little danger of severe hyperbilirubinemia, anemia, or hydrops in utero, and prenatal intervention is not indicated. Infants may sometimes be born with moderate anemia. After delivery, there is a potential danger of hyperbilirubinemia.

About one third of blood group A or B neonates born to a blood group O mother will have a positive direct Coombs test.[175] Measurements of endogenous formation of CO, reflective of heme catabolism, have demonstrated, overall, an increased rate of heme catabolism in affected babies compared with controls.[71,203,204,217] Not all DAT-positive neonates, however, develop severe hyperbilirubinemia. In one study, only 20% of DAT-positive neonates actually developed TB values greater than 12.8 mg/dL (219 µmol/L),[175] whereas in another study, only 19.6% required phototherapy.[149] Despite this apparent clinical mildness, newborns with severe hyperbilirubinemia of early onset who do not respond to phototherapy are occasionally encountered. At the extreme end of the spectrum, kernicterus has been described.[28,193] ABO blood group incompatibility with a negative DAT, not usually predictive of hemolysis or hyperbilirubinemia, may sometimes cause early and rapidly progressing jaundice, reminiscent of DAT-positive hemolytic disease.

Paucity of A and B antigenic sites on neonatal RBCs or weak expression of these antigens in neonates, compared with adults, may explain, in part, absence of clinical disease in most DAT-positive newborns. A or B antigenic sites situated in sites other than the RBC may bind with transplacentally acquired antibodies, limiting their availability to the RBC.

Because many ABO-incompatible, direct Coombs-positive neonates have no evidence of ongoing hemolysis and do not develop early jaundice or hyperbilirubinemia, ABO heterospecificity with a positive DAT does not necessarily indicate ABO *hemolytic disease.* Some or all of the following criteria are necessary to support the diagnosis of ABO hemolytic disease:

1. Indirect hyperbilirubinemia, especially during the first 24 hours of life
2. Mother with blood group O, infant with blood group A or B
3. Spherocytosis on blood smear
4. Increased reticulocyte count
5. Evidence of hemolysis based on increased endogenous production of CO. Unfortunately, a readily available clinical tool for determining end-tidal CO, corrected for ambient CO (ETCOc) levels, is no longer available.

In DAT-negative ABO-heterospecific newborns, an interaction with polymorphism for the $(TA)_7$ sequence in the promoter of the gene encoding UGT1A1, significantly increasing the incidence of TB of at least 15 mg/dL (257 µmol/L) compared with controls, has been described.[113]

It is essential to closely observe any newborn born to a blood group O mother and to perform a TB measurement at the first appearance of jaundice. Routine blood group and DAT determination on umbilical cord blood is an option, which may allow for additional risk determination.

ISOIMMUNIZATION DUE TO ANTIBODIES OTHER THAN RhD
More than 50 RBC antigens may cause hemolytic disease of the newborn.[153] The most important of these with regard to prenatal hemolysis include anti-c, anti-Kell, and anti-E,[91,107] although others may also, infrequently, be problematic. Alloimmunization due to these autobodies can sometimes cause severe hemolytic disease of the fetus requiring prenatal intervention. Fetal surveillance protocols and clinical strategies developed for RhD alloimmunization are useful in monitoring all alloimmunized pregnancies. Similarly, the postnatal management should be based on the principles outlined in the management of the RhD-immunized newborn (see "Therapy for Unconjugated Hyperbilirubinemia" section that follows). Anti-Kell isoimmunization warrants special mention because fetal anemia often predominates the clinical picture. This may be due to erythropoietic suppression in addition to a hemolytic process.[226]

Nonimmune Hemolysis
ERYTHROCYTE ENZYMATIC DEFECTS
The mature human erythrocyte lacks a nucleus and the organelles necessary for protein and lipid synthesis. Most of the protein present within its cell membranes is hemoglobin. Because the uptake and release of oxygen and carbon dioxide by hemoglobin in the tissues does not require energy, the erythrocyte relies on glycolysis (through the anaerobic Embden-Meyerhof pathway and the aerobic pentose phosphate pathway) and not on mitochondrial oxidative phosphorylation to generate adenosine triphosphate (ATP). Thus, defects in the glycolytic enzymatic machinery may have profound effects on erythrocyte function and life span.

GLUCOSE-6-PHOSPHATE DEHYDROGENASE DEFICIENCY
An entity that is highly associated with extreme neonatal hyperbilirubinemia and bilirubin encephalopathy is G6PD deficiency.[110] Because G6PD deficiency has major neonatal public health implications, it is discussed in some detail.

G6PD deficiency is a common enzyme deficiency estimated to affect hundreds of millions of people with a worldwide distribution.[23,253] From its original indigenous distribution, including areas in south Europe, Africa, the Middle East, and Asia, immigration patterns have transformed it into a condition that may now be encountered virtually in any corner of the globe. The condition has been overrepresented in reports of neonates with extreme hyperbilirubinemia and bilirubin encephalopathy, relative to the background frequencies of this condition among the populations of the United States, Canada, the United Kingdom, and Ireland.[28,143,193] In the United States–based Pilot Kernicterus Registry,[28] more than 20% of reported neonates had G6PD deficiency, whereas its overall frequency is estimated at less than 3%.[253]

Function of G6PD. G6PD plays a major part in stabilization of the RBC membrane against oxidative damage. The enzyme catalyzes the first step in the hexose monophosphate pathway, oxidizing glucose-6-phosphate to 6-phosphogluconolactone, thereby reducing nicotinamide adenine dinucleotide phosphate (NADP) to NADPH. NADPH is essential for the regeneration of reduced glutathione from oxidized glutathione, a substance that plays an integral part in the body's antioxidative mechanisms. The pathway is also instrumental in stimulating catalase, another important antioxidant. In the absence of G6PD, NADPH will not become available, reduced glutathione will not be regenerated, and cells may be rendered susceptible to oxidative stress. Unlike other body cells, no alternative source of NADPH is available in the RBC, which explains the extreme vulnerability of the G6PD-deficient RBC to oxidative damage. Oxidative membrane damage incurred may manifest as hemolysis.[253]

Genetics of G6PD Deficiency. Because G6PD deficiency is an X-linked condition, males may be normal hemizygotes or deficient hemizygotes, whereas females may be either normal or deficient homozygotes, or heterozygotes. Because of X-inactivation, heterozygotes have two RBC populations: one G6PD deficient, the other G6PD normal. As X-inactivation may be nonrandom, unequal ratios of normal and enzyme-deficient RBCs may coexist. Heterozygotes may, as a result, have either a normal, intermediate, or deficient phenotype.[70] It was previously thought that heterozygotes had sufficient enzyme activity to protect them from the dangers of G6PD deficiency.[253] However, reports suggest that heterozygotes may not be without risk, and fatal kernicterus has been described in a heterozygote.[97,109,115] The most commonly encountered mutations are G6PD A⁻, found in Africa, southern Europe, and in African Americans. G6PD Mediterranean, regarded as a more severe type than G6PD A⁻, is found in Mediterranean countries, the Middle East, and India. Another variant encountered primarily in Asia is G6PD Canton. Many other mutations have been documented.

G6PD Deficiency and Hemolysis. Most G6PD-deficient individuals lead perfectly normal lives and will, for the most part, be unaware of their inherited condition. However, G6PD deficiency may be associated with severe hemolytic episodes with resultant jaundice and anemia, following exposure to a hemolytic trigger. Classically, these episodes often occur after ingestion of or contact with the fava bean (favism). Medications and chemical substances may be implied, but sometimes no offending trigger may be identified. Beutler[23] has emphasized the role of infections in the pathogenesis of acute hemolysis.

In neonates, extreme hemolytic jaundice may develop suddenly and without previous warning. Some identifiable substances associated with neonatal hemolysis include naphthalene used to store clothes, herbal medicines, henna applications, or menthol-containing umbilical potions. Frequently, the trigger cannot be recognized. The hemolysis may be severe, and the TB concentration may increase exponentially to dangerous levels. G6PD deficiency may, therefore, be the one reason that kernicterus may not be completely preventable. Exchange transfusion may be the only recourse. Early hospital discharge with delayed follow-up may place these patients at risk for severe sequelae.[177,198]

Frequently, hematologic indices typical of hemolysis in older children and adults, including falling hemoglobin and hematocrit values and increasing reticulocyte count, may be absent, despite a clinical picture of hemolysis. However, studies of endogenous CO formation, reflective of the rate of heme catabolism, have demonstrated an important role of increased hemolysis in association with this condition.[162,198] Slusher and colleagues,[198] for example, demonstrated significantly higher levels of COHb in Nigerian G6PD-deficient neonates who developed kernicterus, compared with neonates who were hyperbilirubinemic but did not develop signs of kernicterus.

More frequently and less life-threatening, G6PD-deficient neonates may have a more moderate form of jaundice, which occurs at a rate several-fold that of controls. The jaundice usually responds to phototherapy, although exchange transfusion may also be necessary. These infants have a low-grade

hemolysis, which cannot be implicated as the primary icterogenic factor.[116,120] Diminished bilirubin conjugation has been shown to be of major importance in the pathogenesis of the jaundice.[119] An intriguing interaction has been noted between G6PD deficiency and noncoding area (TA)$_7$ promoter polymorphism in the gene encoding UGT1A1.[118] This polymorphism, also known as UGT1A1*28, is associated with Gilbert syndrome. The incidence of hyperbilirubinemia, defined as a TB of at least 15 mg/dL (257 µmol/L), increased in a stepwise, dose-dependent fashion in G6PD-deficient neonates who were heterozygous or homozygous, respectively, for the polymorphism. This effect was not seen in the G6PD-normal control group. Furthermore, G6PD deficiency alone, in the absence of the promoter polymorphism, did not increase the incidence of hyperbilirubinemia over and above that of G6PD-normal counterparts. In contrast, in Asians, in whom the (TA)$_7$ promoter polymorphism is rare, a similar interaction was noticed between G6PD deficiency and coding area mutations of the *UGT1A1* gene.[100]

Unlike the acute hemolytic form of jaundice, this milder form of jaundice can be predicted by predischarge bilirubin testing. Neonates who had a predischarge TB concentration below the 50th percentile were unlikely to develop subsequent hyperbilirubinemia. However, as the predischarge TB increased progressively above the 50th percentile, the risk for subsequent hyperbilirubinemia increased in tandem.[111]

Testing for G6PD Deficiency. Many qualitative or quantitative screening tests are available that should accurately determine the hemizygous state in males or the homozygous state in females. Because many heterozygotes may have intermediate to normal enzyme activity, the heterozygote state is difficult to determine using standard biochemical tests. Females of high-risk groups (Mediterranean origin, African American, African, Middle Eastern or Asian, and Sephardic Jews) should have close follow-up to detect the development of jaundice despite a normal screening. Also, biochemical tests may give a false-normal result if performed during an acute hemolytic episode because older RBCs may be destroyed, leaving younger cells with higher enzyme activity intact.[96] In such cases, G6PD testing should be performed several weeks after the acute hemolysis has subsided. An alternative method is to analyze DNA for the specific suspected mutation. Some countries have introduced neonatal screening for G6PD deficiency combined with parent education in the hope that identification of an infant with G6PD deficiency should lead to avoidance of known triggers of hemolysis and speed the process of evaluation and treatment should an affected neonate become jaundiced.

The treatment of neonatal hyperbilirubinemia associated with G6PD deficiency should follow the guidelines of the AAP[13] for neonates with hemolytic risk factors.

Pyruvate kinase catalyzes the conversion of phosphoenolpyruvate to pyruvate and the formation of ATP from adenosine diphosphate in the Embden-Meyerhof pathway. Deficiency of this enzyme results in a lack of ATP for erythrocytic metabolic activity and in chronic anemia. Pyruvate kinase deficiency, a condition prevalent in northern European peoples and inherited in an autosomal recessive manner,[150] results in a lack of ATP, an important source of energy for RBC metabolism.[263] In the newborn period, anemia, reticulocytosis, and severe jaundice may ensue, requiring exchange transfusion on occasion. Kernicterus has been reported.[222]

Four isozymes are encoded by two genes, among which 180 mutations have been described.[263] Diagnosis is determined by enzyme assay, which should be performed in cases of hemolysis and hyperbilirubinemia not associated with a positive direct Coombs test or spherocytosis. Molecular studies may also confirm the diagnosis.

Hexokinase catalyzes the conversion of glucose to glucose-6-phosphate, the initial step in glycolysis. Hexokinase deficiency predisposes the erythrocyte to oxidant damage and thus is another cause of hemolysis and neonatal hyperbilirubinemia. Inheritance is autosomal recessive, and the gene has been localized to chromosome 10.

Congenital erythropoietic porphyria is an extremely rare, recessively inherited disorder of heme metabolism in which deficient uroporphyrinogen III cosynthase activity inhibits the conversion of hydroxymethyl bilane to type III uroporphyrinogen. Normal heme synthesis can occur only in the presence of greatly elevated levels of type I uroporphyrinogen and type I coproporphyrinogen. These porphyrins are deposited in massive quantities throughout the cells of the body, including the erythrocytes. The disease may present at birth with anemia, jaundice, and splenomegaly. Pink to brown staining of diapers soaked with porphyrin-rich urine is an early clue to the diagnosis. Because porphyrins are photoreactive, the diapers readily fluoresce under ultraviolet light. The same photoreactive properties of porphyrins lead to hemolysis, hyperbilirubinemia, and cutaneous photosensitivity with subepidermal bullae formation.

Deficiencies of other enzymes in the glycolytic pathway, including glucose phosphate isomerase, are capable of producing severe hemolysis and hyperbilirubinemia in the neonatal period.[222]

ERYTHROCYTE STRUCTURAL DEFECTS
See also Chapter 46.
Defects in erythrocyte membrane and cytoskeletal structure alter the shape and deformability of the cell and result in sequestration within the narrow splenic sinusoids. Hemolysis, hyperbilirubinemia, and splenomegaly are the clinical hallmarks of these disorders.

Hereditary Spherocytosis. Of the hereditary RBC membrane defects that may lead to acute hemolysis and hyperbilirubinemia in the newborn, hereditary spherocytosis is probably the most common.[102] In spherocytosis, the normal biconcave shape of the erythrocyte is altered such that the cell assumes a spherical shape—the shape with the smallest possible diameter for its volume. In addition to a reduction in surface area with consequential diminished oxygen uptake and delivery, the limitation in deformability may result in massive splenic sequestration. This condition may be inherited in both an autosomal dominant and recessive fashion, and frequently there may be a history of acute hyperbilirubinemia in a sibling or a parent. Microvesiculization of the RBC membrane results from deficiency of proteins including ankyrin, band 3, α-spectrin, β-spectrin, and protein 4.2 in that membrane. These osmotically fragile RBCs are trapped in the spleen, the microvesicles aspirated by macrophages, and the cell destroyed. The diagnosis can be made microscopically by demonstrating

spherocytes in the peripheral blood smear, with confirmation by the osmotic fragility test. The latter test may be especially important in differentiating babies with hereditary spherocytosis from those with direct Coombs-positive ABO isoimmunization, a condition that may also result in microspherocytosis. Mutations of at least five genes encoding the previously mentioned proteins have been recognized.

Hereditary spherocytosis is frequently associated with neonatal hyperbilirubinemia. Of 178 affected Italian term, predominantly breast-fed newborns, 112 (63%) developed neonatal hyperbilirubinemia requiring phototherapy. The incidence of hyperbilirubinemia was even higher in those who also had a genetic variation in the promoter of the bilirubin *UGT1A1* gene, similar to that described in G6PD deficiency.[102] Kernicterus has been described.[22]

Hereditary Elliptocytosis, Hereditary Pyropoikilocytosis, Hereditary Ovalocytosis, and Hereditary Stomatocytosis. These are rare conditions affecting the erythrocyte membrane. The diagnosis may be made by microscopic examination of the peripheral blood smear. Hemolysis may occur in the neonatal period and result in anemia and hyperbilirubinemia.

Infantile pyknocytosis is a transient abnormality of erythrocyte morphology associated with hemolysis and neonatal jaundice. Small, irregular, dense RBCs with spiny projections are seen in the peripheral smear and account for more than 5% of the total RBC population. Anemia and hemolysis persist throughout the first month of life and often into the second and third months. Jaundice is most severe during the first 2 weeks of life.

INFECTION
Bacterial infection is a known cause of hemolysis and hyperbilirubinemia. Sepsis causes hyperbilirubinemia by increasing bilirubin concentrations through hemolysis, or by impairing conjugation, thereby resulting in decreased excretion of bilirubin. Several theories have been proposed for the mechanism of hyperbilirubinemia in the septic neonate. Neonatal erythrocytes are particularly susceptible to cell injury and Heinz body formation in response to oxidative stress. In addition, heme oxygenase can be induced by oxidants, which could lead to increased catabolism of heme to bilirubin. Because bilirubin is a protective antioxidant, initially in infection, bilirubin levels may be decreased as a result of its consumption. However, the frequent manifestation of hyperbilirubinemia associated with sepsis suggests that this protective mechanism may be overwhelmed in septicemia. Furthermore, disseminated intravascular coagulation resulting from sepsis may produce hemolysis as erythrocytes traverse the depositions of fibrin within the microvasculature. In addition, conjugated hyperbilirubinemia may result from hepatitis secondary to bacterial, viral, fungal, and protozoal infections.

SEQUESTRATION
Sequestration of blood within body cavities can result in increased bilirubin production as the body metabolizes and recycles the heme released as erythrocytes are catabolized. Birth trauma resulting in the collection of RBCs within the layers of tissue covering the skull and brain (cephalohematoma, subdural hematoma, subgaleal hematoma) or elsewhere (bruising associated with precipitous or

instrument-assisted delivery) has the potential to produce hyperbilirubinemia (see also Chapter 28).

Large hemangiomas, as in Kasabach-Merritt syndrome, may be associated with hemolysis and hyperbilirubinemia in addition to thrombocytopenia and depletion of fibrinogen and other clotting factors.

POLYCYTHEMIA

An increase in RBC mass with resultant increased breakdown of these cells has the potential to overload the already immature capacity of the newborn to eliminate heme degradation products. Polycythemia may be associated with delayed cord clamping, maternal-fetal transfusion, and twin-twin transfusion. Infants of diabetic mothers, especially those who are large for gestational age, are known to be at risk for polycythemia. Although the mechanisms underlying polycythemia in this group are unclear, CO excretion studies have shown that increased RBC breakdown, even in the absence of polycythemia, is the source of the hyperbilirubinemia in these neonates (see Chapter 46).[39,202]

DISORDERS OF HEPATIC UPTAKE

Gilbert syndrome is a benign disorder that affects about 6% of the population and produces a chronic unconjugated hyperbilirubinemia. Both defective hepatic uptake of bilirubin and decreased hepatic UGT1A1 activity have been demonstrated. The basis of the reduced activity of UGT lies in the presence of additional TA repeats in the TATAA box in the promoter region of the gene.[32,157] Because the noncoding, rather than coding, area of the gene is affected, Gilbert syndrome individuals have a normally structured UGT1A1 enzyme, but with diminished expression. The latter leads to a decrease in UGT enzyme activity. Although this disease usually does not manifest until after the second decade of life, some neonates with Gilbert syndrome may exhibit hyperbilirubinemia secondary to diminished uptake of bilirubin.[20] When mutations in both the gene for G6PD and the promoter for UGT occur, the degree of neonatal hyperbilirubinemia has been shown to be dose dependent.[118] In addition, in G6PD-deficient infants who had the wild type $(TA)_6$ (normal) gene promoter, the incidence of hyperbilirubinemia was similar to that in infants who were G6PD normal, with the wild-type promoter (9.7% versus 9.9%). The variant UGT promoter, rather than the rate of heme catabolism as measured by blood COHb, was subsequently shown to be the crucial factor in determining the TB, and had a similar incidence of hyperbilirubinemia (>15 mg/dL [257 μmol/L]) to those infants with and without G6PD deficiency. However, in G6PD-deficient infants who were both heterozygous and homozygous for the Gilbert variant, hyperbilirubinemia was more frequent in a stepwise, dose-dependent sequence (32% versus 50%, respectively).[24,118]

DISORDERS OF CONJUGATION

As described earlier, UGT catalyzes the conjugation of bilirubin in the liver. Disorders of conjugation include both those in which there is a primary alteration in UGT and those in which UGT function is secondarily altered.[47]

Crigler-Najjar Syndrome Type I

Crigler-Najjar syndrome type I is a rare autosomal recessive disease characterized by an almost complete absence of hepatic UGT activity. Because the coding area of the *UGT* gene is mutated, the enzyme produced is structurally abnormal, with no bilirubin conjugating capacity. In the homozygous form, severe unconjugated hyperbilirubinemia develops during the first 3 days of life and progresses in an unremitting fashion, with TB concentrations reaching 25 to 35 mg/dL (428 to 599 μmol/L) during the first month of life. Kernicterus often occurs in the neonatal period, especially when the etiology of the disease is unsuspected and aggressive treatment is not initiated. Stools are pale yellow, and bile bilirubin concentrations are less than 10 mg/dL (171 μmol/L) (normal being 50 to 100 mg/dL [855 to 1710 μmol/L]), with total absence of bilirubin glucuronide in bile. Bilirubin glucuronide formation measured in vitro with liver obtained by biopsy is absent. Formation of most nonbilirubin glucuronides is either severely reduced or absent.

With either direct hepatic enzymatic assay or indirect measurement of glucuronide formation, both parents are found to have partial defects (about 50% normal). Enzyme activity reserve should be sufficient to keep TB concentrations within normal limits. Unless a family is known to be affected by the condition, during the first week of life, the recognition of this disorder may be difficult because of confusion with other types of exaggerated unconjugated hyperbilirubinemia. Persistence of unconjugated hyperbilirubinemia at TB concentrations of greater than 20 mg/dL (342 μmol/L) beyond the first week of life, or repeated need for phototherapy in the absence of obvious hemolysis, should prompt concern for this syndrome.

Indirect methods of diagnosis including microassay of UGT activity from a percutaneous liver biopsy specimen or analysis of bile conjugates have been largely replaced by gene analysis. Figure 48-8 includes many of the mutations associated with the condition. Occurrence of the identical mutation in both parents of an affected homozygous infant suggests parental consanguinity.

The management of these neonates requires maintenance of TB concentrations to less than 20 mg/dL (342 μmol/L) during at least the first 2 to 4 weeks of life. The risk for kernicterus persists into adult life, but aggressive management may diminish this risk while awaiting liver transplantation.[207] Today, nearly all neonates with this disorder are treated with phototherapy as initial therapy or after one or more exchange transfusions. Phototherapy is generally continued throughout the early years of life in the hope that this will prevent the development of kernicterus. Despite attempts to expose older children to phototherapy at the highest intensities and longest durations possible, the response to phototherapy progressively decreases with years of use. This may result from increased skin thickness or a changing distribution of the bilirubin pool. Prompt management of all intercurrent infections, febrile episodes, and other types of illness may help prevent later development of kernicterus. Inducers of UGT, such as phenobarbital, are not effective in Crigler-Najjar syndrome type I disease.

Liver transplantation offers the only definitive treatment for the disease. This procedure should not be delayed indefinitely because phototherapy may become less effective with the passage of time, and intercurrent illnesses may precipitate high levels of TB, with the potential of kernicterus, even in children whose TB concentrations had appeared to be under control and who had appeared to be neurologically intact. In a multicenter report of a world survey, 7 of 21 (33%) transplanted children had already developed some form of brain damage at the time of their transplantation. Average age at transplantation was 9.1 ± 6.9 years (range, 1 to 23 years).[224] Hepatocyte transplantation has been used,[48,75] whereas gene therapy may also have promise for these patients in the future.[185]

Crigler-Najjar Syndrome Type II

Crigler-Najjar syndrome type II (also known as Arias disease) is more common than type I and typically benign. Although unconjugated hyperbilirubinemia occurs in the first days of life, TB levels generally do not exceed 20 mg/dL (342 µmol/L). Fasting, illness, and anesthesia may cause temporary increases in bilirubin to above baseline. The occurrence of kernicterus is rare. Evidence of hemolytic disease is absent (although it may occur coincidentally), stool color is normal, and neonates are otherwise healthy.

Unconjugated hyperbilirubinemia persists into adulthood. Biochemically, hepatic UGT activity is nonexistent and indistinguishable from that found in type I disease. Less than 50% of the daily bilirubin production is excreted in bile, and the monoglucuronide is the predominant form.

Another difference between type II and type I diseases lies in the response to phenobarbital of patients with type II.[208] Jaundiced neonates and adults with type II disease respond readily to oral administration of phenobarbital with a sharp decline in TB concentrations, whereas individuals with type I disease demonstrate no such change. Phenobarbital may be used both as a simple clinical tool to differentiate the two syndrome types. Beyond the neonatal period, there should be no long-term risk for kernicterus unless there is coincidental hemolytic disease.

Crigler-Najjar syndrome type II occurs both as an autosomal recessive and dominant inheritance. The range of expression in one or both parents can be from an asymptomatic defect in conjugation on testing to severe icterus. Other members of the family also may either appear icteric or have detectable low-grade unconjugated hyperbilirubinemia. Screening of the parents and other close relatives for hyperbilirubinemia is a useful method for supporting the diagnosis when it is suspected. Testing of the neonate and the parents for the capacity to form glucuronides of bilirubin were used diagnostically in the past, but these methods have been largely replaced by sequencing of the *UGT* gene.[108]

Transient Familial Neonatal Hyperbilirubinemia (Lucey-Driscoll Syndrome)

Lucey-Driscoll syndrome is a rare familial disorder in which neonates of certain mothers may develop severe unconjugated hyperbilirubinemia during the first 48 hours of life. Kernicterus has been reported in untreated newborns. The sera of these neonates and their mothers contain high concentrations of an inhibitor of UGT when tested in vitro. The serum inhibitory effect gradually declines after delivery coincident with gradual decline in TB.

Pyloric Stenosis

Pyloric stenosis may be associated with unconjugated hyperbilirubinemia at the time vomiting begins. Hepatic UGT activity is markedly depressed in the jaundiced neonates. The

mechanism of diminished UGT activity may be due to presence of the variant $(TA)_7$ *UGT1A1* gene promoter, which is associated in adults with Gilbert syndrome.[214]

Duodenal and jejunal obstruction are also associated with exaggerated unconjugated hyperbilirubinemia. Surgical relief of the obstruction results in a decline of TB concentrations to normal within 2 to 3 days. Lower intestinal obstruction, as in Hirschsprung disease, also may result in unconjugated hyperbilirubinemia, although usually of a milder degree than with upper intestinal tract disease. In this situation, as well as when there is upper intestinal tract obstruction, hyperbilirubinemia may result from increased reabsorption of unconjugated bilirubin from the intestine due to stasis of the intestinal contents (see Chapter 47).

Hypothyroidism

UGT activity in congenital hypothyroidism is deficient and may remain suboptimal for weeks or months. Because about 10% of congenitally hypothyroid neonates may develop prolonged, exaggerated jaundice, testing for thyroid function should be performed in these cases. Treatment with thyroid hormone promptly alleviates the hyperbilirubinemia. The mechanism of this association in the human newborn is unknown, but in rats, hypothyroidism impairs hepatic uptake and reduces hepatic ligandin concentrations. Thyroid hormone is also instrumental in many maturational processes. Its absence may delay hepatic bilirubin enzyme and transport development (see Chapter 49, Part 3). It has also been suggested that thyroid hormone can cause changes in UGT protein expression.[82]

DISORDERS OF EXCRETION

Impaired hepatic excretion of bilirubin from disorders such as hepatocyte injury results in conjugated hyperbilirubinemia and is discussed later in this chapter.

DISORDERS OF ENTEROHEPATIC CIRCULATION

Jaundice Associated with Breast Feeding

Jaundice associated with breast feeding is common. Two pathophysiologic mechanisms have been suggested for the early-onset association of jaundice with breast feeding, although this differentiation is not clear, and overlap may exist between these suggested entities. Breast-feeding failure jaundice or breast-feeding–associated jaundice has been so labeled to distinguish it from breast milk jaundice. Breast-feeding failure jaundice is so labeled because the cause appears to be associated with poor feeding practices and not with any change in milk composition. In contrast, breast milk jaundice is apparently related to a change in the composition or physical structure of the milk. Both types result in an exaggerated enterohepatic circulation of bilirubin—one through "starvation" and the other through altered milk chemistry.

BREAST-FEEDING FAILURE JAUNDICE

Breast-feeding failure jaundice occurs in the first weeks of life in breast-fed newborns. Establishing effective breast feeding may be difficult, especially in first-time mothers, who may find lactation to be an intricate process. Maternal factors, such as lack of proper technique, engorgement, cracked nipples, and fatigue may impair effective breast feeding. Neonatal factors such as ineffective suck also may hamper attempts at breast feeding. Even if the mother is experienced in breast feeding and her baby is interested, her milk supply is usually limited to small amounts of colostrum in the first 24 to 48 hours after birth. All these factors may act in combination, resulting in infrequent or ineffective breast feeding. As a result, there may be little stimulus for milk production. Formula supplementation may further impair successful lactation. Exclusively breast-fed neonates are therefore at risk for being relatively underhydrated and less well nourished than formula-fed counterparts. Poor enteral intake may lead to a state of relative starvation and delayed meconium passage. Intestinal content stasis may lead to increased enterohepatic reuptake of bilirubin, increasing the bilirubin load presented to the liver, leading to unconjugated hyperbilirubinemia. This process is similar to the "starvation jaundice" seen in older human patients as well as other animal species fasted for more than 24 hours.

Prevention of breast-feeding failure jaundice includes encouraging frequent (at least 8 to 12 times per day for the first several weeks)[16] breast feeding, avoiding supplementation with water or glucose solutions,[59] and accessing maternal lactation counseling. Intensive support of the breast-feeding mother is necessary, especially in view of early discharge policies in place at many hospitals. Both during birth hospitalization and after hospital discharge, the newborn should be closely monitored for weight gain, adequate urination and stool formation, and the development of jaundice.

BREAST MILK JAUNDICE

Late breast milk jaundice occurs after the first 3 to 5 days of life and may last into the third week of life or beyond. Epidemiologic studies report that 10% to 30% of breast-fed infants in the second to sixth week of life are affected, with some having hyperbilirubinemia into the third month.[78] Presence of the variant $(TA)_7$ UGT1A1 gene promoter may be associated with prolonged breast milk jaundice.[156]

Typically, the TB level rises steadily, peaking at 5 to 10 mg/dL (86 to 171 µmol/L) at about 2 weeks of age, with a gradual decline over the first several months of life. More severely affected neonates may achieve peak levels as high as 20 to 30 mg/dL (342 to 513 µmol/L). There is no evidence of hemolysis, nor do these neonates appear ill; weight gain and intestinal function are normal. Pregnane-3-α,20-β-diol, a progesterone metabolite found in the breast milk fed to affected neonates, was historically thought to be the cause of this disorder because this substance was shown to be a competitive inhibitor of UGT in vitro. Although milk and urine of mothers of these neonates contain this pregnanediol isomer, the inhibitory effect of this hormone has been questioned. Studies have indicated that the milk associated with this syndrome also contains high concentrations of nonesterified long-chain fatty acids. This suggests that certain of these fatty acids act as inhibitors of hepatic UGT, causing retention of unconjugated bilirubin. It is unlikely that the nonesterified long-chain fatty acids would reach the sites of conjugation in smooth endoplasmic reticulum of hepatocytes without prior esterification. Triglycerides of these long-chain fatty acids do not inhibit in vitro activity of UGT. Neither the pregnanediol nor the fatty acids have ever been substantiated as an inhibitor of hepatic conjugation in vivo, and their role in the cause of the breast milk jaundice syndrome remains questionable.

Studies of the enterohepatic circulation of bilirubin in the rat suggest that milk from mothers of neonates with this syndrome contains β-glucuronidase, an enzyme that could deconjugate bilirubin and, consequently, enhance enteric reabsorption of bilirubin, thereby increasing the hepatic bilirubin load. The presence of this enhancer of intestinal bilirubin absorption in human milk correlates tightly with the presence of mild to moderate unconjugated hyperbilirubinemia in neonates during the second and third weeks of life. With more than 50% of all breast-fed neonates manifesting this effect of breast milk, this phenomenon may be a normal physiologic development comparable to, and an extension of, physiologic jaundice of the early newborn period.

Usually, other than jaundice, the neonates appear healthy, and no abnormal findings are noted. Although not recommended unless TB concentrations reach levels that might be of danger to the infant, interruption of nursing and substitution with formula feeding for 1 to 3 days usually causes a prompt decline of the TB concentration to about half or less of the original level. On resumption of nursing, the TB does not usually increase substantially. Brief interruption of nursing may be useful to confirm the diagnosis, thereby allaying parental anxiety. Failure to respond in this manner indicates that the neonate's jaundice may be unrelated to breast feeding, and other causes should be sought. Supplementation with milk formula may have an effect similar to complete cessation of nursing.[83] An alternative to temporary cessation of breast feeding would be to confirm that the TB is primarily unconjugated, that thyroid function tests are normal, and that there is no evidence of urinary infection. In the situation in which the infant is thriving and the TB does not reach dangerous levels, it may be prudent to observe the infant. It should not be forgotten, however, that rare disorders of bilirubin conjugation may occur in breast-feeding infants and may lead to erroneous diagnosis. Effective nursing practices that prevent early "starvation" in breast-fed newborns may reduce not only the incidence of breast-feeding failure jaundice, but also the severity of breast milk jaundice.[10,146]

Sequelae of Unconjugated Hyperbilirubinemia

The recognition that unconjugated bilirubin may penetrate the brain cell under certain circumstances and its association with neuronal dysfunction and death are reasons for carefully managing newborn infants with significant hyperbilirubinemia.[14,15] There is some evidence that, despite the publication of national guidelines for the prevention and management of hyperbilirubinemia in several countries (United States, Canada, South Africa, Israel and, very recently, the United Kingdom), kernicterus continues to occur in industrialized countries in which the condition was thought to have been "extinct."[28,65,142,193] Acute bilirubin encephalopathy (defined as the acute manifestations of bilirubin-induced neurologic dysfunction, or BIND) and its resultant sequela, kernicterus (defined as chronic and permanent sequelae of BIND) should, for the most part, be preventable conditions. Concerns that risks for acute bilirubin encephalopathy or kernicterus have been exaggerated with regard to term, otherwise healthy neonates have been outweighed by the perpetuation of cases up to present times.[12,164]

There is no single TB concentration that can be regarded as safe or categorically dangerous. The TB concentration, although used clinically to determine the need for phototherapy and exchange transfusion, is a poor predictor of subsequent neurodevelopmental outcome. It is unlikely that in an otherwise healthy, term infant with no obvious hemolytic condition, BIND will occur at TB concentrations below 25 mg/dL (428 μmol/L). In the presence of hemolysis, prematurity, or other risk factors (see later), or in the presence of poor relative health, the danger point may be reached at lower levels of TB.[55,105] In a term infant thought to be actively hemolyzing, a TB concentration of 18 to 20 mg/dL (308 to 343 μmol/L) should probably not be exceeded.[37,43] Until definitive scientific data indicate otherwise, hyperbilirubinemia should be seen as being capable of producing a spectrum of neurologic dysfunction in the newborn, ranging from transient mild encephalopathy to permanent severe neurologic impairment secondary to neuronal necrosis (kernicterus). In addition, it is important to understand that bilirubin metabolism is a dynamic process influenced by many factors. An isolated TB level obtained at one point in time is inadequate to fully assess the risk for sequelae for a particular neonate. Many other factors, including the gestational age and relative health of the newborn, need to be carefully evaluated.

TRANSIENT ENCEPHALOPATHY OR ACUTE BILIRUBIN ENCEPHALOPATHY

Early bilirubin toxicity is transient and reversible. This is suggested by clinical observations of increasing lethargy in tandem with rising TB concentrations, with reversal of lethargy after exchange transfusion. Brainstem auditory evoked response (BAER) may show changes in the wave latency and magnitude, characteristic of early signs of acute bilirubin encephalopathy.[196] BAER signs typically encountered in neonates with moderate unconjugated hyperbilirubinemia (10 to 20 mg/dL [171 to 342 μmol/L]) include prolongation of latencies of waves III and IV-V, and interpeak I-III and I-V, compared with neonates of similar gestational and postnatal ages without hyperbilirubinemia. Prolonged latencies in peak IV-V and interpeak I-V suggest interference with brainstem conduction. These changes in evoked responses reverse with either exchange transfusion or spontaneous decline in TB concentrations.

Long-term follow-up of children with neonatal abnormalities in brainstem responses believed to be due to hyperbilirubinemia are not yet available and the significance of abnormal BAER findings remains unknown.[194,250] An abnormal BAER suggests an injury of the VIII cranial nerve. Bilirubin auditory neuropathy may occur even in the context of normal cochlear function, as measured by otoacoustic emission (OAE), emphasizing the need to perform BAER testing, and not to rely on OAE, in neonates who are suspected of having auditory damage due to hyperbilirubinemia. During the early stages of BIND, a characteristic signal signature can be seen by magnetic resonance imaging (MRI) using T1- and T2-weighted imaging.[85,177] Consequently, the presence of an abnormal BAER, normal OAE, and focal changes in the globus pallidus and medial lobe of the hippocampus by MRI is highly suggestive of acute bilirubin encephalopathy (Fig. 48-13).

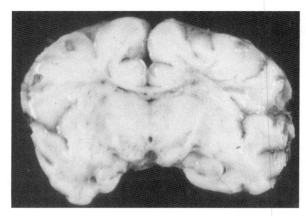

Figure 48-13. See color insert. Acute bilirubin encephalopathy. Coronal section through parietotemporal lobes. Note selective symmetric yellow discoloration in the hippocampus and subthalamic nuclei. Thalamus and globus pallidus are focally stained. (*From Zangen S, et al: Fatal kernicterus in a girl deficient in glucose-6-phosphate dehydrogenase: a paradigm of synergistic heterozygosity,* J Pediatr *154:616-619, 2009.*)

KERNICTERUS

If early acute bilirubin encephalopathy is unrecognized or untreated, it may progress to permanent neurologic impairment. The term *kernicterus* (German *kern*, kernel or nucleus, and *ikteros*, jaundice) has been traditionally used to describe the pathologic findings of bilirubin toxicity within the brain: staining and necrosis of neurons in the basal ganglia, hippocampal cortex, subthalamic nuclei, and cerebellum, followed by gliosis of these areas in survivors (Fig. 48-14). The cerebral cortex is generally spared. About half of all infants with kernicterus observed at autopsy also have extraneural lesions of bilirubin toxicity. These include necrosis of renal tubular cells, intestinal mucosa, and pancreatic cells in association with intracellular crystals of bilirubin. Gastrointestinal hemorrhage may accompany these lesions.[216]

Kernicterus is also used to describe the clinical presentation of worsening encephalopathy. In the term newborn, several phases of kernicterus have been classically described. Phase 1 is marked by poor sucking, hypotonia, and depressed sensorium. Fever, retrocollis, and hypertonia that may progress to frank opisthotonos are seen in phase 2. The hypertonia becomes less pronounced in phase 3, but high-pitched cry, hearing and visual abnormalities, poor feeding, and athetosis are manifest. Seizures may also occur. The usual time course for progression of the disease is about 24 hours. Long-term survivors often demonstrate the classic signs of kernicterus, including choreoathetoid cerebral palsy, upward gaze palsy, sensorineural hearing loss, and dental dysplasia during later infancy and childhood. The intellect may be spared, and mental retardation is not universally encountered. However, infants with normal intelligence frequently have severe physical handicaps, making rehabilitation, education, and independent living unlikely. These sequelae of bilirubin toxicity may also develop in neonates who never manifested clinical signs of acute bilirubin encephalopathy during the newborn period. In addition, earlier epidemiologic studies suggest that

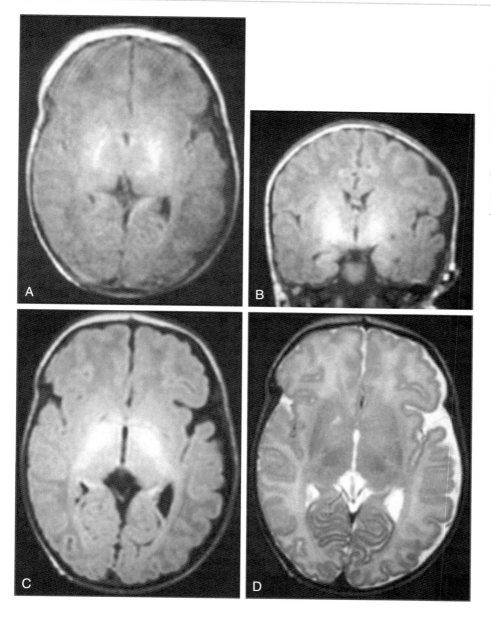

Figure 48-14. Magnetic resonance images of a 21-day-old, preterm male neonate with acute kernicterus. Axial (**A**) and coronal (**B**) T1-weighted and axial FLAIR (**C**) images at the level of the basal ganglia show symmetric, hyperintense globus pallidus involvement. This is not apparent on the axial T2-weighted (**D**) image. *(From Coskun A, et al: Hyperintense globus pallidus on T1-weighted MR imaging in acute kernicterus: is it common or rare? Eur Radiol 15:1263, 2005.)*

some neonates may have sequelae of subclinical bilirubin encephalopathy characterized only by the later development of mild disorders of motor function or abnormal cognitive function, or both.[52,192]

Presentation in preterm neonates is less stereotypical, and these patients may simply appear ill without signs specific for kernicterus. Bilirubin may enter the brain at lower levels of TB than would be expected in term infants. Moreover, bilirubin staining of central nervous system (CNS) structures in premature neonates may not be indicative of overt kernicterus and may result from developmental differences in CNS permeability to bilirubin and in situ bilirubin metabolism. Mortality occurs in about 50% of term newborns but may occur more frequently in the preterm population with kernicterus.[4]

Bilirubin is thought to enter the brain through multiple mechanisms. These include: (1) bilirubin production that overwhelms the normal buffering capacity of the blood and tissues; (2) alterations in the bilirubin-binding capacity of albumin and other proteins resulting in the presence of unconjugated bilirubin in the circulation; (3) increased CNS permeability to bilirubin secondary to disruption of the blood-brain barrier; and (4) other factors that may affect those previously mentioned or act through novel independent mechanisms.

Unconjugated bilirubin is nonpolar and lipid soluble, and its aqueous solubility in plasma water is extremely small, mandating its binding in plasma primarily to albumin. Binding to other components of blood (β-globulin, RBC membranes, and platelets) may also occur when the albumin-binding capacity for bilirubin is exceeded. It has long been believed that bilirubin toxicity occurs when the albumin-binding capacity for bilirubin is saturated and the unbound or "free" bilirubin (bilirubin in aqueous phase) concentration rises in blood. Whether this is, in fact, the basic pathophysiologic mechanism of kernicterus remains unresolved.

The human albumin molecule is capable of binding at least two molecules of bilirubin, with the first molecule more tightly bound than the second. Additional classes of binding sites, if operative in vivo, have much lower affinities than the first two. At a molar ratio of 1, each gram of human albumin binds 8.2 mg of bilirubin. Thus, at an average albumin concentration of 3 g/dL, the first binding site should be capable of binding 25 mg of bilirubin per deciliter of serum or plasma. The second binding site should be capable of binding an additional 25 mg/dL for a total binding capacity of 50 mg/dL.

Various techniques have been proposed to measure albumin binding of bilirubin, but their application and interpretation in clinical management are not generally accepted. The dye-binding methods using 2-(4'-hydroxybenzeneazo) benzoic acid and direct-yellow-7 are based on the measurement of reserve binding sites on the albumin molecule and should be capable of indicating impending risk. The column chromatographic methods (Sephadex G-25), the salicylate displacement spectrophotometric method (saturation index), the RBC uptake method, and the oxidation technique (peroxidase method) should all be capable of detecting small increases in plasma unbound bilirubin or "loosely bound" bilirubin, in theory, denoting increased risk for developing kernicterus.[6,7] However, current laboratory and clinical data are still insufficient to permit a recommendation for the use of either a single method or a combination of methods to guide the clinical management of infants with neonatal unconjugated hyperbilirubinemia. Furthermore, it may be falsely reassuring to assume that in vitro binding capacities will remain reliably static in an in vivo system that changes so dynamically during the first postnatal days.

The bilirubin-binding capacity of albumin is thought to be decreased in sick term and premature human neonates. In addition, the serum albumin concentration is often lower in these patients than in healthy, term counterparts. Theoretically, both of these factors may act to place the sick term or premature neonate at higher risk for kernicterus at lower TB levels than seen in the healthy term newborn.[223,246] There is still debate about whether the bilirubin-binding capacity of albumin decreases as pH drops below 7.4, despite the known solubility decrease of bilirubin with increasing acidity. Numerous agents compete with bilirubin for binding sites on albumin, acting to displace bilirubin and increase the ratio of free to bound bilirubin in the serum. Free fatty acids, which are elevated in sepsis and hypoxemia, are capable of displacing bilirubin. Similarly, intravenous lipid emulsions rarely can contribute to elevated free fatty acids and thus displacement of bilirubin. Sulfisoxazole and other sulfa drugs, indomethacin, and salicylates readily displace bilirubin. Even ampicillin, when injected rapidly, has the potential to act in a similar manner. Benzyl alcohol, once used as a preservative in various medications, has been shown to competitively inhibit bilirubin binding. Finally, certain substances used in the preparation of albumin solutions may act to decrease its bilirubin-binding capacity.[35,242]

Disruption of the blood-brain barrier allows the passage of molecules otherwise prevented from entering the CNS. Hypertonicity of the serum, meningitis, and hypoxemia all increase CNS permeability to bilirubin.[94] It has been reported that unconjugated bilirubin is a substrate for phosphorylated glycoprotein (P-GP)[106,247] and that P-GP in the blood-brain barrier may play a role in limiting the entry of bilirubin into the CNS. P-GP is an integral plasma membrane transport protein, dependent on ATP, which can transport a wide variety of substrates across biologic membranes.

Many other factors may play a role in regulating bilirubin entry into the brain. Kernicterus has been reported to occur in adults with Crigler-Najjar syndrome type I, but only when TB concentrations have reached 45 to 55 mg/dL (770 to 941 μmol/L). This contrasts with the situation in the full-term newborn in which kernicterus may be anticipated at somewhat lower concentrations, suggesting presence of a maturational process in the blood-brain barrier integrity.

In addition to bilirubin produced within the reticuloendothelial system, bilirubin may be produced within the brain. The mammalian brain has two isoforms of HO, HO-1 and HO-2, which convert heme to biliverdin.[69] HO-1 normally shows little baseline activity in the brain but is capable of being rapidly upregulated in response to stress. Most HO activity in the brain is the result of the constitutive enzyme HO-2. HO-1 and HO-2 are distributed in selected areas of the brain, many of which play roles in motor and auditory function. Biliverdin reductase is also found in the brain, catalyzing the conversion of biliverdin to bilirubin. Although bilirubin thus formed is normally rapidly cleared by bilirubin oxidase, it is possible that this fraction of the bilirubin pool does contribute to the development of kernicterus. These enzyme systems are developmentally regulated and may also be influenced by any of the disease states previously mentioned. Because the bilirubin produced and metabolized in situ must be transported out of the brain, interference with this transport mechanism may be another potential mechanism of contributing to kernicterus.

Once bilirubin has gained access to the CNS, there are several postulated mechanisms of neuronal injury: (1) passage through lipid moieties of cell membranes into the lipids of subcellular organelles such as mitochondria, interfering with critical steps in energy metabolism; (2) binding to specific membrane, organelle, or cytoplasmic proteins, and inhibiting their function; and (3) damage and direct interference with the function of DNA.[49]

The neurotoxicity of bilirubin is currently being debated. As described earlier, HO catalyzes the conversion of heme to biliverdin, releasing equimolar amounts of CO. Carbon monoxide may function as a neurotransmitter within the CNS and has been implicated as playing a role in memory. However, CO may also act as a neurotoxin and have deleterious effects, including neuronal necrosis. The deposition of bilirubin in the brain of patients with kernicterus may not be the primary insult, but rather may be a relatively innocuous marker of neuronal damage produced by other means. Bilirubin has antioxidant properties and may, at physiologic levels, provide protection from oxidative injury.[152,262] Whatever the mechanism of bilirubin neurotoxicity, clinical decisions regarding the management of hyperbilirubinemia and the institution of therapy are based on the TB concentration, and given its apparent effectiveness in reducing the incidence of kernicterus, it would be unwise to alter the current approach to therapy.

Diagnosis of Unconjugated Hyperbilirubinemia

About two thirds of the more than 4 million neonates born annually in the United States become clinically jaundiced. Clearly, the number of jaundiced neonates who will develop sequelae of hyperbilirubinemia is substantially less than this. The challenge to the pediatrician is to determine which newborns may become or are already abnormally jaundiced and therefore are at risk for severe sequelae.[137] The recommendations by the AAP for the laboratory evaluation of the jaundiced infant at 35 weeks' gestation or later are listed in Table 48-1.

TOTAL BILIRUBIN (TB) MEASUREMENTS

When the clinical screening examination detects a jaundiced newborn, the mainstay of clinical management includes determination of TB concentrations in the serum or plasma. Direct bilirubin measurements will not contribute much information in the early stages of jaundice but should be performed in cases of prolonged hyperbilirubinemia or of hyperbilirubinemia not responding to therapy, or if a disease process is suspected. In most patients, repeat determinations will be necessary in the acute stage of jaundice to determine the trajectory, the peak bilirubin concentration, and whether indications for instituting therapy have been reached. Following that, an at least daily determination should be performed until a clear pattern of decline is observed. Clinical judgment is necessary to determine whether TB concentrations may be monitored on an ambulatory basis, thereby eliminating the need for prolonged hospitalization, or whether the risk for severe hyperbilirubinemia warrants in-hospital observation. Thus, the clinician must determine whether any individual neonate is at high or low risk for developing severe hyperbilirubinemia or kernicterus. Neonates at high risk for kernicterus include those presenting with jaundice in the first 24 hours of life, pallor, or hepatosplenomegaly, and with documented immune or nonimmune hemolytic conditions.

Bhutani and colleagues, in a study performed in 1999 on a racially diverse population of term healthy newborns, established that a percentile-based bilirubin nomogram using age-in-hours-specific predischarge TB levels can accurately predict an infant's level of risk for developing hyperbilirubinemia (see Fig. 48-9).[27] Infants with a predischarge TB in the 95th percentile or higher (high-risk zone) had a 57% risk for developing severe hyperbilirubinemia (TB of 17 mg/dL [291 μmol/L] or greater). Risk was 13% for infants in the high-intermediate zone (TB between the 75th and 95th percentiles). Infants with TB levels between the 40th and 75th percentiles (low-intermediate risk) had a risk of 2.1%. Infants with TB in the 40th percentile or less had no risk. All TB measurements should be plotted on the Bhutani nomogram, which takes into account the rapidly occurring changes in TB concentrations. It will be clear from a study of the nomogram that an individual TB reading may have different connotations depending on the hour of life at which the blood was sampled. The closer the TB reading to the 95th percentile for hours-of-life, the greater becomes the risk for subsequent hyperbilirubinemia. Conversely, a TB reading below the 40th percentile is usually associated with a low risk for hyperbilirubinemia. A useful method of assessing whether the rate of rise of TB is greater than normal is to plot several TB points on the graph and determine whether the trajectory runs in parallel with the graph or at a more rapid rate or "jumping" to a higher percentile track (Fig. 48-15).

Classification of hyperbilirubinemia as conjugated or unconjugated requires fractionation of serum or plasma bilirubin into direct- and indirect-reacting pigments, respectively. Simple techniques that fail to distinguish direct- from

TABLE 48-1   Laboratory Evaluation of the Jaundiced Infant ≥35 Weeks of Gestation

Indications	Assessments
Jaundice in first 24 hr	TcB and/or TB
Jaundice appears excessive for age	TcB and/or TB
Infant receiving phototherapy or TB rising rapidly (i.e., crossing percentiles [see Fig. 48-15]) and unexplained by history and physical examination	Blood type and Coombs test, if not obtained with cord blood CBC and smear Direct or conjugated bilirubin Optional: reticulocyte count, G6PD, ETCOc, if available Repeat TB in 4 to 24 hr, depending on infant age and TB level
TB concentration approaching exchange levels or not responding to phototherapy	Reticulocyte count, G6PD, albumin, ETCOc (if available)
Elevated direct (or conjugated) bilirubin level	Urinalysis and urine culture Evaluate for sepsis indicated by history and physical examination
Jaundice present at or beyond age 3 weeks, or if the infant is sick	Total and direct (conjugated) bilirubin level If direct bilirubin elevated, evaluate for causes of cholestasis Check results of newborn thyroid and galactosemia screen; evaluate for signs and symptoms of hypothyroidism

CBC, complete blood count; ETCOc, end-tidal carbon monoxide, corrected for inhaled CO; G6PD, glucose-6-phosphate dehydrogenase; TcB, transcutaneous bilirubin; TB, total bilirubin.
From American Academy of Pediatrics Subcommittee on Hyperbilirubinemia: Management of hyperbilirubinemia in the newborn infant 35 or more weeks of gestation, *Pediatrics* 114:297, 2004.

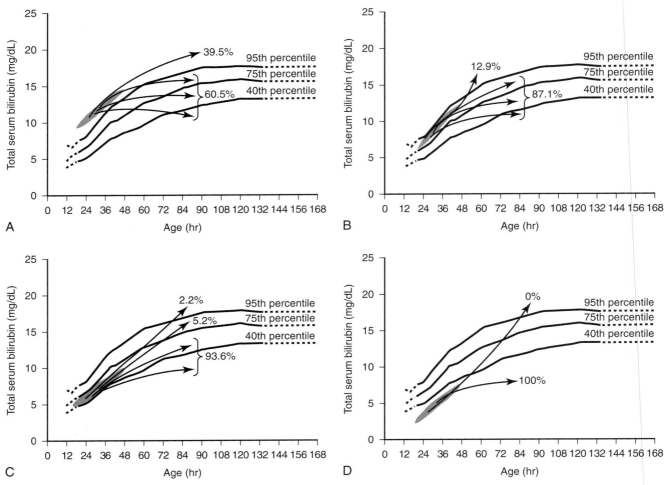

Figure 48–15. Outcome of newborns as defined by the percentage of newborns that remain or move up to the high-risk zone after their risk assessment with the predischarge bilirubin value (represented by the *shaded area*). **A,** Outcome for newborns designated in the high-risk zone (*n* = 172). **B,** outcome of newborns in upper-intermediate-risk zone (*n* = 356). **C,** Outcome of newborns in the lower-intermediate-risk zone (*n* = 556). **D,** Outcome of newborns in the low-risk zone (*n* = 1756). (*From Bhutani VK, et al: Predictive ability of a predischarge hour-specific serum bilirubin for subsequent significant hyperbilirubinemia in healthy term and near-term newborns,* Pediatrics 103:6, 1999.)

indirect-reacting pigment are not recommended, but they may be useful as less expensive methods for screening and frequent repeat determinations, and in emergency situations. The prototype of colorimetric methods is the van den Bergh test, a modification of the Ehrlich diazo reaction. The Jendrassik-Grof method has also been used widely as an automated procedure in many hospital laboratories.

Newer automated methods, such as the Ektachem system, provide greater precision and the ability to measure the covalently bound δ-bilirubin. Compared with the values of direct bilirubin obtained by high-performance liquid chromatography, the Jendrassik-Grof and other diazo methods exaggerate this fraction to variable degrees. These older, nonspecific diazo reaction methods also fail to measure the δ-bilirubin fraction, underestimating total bilirubin by 0.2 to 0.3 mg/dL (3 to 5 μmol/L) in the normal adult. High-performance liquid chromatography probably provides the most accurate measurement of TB but is impractical for routine clinical laboratory use. The Ektachem method has

gained wide acceptance. It uses a dry film system for measurement of TB and subfractions (indirect, direct, and δ) for general clinical laboratory use. The adult upper limit of normal for TB by this method is 1.3 mg/dL (22 μmol/L), and for the conjugated fraction, 0.3 mg/dL (5 μmol/L), of which two thirds is in the form of δ-bilirubin. For newborns younger than 2 weeks, a simpler and less expensive single-film method can be used, omitting measurement of δ-bilirubin, which is not found in this age group.

High levels of direct-reacting bilirubin reflect a different set of pathologic entities that do not respond to the usual interventions for unconjugated hyperbilirubinemia and will be considered later in this chapter. It is useful to consider four groups of newborns when making decisions regarding laboratory evaluation and therapy of unconjugated hyperbilirubinemia: (1) healthy term (more than 37 completed gestational weeks); (2) sick term; (3) healthy premature; and (4) sick premature neonates. Studies to date have dealt almost exclusively with the healthy term newborn. Although unconjugated hyperbilirubinemia is a disease of multiple causes, and neonates should be treated differently on the basis of gestational age and relative state of health, some general comments can be made.

Further laboratory investigation should be considered when TB concentrations are (1) 4 mg/dL (68 μmol/L) or greater in cord blood; (2) increasing at a rate of 0.5 mg/dL (9 μmol/L) or greater per hour over a 4- to 8-hour period; (3) increasing at a rate of 5 mg/dL (86 μmol/L) or greater per day; (4) 13 to 15 mg/dL (222 to 257 μmol/L) or greater in full-term infants at any time; (5) 10 mg/dL (171 μmol/L) or greater in premature neonates at any time; or (6) when clinical jaundice persists beyond 10 to 14 days of life.

Further diagnostic studies should be based on a thorough history and physical examination, which can narrow the differential diagnosis. A careful history from the parents may reveal familial patterns of neonatal hyperbilirubinemia or anemia or ethnic patterns associated with severe neonatal jaundice. Observation of the parents for jaundice and even determination of TB concentrations in them also may be useful in the diagnosis of familial types of hemolytic disease or inherited hepatic dysfunction. Patterns of feeding, the time of onset, and the frequency of breast feeding also may be important. A careful physical examination with special attention to liver and spleen size, skin appearance, and neurobehavioral status should be performed in the evaluation of a jaundiced neonate.

Initial studies that may be indicated include determination of maternal blood group and Rh type, a screen for antibodies directed against minor erythrocyte antigens, determination of neonatal blood group and Rh type, direct Coombs or antiglobulin test, hemoglobin or hematocrit, smear of peripheral blood for RBC morphology, and reticulocyte count. In the presence of significant jaundice with a potential ABO incompatibility (type O mother and type A or B infant), the direct Coombs test should be repeated at least once if originally negative because initial false-negative results have often been noted. It should be borne in mind that hematologic indexes indicative of hemolysis in older children and adults may not be useful in the diagnosis of increased hemolysis in neonates, because of overlap in these indexes between hemolytic and nonhemolytic conditions. An elevated ETCOc level may be indicative of ongoing hemolysis, but a suitable, noninvasive, point-of-care technology is not currently available (see "End-Tidal Carbon Monoxide Measurements," later). Determination of erythrocyte G6PD activity may be useful in cases of unexplained hyperbilirubinemia or hyperbilirubinemia not responding to intense phototherapy. Consideration of the family's ethnic group may be useful in deciding whether to perform a G6PD test. Cord blood should be saved in the event further testing is indicated.

More extensive studies for rarer forms of hemolytic disease and enzyme assays or genetic testing for UGT activity may be deferred until the chronicity of the disease has been established. Studies for hepatocellular disease (such as hepatitis and obstructive biliary disease), including serum glutamic-oxaloacetic transaminase and serum glutamic-pyruvic transaminase, alkaline phosphatase, and cholesterol, need to be performed only when there is a significant elevation of conjugated bilirubin or liver disease.

Until a laboratory method is proved to accurately assess the risk for developing BIND, the need for treatment,

and the progression from phototherapy to exchange transfusion must be based on clinical judgment. Factors that will influence the use of therapeutic modalities available are based on the maturational state of the infant, the severity of the associated pathophysiologic process, and the presence of increased hemolysis, in conjunction with evaluation TB concentrations. The method of management chosen for an individual neonate is determined in part by the TB concentration at which therapy is instituted. The 2004 guideline of the AAP has formulated an established and uniform policy regarding the methods to be used and criteria for initiation of therapy.[13] The risk factors for the development of severe hyperbilirubinemia in infants of 35 weeks' gestation or more are listed in Box 48-2.

Another problem in the assessment of any particular TB concentration involves variation within and between laboratories. In a study by Vreman and colleagues, high interlaboratory and interinstrument variations in the measurements of

---

BOX 48-2 **Risk Factors for Development of Severe Hyperbilirubinemia in Infants ≥35 Weeks of Gestation**

MAJOR RISK FACTORS
Predischarge TB or TcB level in the high-risk zone (see Fig. 48-9)
Jaundice observed in the first 24 hours
Blood group incompatibility with positive direct antiglobulin test, other known hemolytic disease (e.g., G6PD deficiency)
Gestational age 35 to 36 weeks
Previous sibling received phototherapy
Cephalohematoma or significant bruising
Exclusive breast feeding, particularly if nursing poorly and weight loss is excessive
East Asian race

MINOR RISK FACTORS
Predischarge TB or TcB in the high intermediate-risk zone
Gestational age 37 to 38 weeks
Jaundice observed before discharge
Previous sibling with jaundice
Macrosomic infant of diabetic mother
Maternal age ≥25 years
Male sex

FACTORS ASSOCIATED WITH DECREASED RISK OF SIGNIFICANT JAUNDICE*
TB or TcB in the low-risk zone (see Fig. 48-9)
Gestational age ≥41 weeks
Exclusive bottle feeding
Black race
Discharge from hospital after 72 hours

*Listed in order of decreasing importance.
G6PD, glucose-6-phosphate dehydrogenase; TcB, transcutaneous bilirubin; TB, total bilirubin.
From American Academy of Pediatrics Subcommittee on Hyperbilirubinemia: Management of hyperbilirubinemia in the newborn infant 35 or more weeks of gestation, *Pediatrics* 114:297, 2004.

TB were reported.[233] They found that imprecision for a particular method or a given laboratory was acceptable, but inaccuracy was highly variable and should be taken into account in the interpretation of all TB measurements. Another factor contributing to these variations is the lack of appropriate bilirubin standards and consistent handling of clinical specimens. All these observations warrant the need for universal standardization of all bilirubin measurements. Lo and coworkers analyzed specimens of TB from the College of American Pathologists (CAP) Neonatal Bilirubin (NB) and Chemistry (C) surveys using the reference method.[133] They found that the use of different methods in the NB and C surveys, together with the presence of nonhuman protein base and ditaurobilirubin in the survey specimens, accounted for wide variations in accuracy and imprecision between instruments and laboratories. Furthermore, they recommend that survey samples should consist only of human serum enriched with unconjugated bilirubin.

The measurement of unbound or "free" bilirubin concentrations is another potential measure to assess the risk for developing bilirubin neuropathy or encephalopathy. Data are limited, but preliminary studies show that unbound bilirubin levels may be better correlated with BIND than the TB.[173,195,249]

TRANSCUTANEOUS BILIRUBINOMETRY

Visual inspection is the most commonly used means of screening newborns for hyperbilirubinemia. Jaundice progresses cephalocaudally. Digital pressure that blanches the skin diminishes the effects of pigmentation and local cutaneous perfusion and allows the detection of jaundice. Proper lighting is important in detecting subtle levels of jaundice. However, visual assessment is subjective, dependent on observer experience and is notoriously inaccurate.

Transcutaneous bilirubinometry (TcB) is a method using reflectance photometry or transcutaneous colorimetry[259,260] as a noninvasive estimate of TB levels.[147] The technique offers an objective measurement of skin color, from which a reading, reflecting the TB, is derived. Two devices, the BiliChek (Philips Childrens Medical Ventures, Monroeville, PA) and JM-103 Jaundice Meter (Konica Minolta/AirShields JM 103 Jaundice Meter, Draeger Medical AG and Co, Lubeck, Germany)[261] are currently commercially available. They differ in their ease of use and their propensity to be affected by variations in skin color. A number of studies have shown that these instruments provide fairly accurate estimates of TB in term and near-term newborn infants of varying races and ethnicities, generally providing values within 2 to 3 mg/dL (34 to 51 μmol/L) of the TB, if the TB is less than 15 mg/dL (257 μmol/L).[25,66,138,187] The technology tends to under-read the actual TB measurement and should be regarded as a screening mechanism rather than an accurate reflection of the TB. The devices have been evaluated as potential predischarge screening tools[138] to identify infants at risk (i.e., TB level at the 95th percentile or higher). As a result of these studies, an age-in-hours-specific nomogram based on TcB measurements has been established and shown to successfully predict the development of hyperbilirubinemia. However, additional studies are warranted to establish a strong and reliable correlation between TcB and TB at levels of 15 mg/dL (257 μmol/L) and higher, as well as during and after phototherapy and in premature or low-birthweight infants, before its routine use can be advocated.

END-TIDAL CARBON MONOXIDE MEASUREMENTS

Because the breakdown of heme by the rate-limiting enzyme HO produces equimolar quantities of CO and biliverdin, which is immediately reduced to bilirubin, the measurement of CO in the end-tidal breath, corrected for ambient CO (ETCOc), of the newborn can be used as an index of in vivo heme degradation and bilirubin production and, hence, hemolysis.[204] A portable device that allowed automatic sampling and bedside analysis of ETCOc yielded results comparable to gas chromatography and was used to accurately estimate COHb levels in neonates, children, and adults (see Chapter 31).[234] Unfortunately, this device is not currently available.

In a large multicenter study, Stevenson and colleagues found that a measurement of ETCOc at 30 ± 6 hours of age, alone or in combination with a TB measurement, did not improve the predictive ability of the age-in-hours-specific TB level, although it was as good as a measurement of TB alone for this purpose.[203] They did find, however, that the use of an ETCOc measurement in combination with the TB level aids in the following: (1) the discrimination between infants with increased bilirubin production rates and infants with decreased elimination; (2) the identification of infants with increased bilirubin production due to ABO incompatibility or other causes of hemolysis; and (3) the identification of infants with impaired conjugation defects, who have a normal ETCOc level with rising TB levels. In other words, high producers of CO and bilirubin are most likely undergoing a hemolytic process, whereas infants with high TB levels and normal bilirubin production rates most likely have a defect in bilirubin conjugation. The measurement of ETCOc could provide direct information of the rate of bilirubin production. Bhutani and coworkers, using data from this study, constructed an age-in-hours-specific ETCOc nomogram for measurements taken between 4 and 48 hours postnatal age, revealing that an ETCOc in the 75th percentile or less at 30 ± 6 hours of age is 1.7 ppm or less and is considered the threshold of increased bilirubin production.[26]

BILIRUBIN-TO-ALBUMIN MOLAR RATIO

The molar ratio of bilirubin (mg/dL) to albumin (g/dL) correlates with unconjugated bilirubin levels in newborns and, therefore, can be used as a surrogate for unbound bilirubin or residual binding capacity of albumin.[5] Sick infants have an impaired albumin binding of bilirubin and can have ratios of 0.7, and it is recommended that the ratio should not exceed 0.5. In addition, albumin levels and the ability of albumin to bind bilirubin vary significantly in sick infants. It has also been shown that binding increases with increasing gestational and postnatal age. The bilirubin-to-albumin molar ratio (BAMR) may be used as an adjunct to measurements of TB in determining the need for exchange transfusion (Table 48-2).

Therapy for Unconjugated Hyperbilirubinemia

After it has been determined that a patient is at risk for the sequelae of unconjugated hyperbilirubinemia, prompt therapy should be instituted. The current mainstay of treatment is phototherapy, which has been proved to be instrumental in containing the rate of rise of TB and lowering the TB. In cases of failure of phototherapy, or in newborns presenting with

TABLE 48–2   Bilirubin-to-Albumin Molar Ratio (BAMR) as a Determinant of the Need for Exchange Transfusion

Risk Category	BAMR AT WHICH EXCHANGE TRANSFUSION SHOULD BE CONSIDERED	
	TB (mg/dL)/Albumin (g/dL)	TB (μmol/L)/Albumin (μmol/L)
Infants ≥38⁰/₇ wk	8.0	0.94
Infant 35⁰/₇ to 37⁶/₇ wk and well or ≥38⁰/₇ wk if higher risk or isoimmune hemolytic disease or G6PD deficiency	7.2	0.84
Infant 35⁰/₇ to 37⁶/₇ wk if higher risk or isoimmune hemolytic disease or G6PD deficiency	6.8	0.80

If TB is at or is approaching the exchange level, send blood for immediate type and crossmatch. Blood for exchange transfusion is modified whole blood (red blood cells and plasma) crossmatched against the mother and compatible with the infant.
G6PD, glucose-6-phosphate dehydrogenase; TB, total bilirubin.
From American Academy of Pediatrics Subcommittee on Hyperbilirubinemia: Management of hyperbilirubinemia in the newborn infant 35 or more weeks of gestation, *Pediatrics* 114:297, 2004.

extremely high TB concentrations, exchange transfusion will definitively lower the TB to a level that will no longer be of danger to the neonate. Intravenous immunoglobulin (IVIG) and phenobarbital therapy also have a role in the management of hyperbilirubinemia. The intensity and invasiveness of therapy are determined by the many factors discussed thus far, including the gestational age and relative health of the neonate, the current level of TB, and an estimation of the rate of rise in view of the dynamic nature of bilirubin metabolism in the newborn. An example of a clinical pathway for the management of the newborn infant readmitted for phototherapy or exchange transfusion is given in Box 48-3.

BOX 48–3   Examples of a Clinical Pathway for the Management of the Newborn Infant Readmitted for Phototherapy or Exchange Transfusion

TREATMENT
Use intensive phototherapy and/or exchange transfusion as indicated in Figs. 48-21 and 48-22.

LABORATORY TESTS
TB and direct bilirubin level
Blood type (ABO, Rh)
Direct antibody test (Coombs test)
Serum albumin
CBC with differential and peripheral blood smear for RBC morphology
Reticulocyte count
ETCOc (if technology is available)
G6PD screen, if indicated by ethnicity or geographic origin or if poor response to phototherapy
Urinalysis for reducing substances
If history or presentation suggests sepsis, perform blood culture, urine culture, and CSF examination for protein, glucose, cell count, and culture.

INTERVENTIONS
If TB ≥25 mg/dL (428 μmol/L) or ≥20 mg/dL (342 μmol/L) in a sick infant or infant <38 weeks' gestation, obtain a type and crossmatch, and request blood in case exchange transfusion becomes necessary.

In infants with isoimmune hemolytic disease and a TB rising despite intensive phototherapy or rising to within 2 to 3 mg/dL (34 to 51 μmol/dL) of exchange level (see Fig. 48-22), administer IVIG (500 to 1000 mg/kg) over 2 hours and repeat if necessary.
If infant's weight loss from birth is greater than 12% or there is clinical or biochemical evidence of dehydration, recommend formula or expressed breast milk. If oral intake in question, give IV fluids.

FOR INFANTS RECEIVING INTENSIVE PHOTOTHERAPY
Breastfeed or bottle-feed (formula or expressed breast milk) every 2 to 3 hours.
If TB ≥25 mg/dL (428 μmol/L), repeat TB within 2 to 3 hours.
If TB 20 to 25 mg/dL (342 to 428 μmol/L), repeat TB within 3 to 4 hours.
If TB <20 mg/dL (342 μmol/L), repeat TB in 4 to 6 hours.
If TB continues to fall, repeat TB in 8 to 12 hours.
If TB is not decreasing, or is moving closer to level for exchange transfusion, or the TB-to-albumin ratio exceeds levels shown in Table 48-2, consider exchange transfusion.
When TB is below 13 to 14 mg/dL (222 to 239 μmol/L), discontinue phototherapy.
Depending on the cause of the hyperbilirubinemia, it is an option to measure TB **24 hours** after discharge to check for rebound hyperbilirubinemia (see text).

CBC, complete blood count; CSF, cerebral spinal fluid; ETCOc, end-tidal carbon monoxide, corrected for inhaled CO; G6PD, glucose-6-phosphate dehydrogenase; IV, intravenous; IVIG, intravenous immunoglobulin; RBC, red blood cell; TB, total bilirubin.
From American Academy of Pediatrics Subcommittee on Hyperbilirubinemia: Management of hyperbilirubinemia in the newborn infant 35 or more weeks of gestation, *Pediatrics* 114:297, 2004.

PHOTOTHERAPY

Phototherapy is the most widely used form of therapy for the treatment and prophylaxis of neonatal unconjugated hyperbilirubinemia. In nearly all neonates, phototherapy reduces or blunts the rise of TB concentrations (regardless of maturity, the presence or absence of hemolysis, and the degree of skin pigmentation). Given the decades of experience with its use worldwide and the lack of reported serious long-term side effects thus far, short-term phototherapy appears to be safe. The initial report from the Collaborative Study on the Effectiveness and Safety of Phototherapy, undertaken under the auspices of the National Institute of Child Health and Human Development (NICHD), demonstrated that neonates receiving phototherapy require significantly fewer exchange transfusions. More important, these infants had an incidence of gross kernicterus and subsequent neurobehavioral performance that was lower than those who received only exchange transfusions to control hyperbilirubinemia. Furthermore, subsequent follow-up studies revealed no adverse outcome in the infants who received phototherapy in the neonatal period.[36,148,190]

Mechanism of Action

Three independent mechanisms have been proposed to explain the action of phototherapy in reducing TB concentrations in neonates (Fig. 48-16).[257] The first and most important pathway is geometric photoisomerization of the native unconjugated bilirubin IX-α (Fig. 48-17). Unconjugated bilirubin IX-α is normally in the 4Z,15Z configuration. In this form, the −COOH group of each carboxymethyl side chain interacts through three hydrogen bonds with the C=O and N-H group of the pyrrole rings in the opposite half-molecule. As a result, ionization of the two −COOH and two keto groups is inhibited, making the molecule nonpolar and water insoluble. When illuminated by wavelengths (peak, 460 ± 10 nm), light is absorbed by bilirubin and unconjugated bilirubin undergoes Z-to-E (configurational) isomerization at either one or both of the bridge double bonds to yield potentially three isomers: 4E,15Z; 4Z,15E; and 4E,15E. The E configuration spatially precludes hydrogen bonding of the molecule, which therefore remains open or unfolded and free

to ionize. Thus, the E isomer is more polar and soluble than the Z isomer. Because the liver can transport only soluble bilirubin into bile, the E isomers can be excreted without the need for conjugation.

At least two pairs of geometric photoisomers have been identified in vivo. The first pair, photoisomers IA and IB, is presumably the two possible E,Z isomers. The second pair, photobilirubins IIA and IIB, is most likely two rotamers of the 4E,15E isomer. Both pairs are presumably formed rapidly in the skin, subcutaneous tissue, and capillaries. Being more polar, all these isomers partition into the plasma, continuously shifting the equilibrium to promote more isomer formation. These isomers are rapidly taken up by the liver and transported into bile. These photoisomers are destabilized by bile acids, rapidly reverting to native unconjugated bilirubin IX-α in the bile ducts and intestine. The rotameric isomers remain mostly intact and are the major polar photoproducts found in bile. This photoisomerization pathway may be responsible for more than 80% of the augmented bilirubin elimination during phototherapy. Geometric photoisomerization is not, however, the only isomerization pathway open to photoexcited bilirubin. The proximity of the side-chain double bond at C-3 to the adjacent pyrrole ring allows an intramolecular cyclization, again rendering the bilirubin molecule more polar (see Fig. 48-17B). This structural isomer of bilirubin is called *lumirubin*, and it is also excreted into bile without need for hepatic conjugation. Lumirubin, a soluble compound, is the major photoproduct excreted with the bile and urine, and its conversion is the rate-limiting step in the elimination of bilirubin by phototherapy.

The third pathway of phototherapy involves a variety of bilirubin oxidation reactions, resulting from an autosensitized reaction involving singlet oxygen. The products formed by these reactions are multiple but include biliverdin, dipyrroles, and monopyrroles. Many of these products are colorless, nonreactive in the van den Bergh test, and presumably excreted by the liver and kidney without need for conjugation. Compared with the photoisomerization pathway, the oxidation mechanism appears to play a very minor role in photocatabolism of unconjugated bilirubin in vivo (Fig. 48-18).[131,238]

Figure 48-16. General mechanism of phototherapy for neonatal jaundice. *Solid arrows* represent chemical reactions; *broken arrows* represent transport process. Pigments may be bound to proteins in compartments other than blood. Some excretion of photoisomers in urine also occurs. B, bilirubin (Z,Z isomer); LR, lumirubin (E and Z isomers); OxB, bilirubin oxidation products; PB, photobilirubin. (*Modified from McDonagh AF, Lightner DA: "Like a shrivelled blood orange": bilirubin, jaundice, and phototherapy, Pediatrics 75:443, 1985. Used with permission of the American Academy of Pediatrics.*)

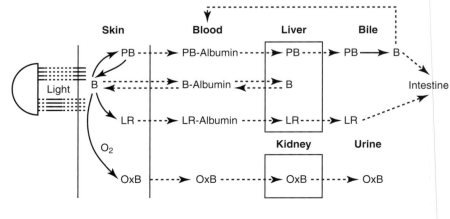

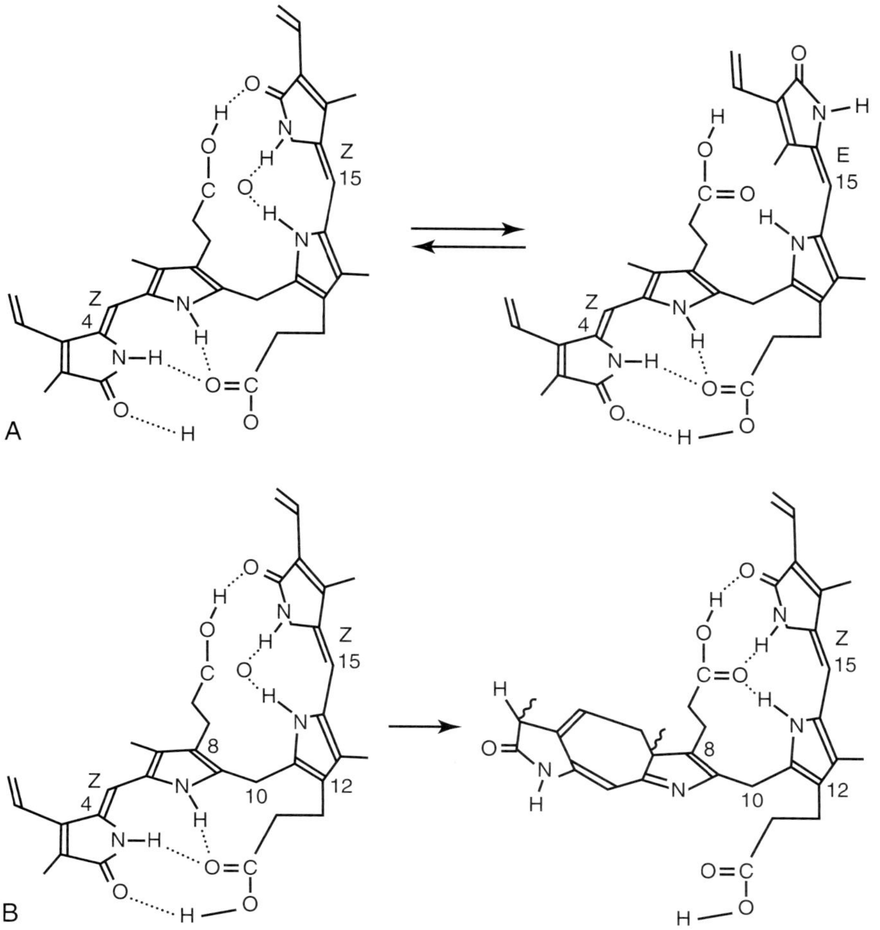

A

Figure 48–17. Isomerization pathways for bilirubin during phototherapy. **A,** Z-E carbon double-bond configurational isomerization of bilirubin. **B,** Intramolecular cyclization of bilirubin to form lumirubin. (*Modified from McDonagh AF, Lightner DA: "Like a shrivelled blood orange": bilirubin, jaundice, and phototherapy,* Pediatrics *75:443, 1985. Used with permission of the American Academy of Pediatrics.*)

B

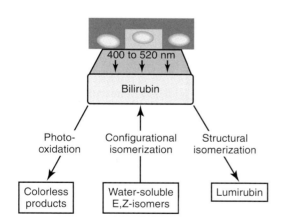

Figure 48–18. The major mechanisms of bilirubin photoalteration. (*Redrawn from Vreman HJ, et al: Light emitting diodes for phototherapy for the control of jaundice. In Holick M editor:* Biology of light 2001, *Proceedings of a Symposium. Boston, 2002, Kluwer Academic, pp 355-367.*)

Technique

Phototherapy is not a standardized practice in the United States at this time, and there exist many different devices capable of delivering phototherapy with varying efficacies. Any physician using one of these devices must be cognizant

of the variables influencing the efficacy of phototherapy and ensure that the device is used appropriately.

The first variable to consider is the wavelength of light used to induce photoisomerization (Fig. 48-19). Bilirubin absorbs light maximally in the blue range (340 to 540 nm), with peak absorption for albumin-bound bilirubin at about 460 nm and for unbound bilirubin at about 440 nm. Daylight and cool white lamps have a spectral emission of 380 to 720 nm with a peak of 578 ± 10 nm and are less effective than blue lamps (F20 T12/B), which have a narrower spectral range and peak between 420 and 480 nm. Special blue lamps (F20 T12/BB and TL52 tubes [Philips, The Netherlands]) emit narrower spectra of light with greater irradiance at the main therapeutic spectrum and have been shown to be most effective. The blue hue that is produced by these lamps can interfere with skin color assessment in jaundiced neonates, and it has been reported to produce dizziness and nausea variably in those caring for these patients. These side effects may be readily tempered by the addition of daylight fluorescent lamps to the phototherapy unit.[54,68] However, incorporation of white fluorescence "dilutes" the blue intensity, thereby dramatically decreasing the effectiveness of phototherapy.[238]

Several studies showed that phototherapy with green light (peak at 525 nm) is as effective as that with blue light and better than white light in reducing bilirubin concentrations. Green light lacks the untoward side effects often

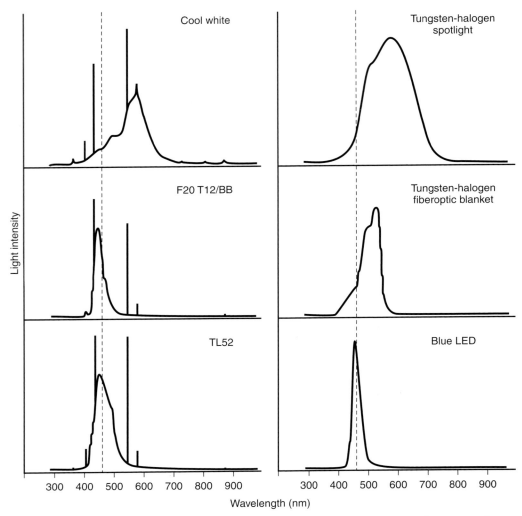

Figure 48–19. Emission spectra of phototherapy devices. The intensities are shown on a linear relative scale. The spectra of the three fluorescent lamps (cool white, and special blue [F20 T12/BB and TL52]), tungsten-halogen (spotlight [Olympic Medical Mini-Bililite, Seattle, WA] and fiberoptic blanket [Biliblanket, Ohmeda, Columbia, OH]), and blue light-emitting diodes (LEDs [neoBLUE, Natus Medical, Inc., San Carlos, CA]) were measured under identical conditions on an S-2000 spectrophotometer (Ocean Optics, Inc., Dunedin, FL). *Dotted line* represents the peak absorption of bilirubin at about 460 nm. *(From Vreman HJ, et al: In vitro efficacy of an LED-based phototherapy device [neoBLUE] compared to traditional light sources, Pediatr Res 53:400A, 2003.)*

associated with intense blue light. However, further study is needed to definitively determine the clinical benefit of green light because green light phototherapy has not been widely adopted.[18,228]

The second variable that influences the efficacy of phototherapy is energy output or irradiance as measured in units of microwatts per square centimeter per nanometer ($\mu W/cm^2/nm$). Effective phototherapy must provide irradiance well above the levels that have been determined to be minimally effective in producing bilirubin degradation while not exceeding levels beyond which no significant increases in response are evident. This also helps avoid potential side effects such as elevation in body temperature. A standard phototherapy unit operating under optimal conditions would provide clinically significant, but minimally effective,

levels of phototherapy (about 6 to 12 $\mu W/cm^2/nm$). In intensive phototherapy, irradiance is increased to 25 $\mu W/cm^2/nm$ or greater. The BiliBed Phototherapy Unit (Medela, Inc., McHenry, IL) can deliver up to 60 $\mu W/cm^2/nm$.

Standard phototherapy lamps are normally positioned within 40 cm from the infant, but should more intensive phototherapy be required, the lamps may be placed within 15 to 20 cm of the patient, provided fluorescent lamps, and not heat-producing halogen lamps with a potential danger of causing thermal injury, are used. Conversely, increasing the distance from the lamp to the skin surface of the neonate results in a theoretical diminution of light energy by a factor equal to the square of the increase in the distance (Fig. 48-20).[139]

The greater the surface area of the newborn exposed, the greater will be the effectiveness of phototherapy. Skin

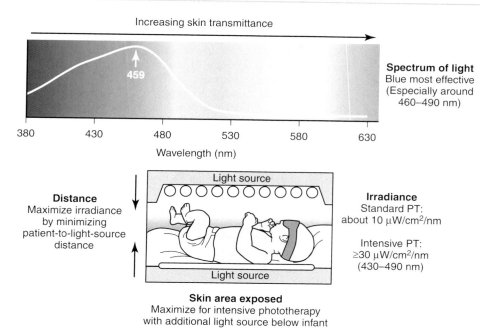

Figure 48-20. See color insert. Important factors in the efficacy of phototherapy (PT). The absorbance spectrum of bilirubin bound to human serum albumin (*white line*) is shown superimposed on the spectrum of visible light. Clearly, blue light is most effective for phototherapy, but because the transmittance of skin increases with increasing wavelength, the best wavelengths to use are probably in the range of 460 to 490 nm. Term and near-term infants should be treated in a bassinet, not an incubator, to allow the light source to be brought to within 10 to 15 cm of the infant (except when halogen or tungsten lights are used), increasing irradiance and efficacy. For intensive phototherapy, an auxiliary light source (fiberoptic pad, light-emitting diode [LED] mattress, or special blue fluorescent tubes) can be placed below the infant or bassinet. If the infant is in an incubator, the light rays should be perpendicular to the surface of the incubator in order to minimize loss of efficacy due to reflectance. (*From Maisels MJ, McDonagh AF: Phototherapy for neonatal jaundice,* N Engl J Med *358:920, 2008.*)

pigmentation does not reduce the effectiveness of phototherapy. With use, fluorescent lamp energy output declines to a degree that varies from one type of lamp to another. A meter for monitoring lamp energy output should be used routinely during treatment to ensure optimal treatment. Although commercially available photometers have been found to vary in their absolute measurement of irradiance because of differences in meter sensitivity (i.e., peak and range) and the emission characteristics of their light sources, they are still useful in determining relative lamp decay. Lamps that have lost more than 20% of the acceptable output should be replaced.

All lamps should be housed behind Plexiglas to reduce the danger to the patient should a lamp explode. Also, it has been shown that Plexiglas provides protection from any harmful ultraviolet irradiation arising from the available light sources. Patients may be cared for on an open warmer or in a crib. Use of a closed incubator may increase the distance of the light source from the infant, thereby attenuating the irradiance delivered to the patient.

The third variable affecting the efficacy of phototherapy is the body surface area of the neonate exposed to light. Ideally, neonates should be naked when under phototherapy; however,

use of diapers, folded back to cover as little of the baby's surface as practically possible, may improve on the obvious disadvantages of leaving the infant unclothed. Positioning of several phototherapy units around the newborn, or placing the baby on a phototherapy mattress in addition to the overhead lights, may increase exposure. A white sheet draped around the periphery of the bed may also act to reflect light onto relatively underexposed areas, thereby increasing the overall light irradiance.

Other conventionally used devices incorporate tungsten-halogen lamps as their light source for use as spotlights. Another technique involves transmission of light through a fiberoptic bundle to a pad or blanket around the infant.[77] The advantage of the latter technology is that the source of light, and therefore heat, will be at a distance from the infant. In infants with severe hyperbilirubinemia, the previously mentioned techniques can be used in combination to increase light intensity (irradiance) and body surface area exposure.[3,67] Too frequently, currently used doses of phototherapy are well below the optimal therapeutic range.[210] The AAP recommends the use of intensive phototherapy, especially for infants readmitted for hyperbilirubinemia, or if the threshold for exchange transfusion is approaching. Intensive phototherapy implies the use of high levels of irradiance in the therapeutic range (usually ≥30 µW/cm²/nm) delivered to as much of the infant's surface area as possible.

Another method of delivering light has been introduced. It involves the use of arrays of blue light-emitting diodes (LEDs), which can deliver high-intensity narrow band light in the absorption spectrum of bilirubin.[235,238] This technology has been incorporated into a new phototherapy device (neoBLUE, Natus Medical, Inc., San Carlos, CA) and shown to be an effective and safe alternative to other modes of phototherapy.[191,238] An LED light source is now also available as a mattress in addition to overhead lights. Advantages of the LED technology include the ability to increase the light intensity to a level higher than many conventional technologies without significantly warming the baby, and the long period during which the lamps remain effective without the need for replacement.

Clinical studies comparing intermittent to continuous phototherapy have yielded conflicting results. Several studies failed to show effectiveness of the intermittent therapy. These results may have resulted from prolonged light-on and light-off cycles—for example, 6- to 12-hour on-off schedules. Photoisomerization of bilirubin occurs primarily in skin layers, and the restoration of the bilirubin pool in the skin takes about 1 to 3 hours. Thus, a prolonged on-off schedule may not be as effective as continuous therapy, but an on-off cycle of less than 1 hour is apparently as effective as continuous treatment. Phototherapy lights should be shut off and eye patches removed during feeding and family visiting for up to 1 hour because this does not significantly reduce phototherapy effectiveness.

Some reports have demonstrated that home phototherapy may be an effective and safe alternative to prolonged hospitalization for healthy full-term neonates with jaundice. Clear advantages of home-centered phototherapy include (1) reduced cost; (2) avoidance of parent-infant separation; and (3) parental satisfaction.[95,183] However, complications of home phototherapy that might result from inadequate nursing supervision include corneal abrasion, eye patch misuse, excessive weight loss, temperature derangement, and ineffective bilirubin reduction. Whether there is any valid indication for phototherapy for those neonates who could be safely managed at home is questionable. Those with valid indications are generally too sick, too small, or too close to the exchange transfusion level to be safely treated at home. The Committee on the Fetus and Newborn (COFN)of the AAP has not endorsed home phototherapy, but it has issued a strict guideline for its use.[11] Because the devices available for home phototherapy may not provide the same degree of irradiance or surface-area exposure as those available in hospital, the Subcommittee on Hyperbilirubinemia of the AAP recommends that home phototherapy should be used only in infants whose bilirubin levels are in the "optional phototherapy" range (see "Indications," below).[13] It is not appropriate for infants with higher bilirubin concentrations or if the TB is approaching the exchange transfusion level. As with hospitalized infants, the TB must be monitored regularly.

Indications

Although not "evidence based," the AAP has issued a comprehensive guideline for the commencement of phototherapy in infants older than 35 weeks' gestation (Fig. 48-21). These guidelines take into account the presence of risk factors as well as prematurity, and also are adapted to the dynamic changes in TB concentrations during the first days of life. Thus, there is no single TB concentration at which phototherapy should be commenced, but each newborn must be assessed individually, taking into consideration postnatal age, gestational age, and other risk factors, enumerated in the legend of Figure 48-21. The TB level at which phototherapy may be discontinued must also be decided in view of these factors. It may be useful to continue plotting the TB concentrations of the hour-specific bilirubin nomogram during phototherapy, and discontinue phototherapy once the TB has decreased below the 75th percentile for hours-of-life, or even closer to the 40th percentile in infants with lower gestational age or in the presence of risk factors. Follow-up for rebound, not necessarily requiring continued hospitalization, should be performed in cases of newborns younger than 37 weeks' gestation, those with positive DAT, and those treated at or before 72 hours' postnatal age.[117]

The AAP guideline does not extend to premature infants younger than 35 weeks' gestational age. However, Maisels and Watchko have suggested therapeutic guidelines for these newborns, both by gestational age and by birthweight (Tables 48-3 and 48-4).[141] Recently published NICE guidelines provide a graph incorporating indications for phototherapy and exchange transfusion for each week of gestational age. (Available at http://www.nice.org.uk/CG98.)

Complications

Several potential complications may occur with the use of phototherapy.[184] The effect of high-intensity light exposure on the eyes of human neonates is uncertain, but animal studies indicate that retinal degeneration may occur after several days of continuous exposure. It is essential therefore that the eyes of all newborns exposed to phototherapy be covered with sufficient layers of opaque material to guard against the possibility of damage. The use of fiberoptic phototherapy does not eliminate the need to cover the patient's eyes.

Phototherapy may produce an increase in body and environmental temperature. Fluid balance, especially in the premature neonate, is a key management issue in the patient being treated with phototherapy. There is increased insensible and intestinal water loss during phototherapy, which must be compensated for by an increase of about 25% above the estimated fluid need without phototherapy. In addition, stools may be slightly looser and more frequent.[21] Fiberoptic phototherapy appears to result in lower insensible water losses and therefore slightly less need for increased maintenance fluids (see Chapter 36). LED-based devices, however, do not release a significant amount of heat, and their use results in less insensible water loss. Term infants treated with LED light in open cribs should have their body temperatures monitored to detect excessive body cooling.

A well-recognized side effect of phototherapy is the *bronze baby syndrome*. In this disorder, the serum, urine, and skin become brown-black (bronze) several hours or more after a neonate is placed under the phototherapy lamps. All reported neonates with this syndrome have recovered without apparent sequelae, except one term neonate who died and was found to have kernicterus on autopsy. In nearly all patients, conjugated hyperbilirubinemia and retention of bile acids have been noted either before light exposure or

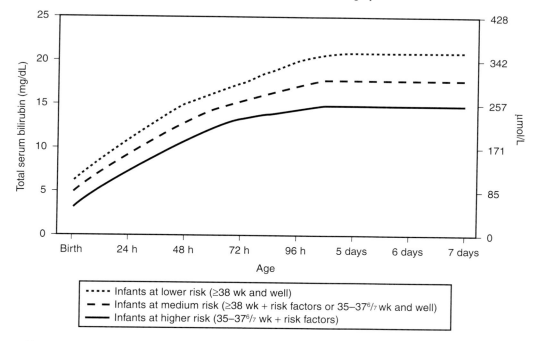

GUIDELINES FOR PHOTOTHERAPY IN HOSPITALIZED INFANTS ≥35 WEEKS
Note: These guidelines are based on limited evidence and the levels shown are approximations. The guidelines refer to the use of intensive phototherapy which should be used when the TSB exceeds the line indicated for each category.

····· Infants at lower risk (≥38 wk and well)
— — Infants at medium risk (≥38 wk + risk factors or 35–37⁶/₇ wk and well)
—— Infants at higher risk (35–37⁶/₇ wk + risk factors)

- Use total bilirubin. Do not subtract direct reacting or conjugated bilirubin.
- Risk factors = isoimmune hemolytic disease. G6PD deficiency, asphyxia, significant lethargy, temperature instability, sepsis, acidosis, or albumin <3.0 g/dL (if measured).
- For well infants 35–37⁶/₇ wk can adjust TSB levels for intervention around the medium risk line. It is an option to intervene at lower TSB levels for infants closer to 35 wk and at higher TSB levels for those closer to 37⁶/₇ wk.
- It is an option to provide conventional phototherapy in hospital or at home at TSB levels 2–3 mg/dL (35–50 μmol/L) below those shown but home phototherapy should not be used in any infant with risk factors.

Figure 48–21. Guidelines for phototherapy in hospitalized infants aged ≥35 weeks of gestation. Infants are designated as higher risk because of the potential negative effects of the conditions listed on albumin binding of bilirubin, the blood-brain barrier, and the susceptibility of the brain cells to damage by bilirubin. (*Adapted from American Academy of Pediatrics Subcommittee on Hyperbilirubinemia: Management of hyperbilirubinemia in the newborn infant 35 or more weeks of gestation,* Pediatrics *114:297, 2004. Used with permission of the American Academy of Pediatrics.*)

after the syndrome has developed. This syndrome has been reproduced in Gunn rats when their smaller bile ducts become obstructed by precipitated bile pigment during phototherapy. Photobilirubin II is shown to be degraded to brown pigments in vitro and when administered to Gunn rats in vivo. It seems likely that the bronze color of the plasma and urine in bronze baby syndrome results from retention of bile pigment photoproducts when their biliary excretion is impaired by concomitant cholestasis. A study in two infants with this syndrome showed an increase in coproporphyrin in the blood, and photoirradiation of this substance produced copper coproporphyrin degradation products similar to those found in neonates with this syndrome. It is generally recommended that phototherapy not be used in neonates with significant conjugated hyperbilirubinemia or other evidence of cholestasis. However, because there have been case reports of newborns who developed kernicterus in the presence of predominantly direct hyperbilirubinemia,

the role of conjugated bilirubin in the pathophysiology of bilirubin encephalopathy is not clear, and affected infants should be assessed for the need for phototherapy on an individual basis.[89]

Congenital erythropoietic porphyria is another syndrome in which phototherapy is contraindicated because it may lead to death. This rare disorder is characterized by hemolysis, splenomegaly, and pink to red urine that fluoresces orange under ultraviolet light. Exposure to visible light of moderate to high intensity and of wavelengths between 400 and 500 nm (blue) produces severe bullous lesions on the exposed skin and accelerated hemolysis. Mixed hyperbilirubinemia with a significant direct-reacting fraction may also be seen in this disease.

Other theoretical dangers of phototherapy include electrical shock or fire from poorly grounded or defective equipment and unproven potential long-term effects on endocrine and sexual maturation and DNA repair mechanisms in skin

TABLE 48-3 Guidelines for the Use of Phototherapy and Exchange Transfusion in Low-Birthweight Infants Based on the Birthweight

Birthweight	TOTAL BILIRUBIN LEVEL, mg/dL (μmol/L)*	
	Phototherapy†	*Exchange Transfusion‡*
≤1500	5-8 (85 to 140)	13-16 (220-275)
1500-1999	8-12 (140 to 200)	16-18 (275-300)
2000-2499	11-14 (190 to 240)	18-20 (300-340)

Note that these guidelines reflect ranges used in neonatal intensive care units. They cannot take into account all possible situations. Lower bilirubin concentrations should be used for infants who are sick—for example, presence of sepsis, acidosis, hypoalbuminemia—or have hemolytic disease.
*Consider initiating treatment at these levels. Range allows discretion based on clinical conditions or other circumstances. Note that bilirubin levels refer to total serum/plasma bilirubin concentrations. Direct reacting or conjugated bilirubin levels should not be subtracted from the total.
†Used at these levels and in therapeutic doses, phototherapy should, with few exceptions, eliminate the need for exchange transfusions.
‡Levels for exchange transfusion assume that bilirubin continues to rise or remains at these levels despite intensive phototherapy.
From Maisels MJ: Jaundice. In Avery GB, et al, editors: *Neonatology: pathophysiology and management of the newborn*, 5th ed, Philadelphia, 1999, Lippincott Williams & Wilkins, p 765.

TABLE 48-4 Guidelines for the Use of Phototherapy and Exchange Transfusion in Preterm Infants Based on the Gestational Age

Gestational Age (wk)	TOTAL BILIRUBIN LEVEL, mg/dL (μmol/L)*		
	Phototherapy	Exchange Transfusion	
		*Sick**	*Well*
36	14.6 (250)	17.5 (300)	20.5 (350)
32	8.8 (150)	14.6 (250)	17.5 (300)
28	5.8 (100)	11.7 (100)	14.6 (250)
24	4.7 (80)	8.8 (150)	11.7 (200)

*Rhesus disease, perinatal asphyxia, hypoxia, acidosis, hypercapnia.
From Ives NK: Neonatal jaundice. In Rennie JM, Robertson NRC, editors: *Textbook of neonatology*, New York, 1999, Churchill Livingstone, p 714.

epithelial cells. However, follow-up studies of phototherapy-treated premature and full-term neonates have failed to demonstrate any increase in morbidity or mortality ascribed to the appropriate use of phototherapy. A multicenter study to determine whether aggressive phototherapy to prevent neurotoxic effects of bilirubin benefits or harms extremely low-birthweight infants (≤1000 g) has recently been completed.[161] Aggressive phototherapy, compared with conservative phototherapy, significantly reduced the mean peak serum bilirubin level, but the primary outcome, a composite of death or neurodevelopmental impairment, was similar between groups. The rate of neurodevelopmental impairment alone was significantly reduced with aggressive phototherapy, but this reduction have been offset by an increase in mortality among infants weighing 501 to 750 g at birth.

No scientific evidence exists indicating that hydration directly lowers TB levels. On the other hand, dehydration is not known to be beneficial to patients in this context, and therefore all neonates should receive appropriate replacement and maintenance fluids. Conjugated bilirubin is water soluble and eliminated from the body in urine, bile, and stool.

Inasmuch as appropriate hydration maintains adequate urine output, bile flow, and stool excretion, fluid administration indirectly assists in the removal of unconjugated bilirubin. Ideally, this fluid is given enterally to stimulate gastrointestinal tract motility. The use of a milk-protein formula may be considered to inhibit enterohepatic reabsorption of bilirubin, thereby lowering the TB.

PHARMACOLOGIC THERAPY

Phenobarbital

In experimental animals, UGT activity can be increased or induced with administration of phenobarbital, ethanol, chloroquine, antihistamines, heroin, and chlorophenothane (also known as DDT). These substances are not specific for any one enzyme but stimulate many hepatic membrane-bound enzyme systems and hepatic protein synthesis in general. Because of the known and potential toxicity of these agents, only phenobarbital has been used with regularity in humans.[220,243]

After the demonstration that phenobarbital administration to a child with Crigler-Najjar syndrome type II disease reduced TB concentrations, phenobarbital administration to pregnant mothers and their offspring was shown to reduce by about 50%, peak serum TB concentrations caused by physiologic jaundice. Studies in newborn rhesus monkeys have demonstrated that the major effect of this therapy is to increase hepatic UGT activity and the conjugation of bilirubin. It also may enhance hepatic uptake of bilirubin in the newborn. The administration of phenobarbital to newborns at the time jaundice is first observed or even immediately after delivery is much less effective than its administration to the mother during pregnancy for at least 2 weeks before delivery. The drug is much less effective in premature neonates. As a prophylactic measure, it would be necessary therefore to administer phenobarbital to large numbers of pregnant women for prolonged periods during pregnancy because the time of delivery could not be predicted with certainty. Even then, the premature neonates most susceptible to the toxic effects of hyperbilirubinemia would receive little or no beneficial effect.

Phenobarbital is potentially addictive, may lead to excessive sedation of the newborn, and has other potent metabolic effects in addition to those on bilirubin metabolism. For these reasons, its use has not achieved wide application but has been reserved largely for specific high-risk populations. For example, in the unexplained severe hyperbilirubinemia of newborns from the Greek coastal islands, the frequency of kernicterus has been significantly reduced by general administration of phenobarbital to pregnant women during the last trimester. A dosage of 60 mg/day is sufficient for maternal administration and 5 mg/kg per day for neonatal treatment. Similar effects have been observed in full-term Korean newborns. Phenobarbital is also useful in the differentiation of Crigler-Najjar syndromes type I and type II. Combining phenobarbital treatment with phototherapy has no advantage, the effect being no greater than that of phototherapy alone.

Metalloporphyrins

Metalloporphyrins, which are synthetic derivatives of heme, have been shown to be effective competitive inhibitors of HO, the rate-limiting enzyme for the degradation of heme to form bilirubin.[212] Originally proposed by Maines in 1981[135] for use in modulating bilirubin production, these compounds have been extensively studied. The first metalloporphyrin to be evaluated for use in preventing neonatal unconjugated hyperbilirubinemia was tin protoporphyrin (SnPP). Administration of this compound was shown to decrease bilirubin concentrations in newborn rats, rhesus monkeys, and adult rats with hemolytic anemia, and it was the first synthetic heme analogue used for the purpose of inhibiting HO in human neonates.[64] Although highly efficacious, the photoreactivity of this metalloporphyrin made it a less desirable drug.[230,237] Whitington and associates' studies demonstrate that SnPP reduces endogenous bilirubin formation without impairing hepatic uptake, excretion, or enteric resorption of bilirubin.[252] In newborn rhesus monkeys, administration of SnPP produced skin ulcerations, whereas in human neonates who also received phototherapy, some mild erythema of the skin was observed.[53,135,252] Human trials with tin mesoporphyrin (SnMP) in preterm neonates have shown a dose-dependent reduction in peak bilirubin levels irrespective of gestational age, and a reduction in the need for phototherapy compared with controls.[121,122,145,180,221] Mild transient erythema in patients

requiring phototherapy was the only side effect noted.[221] In human studies, it has been shown that a single IM dose of 6 μM SnMP per kilogram body weight eliminates the need for phototherapy during the postnatal period.[145,221] The efficacy of SnMP has been well described by several investigators in patients with Crigler-Najjar syndrome,[76,186] but SnMP does contain a foreign metal, it induces the HO-1 promoter,[61,159,264] and it can inhibit other enzymes such as nitric oxide synthase and soluble guanylyl cyclase.[256] An alternative compound, zinc protoporphyrin (ZnPP), has been proposed, but it has a much lower inhibitory potency and is not well absorbed after oral administration. Nevertheless, it is a naturally occurring metalloporphyrin possessing both in vitro and in vivo inhibition of both HO-1 and HO-2 isozymes in studies using neonatal rodents and nonhuman primates.[230] Moreover, ZnPP is minimally photoreactive in vivo.[231,240] Other metalloporphyrins being evaluated for their safety and efficacy are chromium mesoporphyrin (CrMP) and zinc deuteroporphyrin bis glycol (ZnBG), compounds, which are orally absorbed and are potent heme oxygenase inhibitors.[230,237]

Other Nonmetalloporphyrin Inhibitors

Some nonmetalloporphyrin inhibitors of HO have been identified. Originally designed for use in transplantation survival studies, peptide inhibitors have been reported not only to be immunosuppressive in vitro and in vivo[103] but also to inhibit in vitro HO activity dose dependently. However, in mouse studies, it has been found that administration of peptides may upregulate HO-1 messenger RNA and protein in the liver, spleen, and kidney. These findings have precluded human studies investigating the efficacy of peptides for the treatment of hyperbilirubinemia.

Imidazole dioxolanes, inhibitors of cholesterol production,[41,209,241] have also been found to inhibit in vitro[60,126,229,239] and in vivo[160] HO activity, despite being structurally different from metalloporphyrins. It has been demonstrated that these compounds are highly selective for inhibiting the inducible HO-1, but like metalloporphyrins, some imidazole dioxolanes may affect other important enzymes, such as nitric oxide synthase (NOS) and soluble guanylyl cyclase.[126] One of these compounds, Azalanstat, has been reported to effectively inhibit in vivo HO activity, but does so only at a high dose and also can induce HO-1 gene transcription,[160] thus limiting its clinical use.

Miscellaneous Agents

As already discussed, reabsorption of unconjugated bilirubin may contribute to a significant portion of hepatic bilirubin load in the newborn period. Frequent milk feeding (cow or human) may slow the rise of TB levels and enhance the bilirubin-reducing effect of phototherapy. Oral administration of nonabsorbable substances that bind bilirubin in the intestinal lumen and presumably reduce enteric absorption of bilirubin may reduce peak TB concentrations in physiologic jaundice. Orlistat has been used to increase fecal fat excretion, thereby enhancing bilirubin elimination and decreasing the serum unconjugated bilirubin concentrations in Crigler-Najjar syndrome.[92] Feeding breast-fed newborns β-glucuronidase inhibitors (L-aspartic acid or enzymatically hydrolyzed casein) during the first week reduced jaundice without affecting breast feeding deleteriously.[84] Activated charcoal has been used but is effective only when administered during the first

12 hours of life.[58] Agar has also been shown to be effective.[42,169] Further study of this type of therapy is needed before recommendations can be made regarding clinical applications. These pharmacologic agents may be no more effective than frequent milk feeding (every 2 hours).

Intravenous Immunoglobulin

High-dose IVIG (500 to 1000 mg/kg) administered over 2-4 hours has been shown in several small studies to reduce TB levels and the need for exchange transfusion in fetuses and neonates with Rh and ABO immune hemolytic disease.[128,188] Carboxyhemoglobin studies performed 24 hours after IVIG infusion in DAT-positive ABO-heterospecific neonates have demonstrated that, in those infants who responded to IVIG infusion with a decrease in TB, hemolysis was inhibited compared with the preadministration status. Exchange transfusion was avoided in responding newborns, but not in those in whom there was no response. Lack of response was attributed to higher rates of hemolysis, in which case use of a higher dose of IVIG was suggested.[93] The use of IVIG administration should be considered in neonates with DAT-positive immune hyperbilirubinemia who are not responding to intense phototherapy and whose TB concentration is approaching exchange transfusion indications. This dose can be repeated after 12 hours if necessary. Recommendations for IVIG have been included in the revised AAP Practice Parameter (see Box 48-3).

EXCHANGE TRANSFUSION

See Chapter 46, Part 2.

Exchange transfusion, first described by Diamond and associates,[62,63] is the standard mode of therapy for immediate treatment of hyperbilirubinemia to prevent kernicterus and for correction of anemia in erythroblastosis fetalis. Its use in the past decade has actually been reduced as a result of the use of RhoGAM to prevent Rh isoimmune disease, the application of phototherapy, and more recently, the administration of IVIG in cases of isoimmunity. In infants with severe hyperbilirubinemia due to isoimmunity or other hemolytic conditions, especially G6-PD deficiency, exchange transfusion may the only effective method of adequately reducing TB concentrations.

Objectives

With this technique, the equivalent of two neonatal blood volumes (160 mL/kg of body weight) is replaced in aliquots not to exceed 10% of the total blood volume. This results in the replacement of about 85% of the circulating RBCs.[227] Bilirubin concentrations are usually reduced by 50%. Although the procedure is relatively safe when performed by experienced practitioners in term neonates, it nevertheless carries a risk for both mortality (0.1% to 0.5% in term neonates) and morbidity as well as being time consuming and expensive. The procedure usually takes 1 to 2 hours. Slower exchanges should theoretically increase the quantity of bilirubin removed by permitting equilibration of pigment from tissue, but the differences are too small to justify the increased risk of prolonging the duration of the procedure. The indications for exchange transfusion need to be individualized, taking into account gestational age and severity of illness (Fig. 48-22). During acute hospitalization, exchange is recommended if TB rises to the indicated levels despite intensive phototherapy. For readmitted infants, if TB is above the exchange level, serial TBs should be performed every 2 to 3 hours, and if TB remains at or above levels indicated, exchange is recommended after 6 hours of intensive phototherapy.[13]

Indications

In the past, it was regularly recommended that TB, even in healthy term infants, be kept below 20 mg/dL (342 μmol/L) during the first 28 days of life. This has been questioned, and a growing consensus has developed that levels as high as 25 mg/dL (428 μmol/L) are acceptable for otherwise healthy, full-term, asymptomatic infants with no obvious hemolytic condition. When the exchange level is considered, conjugated bilirubin should not be subtracted from the total. Despite the inability of direct-reacting bilirubin to enter the CNS, it is possible that direct-reacting bilirubin can partially displace unconjugated bilirubin from albumin-binding sites to increase the risk for kernicterus.

In the face of rapidly rising TB concentrations, as may be seen in Rh erythroblastosis or other types of hemolytic disease, the decision to perform the exchange transfusion should anticipate the rise (from previous TB concentrations, hemoglobin concentrations, and reticulocyte count), so that the exchange transfusion is underway by the time the critical level is reached.

The indications for exchange transfusion are based on the infant's TB concentrations in combination with postnatal age, gestational age, and other risk factors, such as isoimmune hemolytic disease, G6PD deficiency, asphyxia, lethargy, temperature instability, sepsis, acidosis, and bilirubin-to-albumin molar ratio (BAMR). In 2004, the AAP published a comprehensive guideline for initiating exchange transfusion for term and near-term neonates.[13] Indications for low-birthweight neonates or those with lower gestational ages than those specified in the AAP guideline have also been published.[141]

In the severely affected erythroblastotic neonate, clinical judgment rather than laboratory data should be used to decide whether the neonate requires immediate exchange transfusion after delivery. In this situation, a partial exchange transfusion using packed RBCs, coupled with reduction in blood volume if venous pressure is elevated, and with measures to ensure adequate ventilation and correction of acidosis and shock, will often be life saving. In most exchange transfusions, fresh whole or reconstituted citrate-phosphate-dextrose–anticoagulated blood should be used. If blood older than 5 days must be used, the pH should be checked and sodium bicarbonate added to correct the pH to 7.1. Full correction to pH 7.4 may result in later excessive rebound alkalosis as the citrate is metabolized. Use of heparinized blood avoids additional osmolar loads and may obviate the need to administer calcium or correct for acidosis but may result in hypoglycemia and markedly increased free fatty acid concentrations (see Chapter 49, Part 2).

Technique

Although there are numerous different combinations of blood components that can be used safely and effectively, there is no single combination or component that is superior.[211] RBCs reconstituted with 5% albumin or fresh frozen

GUIDELINES FOR EXCHANGE TRANSFUSION IN INFANTS ≥35 WEEKS
Note: These guidelines are based on limited evidence and the levels shown are approximations.
During birth hospitalization, exchange transfusion is recommended if TSB rises to these levels
despite intensive phototherapy. For readmitted infants, if TSB is above exchange level, repeat
TSB every 2–3 hours and consider exchange if TSB remains above levels indicated after
intensive phototherapy for 6 hours.

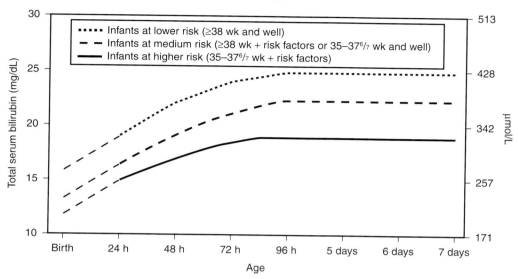

- The dashed lines for the first 24 hours indicate uncertainty due to a wide range of clinical circumstances and a range of responses to phototherapy.
- Immediate exchange transfusion is recommended if infant shows signs of acute bilirubin encephalopathy (hypertonia, arching, retrocollis, opisthotonos, fever, high pitched cry) or if TSB is 25 mg/dL, (85 μmol/L) above these lines.
- Risk factors—isoimmune hemolytic disease, G6PD deficiency, asphyxia, significant lethargy, temperature instability, sepsis, acidosis.
- Measure serum albumin and calculate bilirubin/albumin (B/A) ratio (See legend).
- Use total bilirubin. Do not subtract direct reacting or conjugated bilirubin.
- If infant is well and 35–37⁶/₇ wk (median risk) can individualize TSB levels for exchange based on actual gestational age.

Figure 48–22. Guidelines for exchange transfusion in hospitalized infants aged ≥35 weeks of gestation. Note that these suggested levels represent a consensus of most of the committee but are based on limited evidence and the levels shown are approximations. (*Adapted from American Academy of Pediatrics Subcommittee on Hyperbilirubinemia: Management of hyperbilirubinemia in the newborn infant 35 or more weeks of gestation, Pediatrics 114:297, 2004. Used with permission of the American Academy of Pediatrics.*)

plasma are most frequently used. Mixtures containing a citrate anticoagulant may cause hypocalcemia, but the administration of calcium during the exchange is seldom practiced. Transfused blood should not contain RBC antigens to which the mother has antibodies. Irradiation of blood is recommended for all exchange transfusions, especially if the infant had undergone an intrauterine transfusion, but may be omitted in clinical emergencies.[80] Because the transfused blood is frequently deficient in platelets, the platelet count should be monitored after exchange transfusion, and platelet transfusion should be considered in infants who are severely thrombocytopenic or who have a bleeding tendency.

The administration of salt-poor albumin (1 g/kg) to neonates 1 to 2 hours before exchange transfusion to increase the efficiency of bilirubin removal by shifting more tissue-bound bilirubin into the circulation has been advocated and shown to increase the bilirubin removed by 40%. As the total amount of bilirubin removed during an exchange transfusion

is only a small portion of the total-body pool of bilirubin, this increase may not significantly alter subsequent bilirubin concentrations or the need for additional exchange transfusions. In addition, theoretically, the transient increase in TB concentration after albumin administration could increase, rather than reduce, the risk for kernicterus if there are local phenomena at the brain level that enhance entry of bilirubin into neurons. Finally, constituents of some albumin solutions may act to displace bilirubin from its binding sites, potentially increasing the percentage of free bilirubin present in the plasma. Thus, pretreatment with albumin before exchange transfusion is not routinely recommended.

Complications

The AAP[13] recommends that exchange transfusions be performed only by trained personnel in a neonatal intensive care unit with full monitoring and resuscitation capabilities. Exchange transfusion is an invasive procedure, and complications may be related to the blood transfusion itself, catheter-related complications, and those related to the procedure.[244] The potential complications of exchange transfusion are listed in Box 48-4. Severe hemolysis due to the use of incompatible RBCs may be life-threatening. With modern-day screening for infection, there is only a slight chance of transmission of viral or bacterial infection. Hyperkalemia may result if the transfused blood has been stored for a long period. Rebound hypoglycemia may occur if the glucose load during exchange transfusion is large. Graft-versus-host disease is rare but may occur in premature infants or those who have had in utero transfusions. Umbilical venous catheterization may result in air embolism, hemorrhage, or infection.

Presently, serious complications of exchange transfusion are uncommon. Mortality rates are very low in healthy, term neonates, but are increased for sick or extremely premature infants. In a study of 106 neonates who underwent 140 exchange transfusions between 1980 and 1995, the overall mortality was 2%, but increased to 8% in the subset of infants who were ill.[104] In a smaller series, no serious adverse effects or death occurred among 22 term neonates who had 26 exchange transfusions between 1990 and 1998.[46] In another review of 55 neonates who underwent 66 exchange transfusions between 1992 and 2002,[176] 74% had some form of adverse event, with the most common being thrombocytopenia, hypocalcemia, and metabolic acidosis.

If performed under intensive care facilities and with appropriate expertise, the advantages of performing an exchange transfusion clearly outweigh the potential risk, albeit small, of serious complications. Preparations for emergency situations should be made before initiation of the procedure.

Individualization of Therapeutic Guidelines

The TB level is one of the major criteria to be evaluated when considering the initiation or escalation of treatment for unconjugated hyperbilirubinemia. Although it is believed that it is the unconjugated fraction that presents the danger of kernicterus, the exact ratio of unconjugated and conjugated bilirubin is difficult to assess because its quantitation exhibits

---

BOX 48–4 Potential Complications of Exchange Transfusion

- Thrombocytopenia, particularly with repeat transfusions
- Portal vein thrombosis or other thromboembolic complications
- Umbilical or portal vein perforation
- Acute necrotizing enterocolitis
- Arrhythmia, cardiac arrest
- Hypocalcemia, hypomagnesemia, hypoglycemia
- Respiratory and metabolic acidosis, rebound metabolic alkalosis
- Graft-versus-host disease
- Human immunodeficiency virus, hepatitis B and C infection
- All other potential complications of blood transfusions

---

great variability among laboratories. In view of this, the conjugated bilirubin level should not be subtracted from the TB level unless it constitutes more than 50% of the total. As was stated previously, many variables other than the TB level influence the susceptibility of a particular patient to the sequelae of unconjugated hyperbilirubinemia; these include genotype, gestational age, chronologic age, and the presence of hemolytic or other disease states. Therefore, it is useful to consider four groups of patients at risk for kernicterus and modify treatment on the basis of the category: the healthy term (>37 weeks' estimated gestational age), the sick term, the healthy premature, and the sick premature neonate.

In 1994, the Provisional Committee for Quality Improvement and Subcommittee on Hyperbilirubinemia of the AAP published recommendations for the management of unconjugated hyperbilirubinemia in healthy term neonates.[12] The recommendations were revised in 2004[13] and are detailed in Figures 48-15, 48-21, and 48-22. Whereas the 1994 guidelines did not offer suggestions for the management of newborns with hemolytic conditions, the 2004 guidelines take into account both term and late preterm infants, with and without risk factors. Risk factors to be taken into account for the purpose of deciding whether to institute phototherapy or exchange transfusion include isoimmune hemolytic disease, G6PD deficiency, asphyxia, significant lethargy, temperature instability, sepsis, and acidosis. Jaundice manifesting in the first 24 hours of life is emphasized as an important risk factor, and recommendations for infants with early jaundice are included in the therapeutic guidelines. Therefore, a more conservative approach should be taken to initiating therapy for hyperbilirubinemia (Table 48-5). Similarly, TB levels rising at a rate greater than 0.5 mg/dL per hour (9 μmol/L) or "jumping tracks" on the bilirubin nomogram indicate a state of active hemolysis; such patients should be considered as falling into the "sick," or risk factor, category. It is exceedingly important in these cases to institute and revise therapies on the basis not only of the current level of bilirubin but also of an estimate of the anticipated peak. Thus, early in the patient's course, phototherapy or exchange transfusion may be performed at a relatively lower bilirubin level than for a similar bilirubin level occurring at a later time (see Box 48-3).

Prediction of Hyperbilirubinemia and Postdischarge Follow-up

An examination of the hours-of-life specific bilirubin nomogram will reveal that the TB continues to rise in a steady fashion throughout the first days of life, arriving at its peak at about 4 to 5 days. An infant who is discharged home at or around 48 hours of age will only have started to increase the TB and will reach the peak TB at home. Great responsibility is, therefore, placed on the parents to detect deepening jaundice and to approach the appropriate facilities should hyperbilirubinemia develop. Many cases of kernicterus have developed at home in newborns previously thought to be well and discharged from the newborn nursery as healthy.[28] To assist in discharge planning and in an attempt to detect at least some of the infants with developing hyperbilirubinemia, the AAP[13] has issued guidelines for postdischarge follow-up (Box 48-5). It is recommended that every newborn be seen by a pediatrician within 2 to 3 days of discharge, even those

TABLE 48–5 Guidelines for the Management of Hyperbilirubinemia Based on the Birthweight and Relative Health of the Newborn

| | TOTAL BILIRUBIN LEVEL (mg/dL) | | | |
| | Healthy | | Sick | |
Birthweight	Phototherapy	Exchange Transfusion	Phototherapy	Exchange Transfusion
<1000 g	5-7	Variable	4-6	Variable
1001-1500 g	7-10	Variable	6-8	Variable
1501-2000 g	10-12	Variable	8-10	Variable
2001-2500 g	12-15	Variable	10-12	Variable

BOX 48–5 Postdischarge Follow-up

INFANT DISCHARGED	SHOULD BE SEEN BY:
Before age 24 hr	72 hr
Between age 24 and 47.9 hr	96 hr
Between age 48 and 72 hr	120 hr

From American Academy of Pediatrics Subcommittee on Hyperbilirubinemia: Management of hyperbilirubinemia in the newborn infant 35 or more weeks of gestation, *Pediatrics* 114:297, 2004.

who were not jaundiced at the time of discharge. Clinical judgment should be used when scheduling follow-up, and infants with risk factors for hyperbilirubinemia may be seen earlier than recommended in Box 48-5, as judged clinically necessary.

In a recent update[137a] to the 2004 AAP guidelines, a predischarge measurement of TB or transcutaneous bilirubin is recommended and the risk for hyperbilirubinemia detected on the basis of the infant's age in hours and the bilirubin measurement, which may require readmission to the hospital for treatment. Moreover, all infants should be screened for risk factors when planning for the postdischarge visit.

CONJUGATED HYPERBILIRUBINEMIA

Neonatal jaundice associated with a rise in conjugated bilirubin is indicative of a defect or insufficiency in bile secretion, biliary flow, or both and is always pathologic. It is commonly accompanied by a rise in serum levels of other constituents of bile, such as bile salts and phospholipids. The designation *cholestasis*, meaning reduction in bile flow, is used to describe this group of disorders. The rise of conjugated serum bilirubin may be the result of primary defects in the hepatocellular transport or excretion of bile, or secondary to abnormalities in bile duct function or structure.[17] Sequelae are specific to the many diverse diseases producing this clinical entity, and therefore treatment, when possible, is directed at the underlying disease.

The hepatocellular phase of bile secretion involves the transport of conjugated bilirubin across the hepatic cell membrane at the biliary pole. The lateral cell membrane at this site is folded to form microvilli and becomes part of the canalicular space, surrounded by two or more adjacent hepatocytes. Microvilli and the underlying cytoplasm contain

microfilaments visible by electron microscopy. These structures consist of the contractile protein actin, which is necessary for normal canalicular contraction and microvillous motility, important elements in the generation of intrahepatic bile flow. At the border of the bile canaliculus, hepatocytes are joined in a "tight junction," which under normal circumstances forms an efficient barrier, preventing the contents of the bile canaliculus from entering the perisinusoidal space of Disse or the vascular compartments (Fig. 48-23). The bile

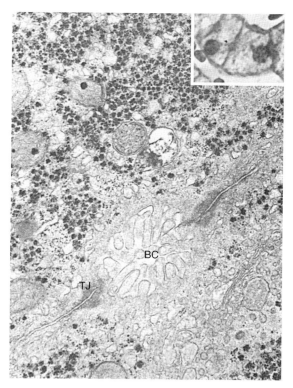

Figure 48–23. Electron micrograph of two adjacent normal hepatocytes. Note the microvillar surface of the bile canaliculus (BC). Tight junctions (TJ) border the canaliculus. *Insert:* A high-power view of two adjacent hepatocytes as seen in the light microscope. In such preparations, bile canaliculi appear as poorly defined condensations of the cell membrane. Eponembedded; ×6000. (*Courtesy of Dr. L. Biempica, Albert Einstein College of Medicine, Bronx, NY.*)

canaliculus is an integral part of hepatocytes. It follows that any hepatocellular injury may result in impairment of the cellular phase of bile excretion and breakdown of the tight junctions, leading to the clinical and laboratory findings of cholestasis.

Hyperbilirubinemia resulting from hepatocellular injury may be associated with other abnormalities that reflect impairment of other hepatocellular functions. These abnormalities include hypoglycemia, fluid retention, and bleeding. On the other hand, injury may selectively impair bile secretion at the biliary pole of hepatocytes, resulting in an isolated laboratory finding of conjugated hyperbilirubinemia. A liver biopsy taken in the early stages of one of the diseases caused by a hepatocellular defect in bile secretion would characteristically show bile pigment granules in hepatocytes and canaliculi, referred to as *intracellular* and *intracanalicular cholestasis*. Bile pigment granules are not seen in either hepatocytes or canaliculi of normal liver parenchyma. In fact, the canalicular lumen is not visualized in routine sections of normal liver parenchyma because it is partially obliterated by microvilli identifiable only by electron microscopy. In cholestasis, there is usually blistering, blunting, or destruction of these microvilli, transforming the bile canaliculus into a widened, round space containing bile (the bile plug). On rare occasions, liver biopsies from patients with conjugated hyperbilirubinemia fail to show any abnormalities when examined with the light microscope.

The ductal phase of bile excretion includes those events that take place in the biliary system distal to the bile canaliculus (Fig. 48-24). The intrahepatic biliary system comprises the bile ductules (the initial portion of which is frequently referred to as the *canals of Hering*); the interlobular (portal) bile ducts, recognized by their constant association with a vein and an arteriole; and the right and left hepatic ducts, which in some individuals may partially extend beyond the liver capsule at the liver hilum. The extrahepatic component includes the common hepatic duct, the cystic duct, the gallbladder, and the common bile duct (choledochus). The extrahepatic biliary system and the major right and left hepatic ducts contain intramural and periductal glandular structures. Although the role of these structures in humans is not clearly understood, information derived from animal experiments suggests they may play an important role in bile duct regeneration or failure to regenerate. This is suggested by the presence of glands or ductules in duct remnants resected during portoenterostomy for biliary atresia (see under specific disorders in the following paragraphs). Most diseases affecting the extrahepatic bile ducts, and occasionally the left and right hepatic ducts, are associated with segmental or diffuse luminal obliteration and are primarily expressions of mechanical disturbance in bile flow.

Diseases involving the intrahepatic ducts, in the absence of concomitant extrahepatic disease, are complex and probably result from a combination of mechanical obstruction to the flow of bile, abnormalities of the biochemical pathways involved in the process of bile secretion, and, in some cases, persistence of infectious agents or viral antigens. In rapidly occurring duct obstruction, dilation of proximal branches is noted. This change may not be present when luminal obliteration is incomplete or when it develops slowly because these cases are frequently complicated by reduction in intrahepatic bile secretion and flow. A constant and characteristic tissue response to complete mechanical obstruction of a major bile duct is dilation and proliferation of proximal portions of the intrahepatic biliary system, including the ductules and canals of Hering, structures that are outside the confines of the portal tracts. A constant accompaniment to bile duct proliferation is an increase in surrounding connective tissue, which eventually leads to fibrous bridging between adjacent portal tracts, causing biliary cirrhosis. Although bile secretory

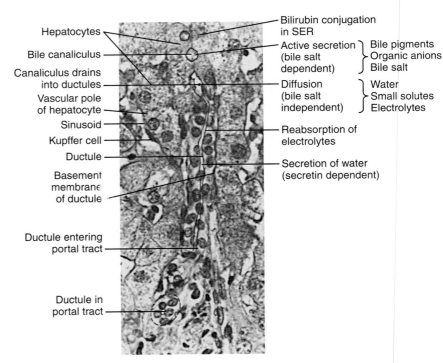

Figure 48–24. Microscopic section of normal liver depicting transition between the bile canaliculus and bile ductule entering the portal tract. Anatomic structures are identified to the *left* of the illustration, and the corresponding physiologic events are listed on the *right*. SER, smooth endoplasmic reticulum.

defects may initially be purely hepatocellular or ductal, any long-standing abnormality in the flow of bile leads to some degree of hepatocellular damage.

Box 48-6 lists diseases that may manifest as conjugated hyperbilirubinemia in the neonatal period. This list is divided into those disorders caused by a primary defect in the hepatocellular phase of bile secretion and those caused by ductal disturbances. In most of these disorders, direct-reacting bilirubin accounts for 50% to 90% of the TB level. A small amount of indirect-reacting bilirubin is always present, reflecting mild hemolysis, defective uptake and excretion, or hydrolysis of conjugated bilirubin. Early in the onset of conjugated hyperbilirubinemia in the neonate, the direct-reacting portion may account for only 10% to 25% of TB. As hepatic conjugation and uptake of bilirubin mature, the indirect-reacting portion decreases, whereas the direct portion increases.[55,98,179]

Causes of Conjugated Hyperbilirubinemia

Conjugated hyperbilirubinemia results from interference with the hepatic excretion of conjugated bilirubin into bile. Idiopathic neonatal hepatitis and biliary atresia together account for about 60% to 80% of all cases of conjugated hyperbilirubinemia. It is possible that similar pathogenetic mechanisms produce a spectrum of disease, with biliary atresia being the final possible, but not the inevitable, outcome. Because of this, it is useful to discuss these two entities simultaneously.[19]

Idiopathic neonatal hepatitis is defined as prolonged conjugated hyperbilirubinemia without the apparent stigmata of a generalized viral illness, the evidence of identifiable infectious agents, or an etiologically specific metabolic abnormality. On liver biopsy, this group is characterized by extensive transformation of hepatocytes into multinucleated giant cells, and it is therefore sometimes referred to as *neonatal giant cell hepatitis*. Giant cell transformation of hepatocytes does not reflect any specific etiology. It is caused by rupture of lateral cell membranes of adjacent hepatocytes, with consequent reduction in the number of bile canaliculi and retention of conjugated bilirubin. It is seen in various inherited metabolic disorders and some infections. Necrosis of hepatocytes and inflammation are usually present, although special stains (e.g., silver impregnation) may be necessary to demonstrate loss of hepatocytes. Necrosis and inflammation may be transient, with giant hepatocytes persisting for many months or even years.[51]

Extrahepatic biliary atresia is defined as a condition in which there is luminal obliteration or apparent absence of all or segments of the extrahepatic biliary system.

BOX 48–6 Diseases That May Manifest as Conjugated Hyperbilirubinemia in the Neonatal Period

HEPATOCELLULAR DISTURBANCES IN BILIRUBIN EXCRETION
Primary Hepatitis
Neonatal idiopathic hepatitis (giant cell hepatitis)
Hepatitis caused by identified infectious agents
- Hepatitis B
- Rubella
- Cytomegalovirus
- *Toxoplasma* organisms
- Coxsackie virus
- Echoviruses 14 and 19
- Herpes simplex and varicella-zoster viruses
- Syphilis
- *Listeria* organisms
- Tubercle bacillus
"Toxic Hepatitis"
Systemic infectious diseases
- *Escherichia coli* (sepsis or urinary tract)
- *Pneumococcus* organisms
- *Proteus* organisms
- *Salmonella* organisms
- Idiopathic diarrhea
Intestinal obstruction
Parenteral alimentation
Ischemic necrosis
Hematologic Disorders
Erythroblastosis fetalis (severe forms)
Congenital erythropoietic porphyria

Metabolic Disorders
α_1-Antitrypsin deficiency
Galactosemia
Tyrosinemia
Fructosemia
Glycogen storage disease type IV
Lipid storage diseases
- Niemann-Pick disease
- Gaucher disease
- Wolman disease
Cerebrohepatorenal syndrome (Zellweger syndrome)
Trisomy 18
Cystic fibrosis
Familial intrahepatic cholestasis: Byler disease
Hemochromatosis
Idiopathic hypopituitarism

DUCTAL DISTURBANCES IN BILIRUBIN EXCRETION
Extrahepatic Biliary Atresia
Isolated
Trisomy 18
Polysplenia-heterotaxia syndrome
Intrahepatic Biliary Atresia
   (nonsyndromatic paucity of bile ducts)
Alagille Syndrome (arteriohepatic dysplasia)
Intrahepatic Atresia Associated with Lymphedema
Extrahepatic Stenosis and Choledochal Cyst
Bile Plug Syndrome
Cystic Disease
Tumors of the Liver and Biliary Tract
Periductal Lymphadenopathy

Differentiation between these two groups of diseases may be difficult in the early stages; however, an early accurate diagnosis is essential for the choice of proper clinical management.[161b] Extrahepatic biliary atresia requires early surgical intervention. Unrelieved by surgery, the defect inevitably leads to death from biliary cirrhosis in the first 3 years of life. The prognosis in idiopathic neonatal hepatitis is uncertain and cannot be predicted on the basis of clinical or laboratory findings. Familial cases have a poor prognosis, with recovery rates of less than 30%. Sporadic cases have a recovery rate of 65% to 83% in various series. The poor prognosis in familial cases may be indicative of a metabolic defect.

The causes of idiopathic neonatal hepatitis and biliary atresia remain undetermined. The long-held view that biliary atresia represents a simple congenital developmental anomaly with failure of canalization is now thought untenable. In most cases, biliary atresia and neonatal hepatitis occur as isolated abnormalities, and both are considered to represent acquired conditions that may be initiated by the same or similar noxious factors. In support of the acquired nature of most cases of biliary atresia is the absence of reported cases in stillborn fetuses and the relatively rare association with other malformations. Similarly, clinical evidence of total obstruction to the flow of bile (such as acholic stools or colorless meconium) is not detected in the early stages of jaundice. The onset of acholic stools and conjugated hyperbilirubinemia is frequently delayed until 2 weeks of life or later. Microscopic changes observed in the extrahepatic biliary system or its fibrous remnant removed during the Kasai procedure (see under "Treatment of Extrahepatic Biliary Atresia," later), strongly suggest a sequence of changes that include acute cholangitis, necrosis, inflammation, attempted regeneration, and obliterative fibrosis (Fig. 48-25).

Clinical and pathologic observations over a long period indicate that some patients fulfill all known criteria for neonatal hepatitis, including surgical demonstration of patent biliary ducts in the early stages of jaundice, and then go on to develop extrahepatic biliary atresia.

Injury to the structures involved in bile secretion (hepatocytes and biliary epithelium) may occur either in utero or in the perinatal period, but the consequences of such injury, and therefore clinically manifested disease, are delayed until some time after birth. Clinical manifestations and eventual outcome may depend on the severity and persistence of lesions in a specific location. Thus, primary injury to hepatocytes may result in clinical manifestations of neonatal hepatitis, whereas injury to major bile ducts and gallbladder may result in biliary atresia. Reovirus type 3 has been implicated as an etiologic factor in extrahepatic biliary atresia as well as in neonatal hepatitis. These studies include an experimental model in which a hepatobiliary disease bearing a strong resemblance to human biliary atresia can be induced in very young mice by infection with reovirus type 3. No studies, however, have definitively proved a role for any of the known hepatotrophic viruses including reovirus type 3 in the etiology of biliary atresia in humans.[81,158]

Other viruses such as cytomegalovirus and rubella virus have been implicated in intrahepatic bile duct destruction and paucity.[73] Patients currently classified as having idiopathic neonatal hepatitis constitute a heterogeneous group that undoubtedly includes various, as yet undefined, metabolic disorders. A metabolic disorder may explain the recurrent incidence of this disease in some families.

Most patients with idiopathic neonatal hepatitis or biliary atresia represent isolated cases without familial incidence or associated anomalies. Neonatal hepatitis has a familial incidence of 10% to 15%, whereas no familial cases of histologically proven extrahepatic biliary atresia have been observed.[77a,130a] Rare occurrences of neonatal hepatitis and biliary atresia in two siblings have been reported. Both neonatal hepatitis and biliary atresia occur more frequently in patients with trisomy 18 than in the general population. Biliary atresia has been observed in

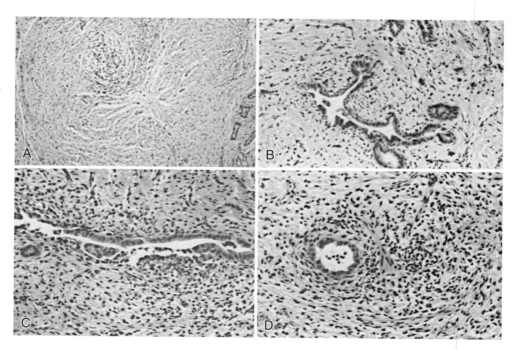

Figure 48–25. Microscopic preparations of fibrous remnant of extrahepatic biliary system resected during Kasai procedure for biliary atresia. **A,** Most distal portion of specimen, showing complete obliteration of lumen by fibrous tissue. **B** to **D,** More proximal segments, illustrating a spectrum of changes that includes necrosis of lining epithelium, acute and chronic inflammation, mural fibrosis with distortion of lumen, and great variation in size of ductlike structures. All micrographs ×60.

association with the polysplenia-heterotaxia syndrome in 10% to 15% of cases. This syndrome is characterized by situs inversus of abdominal organs, intestinal malrotation, multiple spleens, centrally placed liver, and a variety of cardiac, pulmonary, and vascular malformations. The inferior vena cava is frequently absent.

Early clinical manifestations of both idiopathic neonatal hepatitis and biliary atresia may be limited to jaundice. In a small proportion of patients, especially among those who later develop neonatal hepatitis, jaundice may be apparent at birth, documented by increased concentrations of conjugated bilirubin in cord blood. No case of extrahepatic biliary atresia has ever been described in which elevation of direct-reacting bilirubin was found in the cord blood. Jaundice usually becomes apparent between the second and sixth weeks of life. The dark yellow staining of diapers from the presence of bilirubin in the urine often prompts the parents to seek medical advice. Jaundice is frequently first noted by the physician during a well-baby visit. Hepatomegaly may be present in both neonatal hepatitis and biliary atresia. Splenomegaly is more frequently present in neonatal hepatitis, but this is not a constant finding. Its presence in biliary atresia usually signifies cirrhosis. Obstruction to the flow of bile is reflected by acholic stools and may be observed in both neonatal hepatitis and biliary atresia. It is always transient and incomplete in neonatal hepatitis, but its duration is variable and may extend beyond the crucial period during which an accurate diagnosis must be established if surgical correction is needed. Routine clinical and laboratory findings usually do not distinguish between extrahepatic biliary atresia and neonatal hepatitis. A routine series of diagnostic laboratory tests is suggested, however, to establish the severity of hepatic involvement and to screen for possible causes (Box 48-7). The failure of routine tests to distinguish between neonatal hepatitis and biliary atresia has led to a continued search for other distinguishing biochemical characteristics. α-Fetoproteins are frequently present in the sera of patients with neonatal hepatitis but may be absent in patients with biliary atresia.

A reliable method for the evaluation of patency of extrahepatic bile ducts is the use of technetium-99m acetanilidoiminodiacetic acid (IDA) or IDA derivatives such as paraisopropyl iminodiacetic acid or di-isopropyl iminodiacetic acid.[200] These compounds are efficiently extracted by hepatocytes and are excreted with bile into the intestines. When complete obstruction exists, no activity is detected in the intestines. Pretreatment with phenobarbital for 7 days before testing promotes excretion of isotope in neonates with severe intrahepatic cholestasis and thus reduces the chance for a mistaken diagnosis of extrahepatic obstruction. Phenobarbital is given orally at the dose of 5 mg/kg daily. Patients are given nothing by mouth for 1 hour before and 2 hours after injection of the radiotracer to avoid gallbladder contraction and dilution of radiotracer excreted into the intestines. Combining cholescintigraphy with a string test (determination of color and radioactivity count in duodenal fluid) increases the sensitivity and specificity of the diagnosis. Infants with biliary atresia will have a negative hepatobiliary scan at 24 hours or a string radioactive count of less than 197,007 counts per minute.[161a]

Ultrasonography has also been applied in the evaluation of neonatal cholestasis. Although the demonstration of a normal gallbladder is usually indicative of an intrahepatic

---

BOX 48–7 Laboratory Tests Recommended for Evaluation of Neonatal Conjugated Hyperbilirubinemia

LIVER FUNCTION TESTS
TB and direct-reacting bilirubin, total serum protein, and serum protein electrophoresis
SGOT (AST), SGPT (ALT), alkaline phosphatase (and 5'-nucleotidase if alkaline phosphatase elevated), and γ-glutamyl transpeptidase
Cholesterol
Serum and urine bile acid concentrations, if available
α₁-Antitrypsin
Technetium-99m iminodiacetic acid scan
α-Fetoprotein

HEMATOLOGIC TESTS
Complete blood count, smear, and reticulocyte count
Direct Coombs test and erythrocyte G6PD
Platelet count
Prothrombin time and partial thromboplastin time

TESTS FOR INFECTIOUS DISEASE
Cord blood IgM
VDRL; FTA-ABS; complement fixation titers for rubella, cytomegalovirus, and herpesvirus; and Sabin-Feldman dye test titer for toxoplasmosis
HB$_s$Ag in both infant and mother
Viral cultures from nose, pharynx, blood, stool, urine, and cerebrospinal fluid

URINE TESTS
Routine urinalysis, including protein and reducing substances
Urine culture
Bilirubin and urobilinogen
Amino acid screening

LIVER BIOPSY
Light microscopy
Specific enzyme assay (if indicated)

RADIOLOGIC AND ULTRASOUND STUDIES (IF INDICATED)

ADDITIONAL DIAGNOSTIC STUDIES FOR METABOLIC DISORDERS (IF INDICATED)

ALT, alanine transferase; AST, aspartate aminotransferase; FTA-ABS, fluorescent treponemal antibody absorption (test); G6PD, glucose-6-phosphate dehydrogenase; HB$_s$Ag, hepatitis B surface antigen; SGOT, serum glutamic-oxaloacetic transaminase; SGPT, serum glutamic-pyruvic transferase; TB, total bilirubin; VDRL, Venereal Disease Research Laboratory.

---

cause for cholestasis, it may be seen in extrahepatic biliary atresia and is, therefore, not a reliable sign. As intrahepatic bile ducts are usually not dilated in extrahepatic biliary atresia, their presence should suggest another cause.

Histopathologic examination of the liver is an integral part of the evaluation of any patient with persistent conjugated hyperbilirubinemia. It is best performed and analyzed after all other pertinent laboratory data have been gathered. A percutaneous liver biopsy usually yields adequate tissue for microscopic and, if desired, electron microscopic and virologic studies. If a metabolic disorder is suspected, as for example in familial cases, a liver core should be frozen and saved at −70°C for possible subsequent biochemical analysis. In most patients (90% to 95%), liver biopsy establishes or confirms the correct diagnosis, sparing the neonate with neonatal hepatitis an unnecessary surgical procedure. Before the biopsy, the prothrombin time and platelet count must be ascertained and assessed to determine the safety of performing the procedure and the need for correction. A prolonged prothrombin time may be corrected in some patients by administration of vitamin K. In some situations in which a biopsy is urgently required, fresh frozen plasma may be administered before and 6 hours after percutaneous biopsy. Postoperatively, neonates must be observed closely for vital signs or clinical changes that indicate significant bleeding, bile peritonitis, or pneumothorax, the rare but significant complications of the procedure. In the final analysis, the isotope scan and a percutaneous liver biopsy are the only reliable means available without surgical exploration to distinguish between neonatal hepatitis and extrahepatic biliary obstruction.

The liver biopsy in neonatal hepatitis is characterized by marked irregularity in the size of hepatocytes and, in some cases, by numerous giant hepatocytes (Figs. 48-26 and 48-27).

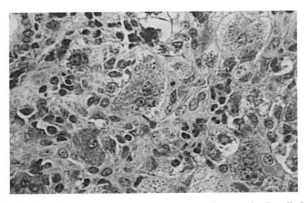

Figure 48–26. Neonatal hepatitis. Note the marked cellular irregularity obliterating the normal orderly plate arrangement. Intracanalicular bile is present. Small cells in sinusoids are Kupffer cells and elements of extramedullary hematopoiesis. Paraffin embedding and hematoxylin-eosin staining; ×60.

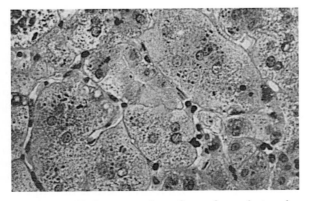

Figure 48–27. High-power view of transformed giant hepatocytes. Most of the intracytoplasmic granules represent bile pigment. Paraffin embedding and hematoxylin-eosin staining; ×200.

Giant cells may contain from 4 to 100 nuclei. The cytoplasm of these giant cells is usually foamy and contains bile pigment. Bile canaliculi appear to be reduced in number and proportion to the number of giant hepatocytes. Necrosis and inflammation are frequently detected. Kupffer cells are swollen and contain bile pigment, lipofuscin, iron, and phagocytosed debris of destroyed hepatocytes. Extramedullary hematopoiesis is almost always present. Although these findings may also be present in biliary atresia, it is the relative absence of bile duct proliferation that distinguishes neonatal hepatitis from biliary atresia. In some cases of neonatal hepatitis, there is evidence of inflammatory injury to portal bile ducts, with epithelial reduplication interpreted as regenerative activity. The aforementioned changes are usually seen in early stages, soon after onset of jaundice. Biopsies taken after 3 months of age may show little necrosis and inflammation and, instead, demonstrate fibrosis or cirrhosis. Giant cell transformation of hepatocytes may persist for months or years.

It has been shown in patients and in animal experiments that soon after obstruction of the common bile duct, ducts and ductules in portal tracts and in periportal zones begin to proliferate. This phenomenon involves most, if not all, portal tracts and is present even at the periphery of the liver, far removed from the site of obstruction. Therefore, in biliary atresia, changes suggesting blockage in the major (mostly extrahepatic) bile ducts are seen. At least three portal tracts should be available for examination. In biliary atresia, all tracts will show some degree of proliferation. In early stages, ductular proliferation may be present without increased fibrosis. The ducts have a varicose appearance and contain focal bile plugs. Later, ducts and ductules frequently appear distorted (Fig. 48-28) because of a discrepancy between the rate of proliferation of biliary epithelium and that of the surrounding fibrous tissue. An associated inflammatory exudate is occasionally seen around proliferated ductules, but a true cholangitis with epithelial necrosis and intramural inflammation is rarely encountered except in association with surgical complications. Other changes within portal tracts include dilated lymphatics and, occasionally, tortuous and thick-walled arterioles. In later stages of extrahepatic biliary atresia, ductular epithelium may disappear, having been replaced by collagen fibers, and this may lead to a secondary paucity of portal bile ducts.

Extensive paucity of bile ducts, whether primary or secondary, is associated with a clinical syndrome resembling that observed in primary biliary cirrhosis, or sclerosing cholangitis, with hypercholesterolemia, xanthomas, and pruritus. Hepatocytes in biliary atresia show intracellular and canalicular cholestasis, with the canalicular component predominating (Fig. 48-29). In about one third of all patients with biliary atresia, there is giant cell transformation of hepatocytes. In most cases, this transformation is primarily centrolobular (around terminal branches of the hepatic vein) and is not associated with necrosis and inflammation. Extramedullary hematopoiesis may also be present.

Treatment of Neonatal Hepatitis

Clinical management of neonatal hepatitis consists of supportive measures because no specific therapy is known. Many neonates have a transient but significant reduction in bile flow, often requiring replacement of fat-soluble

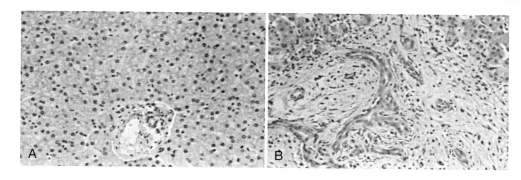

Figure 48–28. A, Portal tract of normal neonate, containing a large, thin-walled vein and single cross section of a bile duct. B, Portal tract from neonate with biliary atresia. Note marked enlargement of tract from fibrosis that surrounds multiple elongated bile ducts. Both micrographs, ×60.

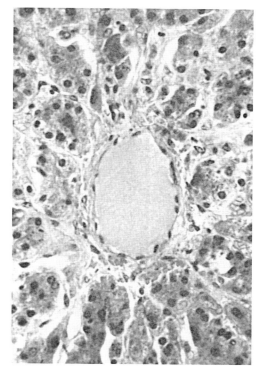

Figure 48–29. Extrahepatic biliary atresia. Central vein surrounded by hepatocytes. Intracanalicular bile plugs are present. In addition, hepatocytes contain intracytoplasmic bile pigment granules. Paraffin embedding and hematoxylin-eosin staining.

vitamins, particularly vitamins D and K. Subclinical rickets is common in these neonates and may contribute to the increase in serum concentrations of alkaline phosphatase. Persistence of acholic or very pale stools without significant lowering of direct-reacting serum bilirubin concentrations after 1 month should be viewed as an indication for repeat clinical study, including liver biopsy. This practice permits detection of patients whose extrahepatic bile ducts sclerose after an initial phase of hepatitis and who are, therefore, suitable candidates for exploratory laparotomy and corrective surgery. On rare occasions, patients with neonatal hepatitis and complete obstruction, as evidenced by acholic stools, may recover rapidly after operative cholangiography that shows normal extrahepatic ducts. This phenomenon is probably the result of flushing out of inspissated bile in the extrahepatic biliary system, with consequent relief of obstruction. This situation may be seen in cystic fibrosis or severe dehydration. Fluctuations in stool color should alert the clinician to the possible existence of a choledochal cyst, which can usually be diagnosed with ultrasound and treated surgically. There are no early reliable criteria on which the prognosis of a particular patient can be based.

Treatment of Extrahepatic Biliary Atresia

When the clinical evaluation indicates complete biliary obstruction or proves inconclusive, the patient should undergo an exploratory laparotomy. On entry of the abdomen and after initial scrutiny of the biliary system, an operative cholangiogram should be performed to confirm and characterize the extrahepatic lesion and define its extent. The classification proposed by the Japanese Society of Pediatric Surgeons divides extrahepatic biliary atresia into three types, based on gross observations during laparotomy:

Type I: Atresia of the common bile duct with patent proximal ducts

Type II: Atresia of the common hepatic duct with patent proximal ducts

Type III: Atresia of the right and left hepatic ducts at the porta hepatis

Operative examination of these neonates should be performed only by surgeons prepared to proceed with corrective procedures if necessary. Reoperation after exploratory laparotomy increases the technical difficulties and delays the institution of corrective measures. Reconstitution of normal biliary drainage by direct anastomosis of grossly identifiable segments of patent bile ducts to the gastrointestinal tract is possible in only a very small proportion of patients with biliary atresia (estimated at 5% to 10%). These include the rare cases of choledochal cyst and occlusion of a short segment of the common bile duct by a valve, a membrane, or fibrosis. In most patients with biliary atresia, there are no grossly visible ducts proximal to the atretic segment. In the past, all these patients were considered inoperable. Untreated patients, although jaundiced, often appear clinically well in the first few months of life, but they deteriorate rapidly after cirrhosis develops, with clinical manifestations of portal hypertension, ascites, hypersplenism, infection, and hemorrhage.[100a,190a]

In 1968, Kasai and associates[122a] described for the first time in the American literature an operative procedure in which the periphery of the transected fibrous tissue of the porta hepatis, devoid of grossly identifiable ducts, was anastomosed to a Roux-en-Y loop of small intestine (portoenterostomy). Kasai's portoenterostomy or variations of this procedure are currently performed in most medical centers.

The immediate goal for surgical correction is the reestablishment of bile drainage, which is now achieved in most neonates when operated on before 3 months of age. Cure rate, however, is still poor. In most operated patients, fibrosis increases with time and eventually progresses to cirrhosis despite adequate bile drainage. It is currently unclear whether progressive liver fibrosis represents continuation of the same type of injury responsible for the initial obliterative process in extrahepatic ducts or if it is the result of ascending cholangitis complicating surgery. In addition to the age at the time of surgery, other factors that influence the outcome include the size and patency of microscopic ducts in the transected porta hepatis and the preservation of intact epithelial lining.[123]

Orthotopic liver transplantation is the definitive therapy for biliary atresia. Survival statistics have steadily improved since 1981, when cyclosporin A and steroid therapy were introduced. Other drugs that produce effective immunosuppression and fewer side effects, such as FK 506, lessen the mortality and morbidity of transplantation, resulting in longer and more productive lives for graft recipients.[190a,218,258]

KNOWN INFECTIOUS CAUSES

In a small proportion of neonates with neonatal hepatitis, a specific infectious agent may be identified either by direct isolation and culture or by serologic tests that detect specific antibodies. In addition, microbial antigens may be identified in liver biopsy using monoclonal antibodies and immunocytochemical staining methods. Among infectious agents reported in association with neonatal hepatitis are organisms such as *Treponema pallidum* and *Listeria* species, and viruses such as rubella and Coxsackie virus, the herpes group of viruses (herpes simplex, varicella-zoster, cytomegalovirus), and adenovirus. The protozoan *Toxoplasma gondii* also has been implicated. Fetal infection may take place in utero either by transplacental spread or by an ascending infection of the amniotic fluid, usually after rupture of membranes. In some cases, infection may occur during delivery by aspiration or swallowing of vaginal contents. Clinically, patients in this group may appear sick and fail to thrive and also may have evidence of CNS and other organ involvement. In many patients, there are stigmata of generalized infection. Laboratory findings are similar to those seen in idiopathic neonatal hepatitis, but stools are not acholic, and therefore biliary atresia usually is not suspected. Although congenital infection with human immunodeficiency virus (HIV) is diagnosed with increasing frequency, cholestasis is rare in the neonatal period.

Liver biopsy may be helpful in the diagnosis of infectious agents, especially in infections with the herpesviruses. These DNA viruses replicate in the nucleus, resulting in intranuclear inclusion bodies that can be seen with the light microscope. Cytomegalic inclusion disease is characterized by marked enlargement of hepatocytes, biliary epithelium, and Kupffer cells caused by intranuclear as well as intracytoplasmic inclusions. In some cases, however, the virus has been isolated from patients in whom liver biopsy showed giant cell transformation of hepatocytes with no evidence of inclusions.[155]

Hepatitis B surface antigen (HBsAg) may be transmitted from mother to infant, probably by aspiration of vaginal contents, including blood, during delivery. With few exceptions, infants born to HBsAg-positive mothers show no antigenemia in cord blood or in the first month of life. Repeated serologic tests indicate that HBsAg appears in the serum of these infants between 5 and 7 weeks of life and reaches a peak at 10 weeks. Antigenemia in the newborn may be associated with liver injury, and both may persist for many months or possibly years. It is necessary, therefore, to closely observe all infants of HBsAg-positive mothers for many years for clinical and laboratory evidence of chronic liver disease. Severe and even fulminant neonatal hepatitis associated with HBsAg has been described in infants of chronic carriers and after neonatal transfusions. Prophylaxis with concurrent administration of hepatitis B immune globulin (HBIG) and hepatitis B vaccine is effective in preventing neonatal infection in more than 90% of exposed newborns. HBIG (0.5 mL IM) should be given within 12 hours of birth. In addition, hepatitis B vaccine should be given IM concurrently within 12 hours of birth at a different anatomic site and repeated at 1 to 2 and 6 months of age (for preterm infants who weigh less than 2000 g at birth, a total of four doses of vaccine should be given according to the immunization schedule for preterm infants, see also appendix C). Concurrent use of HBIG and vaccine does not appear to interfere with vaccine efficacy (see Chapters 23 and 39).[45,201]

Hepatitis C virus (HCV), a single-stranded RNA virus in the flavivirus family, has been found to be the etiologic agent in most cases previously referred to as non-A, non-B hepatitis. Transmission occurs through both the percutaneous and the nonpercutaneous route. The incubation period varies from 2 weeks to 6 months. The signs of acute disease include malaise, fever, elevation in hepatic transaminases, and jaundice. Fulminant hepatitis and acute hepatic failure are rare. Although about three fourths of acute infections are asymptomatic, about one half of affected patients will develop chronic hepatitis, with 20% of these patients progressing to cirrhosis. Progression of the disease is slow, with an average of 10 years to chronic hepatitis, 20 years to cirrhosis, and 30 years to hepatocellular carcinoma. Although infected infants manifest biochemical features of hepatocellular injury, other manifestations of the disease are relatively mild throughout childhood.[30]

The overall risk for vertical transmission of HCV has been shown to be as high as 10% in several studies. Women who are infected with both HCV and HIV and those with HCV viremia are at the greatest risk for transmitting HCV to their offspring.[86,170] The persistence of maternal antibody in the infant is variable but may be as long as 8 to 12 months. Diagnosis in the neonate and infant is made by measuring serial anti-HCV (IgG) titers (using enzyme immunoassays followed by recombinant immunoblot assays detecting antibody against HCV core antigen or other nonstructural proteins) or by directly detecting the presence of HCV ribonucleic acid through the reverse-transcriptase polymerase chain reaction. No proven therapy is currently available to neonates infected with HCV. Combination therapy with peginterferon and ribavirin is recommended for chronic HCV in adults.[206] The safety and efficacy of HCV therapies are currently being investigated in children. HCV has been detected in the breast milk of HCV-infected mothers.

Although theoretically possible, transmission of HCV through breast feeding has not been documented in HCV-positive, HIV-negative mothers. Thus, according to most authorities, breast feeding is not currently contraindicated in HCV-positive, HIV-negative women.[132]

SEPSIS

Microorganisms and their biologic products may have direct toxic effects on the cells and structures responsible for the hepatocellular and ductal phases of conjugated bilirubin excretion. This may be complicated by sepsis-induced hemolysis, further adding to the bilirubin load. Postmortem examination of neonates with severe sepsis has shown centrilobular cholestasis, focal hepatocellular necrosis, and giant cell transformation in some patients. In others, no hepatic lesions can be demonstrated by light microscopy. Severe urinary tract infection, particularly with coliform bacilli, is associated with this syndrome. In this case, generalized septicemia is not an essential feature, and cholestasis may be caused by massive endotoxin release. Antibiotic treatment is followed by prompt relief of hyperbilirubinemia.

HEPATIC METABOLIC DISEASE

Several metabolic disorders result in hepatocellular injury in the neonatal period and give rise to a clinical pathologic syndrome that may resemble neonatal hepatitis or biliary atresia. α_1-Antitrypsin deficiency in the homozygous state (PiZZ) may be manifested by neonatal liver injury. It is estimated that only 10% to 20% of all individuals with this abnormality will have liver disease. Most PiZZ individuals never develop clinical evidence of liver disease, but they may develop pulmonary emphysema as adults. Patients with α_1-antitrypsin deficiency may show all the signs and symptoms of neonatal hepatitis or biliary atresia, including acholic stools. Liver biopsy also may show changes consistent with either one of the aforementioned conditions. Bile duct proliferation may be so pronounced that exploratory laparotomy is performed. Although in older children, periportal hepatocytes frequently contain intracytoplasmic inclusions that give a positive reaction with periodic acid–Schiff stain and resist diastase digestion, these are rarely seen in the neonatal period. Immunocytochemical staining may be helpful in demonstrating granules of α_1-antitrypsin, present in hepatocytes of patients with deficient states, but not in normal phenotypes. Phenotyping of the Pi system should be carried out in all suspected cases. In many infants, neonatal cholestasis may regress before the age of 6 months and reappear later in childhood or adolescence when the patient becomes cirrhotic. The pathogenesis of liver disease associated with this anomaly is not fully understood.[2,167] Recent studies suggest that the liver disease is a result of toxic gain-of-function mutations that cause the α_1-antitrypsin protein to fold aberrantly and be retained in the endoplasmic reticulum of hepatocytes rather than be secreted into the blood.[87,178]

Several defects in carbohydrate, protein, and lipid metabolism occur with conjugated hyperbilirubinemia. Deficient activity of galactose-1-phosphate uridyltransferase is inherited as an autosomal recessive disease with an incidence of about 1 in 50,000. It results in the accumulation of galactose-1-phosphate in the liver, producing hepatomegaly and conjugated hyperbilirubinemia. Other associated findings in galactosemia include hypoglycemia, emesis, failure to thrive, cataracts, and ascites. Mental retardation and cirrhosis occur if dietary treatment is not instituted early. The acute form of tyrosinemia is also an autosomal recessive disease and is characterized by elevations in plasma tyrosine and methionine accompanied by hepatic and renal dysfunction, emesis, and failure to thrive. Dietary tyrosine restriction prevents cirrhosis and early death. Niemann-Pick disease (deposition of sphingomyelin and cholesterol) and Gaucher disease (deposition of glucosylceramide), both autosomal recessive diseases, have also been reported to be associated with conjugated hyperbilirubinemia (see Chapter 50).[88]

TOTAL PARENTERAL NUTRITION–INDUCED HEPATIC INJURY

Prolonged use (≥ 2 weeks) of total parenteral nutrition may produce conjugated hyperbilirubinemia which may persist for some time after cessation of this mode of nutrition. Liver biopsy shows evidence of hepatocellular injury with swelling of hepatocytes, necrosis, cholestasis, and occasional giant cell transformation. Trace elements (specifically manganese and copper) should be removed from the total parenteral nutrition solution if conjugated hyperbilirubinemia occurs.[38,251] Baseline copper levels and monthly monitoring are recommended to avoid copper deficiency.[101]

MECHANICAL OBSTRUCTION

Inspissated Bile (Bile Plug) Syndrome

Obstruction of a major bile duct by thick bile or mucus is known as the *bile plug syndrome* or the *inspissated* (Latin *inspissatus*, thickened) *bile syndrome*. Although it may be seen in cases of cystic fibrosis, most often the cause is obscure. The obstruction usually resolves gradually, with or without phenobarbital therapy. Severe cases may require irrigation of the biliary tree or direct surgical extraction of the plug.

Choledocholithiasis

Choledocholithiasis is most commonly seen in neonates with a history of severe intrauterine hemolysis. The excessive bilirubin load results in the formation of gallstones, which have the potential to block the secretion of conjugated bilirubin. Gallstones may also be seen in patients receiving total parenteral nutrition. The diagnosis is suspected because of the presence of conjugated hyperbilirubinemia, bilirubinuria, acholic stools, and a palpable gallbladder. It is confirmed with ultrasound or radiotracer imaging of the hepatobiliary system. Spontaneous resolution is common, but cholecystectomy may be necessary in cases of cholangitis or progressive elevation of conjugated bilirubin levels.

Cystic Diseases

Cyst formation in the biliary system may result in obstruction of bile flow and produce conjugated hyperbilirubinemia. Congenital hepatic fibrosis is an autosomal recessive disease marked by hamartomatous and fibrotic changes of the interlobular bile ducts. Most cases are associated with cysts of the renal collecting tubules, and the prognosis depends greatly on the degree of renal impairment. *Caroli disease* is the name given to cystic dilation of the major intrahepatic ducts. Cholangitis is a chronic problem, and the outcome is variable. Cysts found along the extrahepatic biliary tree (common hepatic duct, common bile duct, gallbladder) are known as *choledochal cysts*. These are more commonly seen in females and may lead to portal hypertension, cirrhosis, and carcinoma. Complete surgical excision is the definitive treatment. It is believed that these three disease entities may have a common etiology that differentially manifests itself depending on the timing, duration, and location of the insult. Taken together, they are rare causes of conjugated hyperbilirubinemia presenting in the neonatal period.

Masses

Obstruction of the extrahepatic biliary ducts may also rarely occur with tumors such as primary hepatoblastoma and metastatic neuroblastoma, enlarged periductal lymph nodes, and distended loops of bowel. Treatment is directed at the underlying disorder.

MISCELLANEOUS CAUSES OF CONJUGATED HYPERBILIRUBINEMIA

Alagille syndrome (arteriohepatic dysplasia) is an autosomal dominant disease with clinical variability characterized by a paucity of intrahepatic bile ducts in the presence of patent extrahepatic ducts. Other findings include unusual facies, vertebral anomalies, peripheral pulmonary stenosis, posterior embryotoxon (incomplete iridocorneal separation), and retarded mental, physical, and sexual development.[9,255] Mutations in Jagged1 (chromosome 20p12) have been identified in about 70% of patients studied with Alagille syndrome.[56,127,168] Jagged1 is a cell surface ligand for the Notch receptor. The interaction between Jagged1 and Notch is critical for proper cell differentiation during early development. The Alagille syndrome appears to result from haploinsufficiency of Jagged1. Inability to identify a Jagged1 mutation in nearly 30% of patients indicates that additional causal defects are likely.

Early clinical manifestations and laboratory findings are identical to those observed in patients with extrahepatic biliary atresia. Later in the first year of life, however, serum cholesterol concentrations rise well beyond those observed in other forms of infantile liver disease. Levels higher than 1000 mg/dL may be seen in as early as the third month of life. Cutaneous xanthomas are prominent in the later stages of untreated disease, usually after 1 year of age. It is important to recognize this condition before exploratory surgery because the patency of the very narrow and collapsed extrahepatic ducts may be extremely difficult to demonstrate. Not only is portoenterostomy unsuccessful in establishing bile flow in this condition, but also it actually accelerates the progression of liver disease.

A nonsyndromic form of intrahepatic bile duct paucity has also been described. A familial form of cholestasis and paucity of intrahepatic bile ducts is associated with development of lymphedema of the lower extremities around the time of puberty. Although initially described cases in this group were from families of Norwegian extraction, similar cases have been reported from England, France, and Sweden.[1]

Zellweger (cerebrohepatorenal) syndrome is a rare autosomal recessive disease marked by the absence of hepatic and renal peroxisomes. Because peroxisomes have many vital anabolic and catabolic functions within the cell, their absence results in profound cellular dysfunction. In addition to conjugated hyperbilirubinemia, affected patients manifest characteristic facies (high forehead, flat occiput, large fontanelle, shallow orbital ridges, micrognathia), feeding difficulties, hypotonia, seizures, and mental retardation. Death usually occurs early in infancy.

Isolated cases of conjugated hyperbilirubinemia have been described in association with hypoplastic left heart syndrome, severe internal hemorrhage, familial lethal hemochromatosis, and rarely in association with umbilical vein catheterization.

ACKNOWLEDGMENTS

The authors and editors acknowledge the contribution of Kwang-Sun Lee, Rachel Morecki, and Lawrence M. Gartner to previous editions of this chapter, large portions of which remain unchanged.

REFERENCES

1. Aagenaes O: Hereditary recurrent cholestasis with lymphoedema—Two new families, *Acta Paediatr Scand* 63:465, 1974.
2. Adams JA, Hey DJ, Hall RT: Incidence of hyperbilirubinemia in breast- vs. formula-fed infants, *Clin Pediatr* 24:69, 1985.
3. Agati G, et al: Configurational photoisomerization of bilirubin *in vitro*—II. A comparative study of phototherapy fluorescent lamps and lasers, *Photochem Photobiol* 41:381, 1985.
4. Ahdab-Barmada M, Moossy J: The neuropathology of kernicterus in the premature neonate: diagnostic problems, *J Neuropathol Exp Neurol* 43:45, 1984.
5. Ahlfors CE: Criteria for exchange transfusion in jaundiced newborns, *Pediatrics* 93:488, 1994.
6. Ahlfors CE: Measurement of plasma unbound unconjugated bilirubin, *Anal Biochem* 279:130, 2000.
7. Ahlfors CE: Unbound bilirubin associated with kernicterus: a historical approach, *J Pediatr* 137:540, 2000.
8. Akaba K, et al: Neonatal hyperbilirubinemia and mutation of the bilirubin uridine diphosphate-glucuronosyltransferase gene: a common missense mutation among Japanese, Koreans and Chinese, *Biochem Mol Biol Int* 46:21, 1998.
9. Alagille D, et al: Syndromic paucity of interlobular bile ducts (Alagille syndrome or arteriohepatic dysplasia): review of 80 cases, *J Pediatr* 110:195, 1987.
10. Alonso EM, et al: Enterohepatic circulation of nonconjugated bilirubin in rats fed with human milk, *J Pediatr* 118:425, 1991.
11. American Academy of Pediatrics: Committee on Fetus and Newborn. Home phototherapy, *Pediatrics* 76:136, 1985.
12. American Academy of Pediatrics: Practice parameter: Management of hyperbilirubinemia in the healthy term newborn. Provisional Committee for Quality Improvement and Subcommittee on Hyperbilirubinemia, *Pediatrics* 94:558, 1994.
13. American Academy of Pediatrics: Clinical practice guideline: Management of hyperbilirubinemia in the newborn infant ≥35 weeks of gestation. Provisional Committee for Quality Improvement and Subcommittee on Hyperbilirubinemia. *Pediatrics* 114:297, 2004.

14. American Academy of Pediatrics, American College of Obstetricians and Gynecologists: Discharge. In *Guidelines for perinatal care*, Elk Grove Village, IL, 1997, American Academy of Pediatrics, American College of Obstetricians and Gynecologists.
15. American Academy of Pediatrics, American College of Obstetricians and Gynecologists: Hyperbilirubinemia. In *Guidelines for perinatal care*, Elk Grove Village, IL, 1997, American Academy of Pediatrics, American College of Obstetricians and Gynecologists.
16. American Academy of Pediatrics, *American College of Obstetricians and Gynecologists: Guidelines for perinatal care*, 5th ed, Elk Grove Village, IL, 2002, American Academy of Pediatirics, American College of Obstetricians and Gynecologists.
17. Arrese M, et al: Hepatobiliary transport: molecular mechanisms of development and cholestasis, *Pediatr Res* 44:141, 1998.
18. Ayyash H, et al: Green or blue light phototherapy for neonates with hyperbilirubinaemia, *Arch Dis Child* 62:843, 1987.
19. Balistreri WF: Neonatal cholestasis: lessons from the past, issues for the future, *Semin Liver Dis* 7:61, 1987.
20. Bancroft JD, et al: Gilbert syndrome accelerates development of neonatal jaundice, *J Pediatr* 132:656, 1998.
21. Berant M, et al: Phototherapy-associated diarrhea. The role of bile salts, *Acta Paediatr Scand* 72:853, 1983.
22. Berardi A, et al: Kernicterus associated with hereditary spherocytosis and UGT1A1 promoter polymorphism, *Biol Neonate* 90:243, 2006.
23. Beutler E: G6PD deficiency, *Blood* 84:3613, 1994.
24. Beutler E, et al: Racial variability in the UDP-glucuronosyltransferase 1 (UGT1A1) promoter: a balanced polymorphism for regulation of bilirubin metabolism? *Proc Natl Acad Sci U S A* 95:8170, 1998.
25. Bhutani VK, et al: Noninvasive measurement of total serum bilirubin in a multiracial predischarge newborn population to assess the risk of severe hyperbilirubinemia, *Pediatrics* 106:E17, 2000.
26. Bhutani VK, et al: End-tidal carbon monoxide hour-specific nomogram: for early and pre-discharge identification of babies with increased bilirubin production, *J Perinatol* 21:501, 2001.
27. Bhutani VK, et al: Predictive ability of a predischarge hour-specific serum bilirubin for subsequent significant hyperbilirubinemia in healthy term and near-term newborns, *Pediatrics* 103:6, 1999.
28. Bhutani VK, et al: Kernicterus: epidemiological strategies for its prevention through systems-based approaches, *J Perinatol* 24:650, 2004.
29. Blumenthal SG, et al: Changes in bilirubins in human prenatal development, *Biochem J* 186:693, 1980.
30. Bortolotti F, et al: Hepatitis C virus infection and related liver disease in children of mothers with antibodies to the virus, *J Pediatr* 130:990, 1997.
31. Bosma PJ: Inherited disorders of bilirubin metabolism, *J Hepatol* 38:107, 2003.
32. Bosma PJ, et al: The genetic basis of the reduced expression of bilirubin UDP-glucuronosyltransferase 1 in Gilbert's syndrome, *N Engl J Med* 333:1171, 1995.
33. Bratlid D, et al: Effect of serum hyperosmolality on opening of blood-brain barrier for bilirubin in rat brain, *Pediatrics* 71:909, 1983.
34. Brett EM, et al: Delta bilirubin in serum of pediatric patients: Correlations with age and disease, *Clin Chem* 30:1561, 1984.
35. Brodersen R, Stern L: Deposition of bilirubin acid in the central nervous system—A hypothesis for the development of kernicterus, *Acta Paediatr Scand* 79:12, 1990.
36. Brown AK, et al: Efficacy of phototherapy in prevention and management of neonatal hyperbilirubinemia, *Pediatrics* 75:393, 1985.
37. Brown AK, et al: Jaundice in healthy, term neonates: do we need new action levels or new approaches? [comment], *Pediatrics* 89:827, 1992.
38. Brown MR, et al: Decreased cholestasis with enteral instead of intravenous protein in the very low-birth-weight infant, *J Pediatr Gastroenterol Nutr* 9:21, 1989.
39. Bucalo LR, et al: Pulmonary excretion of carbon monoxide in the human infant as an index of bilirubin production. IIc. Evidence for the possible association of cord blood erythropoietin levels and postnatal bilirubin production in infants of mothers with abnormalities of gestational glucose metabolism, *Am J Perinatol* 1:177, 1984.
40. Burchell B, Hume R: Molecular genetic basis of Gilbert's syndrome, *J Gastroenterol Hepatol* 14:960, 1999.
41. Burton PM, et al: Azalanstat (RS-21607), a lanosterol 14 alpha-demethylase inhibitor with cholesterol-lowering activity, *Biochem Pharmacol* 50:529, 1995.
42. Caglayan S, et al: Superiority of oral agar and phototherapy combination in the treatment of neonatal hyperbilirubinemia, *Pediatrics* 92:86, 1993.
43. Cashore WJ: Hyperbilirubinemia: should we adopt a new standard of care? *Pediatrics* 89:824, 1992.
44. Cashore WJ, Oh W: Unbound bilirubin and kernicterus in low-birth-weight infants, *Pediatrics* 69:481, 1982.
45. Centers for Disease Control: Recommendations for protection against viral hepatitis. Recommendation of the Immunization Practices Advisory Committee. Department of Health and Human Services, *Ann Intern Med* 103:391, 1985.
46. Chima RS, et al: Evaluation of adverse events due to exchange transfusions in term and near-term newborns, *Pediatr Res* 49:324, 2001.
47. Chowdhury JR: Hereditary jaundice and disorders of bilirubin metabolism. In Shriver CR editor: *The metabolic basis of inherited disease*, 6th ed, New York, 1989, McGraw-Hill; 1367.
48. Chowdhury JR, et al: Human hepatocyte transplantation: gene therapy and more? *Pediatrics* 102:647, 1998.
49. Chuniaud L, et al: Cytotoxicity of bilirubin for human fibroblasts and rat astrocytes in culture. Effect of the ratio of bilirubin to serum albumin, *Clin Chim Acta* 256:103, 1996.
50. Clarke DJ, et al: Genetic defects of the UDP-glucuronosyltransferase-1 (UGT1) gene that cause familial non-haemolytic unconjugated hyperbilirubinaemias, *Clin Chim Acta* 266:63, 1997.
51. Clayton PT, et al: Familial giant cell hepatitis associated with synthesis of 3 beta, 7 alpha-dihydroxy-and 3 beta,7 alpha, 12 alpha-trihydroxy-5-cholenoic acids, *J Clin Invest* 79:1031, 1987.
52. Connolly AM, Volpe JJ: Clinical features of bilirubin encephalopathy, *Clin Perinatol* 17:371, 1990.
53. Cornelius CE, Rodgers PA: Prevention of neonatal hyperbilirubinemia in rhesus monkeys by tin-protoporphyrin, *Pediatr Res* 18:728, 1984.
54. Costarino AT, et al: Bilirubin photoisomerization in premature neonates under low- and high-dose phototherapy, *Pediatrics* 75:519, 1985.

55. Crawford JM, et al: Formation, hepatic metabolism, and transport of bile pigments: a status report, *Semin Liver Dis* 8:105, 1988.

56. Crosnier C, et al: Mutations in Jagged1 gene are predominantly sporadic in Alagille syndrome, *Gastroenterology* 116:1141, 1999.

57. Cui Y, et al: Hepatic uptake of bilirubin and its conjugates by the human organic anion transporter SLC21A6, *J Biol Chem* 276:9626, 2001.

58. Davis DR, Yeary RA: Activated charcoal as an adjunct to phototherapy for neonatal jaundice, *Dev Pharmacol Ther* 10:12, 1987.

59. De Carvalho M, et al: Frequency of breast-feeding and serum bilirubin concentration, *Am J Dis Child* 136:737, 1982.

60. DeNagel DC, et al: Identification of non-porphyrin inhibitors of heme oxygenase-1, *Neuroscience* 24:2058, 1998.

61. DeSandre GH, et al: The effectiveness of oral tin mesoporphyrin prophylaxis in reducing bilirubin production after an oral heme load in a transgenic mouse model, *Biol Neonate* 89:139, 2006.

62. Diamond LK: Erythroblastosis foetalis or haemolytic disease of the newborn, *Proc Royal Soc Med* 40:546, 1977.

63. Diamond LK, et al: Erythroblastosis fetalis: VII. Treatment with exchange transfusion, *N Engl J Med* 244:39, 1951.

64. Drummond GS, Kappas A: Prevention of neonatal hyperbilirubinemia by tin protoporphyrin IX, a potent competitive inhibitor of heme oxidation, *Proc Natl Acad Sci U S A* 78:6466, 1981.

65. Ebbesen F: Recurrence of kernicterus in term and near-term infants in Denmark, *Acta Paediatr* 89:1213, 2000.

66. Ebbesen F, et al: A new transcutaneous bilirubinometer, BiliCheck, used in the neonatal intensive care unit and the maternity ward, *Acta Paediatr* 91:203, 2002.

67. Ennever JF: Blue light, green light, white light, more light: treatment of neonatal jaundice, *Clin Perinatol* 17:467, 1990.

68. Ennever JF, et al: Rapid clearance of a structural isomer of bilirubin during phototherapy, *J Clin Invest* 79:1674, 1987.

69. Ewing JF, et al: Normal and heat-induced patterns of expression of heme oxygenase-1 (HSP32) in rat brain: hyperthermia causes rapid induction of mRNA and protein, *J Neurochem* 58:1140, 1992.

70. Fairbanks VF, Fernandez MN: The identification of metabolic errors associated with hemolytic anemia, *JAMA* 208:316, 1969.

71. Fallstrom SP, Bjure J: Endogenous formation of carbon monoxide in newborn infants. 3. ABO incompatibility, *Acta Paediatr Scand* 57:137, 1968.

72. Fevery J: Bilirubin in clinical practice: A review, *Liver Int* 28:592, 2008.

73. Finegold MJ, Carpenter RJ: Obliterative cholangitis due to cytomegalovirus: a possible precursor of paucity of intrahepatic bile ducts, *Hum Pathol* 13:662, 1982.

74. Fischer AF, et al: Comparison of bilirubin production in Japanese and Caucasian infants, *J Pediatr Gastroenterol Nutr* 7:27, 1988.

75. Fox IJ, et al: Treatment of the Crigler-Najjar syndrome type I with hepatocyte transplantation, *N Engl J Med* 338:1422, 1998.

76. Galbraith RA, et al: Suppression of bilirubin production in the Crigler-Najjar type I syndrome: studies with the heme oxygenase inhibitor tin-mesoporphyrin, *Pediatrics* 89:175, 1992.

77. Gale R, et al: A randomized, controlled application of the Wallaby phototherapy system compared with standard phototherapy, *J Perinatol* 10:239, 1990.

77a.Garcia-Barceló MM, Yeung MY, Miao XP: Genome-wide association study identifies a susceptibility locus for biliary atresia on m10q24.2, *Hum Mol Genet* 19:2917, 2010.

78. Gartner LM: Neonatal jaundice, *Pediatr Rev* 15:422, 1994.

79. Gartner LM, et al: Effect of milk feeding on intestinal bilirubin absorption in the rat, *J Pediatr* 103:464, 1983.

80. Gibson BE, et al: Transfusion guidelines for neonates and older children, *Br J Haematol* 124:433, 2004.

81. Glaser JH, Morecki R: Reovirus type 3 and neonatal cholestasis, *Semin Liver Dis* 7:100, 1987.

82. Goudonnet H, et al: Differential action of thyroid hormones and chemically related compounds on the activity of UDP-glucuronosyltransferases and cytochrome P-450 isozymes in rat liver, *Biochim Biophys Acta* 1035:12, 1990.

83. Gourley GR: Breast-feeding, neonatal jaundice and kernicterus, *Semin Neonatol* 7:135, 2002.

84. Gourley GR, et al: A controlled, randomized, double-blind trial of prophylaxis against jaundice among breastfed newborns, *Pediatrics* 116:385, 2005.

85. Govaert P, et al: Changes in globus pallidus with (pre)term kernicterus, *Pediatrics* 112:1256, 2003.

86. Granovsky MO, et al: Hepatitis C virus infection in the mothers and infants cohort study, *Pediatrics* 102:355, 1998.

87. Greene CM, et al: Alpha-1 antitrypsin deficiency: a conformational disease associated with lung and liver manifestations, *J Inherit Metab Dis* 31:21, 2008.

88. Greene HL: Glycogen storage disease, *Semin Liver Dis* 2:291, 1982.

89. Grobler JM, Mercer MJ: Kernicterus associated with elevated predominantly direct-reacting bilirubin, *S Afr Med J* 87:1146, 1997.

90. Grundbacher FJ: The etiology of ABO hemolytic disease of the newborn, *Transfusion* 20:563, 1980.

91. Hackney DN, et al: Management of pregnancies complicated by anti-c isoimmunization, *Obstet Gynecol* 103:24, 2004.

92. Hafkamp AM, et al: Orlistat treatment of unconjugated hyperbilirubinemia in Crigler-Najjar disease: a randomized controlled trial, *Pediatr Res* 62:725, 2007.

93. Hammerman C, et al: Intravenous immune globulin in neonatal immune hemolytic disease: does it reduce hemolysis? *Acta Paediatr* 85:1351, 1996.

94. Hansen TW, et al: Effects of sulfisoxazole, hypercarbia, and hyperosmolality on entry of bilirubin and albumin into brain regions in young rats, *Biol Neonate* 56:22, 1989.

95. Heiser CA: Home phototherapy. *Pediatr Nurs* 13:425, 1987.

96. Herschel M, Beutler E: Low glucose-6-phosphate dehydrogenase enzyme activity level at the time of hemolysis in a male neonate with the African type of deficiency, *Blood Cells Mol Dis* 27:918, 2001.

97. Herschel M, et al: Hemolysis and hyperbilirubinemia in an African American neonate heterozygous for glucose-6-phosphate dehydrogenase deficiency, *J Perinatol* 22:577, 2002.

98. Hofmann AF: Current concepts of biliary secretion, *Dig Dis Sci* 34:16S, 1989.

99. Hsia DYY, et al: Erythroblastosis fetalis: VIII. Studies of serum bilirubin in relation to kernicterus, *N Engl J Med* 247:668, 1952.

100. Huang CS, et al: Glucose-6-phosphate dehydrogenase deficiency, the UDP-glucuronosyl transferase 1A1 gene, and neonatal hyperbilirubinemia, *Gastroenterology* 123:127, 2002.

100a. Huang L, Wang W, Liu G, et al: Laparoscopic cholecystochol-angiography for diagnosis of prolonged jaundice in infants, experience of 144 cases, *Pediatr Surg Int* 26:711, 2010.

101. Hurwitz M, et al: Copper deficiency during parenteral nutrition: a report of four pediatric cases, *Nutr Clin Pract* 19:305, 2004.

102. Iolascon A, et al: Hereditary spherocytosis: From clinical to molecular defects, *Haematologica* 83:240, 1998.

103. Iyer S, et al: Characterization and biological significance of immunosuppressive peptide D2702.75-84 (E → V) binding protein. Isolation of heme oxygenase-1, *J Biol Chem* 273:2692, 1998.

104. Jackson JC: Adverse events associated with exchange transfusion in healthy and ill newborns, *Pediatrics* 99:E7, 1997.

105. Jardine DS, Rogers K: Relationship of benzyl alcohol to kernicterus, intraventricular hemorrhage, and mortality in preterm infants, *Pediatrics* 83:153, 1989.

106. Jetté L, et al: Interaction of drugs with P-glycoprotein in brain capillaries, *Biochem Pharmacol* 50:1701, 1995.

107. Joy SD, et al: Management of pregnancies complicated by anti-E alloimmunization, *Obstet Gynecol* 105:24, 2005.

108. Kadakol A, et al: Genetic lesions of bilirubin uridine-diphosphoglucuronate glucuronosyltransferase (UGT1A1) causing Crigler-Najjar and Gilbert syndromes: correlation of genotype to phenotype, *Hum Mutat* 16:297, 2000.

109. Kaplan M, et al: Neonatal hyperbilirubinemia in glucose-6-phosphate dehydrogenase-deficient heterozygotes, *Pediatrics* 104:68, 1999.

110. Kaplan M, Hammerman C: Glucose-6-phosphate dehydrogenase deficiency: a hidden risk for kernicterus, *Semin Perinatol* 28:356, 2004.

111. Kaplan M, et al: Predischarge bilirubin screening in glucose-6-phosphate dehydrogenase-deficient neonates, *Pediatrics* 105:533, 2000.

112. Kaplan M, et al: Bilirubin genetics for the nongeneticist: hereditary defects of neonatal bilirubin conjugation, *Pediatrics* 111:886, 2003.

113. Kaplan M, et al: Gilbert's syndrome and hyperbilirubinaemia in ABO-incompatible neonates, *Lancet* 356:652, 2000.

114. Kaplan M, et al: Differing pathogenesis of perinatal bilirubinemia in glucose-6-phosphate dehydrogenase-deficient versus-normal neonates, *Pediatr Res* 50:532, 2001.

115. Kaplan M, et al: Acute hemolysis and severe neonatal hyperbilirubinemia in glucose-6-phosphate dehydrogenase-deficient heterozygotes, *J Pediatr* 139:137, 2001.

116. Kaplan M, et al: Hyperbilirubinemia among African American, glucose-6-phosphate dehydrogenase-deficient neonates, *Pediatrics* 114:e213, 2004.

117. Kaplan M, et al: Post-phototherapy neonatal bilirubin rebound: a potential cause of significant hyperbilirubinaemia, *Arch Dis Child* 91:31, 2006.

118. Kaplan M, et al: Gilbert syndrome and glucose-6-phosphate dehydrogenase deficiency: a dose-dependent genetic interaction crucial to neonatal hyperbilirubinemia, *Proc Natl Acad Sci U S A* 94:12128, 1997.

119. Kaplan M, et al: Conjugated bilirubin in neonates with glucose-6-phosphate dehydrogenase deficiency, *J Pediatr* 128:695, 1996.

120. Kaplan M, et al: Contribution of haemolysis to jaundice in Sephardic Jewish glucose-6-phosphate dehydrogenase deficient neonates, *Br J Haematol* 93:822, 1996.

121. Kappas A, et al: Direct comparison of Sn-mesoporphyrin, an inhibitor of bilirubin production, and phototherapy in controlling hyperbilirubinemia in term and near-term newborns, *Pediatrics* 95:468, 1995.

122. Kappas A, et al: A single dose of Sn-mesoporphyrin prevents development of severe hyperbilirubinemia in glucose-6-phosphate dehydrogenase-deficient newborns, *Pediatrics* 108:25, 2001.

122a. Kasai M, Kimura S, Asakura Y, et al: Surgical treatment of biliary atresia, *J Pediatr Surg* 3:665, 1968.

123. Kaufman SS, et al: Nutritional support for the infant with extrahepatic biliary atresia, *J Pediatr* 110:679, 1987.

124. Kawade N, Onishi S: The prenatal and postnatal development of UDP-glucuronyltransferase activity towards bilirubin and the effect of premature birth on this activity in the human liver, *Biochem J* 196:257, 1981.

125. King CD, et al: UDP-glucuronosyltransferases, *Curr Drug Metab* 1:143, 2000.

126. Kinobe RT, et al: Selectivity of imidazole-dioxolane compounds for *in vitro* inhibition of microsomal haem oxygenase isoforms, *Br J Pharmacol* 147:307, 2006.

127. Krantz ID, et al: Spectrum and frequency of Jagged1 (JAG1) mutations in Alagille syndrome patients and their families, *Am J Hum Genet* 62:1361, 1998.

128. Kubo S, et al: Can high-dose immunoglobulin therapy be indicated in neonatal rhesus haemolysis? A successful case of haemolytic disease due to rhesus (c + E) incompatibility, *Eur J Pediatr* 150:507, 1991.

129. Langbaum ME, et al: Automated total and neonatal bilirubin values in newborns: is a distinction clinically relevant? *Clin Chem* 38:1690, 1992.

130. Lee CS, et al: Development of jaundice in Korean neonates after cesarean section, *Acta Paediatr Jpn* 39:309, 1997.

130a. Leyva-Vega M, Gerfen J, Thiel BD, et al: Genomic alterations in biliary atresia suggest region of potential disease susceptibility in 2q37.3, *Am J Med Genet A* 152A:886, 2010.

131. Lightner DA, et al: Bilirubin photooxidation products in the urine of jaundiced neonates receiving phototherapy, *Pediatr Res* 18:696, 1984.

132. Lin HH, et al: Absence of infection in breast-fed infants born to hepatitis C virus-infected mothers, *J Pediatr* 126:589, 1995.

133. Lo SF, et al: Performance of bilirubin determinations in US laboratories—revisited, *Clin Chem* 50:190, 2004.

134. Mackenzie PI, et al: Polymorphisms in UDP glucuronosyltransferase genes: functional consequences and clinical relevance, *Clin Chem Lab Med* 38:889, 2000.

135. Maines MD: Zinc protoporphyrin is a selective inhibitor of heme oxygenase activity in the neonatal rat, *Biochim Biophys Acta* 673:339, 1981.

136. Maisels MJ: Jaundice. In Avery GB, Fletcher MA, MacDonald MG editors: *Neonatology: pathophysiology and management of the newborn*, 5th ed, Philadelphia, 1999, Lippincott Williams and Wilkins, p 765.

137. Maisels MJ, et al: Jaundice in the healthy newborn infant: a new approach to an old problem, *Pediatrics* 81:505, 1988.

137a. Maisels MJ, Bhutani VK, Bogen D, et al: Hyperbilirubinemia in the newborn infant ≥35 weeks' gestation: an update with clarifications, *Pediatrics* 124:1193, 2009.

138. Maisels MJ, Kring E: Transcutaneous bilirubinometry decreases the need for serum bilirubin measurements and saves money, *Pediatrics* 99:599, 1997.

139. Maisels MJ, McDonagh AF: Phototherapy for neonatal jaundice, *N Engl J Med* 358:920, 2008.

140. Maisels MJ, Newman TB: Kernicterus in otherwise healthy, breast-fed term newborns, *Pediatrics* 96:730, 1995.

141. Maisels MJ, Watchko JF: Treatment of jaundice in low birth-weight infants, *Arch Dis Child Fetal Neonatal Ed* 88:F459, 2003.

142. Manning D: American Academy of Pediatrics guidelines for detecting neonatal hyperbilirubinaemia and preventing kernicterus, *Arch Dis Child Fetal Neonatal Ed* 90:F450, 2005.

143. Manning D, et al: Prospective surveillance study of severe hyperbilirubinaemia in the newborn in the UK and Ireland, *Arch Dis Child Fetal Neonatal Ed* 92:F342, 2007.

144. Marks GS, et al: Does carbon monoxide have a physiological function? *Trends Pharmacol Sci* 12:185, 1991.

145. Martinez JC, et al: Control of severe hyperbilirubinemia in full-term newborns with the inhibitor of bilirubin production Sn-mesoporphyrin, *Pediatrics* 103:1, 1999.

146. Martinez JC, et al: Hyperbilirubinemia in the breast-fed newborn: a controlled trial of four interventions, *Pediatrics* 91:470, 1993.

147. Masiels MJ: Historical perspectives: transcutaneous bilirubinometry, *NeoReviews* 7:e217, 2006.

148. McDonagh AF, Lightner DA: "Like a shrivelled blood orange"—Bilirubin, jaundice, and phototherapy, *Pediatrics* 75:443, 1985.

149. Meberg A, Johansen KB: Screening for neonatal hyperbilirubinaemia and ABO alloimmunization at the time of testing for phenylketonuria and congenital hypothyreosis, *Acta Paediatr* 87:1269, 1998.

150. Mentzer WC: Pyruvate kinase deficiency and disorders of glycolysis. In Nathan DG, Orkin SH editors: *Nathan and Oski's Hematology of infancy and childhood*, 5th ed. *Philadelphia: WB Saunders Company*; 665, 1998.

151. Michalski C, et al: A naturally occurring mutation in the SLC21A6 gene causing impaired membrane localization of the hepatocyte uptake transporter, *J Biol Chem* 277:43058, 2002.

152. Mireles LC, et al: Antioxidant and cytotoxic effects of bilirubin on neonatal erythrocytes, *Pediatr Res* 45:355, 1999.

153. Moise KJ: Red blood cell alloimmunization in pregnancy, *Semin Hematol* 42:169, 2005.

154. Moise KJ Jr: Management of rhesus alloimmunization in pregnancy, *Obstet Gynecol* 112:164, 2008.

155. Mok JQ, et al: Infants born to mothers seropositive for human immunodeficiency virus. Preliminary findings from a multicentre European study, *Lancet* 1:1164, 1987.

156. Monaghan G, et al: Gilbert's syndrome is a contributory factor in prolonged unconjugated hyperbilirubinemia of the newborn, *J Pediatr* 134:441, 1999.

157. Monaghan G, et al: Genetic variation in bilirubin UPD-glucuronosyltransferase gene promoter and Gilbert's syndrome, *Lancet* 347:578, 1996.

158. Morecki R, et al: Detection of reovirus type 3 in the porta hepatis of an infant with extrahepatic biliary atresia: ultrastructural and immunocytochemical study, *Hepatology* 4:1137, 1984.

159. Morioka I, et al: Systemic effects of orally-administered zinc and tin (IV) metalloporphyrins on heme oxygenase expression in mice, *Pediatr Res* 59:667, 2006.

160. Morisawa T, et al: Inhibition of heme oxygenase activity in newborn mice by Azalanstat, *Can J Physiol Pharmacol* 86:651, 2008.

161. Morris BH, et al: Aggressive vs. conservative phototherapy for infants with extremely low birth weight, *N Engl J Med* 359:1885, 2008.

161a. Moyer V, Freese DK, Whitington PF, et al: Guideline for the evaluation of cholestatic jaundice in infants: recommendations of the North American Society for Pediatric Gastroenterology, Hepatology and Nutrition, *J Pediatr Gastroenterol Nutr* 39(3):306, 2004.

161b. Moyer K, Kaimal V, Pacheco C, et al: Staging of biliary atresia at diagnosis by molecular profiling of the liver, *Genome Med* 2:33, 2010.

162. Necheles TF, et al: The role of haemolysis in neonatal hyperbilirubinaemia as reflected in carboxyhaemoglobin levels, *Acta Paediatr Scand* 65:361, 1976.

163. Newman TB, Maisels MJ: Does hyperbilirubinemia damage the brain of healthy full-term infants? *Clin Perinatol* 17:331, 1990.

164. Newman TB, Maisels MJ: Evaluation and treatment of jaundice in the term newborn: a kinder, gentler approach, *Pediatrics* 89:809, 1992.

165. Nilsen ST, et al: Males with neonatal hyperbilirubinemia examined at 18 years of age, *Acta Paediatr Scand* 73:176, 1984.

166. Nishioka T, et al: Orlistat treatment increases fecal bilirubin excretion and decreases plasma bilirubin concentrations in hyperbilirubinemic Gunn rats, *J Pediatr* 143:327, 2003.

167. Nord KS, Saad S, Joshi VV, McLoughlin LC: Concurrence of alpha 1-antitrypsin deficiency and biliary atresia, *J Pediatr* 111:416, 1987.

168. Oda T, et al: Mutations in the human Jagged1 gene are responsible for Alagille syndrome, *Nat Genet* 16:235, 1997.

169. Odell GB, et al: Enteral administration of agar as an effective adjunct to phototherapy of neonatal hyperbilirubinemia, *Pediatr Res* 17:810, 1983.

170. Ohto H, et al: Transmission of hepatitis C virus from mothers to infants. The Vertical Transmission of Hepatitis C Virus Collaborative Study Group, *N Engl J Med* 330:744, 1994.

171. Okuda H, et al: Dose-related effects of phenobarbital on hepatic glutathione-S-transferase activity and ligandin levels in the rat, *Drug Metab Dispos* 17:677, 1989.

172. Onishi S, et al: Postnatal development of uridine diphosphate glucuronyltransferase activity towards bilirubin and 2-aminophenol in human liver, *Biochem J* 184:705, 1979.

173. Ostrow JD, et al: Reassessment of the unbound concentrations of unconjugated bilirubin in relation to neurotoxicity *in vitro*, *Pediatr Res* 54:98, 2003.

174. Ozmert E, et al: Long-term follow-up of indirect hyperbilirubinemia in full-term Turkish infants, *Acta Paediatr* 85:1440, 1996.

175. Ozolek JA, et al: Prevalence and lack of clinical significance of blood group incompatibility in mothers with blood type A or B, *J Pediatr* 125:87, 1994.

176. Patra K, et al: Adverse events associated with neonatal exchange transfusion in the 1990s, *J Pediatr* 144:626, 2004.

177. Penn AA, et al: Kernicterus in a full term infant, *Pediatrics* 93:1003, 1994.

178. Perlmutter DH: Pathogenesis of chronic liver injury and hepatocellular carcinoma in alpha-1-antitrypsin deficiency, *Pediatr Res* 60:233, 2006.

179. Phillips MJ, et al: Mechanisms of cholestasis, *Lab Invest* 54:593, 1986.

180. Reddy P, et al: Tin-mesoporphyrin in the treatment of severe hyperbilirubinemia in a very-low-birth-weight infant, *J Perinatol* 23:507, 2003.

181. Ritter JK, et al: Cloning of two human liver bilirubin UDP-glucuronosyltransferase cDNAs with expression in COS-1 cells, *J Biol Chem* 266:1043, 1991.

182. Rodgers PA, Stevenson DK: Developmental biology of heme oxygenase, *Clin Perinatol* 17:275, 1990.

183. Rogerson AG, et al: 14 Years of experience with home phototherapy, *Clin Pediatr* 25:296, 1986.

184. Rosenfeld W, et al: Phototherapy effect on the incidence of patent ductus arteriosus in premature infants: prevention with chest shielding, *Pediatrics* 78:10, 1986.

185. Roy-Chowdhury N, et al: Gene therapy for inherited hyperbilirubinemias, *J Perinatol* 21 Suppl 1:S114, 2001.

186. Rubaltelli FF, et al: Congenital nonobstructive, nonhemolytic jaundice: effect of tin-mesoporphyrin, *Pediatrics* 95:942, 1995.

187. Rubaltelli FF, et al: Transcutaneous bilirubin measurement: a multicenter evaluation of a new device, *Pediatrics* 107:1264, 2001.

188. Rübo J, et al: High-dose intravenous immune globulin therapy for hyperbilirubinemia caused by Rh hemolytic disease, *J Pediatr* 121:93, 1992.

189. Sampietro M, Iolascon A: Molecular pathology of Crigler-Najjar type I and II and Gilbert's syndromes, *Pediatrics* 84:150, 1999.

190. Scheidt PC, et al: Phototherapy for neonatal hyperbilirubinemia: six-year follow-up of the National Institute of Child Health and Human Development clinical trial, *Pediatrics* 85:455, 1990.

190a. Schreiber RA, Barker CC, Roberts EA, Martin SR: and the Canadian Pediatric Hepatology Research Group: Biliary atresia in Canada: the effect of centre caseload experience on outcome, *Pediatr Gastroenterol Nutr* 51:61, 2010.

191. Seidman DS, et al: A new blue light-emitting phototherapy device: a prospective randomized controlled study, *J Pediatr* 136:771, 2000.

192. Seidman DS, et al: Neonatal hyperbilirubinemia and physical and cognitive performance at 17 years of age, *Pediatrics* 88:828, 1991.

193. Sgro M, et al: Incidence and causes of severe neonatal hyperbilirubinemia in Canada, *CMAJ* 175:587, 2006.

194. Shapiro SM: Somatosensory and brainstem auditory evoked potentials in the Gunn rat model of acute bilirubin neurotoxicity, *Pediatr Res* 52:844, 2002.

195. Shapiro SM: Bilirubin toxicity in the developing nervous system, *Pediatr Neurol* 29:410, 2003.

196. Shapiro SM, Nakamura H: Bilirubin and the auditory system, *J Perinatol* 21(Suppl 1):S52, 2001.

197. Siegel E, Wason S: Mothball toxicity, *Pediatr Clin North Am* 33:369, 1986.

198. Slusher TM, et al: Glucose-6-phosphate dehydrogenase deficiency and carboxyhemoglobin concentrations associated with bilirubin-related morbidity and death in Nigerian infants, *J Pediatr* 126:102, 1995.

199. Sorrentino D, et al: The hepatocellular uptake of bilirubin: current concepts and controversies, *Mol Aspects Med* 9:405, 1987.

200. Spivak W, et al: Diagnostic utility of hepatobiliary scintigraphy with ^{99m}Tc-DISIDA in neonatal cholestasis, *J Pediatr* 110:855, 1987.

201. Stevens CE, et al: Perinatal hepatitis B virus transmission in the United States. Prevention by passive-active immunization, *JAMA* 253:1740, 1985.

202. Stevenson DK, et al: Pulmonary excretion of carbon monoxide in the human infant as an index of bilirubin production. IV. Effects of breast-feeding and caloric intake in the first postnatal week, *Pediatrics* 65:1170, 1980.

203. Stevenson DK, et al: Prediction of hyperbilirubinemia in near-term and term infants, *Pediatrics* 108:31, 2001.

204. Stevenson DK, et al: Bilirubin production in healthy term infants as measured by carbon monoxide in breath, *Clin Chem* 40:1934, 1994.

205. Stocker R, et al: Antioxidant activities of bile pigments: biliverdin and bilirubin, *Methods Enzymol* 186:301, 1990.

206. Strader DB, et al: Diagnosis, management, and treatment of hepatitis C, *Hepatology* 39:1147, 2004.

207. Strauss KA, et al: Management of hyperbilirubinemia and prevention of kernicterus in 20 patients with Crigler-Najjar disease, *Eur J Pediatr* 165:306, 2006.

208. Sugatani J, et al: The phenobarbital response enhancer module in the human bilirubin UDP-glucuronosyltransferase UGT1A1 gene and regulation by the nuclear receptor CAR, *Hepatology* 33:1232, 2001.

209. Swinney DC, et al: Selective inhibition of mammalian lanosterol 14 alpha-demethylase by RS-21607 *in vitro* and *in vivo*, *Biochemistry* 33:4702, 1994.

210. Tan KL: The pattern of bilirubin response to phototherapy for neonatal hyperbilirubinaemia, *Pediatr Res* 16:670, 1982.

211. Technical Manual Committee: Neonatal and pediatric transfusion practice. In Vengelen-Tyler V, editor: *Technical Manual of the American Association of Blood Banks*, Bethesda, 1999, p. 513-530.

212. Tenhunen R, et al: The enzymatic conversion of heme to bilirubin by microsomal heme oxygenase, *Proc Natl Acad Sci U S A* 61:748, 1968.

213. Tirona RG, et al: Polymorphisms in OATP-C: Identification of multiple allelic variants associated with altered transport activity among European- and African-Americans, *J Biol Chem* 276:35669, 2001.

214. Trioche P, et al: Jaundice with hypertrophic pyloric stenosis as an early manifestation of Gilbert syndrome, *Arch Dis Child* 81:301, 1999.

215. Tukey RH, Strassburg CP: Human UDP-glucuronosyltransferases: metabolism, expression, and disease, *Annu Rev Pharmacol Toxicol* 40:581, 2000.

216. Turkel SB: Autopsy findings associated with neonatal hyperbilirubinemia, *Clin Perinatol* 17:381, 1990.

217. Uetani Y, et al: Carboxyhemoglobin measurements in the diagnosis of ABO hemolytic disease, *Acta Paediatr Jpn* 31:171, 1989.

218. Vacanti JP, et al: The therapy of biliary atresia combining the Kasai portoenterostomy with liver transplantation: a single center experience, *J Pediatr Surg* 25:149, 1990.

219. Valaes T: Bilirubin and red cell metabolism in relation to neonatal jaundice, *Postgrad Med J* 45:86, 1969.

220. Valaes T, et al: Effectiveness and safety of prenatal phenobarbital for the prevention of neonatal jaundice, *Pediatr Res* 14:947, 1980.

221. Valaes T, et al: Control of jaundice in preterm newborns by an inhibitor of bilirubin production: studies with tin-mesoporphyrin, *Pediatrics* 93:1, 1994.

222. Valentine WN: Pyruvate kinase and other enzyme deficiency disorders of the erythrocyte. In Shriver CR, editor: *The metabolic basis of inherited disease,* 6th ed, New York, 1989, McGraw-Hill, p 2341.

223. van de Bor M, et al: Hyperbilirubinemia in low birth weight infants and outcome at 5 years of age, *Pediatrics* 89:359, 1992.

224. van der Veere CN, et al: Current therapy for Crigler-Najjar syndrome type 1: report of a world registry, *Hepatology* 24:311, 1996.

225. van Es HH, et al: Assignment of the human UDP glucuronosyltransferase gene (UGT1A1) to chromosome region 2q37, *Cytogenet Cell Genet* 63:114, 1993.

226. Vaughan JI, et al: Erythropoietic suppression in fetal anemia because of Kell alloimmunization, *Am J Obstet Gynecol* 171:247, 1994.

227. Veall N, Mollison PL: The rate of red-cell exchange in replacement transfusions, *Lancet* 2:792, 1950.

228. Vecchi C, et al: Phototherapy for neonatal jaundice: clinical equivalence of fluorescent green and "special" blue lamps, *J Pediatr* 108:452, 1986.

229. Vlahakis JZ, et al: Imidazole-dioxolane compounds as isozyme-selective heme oxygenase inhibitors, *J Med Chem* 49:4437, 2006.

230. Vreman HJ, et al: Selection of metalloporphyrin heme oxygenase inhibitors based on potency and photoreactivity, *Pediatr Res* 33:195, 1993.

231. Vreman HJ, et al: *In vitro* inhibition of adult rat intestinal heme oxygenase by metalloporphyrins, *Pediatr Res* 26:362, 1989.

232. Vreman HJ, et al: Carbon monoxide excretion as an index of bilirubin production in rhesus monkeys, *J Med Primatol* 18:449, 1989.

233. Vreman HJ, et al: Interlaboratory variability of bilirubin measurements, *Clin Chem* 42:869, 1996.

234. Vreman HJ, et al: Validation of the Natus CO-Stat™ End Tidal Breath Analyzer in children and adults, *J Clin Monit Comput* 15:421, 1999.

235. Vreman HJ, et al: Standardized bench method for evaluating the efficacy of phototherapy devices, *Acta Paediatr* 97:308, 2008.

236. Vreman HJ, et al: Simultaneous production of carbon monoxide and thiobarbituric acid reactive substances in rat tissue preparations by an iron-ascorbate system, *Can J Physiol Pharmacol* 76:1057, 1998.

237. Vreman HJ, et al: Alternative metalloporphyrins for the treatment of neonatal jaundice, *J Perinatol* 21:S108, 2001.

238. Vreman HJ, et al: Phototherapy: current methods and future directions, *Semin Perinatol* 28:326, 2004.

239. Vreman HJ, et al: Azalanstat (RS-1607): Evidence for a novel class of potential heme oxygenase inhibitors, *Pediatr Res* 51:341A(#1980), 2002.

240. Vreman HJ, et al: *In vitro* heme oxygenase isozyme activity inhibition by metalloporphyrins, *Pediatr Res* 43:202A, 1998.

241. Walker KA, et al: Selective inhibition of mammalian lanosterol 14 alpha-demethylase: a possible strategy for cholesterol lowering, *J Med Chem* 36:2235, 1993.

242. Walker PC: Neonatal bilirubin toxicity. A review of kernicterus and the implications of drug-induced bilirubin displacement, *Clin Pharmacokinet* 13:26, 1987.

243. Wallin A, Boreus LO: Phenobarbital prophylaxis for hyperbilirubinemia in preterm infants. A controlled study of bilirubin disappearance and infant behavior, *Acta Paediatr Scand* 73:488, 1984.

244. Watchko JF: Exchange transfusion. In Maisels MJ, Watchko JF editors: *Neonatal Jaundice,* Amsterdam, 2000, Harwood Academic Publishers, 169.

245. Watchko JF: Hyperbilirubinemia and bilirubin toxicity in the late preterm infant, *Clin Perinatol* 33:839, 2006.

246. Watchko JF, Claassen D: Kernicterus in premature infants: current prevalence and relationship to NICHD Phototherapy Study exchange criteria, *Pediatrics* 93:996, 1994.

247. Watchko JF, et al: Brain bilirubin content is increased in P-glycoprotein-deficient transgenic null mutant mice, *Pediatr Res* 44:763, 1998.

248. Watchko JF, Oski FA: Bilirubin 20 mg/dL = vigintiphobia, *Pediatrics* 71:660, 1983.

249. Wennberg RP, et al: Toward understanding kernicterus: a challenge to improve the management of jaundiced newborns, *Pediatrics* 117:474, 2006.

250. Wennberg RP, et al: Abnormal auditory brainstem response in a newborn infant with hyperbilirubinemia: improvement with exchange transfusion, *J Pediatr* 100:624, 1982.

251. Whitington PF: Cholestasis associated with total parenteral nutrition in infants, *Hepatology* 5:693, 1985.

252. Whitington PF, et al: The effect of tin (IV)-protoporphyrin-IX on bilirubin production and excretion in the rat, *Pediatr Res* 21:487, 1987.

253. WHO: Glucose-6-phosphate dehydrogenase deficiency. WHO Working Group, *Bull World Health Organ* 67:601, 1989.

254. Widness JA, et al: Direct relationship of fetal carboxyhemoglobin with hemolysis in alloimmunized pregnancies, *Pediatr Res* 35:713, 1994.

255. Witzleben CL, et al: Bile canalicular morphometry in arteriohepatic dysplasia, *Hepatology* 7:1262, 1987.

256. Wong RJ, et al: Tin mesoporphyrin for the treatment of neonatal hyperbilirubinemia, *NeoReviews* 8:e77, 2007.

257. Wong RJ, et al: Neonatal jaundice: bilirubin physiology and clinical chemistry, *NeoReviews* 8:e58, 2007.

258. Wood RP, et al: Optimal therapy for patients with biliary atresia: portoenterostomy ("Kasai" procedures) versus primary transplantation, *J Pediatr Surg* 25:153, 1990.

259. Yamanouchi I, et al: Transcutaneous bilirubinometry: preliminary studies of noninvasive transcutaneous bilirubin meter in the Okayama National Hospital, *Pediatrics* 65:195, 1980.

260. Yamauchi Y, Yamanouchi I: Transcutaneous bilirubinometry. Interinstrumental variability of TcB instruments, *Acta Paediatr Scand* 78:844, 1989.

261. Yasuda S, et al: New transcutaneous jaundice device with two optical paths, *J Perinat Med* 31:81, 2003.

262. Yeo KL, et al: Outcomes of extremely premature infants related to their peak serum bilirubin concentrations and exposure to phototherapy, *Pediatrics* 102:1426, 1998.

263. Zanella A, et al: Pyruvate kinase deficiency: the genotype-phenotype association, *Blood Rev* 21:217, 2007.

264. Zhang W, et al: Selection of potential therapeutics based on *in vivo* spatiotemporal transcription patterns of heme oxygenase-1, *J Mol Med* 80:655, 2002.

CHAPTER 49

Metabolic and Endocrine Disorders

PART 1

Disorders of Carbohydrate Metabolism

Satish C. Kalhan and Sherin U. Devaskar

The fetus depends entirely on the mother for its nutrient needs, including glucose. At birth, when the maternal supply is discontinued, the neonate must adjust to an independent existence. This transition to the extrauterine environment is often perturbed by alterations in the mother's metabolism or by intrinsic fetal and placental problems that result in changes in the neonate's glucose homeostasis. An understanding of the normal physiologic adaptation of the maternal-fetal nutritional relationship during pregnancy and of fetal glucose homeostasis and glucose metabolism during the transition to extrauterine life serves as a framework for evaluating disordered glucose metabolism in the neonate.

PLACENTAL TRANSPORT OF NUTRIENTS: MATERNAL-FETAL RELATIONSHIP

Although the fetus is entirely dependent on the mother for nutrients, it is hormonally independent of the mother (Fig. 49-1). Because no maternal peptide hormones are transported to the fetus in any significant amount, fetal endocrine and paracrine responses are mediated by the transport of nutrients such as glucose and amino acids to the fetus.

Glucose

Maternal glucose is the major substrate delivered to the human fetus for energy metabolism.[47] Glucose is transported to the fetus along a downward concentration gradient by carrier-mediated transport. In normal pregnancies, the plasma glucose concentration of the fetus is about 70% to 80% of that for the mother. Because maternal-fetal glucose transfer is not saturated by the range of glucose concentrations observed in human pregnancy, even when complicated by diabetes, fetal glucose uptake becomes excessive as the maternal glucose concentration increases. When fetal glucose uptake exceeds the requirements of energy production and growth, the excess glucose is stored as glycogen and triglycerides.

Fatty Acids

The transfer of fatty acids from the mother to the fetus appears to occur only in the free form (i.e., free fatty acids [FFAs]) and to depend on chain length, lipid solubility, and protein binding. A progressive shortening of chain length from C16 to C8 is associated with an increased transfer rate. Protein binding appears to slow the rate of transfer. Contrary to a previously held belief, data suggest that fatty acids are transported in significant amounts from the mother to the fetus.[78] A number of proteins involved in the sequestration and transport of fatty acids have been identified in the human placenta.[25] In addition, a significant amount of nonessential fatty acid appears to be synthesized de novo by the fetus in utero.

Amino Acids

Amino acids are transported to the fetus against a concentration gradient by a carrier-mediated transport process. Amino acids may be transported through the placenta either unchanged or after placental metabolism and processing—for example, leucine can be transferred intact or as its keto analogue α-ketoisocaproic acid. The syncytiotrophoblast is usually considered the main transport epithelium of the term placenta. Amino acids are transported by means of energy-dependent processes through selective amino acid transport systems.

Other Fetal Substrates

β-Hydroxybutyrate and possibly acetoacetate, the major ketone bodies, are transported along a concentration gradient.[3] The concentration of β-hydroxybutyrate in fetal blood is significantly less than that in maternal plasma (<50%);

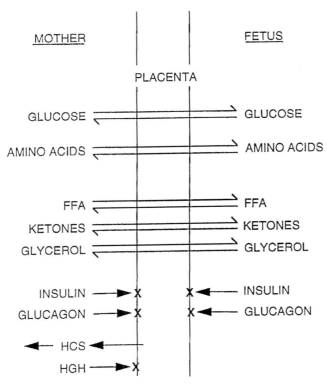

Figure 49–1. Maternal-fetal substrate hormone relationship. FFA, free fatty acids; HCS, human chorionic somatomammotropin; HGH, human growth hormone.

however, a linear correlation between the maternal and fetal concentrations has been reported.

Glycerol

There is a linear correlation between maternal and fetal glycerol levels, in most instances with the fetal level being somewhat lower than the simultaneously determined maternal plasma level.[3]

Lactate

The data on the maternal-fetal lactate relationship in human studies are conflicting. Two studies in sheep clearly demonstrated placental production and fetal utilization of lactate,[11] but the data in human studies showed higher levels of lactate in fetal than in maternal blood. In the few studies in which umbilical artery and vein samples were obtained simultaneously, the data could be interpreted as net fetal production and placental clearance of lactate.

FETAL HORMONES MEDIATING GROWTH

Immunoreactive insulin has been demonstrated in both plasma and pancreatic tissue at as early as 8 weeks of gestation; the source appears to be the fetal pancreas because the placenta is impermeable to insulin. At 13 to 18 weeks of gestation, the fetal insulin response to sustained maternal hyperglycemia is negligible. However, at term, the fetus is capable of a significant

response to prolonged hyperglycemia, although to a lesser degree than adults. When the fetus receives appropriate glucose from the mother, the requirement for an insulin response is minimal. With repeated episodes of hyperglycemia, as in maternal diabetes, a greater insulin response is seen, indicating that B-cell sensitivity is being induced or enhanced. That insulin may modify the growth rate in utero has been shown by the positive correlation between the fetal plasma insulin concentration and fetal weight. Human growth hormone (GH) has been measured at as early as 9 weeks of gestation and increases rapidly between the 11th and 16th weeks. Because the transplacental transfer of GH is negligible, the fetal pituitary appears to be its source in the fetus. At term, fetal plasma GH levels are higher than those of maternal plasma. Unlike those of adults, fetal GH levels are not suppressed during hyperglycemia and actually show a paradoxical rise. Several studies have demonstrated the role of insulin as the growth-promoting hormone of the fetus and that the fetus can sustain normal growth in the absence of GH.

FETAL GLUCOSE METABOLISM

Under normal circumstances (i.e., in an uncomplicated, normal pregnancy), the fetus is entirely dependent on the mother for a continuous supply of glucose for both energy metabolism and the synthesis of other metabolic substrates.[47] The fetal liver contains the full complement of enzymes required for the synthesis and breakdown of glycogen. Hepatic glycogen content is low early in gestation; a slow, continuous increase occurs between 15 and 20 weeks; and a rapid accumulation of glycogen in the liver is observed late. The fetus also has all the key hepatic enzymes involved in gluconeogenesis, although their levels are lower than those in adults.[45] The only exception is cytosolic phosphoenolpyruvate carboxykinase, which, at least in the rat, is not expressed in utero and appears immediately after birth (Fig. 49-2).[34] Data in humans in vivo are not available; however, there is a consensus that in the mammalian species studied, the gluconeogenic capacity is not expressed in utero under unperturbed circumstances and the contribution of gluconeogenesis from lactate, pyruvate, or alanine to glucose is quantitatively negligible.[58] Studies in humans and animals have consistently demonstrated that the fetus does not produce glucose and that maternal glucose is the only source of fetal glucose. Fluctuations in maternal blood glucose are rapidly reflected in parallel changes in fetal glucose concentration. These variations occur even in response to acute hypoglycemia induced by insulin infusion in the mother during sheep pregnancy. However, if maternal hypoglycemia is prolonged, the fetus begins glucose production.[23] Whether such a response can occur in human pregnancy has not been examined and cannot be pursued without violating ethical standards. Glucose is the primary fuel for the fetus, accounting for about 80% of fetal energy consumption. The remaining 20% of fetal energy needs is provided by lactate, amino acids, and other means.

GLUCOSE METABOLISM AFTER BIRTH

At birth, as a result of cutting the umbilical cord, the supply of glucose and other nutrients abruptly ceases, and the newborn infant has to mobilize its depots to meet energy requirements.

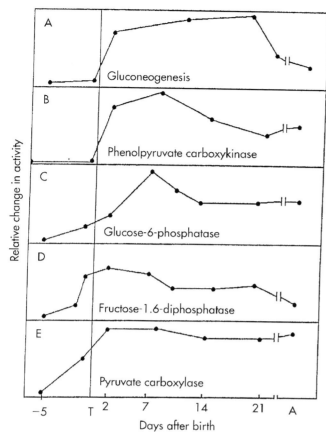

Figure 49–2. Changes in the relative activity of gluconeogenic enzymes in the rat liver during development. *(From Hanson RW, et al: Gluconeogenesis: its regulation in mammalian species, New York, 1976, John Wiley & Sons.)*

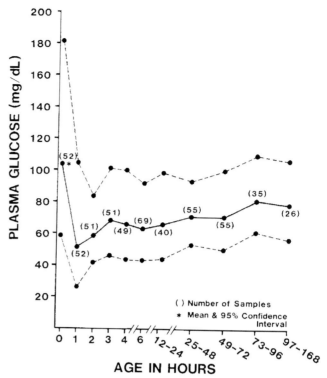

Figure 49–3. Plasma glucose levels in healthy term neonates delivered vaginally with birthweight between 2.5 and 4 kg. *(From Srinivasan G, et al: Plasma glucose values in normal neonates: a new look, J Pediatr 109:114, 1986.)*

Coincident with clamping of the umbilical cord are an acute surge in the levels of circulating epinephrine, norepinephrine, and glucagon and a fall in the levels of insulin. These hormones concomitantly mobilize hepatic glycogen and stimulate gluconeogenesis, resulting in a steady rate of glucose production and maintenance of the plasma glucose concentration.

The plasma glucose concentration in umbilical vein blood is about 80% of the prevailing maternal blood glucose concentration. After birth, the plasma glucose concentration falls in all infants, reaching its lowest value between 30 and 90 minutes after birth. Thereafter, in full-term healthy neonates, the plasma glucose concentration rises and is maintained at a steady level of 40 to 80 mg/dL. Full-term newborn infants can tolerate fasting without a significant change in the blood glucose concentration. Fasting up to 9 hours after a meal did not cause a decrease in the plasma glucose concentration.[21] In full-term infants, the plasma glucose levels obtained at random intervals during the first week after birth have ranged from 40 to 100 mg/dL, with a mean of 80 mg/dL (Fig. 49-3).[83] These levels are higher than those previously reported in fasting infants and reflect changes in feeding practices and the random nature of measurements. The plasma glucose concentration in healthy, asymptomatic, breast-fed babies has been reported to be lower than that in

formula-fed infants[86] during the first 24 hours of life—an average of 2.1 ± 0.07 mmol/L, or 37 mg/dL (range, 1.2 to 3.4 mmol/L, or 21 to 61 mg/dL). The plasma glucose values in infants who are small for gestational age (SGA) and in premature infants are somewhat lower.[37,45] Although no clear definition of hypoglycemia can be described, most investigators consider a plasma glucose level lower than 35 mg/dL to be abnormal, regardless of gestational age (see Chapter 14).

The rates of glucose production and utilization have been measured by a number of investigators with isotopic tracer dilution methods.[21] All these studies demonstrated the ability of newborn infants, both full-term and preterm, to produce glucose at rates significantly higher than those in adults. On average, the neonate produces glucose at rates between 4 and 6 mg/kg per minute. The higher rates of glucose production in the neonate reflect the higher ratio of brain to body weight, the brain being the major glucose-using organ. In the first few days after birth, the rate of glucose production during fasting in full-term infants has been reported to decrease slightly. As the infant grows, the rate of glucose production expressed per unit of body weight decreases, so by adolescence, it approaches the rate of adults.

Hepatic glucose output depends on (1) adequate glycogen stores, (2) sufficient supplies of endogenous gluconeogenetic precursors, (3) a normally functioning hepatic gluconeogenetic and glycogenolytic system, and (4) a normal endocrine system for modulating these processes. At birth, the neonate has glycogen stores that are greater than those in the adult.

However, because of twofold greater basal glucose utilization, the stores begin to decline within 2 to 3 hours after birth. Muscle and cardiac carbohydrate levels fall more slowly. During asphyxia, the energy requirements are met by anaerobic glycolysis, an inefficient mechanism that results in a limited amount of energy and a decrease in glycogen stores. In premature infants, both total carbohydrate and fat content are reduced, and depletion of liver carbohydrates occurs. Endogenous *gluconeogenetic* substrate availability is probably not a limiting factor because the concentration of plasma amino acids is high at birth as a consequence of active placental transport. Similarly, other *gluconeogenetic* precursors, such as lactate, pyruvate, and glycerol, are also increased. Nevertheless, active gluconeogenesis from alanine and lactate has been demonstrated in the human newborn soon after birth.[48,49] Finally, hepatic glucose production is normally regulated; that is, it decreases in response to glucose as well as insulin infusion in both full-term and preterm healthy neonates.[42] However, in sick or stressed neonates, exogenous glucose infusion may not completely suppress endogenous glucose production.

The fall in blood glucose that normally occurs after birth is accompanied by an increased level of GH, a relatively low concentration of immunoreactive insulin, and an increase in plasma glucagon. The neonate shows an attenuated but significant insulin response to a variety of stimuli. After the oral administration of glucose, the insulin response in the normal neonate is similar to that in adults with chemical diabetes, that is, a lag in insulin response and a delayed peak. The premature infant has a minimal and variable insulin response, but the values are markedly increased by the intravenous administration of glucose plus amino acids. The physiologic role of increased GH levels has not been defined; GH values are high during the first 48 to 72 hours and gradually decline but are still elevated at 8 weeks of age. In addition, the newborn shows a paradoxical rise in GH after glucose infusion. Plasma glucagon values at birth are similar to or slightly higher than maternal levels. Glucagon and GH are not suppressed during hyperglycemia. In healthy newborns, intravenous and oral alanine feedings raise plasma glucagon and glucose levels.

Adaptation to prolonged starvation in adult humans is facilitated by the ability of the brain to derive much of its energy from the oxidation of ketone bodies, which decreases the need for gluconeogenesis and spares muscle protein. The enzymes involved in ketone body utilization pathways are present in the brain tissue of human fetuses and newborns. That ketone bodies can be used by the brain of infants and children has been shown by measurements of arteriovenous differences across the brain.

The transition from an intrauterine environment to independent extrauterine life is also characterized by intense lipid mobilization, as shown by a rapid increase in plasma glycerol and FFAs. In addition, there is a shift in the sources of energy for oxidative metabolism, as evidenced by a decline in the respiratory quotient. An increased contribution of fat to oxidative metabolism is reflected in a drop in the respiratory quotient from near 1.0 at birth to a level between 0.8 and 0.85 within a few hours after birth. Evidence of significant lipolysis in the neonate has been obtained by using isotopic tracers to measure glycerol kinetics.[10,68] These studies showed that lipolysis in the neonate occurs at rates almost threefold greater than those in adults, and that the major metabolic fate of glycerol released as a result of lipolysis is conversion to glucose.

Measurement of Glucose

Factors frequently overlooked in the interpretation of glucose concentration are the type of sample and the method of analysis. Whole blood includes red blood cells, which have a glucose concentration lower than that of plasma. Plasma glucose values are higher than those of whole blood by about 14%; the difference may be greater at very low glucose values (<30 mg/dL). Whole-blood glucose content also varies in accordance with the hematocrit. Neonatal red blood cells contain high concentrations of glycolytic intermediates; therefore, whole blood must be deproteinized with zinc hydroxide before analysis. Capillary blood samples should be collected from a warm heel and kept on ice because the rate of in vitro glycolysis is increased in red blood cells at room temperature; whole-blood glucose values may drop 15 to 20 mg/dL per hour if the sample is allowed to stand at room temperature. The most frequently used method for glucose determination in the laboratory is an automatic analysis technique with glucose oxidase or a commercial glucose oxidase immobilized electrode. Plasma or serum glucose concentrations are determined, and the results are very accurate.

In many nurseries, the rapid assessment of whole-blood glucose concentrations is accomplished by a glucose oxidase and peroxidase chromogen test strip method, either alone or with a reflectance colorimeter. However, all test strip methods show significant variations in glucose concentrations compared with laboratory methods, particularly in the low glucose range (<45 mg/dL). Devices and operator techniques vary, with confounding influences of incubation time and the hematocrit. It remains to be determined whether laboratory instrumentation can be moved to the bedside and used effectively, safely, and legally by nursery personnel. There should not be sole reliance on test strip devices, and tests resulting in borderline values (<40 to 45 mg/dL) should be repeated by using standard laboratory methods. Test strips are more reliable at high glucose concentrations and may be useful for screening or identifying a trend when hyperglycemia is suspected.

Continuous glucose monitoring, using a subcutaneously placed microdialysis sensor, has been validated in adults and children with diabetes. The feasibility, safety, and usefulness of these techniques have been examined in babies with low birthweight.[6,8] These data show that such devices can be useful for monitoring asymptomatic hypoglycemia, which may be missed by the current practice of intermittent testing. However, these methods cannot measure glucose levels below 45 mg/dL with confidence, and the variance is large at the high glucose concentrations. Thus far, these techniques have been used only for research studies, and their associated potential risks require further evaluation.

HYPOGLYCEMIA

Perturbations in glucose metabolism after birth caused by failure to adapt to the extrauterine environment, as a result of either alterations in maternal metabolism or intrinsic metabolic problems in the neonate, often result in hypoglycemia. Lengthy debate has occurred among investigators regarding the definition of hypoglycemia.[16] The controversy arises partly because of the spontaneous decrease followed by recovery of the blood glucose concentration after birth and partly because many neonates have very low blood glucose concentrations without any clinical signs or symptoms (i.e., asymptomatic hypoglycemia). Finally, a convincing relationship between asymptomatic hypoglycemia in the neonate and long-term neurologic sequelae has not been demonstrated (see later section, "Prognosis of Neonatal Hypoglycemia"). Attempts have been made to define hypoglycemia by either a statistical approach or correlation of blood glucose concentration with clinical signs and symptoms. Because the clinical signs of hypoglycemia in the neonate are not specific to alterations in glucose concentration, the latter approach has not been successful. The statistical definition of hypoglycemia is based on surveys of large numbers of infants. *Abnormality* is defined as a blood glucose concentration that falls outside a prescribed limit, for example, outside 2 standard deviations from the norm.[16,54] Based on studies of preterm and term neonates conducted in the 1960s, abnormal blood glucose levels were defined as those less than 30 mg/dL in full-term infants during the first 72 hours after birth and less than 20 mg/dL in preterm infants (i.e., infants weighing <2500 g). However, since that time, the intrapartum clinical care of the mother and nutritional clinical management of the neonate have changed markedly, so the glucose concentrations observed several years ago are no longer seen in current clinical practice. In addition, the routine use of intravenous dextrose-containing fluids in preterm infants has confounded the ability to study glucose concentration in these small babies. Using 95% confidence intervals of the mean, Srinivasan and colleagues[83] showed that normal, healthy, full-term infants who were fed early achieved plasma glucose values of higher than 40 mg/dL within 4 hours after birth and higher than 45 mg/dL within 24 hours after birth. In their study, 10% of the neonates had at least one value of less than 35 mg/dL in the first 3 hours (see Fig. 49-3). Others have recommended that serum concentrations of lower than 30 mg/dL in the first 24 hours and lower than 40 mg/dL after 24 hours be considered hypoglycemic. Based on their study of preterm infants, Lucas and coworkers[55] suggested that plasma glucose values of less than 47 mg/dL be considered hypoglycemic.

Although a consensus regarding cutoff values for hypoglycemia has not been reached, most investigators would consider a plasma glucose concentration of lower than 36 mg/dL to be low (hypoglycemia requiring intervention) in a full-term neonate 2 to 3 hours after birth. Care should be taken in interpreting glucose values during the transition period (i.e., the first 2 to 3 hours after birth), when the plasma glucose concentration may drop to low levels followed by spontaneous improvement. If low glucose levels are observed during this time, frequent glucose determinations should be obtained to demonstrate recovery. The definition of hypoglycemia for preterm infants should not be any different from that for full-term infants. Finally, hypoglycemia in the neonate should be described as transient or persistent, and in either or both of these cases, as symptomatic or asymptomatic. Such a description has

implications for both clinical management and long-term consequences.

Transient hypoglycemia implies low glucose values that last only a short time if not corrected and that it is confined to the newborn period. In contrast, persistent and recurrent hypoglycemia implies a form that requires prolonged management (glucose infusions for several days at high rates of infusion) and perhaps pharmacologic intervention. Several of these hypoglycemia syndromes may continue throughout infancy and childhood.

The clinical manifestations of hypoglycemia are nonspecific and similar to those of many disorders in newborn infants (Box 49-1). The clinical signs and symptoms of hypoglycemia should improve with correction of the low glucose concentration. In addition, careful attention should be given to ensure that other associated disorders (e.g., sepsis, asphyxia) are not missed.

Because of its implications for both long-term prognosis and clinical management, it is worthwhile to consider two types of neonatal hypoglycemia: those cases limited to the newborn period (transient hypoglycemia) and those cases continuing over an extended period of time or occurring more than once (persistent or recurrent hypoglycemia) (Box 49-2). Transient hypoglycemia is often a consequence of changes in the metabolic environment in utero or ex utero, whereas persistent or recurrent hypoglycemia arises from intrinsic metabolic problems in the infant. Either type of hypoglycemia may manifest asymptomatically or symptomatically.

Transient Hypoglycemia Caused by Changes in Maternal Metabolism

INTRAPARTUM GLUCOSE ADMINISTRATION

As already discussed, the fetus is entirely dependent on the mother for the supply of glucose, and fetal glucose concentration closely mimics that of the mother.[3] An increase in maternal glucose concentration as a result of exogenous glucose infusion causes an increase in fetal glucose concentration, which in turn causes an increase in fetal insulin levels.

BOX 49–1 **Clinical Symptoms and Signs of Hypoglycemia***

- Abnormal crying
- Irritability
- Apnea, cyanotic spells
- Jitteriness, tremors
- Feeding difficulty
- Lethargy or stupor
- Grunting, tachypnea
- Seizures
- Hypothermia
- Sweating
- Hypotonia, limpness
- Tachycardia

---

*Clinical signs should be alleviated with concomitant correction of plasma glucose levels.

BOX 49–2 Causes of the Two Types of Neonatal Hypoglycemia

I. Transient hypoglycemia
  A. Associated with changes in maternal metabolism
    1. Intrapartum administration of glucose
    2. Drug treatment
      a. Terbutaline, ritodrine, propranolol
      b. Oral hypoglycemic agents
    3. Diabetes in pregnancy: infant of diabetic mother
  B. Associated with neonatal problems
    1. Idiopathic condition or failure to adapt
    2. Intrauterine growth restriction
    3. Birth asphyxia
    4. Infection
    5. Hypothermia
    6. Hyperviscosity
    7. Erythroblastosis fetalis
    8. Other
      a. Iatrogenic causes
      b. Congenital cardiac malformations
II. Persistent or recurrent hypoglycemia
  A. Hyperinsulinism
    1. β-cell hyperplasia, nesidioblastosis-adenoma spectrum, sulfonylurea receptor defect
    2. Beckwith-Wiedemann syndrome
  B. Endocrine disorders
    1. Pituitary insufficiency
    2. Cortisol deficiency
    3. Congenital glucagon deficiency
    4. Epinephrine deficiency
  C. Inborn errors of metabolism
    1. Carbohydrate metabolism
      a. Galactosemia
      b. Hepatic glycogen storage diseases
      c. Fructose intolerance
    2. Amino acid metabolism
      a. Maple syrup urine disease
      b. Propionic acidemia
      c. Methylmalonic acidemia
      d. Hereditary tyrosinemia
      e. 3-hydroxy, 3-methyl glutaric acidemia
      f. Ethylmalonic-adipic aciduria
      g. Glutaric acidemia type II
    3. Fatty acid metabolism
      a. Defects in carnitine metabolism
      b. Acyl-coenzyme dehydrogenase defects
  D. Neurohypoglycemia (hypoglycorrhachia) due to defective glucose transport

Studies in animals have shown that fetal hyperinsulinism, caused by either direct infusion of insulin to the fetus or fetal hyperglycemia, results in an increased metabolic rate in the fetus, fetal hypoxemia, and metabolic acidosis. Similar patterns of change have been demonstrated in human pregnancy.[72] The acute administration of glucose during the intrapartum period—for example, to prevent hypotension during the conduction of anesthesia—has been shown to result in increased glucose, insulin, and lactate levels in the cord blood obtained at delivery.[49,72] Fetal hyperinsulinism leads to hyperinsulinemia and hypoglycemia in the neonate. Similar observations have been reported in diabetic pregnancy. Therefore, caution should be exercised in the administration of glucose to the mother during labor and delivery (see Chapter 25). Blood glucose concentrations in the mother should not be allowed to exceed those observed in the normal physiologic range.

MATERNAL TREATMENT

The antidiabetic drugs tolbutamide and chlorpropamide cross the placenta and produce pancreatic β-cell hyperplasia and increased insulin release. Tolbutamide has a markedly prolonged half-life in the neonate and has been found in higher concentrations in the newborn after delivery than those found in maternal blood. Although they are not used extensively in the United States, these drugs are used in other countries to treat gestational diabetes. Protracted hypoglycemia may occur after birth. Exchange transfusion was required in one infant whose mother received chlorpropamide and in whom hypoglycemia was not responsive to any conventional method of management. Newer formulations of these drugs have been shown to be safer because they do not cross the placenta as readily as the previous products.

Benzothiadiazide diuretics may cause neonatal hypoglycemia by stimulation of fetal β cells or secondary to an elevation in maternal glucose levels. Salicylates may cause hypoglycemia by uncoupling mitochondrial oxidative phosphorylation.

Oral β-sympathomimetic tocolytic drugs such as terbutaline and ritodrine have caused sustained hypoglycemia and elevated cord blood insulin levels in infants delivered within 2 days after termination of tocolytic therapy (see Chapter 16). These agents may cause neonatal hypoglycemia through maternal hyperglycemia and fetal hyperglycemia and hyperinsulinemia.

β-Adrenergic blocking agents such as propranolol cross the mammalian placenta, and their effects on the fetus are easily demonstrated. These drugs are used during pregnancy for the treatment of hypertension, hyperthyroidism, cardiac arrhythmia, and other conditions. They may interfere with the effects of the normal surge in catecholamine levels at birth. In animal studies, propranolol has been shown to impair fetal growth and may cause neonatal hypoglycemia and impair the thermogenic response to cold exposure.

DIABETES IN PREGNANCY: THE INFANT OF A DIABETIC MOTHER

Although perturbations in glucose metabolism in the mother and their consequences to the fetus and neonate constitute the major metabolic disturbances of diabetes in pregnancy, neonatal morbidity involves a number of organ systems. The major neonatal morbidities in infants of diabetic mothers (IDMs) whose maternal diabetes was not rigorously managed are displayed in Box 49-3.

The pathogenesis of the spectrum of fetal and neonatal morbidities in the IDM has now been described by a number of careful studies in human and animal models. Intermittent hyperglycemia in the mother results in hyperglycemia in the fetus, which in turn causes hypertrophy of the fetal pancreatic islets and β cells and increased secretion of insulin. Because

BOX 49–3 Morbidity in Infants of Diabetic Mothers

- Congenital anomalies
- Heart failure and septal hypertrophy of heart
- Hyperbilirubinemia
- Hypocalcemia
- Hypoglycemia
- Macrosomia
- Renal vein thrombosis
- Small left colon
- Unexplained intrauterine demise
- Polycythemia
- Visceromegaly

of the lack of significant transfer of insulin from the mother to the fetus in humans, the circulating insulin in the fetal compartment is mostly of fetal origin. However, two studies have demonstrated that in insulin-dependent diabetes, in the presence of antibodies to insulin, a small amount of insulin exogenously administered to the mother may be transported to the fetus.[5,59] Nevertheless, the newborn IDM has been shown to be hyperinsulinemic, as evidenced by increased levels of insulin and C peptide in the umbilical blood. The consequences of fetal hyperinsulinemia have been documented in experimental animal models. By infusing insulin directly into the normal rhesus monkey fetus through an osmotic pump, Susa and associates[85] showed that fetal hyperinsulinemia resulted in macrosomia, cardiomegaly, and an increase in adipose tissue. In addition, the activity of hepatic enzymes affecting lipid synthesis increased. Chronic

fetal hyperinsulinemia also results in an increase in the metabolic rate and oxygen consumption, leading to relative hypoxemia, which in turn results in an increase in the synthesis of erythropoietin and an increase in red blood cell mass and polycythemia.[12] In addition, hyperinsulinemia has been shown to suppress the production of surfactant in the lung and thus predispose to respiratory distress syndrome after birth (see Chapter 44). An excessive accumulation of glycogen in the liver, adipose tissue, and other tissues has also been observed in IDMs. The sequence of these metabolic events is outlined in Figure 49-4.

Although the excessive transport of glucose from the mother to the fetus has been said to be primarily responsible for fetal metabolic and physiologic perturbations in the IDM, this hypothesis may also include the excessive transport of other nutrients (i.e., amino acids and lipids). An absolute or relative lack of insulin in the mother leads to the increased transport of mixed nutrients to the fetus as a consequence of increased levels of these nutrients in the maternal compartment. The increased concentration of these nutrients in the fetal circulation stimulates fetal insulin secretion, which in turn stimulates excessive fetal growth.

After birth, the newborn IDM whose mother's disease has not received rigorous antepartum management appears to be unable to produce sufficient circulating glucose and alternative fuels. Even the infants of mothers with rigorous management (i.e., those who have maintained normoglycemia throughout gestation) develop significantly lower blood glucose concentrations than those of normal infants. In addition, they do not mobilize fatty acids from adipose tissue; as a result, their circulating levels of FFAs remain low, although a normal increase in plasma glycerol has been observed. Such a metabolic picture

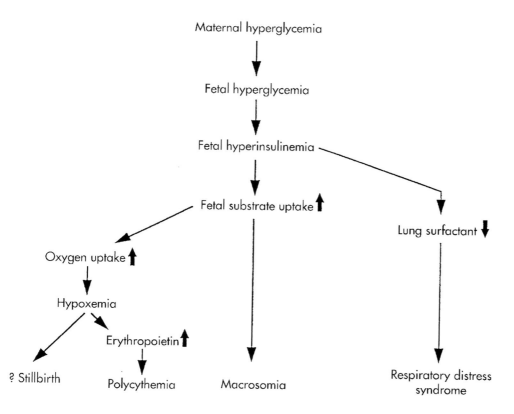

Figure 49–4. Flow diagram of pathogenic events that result in fetal and neonatal morbidity in infants of diabetic mothers. (*From Schwartz R, et al: Infant of the diabetic mother,* J Pediatr Endocrinol 5:197, 1992.)

suggests a persistent insulin action and the lack of a counter-regulatory hormonal response. The latter is confirmed by the lack of an increase in circulating glucagon and catecholamine levels in IDMs during hypoglycemia. The combination of hyperinsulinism and insufficient counter-regulation results in decreased hepatic glucose production, increased peripheral glucose uptake, and impaired lipolysis. When measured by the isotope tracer dilution method, IDMs produce glucose at significantly lower rates than normal infants.[46] In addition, their basal metabolic rates, or rates of oxygen consumption, have been reported to be lower than those of normal infants.

Several of these metabolic and morphologic abnormalities can be reversed with fastidious management of diabetes in the mother. Data from several studies showed that with rigorous management throughout pregnancy, IDMs do not become hypoglycemic and maintain normal rates of glucose production and basal metabolism.

Clinical Manifestations

It should be recognized that the clinical manifestations described here relate to diabetic mothers whose metabolism has not been well controlled. Data from a study[4] in which maternal diabetes was rigorously managed by either an insulin infusion pump or split-dose insulin therapy are shown in Table 49-1. Despite rigorous management and reduced maternal hyperglycemia, significant morbidity may persist.

MACROSOMIA

At birth, these infants are obese, plethoric, and large for gestational age (LGA) and show evidence of excessive fat as well as visceromegaly in the form of a large liver, spleen, and heart (Fig. 49-5). Because the growth of the brain and possibly the kidney is not dependent on insulin, these two organs are normal in size. Careful management of maternal metabolism tends to reduce the incidence of macrosomia but does not prevent it.

CONGENITAL ANOMALIES

The incidence of congenital malformations is increased twofold to threefold in the infants of insulin-dependent diabetic mothers compared with the normal population. The frequency of congenital anomalies is not increased in the infants of gestationally diabetic mothers or in those of diabetic fathers. A developmental morphologic approach, as applied by Mills and colleagues, suggests that congenital malformations in IDMs occur before the seventh week of development.[62] A number of congenital anomalies, including those of the heart, musculoskeletal system, and genitourinary system, have been reported. Caudal agenesis or dysplasia syndrome (Fig. 49-6) is seen with markedly increased frequency, especially in IDMs. This syndrome consists of agenesis or hypoplasia of the femora in conjunction with agenesis of the lower vertebrae and sacrum. Data from animal models show that certain genes belonging to the *PAX* family are involved in enhancing apoptosis, which then results in structural defects, for example, neural tube defects. The frequency of congenital anomalies is significantly increased in mothers with poor metabolic control, as evidenced by increased hemoglobin A_{1c} levels early in gestation,[61] and a significant decrease in congenital malformations has been reported with rigorous metabolic regulation in the periconceptional period (see Chapter 16).[30]

HYPOGLYCEMIA

The pathogenesis of hypoglycemia has been described already. Immediately after birth, there is a significant decrease in plasma glucose concentration, reaching a nadir between 30 and 90 minutes and followed by a spontaneous recovery in most infants. However, in some infants, the plasma glucose level remains persistently low (i.e., <36 mg/dL, often <20 mg/dL), necessitating intervention. Most of these infants are asymptomatic. Irrespective of symptoms, the current recommendation is to correct the hypoglycemia with an appropriate glucose infusion. It should be underscored that hypoglycemia in the newborn does not necessarily reflect the

TABLE 49–1 Neonatal Outcome in Infants of Rigorously Managed Diabetic Mothers			
Parameter	Infants of Diabetic Mother (*N* = 78)	Controls (*N* = 78)	*P*
Birthweight (g)	3454 ± 817	3271 ± 621	—
Gestational age (wk)	37.9 ± 0.95	39.3 ± 1.7	.0001
K score*	0.77 ± 0.95	0.18 ± 0.91	.0001
Macrosomia (>4 kg)	19 (24%)	8 (10%)	.03
Large for gestational age	32 (41%)	12 (15%)	.0002
Hypoglycemia	11 (14%)	1 (1%)	.0025
Hyperbilirubinemia	36 (46%)	18 (23%)	.002
Respiratory distress syndrome	9 (12%)	1 (1%)	.008
Admission to neonatal intensive care unit	21 (27%)	9 (12%)	.01

*The K score is a method of adjusting the birthweight in grams for the infant's gestational age. A K score of 1 represents the 90th percentile for weight; scores of 0 and −1 represent the 50th and 10th percentiles, respectively.
Adapted from Aucott SW, et al: Rigorous management of insulin-dependent diabetes mellitus during pregnancy, *Acta Diabetol* 31:126, 1994.

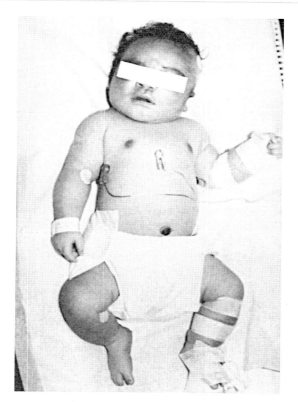

Figure 49–5. Infant of mother with gestational diabetes; the baby was born at 40 weeks of gestation with a birthweight of 4.6 kg. The infant developed hypoglycemia and was treated with intravenous glucose.

magnitude of antepartum metabolic control of the mother and may simply be the consequence of hyperglycemia during labor and delivery.

HYPOCALCEMIA AND HYPOMAGNESEMIA
See Chapter 49, Part 2.
Alterations in calcium and magnesium homeostasis occur in about 50% of infants born to insulin-dependent diabetic mothers. Unlike hypoglycemia, hypocalcemia becomes apparent between 48 and 72 hours after birth. Plasma calcium concentrations of lower than 7 mg/dL are frequently observed. Hypocalcemia has been related to the severity and duration of maternal diabetes. In addition, it may be potentiated by prematurity and asphyxia. The mechanisms of hypocalcemia are probably failure of the IDM to mount an appropriate parathyroid hormone (PTH) response, persistently high levels of calcitonin, and possibly alterations in vitamin D metabolism. Hypomagnesemia (<1.5 mg/dL) has also been frequently observed. It is usually transient, and its pathophysiologic significance remains uncertain.

Both hypocalcemia and hypomagnesemia may be manifested with jitteriness and may require supplemental calcium therapy. However, in most infants, they are transient events that improve spontaneously.

The management strategies for other clinical problems, such as polycythemia (see Chapter 46, Parts 1 and 2), hyperbilirubinemia (see Chapter 48), and renal vein thrombosis

(see Chapter 51), that occur with slightly higher frequency in IDMs are similar to those in otherwise normal infants.

SEPTAL HYPERTROPHY OF THE HEART
Septal hypertrophy and cardiomegaly are specific phenotypic consequences of diabetes in pregnancy and may be manifested with heart failure in the neonate (Fig. 49-7) (see Chapter 45). In addition, data in the asymptomatic infants of gestationally diabetic mothers have shown alterations in diastolic function and decreased passive compliance of the ventricular myocardium. By serially evaluating cardiac growth in utero in the fetuses of diabetic mothers, it has been shown that despite good metabolic control, cardiac hypertrophy developed in late gestation (34 to 40 weeks). Although IDMs with septal hypertrophy may present with obstructive left heart failure, they may also be asymptomatic. Follow-up data show that cardiomyopathy in an IDM is a transient disease and usually disappears spontaneously within 6 months after birth. Otherwise minor functional changes, such as impaired diastolic filling, have been reported in infants of gestational diabetic mothers and are usually not clinically significant.

Management of the Diabetic Mother
See Chapter 16.
Strict metabolic control, improved fetal surveillance, early delivery, and neonatal intensive care have led to improved survival among IDMs. Preconceptional and early postconceptional metabolic control may decrease the incidence of congenital malformations. Improving maternal compliance, preventing ketoacidosis, and recognizing and treating pregnancy-induced hypertension and pyelonephritis are particularly important. Attempts should be made to maintain maternal fasting plasma glucose values at less than 80 mg/dL and 2-hour postprandial plasma glucose values at less than 120 mg/dL.

With appropriate ambulatory support, hospitalization is not required in most mothers. Indications for hospitalization include pregnancy-induced hypertension, acute or chronic polyhydramnios, infections, and poor metabolic control. Early screening for congenital malformations includes a determination of the maternal serum α-fetoprotein level for open neural tube defects and a level II ultrasound at 18 to 20 weeks of gestation (see Chapters 8 and 9). Follow-up ultrasonography is useful in the evaluation of amniotic fluid volume, fetal growth, and placental grading. Tests of fetal well-being begin in the second trimester (28 to 32 weeks of gestation). These tests usually include daily fetal movement counts and biweekly biophysical testing (nonstress testing, biophysical profile, or both) or nonstress testing combined with an amniotic fluid index (see Chapter 10).

Delivery in insulin-dependent women is indicated after documentation of fetal lung maturity by amniocentesis (see Chapter 44, Part 1). With appropriate care and fetal surveillance, most patients are now monitored expectantly for the spontaneous onset of labor at term. Vaginal delivery is preferred, but obstetric factors may justify cesarean delivery. Caution should be exercised in the delivery of a macrosomic fetus at risk for traumatic complications. During labor, glucose and insulin therapy should be adjusted to maintain normoglycemia in the mother.

Delivery should take place in a hospital, where the newborn can be carefully monitored. Glucose values are checked

Figure 49–6. Anteroposterior (*left*) and lateral (*right*) radiographs of sacral agenesis in an infant of a diabetic mother.

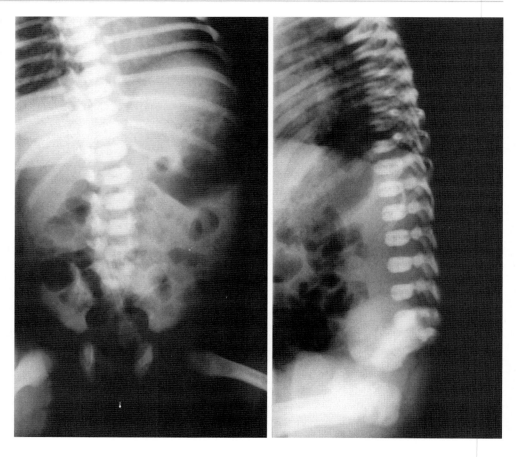

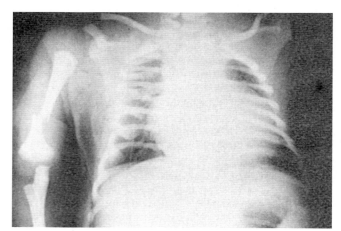

Figure 49–7. Chest radiograph of a vaginally delivered, full-term infant (4.7 kg) of a diabetic mother. The infant had cardiomegaly, hepatomegaly, congested lung fields, and fractures of the right humerus and left clavicle.

during the first 3 hours after birth (typically between 30 and 60 minutes), sporadically before feedings, and any time symptoms are suspected. Feedings may be started as soon as the infant is stable, usually within 2 to 4 hours after birth, and continued at 3- to 4-hour intervals.

Even though physiologic and clinical data clearly demonstrate a marked reduction in fetal and neonatal morbidity and

mortality in pregnancy with diabetes, two studies from the United Kingdom failed to show that such a goal was achieved in clinical practice.[13,41,82] Continuous rigorous surveillance of diabetes throughout the pregnancy and fastidious management of altered metabolism are required.

Prognosis

Improvements in antepartum care, fetal monitoring, rigorous control of maternal metabolism, and maternal education have all resulted in reduced perinatal mortality and morbidity. In addition, control of maternal metabolism during the periconceptional period has resulted in a decreased incidence of congenital malformations in IDMs. However, certain morbidities, such as hypoglycemia, macrosomia, and polycythemia, persist. The long-term consequences of an abnormal intrauterine metabolic environment remain a subject of continued interest. In the rat fetus, intrauterine hyperinsulinism induced by injection of insulin resulted in fetal and neonatal macrosomia. Significantly, this macrosomia persisted for up to 12 weeks after birth—the final time point of the study. In addition, mild hyperglycemia induced by glucose infusion during pregnancy in the rat resulted in glucose intolerance and impaired insulin secretion. Limited data in humans have examined the long-term consequences of an altered intrauterine metabolic environment in the infant and young adult.[70] Even though the IDM may be born macrosomic and obese, most of these changes in body composition tend to reverse during infancy. Long-term follow-up studies have not shown an increased risk for obesity or diabetes in this population.[70] Exceptions were a study by Vohr and colleagues,[90] which demonstrated a correlation between being LGA at birth and having a higher weight-to-height ratio at 7 years of age, and a study of the Pima Indians by Pettitt and coworkers, which demonstrated a high incidence of obesity and diabetes in the children of diabetic mothers. However, the impact of the intrauterine environment could not be separated from genetic predisposition in the latter study.

The risk for the subsequent development of insulin-dependent diabetes in IDMs has been carefully examined in a series of studies from the Joslin Diabetes Center. The cumulative risk for the development of insulin-dependent diabetes mellitus before 20 years of age was 2.1% (20 of 739 mothers) when the mother had diabetes and 5.1% (28 of 840 fathers) when the father had insulin-dependent diabetes.[27,92] The slightly increased risk for diabetes mellitus in IDMs was shown to be independent of risk factors for perinatal morbidity. Diabetes in the father did not influence morbidity in the infant except for the genetic predisposition for diabetes.

Another study revealed that the children of diabetic mothers, with and without macrosomia in the newborn period, had higher body mass indexes, higher blood pressures, and higher glucose and insulin levels on glucose tolerance testing when evaluated at age 18 to 26 years.[75] Other studies have shown impaired insulin signaling and glucose transport and altered mitochondrial number and function in the skeletal muscle of the adult offsprings of diabetic mothers. These data need to be confirmed and their health consequences determined in a large cohort of carefully monitored children.

The evaluation of the neurodevelopmental outcome of IDMs is confounded by the contribution of perinatal events such as birth asphyxia and metabolic acidosis. Recent data from animal models suggest relative iron deficiency in the brain that has been related to functional impairment. Nonetheless, several investigators have examined the impact of alterations in maternal metabolism, specifically changes in blood glucose and ketones, on neurodevelopment in the newborn period and early childhood. In 1969, Churchill and colleagues[14] first reported that diabetic mothers with acetonuria had offspring with lower intelligence quotients (IQs) than controls (mean IQ, 93 versus 102). These subjects were part of the large Perinatal Study, and the infants were given either Bayley mental and motor examinations at 8 months or the Stanford-Binet IQ test at 4 years. In this study, the mean IQ of the offspring of diabetic mothers without acetonuria was equal to that of controls (101). In addition, this association between acetonuria and the IQ of the children was present in both gestational diabetes and insulin-dependent diabetes. Intellectual delay at ages 3 and 5 years in infants born to acetonuric women has been observed. It should be emphasized that acetonuria is also a marker of poor metabolic control. Since these early studies, much improvement in the antepartum management of maternal diabetes has occurred, so the neuropsychological outcome for the IDM should be examined in relation to maternal blood glucose control, alterations in lipid metabolism (e.g., FFAs, ketones), and perinatal events such as neonatal asphyxia and hypoglycemia. Available data[81] show that, when examined as a group, IDMs have mental development indexes and Stanford-Binet test scores that are not significantly different from those of infants of normal mothers. However, when correlation analyses were performed, a negative correlation was observed by Rizzo and colleagues[76] between second- and third-trimester glycemic regulation (hemoglobin A_{1c} and fasting plasma glucose levels) and the newborn behavior dimensions of the Brazelton Neonatal Behavioral Assessment and between third-trimester ketonuria and mental developmental index scores at 2 years of age and Stanford-Binet scores at 3 to 5 years of age. Finally, it was demonstrated in other studies that IDMs who were born with malformations or who were shown to have early growth delay in utero tended to present with developmental impairments.[70]

The impact of neonatal hypoglycemia on later developmental outcome was examined by Haworth and coworkers[39] in a prospective follow-up study of 36 IDMs. They did not find any correlation between neonatal blood glucose levels or the duration of hypoglycemia and neurologic abnormalities.

Transient Hypoglycemia Associated with Neonatal Problems

IDIOPATHIC CONDITION OR FAILURE TO ADAPT

For apparently unknown reasons, a number of infants develop hypoglycemia, and the cases have been designated as idiopathic hypoglycemia or failure to adapt to the extrauterine environment. As maternal obstetric care continues to improve and more contributory factors are identified, the number of cases of idiopathic hypoglycemia continues to decrease. A careful maternal history should be obtained whenever an infant develops hypoglycemia for reasons that are not easily evident. Contributory factors may include maternal obesity and mild glucose intolerance in the mother.

Maternal Obesity

Many infants born to obese mothers without evidence of impaired glucose tolerance develop low blood glucose concentrations in the immediate newborn period. With the increasing incidence of obesity in the general population, the number of such babies continues to increase. The exact mechanism of impaired glucose homeostasis in these infants has not been examined. It is likely to be related to obesity-related insulin resistance of the mother, which also has been correlated with the higher frequency of macrosomia in these infants.

INTRAUTERINE GROWTH RESTRICTION AND INFANTS WHO ARE SMALL FOR GESTATIONAL AGE

See Chapter 14.

Hypoglycemia has been frequently reported in infants who are SGA (<10th percentile in weight for gestational age). However, the reported incidence has been quite variable. Lubchenco and coworkers[54] reported the following frequencies of hypoglycemia (defined as plasma glucose levels lower than 30 mg/dL before the first feeding) in infants who are SGA: 18% in infants born between 42 and 46 weeks of gestation, 25% between 38 and 42 weeks of gestation, and 67% at less than 38 weeks of gestation. Most of the hypoglycemic infants also had a history of fetal distress and birth hypoxia. Other investigators have reported a much lower rate of hypoglycemia. The variation in incidence may reflect different causes of intrauterine growth restriction, such as maternal nutrition, uteroplacental insufficiency, fetal infection, or maternal metabolic perturbations. In addition, because polycythemia and fetal and neonatal hypoxemia are frequently seen in infants who are SGA, polycythemia and hypoxemia by themselves could contribute to the incidence of hypoglycemia. The data from the previous studies are probably overestimated and not applicable to the present-day population. Studies suggest that the incidence of hypoglycemia (blood glucose <30 mg/dL) in infants born SGA to an otherwise healthy population of mothers is much less than previously reported and ranges from 6% to 14%.[77] The age at which hypoglycemia occurred was examined by Holtrop.[44] In that study, 27 (90%) of 30 infants who were SGA developed hypoglycemia during the first 12 hours after birth.

Therefore, the infant who is SGA is at a high risk for neonatal hypoglycemia, particularly when born prematurely, that is, at less than 38 weeks of gestation. Hypoglycemia, which may be either symptomatic or asymptomatic, is usually seen within the first 24 hours after birth. Associated findings include evidence of asphyxia or hypoxia, polycythemia, and hypocalcemia. The incidence of these findings is probably related to the cause of growth restriction.

The relation between neonatal hypoglycemia and so-called symmetric and asymmetric growth restriction has not been specifically addressed. In general, the consensus among investigators is that hypoglycemia is more common among infants with asymmetric growth restriction because that group represents true intrauterine nutrient deprivation.

The pathogenesis of hypoglycemia has been the subject of numerous investigations and speculation in both humans and animal models. Clinical observations in infants who were SGA showed an early recruitment of fat for oxidative metabolism, as evidenced by a lower respiratory quotient and a higher rate of lipolysis, compared with infants who were appropriate sizes for gestational age.[68] This finding led to the speculation of decreased glycogen stores and their early depletion in infants who are SGA. Early depletion of glycogen stores was also postulated based on the higher brain-to-body ratio of infants who are SGA and the dependence of the brain on glucose for oxidative metabolism. The data of Hawdon and colleagues[36-38] contrast with those of these older studies; however, most of the infants they studied were in the fed state or were receiving intravenous glucose. A decreased rate of gluconeogenesis has been proposed as a contributor to hypoglycemia in infants who are SGA based on high levels of *gluconeogenetic* substrates and a lower glucose response to the administration of alanine, a key *gluconeogenetic* amino acid. However, Frazer and coworkers,[29] using isotopic tracer methods, were able to demonstrate the incorporation of alanine carbon into glucose in such infants soon after birth. Other investigators have reported high insulin levels[15] and higher fractional rates of the disappearance of glucose in infants who were SGA, but again these infants were in the fed state or were receiving parenteral nutrients when they were examined. The role of glucagon in the development of hypoglycemia remains unclear. Infants who are SGA have been observed to mount a significant glucagon response to hypoglycemia. However, the response to exogenous glucagon administration has been variable, particularly in relation to plasma amino acids. Hypoglycemic infants who are SGA appear not to show a normal decrease in plasma amino acids in response to intravenous infusion of glucagon. The GH response to hypoglycemia and glucose infusion is reported to be normal.

Studies of the fetal metabolic state by cordocentesis in pregnancies complicated by intrauterine growth restriction have shown a high incidence of hypoxemia, high blood lactate concentrations, and metabolic acidosis.[26,58,64]

A number of approaches have been applied to study intrauterine growth restriction in animal models. They include uterine artery ligation, maternal starvation, maternal hypoxemia, and maternal hypoglycemia. The neonatal metabolic responses varied with the type of experimental model, but all of the models showed growth restriction, hypoglycemia, and depletion of hepatic glycogen stores. The mechanism of hypoglycemia remains unclear. Newborn dogs that had growth restriction as a result of maternal starvation showed lower glucose levels but unchanged glycogenolysis, lower plasma fatty acids, and ketone levels but also lower rates of gluconeogenesis from alanine, and unchanged rates of lipolysis, suggesting that reduced gluconeogenesis and ketogenesis contributed to hypoglycemia. In comparison, growth restriction by ligation of the uterine artery in the rat resulted in lower plasma glucose concentrations and inappropriate hyperinsulinemia as well as lower hepatic glycogen levels. The delayed induction of liver phosphoenolpyruvate carboxykinase in this model suggests delayed appearance of gluconeogenesis. On follow-up, the intrauterine growth-restricted pups in this rat model remained smaller than those of the controls in both weight and length; that is, they showed no evidence of catch-up growth,[66] suggesting that the intrauterine insult had a permanent impact on growth. Maternal treatment with glucocorticoids attenuated neonatal hypoglycemia in the rat model, possibly by stimulating gluconeogenesis. Finally, studies of the adrenergic system and cerebral oxidative metabolism have not demonstrated any significant change, and studies of somatostatin C (insulin-like growth factor-1) have shown decreased levels in the growth-restricted rat fetus.

The management of these infants involves treatment of the associated clinical problems—hypoxia, hyperviscosity, careful monitoring for hypoglycemia, and the early establishment of adequate nutrition. The treatment of hypoglycemia is similar to the one outlined later.

HEPATIC GLUCOSE-6-PHOSPHATASE AND PREMATURITY

Glucose-6-phosphatase is a membrane-bound enzyme associated with the endoplasmic reticulum in the liver and the kidney—the two important glucogenic organs. It catalyzes the breakdown of glucose-6-phosphate into free glucose, the terminal step in both glycogenolysis and gluconeogenesis. Hume and colleagues[44a] have measured the activity and protein content of glucose-6-phosphatase in the liver of newborn infants soon after their deaths and observed that the enzyme activity is low before birth and increases to about 10% of adult values by term gestation. In a series of studies, they have suggested that the low activity of glucose-6-phosphatase, partly influenced by hormonal, nutrient, and other factors, including stress, may contribute to hypoglycemia in premature infants. However, the direct cause-and-effect relationship is difficult to discern from their studies. A severe deficiency of glucose-6-phosphatase certainly can lead to profound hypoglycemia, as in glycogen storage disease type I. Whether a relatively lower activity, as measured by Hume and colleagues[44a] in autopsy samples, can cause hypoglycemia remains to be confirmed.

BIRTH ASPHYXIA

The mechanism of low glucose after birth asphyxia remains unknown. Affected infants often require high rates of glucose infusion to maintain a normal glucose concentration, suggesting either an increased insulin concentration or increased sensitivity to insulin. An inappropriately high insulin concentration relative to prevailing glucose concentration has been reported in a number of case reports and in a prospective study by Davis and associates.[18] Interestingly, high plasma insulin levels in their study were associated with a poor neurodevelopmental outcome. The mechanism of the resulting hyperinsulinemia remains unclear. Because asphyxia also results in an increase in plasma glucagon, interleukin-6, hydrocortisone, and other counter-regulatory hormones, with associated changes in insulin receptor binding, it can also induce an insulin-resistant state. From a clinical perspective, it is important to carefully monitor the plasma glucose concentration in asphyxiated newborn babies and adjust the parenteral glucose infusions accordingly.

INFECTION

See Chapter 39.

Hypoglycemia in association with overwhelming sepsis has rarely been reported in newborn infants. Hyperglycemia is more common than hypoglycemia. The mechanism of hypoglycemia with sepsis is not well defined. Depleted glycogen stores, impaired gluconeogenesis, and increased peripheral glucose utilization may all be contributing factors. The usual response to sepsis in most animal models has been an increase in the rates of glucose production and gluconeogenesis as a result of counter-regulatory hormonal responses. A decrease in these processes is seen only during an agonal stage; therefore, hypoglycemia with sepsis should be considered an indicator of a fulminating infection.

HYPOTHERMIA

See Chapter 30.

The occurrence of hypothermia secondary to hypoglycemia has been well documented and is a useful clinical sign. Studies in which 2-deoxy-D-glucose was used in adults suggest that hypoglycemia, directly or secondarily, may affect a central thermoregulatory center in the hypothalamus that is sensitive to glucose. Hypoglycemia may also be secondary to hypothermia. The normal core temperature in the neonate is between 36.5° and 37.5°C (97.7° to 99.5°F). If the body temperature falls, the heat production increases several times above that of the basal level, resulting in a more rapid depletion of energy stores. Hypoglycemia is also seen in neonates with severe cold injury after prolonged exposure to cold who had rectal temperatures lower than 32°C (89.6°F).

HYPERVISCOSITY

See Chapter 46.

A negative correlation between plasma hematocrit and glucose concentration was reported by Haworth and colleagues[40] in full-term infants with growth restriction. The mechanism

for the lower glucose concentration observed with increased viscosity was examined by Creswell and associates[17] in newborn lambs. Their data showed that newborn lambs made polycythemic by exchange transfusion had lower plasma glucose concentrations; however, there was no change in the rates of glucose production and utilization. The authors suggested that hyperviscosity acts as an independent variable to depress plasma glucose concentration.

ERYTHROBLASTOSIS FETALIS

See Chapter 21 and Chapter 46, Parts 1 and 2.

Previous studies reported an association between erythroblastosis fetalis due to Rh incompatibility and neonatal hypoglycemia. Hypoglycemia was particularly prominent in severely anemic infants and was seen more frequently after exchange transfusion. Because the exchange transfusions were performed with blood containing acid citrate dextrose, the hypoglycemia occurring after exchange transfusion could be the result of glucose-induced hyperglycemia and hyperinsulinemia. Intravenous glucose tolerance tests performed in infants affected by erythroblastosis fetalis who were not anemic showed their blood glucose and insulin levels before and during the test to be similar to those in normal infants. With the use of cordocentesis and the ability to obtain fetal blood samples in an undisturbed state, attempts have been made to examine the effects of fetal anemia and associated hypoxemia on fetal growth and biochemical parameters. The data revealed that only the severely anemic fetuses (i.e., those with hemoglobin concentrations of less than 30% of the normal value) showed decreased growth rates[65] and changes in umbilical venous blood pH. More importantly, no correlations between the severity of anemia and hypoxemia and levels of plasma insulin and C peptide were observed. Therefore, the suggestion of hyperinsulinemia based on the earlier studies has not been substantiated. Furthermore, the current management of Rh immunization has markedly reduced the severity of erythroblastosis fetalis and anemia in the fetus and the newborn infant. Nevertheless, the plasma glucose concentration should be carefully monitored in these infants after birth.

IATROGENIC CAUSES

Reactive hypoglycemia may occur after abrupt cessation of hypertonic glucose infusions, including those used for parenteral nutrition. Marked variability of blood glucose values may also occur as a result of changing rates of glucose infusion.

Refractory hypoglycemia has been associated with an umbilical artery catheter positioned near the origin of the vessels supplying the pancreas (T11 to L1). Direct glucose infusion into the vessels of the pancreas can lead to hyperinsulinemia and hypoglycemia. Hypoglycemia was also reported with a normally positioned catheter at T8 to T9; it responded to catheter repositioning.

Intravenous indomethacin infusion in premature infants with patent ductus arteriosus causes a drop in glucose to potentially hypoglycemic levels. The indomethacin-induced drop in glucose starts as soon as 1 hour after the beginning of intravenous indomethacin administration and is the lowest at 6 to 12 hours.

CONGENITAL CARDIAC MALFORMATIONS

The mean blood glucose concentration in neonates and older children with congenital cyanotic heart disease or congestive heart failure may be lower than that in healthy controls. Glucose disappearance rates and fasting insulin and GH values are normal, but glucose values after glucagon administration are lower than those in healthy children. Although the mechanism is unknown, chronic hypoxia, leading to decreased glycogen stores, may be a contributing factor. Hypoglycemia may also lead to cardiomegaly and congestive heart failure in the absence of congenital malformations. Therefore, the presence of either hypoglycemia or congestive heart failure should be considered when one or the other appears (see Chapter 45).

Persistent or Recurrent Hypoglycemia

HYPERINSULINISM

Nesidioblastosis-Adenoma Spectrum

Persistent neonatal hyperinsulinemic hypoglycemia (PNHH) can result from various pathologic lesions generally included under the heading of *nesidioblastosis-adenoma spectrum*.[67] The concept of nesidioblastosis has been questioned by several investigators because it is a common feature of the immature or developing pancreas in normoglycemic neonates and infants. This disorder is usually seen sporadically, but familial PNHH has been reported in at least 15 families; therefore, autosomal recessive inheritance must be considered. The neonates are usually LGA but may be appropriate for gestational age. At birth, they lack positive physical findings, although some facial dysmorphism has been reported in some of these infants during later infancy and childhood. Hypertrophic cardiomyopathy was reported in one infant. Maternal history is noncontributory, but a careful history may reveal previous neonatal deaths or unexplained seizures or mental restriction in other siblings. The diagnosis has been made at birth in asymptomatic infants and prenatally based on familial history. Most infants present during the first 24 to 48 hours after birth with such severe symptoms as seizure, hypotonia, apnea, and cyanosis. Asymptomatic hypoglycemia has been diagnosed in the siblings shortly after birth. Sudden infant death has also been linked to nesidioblastosis. The diagnosis is suspected when hypoglycemia appears soon after birth, requiring high rates of glucose infusion.

These infants typically have high blood insulin levels; even if they are in the normal range, insulin levels are likely to be inappropriately high in relation to the prevailing glucose concentration. Measurements of C peptide may be useful because it has twice the half-life of insulin. Tolerance tests may be difficult to perform because of the inability of the patient to fast for even short periods. Other measurements, such as branched-chain amino acids and ketones, have been suggested but are difficult to evaluate because of the high glucose infusions required to maintain normoglycemia. Other diagnostic methods (e.g., radiologic imaging of the pancreas) are not very helpful in cases of nesidioblastosis but may occasionally help visualize a pancreatic tumor.

A definitive diagnosis can be made only by pathologic examination and may require immunocytologic and electron-microscopic studies. Two basic lesions have been described: diffuse and focal. The two forms cannot be separated by clinical or laboratory investigations. The focal lesions, called *focal adenomatous hyperplasia*, consist of the confluence of apparently normally organized islets separated by a few exocrine acini but maintaining a normal lobular pancreatic structure.[20] This disorder is associated with the loss of the maternal allele from the imprinted chromosomal region 11p15 and partial mutation of the sulfonylurea receptor (*SUR1*) gene.[19,89] These lesions are quite different from the "true" islet cell adenomas, which are usually seen in adults but rarely in infants. Diffuse nesidioblastosis involves the whole pancreas and is distinguished by islets of irregular size and ductuloinsular complexes that contain hypertrophied insulin cells. In some cases, immunofluorescent and Feulgen techniques show an increased size of the nuclear area and absorbance of the B cells as the only pathologic findings.

With the use of various molecular biologic and genetic epidemiologic methods, the molecular basis for the abnormal insulin secretion in these disorders has been elucidated. As described in Figure 49-8, insulin secretion by the β cells requires an increase in the intracellular adenosine triphosphate (ATP) concentration as a result of glycolysis and the oxidation of glucose. After entry into the β cell, which is facilitated by a specific glucose transporter protein (GLUT2), glucose is phosphorylated to form glucose-6-phosphate. The latter enters the glycolytic pathway to form pyruvate and is oxidized in the tricarboxylic acid cycle. One of the other substrates entering this cycle is glutamate, which forms α-ketoglutarate, a reaction catalyzed by glutamate dehydrogenase. The increase in ATP concentration and the consequent increase in the ratio of ATP to adenosine diphosphate (ADP) affect the ATP-sensitive potassium (K^+) channel (K_{ATP}), resulting in the depolarization of the β-cell membrane. This process in turn results in the activation of voltage-gated calcium channels and the entry of Ca^{2+} into the cell. An increase in the intracellular Ca^{2+} concentration results in the release of insulin into the circulation.

Thomas and coworkers[87] identified two separate *SUR* gene splice site mutations that segregated from the disease phenotype in affected individuals from nine different families with familial PNHH. Both mutations resulted in aberrant processing of the RNA sequence and disruption of the putative second nucleotide binding domain of the SUR protein. The authors concluded that abnormal insulin secretion in PNHH appears to be caused by the mutations in the *SUR* gene.

Since that first report, a number of other families with the same genetic defect and new mutations in the insulin-secretory mechanism have been identified.[24] The K_{ATP} channels consist of *SUR1* and an inward-rectifying K^+ channel ($KIR_{6.2}$). One patient with a nonsense mutation of the $KIR_{6.2}$ gene associated with familial hyperinsulinism has been identified.[87] Another mutation of $KIR_{6.2}$ associated with hyperinsulinemic hypoglycemia has been reported. Other genetic defects described so far are those related to mutations of genes for glucokinase and glutamate dehydrogenase[31,84] and phosphomannose isomerase deficiency. Additional genetic defects causing hypersecretion of insulin may be identified in the future. It is important to note that

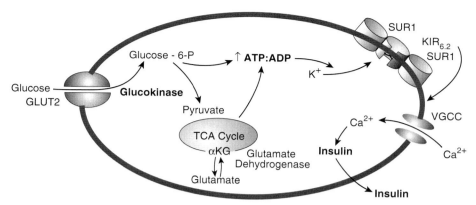

Figure 49–8. Mechanism of glucose-induced insulin secretion by the β cell of the pancreas. Glucose entry into the β cell is facilitated by a specific glucose transporter protein (GLUT2). Intracellular metabolism of glucose through glycolysis and in the tricarboxylic acid (TCA) cycle increases the intracellular concentration of adenosine triphosphate (ATP). The increase in the ratio of ATP to adenosine diphosphate (ADP) affects the ATP-sensitive potassium (K^+) channel, causing an efflux of K^+ and depolarization of the β-cell membrane that in turn activate the voltage-gated calcium (Ca^{2+}) channel (VGCC) and entry of Ca^{2+} into the cell. The increase in free intracellular Ca^{2+} initiates release of insulin. As discussed in the text, mutations of glucokinase, glutamate dehydrogenase, *SUR1*, and *KIR*$_{6.2}$ have thus far been associated with hyperinsulinemic hypoglycemia. αKG, α-ketoglutarate; Glucose-6-P, glucose-6-phosphate; KIR, inward-rectifying potassium channel; SUR, sulfonylurea receptor.

the mutation of glutamate dehydrogenase is manifested with hyperammonemia in addition to hyperinsulinemic hypoglycemia.[84]

Other genetic disorders (e.g., short-chain 3-hydroxyacyl-coenzyme A dehydrogenase) have also been reported to present with hyperinsulinemic hypoglycemia.

The definitive therapy for infants with hypoglycemia in the nesidioblastosis-adenoma spectrum is early subtotal (85%) or total (95% to 98%) pancreatectomy. Total pancreatectomy has been advocated as the procedure of choice, although some infants with recurrent hypoglycemia after subtotal pancreatectomy have been treated successfully with alloxan (mesoxalyl urea). A major advance in the preoperative diagnosis of focal and diffuse lesions was presented by deLonlay-Debeney and coworkers.[20] By using transhepatic pancreatic vein catheterization, they were able to identify the site of hypersecretion of insulin in 17 of 19 neonates with focal adenomatous lesions so that the disorder could be successfully managed by partial pancreatectomy. [18F]-DOPA positron emission tomography has also been used successfully for the identification and localization of focal form of lesions.[35] Zinc protamine glucagon, as intramuscular injections or orally administered starch, has also been used postoperatively. However, in most instances, preoperative medical therapy consisting of various combinations of glucose infusion, diazoxide, glucagon, and somatostatin[43] fails to control hypoglycemia. Continuous somatostatin infusion with the addition of glucagon to correct somatostatin-induced hypoglucagonemia has been used for temporary preoperative medical control. A long-acting somatostatin analogue (octreotide) with 50 to 100 times greater potency than endogenous somatostatin has been used both preoperatively and postoperatively.

Conservative (nonsurgical) management has been successful in some asymptomatic hypoglycemic infants who were diagnosed at birth. Infants with the nesidioblastosis-adenoma spectrum have a high incidence of neurologic damage, which is probably a reflection of the severity of symptomatic hypoglycemia and the delay in diagnosis. Because *SUR1* genes are also expressed in neuronal cells, it has been suggested that the neurologic deficit in these infants may be related to an *SUR1* mutation in the brain. Long-term follow-up data in infants with total pancreatectomy demonstrate variable responses—some develop no pancreatic insufficiency, whereas others develop frank diabetes as well as exocrine pancreatic insufficiency.

Beckwith-Wiedemann Syndrome

The characteristic features of Beckwith-Wiedemann syndrome include macroglossia, omphalocele, and hyperplastic visceromegaly, often also called *congenital overgrowth syndrome*. Since the original description by Beckwith and Wiedemann, a number of other clinical findings of this syndrome have been described,[71] which are listed in Box 49-4. The frequency of these clinical manifestations is variable. Macroglossia, a uniform enlargement of the tongue, is present in more than 80% of cases. Other craniofacial characteristics include midface hypoplasia, a prominent occiput, and nevus flammeus. Characteristic ear creases or pits are present in about 75% of individuals. Anterior abdominal wall defects, which are present in about 80% of cases, include omphalocele, umbilical hernia, and diastasis recti abdominis. Cardiac defects are reported in about 25% of cases; however, no specific cardiac abnormality is prominent.

Most (more than 75%) of these infants are above the 90th percentile in length and weight for gestational age and tend

---

BOX 49–4 Major Findings in Beckwith-Wiedemann Syndrome

CLINICAL FINDINGS
Advanced bone age
Ear anomalies
Pits and/or creases
Facial nevus flammeus
Hemihypertrophy
Macroglossia
Maxillary underdevelopment
Muscular hypertrophy
Neonatal hypoglycemia
Neonatal polycythemia
Prenatal and postnatal gigantism
Prominent occiput
Abdominal wall defects
Diastasis recti abdominis
Omphalocele
Umbilical hernia
Cardiac defects
Clitoromegaly
Cryptorchidism
Tumors (Wilms tumor)
Visceromegaly: Kidney, liver, spleen

PATHOLOGIC FINDINGS
Adrenal cortical cytomegaly and cysts
Hypertrophy and hyperplasia of islets of Langerhans
Medullary dysplasia and medullary sponge kidneys
Nephromegaly with prominent lobulation
Persistent nephrogenesis

---

to remain at the 90th percentile during early infancy and childhood. No differences between male and female infants have been reported.

Hypoglycemia is present in at least half the cases[71] and may be manifested soon after birth. Endocrine evaluation of the few reported cases has not been consistent. However, based on the clinical features of hypoglycemia with low FFAs and ketones and autopsy findings of islet cell hyperplasia, it is believed that hypoglycemia is caused by hyperinsulinism in this syndrome. Plasma GH levels have been reported to be normal, and somatomedin levels were reported to be increased in one infant. These infants may require glucose infusion at high rates in the immediate neonatal period. Spontaneous regression of hypoglycemia is suggested in most infants. Hypocalcemia has also been reported in some instances.

Patients with Beckwith-Wiedemann syndrome are also predisposed to certain malignancies (adrenal carcinoma, nephroblastoma) and appear to have an increased risk for malignancies associated with hemihypertrophy.

Chromosomal studies have been reported in several patients with Beckwith-Wiedemann syndrome. They have ranged from normal chromosomal patterns on unbanded studies to abnormal karyotypes such as duplication of 11p, balanced translocation (11p,22q), duplication of the distal two thirds of 8q, and deletion of the upper half of 12p.[71] It has been

suggested that some of the symptoms of Beckwith-Wiedemann syndrome may be related to the known genes in the area of abnormalities in the chromosomes—genes for insulin and Wilms tumor as well as others—as a contiguous gene syndrome.

Fetal growth is influenced by paternally expressed, growth-promoting *IGF2* and maternally expressed, growth-suppressing *H19* genes. In addition, the cell cycle–regulating gene *CDKN1C* has been demonstrated to be involved in fetal growth. Altered imprinting of these genes on chromosome 11p15.5 has been implicated in the pathogenesis of Beckwith-Wiedemann syndrome. Genetic studies in patients with Beckwith-Wiedemann syndrome have identified three major subgroups of patients: familial, sporadic, and chromosomally abnormal. A large proportion of patients with the familial and sporadic forms of Beckwith-Wiedemann syndrome have no underlying cytogenetic abnormalities. However, 20% of the sporadic cases have been found to involve uniparental disomy for 11p15.5.[57] Altered imprinting of the candidate genes for Beckwith-Wiedemann syndrome (*IGF2* and *H19*) has also been described in the sporadic form.[57] The most frequent abnormality detected in the familial form involves mutations in the *CDKN1C* gene.

ENDOCRINE DISORDERS

Pituitary Insufficiency
Neonatal hypoglycemia associated with anterior pituitary hypofunction may represent a series of separate syndromes, with defects ranging from no structural abnormalities in the brain to septo-optic dysplasia, craniofacial defects, and anencephaly. Although this disorder is considered rare, the true incidence is unknown because it usually goes unrecognized as a result of the absence of characteristic physical findings in the newborn.

CLINICAL AND LABORATORY MANIFESTATIONS
Symptoms of hypoglycemia may begin during the first hours of postnatal life and are marked by their severity. They include sudden and profound limpness, convulsions, apnea, cardiovascular collapse, and cardiac arrest. The infants are of normal length and weight and born at or after term. Males predominate at a ratio of 2:1. The physical examination may be unrevealing; however, some male infants have a microphallus, poorly developed scrotum, small and undescended testes, or some combination of these features. Facial abnormalities consisting of a cleft lip and palate, a poorly developed nasal septum, hypotelorism or hypertelorism, abnormalities of antidiuretic hormone secretion, or widely spaced nipples have been described. Although the infants are of normal size at birth, growth restriction and delayed bone age may be found in children as young as 6 to 8 weeks of age.

Serum GH values are not measurable or in the normal adult range, in contrast to the elevated values usually found in normal newborns. The paradoxical increase in GH during glucose infusion in normal newborns does not occur when hypoglycemia is associated with pituitary deficiency. The cortisol concentration may be low (see Appendix B) at the time of symptomatic hypoglycemia. Hypothyroidism is common. A deficiency in hypothalamic hormones has been shown by a rise in thyroid-stimulating hormone (TSH), or thyrotropin, after stimulation with thyrotropin-releasing hormone (TRH) and by increased prolactin levels with a poor luteinizing hormone (LH) response after stimulation with releasing hormone. The adrenals respond to adrenocorticotropic hormone (ACTH) stimulation, but a deficiency in ACTH may be demonstrated by the use of metyrapone.

PATHOLOGY

At postmortem examination, the pituitary gland may be hypoplastic or aplastic, the thyroid and adrenal glands small, and the cellular architecture of the adrenals disorganized, with atrophy or absence of the fetal cortex. Multiple congenital anomalies of the central nervous system (CNS), including holoprosencephaly and arrhinencephalia, may be found. Radiographic studies have demonstrated the absence of the septum pellucidum and massa intermedia. Hypoplasia or aplasia of the adenohypophysis without cerebral or facial anomalies may also occur. There may be different expressions of the same syndrome, depending on the extent of pituitary hypoplasia or other CNS anomalies, or both.

PATHOGENESIS

The underlying pathogenic mechanisms remain unclear, although aplasia of the anterior pituitary was found in siblings of three patients and in two patients with familial histories of consanguinity. This finding is consistent with a possible autosomal recessive inheritance. Whether the disorder is caused by failure of the pituitary to form or by degeneration of the pituitary is unknown. It is also possible that abnormalities of the hypothalamus with a deficiency in hypophysiotropic releasing hormones is responsible for the multiple endocrinopathies observed in these infants. The pathophysiologic relationships among pituitary hypoplasia, CNS anomalies, and other pituitary hypofunctions are unknown. The exact mechanism of hypoglycemia in these disorders remains undefined.

TREATMENT

Therapy consists of replacement with synthetic GH. Cortisol is replaced cautiously, with maintenance doses of hydrocortisone for proven hypoadrenalism. Thyroxine (T_4) replacement is started once hypothyroidism is documented.

Cortisol Deficiency

Familial isolated glucocorticoid deficiency has been described in a family of five siblings; in two of the infants, glucocorticoid production was normal initially and deficient at a later age. This finding suggests that in some families there may be a degenerative process in the adrenal gland.

Maternal steroid therapy resulting in neonatal subclinical adrenal insufficiency was reported in an infant with cushingoid facies, transient hypoglycemia, and a poor response to intravenous corticotropin at 20 hours. However, maternal steroid therapy, such as that for chronic asthma, only rarely has been related to neonatal adrenal insufficiency and hypoglycemia.

ACTH unresponsiveness is a hereditary disorder in which the adrenal glands fail to produce adequate cortisol but aldosterone secretion is normal and ACTH levels are increased. There are feeding problems, a failure to thrive, and

regurgitation in the neonatal period; hypoglycemia, convulsions, and shock or even death may occur in infancy or early childhood. The syndrome is characterized by hyperpigmentation, normal serum electrolyte concentrations, and an unusually severe, untoward response to illness or stress. There is often a history of affected siblings, and an autosomal recessive mode of inheritance has been suggested. The pathogenesis of this syndrome is poorly understood. The differentiation of the zones of the adrenal cortex in utero requires ACTH except for the zona glomerulosa, which is primarily under renin-angiotensin control. The histologic examination of the adrenal glands of patients with ACTH unresponsiveness has revealed an intact zona glomerulosa and atrophy of the zona fasciculata and zona reticularis. An abnormality at the site (or sites) of ACTH action or cortisol biosynthesis has been postulated.

Adrenal hemorrhage is discussed in Chapter 28.

Congenital adrenal hyperplasia (see Part 4 of this chapter) may be diagnosed in the neonatal period because of the presence of hypoglycemia. The diagnosis is difficult in male infants when there are no positive physical findings. Family history may reveal previously unexplained neonatal deaths.

Congenital Glucagon Deficiency

Two male infants have been reported with glucagon deficiency; the disorder became evident on the second to third day of postnatal life, with repeated convulsive movements, hypotonia, weak crying, and poor sucking. In both infants, the diagnosis was based on a low basal glucagon concentration and a strong hyperglycemic response to glucagon. In one of the infants, the response to glucagon was lacking, and in the other, there was a lack of response to hypoglycemia and alanine infusion. The parents of this second infant were closely related and had partly deficient glucagon secretion; two siblings of this infant died before 5 months of age with probable hypoglycemia. Therefore, an autosomal recessive inherited disorder is suggested.

Epinephrine Deficiency

This disorder is extremely rare. In infants who are SGA, it has been described secondary to adrenal hemorrhage. The diagnosis may be suspected in an infant who has been acutely ill (i.e., hypotensive) during the perinatal period and can be confirmed by measuring plasma or urine catecholamine levels. Some of these infants may develop adrenal calcification, which may be identified on follow-up.

INBORN ERRORS OF CARBOHYDRATE METABOLISM

Galactosemia
See Chapter 50.

Hepatic Glycogen Storage Disease
See Chapter 50.

Fructose Intolerance
See Chapter 50.

Fructose is the main sweetening agent in nature, occurring mostly in fruits, vegetables, and honey, and is often added as a sweetener to foods and beverages in the form of disaccharide sucrose. In humans, the liver is the main site of fructose metabolism, with significantly less important sites being the kidney, gut, and other tissues. Absorption of fructose in the gut does not appear to require an active transport system. Fructose is rapidly metabolized, disappearing from the circulation almost twice as fast as glucose. Fructose is metabolized by specific enzymes that convert it into intermediates of the glycolytic-gluconeogenetic pathway. The key enzymes associated with disorders of fructose metabolism have been identified. Fructose is first phosphorylated to fructose-1-phosphate by fructokinase. Fructose-1-phosphate is split into dihydroxyacetone phosphate and glyceraldehyde by the action of aldolase. Glyceraldehyde is converted to glyceraldehyde-3-phosphate by the action of triokinase. Dihydroxyacetone phosphate and glyceraldehyde-3-phosphate are the intermediates in the glycolytic-gluconeogenetic pathway. Additionally, fructose-1,6-bisphosphatase is a key gluconeogenetic enzyme that catalyzes the conversion of fructose-1,6-biphosphate into fructose-6-phosphate.

It has been suggested that intravenous fructose be used for the treatment of hypoglycemia in both adults and newborn infants because of the lack of hyperglycemia associated with its administration and therefore the lack of reactive hypoglycemia. However, caution should be exercised because the metabolism of fructose in the liver causes increased lactate formation, high-energy phosphate depletion, increased uric acid formation, and inhibition of protein synthesis. The use of fructose in the treatment of hypoglycemia in the neonate, or for that matter in an adult, is not recommended.

Essential fructosemia is a rare and harmless disorder characterized by the appearance of fructose in the urine. This disorder is the consequence of a deficiency of fructokinase, which results in an inability to metabolize fructose.

Hereditary fructose intolerance, or aldolase-B deficiency, results in an inability to split fructose-1-phosphate into triose phosphates. The enzymatic activity contributing to the formation of fructose-1,6-biphosphate from triose phosphates is also reduced.

Affected babies can breastfeed without any ill effects, and symptoms do not appear until fructose or sucrose is introduced in the diet (e.g., cow milk formulas with added sucrose) or at weaning, when fruits and vegetables are introduced. Clinical manifestations include hypoglycemia after the ingestion of meals containing fructose, lethargy, nausea, vomiting, pallor, sweating, and evidence of liver dysfunction such as jaundice, hepatomegaly, a bleeding tendency, and proximal renal tubular dysfunction. The symptoms are reported to be much worse in younger infants than older children. Genetically, it is a heterogeneous disorder with wide variation in manifestations. Treatment consists of the complete elimination of all sources of fructose from the diet, including foods and medications.

Fructose-1,6-bisphosphatase deficiency should actually be called a defect in gluconeogenesis rather than a disorder of fructose metabolism because these infants can tolerate fructose in their diets. Fructose-1,6-bisphosphatase is the key regulatory enzyme in the gluconeogenetic pathway involved in the formation of fructose-6-phosphate, the immediate precursor of glucose-6-phosphate, and finally glucose. A deficiency of this enzyme results in an inability to make glucose from all gluconeogenetic precursors (i.e., pyruvate, amino

acids, and glycerol) and therefore results in hypoglycemia when gluconeogenesis is the major source of glucose, such as that occurring during fasting. These infants can present in the neonatal period with hypoglycemia and severe metabolic acidosis. The clinical manifestations are related to hypoglycemia and acidosis and include lethargy, tachycardia, apnea, hypotonia, and tachypnea. Laboratory findings include hypoglycemia during fasting (i.e., when glycogen stores are low), high plasma lactate, alanine, and ketones with metabolic acidosis. The defect is inherited as an autosomal recessive disorder and is seen more often in girls than boys.

Treatment is aimed at the maintenance of plasma glucose through frequent feedings and avoidance of prolonged periods of fasting. A therapeutic regimen consisting of the continuous nighttime administration of glucose by the nasogastric route, as in glycogen storage disease, should be successful.

Hereditary fructose intolerance may manifest in the neonatal period if the susceptible infant is fed a sucrose-containing formula or given table sugar, fruits, or fruit juices. Symptoms include vomiting, failure to thrive, excessive sweating, and unconsciousness or convulsions. Hypoglycemia is frequently seen, as are fructosemia and fructosuria, after the ingestion of fructose.

NEUROHYPOGLYCEMIA (HYPOGLYCORRHACHIA) CAUSED BY DEFECTIVE GLUCOSE TRANSPORT

Glucose is transported from the blood to the brain and cerebrospinal fluid by a carrier-facilitated diffusion process in which the combination of glucose and a plasma membrane carrier protein facilitates its rapid transfer across the membrane and into the cell. At least five such membrane carrier proteins, designated glucose transporters, have been identified in various tissues. The transport protein (designated GLUT1) that facilitates glucose transport across brain microvessels has the same properties as the one that transports glucose into red blood cells, which has allowed investigators to infer glucose transport into the brain by studying the GLUT1 protein in red blood cells.[28] DeVivo and colleagues[22] described two children who presented with seizures and developmental delay. In both infants, the seizures appeared at about 2 months of age. Repeated laboratory studies showed low glucose and lactate in the cerebrospinal fluid in the presence of normal blood glucose levels. A detailed evaluation revealed no other abnormalities, such as meningitis or intracranial hemorrhage, as a possible cause. The glucose levels in the cerebrospinal fluid ranged between 18 and 35 mg/dL when the blood glucose concentration ranged between 86 and 120 mg/dL. The investigators suspected a defect in glucose transport from the blood to the brain and demonstrated a decreased density of GLUT1 protein in the patients' red blood cells. In addition, immunobinding studies suggested subtle biochemical alterations in the GLUT1 protein of one of the patients. Since this original description, 16 other infants have been identified.[50] Seidner and coworkers[80] identified two distinct classes of mutation as the molecular basis for the functional defect of glucose transport: the hemizygosity of GLUT1 and a nonsense mutation resulting in truncation of the GLUT1 protein. These patients are of clinical importance and point to the need to measure cerebrospinal fluid glucose and lactate levels in those with seizure disorders. Because the brain can use ketones for oxidative metabolism, and the transport of ketones across the blood-brain barrier is not mediated by GLUT1 proteins, attempts have been made to treat this disorder with a ketogenic diet.[50]

Management of Neonatal Hypoglycemia

The clinical management of neonatal hypoglycemia should include (1) anticipation of the group at high risk, (2) correction of hypoglycemia, and (3) investigation and treatment of the cause of hypoglycemia. Often, it is not possible to identify the cause of hypoglycemia, and the treatment remains limited to correction of the low blood glucose concentrations.

Because hypoglycemia is asymptomatic in a large number of neonates, it has become an accepted practice to monitor blood glucose in newborn infants who are at risk for hypoglycemia. This monitoring practice includes (1) infants who are LGA (>90th percentile) or SGA (<10th percentile), (2) macrosomic infants with birthweight greater than 4000 g, (3) IDMs, and (4) acutely ill infants in the intensive care unit with septicemia, asphyxia, respiratory distress, prematurity, and other illnesses. In the last category, the symptoms of hypoglycemia are overshadowed by those of the acute clinical problems. In addition, blood glucose should be routinely monitored in small preterm infants who are receiving total parenteral nutrition even if they appear clinically well and stable. Glucose monitoring in healthy infants born at term gestation is not recommended.

In asymptomatic infants at risk for hypoglycemia, blood glucose should be determined during the first few hours after birth until feeding is established; thereafter, blood glucose should be monitored randomly before feeding. Although the routine for monitoring glucose immediately after birth varies from institution to institution, a rational approach can be outlined based on physiologic changes in plasma glucose in healthy, full-term infants. As discussed previously, the blood glucose levels in all neonates decline, reaching a nadir between 30 and 60 minutes after birth, and then rise to reach a stable plateau between 90 and 180 minutes after birth. Therefore, a blood glucose measurement obtained during these time periods necessitates a follow-up measurement to document whether the glucose level is decreasing or returning to normal, stable levels. If two consecutive blood glucose concentrations obtained 15 minutes apart 2 hours after birth are less than 45 mg/dL, the infant should be closely monitored; if the values are less than 36 mg/dL, the infant is considered to have hypoglycemia, and intervention strategies are initiated. It should be emphasized that these thresholds are arbitrary values derived from data from otherwise normal infants.[16] There are no clearly defined values for hypoglycemia during the initial period of transition (birth to 2 hours). Various cutoff values for the definition of hypoglycemia have been proposed, ranging from 30 to 45 mg/dL. Furthermore, all bedside measurements of blood glucose concentration obtained by enzyme-strip methods should be considered only as screening results and confirmed by appropriate laboratory measurements. The enzyme-strip methods are not particularly accurate in the low blood glucose range, which is commonly observed in the newborn nursery or in the neonatal intensive care unit.

The treatment strategies for hypoglycemia depend on whether it is transient or persistent and asymptomatic or symptomatic. All infants with symptomatic hypoglycemia, regardless of cause or age, should be treated with parenteral glucose infusion. The greatest variance in the management of hypoglycemia is seen in the asymptomatic infant diagnosed soon after birth (i.e., during the first 2 hours). This type of hypoglycemia is often transient and recovers spontaneously. However, in clinical practice, it is often treated with early feedings. Controlled studies examining the benefits or impact of this early feeding on recovery from hypoglycemia have not been performed. It has been suggested that as many as 10% of the healthy infants who are the appropriate size for gestational age develop transient asymptomatic hypoglycemia, which in most cases is managed by the initiation of early, normal feeding. Symptomatic infants should be treated only by parenteral glucose and not by oral feeding.

Persistent hypoglycemia is ascribed to the group of infants who continue to require high rates of intravenous glucose administration over several days to maintain normal glucose concentrations. Such persistent hypoglycemia is often related to hyperinsulinemia and may require pharmacologic interventions, as discussed later.

INTRAVENOUS GLUCOSE INFUSIONS

Parenteral glucose is administered at a rate of 6 to 8 mg/kg per minute, corresponding to 3.6 to 4.8 mL/kg per hour of a 10% dextrose solution. This infusion rate is based on the rate of endogenous glucose production in healthy newborn infants. The aim of therapy is to maintain the plasma glucose concentration at a level higher than 45 mg/dL. Plasma glucose levels are monitored frequently (every 1 to 2 hours) until they are stable and then less frequently (every 4 to 6 hours). If the glucose concentrations do not increase to normal levels, the rate of infusion should be increased by 1 to 2 mg/kg per minute every 3 to 4 hours while monitoring the glucose response. Infants with severe hypoglycemia and those who require high rates of glucose infusion may benefit from having a securely placed intravenous line such as a central line or an umbilical vein catheter placed above the liver. Caution should be exercised in administering glucose through the umbilical artery catheter—if the catheter is placed near the celiac axis, the administered glucose may preferentially perfuse the pancreas and thus inadvertently cause an increased insulin response and hypoglycemia.

In symptomatic infants and when there is a need to rapidly increase the plasma glucose level, a minibolus of 200 mg/kg (2 mL/kg of 10% dextrose in water) may be given over 1 minute (Fig. 49-9).[53] However, any glucose bolus must be administered through a secure intravenous line so that a constant-rate infusion of glucose may follow. In fact, in most instances, an attempt should be made to first start the intravenous infusion and then give the intravenous bolus infusion for the immediate correction of low plasma glucose.

Feedings may be initiated when the blood glucose level has been stable for a reasonable time period (3 to 6 hours). Some investigators suggest that the feeding should be given only as a constant-rate nasogastric drip to avoid hormonal excursion. Although such a concept is theoretically logical, there are no observed data to support it. Nevertheless, infants

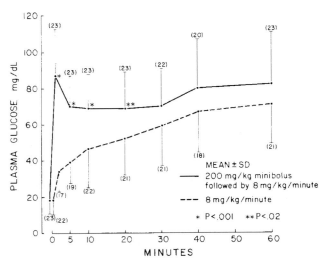

Figure 49–9. A comparison of the results of two treatment regimens for hypoglycemic neonates. A group of 23 hypoglycemic infants were treated with 200 mg/kg of glucose given in a minibolus, followed by a constant glucose infusion of 8 mg/kg per minute; a separate group of 22 hypoglycemic neonates received only the constant glucose infusion (8 mg/kg per minute). (*From Lilien LD, et al: Treatment of neonatal hypoglycemia with minibolus and intravenous glucose infusion, J Pediatr 97:25, 1980.*)

with persistent hypoglycemia, those who are symptomatic, and those who require high rates of glucose infusion are best managed exclusively by parenteral glucose infusion and without oral feeding until their plasma glucose concentrations have stabilized.

The infant can be weaned from parenteral glucose infusion after the plasma glucose concentration has been stable at about 50 to 70 mg/dL for 2 to 3 days. Glucose infusions can be decreased every 3 to 4 hours as long as the blood glucose concentration remains stable. The concentration of glucose in the blood should be monitored with each change in the rate of intravenous glucose infusion. Such a regimen leads to the successful discontinuation of glucose infusion in almost all infants.

If the infant continues to require high rates of intravenous glucose infusion, a diagnosis of hyperinsulinism should be considered and pharmacologic intervention planned. The following pharmacologic agents are used for the treatment of hypoglycemia.

GLUCAGON

Except for the rare patient with a deficiency of this peptide, glucagon is seldom used to increase the plasma glucose concentration at an acute rate. It has been used most often for the diagnosis of hepatic glycogen storage disease, a condition in which no or a minimum increase in plasma glucose concentration is seen in response to glucagon. This single-chain peptide is secreted primarily by the alpha cells of the pancreas. Glucagon increases the blood glucose concentration by increasing both glycogenolysis and gluconeogenesis. An acute administration of glucagon, for example, 150 to 300 μg/kg

given intravenously or intramuscularly, results in an increase in blood glucose by more than 50% in most normal infants. However, the effect is transient, and the administration of glucagon should be followed by intravenous glucose infusion to maintain blood glucose levels. Long-acting glucagon preparations (zinc protamine glucagon) have been used for glucagon deficiency states or in combination with somatostatin for the treatment of nesidioblastosis.

EPINEPHRINE

Although the use of epinephrine to increase blood glucose concentration was recommended in the past, it is rarely used because of its other systemic effects. Its absolute indication would be in the rare infant with epinephrine deficiency. Epinephrine acts by increasing hepatic glucose output through glycogenolysis and decreasing peripheral glucose uptake, mostly in muscle. In addition, epinephrine suppresses insulin secretion and increases lipolysis so that the blood levels of FFAs and glycerol can increase after epinephrine administration.

DIAZOXIDE

Diazoxide is a benzothiadiazine derivative that is structurally closely related to the thiazide diuretics yet has none of the diuretic effects of thiazides. Initially introduced as an effective antihypertensive agent, it is more often used for the treatment of hypoglycemia due to hyperinsulinism. Diazoxide has been shown to cause decreased insulin secretion, both in vivo and in vitro, and catecholamine release. The combined effect of decreased insulin secretion and increased epinephrine release results in an increase in hepatic glucose production and a decrease in the peripheral utilization of glucose. In addition, increased lipolysis results in an increase in plasma levels of FFAs and glycerol. The drug is eliminated for the most part by glomerular filtration, and hepatic transformation is quantitatively less important than renal excretion. Ninety percent of circulating diazoxide is bound to albumin. The estimated half-life in adults is 20 to 30 hours. Serum levels have not been related to the hypotensive effects of the drug. The usual effective dose for the management of hyperinsulinemic hypoglycemia in the newborn is 5 to 20 mg/kg per day, administered orally in an 8- to 12-hour dose. The drug has been used effectively for long periods without any significant side effects, which include sodium and water retention, expansion of plasma volume and edema, hypertrichosis lanuginosa, thrombocytopenia, anorexia, vomiting, and sometimes extrapyramidal symptoms. However, these side effects are relatively uncommon except for hypertrichosis lanuginosa and fluid retention.

SOMATOSTATIN

Somatostatin, a tetradecapeptide (a peptide containing 14 amino acids), was originally isolated from the rat hypothalamus and shown to inhibit the release of GH. Subsequent work has shown the presence of a number of somatostatin-related peptides distributed widely in the body, including the hypothalamus, nervous tissue, gut, and endocrine and exocrine glands (including the pancreas). When administered exogenously, somatostatin inhibits the secretion of glucagon, insulin, GH, and thyrotropin. In addition, it has a number of physiologic effects on the gut, in particular the inhibition of exocrine secretion, changes in gut motility, and reduction of splanchnic blood flow. It has been used extensively in physiologic studies to examine the role of insulin and glucagon in the regulation of glucose metabolism. Infused into a normal human, it suppresses the secretion of both insulin and glucagon, causing a fall in plasma glucose due to the suppression of glucagon secretion, followed by a transient increase. The ability of somatostatin to suppress hormone secretion has been used in the short-term treatment of a variety of hyperfunctioning endocrine tumors, such as insulinomas, glucagonomas, gastrinomas, and GH-secreting adenomas. In the neonate, somatostatin has been used to treat nesidioblastosis (hyperinsulinemic hypoglycemia) as an emergency measure, with variable success, and evaluate the usefulness of pancreatectomy.

The clinical use of somatostatin has been hampered by its short half-life of less than 3 minutes and a short duration of action. Therefore, attempts have been made to synthesize long-acting analogues. Octreotide, the first somatostatin analogue introduced for clinical use, is significantly more potent in its hormone-suppressive effect. After subcutaneous injection, its elimination half-life is reported to be 2 hours. It has been used with some success in the management of islet cell tumors, insulinomas, and nesidioblastosis. However, the response has been variable because octreotide receptors are not consistently expressed in all of these conditions.

GROWTH HORMONE

Treatment with GH should be used only when its deficiency or hypopituitarism has been confirmed.

GLUCOCORTICOIDS

In the past, steroids were widely used in hypoglycemic infants. With the advent of diazoxide and octreotide, together with recognition of the side-effect profile of steroids, such therapy is used less frequently.

PANCREATECTOMY

Subtotal (85% to 90%) or total removal of the pancreas is recommended in cases of persistent hypoglycemia due to pancreatic nesidioblastosis when hyperinsulinemia has been demonstrated and aggressive medical therapy with glucose and diazoxide has been unsuccessful. Total pancreatectomy is preferred because of the high incidence of hypoglycemia at follow-up, which may require treatment with diazoxide and somatostatin. Most of these infants develop insulin-dependent diabetes during puberty.

Prognosis of Neonatal Hypoglycemia

The long-term impact of hypoglycemia in the newborn has remained a subject of controversy and debate. The controversy stems in part from the common belief (not based on scientific data) that the brain of the newborn infant can tolerate a significantly lower blood glucose concentration than that of the adult. This belief was supported by the lower mean blood glucose concentrations observed in asymptomatic and otherwise healthy full-term neonates and the even lower mean glucose concentrations observed in preterm neonates.

The brain is an obligatory consumer of glucose which is transported to the brain by specific glucose transporter proteins that are not under the influence of hormonal regulation by insulin. It has been speculated that the availability and utilization of alternative energy sources (i.e., ketones and lactate) may explain the apparent tolerance of lower plasma glucose concentrations by the neonate. Although the fetal and neonatal brain has been shown to have the ability to use ketones as alternative fuels, clinical data regarding the quantitative contribution of ketones to neonatal brain metabolism have not been secured.

Neuropathologic studies in animals have demonstrated the injurious effect of hypoglycemia in both adults and newborns. It has been shown that insulin-induced hypoglycemia in newborn rat pups results in the generalized diminution of brain weight, cellularity, and protein content. Studies in newborn infants who had died after prolonged hypoglycemia showed acute degeneration of neurones and glial cells and fragmentation of nuclei throughout the CNS.[2] These findings are not specific to hypoglycemia and are also seen in severe hypoxia. Therefore, in the limited number of human studies, it has been difficult to correlate clinical hypoglycemia with the neuropathologic findings. The magnetic resonance neuroimaging of infants who had hypoglycemia in the newborn period showed dilation of the lateral ventricles, cerebral edema, and a loss of gray and white matter differentiation. A consistent involvement of the occipital lobes or parieto-occipital cortex was reported in 825 of the infants.[1] Mechanisms of the vulnerability of the occipital region to hypoglycemic injury are unclear but are similar to those reported in animal studies. It is important to underscore that all the infants who had neuroimaging studies had symptomatic hypoglycemia and that no clinical correlate of these occipital cortex injuries have been reported thus far.[63,88] Studies in rhesus monkeys after 10 hours of hypoglycemia in the newborn period demonstrated motivational and adaptability problems at 8 months of age. However, if special attention was devoted to these animals, there were no cognitive or behavioral deficits.[79]

The associated clinical problems of hypoxemia, birth trauma, respiratory distress, prematurity, and other conditions make it difficult to assess the long-term effects of hypoglycemia in the human neonate. The problem has been confounded by incomplete follow-up, the lack of adequate control groups, and the lack of a uniform definition of hypoglycemia. A few broad conclusions can be drawn. Transient asymptomatic hypoglycemia in an otherwise healthy neonate has been associated with a good prognosis. Several studies of small groups of subjects have suggested that symptomatic hypoglycemia in the infant results in long-term neurologic damage. However, these data should be interpreted with caution because of a number of confounding variables. Griffiths and colleagues[33] retrospectively compared 41 hypoglycemic neonates with 41 controls and found evidence of cerebral damage in 6 (14.6%) members of the hypoglycemia group. However, 5 (12.2%) of the controls also had evidence of cerebral damage. There were no differences in IQ, locomotor scores, behavioral disorders, or history of convulsion in infancy and childhood. None of the 12 infants with asymptomatic hypoglycemia showed cerebral sequelae. This study was performed in infants who were admitted to the intensive care unit for other reasons or who had birthweight of less than 2000 g, and follow-up data were obtained in only 41 of the 115 hypoglycemic infants.

Koivisto and coworkers[51] monitored 151 infants treated for neonatal hypoglycemia for 1 to 4 years and compared them with 56 control infants without hypoglycemia or other demonstrable diseases. They reported that 4 of the 8 (50%) children with convulsions had evidence of cerebral damage, including infantile spasms, severe hypotonia, and cataracts, and one was classified as doubtful. Of the 77 children with symptomatic hypoglycemia but no convulsions, 9 (11.7%) exhibited pathologic conditions. In the group of 66 children with asymptomatic hypoglycemia, 4 (6.1%) were classified as pathologic on the basis of ophthalmologic findings only. Among controls, 3 (5.4%) of 56 exhibited pathologic conditions. There was a statistically significant impact of symptomatic hypoglycemia on long-term neurologic outcome compared with controls.

Pildes and associates[73] investigated the effects of treated hypoglycemia in 39 infants monitored prospectively for 5 to 7 years compared with 41 nonhypoglycemic controls. They observed that mean head circumference remained smaller in the hypoglycemia group than it did in controls. The incidence of neurologic abnormality at ages 2, 3, and 6 years was higher (35.7% [5 of 14]) in hypoglycemic children, and the incidence of IQ scores below 86 at age 5 to 7 years was higher (52% [13 of 25] of the hypoglycemic children versus 22% [6 of 27] of the controls). This study suffered from incomplete follow-up and lack of control for potential confounding variables. Finally, although the number of infants with low IQ scores was statistically significantly higher in the hypoglycemia group, the mean IQ scores were not different between the hypoglycemia group and controls. In summary, although they are suggestive of neurologic sequelae, the data on the long-term neurologic consequences of symptomatic hypoglycemia remain for the most part inconclusive because of the number of problems identified with each study.

Evaluation of physical growth and psychomotor development of preterm (≤34 weeks of gestation) and SGA (<10th percentile) neonates who had recurrent episodes of hypoglycemia demonstrated neurodevelopmental and physical growth deficits until 5 years of age.

Until recently, brain injury patterns identified on early MRI scans and their relationships to the nature of the hypoglycemic insult and neurodevelopmental outcomes have been poorly defined. Burns[11a] studied 35 term infants with early brain MRI scans after symptomatic neonatal hypoglycemia (median glucose level: 1 mmol/L) without evidence of hypoxic-ischemic encephalopathy. They reported that white matter abnormalities occurred in 94% of infants with hypoglycemia, being severe in 43%, with a predominantly posterior pattern in 29% of cases. Cortical abnormalities occurred in 51% of infants; 30% had white matter hemorrhage, 40% basal ganglia/thalamic lesions, and 11% an abnormal posterior limb of the internal capsule. Three infants had middle cerebral artery territory infarctions. Twenty-three infants (65%) demonstrated impairments at 18 months, which were related to the severity of white matter injury and involvement of the posterior limb of the internal capsule. They concluded that the patterns of injury associated with symptomatic neonatal hypoglycemia were more varied than described previously. White matter injury was not confined to the posterior regions; hemorrhage, middle cerebral artery infarction, and basal ganglia/thalamic abnormalities were seen, and cortical involvement was common. Early MRI findings were more instructive than the severity or duration of hypoglycemia for predicting neurodevelopmental outcomes.

Only one study has examined the effects of hypoglycemia in the preterm neonate. Lucas and colleagues[55] examined the neurodevelopmental outcome of 661 preterm infants weighing less than 1850 g at birth in a multicenter, randomized, controlled trial of feeding. Moderate hypoglycemia (a plasma glucose concentration < 46.8 mg/dL) occurred in 433 infants and was found in 104 infants on 3 to 30 separate days. The number of days on which moderate hypoglycemia occurred was strongly related to reduced mental and motor developmental scores at a corrected age of 18 months, even after statistical adjustments for a wide range of factors known to influence development. When hypoglycemia was recorded on 5 or more separate days, the incidence of neurodevelopmental impairment was 42% (13 of 31). This study was significant because it showed that even moderate degrees of hypoglycemia (i.e., about 47 mg/dL), when frequently observed, could be correlated with abnormal neurodevelopmental outcome. A longer follow-up showed only a decrease in arithmetic and motor scores at 7½ to 8 years of age, suggesting that either the earlier observations were transient or any improvement over time was the result of adaptation.[56]

HYPERGLYCEMIA

A high blood glucose concentration is less frequently observed in newborn infants than hypoglycemia. This partially results from the ability of normal infants, both preterm and full-term, to adapt to exogenous glucose administration by (1) decreasing or suppressing endogenous glucose production and (2) increasing glucose uptake in the periphery. The net effect of such an adaptive response is the maintenance of normal blood glucose concentrations, even during high rates of glucose infusion. The definition of hyperglycemia in the newborn remains unclear. Obviously, hyperglycemia should be defined in the context of its clinical implications. Similar to other situations in older infants and adults, hyperglycemia increases blood osmolarity and may cause electrolyte disturbances, osmotic diuresis, and the associated loss of electrolytes in the urine. Because renal function in the neonate is significantly different from that in adults, all of the effects of hyperglycemia may not be seen. Specifically, the plasma glucose level at which renal glycosuria may occur is highly variable, depending on the maturity of renal function, so that renal glycosuria may be seen in extremely immature infants at plasma glucose levels that would be considered within the normal range. In general, most clinicians consider a plasma glucose range of higher than 180 to 200 mg/dL to represent hyperglycemia. Whether such hyperglycemia requires treatment depends on the associated abnormalities. Studies have demonstrated that even in the presence of significant hyperglycemia (a blood glucose concentration of 197 ± 15 mg/dL, mean ± SEM), the amount of glucose excreted or lost in the urine was less than 1% of the infused glucose. In addition, there was no significant diuresis, suggesting that such hyperglycemia (and minimum glycosuria) does not require the adjustment of intravenous fluids or insulin therapy. It should be emphasized that a change in blood glucose concentration from 90 mg/dL to 180 mg/dL results in a change in blood osmolarity of 5 mOsm/L, which is relatively small compared with the normal range of plasma osmolarity (280 to 300 mOsm/L). The clinical circumstances in which hyperglycemia is observed in the newborn are described here.

Hyperglycemia in the infant with low birthweight is probably the most commonly observed perturbation of glucose metabolism in neonatal intensive care units. In the past, it was often attributed to the "immaturity" of glucose homeostasis in the infant with low birthweight or to the inability of the neonate to tolerate exogenous glucose infusion. However, studies have demonstrated that glucose metabolism, even in an infant with extremely low birthweight, is comparable to that in the full-term infant. These studies showed that (1) infants with low birthweight produce glucose at rates similar to those in full-term infants; (2) hepatic glucose production is regulated both by glucose and insulin and is suppressed in response to exogenous glucose infusion, hyperglycemia, or increased insulin levels; (3) hepatic glucose production is completely suppressed when glucose and amino acids are infused simultaneously, as in parenteral nutrition; (4) intravenous lipids do not cause any change in glucose production; and (5) peripheral glucose uptake increases normally in response to an increase in circulating insulin levels. The reasons for the observed hyperglycemia in the infant with low birthweight appear to involve stress related to the clinical problems. That hyperglycemia is not related to low circulating insulin levels was demonstrated by Lilien and associates,[52] showing that circulating insulin levels in hyperglycemic infants were appropriately increased and that there was a good linear correlation between plasma glucose and insulin levels in both normoglycemic and hyperglycemic infants.

In conclusion, hyperglycemia in the infant with low birthweight is most likely related to the secretion of glucose counter-regulatory hormones as a result of stress or to the release of cytokines in infected infants. In fact, the levels of circulating catecholamines were noted to be high in infants with low birthweight and were attributed to clinical manipulations such as ventilatory support. Therefore, a high glucose concentration in an infant with low birthweight should be considered an indicator of clinical problems not primarily related to glucose metabolism. In addition to having their blood glucose concentrations managed, these infants must be evaluated for the possible cause of hyperglycemia, which in most could be systemic septicemia.

DIABETES MELLITUS IN THE NEWBORN

Neonatal diabetes mellitus, a relatively rare condition, is often manifested as hyperglycemia, glycosuria, dehydration, weight loss, and the presence or absence of ketonemia, ketonuria, or metabolic acidosis. Most of these infants are born SGA (Fig. 49-10). The time of presentation for the infants reported in the literature has been between the second day of birth and 6 weeks of age. Plasma insulin levels during the basal state and in response to a glucose load have been reported to be low. Previously, neonatal diabetes was only a rare case report in the literature; however, clinical and genetic studies have made major contributions toward our understanding of this disorder. Based on studies of large groups of reported infants, two clinical phenotypes can be recognized—transient diabetes and permanent diabetes.

Most patients with transient neonatal diabetes have intrauterine growth restriction, underscoring the important role

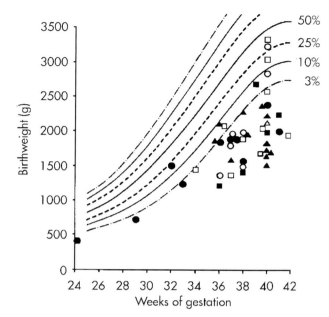

Figure 49–10. Birthweight of 45 infants with neonatal diabetes mellitus. *Closed symbols* denote girls; *open symbols* denote boys; circles, transient diabetes; triangles, transient diabetes with later recurrence; squares, permanent diabetes. (*From Von Mühlendahl KE, et al: Long-term course of neonatal diabetes,* N Engl J Med 333:704, 1995.)

of insulin in fetal growth. In a large French cohort of 29 infants reported by Metz and coworkers,[60] gender distribution was similar, and intrauterine growth restriction was present in 74% of the patients with the disorder. The median age at diagnosis was 6 days (range, 1 to 81 days). Birth defects were reported in 2 patients, one with macroglossia and the other with a congenital heart defect. Mean insulin and C peptide levels were low at the time of diagnosis.

Transient neonatal diabetes gets its name from the observation that remission occurs after a variable period, and the infants do not require insulin therapy. However, diabetes may manifest later, particularly around puberty. Three genetic anomalies on chromosome 6 have been identified to be associated with the condition. They are paternal uniparental isodisomy of chromosome 6, unbalanced paternal duplications of 6q24, and methylation defects at 6q24, all implying a disorder of imprinting whereby the expression of a gene or genes is affected by parental origin. These anomalies were reported in 11 of 19 patients examined by Metz and colleagues.[60] Patients with anomalies of chromosome 6 could be offered genetic counseling. With uniparental disomy, the risk for recurrence in a sibling or child of the index patient is small, whereas the risk for transmitting the disease to the children of a man with 6q trisomy would be high.

In contrast to the so-called transient diabetes, infants with permanent neonatal diabetes present a little later, usually within the first 3 months, and require insulin treatment for life. Some of these patients have been successfully switched to oral sulfonylureas.[91] Mutations in genes encoding glucokinase account for a minority of patients. Another rare form of autosomal recessive diabetes has been mapped to chromosome 10p12.1-p13. Gloyn and associates[32] have identified six novel heterozygous missense mutations in 10 of the 29 patients with permanent diabetes. Four of these 10 patients also had severe developmental delay and muscle weakness. The authors hypothesized that an activating mutation in the gene encoding the inward-rectifying potassium channel Kir$_{6.2}$, a subunit of the K$_{ATP}$ channel, causes monogenic diabetes because the inactivating mutation in this gene leads to uncontrolled insulin secretion and hyperinsulinemic hypoglycemia (see Fig.49-8). The authors confirmed this hypothesis by expressing the mutation in *Xenopus laevis* oocytes.[69] Since K$_{ATP}$ channels and their Kir$_{6.2}$ pore-forming subunits are expressed in the skeletal muscle and neurons throughout the brain, it was speculated that the severe developmental delay observed in some of the patients may be related to the altered activity of these channels in the brain and skeletal muscle.

With the development of sophisticated molecular techniques, it is likely that additional mutations or defects in β-cell function and insulin synthesis and secretion will be identified as the causes of diabetes mellitus in the neonate.

Treatment includes correction of fluid-electrolyte disturbances and hyperglycemia. These infants are often extremely sensitive to insulin and respond well to a daily insulin dose of 3 to 4 U/kg of body weight. Insulin dosage must be adjusted based on plasma glucose concentration, glycosuria, or both. Because of the risk for hypoglycemia, careful and frequent monitoring of plasma glucose levels should be performed.

Diabetes mellitus due to pancreatic lesions is extremely rare and is usually manifested soon after birth. The metabolic abnormalities are the result of either the absence of a pancreas (or pancreatic hypoplasia) or the congenital absence of insulin-secreting B cells. Both lesions result in a lack of insulin secretion. Because insulin is a primary growth-promoting hormone in utero, these infants are severely growth restricted at birth. They rapidly become hyperglycemic soon after birth, often to extremely high levels, and require immediate insulin therapy. There may be other associated congenital abnormalities, such as congenital heart defects. In infants with pancreatic hypoplasia, the insufficiency of the exocrine pancreas has also been reported. Very few infants have been reported to survive, primarily because of associated lethal congenital anomalies.

INSULIN THERAPY IN THE BABY WITH LOW BIRTHWEIGHT

Intravenous insulin in infants with low birthweight has been used by several investigators to (1) treat hyperglycemia and (2) enhance the delivery and assimilation of nutrients and consequently accelerate growth. The rationale for such an approach is based on the observation that hyperglycemia and the inability to use glucose and other nutrients may be related to resistance to insulin action in those infants, resulting from either so-called immaturity or a heightened counter-regulatory "stress" response, that is, increased levels of catecholamines, glucagon, growth hormone, and cortisol. Data from studies in critically ill adults in intensive care units and some studies in extremely low-birthweight babies have demonstrated a correlation between hyperglycemia and adverse outcome, risk for organ failure, risk for death, and prolonged length of stay in the intensive care unit.

In addition, when carefully undertaken with frequent monitoring of the plasma glucose concentration, insulin administration in infants with low birthweight is considered safe.

Insulin, the critical glucoregulatory hormone, is also the major growth factor for the fetus and anabolic hormone after birth. It stimulates protein and fat accretion by stimulating whole-body protein synthesis and de novo lipogenesis, thereby suppressing lipolysis. Insulin affects these processes either directly or by regulating the production of insulin-like growth factor-1 and insulin-like growth factor binding proteins.

The usual dose for a continuous intravenous infusion is 0.04 to 0.10 units/kg per hour administered in a minimum volume (0.04 to 0.1 mL) of isotonic saline solution. The intravenous tubing is flushed with the insulin solution to saturate the binding sites on the tubing so that insulin cannot stick to the plastic tubing. The dose should be adjusted with increasing caloric intake, with the goal being to maintain the blood glucose concentration at a level between 100 and 150 mg/dL.[9] The higher glucose levels are suggested to maintain an adequate margin of safety.

Limited information published in the literature on the use of intravenous insulin has given equivocal results. In a retrospective review of their 34 insulin-treated infants and 42 controls, Binder and associates[9] did not observe an impact of insulin administration on energy intake or growth. Nonetheless, insulin administration did reduce glucose intolerance. In contrast, it also has been shown that the delivery of significantly greater amounts of calories as glucose with insulin administration results in greater weight gain. Whether this weight gain represents an increase in lean body mass or an increase in lipid synthesis is not known. However, based on physiologic observations in adults, it is likely that the increased assimilation of glucose with insulin results in the increased synthesis of fat from glucose.

A large multicenter, international study of early insulin therapy for 7 days in infants with very low birthweight failed to show significant differences in the intended primary outcome measures, that is mortality at the expected date of delivery, and secondary measures such as somatic growth, incidence of sepsis, retinopathy, intracranial lesions at 28 days of age, and length of stay in the intensive care unit.[7] However, an intention-to-treat analysis showed statistically significant higher mortality at 28 days in the early insulin group ($P = .04$). Lack of a significant effect on primary outcome, and subsequent observation of an increased incidence of brain parenchymal lesions (periventricular leukomalacia and evidence of porencephalic cysts), in the intervention group caused the data safety monitoring board to suspend the study. It is significant to note that 36% of patients in the conventional group were also treated with insulin.

In addition, it has been noted that the control of plasma glucose during periods of high energy intake and clinical deterioration requires the frequent adjustment of insulin infusion and is extremely time consuming. Similar experiences have been reported by others. It is for this reason that insulin therapy has been used sparingly, and only then to treat hyperglycemia. When administering insulin to the neonate, frequent glucose monitoring and adjustment in the rate of glucose infusion are required to prevent hypoglycemia.

In a carefully performed study of four infants, Poindexter and colleagues[74] showed that exogenous insulin administration was associated with a high rate of glucose infusion and high plasma lactate levels. Plasma insulin levels in their study had increased 10-fold (from 7 to 79 μU/mL), and the rate of glucose infusion had to be increased from 6.8 to 15.7 mg/kg per minute. These data point to the importance of careful monitoring when insulin therapy is used for the management of hyperglycemia in the infant with low birthweight.

The large clinical trial also raises the issue as to why multicenter trials are unsuccessful when compared with small, single center trials. This may be due, in part, to the difficulty in achieving the targeted goals in several centers, particularly when caring for critically sick babies with low birthweight in the intensive care unit. For example, in the study of Beardsall and associates,[7] the nutrient intake, particularly protein intake, remained low during the period of insulin therapy, and a significant number of subjects in the control group (36%) were also treated with insulin. Additionally, the outcomes measured, that is, death before the expected date of delivery, sepsis, length of stay, and so forth, are complex with multiple factors and may not be expected to be influenced by insulin treatment of 1 week's duration.

REFERENCES

1. Alkalay AL, et al: Brain imaging findings in neonatal hypoglycemia: case report and review of 23 cases. *Clin Pediatr* 44:783, 2005.
2. Anderson JM, et al: Pathological changes in the nervous system in severe neonatal hypoglycemia, *Lancet* 13:372, 1966.
3. Ashmead GG, et al: Maternal-fetal substrate relationships in the third trimester in human pregnancy, *Gynecol Obstet Invest* 35:18, 1993.
4. Aucott SW, et al: Rigorous management of insulin-dependent diabetes mellitus during pregnancy, *Acta Diabetol* 31:126, 1994.
5. Bauman WA, et al: Transplacental passage of insulin complexed to antibody, *Proc Natl Acad Sci U S A* 78:4558, 1981.
6. Baumeister FAM, et al: Glucose monitoring with long-term subcutaneous microdialysis in neonates, *Pediatrics* 108:1187, 2001.
7. Beardsall K, et al: Early insulin therapy in very-low-birth-weight infants, *N Engl J Med* 359:1873, 2008.
8. Beardsall K, et al: The continuous glucose monitoring sensor in neonatal intensive care, *Arch Dis Child Fetal Neonatal Ed* 90:R307, 2005.
9. Binder ND, et al: Insulin infusion with parenteral nutrition in extremely low birth weight infants with hyperglycemia, *J Pediatr* 114:273, 1989.
10. Bougneres PF, et al: Lipid transport in the human newborn: palmitate and glycerol turnover and the contribution of glycerol to neonatal hepatic glucose output, *J Clin Invest* 70:262, 1982.
11. Burd LI, et al: Placental production and foetal utilisation of lactate and pyruvate, *Nature* 254:710, 1975.
11a. Burns CM, Rutherford MA, Boardman JP, et al: Patterns of cerebral injury and neurodevelopmental outcomes after symptomatic neonatal hypoglycemia, *Pediatrics* 122:65, 2008.
12. Carson BS, et al: Effects of a sustained insulin infusion upon glucose uptake and oxygenation of the ovine fetus, *Pediatr Res* 14:147, 1980.
13. Casson IF, et al: Outcomes of pregnancy in insulin dependent diabetic women: results of a five year population cohort study, *BMJ* 315:275, 1997.
14. Churchill JA, et al: Neuropsychological deficits in children of diabetic mothers, *Am J Obstet Gynecol* 105:257, 1969.
15. Collins JE, et al: Hyperinsulinaemic hypoglycaemia in small for dates babies, *Arch Dis Child* 65:1118, 1990.
16. Cornblath M, et al: Controversies regarding definition of neonatal hypoglycemia: suggested operational thresholds, *Pediatrics* 105:1141, 2000.
17. Creswell JS, et al: Hyperviscosity in the newborn lamb produces perturbation in glucose homeostasis, *Pediatr Res* 15:1348, 1981.
18. Davis D, et al: Inappropriately high plasma insulin levels in suspected perinatal asphyxia, *Acta Paediatr* 88:76, 1999.
19. de Lonlay P, et al: Somatic deletion of the imprinted 11p15 region in sporadic persistent hyperinsulinemic hypoglycemia of infancy is specific of focal adenomatous hyperplasia and endorses partial pancreatectomy, *J Clin Invest* 100:802, 1997.
20. deLonlay-Debeney P, et al: Clinical features of 52 neonates with hyperinsulinism, *N Engl J Med* 340:1169, 1999.
21. Denne SC, et al: Glucose carbon recycling and oxidation in human newborns, *Am J Physiol* 251:E71, 1986.
22. DeVivo DC, et al: Defective glucose transport across the blood-brain barrier as a cause of persistent hypoglycorrhachia, seizures, and developmental delay, *N Engl J Med* 325:703, 1991.
23. DiGiacomo JE, et al: Fetal glucose metabolism and oxygen consumption during sustained hypoglycemia, *Metabolism* 39:193, 1990.
24. Dunne MJ, et al: Familial persistent hyperinsulinemic hypoglycemia in infancy and mutations in the sulfonylurea receptor, *N Engl J Med* 336:703, 1997.
25. Duttaroy AK: Transport of fatty acids across the human placenta: a review, *Prog Lipid Res* 48:52, 2009.
26. Economides DL, et al: Blood glucose and oxygen tension levels in small-for-gestational-age fetuses, *Am J Obstet Gynecol* 160:385, 1989.
27. El-Hashimy M, et al: Factors modifying the risk of IDDM in offspring of an IDDM parent, *Diabetes* 44:295, 1995.
28. Fishman RA: The glucose transporter protein and glucopenic brain injury, *N Engl J Med* 325:731, 1991.
29. Frazer TE, et al: Direct measurement of gluconeogenesis from $[2,3^{-13}C_2]$alanine in the human neonate, *Am J Physiol* 240:E615, 1981.
30. Fuhrmann K, et al: Prevention of congenital malformations in infants of insulin-dependent diabetic mothers, *Diabetes Care* 6:219, 1983.
31. Glaser B, et al: Familial hyperinsulinism caused by an activating glucokinase mutation, *N Engl J Med* 338:226, 1998.
32. Gloyn AL, et al: Activating mutations in the gene encoding the ATP-sensitive potassium-channel subunit $Kir_{6.2}$ and permanent neonatal diabetes, *N Engl J Med* 350:1838, 2004.
33. Griffiths AD, et al: Assessment of effects of neonatal hypoglycemia: a study of 41 cases with matched controls, *Arch Dis Child* 46:819, 1971.
34. Hanson RW, et al: *Gluconeogenesis: its regulation in mammalian species*, New York, 1976, John Wiley & Sons.
35. Hardy OT, et al: Accuracy of [^{18}F]Fluorodopa positron emission tomography for diagnosing and localizing focal congenital hyperinsulinism, *J Clin Endocrinol Metab* 92:4706, 2007.
36. Hawdon JM, et al: Hormonal and metabolic response to hypoglycaemia in small for gestational age infants, *Arch Dis Child* 68:269, 1993.
37. Hawdon JM, et al: Metabolic adaptation in small for gestational age infants, *Arch Dis Child* 68:262, 1993.
38. Hawdon JM, et al: The role of pancreatic insulin secretion in neonatal glucoregulation: II. Infants with disordered blood glucose homeostasis, *Arch Dis Child* 68:280, 1993.

39. Haworth JC, et al: Prognosis of infants of diabetic mothers in relation to neonatal hypoglycaemia, *Dev Med Child Neurol* 18:471, 1976.

40. Haworth JC, et al: Relation of blood glucose to haematocrit, birthweight, and other body measurements in normal and growth-restricted newborn infants, *Lancet* 28:901, 1967.

41. Hawthorne G, et al: Prospective population based survey of outcome of pregnancy in diabetic women: Results of the Northern Diabetic Pregnancy Audit, 1994, *BMJ* 315:279, 1997.

42. Hertz DE, et al: Intravenous glucose suppresses glucose production but not proteolysis in extremely premature newborns, *J Clin Invest* 92:1752, 1993.

43. Hirsch HJ,, et al: Hypoglycemia of infancy and nesidioblastosis: Studies with somatostatin, *N Engl J Med* 296:1323, 1977.

44. Holtrop PC: The frequency of hypoglycemia in full-term large and small for gestational age newborns, *Am J Perinatol* 10:150, 1993.

44a. Hume R, Burchell A: Abnormal expression of glucose-6-phosphatase in preterm infants, *Arch Dis Child* 68:202, 1993.

45. Kalhan S, et al: Gluconeogenesis in the fetus and neonate, *Semin Perinatol* 24:94, 2000.

46. Kalhan SC, et al: Attenuated glucose production rate in newborn infants of insulin-dependent diabetic mothers, *N Engl J Med* 296:375, 1977.

47. Kalhan SC, et al: Glucose production in pregnant women at term gestation: sources of glucose for human fetus, *J Clin Invest* 63:388, 1979.

48. Kalhan SC, et al: Estimation of gluconeogenesis in newborn infants, *Am J Physiol* 281:E991, 2001.

49. Kenepp NB, et al: Fetal and neonatal hazards of maternal hydration with 5% dextrose before caesarean section, *Lancet* 22:1150, 1982.

50. Klepper J, et al: Defective glucose transport across brain tissue barriers: a newly recognized neurological syndrome, *Neurochem Res* 24:587, 1999.

51. Koivisto M, et al: Neonatal symptomatic and asymptomatic hypoglycemia: a follow-up study of 151 children, *Dev Med Child Neurol* 14:603, 1972.

52. Lilien LD, et al: Hyperglycemia in stressed small premature neonates, *J Pediatr* 94:454, 1979.

53. Lilien LD, et al: Treatment of neonatal hypoglycemia with minibolus and intravenous glucose infusion, *J Pediatr* 97:25, 1980.

54. Lubchenco LO, et al: Incidence of hypoglycemia in newborn infants classified by birth weight and gestational age, *Pediatrics* 47:831, 1981.

55. Lucas A, et al: Adverse neurodevelopmental outcome of moderate neonatal hypoglycaemia, *BMJ* 297:1304, 1988.

56. Lucas A, et al: Outcome of neonatal hypoglycaemia, *BMJ* 318:194, 1999.

57. Maher ER, et al: Beckwith-Wiedemann syndrome: imprinting in clusters revisited, *J Clin Invest* 105:247, 2000.

58. Marconi AM, et al: An evaluation of fetal glucogenesis in intrauterine growth-restricted pregnancies, *Metabolism* 42:860, 1993.

59. Menon RK, et al: Transplacental passage of insulin in pregnant women with insulin-dependent diabetes mellitus, *N Engl J Med* 323:309, 1990.

60. Metz C, et al: Neonatal diabetes mellitus: chromosomal analysis in transient and permanent cases, *J Pediatr* 141:483, 2002.

61. Miller E, et al: Elevated maternal hemoglobin A_{1c} in early pregnancy and major congenital anomalies in infants of diabetic mothers, *N Engl J Med* 304:1331, 1981.

62. Mills JL, et al: Malformations in infants of diabetic mothers occur before the seventh gestational week: implications for treatment, *Diabetes* 28:292, 1979.

63. Murakami Y, et al: Cranial MRI of neurologically impaired children suffering from neonatal hypoglycemia, *Pediatr Radiol* 29:23, 1999.

64. Nicolaides KH, et al: Blood gases, pH, and lactate in appropriate- and small-for-gestational-age fetuses, *Am J Obstet Gynecol* 161:996, 1989.

65. Nicolini U, et al: Maternal-fetal glucose gradient in normal pregnancies and in pregnancies complicated by alloimmunization and fetal growth retardation, *Am J Obstet Gynecol* 161:924, 1989.

66. Ogata ES, et al: Altered growth, hypoglycemia, hypoalaninemia, and ketonemia in the young rat: postnatal consequences of intrauterine growth retardation, *Pediatr Res* 19:32, 1985.

67. Parimi P, Kalhan SC: Persistent hyperinsulinemic hypoglycemia of infancy. In Fanaroff AA, et al, editors: *Year book of neonatal-perinatal medicine*. St. Louis, 1999, Mosby-Year Book, p 281.

68. Patel D, et al: Glycerol metabolism and triglyceride fatty acid cycling in the human newborn: effect of maternal diabetes and intrauterine growth retardation, *Pediatr Res* 31:52, 1992.

69. Peake JE, et al: X-linked immune dysregulation, neonatal insulin dependent diabetes, and intractable diarrhoea, *Arch Dis Child* 74:F195, 1996.

70. Persson B, et al: Follow-up of children of insulin-dependent and gestational diabetic mothers' neuropsychological outcome, *Acta Paediatr Scand* 73:348, 1984.

71. Pettenati MJ, et al: Wiedemann-Beckwith syndrome: presentation of clinical and cytogenetic data on 22 new cases and review of the literature, *Hum Genet* 74:143, 1986.

72. Philipson EH, et al: Effects of maternal glucose infusion on fetal acid-base status in human pregnancy, *Am J Obstet Gynecol* 157:866, 1987.

73. Pildes RS, et al: A prospective controlled study of neonatal hypoglycemia, *Pediatrics* 54:5, 1974.

74. Poindexter BB, et al: Exogenous insulin reduces proteolysis and protein synthesis in extremely low birth weight infants, *J Pediatr* 132:948, 1998.

75. Pribylova H, et al: Long-term prognosis of infants of diabetic mothers: relationship between metabolic disorders in newborns and adult offspring, *Acta Diabetol* 33:30, 1996.

76. Rizzo T, et al: Correlations between antepartum maternal metabolism and intelligence of offspring, *N Engl J Med* 325:911, 1996.

77. Robertson PA, et al: Neonatal morbidity according to gestational age and birth weight from five tertiary care centers in the United States, 1983 through 1986, *Am J Obstet Gynecol* 166:1629, 1992.

78. Ruyle M, et al: Placental transfer of essential fatty acids in humans: venous-arterial difference for docosahexaenoic acid in fetal umbilical erythrocytes, *Proc Natl Acad Sci U S A* 87:7902, 1990.

79. Schrier AM, et al: Neonatal hypoglycemia in the rhesus monkey: effect on development and behavior, *Infant Behav Dev* 13:189, 1990.

80. Seidner G, et al: GLUT-1 deficiency syndrome caused by haploinsufficiency of the blood-brain barrier hexose carrier, *Nat Genet* 18:188, 1998.

81. Sells CJ, et al: Long-term developmental follow-up of infants of diabetic mothers, *J Pediatr* 125:S9, 1994.

82. Simmons D: Persistently poor pregnancy outcomes in women with insulin dependent diabetes, *BMJ* 315:263, 1997.

83. Srinivasan G, et al: Plasma glucose values in normal neonates: A new look, *J Pediatr* 109:114, 1986.

84. Stanley CA, et al: Hyperinsulinism and hyperammonemia in infants with regulatory mutations of the glutamate dehydrogenase gene, *N Engl J Med* 338:1352, 1998.

85. Susa JB, et al: Chronic hyperinsulinemia in the fetal rhesus monkey: Effects of physiologic hyperinsulinemia on fetal growth and composition, *Diabetes* 33:656, 1984.

86. Swenne I, et al: Inter-relationship between serum concentrations of glucose, glucagon and insulin during the first two days of life in healthy newborns, *Acta Paediatr* 83:915, 1994.

87. Thomas PM, et al: Mutations in the sulfonylurea receptor gene in familial persistent hyperinsulinemic hypoglycemia of infancy, *Science* 268:426, 1995.

88. Traill Z, et al: Brain imaging in neonatal hypoglycemia, *Arch Dis Child Fetal Neonatal Ed* 79:F145, 1998.

89. Verkarre V, et al: Paternal mutation of the sulfonylurea receptor (SUR1) gene and maternal loss of 11p15 imprinted genes lead to persistent hyperinsulinism in focal adenomatous hyperplasia, *J Clin Invest* 102:1286, 1998.

90. Vohr BR, et al: Somatic growth of children of diabetic mothers with reference to birth size, *J Pediatr* 97:196, 1980.

91. Von Muhlendal KE, et al: Long-term course of neonatal diabetes, *N Engl J Med* 333:704, 1995.

92. Warram JH, et al: Differences in risk of insulin-dependent diabetes in offspring of diabetic mothers and diabetic fathers, *N Engl J Med* 311:149, 1984.

PART 2

Disorders of Calcium, Phosphorus, and Magnesium Metabolism

Jacques Rigo, Mohamed W. Mohamed, and Mario De Curtis

Ninety-eight percent of the calcium, 80% of the phosphorus, and 65% of the magnesium in the body are in the skeleton; these elements are also constituents of the intracellular and extracellular spaces. The metabolic homeostasis of calcium, phosphorus, and magnesium and mineralization of the skeleton are complex functions that require the intervention of various parameters; an adequate supply of nutrients; the development of the intestinal absorption process; and the effects of several hormones, such as parathormone, vitamin D, and calcitonin, as well as optimal renal and skeletal controls.[98] Bone formation requires protein and energy for collagen matrix synthesis, and an adequate intake of calcium and phosphorus is necessary for correct mineralization.[97] During development, nutrients are transferred mainly across the placenta. From the analysis of stillbirths and deceased neonates, it has been calculated that during the last trimester of gestation, the daily accretion per kilogram of body weight represents around 120 mg of calcium, 70 mg of phosphorus, and

3 mg of magnesium.[118] Therefore, at birth, the whole-body content of a term infant represents about 30 g of calcium, 16 g of phosphorus, and 0.75 g of magnesium. After birth, the use of the gastrointestinal tract to provide nutrients for growth causes a reduction in calcium availability for bone accretion,[114] promoting the occurrence of relative osteopenia in preterm infants and to a lesser extent in term infants. Thus, during infancy, absolute values of whole-body mineral accretion per day are similar to the relative values per kilogram of body weight during fetal life. In addition to their roles in bone formation, calcium, phosphorus, and magnesium play important roles in many physiologic processes, such as transport across membranes, activation and inhibition of enzymes, intracellular regulation of metabolic pathways, secretion and action of hormones, blood coagulation, muscle contractility, and nerve conduction. The 20% of phosphorus not complexed within bone is present mainly as adenosine triphosphate, nucleic acids, and cell and organelle membranes. Magnesium, an essential intracellular cation, is critical in energy-requiring metabolic processes, protein synthesis, membrane integrity, nervous tissue conduction, neuromuscular excitability, muscle contractility, hormone secretion, and intermediary metabolism.

CALCIUM, PHOSPHORUS, AND MAGNESIUM PHYSIOLOGY

Calcium Physiology

SERUM CALCIUM

Serum calcium represents a minimum fraction of total-body calcium because only about 1% of calcium is present in extracellular fluid and soft tissues. In the circulation, calcium is distributed among three interconvertible fractions. About 50% of total serum calcium is in ionized form at the normal serum protein concentration and represents the biologically active component of the total serum calcium concentration. Another 8% to 10% is complexed to organic and inorganic acids (e.g., citrate, lactate, bicarbonate, sulfate, and phosphate); together, the ionized and complexed calcium fractions represent the diffusible portion of circulating calcium. About 40% of serum calcium is protein bound, primarily to albumin (80%) but also to globulins (20%).[55] Ionized calcium is the only physiologically active fraction. The protein-bound calcium is not biologically active but provides a rapidly available reserve of calcium. Under normal circumstances, the serum calcium concentration is tightly regulated by parathyroid hormone (PTH) and calcitriol (1,25-dihydroxy vitamin D_3; $1,25[OH]_2D_3$), which increase serum calcium (Fig. 49-11), and by calcitonin, which decreases serum calcium.

Serum total and ionized calcium concentrations are relatively high at birth but decrease sharply during the first hours of life to reach a nadir at 24 hours and increase progressively thereafter up to the end of the first week of life (Table 49-2). Sudden changes in the distribution of calcium between ionized and bound fractions may cause symptoms of hypocalcemia even in children with functioning hormonal mechanisms for the regulation of the ionized calcium concentration. Increases in the extracellular fluid concentration of anions such as phosphate, citrate, or bicarbonate increase the proportion of bound calcium and decrease ionized calcium. Alkalosis

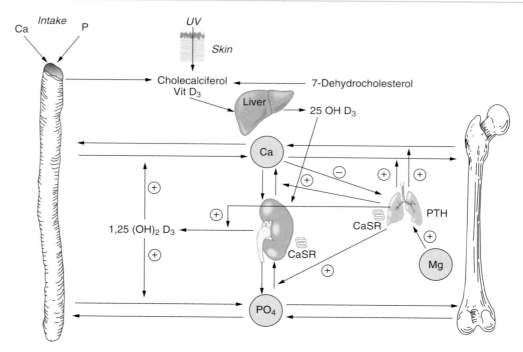

Figure 49–11. Regulation of calcium (Ca) and phosphate (PO_4) homeostasis. Parathyroid hormone (PTH) increases Ca release from bone, Ca resorption in the kidney, and $1,25(OH)_2D_3$ excretion from the kidney. PTH production is stimulated by low Ca and inhibited by low Mg and high $1,25(OH)_2D_3$. Vitamin D increases Ca release from bone and Ca and PO_4 absorption from the intestine. Vitamin D production is stimulated by high PTH and low PO_4. CaSR, calcium-stimulating response; OH, hydroxylase; P, phosphorus; UV, ultraviolet light; Vit, vitamin.

TABLE 49–2 Evolution of Serum Calcium Concentrations (mmol/L*) during the First 10 Days of Life in Term and Preterm Infants

Age	TERM		PRETERM	
	Mean	95% Confidence Interval	Mean	95% Confidence Interval
Birth (cord blood)	2.55	2.25-2.85	2.24	1.58-2.90
24 hr	2.25	1.95-2.55	1.94	1.64-2.24
48 hr	2.39	2.14-2.64	1.85	1.47-2.23
120 hr	2.46	2.25-2.68	2.22	1.84-2.60
240 hr	2.48	2.26-2.69	2.45	2.45-2.89

*Conversion to mg/dL: 0.2495 × mg/dL = mmol/L.

increases the affinity of albumin for calcium and thereby decreases the concentration of ionized calcium. In contrast, acidosis increases the ionized calcium concentration by decreasing the binding of calcium to albumin. Although it is conventional to measure the total serum calcium concentration, more physiologically relevant information is obtained by direct measurement of the ionized calcium concentration. This measurement is particularly important when evaluating patients who have abnormal circulating proteins and after blood transfusion for the correction of acidosis and hyperventilation. For example, total serum calcium decreases about 1 mg/dL, or 0.25 mmol/L, for each 1 g/dL of decrease in serum albumin, without any change in ionized calcium. When it is not possible or practical to determine the ionized calcium concentration directly, a corrected total calcium concentration can be derived by using one of several proposed algorithms that are based on albumin or total protein concentrations.[55]

PLACENTAL TRANSPORT

During pregnancy, there is an active calcium transfer from the mother to the fetus, reaching a peak of 120 to 150 mg/kg of fetal weight per day during the third trimester. To meet the high demand for mineral requirements of the developing skeleton, the fetus maintains higher blood calcium and phosphorus levels than the ambient maternal levels. This process is the result of the active transport of calcium across the placenta by a calcium pump in the basal membrane that maintains a gradient of maternal-to-fetal calcium of 1:1.4. The main regulator of fetal ionized calcium appears to be parathormone-releasing protein (PTHrP), which is produced by the placenta as well as by the fetal parathyroid glands.[120] Animal data suggest that both PTH and PTHrP act in the regulation of fetal mineral metabolism. PTHrP regulates placental calcium transfer, fetal blood calcium, and differentiation of the cartilaginous growth plate into endochondral bone. By contrast, PTH may play a more dominant role than PTHrP in regulating fetal blood calcium. Blood calcium and PTH levels are rate-limiting determinants of skeletal mineral accretion, and the lack of both PTH and PTHrP induces fetal growth restriction.[62]

The role of vitamin D in fetal physiology is not well understood. Cord concentrations of 25-hydroxyvitamin D and 1,25-dihydroxyvitamin D correlate significantly with those found in the maternal circulation, suggesting that the vitamin D pool of the fetus depends entirely on that of the mother. Fetomaternal relationships of 1,25-dihydroxyvitamin D concentrations are still debated, although a significant correlation was reported in infants. Most of the 1,25-dihydroxyvitamin D found in fetal plasma is due to fetal kidney hydroxylation activity; nevertheless, cord blood concentrations of 1,25-dihydroxyvitamin D in fetal plasma from infants with renal agenesis (Potter syndrome) are still one third of those observed in healthy newborns. Thus, it has been demonstrated that the placenta is able to synthesize and metabolize 1,25-dihydroxyvitamin D through the activity of 25-hydroxyvitamin D-1α hydroxylase and 1,25-dihydroxyvitamin D-24 hydroxylase, two key enzymes for vitamin D metabolism.[12] It has been suggested that methylation of the vitamin D-24-hydroxylase gene plays an important role in maximizing active vitamin D bioavailability at the fetomaternal interface.[84] The effect of 1,25-dihydroxyvitamin D on placental calcium transfer could be related to the expression of the placental calcium transporter PMCA3 messenger RNA (mRNA).[69] In addition, active transplacental calcium and phosphate transfer is at least partly dependent on insulin-like growth factor-1 (IGF-1), itself a stimulating factor of fetal and placental 1,25-dihydroxyvitamin D synthesis. Fetal IGF-1 is frequently downregulated in conditions leading to intrauterine growth restriction (IUGR).[15]

Bone mass of the newborn may be related to the vitamin D status of the mother. The results of dual-energy x-ray absorptiometry (DEXA) show that vitamin D status in winter is correlated with a marked reduction in total bone mineral content in newborn infants. Whole-body bone mineral content values could be 20% lower in countries in which milk products are not supplemented with vitamin D than in countries in which milk products are supplemented.[107] Studies of malnourished populations show that infants of mothers severely deficient in vitamin D may be born with rickets and can suffer fractures in the neonatal period.[16,107]

INTESTINAL ABSORPTION

Calcium absorption is the main determinant of its retention; consequently, it has a significant impact on bone mineral content. Calcium absorption occurs in the small intestine by both active and passive processes. Ionization of calcium compounds, which requires an acid pH, develops in the stomach and is a prerequisite for absorption. Vitamin D is essential for the active absorption of calcium, which involves carriers such as calcium-binding proteins.

After birth, calcium absorption limits the rate of bone mineralization for growth. There may be a reduction in calcium bioavailability, although the absorption rate is higher than that during all other periods of life.[25] The average reported absorption of calcium in the newborn is about 60% of its intake. The absorption of calcium added to human milk with commercially available fortifiers parallels that of the calcium endogenous to human milk. Its absorption occurs in the small intestine by two main routes—either through or between cells.[80] Movement through the cell takes place by active transport. Calcium enters the cell across the brush border membrane down a chemical gradient through a chan-

nel or carrier. It moves across the cell bound to a cytosolic calcium-binding protein (calbindin D_{9k}) and is extruded against a gradient by using a calcium–adenosine triphosphatase pump. Active transport is dependent on vitamin D. The major role of vitamin D in transcellular calcium transport involves the biosynthesis of calcium-binding protein. However, it also appears that vitamin D could modulate the entry and extrusion of calcium from intestinal cells. At present, the rate-limiting step of calcium transport is still controversial. Another less likely manner of calcium absorption involves pinocytosis. Calcium is engulfed by membrane vesicles and moves across the cell, fusing with the plasma membrane and releasing calcium into the extracellular space. Passive calcium transport is driven by chemical gradients that represent movement of calcium among the cells (paracellular transport). It accounts for most of the calcium absorption, particularly in premature infants, in whom the transport, which is transcellular and dependent on vitamin D, is not completely expressed.[23,24] In addition to vitamin D status, various other factors affect calcium absorption.[9,24] Ionization of calcium compounds, which requires an acid pH, occurs in the stomach and is a prerequisite for absorption. Therefore, low availability could be the result of an insoluble fraction of calcium intake or the precipitation of calcium in the gut. Calcium chloride, citrate, and carbonate have higher solubilities than calcium phosphate, which should be avoided in formulas.[9] By contrast, the higher solubility of organic calcium, such as that found in calcium gluconate or glycerophosphate, improves its absorption.[9] The quantity and quality of fat intake may also influence calcium absorption through the formation of calcium soap. It has been suggested that the free palmitate content in the gastrointestinal tract after the hydrolysis of triglyceride may impair calcium absorption.[27] The lower bioavailability of calcium in preterm formulas than that found in human milk would be partly due to palmitate, which is predominantly esterified at the glycerol 1,3 positions (Sn-1, Sn-3) in preterm formulas, in contrast to human milk. However, human milk contains a bile salt–stimulated lipase that is not specific to the Sn-1 and Sn-3 positions. The improvement of calcium absorption with the use of medium-chain triglycerides is probably the result of the reduction of total saturated long-chain fatty acid content in formula. At present, with the use of a well-absorbed fat blend (±85% fat absorption), the influence of calcium soap formation and the β-palmitate content formula could be relatively minimal in clinical practice. A relatively low gastrointestinal pH content or the lactose and casein content of the formula may also have an additional positive effect on calcium absorption.[25,126] In light of the considerable requirements of preterm infants, all these factors probably play a significant role in the amount of calcium retained and deposited in the skeleton.

Medications also interfere with calcium absorption; for example, glucocorticoids inhibit intestinal transfer. Some anticonvulsants can also inhibit calcium absorption either directly (phenytoin) or indirectly through interference with vitamin D metabolism (phenobarbital and phenytoin). In newborn infants, a significant amount of calcium is secreted in the intestinal lumen through digestive fluid. With the use of stable isotopes, endogenous fecal calcium excretion and true calcium absorption may be evaluated. Considering that fecal calcium excretion may represent about 15 mg/kg per day in preterm infants, the true calcium absorption rate is significantly higher than the apparent rate measured by conventional metabolic balances.[48] Numerous metabolic balance studies have been performed in preterm infants fed human milk or a formula (Table 49-3)[23,27,95,98,100] to evaluate apparent calcium absorption. In preterm infants fed human milk, calcium absorption ranges from 60% to 70%, depending on the calcium intake, whereas calcium retention is related to the phosphorus supply. Supplementation of human milk with phosphorus alone normalizes calciuria and allows calcium retention to reach about 35 mg/kg per day. When calcium and phosphorus are provided together or as human milk fortifiers, calcium retention and absorption rates parallel that of human milk, reaching 60 mg/kg per day. The use of

new human milk fortifiers containing highly soluble calcium glycerophosphate improves calcium retention to 90 mg/kg per day (see Table 49-3).[98] In formula-fed infants, the percentage of net calcium absorption is less than that with human milk, ranging from 35% to 60%. Most of the difference probably results from the various factors affecting calcium solubility and absorption. At present, the use of a preterm formula with a high mineral content does not necessarily improve mineral retention.[95] Indeed, because of the poor solubility of calcium salts, especially calcium phosphate, the calcium content measured in formulas may be significantly lower than the claimed value, and an additional loss due to precipitation may occur before feeding.[95] In metabolic studies, the actual amount of calcium provided by feeding needs to be measured. As shown in Table 49-3, calcium retention

TABLE 49-3   Calcium, Phosphorus, and Magnesium Absorption and Retention in Preterm Infants Fed Human Milk (without or with a Human Milk Fortifier) and Preterm Formulas*

	HUMAN MILK AND HUMAN MILK FORTIFIER			PRETERM FORMULAS			
	N = 36	N = 22	N = 23	N = 31	N = 37	N = 27	N = 20
Postnatal age (days)	26.4 ± 9.6	30.4 ± 1.8	29.7 ± 8.1	23.3 ± 12.8	32.7 ± 15.1	32.5 ± 10.5	32.7 ± 8.9
Body weight (g)	1788 ± 284	1677 ± 209	1662 ± 231	1945 ± 286	1941 ± 245	1764 ± 244	1648 ± 114
CGA† (wk)	34.6 ± 1.6	34.4 ± 1.1	34.0 ± 1.3	34.7 ± 1.6	35.0 ± 1.8	33.8 ± 1.6	33.9 ± 1.3
Calcium (mg/kg/day)							
Intake	56.4 ± 9.0	85.5 ± 7.6	138.4 ± 27.9	80.5 ± 6.7	101.0 ± 8.0	134.5 ± 7.3	165.9 ± 9.5
Stool	21.0 ± 10.3	26.2 ± 16.4	56.3 ± 28.7	39.7 ± 11.1	46.8 ± 15.1	72.6 ± 21.9	103.2 ± 22.7
Absorption	35.3 ± 8.8	59.3 ± 16.4	82.0 ± 26.6	40.8 ± 13.8	54.2 ± 13.0	61.8 ± 17.8	62.7 ± 21.9
Urine	7.0 ± 6.4	5.8 ± 4.5	5.0 ± 4.0	2.1 ± 1.5	3.2 ± 2.4	4.9 ± 3.2	4.9 ± 3.9
Retention	28.3 ± 9.3	53.4 ± 15.6	77.1 ± 25.4	38.8 ± 13.9	50.9 ± 13.1	57.0 ± 18.1	57.8 ± 21.8
Net absorption (%)	63.5 ± 15.2	69.4 ± 18.8	59.9 ± 17.3	50.2 ± 15.1	53.9 ± 13.1	46.4 ± 14.6	37.8 ± 13.0
Phosphorus (mg/kg/day)							
Intake	40.3 ± 12.2	55.6 ± 15.0	84.7 ± 7.4	59.2 ± 6.5	68.7 ± 7.6	86.2 ± 11.7	94.5 ± 6.3
Stool	3.0 ± 1.6	3.7 ± 1.8	5.5 ± 2.4	6.6 ± 3.5	5.4 ± 2.4	13.1 ± 8.3	34.4 ± 10.1
Absorption	37.4 ± 12.6	51.9 ± 15.8	79.2 ± 7.7	52.5 ± 7.3	63.3 ± 7.1	73.2 ± 10.6	60.1 ± 14.4
Urine	7.9 ± 8.2	6.3 ± 9.6	19.4 ± 8.9	14.2 ± 5.8	18.1 ± 7.3	22.3 ± 11.0	8.8 ± 10.6
Retention	29.4 ± 9.1	45.5 ± 14.9	59.8 ± 11.7	38.4 ± 7.6	45.2 ± 7.0	50.9 ± 8.1	51.3 ± 8.2
Net Absorption (%)	91.7 ± 4.8	92.3 ± 5.0	93.4 ± 3.2	88.6 ± 6.1	92.1 ± 3.2	85.1 ± 8.9	63.1 ± 11.5
Magnesium (mg/kg/day)							
Intake	5.9 ± 1.5	5.8 ± 1.8	7.3 ± 1.5	9.1 ± 2.1	9.4 ± 2.1	12.3 ± 2.4	8.1 ± 2.3
Stool	3.1 ± 1.6	2.9 ± 1.2	4.7 ± 1.7	4.9 ± 3.1	4.9 ± 2.1	6.8 ± 2.3	4.3 ± 1.7
Absorption	2.8 ± 0.9	2.9 ± 1.2	2.5 ± 1.9	4.2 ± 2.1	4.5 ± 1.7	5.5 ± 2.2	3.8 ± 1.7
Urine	1.0 ± 0.7	0.6 ± 0.6	0.5 ± 0.5	1.0 ± 0.9	1.3 ± 0.9	1.9 ± 1.0	0.9 ± 0.9
Retention	1.8 ± 1.2	2.3 ± 1.0	2.0 ± 1.8	3.1 ± 1.9	3.2 ± 1.9	3.6 ± 2.0	2.9 ± 1.1
Net absorption (%)	48.8 ± 17.3	50.2 ± 15.6	33.0 ± 26.8	48.5 ± 23.5	48.5 ± 17.3	44.8 ± 15.2	47.3 ± 13.2

*In human milk groups, calcium and phosphorus absorption and retention are related to intake, in contrast to formula groups, in which a plateau is reached rapidly due to a decrease in net absorption (%). Magnesium absorption and retention are similar in human milk and formula groups and are related to intake.
†Gestational age at the time of the balance study.
CGA, corrected gestational age.

limited to 90 mg/kg per day could presently be expected in preterm infants fed a preterm formula with a highly soluble calcium content. Nevertheless, those values are still relatively far from the reference values calculated during the last trimester of gestation (120 to 130 mg/kg per day), which is still considered the target mineral accretion rate for infants with very low birthweight (VLBW).

RENAL EXCRETION

Under normal circumstances, calcium status is maintained by a balance between its intestinal absorption and renal excretion. Urinary excretion is the result of glomerular filtration followed by the sum of the processes of tubular reabsorption and secretion. About 70% of the filtered load of calcium is reabsorbed in the proximal tubule and 20% in the thick ascending limb of the loop of Henle in association with Na^+ reabsorption. Although it is responsible for only 5% to 10% of Ca^{2+} reabsorption, the major regulation of Ca^{2+} reabsorption occurs in the distal convoluted tubule by a mechanism independent of Na^+ reabsorption but regulated by PTH and $1,25(OH)_2D_3$. Calcium reabsorption is increased by both PTH and $1,25(OH)_2D_3$. It is also regulated by ionized calcium concentration, phosphate concentration, and acid-base status and increases with Ca^{2+} depletion and alkalosis but decreases with hypercalcemia, phosphate depletion, and acidosis. The effects of diuretics on renal calcium excretion vary considerably. Furosemide markedly increases renal calcium losses and is a risk factor for neonatal nephrocalcinosis. Thiazides increase renal tubular calcium reabsorption, thereby reducing calciuria (see Chapter 51).[89,113]

The ability of the kidney to dispose of excess calcium represents a major homeostatic mechanism. Under normal circumstances, nearly all filtered calcium (98%) is reabsorbed in the renal tubule. However, preterm and term infants differ from the adult in three main aspects: (1) Renal function is far from being completely developed. (2) Mineral requirements for growth are very high. (3) Renal calcium load results solely in the difference between net absorption and net bone and soft tissue retention. Considering that calcium soft tissue retention is negligible, renal calcium load is highly dependent on bone calcium deposition associated with phosphorus in the form of hydroxyapatite $[Ca_{10}(PO_4)_6(OH)_2]$ containing a molar calcium-to-phosphorus ratio of 1.67 (2.15 wt/wt). Therefore, the main determinant of the urinary loss of calcium in preterm and term neonates is relative to phosphorus depletion,[64,113] which has been illustrated in balance studies performed in growing preterm infants fed human milk. When human milk is provided exclusively, there is an increase in the urinary excretion of calcium associated with very low urinary phosphate excretion. In contrast, when human milk is supplemented with phosphate, significant phosphaturia appears at the same time that calciuria decreases to a minimum level. Therefore, hypercalciuria can be explained by a relative phosphate depletion that cannot meet the phosphate demand necessary for skeletal mineralization (Fig. 49-12).

INTAKE

Mature human milk contains approximately 340 mg of calcium per liter, corresponding to 50 mg per 100 kcal. Considering the smaller amount of calcium absorption with the use of formula, the guidelines of a recent Life Sciences Research Office Report on term infant formula nutrient requirements and those of the Scientific Committee on Food of the European Commission for infant formulas during the first 6 months of life recommended a content of 50 to 140 mg of calcium per 100 kcal.[38,92]

For preterm infants, recommendations are based on fetal accretion rates. In 1985, the American Academy of Pediatrics recommended that formulas contain 140 to 160 mg of calcium per 100 kcal.[3] More recently, the Life Sciences Research Office recommended a calcium content of 123 to 185 mg per 100 kcal for preterm infant formula, and an international expert panel suggested a similar value of 90 to 180 mg per 100 kcal.[10,58] However, the European Society for Pediatric Gastroenterology, Hepatology, and Nutrition (ESPGHAN) committee of nutrition considers that those calcium needs are based on data obtained in infants fed preterm formulas with low calcium bioavailability. It suggests that after birth, bone metabolism is designed to accelerate bone turnover, reducing calcium requirements, and that the relative osteopenia observed in preterm infants could be considered at least partially physiologic. Because a calcium retention level ranging from 60 to 90 mg/kg per day ensures appropriate mineralization and decreases the risk for fracture in infants with VLBW, the ESPGHAN Committee on Nutrition recommended the use of highly bioavailable calcium salts providing a calcium content of 110 to 130 mg per 100 kcal.[39]

Phosphorus Physiology

Unlike calcium, phosphorus remains in the soft tissues, mainly in the form of phosphate esters, and in extracellular fluid in the form of inorganic phosphate ions. It represents about 15% of the whole-body content. Given its widespread distribution, phosphorus plays a critical role in many biologic processes, including energy metabolism, membrane composition, nucleotide structure, cellular signaling, and bone mineralization. It is, therefore, not surprising that a deficiency of phosphorus results in clinical disease, including muscle weakness, impaired leukocyte function, and abnormal bone metabolization.

SERUM PHOSPHORUS

In serum, about two thirds of phosphorus is organic (lipid phosphorus and phosphoric ester phosphorus) and one third inorganic. In routine clinical practice, only inorganic phosphorus is measured. About 85% of the inorganic phosphorus is ionized, circulating as monohydrogen or dihydrogen phosphate; 5% is complexed with sodium, magnesium, or calcium; and 10% is protein bound. Because so many phosphorus species are present, depending on pH and other factors, the serum concentration is conventionally expressed as the mass of the elemental phosphorus (mmol/L, or mg/dL). In contrast to calcium, the serum phosphorus concentration varies widely depending mainly on intake and renal excretion but is also influenced by age, gender, pH, and a variety of hormones. At birth, the mean serum phosphorus concentration is relatively low (2.6 mmol/L, or 6.2 mg/dL) but thereafter rises rapidly to reach 3.4 mmol/L, or 8.1 mg/dL, owing to both endogenous phosphorus release and low renal excretion.[64,113] Serum phosphorus subsequently varies. The diet partially determines the serum phosphorus content: It is higher in formula-fed than breast-fed infants. Serum phosphorus is inversely related to serum calcium concentration. After the neonatal period, the serum phosphorus concentration progressively decreases to 2.1 mmol/L, or 5 mg/dL, at the age of 1 to 2 years; 1.8 mmol/L, or

Figure 49–12. Metabolism of calcium (Ca) and phosphorus (P) in term infants with feeding.

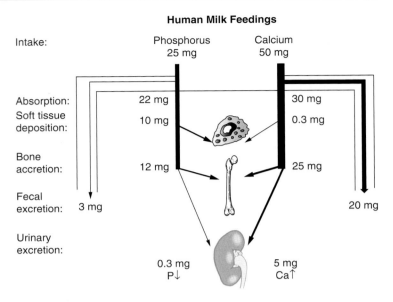

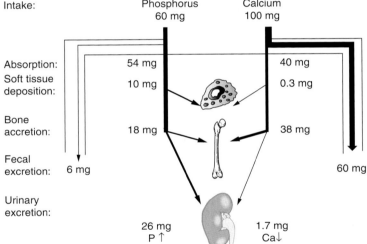

4.4 mg/dL, in middle childhood; and 1.5 mmol/L, or 3.5 mg/dL, at the end of adolescence.[89]

PLACENTAL TRANSPORT

During pregnancy, there is transfer of phosphorus from the mother to the fetus that reaches a peak of 60 to 75 mg/kg per day during the third trimester; 75% is retained for bone mineralization, and 25% is retained in other tissues. The transplacental transport of phosphorus is an active process against a concentration gradient and is sodium dependent. Both $1,25(OH)_2D_3$ and fetal PTH may be involved in the regulation of placental phosphorus transfer.

INTESTINAL ABSORPTION

Intestinal phosphorus absorption takes place primarily in the duodenum and jejunum and to a lesser extent in the ileum and colon. It occurs by two mechanisms: an active, sodium-dependent transcellular process localized to the mucosal surface, and passive diffusion through the paracellular pathway. It

depends on both the absolute amount of dietary phosphorus and the relative concentrations of calcium and phosphorus (an excessive amount of either can decrease the absorption of the other). Vitamin D may stimulate active phosphorus absorption, although it is largely independent of vitamin D intake. The efficiency of this absorption is high (close to 90% of intake) regardless of the type of milk given.[89,113] However, the use of poorly soluble calcium salt such as calcium triphosphate in formulas is associated with a significant reduction in phosphorus absorption.[80,98] In contrast to calcium, a small amount of phosphate is secreted in the intestinal lumen through digestive fluid.

RENAL EXCRETION

The kidney contributes to a positive phosphate balance during growth by the reabsorption of a relatively high fraction of filtered inorganic phosphate (99% in newborns, 95% in infants fed human milk, and 80% in adults). Preterm infants have an increased fractional excretion of phosphate and are at a greater risk for developing signs and symptoms of phosphate deficiency. The bulk of filtered phosphate is reabsorbed in the proximal tubule through a sodium-dependent transporter, the Na^+-phosphate cotransporter. A change from breast milk with a low phosphate content to a formula with a high content is associated with a rapid downregulation of Na^+-phosphate cotransporter-2 mRNA and protein in the brush border membrane. The age-related decrease in phosphate reabsorption observed after the weaning period appears to be correlated with the smaller phosphate needs of adult and older animals than those of growing animals. It is surprising that the fractional reabsorption of phosphate is higher in growing than fully grown animals and humans.[52] The kidney is the major determinant of the plasma phosphate concentration. There is no extrarenal mechanism for regulating plasma phosphorus except the net input of phosphorus into extracellular fluid from all sources. Because the intestinal absorption of phosphorus is very efficient and fairly unregulated, renal phosphorus excretion plays an important role in maintaining its balance. Filtered load depends on the plasma phosphorus level and glomerular filtration rate (GFR). Tubular reabsorption is an active and saturable process that gives rise to a maximal rate of tubular reabsorption (T_m). There is a plasma minimal threshold below which phosphorus reabsorption is almost complete and urinary excretion close to zero and a maximal threshold above which all tubular reabsorptive systems are saturated, so each additional increment in filtered load is associated with a parallel increment in excretion.[64,89,113] In the intermediate zone, there is a functional relationship between GFR and T_m, known as the *glomerulotubular balance*, in which a change in GFR is compensated for by a change in T_m in order to regulate phosphorus excretion. In preterm infants, the minimal and maximal threshold levels are 1.75 mmol/L (5.4 mg/dL) and 2.45 mmol/L (7.6 mg/dL), respectively (Fig. 49-13).[113] The level of PTH activity in plasma is probably the single most important physiologic regulator of phosphorus excretion. PTH inhibits phosphorus reabsorption, but its activity appears to be limited to the intermediate zone between the minimal and maximal plasma threshold levels. In contrast, $1,25(OH)_2$ vitamin D synthesis, stimulated by a decrease in plasma phosphorus concentration, has an indirect effect on phosphorus reabsorption by its effect on mineral absorption and mobilization from bone, resulting in an increase in plasma calcium concentration and the suppression of PTH release. During early postnatal life, the phosphate response to PTH is blunted, whereas PTH increases tubular calcium reabsorption. Together, these actions result in the retention of both calcium and phosphate in infants, which is favorable for growth. The role of newly discovered phosphatonin peptides such as FGF23 in the regulation of phosphorus excretion during early life remain to be established. FGF23 principally functions as a phosphaturic factor and counter-regulatory hormone for $1,25(OH)_2$ vitamin D production. Excess FGF23 secreted by osteocytes in bone causes hypophosphatemia through inhibition of Na-phosphate cotransporter-2. Excess FGF23 also suppresses $1,25(OH)_2$ vitamin D through inhibition of 25-hydroxyvitamin D-1α-hydroxylase and stimulation of 24-hydroxylase, which inactivate $1,25(OH)_2$ vitamin D in the proximal tubule of the kidney. In contrast, deficiency of FGF23 results in the opposite renal phenotype consisting

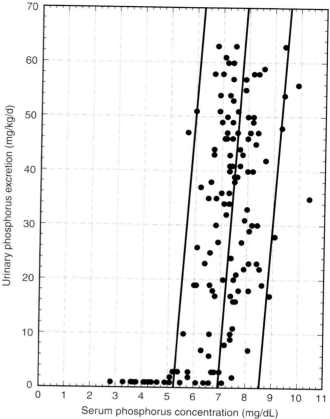

Figure 49–13. Relationship between urinary excretion of phosphorus and serum phosphate level ($n = 198$) in preterm infants. Regression lines represent the minimal, mean, and maximal plasma phosphate concentration thresholds for tubular reabsorption of phosphate. Points to the left of the minimal threshold were considered hypophosphatemia associated with phosphorus depletion. Points to the right of the maximal threshold were considered hyperphosphatemia due to low glomerular filtration rates and relative phosphorus overload.

of hyperphosphatemia and elevated production of $1,25(OH)_2$ vitamin D. Downregulation of FGF23 could promote the relative hyperphosphatemia and the relative increase in $1,25(OH)_2$ vitamin D promoting bone mineralization during early rapid growth in the neonatal period.[91] Absorbed phosphate enters the extracellular phosphate pool, which is in equilibrium with bone and soft tissue. In adults with neutral phosphorus balance, the amount of phosphorus excreted by the kidney is equal to the net amount absorbed by the intestine; in growing infants, it is less than the net amount absorbed owing to the deposition of phosphorus in soft tissues and bone. In growing infants, phosphorus will preferentially go to soft tissue with a weight-to-weight nitrogen-to-phosphorus ratio of 15:1 and to bone with a weight-to-weight calcium-to-phosphorus ratio of 2.15:1. The residual phosphorus constitutes the renal phosphorus load influencing plasma concentration and urinary excretion. In the face of a limited total phosphorus supply, bone mineral accretion may be limited, leading to significant calcium excretion associated

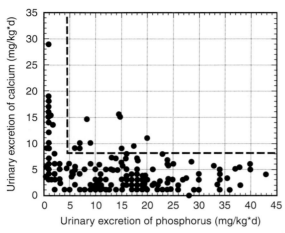

Figure 49–14. Relationship between urinary excretion of calcium and urinary excretion of phosphorus in preterm infants ($n = 198$). Hypercalciuria (>8 mg/kg/day) is related to low phosphate excretion (<3 mg/kg/day). Conversely, urinary excretion of calcium below 8 mg/kg/day is usually observed in preterm infants with phosphorus excretion over 4 mg/kg/day.

with very low urinary excretion of phosphorus (Fig. 49-14). This particular situation is illustrated in Figure 49-12, showing calcium and phosphorus metabolism in term infants fed human milk or formula.

INTAKE

Mature human milk contains about 140 mg of phosphorus per liter, corresponding to 21 mg per 100 kcal. The recent guidelines for infant formulas in the first 6 months of life recommend minimal and maximal contents of 20 and 70 mg/100 kcal, respectively.[38,92] However, to avoid the occurrence of hypocalcemia or hypercalcemia resulting from an unbalanced diet containing the minimal calcium combined with the maximal phosphorus content (or inversely), the Life Sciences Research Office and the Scientific Committee on Food of the European Commission recommend that the calcium-to-phosphorus ratio be maintained at more than 1.1:1 but less than 2.0:1.

For preterm infants, the recommendations are based on fetal accretion rates. In 1985, the American Academy of Pediatrics recommended 95 to 108 mg of phosphorus per 100 kcal for preterm formulas, whereas more recently, the Life Sciences Research Office and the International Expert Panel recommended similar values, with a calcium-to-phosphorus ratio maintained at more than 1.7:1 but less than 2.0:1.[3,10,58] Considering a nitrogen retention ranging from 350 to 450 mg/kg per day and a calcium retention from 60 to 90 mg/kg per day, the ESPGHAN Committee on Nutrition recommended an adequate intake of 65 to 90 mg/kg per day of a highly absorbable source of phosphate (90%) with a calcium-to-phosphorus ratio between 1.5 and 2.0.[3]

Magnesium Physiology

To less of an extent than calcium and phosphorus, the skeleton represents the largest magnesium store (60%), which is divided into two compartments: one firmly bound to apatite

and nonmobilizing, and the other absorbed to the surface of the mineral crystals and contributing to magnesium homeostasis.[63]

The remaining magnesium is distributed in skeletal muscle, the nervous system, and other organs with a high metabolic rate. Magnesium is the second most abundant intracellular cation, playing a crucial role in many physiologic functions. It is critical in energy-requiring metabolic processes, protein synthesis, membrane integrity, nervous tissue conduction, neuromuscular excitability, muscle contraction, hormone secretion, and intermediate metabolism.

SERUM MAGNESIUM

In serum, about one third of the magnesium is bound to protein, mainly albumin; the remaining two thirds is ultrafilterable, being about 92% free and 8% complexed to citrate, phosphate, and other compounds.[7,63] The plasma magnesium concentration is elevated in preterm and term infants (0.8 ± 0.16 mmol/L, or 2.0 ± 0.4 mg/dL) and decreases soon after infancy to adult values.[59] The sum of ionized and complexed magnesium constitutes its diffusible or ultrafilterable form. Although the concentration of this form of magnesium in plasma remains almost constant (0.45 ± 0.1 mmol/L, or 1.1 ± 0.2 mg/dL), the proportion of this diffusible form in relation to total magnesium increases progressively with age (preterm newborn infants, 52%; term newborns, 62%; infants, 66%; and children, 70%). The concentration of magnesium in red blood cells (about 2.5 mmol/L) appears to be genetically controlled and represents an acceptable indicator of magnesium content in other tissues.[7,67]

PLACENTAL TRANSPORT

Magnesium freely crosses the placental barrier and accumulates in the fetus mainly during the first trimester of pregnancy.[7] Placental transfer continues throughout gestation, at a daily rate of 3 to 5 mg.[77] The transfer of magnesium across the placenta depends on an active transport mechanism different from that of calcium, which is necessary to maintain higher fetal than maternal concentrations. There is currently no clear information on the regulation of placental transport.[115] Obviously, situations of magnesium excess or deficiency in the mother are also reflected in the fetus.[77]

INTESTINAL ABSORPTION

About 40% of ingested magnesium is absorbed in the gut, mainly in proximal parts of the small intestine. Newborn infants, especially preterm infants, have an increased capacity for intestinal absorption of magnesium.[7,63] Net magnesium absorption is the sum of the absorbed magnesium from ingested foods and digestive fluids. There are two mechanisms of absorption: One is passive and the other active and saturable. Passive absorption occurs by means of a paracellular pathway, following a favorable electrochemical gradient as a function of water and solute movement, and appears to be proportional to dietary intake. Regulated, active transport depends on a saturable carrier present in the luminal membrane and operates only under conditions of low magnesium intake. The factors regulating the intestinal absorption of magnesium are largely unknown. The magnesium concentration in the digestive tract is the most important determinant of the amount of magnesium absorbed; nevertheless, food elements capable of influencing magnesium absorption should be taken into account in the investigation of cases of low magnesium intake. Substances that increase magnesium solubility favor its absorption, whereas substances that form insoluble complexes decrease its likelihood. Data show that no competition exists between magnesium and calcium for absorption because calcium supplementation does not decrease magnesium absorption. In contrast, phosphates can inhibit magnesium absorption through the formation of insoluble magnesium complexes in the intestine. Magnesium absorption in the gut is not stimulated by $1,25(OH)_2$ vitamin D.

RENAL EXCRETION

The kidney plays a major role in magnesium homeostasis. It conserves magnesium in response to a deficiency and increases excretion in proportion to the load presented to the kidney.[63] About 70% to 80% of serum magnesium is filtered through the glomerular membrane, but only 5% to 15% of the filtered magnesium is reabsorbed along the proximal tubule, which is considerably less than the amount of fractional reabsorption of sodium or calcium. The primary site for magnesium reabsorption is the thick ascending limb of the loop of Henle, where about 65% of the filtered magnesium is reabsorbed. At this site, magnesium reabsorption is associated with NaCl cotransport. Reabsorption takes place transcellularly, following the favorable transepithelial magnesium concentration gradient, resulting from water absorption. The thick ascending limb of the loop of Henle has a major role in the reabsorption of magnesium, absorbing 70% to 80% of the filtered magnesium. This reabsorption is mainly passive and depends on the favorable transepithelial electric gradient. The distal convoluted tubule reabsorbs only the remaining 10% to 15%, but the reabsorption is especially important because it determines the final amount of magnesium present in the urine. In this part of the nephron, magnesium is transcellularly reabsorbed by an active mechanism.[30] Analyzing magnesium intake and urinary excretion, one can observe that there is an average volume of elimination of about one third of the dietary magnesium in the urine. When the magnesium intake is severely restricted in humans with normal kidney function, urine output decreases. Supplementing a normal intake increases urinary excretion without altering normal serum levels as long as renal function is normal and the amounts given are not excessive. Overall, the tubular reabsorption of magnesium is a process that is quantitatively limited; the maximal rate of this reabsorption appears to be lower than that of calcium and phosphorus.[71]

Renal homeostasis of magnesium is regulated by many hormonal and nonhormonal factors. The hormonal factors interact to modify the transepithelial electric gradient, tubular permeability at the level of the loop of Henle, or mechanism of active transport at the level of the distal convoluted tubule. PTH, calcitonin, glucagon, vasopressin, and insulin all increase the tubular reabsorption of magnesium. The role of aldosterone is misunderstood, but magnesium reabsorption follows sodium reabsorption; it increases under conditions of volume depletion and decreases under conditions of volume expansion. The nonhormonal factors include the concentration of magnesium in the tubular lumen, acid-base equilibrium, and plasma concentrations of potassium and inorganic phosphate. The tubular reabsorption of magnesium is closely linked to that of calcium. It has been recently shown that epithelial cells of the loop of Henle loop and the distal convoluted tubule have receptors that sense the extracellular concentrations of both Mg^{2+} and Ca^{2+}. Metabolic acidosis also increases the urinary excretion of magnesium.[63] Daily urinary excretion in normal children oscillates between 1.6 and 2.8 mg/kg of body weight daily. Normal values for the ratio of urinary magnesium to urinary creatinine (mg/mg) change with age.[6,71] An increased value observed during infancy does not represent a higher excretion of magnesium but is related to the diminished excretion of creatinine per unit of lean body mass during this age period.

INTAKE

Mature human milk contains about 26 mg of magnesium per liter, corresponding to 3.9 mg per 100 kcal. Guidelines for infant formulas during the first 6 months of life[38,92] recommend minimal and maximal contents of 4 to 5 mg and 15 to 17 mg/100 kcal, respectively. For preterm infants, the recommendations are based on fetal accretion rates, and values similar to those at term have been suggested (6.8 to 17 mg/100 kcal and 7.9 to 15 mg/kg per day, respectively).[10,39,58]

HORMONAL REGULATION

Parathyroid Hormone

The four parathyroid glands, through the secretion of PTH, regulate serum calcium concentrations and bone metabolism. PTH is synthesized as a larger (115–amino acid) precursor (prepro-PTH) but is stored and secreted mainly as an 84–amino acid peptide, with the 1-34,N-terminal portion conferring bioactivity.[70,103]

EFFECTS

The effects of PTH on mineral metabolism are initiated by the binding of PTH to the type 1 PTH receptor in the target tissues. Another PTH receptor (type 2) has been found in the brain and intestine. Its main ligand is a peptide different from PTH; the functions of this receptor are not known. As a result, PTH regulates large calcium fluxes across bone, kidneys, and intestine (see Fig. 49-11). PTH increases serum calcium concentrations directly by increasing bone resorption and renal calcium reabsorption and indirectly by increasing renal synthesis of $1,25(OH)_2D_3$, thereby increasing intestinal calcium absorption. PTH also lowers serum phosphorus concentrations through its phosphaturic action on the renal proximal tubule. This action minimizes the possibly adverse effect of hyperphosphatemia related to bone resorption on calcium homeostasis.

REGULATION OF SECRETION

Serum calcium concentration regulates PTH secretion; high concentrations inhibit the secretion of PTH, and low concentrations stimulate it. Low or falling serum calcium concentrations act within seconds to stimulate PTH secretion, initiated by means of a calcium-sensing receptor on the surfaces of parathyroid cells. This receptor is a heptahelical molecule, like the receptors for light, odorants, catecholamines, and many peptide hormones. The calcium-sensing receptor is expressed in the parathyroid glands, where it regulates PTH secretion, and in the kidneys, where it regulates tubular calcium reabsorption. Decreases in ionized calcium of as little as 0.4 mmol/L stimulate PTH secretion, and increases suppress it (although usually not completely). Acute decreases in magnesium concentrations also stimulate PTH secretion, and increases depress it. However, chronic magnesium deficiency paradoxically decreases PTH secretion, probably by altering the calcium-sensitive, magnesium-dependent adenylate cyclase involved in PTH secretion.

Slower regulation of PTH secretion occurs over a period of hours as a result of cellular changes in PTH mRNA. Vitamin D and its metabolites 25-hydroxyvitamin D and 1,25-dihydroxyvitamin D, acting through vitamin D receptors, decrease the level of PTH mRNA, and hypocalcemia increases it. The slowest regulation of PTH secretion occurs over days or even months and reflects changes in the growth of the parathyroid glands. Metabolites of vitamin D directly inhibit the mass of parathyroid cells; hypocalcemia stimulates the growth of parathyroid cells independent of the contrary action of vitamin D metabolites.

Both activating and inactivating calcium-sensing receptor (CaSR) mutations have been identified. Loss-of-function CaSR mutations elevate the set point for both PTH secretion and tubular calcium reabsorption, causing hypercalcemia. The associated clinical syndromes are familial benign hypocalciuric hypercalcemia and neonatal severe hyperparathyroidism. Gain-of-function CaSR mutations decrease the set point for both PTH secretion and tubular calcium reabsorption in response to hypocalcemia. The associated clinical syndrome is autosomal dominant hypocalcemic hypercalciuria. These syndromes are discussed later. Some cases of nonfamilial idiopathic hypoparathyroidism may also be caused by gain-of-function CaSR mutations.

The human calcium receptor gene contains seven exons and is located at 3q13.3-21. In the parathyroid gland, the calcium receptor mediates inhibition by extracellular Ca^{2+} concentration of PTH secretion, of *PTH* gene expression, and of parathyroid cellular proliferation. In the kidney, the receptor mediates the direct inhibition of the reabsorption of divalent cations in the thick cortical ascending limb of the loop of Henle.[102]

FETAL PARATHYROID FUNCTION

Human parathyroid glands are functionally active as early as 12 weeks of gestation. However, fetal parathyroid glands are functionally suppressed by high intrauterine calcium concentrations, and PTH levels in cord blood are frequently below the detection limit.[109] PTH does not appear to cross the placenta in either direction, and the role of fetal PTH in maternal-fetal calcium transport is not clearly established. Nevertheless, fetal PTH levels contribute importantly to fetal ionized calcium levels and mineralization of the bone matrix.[62] In contrast, a midregion fragment of PTHrP, produced by the fetal parathyroid glands and various fetal tissues, appears mainly responsible for regulating the maternal-fetal calcium gradient. It has been shown that PTHrP directly affects adenosine triphosphate–dependent calcium transport across the basal plasma membrane of the human syncytiotrophoblast at a concentration within the physiologic range

(5 pg/mL).[121] Therefore, both PTH and PTHrP act synergistically during fetal life to promote calcium transfer, high blood calcium concentration, bone development, and matrix mineralization.

Maternal hyperparathyroidism results in maternal hypercalcemia, which leads to fetal hypercalcemia and suppression of fetal and neonatal parathyroid glands. Conversely, untreated maternal hypoparathyroidism leads to maternal hypocalcemia, fetal hypocalcemia, and secondary fetal and neonatal hyperparathyroidism.

NEONATAL PARATHYROID FUNCTION

After birth, with the abrupt termination of the maternal calcium supply, serum calcium in the newborn decreases, and serum PTH increases correspondingly. Both term and preterm infants may show a PTH response to falling serum calcium. Infants with VLBW have a decreased PTH surge compared with full-term infants. Infants of diabetic mothers may have impaired PTH production during the beginning days of life. Infants with birth asphyxia may also have decreased PTH responses to hypocalcemia.

PARATHYROID HORMONE REFERENCE VALUES

Current assays for serum PTH are conducted at two sites that are designed to detect both amino-terminal and carboxy-terminal epitopes of the peptide. The better assays are those that are well standardized, do not cross-react with PTH-related peptide, and are sufficiently sensitive so that normal values can be distinguished from subnormal values. PTH molecules that are reactive in these two-site immunoassays are considered intact, but some have no bioactivity. For example, a loss of only six amino acids to yield PTH (7-84) eliminates all bioactivity but does not affect the immunoreactivity measured in most or all of these assays.

In full-term newborns, serum PTH concentrations tend to be low in cord blood but increase within the first 48 hours of life in response to the decrease in serum calcium. In preterm infants, the serum immunoreactive, intact PTH concentrations increase immediately after birth, indicating that, in them, the secretion of the hormone responds physiologically to the hypocalcemic stimulus. This increase in immunoreactive PTH concentration could be blunted when premature infants receive calcium by infusion, with the calcium load buffering the postnatal depression of serum calcium. By day 10, the serum concentrations of intact PTH return to euparathyroid values (Table 49-4).[107] The multiplication factor for serum PTH from picograms per deciliter to picomoles per liter (pg/dL to pmol/L) is 0.11.

Vitamin D

SYNTHESIS AND METABOLISM

Vitamin D is synthesized endogenously in the skin (cholecalciferol or vitamin D_3) after sunshine exposure to high-energy ultraviolet photons (ultraviolet B, 290 to 315 nm) or is absorbed from dietary sources in the duodenum and jejunum as either vitamin D_3 (from animal sources) or vitamin D_2 (ergocalciferol [from vegetable sources]). Regardless of its origin, vitamin D_2 and D_3 are transported bound to the vitamin D–binding protein to the liver, where it is hydroxylated at

	PTH(1-84) (pmol/L)	cPTH (pmol/L)	DBP (μmol/L)
TABLE 49–4 Evolution of Intact Parathyroid Hormone (1-84), Carboxy-Terminal Parathyroid Hormone, and Vitamin D–Binding Protein Concentrations in 15 Preterm Infants			
Cord serum	11 ± 3	48 ± 8	4.43 ± 0.37
Day 1	66 ± 11*	125 ± 15*	4.40 ± 0.34
Day 2	87 ± 11*	168 ± 5*	4.96 ± 0.23
Day 5	67 ± 9*	152 ± 16*	6.21 ± 0.26*
Day 10	23 ± 4	69 ± 6	6.03 ± 0.30*
Day 30	38 ± 7	80 ± 11	5.16 ± 0.23

*Significantly different from cord serum, $P < .05$.
cPTH, carboxy-terminal PTH; DBP, vitamin D–binding protein; PTH, parathyroid hormone.
From Salle BL, et al: Perinatal metabolism of vitamin D, *Am J Clin Nutr* 71:1317S, 2000.

carbon 25 to form vitamin D_3 (25[OH]D_3, or calcidiol), the most abundant vitamin D metabolite. The generation of calcidiol is not regulated, and circulating concentrations of 25[OH]D_3 provide a useful index of vitamin D status (reflecting both dietary intake and sunshine exposure). Subsequently in the kidney, 25[OH]D_3 is further hydroxylated at carbon 1 to form the final active metabolite, 1,25(OH)$_2D_3$, or calcitriol. This last transformation is tightly regulated and is the rate-limiting step in vitamin D metabolism. 1,25(OH)$_2D_3$ can also be synthesized by various cells, including monocytes and skin cells, as well as by the placenta during pregnancy. However, this local production of 1,25(OH)$_2D_3$ is not associated with calcium homeostasis but could contribute to regulating cell growth.[50]

EFFECTS

Normal vitamin D status is necessary to maintain calcium and phosphorus homeostasis. The effects of 1,25(OH)$_2D_3$ (calcitriol) on target tissues are initiated by its binding to a steroid receptor (vitamin D receptor) distributed in numerous tissues, leading to the synthesis of a variety of proteins. Therefore, 1,25(OH)$_2D_3$ acts on the small intestine, increasing the absorption of calcium and phosphorus by the synthesis of calcium-binding (calbindin-D) proteins; on bone, mobilizing calcium and phosphorus by increasing the number of osteoclasts; and on the kidney, increasing calcium reabsorption in the distal nephron segments by increasing the expression of the epithelial calcium influx channel. There is a natural polymorphism in the genotype of the vitamin D receptor that contributes to skeletal metabolism in early childhood and to the genetic determinant of the peak bone mass.

REGULATION OF SECRETION

In contrast to hepatic 25-hydroxylation, renal 1-hydroxylation, which leads to the active metabolite, appears to be tightly regulated. The main factors increasing the synthesis of calcitriol through stimulation of renal 25(OH)D_3-1α-hydroxylase are PTH, PTHrP, hypocalcemia, hypophosphatemia, and other

hormonal factors, such as IGF-1, estrogen, prolactin, and growth hormone. The production of calcitriol is inhibited by elevated serum levels of calcium and phosphorous, but also by the newly discovered phosphatonin peptides implicated in phosphorus homeostasis. Thus, an increase in FGF23 production suppresses 1,25(OH)$_2$ vitamin D through inhibition of 25-hydroxyvitamin D-1α-hydroxylase and stimulation of 24-hydroxylase inactivating 1,25(OH)$_2$ vitamin D in the proximal tubule of the kidney.[91]

FETAL VITAMIN D FUNCTION

Serum 25-hydroxyvitamin D concentration depends on vitamin D intake and production. The production of vitamin D is influenced by geographic location, season, skin pigmentation, and latitude. Vitamin D deficiency is very common during pregnancy, especially in areas with a prolonged winter season. It is lower in black pregnant women in contrast to white pregnant women. In the northern United States, about 45% of black pregnant women are vitamin D deficient (25-hydroxyvitamin D <37.5 nmol/L) as opposed to 5% of white women in late pregnancy. On the other hand, 50% to 60% of white and black pregnant women are vitamin D insufficient (25-hydroxyvitamin D: 37.5 to 80 nmol/L).[20]

1,25-Dihydroxyvitamin D concentration increases from the beginning of pregnancy. In humans, a proportion of the circulating active metabolite appears to be derived from maternal decidual cells, but increased 1,25-dihydroxyvitamin D synthesis by the mother's kidneys is not excluded. In addition, serum concentrations of vitamin D–binding protein increase during pregnancy.[108]

Cord concentrations of the major vitamin D metabolites are consistently lower than those measured in the mother's serum. Placental vein 25-hydroxyvitamin D concentrations correlate significantly with those found in the maternal circulation, suggesting that calcidiol easily diffuses across the placental barrier and that the vitamin D pool of the fetus depends entirely on that of the mother. The fetomaternal relations of 1,25-dihydroxyvitamin D concentrations are more complex, but a correlation between fetal and maternal concentrations was found in both full-term and preterm infants. Nevertheless, most of the 1,25-dihydroxyvitamin D in fetal plasma is due to fetal kidney activity, as suggested by studies in fetal plasma from infants with renal agenesis. Actually, the precise role of the placental 1,25-dihydroxyvitamin D activity in the mineral homeostasis during the fetal life needs to be evaluated.

In malnourished populations with vitamin D deficiency, osteomalacia in the mother and abnormal skeletal metabolism in the fetus and infant have been reported. Infants of severely malnourished mothers may be born with rickets and can suffer fractures during the neonatal period. Therefore, bone mass of the newborn may be related to the vitamin D status of the mother. Comparison of the results of DEXA from different countries shows that infant whole-body bone mineral content values are lower in countries in which milk products are not supplemented with vitamin D than in those in which milk products are supplemented. In contrast, vitamin D supplementation of malnourished mothers results in improved growth of the fetus and child in terms of both birthweight and subsequent linear growth during infancy. Moreover, maternal vitamin D status during pregnancy may have influence on the fetal skeletal development starting as early as 19 weeks' gestation[68] and can persist long after infancy. At the age of 9 years, children whose mothers had deficient or insufficient concentrations of 25-hydroxyvitamin D in late pregnancy had a reduced bone size and bone mineral content.[56]

It is worth mentioning that maternal vitamin D deficiency has been linked to other short- and long-term health problems in offspring, including type 1 diabetes and childhood asthma.[26,33,37] Moreover, it appears that vitamin D insufficiency during pregnancy is potentially associated with an increased risk for preeclampsia,[19] insulin resistance, and gestational diabetes mellitus,[29,65] primary cesarean delivery,[75] and bacterial vaginosis.[18]

Current guidelines recommend a vitamin D supplement of 200-400 IU/day during pregnancy, with increased doses of 1000 IU/day reserved for at-risk populations (particularly in the 3rd trimester). Future guidelines may suggest that doses of 2000-4000 IU/day for all pregnant women during the 2nd and 3rd trimester are safe and more effective in preventing complications associated with vitamin D deficiency in pregnancy.[56a]

NEONATAL VITAMIN D: FUNCTION AND RECOMMENDATIONS

Plasma 25(OH) D_3 concentration is a useful vitamin D biomarker reflecting vitamin D supply and use over a period of time. Unfortunately, the cutoff used for serum 25(OH) D_3 concentrations varies among researchers, leading to various prevalence of vitamin D deficiency or insufficiency. Nevertheless, several surveys show a high rate of poor maternal vitamin D status throughout the world, particularly in countries without vitamin D supplementation, with poor sun exposure, extensive clothing, or with deeply pigmented skin. Thus, the rate of cord blood vitamin D insufficiency (<20 nmol/L; <8.3 ng/mL) may reach up to 70% in European populations.[86]

The concentration of vitamin D is low in human milk (20 to 60 IU/L), and lower than that in regular formulas (400 to 600 IU/L). In breast-fed infants not receiving vitamin D supplements, vitamin D stores could be depleted within 8 weeks of delivery, suggesting the need for vitamin D supplementation.[45] A minimum daily intake of 400 IU (10 μg/day) of vitamin D is recommended by the American Academy of Pediatrics for all infants beginning soon

after birth, including those who are exclusively breastfed.[5] Moreover, in breast-fed full-term infants born to mothers who are vitamin D deficient, maternal supplementation with vitamin D could be required to increase the human milk vitamin D concentration and in turn improve infant vitamin D status. In addition, vitamin D is metabolized in the liver, and anticonvulsants such as phenobarbital and diphenylhydantoin increase its hepatic catabolism and requirements.

In preterm infants, as a result of the decrease in serum calcium during the first days of age, the postnatal surge in PTH induces increased synthesis of $1,25(OH)_2D_3$ during the first days day of life. Provision of 1000 IU of vitamin D_3 increases the 25-hydroxyvitamin D pool of the newborn at birth, followed by rapid renal synthesis of 1,25-dihydroxyvitamin D during the early postnatal days (Fig. 49-15). In infants with VLBW (<1500 g), immaturity of the vitamin D activation pathway, either alone or in combination with other abnormalities, particularly transient hypoparathyroidism, hypercalcitoninemia, and end-organ resistance to hormonal effects, may promote late neonatal hypocalcemia. However, after 28 weeks of gestation, activation of vitamin D is operative as early as 24 hours after birth. Vitamin D supplementation just after birth improves its nutritional status, as evidenced by rises in both plasma 1,25- and 25-hydroxyvitamin D concentrations.

In countries with high vitamin D status, plasma 25-hydroxyvitamin D remained normal for 6 months while infants received about 400 IU/day (<10 μg/day). By contrast, in France and other countries where dairy products are not enriched with vitamin D, sunshine exposure is restricted,[16] and mean cord concentrations of 25-hydroxyvitamin D are low, the administration of vitamin D (from 1000 IU/day, or 25 μg/day) resulted in a rapid increase in circulating concentrations of total 1,25-dihydroxyvitamin D by 5 days of age, promoting calcium absorption and mineral accretion rates during the neonatal period.[23,114] Therefore, vitamin D recommendations may differ significantly between North American (400 IU/day) and European (800 to 1000 IU/day) countries.[39]

REFERENCE VALUES

New information on the additional role of vitamin D on glucose homeostasis, immune system, cardiovascular disease, and cancer has resulted in defining vitamin D deficiency in adults as a 25-OH-D concentrations of <50 nmol/L and vitamin D insufficiency as a 25-OH-D concentration of 50 to

Figure 49-15. Mean (±SEM) serum total 25-hydroxyvitamin D [25(OH)D] and 1,25-dihydroxyvitamin D [1,25(OH)$_2$D] concentrations as a function of age in 15 preterm infants (birthweight, 1578 ± 78 g; gestational age, 31.7 ± 0.5 wk) who received 1000 IU/d of vitamin D (25 μg/d) from birth. Significantly different from cord serum: *P < .05, **P < .01, ***P < .001. (*From Salle BL, et al: Perinatal metabolism of vitamin D,* Am J Clin Nutr 71:1317S, 2000.)

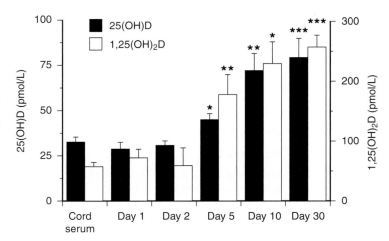

80 nmol/L. At the present time, however, consensus has not been reached with regard to the concentration of 25-OH-D to define vitamin D insufficiency for infants and children. Universal units of measure for 25-OH-D and 1,25-OH2-D are in nanomoles per liter (nmol/L). Conversion to nanogram per milliliter (ng/mL) is made by dividing the value expressed in nmol/L by 2.496. Thus, 80 nmol/L becomes 32 ng/mL.[5]

Calcitonin

SYNTHESIS AND METABOLISM

Calcitonin is a 32–amino acid peptide secreted by the thyroidal C cells, which also produce the calcitonin gene–related protein (CGRP). Calcitonin is also produced in other tissues, notably pituitary cells and other neuroendocrine cells in which calcitonin has a local paracrine effect but does not contribute to its peripheral effect. Both the *calcitonin/CGRP* and *PTH* genes are located on chromosome 11. The primary RNA transcript of the *calcitonin/CGRP* gene encodes two distinct peptides, calcitonin and calcitonin gene–related peptide-α (CGRPα). Cell-specific alternative RNA processing results in calcitonin being produced almost exclusively by the thyroidal C cell, and in CGRPα being produced throughout the central and peripheral nervous systems, acting as a vasodilator and a neuromodulator. The physiologic effects of CGRPα on bone are unclear.[49]

EFFECTS

The CaSR regulates serum calcium by suppressing the secretion of PTH; it also regulates renal tubular calcium excretion. It has recently been recognized that CaSR mRNA is also expressed by the C cells of the thyroid, the source of calcitonin. The CaSR has a dual physiologic response to acute increases in ionized calcium, which includes the inhibition of PTH release, the stimulation of calcitonin release, and the reverse effects in response to a decrease in calcium.[42]

The effects of calcitonin are independent of PTH and vitamin D action. Both ends of the molecule contain species-invariant residues that are required for its binding to receptors coupled with high-affinity G proteins on the osteoclast. Calcitonin inhibits extracellular Ca^{2+} sensing, a potent antiresorptive signal, and by implication, calcitonin withdrawal should enhance Ca^{2+} sensing and limit resorption. The principal effect of calcitonin is to decrease osteoclastic bone resorption and the amount of calcium and phosphorus released from bone. Additionally, calcitonin increases calcium and phosphorus excretion, so the overall effect of calcitonin is to decrease serum calcium and phosphorus concentrations. With regard to magnesium, calcitonin may decrease both its release from bone and renal tubular reabsorption. In humans, serum calcitonin rises during pregnancy, growth, and lactation. It is during these periods of calcium stress that a tonic antiresorptive hormone will best exert its effects to limit skeletal loss and promote mineral accretion. An additional effect of calcitonin is its stabilizing effect on bone microarchitecture, which precedes the changes in bone mineral density observed in its therapeutic use for Paget disease, hypercalcemia of malignancy, and osteogenesis imperfecta. Calcitonin has a very short half-life and is cleared mainly by the kidney. In general, however,

the precise physiologic role of calcitonin in humans is still not well understood.[124]

REGULATION OF SECRETION

Secretion of calcitonin varies with acute changes in serum calcium concentrations: it increases when serum calcium increases and decreases when serum calcium falls. Under usual circumstances, calcitonin is secreted only when serum calcium reaches about 2.37 mmol/L (9.5 mg/dL). When serum calcium exceeds such concentrations, serum calcitonin and calcium concentrations are directly correlated. The calcitonin response to chronic changes in calcium is still controversial.

FETAL CALCITONIN FUNCTION

The role of calcitonin in fetal mineral metabolism has not been extensively examined. Calcitonin is expressed by human thyroidal C cells early in gestation, and it circulates in fetal blood at levels that are higher than those in the mother. In animal studies, the pharmacologic administration of calcitonin or calcitonin antiserum altered the serum calcium of fetal rats in predictable and opposite directions. However, fetal thyroidectomy with subsequent thyroxine replacement did not appear to affect fetal blood calcium, indicating that the physiologic amounts of calcitonin derived from the fetal thyroid may not be required to maintain normal serum calcium. In a study using a *calcitonin/CGRP* gene knockout model in mice, McDonald and colleagues[74] suggested that calcitonin and CGRP are not needed for normal fetal calcium metabolism—they may instead regulate some aspects of fetal magnesium metabolism. In human pregnancy, calcitonin concentrations are elevated in the fetus presumably because of the high fetal serum calcium concentrations, but the contributions of calcitonin to normal skeletal growth and reduced bone remodeling during fetal life have not been demonstrated.

NEONATAL CALCITONIN FUNCTION

At birth, serum calcitonin concentrations are higher in cord blood than maternal blood, and they increase further in the first 24 hours of life. Serum calcitonin may be higher in preterm than full-term infants and higher in hypocalcemic preterm infants than normocalcemic ones. Serum calcitonin is also higher in asphyxiated than nonasphyxiated, full-term infants. The physiologic importance of the postnatal increase of calcitonin is unclear. On the one hand, it may protect the skeleton from excessive bone resorption; on the other hand, it may contribute to neonatal hypocalcemia in some infants. It is uncertain whether calcitonin plays a specific role in neonatal hypocalcemia. Excess calcitonin would not explain the hyperphosphatemia commonly associated with neonatal hypocalcemia.

BONE DEVELOPMENT

Ontogenesis

The perinatal development of bone occurs through two separate but interrelated processes: intramembranous and endochondral.[98] In both mechanisms, bone is made in a precursor area occupied by fibrous mesenchyme or in an area of cartilaginous tissue. Intramembranous bone is the first to begin ossification. It does not have cartilaginous precursors, occurring largely in the bone of the skull, maxilla, and mandible, and results in mesenchymal cell differentiation to produce preosteoblasts and then osteoblasts, with the subsequent formation of an organic bone matrix (osteoid). The elaborated bony trabeculae then fuse to form the primary spongiosa. Osteoblasts cover the surface of the spongiosa and deposit new layers of the bone matrix while new bone is being removed from other surfaces by a special group of multinucleated phagocytic cells called *osteoclasts*. During development, the structure of the fibrous mesenchyme is continuously formed, allowing growth, whereas the osteoblastic and osteoclastic activities induce a remodeling process, with the net result of membranous bone formation and mineral deposition.

In contrast, all bones of the appendicular and axial skeleton grow by the transformation of growth plate cartilage into bone through a series of cell and matrix changes referred to as *endochondral ossification*. During development, the cartilaginous template increases in size by appositional and interstitial chondrocyte growth and by the continuous synthesis of a hyaline matrix. As the cartilage model continues to grow, the central chondrocytes hypertrophy and increase their cellular volumes. Calcium salts begin to precipitate in the matrix partitions separating the hypertrophic cells, and capillary buds penetrate the perichondrium and begin to invade the hypertrophic cell area. Osteoblasts appear in the wake of the capillary invasion and begin to lay down a thin collar of osteoid around the midsection of the cartilage model. Therefore, a medullary cavity is formed in the area that will become the midshaft of the long bone, establishing the first center of ossification. The perichondrium is called the *periosteum*. In this vascularized environment, the osteoblasts deposit layers of osteoid on the residual calcified cartilage, and bone tissue gradually replaces the formerly solid mass of cartilage. The cartilage, which is left at either end of the bone, forms the growth plate, permitting longitudinal growth of the bone. At the distal (epiphyseal) end of the growth plate the chondrocytes proliferate, lengthening the bone. Proximal to these cells, the cartilage becomes calcified. The calcified cartilage is partially resorbed by osteoclasts and subsequently replaced by woven bone. There is further remodeling in which woven bone is progressively replaced with lamellar bone. For long bone, the key features of its formation include the development of the primary ossification site, the appearance of a tubular diaphysis and marrow cavity, the location and geometry of the growth plate, and finally the appearance and location of the secondary ossification center, which develops mostly after term in the human neonate.

Detailed qualitative descriptions of metaphyseal bone histology during early development have been available for decades. More recently, histomorphometric data from femoral metaphyses in a group of 35 fetuses and newborns with gestational ages ranging from 16 to 41 weeks established morphometric reference data and provided the opportunity to gain insight into long-bone growth in humans. Despite a rapid rate of net bone gain, osteoid indexes were relatively low, indicating that mineralization occurred very rapidly after bone deposition and then suggesting that modeling, not remodeling, is the predominant mechanism responsible for the development of femoral metaphyseal cancellous bone in utero.[107] Therefore, during fetal life, various environmental factors are specifically oriented to promote growth, high mineral transfer, and increases in the physical mineral density of the skeleton.

Factors Affecting Growth and Mineralization

During gestation, the fetus receives an ample provision of nutritional supply through the placenta. Nitrogen, energy, minerals, and vitamins allow a high velocity of body length growth, representing about 1.2 cm per week during the last trimester of gestation. The fetus maintains its hypercalcemic state in a high calcitonin and estrogen environment, promoting the modeling-to-remodeling ratio in favor of modeling and thus increasing endocortical bone. In addition, according to the mechanostat theory of bone development, fetal bone is also driven by the mechanical force applied to the fetal skeleton during the intrauterine resistance training provided by regular fetal kicks against the uterine wall.[93,94] Consequently, at term, the newborn skeleton has a high physical density (bone mass divided by bone volume), with elevated cortical thickness and relatively small marrow cavities.

Various factors influence the processes of growth, mineralization, and bone structure. Growth is directly related to protein and energy supplies but also to the hormonal environment comprising insulin, IGF-1, and IGF-2, among others. Bone formation, mineralization, and structure are related to mineral supply and hormonal factors such as PTH, recombinant PTH, vitamin D, and calcitonin, as well as others, such as genetics and physical activity. Several factors have been found to have a significant impact on newborn bone mineral content and developing fetal bone.[81] Reduced calcium supply, vitamin D deficiency, ethanol consumption, and smoking during pregnancy are all factors affecting fetal skeletal development in addition to low weight related to gestation and diabetes in the mother.

Evaluation of Fetal Mineral Accretion

From cadaver analysis, the whole-body calcium accretion rate and bone composition have been determined and histomorphometric evaluation performed. At present, about 163 whole-body carcass analyses have been performed in deceased fetuses and newborn infants, allowing the estimation of intrauterine whole-body composition and the calculation of weight gain composition.[118] From these studies, it appears that in preterm and term infants who are appropriate for gestational age, whole-body calcium accretion was exponentially related to gestational age and linearly related to body weight. Similar values have been obtained with the use of neutron activation techniques.[36]

DEXA is becoming the most accurate and precise noninvasive technique for assessing bone mineralization in vivo. Validation of its use in subjects with low body mass has supported its increasing use in preterm and term infants.[118] After this validation study, normative data for bone mineral content (BMC) and projected bone area in 106 healthy preterm and term infants near birth were established to get reference intrauterine values (Fig. 49-16). BMC and bone area were positively related to body weight, body length, and gestational age.

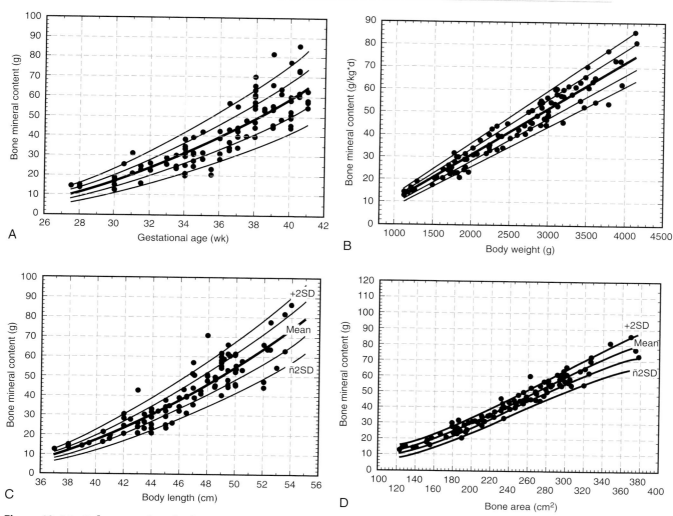

Figure 49–16. Reference values for bone mineral content related to gestational age (**A**), body weight (**B**), body length (**C**), and projected bone area (**D**) determined at birth in preterm and term infants (*n* = 106). *(From Rigo J, et al: Reference values of body composition obtained by dual energy X-ray absorptiometry in preterm and term neonates,* J Pediatr Gastroenterol Nutr *27:184, 1998.)*

However, in multivariate analysis, body weight was the major and also the only predictor of those parameters. The conversion equation for BMC to calcium allowed the calcium content to be compared with the data obtained from carcass analysis or with neutron activation analysis.[96] The perfect agreement between the in vivo calcium estimations and reference values suggests that the translation equation calculated in newborn piglets may be applied to newborn infants scanned with identical equipment soon after birth. However, the validity of the conversion of BMC to calcium content after the first few days of life was not confirmed in view of the major changes in bone growth and mineral deposition that occur after birth. Normative data for preterm and term infants are extremely limited and the results frequently difficult to compare because of the different equipment and software used.[46,60,88,107]

Isolated femurs obtained from human fetuses and newborn infants deceased near birth have been analyzed for chemical composition[34] and histomorphometric evaluation.[44,108] From those studies, it appears that the ratios of calcium to nitrogen and the mineralized bone volume to the total (mineralized and nonmineralized) femoral volume increase progressively during the second part of gestation. These and other data[96] suggest that during the last trimester of gestation, there is disproportionate mineral accretion. The ratio of mineralized to total bone volume increases continuously, leading to a progressive change in volumetric bone mineral density.

Quantitative ultrasound (QUS) has been proposed as a diagnostic tool to evaluate bone mineralization in newborn infants. It measures the speed of sound (SOS) propagation through the bone, which reflects, in addition to bone density, other bone properties such as cortical thickness, elasticity, and microstructure, thus providing more a complete picture of the bone strength. QUS has the advantage of being nonionizing, inexpensive, and portable. However, the values of SOS can be influenced by the operator's experience, humidity, and

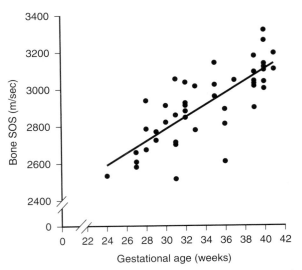

Figure 49–17. Cross-sectional relationship between tibial speed of sound (SOS) and gestational age (r = 0.78, P < .0005). *(From Nemet D, et al: Quantitative ultrasound measurements of bone speed of sound in premature infants,* Eur J Pediatr *160:736, 2001.)*

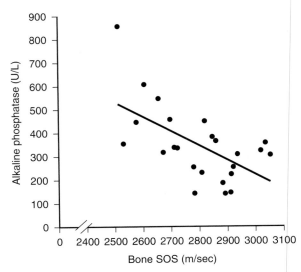

Figure 49–18. Cross-sectional relationship between tibial speed of sound (SOS) and serum alkaline phosphatase in premature infants (r = −0.59, P < .005). *(From Nemet D, et al: Quantitative ultrasound measurements of bone speed of sound in premature infants,* Eur J Pediatr *160:736, 2001).*

temperature. At birth, there is a significant correlation between tibial SOS values and gestational age (Fig. 49-17), birthweight, and birth length. The SOS values are significantly lower in preterm infants at birth compared with term infants and appear to fall when measured longitudinally in preterm infants. This indicates less mineral content in preterm infants than in term infants. The correlation between SOS values and biochemical markers of osteopenia of prematurity is controversial. Although some studies showed an inverse relation between alkaline phosphatase and SOS values (Fig. 49-18),[8,82] others failed to show this relationship.[72] QUS has potential use to assess bone health in the newborn, but it is not widely available, nor has it gained traction in clinical use.

Physiologic Skeletal Changes in the Early Postnatal Period

TERM INFANTS

At birth, there is an abrupt interruption of the nutrient supply from the mother through the placenta, and nutritional support is progressively provided by the gastrointestinal route. As a result, the relatively hypercalcemic fetus becomes a relatively hypocalcemic newborn, inducing a stimulation of PTH secretion. Therefore, there is a large reduction in calcium availability for bone mineralization compared with the prenatal situation. Indeed, in normal term infants fed human milk or a regular term formula, the calcium retention falls dramatically from 100 mg/kg per day to 20 to 30 mg/kg per day, whereas the growth rate remains relatively similar and close to 30 g/day. The hormonal environment changes postnatally because the placental supply of estrogen and many other hormones has been cut off. In addition, mechanical

stimulation is likely to be lower postnatally. The infant's movements typically occur without much resistance, thus putting smaller loads on the skeleton.[76,93,94] Therefore, there is a need for postnatal adaptation of the skeleton, and some of the factors implied in the fetal modeling-to-remodeling ratio disappear, inducing an increase in endosteal bone resorption. The physical density of long bones such as the femoral diaphysis decreases by about 30% during the first 6 months of life. This change is mostly the result of an increase in marrow cavity size, which is faster than the increase in the cross-sectional area of the bone cortex.

In term infants, these postnatal changes have been classically called *physiologic osteoporosis of infancy*, but they appear to occur without an increase in bone fragility. This phenomenon is well illustrated by the evolution of bone mineral apparent density (BMAD, g/cm^3) during fetal life, in which there is a continuous increase that contrasts with that obtained from birth to the first months of life, at which time a rapid reduction in BMAD is observed (Fig. 49-19).

INFANTS WITH VERY LOW BIRTH WEIGHT

The goal of feeding regimens for infants with VLBW is to obtain a prompt postnatal resumption of growth to a rate approximating intrauterine growth (see Chapter 35). In practice, at birth there is an abrupt interruption of the nutrient supply from the mother through the placenta, and the nutritional support needs to be provided by parenteral and enteral routes. From preterm to term birth, the mineral supplies are far from those provided during fetal life, whereas length and skeletal growth remain relatively high. In addition, postnatal adaptations of the skeletal system to extrauterine conditions also occur in premature infants, with the difference being that they take place earlier than they do in term babies.[98] The process of birth interrupts active fetal bone mineralization and,

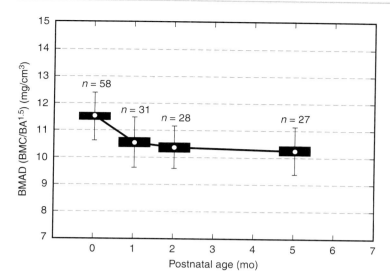

Figure 49–19. Change in bone mineral apparent density (BMAD) according to postnatal age in healthy term infants ($n = 144$). BMC, bone mineral content; BA, bone area.

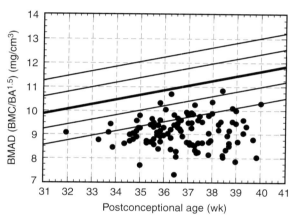

Figure 49–20. Comparison between bone mineral apparent density (BMAD) at discharge in infants with very low birthweight (•, $n = 108$) and reference values (regression lines, $n = 106$). BMC, bone mineral content; BA, bone area.

combined with the reduction in calcium availability, contributes to a reduction in bone physical density. These postnatal changes have been classically called *preterm osteopenia*, but contrary to those observed in term infants, these changes can be accompanied by an increase in bone fragility and the risk for fracture. In this situation, there is a sharp postnatal decrease in BMAD during the early postnatal weeks of life up to discharge near term (Fig. 49-20). The mechanisms of postnatal adaptation of the skeleton are not entirely clear, but it is probably of questionable benefit to require identical mineral supplies and retention in a fetus and preterm infant at similar postconceptional ages. Therefore, because of the difference between intrauterine and extrauterine conditions, the care of premature infants should not require the determination of intrauterine calcium accretion rates. Indeed, in the long run, the skeletons of these infants will adapt to the remodeling stimulation and the mechanical requirements, two factors that could reduce the nutritional requirements for calcium.

CLINICAL CONDITIONS ASSOCIATED WITH CALCIUM DISTURBANCES

Neonatal Hypocalcemia

Neonatal hypocalcemia has been variously defined as a calcium level of less than 2 mmol/L (1 mmol/L = 4 mg/dL), less than 1.87 mmol/L, or less than 1.75 mmol/L. This variance in definition is at least partially due to the lack of clinical signs in many neonates, even at a very low serum total calcium concentration.

A better definition of neonatal hypocalcemia would be based on the metabolically active component of calcium, ionized calcium, because changes in ionized calcium concentration are more likely to have physiologic significance. Under conditions of normal acid-base status and normal albumin levels, the serum total calcium level and Ca^{2+} are linearly correlated, so total serum calcium measurements remain useful as a screening test. However, because Ca^{2+} is the physiologically relevant fraction, in sick infants, it is preferable to directly determine Ca^{2+} in freshly obtained blood samples (see Appendix B).

Neonates at the greatest risk for symptomatic or asymptomatic neonatal hypocalcemia, such as the infants of diabetic mothers or preterm or asphyxiated neonates, are frequently sick for a multitude of reasons, and the contribution of neonatal hypocalcemia to signs related to their primary illness can be easily obscured. From a clinical viewpoint, because Ca^{2+} concentrations are maintained within narrow ranges under normal circumstances, the potential risk for disturbances of physiologic function increases as the Ca^{2+} concentration decreases. A useful approach to the classification of neonatal hypocalcemia is by time of onset. The early and late forms of hypocalcemia have different causes and occur in different clinical settings.

EARLY HYPOCALCEMIA

Refer to Boxes 49-5 and 49-6.

Term Infants

Early neonatal hypocalcemia occurs during the first 4 days of life and represents an exaggeration of the normal fall in serum calcium concentration that occurs during the first 24 to

---

BOX 49–5 Causes of Neonatal Hypocalcemia

EARLY HYPOCALCEMIA (1-4 DAYS OF AGE)
Prematurity
Maternal diabetes
Perinatal stress, asphyxia
Intrauterine growth restriction
Maternal anticonvulsants

LATE HYPOCALCEMIA (5-10 DAYS OF AGE)
Hyperphosphatemia (high phosphate load, advanced renal insufficiency)
Hypomagnesemia
Vitamin D deficiency
Parathyroid hormone resistance (transient neonatal pseudohypoparathyroidism)
Hypoparathyroidism
Primary: parathyroid agenesis, 22q11 deletion, parathyroid hormone gene mutation
Secondary: maternal hyperparathyroidism
Calcium-sensing receptor defects, autosomal dominant hypocalcemic hypercalciuria
Acquired or inherited disorders of vitamin D metabolism
Neonatal hypocalcemia associated with skeletal dysplasia
Other causes (alkalosis, citrated blood transfusions, phototherapy, viral gastroenteritis, lipid infusions)

BOX 49–6 Diagnostic Steps for Hypocalcemia

HISTORY
Family
Pregnancy (diabetes mellitus, hyperparathyroidism, intrapartum events, fetal distress, asphyxia)
Nutritional supplies of the newborn infant

PHYSICAL EXAMINATION
Jitteriness, apnea, cyanosis
Seizures
Associated features (prematurity, dysmorphism, congenital heart defect)

INVESTIGATIONS
Total serum and ionized calcium, magnesium, phosphorus, glucose
Acid-base balance
Chest radiograph (e.g., thymic shadow, aortic arch position)
Urinary calcium, magnesium, phosphorus, creatinine, drug screen
Vitamin D metabolites
Parathyroid hormone
Calcitonin
Others (e.g., malabsorption, lymphocyte count, T-cell numbers and function, maternal and family screening, molecular genetic studies)
Genetic studies for 22q11 deletion

---

48 hours of life. At birth, there is an interruption of maternal calcium supply, and the serum calcium concentration in infants is maintained by either the increased calcium flux from bone or sufficient exogenous calcium intake. Trabecular bone, which is richly vascularized, represents the main source of potentially rapidly mobilized calcium. Because intestinal calcium absorption is correlated with intake and dietary calcium is usually low on the first day of life, the serum calcium concentration decreases on the first day of life.[55,104]

Normal serum concentrations for Ca^{2+} in full-term newborns reach a nadir at about 24 hours of age (1.10 to 1.36 mmol/L, or 4.4 to 5.4 mg/dL) and rise slowly thereafter. In full-term infants, hypocalcemia can be best defined as an ionized calcium concentration of less than 1.10 mmol/L (4.4 mg/dL), which is the standard nadir in normal infants. This concentration represents 2 standard deviations below the mean at 24 hours. This definition is a statistical one and is based on assumptions of normal distributions of physiologic variables. Further investigation needs to define physiologically important limits for term and preterm neonates. If an ionized calcium measurement is not available, the traditional definition—a total serum calcium concentration of less than 2.0 mmol/L (8.0 mg/dL)—can be used. Characteristically, early neonatal hypocalcemia occurs most frequently in preterm infants, asphyxiated infants, infants of diabetic mothers, and those with significant IUGR, and infants of mothers treated with anticonvulsants during pregnancy.

In preterm infants, the reference values for ionized calcium are available only for large, moderately premature infants who show values very similar to those for full-term infants. These cutoff values might not apply to smaller infants, given insufficient physiologic data on ionized calcium. At present, the traditional cutoff point, a total calcium content of less than 1.75 mmol/L (7.0 mg/dL), remains reasonable in infants with VLBW.

Preterm Infants

The frequency of hypocalcemia varies inversely with birthweight and gestational age. In preterm infants, the postnatal decrease in the serum calcium level typically occurs more rapidly than it does in term infants, the magnitude of the depression being inversely proportional to gestation. Many infants with low birthweight and nearly all those with extremely low birthweight (ELBW) exhibit total calcium levels of less than 7.0 mg/dL by day 2. However, the fall in Ca^{2+} is not proportional to that in total calcium concentration, and the ratio of ionized to total calcium is higher in these infants. The reason for the maintenance of Ca^{2+} is uncertain but is probably related to low serum protein concentration and pH associated with prematurity. The sparing effvect of Ca^{2+} may partially explain the frequent lack of signs in preterm infants with low total calcium levels.

Early neonatal hypocalcemia apparently results from the abrupt interruption of the placental supply and the low intake provided by oral and parenteral nutrition and also by the insufficient release of PTH by immature parathyroid glands or the inadequate responsiveness of the renal tubular cells to PTH. An exaggerated rise in calcitonin secretion in premature infants may play a contributory role.[55] In infants with VLBW, the high renal sodium excretion probably aggravates calciuric losses, and relative end-organ resistance to $1,25(OH)_2D_3$ may exist.

Hypocalcemia is temporary, and the serum calcium concentration gradually reverts to normal after 1 to 3 days. Factors contributing to serum calcium normalization include increased calcium intake with feedings, increased renal phosphorus excretion, and improved parathyroid function. Calcium supplementation may hasten the restorative process.

Maternal Diabetes

See Chapter 16.

Infants of diabetic mothers (IDMs) demonstrate an exaggerated postnatal drop in circulating calcium levels compared with controls of gestational age. Prematurity and birth asphyxia are frequently associated problems that independently increase the risk for hypocalcemia. In IDMs, hypocalcemia appears to be related to hypomagnesemia, the maternal form of which is caused by urinary magnesium losses with diabetes and leads to fetal magnesium deficiency and secondary functional hypoparathyroidism in the fetus and newborn. Hypocalcemia in IDMs is also correlated with the severity of maternal diabetes, which is classified by White's criteria. The natural history is usually similar to that of early neonatal hypocalcemia in preterm infants, but hypocalcemia sometimes persists for several additional days. Improved metabolic control for pregnant diabetic women has markedly diminished the occurrence and severity of early neonatal hypocalcemia in IDMs. The incidence of hypocalcemia is also increased in the infants of gestational diabetic mothers, and the role of hypomagnesemia has been demonstrated.[14]

Perinatal Asphyxia

In asphyxiated infants, the following factors may contribute to early hypocalcemia: a decreased calcium intake due to delayed feedings, an increased endogenous phosphorus load resulting from the reduction of the glomerular filtration rate, and an increased serum calcitonin concentration. Hyperphosphatemia may induce relative PTH resistance. Theoretically, the correction of acidosis with alkali may further aggravate hypocalcemia by inducing decreased calcium flux from bone to the extracellular fluid and by lowering the ionized calcium concentration.

Maternal Anticonvulsants

Anticonvulsants such as phenobarbital and diphenylhydantoin increase the hepatic catabolism of vitamin D and predispose to vitamin D deficiency in the absence of its appropriate supplementation. The infants of epileptic mothers may be at an increased risk for neonatal hypocalcemia. This complication can be prevented by maternal vitamin D supplementation (1000 IU/day) during pregnancy.

LATE HYPOCALCEMIA

Hypocalcemia is conventionally defined as late when it occurs after the first 4 days of life. Late neonatal hypocalcemia usually develops at about 1 week of age (see Box 49-5) and more frequently in term than preterm infants, and it is not correlated with maternal diabetes, birth trauma, or asphyxia. In some instances, the clinical distinction between early and late hypocalcemia may not be clear.

Phosphate Loading

Hypocalcemia induced by an elevated phosphorus supply usually occurs at the end of the first week of life. Late-onset hypocalcemia is considered to be a manifestation of relative resistance of the immature kidney to PTH. In these infants, the renal tubular cells are unable to respond appropriately to PTH, leading to renal retention of phosphorus and hypocalcemia. These biochemical features strongly resemble those of pseudohypoparathyroidism.[55,64,113] The normally low neonatal GFR may also play a role in limiting the ability to excrete the phosphorus load. Late hypocalcemia was frequently observed in infants fed cow's milk or evaporated milk because of their high phosphorus content. With the introduction of adapted infant formulas, late hypocalcemia, although not abolished, has become uncommon. However, even with current formulas, the formula-fed infants have lower serum ionized calcium and higher serum phosphorus in the first week of life than breast-fed infants. These differences correlate with the absolute phosphorus amount but not with the different calcium-to-phosphorus ratios in formulas. The phosphate load increases calcium bone deposition, leading to hypocalcemia. The normal response to hypocalcemia is an increase in PTH secretion, inducing an increase in both the urinary excretion of phosphate and the tubular resorption of calcium. The pathogenesis of this "transient hypoparathyroidism" in late neonatal hypocalcemia is poorly understood. The inadequate secretion of PTH, immaturity of PTH receptors, or transient change in the threshold of CaSR may play an important role.[120] Serum calcium levels frequently increase when these infants are given human milk, lower-phosphate formulas, and calcium supplements. After several days to weeks, serum PTH usually increases, and the infants are able to tolerate a higher dietary phosphate load. Some of these infants have a persistent or recurrent inability to mount an adequate PTH response to a hypocalcemic challenge and may have a form of congenital hypoparathyroidism.

Hypomagnesemia

Neonatal hypocalcemia usually accompanies hypomagnesemia because magnesium deficiency inhibits the secretion of PTH and reduces responsiveness to its action. Depression of the serum magnesium levels in newborns is due to primary hypomagnesemia with secondary hypocalcemia or transient hypomagnesemia.[55,104]

Primary hypomagnesemia with secondary hypocalcemia presents in infancy with persistent hypocalcemia and seizures that cannot be controlled with anticonvulsants or calcium gluconate. It is a rare autosomal recessive disorder resulting from primary defects in the intestinal transport of magnesium. The gene has been segregated to chromosome 9.[30] Serum magnesium is frequently less than 0.8 mg/dL (normally, 1.6 to 2.8 mg/dL), and circulating levels of PTH are low despite the presence of hypocalcemia. The administration of magnesium to these infants leads to spontaneous parallel increases in serum PTH levels, serum calcium levels, and renal phosphate clearance.

Transient neonatal hypomagnesemia often occurs in association with hypocalcemia. The decrease in the serum magnesium level is usually less severe (0.8 to 1.4 mg/dL) than that in magnesium transport defects. In many infants with transient hypomagnesemia, the serum magnesium level increases spontaneously as the serum calcium level returns to normal after the administration of calcium supplements.

Transient hypomagnesemia secondary to renal magnesium wasting can be caused by the administration of loop diuretics, aminoglycosides, amphotericin B, urinary tract obstruction, or the diuretic phase of acute renal failure. The disorder may be mistaken for a form of neonatal hypoparathyroidism because of tetany and hypocalcemia or confused with Bartter syndrome (hypokalemic alkalosis with hypercalciuria) because of secondary potassium wasting. The diagnosis can be made by finding low serum magnesium levels with inappropriately high urinary magnesium excretion. A common laboratory feature of magnesium depletion is hypokalemia. Attempts to restore the potassium deficit with potassium therapy alone are usually not successful without simultaneous magnesium therapy.

Neonatal Hypoparathyroidism

The biochemical characteristics of hypoparathyroidism are hypocalcemia and hyperphosphatemia in the presence of normal renal function. Serum PTH concentrations are low or undetectable. The causes of hypoparathyroidism are diverse, representing disruptions of one or more of the steps in the development and maintenance of PTH secretion.[70]

SECONDARY HYPOPARATHYROIDISM RELATED TO MATERNAL DISEASES

This transient condition may occur in the offspring of mothers with hyperparathyroidism or hypercalcemia from any cause. Maternal history may not be contributory because the maternal disease (usually a benign adenoma) may be asymptomatic and discovered only after the diagnosis is made in the newborn. Maternal hypercalcemia leads to fetal hypercalcemia and secondary fetal hypoparathyroidism. This condition resolves spontaneously in days to weeks, and supportive therapy with calcium, $1,25(OH)_2D_3$, or both usually suffices, but it may be temporally exacerbated by the feeding of high-phosphate diets.

DEVELOPMENTAL DEFECTS IN THE PARATHYROID GLANDS

The isolated absence of parathyroid gland development may be inherited in an X-linked or autosomal recessive fashion. The most well described example is DiGeorge syndrome (and the closely related velocardiofacial syndrome). Manifestations of these syndromes include incomplete development in the branchial arches, resulting in varying degrees of parathyroid and thymic hypoplasia; conotruncal cardiac defects; facial malformations; and learning disabilities. Both syndromes are associated with rearrangements and microdeletions affecting an unknown gene or genes on the short arm of chromosome 22q11. The constellation of abnormalities in DiGeorge syndrome has been referred to as CATCH 22 (cardiac defects, abnormal facies, thymic hypoplasia, cleft palate, hypocalcemia). The presence of hypocalcemia with congenital abnormalities should prompt detailed genetic analysis, but it should be remembered that the calcium content may return to a normal level spontaneously (transient congenital hypoparathyroidism).

Isolated agenesis of the parathyroid glands in one family has been attributed to a recessive deletion in the gene on chromosome 6 that normally encodes a transcription factor.[70]

DEFECTS IN THE PARATHYROID HORMONE MOLECULE

A few cases of familial hypoparathyroidism have been described in which the cause was a mutation in the gene for PTH that resulted in the synthesis of a defective PTH molecule and undetectable amounts of PTH in serum.

DEFECTIVE REGULATION OF PARATHYROID HORMONE SECRETION

Hypocalcemia and hypercalciuria are the chief features of autosomal dominant hypercalciuric hypocalcemia, which is caused by activating mutations of the parathyroid and renal CaSR. These mutations cause excessive calcium-induced inhibition of PTH secretion. Hypocalcemia is usually mild and asymptomatic. When it is mild, it should be treated cautiously, if at all, because raising serum calcium concentrations further increase urinary calcium excretion and may cause nephrocalcinosis.[87]

Hypocalcemia Resulting from Vitamin D Disorder

Maternal vitamin D deficiency is the major risk for neonatal vitamin D deficiency presenting as hypocalcemia. Vitamin D deficiency is unusual in countries in which it is common practice to supplement the diet with vitamin D dairy products and other foods. However, it occurs in women in whom both sunlight exposure and the dietary intake of vitamin D are inadequate. At high risk are immigrants from the Middle East or South Asia who continue to wear traditional clothing. Therefore, if daily vitamin D supplementation during the duration of pregnancy can be undertaken, the amount given should be 400 IU/day (10 μg/day). In countries in which dairy products are not supplemented with vitamin D and sunshine exposure is low (e.g., in northern countries), or when presentation for antenatal care is delayed, 1000 IU/day (25 μg/day) should be given during the last 3 months of pregnancy, or 100,000 IU (2500 μg/day) in one dose at the beginning of the last trimester.[107] Breast-fed infants of strictly vegetarian mothers are also susceptible to early-onset hypocalcemic rickets. Daily supplementation of 400 IU for infants and 800 IU for pregnant and lactating women is considered sufficient to prevent neonatal rickets. The vitamin D requirements of preterm infants are influenced by body stores at birth, which in turn are related to the length of gestation and maternal stores. These factors should be taken into consideration when vitamin D supplementation policies are developed in each country. A daily dose of vitamin D of 400 IU (10 μg), independent of that contained in low-birthweight formulas, appears satisfactory in the United States. In contrast, a daily dose of vitamin D of 1000 IU (25 μg) has been recommended in the European Union, as in countries with poor maternal stores.[107]

Infantile Osteopetrosis

Autosomal recessive ("malignant") osteopetrosis is a rare congenital disorder related to bone resorption abnormalities that may be fatal without hematopoietic stem cell transplantation. It is believed to arise as a result of the failure of osteoclasts to resorb immature bone, which leads to abnormal bone marrow cavity formation and to the clinical signs and symptoms of bone marrow failure. Impaired bone remodeling associated with the dysregulated activity of osteoclasts for such a condition may cause bony narrowing of the cranial nerve foramina, which in turn typically results in cranial nerve (especially optic nerve) compression. Abnormal remodeling of primary woven bone to lamellar bone results in brittle bone that is prone to fracture. Therefore, fractures, visual impairment, and bone marrow failure are the classic features of this disease.[28] Mutations in the *ATP6i* (*TCIRG1*) gene, encoding the α_3 subunit of the vacuolar proton pump, which mediates the acidification of the bone-osteoclast interface, are implicated in about 50% of the patients affected by this disease.[117] Osteopetrosis can present as late neonatal hypocalcemia (mean age at presentation, 12 days) and is diagnosed easily from its typical radiographic features.

Other Causes of Neonatal Hypocalcemia

Bicarbonate therapy, as well as any form of metabolic or respiratory alkalosis, decreases ionized calcium levels and bone resorption of calcium. Transfusion and plasmapheresis with citrated blood can form nonionized calcium complexes, thus decreasing Ca^{2+}. Furosemide and xanthine therapy promotes calciuresis as well as nephrolithiasis. Phototherapy appears to be an additional possible cause of neonatal hypocalcemia, although the mechanism is still uncertain. Lipid infusions may increase serum free fatty acid levels, which form insoluble complexes with calcium. Most of these effects are transient, and cessation of therapy is associated with a return to normal serum calcium levels.

CLINICAL MANIFESTATIONS OF HYPOCALCEMIA

The clinical manifestations of neonatal hypocalcemia in infants may be easily confused with other neonatal disorders (e.g., hypoglycemia, sepsis, meningitis, asphyxia, intracranial bleeding, narcotic withdrawal). The neonate with hypocalcemia may be asymptomatic; the less mature the infant, the more subtle and varied the clinical manifestations. In the neonatal period, the main clinical signs of hypocalcemia are jitteriness (increased neuromuscular irritability and activity) and generalized convulsions, although focal seizures have also been reported. Infants may also be lethargic, eat poorly, vomit, and have abdominal distention. The degree of irritability does not appear to correlate with serum calcium values. Furthermore, hypocalcemia may be asymptomatic. Therefore, suspicion of hypocalcemia should be confirmed by the measurement of total serum calcium and Ca^{2+}. The diagnostic workup for hypocalcemia (see Box 49-6) includes a history, physical examination, and relevant investigations. In clinical practice, the diagnosis of hypocalcemia is based on the determination of ionized or total calcium. Serum magnesium should also be measured because hypomagnesemia may coexist and cause identical signs. The measurement of calcium-regulating hormones is not routinely recommended unless hypocalcemia is prolonged, refractory, or recurrent. Chest radiographic examination for a thymic silhouette is indicated if DiGeorge syndrome is suspected. The measurement of electrocardiographic QT intervals, corrected for heart rate, is also of little value for the prediction of neonatal hypocalcemia. Assays of calciotropic hormones and 25(OH)D may be useful in the diagnosis of uncommon causes of neonatal hypocalcemia, such as primary hypoparathyroidism, malabsorption, and disorders of vitamin D metabolism. Molecular genetic studies may be needed to confirm a specific diagnosis and have potentially important clinical relevance for the patient's clinical

outcome. Other investigations, which are listed in Box 49-6, may be important in the differential diagnosis and understanding of the pathophysiology of hypocalcemia

TREATMENT

Early Neonatal Hypocalcemia

The choice of treatment for early neonatal hypocalcemia is complicated by several factors, among them that (1) the condition may coexist with other neonatal complications (e.g., asphyxia, hypoglycemia) that cause similar signs; (2) it may be associated with seizures, which may have a different etiology; and (3) it may remain asymptomatic and in most newborns is a self-limited disorder.

SYMPTOMATIC HYPOCALCEMIA

The treatment of symptomatic hypocalcemia consists of the administration of calcium salts. Calcium gluconate is preferred over calcium chloride, which can cause metabolic acidosis. A 10% solution contains about 9.4 mg of elemental Ca per milliliter. In case of seizures, 2 mL/kg of calcium gluconate (about 18 mg/kg of elemental calcium) is given intravenously over 10 minutes, accompanied by heart rate monitoring. The infusion should be temporarily discontinued if bradycardia occurs. Toxic reactions may be avoided if the maximal intravenous dose of calcium gluconate administered at any one time does not exceed 2 mL/kg; doses above 3 mL/kg should be administered with caution. After the resolution of seizures, intravenous calcium solution may be continued at a dose of 1.87 mmol/kg (75 mg/kg) of elemental calcium per day until the serum calcium concentrations have remained consistently in the normal range. Thereafter, the intravenous calcium solution can be reduced in a stepwise fashion (i.e., 50% for 24 hours, 25% for another 24 hours) and then discontinued.

Complications of intravenous calcium therapy include extravasation into soft tissues (with calcium deposition and sometimes cutaneous necrosis) and bradycardia. Particular care should be exercised when calcium is infused into an umbilical venous catheter with the tip close to (or in) the heart. Because of the many potential risks, arterial infusions of calcium in high concentrations should be avoided. However, parenteral nutrition solutions containing standard mineral (including calcium) content can be safely infused through appropriately positioned umbilical venous or arterial catheters. The direct administration of calcium preparations with bicarbonate or phosphate solution results in precipitation and must be avoided.

As an alternative, if infants can tolerate oral fluids, the intravenous form of calcium gluconate can be given orally at the same dose after the initial correction. All calcium preparations are hypertonic, and there is the theoretical potential for precipitating necrotizing enterocolitis in infants at risk for this condition. The duration of supplemental calcium therapy varies with the course of hypocalcemia. As few as 2 or 3 days of therapy are usually required. However, the requirement for calcium therapy may be prolonged in the case of hypocalcemia caused by malabsorption or hypoparathyroidism. The serum calcium concentration should be measured daily during the first few days of treatment and for 1 or 2 days after its discontinuation until the serum calcium and Ca^{2+} concentrations are stabilized. Persistent hypocalcemia needs further investigation. A poor response to calcium therapy may often result from concurrent magnesium deficiency. The treatment of early neonatal hypocalcemia with vitamin D metabolites and exogenous PTH offers no practical advantage.

ASYMPTOMATIC HYPOCALCEMIA

In asymptomatic hypocalcemia, opinions vary on the need for and intensity of therapy. Some authors do not favor treatment because in most cases, hypocalcemia resolves spontaneously with time. However, hypocalcemia has potentially adverse effects on both the cardiovascular system and the central nervous system (CNS). It is common to treat asymptomatic full-term infants with an ionized calcium concentration of less than 1.10 mmol/L (4.40 mg/dL). For totally asymptomatic preterm infants, a cutoff point of 1.50 mmol/L (6.0 mg/dL) of total serum calcium is considered; however, clinical practice is extremely variable. The treatment of asymptomatic hypocalcemia can be instituted with oral or intravenous calcium salts by using the regimen indicated previously.

Late Neonatal Hypocalcemia

There is usually little debate regarding the treatment of late hypocalcemia. Because serum calcium is not routinely measured after the first few days of life, late hypocalcemia is usually symptomatic when diagnosed. In phosphorus-induced hypocalcemia, a low-phosphorus formula (or human milk) and oral calcium supplementation are indicated to decrease phosphorus absorption and increase calcium absorption.

In hypomagnesemia, the magnesium deficiency usually has to be corrected before hypocalcemia can be treated successfully. Magnesium may be administered intramuscularly or intravenously as a 50% solution of magnesium sulfate in a dose of 25-50 mg/kg (0.05-0.1 mL/kg). Intravenous infusions should be administered slowly with electrocardiographic monitoring to detect acute rhythm disturbances, which may include prolongation of atrioventricular conduction time and a sinoatrial or atrioventricular block. The magnesium dose may be repeated every 8-12 hours, depending on the clinical response and the (monitored) serum magnesium levels. Many infants with transient hypomagnesemia respond sufficiently to one or two injections of magnesium.

Infants with normal intestinal absorption who develop late hypocalcemia with vitamin D deficiency rickets usually respond within 4 weeks to 1000 to 2000 IU/day of oral vitamin D. These infants should receive at least 40 mg/kg per day of elemental calcium in order to prevent hypocalcemia because unmineralized osteoid is able to mineralize when vitamin D is provided ("hungry bones" syndrome).

Hypoparathyroidism requires therapy with vitamin D or one of its metabolites; $1,25(OH)_2D_3$ (or 1 α-hydroxyvitamin D_3, a synthetic analogue that undergoes hepatic 25-hydroxylation) has the advantage of a shorter half-life, and treatment may be more easily tailored to the individual patient. In the CaSR mutation, the need for therapeutic correction of hypocalcemia remains an open question considering that hypercalciuria and nephrocalcinosis may be deleterious to renal function.[66] Attention should be directed toward a number of concomitant treatments. Because thiazide diuretics can increase renal calcium reabsorption, the inadvertent institution or discontinuation of these drugs may increase or decrease, respectively, the plasma calcium level. In contrast, furosemide and other loop diuretics can increase the renal clearance of calcium and depress serum calcium levels. The administration of glucocorticoids antagonizes the action of vitamin D (and the analogues) and may also precipitate hypocalcemia. The development of hypomagnesemia may also interfere with the effectiveness of treatment with calcium and vitamin D.[55]

PREVENTION OF NEONATAL HYPOCALCEMIA

The most effective prevention of neonatal hypocalcemia includes the prevention of prematurity and birth asphyxia, the judicious use of bicarbonate therapy, and mechanical ventilation, for example, during the intentional induction of alkalosis in the treatment of persistent pulmonary hypertension, although this therapy has fallen out of favor. Maintenance of normal maternal vitamin D status with exogenous vitamin D supplements, if needed, may be helpful in maintaining normal fetal vitamin D status and may prevent late hypocalcemia in some neonates. The pharmacologic prevention of neonatal hypocalcemia, especially in infants with VLBW, is based on the prophylactic use of calcium salts, phosphorus salts, and vitamin D supplementation from the first day of life, with a regular survey of serum concentrations and urinary excretion.

Neonatal Hypercalcemia

Hypercalcemia is defined as a pathologic elevation in plasma ionized Ca^{2+} concentration greater than 1.35 mmol/L (5.4 mg/dL) with or without a simultaneous elevation in total calcium concentration of greater than 2.75 mmol/L (11.0 mg/dL).[55,101,102] Neonatal hypercalcemia is relatively uncommon, but it needs to be recognized because it can result in significant morbidity or mortality. The clinical symptoms of sustained hypercalcemia are not specific. Infants with mild increases in serum calcium (2.75 to 3.25 mmol/L, or 11 to 13 mg/dL) often fail to show specific symptoms of hypercalcemia. Nonspecific signs and symptoms such as anorexia, vomiting, and constipation (but rarely diarrhea) may occur with moderate to severe hypercalcemia. The presence of seizures, bradycardia, or arterial hypertension is very exceptional. On physical examination, infants may appear dehydrated, lethargic, and hypotonic. Those with chronic hypercalcemia may present with failure to thrive as the principal source of physical distress. Renal function is generally impaired, and polyuria and hypercalciuria are observed. However, renal complications such as nephrocalcinosis, nephrolithiasis, and hematuria may be the earliest clinical manifestations of hypercalcemia.

IATROGENIC HYPERCALCEMIA

Refer to Boxes 49-7 and 49-8.

Iatrogenic hypercalcemia is the most common type of hypercalcemia in the newborn and should be considered before starting extensive investigation of rare syndromes. It may result from excessive intravenous calcium administration during total parenteral nutrition or exchange transfusion. Other causes of iatrogenic hypercalcemia are the use of extracorporeal membrane oxygenation, which can cause transient hypercalcemia in up to 30% of infants, and vitamin D intoxication

BOX 49–7 Causes of Neonatal Hypercalcemia

IATROGENIC
Calcium salts, vitamin A
Hypophosphatemia (prematurity)
Hypervitaminosis D
Thiazide diuretics

DISORDERS OF PARATHYROID FUNCTION
Maternal hypocalcemia, hypoparathyroidism
Mutation of the parathyroid hormone–related protein receptor
 ▪ Jansen metaphyseal chondrodysplasia
Calcium-sensing receptor defects
 ▪ Familial hypocalciuric hypercalcemia
 ▪ Neonatal severe hyperparathyroidism

IDIOPATHIC INFANTILE HYPERCALCEMIA

HYPERPROSTAGLANDIN E SYNDROME

SEVERE INFANTILE HYPOPHOSPHATASIA

OTHER CAUSES
Congenital carbohydrate malabsorption
Distal renal tubular acidosis
Tumor-related hypercalcemia
Congenital hypothyroidism
Williams syndrome
Subcutaneous fat necrosis
Blue diaper syndrome

BOX 49–8 Diagnostic Steps in Hypercalcemia

HISTORY
Familial or maternal calcium or phosphorus disease
Traumatic birth
High maternal or neonatal supplies of vitamin D and/or A
Drugs during pregnancy (thiazide, lithium)

PHYSICAL EXAMINATION
Growth restriction
Lethargy, dehydration
Seizures, hypertension
Associated features (e.g., elfin facies, congenital heart disease, mental retardation, subcutaneous fat necrosis)

INVESTIGATIONS
Total and ionized calcium, phosphorus, magnesium, alkaline phosphatase
pH, total protein, creatinine
Urinary calcium, phosphorus, creatinine, cyclic adenosine monophosphate
Chest and long-bone radiographs
Renal ultrasound
Parathyroid hormone, 25-OH vitamin D, 1,25-OH vitamin D
Ophthalmologic evaluation, electrocardiography (QT interval)
Others: parathormone-releasing hormone, parental serum calcium and phosphorus concentrations, vitamin A
Molecular genetic studies

from the administration of excessive vitamin D supplements. Vitamin A toxicity is rare and can cause severe hypercalcemia. As vitamin A is metabolized by the kidney, renal insufficiency causes toxic accumulation, which probably directly acts on bone to cause increased resorption and hypercalcemia. Moderate hypercalcemia may also be the result of phosphorus deficiency in premature infants receiving unbalanced calcium and phosphorus regimens in oral and parenteral nutrition. In this situation, hypercalcemia is accompanied by hypophosphoremia. Infants with VLBW who are fed mineral-unsupplemented human milk may develop hypophosphatemic hypercalcemia. The low phosphorus concentration in human milk causes phosphorus deficiency, leading to an increased calcium concentration and hypercalciuria. The absorbed phosphorus is preferentially oriented for soft tissue formation, whereas the remaining phosphorus is insufficient to allow calcium deposition. Hypophosphatemia stimulates renal synthesis of calcitriol, which activates the intestinal absorption and skeletal resorption of calcium and phosphorus. Phosphorus supplementation and the use of human milk fortifiers can prevent hypophosphatemia and hypercalcemia. Similar situations have been reported in infants on parenteral nutrition, providing an unbalanced calcium-to-phosphorus ratio. Additionally, thiazide diuretics reduce renal calcium excretion and may represent a contributing factor.

CONGENITAL HYPERPARATHYROIDISM

Neonatal hyperparathyroidism is defined as symptomatic hypercalcemia with skeletal manifestations of hyperparathyroidism during the first 6 months of life. It may present in the first few days of life with PTH-dependent hypercalcemia, hypotonia, constipation, and respiratory distress.

Secondary Hyperparathyroidism
In many cases, a thorough investigation of the infant's mother will disclose previously known but poorly treated hypoparathyroidism, pseudohypoparathyroidism, or clinically unsuspected hypocalcemia, as seen in mothers with renal tubular acidosis that had induced severe secondary hyperparathyroidism in the developing fetus during pregnancy. The clinical presentation is variable and may depend on the severity of maternal hypocalcemia. Neonatal hypercalcemia is not a constant manifestation of this condition, whereas there is usually some radiologic evidence of metabolic bone disease. Secondary hyperparathyroidism is a transient condition with a good prognosis provided that supportive measures are instituted. Bone disease usually resolves by 6 months of age.

Primary Hyperparathyroidism
In other cases, heterozygous or homozygous loss-of-function mutations in the *CASR* gene cause neonatal hyperparathyroidism.[54,70,87]

The main forms of primary familial hyperparathyroidism presenting in infancy are autosomal dominant familial hypocalciuric hypercalcemia (FHH), resulting from an inactivating mutation of the *CASR* gene; neonatal severe hyperparathyroidism (NSHPT) in children with homozygous or double heterozygous mutations of the *CASR* gene; and sporadic neonatal hyperparathyroidism due to a de novo heterozygous *CASR* mutation. In many families, NSHPT and FHH are the homozygous and heterozygous manifestations, respectively, of the same genetic defect.

FAMILIAL HYPOCALCIURIC HYPERCALCEMIA

FHH is characterized by lifelong and generally asymptomatic, modest elevations in serum calcium levels, with relative hypocalciuria and PTH levels that are not suppressed by hypercalcemia and are inappropriately normal. Hypercalcemia is accompanied by borderline hypermagnesemia and hypophosphatemia. The low urinary excretion of calcium is inappropriate considering the presence of hypercalcemia. Therefore, loss-of-function *CASR* mutations cause an increase in the set point for serum Ca^{2+}-responsive PTH release and elevate the renal calcium reabsorption at any given level of serum calcium, leading to hypercalcemia and hypocalciuria.

NEONATAL SEVERE HYPERPARATHYROIDISM

In contrast, individuals who are homozygous for *CASR* mutations have NSHPT, a disorder characterized by marked hypercalcemia, skeletal demineralization, and parathyroid hyperplasia, which can be fatal without parathyroidectomy.

NSHPT is generally manifested in the first few days of life with failure to thrive, hypotonia, constipation, and respiratory distress. Bony abnormalities are major and include undermineralization, subperiosteal erosion, metaphyseal destruction, and multiple fractures of both the long bones and ribs. It is often a life-threatening disorder, with a mortality rate of more than 25% in historical series. Children who survive NSHPT but remain hypercalcemic may feed poorly, with resulting failure to thrive; hypotonia; and developmental delay, and may be at risk for subsequent neurodevelopmental deficits. After the infant is rendered aparathyroid by surgical treatment, there is a dramatic fall in the serum calcium level, necessitating vitamin D and calcium therapy. Constitutional symptoms quickly reverse, with resolution of the bony abnormalities over about 6 months. Subtotal parathyroidectomy is often ineffective. Total parathyroidectomy with partial autotransplantation could be performed, leaving a minimal amount of parathyroid tissue necessary for normal calcium homeostasis. It has been suggested that the use of pamidronate may be helpful to stabilize life-threatening demineralization before parathyroidectomy in rescue situations.[123]

Williams Syndrome

Williams syndrome (also known as *Williams-Beuren syndrome*) is a multisystem disorder now recognized to be caused by a microdeletion of chromosome 7.[4] It is present at birth and affects boys and girls equally. Williams syndrome is characterized by dysmorphic, elfin facies (100%); cardiovascular disease (most commonly supravalvar aortic stenosis 80%); mental retardation (75%); a consistent cognitive profile (90%); and idiopathic hypercalcemia (15%). The microdeletion codes for the structural protein elastin explain some of the characteristics of Williams syndrome. The pathogenesis of other characteristics, such as hypercalcemia, mental retardation, and unique personality traits, remains unexplained.

Idiopathic infantile hypercalcemia (IIH) is an intriguing feature of Williams syndrome that can contribute to the presence of extreme irritability, vomiting, constipation, and muscle cramps associated with this condition. IIH usually occurs during the first year of life, with a peak between 5 and 8 months. Hypercalciuria in some infants may lead to nephrocalcinosis.[73,90] Symptomatic hypercalcemia usually resolves during childhood, but lifelong abnormalities of calcium and vitamin D metabolism may persist. The mechanisms responsible for hypercalcemia are not uniform. Some of these infants have elevated vitamin D metabolites, suggesting vitamin D intoxication or subtle renal dysregulation of vitamin D metabolism, both of which would account for the increased intestinal calcium absorption. In others, the vitamin D levels are normal, suggesting an increased sensitivity to vitamin D, again accounting for increased gut absorption. Recently, some infants have been found to have elevated PTHrP levels at the time of the onset of hypercalcemia. Its inheritance pattern is still questioned. The pedigree is consistent with autosomal recessive inheritance, but the presence of hypercalciuria among other family members suggests more complex inheritance.

Subcutaneous Fat Necrosis

See Chapter 28.

Subcutaneous fat necrosis is common in full- or late-term newborns who experience a traumatic or difficult delivery. Fat necrosis occurs in tissues that sustain direct trauma, such as those on which forceps or vacuum extraction is used. It is characterized by multiple indurated plaques or nodules with or without erythema on the cheeks, buttocks, posterior trunk, or extremities. Many lesions become calcified or fluctuant with liquefied fat. The cause of this disorder is unknown, but it may be initiated by ischemic injury, hypoxia, or hypothermia. Subcutaneous fat necrosis may be clinically occult, with spontaneous resolution over several weeks to as long as 6 months.[35,122] Hypercalcemia is uncommon, but it is the most frequently reported and serious complication of subcutaneous fat necrosis. Hypercalcemia usually appears when the subcutaneous fat necrosis begins to resolve, but it has been associated with long-term intellectual impairment and may be fatal if unrecognized, requiring the need for long-term monitoring of total and ionized calcium levels after the onset of skin lesions.

The pathogenesis of hypercalcemia is not fully understood. Three hypotheses have been proposed. In the first, the calcium is released from the resolving subcutaneous plaques, but most individuals do not develop hypercalcemia or have calcium deposition in the subcutaneous fat necrosis lesions. In the second, the elevated levels of PTH and prostaglandin E_2 stimulate bone resorption, but most patients have levels within the normal range. Elevated prostaglandin levels may be the result of emesis and therapy with furosemide. The third, the most widely accepted theory, proposes that the elevated $1,25(OH)_2D_3$ secreted from the granulomas of subcutaneous fat necrosis lesions stimulates intestinal calcium uptake. PTH normally stimulates the production of $1,25(OH)_2D_3$ from $25(OH)D_3$ by the kidney. The findings of low-normal PTH concentrations and elevated $1,25(OH)_2D_3$ support the hypothesis of the extrarenal production of $1,25(OH)_2D_3$.

Other Causes of Hypercalcemia

Congenital carbohydrate malabsorption can cause hypercalcemia during the first few months of life. Case reports have been provided for congenital lactase, glucose-galactose, or sucrase-isomaltase deficiency with hypercalcemia and neph-rocalcinosis.[17,85] The etiology of hypercalcemia is unclear, but it is thought to be related to an increase in intestinal calcium absorption secondary to increased gut lactose or galactose or to metabolic acidosis, or both.

Distal renal tubular acidosis is another disorder associated with hypercalcemia and nephrocalcinosis. Metabolic acidosis also has a significant effect on calcium homeostasis. In chronic metabolic acidosis, the buffering of acidosis by bone salts is markedly enhanced. Bone demineralization results from the release of calcium carbonate from the bone to neutralize excess hydrogen ions. In addition to its other effects, metabolic acidosis reduces the urinary citrate concentration and increases the risk for the formation of insoluble calcium oxalate or phosphate crystals.

Severe infantile hypophosphatasia is an autosomal recessive disorder associated with a marked deficiency in serum and tissue alkaline phosphatase, skeletal demineralization and bone deformity, and hypercalcemia.[119] This disorder presents with a spectrum of clinical manifestations. The most severe form presents with polyhydramnios; extreme skeletal hypomineralization; short, deformed limbs; and fetal death. Less severe forms are carried to term, but the infant has hypercalcemia, severe rachitic changes, and undermineralized bone on radiograph. These less severe forms are generally lethal early in life. An additional clinical form, transmitted as an autosomal dominant trait characterized by perinatal symptoms but a better clinical course, has been described.[79]

Jansen metaphyseal chondrodysplasia arises from a heterozygous mutation in the PTH/PTHrP receptor. The receptor is found in the kidney, bone, and growth plate. The constitutive activity in bone causes hypercalcemia due to increased bone resorption and is lifelong. The aberrant receptor in the growth plate alters its function, resulting in postnatal-onset, short-limbed dwarfism. As infants, they are of normal length and appearance. However, in childhood, the phenotype becomes more apparent, with prominent hypertelorism, mandibular hypoplasia, and a progressive and disproportionately short stature. At birth, these infants have obvious bony lesions on radiograph, consisting of rachitic changes, radiolucencies, and irregularities of the metaphyses of the long bones.

Blue diaper syndrome is a rare familial disease in which hypercalcemia and nephrocalcinosis are associated with a defect in the intestinal transport of tryptophan. The mechanism of hypercalcemia is uncertain, although oral tryptophan loading in humans and experimental animals produces an increase in the serum calcium level. The bacterial degradation of tryptophan in the intestine leads to excessive indole production, which is converted to indican in the liver and causes indicanuria. The oxidative conjugation of two molecules of indican forms the water-insoluble dye indigo blue (indigotin), which causes a peculiar bluish discoloration of the diaper. The clinical course is characterized by failure to thrive, recurrent unexplained fever, infections, marked irritability, and constipation. Treatment consists of glucocorticoid administration and low calcium and low vitamin D diets.

Tumor-related hypercalcemia has been found in infants with increased levels of PTHrP, which is thought to be the causative agent of hypercalcemia.

Congenital hypothyroidism has also been associated with hypercalcemia, but the mechanism for its action has yet to be thoroughly clarified.

CLINICAL MANIFESTATIONS

Most infants are asymptomatic when diagnosed. Those with mildly elevated levels of calcium often fail to manifest specific symptoms of hypercalcemia. Infants with chronic hypercalcemia may present with failure to thrive as the principal source of physical distress. There are nonspecific signs and symptoms such as anorexia, vomiting, and constipation (but rarely diarrhea); polyuria may occur with moderate to severe hypercalcemia. In severe hypercalcemia, infants are often dehydrated, lethargic, and hypotonic. Alternatively, they may present with seizures. Clinically, these infants can have bradycardia, a short QT interval, and hypertension. However, renal complications such as nephrocalcinosis, nephrolithiasis, and hematuria may be the earliest clinical manifestations of hypercalcemia. Otherwise, the physical examination is usually normal except for the infants with subcutaneous fat necrosis, Williams syndrome, Jansen metaphyseal chondrodysplasia, and hypophosphatasia.

In clinical practice, the following approach may be useful. First, the possibility of iatrogenic hypercalcemia should be excluded. Second, a maternal history of calcium-phosphorus disease or excessive vitamin D intake during pregnancy should be investigated. Third, the signs of clinical syndromes associated with hypercalcemia, such as blue diapers, fat necrosis, and elfin facies, should be sought. Fourth, the initial laboratory evaluation should include serum calcium, phosphorus, alkaline phosphatase, PTH, the urinary calcium-to-creatinine ratio, and tubular reabsorption of phosphorus. In most cases, these tests allow the differentiation of hypercalcemia caused by parathyroid disorders from nonparathyroid conditions. In hyperparathyroidism, the serum phosphorus concentration is low; renal tubular phosphorus reabsorption is decreased, usually to less than 85%; and the serum PTH concentration is elevated. Finally, additional tests may be performed: A serum $25(OH)D_3$ determination may be useful when an excess of vitamin D is suspected; long-bone radiographs identify demineralization, osteolytic lesions, or both (hyperparathyroidism), or osteosclerotic lesions (occasionally with vitamin D excess); measurements of serum and urinary calcium in parents allow a diagnosis of familial hypocalciuric hypercalcemia; and renal sonography detects nephrocalcinosis.

TREATMENT

The treatment of neonatal hypercalcemia depends on the severity of the presentation. Conservative management is appropriate in the case of mild hypercalcemia in a preterm infant resulting from an inappropriate mineral supply, hypoalbuminemia, or chronic acidosis, with special emphasis on the phosphorus supply when hypercalcemia is associated with hypophosphatemia. Hypercalcemia seen in newborns exposed to maternal hypocalcemia is usually mild and transient, and treatment consists of no more than supplying the appropriate amounts of calcium and phosphorus in the milk.

Infants with moderate to severe hypercalcemia need more aggressive treatment. The initial steps are not specific: (1) discontinue oral and intravenous calcium and vitamin D supplementation and dietary restriction; (2) increase the urinary excretion of calcium by maximizing glomerular filtration with the administration of intravenous fluids, which consist of standard saline at about twice the maintenance requirements; and (3) encourage calcium excretion with furosemide after rehydration but with particular attention to maintaining electrolyte homeostasis.

More specific therapy comprises the use of glucocorticoids, calcitonin, bisphosphonate, dialysis, and total parathyroidectomy. Glucocorticoids (2 mg/kg of prednisone) decrease intestinal calcium absorption, decrease bone resorption, and increase renal excretion. They may be useful during a short period, mainly in cases of an excess of vitamin D, but are relatively ineffective in cases of hyperparathyroidism. Calcitonin (4 to 8 IU/kg subcutaneously every 12 hours, up to a maximum of 8 IU/kg every 6 hours) reduces the serum calcium concentration, but its effectiveness declines after a few days. Bisphosphonate therapy is limited in newborn infants. However, pamidronate (0.5 to 2.0 mg/kg) has been used in the treatment of subcutaneous fat necrosis and could be an ideal agent to stabilize cases of NSHPT, as recently suggested. A calcimimetic drug that reduces PTH secretion, approved by the U.S. Food and Drug Administration for chronic secondary hyperparathyroidism in dialyzed patients, could be of major interest in primary hyperparathyroidism but needs to be evaluated during infancy.[120] Dialysis could be prescribed with a low-calcium dialysate (1.25 mmol/L) in the face of severe and unremitting hypercalcemia. Total parathyroidectomy with partial autotransplantation could be a rescue treatment in the severe form of NSHPT.

In the chronic phase, dietary restriction with the use of a special formula without vitamin D supplementation is the mainstay of treatment. If the dietary regimen is insufficient, corticosteroids can be used with caution. Cellulose phosphate binders have been occasionally used in children, but there is limited experience in neonates, and they may contain unwanted free phosphate.

Nephrocalcinosis in Preterm Infants

Nephrocalcinosis refers to deposits of calcium crystals diffusely located in the parenchyma of the kidney. The incidence is particularly high in infants with VLBW and ELBW. However, it varies widely between 1.7% and 64% depending on different study populations, ultrasonographic criteria, and equipment.[53,110] Ultrasonography has been found to be a sensitive and reliable method for the detection of nephrocalcinosis. It shows either bright reflections of 1 ± 2 mm without acoustic shadowing, defined as white flecks, or bright reflections larger than 2 mm with or without acoustic shadowing, defined as white dots. The etiology of nephrocalcinosis in preterm neonates has not been fully clarified. It develops as the result of an imbalance between stone-inhibiting and stone-promoting factors. Because of its hypercalciuric effect, furosemide therapy is most frequently mentioned as a provocative factor. Treatment with aminoglycosides, corticosteroids, and xanthines may also contribute to stone formation, and neonates with lower birthweight, shorter gestational age, and transient renal failure appear to run a higher risk. Moreover, preterm neonates receive a high intake of calcium, phosphorus, and vitamin D during the first months of life to prevent rickets of prematurity, with frequent calcium-phosphorus imbalance owing to poor solubility in parenteral nutrition and broad variability of intestinal absorption rates in enteral nutrition. Immature kidneys have relatively better developed deep nephrons, with a long Henle loop and probably a low urinary flow velocity. Therefore, conditions are favorable for the formation of crystals, which then stick to the surface and grow. Preterm neonates who develop nephrocalcinosis have a high urinary calcium-to-creatinine ratio, and an accompanying high intake of ascorbic acid might contribute to the high urinary oxalate-to-creatinine ratio, which is a potent lithogenic factor. In contrast, a low urinary citrate-to-calcium ratio, considered a lithoprotective factor, has been reported in infants with ELBW, suggesting that supplementation with alkaline citrate may have a beneficial effect in the prevention of nephrocalcinosis.[116]

The short- and long-term evolution of nephrocalcinosis has not been clearly defined. Ultrasonographic abnormalities that develop during the first months of life disappear in most patients within months to years. A study showed persistent nephrocalcinosis at 30 months of age in former preterm infants diagnosed with neonatal nephrocalcinosis.[111] Although proximal tubular function is unaffected in children with neonatal nephrocalcinosis, high blood pressure and impaired glomerular and distal tubular function might occur more frequently than in healthy term children.[111]

The long-term outcome of nephrocalcinosis in preterm neonates has not been defined, but small-scale studies suggest a decrease in renal function.[57] In contrast, nephrocalcinosis was not a prognosis factor for long-term (3 to 18 years) renal disease in infants with ELBW who had neonatal renal failure.[1]

CLINICAL CONDITIONS ASSOCIATED WITH MAGNESIUM DISTURBANCES

Hypomagnesemia

Hypomagnesemia occurs when serum magnesium concentrations fall below 0.66 mmol/L (1.6 mg/dL), although clinical signs often do not develop until they fall below 0.49 mmol/L (1.2 mg/dL). The signs of hypomagnesemia are the same as those of hypocalcemia: irritability, tremors, and seizures. Because serum magnesium does not reflect total-body magnesium, there is no strict correlation between the clinical signs and serum magnesium concentrations. Hypomagnesemia and hypocalcemia frequently coexist.

ETIOLOGY

Refer to Box 49-9.

Maternal Diabetes

In diabetes, glycosuria causes polyuria and increased urinary magnesium losses. The severity and prevalence of hypomagnesemia in the infants of insulin-dependent diabetic mothers are directly related to the severity of maternal diabetes, which is thought to reflect the severity of maternal magnesium deficiency. The incidence of hypomagnesemia is also increased in infants of gestational diabetic mothers.[14] Hypomagnesemia in IDMs (and infants of gestational diabetic mothers) is associated with neonatal hypocalcemia and decreased parathyroid

BOX 49–9   Neonatal Hypomagnesemia and Hypermagnesemia

NEONATAL HYPOMAGNESEMIA
Decreased magnesium supply
- Maternal magnesium deficiency
- Intrauterine growth restriction
- Maternal diabetes, insulin-dependent and gestational
- Malabsorption syndrome
- Extensive small intestine resection
- Intestinal fistula or diarrhea
- Hepatobiliary disorders
- Defect of intestinal magnesium transport: primary hypomagnesemia with hypocalcemia

Magnesium loss
- Exchange transfusion with citrated blood
- Decreased renal tubular reabsorption
- Primary:
  Infantile isolated renal magnesium washing (dominant and recessive)
  Hypomagnesemia with hypercalciuria and nephrocalcinosis
- Secondary:
  Extracellular fluid compartment expansion, osmotic diuresis
- Drugs (e.g., loop diuretics, aminoglycosides)
- Other causes
- Increased phosphate intake
- Maternal hyperparathyroidism

NEONATAL HYPERMAGNESEMIA
Increased magnesium supply
- Maternal treatment with magnesium sulfate
- Neonatal magnesium therapy: asphyxia, pulmonary hypertension
- Parenteral nutrition
- Antacids, enema

---

function. Cord serum magnesium concentrations and its stores are decreased. Magnesium supplementation improves both serum calcium and PTH.

Intrauterine Growth Restriction
Some infants with IUGR manifest hypomagnesemia at birth. This manifestation may represent conditions in which maternal supply, placental transfer of magnesium, or both are deficient. Hypomagnesemia is seen especially in infants with IUGR born from young, primiparous, toxemic mothers.

Neonatal Hypoparathyroidism
PTH and serum magnesium concentrations are interrelated, so it may not be clear whether hypomagnesemia is the cause or the effect of hypoparathyroidism. A magnesium infusion test may help resolve the issue. If PTH increases after the magnesium load, magnesium deficiency with secondary functional hypoparathyroidism is likely. If PTH does not increase, hypoparathyroidism is probably unrelated to the deficiency.

Inherited Disorders of Renal Magnesium Handling
The genetic basis and cellular defects of a number of primary magnesium wasting diseases have been elucidated during the past decade.[30,31]

PRIMARY HYPOMAGNESEMIA WITH SECONDARY HYPOCALCEMIA
This is a rare autosomal recessive disorder resulting from primary defects in the intestinal transport of magnesium, with the responsible gene mapping to the long arm of chromosome 9. It presents in early infancy with persistent hypocalcemia and seizures that cannot be controlled with anticonvulsants, calcium gluconate, or both. Serum magnesium is frequently less than 0.8 mg/dL (normal, 1.6 to 2.8 mg/dL), and circulating levels of PTH are low despite the presence of hypocalcemia. In older children with inadequate magnesium control, clouded sensorium, disturbed speech, and choreoathetoid movements have been observed. The administration of magnesium to these infants leads to spontaneous parallel increases in serum PTH levels, serum calcium levels, and renal phosphate clearance. The prognosis is favorable if a diagnosis is made early enough.

INFANTILE ISOLATED RENAL MAGNESIUM WASTING (DOMINANT)
Hypomagnesemia as the result of isolated renal magnesium loss is an autosomal dominant condition associated with few symptoms other than chondrocalcinosis. Patients always have hypocalciuria and variable but usually mild hypomagnesemic symptoms.

INFANTILE ISOLATED RENAL MAGNESIUM WASTING (RECESSIVE)
There is evidence of a variant form of hypomagnesemia that is more consistent with isolated renal magnesium loss with autosomal recessive inheritance. Patients also have variable symptoms, but they usually have normal urinary calcium excretion.

HYPOMAGNESEMIA WITH HYPERCALCIURIA AND NEPHROCALCINOSIS
A distinct syndrome of hypomagnesemia with hypercalciuria and nephrocalcinosis (HHN) has been described. The HHN syndrome is an autosomal recessive disorder that is characterized by renal magnesium wasting and results in persistent hypomagnesemia and marked hypercalciuria, leading to early nephrocalcinosis. It is distinguished from other conditions by the absence of infantile hypocalcemic tetany and normal plasma potassium.

Other Causes of Hypomagnesemia
Secondary defects in the renal tubular reabsorption of magnesium may result from extracellular fluid expansion caused by excessive glucose, sodium, or fluid intake or by osmotic diuresis. Loop diuretics such as furosemide and high doses of aminoglycosides such as gentamicin may cause magnesuria. Any severe malabsorption syndrome can cause magnesium deficiency. In the neonatal period, multiple exchange blood transfusions, with citrate as an anticoagulant, result in the complexing of citrate with magnesium, which leads to hypomagnesemia.

CLINICAL MANIFESTATIONS

Hypomagnesemia in the neonatal period is usually transient (except for malabsorption syndromes) and asymptomatic, but it can cause hyperexcitability and occasionally severe, intractable hypocalcemic seizures that are unresponsive to calcium infusion and anticonvulsants. Hypomagnesemia should be considered in any patient with hypocalcemia that does not respond clinically or biochemically to calcium or vitamin D therapy.

TREATMENT

Hypomagnesemia should not be treated with calcium or vitamin D, which may cause a further decrease in serum magnesium. The administration of magnesium salts is the treatment of choice. The average amount of magnesium sulfate required in the neonate is a 50% solution of magnesium sulfate, 0.05 to 0.1 mL/kg (0.1 to 0.2 mmol/kg, or 2.5 to 5.0 mg/kg of elemental magnesium), given intramuscularly or by slow intravenous infusion over 15 to 20 minutes. Repeated doses may be required every 8 to 12 hours. Possible complications of intravenous infusion include systemic hypotension and prolongation or even blockade of sinoauricular or atrioventricular conduction.

Concomitant oral magnesium supplements can be started if oral fluids are tolerated. A 50% solution of magnesium sulfate can be given at a dose of 0.2 mL/kg per day. In specific magnesium malabsorption, daily oral doses of 1 mL/kg per day may be required. Daily serum magnesium concentrations should be measured until the values are stable to evaluate efficacy and safety. Oral magnesium salts are not well absorbed, and large doses may cause diarrhea. The maintenance magnesium supplement should be diluted fivefold to sixfold to allow for more frequent administration, maximizing gut absorption and minimizing side effects.

Neonatal seizures due to hypocalcemia and hypomagnesemia do not have a uniformly favorable outcome. Neurologic abnormalities at follow-up have been found in about 22% of patients.

Hypermagnesemia

Hypermagnesemia is defined as a serum magnesium concentration of greater than 1.15 mmol/L (2.8 mg/dL). Hypermagnesemia is invariably an iatrogenic event caused by excessive magnesium administration. Because magnesium balance is regulated mainly by the kidneys, decreased renal function can be a contributing factor.

ETIOLOGY

Refer to Box 49-9.

Maternal Treatment with Magnesium Sulfate

Magnesium sulfate is used to prevent seizures in preeclampsia and as a tocolytic agent (see Chapters 15 and 17). Maternal hypermagnesemia results in fetal and neonatal hypermagnesemia. Concomitant maternal hypocalcemia may also occur secondary to decreased serum PTH concentrations. With the current treatment of preeclampsia, the neonatal serum magnesium concentration usually does not rise to a potentially dangerous level and gradually returns to normal after a few days.

Excessive Magnesium Administration

Treatment with magnesium-containing antacids for the prevention and treatment of stress ulcers has been reported to cause hypermagnesemia. Excessive magnesium administration with total parenteral solution is a potential cause of hypermagnesemia, especially in sick neonates.

High doses of intravenous magnesium sulfate have been used in the treatment of persistent pulmonary hypertension in the newborn. At high doses, magnesium appears to reverse the hypoxia-induced increase in pulmonary arterial pressure.

CLINICAL MANIFESTATIONS

Hypermagnesemia should be suspected in depressed infants born to mothers who have been treated with magnesium sulfate. In most cases, hypermagnesemia is associated only with hypotonia. However, in extreme cases severe neuromuscular depression (a curare-like effect) and respiratory failure (CNS depression) may occur. In adults, the signs may include neuromuscular depression and hypotension (usually at magnesium concentrations of greater than 1.64 to 2.46 mmol/L, or 4 to 6 mg/dL), difficult urination (greater than 2.05 mmol/L, or 5 mg/dL), CNS depression (greater than 2.46 to 3.28 mmol/L, or 6 to 8 mg/dL), and respiratory depression and coma (greater than 4.92 to 8.33 mmol/L, or 12 to 17 mg/dL).

Serum calcium concentrations may be normal, decreased, or increased in hypermagnesemic neonates. Hypermagnesemia may suppress PTH and $1,25(OH)_2D_3$ production and may result in lower serum calcium concentrations. Rickets has been reported when maternal magnesium therapy is prolonged (e.g., in tocolysis to prevent preterm delivery).

TREATMENT

In most cases of neonatal hypermagnesemia, supportive treatment is sufficient because an excess of magnesium is gradually removed through urinary excretion. Calcium is a direct antagonist of magnesium, and intravenous calcium given at the same dosage as that given for the treatment of hypocalcemia may be useful for acute therapy. Optimal hydration is important to ensure adequate urinary flow. Loop diuretic therapy may increase magnesium excretion. In cases of severe CNS depression, exchange blood transfusions may be used to lower the increased serum magnesium concentration. Citrated donor blood is particularly useful because the complexing action of citrate expedites the removal of magnesium from the infant. Peritoneal dialysis and hemodialysis may be considered in refractory patients. Supportive measures such as cardiorespiratory assistance and adequate hydration may be needed.

OSTEOPENIA OF PREMATURITY

Premature babies are at increased risk for developing bone disease by reduced bone mineral content. Increased survival of infants with VLBW has been associated with an increased incidence of osteopenia of prematurity, which is also called *metabolic bone disease* or *rickets of prematurity*. The incidence is inversely proportional to gestational age and birthweight, and two decades ago, it was estimated to be 50% in infants weighting less than 1000 g and 23% to 32% in infants weighting less than 1500 g; however, the current incidence is difficult to estimate because the nutritional strategy has changed. Maximizing calcium and phosphorus intake from parenteral and enteral nutrition, early initiation of feeding, and decreased use of paralysis during mechanical ventilation probably have decreased the incidence of the disease.

Etiology

From birth, premature babies begin the process of physiologic postnatal adaptation, which is characterized by an increase in bone remodeling, with a progressive increase in marrow cavity size and a concomitant reduction in physical density. The reasons for the postnatal adaptation of the skeleton are not entirely clear, but it is obvious that the skeleton is exposed to different conditions before and after birth. First, in utero mechanical stimulation is likely to be higher. In utero movement offers more resistance against the uterine wall than spontaneous movements occurring after birth in infants with VLBW.[94] Second, the hormonal situation is different postnatally because the placental supply of estrogen and many other hormones has been cut off. Third, mineral supplies differ greatly from those provided during fetal life, while length and skeletal growth rates remain relatively high during the last trimester of gestation.[98] During the last trimester of gestation, the daily accretion rate per kilogram of body weight represents around 120 mg of calcium and 70 mg of phosphorus, which contrasts with the 40 to 90 mg of calcium and 30 to 60 mg of phosphorus retention obtained by metabolic balance studies in preterm infants fed fortified human milk or preterm formula.

Although vitamin D deficiency can cause rickets, it is not the primary cause of osteopenia of prematurity; vitamin D supplementation alone does not reduce the incidence of rickets. Adequate serum concentrations of $25(OH)D_3$ and $1,25(OH)_2D_3$ can be achieved with supplementation of 400 to 1000 IU/day of vitamin D. The role of maternal vitamin D status in the development of osteopenia of prematurity is not clear, although low maternal vitamin D status is associated with reduced bone mineralization of offspring in term infants.

Additional risk factors for bone disease in preterm infants include prolonged parenteral nutrition, feeding with unsupplemented human milk, fluid restriction, chronic illness, and the use of hypercalciuric drugs such as furosemide for the treatment of bronchopulmonary dysplasia and methylxanthines for the treatment of apnea and bradycardia, both of which increase calcium loss. The use of postnatal steroids can decrease bone formation. In addition, immobility, especially for prolonged periods of sedation during mechanical ventilation, could enhance calcium loss and demineralization. There is evidence that placental insufficiency has a role in the development of osteopenia of prematurity. There is an increased incidence of osteopenia of prematurity in infants with IUGR[51] or born to mothers with preeclampsia.[22] Severe demineralization has also been reported in infants born to a mother with severe chorioamnionitis.[106]

Development of osteopenia of prematurity in preterm infants may be associated with genetic polymorphisms. Candidate genes associated with adult osteoporosis have been evaluated for bone disease in infants in VLBW. A correlation between osteopenia of prematurity and thymine-adenine repeat [(TA)n] allelic variant in the estrogen receptor gene has been described.[21] A summary of the risk factors that contribute to the development of osteopenia of prematurity is illustrated in Figure 49-21.

The rate of rickets is inversely related to birthweight. Despite the differences in incidence according to reference criteria, significant bone demineralization was diagnosed by DEXA at term in more than 50% of infants with a birthweight of less than 1500 g and close to 100% of those with a birthweight of less than 1000 g.

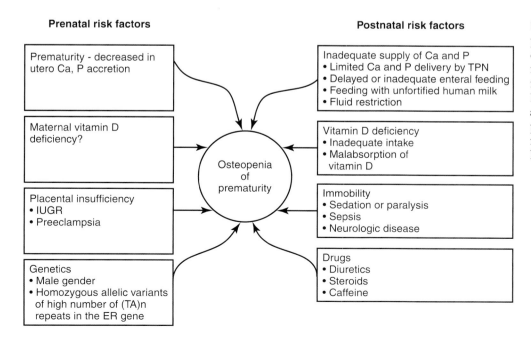

Prenatal risk factors

Prematurity - decreased in utero Ca, P accretion

Maternal vitamin D deficiency?

Placental insufficiency
• IUGR
• Preeclampsia

Genetics
• Male gender
• Homozygous allelic variants of high number of (TA)n repeats in the ER gene

Osteopenia of prematurity

Postnatal risk factors

Inadequate supply of Ca and P
• Limited Ca and P delivery by TPN
• Delayed or inadequate enteral feeding
• Feeding with unfortified human milk
• Fluid restriction

Vitamin D deficiency
• Inadequate intake
• Malabsorption of vitamin D

Immobility
• Sedation or paralysis
• Sepsis
• Neurologic disease

Drugs
• Diuretics
• Steroids
• Caffeine

Figure 49–21. Prenatal and postnatal risk factors for development of osteopenia of prematurity. Ca, calcium; IUGR, intrauterine growth restriction; P, phosphorus; (TA)n, thymine-adenine repeat; TPN, total parenteral nutrition; VDR, vitamin D receptor; COLIA1, collagen I-α1.

Diagnosis

CLINICAL SYMPTOMS

Clinical symptoms of osteopenia are rare in infants with VLBW because of the widespread use of well-balanced parenteral solutions, human milk fortifiers, and preterm formulas. Fractures, which represent the major symptom and were detected in up to 24% of infants with VLBW in the late 1980s, have diminished.[61]

BIOCHEMICAL FEATURES

Biochemical features are relatively nonspecific. Usually serum calcium concentrations are within the normal range and serum phosphorus concentrations are normal or low at the time of diagnosis. The occurrence of a prolonged reduction of serum phosphorus during the early weeks of life could be predictive of the occurrence of osteopenia because infants with ELBW are at risk for low renal phosphate reabsorption (tryptophan and GFR values), leading to urinary phosphate excretion even in the presence of low serum phosphate levels. Therefore, the absence of or very low urinary phosphate excretion also needs to be considered as an indicator of phosphate depletion. Alkaline phosphatase is frequently used to screen for osteopenia of prematurity despite conflicting evidence about its sensitivity and specificity.[47] Alkaline phosphatase of more than five times the upper adult limit of normal has been suggested as indicator of rickets. Radiologic changes of osteopenia were detected in one study when the alkaline phosphatase was greater than 750 IU/L.[43] The peak alkaline phosphatase level is inversely related to the serum phosphorus concentration.[78] Therefore, the combination of alkaline phosphatase and serum phosphorus concentration could be more useful to screen for osteopenia of prematurity than alkaline phosphatase alone. Alkaline phosphatase level higher than 900 lU/L has predicted radiographic osteopenia by DEXA scan with 88% sensitivity and 71% specificity, but the sensitivity is much higher with concomitant lower serum phosphorus concentrations (<1.8 mmol/L).[13] Other studies have found that neither alkaline phosphatase nor serum phosphorus can predict bone mineralization outcome in premature infants.[40] Therefore, following sequential levels of alkaline phosphatase rather than a single level could be more useful to screen and to monitor treatment of osteopenia of prematurity.

HORMONAL FEATURES

In preterm infants, the serum PTH, serum $25(OH)D_3$, and serum $1,25(OH)_2D_3$ concentrations increase during the first month of life. Both 25- and 1,25-hydroxylation mechanisms are functionally active in preterm infants. Both the $25(OH)D_3$ and $1,25(OH)_2D_3$ levels are related to the mother's vitamin D status at birth as well as to the vitamin D supply to the newborn during the first weeks of life. In infants with VLBW supplemented with vitamin D, osteopenia does not appear to be related to the hormonal status.

RADIOLOGIC FEATURES

Standard radiographs do not allow an accurate assessment of bone demineralization. Bone mineral density must decrease by 30% or more to be diagnosed by this method, and interobserver variability is considerable. However, standard radiographs can detect fractures, and a wrist radiograph at 6 to 8 weeks of age remains a practical assessment of the presence of overt rickets. Radiographs must be carefully examined because fractures, especially line fractures, are easily missed. DEXA is the current standard in whole-body mineral measurement, and normative data are available. DEXA equipment is not portable, so performing a scan involves transportation of the infant, which may not be feasible for very small and sick infants who are at the greatest risk for metabolic bone disease. Ultrasound quantification by the measurement of SOS is presently under evaluation,[83,105] as discussed earlier.

Prevention and Treatment

Calcium and phosphorus requirements in preterm infants are usually based on demands for matching intrauterine bone mineral accretion rates and the maintenance of serum calcium and phosphorus concentrations comparable to those of normal term infants. However, more recent consideration of bone physiology suggests that the process of postnatal adaptation could modify the requirement, considering that the remodeling stimulation by itself provides part of the mineral requirement necessary for postnatal bone turnover. Under extrauterine conditions, the care of premature infants should not necessarily aim to achieve intrauterine calcium accretion rates. Subsequently, the skeletons of these infants will adapt to the mechanical requirements whether intrauterine calcium accretion rates are achieved or not.[2]

PARENTERAL NUTRITION

See Chapter 35.

Inadequate calcium and phosphorus intake has been associated with diminished bone mineralization in parenterally fed premature infants. This deficiency occurs when protein and energy are adequate for growth but calcium and phosphorus are insufficient to sustain appropriate skeletal mineralization. Calcium and phosphorus cannot be provided through parenteral solutions at the concentrations needed to support in utero accretion because of precipitation. The solubility of calcium and phosphorus in parenteral solutions depends on the temperature, type, and concentration of amino acids; dextrose concentrations; pH of the calcium salt; sequence of the addition of calcium and phosphorus to the solution; calcium-to-phosphorus ratio; and presence of lipids. More acidic pediatric amino acid solutions improve calcium and phosphorus solubility. With a range of fluid intake of 120 to 150 mL/kg per day, it is advisable to supply a calcium content of 50 to 60 mg/dL (1.25 to 1.5 mmol/dL) and a phosphorus content of 40 to 45 mg/dL (1.25 to 1.5 mmol/dL), corresponding to a calcium-to-phosphorus ratio of 1.3:1 by weight and 1:1 by molar ratio in the total hyperalimentation solution. This quantity of calcium provided by the parenteral route is about 60% to 75% of that deposited by the fetus during the last trimester of gestation (100 to 120 mg/kg per day) but similar to or higher than that obtained in enteral nutrition with presently available preterm formulas. Administering sufficient amounts of calcium and phosphorus in hyperalimentation solutions is no longer a problem in countries in which organic phosphate preparations are available. The use of calcium glycerophosphate has the additional benefit of a much lower content of aluminum. However, information on bone mineralization in infants with ELBW receiving what appears to be adequate calcium and phosphate intake is still limited.[99]

ENTERAL NUTRITION

See Chapter 35.

The exclusive use of human milk without phosphorus and mineral fortification promotes the occurrence of osteopenia and rickets in infants with VLBW. Both liquid and powdered human milk fortifiers are commercially available. Their use has dramatically reduced the incidence of fractures and radiologically diagnosed osteopenia. A similar reduction has also been observed in preterm infants fed preterm formulas. In contrast, a significant reduction in BMC related to gestational age, body weight, and bone area as well as BMAD is still observed in most infants with VLBW at the time of discharge.[32,98]

Although both the absorption and retention rates of calcium and phosphorus are higher in infants than adults, intestinal absorption of minerals remains a limiting factor of mineral accretion. The range of calcium and phosphorus contents is wide in preterm formulas (70 to 140 mg/100 kcal and 50 to 108 mg/100 kcal, respectively). However, standard balance studies have reported that absorption rates are about 60% for calcium in human milk but tend to decrease up to 35% in formulas containing the highest calcium content (see Table 49-3). In contrast, phosphorus is generally well absorbed (80% to 90%), but phosphorus retention is related to calcium and protein accretion. These figures are similar to those obtained with stable-isotope techniques, taking into consideration the endogenous intestinal calcium secretion. The high fecal calcium excretion observed in preterm infants fed high-calcium preterm formulas is not necessarily beneficial because it has been related to impaired fat absorption, stool hardness, and prolonged gastrointestinal transit time.

MONITORING MINERAL SUPPLEMENTATION

As stated previously, there are very few markers of adequate bone mineralization during the early weeks of life in newborn infants. BMC can be measured accurately by DEXA, but in clinical practice, it is performed in very few centers.

An ideal approach to assess the adequacy of mineral intake may involve the following recommendations:

1. Calcium and phosphorus need to be provided together from the first hours of life in a well-balanced parenteral solution when necessary.
2. Vitamin D supplementation (400 to 1000 IU orally or 160 to 320 IU parenterally) according to maternal status and seasonal variation may be provided from the first day of life.
3. Serum phosphorus concentrations should be regularly determined and maintained above 6 mg/dL (2 mmol/L). Serum phosphorus is much more loosely regulated than serum calcium and may be an effective indicator of the adequacy of mineral intake.
4. Urinary calcium and phosphorus should be measured. Because phosphorus excretion is inversely related to calcium excretion, the simultaneous presence of both calcium and phosphorus in spot urine samples in a ratio of less than 0.5 indicates that both are provided in sufficient amounts.

Conversely, the absence of either calcium or phosphorus from urine samples indicates a deficiency of one of these minerals and that maximal tubular reabsorption is in effect.
5. Serum alkaline phosphatase should be measured. It is of limited absolute value given its wide fluctuation, but marked elevations (more than five times the normal rate, or more than 1200 IU) may indicate the presence of rickets and the risk for subsequently reduced linear growth.

MECHANICAL STIMULATION PROGRAM

Reduced mechanical stimulation against resistance and reduction of spontaneous movements occurring after birth in infants with VLBW frequently sedated for prolonged periods enhances calcium losses and demineralization. It has been reported that a gentle program of physiotherapy, including passive mobilization and the stimulation of active mobilization against resistance, improves bone mineral density in VLBW infants.[2] However, available data are inadequate to justify the standard use of physical activity programs in preterm infants or to predict the long-term effect of such interventions.[112]

Outcome

Catch-up mineralization is rapidly observed after discharge in infants with VLBW.[11] At 6 months of corrected age, spine and total bone mineral density, corrected for anthropometric values, are in the range of normal term newborn infants. In fact, the catch-up mineralization observed after discharge is quite similar to that observed after the initial acceleration of growth during adolescence. Nevertheless, peak bone mass may be less during adulthood.[125] Therefore, Fewtrell and coworkers found that at 8 to 12 years of age, formerly preterm infants were shorter, were lighter, and had lower BMCs than controls. However, BMC was appropriate for the body size achieved and was not affected by early dieting or human milk feeding.[41]

Osteopenia or rickets of prematurity appears to be a self-resolving disease, although the potential long-term consequences on the attainment of peak bone mass are not clearly known. Even if BMC improves spontaneously in most infants, this discovery does not imply that a period of demineralization is acceptable. Although the long-term consequences are unclear, the benefits of prevention and treatment include avoidance of fractures and possibly improved linear growth and peak bone mass.

ACKNOWLEDGMENTS

The authors and editors acknowledge the important contributions of S. De Marini and R. C. Tsang to the previous editions of this chapter, portions of which remain unchanged.

REFERENCES

1. Abitbol CL, et al: Long-term follow-up of extremely low birth weight infants with neonatal renal failure, *Pediatr Nephrol* 18:887, 2003.
2. Aly H, et al: Physical activity combined with massage improves bone mineralization in premature infants: a randomized trial, *J Perinatol* 24:305, 2004.

3. American Academy of Pediatrics, Committee on Nutrition: Nutritional needs of low birth weight infants, *Pediatrics* 75:976, 1985.

4. American Academy of Pediatrics, Committee on Genetics Health Care Supervision for Children with Williams Syndrome, *Pediatrics* 107:1192, 2001.

5. American Academy of Pediatrics: Wagner CL, Greer FR; Section on Breastfeeding; Committee on Nutrition: Prevention of rickets and vitamin D deficiency in infants, children, and adolescents, *Pediatrics* 122:1142, 2008.

6. Ariceta G, et al: Renal magnesium handling in infants and children, *Acta Paediatr* 85:1019, 1996.

7. Ariceta G, Rodriguez-Soriano J: Magnesium. In Preedy VR, Grimble G, Watson R, editors: *Nutrition in the Infant: problems and Practical Procedures*, 1st ed, London, 2001, Greenwich Medical Media, p 149.

8. Ashmeade, et al: Longitudinal measurements of bone status in preterm infants, *Acta Paediatr* 97:1625, 2008.

9. Atkinson SA, Tsang RC: Calcium, magnesium, phosphorus, and vitamin D. In Tsang R, et al, editors: *Nutrition of the preterm infant*, 2nd ed, Cincinnati, Ohio, 2005, Digital Education Publishing, p 245.

10. Atkinson SA: Calcium and phosphorus needs of premature infants, *Nutrition* 10:66, 1994.

11. Avila-Diaz M, et al: Increments in whole body bone mineral content associated with weight and length in pre-term and full-term infants during the first 6 months of life, *Arch Med Res* 32:288, 2001.

12. Avila E, et al: Regulation of vitamin D hydroxylases gene expression by 1,25-dihydroxyvitamin D3 and cyclic AMP in cultured human syncytiotrophoblasts, *J Steroid Biochem Mol Biol* 103:90, 2007.

13. Backström MC, et al: Bone isoenzyme of serum alkaline phosphatase and serum inorganic phosphate in metabolic bone disease of prematurity, *Acta Paediatr* 89:867, 2000.

14. Banerjee S, et al: Lower whole blood ionized magnesium concentrations in hypocalcemic infants of gestational diabetic mothers, *Magnes Res* 16:127, 2003.

15. Baschat AA: Fetal responses to placental insufficiency: an update, *Br J Obstet Gynaecol* 111:1031, 2004.

16. Bassir M, et al: Vitamin D deficiency in Iranian mothers and their neonates: a pilot study, *Acta Paediatr* 90:577, 2001.

17. Belmont JW, et al: Congenital sucrase-isomaltase deficiency presenting with failure to thrive, hypercalcemia, and nephrocalcinosis, *BMC Pediatr* 25:2, 2002.

18. Bodnar LM, et al: Maternal vitamin D deficiency is associated with bacterial vaginosis in the first trimester of pregnancy, *J Nutr* 139:1157, 2009.

19. Bodnar LM, et al: Maternal vitamin D deficiency increases the risk of preeclampsia, *J Clin Endocrinol Metab* 92:3517, 2007.

20. Bodnar LM, et al: High prevalence of vitamin D insufficiency in black and white pregnant women residing in the northern United States and their neonates, *J Nutr* 137:305, 2007.

21. Bosley AR at al: Influence of genetic polymorphisms on bone disease of preterm infants, *Pediatr Res* 60:607, 2006.

22. Bosley AR, et al: Aetiological factors in rickets of prematurity, *Arch Dis Child* 55:683, 1980.

23. Bronner F, et al: Net calcium absorption in premature infants: results of 103 metabolic balance studies, *Am J Clin Nutr* 56:1037, 1992.

24. Bronner F, Stein WD: Calcium homeostasis—an old problem revisited, *J Nutr* 125:1987S, 1995.

25. Bronner F, Pansu D: Nutritional aspects of calcium absorption, *J Nutr* 129:9, 1999.

26. Camargo CA, et al: Maternal intake of vitamin D during pregnancy and risk of recurrent wheeze in children at 3 y of age, *Am J Clin Nutr* 85:788, 2007.

27. Carnielli VP, et al: Feeding premature newborn infants palmitic acid in amounts and stereoisomeric position similar to that of human milk: effects on fat and mineral balance, *Am J Clin Nutr* 61:1037, 1995.

28. Chen CJ, et al: Malignant infantile osteopetrosis initially presenting with neonatal hypocalcemia: case report, *Ann Hematol* 82:64, 2003.

29. Clifton-Bligh RJ, et al: Maternal vitamin D deficiency, ethnicity and gestational diabetes, *Diabetes Med* 25:678, 2008.

30. Cole DEC, Quamme GA: Inherited disorders of renal magnesium handling, *J Am Soc Nephrol* 11:1937, 2000.

31. Dai LJ, et al: Magnesium transport in the renal distal convoluted tubule, *Physiol Rev* 81:51, 2001.

32. De Curtis M, Rigo J: Enteral nutrition in preterm infants. In Guandalini S, editors: *Textbook of pediatric gastroenterology and nutrition*, London, 2004, Taylor & Francis, p 599.

33. Devereux G, et al: Maternal vitamin D intake during pregnancy and early childhood wheezing, *Am J Clin Nutr* 85:853, 2007.

34. Dickerson JWT: Changes in composition of the human femur during growth, *Biochem J* 82:56, 1962.

35. Dudink J, et al: Subcutaneous fat necrosis of the newborn: hypercalcemia with hepatic and atrial myocardial calcification, *Arch Dis Child Fetal Neonatal Ed* 88:F343, 2003.

36. Ellis KJ, et al: Body elemental composition of the neonate: new reference data, *Am J Hum Biol* 5:323, 1993.

37. Erkkola M, et al: Maternal vitamin D intake during pregnancy is inversely associated with asthma and allergic rhinitis in 5-year-old children, *Clin Exp Allergy* 39:875, 2009.

38. European Commission, Scientific Committee on Food: *Report of the Scientific Committee on Food on the Revision of Essential Requirements of Infant Formulae and Follow-on Formulae* (website). http://ec.europa.eu/food/fs/sc/scf/index_en.html. Accessed July 23, 2010.

39. European Society for Paediatrics Gastroenterology, Hepatology and Nutrition (ESPGHAN); Committee on Nutrition; Agostoni C, et al: Enteral nutrient supply for preterm infants, *J Pediatr Gastroenterol Nutr* 50:1-9, 2010.

40. Faerk J, et al: Bone mineralisation in premature infants cannot be predicted from serum alkaline phosphatase or serum phosphate, *Arch Dis Child Fetal Neonatal Ed* 87:F133, 2002.

41. Fewtrell MS, et al: Neonatal factors predicting childhood height in preterm infants: evidence for a persisting effect of early metabolic bone disease? *J Pediatr* 137:668, 2000.

42. Fudge NJ, Kovacs CS: Physiological studies in heterozygous calcium sensing receptor (CaSR) gene-ablated mice confirm that the CaSR regulates calcitonin release in vivo, *BMC Physiol* 4:5, 2004.

43. Glass EJ, et al: Plasma alkaline phosphatase activity in rickets of prematurity, *Arch Dis Child* 57:373, 1982.

44. Glorieux FH, et al: Dynamic histomorphometric evaluation of human fetal bone formation, *Bone* 12:377, 1997.

45. Greer FR: Vitamin D deficiency-it's more than rickets, *J Pediatr* 143:422, 2003.

46. Hammami M, et al: Phantoms for cross-calibration of dual energy X-ray absorptiometry measurements in infants, *J Am Coll Nutr* 21:328, 2002.

47. Harrison CM, et al: Osteopenia of prematurity: a national survey and review of practice, *Acta Paediatr* 97:407, 2008.

48. Hillman LS, et al: Measurement of true absorption, endogenous fecal excretion, urinary excretion, and retention of calcium in term infants by using a dual-tracer, stable-isotope method, *J Pediatr* 123:444, 1993.

49. Hoff AO, et al: Increased bone mass is an unexpected phenotype associated with deletion of the calcitonin gene, *J Clin Invest* 110:1849, 2002.

50. Holick MF: Vitamin D: Photobiology, metabolism, mechanism of action, and clinical applications. In Favus MJ, editors: *Primer on the Metabolic Bone Diseases and Disorders of Mineral metabolism*, Philadelphia, 1999, Lippincott Williams & Wilkins, p 92.

51. Holland PC, et al: Prenatal deficiency of phosphate, phosphate supplementation, and rickets in very-low-birthweight infants, *Lancet* 335:697, 1990.

52. Holtback U, Aperia AC: Molecular determinants of sodium and water balance during early human development, *Semin Neonatol* 8:291, 2003.

53. Hoppe B, et al: Nephrocalcinosis in preterm infants: a single center experience, *Pediatr Nephrol* 17:264, 2002.

54. Houillier P, Paillard M: Calcium-sensing receptor and renal cation handling, *Nephrol Dial Transplant* 18:2467, 2003.

55. Hsu SC, Levine MA: Perinatal calcium metabolism: physiology and pathophysiology, *Semin Neonatol* 9:23, 2004.

56. Javaid MK, et al: Maternal vitamin D status during pregnancy and childhood bone mass at age 9 years: a longitudinal study, *Lancet* 367:36, 2006.

56a. Johnson DD, Wagner CL, Hulsey TC, et al: Vitamin D deficiency and insufficiency is common during pregnancy, *Am J Perinatol* Jul 16, 2010 (Epub ahead of print).

57. Jones CA, et al: Renal calcification in preterm infants: follow up at 4-5 years, *Arch Dis Child Fetal Neonatal Ed* 76:F185, 1997.

58. Klein CJ: Nutrient requirements for preterm infant formulas, *J Nutr* 132:1395S, 2002.

59. Koo WW, Tsang RC: Mineral requirements of low-birth-weight infants, *J Am Coll Nutr* 10:474, 1991.

60. Koo WW, et al: Dual-energy X-ray absorptiometry studies of bone mineral status in newborn infants, *J Bone Min Res* 11:997, 1996.

61. Koo WWK, Steichen JJ: Osteopenia and rickets of prematurity. In Polin RA, Fox WW, editors: *Fetal and neonatal physiology*, Philadelphia, 1998, WB Saunders, p 2335.

62. Kovacs CS, et al: PTH regulates fetal blood calcium and skeletal mineralization independently of PTHrP, *Endocrinology* 142:4983, 2001.

63. Laires MJ, et al: Role of cellular magnesium in health and human disease, *Front Biosci* 1:262, 2004.

64. Langhendries JP, et al: Phosphorus intake in preterm babies and variation tubular reabsorption for phosphate per liter glomerular filtrate, *Biol Neonate* 61:345, 1992.

65. Lapillonne A: Vitamin D deficiency during pregnancy may impair maternal and fetal outcomes, *Med Hypotheses* 74:71-75, 2009.

66. Lienhardt A, et al: Activating mutations of the calcium-sensing receptor: management of hypocalcemia, *J Clin Endocrinol Metab* 86:5313, 2001.

67. Lönnerdal B: Effects of milk and milk components on calcium, magnesium and trace element absorption during infancy, *Physiol Rev* 77:643, 1997.

68. Mahon P, et al: Low Maternal vitamin D status and fetal bone development: cohort study, *J Bone Miner Res* 24:663-668, 2009.

69. Martin R, et al; SWS Study Group: Placental calcium transporter (PMCA3) gene expression predicts intrauterine bone mineral accrual, *Bone* 40:1203, 2007.

70. Marx SJ: Hyperparathyroid and hypoparathyroid disorders, *N Engl J Med* 343:1863, 2000.

71. Matos V, et al: Urinary phosphate/creatinine, calcium/creatinine, and magnesium/creatinine ratios in a healthy pediatric population, *J Pediatr* 131:252, 1997.

72. McDevitt H, et al: Quantitative ultrasound assessment of bone health in the neonate, *Neonatology* 91:2, 2007.

73. McTaggart SJ, et al: Familial occurrence of idiopathic infantile hypercalcemia, *Pediatr Nephrol* 13:668, 1999.

74. McDonald KR, et al: Ablation of calcitonin/calcitonin gene-related peptide-α impairs fetal magnesium but not calcium homeostasis, *Am J Physiol Endocrinol Metab* 287:E218, 2004.

75. Merewood A, et al: Association between vitamin D deficiency and primary cesarean section, *J Clin Endocrinol Metab* 94:940, 2009.

76. Miller ME: The bone disease of preterm birth: a biomechanical perspective, *Pediatr Res* 53:10, 2003.

77. Mimouni F, Tsang RC: Perinatal magnesium metabolism: personal data and challenge for the 1990s, *Magnes Res* 4:109, 1991.

78. Mitchell SM, et al: High frequencies of elevated alkaline phosphatase activity and rickets exist in extremely low birth weight infants despite current nutritional support, *BMC Pediatr* 9:47, 2009.

79. Moore CA, et al: Mild autosomal dominant hypophosphatasia: in utero presentation in two families, *Am J Med Genet* 86:410, 1999.

80. Namgung R, Tsang RC: Neonatal calcium, phosphorus and magnesium homeostasis. In Polin RA, Fox WW, editors: *Fetal and Neonatal physiology*, Philadelphia, 1998, WB Saunders, p 2308.

81. Namgung R, Tsang RC: Factors affecting newborn bone mineral content: In utero effects on newborn bone mineralization, *Proc Nutr Soc* 59:55, 2000.

82. Nemet D, et al: Quantitative ultrasound measurements of bone speed of sound in premature infants, *Eur J Pediatr* 160:736, 2001.

83. Nemet D, et al: Quantitative ultrasound measurements of bone speed of sound in premature infants, *Eur J Pediatr* 160:736, 2001.

84. Novakovic B, et al: Placenta-specific methylation of the vitamin D 24-hydroxylase gene: implications for feedback autoregulation of active vitamin D levels at the fetomaternal interface, *J Biol Chem* 284:14838, 2009.

85. Pahari A, et al: Neonatal nephrocalcinosis in association with glucose-galactose malabsorption, *Pediatr Nephrol* 18:700, 2003.

86. Pawley N, Bishop NJ: Prenatal and infant predictors of bone health the influence of vitamin D, *Am J Clin Nutr* 80(6 Suppl):1748S, 2004.

87. Pearce SH: Clinical disorders of extracellular calcium sensing and the molecular biology of the calcium-sensing receptor, *Ann Med* 34:201, 2002.

88. Picaud JC, et al: First all-solid pediatric phantom for dual energy x-ray absorptiometry measurements in infants, *J Clin Densitom* 6:17, 2003.

89. Portal AA: Calcium and phosphorus. In Avner ED, et al, editors: *Pediatric nephrology*, 5th ed, Philadelphia, 2004, Lippincott Williams & Wilkins, p 209.

90. Pronicka E, et al: Persistent hypercalciuria and elevated 25-hydroxyvitamin D3 in children with infantile hypercalcemia, *Pediatr Nephrol* 11:2, 1997.

91. Quarles LD: Endocrine functions of bone in mineral metabolism regulation, *J Clin Invest* 118:3820, 2009.

92. Raiten DJ, et al: Life Sciences Research Office Report. Executive summary for the report: assessment of nutrient requirements for infant formulas, *J Nutr* 128:2059S, 1998.

93. Rauch F, Schoenau E: The developing bone: slave or master of its cells and molecules? *Pediatr Res* 50:309, 2001.

94. Rauch F, Schoenau E: Skeletal development in premature infants: a review of bone physiology beyond nutritional aspects, *Arch Dis Child Fetal Neonatal Ed* 86:F82, 2002.

95. Rigo J, et al: Nutritional needs of premature infants: current issues, *J Pediatr* 149:s80, 2006.

96. Rigo J, et al: Reference values of body composition obtained by dual energy X-ray absorptiometry in preterm and term neonates, *J Pediatr Gastroenterol Nutr* 27:184, 1998.

97. Rigo J, et al: Premature bone. In Bonjour JP, Tsang RC, editors: *Nutrition and bone development*. Nestlé Nutrition Workshop Series, vol 41, Philadelphia, 1999, Vevey/Lippincott-Raven, p 83.

98. Rigo J, et al: Bone mineral metabolism in the micropremie, *Clin Perinatol* 27:147, 2000.

99. Rigo J, De Curtis M: Parenteral nutrition in premature infants. In Guandalini S, editor: *Textbook of pediatric gastroenterology and nutrition*, London, Taylor & Francis, 2004, p 619.

100. Rigo J, et al: Enteral calcium, phosphate and vitamin D requirements and bone mineralization in preterm infants, *Acta Paediatr* 96:969, 2007.

101. Rodd C, Goodyer P: Hypercalcemia of the newborn: etiology, evaluation, and management, *Pediatr Nephrol* 13:542, 1999.

102. Rodriguez SJ: Neonatal hypercalcemia, *J Nephrol* 16:606, 2003.

103. Root AW: Disorders of calcium and phosphorus metabolism. In Rudolph CD, et al, editors: *Rudolph's pediatrics*, New York, 2002, McGraw-Hill, p 2142.

104. Rubin LP: Disorders of calcium and phosphorus metabolism. In Taeusch HW, Ballard RA, editors: *Avery's diseases of the newborn*, 7th ed, Philadelphia, 1998, WB Saunders Co, p 1189.

105. Rubinacci A, et al: Quantitative ultrasound for the assessment of osteopenia in preterm infants, *Eur J Endocrinol* 149:307, 2003.

106. Ryan S, et al: Mineral accretion in the human fetus, *Arch Dis Child* 63:799, 1988.

107. Salle BL, et al: Perinatal metabolism of vitamin D, *Am J Clin Nutr* 71:1317S, 2000.

108. Salle BL, et al: Human fetal bone development: histomorphometric evaluation of the proximal femoral metaphysis, *Bone* 30:823, 2002.

109. Saxe A, et al: Parathyroid hormone and parathyroid hormone-related peptide in venous umbilical cord blood of healthy neonates, *J Perinat Med* 25:288, 1997.

110. Schell-Feith EA, et al: Etiology of nephrocalcinosis in preterm neonates: association of nutritional intake and urinary parameters, *Kidney Int* 58:2102, 2000.

111. Schell-Feith EA, et al: Preterm neonates with nephrocalcinosis: natural course and renal function, *Pediatr Nephrol* 18:1102, 2003.

112. Schulzke SM, et al: Physical activity programs for promoting bone mineralization and growth in preterm infants, *Cochrane Database Syst Rev* 2:CD005387, 2007.

113. Senterre J, Salle B: Renal aspects of calcium and phosphorus metabolism in preterm, *Biol Neonate* 53:220, 1988.

114. Senterre J: Osteopenia versus rickets in premature infants. In Glorieux FH, editor: *Rickets*. Nestlé Nutrition Workshop Series, vol 21, New York, 1991, Vevey/Raven Press, p 145.

115. Shaw AJ, et al: Evidence for active maternofetal transfer of magnesium across the in situ perfused rat placenta, *Pediatr Res* 27:622, 1990.

116. Sikora P, et al: Hypocitraturia is one of the major risk factors for nephrocalcinosis in very low birth weight infants, *Kidney Int* 63:2194, 2003.

117. Sobacchi C, et al: The mutational spectrum of human malignant autosomal recessive osteopetrosis, *Hum Mol Genet* 10:1767, 2001.

118. Sparks JW: Human intrauterine growth and nutrient accretion, *Semin Perinatol* 8:74, 1984.

119. Spentchian M, et al: Severe hypophosphatasia: characterization of fifteen novel mutations in the ALPL gene, *Hum Mutat* 22:105, 2003.

120. Stewart AF: Translational implications of the parathyroid calcium receptor, *N Engl J Med* 351:324, 2004.

121. Strid H, et al: Parathyroid hormone-related peptide (38-94) amide stimulates ATP-dependent calcium transport in the basal plasma membrane of the human syncytiotrophoblast, *J Endocrinol* 175:517, 2002.

122. Tran JT, Sheth AP: Complications of subcutaneous fat necrosis of the newborn: a case report and review of the literature, *Pediatr Dermatol* 20:257, 2003.

123. Waller S, et al: Neonatal severe hyperparathyroidism: genotype/phenotype correlation and the use of pamidronate as rescue therapy, *Eur J Pediatr* 63:589, 2004.

124. Zaidi M, et al: Calcitonin and bone formation: a knockout full of surprises, *J Clin Invest* 110:1769, 2002.

125. Zamora SA, et al: Lower femoral neck bone mineral density in prepubertal former preterm girls, *Bone* 29:424, 2001.

126. Ziegler EE, Fomon SJ: Lactose enhances mineral absorption in infancy, *J Pediatr Gastroenterol Nutr* 2:288, 1983.

PART 3

Thyroid Disorders
Susan R. Rose

Many physiologic factors influence fetal and neonatal thyroid function. They include embryogenesis of the thyroid, fetal-maternal relationships and the dynamic alteration of thyroid function with birth, the action of thyroid hormones, the synthesis and transport of these hormones, and mechanisms regulating thyroid function. Thyroid hormone abbreviations are defined in Table 49-5. To provide the background necessary to

TABLE 49–5	Abbreviations Related to Thyroid Hormones

ACTH, adrenocorticotropic hormone

CH, congenital hypothyroidism

DIT, diiodothyronine (diiodotyrosine)

FT_4, free T_4

FT_3, free T_3

GH, growth hormone

IQ, intelligence quotient

KI, potassium iodide

MIT, monoiodothyronine (monoiodotyrosine)

MTZ, methimazole

PTU, propylthiouracil

rT_3, reverse T_3 (3,3′,5′-L-triiodothyronine)

SGA, birth small for gestational age

T_4, thyroxine (tetraiodothyronine)

T_3, triiodothyronine (3,5,3′-L-triiodothyronine)

T_3U (T_3RU), T_3 resin uptake to estimate thyroid binding

TBG, thyroid (thyroxine)-binding globulin

TBII, TSH-binding/inhibiting immunoglobulins

TG, thyroglobulin

TGAb, thyroglobulin antibodies

TH, thyroid hormone

TPOAb, thyroid peroxidase (formerly microsomal) antibodies

TRAb, TSH-receptor antibodies

TRH, thyrotropin-releasing hormone, TSH-releasing hormone (L-pyroglutamyl-L-histidyl-L-prolineamide)

TSH, thyrotropin

TSI, TSH receptor-stimulating immunoglobulins

TTR, transthyretin (formerly T_4-binding prealbumin)

understand thyroid disorders in infants, this chapter begins with sections on thyroid physiology and laboratory tests. Embryology and fetal development of thyroid function are then described. Finally, clinical conditions of altered thyroid function are discussed.

PHYSIOLOGIC ACTION OF THYROID HORMONES

Functions of the Thyroid Gland

The principal functions of the thyroid gland are to synthesize, store, and release the thyroid hormones thyroxine (T_4) and triiodothyronine (T_3) into the circulation. The major secretory product of the thyroid is T_4. Thyroidal secretion of T_3 accounts for only about 20% of its production.

The remaining 80% is derived from peripheral deiodination of T_4. Therefore, T_4 acts as a prohormone for T_3 because T_4 has negligible intrinsic metabolic activity in most tissues. Most of the physiologic effects of thyroid hormone are mediated by T_3 through its interaction with the thyroid response element on DNA.[3]

Neurologic Effects

Congenital thyroid hormone deficiency results in cretinism (severe mental retardation) if not treated. This effect is prevented by thyroid hormone replacement early in life. Newborn screening for thyroid deficiency was initiated in Quebec in 1974. Intellectual development is normal in children with congenital hypothyroidism who are treated early and aggressively and is significantly better in those treated early (by 7 days of age) and with higher thyroid hormone doses (12 μg/kg per day) than in those started on therapy later or treated with lower doses.[9]

Prenatal and postnatal maturation of the brain, retina, and cochlea is thyroid hormone dependent.[23] Thyroid hormone modulates expression of thyroid hormone–responsive target genes at precise times during development, controlled by an interplay of deiodinases, thyroid receptor expression, transporters, cofactors, and transcription factors.[3,7] T_3 promotes the neural differentiation of embryonic stem cells. Genes involved in neural migration are also regulated by thyroid hormone.[4,7]

Thyroidectomy in neonatal monkeys results in defective growth and development of the brain. The degree of mental retardation in cretinism is related to the severity and duration of the hypothyroid state of the infant. The brain is susceptible to a lack of thyroid hormone during its rapid growth and maturation. Defective growth and permanent damage do not occur if hypothyroidism begins after morphologic maturation of the brain is completed (i.e., after a postnatal age of 2 to 3 years).

Thyroid hormone also affects peripheral nerves. In hypothyroidism, relaxation phase of the ankle and knee-jerk reflexes is prolonged; in hyperthyroidism, sympathetic and autonomic responses may be exaggerated.

Cellular Metabolism

One of the principal actions of thyroid hormone is to stimulate rate of cellular oxidation in a large variety of tissues, leading to increased oxygen consumption, liberation of carbon dioxide, and production of heat. In hypothyroidism, the basal metabolic rate is reduced, but in hyperthyroidism, it is increased. The action of thyroid hormone may be mediated through increased protein synthesis. T_3 binds to the thyroid response element in the cell nucleus, leading to enhancement of polymerase activity, which in turn leads to increased cellular messenger RNA (mRNA) and corresponding proteins.[3] Synthesis of membranous sodium-potassium adenosine triphosphatase (ATPase) is enhanced by this mechanism. A large portion of oxygen consumption depends on sodium pump activity. T_3 has direct effects on the mitochondria in vitro and probably in vivo.[53] T_4 in cell culture induces phosphorylation of mitogen-activated protein kinase. Thyroid hormone enhances response of β-receptors to catecholamines without increasing the number of receptors.

Clinically, the calorigenic action of thyroid hormone affects circulation by increasing heart rate, stroke volume, and cardiac output. The pulse pressure is widened mainly by a decrease in the diastolic pressure and by some elevation in the systolic pressure. Circulation time is shortened. In hypothyroidism, the electrocardiogram (EKG) may show decreased voltage for all complexes, prolongation of the PR interval, and depression or inversion of the T wave. However, effects on the EKG may be secondary to myxedema of the myocardium.

Protein and Lipid Metabolism

Negative nitrogen balance occurs in hyperthyroidism unless the patient is protected by adequate caloric intake to provide for the increased energy requirements. In severe hypothyroidism, there is deposition of a mucoprotein containing hyaluronic acid in extracellular myxedematous fluid. Thyroid hormone influences the incorporation of creatinine into the phosphocreatine cycle. In hypothyroidism, there is an excessive storage of creatine, whereas in hyperthyroidism, the urinary excretion of creatine is increased. However, the total excretion of creatine and creatinine is not affected by thyroid hormone. Therefore, thyroid hormone changes the urinary creatine-creatinine balance; creatine accounts for 10% to 30% in the normal child, 0% to 10% in those with hypothyroidism, and 25% to 65% in those with hyperthyroidism.

Effects of thyroid hormone on lipid metabolism are seen in the increased serum total cholesterol and low-density lipoprotein (LDL) cholesterol concentrations in hypothyroidism. The total neutral fats, fatty acids, apolipoprotein B, and phospholipids of the serum are also increased in hypothyroidism.[26]

Carbohydrates, Calcium, Vitamin D, Water Balance, and Liver Function

The rate of glucose absorption and use is increased by thyroid hormone. In hypothyroidism, hypercalcemia may occur, the serum carotene level may be high, and the glucuronic acid conjugation mechanism of the liver may be impaired. In infants, hyperbilirubinemia associated with primary hypothyroidism is almost entirely indirect; in hypothalamic-pituitary hypothyroidism, it is both direct and indirect. Retention of water in the extracellular compartment occurs in hypothyroidism, producing the myxedematous fluid.

In hyperthyroidism, calcium balance tends to be negative; urinary and fecal calcium excretion is enhanced. Demineralization of bone occurs, and efflux of calcium from the bones leads to higher plasma ionized calcium and phosphate and lower circulating $1,25(OH)_2D_3$, which in turn results in decreased calcium absorption from the intestine.

Growth and Development

A principal action of thyroid hormone is its effect on growth and development. These effects may be tissue specific and synergistic with other hormones. Prenatal growth is highly dependent on nutrition and insulin secretion. Postnatal linear growth is dependent on thyroid hormone and growth hormone (GH), which are mediated through

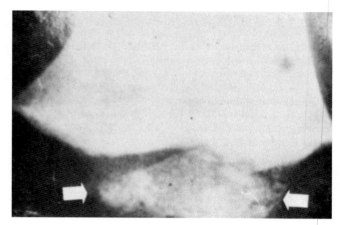

Figure 49-22. Epiphyseal dysgenesis of the distal femoral center.

insulin-like growth factor type 1 and its receptor. Similar synergistic effects between thyroid hormone and growth hormone can be observed in skeletal maturation. Thyroid hormone exerts its effects together with multiple hormones and growth factors. When primary hypothyroidism occurs, dental eruption, linear growth, and skeletal maturation are retarded. Retardation of skeletal maturation may be severe and is associated with immature skeletal proportions and facial contours, which contribute to the characteristic body configuration of hypothyroidism (long torso compared to short length of arms and legs) that is different from that seen in stunted growth caused by isolated GH deficiency. Ossification of cartilage is also disturbed in hypothyroidism, leading to epiphyseal dysgenesis in radiographs of the ossifying epiphyseal centers (Fig. 49-22). Growth rate and adult height are normal in children with congenital hypothyroidism in whom thyroid hormone therapy is consistently maintained.[34]

Calcitonin

In addition to the classic thyroid hormones (T_4 and T_3), a calcium-lowering hormone, thyrocalcitonin (i.e., calcitonin), is secreted by the parafollicular cells of the thyroid. Although calcitonin has hypocalcemic and hypophosphatemic actions when administered to humans, its physiologic role is not yet clearly understood. In normal newborn infants, a physiologic nadir in serum calcium concentration occurs at 24 to 48 hours of age, potentially related to delayed responsiveness of calcitonin. Thyroidectomy does not lead to hypercalcemia because there is secretion of calcitonin from extrathyroidal organs such as the brain, thymus, lung, gastrointestinal tract, and bladder.

SYNTHESIS, RELEASE, TRANSPORT, AND USE OF THYROID HORMONES

The biologically active thyroid hormones T_4 (also known as L-thyroxine) and T_3 are iodinated amino acids. Their synthesis starts within the follicular cells.

Iodine Metabolism

Iodine is supplied to the body mainly through dietary intake, but it can be absorbed readily from the skin, lungs, and mucous membranes. Application of iodine-containing ointment or lotion to the skin, common during procedures with premature or sick infants, causes very high levels of iodide in circulation and promptly blocks thyroid hormone release from the thyroid gland. Although some organic iodine compounds, including T_4 and T_3, can be absorbed unchanged from the gastrointestinal tract, most are reduced and absorbed as inorganic iodide. One fourth to one third of ingested iodide is taken up by the thyroid; this is the basis for radioiodine uptake studies.

This iodide-trapping mechanism involves an active transport process (an iodide pump [iodide symporter]) that requires oxidative phosphorylation. The iodide pump is a major rate-limiting step in thyroid hormone biosynthesis and, when it is defective, is a rare cause of congenital goitrous hypothyroidism.[15] The iodide pump is present at both the basal and apical surfaces of follicular cells. At the basal cell surface, the pump concentrates iodide in the cells by transporting them from the extracellular space. At the apical cell surface, the pump pushes iodide into the follicular lumen as a secondary reservoir. The mechanism is capable of maintaining intrathyroidal iodide concentration at a 20-fold to 100-fold higher level than that of serum. Some anions—bromide (Br^{2-}), nitrate (NO_2^-), thiocyanate (SCN^{2-}), perchlorate (ClO_4^{2-}), and technetium pertechnetate (TcO_4^{2-})—are capable of competitively inhibiting iodide transport.

Iodide is immediately oxidized to an active form for iodination of thyroglobulin (TG) by a peroxidase enzyme system.[15] TG, a glycoprotein, is synthesized by the ribosomes of the follicular cells. Iodation of TG (organification) appears to occur at the cell colloid-lumen interface. Almost all the iodine taken up by the thyroid is rapidly incorporated into the 3 and the 5 positions of the many tyrosyl residues of TG to form monoiodothyronine (MIT) and diiodothyronine (DIT). Once it is organically bound to tyrosyl residues, iodine can no longer be readily released from the thyroid. Defects in iodide oxidation or organification can be seen in several types of goitrous cretinism.

Synthesis of Triiodothyronine and Thyroxine

The synthesis of T_3 requires the coupling of an MIT and a DIT molecule, accompanied by elimination of an alanine residue. T_4 is formed by the coupling of two DIT molecules. These reactions occur within the structure of TG and involve oxidative processes, probably catalyzed by thyroid peroxidase as well.

Secretion of Triiodothyronine and Thyroxine

Secretion of T_4 and T_3 into the circulation requires the liberation of these moieties from TG.[45] TG molecules pass from the lumen of the follicles into the follicular cells (endocytosis), where colloid droplets are ingested by lysosomes and undergo proteolysis. Congenital hypothyroidism may result from abnormal TG synthesis or metabolism. Of the about 125 tyrosyl residues in TG, only about 10 form iodothyronines, and

another 20 consist of MIT and DIT. After proteolysis of TG, the freed MIT and DIT are deiodinated by iodotyrosine deiodinase, and the liberated iodide is recycled by the thyroid for reiodination of new TG. A defect in the deiodination mechanism of freed iodotyrosines results in depletion of iodine by release from the thyroid gland into the circulation and then excretion into the urine, resulting in goitrous cretinism.

Serum Protein Binding or Transport

The thyroid is the only source of T_4, and its blood concentration is 50 to 100 times greater than that of T_3. T_4 and T_3 secreted into the circulation are transported by loose attachment, through noncovalent bonds, to the plasma proteins. Three proteins play a role in the transport system. More than 75% of T_4 is normally bound to thyroxine-binding globulin (TBG). A second carrier protein is TTR (formerly called T_4-binding prealbumin); about 15% of T_4 is bound to TTR. A third protein is serum albumin, a high-capacity, low-affinity, iodothyronine-binding protein that usually transports less than 10% of the circulating T_4. While T_4 binds with all three proteins, T_3 binds only with TBG and albumin, and its binding affinity is much less than that of T_4. The free T_4 (FT_4) concentration more accurately indicates the metabolic status of the individual than total T_4 or T_3 does because only the free hormones can enter the cells to exert their effects. If the capacity of TBG is increased, a rise in the concentration of total hormones will follow, and the concentration of free hormones will be maintained without significant change.

Monodeiodination of Thyroxine

Monodeiodination of T_4 occurs in many tissues through the action of three distinct deiodinase enzymes. Type I deiodinase, or 5'-monodeiodinase, is found in peripheral tissues such as the liver and kidney. Deiodination at the 5' position of T_4 in peripheral tissues generates T_3, the iodothyronine that mediates the metabolic effects of thyroid hormone. Eighty percent of circulating T_3 is produced by the monodeiodination of T_4. However, the relative serum levels of T_4 and T_3 do not reflect the intracellular proportions of the hormones. The tissue distribution of T_3 may differ greatly from that of T_4 from tissue to tissue. The plasma half-life of T_3 is one day, compared with 6.9 days for T_4. However, the plasma half-life of T_4 is much shorter (3.6 days) in neonates. Most T_3 is localized in cells, whereas T_4 is found mainly in the extracellular space. The metabolic effects of T_3 are mediated through binding to specific receptors in the DNA response element that regulates transcription. It also interacts with membranous, mitochondrial, and cytosolic binding sites. The direct binding of T_4 in fetal neural tissue may be important in early neural development in order to permit intracellular deiodination to T_3.

Neural tissue requires FT_4 (and does not bind T_3). Intracellularly, the FT_4 is converted to FT_3 by type II deiodinase. Type II deiodinase regulates T_3 production from T_4 in the pituitary, neuroglial cells, and astrocytes and is involved in the control of TSH secretion.[44]

Type III deiodinase, or 5-deiodinase, regulates peripheral deiodination of T_4 at the 5 position on the thyronine molecule instead of 5' and generates reverse T_3 (rT_3). Serum rT_3

concentration parallels that of T_3 in normal circumstances but not in fetal life, starvation, or patients with severe nonthyroidal illnesses (e.g., euthyroid sick syndrome, nonthyroidal illness syndrome). rT_3 is generally metabolically inactive, although weak nuclear binding activity has been reported.

REGULATION OF THYROID FUNCTION

Control of thyroid hormone secretion is centered in the hypothalamic-pituitary-thyroid axis. Basophilic cells of the anterior pituitary gland synthesize and store thyrotropin (TSH), a glycoprotein capable of rapidly increasing intrathyroidal cyclic adenosine monophosphate (cAMP). TSH release from the pituitary causes an increased uptake of iodine by the thyroid, accelerates virtually all steps of iodothyronine synthesis and release, and increases the size and vascularity of the thyroid. These changes are mediated by activation of adenylate cyclase and tyrosine kinase. Human chorionic gonadotropin (hCG) weakly competes with TSH for receptors on thyroid follicular cells. Hyperthyroidism seen in patients with choriocarcinoma can be explained by this mechanism. Similarly, certain immunoglobulins—among them TSH-binding inhibiting immunoglobulins and TSI (discussed later)—found in autoimmune thyroid diseases, compete with TSH for binding to TSH receptors. Graves disease can be explained by this mechanism.

Secretion and plasma levels of TSH are inversely related to circulating levels of FT_3 and FT_4. The inhibitory feedback action of FT_3 and FT_4 involves a direct action of these hormones on the pituitary gland without involving the hypothalamus. Therefore, secretion of TSH is regulated directly by the ambient intrapituitary T_3 concentration and intrapituitary deiodination of T_4 to T_3 by type II monodeiodinase activity.[44] A progressive decline in the T_4 secretion rate with increasing age partially reflects maturational changes in thyrotropin-releasing hormone (TRH) and TSH secretion.[16,17]

The hypothalamus secretes TRH, a tripeptide that stimulates release of TSH by the pituitary gland. Although precise anatomic locations of TRH biosynthesis are not known, TRH synthetase is found in the median eminence and ventral and dorsal hypothalamus. When TRH is infused, it rapidly stimulates release of TSH into the circulation, and plasma TSH reaches a peak value in 20 to 30 minutes. Plasma half-life of TRH is extremely short, probably not exceeding 4 minutes. Production of TRH is modulated by both peripheral and hypothalamic thermal receptors. Exposure to a cold environment increases TRH synthetase activity. This activity is reduced in hypothyroid animals and increased in hyperthyroid animals. The hypothalamus may regulate the setpoint of feedback control as a thermostat through TRH, with iodothyronines playing a positive-feedback role in TRH synthesis. This control probably operates in neonates whose circulating TSH becomes rapidly elevated after parturition. After administration of TRH, there is an increase in the secretion of TSH, prolactin, and GH in normal neonates and older patients with pituitary tumors.

A circadian variation of circulating TSH has been found in normal children and adults.[44] A peak TSH concentration (about 3 to 4 mU/L) develops between 10:00 PM and 4:00 AM

and is about twofold higher (50% to 300% higher) than the afternoon (2:00 PM to 6:00 PM) nadir values. This nocturnal TSH surge is not directly related to sleep; it is blunted or absent in central (secondary or tertiary) hypothyroidism but maintained in primary hypothyroidism. The circadian pattern of TSH is not yet present in neonates but has been noted to be present in infants as young as 4 months of age.

In most children with idiopathic hypopituitarism, TSH release after TRH administration is normal, indicating impaired TRH secretion rather than a primary TSH deficiency.[55] TRH-mediated TSH release can be augmented by administration of theophylline or estradiol and may be blunted by the administration of L-dopa, somatostatin, or glucocorticoids. However, clinically significant hypothyroidism rarely occurs after prolonged administration of glucocorticoids or adrenocorticotropic hormone (ACTH).

In addition to hypothalamic-pituitary regulation, the thyroid is responsive to an intrinsic autoregulatory mechanism, intrathyroidal iodide, which compensates for fluctuation in dietary iodine intake. However, iodide trapping by the follicular cells is modulated by variations in dietary iodine intake within the physiologic range.

LABORATORY TESTS USED IN THE DIAGNOSIS OF THYROID DISEASE IN INFANCY AND CHILDHOOD

Concentration of Circulating Thyroid Hormones

With the development of sensitive methods, more tests to determine thyroid function and disease have become available in hospitals and reference laboratories (Table 49-6). Concomitantly, many previously used thyroid function tests are now obsolete, such as the protein-bound iodine test.

Total plasma or serum TSH, T_4, T_3, and rT_3 can be determined by specific competitive assays. These procedures require a very small quantity of blood (<50 μL), an advantage exploited for screening neonates for hypothyroidism. Determination of TSH is the most sensitive test to detect primary hypothyroidism, or thyroid gland failure.[5]

Thyroxine

The plasma pool of T_4 constitutes a large protein-bound reservoir; this pool turns over slowly. Therefore, T_4 measurement usually reflects the adequacy of the hormonal supply. The normal level of T_4 is age dependent in infancy and childhood, particularly during the neonatal period. T_4 reaches a peak concentration shortly after birth and declines slowly, gradually approaching the adult normal range in puberty.[16] The range of normal levels for each age group is also wide. Normal adult values of serum T_4 by radioimmunoassay are about 8.3 ± 2.4 μg/dL (see Appendix B). However, it should be kept in mind that more than 99% of circulating T_4 is bound to serum thyroid hormone–binding proteins. Any change or abnormality in the concentration of these proteins, particularly TBG, can affect the T_4 level. Several clinical situations and pharmacologic agents can alter the levels of TBG or transthyretin (TTR).

TABLE 49-6	Laboratory Tests Used for the Diagnosis of Thyroid Disorders and Assessment of Thyroid Function in Infancy and Childhood

Serum Tests

Thyrotropin (TSH)

Thyroid hormones: thyroxine (T_4), free T_4 by analogue methods (initial screen) and direct dialysis (definitive method), triiodothyronine (T_3)

Thyroid hormone-binding protein: thyroid-binding globulin (TBG)

Thyroid autoantibodies: thyroglobulin antibodies (TGAb), thyroperoxidase (microsomal) antibodies (TPOAb), TSH-receptor antibodies (TRAb) by TBII or TSI methods

Thyroglobulin (TG)

Imaging Tests

Thyroid scan with ^{99m}Tc-pertechnetate or ^{123}I-iodide

Thyroid ultrasound

Miscellaneous Tests

Assessment of skeletal maturation

In vivo isotopic tests: ^{123}I-iodide uptake test; perchlorate discharge test at 2 hours after isotope ingestion

Thyrotropin-releasing hormone (TRH) stimulation test

TSH surge test

Urinary iodine excretion

Drug Effects on Thyroid Concentrations

Certain anticonvulsants not only bind competitively to TBG but also interfere with T_4 assays, without greatly influencing the TSH level in a person with an otherwise normal thyroid reserve. These drugs include phenytoin, valproate, primidone, and carbamazepine. As much as twice the dose of drugs such as carbamazepine may be required in a patient receiving T_4 therapy. In addition, T_4 dose requirement may double in a patient receiving carbamazepine. Other drugs, such as furosemide, salicylate, and L-asparaginase, compete with thyroid hormone for binding with plasma proteins and can alter the levels of T_4, T_3, FT_4, and FT_3. Phenobarbital increases hepatic binding of T_4 and its disposal without altering circulating levels of thyroid hormone. Propylthiouracil (PTU), propranolol, dexamethasone, and some cholecystographic dyes inhibit peripheral conversion of T_4 to T_3. This effect of PTU is separate from its action on thyroid hormone biosynthesis by the thyroid gland. Administration of T_3 results in a decrease in T_4 because it suppresses endogenous T_4 secretion.

Amiodarone, an antiarrhythmic drug, contains covalently bound iodine and can alter thyroid test results.[6] It inhibits the hepatic conversion of T_4 to T_3 and decreases the clearance of T_4. FT_4 and rT_3 are increased, and T_3 and FT_3 are decreased.

Because of its high content of iodine, amiodarone can also result in either hypothyroidism or hyperthyroidism and may cause congenital goitrous hypothyroidism when it is administered to pregnant women. This effect is analogous to direct exposure of the fetus or infant to high doses of iodine.

Triiodothyronine

When TSH becomes elevated, the percentage of T_3 produced by the thyroid gland is increased. Serum concentration of T_3 can vary from day to day. Because of the overall small quantity of T_3 in serum, its level may not fall below the normal range until T_4 is critically low. Therefore, serum T_3 is not very useful in evaluation of patients for possible hypothyroidism. T_3 is physiologically low in the fetus and cord blood, but rises promptly after birth to levels greater than those in older children and adults. T_3 and FT_3 are also low during nonthyroidal illness. Normal serum T_3 concentrations vary among laboratories but generally range from about 100 to 220 ng/dL in children and 80 to 200 ng/dL in adults.[5]

Reverse Triiodothyronine

Most hormonally inactive rT_3 is derived from deiodination of T_4 and represents a deiodination rate similar to that of T_4-to-T_3 conversion in normal adults. Serum half-life is very short, less than one half that of T_3. Concentration of rT_3 usually parallels that of T_3. However, rT_3 is disproportionately high in the fetus, in the early neonatal period, and in severe nonthyroidal illness, probably reflecting altered tissue metabolism of T_4.[5] Normal adult serum level of rT_3 is 30 to 80 ng/dL.

Free Hormones

FT_4 in serum can be estimated by direct dialysis. This method depends on the FT_4 concentration being governed by equilibrium in levels of binding proteins, protein-bound T_4, and FT_4, following the law of mass action. In clinical settings, FT_4 does not depend on the T_4-binding capacity as such because a change in such a capacity is soon compensated for by a change in the amount of T_4 released from the thyroid. To estimate FT_4, serum is placed in a dialysis cell on one side of a semipermeable dialysis membrane, with a buffer solution on the other side. T_4 equilibrates across the membrane. Bound T_4 remains with serum, and free T_4 crosses the membrane and enters the buffer solution. T_4 is measured in the buffer solution, and the amount corresponds to the level of endogenous FT_4. FT_3 levels in the serum can be measured in the same dialysate as that used for FT_4. Other analogue methods for determining FT_4 have been introduced.

The principle of analogue methods is that the rate of binding of labeled hormones to antibodies depends on the FT_4 concentration during a timed incubation. Analogue methods are less expensive, can be performed more rapidly than the direct dialysis method, and are acceptable for routine testing in children. However, FT_4 analogue methods may not provide an accurate assessment of FT_4 in some neonates, patients receiving medications that interfere with T_4 binding, chronically or critically ill neonates or children, or patients with very low levels of TBG.[51]

When hypothalamic or pituitary hypothyroidism is suspected, the definitive test to measure the FT_4 is by direct dialysis. This test is readily available in specialized commercial laboratories. Because there is a delay in obtaining results, the specimen should be collected and T_4 therapy started. If there is an associated ACTH or cortisol deficiency, hydrocortisone therapy should be started at least 6 to 8 hours before T_4 therapy is initiated.[19]

Measurement of FT_3 is not currently part of standard care. In the future, FT_3 measurements may be shown to be useful in assessing hypothyroidism. Currently, FT_3 may be useful when the diagnosis of thyrotoxicosis is suspected and TSH is suppressed but values for T_4, T_3, or both are normal. The approximate serum values for normal adults are 1.0 to 2.4 ng/dL for FT_4 and 240 to 620 pg/dL for FT_3. The range of normal values for infants and young children is probably higher than that for adults, but exact ranges have not been established.

Proteins That Bind to Thyroid Hormones

Because concentrations of T_4 and T_3 are affected by those of thyroid hormone–binding proteins and by the degree of their saturation at the binding site, T_4 must be interpreted with a simultaneous evaluation of these proteins. The simplest approach is to measure TSH and FT_4 (by dialysis or analogue methods) and not measure T_4 at all, avoiding the issue of changes in levels of thyroid hormone–binding proteins.

The alternative approach is to determine T_3U, which is a rapid, indirect assessment of the binding proteins. However, it may not be accurate in the same clinical conditions as those described previously for the FT_4 analogue methods. The T_3U value is then multiplied by the total T_4 value to give the FT_4 index, which is essentially a mathematically corrected T_4 value for the degree of saturation of the thyroid hormone–binding proteins. Direct dialysis is the best FT_4 method, especially in infants. Analogue methods are very cost-effective in measuring FT_4 and will probably replace methods that measure the FT_4 index.

In general, when TBG is increased in a euthyroid individual, T_4 is elevated and T_3U is low, but FT_4 is about normal. The reverse situation is observed in individuals with low TBG, but again FT_4 is normal. The administration of a drug that competes with T_4 for TBG-binding sites results in low T_4 and high T_3U but normal FT_4.

Serum TBG is determined by radioimmunoassay in commercial laboratories, and its measurement is useful in the quantitation of abnormal levels of TBG. Because most T_4 is bound to TBG, these measurements give a good approximation of the T_4-binding protein capacity. The binding capacity of TBG is increased in many clinical situations, including those during pregnancy and in neonates. It may also be increased in patients with hypothyroidism, liver disease, porphyria, or AIDS.

Pharmacologic agents that increase TBG levels include estrogens, methadone, and heroin. The concentration of TBG may be decreased in preterm infants and in hyperthyroidism, hypercortisolism, acromegaly, diabetic ketoacidosis, chronic hepatic diseases, alcoholism, nephrotic syndrome, other chronic renal diseases, and protein-calorie malnutrition. Drugs that decrease TBG levels include androgens, anabolic steroids, danazol, glucocorticoids, and L-asparaginase. Pharmacologic agents that compete with T_4 for TBG-binding sites include salicylates, phenytoin, and possibly other anticonvulsants, hypolipemic agents, sulfonylureas, diazepam, heparin, and fenclofenac. These agents give falsely low T_4 and falsely high T_3U values. TSH and FT_4 determinations by direct dialysis method are usually normal. The normal value for TBG in adults is about 1.2 to 2.8 mg/dL.

Thyrotropin

Measurements of TSH and FT_4 are the most important tools for screening thyroid function. Serum TSH is measured by specific competitive-binding isotopic and nonisotopic methods, and values are expressed in milliunits per liter (mU/L) of an international reference standard. TSH is the most sensitive test for primary hypothyroidism at any age and is used in many neonatal thyroid screening programs. Serum TSH is also an indicator of the adequacy of thyroid hormone replacement therapy and is used in assessment of the hypothalamic-pituitary-thyroid axis by the TSH surge test and the TRH test (see later discussions). The normal adult value is 0.2 to 3.0 mU/L.[5] TSH is elevated in primary hypothyroidism. A surge of TSH release also occurs at parturition and reaches a peak within 2 hours after birth. TSH in the cord serum and the infant's serum after the first day of postnatal life is usually less than 20 mU/L. Therefore, TSH is the most important test to screen for primary congenital hypothyroidism. The target range for TSH during thyroid hormone therapy for primary hypothyroidism is 0.5 to 2 mU/L. The highly sensitive TSH assay can also be used in identifying individuals with thyrotoxicosis in whom TSH is suppressed to less than 0.01 mU/L.

Thyroid Autoantibodies

Numerous methods have been used for detection of a large variety of thyroid antibodies. Assays for thyroglobulin antibodies (TGAb) and thyroperoxidase (microsomal) antibodies (TPOAb) are widely available. These antibodies are found in Hashimoto thyroiditis and in about 2% of the adult population. TSH receptor stimulating and blocking antibodies may be detected in the sera of patients with autoimmune thyroid diseases and are known as TSH receptor antibodies (TRAb). TRAb that are stimulatory are found in the sera of patients with active Graves disease and are known as TSI. TRAb that are inhibitory are called TBII.

Mothers with primary hypothyroidism and Hashimoto thyroiditis may have circulating serum TBII or antibodies that block the TSH receptor. These mothers give birth to children with a transient form of congenital hypothyroidism as a result of the transplacental transfer of TBII. The disease may recur in infants of subsequent pregnancies if the high-affinity antibody persists in the mother's circulation. The half-life of immunoglobulins in the neonate is about 2 weeks, and TRAb usually disappear from the serum of affected infants by 6 to 8 weeks of age.

Mothers with Graves hyperthyroidism may have TBII but more commonly have TSI. These mothers give birth to children with a transient form of hyperthyroidism as a result of the transplacental transfer of TSI. This disease may also recur in infants of subsequent pregnancies if the high-affinity antibody persists in the maternal circulation. Hyperthyroidism in the affected infant may persist for 2 to 6 months.

Thyroglobulin

It was previously believed that TG was present only in the thyroid gland. With the development of radioimmunoassay for TG, it is now known that some of it appears in the circulation. The mean value of TG for normal adults is 5 ng/mL, with a range from less than 1 to about 30 ng/mL. The median value for preterm infants at birth is high (102 ng/mL), rapidly decreases during the first 30 days of life for reasons not yet understood, and further decreases during infancy and childhood to the adult mean value by 20 years of age.

In athyreotic cretinism, TG is not detectable. However, in the form of autoimmune congenital hypothyroidism caused by antibodies that block the TSH receptor, TG may be detectable even when the radioactive iodine scan suggests an absent thyroid gland. Ultrasound identifies the thyroid gland; TG levels may be elevated when the thyroid gland is hyperactive, as in endemic goiter, subacute thyroiditis, toxic nodular goiter, and Graves disease. TG cannot be reliably measured in Hashimoto thyroiditis because of the possible presence of TGAb. TG levels are often greatly increased in papillary-follicular carcinoma but not in medullary or anaplastic carcinoma of the thyroid. TG levels are useful not only in the differential diagnosis, but also in follow-up studies to monitor patients for recurrence of papillary-follicular carcinoma.

Thyroid Imaging

The development of sensitive and specific assays to quantitate thyroid hormone and TSH has largely obviated the need for radioiodine uptake studies in childhood. As a result, radioactive thyroid scans are rarely performed in infants and children. Measurement of TG concentration can identify the presence or absence of thyroid glandular tissue. Ultrasonography of the thyroid gland is useful for visualization of normal-sized glands and goiters. It is also used to distinguish solid and cystic nodules of the thyroid. Ultrasonography can identify dysgenetic thyroid glands.[37] Slower correction of TSH may be seen with dysgenetic glands than with eutopic glands. Ultrasonography should be used as the first imaging tool, with a scan performed to distinguish agenesis from ectopia. However, hypoplastic or ectopic glands may be missed by this technique. When a scan is necessary, ^{123}I or ^{99m}Tc should be used to reduce radiation exposure to the child. The half-life of ^{123}I is 13.3 hours, compared with 8 days for [131]I.

Radioiodine uptake studies are invaluable for diagnosing certain inborn errors of thyroid hormone synthesis, such as the iodide-trapping defect and the iodide oxidation or organification defect. ^{99m}Tc-pertechnetate can also be used for iodide-trapping studies because this anion is trapped by the thyroid in a manner similar to iodine, but is not organified and is therefore discharged early from the thyroid gland. In addition to the thyroid gland, the salivary glands, gastric mucosa, uterus, small intestine, mammary glands, and placenta are capable of concentrating iodine. In patients with goitrous cretinism caused by iodide-trapping defects, the ability of salivary glands to trap iodide can be exploited for diagnostic purposes. The trapping defect is shared by the

thyroid and the salivary glands in these patients. The perchlorate discharge test is performed during the radioiodine uptake test to detect the presence of a defect in the oxidation of iodide to iodine (see "Congenital Hypothyroidism").

Thyrotropin-Releasing Hormone

In 2002, the TRH test became commercially unavailable in the United States. Historically, TRH was the first identified hypothalamic neuropeptide and had been used in clinical assessment since the 1960s. The following section regarding the TRH test is retained in this chapter for reference in the event that the TRH test again becomes a tool available to the clinician.

Given current ultrasensitive TSH assays, the TRH test is required only when TSH is mildly elevated (4.5 to 10 mU/L) to help determine whether the child has mild primary hypothyroidism (as opposed to central hypothyroidism) or for the assessment of possible thyroid hormone resistance. A suppressed basal TSH value is significant and sufficient for the diagnosis of hyperthyroidism, and a basal TSH concentration of higher than 10 mU/L (after the first week of age) is significant and sufficient for the diagnosis of primary hypothyroidism.

A bolus infusion of TRH (7 μg/kg of body weight) results in increased TSH that peaks at 20 to 30 minutes. A peak increment of 10 to 30 mU/L is seen in healthy children, with a decline to basal TSH levels by 2 to 3 hours. Serum T_3 levels peak at 3 to 4 hours and T_4 levels at 6 to 9 hours after TRH. Therefore, the TRH test can be used to examine responsiveness of both TSH to TRH and of thyroid gland to TSH, when necessary. Patients with primary hypothyroidism have an exaggerated TSH response. Patients with hyperthyroidism and those receiving T_4 replacement do not respond to TRH stimulation because of chronic suppression of TSH by thyroid hormone.[19]

The TRH test may be helpful in confirming central hypothyroidism (pituitary or hypothalamic) in some patients. Those with secondary (pituitary) hypothyroidism do not respond to TRH.[19] In some patients with tertiary hypothyroidism (hypothalamic TRH deficiency), a delayed response of TSH to TRH stimulation is seen, so TSH at 60 minutes is higher than that present at 20 to 30 minutes. However, many patients with tertiary hypothyroidism have a normal response to TRH.

Thyroid-Stimulating Hormone Surge Test

Central hypothyroidism is diagnosed in infants who have low or low-normal FT_4, no TSH elevation, and other common features of hypopituitarism (e.g., hypoglycemia, microphallus). More subtle central hypothyroidism (FT_4 in the lowest third of the normal range) can be confirmed in children older than 1 year by the TSH surge test.[44] This test is not useful in infants younger than 6 months, before development of the circadian pattern of TSH secretion.

The TSH surge test is performed by obtaining blood for TSH assay at the usual time of the nadir of the circadian variation of TSH (the mean of two or three samples between 10:00 AM and 6:00 PM) and again at the usual time of peak TSH secretion (the mean of the three highest sequential samples between 10:00 PM and 4:00 AM). The mean nadir and peak TSH values are calculated. Normal night-time (peak) TSH values are 50% to 300% higher than those (nadir) obtained during the day. Blunting or absence of this rise confirms central hypothyroidism.[44] At age over 2y, with FT4 below 1.2 mg/dL, 8 AM to 4 PM TSH ratio below 1.3 also confirms central hypothyroidism.[44a]

EMBRYOGENESIS

The major portion of the human thyroid originates from the median anlage, the tissue that arises from the pharyngeal floor (toward the back of the future tongue) and is identifiable in the 17-day-old embryo.[40] The median anlage is initially in close contact with the endothelial tubes of the embryonic heart. With the descent of the heart, the rapidly growing median thyroid is progressively pulled caudally until it reaches its final position in front of the second to sixth tracheal ring by 45 to 50 days of gestation. The pharyngeal region contracts to become a narrow stalk called the *thyroglossal duct*, which subsequently atrophies. The descent of the heart may influence the downward movement of the thyroid because of topographic contact. The median anlage usually grows caudally so that no lumen is left in the tract of its descent. An ectopic thyroid gland or persistent thyroglossal duct or cyst results from abnormalities of thyroid descent. Lateral parts of the descending median anlage expand to form the thyroid lobes and the isthmus.[40]

The second source of thyroid tissue is composed of a pair of ultimobranchial bodies arising from the caudal extension of the fourth pharyngeal pouch. These bodies are initially connected to the pharynx by the pharyngobranchial duct (late seventh week). The pharyngeal connection is subsequently lost, and the ductal lumen becomes obliterated. The ultimobranchial bodies are incorporated into the expanding lateral lobes of the median anlage. They contribute little to the future size of the thyroid, and their differentiation appears to require the influence of the median anlage. Parafollicular or C cells arise from the ultimobranchial bodies in mammals and are the source of calcitonin.

By the latter part of the 10th week of gestation, the histogenesis of the thyroid is virtually complete, although the follicles do not contain colloid.[40] A single layer of endothelial cells surrounds the follicular lumen. T_4 has been detected in the serum of a 78-day-old fetus. At this age, the fetal thyroid is capable of trapping and oxidizing iodide.[19] Therefore, the fetal thyroid begins to secrete thyroid hormone and contributes to the fetal circulation of thyroid hormone by the beginning of the second trimester.

At the same time as the development of the thyroid gland, the fetal pituitary and hypothalamus are also forming and beginning to function. The anterior pituitary gland is derived from the Rathke pouch, which originates at the roof of the pharynx. Histologic differentiation of pituitary cells can be observed by 7 to 10 weeks of gestation, and TSH can be detected in fetal blood by 10 to 12 weeks.[28] The hypothalamus develops from the ventral portion of the diencephalon. TRH has been found in fetal whole-brain extracts by 30 days and in the hypothalamus by 9 weeks of gestation.

Knowledge regarding the genetic basis of normal thyroid physiology and disease has been rapidly developing and will continue to advance (Table 49-7).[27] For additional updates, the reader can consult the following websites: www.ncbi.nlm.nih.gov/PubMed, www.ncbi.nlm.nih.gov/Omim, and www.uwcm.ac.uk/uwcm/mg/hgmd0.html.

THYROID FUNCTION: FETAL-MATERNAL RELATIONSHIP

In considering the fetal-maternal relationship, the placenta is of major importance. TSH does not cross the placental barrier, whereas TRH does. Although there is some maternal-to-fetal transport of T_4 during the third trimester, transfer during the first trimester from the mother to the fetus may be greater because fetal brain development appears to depend on maternally derived T_4. Maternal hypothyroidism during early gestation can lead to neurologic damage of the fetus.[30] Because the placenta rapidly deiodinates T_4 into biologically inactive rT_3 and DIT, transplacental transfer of maternal T_4 during later stages of pregnancy is limited. However, this T_4 transfer in a fetus with a total inability to synthesize T_4 results in a fetal T_4 concentration that is 25% to 50% of that found in normal neonates. Therefore, in a mother with normal thyroid function, the hypothyroid fetus is somewhat protected. The mother with hypothyroidism and a normal fetus may have a relative thyroid deficit in the first trimester of gestation, whereas the mother with hypothyroidism and a hypothyroid fetus may experience a more significant deficit.[20]

Iodine deficiency may be a factor contributing to concurrent maternal and fetal hypothyroidism. The ideal allowance of iodine for pregnant women is 250 to 300 μg daily.[14,21] Iodides cross the placenta readily. Iodine in excess can also cause problems in the fetus. Iodides and iodine, when given in large quantities, produce a transient inhibition of T_4 synthesis by diminishing iodination, probably through effects on thyroidal autoregulation. Therefore, iodine given to the mother in large amounts causes goiter in the offspring (Fig. 49-23). Even iodine applied topically to the mother, such as the vaginal application of povidone-iodine, can adversely affect thyroid function of the newborn and may cause transient primary hypothyroidism.

Other clinically important compounds that can affect fetal thyroid function by crossing the placenta from the mother to the fetus are antithyroid drugs, environmental goitrogens, endocrine disruptors, and thyroid antibodies.[19,32] Antithyroid drugs include perchlorates and thionamide compounds such as thiourea, thiouracil, PTU, methimazole, and carbimazole. Transplacental transfer of these drugs can result in fetal goiter with or without hypothyroidism. Transfer of TSI across the placenta to the fetus can cause transient neonatal thyrotoxicosis (see "Thyrotoxicosis," later); the placental transfer of TBII can cause transient neonatal hypothyroidism.

Thyroid hormone can be detected in the amniotic fluid. However, T_4, FT_4, T_3, and TSH levels in the amniotic fluids correlate poorly with maternal or fetal serum levels. Although more invasive, cordocentesis provides levels that more accurately represent the fetal thyroid hormone status.[47] More than 20 case reports of highly elevated amniotic or fetal blood TSH concentrations (samples obtained between 24 and 38 weeks of gestation) in fetuses found to have large goiters

TABLE 49–7   Inherited Disorders of Thyroid Metabolism

Hypothalamic-Pituitary Development	Gene	Inheritance
Combined pituitary hormone deficiency	Mutations of *LHX3, HESX1, PROP1, POU1F1*	AR or AD
TRHR	Loss-of-function TRHR mutation	AR
TSH deficiency	TSH β-subunit mutation	AR
TSHR	Loss-of-function TSHR mutation Resistance to TSH with normal TSHR Gain-of-function TSHR mutation *GNAS1* mutations	AR or AD AD AD
Thyroid Gland Development	*TITF1* (haploinsufficiency) Mutations of *FOXE1, PAX8* *TTF2, NKX2-1, HHEX, BCL2*	AR or AD
Organification		
Iodide transport	Iodide symporter NIS *SLC5A5*	AR
TPO	TPO mutations *THOX2*	AR
Pendred syndrome	Pendred syndrome mutations	AR
Thyroid NADPH oxidase	*DUOX1* and *DUOX2* mutations	
TG	TG mutations	AR or AD
Iodide cycling	Defect not known	?AR
Thyroid Hormone Transport		
TBG	TBG deficiency, partial or complete X-linked recessive TBG excess	X-linked recessive X-linked recessive
TTR	TTR mutations	AD
Albumin	Albumin mutations	AD
Generalized Thyroid Hormone Resistance	THR mutations THR-β	AD

AD, autosomal dominant; AR, autosomal recessive; GNAS, gene encoding G$_s$-protein α subunit; NADPH, reduced nicotinamide-adenine dinucleotide phosphate; TBG, thyroxine-binding globulin; TG, thyroglobulin; THR, thyroid hormone receptor; TPO, thyroid peroxidase; TRHR, thyrotropin-releasing hormone receptor; TSH, thyrotropin; TSHR, TSH receptor; TTR, transthyretin.
Adapted from Knobel M, Medeiros-Neto G: An outline of inherited disorders of the thyroid hormone generating system, *Thyroid* 13:771, 2003.

by ultrasonography have led to prenatal therapy by means of the intra-amniotic injection of thyroid hormone (T$_4$ or T$_3$). Treatment effects have included reduction of fetal goiter, reduction of polyhydramnios, and reduction or normalization of TSH.

T$_4$ is detectable in fetal serum by the 12th week of gestation.[47] Thereafter, both T$_4$ and FT$_4$ increase linearly in relation to gestational age. Mean cord concentration of T$_4$ between 20 and 30 weeks of gestation is 5.5 ± 1.6 μg/dL. Normal ranges have been published for thyroid hormone concentrations in third-trimester amniotic fluid.[47] At term, the T$_4$ reaches 12.6 ± 4.0 μg/dL in umbilical cord serum, which is 10% to 20% lower than the corresponding value in maternal serum. FT$_4$ in cord blood is equal to or higher than that in maternal blood. Fetal T$_4$ metabolism differs markedly from that of postnatal life. In the fetus, T$_4$ is metabolized predominantly to rT$_3$ rather than T$_3$.

The concentration of rT$_3$ in the fetus exceeds 250 ng/dL early in the third trimester and progressively decreases to 150 to 200 ng/dL at term.[28] By the third to fifth day after birth, a rapid decrease occurs in rT$_3$, which reaches adult levels by 1 to 2 months of age. Compared with T$_3$, rT$_3$ has minimum metabolic activity. Therefore, serum concentrations and production rates of rT$_3$ are much higher in the fetus, whereas both T$_3$ and FT$_3$ in the fetal circulation are lower than those in the adult. T$_3$ and FT$_3$ in cord blood have been shown to be 30% to 50% of the maternal concentrations at term.

TSH is also present in the 12-week-old fetus and rapidly rises thereafter, in parallel with the increasing FT$_4$. TSH does not correlate with fetal T$_4$ or maternal FT$_4$. TSH is higher in the fetus than in the mother. At term, the fetal value of TSH is more than twice that found in the mother. These findings suggest that fetal TSH regulates fetal thyroid function.

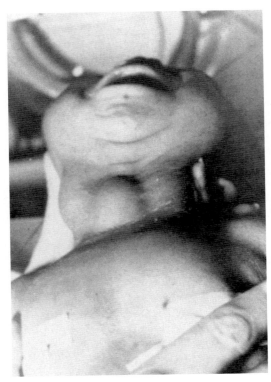

Figure 49–23. Iodine-induced goiter in a neonate. The lateral bulging of the neck is caused by enlarged lateral lobes of the thyroid.

T_4-binding proteins can also be detected in the 12-week-old fetus. During early fetal life, T_4 appears to be bound mainly to TTR and albumin. Fetal TBG increases rapidly and by midgestation reaches a level approaching that in a full-term infant. During early gestation, the rise in fetal TBG parallels the increase in T_4 bound to TBG. The binding capacity of TBG in premature and full-term infants is about 1.5 times that in the normal adult but lower than that in the mother. The high TBG in the neonate is caused by transplacental transfer of estrogens from the mother and to a large extent accounts for the high T_4 in infants. TBG remains essentially unchanged during the first 5 days of life. TTR is low in both newborn and maternal sera and plays a minor role after midgestation.

Shortly after birth, transient but marked hyperactivity occurs in the thyroid function of neonates (Tables 49-8 and 49-9). Within the first minutes of life, there is a dramatic release of TSH, reaching a peak level of about 100 mU/L at 30 minutes of age. This hypersecretion of TSH persists during the next 6 to 24 hours. Evidence shows that this acute rise in TSH may be stimulated at least partially by a drop in the body temperature of the fetus with birth. In response to the postnatal TSH surge, T_4, FT_4, and T_3 increase progressively during the first hours of extrauterine life, reaching a peak at about 48 hours of age. The increases in T_3 and FT_3 are more marked than those of T_4 and FT_4 during this period because of increased peripheral conversion of T_4 to T_3. Therefore, neonates experience a physiologic hyperthyroid state during the first few days of life. The absence of this chemically hyperthyroid state constitutes strong evidence of congenital hypothyroidism. Concentrations of thyroid hormone remain elevated during the first 2 weeks of life and fall gradually thereafter, with FT_4 reaching high-normal adult values by 4 to 6 weeks of age. True adult levels of T_4 and T_3 are not reached until puberty probably because TBG levels in children remain elevated compared with adults until mid-puberty (Table 49-8 and 49-9).

The postnatal TSH surge occurs even in preterm infants and those who are small for gestational age (SGA), although the changes in TSH and iodothyronines are less than those in healthy full-term infants. In preterm infants, T_4 concentrations may decline for a week and then gradually rise, remaining lower than those of full-term infants during the first weeks of life.[18] FT_4 is usually in the normal range for adults, although it is low compared with that in healthy full-term infants. T_4 varies in relation to TBG values. TSH returns to normal adult values after 3 to 10 days of postnatal life regardless of gestational age (see Tables 49-8 and 49-9) (see later section, "Transient Disorders of Thyroid Function").

In human milk, T_4 is present in very small amounts. The concentrations of T_3 and rT_3 in human milk vary from specimen to specimen. The T_3 concentration in breast milk is insufficient to prevent the detrimental effects of hypothyroidism, although it may alleviate the symptoms in certain cases.

The iodine kinetics in infants and children are different from those in adults. The thyroid weighs about 2 g at birth, which is about one tenth of its adult weight. The 24-hour ^{123}I uptake by the thyroid in the infant after 1 month of age is similar to that in the adult. Therefore, the concentration of ^{123}I per gram of thyroid tissue in the infant is greater than that in the adult. The thyroid of the infant is more susceptible than that of the adult to damage by radiation and to the blocking effects of iodine and other goitrogens. T_4 turnover rate is also higher in infants and children than that in adults, which accounts for their greater thyroid hormone requirements per unit of body weight.

CONGENITAL HYPOTHYROIDISM

Congenital hypothyroidism is a deficiency in thyroid hormone present at or before birth.[29] Prompt diagnosis is critical because a delay in treatment can lead to irreversible brain damage or cretinism. However, overt signs of hypothyroidism are rarely present at birth, and 95% of affected babies are asymptomatic. Dynamic changes in thyroid function after birth, limited dependence of peripheral tissues on thyroid hormone until late in fetal life, and deprivation of maternal hormones and factors acquired by transplacental transfer contribute to the difficulty in establishing a diagnosis. Newborn screening for hypothyroidism was first performed and consequently established in 1972 in Quebec, Canada, to permit early identification of infants at risk and allow prompt institution of thyroid hormone replacement therapy (see "Neonatal Screening for Hypothyroidism," later).[1,29]

TABLE 49-8 Representative Serum Values of Total and Free Thyroid Hormones, Thyroxine-Binding Globulin, and Thyrotropin in Cord Blood and Early Neonatal Period Compared with Adult and Maternal Values*

Reference	Source of Serum or Age of Infant	N	Thyroxine (T₄) (μg/dL)	Free T₄ (ng/dL)	Triiodothyronine (T₃) (ng/dL)	Free T₃ (ng/dL)	Thyroxine-Binding Globulin (TBG) (mg/dL)	Thyrotropin (TSH) (μ/L)
Erenberg, et al								
	Cord blood	26	11.9 ± 0.4	2.9 ± 0.1	50.5 ± 3.6	146 ± 12	5.4 ± 0.5	
	60 min	8-12			293	863		
	4 hr	10-21	16.2		419	1260		
	36-48 hr	9		7.0				
	60-72 hr	7-19		6.0	220	620		
	5 days	6	12.6					
	Pregnant women	17	14.3 ± 0.7	2.7 ± 0.2	173 ± 8	398 ± 30		8.7 ± 0.6
	Adults	40	8.3 ± 0.4	2.4 ± 0.1	122 ± 5	378 ± 27		3.5 ± 0.7
Abuid, et al								
	Cord blood	27-30	10.9 ± 0.3	2.2 ± 0.1	48 ± 3	130 ± 10		8.5 ± 0.7
	3 days	23-26	17.2 ± 0.5	4.9 ± 0.3	125 ± 8	410 ± 20		7.3 ± 1.0
	6 wk	15	10.3 ± 0.4	2.1 ± 0.1	163 ± 6	400 ± 20		<5
	Mothers at term	8	12.8 ± 1.4	1.4 ± 0.2	145 ± 12	310 ± 40		
	Adults	11	8.8 ± 0.5	1.9 ± 0.1	112 ± 5	290 ± 20		0.5 to 4.8

*T₄, T₃, TBG, and TSH were measured by radioimmunoassay methods, and free T₄ and free T₃ by assessment of the dialyzable fractions. All values are the mean or mean ± SEM.
Data from Abuid J, et al: Total and free tri-iodothyronine and thyroxine in early infancy, *J Clin Endocrinol Metab* 39:263, 1974; Erenberg A, et al: Total and free thyroid hormone concentrations in the neonatal period, *Pediatrics* 53:211, 1974.

TABLE 49–9 Normal Range for Thyroxine, Triiodothyronine, Thyroxine-Binding Globulin, and Thyrotropin in Infancy and Childhood*

Age	TOTAL T_4 (μg/dL) Mean	Range	TOTAL T_3 (ng/dL) Mean	Range	TBG (mg/dL) Mean	Range	TSH (mU/L) Mean	Range
Cord blood	10.2	7.4-13.0	45	15-75	5.6	—	9.0	<2.5-17.4
1-3 days	17.2	11.8-22.6	124	32-216	5.0	—	8.0	<2.5-13.3
1-2 wk	13.2	9.8-16.6	250	—	—	—	—	—
2-4 wk	11.0	7.0-15.0	160	160-240	—	—	4.0	0.6-6.0
1-4 mo	10.3	7.2-14.4	163	117-209	—	—	<2.5	<2.5
4-12 mo	11.0	7.8-16.5	176	110-280	4.4	3.1-5.6	2.1	0.5-4.8
1-5 yr	10.5	7.3-15.0	168	105-269	4.2	2.9-5.4	2.0	0.5-4.8
5-10 yr	9.3	6.4-13.3	150	94-241	3.8	2.5-5.0	2.0	0.5-4.8
10-15 yr	8.1	5.6-11.7	113	83-213	3.3	2.1-4.6	1.9	0.5-4.8
Adult	8.4	4.3-12.5	125	70-204	3.5	2.1-5.5	1.8	0.2-4.8

*T_4, T_3, TSH, and TBG are measured by radioimmunoassay. Range equals mean ± 2 SD.
T_4, thyroxine; T_3, triiodothyronine; TBG, thyroxine-binding globulin; TSH, thyrotropin.
From LaFranchi SH: Hypothyroidism, *Pediatr Clin North Am* 26:33, 1979.

Etiology and Pathogenesis

The etiologic classification of congenital hypothyroidism:
I. Primary hypothyroidism
  A. Defective embryogenesis of thyroid
    1. Agenesis (athyreosis)
    2. Dysgenesis
      a. Thyroid remnant in normal location (hypoplasia)
      b. Maldescent or ectopic thyroid gland (ectopia)
  B. Inborn error of hormone synthesis or metabolism (familial dyshormonogenesis)
    1. Iodide-trapping defect
    2. Iodide organification (oxidation) defect
      a. Without deafness
      b. With deafness (Pendred syndrome)
    3. Coupling defect of iodotyrosines
    4. Deiodination defect
      a. Generalized
      b. Limited to thyroid gland
      c. Limited to peripheral tissues
    5. TG synthetic defects
    6. Goiter with calcification
    7. Peripheral tissue resistance to thyroid hormone
    8. Unresponsiveness of thyroid to TSH
  C. Goitrous cretinism caused by maternal ingestion of goitrogens
  D. Iodine deficiency (endemic goiter)
II. Central hypothyroidism
  A. Genetic mutation or deletion (see Table 49-7)
    1. Isolated deficiency of TSH β-subunit
    2. Abnormality of hypothalamic-pituitary development, with multiple pituitary hormone deficiencies
  B. Midline congenital defect (septo-optic dysplasia, holoprosencephaly, cleft lip, single central incisor)
  C. Acquired birth injury (usually hypothalamic TRH deficiency) (birth injury, hemorrhage, hydrocephalus, meningitis, trauma, nonaccidental injury)

DEFECTIVE EMBRYOGENESIS OF THE THYROID

In contrast to the clear preponderance of thyroid disorders in females compared with males during childhood and adult life, the gender difference in incidence of congenital hypothyroidism is much less obvious. In North America, the female-to-male ratio is about 2:1, as detected by neonatal screening programs.[1] The relative incidences of each type of congenital hypothyroidism vary widely in different geographic locations.

In nongoitrous regions, defective embryogenesis of the thyroid accounts for 80% to 90% of nonendemic congenital hypothyroidism. Loss-of-function mutations of the TSH receptor gene lead to hypoplasia of the thyroid gland and TSH elevation (see Table 49-7).[27] Mutations in transcription factors (such as *PAX8* and *TTF2*) may be responsible for some cases of congenital hypothyroidism. Failure in the anatomic development of the thyroid gland may be complete or partial. Residual thyroid tissue in the normal position or in ectopic location is detected in 60% to 80% of infants and children with hypothyroidism. An ectopic thyroid is usually composed of a remnant of undescended thyroid tissue that is usually situated in the midline. Undescended thyroid is located at the base of the tongue in about half of the cases, between the tongue and the hyoid bone in about one fourth, and between the hyoid bone and the normal location in the remaining one fourth. Ectopic tissue is often capable of undergoing compensatory hypertrophy when hormone production becomes inadequate, and thus may be found as a midline mass. Etiology of defective embryogenesis of the thyroid is unknown. Dysgenesis of the thyroid can be a familial condition. The ectopic or dysgenetic tissue may show a transient iodine organification defect.

Neonates with congenital hypothyroidism do not have an increased incidence of TGAb or TPOAb, nor do mothers with these autoimmune antibodies appear to have a higher risk for giving birth to children with congenital hypothyroidism.

However, these antibodies, as well as inhibiting TRAb, are associated with transient neonatal hypothyroidism.[19] Some types of maternal autoimmune antibodies against the thyroid may play a role in pathogenesis of the thyroid gland. One mother with both TSI and TBII was reported to have given birth to euthyroid, hyperthyroid, and hypothyroid children in three successive pregnancies.

FAMILIAL DYSHORMONOGENESIS

Genetically determined errors of T_4 synthesis or metabolism involve a deficiency of one or more enzymes necessary at various stages of the biosynthetic and metabolic pathways. Impaired secretion of T_4 and T_3 results in hypersecretion of TSH, usually leading to compensatory hyperplasia of the thyroid. The familial forms of congenital hypothyroidism are usually referred to as *familial dyshormonogenesis*. Hypothyroidism, goiter, or both may be present in the newborn and infant, depending on the degree and time of onset of the hormonal deficiency. Family members of children with familial dyshormonogenesis often have less severe defects manifested by goiter without associated hypothyroidism. Genetic defects in TG and thyroperoxidase synthesis have been reported in a few patients with familial dyshormonogenesis.

Hypothyroidism caused by a defect in the trapping of iodide can be confused with athyreosis because of the failure of administered radioiodine to be concentrated in the neck (point mutation in *SLC5A5*, sodium-iodide symporter). However, a goiter is clearly present in these patients, and salivary glands fail to concentrate radioiodine. A partial defect in iodine trapping results in decreased but not absent radioiodine uptake by the thyroid and salivary glands. The iodine-trapping defect is an autosomal recessive trait.[15]

There are specific types of defects in the oxidation or organification of iodide. Among them, the thyroperoxidase enzyme is deficient or defective, or cofactors that are required for activation of the enzyme or for the hydrogen peroxide generating system are defective (mutations in thyroperoxidase or *THOX2*).[15,33] These defects are usually associated with more severe hypothyroidism. In Pendred syndrome, patients have goiter with mild hypothyroidism or euthyroidism and congenital deafness. Many have an abnormal radioiodide discharge from the thyroid after perchlorate administration, indicative of defective iodide oxidation. However, peroxidase activity and hydrogen peroxide generation have been reported to be normal. TG is normal in quantity and low in iodine and hormone content. The mRNA encoding the 3′ region of TG may be abnormal, reducing efficiency of iodination and iodotyrosyl coupling. Chromosomal location reported for Pendred syndrome is 7q31. The sensorineural hearing defect is caused by a Mondini malformation of the cochlea. Incidence of this disorder is estimated to be about 1.5 to 3 per 100,000 schoolchildren. The defects are transmitted as autosomal recessive traits.

Mode of transmission of other inborn errors of thyroid hormone synthesis or metabolism has not been clearly established, although autosomal recessive inheritance and single gene mutations have been reported for most entities. In the coupling defect of iodotyrosines, T_4 and T_3 are decreased and MIT and DIT are increased in both serum and the thyroid gland (gene mutation not yet identified). In patients with iodothyronine deiodinase defects, there is a rapid turnover of thyroid iodine and wasting of iodotyrosines into the urine. The defect may be generalized, or it may be limited to intrathyroidal or peripheral deiodination. Defects in TG synthesis are suspected in patients with abnormal iodoproteins in their sera. Absent serum TG in neonates and mutations in the TG gene (8q24, stopping synthesis or causing conformational changes in the molecule) have been reported in these patients. Other rare types of familial dyshormonogenesis include a large kindred with goiter characterized by extensive intrathyroidal calcification. Transmission pattern suggests an autosomal dominant trait.

Generalized resistance to thyroid hormone by peripheral tissues (without resistance by the pituitary) has been reported (3q24, thyroid hormone receptor-β). Affected members of a family had deaf-mutism, goiter, delayed skeletal maturation with stippled epiphyses, and increased levels of thyroid hormone. Patients were reported to be clinically hypothyroid and required frequent thyroid hormone replacement therapy. However, the TSH response to TRH stimulation was normal.

Unresponsiveness of the thyroid gland to TSH has been reported in some children with congenital hypothyroidism without goiter. Serum TSH was elevated, and exogenous TSH stimulation caused no thyroid response (no increased radioiodine uptake or serum iodothyronine levels). Loss-of-function germline mutations of both alleles of the gene for the TSH receptor have been reported to cause resistance to the action of TSH and hypothyroidism.[35] The mutations were located in the extracellular, TSH-binding domain of the TSH receptor. The TSH receptor is coupled to the protein that binds to guanine nucleotide, or G protein. In these mutations, the TSH receptor does not activate G protein, and the effector adenylate cyclase (cAMP) signaling pathway remains inactive (*GNAS* mutations).[42] Some patients with these mutations may also have resistance to other hormones mediated by G protein (parathyroid hormone, growth hormone–releasing hormone, luteinizing hormone, follicle-stimulating hormone), as in pseudohypoparathyroidism type Ia.

MATERNAL INGESTION OF GOITROGENS

Maternal ingestion of antithyroid drugs, especially iodides, thiocarbamides, and potassium perchlorate, can cause neonatal goitrous hypothyroidism. Expectorants are an example of over-the-counter drugs containing iodides. Although correlation between dosages of these drugs and incidence of neonatal goiter is poor, prolonged administration of large doses of these drugs increases the risk for goitrous congenital hypothyroidism. Administration of large quantities of an inorganic iodide to the mother, usually as a perinatal or neonatal antiseptic, also causes neonatal goiter filled with colloid (see Fig. 49-23). Administration of amiodarone, an antiarrhythmic drug that contains two atoms of iodine, has resulted in goitrous congenital hypothyroidism in 11 of 64 (17%) treated pregnancies.[6] Radioiodine treatment given to pregnant women after 11 to 12 weeks of gestation has resulted in congenital hypothyroidism in the offspring. It is worthy of note that the hypothyroidism was not obvious at birth in most instances.

IODINE DEFICIENCY

Endemic goiter and cretinism are still prevalent in large geographic areas where dietary iodine is deficient. In iodide-sufficient regions, no more than 3% of newborns have transient TSH elevation. There are two severe types of endemic cretinism: myxedematous cretinism with metabolic symptoms of hypothyroidism and neurologic cretinism with dominant neurologic disorders. Despite the prevalence of intellectual impairment in endemic iodine-deficient regions, incidence of goiter in neonates is relatively low in these areas. Many individuals living in the same environment do not develop goiter. These observations suggest that other environmental factors may be superimposed on iodine deficiency. For instance, selenium deficiency leads to the inadequate use of iodine.[25] Iodine deficiency results in altered iodine metabolism, and the production of T_3 is increased relative to T_4. Reduced maternal T_4 levels early in gestation may deprive the developing fetal brain of T_4, which may be the essential iodothyronine for early brain maturation.

Many countries have initiated salt iodination. However, there is some concern that maternal iodine deficiency may be reappearing in developed countries despite salt iodination because diet-conscious young women may avoid iodine-supplemented salt and breads.[21] Iodine supplementation before or during pregnancy may normalize thyroid function in the mother and newborn. The recommended iodine intake for pregnant women is 200 μg daily, and in infants, the recommended intake is 40 μg daily.[21] Urinary iodine assay can be used to assess the adequacy of iodine uptake. Cochrane review indicated that there are insufficient data to support routine supplemental iodine in preterm infants.[24]

CENTRAL HYPOTHYROIDISM

Secondary (pituitary) and tertiary (hypothalamic) hypothyroidism are not commonly recognized in neonates. Central hypothyroidism can be confirmed in children and adults by the TSH surge test.[44,55] However, circadian variation of TSH secretion does not mature until about 4 to 6 months of age. Infants with central hypothyroidism can be detected through neonatal thyroid screening programs when T_4 measurements are included with TSH as the neonatal screening test (see Appendix Fig. B-6). Most of these patients have TRH deficiency, causing low-normal T_4 and low or normal TSH levels. They respond to TRH infusion with a sharp rise in serum TSH.

Secondary hypothyroidism may be suspected in infants with low T_4 and FT_4 and low TSH.[19] However, many infants with central hypothyroidism have normal TSH and are missed until they are older than one year.[35a] A low FT_4 by direct dialysis is the confirmatory test that determines the need for continued treatment when the diagnosis is suspected on the basis of initial tests. When available, the TRH infusion test may be used to distinguish hypothalamic TRH deficiency from pituitary TSH deficiency.

Pituitary TSH deficiency is rare in neonates (1 in 100,000).[4] However, autosomal recessive disorders that cause severe hypothyroidism as a result of congenital TSH deficiency have been reported. Mutations have been identified in the β-subunit of TSH, the TRH gene, and the TRH receptor gene.[41] Congenital TSH and growth hormone deficiencies may occur as the result of a difficult birth or anoxia.[39] Multiple pituitary hormone deficiencies suggest a genetic defect in the cascade leading to fetal pituitary formation, such as PROP1, LHX3, or POU1F1. When present, pituitary aplasia may be associated with anencephaly or other severe malformations of the brain. These patients rarely survive beyond the neonatal period.

Other midline facial, cranial, or intracranial defects should suggest the possibility of hypopituitarism, including altered functioning of the hypothalamic-pituitary-thyroid axis. Septo-optic dysplasia, often associated with pituitary hormone deficiencies, can be manifested as secondary or (more commonly) tertiary hypothyroidism. A genetic mutation in HESX1 has been described in septo-optic dysplasia. Clinical symptoms of hypopituitarism, such as neonatal hypoglycemia (from growth hormone and ACTH deficiencies), polyuria (from antidiuretic hormone deficiency), or a small phallus in boys (from gonadotropin deficiency), whether or not accompanied by the presence of blindness, congenital nystagmus, or midline defects of the brain, should alert the physician to suspect septo-optic dysplasia.

Neonatal Screening for Hypothyroidism

Every state in the United States and every province in Canada have legislatively mandated the screening of newborns for congenital hypothyroidism.[1] Screening programs have also been established in Western Europe, parts of Eastern Europe, Japan, Australia, and parts of Asia, South America, and Central America. However, many countries still do not have a nationwide program for neonatal thyroid screening (see Table 49-10).

Most programs currently use the filter paper spot technique.[1] Capillary blood specimens from a heel stick are obtained at 24 hours to 5 days of age. The filter paper designed for this purpose bears printed circles. Blood samples are placed in these circular areas to fill and saturate the areas. Most programs throughout the world screen for primary hypothyroidism with the measurement of TSH only.[19] In some U.S. states and some Canadian provinces, initial screening measures T_4. Those samples with T_4 values that fall within the lowest 10th percentile of that day's T_4 determinations are tested for TSH. These methods effectively screen for congenital hypothyroidism for the following reasons: (1) they are easily incorporated into the existing metabolic-genetic screening programs (e.g., phenylketonuria screening); (2) primary T_4 with confirmatory TSH screening (T_4 + TSH) also rapidly identifies those infants with central hypothyroidism or TBG deficiency; (3) selectivity is high because TSH measurements discriminate between affected and nonaffected infants, with a low recall rate (0.3% to 1%); (4) cases of mild congenital hypothyroidism are identified by primary TSH screening, and most cases are also identified by T_4 + TSH screening.

Both methods of screening (primary TSH and primary T_4 + TSH) appear to be capable of detecting almost all infants with primary congenital hypothyroidism, the only form of congenital hypothyroidism that carries a high risk for mental retardation if not detected early and treated adequately. Although a TSH level of greater than 50 mU/L is highly suggestive of congenital hypothyroidism, some affected infants have TSH values between 25 and 50 mU/L. These infants require prompt serum confirmation testing because many will be shown to have primary congenital hypothyroidism. The practice of early hospital discharge (before 48 hours of age) has led to a higher rate of indeterminate results. Infants screened before 48 hours of age require recheck of the newborn screen by the primary care physician at 2 weeks. Preterm infants screened prior to 48 hours of age have an elevated false positive rate.[47a] From mass screening programs in North America, overall incidence of congenital hypothyroidism appears to be about 1 in 3500 to 4000 births.

TABLE 49-10 International Studies Showing Geopolitical Trends in Rising Awareness of Need for Neonatal Thyroid Screening

Author	Date	Country	Date of Screening	Method	No. of Subjects Screened	Incidence	No. of Cases of CH	Observations
Golbahar	2010	Bahrain		Cord TSH	17,802	1:2967	6	one hospital
Adeniran	2010	Nigeria	2005	T4, T3, TSH	114			pilot study
Magalhaes	2009	Sao Paulo, Brazil	1997-2005		194,090	1:2595	76	one city
Zhan	2009	China	1985-2007		18.8 million	1:2047	9198	
Sranieri	2009	Mato Grosso, Brazil	2003-2004		66,337	1:9448		one state, at 8-30 days
Zarina	2008	Malasia	2004-2006	Cord TSH	13,875	1:6938	2	one hospital, high sample rejection rate
Afroze	2008	Pakistan	2008		3200	1:1600	2	one hospital
Rendon-Macias	2008	Mexico	2000-2004	Cord TSH	2.78 mllion	1:2926	1286	
Tahirovic	2008	Bosnia and Herzegovina	1999-2007	TSH	87,061	1:3957	22	
Gijurkova	2008	Macedonia	2002-2007	TSH	78,514	1:2804	28	
Hardy	2008	United Arab Emirates	1998-2004	Cord T4 and TSH	1778	1:1778	13	1 hospital
Ordookhani	2008	Iran		Cord TSH and then T4	50,409	1:5601	9	2 cities
Rashmi	2007	India		Cord TSH	1590			
Saglam	2007	Turkey		TSH and then T4	11,770	1:2354	5	1 city
Hopfner	2007	Germany	1988-1992			1:3313		
Maniatis	2006	Colorado, USA	1996-2004	T4, then TSH Same, 2nd screen	494,324 471,877	1:2703 1:2174	185 42	2nd screen identified 1 of 11,111 babies
Lanting	2005	Netherlands	1995-2000	T4, then TSH	1,118,079	1:3005 (1:16,404)	393 primary hypothyroidism (66 central hypothyroidism)	
Tylek-Lemanska	2005	Poland	1999-2001	TSH	3854	1:241	16	1 province possible iodine deficiency

Continued

TABLE 49–10 International Studies Showing Geopolitical Trends in Rising Awareness of Need for Neonatal Thyroid Screening—cont'd

Author	Date	Country	Date of Screening	Method	No. of Subjects Screened	Incidence	No. of Cases of CH	Observations
Wu	2005	Hunan, China	1997-2003	TSH	106,224	1;1562	68	Above national average of 1:3009
Chen	2005	Zhejiang, China	1999-2004	TSH, T_3, T_4	1,112,784	1:1457	764	
Skordis	2005	Cyprus	1990-2000	TSH	109,532	1:1800	61	3 cities
Simsek	2005	Turkey	2000-2002	TSH	18,606	1:2326	6	1 hospital
Panamonta	2003	Thailand	2000-2002	TSH	9558	1:3186	6	
Al-Hosani	2003	United Arab Emirates	1995-2000	TSH	138,718	1:1570	88	
Daher	2003	Lebanon	1998-2002	TSH	9117	1:1823	5	8 hospitals
Ordookhani	2003	Iran	1998-2001	Cord TSH	20,107	1:914	22	Late diagnosis associated with lower IQ
Al Shaikh	2003	Oman	Feasibility	NA, 1 hospital	NA	14 by screen; 31 at 9 mo		Need universal iodine supply
Bhatara	2002	India	Regional	TSH / T_4	12,407 / 25,244	1:2481 / 1:2804	5 / 9	
Olivieri	2002	Italy	1991-1998	TSH	NA	NA	1420	Congenital malformations increased in infants with CH
Churesigaew	2002	Thailand	1995-2000	TSH, then T_4	62,681	1:4178	15	2:1 female-to-male ratio, 1 hospital
Foo	2002	N. Ireland	1983-1993	TSH	NA	NA	131	
Henry	2002	Saudi Arabia	1985-2000	Cord TSH	121,404	1:2759	44	1.8:1 female-to-male ratio
Kurinczuk	2002	W. Australia	1981-1987 1988-1998	T_4	356,000	1:5747 1:2845	126	Increased birth defects in females
Asakura	2002	Japan	1979-1997	Simultaneous TSH and T_4, FT_4	1,284,130	1:1946 1:160,516	250 primary 8 central hypothyroidism	
Connelly	2001	Victoria	1977-1988	T_4	704,723	1:3541	199	
Castanet	2001	France	1978 (1st 19 yr)	NA	14,416,428	1:3560	4049	
Feleke	2000	Ethiopia	Feasibility 1996-1997	TSH, then T_4	4206	None in 4206		

Mandel	2000	Massachu-setts	1993-1996	T_4, then TSH	311,282	1:2638	118	
Waller	2000	California	1990-1998	T_4, then TSH	5,049,185	1:2796	1806	
Mikelsaar	1999	Estonia	NA	TSH	NA	1:2860	NA	Need universal iodine prophylaxis. Transient TSH elevation in 17.7% of infants
Vela	1999	Mexico	2 yr	TSH	1,140,364	1:2517	453	26% of infants screened
Wu	1999	Malaysia	8 mo in 1995	Cord TSH	11,000	1:3666	3	26% of recalls not traceable 48% no response to recall
King	1999	Oklahoma	1979	T_4, then TSH	46,740	1:3339	14 159 since 1979	1 of 64 infants; abnormal T_4, normal TSH 1 of 82, abnormal TSH on screen
Joseph	1999	Singapore	1981 pilot 1990 nat'l	Cord TSH	400,000	1:3000	About 133	
Fan	1999	China	1981	NA	1,100,000	1:5469	201	
Ojile	1998	Nigeria	Pilot	Cord TSH	NA	14/1000	NA	Suggest iodine deficiency
Law	1998	Wales	1982-93, 12 yr	NA	445,944	1:3279	136	1.9:1 female-to-male ratio
Hunter	1998	NW USA, regional	1975-1995	T_4, then TSH	1,747,805	1:3884 1:60,269	450 Central hypothyroidism	
Kaiserman	1997	Israel	1979-1987	TSH	657,384	1:3354	196	
Roberts	1997	Atlanta	1979-1992	T_4, then TSH	485,000	1:5000 1:48,500	87 primary 10 central hypothyroidism	
Ray	1997	Scotland	1979-1993	TSH	1,029,600	1:4400		

CH, congenital hypothyroidism; FT_4, free T_4; IQ, intelligence quotient; NA, not applicable; T_4, thyroxine; TSH, thyrotropin.

Incidence of congenital hypothyroidism (including dyshormonogenesis) is greatly increased in Down syndrome, as are acquired autoimmune diseases of the thyroid gland, pancreas, stomach, and adrenal gland.[22] Obvious congenital hypothyroidism occurs in 1 of about 140 subjects with Down syndrome. T_4 concentrations in 284 newborns with Down syndrome were significantly decreased compared with those in controls.[50] Many additional children with Down syndrome have mildly elevated TSH (5 to 15 mU/L) and low-normal FT_4 values. TSH bioactivity appears to be normal, suggesting that these children with Down syndrome and mild TSH elevation have mild tissue hypothyroidism. If TSH elevation persists up to 4 weeks of age, the child's mental development may be best protected by initiating thyroid hormone replacement, as in transient hypothyroidism.[1]

There is a female preponderance of 2:1 in the incidence of congenital hypothyroidism in North America, with aplastic or hypoplastic thyroid gland in about one third of the cases. The prevalence of nonendemic, goitrous congenital hypothyroidism depends on frequency of the defective gene in the population but usually occurs in 10% to 20% of infants with primary hypothyroidism. Ectopic thyroid tissue occurs in 33% to 50% of congenital hypothyroidism cases. Ascertainment depends on sophistication of imaging methods. Infants with central hypothyroidism constitute less than 5% of the detected cases. In the United States, combined incidence of secondary and tertiary hypothyroidism is about 1 in 80,000 to 100,000 births, and that of goitrous hypothyroidism is about 1 in 30,000 births. There are geographic differences in prevalence of transient hypothyroidism that may be related to iodine intake. In areas with an adequate iodine supply, most infants with transient hypothyroidism were born to mothers who received goitrogens during pregnancy. Some cases result from placental transmission of maternal antibodies.

Screening programs that measure T_4 also identify infants with TBG deficiency. This predominantly X-linked trait (Xq22.2) occurs as frequently as 1 in 5000 to 10,000 births. TBG deficiency has no clinical importance but leads to abnormal laboratory tests. T_4 and TSH concentrations are low, T_3U is elevated, and FT_4 is normal. Diagnosis can be confirmed by low TBG concentration on specific radioimmunoassay. Infants with normal FT_4 and TSH levels should not be treated with thyroid hormone.[19]

Clinical Manifestations

Even in athyreotic infants, classic clinical features of congenital hypothyroidism are usually absent at birth and appear only gradually over about 6 weeks. In patients with a functional remnant of thyroid tissue and in those with familial dyshormonogenesis, clinical manifestations may be delayed several months or years, depending on the functional state of the thyroid.[19] Early manifestations include lethargy, inactivity, hypotonia, periorbital edema, large anterior and posterior fontanelles, feeding difficulty, respiratory distress, pallor, prolonged icterus, perioral cyanosis, mottled skin, poor or hoarse crying, constipation, and hypothermia.[19]

Feeding difficulty is often first noted by the mother or a nurse; the infant readily falls asleep after sucking for a short period, necessitating repeated stimulation and a prolonged period to complete the feeding. Respiratory distress associated with myxedema of the airway is characterized by noisy breathing, nasal stuffiness, and intermittent cyanosis, especially in the perioral area. Respiratory symptoms may lead to suspicion of congenital anomalies of the airway or congenital heart disease. After the first week of life, prolonged physiologic jaundice may be an indication of hypothyroidism. Jaundice may appear to be further prolonged when carotenemia is superimposed after feeding the infant a diet high in carotene. In primary hypothyroidism, indirect hyperbilirubinemia predominates, whereas in central hypothyroidism, there is a mixture of indirect and direct hyperbilirubinemia. Serum creatinine may be elevated.

Classic features of congenital hypothyroidism in the infant usually become apparent after about 6 weeks of age (Fig. 49-24). They include typical facies, characterized by a depressed nasal bridge, a relatively narrow forehead, puffy eyelids; thick, dry, cold skin; long and abundant coarse hair; large tongue, abdominal distention, umbilical hernia, hyporeflexia, bradycardia, hypotension with narrow pulse pressure, anemia, and widely patent cranial sutures.[19]

Lingual thyroid tissue can occasionally be seen in infants and children as a discrete round mass at the base of the tongue (Fig. 49-25). The base of the tongue must be firmly depressed to visualize the lingual thyroid. Because ectopic

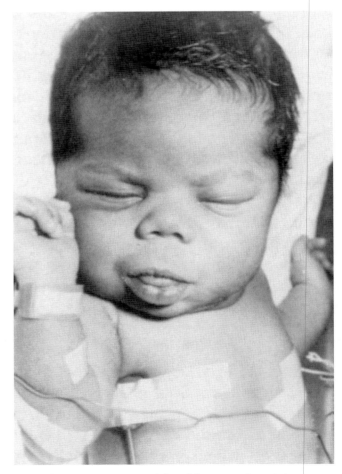

Figure 49-24. Typical facial features of cretinism.

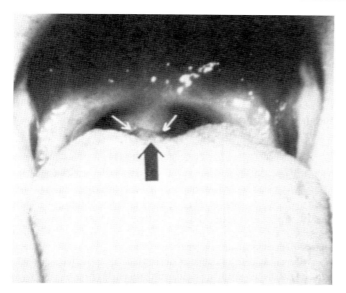

Figure 49–25. Visualization of a lingual thyroid.

thyroid tissue may function normally at birth, the ectopic gland of a child may not be detected by newborn screening and may present during childhood or adolescence with a lingual mass associated with speech and feeding problems. In some instances, the sublingual thyroid is palpable as a round midline mass deep under the mandible or is visualized by ultrasonography.

Neonatal goiters may be extremely large, asymmetric, and confused with hygroma or other cervical masses (see Fig. 49-23). Alternatively, the goiter may be quite small and escape notice. The thyroid can be palpated in infants by placing them in the prone position, gently extending the neck, identifying the thyroid cartilage, and palpating inferiorly and laterally for the thyroid isthmus and lobes. The normal size of each thyroid lobe is about equal to the volume of the distal segment of the patient's thumb.

In infants with central hypothyroidism, there is no thyroid enlargement. Onset of symptoms tends to be gradual because some T_4 production continues. As a result, prognosis for mental development remains good. However, signs of other pituitary hormone deficiencies, congenital midbrain defects, or both are typically present. These signs may include neonatal hypoglycemia, a small penis, hypospadias, undescended testes, wandering nystagmus, cleft lip or palate, and combined direct and indirect hyperbilirubinemia. Growth failure gradually becomes evident in these patients.[35a,44]

Laboratory Manifestations

When the diagnosis of congenital hypothyroidism is suspected, thyroid function tests should be performed. It is advisable to assess FT_4, TSH, and TG levels.[1] Measurements of T_3, rT_3, FT_3, and T_3U are not currently indicated. Elevated serum TSH value is the most sensitive and specific test to confirm the diagnosis of primary hypothyroidism. The normal value for TSH in cord blood is higher than that at any other age (see Tables 49-8 and 49-9). The physiologic TSH surge occurs during the first 6 hours of life, as noted earlier,

and concentration of TSH may remain higher than 10 mU/L during the first 24 to 48 hours of life. Infants whose specimens were collected before 24 hours of life and who have mildly elevated TSH values very likely will have normal thyroid function tests on repeated testing.[47a]

The typical laboratory findings for primary hypothyroidism are an elevated TSH, with T_4 and FT_4 values in the low or low-normal range. A low or undetectable TG concentration with TSH elevation confirms a dysgenetic or absent thyroid gland, whereas a high TG with TSH elevation suggests an organification defect. In central hypothyroidism, TSH is usually normal, T_4 is low-normal, and FT_4 is in the lowest third of normal. In the latter, further investigation should include assessment of FT_4 by direct dialysis and measurement of TBG to confirm the diagnosis.

In infants with acute or chronic illness including respiratory distress syndrome, the euthyroid sick syndrome or nonthyroidal illness syndrome may be present and affects thyroid function test results but does not produce hypothyroidism.[18] Typical laboratory findings in nonthyroidal illness are low or normal serum T_4, normal FT_4 by direct dialysis, and normal TSH. Total T_3 can be very low, and rT_3 is elevated. In certain types of hypothyroidism, such as iodine-deficient cretinism, the preferential synthesis of T_3 may occur. Therefore, a normal or high T_3 concentration alone does not exclude hypothyroidism any more than does a normal T_4 concentration.

When a confusing situation arises, such as borderline values in screening tests, a repeated measurement of TSH and FT_4 determination by direct dialysis may be helpful. The TRH stimulation test may be helpful if available.

Retardation of bone maturation is present in about half of the newborns with primary hypothyroidism and may suggest the fetal age at which a deficiency developed in the delivery of thyroid hormone to responsive tissues. Therefore, assessment of bone age is useful in the newborn.[1] However, radiographic examination of the hand and wrist (most often used in estimating bone age in children older than 2 years) is not helpful during the neonatal period because the first wrist ossification center, the hamate, does not appear in the normal infant until 3 to 4 months of age. Retardation of bone maturation in neonates is best assessed by radiographs of the knee and foot. The ossification centers of the calcaneus and talus appear at about 26 to 28 weeks of gestation, and those of the distal femur at about 34 to 36 weeks. The proximal tibial epiphyses appear at about 35 weeks of gestation. Absence of the distal femoral epiphyses in a newborn weighing 3000 g or more or absence of the distal femoral and proximal tibial epiphyses in an infant weighing 2500 to 3000 g at birth suggests an intrauterine thyroid hormone deficiency.

Ossification of the cartilage of the epiphyses is also disturbed in hypothyroidism. Ossification normally begins from the center of the cartilage and extends peripherally in an orderly manner. In hypothyroidism, calcification of epiphyseal centers starts from multiple irregular foci scattered within the developing cartilage. The irregular calcification pattern appears on the radiograph as stippled or fragmented ossification centers and is referred to as *epiphyseal dysgenesis* (see Fig. 49-22). This finding is highly characteristic of hypothyroidism and provides a strong clue for the diagnosis. Abnormal changes occur in the epiphyseal cartilage secondary to thyroid hormone deficiency before calcification, so even after hypothyroidism is treated, the characteristic pattern of calcification appears in all the centers that normally would have calcified during the period of deficiency. Stippled epiphyses may also occur in thyroid hormone resistance. The only other disorder with stippled epiphyses is multiple epiphyseal dysplasia, and thyroid function is normal in this familial disease.

In severe myxedema, low voltage of all complexes in the EKG and electroencephalogram may be seen, and cardiomegaly, reflecting myxedema of the heart, may be identified on a radiograph of the chest. Measurements of serum cholesterol levels and basal metabolic rates are not reliable diagnostic aids in the assessment of thyroid function during the neonatal period.

Interpretation of Scanning Results

An enlarged, lingual, or dysgenetic thyroid may be identifiable by ultrasound.[37] The use of ^{123}I or ^{99m}Tc-pertechnetate is recommended when practical to distinguish dysgenesis from ectopia. Within 2 hours, a definitive diagnosis of ectopic dysgenesis or athyreosis compared with antibody-induced hypothyroidism (TRAb) can be made, the family counseled, and treatment started after serum is collected for thyroid tests. Furthermore, when goiter is present, the family can be counseled about autosomal recessive disease and its probability of recurrence, and additional tests can be performed on DNA from the patient and family without a delay in initiating therapy.[29] However, initiation of thyroid hormone replacement therapy should not be delayed so that a scan may be obtained. Ultrasound may be performed and the scan can be delayed until after the age of 2 or 3 years, a time when thyroid hormone therapy can be safely withheld for 4 to 6 weeks.

^{99m}Tc can be intravenously administered by means of the same venous access used to collect blood for confirmatory thyroid function tests. Radioiodine should be administered through a nasogastric tube and the tube flushed with water to prevent any loss of the tracer. The presence of a defective iodine-trapping mechanism can be suspected in infants with goiter when there is a failure of radioiodine to be concentrated in the thyroid within 2 to 4 hours after oral administration of the tracer. The defect can be demonstrated by comparing radioiodine concentrations in simultaneously obtained samples of saliva and plasma 1 to 2 hours after the administration of the tracer. In the normal infant, salivary level is at least 10-fold and usually 20-fold greater than that in plasma. Radioiodine fails to be concentrated in the salivary glands of patients with defective iodine trapping.

In patients with one of the iodide oxidation defects, iodide taken up by the thyroid is readily released from the gland because it cannot be rapidly oxidized to iodine, especially in the presence of a competitive inhibitor. When thyroid uptake of radioiodine is measured 2, 4, 6, and 24 hours after oral administration of radioiodine in these patients, uptake may be normal or elevated during the early hours but rapidly declines within 24 hours. In normal infants, thyroid uptake of radioiodine gradually increases during the first 4 to 6 hours and plateaus at a level equal to 15% to 30% of the administered dose at the end of 24 hours.

When rapid oxidation of inorganic iodide to iodine fails to take place in the thyroid, an anion such as perchlorate can competitively inhibit the iodide accumulation, leading to a net loss of iodide from the gland. The perchlorate discharge test involves measurement of ^{123}I-iodide uptake at 2 hours, after which sodium or potassium perchlorate is given orally in doses of 10 mg/kg of body weight. Thyroid uptake is measured every 15 to 30 minutes for 2 hours. If the uptake decreases by more than 20% of the initial value, a defect in iodide oxidation is confirmed.

Immaturity of the oxidation system is suggested by reports of infants with transient thyroid dyshormonogenesis. They had positive perchlorate discharge tests at birth but normal thyroid function and uptake when tests were repeated after 2 years of age once thyroid hormone replacement therapy was discontinued. The defect may be temporary in ectopic thyroid tissue. These factors may constitute additional reasons to wait until the age of 2 or 3 years to perform the perchlorate discharge test.

Differentiation among other types of familial dyshormonogenesis is more difficult and often technically impossible to achieve during infancy. Studies required for the differential diagnosis usually involve the administration of radioactive substances in doses greater than those considered safe for infants. Studies of iodine kinetics in blood specimens obtained after the administration of radioiodine, in tissue culture specimens obtained by biopsy, or in both may be necessary for differential diagnosis. Therefore, in most instances, patients should be treated for a few years, with a definitive study undertaken at a later date. In the future, additional specific mutations will be known, and diagnosis may be confirmed by DNA analysis.

Diagnosis of hypothyroidism caused by maternal ingestion of goitrogens or neonatal exposure to iodine is usually established from the history and confirmed by its self-limited course. Thyroid hormone therapy should be administered in standard doses (see "Treatment" section, later). Therapy may be withdrawn at 3 years of age and thyroid function reevaluated off therapy.[1] Perchlorate discharge test may be positive both in iodine-induced goiter and after administration of antithyroid drugs. Urinary iodine concentration is elevated in infants with transient hypothyroidism caused by iodine excess.

In iodine deficiency, there is a decreased ratio of T_4 to T_3. When goiter is present, there should be an elevation of serum TSH and a decrease in serum T_4 levels after birth. Urinary concentration of iodine is low (<12 mg/dL) in these infants, and radioiodine uptake is increased.

TRANSIENT DISORDERS OF THYROID FUNCTION

Several causes of transient neonatal thyroid dysfunction must be distinguished from permanent disorders of thyroid function. The results of neonatal screening tests from these patients may mimic those found in permanent hypothyroidism and may lead to an erroneous diagnosis.

Transient Primary Neonatal Hypothyroidism

Transient hypothyroidism may occur in apparently healthy full-term infants. Thyroid function in patients with transient primary hypothyroidism reverts to normal either very promptly and spontaneously or after several months of T_4 therapy. If FT_4 is low or steadily decreases or TSH remains higher than 5 mU/L on serial testing within the first month of life, the infant should be treated with T_4 until 3 years of age to protect brain development. Persistent TSH elevation (beyond 4 weeks of age) is undesirable for brain development. Of course, one cannot know whether the case of hypothyroidism was transient until later.[10]

The incidence of transient primary hypothyroidism is higher in geographic areas where the dietary supply of iodine is insufficient. Premature infants are more susceptible, and incidence increases with decreasing gestational age.[18] The T_4 levels are low and TSH levels usually increased, but these test results may overlap with the normal range. FT_4 levels fall into the range seen in neonates with congenital hypothyroidism during the first 1 to 2 weeks of life. In many cases, the T_4, T_3, and TSH levels in the cord blood of affected infants have been found to be normal, suggesting that hypothyroidism developed only after birth. The condition is frequently associated with transient hypothyroxinemia of prematurity, which confounds the diagnosis. Transient hypothyroidism may develop after low Apgar scores are observed. Low urinary iodine concentration suggests inadequate dietary iodine availability as the causative factor. Iodine supplementation of the diet may successfully correct hypothyroidism and goiter in these infants.

The transplacental passage of antithyroid drugs from the mother may cause transient hypothyroidism with goiter in the neonate. Excessive supply of iodine may also cause transient hypothyroidism. Premature infants appear to be more susceptible to iodine-induced transient hypothyroidism. The excessive application of iodine-containing antiseptics to mucous membranes (e.g., omphalocele) or intact skin has also caused transient hypothyroidism in infants. Yet another cause of transient neonatal hypothyroidism may be the transplacental transfer of maternal inhibiting TRAb. These antibodies may persist in the infant's circulation for 2 to 3 months until they are metabolized. No goiter is present, and no image is seen on the thyroid scan, although thyroid tissue can be seen on an ultrasonogram.

Transient Hyperthyrotropinemia

Transient hyperthyrotropinemia is characterized by elevated serum TSH concentrations during the neonatal period despite normal T_4 and FT_4 levels. This condition probably represents mild transient or permanent primary hypothyroidism.[10] The basis for this statement is the sensitivity of modern TSH assays. TSH concentrations are the most sensitive indicators that the hypothalamic-pituitary axis is experiencing less T_4 than the body perceives to be optimal. The hypothalamic-pituitary-thyroid axis is finely tuned to maintain a fairly stable level of FT_4 within any individual. Divergence from this individual optimal setpoint because of illness or malfunctioning of the thyroid gland results in TSH elevation except when the hypothalamus or pituitary is unable to respond (in central hypothyroidism or rare pituitary resistance to FT_4 feedback). There may be a delayed rise in TSH, particularly in infants with very low birthweight.[1]

If left untreated, the high TSH levels may persist for a few days to several months or years.[1,2] The infants appear to be asymptomatic, and the cause of the condition is unknown. This disorder is very likely to be missed because, until recently, newborn screening programs in the United States initially used T_4, with TSH not measured unless initial T_4 fell into the lowest 10% level of each assay.[19] Transient TSH

elevation has been reported in infants born to mothers who received antithyroid medications or iodine and in neonates with iodine deficiency. The incidence of transient neonatal TSH elevation appears to be higher in infants with Down syndrome.

In the case of persistence of TSH elevation above 5 mU/L, these patients may have permanent congenital hypothyroidism, transient neonatal hypothyroidism, or acquired autoimmune thyroid disorders.[10] Because untreated hypothyroidism can result in developmental loss, it will benefit the infant's brain development to initiate thyroid hormone replacement therapy by 4 to 6 weeks of age in cases of continued mild TSH elevation, rather than continue to monitor the levels without treatment while waiting for the resolution of TSH elevation. Treatment should be continued until the age of 3 years, when thyroid function can be reevaluated. If increased TSH persists at this older age, a thyroid scan or ultrasound examination should be performed to exclude ectopic thyroid dysgenesis or goiter from mild familial dyshormonogenesis.[19]

Transient Hypothyroxinemia

Transient hypothyroxinemia is seen in many preterm infants,[18] related to immaturity of the hypothalamic-pituitary axis. Serum T_4 and FT_4 levels are low in comparison with those of full-term infants, but TSH levels are normal. Serum TBG levels are only slightly low in preterm infants and do not account for the degree of hypothyroxinemia. When dietary supply of iodine is slightly deficient, low T_4 and FT_4 levels in preterm infants may be accompanied by high TSH levels and exaggerated TSH responses to TRH stimulation. Therefore, preterm infants living in iodine-deficient areas are exposed to the combined risk for transient tertiary and primary hypothyroidism. Prevalence of transient hypothyroxinemia may be as high as 1 in 6000 births in certain regions.

Low T_4 has been associated with a higher risk for intraventricular hemorrhage or death in premature infants. Serious illness is also a cause of low T_4 values.[18] With gestational ages of less than 30 weeks, there may be low TBG. After 30 weeks of gestation, TBG reaches the concentration present at term and does not account for the serum concentrations of T_4.

In preterm infants, the T_4 levels usually increase on repeated evaluations and become normal by 3 to 4 months of age.[18] By 6 months of age, all infants had T_4 levels in the normal range, thus documenting the transient nature of the defect. Developmental attainment at 1 year of age was equal to that in a matched control group who did not have low T_4 levels. No clear effect of T_4 administration on developmental outcome was found. It is recommended that thyroid screening in preterm infants be performed at 5 days of age and repeated at 2, 4, and 6 weeks of age.[18] Therapy for hypothyroxinemia in preterm infants born at less than 28 weeks of gestation led to improvement in mental outcome and less adverse medical outcome than those not treated. However, those preterm infants born at greater than 28 weeks of gestation had increased morbidity with thyroid hormone therapy. A placebo-controlled study in infants born at less than 30 weeks of gestation did not show beneficial effects of T_3 therapy plus hydrocortisone compared with placebo on risk for death or ventilator dependence at 1 or 2 weeks of age.[8]

Therefore, in the absence of TSH elevation, pragmatic treatment with thyroid hormone is not currently indicated in full-term or preterm infants with transient hypothyroxinemia or respiratory distress.[18] A Cochrane review has recommended controlled trials to further assess thyroid hormone therapy in very preterm infants with hypothyroxinemia.[38]

EUTHYROID SICK SYNDROME

In acutely ill patients, serum T_3 is decreased. Current hypothesis is that alterations in thyroid hormone occur as an adaptive response to decreased basal metabolic rates in severely ill patients. The syndrome has been recognized in sick infants and children.[11,12] These patients may have severe nonthyroidal illnesses that are either acute or chronic.

The consistent finding is an abnormally low serum T_3 level, accompanied by an increase in the rT_3 level. T_4 may be low or normal and FT_4 may be normal, depending on metabolic clearance rate of T_4. Serum TBG may be low or normal, and TSH is normal. In preterm infants, T_4, FT_4, and T_3 levels are naturally lower than those in term infants, and rT_3 is high.[18] Therefore, thyroid tests in preterm infants may present a confusing situation when the infants are ill from nonthyroidal diseases.

In the neonatal period, preterm infants with respiratory distress syndrome are the most frequently encountered patients with euthyroid sick syndrome.[18,49] In children, a variety of nonthyroidal illnesses have been associated with this syndrome, including severe gastroenteritis, acute leukemia, anorexia nervosa, renal disease, burns, and surgical stress. An alteration in T_4 metabolism to favor production of rT_3 over T_3 appears to occur rapidly. Euthyroid sick syndrome is found in patients with acute metabolic stress (e.g., diabetic ketoacidosis) and occurs in all pediatric patients who undergo cardiac surgery. There is a sharp rise in rT_3 and a less dramatic fall in T_3 by 2 hours after cardiac surgery. Reverse T_3 returns to normal before T_3, and there is an inverse relationship between the severity of illness and the T_3 level.

In euthyroid sick syndrome, abnormal thyroid function gradually reverts to normal function as the patient's primary illness improves.[19] During recovery, TSH may be transiently elevated (up to 15 mU/L). Treatment with thyroid hormone is not indicated in these patients. However, preterm infants at risk should be monitored by serial determinations of FT_4 and TSH, and T_4 treatment should be initiated if there is a progressive increase in serum TSH and decrease in FT_4.[28] T_4 treatment should probably be initiated if the illness state is expected to be persistent and TSH remains elevated for a month or longer.

Differential Diagnosis

Errors in diagnosis of congenital hypothyroidism usually result from a failure of the newborn screening program (no specimen collected or a laboratory error), from a clinical failure to suspect the condition, or from the misdiagnosis of other disorders as hypothyroidism.[1] These errors typically arise when the diagnosis is based on a few suggestive clinical features, and laboratory data are incorrectly interpreted. It is necessary to perform newborn screening even in sick newborns so that clear-cut abnormalities cannot be missed. Repeated screening is then indicated as the illness resolves.[18]

During the early neonatal period, respiratory difficulty, pallor, and cyanosis in hypothyroid infants must be differentiated from other common causes of respiratory distress and from congenital heart disease. Lethargy, inactivity, hypotonia, and feeding difficulty may be mistaken for manifestations of sepsis or brain damage from a variety of causes. The prolonged jaundice in hypothyroidism must not be confused with icterus caused by hemolytic anemia, septicemia, or hepatic disease. The coarse facial features, macroglossia, and dry skin of hypothyroidism can mislead one to suspect Hurler syndrome, chondrodystrophy, or Down syndrome. A large goiter must not be confused with a hygroma, cyst, or tumor of the neck. A lingual thyroid, when visible or obstructing the airway, may be mistaken for a tumor of the pharyngeal area. Although epiphyseal dysgenesis may resemble osteochondritis deformans in its radiographic appearance, the latter does not occur during the neonatal period.

Treatment

All hypothyroid infants, with or without goiter, should be rendered euthyroid as promptly as possible by thyroid hormone replacement therapy.[46] When there is low T_4 and elevated TSH on screening tests, thyroid hormone replacement therapy for neonatal congenital hypothyroidism must be started as soon as blood is collected for serum confirmation tests.[1] A delay of 8 days in the initiation of thyroid hormone therapy can be detected later as a lower score on IQ testing.[9] The half-life of serum T_4, including T_4 acquired from the mother, is short in infants (3 to 4 days) compared with adults (about 6 days). Neonates with a euthyroid goiter should be regarded as having mild congenital hypothyroidism (elevated TSH with normal FT_4). For example, those with mild TSH elevation and normal FT_4 may be monitored with serial TSH and FT_4 tests and not treated for up to 4 weeks. However, if TSH remains elevated, thyroid hormone therapy should be started. An infant with an ectopic thyroid gland should be treated without delay because overt hypothyroidism is virtually inevitable at a later age. In rare instances in which the diagnosis of congenital hypothyroidism cannot be established expeditiously because of confounding laboratory results, it is the safest course to fully treat the infant for the first 2 to 3 years of life and then reevaluate. Breast feeding can continue. Specifically, human breast milk does not contain enough T_4 to alter thyroid hormone levels in the infant. At 3 years of age, after the brain has substantially completed its growth, treatment can be withdrawn or decreased by 50% and the patient studied 4 to 6 weeks later.

Although most infants with congenital hypothyroidism are asymptomatic and identified on neonatal screening tests, they must be treated vigorously at the youngest possible age.[9] There is increasing evidence that the previously recommended doses of thyroid hormone replacement are inadequate for some infants. Inadequate thyroid hormone treatment, either by the physician's direction or because of poor compliance, appears to be a significant contributor to lower intelligence in older children who were treated from the first 2 months of life.

Asymptomatic infants and those with minimal clinical manifestations of congenital hypothyroidism can be given sodium-L-thyroxine, 12 to 15 μg/kg per day (administered orally once per day), beginning as soon as the diagnosis is established (optimally by 2 weeks of age).[1] The pill should be crushed or a brand used that dissolves easily in liquid and suspended in a small amount of formula, breast milk, or water (not the whole bottle). The suspension can be provided by way of a cross-cut nipple and followed later by the feeding. The initial dose of T_4 does not need to exceed 50 μg/day. T_4 increases to more than 10 μg/dL and FT_4 to more than 2 ng/dL within 3 to 7 days. At 1 month of age, the thyroid hormone dose may need to be decreased to 37.5 μg/day or on rare occasions to 25 μg/day if FT_4 exceeds 2.5 ng/dL, TSH is below 0.05 mU/L, or clinical symptoms of thyrotoxicosis develop. The target for TSH concentrations should be between 0.5 and 2.0 mU/L during thyroid hormone replacement therapy for primary hypothyroidism.[5]

In preterm infants, the same starting dose of T_4 (12 to 15 μg/kg per day) is recommended to promptly increase T_4 to normal. The dose may need to be decreased, as described, once T_4 values reach the desired normal level.[1]

No adverse effects from this dose of T_4 replacement therapy were found in infants during their first year of life as long as they were frequently monitored, including FT_4 and TSH determinations. Sodium-L-thyroxine is the drug of choice because the cerebral cortex derives about 80% of the required T_3 directly from the monodeiodination of circulating T_4.[1] T_3 and desiccated thyroid are no longer recommended for the treatment of congenital hypothyroidism. No advantage is observed with a combined T_3 and T_4 preparation.

In treatment of infants with severe myxedema with fluid retention, possible complications should be kept in mind. Cardiac insufficiency caused by overtaxing the myxedematous heart through too rapid a mobilization of the myxedema fluid into the circulation is well known in the adult. This complication in older children and adults is prevented by administering a small dose of thyroid hormone at first and gradually increasing the dosage. However, infants generally tolerate a rapid restoration to the euthyroid state better than adults, and a prompt restoration of T_4 to a normal value is important for the recovery of brain development and maturation. Nevertheless, excessive thyroid hormone therapy must be avoided, and the dose must be adjusted judiciously if there is evidence of severe myxedema, particularly of the heart. Aspiration of food rarely occurs in otherwise normal infants after therapy has been started. There is aspiration only in cases of severe myxedema from an impairment in swallowing (caused by myxedema of the pharyngeal area), compounded by an increased appetite as the euthyroid state is restored. Therefore, when myxedema is severe, the infant should be fed carefully and slowly during the early phase of treatment.

After replacement therapy is initiated, the dose of T_4 should be adjusted so that T_4 and FT_4 levels are maintained at high-normal adult values (>10 μg/dL and >2 ng/dL, respectively).[1] Thereafter, thyroid function test values should be kept at age-appropriate levels, which differ in children from those in adults (see Tables 49-8 and 49-9). With thyroid hormone replacement therapy, TSH is maintained between 0.5 and 2.0 mU/L during the first 2 years of life.[5] Sodium-L-thyroxine is less well absorbed in adults during food intake and when an infant is fed a soy formula (compared with cow's milk). For these reasons, the optimal time at which T_4 should be given is at least one-half hour before a feeding. However, from a practical point of view, infants can be given their thyroid medicine in a small amount of formula, with dosing adjusted on this regimen.

During the first years of life, patients should be monitored frequently—at least every 2 months during the first 6 months of life, every 3 months during the next 2 years, and then twice a year—to assess clinical progress, FT_4, and TSH.[1] Because poor compliance and noncompliance have major sequelae, the initial and ongoing counseling of parents is of great importance.

Between 2 and 6 years of age, the average dose of sodium-L-thyroxine required to initiate treatment is about 5 μg/kg per day; from 6 to 12 years of age, it is 4 μg/kg per day. Thereafter, an initial dose of 2 to 3 μg/kg per day should be adequate. In adults, the average thyroid hormone dose is 1.6 μg/kg per day (the average adult dose is 112 μg daily). These doses approximate 100 μg/m² per day. The treatment of each patient must be individualized. The dosage should be adjusted so that a clinically euthyroid state—TSH between 0.5 and 2.0 mU/L and FT_4 levels in the upper part of the normal range—can be maintained.

Clinical observation should be supplemented by monitoring of the growth curve, FT_4, and TSH. Patients with permanent congenital hypothyroidism (e.g., dysgenesis, dyshormonogenesis) require lifetime substitution therapy. Therapy should be continued consistently until formally re-evaluated under physician supervision at 3y of age.[26a] After 3 years, if there is uncertainty about whether the disease is permanent or transient, or if the dose of T_4 has not required increase because TSH has remained in the target range of 0.5 to 2.0 mU/L, discontinuation of T_4 therapy for 4 to 6 weeks, with monitoring of the TSH, should distinguish transient from permanent congenital hypothyroidism.

Goitrous cretinism caused by the maternal ingestion of goitrogens is a self-limited condition.[19] The blocking effect of antithyroid drugs usually disappears several days after birth. Therefore, if the goiter is small, TSH is not elevated, and the patient is euthyroid, no treatment is required. However, if the patient is hypothyroid and TSH is elevated or if the goiter is large, it is safer to treat the infant until the age of 3 years, as described previously. Shrinkage of the goiter may be hastened by substitution therapy, and treatment can be withdrawn after the thyroid returns to a normal size. Occasionally, the goiter is huge, and asphyxia may occur in the neonate from a goiter that encircles the trachea. This complication is most often seen in iodide-induced goiter and constitutes a medical emergency.

Although PTU is secreted in breast milk, the amount is so small that there should be no effects resulting from the transmission of PTU to the breast-feeding infant. If there is concern, serum TSH should be monitored initially each week for about 4 weeks. Methimazole (MTZ) therapy for mothers is not widely used because its biopotency in the fetus is about four times that of PTU. Nursing mothers are usually not treated with MTZ after delivery. Iodides are secreted into breast milk and could cause iodide-induced hypothyroidism in the breast-fed infant. Those with endemic goiter and hypothyroidism should be given substitution therapy for an indefinite period unless iodine prophylaxis can be ensured in the specific geographic location.

Prenatal diagnosis and intrauterine treatment of congenital hypothyroidism have been successful in only a few instances. Measurements of iodothyronines in amniotic fluid are unreliable. Determination of TSH in amniotic fluid or fetal blood collected by cordocentesis offers better hope for the diagnosis of congenital hypothyroidism at present (see "Thyroid Function: Fetal-Maternal Relationship," earlier). Maternal administration of TRH results in increased fetal TSH and T_3 and does not inhibit the postnatal surge of TSH. The maternal administration of oral T_4 has not yet proved effective in treating the fetus. Prenatal diagnosis and treatment of congenital hypothyroidism await further developments.

Prognosis

Shortly after adequate substitution therapy is instituted, all clinical manifestations of hypothyroidism disappear. If growth restriction was present before treatment, accelerated linear growth occurs. After a period of catch-up growth, an optimal rate of growth is maintained. Goiter or a hypertrophied ectopic thyroid gradually shrinks in size when the patient is properly treated. Coarse hair is gradually lost and replaced by finer, normal hair over several months. If there was a delay in skeletal maturation at diagnosis, treatment is associated with an acceleration in bone maturation after a latent period of a few months. Thereafter, osseous development parallels the chronologic and height ages. When hypothyroidism is treated with a slightly excessive dose of thyroid hormone for a prolonged period, bone maturation may gradually exceed the chronologic age even though the patient fails to show overt signs of hyperthyroidism or has clearly elevated T_4. With substitution therapy, epiphyseal dysgenesis (see Fig. 49-22) appears in ossification centers that failed to calcify while the patient was hypothyroid, and then the calcification coalesces to form a normal epiphysis.

Although the prognosis for physical recovery is good, including stature,[34] the prognosis for normal mental and neurologic performance is less certain for infants whose disorders were not detected early by newborn screening. There have been some reports in which a low to normal IQ score was correlated with severe hypothyroidism at birth and intrauterine hypothyroidism (evidenced by retarded bone maturation at birth) even when replacement therapy was begun within the first 2 months of life. More than 80% of infants given replacement therapy before 3 months of age had an IQ score of greater than 85. However, 77% of these infants showed some signs of minimal brain damage, including impairment of arithmetic ability, speech, or fine motor coordination in later life.[48]

Of course, the current goal for therapy is to start thyroid hormone treatment by 1 week of age to optimize long-term outcomes. Auditory brainstem evoked potentials were abnormal in 25% of 37 patients with congenital hypothyroidism treated early. The processing of visuospatial relationships remained affected in adolescents with congenital hypothyroidism.

Current follow-up studies of patients treated within the first few weeks of postnatal life after identification by neonatal screening indicated that neurologic function was normal, with a few minor exceptions. The best outcome occurs with thyroid hormone therapy started at 12 to 15 μg/kg per day by 1 week of age.[9] There are only minor differences in intelligence, school achievement, and neuropsychological test scores in affected congenital hypothyroidism adults treated early with thyroid hormone compared with control groups of

classmates and siblings.[36] Residual defects may include visuospatial processing, sensorimotor defects, and selective memory. A threshold effect of congenital hypothyroidism severity interacts with the effects of dose and age at onset of thyroid hormone therapy. Otherwise, neurologic and intellectual outcomes do not correlate well with the degree of T_4 deficiency found in neonatal screening.

Prior observations and lack of clinical manifestations of hypothyroidism in most neonates led to the current concept that the transplacental transfer of maternal T_4 in the first trimester may protect the brain during early development. For the same reason, maternal hypothyroidism during fetal development can have persistent neurodevelopmental effects on the child.[30] Serum T_4 concentrations at term in athyreotic babies are 25% to 50% of those found in normal neonates. Although they are low, these levels may offer some protection for the fetal brain. It is thought that the low to normal intelligence of patients with congenital hypothyroidism treated early in life results most often from inadequate treatment or poor compliance. During thyroid hormone therapy, recurrent episodes of insufficiently suppressed TSH (>5 mU/L) four or more times after the age of 6 months constitute the most important variable associated with school delay.[31] Thyroid hormone treatment regimens used today are more aggressive in targeting the early correction of TSH than the regimens used 20 or even 10 years ago. Therefore, current newborns with congenital hypothyroidism may have an even better intellectual and neurologic prognosis than those adults with congenital hypothyroidism who are currently being studied.

GOITER

Most neonatal goiters result from maternal ingestion of goitrogens, maternal iodine deficiency, maternal antibodies, or maternal thyroid medications. Prominent goiter is only present at birth in infants with familial dyshormonogenesis. Most of the euthyroid goiters of newborns are caused by compensatory hypertrophy of the thyroid mediated by TSH stimulation and therefore are indicative of mild TSH elevation. These infants should be investigated etiologically and treated appropriately.

Congenital neoplasms of the thyroid rarely occur but may include a Hürthle cell tumor, adenocarcinoma, and teratoma of the thyroid. Teratoma may be suggested by calcification within the thyroid gland. Neoplasm can be suspected when a nodular goiter or hard mass is present in the thyroid. A radioiodine or technetium thyroid scan reveals a cold nodule in the area corresponding to the location of the neoplasm where the uptake of the radioisotope is lacking. A diagnosis of neoplasm should be confirmed by biopsy.

THYROTOXICOSIS
Etiology and Pathogenesis

Neonatal thyrotoxicosis is caused by transplacental transfer of TRAb and TSI from the mother. The disease occurs in the neonate of a mother known to have active Graves disease either before or during pregnancy, Graves disease previously treated with thyroidectomy or radioiodine ablation, or Hashimoto disease. However, mothers with detectable TSI may give birth to normal infants, especially when maternal TSI activity is low. Family studies, observation of twins, and age-specific incidence rates suggest that this disease occurs randomly in a genetically preselected population. Measurement of TSI in third-trimester serum or cord blood can be prognostic of risk for thyrotoxicosis in the newborn.

Neonatal thyrotoxicosis may also occur in infants without detectable TSI. In these infants, the pathogenesis may be familial syndrome of isolated pituitary resistance to thyroid hormone with mild thyrotoxicosis, autosomal dominant inherited germline mutations in the TSH receptor, mutations in the TSH receptor that cause constitutive activation of the receptor, or TSH-independent activation. Mutations in the transmembrane domains of the receptor keep it in the activated state so that G protein and adenylate cyclase can be continuously activated, causing hyperthyroidism. In these cases, TSI does not play a role.

Clinical Manifestations

When neonatal thyrotoxicosis occurs in the infant born to a mother with untreated, active Graves disease, clinical manifestations of hyperthyroidism may become apparent within the first 24 hours of life. Infants may be born prematurely from such a mother. Prenatal diagnosis may be possible in the event of fetal goiter, elevated maternal TSI titer, or elevated maternal DIT.[54] Irritability, excessive movement, tremor, flushing of the cheeks, sweating, increased appetite, weight loss or lack of weight gain, supraventricular tachycardia, goiter, and exophthalmos may be observed in the newborn.[19] Unique to the neonate with severe Graves disease is generalized enlargement of the reticuloendothelial system, causing generalized lymphadenopathy, hepatosplenomegaly, thrombocytopenia, and hypoprothrombinemia. Although a goiter is inevitably present in neonatal thyrotoxicosis, its size varies considerably; it may be small and escape notice on a cursory examination, or it may be large enough to cause tracheal compression. In addition, the goiter may increase in size during the early neonatal period. Exophthalmos is usually mild when present. In severe neonatal thyrotoxicosis, hyperthermia, arrhythmia, and high-output cardiac failure may occur. If the condition remains untreated, death may result.[19]

In most cases, the course of neonatal hyperthyroidism is self-limited because of the gradual depletion of transplacentally acquired TSI. The signs and symptoms subside spontaneously after 3 weeks to 6 months, depending on the severity of the disease. The severity of hyperthyroidism is probably related to the titer of TSI in the plasma of the neonate. However, goiter may persist for some time after all signs of hyperthyroidism disappear. The thyroid gradually returns to its normal size. In rare instances, neonatal thyrotoxicosis may not be a transient disorder and may persist for years.

In the infant born to a mother who received antithyroid medications for the treatment of Graves disease during the latter part of pregnancy, the onset of clinical manifestations may be modified by transplacental acquisition of the antithyroid agent as well as TSI. At birth, the infant may be euthyroid or even hypothyroid, and the presence of a goiter may be the only abnormal feature. Because the plasma half-life of antithyroid agents is short compared with the half-life of TSI, the typical manifestations of neonatal thyrotoxicosis may appear several days to 2 weeks after birth. If the infant is born in a hypothyroid state, a period of euthyroidism may follow within a few days, and thyrotoxicosis may not occur until 5 to 14 days after birth. Although neonatal Graves disease is a disease mediated by monoclonal antibodies, polyclonal antibodies are sometimes produced by the mother and cause atypical disease in the infant. Late-onset hyperthyroidism may not develop until 1 to 2 months of age if a high-affinity TBII in low concentrations initially predominates; once it is metabolized, a second population of TRAb prevails to cause late-onset hyperthyroidism.

Diagnosis and Differential Diagnosis

A maternal history of Graves disease before or during pregnancy is important in the diagnosis of neonatal thyrotoxicosis. Information concerning both prior and current treatment of maternal hyperthyroidism must also be obtained. The infant should be examined sequentially for signs of thyrotoxicosis, and the neck should be palpated carefully to detect a goiter. Determination should be obtained of TSI in infant serum or cord blood, in addition to that of TSH and FT_4; unmeasurable TSH supports the presence of thyrotoxicosis.[5,29] Data should be interpreted in relation to clinical features and age of the neonate. Determination of radioiodine uptake by the thyroid has little value during the neonatal period. A higher titer of TSI in cord blood or neonatal serum strongly supports the diagnosis of neonatal thyrotoxicosis. Serial determinations of TSI in the neonate also help monitor disease activity and contribute to the decision to decrease or terminate therapy.

In the euthyroid or hypothyroid neonate born to a mother who received antithyroid medication during the latter part of pregnancy, it is almost impossible to predict whether thyrotoxicosis will ensue. Therefore, serial examinations of the infant must be undertaken during the first 10 days of life. Although neonatal thyrotoxicosis can be confused with various neurologic disorders, narcotic withdrawal in the infant of an addicted mother, congenital heart disease, or sepsis, a positive maternal history of Graves disease and presence of goiter should readily alert the physician to the correct diagnosis. In normal neonates and infants, the thyroid gland is difficult to palpate. Therefore, an easily palpable thyroid in such an infant should generally be regarded as a goiter.

Persistent neonatal thyrotoxicosis may result from a TSH receptor activating mutation.[52] Rare cases of hyperthyroxinemia are characterized by the syndrome of total or partial loss of peripheral tissue sensitivity to thyroid hormone, called *generalized resistance to thyroid hormone*. Prenatal thyroid hormone resistance may present with growth retardation and goiter that may improve with maternal T_3 therapy. In these patients, FT_4 is elevated and TSH is measurable within the normal range (i.e., not suppressed as expected), but there is no clinical manifestation of hyperthyroidism.[29] Hyperthyroxinemia may also reflect elevated TBG production, in which case FT_4 is normal, and no therapy is needed.[29]

Treatment

The treatment of thyrotoxicosis in a neonate is similar to that in an older child and involves use of antithyroid drugs.[19,43a,43b] Care should be exercised not to induce hypothyroidism with excessive medication. Iodine (Lugol solution) and an antithyroid drug, MTZ, are typically used. Lugol solution can be given in KI doses of 8 mg three times daily. Although iodine rapidly inhibits the release of T_4 from the thyroid, its effects tend to disappear after several weeks. MTZ is given in doses of 0.3 to 1mg/kg per day in one or two divided doses. PTU is no longer recommended for use in children.[43a] Circulating T_4 has a half-life of 3 to 4 days in neonates and about 6 days in adults. Therefore, little or no clinical response to antithyroid drugs can be expected during the first few days of therapy. When FT_4 decreases, TSH increases (although this increase may be delayed despite low FT_4 values), and TRAb decreases over 1 to 4 months. When TSH increases, the dose of MTZ should be reduced or discontinued to determine whether the disease has a self-limited course.[19]

The TSH response to a hypothyroid state induced by the excessive treatment of thyrotoxicosis may be diminished for several months or longer in these infants. Therefore, lack of TSH elevation cannot be relied on to indicate the excessive treatment of thyrotoxicosis. The addition of T_4 therapy to maintain FT_4 just above the mean for the assay may be required to avoid the consequences of infantile hypothyroidism. Monitoring of TSI may facilitate decision making about when to discontinue antithyroid therapy with MTZ. Antithyroid therapy should be discontinued by 6 months of age.

Most signs and symptoms of hyperthyroidism, including the cardiovascular manifestations, are closely related to increased adrenergic response.[19] Therefore, β-adrenergic blocking drugs can alleviate many of the potentially life-threatening, serious manifestations of neonatal thyrotoxicosis. In contrast to antithyroid drugs, these agents can rapidly diminish the severity of thyrotoxicosis, and their effects are evident within a few hours. Propranolol hydrochloride, together with iodine and MTZ, may be used in the treatment of severe neonatal thyrotoxicosis. Propranolol hydrochloride is given orally in a dose of 2 mg/kg per day in two or more divided doses.

Digitalization may be necessary in neonates with cardiac failure. Under these circumstances, reserpine may be contraindicated or must be used with extreme caution. In life-threatening cases, addition of pharmacologic steroids (hydrocortisone, 100 mg/m^2) reduces the production of thyroid hormone. A large goiter compressing the trachea and resulting in asphyxia must be treated surgically by splitting the isthmus.

The euthyroid or hypothyroid infant born to a mother who received antithyroid medications during pregnancy should be managed as described in the section on congenital hypothyroidism. If the infant has already received thyroid hormone, such therapy should be decreased as soon as thyrotoxic manifestations occur, and the appropriate management of hyperthyroidism must be initiated.

In the future, pregnant women with Graves disease may be screened for fetal hyperthyroidism. Prenatal therapy may be possible with the use of oral maternal PTU and adjustment of the dose to normalize fetal TSH, cardiac function, and maternal serum compound W (DIT representing fetal thyroid hormone status). Serial ultrasound monitoring of the fetal thyroid size may be used to detect goiter, suggesting maternal overtreatment and the need for a reduction in PTU dosage.[13]

Prognosis

Before the use of β-adrenergic blocking drugs, neonatal thyrotoxicosis carried a mortality rate of more than 15% if it was not recognized and treated promptly. In most instances, the syndrome has a self-limited duration, and no sequelae have been recognized. A goiter may resolve slowly over several months. Premature closure of all cranial sutures may occur. It is advisable to obtain a radiograph of the skull at 6 to 12 months of age in infants with history of thyrotoxicosis to evaluate this possibility.

FAMILIAL ABNORMALITIES OF THYROXINE-BINDING PROTEINS

Genetic disorders resulting in either increased or decreased levels of T_4-binding proteins have been reported. Affected individuals are healthy and asymptomatic because a change in the level of T_4-binding proteins does not lead to an alteration of FT_4. The disorders are usually discovered fortuitously by the measurement of T_4, which reveals unexpectedly high or low values. Therefore, the only clinical significance of these conditions lies in the abnormal T_4 level, possibly leading to an erroneous diagnosis. The TSH levels are normal in these individuals.

Decreased Thyroxine-Binding Globulin

In several families, affected males had no detectable TBG. Moreover, there was no male-to-male transmission of the trait. The most common form of TBG deficiency is transmitted as an X-linked trait. A female member of one of these families had no detectable TBG and a sex chromosome constitution of XO (Turner syndrome).[43] A single TBG gene has been shown to be present on the long arm of the X chromosome. However, in another family, a deficiency of TBG was found in three males and three females from two generations. The mode of transmission in this family suggested an autosomal dominant trait. Therefore, the level of TBG may be controlled by more than one gene. Prevalence of this disorder is about 1 in 5000 to 10,000 births. In the X-linked form, the affected homozygous males may have a complete lack of TBG or may have partial deficiency, and their heterozygous mothers often have decreased levels of TBG.[43]

Increased Thyroxine-Binding Globulin

Studies in families with increased TBG suggest that the trait is inherited as an autosomal dominant gene. In another family, the affected males transmitted the trait to female but not male offspring, suggesting that the trait is X-linked.

Increased Transthyretin

Families with increased levels of TTR have been reported and specific gene mutations identified. Serum T_4 and FT_4 index (FT_4I) were elevated, but FT_4 and FT_3 were normal.

Familial Dysalbuminemic Hyperthyroxinemia

There have been several reports of individuals who had levels of circulating T_4 that fell into the thyrotoxic range. Despite their high T_4, these individuals are asymptomatic and euthyroid. T_4 and FT_4I are increased. FT_4 is normal when measured by direct dialysis method but increased when determined by analogue assay. T_3 and rT_3 are normal, as are basal TSH and TSH response to TRH. These individuals may be confused with those with hyperthyroidism. However, the TRH test and normal TSH can distinguish between these two conditions. Familial dysalbuminemic hyperthyroxinemia is caused by enhanced binding of T_4 by abnormal serum albumin. The albumin in affected individuals appears to bind T_4 with greater affinity than normal albumin and only slightly less so than TTR. The condition appears to be an autosomal dominant trait, and its prevalence is estimated to be about 1 in 10,000 births. No clinical consequences are observed, and no therapy is required.

REFERENCES

1. American Academy of Pediatrics, Rose SR, et al: Update of newborn screening and therapy for congenital hypothyroidism, *Pediatrics* 117:2290, 2006.
2. Andersen S, et al: Biologic variation is important for interpretation of thyroid function tests, *Thyroid* 13:1069, 2003.
3. Anderson GW, et al: Control of thyroid hormone action in the developing rat brain, *Thyroid* 13:1039, 2003.
4. Asakura Y, et al: Hypothalamo-pituitary hypothyroidism detected by neonatal screening for congenital hypothyroidism using measurement of thyroid-stimulating hormone and thyroxine, *Acta Paediatr* 91:172, 2002.
5. Baloch Z, et al: Laboratory medicine practice guidelines: laboratory support for the diagnosis and monitoring of thyroid disease, *Thyroid* 13:3, 2003.
6. Bartalena L, et al: Effects of amiodarone administration during pregnancy on neonatal thyroid function and subsequent neurodevelopment, *J Endocrinol Invest* 24:116, 2001.
7. Bernal J, et al: Perspectives in the study of thyroid hormone action on brain development and function, *Thyroid* 11:1005, 2003.
8. Biswas S, et al: Pulmonary effects of triiodothyronine (T3) and hydrocortisone (HC) supplementation in preterm infants less than 30 weeks gestation: results of the THORN trial—thyroid hormone replacement in neonates, *Pediatr Res* 53:48, 2003.
9. Bongers-Schokking JJ, et al: Influence of timing and dose of thyroid hormone replacement on development in infants with congenital hypothyroidism, *J Pediatr* 136:292, 2000.
10. Calaciura F, et al: Subclinical hypothyroidism in early childhood: a frequent outcome of transient neonatal hyperthyrotropinemia, *J Clin Endocrinol Metab* 87:3209, 2002.
11. Carrascosa A, et al: Thyroid function in 76 sick preterm infants 30-36 weeks: results from a longitudinal study, *J Pediatr Endocrinol Metab* 21:237, 2008.
12. Clemente M, et al: Thyroid function in preterm infants 27-29 weeks of gestational age during the first four months of life: results from a prospective study comprising 80 preterm infants, *J Pediatr Endocrinol Metab* 20:1269, 2007.
13. Cohen O, et al: Serial in utero ultrasonographic measurements of the fetal thyroid: a new complementary tool in the management of maternal hyperthyroidism in pregnancy, *Prenat Diagn* 23:740, 2003.
14. Delange F: Iodine requirements during pregnancy, lactation and the neonatal period and indicators of optimal iodine nutrition, *Public Health Nutr* 10:1571, 2007.
15. de Vijlder JJ: Primary congenital hypothyroidism: defects in iodine pathways, *Eur J Endocrinol* 149:247, 2003.
16. Elmlinger MW, et al: Reference intervals from birth to adulthood for serum thyroxine (T4), triiodothyronine (T3), free T3, free T4, thyroxine binding globulin (TBG) and thyrotropin (TSH), *Clin Chem Lab Med* 39:973, 2001.
17. Fisher DA, et al: Maturation of human hypothalamic-pituitary-thyroid function and control, *Thyroid* 10:229, 2000.
18. Fisher DA: Thyroid function and dysfunction in premature infants, *Pediatr Endocrinol Rev* 4:317, 2007.
19. Foley TP Jr: Thyroid disease. In Kappy MS, et al, editors: *Wilkins' diagnosis and treatment of endocrine disorders in childhood and adolescence*, 4th ed, Springfield, IL, 1994, Charles C Thomas.
20. Glinoer D: Potential consequences of maternal hypothyroidism on the offspring: evidence and implications, *Horm Res* 55:109, 2001.
21. Glinoer D: Clinical and biological consequences of iodine deficiency during pregnancy, *Endocr Dev* 10:62, 2007.
22. Hasanhodzić M, et al: Down syndrome and thyroid gland, *Bosn J Basic Med Sci* 6:38, 2006.
23. Heindel JJ, Zoeller RT: Thyroid hormone and brain development: translating molecular mechanisms to population risk, *Thyroid* 13:1001, 2003.
24. Ibrahim M, et al:. Iodine supplementation for the prevention of mortality and adverse neurodevelopmental outcomes in preterm infants, *Cochrane Database Syst Rev* 19:CD005253, 2006.
25. Iijima K, et al: Cadmium, lead, and selenium in cord blood and thyroid hormone status of newborns, *Biol Trace Elem Res* 119:10, 2007.
26. Ineck BA, Ng TM: Effects of subclinical hypothyroidism and its treatment on serum lipids, *Ann Pharmacother* 37:725, 2003.
26a. Kemper AR, et al: Discontinuation of thyroid hormone treatment among children in the United States with congenital hypothyroidism: findings from health insurance claims data, *BMC Pediatr* 10:9, 2010.
27. Knobel M, Medeiros-Neto G: An outline of inherited disorders of the thyroid hormone generating system, *Thyroid* 13:771, 2003.
28. Kratzsch J, et al: Thyroid gland development and defects, *Best Pract Res Clin Endocrinol Metab* 22:57, 2008.
29. LaFranchi SH, et al: How should we be treating children with congenital hypothyroidism? *J Pediatr Endocrinol Metab* 20:559, 2007.
30. Lavado-Autric R, et al: Early maternal hypothyroxinemia alters histogenesis and cerebral cortex cytoarchiture of the progeny, *J Clin Invest* 111:1073, 2003.
31. Leger J, et al: Influence of severity of congenital hypothyroidism and adequacy of treatment on school achievement in young adolescents: a population-based cohort study, *Acta Paediatr* 90:1249, 2001.
32. Mastorakos G, et al: The menace of endocrine disruptors on thyroid hormone physiology and their impact on intrauterine development, *Endocrine* 31:219, 2007.
33. Moreno JC, et al: Inactivating mutations in the gene for thyroid oxidase 2 (THOX2) and congenital hypothyroidism, *N Engl J Med* 347:95, 2002.
34. Morin A, et al: Linear growth in children with congenital hypothyroidism detected by neonatal screen and treated early: a longitudinal study, *J Pediatr Endocrinol Metab* 15:973, 2002.
35. Nagashima T, et al: Novel inactivating missense mutations in the thyrotropin receptor gene in Japanese children with resistance to thyrotropin, *Thyroid* 11:551, 2001.

35a. Nebesio TD, et al: Newborn screening results in children with central hypothyroidism, *J Pediatr* 156:990, 2010.

36. Oerbeck B, et al: Congenital hypothyroidism: influence of disease severity and L-thyroxine treatment on intellectual, motor, and school-associated outcomes in young adults, *Pediatrics* 112:923, 2003.

37. Ogawa E, et al: Ultrasound appearance of thyroid tissue in hypothyroid infants, *J Pediatr* 153:101, 2008.

38. Osborn DA: Thyroid hormones for preventing neurodevelopmental impairment in preterm infants, *Cochrane Database Syst Rev*; CD005945, CD005946, CD005948, 2007.

39. Pereira DN, Procianoy RS: Effect of perinatal asphyxia on thyroid-stimulating hormone and thyroid hormone levels, *Acta Paediatr* 92:339, 2003.

40. Pintar JE: Normal development of the hypothalamic-pituitary-thyroid axis. In Braverman LE, et al, editors: *Werner and Ingbar's the thyroid*, 6th ed, Philadelphia, 1991, Lippincott.

41. Pohlenz J, et al: Congenital secondary hypothyroidism caused by exon skipping due to a homozygous donor splice site mutation in the TSH beta-subunit gene, *J Clin Endocrinol Metab* 87:336, 2002.

42. Pohlenz J, et al: A new heterozygous mutation (L338N) in the human Gs alpha (GNAS1) gene as a cause for congenital hypothyroidism in Albright's hereditary osteodystrophy, *Eur J Endocrinol* 148:463, 2003.

43. Reutrakul S, et al: Three novel mutations causing complete T4-binding globulin deficiency, *J Clin Endocrinol Metab* 86:5039, 2001.

43a. Rivkees SA, et al: Propylthiouracil (PTU) hepatotoxicity in children and recommendations for discontinuation of use, *Int J Pediatr Endocrinol* 2009: 132041, 2009.

43b. Rivkees SA, et al: Adverse events associated with methimazole therapy of graves' disease in children, *Int J Pediatr Endocrinol* 2010: 176970, 2010.

44. Rose SR: Disorders of thyrotropin synthesis, secretion, and function, *Curr Opin Pediatr* 12:375, 2000.

44a. Rose SR: Improved diagnosis of mild hypothyroidism using time-of-day normal ranges for thyrotropin, *J Pediatr* 2010 (epub in advance of print).

45. Savin S, et al: Thyroid hormone synthesis and storage in the thyroid gland of human neonates, *J Pediatr Endocrinol Metab* 16:521, 2003.

46. Selva KA, et al: Initial treatment dose of L-thyroxine in congenital hypothyroidism, *J Pediatr* 141:786, 2002.

47. Singh PK, et al: Establishment of reference intervals for markers of fetal thyroid status in amniotic fluid, *J Clin Endocrinol Metab* 88:4175, 2003.

47a. Slaughter J, et al: The effects of gestational age and birth weight on false-positive newborn screening rates, *J Pediatr* 2010, in press.

48. Song SI, et al: The influence of etiology and treatment factors in intellectual outcome on congenital hypothyroidism, *J Dev Behav Pediatr* 22:376, 2001.

49. Tanaka K, et al: Serum free T4 and thyroid stimulating hormone levels in preterm infants and relationship between these levels and respiratory distress syndrome, *Pediatr Int* 49:447, 2007.

50. Van Trotsenburg AS, et al: Lower neonatal screening thyroxine concentrations in Down syndrome newborns, *J Clin Endocrinol Metab* 88:1512, 2003.

51. Wang R, et al: Accuracy of free thyroxine measurements across natural ranges of thyroxine binding to serum proteins, *Thyroid* 10:31, 2000.

52. Watkins MG, et al: Persistent neonatal thyrotoxicosis in a neonate secondary to a rare thyroid-stimulating hormone receptor activating mutation: case report and literature review, *Endocr Pract* 14:479, 2008.

53. Weitzel JM, et al: Regulation of mitochondrial biogenesis by thyroid hormone, *Exp Physiol* 88:121, 2003.

54. Wu SY, et al: Compound W: a potential marker in maternal serum for assessing fetal thyroid function, *Compr Ther* 21:594, 1995.

55. Yamakita N, et al: Usefulness of thyrotropin (TSH)-releasing hormone test and nocturnal surge of TSH for diagnosis of isolated deficit of TSH secretion, *J Clin Endocrinol Metab* 86:1054, 2001.

PART 4

Disorders of Sex Development

Rayzel M. Shulman, Mark R. Palmert, and Diane K. Wherrett

Genetic sex is determined at the time of fertilization, but carrying out the encoded genetic directives that lead to sexual differentiation takes place over 14 weeks of embryonic and fetal development. An error or fault in this process may result in a disorder of sex development (DSD), defined as a discrepancy in the genetic, gonadal, or genital makeup of an individual. This part reviews (1) normal fetal sexual differentiation; (2) an approach to the recognition and diagnosis of neonates who may have a DSD; and (3) the classification, clinical features, and general management principles of DSDs, with the focus on perinatal issues.

FETAL SEXUAL DIFFERENTIATION AND DEVELOPMENT

Genetic Control of Fetal Gonadal Development and Differentiation

The embryo and early fetus, regardless of genetic sex (i.e., 46,XX or 46,XY), are bipotential (i.e., sex indifferent) with respect to their possible sexual differentiation, having the anatomic and biochemical apparatus necessary for both male and female development. For normal male differentiation to occur, a succession of genetic and hormonal signals must be intact and occur normally.[41] The classic teaching is that there is an innate tendency of the embryo and early fetus to differentiate along female lines; that is, female differentiation occurs if the signals for male differentiation are absent. However, evidence is growing that describes an active process involved in female differentiation.[75]

Y CHROMOSOME AND ROLE OF *SRY* GENE

The differentiation of the bipotential gonad is the event that determines the sexual differentiation of the fetus. The presence of the *SRY* gene on the Y chromosome causes the bipotential gonad to differentiate as a testis, and male phenotypic development follows. The presence of one, two, or more X chromosomes does not alter this process; however, the presence of more than one X chromosome (e.g., 47,XXY syndrome) results in eventual meiotic failure, loss of germ cells, and infertility. Candidate genes for an X-linked female determining factor are being investigated.[9]

Early ovarian differentiation does not require two X chromosomes and thus proceeds in 45,X fetuses. Later on, in ovarian differentiation, two X chromosomes are necessary for normal formation of primordial follicles. If part or all of the second X chromosome is missing, ovarian development fails, beginning from about 15 weeks on, because the abnormal primordial follicles and oocytes degenerate rapidly through the remainder of gestation (postfertilization). The resulting gonad appears as an elongated, whitish streak that microscopically shows whorls of fibrous tissue lacking in germ cells or epithelial elements. This "streak" gonad is characteristic of the gonadal dysgenesis syndromes.

Y chromosome fetuses that fail to undergo testicular differentiation are believed to experience the same gonadal changes to form streak gonads, but unlike gonadal dysgenesis in patients with X chromosome abnormalities, these structures carry a high risk for the development of gonadal tumors.[19] These tumors may result from the persistence of residual XY germ cells that did not degenerate or from tumorigenic loci on the Y chromosome.

AUTOSOMAL AND X-LINKED GENES

Although the presence or absence of the *SRY* gene determines the differentiation of the bipotential gonad, additional genes that are both autosomal and X-linked and located upstream and downstream from the *SRY* gene are involved in gonadal development and differentiation (Fig. 49-26).[20] Several of these genes have in common the encoding of a type of protein that functions as a transcription factor or transcription regulatory protein, which activates or represses the expression of other target genes, often in multiple tissues, thereby influencing or controlling a diverse program of cellular differentiation and proliferation during embryonic and fetal development. When gene mutation occurs, an alteration in the functional domain of the transcription factor can lead to abnormal or changed regulation (e.g., from a repressor to an activator) of downstream genes, resulting in abnormal cell differentiation or growth or neoplastic transformation. It is the occurrence of such mutations and the resulting pathologic conditions that have led to the identification and functional understanding of many of these genes.

Embryology and Endocrinology

The bipotential gonads and the anlagen for the genital ducts and external genitalia are derived from the mesodermal germ layer; the exception is the urogenital sinus epithelium, which is of endodermal origin. The bipotential gonadal and genital tissues undergo morphogenesis during the embryonic period, which extends from the end of the third week, or about age 20 days, through the seventh o eighth week of gestational age. Sexual differentiation occurs in the fetal period beginning in the seventh week, when the bipotential gonad begins to differentiate as either a testis or an ovary, and proceeding until 12 to 14 weeks of fetal age, when differentiation of the internal genital ducts and external genitalia along male or female lines is largely complete.

Female development

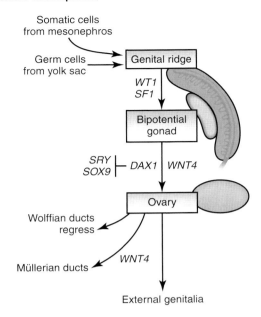

Male development

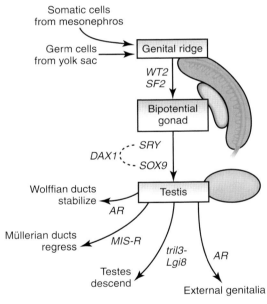

Figure 49–26. Possible roles of key genes in human fetal sexual development. The development of the genital ridge and bipotential gonad is under similar control in the two sexes. An ovary develops in the absence of *SRY* and *SOX9* action, possibly because of the antitestis effects of *DAX1* and *WNT4*. Steroidogenesis is delayed in the ovary by the action of *WNT4*, which is also needed for the development of the müllerian ducts. A testis develops as a result of *SRY* and *SOX9* action, complemented by *DAX1*. The regression of the müllerian ducts is mediated by müllerian inhibiting substance and its receptor (R), whereas the androgenic stabilization of the wolffian ducts and the differentiation of the external genitalia are mediated by the androgen receptor (AR). (*From Hughes IA: Female development—all by default?* N Engl J Med 351:748, 2004.)

DEVELOPMENT OF THE GONADS

The gonadal blastema begins to form at 4 to 4½ weeks in the genital ridge, located bilaterally on the medial aspect of each mesonephros. The somatic component of the gonad is made up of cells from the coelomic epithelium and the underlying mesenchyme or adjacent mesonephros.[66] The germinal component comprises the primordial germ cells, which are mitotically active and migrate from the yolk sac endoderm at 24 days to reach the genital ridge at 4½ to 6 weeks, thereby forming the indifferent gonad (Fig. 49-27).[47]

Sex differentiation of the gonad begins at 7 weeks and denotes the onset of fetal sexual differentiation. The gonad differentiates as a testis if the *SRY* gene and its pathway are present and as an ovary if it is absent. The sex differences that appear in the developing gonad at this time include differentiation of cord somatic cells, changes in germ cell mitotic and meiotic activity, hormone production by the cord and interstitial (mesenchymal) cells, and development of the outer cortex. These differences are detailed in Table 49-11, and an overview is schematically represented in Figure 49-27.

TESTICULAR DIFFERENTIATION

Testicular differentiation begins at 7 to 8 weeks, when the sex cords form loops in the cortex and differentiate as the seminiferous cords; in the hilum, they anastomose to form the rete cords. From 8 weeks on, the seminiferous cords become coiled and thickened and contain 8 to 10 layers of Sertoli cells, whereas the spermatogonia remain located near the basement membrane of the cords. Leydig cells appear in the interstitium between the seminiferous cords at 7½ to 8 weeks. They increase strikingly in number during the third month, occupy half the volume of the testis at 13 to 14 weeks, and then show a significant fall in number. Some Leydig cells are present postnatally but histologically disappear after 3 to 6 months because of the physiologic lowering of gonadotropin stimulation.[27] As the fetus elongates, the testis descends and occupies a more caudal position. In the sixth and seventh months, the cremaster muscle differentiates in the caudal testicular ligament to form the testicular gubernaculum, which penetrates the inguinal canal and is anchored to the connective tissue of the scrotum. The testis descends behind the peritoneum and reaches the scrotum by the eighth or ninth month; the inguinal canal closes after testicular descent is complete.

OVARIAN DIFFERENTIATION

Ovarian differentiation begins at 7 weeks, as outlined previously and in Table 49-11. The sex cords in the ovary show germ cells (oogonia) undergoing repeated mitotic divisions from 7 weeks through about the fifth month. Most oogonia differentiate into oocytes between about 10 and 24 weeks; in so doing, they enter meiosis, proceeding through the first meiotic prophase. After reaching the meiotic prophase, many oocytes become surrounded by a single layer of granulosa cells to form the primordial follicles from about 15 weeks through term. Two X chromosomes are needed for differentiation of the primordial follicle. Oocytes that are not enclosed in a follicle degenerate. During ovarian differentiation, the number of germ cells greatly increases to several million oogonia and oocytes by the fifth month. Most germ cells degenerate thereafter either before or during the primordial follicle stage, leaving about 150,000 oocytes in each ovary at birth.

DEVELOPMENT OF THE GENITAL DUCTS

The internal genital ducts, unlike the gonads, develop from separate anlagen, from the mesonephric or wolffian ducts in the male and from the paramesonephric or müllerian ducts in the female. The wolffian ducts are formed in 26- to 32-day-old embryos; the müllerian ducts begin development at about 37 days in close association with the wolffian ducts, which serve as a guide to the caudal progression of the müllerian ducts. In the absence of the wolffian ducts, the müllerian ducts do not develop.

In the male fetus, the müllerian ducts begin to regress at 7 to 7½ weeks, shortly after the Sertoli cells have differentiated and begun to produce antimüllerian hormone (AMH), otherwise known as *müllerian-inhibiting substance*, and before the onset of local testosterone production by Leydig cells. Regression is complete by 9 weeks. Differentiation of the wolffian ducts is testosterone dependent and begins at about 8½ weeks. The wolffian ducts differentiate into the epididymis and vas deferens, and beginning at 10½ weeks, the seminal vesicles and their ejaculatory ducts develop at the caudal end from lateral outpouchings.

In the female fetus, müllerian duct differentiation occurs in the absence of AMH and does not require the presence of any ovarian hormone. The müllerian ducts form the fallopian tubes, uterus, and upper portion of the vagina beginning in the third month, stimulated in part by epidermal growth factor. The wolffian ducts degenerate in the absence of local testosterone and disappear by 13 weeks. The fallopian tubes later descend with the ovaries and are included in a fold of peritoneum called the *broad ligament*. At birth, the position of the uterus is vertical, and uterine development is disproportionate in that the uterine cervix is twice as large as the fundus; it remains so until puberty. Maternal estrogens stimulate uterine growth in utero, so its size at birth is larger than it is at several months of age; endometrial hyperplasia may occasionally result in transient neonatal uterine bleeding. The development of the vagina depends on the caudal müllerian ducts contacting the endodermal epithelium of the urogenital sinus. At this junction, a multilayered, solid epithelial cord known as the *vaginal plate* is formed; it disintegrates beyond 4 months to form the vaginal lumen. It is not clear whether the lower portion of the vagina is derived from the urogenital sinus, with the upper portion of müllerian origin, or the vagina originates entirely from the urogenital sinus.

DEVELOPMENT OF THE EXTERNAL GENITALIA

The external genitalia in both sexes, like the gonads, are derived from common anlagen (Fig. 49-28). Their inherent development is along female lines unless systemic androgens, specifically dihydrotestosterone (DHT), induce male differentiation. The genital tubercle forms early in the fourth week at the cranial end of the cloacal membrane, and on each side, the labioscrotal swellings and urogenital folds develop. Fusion of the urorectal septum with the cloacal membrane in the seventh week creates a dorsal anal membrane and a ventral urogenital membrane, which rupture in the eighth week to form the anus and urogenital orifice.

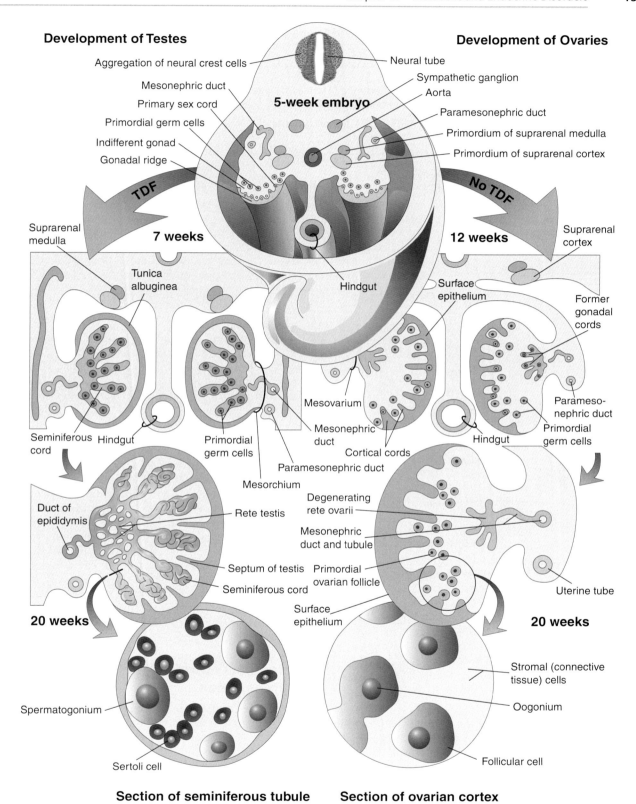

Figure 49–27. Schematic illustration showing differentiation of the indifferent gonads of a 5-week embryo (*top*) into ovaries or testes. *Left side* shows the development of testes resulting from the effects of the testis-determining factor (TDF) located on the Y chromosome. *Right side* shows the development of ovaries in the absence of TDF. (*From Moore KL, Persaud TVN: The developing human: clinically oriented embryology, 8th ed, Philadelphia, 2008, Saunders.*)

TABLE 49–11 Descriptive Features of Testicular and Ovarian Differentiation at 7 Weeks of Gestation

Gonadal Cells	Testicular Differentiation	Ovarian Differentiation
Cord somatic cells	Differentiate as Sertoli cells Synthesize antimüllerian hormone (AMH) at 7½ weeks Unable to aromatize androgens to estrogens	Differentiate as granulosa cells Do not synthesize AMH at this age Able to aromatize androgens to estrogens
Germ cells	Reduced mitotic activity results in small number of spermatogonia Meiosis is inhibited until puberty	High mitotic activity results in large number of oogonia Meiosis is promoted within several weeks
Interstitial cells	Differentiate as Leydig cells Synthesize testosterone de novo at 8 wk	Remain undifferentiated until 15 wk Lack steroidogenic capability at this age
Outer cortex	Sex cords lose connection with surface epithelium Mesenchymal tissue forms tunica albuginea that lacks germ cells	Sex cords retain connection with surface epithelium Thickened zone that contains germ cells

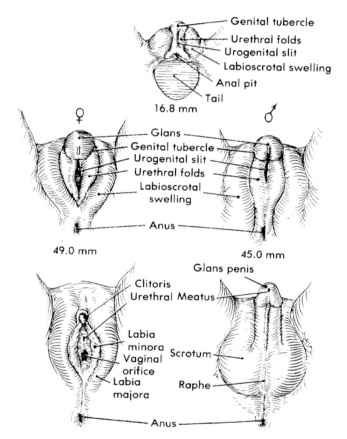

Figure 49–28. Differentiation of the external genitalia in the male and female fetus from the common primordia. *Top,* The indifferent genitalia are shown at about 48 days. The tail of the embryo has been cut away to uncover the genitalia. *Middle,* The genitalia at about 9½ weeks. In the male, anogenital lengthening and midline fusion have begun. *Bottom,* Newborn genitalia. Genitalia differentiation is complete by about 14 weeks of gestation. However, growth during the second and third trimesters accounts for the difference in phallic size. (*From Grumbach MM, et al: Disorders of sexual differentiation. In Wilson JD, et al: Williams textbook of endocrinology, 10th ed, Philadelphia, 2003, Saunders, p 73.*)

Abnormal development of the urorectal septum results in anorectal malformations.

In the male fetus, the indifferent stage of the external genitalia lasts until the ninth week, when, in the presence of systemic androgens, masculinization begins with lengthening of the anogenital distance (see Fig. 49-28). The urogenital and labioscrotal folds fuse in the midline, beginning caudally and progressing anteriorly. The urethra develops with fusion of the urogenital folds, which forms both the membranous urethra in the perineum and the penile urethra along the ventral surface of the phallus. Midline fusion of the labioscrotal folds forms the scrotal raphe, whereas the penile raphe represents the fused portions of the urogenital folds. These processes are complete in the 14-week fetus.

In the 9-week female fetus, the anogenital distance does not increase, and the urogenital folds and labioscrotal swellings do not fuse (see Fig. 49-28). The labioscrotal swellings develop predominantly in their caudal portions but less so than in male fetuses, and they remain unfused as they are transformed into the labia majora. The urogenital folds develop into the labia minora. The epithelium of the vaginal vestibule between the labia minora and the hymen is endodermal, being derived from the urogenital sinus, whereas the epithelium between the labia minora and majora is ectodermal in origin.

Hormonal Control of Fetal Sex Differentiation

The fetal testes play a major role in male sex differentiation by producing two hormones, AMH and testosterone, which are major determinants of internal and external genital differentiation. On the other hand, the fetal ovaries play a negligible or no role in female sex differentiation, although they may have some steroidogenic capacity.

FETAL GONADAL ENDOCRINE FUNCTION

AMH is a large glycoprotein (molecular weight, 140,000 d) produced by the fetal Sertoli cells beginning at 7½ weeks that induces irreversible involution of the müllerian ducts. Regression of the müllerian ducts can be induced by AMH only during a fetal age of 44 to 70 days. The gene coding for AMH is located on chromosome 19p13.3, and for the AMH receptor on chromosome 12.

The other major hormone produced by the fetal testis is testosterone (Fig. 49-29). It is synthesized by the Leydig cells beginning at 8 weeks, and testicular production achieves peak serum testosterone levels at 10 to 15 weeks. In the second half of gestation, males show a gradual decline and females a rise in serum testosterone levels, so by the third trimester, males have similar or only slightly higher levels than females.[68]

The control of the fetal testicular synthesis of testosterone between 8 and 14 weeks is uncertain. The prime candidate has been human chorionic gonadotropin (hCG) of placental or fetal origin, which binds to fetal testes beginning at 8 weeks. From 14 weeks on, the fetal testes are able to respond to hCG with the production of testosterone. In the second and third trimesters, fetal serum luteinizing hormone (LH) levels correlate with the maintenance and subsequent decline of serum testosterone.[6] Follicle-stimulating hormone (FSH) receptors are present in fetal testes from 8 weeks on and may play a role in Sertoli cell or seminiferous tubule development.

The fetal ovary in the first trimester is hormonally quiescent, lacking hCG and FSH binding and the enzymes necessary for steroid synthesis. Starting at 8 weeks, the fetal ovary has aromatase activity and is capable of converting androstenedione or testosterone to estrone or estradiol, but actual production has not been demonstrated. Most estrogen that is present in the fetus is produced by placental aromatase. Amniotic fluid levels of estradiol at 12 to 16 weeks are slightly higher in females, raising the possibility of ovarian synthesis of estrogen. If it is synthesized, estradiol could play a local role in ovarian differentiation.[4]

CONTROL OF GENITAL DIFFERENTIATION: ROLES OF ANTIMÜLLERIAN HORMONE AND TESTOSTERONE

In the absence of testes, female sex differentiation occurs regardless of whether an ovary or no gonad is present; a male fetus castrated early also undergoes female sex differentiation. This activity is in keeping with the inherent tendency of the fetus to develop along female lines.

Male sex differentiation requires bilateral testes that produce AMH from the Sertoli cells and testosterone from the Leydig cells. AMH acts locally to cause regression of only the ipsilateral müllerian duct. If only one testis is present, müllerian duct development occurs on the contralateral side. Testosterone does not cause müllerian duct regression. A 46,XX female with müllerian duct regression due to a *WNT4* mutation suggests that müllerian duct regression can be controlled by proteins other than AMH.[26]

Testosterone produced by the fetal testes is secreted both locally, where it stimulates differentiation of the ipsilateral wolffian duct, and systemically, where it serves as a prohormone in the masculinization of the external genitalia. If only one testis is present, the contralateral wolffian duct fails to differentiate, indicating that the systemically circulating testosterone levels are inadequate for the stimulation of wolffian differentiation. Therefore, testosterone derived from maternal sources or the fetal adrenals, as in congenital adrenal hyperplasia (CAH), does not induce wolffian development.

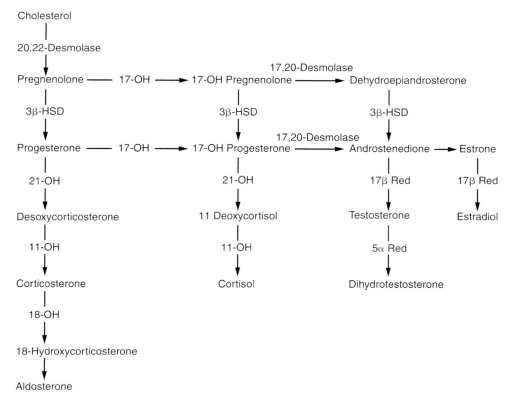

Figure 49–29. Steroid biosynthetic pathway in adrenal and gonadal tissues. 11-OH, 11β-hydroxylase; 17-OH, 17α-hydroxylase; 18-OH, 18-hydroxylase; 21-OH, 21-hydroxylase; 3βHSD, 3β-hydroxysteroid dehydrogenase; 17β, 17β-reductase; 5α, 5α-reductase.

Although the wolffian ducts are stabilized through the effects of testosterone, the external genitalia and urogenital sinus are stimulated to undergo male differentiation by DHT, which is formed in peripheral tissues (external genitalia, liver, kidney, and bone marrow) through the conversion of testosterone by 5α-reductase. Testosterone is a weaker androgen than DHT and does not stimulate male external genital differentiation, serving instead as a prohormone for DHT in this tissue. Systemic testosterone derived from the fetal adrenals, as in CAH, or from maternal sources can induce variable masculinization of the external genitalia when it is metabolized to DHT.

The absence of one testis is usually associated with incomplete masculinization of the external genitalia, suggesting that two testes are generally required to provide adequate systemic levels of testosterone and thus adequate DHT. The period in which DHT can induce male differentiation extends up to 12 to 14 weeks. A deficiency in androgen receptor binding results in androgen insensitivity, which may be partial or complete. In terms of fetal sex differentiation, the androgen-mediated events of wolffian duct differentiation, masculinization of the external genitalia, and growth of genital structures are either impaired or completely fail to occur, depending on the extent of the receptor binding deficiency.

A CLINICAL APPROACH TO THE INFANT WITH GENITAL AMBIGUITY

The evaluation of the neonate with a suspected DSD requires prompt attention and a team approach. Depending on the institution, the team may include neonatology, pediatric endocrinology, genetics, pediatric urology, pediatric gynecology, pediatric surgery, psychology, psychiatry, nursing, and social work. Appropriate initial assessment and management of the newborn with a DSD is essential to helping the family cope with this difficult situation. This evaluation needs to begin as soon as possible and should be approached systematically.

Definition of Ambiguous Genitalia

Most individuals with a DSD have some abnormality of their external genitalia that makes them identifiable at birth. An evaluation of a DSD is needed for patients who have any of the following: male-appearing genitalia with a micropenis, severe hypospadias or bilateral cryptorchidism; the presence of two defects, such as hypospadias and unilateral cryptorchidism; infants with female-appearing genitalia, the presence of posterior labial fusion, clitoromegaly, or a labial or inguinal mass that might represent a gonad; or discordance between the prenatal karyotype and genital examination findings.[35]

History

Most DSDs are either isolated occurrences or inherited as an autosomal recessive or X-linked trait. The family may not know the specifics about other family members with DSDs but may be aware of a family history of a trait that could be a manifestation of a DSD such as infertility, amenorrhea, or hypospadias. Considering CAH, the family should be asked about other infants with unexplained deaths. Consanguinity or a genetically homogeneous population increases the chance of autosomal recessive conditions. The infant's mother should be asked about any medications taken during pregnancy, especially androgens or progestins. In the case of a masculinized female infant, the mother should be questioned about and examined for virilization.

Physical Examination

Considerable information can be obtained by performing a careful physical examination. Specifically, inferences can be made regarding gonadal development and status and the degree of androgen effects. Examples of the wide range of disorders that may cause genital abnormalities are shown in Table 49-12. A schematic representation of varying degrees of virilization, graded using a scale developed by Prader, in males and females is shown later in Figure 49-40.

DELIVERY ROOM OR NURSERY EXAMINATION OF ALL NEWBORNS

Every newborn must have a careful genital examination in the delivery room or nursery. The purposes of the examination are to verify the gender assignment; avoid missing the diagnosis of a DSD, particularly in females with CAH, and recognize mild abnormalities that are not likely to affect gender assignment but require follow-up, such as mild hypospadias or unilateral cryptorchidism. The findings of a normal genital examination are listed in Box 49-10. The genitalia do not need to be overtly ambiguous to qualify for a diagnostic evaluation. Neonates with overtly ambiguous genitalia should have gender assignment deferred. The parents of the neonate should be informed that most of the diagnostic evaluation can be performed in 2 to 3 days, at which time the appropriate gender assignment can usually be made.

GONADAL DESCENT AND SIZE

Gonads should be carefully palpated in the scrotum or labial area and along the inguinal canal. Only a gonad containing testicular tissue (testis or ovotestis) can descend to a position where it is palpable (an ovary almost never descends). A small gonad (longest diameter <8 mm) may be dysgenetic, rudimentary, or due to lack of gonadotropin stimulation. The ability to detect gonads in the inguinal area can be enhanced by applying soap or oil to the skin and the examiner's fingers to decrease friction. With the infant supine, glide two or three fingers with gentle to firm pressure along the inguinal canal toward the scrotum, repeating this action numerous times if necessary. The gonad will be felt "popping" under the fingers. With this technique, less accessible or small gonads can be palpated that would otherwise be missed. Additionally, sit the infant in a frog-leg position and, particularly with crying or increased intra-abdominal pressure, the testis may descend into the lower inguinal or scrotal region.

PENIS SIZE

It is important to assess both the length and the amount of erectile tissue of the penis. A penis that appears small must be measured fully stretched, pressing the ruler down against the pubic ramus, depressing the suprapubic fat pad completely, and measuring to the tip of the glans only, ignoring

TABLE 49–12   Associations of Genital Abnormalities

Abnormal Characteristics	Examples of Associated Disorders
Male-Appearing Genitalia	
Micropenis	Growth hormone or luteinizing hormone deficiency Testosterone deficiency (in second and third trimesters) Partial androgen insensitivity Syndrome: idiopathic
Hypospadias (more severe)	Disorders of gonadal development 46,XX DSD Ovotesticular DSD 46,XX or 46,XX DSD Syndrome: idiopathic
Impalpable gonads	Anorchia Persistent müllerian duct syndrome 46,XX DSD with 21- or 11β-hydroxylase deficiency Cryptorchidism
Small gonads	47,XXY, 46,XX DSD Dysgenetic or rudimentary testes
Inguinal mass (uterus or tube)	Persistent müllerian duct syndrome, dysgenetic testes
Female-Appearing Genitalia	

Clitoromegaly	XX with 21- or 11β-hydroxylase or
	  3β-hydroxydehydrogenase deficiency
	Other 46,XX DSD
	Gonadal dysgenesis, dysgenetic testes,
	  ovotesticular DSD
	46,XY DSD
	Tumor infiltration of clitoris
	Syndrome: idiopathic

Posterior labial fusion	As for clitorimegaly
Palpable gonad(s)	Gonadal dysgenesis, dysgenetic testes, ovotesticular DSD 46,XY DSD
Inguinal hernia or mass	As for palpable gonad(s)

DSD, disorder of sex development.

BOX 49–10   Findings That Constitute a Normal Genital Examination in the Newborn

FEMALE NEWBORN
Vaginal opening fully visible: 3- to 4-mm slit or stellate orifice with heaped-up mucosa (i.e., no posterior labial fusion)
Clitoris width 2 to 6 mm
Absence of gonads in labia majora or inguinal region

MALE NEWBORN
Urethra at tip of glans (which may be inferred by a fully developed foreskin)
Penis of normal stretched length (2.5 to 5 cm) and diameter (0.9 to 1.3 cm)
Bilateral testes of normal size (8 to 14 mm) in the scrotal sacs

---

any excess foreskin (Fig. 49-30). An excellent ruler can be made by placing marks 0.5 cm apart on a wooden stick such as a tongue blade or a flexible strip. The width is measured at the midshaft of the stretched penis. A micropenis is arbitrarily defined as a penis with a normally formed urethra that opens at the tip of the glans in which the stretched length is less than 2.5 cm in the full-term neonate. The length criteria must be adjusted to take into account the smaller phallus in the premature neonate (Fig. 49-31). The definition of a micropenis can also be used to describe a rare condition in which the penile corpora cavernosa are absent or severely deficient in size (Table 49-13), resulting in an abnormally thin penis.

CLITORIS SIZE

A clitoris that appears enlarged is best assessed by measurement of the width (diameter) of the paired corpora cavernosa that compose the erectile shaft of the clitoris. With clitoral

Figure 49–30. **A,** A 2-month-old boy with micropenis and cryptorchidism caused by luteinizing hormone and follicle-stimulating hormone deficiency. The scrotum is compact or "unlived in," and the testes are inguinal. **B,** Centimeter markings are inked on a wooden tongue blade, which is placed near the penis and depressed down on the pubic ramus. The penis is maximally stretched, with the measurement made to the tip of the glans (measurement here is 1.7 cm).

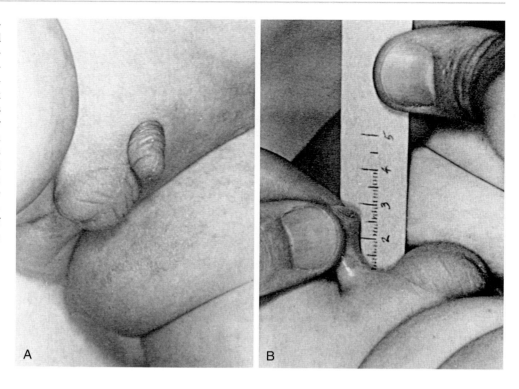

enlargement due to edema or birth trauma, a normal corporal width (<6 mm) is present,[53] whereas clitoral enlargement due to androgen stimulation (occurring in the second and third trimesters) results in increased corporal growth (>6 mm). The width of the clitoris is measured by gently but firmly pressing the shaft of the clitoris between the thumb and forefinger to exclude excess skin and subcutaneous tissue, thereby measuring predominantly the width of the corpora cavernosa (see Table 49-13).

URETHRAL OPENING

If the foreskin is fully formed, the urethra is almost always at the tip of the glans; on rare occasions, the foreskin covers hypospadias on the glans. In boys, hypospadias can vary from mild (off the center of the glans) to severe (at the base of the penis or on the perineum). The prepuce in the hypospadiac penis is usually deficient ventrally and thus appears hooded. Chordee (ventral curvature of the penis) is caused by fibrotic contracture in the area of failed urethral development. The presence of severe hypospadias in a male infant indicates deficient testosterone or DHT action in the first trimester. In girls, the urethral meatus is normally a 1-mm pinhole-like or flat opening located just ventral to the vagina. Androgen exposure at 8 to 14 weeks of fetal age moves the urethral meatus ventrally on the perineum or the shaft of the phallic structure.

VAGINAL OPENING

The vaginal orifice, a 3- to 4-mm slit or stellate opening surrounded by heaped-up mucosa, is normally visible when the examiner lifts up the labia majora. The presence and direct visualization of the vaginal opening indicate the absence of androgen effects and the presence of a distal vagina

(of urogenital sinus origin); whether a uterus (of müllerian duct origin) is also present cannot be inferred from this finding. Conversely, at 8 to 14 weeks of fetal age, exposure of the female fetus to androgens or incomplete androgen stimulation of the male fetus results in variable masculinization. This process can be mild to moderate, with posterior midline fusion of the labia majora that partially or completely covers the vaginal opening, thereby preventing its direct visualization. With severe masculinization, there is formation of a common urogenital sinus (resulting from the internal junction of the vagina and urethra) that is seen as a single 1- to 2-mm flat orifice on the perineum or shaft of the phallus.

LABIOSCROTAL DEVELOPMENT

The labia majora are normally unfused in the female. Partial or complete midline fusion indicates androgen exposure at 8 to 14 weeks of fetal age and predicts ventral placement of the urethral meatus on the perineum or phallus. The scrotum in the male is normally completely fused, with a midline raphe. A compact or "unlived in" scrotum indicates the lack of testes or undescended testes. In the male, incomplete or absent midline fusion indicates deficient or absent androgen effects at 8 to 14 weeks of fetal age and predicts a perineal location of the urethral meatus.

ASSOCIATED DYSMORPHOLOGY

A thorough physical examination should be done to identify any other dysmorphic features. Genital abnormalities are often part of dysmorphic syndromes and are frequently associated with other midline defects. Examples include the presence of the Turner phenotype in gonadal dysgenesis and camptomelic dwarfism (bowing and angulation of the lower limbs, flat facies, shortened vertebrae) in XY gonadal dysgenesis. Some

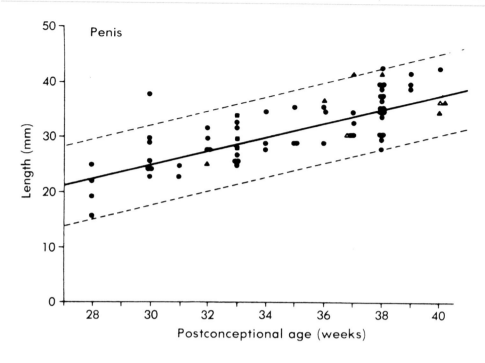

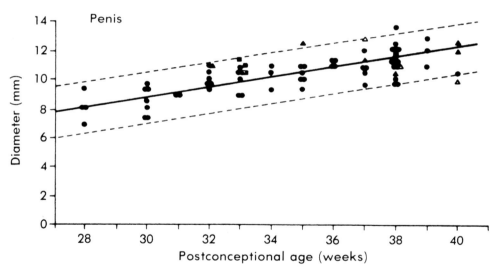

Figure 49–31. Stretched penile length (mean ± 2 SD) (**A**) and penile diameter (mean ± 2 SD) (**B**) in 63 normal premature and full-term male infants (●), two infants who were small for gestational age (△), seven infants who were large for gestational age (▲), and four twins (■). (*From Feldman KW , et al: Fetal phallic growth and penile standards for newborn male infants,* J Pediatr 86:395, 1975).

DSD patients appear phenotypically normal at birth, including many (but not all) cases of gonadal dysgenesis, XX male, 46,XY male with persistent müllerian ducts, and complete androgen insensitivity syndrome (cAIS).

Discussion with Family and Professional Staff

It is important to recognize that the birth of an infant with a DSD is a major stress for the family. A physician experienced in the evaluation of DSD should meet with the family as soon as possible to discuss the situation, ensuring confidentiality and privacy. Both parents should be present if possible. As part of the discussion, the infant's genitalia should be examined with the parents. Parents are frequently afraid to look at

their child's genitalia. Showing the anatomic abnormalities to the family in a calm and professional manner helps the family bond with their child. Outline what will happen (procedures, consultations) and the time frame in which the results will be available. Review with the parents what they plan to tell relatives and friends, which is often a source of great anxiety. Many families and cultures have strong feelings about gender assignment, and these feelings need to be known by the health professionals. Reassure the family that when the data from the tests are available there will be much more information that will help determine the appropriate gender assignment. In most cases, the correct gender assignment will be apparent when the test results become available; in some cases, the gender assignment is not clear, and the options will need to be discussed with the parents.

TABLE 49–13 Anthropometric Measurements of the External Genitalia

Sex	Population	Age	Stretched Penile Length, Mean ± SD, cm (Males), or Clitoral Length, Mean ± SD, mm (Females)	Penile Width, Mean ± SD, cm (Males), or Clitoral Width, Mean ± SD, mm (Females)	Mean Testicular Volume, mL (Males), or Perineum Length, Mean ± SD, mm (Females)
M	United States	30 wk GA	2.5 ± 0.4		
M	United States	Term	3.5 ± 0.4	1.1 ± 0.1	0.52 (median)
M	Japan	Term to 14 yr	2.9 ± 0.4 - .8.3 ± 0.8		
M	Australia	24-36 wk GA	2.27 + (0.16 GA)		
M	China	Term	3.1 ± 0.3	1.07 ± 0.09	
M	India	Term	3.6 ± 0.4	1.14 ± 0.07	
M	North America	Term	3.4 ± 0.3	1.13 ± 0.08	
M	Europe	10 yr	6.4 ± 0.4		0.95-1.20
M	Europe	Adult	13.3 ± 1.6		16.5-18.2
F	United States	Term	4.0 ± 1.24	3.32 ± 0.78	
F	United States	Adult nulliparous	15.4 ± 4.3		
F	United States	Adult	19.1 ± 8.7	5.5 ± 1.7	31.3 ± 8.5

GA, gestational age.
From Lee PA; International Consensus Conference on Intersex organized by the Lawson Wilkins Pediatric Endocrine Society and the European Society for Paediatric Endocrinology: Consensus statement on management of intersex disorders. International Consensus Conference on Intersex (see comment), *Pediatrics* 118:e488, 2006.

Below are examples of scripts for answering questions commonly asked by families with children with a new diagnosis of a DSD. These are taken largely from the Clinical Guideline for the Management of DSD in Childhood, published by the Consortium on the Management of Disorders of Sex Development.

Q: Is my child a boy or a girl?
A: Your question is very important. We wish we could tell you right this minute, but we really can't tell yet. We will have more information after we conduct some tests. It's hard for parents to wait for these test results so we will try to update you every day, and you can call (give contact person's name). Although your baby has a condition you probably haven't heard much about, it isn't that uncommon. We've encountered this before, and we'll help you through this time of confusion. As soon as the tests are completed, we will be able to talk with you about the gender in which it makes most sense to raise your child, and we'll give you a lot more information, too, since quite a lot is known about these variations and we are learning more each day. We want to reassure you that our focus is on supporting you and your child in this time of uncertainty.[28]

Q: What do we tell our friends and family while we wait for the gender assignment?

The following script may be most appropriate for talking to close family and friends. When discussing the situation with others, you may feel more comfortable just letting them know that the baby is in the hospital for tests.

A: This is important. We strongly recommend being open and honest with your friends and family about your child's situation. Even if you don't intend to, lying or withholding information will create a sense of shame and secrecy. Though it can be awkward to talk with family and friends about a child's sex development, being honest signals that you are not ashamed—because you have nothing to be ashamed of—and it also allows others to provide you with the love and support you may need. Isolating yourself at this time will probably make you feel unnecessarily stressed and lonely. Talking about it will help you feel connected with others. . . . So here is what you can tell people: Our baby was born with a kind of variation that happens more often than you hear about. Our doctors are doing a series of tests to figure out whether our baby is probably going to feel more like a boy or a girl. We expect to have more information from them within (specify realistic timeframe), and then we'll send out a birth announcement with the gender and the name we've chosen. Of course, as is true with any child, the various tests the doctors are doing are not going to tell us for sure who our baby will turn out to be. We're going to go on that journey together. We appreciate your love and support and we're looking forward to introducing you to our little one in person soon. It also helps to let your friends and family know whether your baby is healthy or whether there are some health concerns. Finally, take some pictures of your baby's face and share those pictures with others![28]

Because of the stress produced by having a child with DSD, support from a behavioral scientist (social worker, psychologist, psychiatrist) may be helpful for the family. It may be helpful for families to be informed about relevant credible resources listed at the end of this section.[35]

In addition to discussions with the family, it is important to keep the hospital staff who have contact with the family fully informed about the information that has been given to the parents. This professional candor reduces the possibility of the hospital staff personnel making insensitive comments to family members and is especially important in cases in which gender assignment must be delayed.

Initial Diagnostic Evaluation

In cases in which gender assignment is pending, all relevant tests should be obtained as soon as possible. A summary of the initial evaluation is shown in Box 49-11.

BOX 49–11	Initial Diagnostic Evaluation of Disorder of Sex Development in the Neonate
History	Maternal androgens, drugs, teratogens; affected relatives; siblings who died in infancy; consanguinity
Physical	Genitalia, gonads, hyperpigmentation, Turner stigmata, dysmorphic features
Chromosomes	Rapid test for X and Y chromosomes (fluorescent in situ hybridization [FISH], karyotype)
Anatomic	Endoscopy, retrograde genitogram; ultrasound
Biochemical	
If patient is:	Obtain serum levels at appropriate ages for:
XX with müllerian ducts	17-OHP, 11-deoxycortisol, 17-hydroxypregnenolone, testosterone
XX without müllerian ducts	Testosterone, estradiol, LH, FSH
XY with müllerian ducts	Testosterone, estradiol, LH, FSH
XY without müllerian ducts	Testosterone, dihydrotestosterone (DHT), LH, FSH, and if testosterone/DHT is increased or testosterone is normal to low, obtain androstenedione, dehydroepiandrosterone, 17-OHP, progesterone, and 17-hydroxypregnenolone
Basal hormone studies if done at:	
0 to 36 hr	Testes are active because of prior in utero hCG stimulation; testosterone and DHT levels are increased
0.5 to 4 mo	Pituitary-testicular axis is physiologically active; LH, FSH, testosterone, and DHT are increased (peak levels occur at 1 to 2 mo in term infant and later in premature infant)
Any age	Adrenal steroids are abnormal in untreated congenital adrenal hyperplasia

CHROMOSOMES

Fluorescence in situ hybridization (FISH) for X and Y markers may be available within 24 to 48 hours. Results reveal the number of X and Y chromosomes present. Most cytogenetic laboratories can provide a peripheral blood karyotype result within 2 or 3 days for cases of DSD. In cases in which the gender assignment is not clear, the laboratory should be personally contacted and asked to expedite the chromosome result.

BIOCHEMISTRY

Interpretation of biochemistry tests is dependent on the timing of the sample and understanding of the normal levels of hormones at that time. A blood sample should be obtained between 24 and 48 hours after the time of the neonatal surge of androgens, for measurement of testosterone and 17-hydroxyprogesterone (17-OHP). It is desirable to draw extra blood so that the laboratory can save the serum for analysis of other hormones that may be indicated as the evaluation continues. Increased serum levels of testosterone occur physiologically in neonates with functioning testes at 12 to 36 hours and at 2 weeks to 4 to 6 months of age (Fig. 49-32). The level may also increase pathologically at any time from the adrenal secretion of androgens in

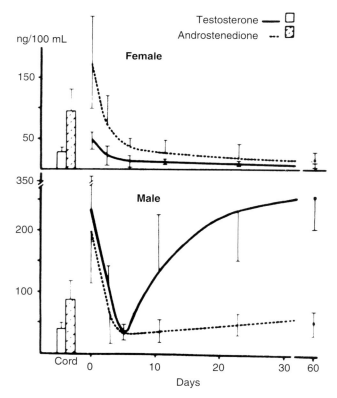

Figure 49–32. Pattern of testosterone and androstenedione plasma levels during the first 60 days of life in normal neonates. The curves join the mean values (± 1 SD) between the different age groups. (*From Forest MG , et al: Pattern of plasma testosterone and delta 4-androstenedione in normal infants: evidence for testicular activity at birth,* J Clin Endocrinol Metab 41:977, 1975. ©1975 The Endocrine Society.)

cases of CAH. Decreased levels of testosterone occur if Leydig cells are deficient or absent, LH activity is impaired, or there is a testosterone biosynthetic defect. Blood samples are also diagnostically useful at 1 or 2 months of age to assess the peak of hypothalamic-pituitary-testicular axis function in infancy.

The measurement of serum AMH has been shown to correlate with Sertoli cell function.[8] An increased level of 17-OHP suggests 21- or 11β-hydroxylase deficiency and implies that any increased levels of testosterone were of adrenal rather than testicular origin in a 46,XX patient. The 17-OHP levels in premature infants are higher than those in full-term infants.[34] In CAH with 21-hydroxylase deficiency, the levels of 17-OHP are often 10 to 50 times the upper limit of the normal level, making the test virtually diagnostic. Inhibin B levels have been shown to rise in males in the first week of life. Its measurement is therefore useful for identifying the presence of Sertoli cells and of functional testes in newborn boys with nonpalpable gonads.[9] Other tests that may be useful, depending on the clinical presentation, are measurements of LH, FSH, estradiol, precursors of testosterone, and DHT.

ULTRASONOGRAPHY

Ultrasound examination can usually determine the presence or absence of the uterus. If no uterus is seen, it suggests that there is testicular tissue producing AMH. If a uterus is present, it suggests either bilateral ovaries, dysgenetic gonads that failed to produce AMH, or an AMH receptor defect. Intrapelvic gonads can sometimes be located. Fetal ultrasonography can identify abnormal genitalia in utero.[55] Adrenal ultrasonography has a sensitivity of 92% and a specificity of 100% for diagnosing CAH when read by an experienced pediatric radiologist.[2] Ovaries may be difficult to identify on ultrasound.

GENITOGRAPHY

Genitography is used to determine the presence or absence of a urogenital sinus and the anatomy of the urethra and vagina. Visualization of the cervix confirms the presence of müllerian duct structures. If radiographs show filling of a fallopian tube, the gonad on that side has failed to produce AMH. Endoscopy may be needed to direct where the radiopaque contrast material is to be injected; otherwise, small vaginal openings into the urethra may be missed.

HUMAN CHORIONIC GONADOTROPIN STIMULATION TEST

A short hCG stimulation test can be used to determine whether functioning Leydig cells are present. One example of a protocol for doing the test is as follows: for full-term infants, 500 units of hCG is given intramuscularly every other day for three injections. The testosterone level is measured on the day after the last injection and compared with the baseline value. There are a number of protocols but no consensus about the best way to do the test. Normal or low levels of testosterone in response to hCG should be interpreted in relation to LH, FSH, and AMH values.[50] A significant rise in testosterone concentration

confirms the presence of Leydig cells and, by implication, testicular tissue.

Refining the Diagnosis

After the chromosome results are available, the initial diagnosis can be confirmed or refined. An approach that can be used to arrive at a final (differential) diagnosis is charted for 46,XY DSD in Figure 49-33 and for 46,XX DSD in Figure 49-34. Details on the specific diagnoses are discussed later.

Gender Assignment in Newborns

The decision about gender assignment is complex and stressful. It should therefore be made expeditiously by a thorough assessment by a multidisciplinary team including the family, medical genetics, cytogenetics, gynecology, pediatric urology, endocrinology, and psychiatry, psychology, or social work.[57] Guiding factors include the diagnosis, appearance of the genitals, surgical options, need for lifelong sex-hormone replacement therapy, potential for fertility, and the views of the family and their cultural practices.[35] In addition, the prospect for a gender identity congruent with sex of rearing and good sexual function should be considered.

Most 46,XX patients with CAH identify as females regardless of degree of genital virilization.[7] About 60% of patients with 5α-reductase deficiency and 17β-hydroxysteroid dehydrogenase deficiency assigned female in infancy, and all those assigned male, identify as males.[15] For individuals with cAIS assigned female in infancy, all continued to live as female.[40] Among both males and females with partial AIS (pAIS) and partial gonadal dysgenesis, about 75% were satisfied with their initial sex assignment. In the case of infants with markedly ambiguous genitalia, including a micropenis and perineoscrotal hypospadias, the decision about sex of rearing should be made after thorough discussion of the results of all investigations, diagnosis, etiology, prognosis, and surgical options.[45] The gender assignment in XY infants with small phalluses remains controversial, but these infants are increasingly being assigned male gender because of lack of need for medical or surgical intervention and potential for fertility.[40] The availability of intracytoplasmic sperm injection has also created the possibility of fertility for males with a very low sperm count. If the phallus is small and associated with hypospadias, partial androgen resistance is a possible diagnosis. Androgen sensitivity can be assessed by the response of the penis to an intramuscular injection of testosterone. If the response is poor, the choice of gender assignment becomes very difficult and must be approached on a case-by-case basis, with extensive discussion with the family.

Nomenclature of Disorders of Sex Development

An improved understanding of the molecular and genetic causes of DSDs and increased awareness about patient sensitivity led to the development of an updated nomenclature for this group of disorders (Table 49-14).[35]

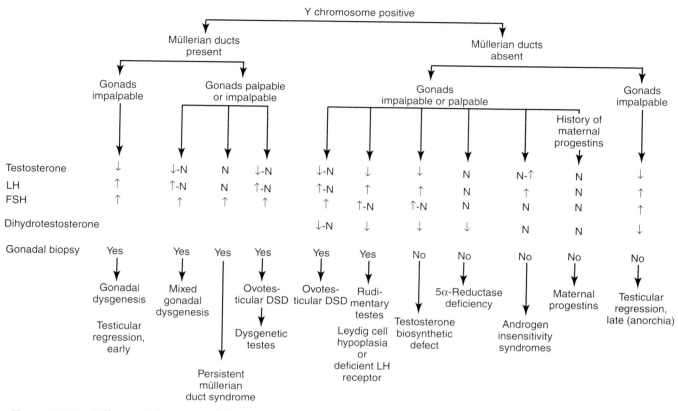

Figure 49–33. Differential diagnosis of disorder of sex development (DSD): presence of the Y chromosome. Ovotesticular DSD may demonstrate either the presence or absence of müllerian ducts. FSH, follicle-stimulating hormone; LH, luteinizing hormone; N, normal range; ↓, decreased; ↑, increased.

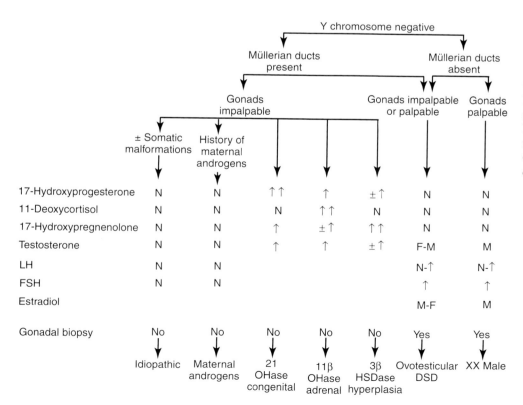

Figure 49–34. Differential diagnosis of disorders of sex development (DSD): absence of the Y chromosome. F, Female range; FSH, follicle-stimulating hormone; HSDase, hydroxysteroid dehydrogenase; LH, luteinizing hormone; M, male range; N, normal range; OHase, hydrogenase; ↓, decreased; ↑, increased.

TABLE 49–14   A Proposed Classification of Causes of Disorders of Sex Development (DSDs)

Sex Chromosome DSD	46,XY DSD	46,XX DSD

A: 47,XXY (Klinefelter syndrome and variants)
B: 45,X (Turner syndrome and variants)
C: 45,X/46,XY (mixed gonadal dysgenesis)
D: 46,XX/46,XY (chimerism)
	A: Disorders of gonadal (testicular) development
	  1. Complete or partial gonadal dysgenesis (e.g. *SRY, SOX9, SF1, WT1, DHH*)
	  2. Ovotesticular DSD
	  3. Testis regression
		A: Disorders of gonadal (ovarian) development
		  1. Gonadal dysgenesis
		  2. Ovotesticular DSD
		  3. Testicular DSD (e.g. *SRY+, dup SOX9*, RSP01)

	B: Disorders in androgen synthesis or action
	  1. Disorders of androgen synthesis
	  LH receptor mutations
	  Smith-Lemli-Opitz syndrome
	  Steroidogenic acute regulatory protein mutations
	  Cholesterol side-chain cleavage (*CYP11A1*)
	  3β-hydoxysteroid dehydrogenase 2 (*HSD3B2*)
	  17α-hydroxylase/17,20-lyase (*CYP17*)
	  P-450 oxidoreductase (*POR*)
	  17β-hydoxysteroid dehydrogenase (*HSD17B3*)
	  5α-reductase 2 (*SRD5A2*)
	  2. Disorders of androgen action
	  Androgen insensitivity syndrome
	  Drugs and environmental modulators
		B: Androgen excess
		  1. Fetal
		  3β-hydoxysteroid dehydrogenase 2 *HSD3B2*
		  21-hydroxylase (*CYP21A2*)
		  P-450 oxidoreductase (*POR*)
		  11β-hydroxylase (*CYP11B1*)
		  Glucocorticoid receptor mutations
		  2. Fetoplacental
		  Aromatase (*CYP19*) deficiency
		  Oxidoreductase (*POR*) deficiency
		  3. Maternal
		  Maternal virilizing tumors (e.g., luteomas)
		  Androgenic drugs

	C: Other
	  1. Syndromic associations of male genital development (e.g., cloacal anomalies, Robinow, Aarskog, hand-foot-genital, popliteal pterygium)
	  2. Persistent müllerian duct syndrome
	  3. Vanishing testis syndrome
	  4. Isolated hypospadias (*CXorf6*)
	  5. Congenital hypogonadotropic hypogonadism
	  6. Cryptorchidism (*INSL3, GREAT*)
	  7. Environmental influences
		C: Other
		  1. Syndromic associations (e.g., cloacal anomalies)
		  2. Müllerian agenesis, hypoplasia (e.g., MURCS)
		  3. Uterine abnormalities (e.g., MODY5)
		  4. Vaginal atresia (e.g., McKusick-Kaufman)
		  5. Labial adhesions

From Hughes IA: Disorders of sex development: a new definition and classification, *Best Pract Res Clin Endocrinol Metab* 22:119, 2008.

DISORDERS OF SEX DEVELOPMENT

Sex Chromosome Disorder of Sex Development

Abnormality in number or parts of sex chromosomes leads to failure of testes or ovaries to undergo normal development.

45,X (TURNER SYNDROME AND VARIANTS)

Loss of the second X chromosome results in a syndrome consisting of a phenotypic female with bilateral streak gonads and accompanying somatic abnormalities. Variant forms include partial deletions of the second X chromosome, such as deletion of the short arm of the X chromosome (XXp−) or

the long arm of the X chromosome (XXq−), or various forms of X chromosome mosaicism (e.g., 45,X/46,XX).

In fetuses with 45,X gonadal dysgenesis, normal ovarian differentiation occurs at up to 13 to 15 weeks of gestation, followed by rapid degeneration and atresia of the primordial ovarian follicles. In affected neonates and infants, the late stages of this process are usually evident, with scattered primordial ovarian follicles in varying states of degeneration seen histologically. The final result is the streak gonad, which usually appears by childhood; it is an elongated, whitish streak consisting of whorls of connective tissue, suggestive of ovarian stroma, that contain no germinal elements or endocrine or other epithelial elements.

Affected patients have normal müllerian duct development, an absence of wolffian ducts, and phenotypically female external genitalia. Because the genitalia are normal, the identification of neonates is limited to those who have the accompanying Turner somatic abnormalities, as listed in Box 49-12. The cardiovascular and lymphatic abnormalities, particularly lymphedema of the dorsa of the feet or hands (Fig. 49-35), are diagnostically the most useful and may be pathogenetically related. In the 45,X fetus, impaired drainage of the lymph channels leads to stasis of lymph fluid, with distention of lymphatics, peripheral lymphedema, increased venous fluid volume, and large veins. Large nuchal cystic hygromas and generalized edema occur frequently in utero. Distention of the cardiac lymphatics is hypothesized to compress the ascending aorta, altering flow in the left atrioventricular canal and affecting pulmonary venous return and consequently resulting in cardiovascular malformations. A strong association is observed between the presence of a webbed neck and the occurrence of aortic coarctation, partial anomalous pulmonary

---

BOX 49–12 Features of Turner Phenotype in the Neonate

- Intrauterine growth restriction
- Head and facies: low-set ears, low nuchal hairline, asynchronous growth of scalp hair, epicanthus, folds below lower lids, micrognathia, high palate
- Lymphatic: lymphedema of dorsa of hands and feet, hypoplasia of nails, loose neck folds (cutis laxa) or cystic hygroma, ascites, pleural or pericardial effusion, gross edema
- Cardiovascular: coarctation of aorta, bicuspid aorta, aortic stenosis, hypoplastic left heart, partial anomalous pulmonary venous drainage, ventricular septal defect, patent ductus arteriosus, and secundum atrial septal defect
- Urinary tract: rotated or horseshoe kidneys, renal hypoplasia, duplications
- Skeletal: short fourth metacarpals, shield chest

Modified from Gordon RR, et al: Turner's infantile phenotype, *Br Med J* 1:483, 1969.

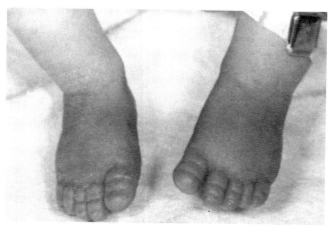

Figure 49–35. Lymphedema of the dorsa of the feet with hypoplasia of the nails in a newborn with 45,X gonadal dysgenesis (Turner syndrome).

venous drainage, a hypoplastic left heart, and secundum atrial septal defect.

The cause of monosomy X is unknown. The mean maternal and paternal ages are not raised, so non-disjunction is not thought to be important; a postfertilization abnormality is thought to be the most likely etiology. The single X is of maternal origin in about 80% of cases. The clinical features of Turner syndrome seem to be related to the haploinsufficiency of the short stature homeobox-containing gene (*SHOX*) and to the lymphogenic gene that causes lymphatic hypoplasia and as a result, soft tissue and visceral anomalies.[54] The parental origin of the missing short arm of the X chromosome may be associated with some of the phenotypic features in Turner syndrome, suggesting possible X chromosome gene imprinting.[65] A few familial cases have been reported. The incidence of the 45,X karyotype in spontaneous abortuses is very high, generally estimated to be 6% to 10%. However, the mean incidence of living 45,X newborns is only about 1 in 5000 female births, suggesting that more than 99% of 45,X fetuses abort. The reasons for this high mortality rate are unclear, but dysfunction of the 45,X placenta or fetal hypoalbuminemia, generalized edema, serous effusions, and cardiovascular abnormalities may play a role.

Individuals with X chromosome mosaicism or partial deletion of the second X chromosome tend to have fewer somatic and gonadal manifestations than those with the 45,X karyotype. In cases of mosaicism, the relative proportions of 46,XX to 45,X cells may determine the extent to which the normal development of gonadal and somatic tissues can occur. Individuals having only a partial deletion of the X chromosome may also manifest a modified phenotype, depending on the part of the X chromosome that is deleted. Genes related to ovarian development and Turner somatic abnormalities are located on both Xp and Xq. The combined incidence of 45,X, partial deletion, and mosaic Turner syndrome is about 1 in 2000 female newborns.

About 40% to 50% of patients with this diagnosis have a partial deletion or mosaicism of the X chromosome; at least 30 cells should be assessed for the possibility of mosaicism. The diagnosis is established by demonstration of a partial or complete deletion of one of the X chromosomes. The differential diagnosis includes XYp− gonadal dysgenesis and structural abnormalities of the Y chromosome, which may also have a Turner somatotype but carry a different prognosis. There is no increased risk for gonadal tumor development in the unequivocal absence of Y chromosome material; however, it may be difficult to establish fully because of the possibility of occult Y chromosome material.[3] Y chromosome material is associated with about a 12% risk for gonadoblastoma.[17] In one study of 171 patients with Turner syndrome, 8% were found to have Y chromosome material.[42]

The Turner phenotype is therefore not a reliable predictor of either the karyotype or the cause of gonadal dysgenesis. In Turner syndrome, serum FSH is elevated from an age of 2 weeks to about 2 to 3 years. The neonatal changes in FSH secretion are qualitatively similar to those of normal girls.[23] The antenatal diagnosis of Turner syndrome has been made after ultrasound identification of a cystic hygroma and pleural effusion.[13] Clinical practice guidelines exist that outline the required screening investigations in individuals with a new diagnosis of Turner syndrome. These include a cardiovascular evaluation by a specialist, renal ultrasound, hearing evaluation, and referral to appropriate support groups.[10] In studies of patients with Turner syndrome, a 15% to 35% incidence of heart anomalies is found. The most common cardiovascular malformations are left sided and include aortic valve abnormality (bicuspid valve, stenosis, regurgitation) in 72% and aortic coarctation in 39%. Ultrasound evaluation of the urinary tract may be performed to establish the presence of an abnormality that may predispose the patient to urinary tract infection or obstruction. Feeding difficulties in infancy, caused by oral-motor dysfunction, may result in a lower rate of weight gain. Patients who are not recognized in infancy come to medical attention later, usually because of short stature or failure of secondary sexual development. The prognosis is primarily for the absence of any ovarian function, but 5% to 15% of patients do show variable secondary sexual development; a very small number of pregnancies have been reported.

47,XXY (KLINEFELTER SYNDROME AND VARIANTS)

The major clinical manifestations of Klinefelter syndrome develop with the onset of puberty, and most patients are recognized at that time or later. The constant features are small testes with histologic evidence of impaired spermatogenesis. Infants with 47,XXY Klinefelter syndrome occasionally have small testes or a micropenis that might permit their recognition, and cases with hypospadias have been reported. Other congenital abnormalities seen in this syndrome included a cleft palate, cryptorchidism, and an inguinal hernia. The fetal testes at midgestation are normal. Testicular histology in the first year of life has varied from normal to abnormal manifestations, with decreased to absent spermatogonia.

The incidence of the 47,XXY karyotype in live newborn males is about 1 in 1000; if Klinefelter variants are added, the overall incidence is about 1 in 800. Increased maternal age is associated with an additional X chromosome, although this effect is not as marked as it is in autosomal trisomies. Among the variant forms of Klinefelter syndrome, patients with 48,XXXY and 49,XXXXY karyotypes are more likely to be recognized early in life. All have somatic abnormalities and mental retardation, and many have a hypoplastic penis. All males with the 49,XXXXY karyotype have cryptorchidism, and 14% have cardiac defects.

45,X/46,XY (MIXED GONADAL DYSGENESIS)

This group of disorders is characterized by the presence of dysgenetic and often asymmetric gonads. The streak gonad represents the end result of failed gonadal (ovarian or testicular) differentiation. *Mixed gonadal dysgenesis* is a term used to describe individuals with a unilateral, functioning testis and a contralateral streak gonad.

Ninety percent of prenatally diagnosed cases have a normal male phenotype, whereas those diagnosed postnatally show variable phenotypes.[70] Most have some degree of virilization of the external genitalia, ranging from clitoromegaly or partial labial fusion to normal male external genitalia. Slightly more than half have a urogenital sinus. All have some müllerian development consisting of an upper vagina, a uterus, and a fallopian tube, usually on the side with the streak or absent gonad. An epididymis or vas deferens is present on the testicular side in 50% of cases, and the testis is

most frequently located in the inguinal canal. Normal to diminished or absent testosterone responses have been reported with hCG stimulation, and gonadotropins are normal or elevated. Gonadal tumors occur in 22%, affecting either the testis or the streak gonad. Diagnostic overlap with ovotesticular DSD, previously referred to as *true hermaphroditism*, may occur in infants if the apparent streak gonad still contains degenerating primordial ovarian follicles that suggest ovarian tissue rather than a streak gonad.

In 45,X/46,XY, Turner somatic features such as lymphedema, cardiovascular abnormalities, or short stature are frequently seen and reflect the presence of 45,X cell lines. The prevalence of the XY cell line in the gonad and the extent of structural abnormality of the Y chromosome determine the degree of testicular development and masculinization.

Appropriate gender assignment in the newborn period should be based on functional considerations and fertility. Dysgenetic gonads should be removed in infancy because of the increased risk for tumor formation.[19] The scrotal testis may be normal prepubertally, but many adults show a loss of germ cells and accompanying tubular sclerosis; a few have spermatocytes.

46,XX/46,XY (CHIMERISM)

The most common phenotype is that seen in ovotesticular DSD, discussed next.

Ovotesticular Disorder of Sex Development

Formerly known as true hermaphroditism, ovotesticular DSD is defined as the coexistence of ovarian and testicular tissue either in the same gonad or in opposite gonads. The ovarian tissue must contain ovarian follicles or corpora albicantia because fibrous stroma alone does not define ovarian tissue. The testicular tissue must contain seminiferous tubules or spermatozoa. Several karyotypes are seen in ovotesticular DSD. About three fifths are 46,XX; one fifth 46,XY or 45,X/46,XY; and the remaining one fifth show mosaicism or chimerism, being 46,XX/46,XY or 46,XX/47,XXY. The most frequently occurring gonadal combinations are an ovary and a testis or an ovary and an ovotestis. An ovotestis accounts for 44% of all gonads in this condition, an ovary 34%, and a testis 22%. Less than 1% of patients have a unilateral streak gonad or a tumor. Ovarian tissue occurs more often on the left side and testicular tissue more often on the right side.

The internal genital ducts reflect the gonadal constitution. On the side with an ovary, a fallopian tube is almost always seen, and on the side with a testis, the vas deferens and epididymis are almost always present. On the side with an ovotestis, a vas deferens is seen 35% of the time and a fallopian tube, often closed at the fimbriated end, 65% of the time. A uterus is described in about 86% of the patients, but it is usually hypoplastic, unicornuate, or otherwise maldeveloped.

The external genitalia are usually ambiguous, although some cases have been reported with normal male or female appearances. The urethra most often opens on the perineum as a urogenital sinus. The phallus is usually larger than a normal clitoris (Fig. 49-36) and often has chordee; it is frequently of sufficient size to give the genitalia a masculine appearance. Gonads are descended or palpable in 61% of patients, more frequently on the right side; about 60% are

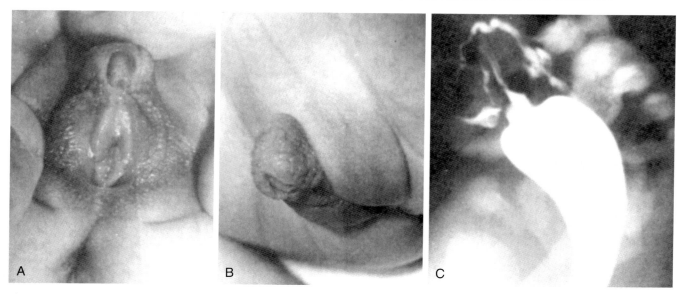

Figure 49-36. **A,** A 46,XX neonate with ovotesticular disorder of sex development was noted at birth to have clitoromegaly (1.8 × 0.8 cm), with a slightly rugose and full labia majora. **B,** The genitalia were otherwise those of a normal female; the gonads were impalpable, and a uterine cervix was present on endoscopy. **C,** A genitogram showed the presence of a 5-cm vagina, above which contrast media entered the uterus and the bilateral fallopian tubes. The serum testosterone level was high normal for a female at 60 ng/dL on day 1 of life; was abnormally elevated to 75 ng/dL and 134 ng/dL at ages 2 and 5 weeks, respectively; and increased to 389 ng/dL after stimulation with human chorionic gonadotropin (hCG). Bilateral gonads spontaneously descended into the inguinal region at age 5 weeks (before hCG stimulation) and were found to be ovotestes on biopsy.

ovotestes, and most of the remainder are testes, but only rarely does an ovary descend. The ovotestis is more likely to descend if it contains a greater proportion of testicular tissue. The ovarian portion of the ovotestis tends to be firm and convoluted and is histologically normal except for a reduction in the number of primordial follicles. The testicular portion tends to be soft, smooth, and histologically normal in infants, but it becomes abnormal in more than 90% of adults, marked as it is by tubular atrophy with undifferentiated germ cells and the absence of spermatogenesis. In intact testes, the histology is similar, with spermatogenesis seen in only 12% of the patients. The testosterone response to hCG stimulation is usually low but can be normal, depending on the amount of testicular tissue present. Gonadal tumors occur in 3% of the patients and are more frequent in those who are Y chromosome positive. Renal abnormalities have been noted in 5% of 150 cases.

Most cases of ovotesticular DSD are 46,XX and on karyotype have no separate Y chromosome material. Explanations include an autosomal or X-linked mutation that turns on a gene downstream from the *SRY* gene that induces testicular differentiation, the translocation of Y chromosome material to an autosome, and chromosome mosaicism in gonadal tissue. Familial cases of 46,XX DSD with male phenotype, 46,XX ovotesticular DSD, or both show phenotypic similarity, typically having ambiguous genitalia, and lack the *SRY* gene or other Y sequences, indicating that these conditions are closely related.

Most cases of ovotesticular DSD are potentially recognizable in the neonatal period because of ambiguous genitalia. The definitive diagnosis requires a gonadal biopsy, but it is preferably delayed until after the neonatal period. Fertility is often impaired in this condition for both males and females. Gender assignment is guided by the same principles outlined for other DSDs. See "Gender Assignment in Newborns," earlier.

46,XY Disorder of Sex Development
DISORDERS OF GONADAL (TESTICULAR) DEVELOPMENT
Complete and Partial Gonadal Dysgenesis
In testicular dysgenesis, the underlying defect is disordered testicular differentiation or development that results in anatomically or histologically abnormal testes and secondary impairment of hormonogenesis or spermatogenesis. Dysgenetic testes are defined by the following characteristics: a failure to induce regression of the ipsilateral müllerian duct structures, an association with incomplete masculinization of the genitalia, variably abnormal histology, and an increased predisposition toward the development of tumors originating from the germinal structures. The testes may be of normal or small size and are usually cryptorchid. The karyotype is typically 46,XY, but other karyotypes are also seen. Dysgenetic testicular tissue can be seen in ovotesticular DSD.

Individuals with complete gonadal dysgenesis (Swyer syndrome) have a 46,XY karyotype, absent testes, female-appearing external genitalia, normal müllerian structures, and streak gonads similar to those of Turner syndrome.[72] A mutation in the *SRY* gene has been reported in 20% to 67% of those with complete gonadal dysgenesis.[35] XY gonadal dysgenesis occurring in families has been described and attributed to mutations in the *SRY* gene that resulted in the reduction rather than loss of DNA binding. The reduced binding presumably leads to variability in sex reversal, allowing some individuals to have near-normal gonadal development. Most cases occur sporadically, but family aggregates have been reported, some involving two or three generations, that are compatible with either X-linked recessive, autosomal recessive, or autosomal dominant and male-limited inheritance.

The clinical recognition of 46,XY gonadal dysgenesis may be possible in the newborn period in infants with clitoromegaly. A neonate occasionally presents with edema of the feet. There is a very high risk for the development of gonadal tumors in XY gonadal dysgenesis. Prophylactic removal of the streak or dysgenetic gonads is indicated in infancy. The gender assignment is most commonly female. Gonadal dysgenesis associated with a Y chromosome is significantly different from the Y-negative forms described previously. Both forms have in common the presence of bilateral or unilateral streak gonadal tissue, the association of the Turner phenotype in some, and a similarity in the gonadotropin sex steroid profiles. However, the streak gonads in patients with Y-positive gonadal dysgenesis differ in important ways.

1. The combination of a streak or dysgenetic gonad and a Y chromosome carries a significant risk for tumor development (Y-negative streak gonads have no increased risk for tumor formation).
2. The streak gonads may show residual dysgenetic tubular elements and develop calcification.
3. Androgen or estrogen production may occur from gonadotropin stimulation of theca or lutein cells lying within a tumor (or occasionally within the streak gonad), causing virilization or feminization.

The causes of Y-positive gonadal dysgenesis are heterogeneous and include a small deletion of distal Yp (the short arm of chromosome Y) with loss of the *SRY* gene, an X chromosome or autosomal mutation that interferes with or prevents testicular differentiation, and Y chromosome abnormalities or mosaicism. A structurally abnormal Y chromosome frequently results in 45,X/46,XY or 45,X/47,XYY mosaicism. When the result is two streak gonads, a female phenotype is usually seen. Varying degrees of testicular development, reflecting the relative prevalence of the XY cell lines, may result in ambiguous or predominantly male genital development. The finding of genital ambiguity, Turner somatic stigmata, or associated malformations allows many patients to be identified in the neonatal period.

Yp gonadal dysgenesis is due to an abnormal X-Y recombination involving the distal ends of Xp and Yp. This may result in translocation and thus loss of the *SRY* gene from the Y to the X chromosome. The resulting XYp− individual has bilateral streak gonads and a female phenotype; most have lymphedema or other Turner somatic features thought to be caused by the loss of certain Yp genes. The incidence of these XY females (1 in 100,000) is much lower than that of their reciprocal XX males (1 in 20,000); it is speculated that the edema associated with Yp deletions has lethal effects on many affected fetuses. Y autosome translocations may also result in loss of the *SRY* gene.

The risk for tumor development in those with mutations in *SRY* is up to 50%.[72] The gonadoblastoma locus on the Y chromosome (*GBY*) must be present for malignant transformation to occur. Testis-specific protein on the Y chromosome (*TSPY*) is a likely candidate gene responsible for malignant transformation.[38] The most common tumor is a gonadoblastoma, which may arise in a streak gonad or a dysgenetic testis, is frequently bilateral, and occurs from the first year of life up to the fourth decade. Although pure gonadoblastomas do not metastasize, they are frequently associated with dysgerminomas or other malignant germ cell tumors. The risk for a tumor is the greatest for poorly differentiated gonadal tissue and an intra-abdominal or inguinal position; only rarely is there tumor formation in a scrotal testis. Unexpected testosterone or estrogen formation may signal tumor development. Total gonadectomy is recommended for those reared as females and considered for undescended gonadal tissue for those reared as males.

MUTATION AND DELETION OF *WT1*: DENYS-DRASH, FRASER, AND WAGR SYNDROMES

The Wilms tumor suppressor gene (*WT1*), which is on chromosome 11p13, encodes a transcription factor that is expressed in the urogenital embryonic tissues that develop into the kidney and gonad. A mutation or deletion of *WT1* causes abnormal gonadal development, as seen in Denys-Drash syndrome (nephropathy, genital abnormalities, Wilms tumor), WAGR syndrome (Wilms tumor, *a*niridia, *g*enitourinary malformations, mental *r*etardation), and Fraser syndrome (gonadal dysgenesis and chronic renal failure). Therefore, *WT1* appears to be required for the early commitment and maintenance of gonadal tissue and to exert its effects upstream from the *SRY* gene (see Fig. 49-26). Both 46,XY and 46,XX individuals may be affected. Although many patients present at birth with ambiguous genitalia ranging from clitoromegaly with labial fusion to hypospadias with undescended testes, others have external genitalia that are phenotypically normal male or female but may be inappropriate for the karyotype. Their underlying DSD defect is in the development of the gonads, which anatomically show wide variation ranging from streak gonads (complete gonadal dysgenesis) to dysgenetic or rudimentary testes or ovaries to ovotestes; gonadoblastomas have developed in some of the dysgenetic gonads. The internal genital ducts usually reflect the gonadal makeup; müllerian duct structures are usually present.

MUTATION OF *SOX9* (*SRY*-LIKE HMG BOX-RELATED GENE 9)

SOX9 mutation is a cause of camptomelic dwarfism and XY gonadal dysgenesis. In the presence of *SRY*, *SOX9* expression is repressed in the female gonad but is upregulated in the developing testis and is crucial in the pathway for testis development. *SOX9* is also responsible for synthesis of collagen type II, and mutations of *SOX9* result in camptomelic dysplasia.[14] Camptomelic dysplasia is a cartilage and skeletal malformation syndrome with congenital angulation and bowing of long bones that is associated with 46,XY complete gonadal dysgenesis in about three fourths of the XY cases. Testicular development in the XY patients ranges from streak gonads to dysgenetic testes to normal testes; the external genitalia show a gradation of defects, from the female phenotype in those with complete gonadal dysgenesis to ambiguous genitalia to a normal male phenotype. The internal genital ducts reflect the gonadal makeup. Patients who have more severe skeletal dysplasia die in the first months of life from respiratory failure, but less severely affected patients may live into adulthood. The mode of inheritance is now recognized to be autosomal dominant, with haploinsufficiency for *SOX9* on chromosome 17 as the cause of both camptomelic dysplasia and gonadal or testicular dysgenesis.

DUPLICATION OF DOSAGE-SENSITIVE SEX REVERSAL
Duplication of the dosage-sensitive sex reversal, adrenal hypoplasia congenita critical region, on the X chromosome, gene 1 (*DAX1*), located on the short arm of the X chromosome, overrides the *SRY* gene and impairs or prevents testicular development, resulting in partial or complete XY gonadal dysgenesis. Affected patients have either ambiguous genitalia or a female phenotype and may also exhibit adrenal insufficiency. Familial cases have been reported.

STEROIDOGENIC FACTOR-1
The steroidogenic factor-1 (*SF1*) gene codes for a nuclear hormone receptor and regulates the expression of other genes involved in sexual development.[41] Mutations in *SF1* can be associated with 46,XY DSD and normal adrenal function and lead to impaired Leydig cell function and androgen biosynthesis.[37]

46,XY Ovotesticular Disorder of Sex Development
See earlier section, "Ovotesticular Disorder of Sex Development."

Gonadal Regression
EARLY REGRESSION WITH GENITAL AMBIGUITY (XY GONADAL AGENESIS)
This condition is characterized by the complete absence of testes, including the absence of gonadal streaks, and associated with the almost complete absence of both müllerian and wolffian duct derivatives and female or partially masculinized genitalia (clitoromegaly and posterior labial fusion). The gonadal and genital features may be explained by very early regression of the developing fetal testes between about 8 and 10 weeks. Testicular failure must have occurred after the initial production of AMH by Sertoli cells but before the Leydig cells could produce sufficient testosterone for a reasonable time. It has been suggested that testicular regression is part of the clinical spectrum of 46,XY gonadal dysgenesis.

Other XY individuals have testes with quite well developed wolffian structures but incomplete masculinization of the external genitalia. Testicular regression presumably occurred slightly later than it did in those patients with the absence of internal genital ducts. Affected siblings have been reported, raising the possibility of autosomal recessive inheritance. In another family, there were subjects from two generations affected, with X-linked or autosomal dominant, sex-limited inheritance suggested. The differential diagnosis includes Leydig cell hypoplasia.

LATE REGRESSION: CONGENITAL ANORCHIA (VANISHING TESTES SYNDROME)
Many cases have been reported of cryptorchid 46,XY males who on exploration were found to have bilateral anorchia but with normal wolffian structures, the absence of müllerian

structures, and normal male external genitalia. The vas deferens ends blindly, often without an epididymis, in either the inguinal canal or upper scrotum (sometimes palpable as a small knot of tissue), which is retroperitoneally near the usual location of the internal inguinal ring, or in the iliac fossa. Neonates and infants with congenital anorchia fail to show any rise in testosterone during either endogenous LH or exogenous hCG stimulation, and they lack AMH. In the 46,XY individual with a male phenotype, these findings are usually but not always diagnostic. If uncertainty exists, laparoscopy or surgical exploration may be necessary. The cause of congenital anorchia is not established, but infections, teratogens, immune mechanisms, or hereditary factors may play a role.[5] About half of those with congenital anorchia also have micropenis.[76] The possibility that bilateral congenital anorchia is part of a continuum with early testicular regression has been suggested.

DISORDERS OF ANDROGEN SYNTHESIS OR ACTION

In these disorders, there is abnormal differentiation of either the internal genital ducts or the external genitalia in a 46,XY individual who has bilateral testes with intact tubular elements (seminiferous tubules with Sertoli and germinal cells). Disordered synthesis or action of testosterone is the underlying cause of the observed abnormalities. Some cases of dysgenetic testes and rudimentary testes overlap phenotypically with this category, but their underlying cause is testicular dysgenesis and not a primary disorder of the testicular hormone synthesis. In patients with 46,XY DSD who are severely undermasculinized, a blind, distal vaginal pouch is present. It appears when a lack of androgen stimulation permits the urovaginal septum to persist.

Androgen Biosynthesis Defect
Five enzymatic steps are involved in the synthesis of testosterone from cholesterol (Fig. 49-37). A defect in any one results in decreased to absent androgen synthesis and 46,XY DSD. Three of these enzymes are also necessary for the adrenal biosynthesis of cortisol: cholesterol side-chain cleavage enzyme (20,22-desmolase), 17α-hydroxylase, and 3β-hydroxysteroid dehydrogenase. Their defects result in accompanying cortisol deficiency with or without aldosterone deficiency (see later section, "Congenital Adrenal Hyperplasia"). The remaining two testosterone biosynthetic enzymes, 17,20-desmolase and 17β-hydroxysteroid dehydrogenase, are not needed for cortisol synthesis. Their deficiencies primarily cause impaired testosterone synthesis that leads to abnormal male differentiation and hypogonadism. Clinical diagnoses are made by finding biochemical evidence of disorders along the testosterone biosynthetic pathway, often accentuated by hCG stimulation testing.

17,20-DESMOLASE (17,20-LYASE) DEFICIENCY
17,20-Desmolase is necessary to form the C19 steroids DHEA and androstenedione, which are precursors of both testosterone and estradiol (see Fig. 49-29). 46,XY individuals who have 17,20-desmolase deficiency show incomplete masculinization ranging from mild hypoplasia of male genitalia to significant ambiguity to female-appearing genitalia, depending on the severity of the defect. Some of those with a female phenotype may be recognized early because of an inguinal or

Figure 49-37. Pathway of testicular steroidogenesis. *Bold arrows* indicate a predominant Δ^5 pathway of steroid production. *Dotted lines* denote a "backdoor" pathway to dihydrotestosterone (DHT) synthesis postulated to be specific to the fetus. The steroidogenic enzymes and their cognate genes are shown. hCG, human chorionic gonadotrophin; LH, luteinizing hormone; LHR, LH receptor; StAR, steroidogenic acute regulatory protein; HSD, hydroxysteroid dehydrogenase deficiency; RD5A1, 5α-reductase type 1; RD5A2, 5α-reductase type 2; AKRIC, aldoketo reductase. (*From Hughes IA: Disorders of sex development: a new definition and classification,* Best Pract Res Clin Endocrinol Metab 22:119, 2008.)

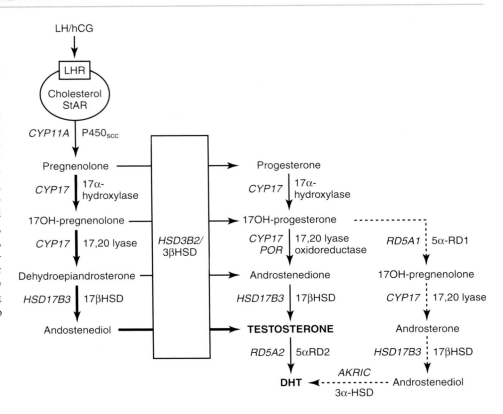

labial gonad or gonads; others are diagnosed later because of delayed puberty. The inheritance is autosomal recessive. If a 46,XY neonate is assigned a female gender, the testes should be removed before puberty. Affected 46,XX patients appear normal in infancy but have delayed puberty because of inadequate estradiol production.

17β-HYDROXYSTEROID DEHYDROGENASE DEFICIENCY
17-Ketosteroid reductase catalyzes the only reversible step involved in testosterone and estradiol synthesis, the interconversion of androstenedione and testosterone and of estrone and estradiol (see Fig. 49-29). It is present in both gonadal and peripheral tissues but only minimally so in adrenocortical tissue. Its deficiency is associated primarily with diminished testosterone synthesis with a decreased plasma testosterone-to-androstenedione ratio. This results in failure of male differentiation in utero.

Of those who are identified in the neonatal period, most affected 46,XY patients have slightly masculinized genitalia (clitoromegaly, posterior labial fusion); a few have more masculinization. The epididymis and vas deferens are well developed, and in many patients, the testes are descended in the inguinal canal or labioscrotal folds. Because the degree of undermasculinization of the external genitalia can be severe, the diagnosis may not be possible in infancy. The inheritance of 17-ketosteroid reductase deficiency is autosomal recessive. It has a high prevalence in the Arab population in the Gaza Strip, Lebanon, Syria, and Turkey.

Untreated 46,XY patients undergo significant masculinization at puberty and may have an accompanying change in gender identity from female to male (a similar change in gender identity is seen in patients with untreated 5α-reductase deficiency).

5α-REDUCTASE DEFICIENCY
5α-Reductase is located peripherally in the tissues of the urogenital sinus, external genitalia, liver, prostate, hair follicles, and sebaceous glands, where it catalyzes the conversion of testosterone to its 5α-reduced product, DHT. Its deficiency in the 46,XY fetus results in failure of the external genitalia to undergo male differentiation. Affected males have normally developed testes that may be descended, absent müllerian duct structures, and male internal ducts (stimulated by testosterone) but phenotypically female or ambiguous external genitalia. Most patients are potentially recognizable at birth, with apparent clitoromegaly, a single perineal orifice that is a urogenital sinus, and posterior labial fusion (Fig. 49-38). A few patients have hypospadias or a micropenis. Most are reared as females; however, in some cultures in which the disorder is widely known and recognized, individuals may be recognized as a third gender. At puberty, noncastrated individuals show striking virilization due to the increase in testosterone, and about 60% change gender as adults.[15] Many undergo a change in gender identity from female to male. DHT-dependent secondary sexual characteristics such as acne, body and facial hair, and prostatic enlargement develop minimally or not at all. The inheritance of primary 5α-reductase deficiency is autosomal recessive.

LEYDIG CELL HYPOPLASIA
Patients with testicular unresponsiveness to hCG and LH fail to undergo male genital differentiation. It is due to an autosomal recessive inactivating mutation in the LH receptor.[62]

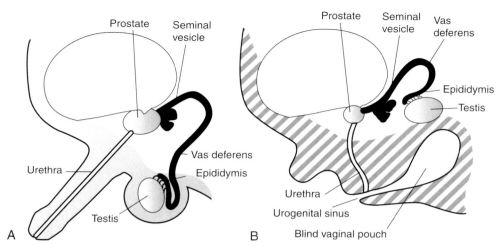

Figure 49–38. **A,** Male differentiation of the external genitalia and urogenital sinus structures is stimulated by dihydrotestosterone (DHT) (*gray areas*), whereas wolffian duct differentiation is stimulated by testosterone (*solid black area*). **B,** 5-Reductase deficiency results in impaired male differentiation of DHT-responsive tissues (*gray bars area*). The external genitalia appear female, and the vesicovaginal septum develops to create a distal, blind vaginal pouch opening into a urogenital sinus. The wolffian duct differentiation is normal (*solid black area*). (*From Imperato-McGinley J, et al: Male pseudohermaphroditism: the complexities of male phenotypic development,* Am J Med 61:251, 1976.)

Primary agenesis or hypoplasia of the Leydig cells is a possible alternative explanation. In the complete absence of hCG binding, a female phenotype with a blind vaginal pouch but no wolffian ducts is seen. Other patients have shown clitoromegaly, posterior labial fusion, or perineal hypospadias with good development of the epididymis and vas deferens, suggesting an incomplete defect. AMH is produced, so müllerian structures are absent. The testes are usually cryptorchid and small postpubertally, although possibly of normal size in infancy. The characteristic findings are a low basal level of testosterone and its precursors, the failure of testosterone response to hCG stimulation, and a marked paucity or absence of Leydig cells on biopsy of the testes. The seminiferous tubules and Sertoli cells are normal, but spermatogenic arrest or absence is seen. The differential diagnosis includes XY gonadal agenesis, rudimentary testes, and those forms of 46,XY DSD involving deficient androgen synthesis or action.

Defect in Androgen Action
ANDROGEN INSENSITIVITY SYNDROMES
The androgen insensitivity syndromes are disorders in which peripheral tissues are partially to completely incapable of responding to stimulation by any androgen because of an androgen receptor or postreceptor defect.[33] Many mutations in the X-linked, androgen receptor gene have been described, leading to variable phenotypes in this disorder.[74] Androgen-mediated events, such as masculine differentiation in utero or virilization during puberty, fail to occur or are impaired to a variable extent, depending on the completeness of the defect.

COMPLETE ANDROGEN INSENSITIVITY SYNDROME
Affected individuals have a 46,XY karyotype with bilateral testes but a failure in wolffian duct development and complete absence of any masculinization of the external genitalia.

They have female-appearing external genitalia with a distal vaginal pouch. The müllerian structures are absent, but microscopic remnants have been reported, possibly from the interference of high, unopposed levels of estrogen with the action of AMH. The testes are of normal size and may be descended into the inguinal canal or labia majora, and more than half of these individuals have an inguinal hernia, which may lead to their clinical recognition in infancy. At puberty, these individuals undergo female breast development and acquire a female habitus due to the testicular production of estradiol and the peripheral conversion of testosterone to estradiol; however, they have primary amenorrhea. No masculinization is seen, and gender identity remains female.

Studies of genital skin fibroblasts derived from patients with cAIS reveal that most have an absence of functional androgen receptors, which is determined by the absence of specific binding of DHT, thus confirming the biochemical cause of their androgen unresponsiveness. The occurrence of cAIS is familial in about 30% of the cases, and a family history of infertile female relatives is sometimes found. Spontaneous mutations are thought to account for the sporadic cases. Screening for the syndrome in an at-risk fetus can be carried out in utero by ultrasound examination of the genitalia and determination of the karyotype. The diagnosis is inferred in the phenotypically female neonate by establishing the absence of a uterine cervix and the presence of a Y chromosome. Both plasma testosterone and LH have been shown to be low at 30 days of age, suggesting that the expected postnatal testosterone rise requires the hypothalamic-pituitary axis to be responsive to testosterone.[11]

The differential diagnosis includes other causes of 46,XY DSD; hCG stimulation testing may be needed to rule out these possibilities. The gender is unequivocally female. There is a 2% increased risk for germ cell malignancy, probably related to the intra-abdominal location of the testes. For this reason, gonadectomy is indicated, however, the timing remains controversial because testosterone is converted to estradiol peripherally and allows for spontaneous development of secondary sexual characteristics.[16] Virtually all malignant tumors have occurred postpubertally.

PARTIAL ANDROGEN INSENSITIVITY SYNDROME

Affected 46,XY individuals have bilateral testes and absent müllerian ducts but incomplete masculinization of their external genitalia, ranging from female-appearing genitalia with clitoromegaly or posterior labial fusion to phenotypically normal male-appearing genitalia. Many have perineal, penoscrotal, or penile hypospadias (Fig. 49-39), and others have a micropenis. There also is wolffian duct development, but it is often incomplete, which may not correlate with the extent of external genital masculinization. At puberty, both masculinization and feminization are seen, the extent depending on the severity of the androgen insensitivity.

The causes of pAIS are heterogeneous. Most individuals have qualitatively abnormal receptors with variable function.[12] Others have reduced amounts of normal receptors, and a few have postreceptor defects. There is an X-linked recessive inheritance of the receptor-related mutations. The phenotype in pAIS is variable and does not necessarily correlate with the genotype.[17]

Except for very few individuals with a normal male phenotype, all individuals with pAIS are infertile. The risk for development of gonadal tumors is not known, but intratubular germ cell neoplasia (a precancerous lesion) frequently occurs in patients with pAIS at as early as 2 months of age. Monitoring for the development of a testicular tumor is needed if the testes are not removed.[16] The testes are removed in those reared as females.

OTHER

Disorders of Antimüllerian Hormone and Antimüllerian Hormone Receptor (Persistent Müllerian Duct Syndrome)

Isolated AMH deficiency or AMH receptor abnormalities result in failure of the müllerian ducts to regress. The clinical picture in the 46,XY individual is that of a phenotypic male with bilateral fallopian tubes, a uterus (occasionally hypoplastic or absent), wolffian duct development, and bilaterally normal testes. Two clinical forms are seen. The typical clinical presentation is in a male with bilateral cryptorchidism and inguinal hernias and normal male external genitalia. During surgery for hernia repair, a uterus and fallopian tubes are found in the inguinal canal. Alternatively, one testis is at least partially descended and accompanied by a fallopian tube and uterus that easily enter the inguinal canal. In addition, about one third have transverse ectopia, the opposite testis being pulled to the side with the inguinal hernia, so that both testes are in the same inguinal canal. Such patients may have an inguinal mass or the appearance of an incarcerated hernia without evidence of intestinal obstruction. Less commonly, the uterus is fixed in the pelvis, and the testes are in an ovarian position. The vas deferens and epididymis

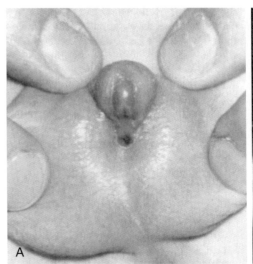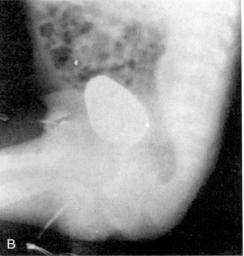

Figure 49–39. **A,** This 46,XY infant with partial androgen insensitivity had ambiguous genitalia at birth (phallus, 1.8 × 0.8 cm; penoscrotal hypospadias; 1-cm testes in scrotum and the absence of a uterine cervix). **B,** Genitogram performed after endoscopy shows a 2-cm utriculus, or blind pouch, opening into the urethra just below the verumontanum; no evidence of a uterus was found. Serum testosterone was elevated at 475 ng/dL at age 40 hours and increased to 1517 ng/dL at age 7½ weeks, with elevated serum luteinizing hormone of 23 mIU/mL at age 7½ weeks. Androgen receptor binding in genital skin fibroblasts showed no demonstrable abnormality, which is often found in partial defects. The parents insisted on male gender. Testosterone therapy did not increase penile size until the dose was increased fourfold above physiologic replacement. Repair of hypospadias was performed in infancy. A younger brother was born with a similar defect.

are typically enmeshed in the uterine wall and mesosalpinx, making it difficult to bring the testes down into the scrotum.

Persistent müllerian duct syndrome is due to a mutation in either the *AMH* gene or its receptor and is inherited according to an autosomal recessive pattern.[18] The gender assignment is male. Orchiopexy should be performed early in infancy to improve testicular outcome. Achieving testicular descent into the scrotum usually requires extensive dissection to free the spermatic cord. The müllerian structures do not need to be removed because they do not develop malignancy and there is a strong risk for damaging the vas deferens. Spermatogenesis is intact, but many patients are infertile, possibly because of abnormal epididymal development, cryptorchidism, or injury to the vas deferens. Intracytoplasmic sperm injection may produce fertility in some of these cases. There is no evidence of an increased risk for testicular tumors compared with other causes of cryptorchidism.

Environmental Influences: Endocrine Disrupting Chemicals

Attention has been drawn to the study of endocrine disrupting chemicals (EDCs), substances that influence the function of an endocrine system and cause adverse health effects.[1] Specifically, there have been concerns about the effects of pesticides, industrial chemicals, and natural plant compounds on sex development. These stem from results of laboratory and animal experiments and have yet to be shown definitively to apply to humans. The effects of EDCs on sex differentiation and development in humans remain unknown. Further studies of these chemicals are needed to gain a better understanding of their role, if any, in human sexual development.

46,XX Disorder of Sex Development

DISORDERS OF GONADAL (OVARIAN) DEVELOPMENT

Gonadal Dysgenesis

Patients with XX gonadal dysgenesis have bilateral streak gonads or hypoplastic ovaries with intact müllerian duct structures and female external genitalia. They differ from patients with Turner syndrome in that they usually have normal stature, an absence of Turner stigmata, no abnormality of the X chromosome, and frequently a familial condition. An abnormality of an autosomal gene that regulates germ cell migration, formation of the bipotential gonad, or ovarian differentiation may be the cause. Familial cases occur frequently. Associated defects are seen in some families, including sensorineural hearing loss (Perrault syndrome), neurologic abnormalities, and renal disease. Isolated instances of clitoromegaly have been described, resulting from testosterone production by either hilar cells or luteinized gonadal stromal cells in a streak gonad. The differential diagnosis includes defects in estradiol synthesis, Slotnick-Goldfarb syndrome (streak gonad plus a hypoplastic ovary that may present as a neonatal ovarian cyst), Malouf syndrome (ovarian dysgenesis, dilated cardiomyopathy, ptosis, broad nasal bridge), and Denys-Drash and Fraser syndromes.

46,XX Ovotesticular Disorder of Sex Development

See earlier section, "Ovotesticular Disorder of Sex Development."

Testicular Disorder of Sex Development (46,XX Male)

Individuals with 46,XX male phenotype have bilateral testes but absence of a Y chromosome on karyotype analysis. Most have normal male internal and external genitalia, but 10% to 20% have ambiguous genitalia because of decreased fetal testosterone production. The testes are of normal size but may be cryptorchid. As with Klinefelter syndrome, the detrimental influence of the second X chromosome results in the absence of spermatogonia, hyalinization of the tubules, and small testes in adults. The testicular histology is almost normal in the first year of life, but after 1 year of age, the spermatogonia are lacking. Most if not all XX males inherit one maternal and one paternal X chromosome. The incidence is about 1 in 20,000 male births. The most common cause is an abnormal X-Y interchange, occurring during paternal meiosis and involving a crossover of variable amounts of adjacent Y sequences to the distal end of the paternal short arm of the X chromosome. Most *SRY*-positive individuals have a normal male phenotype and no disability except infertility. A few have lost more of the X chromosome sequence, resulting in short stature or mental retardation; others with a very small Y interchange have hypospadias or other incomplete male genital development, which is thought to be caused by altered *SRY* gene expression.

A few XX males are found to have no *SRY* gene and no detectable Y sequences. Most of these *SRY*-negative and Y-negative individuals have ambiguous genitalia. The cause is believed to be autosomal, possibly involving a mutation that turns on a gene downstream from the *SRY* gene that leads to testicular differentiation. A mutation in an X-linked gene, unrecognized 46,XX/46,XY mosaicism, and a duplication of *SOX9*[25] are other possible explanations. Gonadal tumors have not been reported.

ANDROGEN EXCESS

The external genital ambiguity is almost always androgen induced; most cases are caused by fetal CAH, and a few result from a maternal androgen source. However, in rare cases, a source of androgens is not found, and an error in morphogenesis is presumed to be the cause.

Androgen exposure between 8 and 14 weeks of fetal age results in variable male differentiation of the external genitalia—that is, labioscrotal fusion, regression of the urovaginal septum to form a urogenital sinus, ventral displacement of the urethral (urogenital) meatus toward or on the phallus, and male phallus differentiation. See Figure 49-40 for a schematic representation of the degrees of virilization adapted from a scale developed by Prader.[73] Androgen exposure occurring beyond 12 or 14 weeks produces growth but not differentiation of the external genitalia—namely clitoral hypertrophy, defined in the neonate by a clitoral width of greater than 6 mm. Most 46,XX DSDs are identified at birth because of genital ambiguity, but the more severely affected neonates may be initially missed, being incorrectly identified as males with hypospadias or undescended testes. The major reason to identify 46,XX DSDs in the immediate neonatal period is that CAH, if present, is potentially life-threatening.

Congenital Adrenal Hyperplasia

CAH comprises a group of disorders in which there is an inherited defect in one of the enzymes required for the adrenocortical synthesis of cortisol from cholesterol. Each of the

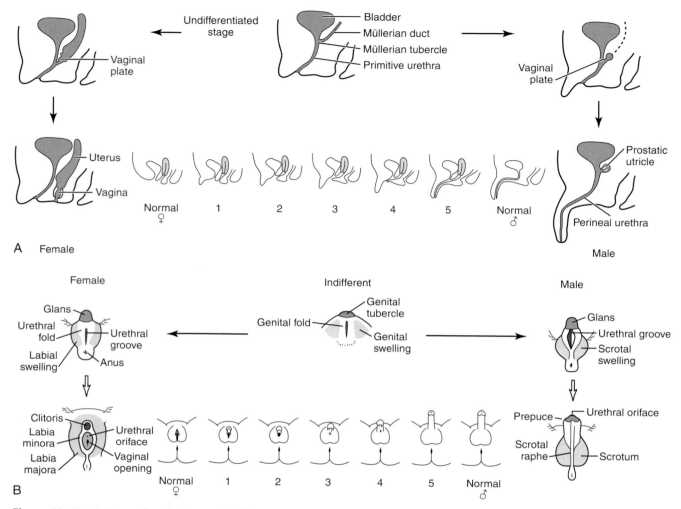

Figure 49-40. A, Normal and abnormal differentiation of the urogenital sinus and external genitalia (cross-sectional view). Diagrams of normal female and male anatomy flank a series of schematic representations of different degrees of virilization of females, graded using the scale developed by Prader. Note that the uterus persists in virilized females even when the external genitalia have a completely masculine appearance (Prader grade 5). B, Normal and abnormal differentiation of the external genitalia (external view). (*From White PC, Speiser PW: Congenital adrenal hyperplasia due to 21-hydroxylase deficiency, Endocr Rev 21:245, 2000.*)

enzyme defects leads to impaired cortisol production that causes a secondary increase in adrenocorticotropic hormone (ACTH). The elevated ACTH stimulates increased adrenocortical steroidogenic activity in an attempt to normalize cortisol production. Clinical problems arise as a consequence of impaired synthesis of the steroid hormones (glucocorticoids, mineralocorticoids, or gonadal sex steroids) beyond the enzymatic block and overproduction of the precursor steroids or their side products before the block (Fig. 49-41). Adrenal enzyme defects not involving cortisol synthesis are excluded from the CAH designation.

The five enzymes or enzymatic steps involved in the synthesis of cortisol from cholesterol are cholesterol side-chain cleavage enzyme complex (or 20,22-desmolase), 3β-hydroxysteroid dehydrogenase (3βHSD), 17α-hydroxylase, 21-hydroxylase, and 11β-hydroxylase (see Fig. 49-29). All except 3βHSD are

members of the cytochrome P-450 group of oxygenases. Except for 17α-hydroxylase, these enzymes are also necessary for mineralocorticoid (aldosterone) biosynthesis. The first three enzymes are present in gonadal tissue, where they are necessary for synthesis of the sex steroids. A deficiency in males results in inadequate testosterone formation and incomplete male sex differentiation; in females, it results in deficient estrogen synthesis, which is clinically significant at puberty.

The 21- and 11β-hydroxylases are found predominantly in the adrenal cortex and only minimally in gonadal tissue and are not necessary for the synthesis of sex steroids. However, their deficiencies (and to a lesser extent the deficiency of 3βHSD) result in excess formation of precursor steroids, which yield an increased production of androgens that induce masculinization of affected female fetuses in utero. By this mechanism, 46,XX DSD occurs, and affected females

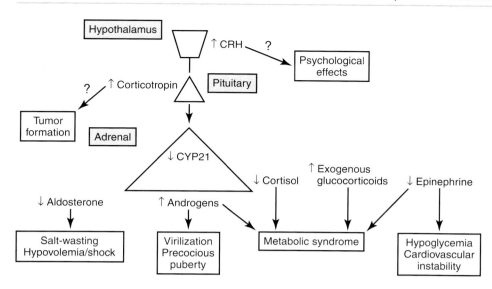

Figure 49–41. Endocrine imbalances characteristic of congenital adrenal hyperplasia. Potential clinical manifestations are given in the text boxes. (*From Merke DP, Bornstein SR: Congenital adrenal hyperplasia,* Lancet 365:2125, 2005.)

should be identifiable at birth by their abnormal genitalia. Affected males who have 21- or 11β-hydroxylase deficiency do not manifest recognizable penile enlargement or other virilization at birth but develop these symptoms postnatally if untreated. On the other hand, affected males with 3βHSD deficiency do have genital ambiguity at birth because of testosterone deficiency. Finally, all five enzyme deficiencies are clinically important because of the associated adrenal glucocorticoid deficiency (with or without mineralocorticoid deficiency). This condition is life-threatening and needs to be recognized and managed early.

21-HYDROXYLASE DEFICIENCY

21-Hydroxylase enzyme deficiency is the most common cause of CAH, accounting for 95% of all cases. Two forms are seen in neonates: a simple virilizing form, in which the enzyme deficiency is partial, and a salt-losing form, in which the enzyme deficiency is more complete. A third form, late-onset or nonclassic 21-hydroxylase deficiency, represents a mild enzyme deficiency that does not have clinical manifestations in the fetus, neonate, or infant. Both of the classic forms are characterized by abnormal virilization of the female fetus. In the simple virilizing form, the salt loss is mild, so adrenal insufficiency does not tend to occur except in stressful circumstances. In the salt-losing form, there is adrenal insufficiency under basal conditions that tends to manifest in the neonatal period or soon thereafter as an adrenal crisis. Seventy percent of all reported cases of CAH are salt wasting and 30% are not salt wasting. The incidence of the classic form estimated from data from 13 countries (United States, France, Italy, New Zealand, Japan, United Kingdom, Brazil, Switzerland, Sweden, Germany, Portugal, Canada, and Spain) is 1 in 15,000 live births, and the carrier frequency of classic CAH is about 1 in 60 individuals.[43]

Simple Virilizing Form. The simple virilizing form is due to a partial deficiency in the 21-hydroxylase enzyme. 21-Hydroxylase is necessary for the conversion of 17-OHP to 11-deoxycortisol (compound S) and of progesterone to 11-deoxycorticosterone (DOC). A deficiency of this enzyme results in an impairment of cortisol and aldosterone biosynthesis, which is compensated

for by the increased secretion of ACTH and angiotensin. This process causes overproduction of the steroids before the enzyme block and a secondary increased secretion of adrenal androgens, which are converted in peripheral tissues to testosterone and DHT, where they cause abnormal virilization (see Fig. 49-41).

Affected fetuses produce increased amounts of androgens beginning in the first trimester. In the female fetus, it leads to varying degrees of male differentiation of the external genitalia and urogenital sinus, but the internal genital ducts develop normally along female lines without any wolffian duct development because its development requires high local and not systemic levels of androgen. At birth, the spectrum of masculinization in females ranges from mild clitoromegaly, usually with some posterior labial fusion, to perineal or penile hypospadias to occasionally complete male differentiation, with the urethra opening at the tip of a male-sized phallus; the latter phenotype may have a normal male appearance except that the gonads are impalpable. The extent of male differentiation in female fetuses tends to reflect the severity of the enzyme defect. Females with the simple virilizing form often show less extensive male differentiation than those with the salt-losing type. In the male fetus, the increased secretion of adrenal androgens is insignificant compared with the fetal production of testicular androgens. The external genitalia are usually normal at birth; some enlargement of the penis may occur, but it is rarely recognizable as such. Female and male neonates may have increased pigmentation of the genitalia or areolae.

Patients with untreated, simple virilizing 21-hydroxylase deficiency continue to produce excess androgens postnatally, resulting in accelerated growth and skeletal maturation and the appearance of androgen-induced sexual changes. Patients with mild CAH generally do not develop symptoms of adrenal insufficiency unless they are exposed to major stress or significant salt depletion (reduced salt intake, vomiting, excessive sweating). A few patients with either form have received medical attention because of recurrent hypoglycemic episodes or seizures, usually occurring during common infections.

Salt-Wasting Form. The salt-wasting form is due to a severe deficiency of the 21-hydroxylase enzyme that results in significant impairment of cortisol and aldosterone synthesis that cannot be compensated for by the increased levels of ACTH and angiotensin. The development of cortisol and aldosterone deficiency, usually in the first weeks of life, results in acute adrenal insufficiency and sodium wasting (see Fig. 49-41). Females with the salt-losing form of CAH may show more complete masculinization of the external genitalia, and some are incorrectly identified as males at birth (Fig. 49-42). Males generally receive medical attention when they develop a salt-losing crisis due to adrenal insufficiency. The symptoms or signs of adrenal insufficiency are not present at birth and rarely occur before 3 to 4 days of age. About half of the untreated patients with salt-losing CAH have onset of adrenal crisis between 6 and 14 days of age; by 1 month of age, more than three fourths have developed adrenal crisis. Less severely affected individuals may present in the following months, usually in association with a stressful condition causing decreased salt intake or increased salt losses, and a few escape crisis entirely. The early symptoms and signs of adrenal crisis are nonspecific and include lethargy, a poor appetite, regurgitation of feedings, failure to thrive, and weight loss. Hyperkalemia, hyponatremia, and metabolic acidosis may be seen early. The regurgitation of feedings may progress to projectile vomiting. Severe symptoms and signs may occur within 1 to 2 days, including dehydration (with accompanying azotemia), hypotension, muscle weakness, obtundation, a gray or cyanotic appearance, cold and clammy skin, hyperkalemic cardiac conduction abnormalities, and hyponatremic or hypoglycemic seizures.

The development of acute adrenal crisis is partially caused by hypoaldosteronism, which results in renal sodium wasting, with depletion of total-body sodium content and an impaired ability to secrete potassium and hydrogen ions in the distal tubule. The decreased total-body sodium content results in hyponatremia, hypovolemia, and decreased tissue perfusion, which account for many of the early symptoms and eventually result in hypotension and shock.

Hypocortisolemia represents the other major component of adrenal insufficiency and results in impairment of cardiovascular, metabolic, and other systemic functions. Among the cardiovascular effects associated with glucocorticoid deficiency are decreased stroke volume and cardiac output, decreased blood pressure, and decreased vascular tone or reactivity. Depletion of the renin substrate occurs in the presence of cortisol deficiency and impairs the renin-angiotensin axis, leading to circulatory failure. Norepinephrine raises the peripheral blood pressure only in the presence of cortisol, suggesting that cortisol exerts a permissive action. There is also an impaired ability of the urine to be concentrated because of the reduced responsiveness of the renal collecting tubules to vasopressin.

Cortisol deficiency is associated with an inability to maintain and mobilize normal hepatic glycogen stores, which during a period of starvation may lead to hypoglycemia. Fat becomes the primary source of energy, a condition that may lead to lipid depletion. Cortisol is normally important for the mobilization of increased glucose production by the liver by both inducing gluconeogenic enzymes and exerting its permissive effects on epinephrine and glucagon-induced glycogenolysis. Cortisol deficiency is associated with impaired muscle activity; normochromic, normocytic anemia; and eosinophilia.

Hormonal Abnormalities. The hormonal abnormalities include a serum level of cortisol that is normal or low with an inadequate rise in response to ACTH administration. ACTH levels in untreated patients with either form of CAH are elevated, but more so in the patients with salt-losing CAH. Plasma renin activity is also elevated, especially in salt-losing CAH. However, in contrast to the simple virilizing form, in salt-losing CAH, there is no increase in aldosterone production in response to sodium restriction or ACTH administration.

Of the steroids preceding the enzyme block, 17-OHP is the most strikingly elevated. Serum concentrations are increased 40 to 400 times above the upper limit of normal values and occasionally higher. Androstenedione can be up to 40 times higher than the normal limit. About 15% of the androstenedione produced is metabolized in peripheral tissues to testosterone, with the adrenals synthesizing very little testosterone. Serum testosterone levels in affected children can be elevated by 20 times the normal range.

Pathology. Pathologically, the adrenal glands are characteristically hyperplastic and enlarged. The effects of excessive ACTH stimulation are seen microscopically. The zona glomerulosa, from which mineralocorticoids are produced, is two to four times wider in the simple virilizing form of CAH but is either normal or absent in the salt-losing form.

Diagnosis. The diagnosis of 21-hydroxylase deficiency in a neonate or infant should be considered in females with any masculinization of the external genitalia, in presumed males with impalpable gonads (including males with hypospadias), in females or males who develop symptoms or signs of adrenal insufficiency or crisis (females should be recognized by their genital abnormalities), and in those who have a family history of CAH or an unexplained death in infancy.

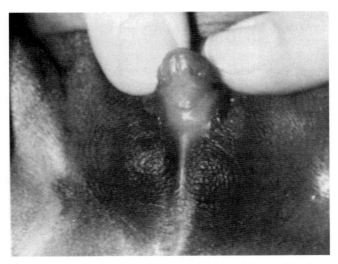

Figure 49–42. A 4-week-old 46,XX neonate with salt-losing 21-hydroxylase deficiency was erroneously thought to be a male with penile hypospadias at birth. There was a small phallus (2.3 × 0.8 cm) and impalpable gonads.

For 21-hydroxylase deficiency, the most useful diagnostic test is the determination of an increased level of serum 17-OHP (more than 80 times higher than normal in a full-term infant).

Newborn Screening. Many jurisdictions have newborn screening programs that include the measurement of 17-OHP and allow the early identification of infants with CAH. Their justification lies in the increased mortality that occurs in infants who are not diagnosed and die of salt-losing crisis or sudden infant death and the increased morbidity that results from adrenal insufficiency, incorrect gender assignment, and premature virilization.[22] Caution is needed in interpreting the values of 17-OHP on newborn screening tests, particularly in the first week of life because many affected neonates show normal levels of 17-OHP on the first day of life and only mild elevation in the first several days before the levels become very high. Conversely, the levels in unaffected full-term neonates may be elevated in cord serum and are high in peripheral serum in the first 12 hours of life before declining to the normal range after 24 hours of age. Levels in premature[34] and sick neonates may overlap with those found in many affected infants in the first few days of life. Many jurisdictions with newborn screening programs have cutoff values that are adjusted according to gestation age or weight, or both.

The method of detection is based on finding an increased level of 17-OHP in blood collected on filter paper at 2 to 5 days of age. False-positive results are usually associated with prematurity (presumably caused by decreased metabolic clearance of 17-OHP) or low birthweight and, less often, with serious illness (probably caused by increased 17-OHP production associated with stress), age less than 24 hours (fetoplacental contribution of 17-OHP), or technical problems.

The overall incidence of 21-hydroxylase deficiency in screened neonates is about 1 in 15,000, ranging from 1 in 11,000 to 1 in 21,000 for most programs. As expected, the male-to-female ratio is about 1:1; salt losers have about a 72% incidence. Although females identified by screening often have variable masculinization of the external genitalia, one third to one half were missed clinically, including some of them inappropriately assigned to male gender. In addition, identification at 5 to 21 days of age has prevented adrenal crisis in many affected but unrecognized neonates. Such screening clearly improves the detection of 21-hydroxylase deficiency in neonates for whom the diagnosis might otherwise have been missed.

In response to administration of synthetic ACTH (Cortrosyn, 35 μg/kg to a maximum of 250 μg intravenously), 17-OHP levels can be plotted on a nomogram to predict the genotype.[49] The measurement of plasma ACTH or serum cortisol is not useful in defining the enzyme defect of CAH but may have value when other causes of adrenal insufficiency are considered.

Despite a negative result of newborn screening, if the diagnosis of CAH is suspected clinically, testing should be done. The diagnosis of the salt-losing form of CAH is based on obtaining clinical or biochemical evidence for sodium wasting. There is typically a clinical diagnosis that is based on the presence of varying degrees of hyponatremia, hyperkalemia, or hypovolemia and its clinical consequences. High urinary sodium concentrations in the presence of normal or low serum sodium concentrations may indicate that an infant is a salt loser. The measurement of aldosterone or plasma renin activity in the untreated state is not diagnostically useful because of the overlap with levels seen in untreated patients with simple virilization.[32] Patients with mild, salt-losing CAH may show normal electrolytes and lack the clinical signs of hypovolemia. Their diagnosis is made biochemically by finding an increased level of plasma renin activity during physiologic glucocorticoid replacement therapy; mineralocorticoid replacement should be added.

Ultrasonography. An experienced pediatric radiologist reading an adrenal ultrasound can identify enlargement and lobulation of the adrenal glands with stippled echogenicity, findings consistent with CAH. Adrenal ultrasonography has been shown to have a sensitivity of 92% and a specificity of 100% for diagnosing CAH.[2]

Treatment. The goals of the treatment of CAH are to normalize ACTH secretion, thereby lowering ACTH-stimulated precursor steroids and their side products, and provide replacement or correction of end product (cortisol, aldosterone, gonadal sex steroid) deficiencies. The two goals are closely interrelated. Normalization of ACTH secretion requires both cortisol replacement and the correction of hypovolemia, with adjustments made during medical stress. Insufficient replacement permits increased ACTH and sodium wasting, and excessive replacement produces a cushingoid state, growth suppression, and hypertension.

In the simple virilizing form of 21-hydroxylase deficiency, normalization of ACTH requires only cortisol replacement. The addition of mineralocorticoid therapy may decrease the amount of cortisol that is needed. The adequacy of cortisol replacement is monitored by the measurement of serum 17-OHP and androstenedione.

In the salt-losing form of 21-hydroxylase deficiency, normalization of ACTH requires the correction of sodium wasting and hypovolemia in addition to the physiologic replacement of cortisol. Hypovolemia is monitored by the measurement of plasma renin activity. Increased levels indicate the presence of hypovolemia caused by sodium wasting, and subnormal levels indicate sodium retention caused by excessive mineralocorticoid replacement.

With regard to maintenance cortisol replacement, allowance must be made for differences in potency, absorption, and duration of action among the available preparations. Hydrocortisone is the oral preparation of choice. Oral replacement doses in CAH usually range from 12 to 20 mg/m² per day given in three divided doses. One study using once-daily dexamethasone at a dose of 0.27 mg/m²/d showed normal growth.[64]

Increases in the dose of hydrocortisone (or other glucocorticoid) should be made during periods of stress, with doubling or tripling of the dose during moderate and severe illnesses. Major illnesses, surgery, or trauma should be covered by the intramuscular or intravenous administration of hydrocortisone at three to six times the maintenance dose to avoid adrenal crisis. At the initiation of therapy, the hydrocortisone dose may be prescribed at maintenance levels or at three times the maintenance dose if stress is present.

For infants who require maintenance mineralocorticoid replacement therapy, it is provided orally.

9α-Fludrocortisone acetate (Florinef Acetate), 0.05 to 0.30 mg, is administered daily. Sodium supplementation (1 to 5 mEq/kg per day) may be needed in the first 1 to 2 years, in part because the renal tubules are less able to conserve sodium. Measurements of blood pressure and the level of plasma renin activity are used to adjust the mineralocorticoid dosage and sodium supplementation. Unlike hydrocortisone or other glucocorticoids, the dose of Florinef Acetate does not change with increases in body size or during stress. As infancy progresses, mineralocorticoid requirements diminish; salt supplementation should be discontinued, and the dose of Florinef Acetate may need to be lowered.

In acute salt-losing adrenal crisis, fluid replacement (beginning with 20 mL/kg of body weight of 0.9% saline), sodium replacement, continuous glucose infusion, glucocorticoid therapy at 50-100 mg/m² (initially given intravenously as the phosphate or succinate ester of hydrocortisone), and mineralocorticoid replacement (Florinef Acetate, 0.1 to 0.2 mg orally every 12 to 24 hours) are needed. Acidosis, hypoglycemia, and hyperkalemia may be present and should be managed, and the patient should be monitored for potassium toxicity. In patients stable enough for diagnostic testing, glucocorticoid therapy may be withheld until the tests are completed. However, therapy should be administered if blood pressure or other functions are not correctable with fluid, saline, glucose, and mineralocorticoid replacement.

Gender Assignment. See the earlier section, "Gender Assignment in Newborns," for a full discussion. Here we discuss gender assignment issues specific to CAH. Female gender assignment is usually recommended in 46,XX CAH individuals regardless of the extent of masculinization of their genitalia. This recommendation is based on the observation that these patients have normal ovaries and müllerian structures and have the potential to lead normal, fertile lives as females. Surgical correction and its timing in females with masculinized external genitalia are controversial. If done, it is usually performed when a reasonable body size has been achieved, commonly in the first 2 to 6 months. Females with CAH have been shown to engage in more masculine play activities.[58] Mixed results have been reported about whether females with CAH have a more masculine pattern on cognitive function tests.[39] Although lower rates of heterosexual orientation,[44] marriage, and fertility have been reported, they generally identify as females and do not have gender dysphoria. Gender identity in girls with CAH is not related to the degree of genital virilization or the age at which genital reconstructive surgery was done.[44] Observed psychological differences have been attributed to insufficient androgen suppression, inadequate vaginal introitus, and possible effects of in utero androgen exposure on the central nervous system.

Genetics. 21-Hydroxylase deficiency is inherited as an autosomal recessive disorder. Genotyping studies of families have established a genetic link with the gene responsible for 21-hydroxylase deficiency. Molecular genetic studies show that two 21-hydroxylase genes are present on each chromosome 6. However, the first gene is nonfunctional (a pseudogene); only the second one is functional. These two genes are named *CYP21P* and *CYP21*, respectively.

Diverse mutational abnormalities of the *CYP21* gene have been described for 21-hydroxylase deficiency, including point mutations, gene conversions (transfer of an abnormal sequence from the pseudogene to the active gene), and deletions. Point mutations and small-gene conversions represent most *CYP21* mutations. They may have mild or severe consequences, affecting messenger RNA stability, enzyme conformation, and function. Gene deletions and large-gene conversions account for the remaining *CYP21* changes, which usually result in defective or absent messenger RNA. Patients with salt wasting have the most deleterious mutations and almost no residual enzyme activity, although there is an overlap among phenotype-genotype correlations. Genotyping to identify the mutation is available.[75]

Prenatal Diagnosis and Treatment. The prenatal diagnosis of 21-hydroxylase deficiency is advocated by many for the affected female fetus because therapy is available to minimize or prevent masculinization of the external genitalia. It is, however, considered experimental by others. To be effective, therapy must be initiated by 8 weeks of gestation. A gene-specific diagnosis in utero can be made on cells obtained by chorionic villus sampling or amniotic fluid analysis.[51] This has replaced the method of making the diagnosis by measuring hormone levels.

If undertaken, the in utero treatment of the female fetus with 21-hydroxylase deficiency requires sufficient glucocorticoid replacement to suppress fetal ACTH and androgen, reducing levels to normal or less than normal; any fetal sodium wasting is presumably corrected by the maternal-placental unit. Dexamethasone given to the mother readily crosses the placenta, and the generally recommended dose (20 μg/kg per pre-pregnancy body weight per day given in three divided doses, preferably not exceeding 1.5 mg/day) is usually effective in limiting or preventing adrenal masculinization of the fetal external genitalia, indicating that dexamethasone can suppress fetal ACTH. Treatment of the fetus at risk is begun optimally when the pregnancy is confirmed and before 9 weeks after the last menstrual period. Because one in four fetuses will be affected and only affected female fetuses need to be treated, there is a seven out of eight chance that continuation of treatment is unnecessary. An algorithm for the diagnosis and prenatal treatment of fetuses at risk for CAH is shown in Figure 49-43. If chorionic villus sampling and amniocentesis are not performed, fetal sex determination by ultrasonography performed later in the second trimester should identify the males and result in continuation of therapy to term only in the females. Among the maternal side effects that are occasionally seen are those of glucocorticoid excess (weight gain, edema, glucose intolerance, and hirsutism); the dexamethasone-induced suppression of the maternal hypothalamic-pituitary-adrenal axis needs to be managed during delivery or other major stress. Untoward effects have not been encountered in the newborns or their mothers.[51] The risks for long-term effects on brain development or psychosexual outcome, if any, are currently being investigated.

11β-HYDROXYLASE DEFICIENCY (HYPERTENSIVE CONGENITAL ADRENAL HYPERPLASIA)

A deficiency of 11β-hydroxylase (cytochrome P-450c11) results in impaired synthesis of cortisol and aldosterone, abnormal virilization from increased androgens formed from the cortisol precursors, and low-renin hypertension from increased formation of DOC, a moderately potent mineralocorticoid. It is the second most common form of CAH, accounting for about 5% of the cases.

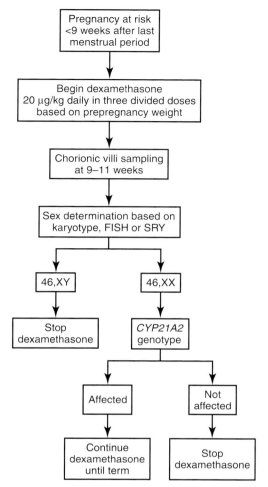

Figure 49–43. Simplified algorithm of treatment, diagnosis, and decision making for prenatal treatment of fetuses at risk for 21-hydroxylase deficiency congenital adrenal hyperplasia. (*From Nimkarn S, New MI: Prenatal diagnosis and treatment of congenital adrenal hyperplasia owing to 21-hydroxylase deficiency, Nat Clin Pract Endocrinol Metab 3:405, 2007.*)

The clinical presentation of 11β-hydroxylase deficiency is varied, and not all the patients develop hypertension. Classically, females are born with virilization ranging from clitoral enlargement to extensive masculinization of the external genitalia, which may lead to incorrect gender assignment; male neonates may have a somewhat larger penis, but this is not routinely recognizable. There may be hyperpigmentation of the genitalia and the areolae. Sodium retention and volume-induced hypertension develop in 50% to 80% of the classic cases. Severe hypertension may occur as early as the first 4 days of life, but more often blood pressure is normal in neonates. The relative severities of the hypertension, virilization, and biochemical findings do not always correlate. Serum sodium levels tend to be in the upper-normal range or minimally elevated, but hypokalemia is inconsistently present.

In exception to the classic presentations, some affected and untreated neonates present with salt losing, which may lead to diagnostic confusion with 21-hydroxylase deficiency.

The cause of their salt-losing conditions is unclear, but possibilities include a combination of physiologic renal immaturity of sodium reabsorption, more severe aldosterone deficiency and less adequate DOC, and the presence of precursor steroids with mineralocorticoid antagonist properties.

The characteristic biochemical abnormality that is observed is an increased level of serum 11-deoxycortisol (compound S), with concentrations usually more than 5 times the upper limit of the normal range. Serum DOC concentrations have also been elevated to more than 10 times the upper limit of normal. Serum 17-OHP, androstenedione, and urinary 17-ketosteroids are also increased and may cause diagnostic confusion with 21-hydroxylase deficiency.

11β-Hydroxylase deficiency should be considered in 46,XX neonates with masculinization of the external genitalia, in salt-losing neonates, in any patient beyond the neonatal period with abnormal virilization, and in hypertensive patients. The diagnosis is supported by the finding of increased levels of serum 11-deoxycortisol and DOC, demonstrating their suppressibility with cortisol replacement therapy, and ACTH stimulation testing showing elevation in 11-deoxycortisol.

11β-Hydroxylase deficiency is autosomal recessive. Two 11β-hydroxylase genes have been identified, which are located on the long arm of chromosome 8; they are linked and show greater than 90% sequence homology. The *CYP11B1* gene is responsible for 11β-hydroxylase deficiency, and the *CYP11B2* gene encodes for aldosterone synthase.[59] Prenatal diagnosis by genotyping of the *CYP11B1* gene by chorionic villus sampling is available.[52]

Treatment of the fetus suspected of having 11β-hydroxylase deficiency is the same as that for 21-OHD. Treatment consists of cortisol replacement therapy, as outlined for 21-hydroxylase deficiency. Glucocorticoid replacement reduces ACTH and precursor steroids toward normal levels, with cessation of virilization. Decreased DOC formation leads to the correction of hypertension in most affected patients. Glucocorticoid therapy is adjusted based on the patient's growth; blood pressure; and levels of serum 11-deoxycortisol, DOC, androstenedione, and plasma renin activity. The gender is usually assigned in agreement with the gonadal sex because normal sexual function and fertility can be attained.

3β-HYDROXYSTEROID DEHYDROGENASE DEFICIENCY

3βHSD type 2 is required for the formation of all three classes of steroids—the glucocorticoids, mineralocorticoids, and sex steroids. Severe deficiency can result in genital ambiguity for both sexes: males with severe penile or perineal hypospadias and females with minimum virilization at birth, with posterior labial fusion and clitoral hypertrophy but normal placement of the urethral meatus. Salt-losing adrenal crisis results from impaired cortisol and aldosterone biosynthesis in the adrenal gland, and the incomplete male genital differentiation results from decreased testosterone biosynthesis in the testes. Mild prenatal virilization in females is thought to result from increased precursor steroid formation; that is, the increased amounts of DHEA are probably converted by peripheral 3βHSD type 1 in the liver, skin, and other tissues. 3βHSD type 2 is required for the formation of biochemically active androgens that induce mild masculinization of the genitalia in the female.

The characteristic biochemical finding in the untreated patient is a marked elevation of ACTH-stimulated 17-hydroxypregnenolone and ratios of 17-hydroxypregnenolone to cortisol.[56] Aldosterone levels are low, and plasma renin activity is increased. A diagnosis can be made on baseline or ACTH-stimulated steroid levels, or both.

Clinical heterogeneity is seen in 3βHSD deficiency, as in the 21- and 11β-hydroxylase deficiency disorders. Multiple gene defects in the *HSD3B2* gene have been described.[69] Sodium wasting varies by degree, ranging from severe to mild to none. The severity of the defect also varies, with some patients having no genital ambiguity at birth but presenting with adrenal insufficiency and some having delayed virilization.

Treatment is the same as that for 21-hydroxylase deficiency; serum levels of 17-hydroxypregnenolone and DHEA serve as guides for the adequacy of glucocorticoid replacement. Mineralocorticoid therapy is monitored by means of measurements of plasma renin activity. There is autosomal recessive inheritance.

CONGENITAL LIPOID ADRENAL HYPERPLASIA

The first step in steroid hormone biosynthesis is the transport of cholesterol into the mitochondria mediated by the steroidogenic acute regulatory (*StAR*) protein. Mutations in this gene cause an autosomal recessive condition known as congenital lipoid adrenal hyperplasia.[46]

It is a rare but serious disorder; many patients have died within the first few months of life. The clinical course for most cases has been the development of severe adrenal insufficiency, sometimes occurring in the first days of life but in milder cases beginning beyond several weeks of age. Sodium wasting has often been extreme, and hypoglycemia may occur. Affected 46,XX females have normal female genitalia; XY males have female or ambiguous external genitalia, often with a blind vaginal pouch, and the testes may be descended. Hyperpigmentation and respiratory problems may occur.

The adrenal glands are enlarged, with a characteristically enormous accumulation of lipid, thus the name *congenital lipoid adrenal hyperplasia*. The testes and Leydig cells show analogous pathology in some but not all males. There may be wolffian duct development, presumably resulting from the partial testicular production of testosterone. Biochemically, there is decreased to absent production of all adrenal and gonadal steroids, depending on the severity of the defect, and an accumulation of cholesterol and its esters in the adrenals and gonads. Prenatal diagnosis by molecular genetic testing for mutations in the *StAR* gene are now available.[29]

The second step in steroid hormone biosynthesis is the conversion of cholesterol to pregnenolone by the cholesterol side-chain cleavage enzyme (P-450scc). A deficiency in this enzyme (SCC deficiency) results in impaired synthesis of all adrenal and gonadal steroids. P-450scc activity is needed to produce placental progesterone, a hormone that is needed to maintain a pregnancy. For this reason, it was thought that SCC deficiency would lead to spontaneous abortion. There are some rare reports of SCC deficiency with variability in timing of presentation of adrenal failure and not all were found to have adrenal hyperplasia.[30]

SCC deficiency should be considered in cases of adrenal insufficiency and hyperpigmentation and in cases of XY males with ambiguous genitalia. The diagnosis is based on the demonstration of a deficiency of the glucocorticoids, mineralocorticoids, and androgens. Treatment includes cortisol, mineralocorticoid, and salt replacement therapy, as outlined for 21-hydroxylase deficiency. This therapy should be administered aggressively in infancy to reduce the high mortality risk.

17α-HYDROXYLASE DEFICIENCY

17α-hydroxylase/17,20-lyase (P-450c17) deficiency is manifested clinically as hypertension and hypogonadism. Biochemically, it results in impaired conversion of pregnenolone and progesterone to their 17α-hydroxy product. The consequence is reduced cortisol, androgen, and estrogen production. Increased ACTH stimulation produces increased progesterone and its products DOC, corticosterone, and 18-hydroxycorticosterone. The increased mineralocorticoids produce low-renin hypertension (frequently severe and often associated with hyperkalemic alkalosis and borderline hypernatremia), which often develops in infancy. Adrenal insufficiency usually does not develop because of the mineralocorticoid and glucocorticoid properties of DOC and corticosterone. Affected XX females have normal genitalia at birth but fail to undergo secondary sexual development at puberty. The 46,XY males have phenotypically female to variably masculinized external genitalia, often with a distal vagina, variable testicular descent, and the frequent occurrence of inguinal hernia, which may lead to their identification. The internal genital ducts are appropriate for the gonadal sex, except that wolffian duct development may be incomplete. The differential diagnosis for XY individuals includes AIS and other causes of 46,XY DSD.

Cortisol replacement therapy corrects these abnormalities and hypertension; in most, aldosterone secretion returns to a normal level, although in several cases, it has remained abnormally low. Serum levels of testosterone are low and show a poor rise after hCG stimulation. Several different mutations of *CYP17* have been found, with the consequent enzyme deficiencies varying from partial to complete.

Cortisol replacement is given as described for 21-hydroxylase deficiency, but mineralocorticoid therapy is not necessary unless aldosterone secretion fails to return to a normal level.

P-450 OXIDOREDUCTASE DEFICIENCY

The P-450 oxidoreductase deficiency (POR) enzyme acts as a cofactor for P-450 microsomal enzymes including 17-hydroxylase/17,20-lyase, P-450c21 (21-hydroxylase), and P-450aro (aromatase), which are involved in steroid biosynthesis.[67] Because of the complexity of function of the enzyme, deficiency manifests as a wide spectrum of biochemical and clinical features.

Biochemical abnormalities can include elevated 17-OHP and low androgen levels; cortisol may be normal but is poorly responsive to adrenocorticotropic hormone. These indicate partial deficiencies in 21-hydroxylase, 17-hydroxylase, and 17,20-lyase (Fig. 49-44).

Clinical features are a result of abnormalities in steroid hormones, skeletal development, and drug metabolism. Abnormal genital development can be seen in both sexes; males can be undervirilized, and females can be virilized. In

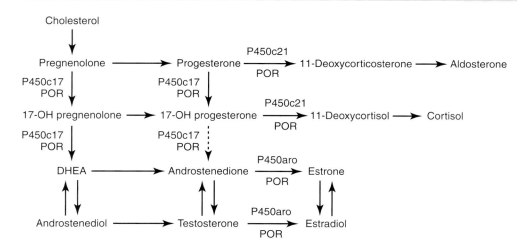

Figure 49–44. Simplified steroid biosynthetic pathway indicating the steps where POR acts as a cofactor. *(From Scott RR, Miller WL: Genetic and clinical features of P450 oxidoreductase deficiency,* Horm Res 69:266, 2008.)

pregnancy, maternal virilization and low maternal estriol and estrone levels may be seen.

Most have associated skeletal malformations, termed *Antley-Bixler syndrome* (ABS). ABS is a syndrome that includes craniosynostosis, midface hypoplasia, choanal atresia or stenosis, radiohumeral or radioulnar synostosis, femoral bowing, and joint contractures and has been found to be caused by POR deficiency.[31] Both autosomal recessive inheritance and an autosomal dominant mutation in fibroblast growth factor receptor-2 (*FGFR2*) gene have been proposed as a cause of ABS.

Since 2004, when the POR mutation was first described, 50 cases have been reported. A number of different mutations have been described, all of which cause apparent partial deficiency of 21-hydroxylase and 17α-hydroxylase/17,20-lyase. Functional assays assessing POR function have been able to link genotype with phenotype.[67] The diagnosis of POR can be made by mutation analysis.

Initial management should include an ACTH stimulation test for cortisol production, with hydrocortisone replacement given if cortisol production is found to be insufficient. Aldosterone deficiency causing salt-wasting is possible because 17-hydroxolase activity is influenced by POR. In infants, the risk for upper airway obstruction caused by skeletal abnormalities, including choanal obstruction, should be assessed. Because some hepatic P-450 enzymes are dependent on POR, effects on drug metabolism due to POR deficiency are possible. Insufficient information is currently available to describe the clinical implications.

Placental Aromatase (CYP19) Deficiency

Placental-fetal aromatase (*CYP19*) is a cytochrome P-450 enzyme that is necessary for the conversion of androgens to estrogen. Placental aromatase deficiency can cause maternal and fetal virilization because of an inability to convert fetal adrenal androgens.[36] There is wide phenotypic variation observed due to mutations in *CYP19*.

Maternally Derived Androgenic Substances

Masculinization of the female fetus occasionally occurs from exposure to androgens or certain other agents derived from the maternal circulation. The extent of masculinization is related to the compound, dosage, duration, and timing of exposure. Exposure at 8 to 14 weeks of gestation may result in midline fusion of the labioscrotal folds; opening of the vagina and urethra into a common urogenital sinus; and (in more severe cases) development of a penile urethra, prostate, and possibly seminal vesicles. Exposure beginning after 12 to 14 weeks results in only clitoromegaly and hypertrophy of the labia majora but no midline fusion and no development of a urogenital sinus. Maternally derived androgens do not usually stimulate wolffian duct development, and the müllerian duct structures and bilateral ovaries develop normally in the absence of AMH. A considerable number of female fetuses do not undergo masculinization because the placenta aromatizes most maternal androgens before they cross over to the fetus, and the high maternal levels of globulin binding to sex steroids favor the concentration of these androgens on the maternal side.

Maternal androgens may be of ovarian, adrenal, or exogenous origin. The Krukenberg tumor and luteoma of pregnancy cause increased androgen production. Maternal androgen-secreting tumors of the ovary rarely occur in pregnancy. Several cases of maternal adrenocortical tumor are reported; maternal virilization in some has been mild compared with that in neonates or that not recognized until years later. Other cases of 46,XX DSD have been reported in association with maternal CAH and maternal polycystic ovarian disease. The measurement of the maternal serum levels of testosterone and DHEA or its sulfate is diagnostically useful even in the absence of maternal virilization. The maternal ingestion of synthetic progestins and androgens may cause abnormal masculinization of the female fetus. In the male fetus, progestin exposure at 8 to 14 weeks of gestation may result in hypospadias. Because these medications have often been given for only part of the pregnancy, the extents of clitoral enlargement, urethral displacement, and labioscrotal fusion are often discordant, contrasting with the other causes of 46,XX DSD. The mother may rarely show mild androgenization. Advanced skeletal maturation may occur in offspring exposed to the more androgenic substances.

The masculinization of females that occurs with androgen or other drug exposure in utero does not progress postnatally. Biochemical studies of the neonate show normal levels of androgens or their metabolites and of 17-OHP. The surgical correction of midline labioscrotal fusion or major clitoromegaly is usually performed by 12 to 18 months of age; mild clitoromegaly may not need to be corrected because the clitoris will become less prominent as the body size increases.

OTHER

Dysgenesis of External Genital Primordia

On rare occasions, the external genitalia of a 46,XX fetus may have a masculinized appearance because of an error in morphogenesis occurring at 4 to 7 weeks of fetal age rather than abnormal androgen exposure at 8 to 12 weeks. The formation of the urorectal septum and differentiation of the cloacal membrane into the urogenital and anal membranes, followed by their breakdown into the urogenital sinus and anus, are critical for the development of the indifferent external genitalia (at 7 weeks) and the lower genital, urinary, and intestinal tracts. In cloacal dysgenesis (Fig. 49-45), a small phallus-like structure develops from the genital tubercle (there is variable formation of a phallic urethra and corpora tissue), and the labioscrotal swellings may or may not develop; the absence of a urogenital groove makes for a more male-appearing perineum. Associated abnormalities include an imperforate anus, the absence of urethral and vaginal outlets (unless a phallic urethra forms), and urinary tract and müllerian (uterine and vaginal) anomalies (these anomalies are not found in any of the traditional forms of 46,XX DSD). The ovaries are usually normal. These abnormalities may be seen in the VATER association (vertebral abnormalities, anal atresia, tracheoesophageal fistula with esophageal atresia, radial and renal dysplasia). Pulmonary hypoplasia is often an associated condition, and obstructive

uropathy may infrequently be associated with Eagle-Barrett (prune-belly) syndrome. Less severe clinical forms are reported associated with a small phallus, partial vaginal outlet obstruction, and other urinary and genital tract anomalies.

Müllerian and Vaginal Dysgenesis

There is a frequent association of abnormal to absent müllerian duct structures with vaginal agenesis in 46,XX females with normal ovaries known as Mayer-Rokitansky-Küster-Hauser (MRKH) syndrome. MRKH syndrome is further classified as type 1 (isolated) or Rokitansky sequence and type II or MURCS association (müllerian duct aplasia, renal dysplasia, and cervical somite anomalies). It is sometimes also referred to as CAUV (congenital absence of the uterus and vagina), MA (müllerian aplasia), or GRES (genital renal ear syndrome).[48] A disturbance in mesodermal organization partially involving the formation of the caudal segments of the müllerian ducts in the fourth and fifth weeks of embryogenesis is suggested; the possibilities of both teratogenic and pleiotropic genetic causes have been raised. The differential diagnosis includes cAIS. Some patients have an abnormal karyotype. An examination to determine the presence or absence of a vaginal orifice (absent in this disorder), the occasional occurrence of hydrometra, and the presence of somatic abnormalities help to identify affected neonates. Vaginal construction is necessary; the extent of the uterine malformation needs to be assessed. About 70% of female patients with unilateral renal agenesis have ipsilateral müllerian duct abnormalities.

It has been proposed that MRKH syndrome is caused by a developmental field defect. The *WNT4* gene is important in

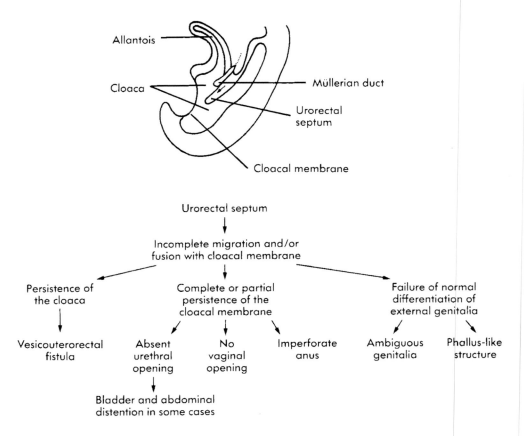

Figure 49–45. Diagram showing proposed mechanism for urorectal septum malformation sequence. The resulting cloacal dysgenesis leads to malformation of the external genital primordia and other accompanying abnormalities. In the affected 46,XX fetus, the genital tubercle (between the cloaca and allantois) forms a small phallus-like structure. This development, coupled with the failure to form a urogenital groove, produces ambiguous or male-appearing external genitalia. (*From Escobar LF , et al: Urorectal septum malformation sequence: report of six cases and embryological analysis,* Am J Dis Child 141:1021, 1987.)

the development and maintenance of müllerian duct formation and ovarian steroidogenesis. For this reason, WNT4 deficiency had been proposed as a cause of MRKH syndrome. However, it is now known to be responsible for a clinically distinct phenotype. Currently, no single gene mutation has been implicated as an explanation for the MRKH syndrome.

Common Presenting Problems

HYPOSPADIAS

Hypospadias is a condition of failed male urethral differentiation in which the urethral meatus lies somewhere proximal to the tip of the glans penis. It occurs between 9 and 14 weeks of gestation. In mild cases, the meatus opens on the ventral surface of the glans, corona, or upper penile shaft, and in severe cases, on the lower shaft, penoscrotal junction, or perineum. Hypospadias is the second most common genital abnormality (after cryptorchidism) in male newborns, with an incidence in different series ranging between 0.3% and 0.8%. About 87% of the cases are glandular or coronal, 10% penile, and 3% penoscrotal or perineal.

Other anomalies that may accompany hypospadias include meatal stenosis, hydrocele, cryptorchidism (8% to 10% of cases), and inguinal hernia (8% of cases). More severe forms of hypospadias are often associated with a shawl scrotum or incompletely translocated labioscrotal folds and with a prostatic utricle. Patients with severe hypospadias, urinary tract symptoms, a family history of ureteral reflux, or multiple congenital anomalies are also more likely to have significant abnormalities and should have a uroradiographic evaluation.

Eight percent of patients with hypospadias have a similarly affected brother or father; this figure reaches 16.7% for individuals with penoscrotal or perineal hypospadias. This familial tendency is thought to result from a polygenic mode of inheritance. *CXorf*, a gene on the X chromosome, has been identified as a causative gene for hypospadias.[21] Additional studies investigating other candidate genes involved in male genital development are underway. Mild hypospadias (glandular to penile) without other genital abnormalities or dysmorphic features is very unlikely to be associated with an identifiable endocrinopathy, intersex, or chromosomal abnormality. Severe hypospadias (penoscrotal or perineal) (see Fig. 49-39) is associated with about a 15% risk for such problems occurring. The addition of other genital abnormalities (cryptorchidism or abnormally small penis) (see Fig. 49-42) increases the risk for the occurrence of a DSD or endocrinopathy to 35% in mild and 79% in severe hypospadias.

The differential diagnosis of hypospadias includes female neonates with CAH, other DSDs, various syndromes (e.g., Smith-Lemli-Opitz, Beckwith-Wiedemann), and unknown causes. Rare causes of hypospadias include a deficiency in testosterone production due to the decreased conversion of testosterone to DHT (5α-reductase deficiency), decreased function of the androgen receptor protein (pAIS), and maternal exposure to progestins; they occur between 8 and 14 weeks of gestation. In a study of 48 patients with hypospadias, no androgen production defects could be identified.[24]

The evaluation of hypospadias in the newborn includes a history of possible maternal progestin or estrogen exposure; family history of hypospadias, endocrine disorders, or DSDs; examination to evaluate hypospadias (phallus length, urethral meatus location, chordee, scrotal folds); determination of the presence of gonads and a uterus; determination of an anatomic abnormality of the kidneys; and identification of somatic abnormalities. The major concern in the evaluation of hypospadias is to rule out CAH in a virilized female; if both gonads are impalpable, this possibility must be seriously considered (see Fig. 49-42). If hypospadias is mild and not associated with other abnormalities, diagnostic studies are usually not needed. The surgical repair of hypospadias is performed ideally after 6 months of age by an experienced surgeon. Multistage procedures may be required for severe forms of hypospadias.

MICROPENIS

For a description of how to examine and interpret penis size please see earlier section, "Penis Size" under "Physical Examination." A micropenis is caused by a deficiency in the factors (testosterone or DHT and possibly growth hormone [GH]) needed for normal penile growth to occur after 14 weeks of gestation, when formation of the urethra is complete. The major causes include hypopituitarism (LH deficiency with or without GH deficiency, 30%), primary hypogonadism (25%), pAIS (2%), and idiopathic or undiagnosed causes (43%). The association of a micropenis with early neonatal hypoglycemia (GH and ACTH-cortisol deficiencies), cryptorchidism (LH deficiency) (see Fig. 49-30), persistent neonatal jaundice (hypothyroidism, ACTH-cortisol deficiency), or cleft palate should immediately raise the possibility of congenital hypopituitarism. Other congenital malformations (e.g., septo-optic dysplasia) and chromosome abnormalities are occasionally associated. The complete absence of the penis may rarely occur. The diagnostic evaluation of a micropenis includes the assessment of GH, testosterone, LH, and FSH status and consideration of testing for hypopituitarism. An hCG stimulation test may be performed if testosterone levels are low to assess biosynthetic defects. The karyotype may need to be determined. A course of testosterone therapy to assess penile responsiveness may be administered to exclude significant androgen insensitivity. Testosterone therapy should be planned to normalize penis size and consequently promote a positive body image in childhood.

CRYPTORCHIDISM

Cryptorchidism, or testicular maldescent, is present when one or both testes have failed to descend completely into the scrotum (to a position 4 cm or more below the pubic crest in full-term males weighing more than 2.5 kg). Because the testes normally descend after 7 months of fetal age through the first several months of postnatal age, most affected newborns are found to be normal when they are reevaluated. The incidence of cryptorchidism at birth is about 3.7% in full-term males and 21% in premature males, approaching 100% in the very premature. However, the postnatal completion of testicular descent is seen in 50% of the full-term cryptorchid males by 6 weeks of age and in 67% of the full-term and 73% of the premature cryptorchid males by 3 months of age. A few additional individuals attain full descent by 6 to 9 months of age. The net result is that about 75% of full-term and 90% of premature cryptorchid newborns have full testicular descent by the age of 9 months without therapeutic intervention. Spontaneous testicular descent is very rare after 9 months of age. The incidence of cryptorchidism is about 1% at 1 year of age. In addition to prematurity and low birthweight, other factors associated with an increased incidence of cryptorchidism are birth by cesarean delivery and maternal obesity.

The mechanism of testicular descent is a complex process involving hormonal, mechanical, and genetic factors.[72] Factors thought to affect descent include the gubernaculum, attachment of the epididymis to the testis, rising abdominal pressure, AMH, testosterone or DHT, the genitofemoral nerve, and possibly LH and FSH. Cryptorchidism frequently occurs with disorders of the hypothalamic-pituitary-testicular hormone axis, with dysgenetic testes, and with anatomic defects of the epididymis and the abdominal wall. Cryptorchidism is seen with a higher incidence in patients with umbilical hernia (6%), gastroschisis (15%), omphalocele (33%), and Eagle-Barrett (prune-belly) syndrome (100%), in which intra-abdominal pressure may be important. It is also seen in individuals with meningomyelocele (25%), particularly when the defect is above L2, and in those with cerebral palsy (41%). True cryptorchidism is associated with lower LH and testosterone levels during the pituitary-testicular hormonal surge at ages 1 to 3 months and occurs frequently in cases of hypopituitarism or hypogonadotropism, Prader-Willi syndrome, primary hypogonadism, and androgen insensitivity. A role for AMH is suggested by the association with persistence of the müllerian ducts. An association is also seen with trisomies 13 and 18 and with Aarskog, Noonan, Robinow, Smith-Lemli-Opitz, and other syndromes. Familial cases are reported, and cryptorchidism is found in 6.2% of the brothers and 1.5% to 4% of the fathers of affected patients.

Associated anomalies include an inguinal hernia in many patients, abnormal epididymal formation in 36% to 66%, and hypospadias in about 3%. There are major upper urinary tract anomalies in about 3% of patients, but routine invasive diagnostic studies are not warranted. Some complications of cryptorchidism include (1) progressive histologic deterioration, with changes beginning after 6 months of age; (2) impaired spermatogenesis, with a decrease in the number of germ cells after the first year of life (and later reduced fertility potential); (3) an increased (4-fold to 10-fold) risk for cancer in the undescended testis and also in the contralateral testis in unilateral cryptorchidism; (4) trauma to the testis that is relatively fixed in position; (5) torsion; (6) symptomatic inguinal hernia; and (7) psychological factors related to altered body image. An associated inguinal hernia may require repair in early infancy if it is large enough to permit the abdominal contents to enter or if it causes symptoms.

If both testes are impalpable, the differential diagnosis includes an XX female with CAH or other severe virilizing disorder; anorchia, which occurs in 1% of bilaterally cryptorchid patients; and intra-abdominal testes, which are either normal (as in persistent müllerian duct syndrome) or dysgenetic (as in mixed gonadal dysgenesis or testicular dysgenesis). The evaluation of the infant with impalpable testes includes the determination of CAH and sex chromosomes. Hormone studies, both basal hormones (LH, FSH, and testosterone between 2 weeks and 3 months of age) and the testosterone response to hCG, may provide information about the presence of functioning Leydig cells. The measurement of AMH, ultrasound, magnetic resonance imaging, and laparoscopy have been useful in locating intra-abdominal testes, but laparotomy with exploration to the ends of the spermatic blood vessels is definitive in cases that are not otherwise resolved. The presence of wolffian structures suggests that torsion, vascular accident, or other late in utero degeneration has occurred. Alternatively, a dysgenetic testis may be present. Parental counseling should be undertaken in anticipation of this likelihood.

Because of the early appearance of histologic changes in the cryptorchid testis and initial findings that early treatment improves the histologic outcome, the correction of cryptorchidism is recommended between 6 and 12 months of age, or as soon as possible after diagnosis, if that occurs later.[61] Because spontaneous descent may occur up to 6 to 9 months of age, treatment before that time is not indicated unless the testis is ectopic or has other associated abnormalities. Orchiopexy is optimally performed by an experienced surgeon because the risk for subsequent loss of the testis is high. Hormonal treatment with gonadotropin-releasing hormone is no longer recommended because of its poor efficacy and potentially serious side effects.[69]

CLITOROMEGALY

For a description of how to examine clitoral size, see the earlier section, "Clitoris Size" under "Physical Examination." *Clitoromegaly* is defined as the appearance of clitoral enlargement regardless of cause. The clitoris may be prominent (protruding from between the labia majora), swollen, widened, or elongated. The causes are listed in Box 49-13. The clitoris must be measured to determine whether the paired corpora cavernosa are abnormally enlarged and to rule out the extremely rare finding of a tumor. More commonly, the corpora cavernosa are of normal size and have no evidence of a tumor, making clitoromegaly a benign finding. No further diagnostic evaluation is necessary, and the parents should be reassured that their newborn girl is normal. If the corpora cavernosa are enlarged, a DSD is more likely, and an evaluation should be performed. The assessment should include other signs of androgenization or incomplete masculinization (posterior labial fusion, ventral placement of the urethra,

---

BOX 49–13 Causes of Clitoromegaly in the Neonate

CORPORA CAVERNOSA OF NORMAL SIZE
- Normal variation such as prominent clitoral hood or infant who is small for gestational age
- Swelling, edema, or both due to bruising (e.g., breech presentation)

CORPORA CAVERNOSA ENLARGED DUE TO ANDROGEN STIMULATION
- 46,XX DSD, particularly 21-hydroxylase deficiency
- 46,XY DSD
- Gonadal dysgenesis, dysgenetic testes
- Ovotesticular DSD
- Tumor infiltration of clitoris (neurofibromatosis, lymphoma)

DSD, disorder of sex development.

or hypospadias); determination of whether the gonads are palpable; determination of the presence or absence of a uterus; and measurement of androgens and 17-OH progesterone levels. A karyotype may also be warranted.

RESOURCES FOR FAMILIES

AboutKidsHealth: Sex Development, http://www.aboutkidshealth. ca/HowTheBodyWorks/Sex-Development-Introduction. aspx?articleID=7671&categoryID=XS

Accord Alliance, http://www.accordalliance.org

Handbook for parents: Consortium on the Management of Disorders of Sex Development, http://www.dsdguidelines.org/files/parents.pdf

Intersex Society Of North America, http://www.isna.org

REFERENCES

1. Acerini CL, Hughes IA: Endocrine disrupting chemicals: a new and emerging public health problem? *Arch Dis Child* 91:633, 2006.
2. Al-Alwan I, et al: Clinical utility of adrenal ultrasonography in the diagnosis of congenital adrenal hyperplasia, *J Pediatr* 135:71, 1999.
3. Alvarez-Nava F, et al: Molecular analysis in Turner syndrome, *J Pediatr* 142:336, 2003.
4. Ammini AC, et al: Human female phenotypic development: role of fetal ovaries, *J Clin Endocrinol Metab* 79:604, 1994.
5. Aynsley-Green A, et al: Congenital bilateral anorchia in childhood: a clinical, endocrine and therapeutic evaluation of twenty-one cases, *Clin Endocrinol (Oxf)* 5:381, 1976.
6. Beck-Peccoz P, et al: Maturation of hypothalamic-pituitary-gonadal function in normal human fetuses: circulating levels of gonadotropins, their common alpha-subunit and free testosterone, and discrepancy between immunological and biological activities of circulating follicle-stimulating hormone, *J Clin Endocrinol Metab* 73:525, 1991.
7. Berenbaum SA, Bailey JM: Effects on gender identity of prenatal androgens and genital appearance: evidence from girls with congenital adrenal hyperplasia, *J Clin Endocrinol Metab* 88:1102, 2003.
8. Bergada I, et al: Time course of the serum gonadotropin surge, inhibins, and anti-mullerian hormone in normal newborn males during the first month of life, *J Clin Endocrinol Metab* 91:4092, 2006.
9. Blecher SR, Erickson RP: Genetics of sexual development: a new paradigm, *Am J Med Genet* [Research Support, Non-U.S. Gov't Review] *Part A,* 143:3054, 2007.
10. Bondy CA: Care of girls and women with Turner syndrome: a guideline of the Turner Syndrome Study Group, *J Clin Endocrinol Metab* 92:10, 2007.
11. Bouvattier C, et al: Postnatal changes of T, LH, and FSH in 46,XY infants with mutations in the AR gene, *J Clin Endocrinol Metab* 87:29, 2002.
12. Brinkmann AO: Molecular basis of androgen insensitivity, *Mol Cell Endocrinol* 179:105, 2001.
13. Brookhyser KM, et al: Third trimester resolution of cystic hygroma and pleural effusion in a fetus with Turner syndrome, *Am J Perinatol* 10:297, 1993.
14. Carrillo AA, Berkovitz GD: Genetic mechanisms that regulate testis determination, *Rev Endocr Metabol Dis* 5:77, 2004.
15. Cohen-Kettenis PT: Gender change in 46,XY persons with 5alpha-reductase-2 deficiency and 17beta-hydroxysteroid dehydrogenase-3 deficiency, *Arch Sex Behav* 34:399, 2005.
16. Cools M, et al: Germ cell tumors in the intersex gonad: old paths, new directions, moving frontiers, *Endocr Rev* 27:468, 2006.
17. Deeb A, et al: Correlation between genotype, phenotype and sex of rearing in 111 patients with partial androgen insensitivity syndrome, *Clin Endocrinol (Oxf)* 63:56, 2005.
18. di Clemente N, Belville C: Anti-Mullerian hormone receptor defect, *Best Pract Res Clin Endocrinol Metab* 20:599, 2006.
19. Fallat ME, Donahoe PK: Intersex genetic anomalies with malignant potential [review], *Curr Opin Pediatr* 18:305, 2006.
20. Federman DD: Three facets of sexual differentiation [see comment], *N Engl J Med* 350:323, 2004.
21. Fukami M, et al: CXorf6 is a causative gene for hypospadias, *Nat Genet* 38:1369, 2006.
22. Grosse SD, Van Vliet G: How many deaths can be prevented by newborn screening for congenital adrenal hyperplasia? [see comment], *Horm Res* 67:284, 2007.
23. Heinrichs C, et al: Blood spot follicle-stimulating hormone during early postnatal life in normal girls and Turner's syndrome, *J Clin Endocrinol Metab* 78:978, 1994.
24. Holmes NM, et al: Lack of defects in androgen production in children with hypospadias, *J Clin Endocrinol Metab* 89:2811, 2004.
25. Huang B, et al: Autosomal XX sex reversal caused by duplication of SOX9, *Am J Med Genet* 87:349, 1999.
26. Hughes IA: Female development-all by default? [comment], *N Engl J Med* 351:748, 2004.
27. Huhtaniemi I, Pelliniemi LJ: Fetal Leydig cells: cellular origin, morphology, life span, and special functional features, *Proc Soc Exp Biol Med* 201:125, 1992.
28. Intersex Society of North America: *Clinical Guidelines for the Management of Disorders of Sex Development In Childhood* (website). http://www.dsdguidelines.org/htdocs/clinical/scripts.html. Accessed November 2008.
29. Jean A, et al: Prenatal diagnosis of congenital lipoid adrenal hyperplasia (CLAH) by estriol amniotic fluid analysis and molecular genetic testing, *Prenat Diagn* 28:11, 2008.
30. Kim CJ, et al: Severe combined adrenal and gonadal deficiency caused by novel mutations in the cholesterol side chain cleavage enzyme, P450scc, *J Clin Endocrinol Metab* 93:696, 2008.
31. Ko JM, et al: A case of Antley-Bixler syndrome caused by compound heterozygous mutations of the cytochrome P450 oxidoreductase gene, *Eur J Pediatr* 168:877-80, 2009.
32. Koshimizu T: Plasma renin activity and aldosterone concentration in normal subjects and patients with salt-losing type of congenital adrenal hyperplasia during infancy, *Clin Endocrinol (Oxf)* 10:515, 1979.
33. Lee DK, Chang C: Endocrine mechanisms of disease. Expression and degradation of androgen receptor: mechanism and clinical implication, *J Clin Endocrinol Metab* 88:4043, 2003.
34. Lee JE, et al: Corrected 17-alpha-hydroxyprogesterone values adjusted by a scoring system for screening congenital adrenal hyperplasia in premature infants, *Ann Clin Lab Sci* 38:235, 2008.
35. Lee PA; International Consensus Conference on Intersex organized by the Lawson Wilkins Pediatric Endocrine Society and

the European Society for Paediatric Endocrinology. Consensus statement on management of intersex disorders. International Consensus Conference on Intersex, *Pediatrics* 118:e488, 2006.

36. Lin L, et al: Variable phenotypes associated with aromatase (CYP19) insufficiency in humans, *J Clin Endocrinol Metab* 92:982, 2007.

37. Lin L, et al: Heterozygous missense mutations in steroidogenic factor 1 (SF1/Ad4BP, NR5A1) are associated with 46,XY disorders of sex development with normal adrenal function, *J Clin Endocrinol Metab* 92:991, 2007.

38. Looijenga LH, et al: Tumor risk in disorders of sex development (DSD), *Best Pract Res Clin Endocrinol Metab* 21:480, 2007.

39. Malouf MA, et al: Cognitive outcome in adult women affected by congenital adrenal hyperplasia due to 21-hydroxylase deficiency, *Horm Res* 65:142, 2006.

40. Mazur T: Gender dysphoria and gender change in androgen insensitivity or micropenis, *Arch Sex Behav* 34:411, 2005.

41. MacLaughlin DT, Donahoe PK: Sex determination and differentiation.[see comment] [erratum appears in N Engl J Med 351:306, 2004], *N Engl J Med* 350:367, 2004.

42. Mazzanti L, et al: Gonadoblastoma in Turner syndrome and Y-chromosome-derived material, *Am J Med Genet A* 135:150, 2005.

43. Merke DP, Bornstein SR: Congenital adrenal hyperplasia, *Lancet* 365:2125, 2005.

44. Meyer-Bahlburg HF, et al: Sexual orientation in women with classical or non-classical congenital adrenal hyperplasia as a function of degree of prenatal androgen excess, *Arch Sex Behav* 37:85, 2008.

45. Migeon CJ, et al: Ambiguous genitalia with perineoscrotal hypospadias in 46,XY individuals: long-term medical, surgical, and psychosexual outcome, *Pediatrics* 110:e31, 2002.

46. Miller WL: Disorders of androgen synthesis—from cholesterol to dehydroepiandrosterone, *Med Princ Pract* 1:58, 2005.

47. Moore KL, Persaud TVN: *The developing human: clinically oriented embryology,* 7th ed, Philadelphia, 2003, Saunders.

48. Morcel K, et al: Mayer-Rokitansky-Kuster-Hauser (MRKH) syndrome, *Orphanet J Rare Dis* 2:13, 2007.

49. New MI, et al: Genotyping steroid 21-hydroxylase deficiency: hormonal reference data, *J Clin Endocrinol Metab* 57:320, 1983.

50. Nicolino M, et al: Clinical and biological assessments of the undervirilized male, *BJU Int* 93(Suppl 3):20, 2004.

51. Nimkarn S, New MI: Prenatal diagnosis and treatment of congenital adrenal hyperplasia owing to 21-hydroxylase deficiency, *Nat Clin Pract Endocrinol Metab* 3:405, 2007.

52. Nimkarn S, New MI: Steroid 11beta-hydroxylase deficiency congenital adrenal hyperplasia, *Trends Endocrinol Metab* 19:96, 2008.

53. Oberfield SE, et al: Clitoral size in full-term infants, *Am J Perinatol* 6:453, 1989.

54. Ogata T , et al: Turner syndrome and Xp deletions: clinical and molecular studies in 47 patients, *J Clin Endocrinol Metab* 86:5498, 2001.

55. Pajkrt E, Chitty LS: Prenatal gender determination and the diagnosis of genital anomalies, *BJU Int Suppl* 3:12, 2004.

56. Pang S, et al: Carriers for type II 3beta-hydroxysteroid dehydrogenase (HSD3B2) deficiency can only be identified by HSD3B2 genotype study and not by hormone test, *Clin Endocrinol (Oxf)* 58:323, 2003.

57. Parisi MA, et al: A Gender Assessment Team: experience with 250 patients over a period of 25 years, *Genet Med* 9:348, 2007.

58. Pasterski V, et al: Increased aggression and activity level in 3- to 11-year-old girls with congenital adrenal hyperplasia (CAH), *Horm Behav* 52:368, 2007.

59. Peter M, et al: Disorders of the aldosterone synthase and steroid 11beta-hydroxylase deficiencies, *Horm Res* 51:211, 1999.

60. Richter-Unruh A, et al: Novel insertion frameshift mutation of the LH receptor gene: problematic clinical distinction of Leydig cell hypoplasia from enzyme defects primarily affecting testosterone biosynthesis, *Eur J Endocrinol* 152:255, 2005.

61. Ritzen M: Undescended testes: a consensus on management, *Eur J Endocrinol* 159:S87-S90, 2009.

62. Rivkees SA, Crawford JD: Dexamethasone treatment of virilizing congenital adrenal hyperplasia: the ability to achieve normal growth, *Pediatrics* 106:767, 2000.

63. Sagi L, et al: Clinical significance of the parental origin of the X chromosome in turner syndrome, *J Clin Endocrinol Metab* 92:846, 2007.

64. Satoh M: Histogenesis and organogenesis of the gonad in human embryos, *J Anat* 177:85, 1991.

65. Scott RR, Miller WL: Genetic and clinical features of p450 oxido-reductase deficiency, *Horm Res* 69:266, 2008.

66. Siiteri PK, Wilson JD: Testosterone formation and metabolism during male sexual differentiation in the human embryo, *J Clin Endocrinol Metab* 38:113, 1974.

67. Simard J, et al: A new insight into the molecular basis of 3beta-hydroxysteroid dehydrogenase deficiency, *Endocr Res* 26:761, 2000.

68. Telvi L, et al: 45,X/46,XY mosaicism: report of 27 cases, *Pediatrics* 104:304, 1999.

69. Thorsson AV, et al: Efficacy and safety of hormonal treatment of cryptorchidism: current state of the art, *Acta Paediatr* 96:628, 2007.

70. Uehara S, et al: Complete XY gonadal dysgenesis and aspects of the SRY genotype and gonadal tumor formation, *J Hum Genet* 47:279, 2002.

71. White PC, Speiser PW: Congenital adrenal hyperplasia due to 21-hydroxylase deficiency, *Endocr Rev* 21:245, 2000.

72. Wilhelm D, Koopman P: The makings of maleness: towards an integrated view of male sexual development, *Nat Rev Genet* 7:620, 2006.

73. Yao HH: The pathway to femaleness: current knowledge on embryonic development of the ovary, *Mol Cell Endocrinol* 230:87, 2005.

74. Zenaty D, et al: Bilateral anorchia in infancy: occurrence of micropenis and the effect of testosterone treatment, *J Pediatr* 149:687, 2006.

75. Zeng X, et al: Detection and assignment of CYP21 mutations using peptide mass signature genotyping, *Mol Genet Metab* 82:38, 2004.

CHAPTER 50

Inborn Errors of Metabolism

Arthur B. Zinn

This chapter is a guide for the practicing physician in recognizing and caring for the neonate who might have an inherited metabolic disease. The chapter presents a practical approach to recognizing representative entities belonging to the biochemical groups of metabolic disorders expressed in the neonatal period. Key clinical and laboratory findings that are components of these diseases are discussed (see also references 11, 18, and 45). A metabolic approach to the dysmorphic child also is presented because a small percentage of dysmorphic children have inborn errors of metabolism.

The main problems facing the physician caring for the sick newborn infant are to know when to consider the possibility of a metabolic disorder and what to do to determine quickly and efficiently whether a child has a metabolic disease. After a tentative diagnosis is reached, several reference sources can provide appropriate information about specific diseases.[22,23,84]

Two ongoing, complementary approaches to providing medical care for neonates with inborn errors of metabolism are (1) prospective care of the healthy newborn infant and (2) reactive care of the clinically abnormal newborn infant. Prospective care seeks to identify neonates who have a specific metabolic disorder before clinical manifestations of that disorder develop. The aim of the prospective approach is to prevent the morbidity or mortality that often occurs in the period before recognition, diagnosis, and initiation of therapy for what might be a preventable or treatable disease. The reactive approach aims to arrest or minimize the sequelae of the disease state after the affected child becomes ill or is recognizably abnormal.

This chapter outlines several common misconceptions about inborn errors of metabolism, addresses prospective recognition of inborn errors, including newborn screening programs, and discusses reactive recognition and care of the abnormal newborn infant. In 1983 the US Orphan Drug Act was passed and has generated new therapies for inborn errors of metabolism.[92a]

COMMON MISCONCEPTIONS

Metabolic diseases of infancy are a difficult subject for many physicians and others caring for newborns. Several misconceptions contribute to this difficulty. Eight of these misconceptions are stated below. These misconceptions are expressed in an exaggerated, tongue-in-cheek way to emphasize that, on reflection, most physicians would not acknowledge that these ideas are true. Nevertheless, experience suggests that in the intense atmosphere generated in response to the sick neonate, these misconceptions often influence the care of the child with an inborn error of metabolism.

Misconception 1

Inherited metabolic diseases are rarely a cause of disease in the neonate and should therefore be considered diagnostically as a last resort.

Although individual metabolic diseases are relatively rare, inherited metabolic diseases collectively represent a more common cause of disease in the neonatal period. The estimated incidence in the general population of inherited metabolic diseases varies by more than an order of magnitude, ranging from 1 case per 10,000 live births for phenylketonuria (PKU) to 1 case per 200,000 for homocystinuria. About 100 inherited metabolic disorders are identifiable in the neonatal period.

Assuming that most of these disorders have an incidence closer to the lowest incidence rather than the highest, the overall incidence of metabolic disease is about 1 case per 2000 persons. Newborn screening programs have found an incidence of approximately 1 in 4000 for a subset of these diseases. There is good reason to believe that this estimate of the incidence of metabolic disease in neonates is an underestimate, because many metabolic diseases are underdiagnosed and many diseases are yet to be identified.

Misconception 2

The possibility of a genetic metabolic disease should be considered only when there is a family history of the disease.

Most neonates with an inborn error of metabolism do not have a similarly affected sibling or relative.

The reasons for this pattern follow from the rules of mendelian inheritance. Most inborn errors of metabolism are inherited as autosomal recessive traits, for which the odds are 3:1 in each pregnancy that two heterozygous parents will have an unaffected child. Small family sizes in developed countries make it unlikely to see two affected offspring in a sibship. In a family of two siblings, the odds are about 6% that both siblings will have the disease. In a family of three children, the odds are about 14% that two of the three siblings will be affected and about 2% that all three siblings will be affected.

There often is no forewarning of the birth of a sick boy with an X-linked disorder because he may have one or more healthy older sisters; heterozygous females do not express most X-linked disorders. Many X-linked disorders are the result of new mutations, and the birth of a sick newborn would not be anticipated. Similarly, because many autosomal dominant disorders are also the result of new mutations, a positive family history would not be expected.

Misconception 3

It is difficult to know when to suspect that a sick newborn infant may have a metabolic disorder because presentation of such disorders often mimics that of sepsis in the newborn infant.

Three responses to this point may be made. First, the clinical manifestations of many metabolic diseases are similar to the presentation of many neonatal infections, but this does not mean that the physician should not investigate the possibility of a metabolic disorder. The "sepsis workup" is a broadly focused approach to identifying a putative infection. The metabolic evaluation should be considered for most infants as part of the evaluation for suspected sepsis. Second, a neonate with a metabolic disease may be at greater risk of sepsis than other newborn infants, and the presence of documented sepsis does not exclude the possibility of an underlying metabolic disorder. Galactosemia is a well-documented example of a metabolic disease that predisposes an infant to serious infection. Third, many metabolic diseases do not have sepsis-like features.

Misconception 4

Many metabolic diseases are detectable in the neonatal period, and it is difficult to remember the presentation of each one.

Many metabolic diseases occur in the neonatal period, and it is impossible to remember the pattern of presentation of each; however, the great redundancy in clinical presentations simplifies evaluation. Relatively few algorithms are required to evaluate diseases that have overlapping phenotypes. Algorithms that have clear and multiple branch points are available to facilitate the clinical and laboratory evaluation of patients in whom a metabolic disease is suspected.

Misconception 5

The biochemical pathways and nomenclature of inborn errors of metabolism are impossible to remember.

The biochemical pathways and nomenclature of inborn errors of metabolism are often overwhelming for the expert in metabolic disorders as well as for the practitioner, but detailed knowledge of the pathways and nomenclature is not the important part of the metabolic evaluation. The important aspect of the metabolic evaluation is the development of general approaches to different clinical or laboratory findings that can rapidly reveal whether a metabolic problem exists and, if so, help direct the patient's care.

Misconception 6

It is difficult to diagnose a metabolic disease.

The examination of patients with suspected metabolic disease must be staged, progressing from broad screening tests, which should be available in all settings where care is given to sick neonates, to highly specialized tests, which may be available in only a handful of centers. The idea of a staged evaluation is perhaps best illustrated by the congenital hyperammonemias. The ability to diagnose hyperammonemia should be available in most settings, but the subsequent delineation of a specific cause of hyperammonemia and care of the patient are probably best reserved to a few specialized centers. The job of the physician faced with a sick newborn infant is to think of the possibility of hyperammonemia and to measure the blood ammonia level before the patient is irreversibly damaged by the effects of a disease.

Misconception 7

Metabolic test results take forever to return.

There is often a sense of frustration on the part of physicians, especially house officers, who believe that they order many metabolic studies but rarely learn the results of these studies or find an answer. Some metabolic tests do take a long time to perform. It is important to stage the evaluation. It is generally best to begin with relatively broad-based screening tests that come back quickly and can then be followed by more specific diagnostic studies that usually take longer to perform. The aim is to use the screening studies to obtain preliminary indications on which to base further evaluation and care.

Misconception 8

Relatively few metabolic diseases can be treated, so why spend a great deal of effort looking for something that you cannot fix?

A number of metabolic disorders can be treated, often successfully. The approach to the differential diagnosis should give greater consideration to detecting potentially treatable entities. The initial screening studies should permit identification of classes of disease for which there are therapies. For example, the congenital hyperammonemias are a group of disorders for which generic therapy is available; therapy can be modified after a more specific diagnosis is made. It is also important to establish a diagnosis for the sake of the parents, who almost always seek to understand why they have a sick baby, and for the purpose of formal genetic counseling.

PROSPECTIVE APPROACHES

There are two types of prospective care. The first type is the screening of a high-risk segment of the population—the siblings or other at-risk relatives of patients known to have a particular metabolic disorder. The second type is screening of the entire population or specific subset of newborn infants. The former is of much more limited scope than the latter, but both require the attention of a pediatrician or neonatologist.

The Newborn Infant at High Risk for a Particular Metabolic Disorder

Neonates at high risk for metabolic disorders are the siblings or other at-risk relatives of patients with a known metabolic disorder. These infants include those at risk for diseases for which there is no prenatal diagnosis and those who are at risk for diseases for which prenatal diagnosis is available but whose parents did not wish to have such testing performed. Also included are patients for whom prenatal testing was performed and who require postnatal confirmation of the prenatal test result. Postnatal confirmation is required for a positive or a negative prenatal test result. Postnatal confirmation is especially important for avoiding the unlikely situation of a false-negative prenatal test result that could lead to failure to treat an affected patient.

Management of pregnancies and neonates at high risk requires a coordinated effort among the obstetrician, the geneticist, the metabolic expert (if different from the geneticist), and the pediatrician. The first decision is to determine where the at-risk baby will be delivered. If the baby will not be delivered at a center where a metabolic expert is available, the indications for transfer after birth must be developed before birth. Regardless of where the baby is delivered, a detailed plan must be prepared and made available to all personnel caring for the newborn. The plan should include specific details of what tests will be needed to identify the disease, how the tests will be performed, where the samples for testing are to be sent after they are obtained, and who will follow up on the test results and inform the family.

Newborn Screening Programs

Newborn screening is an important issue for all physicians caring for neonates because it combines a number of significant medical and legal issues. These issues will become progressively more complex and diverse as an increasing number of inborn errors of metabolism become amenable to newborn screening and as the role of physicians in the administration and follow-up of such testing becomes greater.[1,49,52,81,101]

Although there is ongoing discussion and some debate about which medical conditions should be screened and how they are to be screened, there is a consensus about the goals of mass newborn screening. The medical requirements of an acceptable mass screening program for a particular disease include the following:

- The availability of a reliable screening test with a low false-negative rate
- A test that is simple and inexpensive, because many tests will be performed for each case identified
- A rapid screening test that can provide results quickly enough to permit effective intervention
- A definitive follow-up test that is available for unambiguous identification of true-positive results and elimination of false-positive results
- A disorder of a sufficiently deleterious nature that, if untreated, would result in significant morbidity or death
- An effective therapy that significantly alters the natural history of the disease

Relatively few metabolic disorders satisfy all these requirements. These criteria have probably been demonstrated, in a strict sense, only for biotinidase deficiency and PKU. On the other hand, neonates with classic galactosemia or maple syrup urine disease (MSUD), for example, often become very sick within the first few days of life before the results of newborn screening tests are available, thereby compromising the benefit of the screening program. Ascertainment and diagnosis of these disorders depend on specific biochemical testing of a sick infant (see "Specialized Biochemical Testing").

PRINCIPLES OF SCREENING PROGRAMS

A few principles apply to all screening programs. First, all screening tests are subject to false-positive results because of normal biologic variation, genetic heterogeneity, and human error. Accordingly, all positive screening results must be confirmed by definitive analysis. It is important that all patients who require therapy receive it and, conversely, that patients who do not require therapy not be treated.

Second, all positive results must be considered medical emergencies. Many positive results turn out to be falsely positive, but the concept underlying newborn screening is that identification of the few affected patients is crucial. In addition to the potential tragedy of misdiagnosis of the individual neonate, lack of attention that permits delayed care of a single affected patient can seriously jeopardize the public's confidence in and the cost-benefit structure of an entire statewide screening program and can compromise the continuation of such programs.

Third, the disorders that are part of newborn screening programs are the result of autosomal recessive traits, which exhibit variable clinical expression even within families. Thus the siblings of a patient identified by a screening program should be biochemically evaluated for the same disorder because they could be affected although they appear free of symptoms.

Fourth, all patients should be referred to an experienced specialist for definitive diagnosis because these disorders are characterized by clinical and genetic heterogeneity, which can significantly affect care of the patient and genetic counseling for the family.

There is considerable variation in the screening programs of different states in the United States and in various nations.

All states and U.S. territories screen for PKU. Until relatively recently, most states performed newborn screening for three to six metabolic disorders (including PKU, homocystinuria, MSUD, and galactosemia), one endocrine disorder (congenital hypothyroidism), and the hemoglobinopathies. The requirements and procedures for the screening programs for congenital hypothyroidism and the hemoglobinopathies are discussed in Part 3 of Chapter 49 and in Chapter 46, respectively.

Since the 1990s, intensive efforts have been made to expand the scope of newborn screening.[49,52,69,101] These efforts started from the premise that the available newborn screening tests were relatively inefficient and not easily generalized to detect new diseases either within the current categories of disease or in new categories of metabolic disease. Testing programs employed separate tests for each disease of interest.

SCREENING TECHNIQUES

Most state screening programs had focused primarily on the classic disorders of amino acid metabolism, which can be evaluated by bacterial inhibition assays. These assays cannot be easily adapted to screen for the more recently described disorders of organic acid metabolism and fatty acid oxidation. Similarly, the standard methods being used to diagnose the organic acidemias and fatty acid oxidation defects—gas chromatography, or combined gas chromatography and mass spectrometry (GC/MS)—could not be upgraded to large-scale newborn screening programs because they require tedious sample preparation and long analysis times.

Tandem mass spectrometry (MS/MS) circumvents these limitations of the bacterial inhibition assay, gas chromatography, and GC/MS methods. In brief, MS/MS permits analysis of a broad range of metabolites in hundreds of blood samples per day. Most states have adopted, or are in the process of adopting, the MS/MS approach to newborn screening as part of their program.

Newborn screening by MS/MS starts, as did the traditional screening programs, by collecting by heel stick a small blood sample and applying it to a standardized paper card. The period for appropriate collection remains between 1 and 3 days postpartum. Samples collected from either premature infants or sick newborns are potentially more difficult to interpret and are subject to greater false-positive and false-negative rates. The blood samples are shipped to a centralized laboratory where a standardized amount of the specimen card is punched out, following which the metabolites of interest are extracted from the punch, subjected to specific chemical modifications to make them compatible for subsequent MS/MS analysis, and automatically introduced into and analyzed by the MS/MS system.

As opposed to traditional screening protocols that required different analytic approaches for each disorder, the current MS/MS techniques permit analysis of a large number of metabolites belonging to a particular category of disease—hence, many disorders—in each sample. Hundreds of samples can be prepared for analysis, analyzed, and interpreted each day. The analysis is performed by state-of-the-art mass spectrometers that permit highly sensitive, accurate, and concurrent identification of multiple metabolites. Computer software permits pattern recognition using several related metabolites, thereby improving the reliability of the testing. In summary, the MS/MS technology is ideally suited for newborn screening of many samples for many possible disorders.

As with traditional newborn screening programs, the current MS/MS screening programs must determine the normal range for the different metabolites they analyze in their system. More importantly, the programs must set cutoffs above or below which they identify a case as at-risk. This is a difficult, ongoing task. Programs that set their cutoffs too high have an unacceptable false-negative rate, and programs that set their cutoffs too low have an unacceptable false-positive rate.

Pilot programs in the United States and elsewhere have demonstrated that MS/MS programs can detect PKU, MSUD, and homocystinuria as well as or better than the traditional screening approaches.[1,49,69,81,101] Nevertheless the practitioner must still be aware that the MS/MS-based screening programs have similar problems with false-positive and false-negative results as their older counterparts, although they appear to have lower false-positive rates. The practitioner must still determine whether a particular result is truly positive or falsely positive as rapidly and safely as possible. The expanded newborn screening programs have found that approximately 1 in 4000 newborns have an identifiable inborn error of metabolism.

SCREENING FOR DISORDERS

Most states in the United States and many other countries have adopted MS/MS screening to analyze disorders of amino acid metabolism (including several urea cycle disorders), organic acid metabolism, and fatty acid oxidation. The amino acid disorders and urea cycle disorders are detected by analyzing for increased blood concentrations of specific amino acids or combinations of amino acids. Most programs do not screen for disorders that are associated with reduced concentrations of specific amino acids. Similarly, the organic acidemias and fatty acid oxidation disorders are detected by analyzing for increased blood concentrations of specific acylcarnitines, namely, the esters formed between carnitine and the accumulated acids in the various organic acidemias and fatty acid oxidation disorders. As in the case of the amino acid disorders, many programs evaluate samples for combinations of particular acylcarnitines to increase the reliability of their results. Screening for the plasma membrane carnitine uptake defect is an exception to the rule, because it looks for a reduced (rather than increased) concentration of free carnitine.

Table 50-1 lists abnormal laboratory findings, along with the disorders associated with those findings, and the additional testing recommended to evaluate the significance of the findings. In the case of the amino acid disorders, a particular abnormal laboratory finding can be associated with more than one disorder because different enzymatic defects can lead to excessive accumulation of that metabolite.

This is also true for the disorders detectable by acylcarnitine analysis, but in addition, there is some ambiguity in identifying several of the acylcarnitines evaluated in the program. For example, C4 (an acylcarnitine that contains an acid group with four carbons) can be either butyrylcarnitine (wherein the four carbons are arranged in a linear pattern) or

TABLE 50–1 **Differential Diagnosis and Follow-up for Abnormal Laboratory Findings Commonly Reported by Newborn Screening Programs**

Abnormal Laboratory Finding*	Associated Disorders	Follow-up Studies†
Amino Acids		
Glycine	Nonketotic hyperglycinemia (NKHG)	Plasma amino acids Cerebrospinal fluid amino acids Urine organic acids
Leucine (and valine)	Maple syrup urine disease (MSUD)	Plasma amino acids Urine organic acids
Methionine	Homocystinuria	Plasma amino acids Plasma total homocysteine Urine amino acids
Phenylalanine	Phenylketonuria (PKU)	Plasma amino acids Urine biopterins
Tyrosine	Tyrosinemia type I Tyrosinemia type II	Plasma amino acids Urine organic acids (succinylacetone)
Urea Cycle Defect		
Arginine	Arginase deficiency	Plasma amino acids Plasma ammonia
Argininosuccinic acid	Argininosuccinate lyase deficiency	Plasma amino acids Urine amino acids Plasma ammonia
Citrulline	Argininosuccinate synthetase deficiency Argininosuccinate lyase deficiency Citrin deficiency	Plasma amino acids Plasma ammonia
Acylcarnitines‡		
C0 ($\downarrow$)	Carnitine transporter deficiency	Plasma carnitine analysis with acylcarnitine profile Urine carnitine analysis Urine organic acids
C3	Methylmalonic acidemia (MMA) or cofactor (vitamin B_{12}) biosynthesis defect Multiple carboxylase deficiency (MCD) Propionic acidemia (PA)	Plasma carnitine analysis with acylcarnitine profile Plasma total homocysteine Plasma amino acids Urine organic acids
C4	Isobutyryl-CoA dehydrogenase deficiency Short-chain acyl-CoA dehydrogenase (SCAD) deficiency	Plasma carnitine analysis with acylcarnitine profile Urine organic acids
C5	Isovaleric acidemia (IVA) 2-Methylbutyryl-CoA dehydrogenase deficiency	Plasma carnitine analysis with acylcarnitine profile Urine organic acids
C5-3OH,3M-DC	3-Hydroxy-3-methylglutaryl-CoA lyase deficiency	Plasma carnitine analysis with acylcarnitine profile Urine organic acids
C5-OH	Biotinidase deficiency β-Ketothiolase deficiency 3-Methylcrotonyl-CoA carboxylase deficiency Multiple carboxylase deficiency Maternal 3-methylcrotonyl-CoA carboxylase deficiency	Plasma carnitine analysis with acylcarnitine profile Urine organic acids Biotinidase analysis Maternal urine organic acids and carnitine analysis

Continued

TABLE 50–1 Differential Diagnosis and Follow-up for Abnormal Laboratory Findings Commonly Reported by Newborn Screening Programs—cont'd

Abnormal Laboratory Finding	Associated Disorders	Follow-up Studies
C5-DC	Glutaric aciduria type I (GAI)	Plasma carnitine analysis with acylcarnitine profile Urine organic acids
C8 and C10 (and C10:1)	Medium-chain acyl-CoA dehydrogenase (MCAD)	Plasma carnitine analysis with acylcarnitine profile Urine organic acids Mutational analysis (MCAD)
C14 and C16 (and C14:1)	Very-long-chain acyl-CoA dehydrogenase (VLCAD) deficiency	Plasma carnitine analysis with acylcarnitine profile Urine organic acids
C16 and C18	Carnitine-acylcarnitine translocase (CACT) deficiency Carnitine palmitoyltransferase II (CPT II) deficiency	Plasma carnitine analysis with acylcarnitine profile Urine organic acids
C16-OH	Long-chain 3-hydroxyacyl-CoA dehydrogenase (LCHAD) deficiency	Plasma carnitine analysis with acylcarnitine profile Urine organic acids Mutational analysis (LCHAD)
C4-DC, C5-OH, C6 - C16	Multiple acyl-CoA dehydrogenase deficiency (glutaric aciduria type II, GAII)	Plasma carnitine analysis with acylcarnitine profile Urine organic acids

*All abnormal findings reflect increased blood concentrations except where otherwise indicated.
†The studies listed are those that should be done at the first encounter following receipt of the abnormal newborn screening result. Additional, more specific, confirmatory studies such as enzyme analysis or in vitro cell studies using blood cells, cultured skin fibroblasts, or organ biopsies are generally obtained after the results of the initial confirmatory tests are available.
‡The acylcarnitines associated with these disorders are designated by a capital C followed by the number of carbons contained within the fatty acyl group attached to the carnitine; for example, C8 refers to octanoylcarnitine. A colon followed by an arabic numeral indicates one or more unsaturated carbons in the fatty acylcarnitine ester; for example, C10:1 refers to a monounsaturated C10 acylcarnitine. An OH in the designation indicates a hydroxylated acylcarnitine; for example, C5-OH refers to a monohydroxylated 5-carbon acylcarnitine. DC following the carbon number indicates a dicarboxylic acylcarnitine; for example, C5-DC refers to a dicarboxylic 5-carbon acyl group.
↓, decreased.

isobutyrylcarnitine (wherein the four carbons are arranged in a branched pattern). The diseases associated with these two acylcarnitines are quite different, and further studies are required to determine which metabolite, or which disorder, is present.

The confirmatory studies listed in Table 50-1 are readily available in most clinical settings, and discussed in detail later (see "Specialized Biochemical Testing"). The confirmatory studies cited include tests that have a relatively rapid turnaround time, generally 1 to 2 weeks, hopefully leading to rapid confirmation or elimination of a possible diagnosis. Additional, more refined studies, including specific enzyme analysis, whole cell studies, or genetic mutational analysis, are often required to definitively establish a specific diagnosis, but these generally have a longer turn-around time.

The abnormal laboratory findings listed in Table 50-1 permit the diagnosis of more than 20 genetic disorders, including amino acid disorders that encompass several urea cycle disorders, organic acidemias, and fatty acid oxidation disorders. The list of metabolites provided in Table 50-1 is not comprehensive. Many other metabolites have been identified or can theoretically be identified, but they are not

listed because of the rarity or uncertain clinical phenotype of the associated disorder. Not all states test for this particular list of metabolites; some test for fewer and others for more. Practitioners should be familiar with the scope of their local newborn screening program. In any event, the laboratory findings listed in Table 50-1 should provide all practitioners with a foundation for interacting with their local program.

Table 50-2 provides basic information about the disorders cited in Table 50-1, including the name of each disorder along with its common abbreviation (if one is available), the underlying enzymatic defect, the clinical features and natural history, the general approach to treatment, and the prognosis. The frequency of these disorders ranges between approximately 1 in 15,000 for PKU and medium-chain acyl-CoA dehydrogenase (MCAD) deficiency to 1 in 200,000 for MSUD; some disorders have been reported in only a few single-case reports. In addition to their rarity, most of these disorders are characterized by a high degree of clinical variability, making it difficult to provide a succinct but accurate summary. Hopefully, the information will provide the practitioner with a reasonable place to start when confronted with a patient who has an abnormal newborn screening result, following which

(text continued on page 1635)

TABLE 50–2 Inborn Errors of Metabolism That Can Be Ascertained by Tandem Mass Spectrometry-Based Newborn Screening Programs*

Disorder	Defect	Clinical Features and Natural History	Treatment	Prognosis with Treatment
Amino Acid Disorders				
Homocystinuria	Cystathionine β-synthetase deficiency	Generally asymptomatic at birth Developmental delay, dislocated lens, skeletal deformities, and thromboembolic episodes	Dietary protein restriction Selective amino acid restriction (methionine) Vitamin B_6 supplementation plus betaine, folate, and vitamin B_{12}	Patients with vitamin B_6-responsive form of disease have fewer complications and later age of onset of complications than do patients with vitamin B_6-nonresponsive form
Maple syrup urine disease (MSUD)	Branched-chain α-keto acid dehydrogenase deficiency	Patients might present before newborn screening results are available Difficulty feeding, vomiting, lethargy progressing to coma, opisthotonic posturing, and possibly death Ketoacidosis	Emergency treatment might be indicated for symptomatic neonates Chronic care includes: Dietary protein restriction Selective branched-chain amino acid restriction (leucine, isoleucine, valine) Thiamine supplementation for thiamine-responsive patients	Improved intellectual outcome can be expected if treatment is initiated before first crisis, but there is developmental delay in the severe cases Recurrent episodes of ketoacidosis
Nonketotic hyperglycinemia (NKHG)	Glycine cleavage enzyme deficiency	Patients might present before newborn screening results are available Hypotonia, apnea, intractable seizures, and lethargy progressing to coma Burst-suppression EEG pattern Hiccups (characteristic) Transient forms very rare	Various drugs can lower plasma glycine, but none lower CSF glycine or improve clinical outcome Dextromethorphan for seizures	Intractable seizures and poor intellectual development in patients who survive the neonatal period, except in rare instances
Phenylketonuria (PKU)	Phenylalanine hydroxylase deficiency or	Generally asymptomatic at birth After a few months, microcephaly, seizures, and pale pigmentation develop, followed in later years by abnormal posturing, mental retardation, and behavioral or psychiatric disturbances	Dietary protein restriction Selective amino acid restriction (phenylalanine)	Normal development can be expected (although a mild decrease in IQ and behavioral difficulties relative to nonaffected sibs might be seen) if diet is instituted early
	Tetrahydrobiopterin (BH_4) biosynthesis or recycling defect	Patients with BH_4 defects have additional problems secondary to dopamine and serotonin deficiency	Biopterin defects require special care	Patients with biopterin defects have a more guarded prognosis

Continued

TABLE 50-2 Inborn Errors of Metabolism That Can Be Ascertained by Tandem Mass Spectrometry-Based Newborn Screening Programs—cont'd

Disorder	Defect	Clinical Features and Natural History	Treatment	Prognosis with Treatment
Tyrosinemia type I	Fumarylacetoacetate hydrolase deficiency	Patients might present before newborn screening results are available Severe liver failure associated with jaundice, ascites, and bleeding diathesis Peripheral neuropathy and seizures can develop Renal Fanconi syndrome leading to rickets Survivors develop chronic liver disease with increased risk of hepatocellular carcinoma	Emergency treatment might be indicated for symptomatic neonates Chronic care includes: Dietary protein restriction Selective amino acid restriction (phenylalanine and tyrosine) Administration of selective enzyme inhibitor (NTBC) Liver transplantation when indicated to prevent hepatocellular carcinoma	Liver disease could progress despite dietary treatment NTBC treatment improves liver, kidney, and neurologic function, but it does not eliminate risk for hepatocellular carcinoma Liver transplantation might still be required
Tyrosinemia type II	Tyrosine aminotransferase	Corneal lesions and hyperkeratosis of the soles and palms	Selective amino acid restriction (tyrosine)	Good
Urea Cycle Disorders				
Argininosuccinic acidemia	Argininosuccinic acid lyase deficiency	Patients might present before newborn screening results are available Anorexia, vomiting, lethargy, seizures, and coma, possibly leading to death Hyperammonemia	Emergency treatment might be indicated for symptomatic neonates Chronic care includes: Dietary protein restriction Essential amino acid supplementation Arginine or citrulline supplementation Alternative pathway drugs for removing NH_3 (sodium benzoate and phenylbutyrate)	Improved intellectual outcome could be expected if treatment is initiated early, but there is developmental delay in the severe cases Recurrent hyperammonemic episodes
Argininemia	Arginase deficiency	Rarely symptomatic in neonatal period Progressive spastic diplegia or tetraplegia, opisthotonus, seizures Low risk of symptomatic hyperammonemia	Dietary protein restriction Selective amino acid restriction (arginine) Alternative pathway drugs for removing NH_3 (sodium benzoate and phenylbutyrate)	Uncertain, but might improve neurologic outcome

Disorder	Enzyme Deficiency	Clinical Features	Treatment	Outcome
Citrullinemia	Argininosuccinate synthetase deficiency	Patients might present before newborn screening results are available Anorexia, vomiting, lethargy, seizures, and coma, possibly leading to death Hyperammonemia	Emergency treatment might be indicated for symptomatic neonates Chronic care includes: Dietary protein restriction Essential amino acid supplementation Arginine or citrulline supplementation Alternative pathway drugs for removing NH₃ (sodium benzoate and phenylbutyrate)	Improved intellectual outcome can be expected if treatment is initiated early, but there is developmental delay in the severe cases Recurrent hyperammonemic episodes
Organic Acidemias				
Glutaric acidemia type I (GAI)	Glutaryl-CoA dehydrogenase deficiency	Rarely symptomatic in neonatal period, although macrocephaly may be present Progressive macrocephaly, ataxia, dystonia and choreoathetosis, developmental regression, seizures, and strokelike episodes, possibly exacerbated by infection or fasting	Dietary protein restriction Selective amino acid restriction (lysine, tryptophan) Riboflavin and carnitine supplementation	Improved intellectual outcome if treatment is initiated early, but poor neurologic outcome if treatment is started after acute neurologic injury occurs Treatment might slow neurologic deterioration
Glutaric acidemia type II (GAII)	Electron transfer flavoprotein (ETF) deficiency or ETF dehydrogenase deficiency	Commonly manifests in neonatal period Hypotonia, hepatomegaly, abnormal odor, with or without congenital anomalies including facial dysmorphism and cystic kidney disease Metabolic acidosis and hypoglycemia Generally lethal Late-onset forms variable, rarely have structural birth defects	Emergency treatment might be indicated for symptomatic neonates Chronic care includes: Dietary protein restriction Selective amino acid restriction (isoleucine, methionine, threonine, and valine) Carnitine supplementation	Treatment for neonatal-onset forms invariably unsuccessful Dietary fat and protein restriction and riboflavin and carnitine supplementation might help patients with late-onset disease
3-Hydroxy-3-methylglutaric aciduria	3-Hydroxy-3-methylglutaryl-CoA lyase deficiency	Generally does not manifest in neonatal period Episodic hypoglycemia leading to developmental delay	Dietary protein restriction Selective amino acid restriction (leucine) Low-fat diet	Improved intellectual outcome may be expected if treatment is initiated early, but there is developmental delay in the severe cases Recurrent hypoglycemic episodes decrease in frequency and severity over time

Continued

TABLE 50–2 Inborn Errors of Metabolism That Can Be Ascertained by Tandem Mass Spectrometry-Based Newborn Screening Programs—cont'd

Disorder	Defect	Clinical Features and Natural History	Treatment	Prognosis with Treatment
Isobutyric acidemia	Isobutyryl-CoA dehydrogenase deficiency	Uncertain because number of cases is small	Dietary protein restriction Selective amino acid restriction (valine)	Unknown
Isovaleric acidemia (IVA)	Isovaleryl-CoA dehydrogenase deficiency	Patients might present before newborn screening results are available Vomiting, lethargy and coma, possibly death Abnormal odor Thrombocytopenia, leukopenia, anemia Ketoacidosis Hyperammonemia	Emergency treatment might be indicated for symptomatic neonates Chronic care includes: Dietary protein restriction Selective amino acid restriction (leucine) Glycine and carnitine supplementation	Improved intellectual outcome if diagnosed and treated early If treated appropriately, most have normal development Recurrent metabolic episodes
β-Ketothiolase deficiency	Mitochondrial acetoacetyl-CoA thiolase deficiency	Patients might present before newborn screening results are available Vomiting, lethargy and coma, possibly death Abnormal odor Thrombocytopenia, leukopenia, anemia Possible basal ganglia damage Ketoacidosis Hyperammonemia	Dietary protein restriction Selected amino acid restriction (isoleucine) Avoidance of fasting Bicarbonate therapy and intravenous glucose in acute crises Carnitine supplementation	Highly variable clinical course Improved intellectual outcome if diagnosed and treated early If treated appropriately, some patients have normal development Recurrent metabolic episodes
2-Methylbutyric acidemia	2-Methylbutyryl-CoA dehydrogenase deficiency	Uncertain because number of cases is small	Dietary protein restriction Selected amino acid restriction	Uncertain
3-Methylcrotonyl-glycinuria	3-Methylcrotonyl-CoA carboxylase deficiency	Neonatal form: Hypoglycemia and metabolic acidosis Maternal form: Transplacental transport of 3-methylcrotonyl glycine from generally asymptomatic mother to fetus	Neonatal form: Dietary protein restriction Selected amino acid restriction (leucine) Carnitine and glycine supplementation Maternal form: Mother might benefit from carnitine supplementation if she has carnitine insufficiency	Neonatal form: Generally good Maternal form: Mother might benefit from carnitine supplementation

Disorder	Enzyme/Defect	Clinical Features	Treatment	Outcome
2-Methyl-3-hydroxybutyric acidemia	2-Methylbutyryl-CoA dehydrogenase deficiency	Uncertain because number of cases is small	Dietary protein restriction; Selected amino acid restriction	Uncertain
Methylmalonic acidemia (MMA)	Methylmalonyl-CoA mutase deficiency or Vitamin B_{12} (cobalamin) metabolism defect	Patients might present before newborn screening results are available; Vomiting, lethargy and coma, possibly death; Seizures and risk of basal ganglia infarcts; Thrombocytopenia, leukopenia, anemia; Ketoacidosis; Hyperammonemia	Emergency treatment might be indicated for symptomatic neonates; Chronic care includes: Dietary protein restriction; Selective amino acid restriction (isoleucine, methionine, threonine, and valine); Carnitine supplementation; Antibiotic suppression of gut flora (metronidazole); Liver and/or kidney transplantation might be considered; Cobalamin defects require special treatment	Improved intellectual outcome if diagnosed and treated early; If treated appropriately, most have normal development; Recurrent metabolic episodes; Renal failure often develops despite appropriate therapy
Propionic acidemia (PA)	Propionyl-CoA carboxylase deficiency	Patients might present before newborn screening results are available; Vomiting, lethargy and coma, possibly death; Seizures and risk of basal ganglia infarcts; Thrombocytopenia, leukopenia, anemia; Ketoacidosis; Hyperammonemia	Emergency treatment might be indicated for symptomatic neonates; Chronic care includes: Dietary protein restriction; Selective amino acid restriction (isoleucine, methionine, threonine, and valine); Carnitine supplementation; Antibiotic suppression of gut flora (metronidazole and neomycin); Liver transplantation might be considered	Improved intellectual outcome if diagnosed and treated early; If treated appropriately, most have normal development; Recurrent metabolic episodes
Biotinidase deficiency	Biotinidase deficiency	Generally does not manifest in neonatal period; Skin rash and alopecia, optic atrophy, hearing loss, seizures, and developmental delay; Metabolic ketoacidosis	Biotin supplementation	Excellent if diagnosed and deficiency treated before irreversible neurologic damage occurs

Continued

TABLE 50–2   Inborn Errors of Metabolism That Can Be Ascertained by Tandem Mass Spectrometry-Based Newborn Screening Programs—cont'd

Disorder	Defect	Clinical Features and Natural History	Treatment	Prognosis with Treatment
Multiple carboxylase deficiency	Holocarboxylase synthetase deficiency	Commonly manifests in neonatal period Lethargy leading to coma and possibly death Skin rash, impaired T cell immunity, seizures, and developmental delay Metabolic ketoacidosis and hyperammonemia	Biotin supplementation	Most patients respond to some degree to biotin supplementation, but others show poor or no response to biotin supplementation and have significant residual neurologic impairment
Fatty Acid Oxidation				
Carnitine transporter deficiency	Carnitine transporter deficiency	Commonly manifests in neonatal period Cardiomyopathy, skeletal myopathy, and inability to tolerate prolonged fasting	Carnitine supplementation Avoid fasting Low-fat diet	Good response to treatment, often associated with reversal of cardiomyopathic changes
Carnitine/acylcarnitine translocase deficiency	Carnitine/acylcarnitine translocase deficiency	Commonly manifests in neonatal period Lethargy leading to coma, hepatomegaly Cardiomyopathy with ventricular arrhythmia, skeletal myopathy, and early death Hypoketotic hypoglycemia and hyperammonemia	Avoid fasting High-carbohydrate, low-fat diet Nightly cornstarch supplementation Carnitine supplementation	Severe neonatal cases generally have poor outcome and early death Patients with later onset might respond to treatment, but they often succumb to chronic skeletal-muscle weakness or cardiac arrhythmias
Carnitine palmitoyl-transferase type II (CPT II) deficiency	CPT II deficiency	Commonly manifests in neonatal period Coma, cardiomyopathy and ventricular arrhythmias, hepatic disease, and congenital malformation (brain and cystic renal disease) Hypoketotic hypoglycemia Late-onset forms (child or adult) characterized by weakness and exercise-induced rhabdomyolysis	Avoid fasting High-carbohydrate, low-fat diet supplemented with MCT oil Nightly cornstarch supplementation Carnitine supplementation	Severe neonatal cases generally have poor outcome and early death Patients with late-onset disease generally do well

Disorder		Clinical Features	Treatment	Outcome
Long-chain-3-hydroxyacyl-CoA dehydrogenase (LCHAD) deficiency	LCHAD deficiency	Sometimes manifests in neonatal period Cardiomyopathy, hypotonia, hepatic disease, and hypoketotic hypoglycemia Patients later develop rhabdomyolysis, peripheral neuropathy, and pigmentary retinopathy and are at risk for sudden death Heterozygous pregnant women are at risk for acute fatty liver of pregnancy if they are carrying a homozygous fetus	Avoid fasting High-carbohydrate, low-fat diet supplemented with MCT oil Nightly cornstarch supplementation Carnitine supplementation	Early diagnosis and treatment generally leads to improved outcome, but no change in risk of peripheral neuropathy and visual impairment
Medium-chain acyl-CoA dehydrogenase (MCAD) deficiency	MCAD deficiency	Generally does not manifest in neonatal period Recurrent episodes of vomiting, coma, seizures, and possibly sudden death associated with prolonged period of fasting Cardiomyopathy not generally seen Hypoketotic or nonketotic hypoglycemia	Avoid fasting High-carbohydrate, low-fat diet (controversial) Nightly cornstarch supplementation Carnitine supplementation	Excellent intellectual and physical outcome generally seen if treatment is initiated before irreversible neurologic damage occurs
Short-chain acyl-CoA dehydrogenase (SCAD) deficiency	SCAD deficiency	Generally does not manifest in neonatal period Highly variable presentation primarily associated with failure to thrive, developmental delay, Hypoglycemia uncommon Many patients detected by newborn screening program have been asymptomatic	Avoid fasting High-carbohydrate, low-fat diet Nightly cornstarch supplementation Carnitine supplementation	Efficacy of treatment is unknown and metabolic acidosis
Very-long-chain acyl-CoA dehydrogenase (VLCAD) deficiency	VLCAD deficiency	Commonly manifests in neonatal period Lethargy leading to coma, hepatomegaly, cardiomyopathy with ventricular arrhythmia, skeletal myopathy, and early death Hypoketotic hypoglycemia Later-onset forms (childhood or adult) characterized primarily by weakness and exercise-induced rhabdomyolysis	Avoid fasting High-carbohydrate, low-fat diet supplemented with MCT oil Nightly cornstarch supplementation Carnitine supplementation	Severe neonatal cases generally have poor outcome Patients with late-onset disease respond to treatment and do well

Continued

TABLE 50–2 Inborn Errors of Metabolism That Can Be Ascertained by Tandem Mass Spectrometry–Based Newborn Screening Programs—cont'd

Disorder	Defect	Clinical Features and Natural History	Treatment	Prognosis with Treatment
Other				
Galactosemia	Galactose-1-phosphate uridyltransferase deficiency	Early onset characterized by lethargy, poor feeding, jaundice, and possibly sepsis (especially with *Escherichia coli*) Chronic problems include growth failure, cirrhosis, cataracts, seizures, mental retardation, and (in females) ovarian failure	Strict dietary galactose restriction must be started immediately	Improved intellectual outcome and milder problems if diagnosed and treated early Ovarian failure develops despite appropriate therapy Recurrent metabolic episodes

*This table does not provide a complete listing of all the inborn errors that have been identified or might be identified by tandem mass spectrometry. The last inborn error listed, galactosemia, is not detected currently using tandem mass spectrometry, but it is included in the table because it is part of current screening programs. It is important to note that all these disorders are characterized by considerable clinical variability and that treatment must be individualized for each patient.

CSF, cerebrospinal fluid; MCT, medium-chain triglycerides; NTBC, 2-(2-nitro-4-trifluoro-methylbenzoyl)-1,3-cyclohexanedione.

he or she can turn to other resources after a diagnosis is established.

HANDLING TEST RESULTS

The first obligation of the practitioner who receives an abnormal newborn screening report is to inform the parents of the result. The practitioner should explain that the results are provisional and that confirmation is required. The physician must aim for an appropriate balance between his or her own natural desire to reassure the parents that the result might be falsely positive and the desire to instill a sense of appropriate concern in the parents so that they can carry through with appropriate follow-up evaluation. The practitioner's burden is generally more straightforward when the abnormal metabolite is associated with only a single disorder, but the principles of reassurance and follow-up are the same for metabolites that can be found in more than one disorder (see Table 50-1). The physician should then assess the newborn's clinical status and arrange to see the family as expeditiously as possible.

The primary physician should either see the patient or refer the patient to a metabolic disorders specialist for further evaluation and care. It is often best that the primary physician see the patient as soon as possible to assess the patient's status and then work with the metabolic disorders specialist to develop an expeditious plan for evaluation. Confirmatory testing should be initiated as soon as possible.

The decisions about when to initiate treatment and how to treat are based on the nature of the laboratory abnormality found, the quantitative degree of the abnormality, the program's prior experience with false positives for that metabolite, and the patient's clinical status. In general, starting a treatment immediately after the initial confirmatory studies are obtained is both safe and unlikely to compromise the ability to establish a diagnosis. However, this option is predicated on the ability of the physician to make certain that the diagnostic samples are collected properly, sent to the appropriate laboratory, and received in satisfactory condition by the laboratory. Failure to do this before starting treatment might significantly delay the time required to establish a diagnosis and initiate appropriate treatment.

Most of the disorders identified are treated, at least in part, by some form of dietary restriction. A family's desire to continue breast feeding while the diagnostic studies are in progress should be carefully considered in all cases. However, depending on the disorder under consideration and the patient's clinical status, the default position should be in favor of stopping, or at least interrupting, breast feeding until a provisional diagnosis has been established. It is generally a matter of days to a week before the results of the initial confirmatory studies are available, when a more definitive decision can be made about the advisability of breast feeding. Similar reasoning should be exercised about starting vitamin or cofactor supplementation.

EFFECT OF SCREENING PROGRAMS

The impact of the expanded newborn screening programs is still being determined. There have clearly been many instances when the programs have led to the early recognition of an as-yet unaffected newborn, followed by the introduction of appropriate treatment. In some cases, this has meant

that a newborn with one of the organic acidemias or urea cycle defects that can manifest with an acute neurologic intoxication syndrome in the first few days of life does not suffer an insult that produces severe, irreversible neurologic damage. In other cases, the newborn screening result becomes available after a newborn is already ill, but the result provides a rapid diagnosis for the illness and leads to earlier introduction of appropriate therapy, thereby improving the patient's outcome.

However, it is not yet clear whether early recognition and institution of appropriate treatment changes the long-term prognosis for many of these diseases, such as recurrent hyperammonemic crises in the urea cycle defects or renal failure in methylmalonic acidemia. There may also be negative consequences to these new programs. For example, the screening programs could produce undesirable effects on the family of a child with a false-positive result, including increased hospitalization of the child, parental stress, and parent-child dysfunction.[97] Carefully organized multicenter studies are needed to determine the long-term benefits of the expanded newborn programs.

In addition to the current MS/MS newborn screening programs for amino acid and acylcarnitine analysis, new methods for evaluating other groups of inborn errors of metabolism, including the lysosomal storage disorders, are under development. It seems reasonable to anticipate that many of these methods will be introduced over the next several years, further expanding the responsibility and role of the pediatrician and neonatologist in caring for children with metabolic disorders.

Separate summaries of several disorders that were part of the traditional screening programs and that are now evaluated by MS/MS programs (i.e., homocystinuria, MSUD, and PKU) are provided next because they are useful paradigms for understanding the benefit of the newborn screening programs and how they work.[39] A summary is also provided for MCAD deficiency because it is the most common of the fatty acid oxidation disorders that are now evaluated by MS/MS programs, and it is one of the paradigms for this group of disorders. Summaries are also provided for biotinidase deficiency and galactosemia, which are disorders that are primarily evaluated by methodologies other than MS/MS. Other disorders that are now part of expanded newborn screening programs are discussed elsewhere in this chapter, including fatty acid β-oxidation disorders (see "Hypoglycemia"), nonketotic hyperglycinemia (see "The Sick Newborn Infant"), organic acidemias (see "Metabolic Acidosis"), tyrosinemia type I (see "Hepatic Dysfunction"), and urea cycle defects (see "Hyperammonemia").

Screening for Specific Disorders
BIOTINIDASE DEFICIENCY

Biotinidase is an enzyme necessary for recycling biotin, a vitamin cofactor required for four critical intracellular carboxylation reactions: acetyl-coenzyme A (acetyl-CoA) carboxylase, β-methylcrotonyl-CoA carboxylase, propionyl-CoA carboxylase, and pyruvate carboxylase. Hence biotinidase deficiency is one cause of multiple carboxylase deficiency.[39,102] These carboxylase reactions are involved in fatty acid biosynthesis, branched-chain amino acid metabolism, and gluconeogenesis.

Biotinidase deficiency is characterized by a variable clinical presentation but can lead to severe metabolic decompensation in the newborn period; features include ketoacidosis, hypotonia, seizures, and coma. Some children also have significant dermatologic findings (including rash and alopecia) and immunodeficiency. If untreated, older children could have significant developmental delay. This disorder can be treated successfully with biotin supplementation (5 to 20 mg/day PO). Some residual neurologic deficits could persist if treatment does not begin before the onset of symptoms.

Serum biotinidase activity is the gold standard for newborn screening of biotinidase deficiency.[39,102] The disorder can also be detected using MS/MS to measure the blood concentration of C5-OH (3-hydroxyisovalerylcarnitine), the acylcarnitine that is formed secondary to the deficiency of β-methylcrotonyl-CoA carboxylase. However, the sensitivity of the MS/MS approach is unknown, and it might not provide a reliable method for newborn screening. A positive screening result should be confirmed by quantitative serum biotinidase analysis and by performing plasma carnitine analysis and urine organic acid analysis, looking for the characteristic plasma acylcarnitine pattern and organic aciduria that is present in a small percentage of affected patients.

Care must be exercised in collecting and processing the serum specimen used for biotinidase analysis because biotinidase is quite labile at room temperature. It is best to obtain a concurrent control from one or both parents to establish that the sample has been processed properly (i.e., eliminate the chance of a false-positive result).

GALACTOSEMIA

Classic galactosemia is the consequence of galactose-1-phosphate uridyltransferase (GALT) deficiency. Classic galactosemia can manifest in the newborn period with lethargy, poor feeding, jaundice, cataracts, and in some cases, *Escherichia coli* sepsis.[19,39] If unrecognized, this disorder can lead to early death or a chronic course characterized by cirrhosis, cataracts, seizures, and mental retardation. The mainstay of therapy for classic galactosemia is strict dietary lactose restriction.[19,39,98] Diet therapy is difficult to sustain because lactose is a ubiquitous food additive. Dietary galactose restriction should be started as early as possible (preferably within the first few days after birth) to have the best chance of precluding the development of speech and learning problems. However, even children treated early often have mild growth failure, learning disabilities, and verbal dyspraxia. Affected girls almost invariably develop premature ovarian failure.[32,82] This observation serves as a caution to those caring for children with galactosemia that long-term follow-up is mandatory and further improvements in treatment are required.

There are two other forms of galactosemia: uridine diphosphate galactose-4'-epimerase deficiency and galactokinase deficiency. In most cases, epimerase deficiency is a benign condition that does not require treatment. The rarer, systemic form of epimerase deficiency produces a clinical picture similar to classic galactosemia. Galactokinase deficiency is also rare, and produces nuclear cataracts but none of the other manifestations of classic galactosemia. Early

recognition and treatment of this disorder is generally successful.

One approach to screening measures GALT activity. This assay can detect transferase deficiency without regard to prior dietary intake of galactose. It does not evaluate for either epimerase deficiency or galactokinase deficiency. Another approach is to measure galactose and galactose-1-phosphate (the substrate for GALT), which depend on prior dietary galactose intake, and evaluate for all three enzyme deficiencies. Most U.S. states use a combination of these approaches. Because of the rapid onset of symptoms of classic galactosemia and the presence of lactose in breast milk and most artificial formulas, screening programs for galactosemia must provide rapid results. Often, however, the screening results are not available before the affected neonate becomes ill; initial evaluation of a sick newborn should therefore include testing for the presence of urinary reducing substances (see "Specialized Biochemical Testing"). A newborn identified by newborn screen as possibly having classic galactosemia should have definitive biochemical testing by measuring whole blood or erythrocyte GALT activity and erythrocyte red cell galactose-1-phosphate. In addition, genetic analysis for the common GALT mutations is often helpful in interpreting the results of the GALT activity measurements and making treatment decisions. Following initiation of these studies, lactose should be withdrawn from the diet pending results of the laboratory investigations.

Widespread neonatal testing of erythrocyte transferase activity in various populations has revealed considerable genetic heterogeneity of this enzyme deficiency.[19] Some individuals have a partial enzyme deficiency that does not result in significant impairment of galactose metabolism or any discernible clinical disorder; there is no evidence of a need for dietary treatment of these cases. In other cases with partial enzyme activity, erythrocyte galactose-1-phosphate concentrations are increased, and minimal symptoms can develop. These cases can be managed with less-severe restriction of dietary lactose intake.

HOMOCYSTINURIA

Several inborn errors of metabolism produce homocystinuria.[39,65] The most common of these disorders is caused by cystathionine β-synthase deficiency, an autosomal recessive trait. Cystathionine β-synthase is a pyridoxine (vitamin B$_6$)-dependent enzyme. Rare disorders that also lead to homocystinuria include defects in folate or cobalamin metabolism. Screening programs for homocystinuria are based on detection of elevated blood levels of methionine, the precursor of cystathionine. Hypermethioninemia is characteristic of cystathionine β-synthase deficiency, but may not be associated with other causes of homocystinuria.

False-positive and false-negative results do occur in screening programs for homocystinuria.[39,65] False-positive results are generally the consequence of artifacts (e.g., poor quality of sample), but they may also result from nongenetic causes of hypermethioninemia, such as parenteral administration of amino acids or generalized liver disease or, rarely, from a genetic cause such as hereditary tyrosinemia, galactosemia, or citrin deficiency (see "Hepatic Dysfunction"). False-negative results are produced by the milder variants of cystathionine β-synthase deficiency, especially the pyridoxine-responsive form, which might not exhibit hypermethioninemia in the neonatal period.

The diagnosis of homocystinuria should be confirmed in patients with a positive newborn screening test by measuring total plasma homocysteine, plasma amino acids including free homocysteine, and urine amino acids including homocysteine. The diagnosis of cystathionine β-synthase deficiency can be confirmed by measuring the enzyme activity in cultured skin fibroblasts or genetic testing.

Cystathionine β-synthase deficiency rarely manifests in the neonatal period, but it can cause lethargy, poor feeding, and thromboembolic phenomena when it does.[39,65] If untreated, the disorder can lead to musculoskeletal anomalies suggestive of a marfanoid habitus, ectopia lentis, thromboembolic vascular disease, behavioral or psychiatric problems, and mental retardation. Patients with pyridoxine-responsive defects tend to have milder disease than do patients with pyridoxine-nonresponsive defects. All patients should undergo a pyridoxine challenge test to determine whether they are pyridoxine responsive.

Patients with pyridoxine-responsive forms of homocystinuria might require only daily vitamin B_6 supplementation and mild methionine restriction, whereas nonresponders probably require a strict low-methionine diet with cysteine supplementation (cysteine is the product of the cystathionine β-synthase reaction). Patients might also benefit from folate, vitamin B_{12}, and betaine supplementation, which augment the remethylation of homocysteine to methionine, thereby reducing the toxic effects of excessive homocysteine. The outcome for vitamin B_6-responsive patients appears to be good, but the outcome for nonresponders has often been less satisfactory because of the irreversible damage caused by the presenting episode, the therapeutic inadequacy of the present dietary management, or both.

MAPLE SYRUP URINE DISEASE

MSUD is an inborn error of branched-chain amino acid metabolism caused by deficiency of branched-chain α-ketoacid dehydrogenase, which is involved in isoleucine, leucine, and valine metabolism.[39] The classic clinical variant of this disorder manifests in the neonatal period and can lead to serious consequences if it is not recognized and treated within the first week of life. Untreated, the severe neonatal form leads to ketoacidosis and hypoglycemia, lethargy, seizures, and often death. If the patient recovers from this initial episode, the disorder can lead to growth failure and mental retardation.

Treatment requires intensive management of the presenting and subsequent acute episodes and meticulous long-term management that entails a diet containing reduced amounts of the branched-chain amino acids (i.e., isoleucine, leucine, and valine) and, in some cases, supplementation with pharmacologic amounts of thiamine. Thiamine is a cofactor for the branched-chain α-ketoacid dehydrogenase complex; a minority of patients have thiamine-responsive defects.

Screening programs for MSUD are based on the presence of hyperleucinemia. There are relatively few false-positive results. However, there was a relatively high frequency of false-negative results in the traditional screening programs. The rate of false-negative results has been reduced by the use of MS/MS technology because it is more sensitive and can concurrently measure isoleucine, leucine, and valine, thereby permitting the use of amino acid ratios to identify at-risk newborns.

The response to a positive screening result must be rapid because onset of this disease is often within the first week of life. Positive screening results might not be received from the newborn screening program until after the patient is in the neonatal intensive care unit. Bedside detection of the characteristic odor of maple syrup by an alert parent or nurse might be the first evidence of this disorder. The diagnosis should be established by specific blood and urine testing for the characteristic aminoacidopathy (i.e., increased plasma concentrations of allo-isoleucine, isoleucine, leucine, and valine) and the characteristic urinary organic acid pattern (see "Specialized Biochemical Testing"). Definitive enzyme analysis can be performed with leukocytes or cultured skin fibroblasts, but institution of treatment should not be delayed pending definitive analysis.[39,58] Treatment should be started immediately and should include vigorous correction of metabolic acidosis and hypoglycemia. Hemodialysis may be required. Once the infant is stable, the offending amino acids should be carefully reintroduced, either parenterally or orally (see "Metabolic Acidosis").

Treatment has prolonged the life expectancy and the quality of life for patients with MSUD, but the prognosis for intellectual outcome remains guarded because most patients experience recurrent episodes of ketoacidosis.[58] The key factor that correlates with ultimate intellectual outcome is the age of initiation of therapy; initiation of therapy after 10 days of age is rarely associated with normal intellectual outcome.

MEDIUM-CHAIN ACYL-CoA DEHYDROGENASE DEFICIENCY

Medium-chain acyl-CoA dehydrogenase (MCAD) deficiency is the most common inherited disorder of fatty acid oxidation, with an incidence of approximately 1 in 15,000.[34,39,50,78] It has a highly variable clinical presentation, even within families. It appears only rarely in the newborn period. Most patients present between 3 and 24 months of age, but others remain asymptomatic until they are much older, even in adulthood. The initial retrospective studies on MCAD deficiency found that in almost one fourth of patients, the diagnosis followed sudden, unexplained death.

The typical presentation is that of an infant who has unexplained progressive vomiting, hepatomegaly, lethargy leading to coma, and seizures associated with an infectious illness or a period of prolonged fasting. The characteristic laboratory finding is nonketotic or hypoketotic hypoglycemia; signs of liver dysfunction may also be present. Older patients could have a more indolent course that is associated with failure to thrive, developmental delay, or chronic muscle weakness. A significant proportion of patients are asymptomatic. MCAD deficiency is not infrequently diagnosed in an "unaffected" older sibling after his or her younger sibling comes to medical attention for an acute metabolic crisis or a positive newborn screening result for MCAD deficiency.

The diagnosis of MCAD deficiency is confirmed by plasma carnitine analysis with an acylcarnitine profile, urine organic acid analysis, and urine acylglycine analysis.[39,50] The plasma total and free carnitine concentration can vary with the phase of the illness. The plasma acylcarnitine profile typically shows increased amounts of C6, C8, and C10 acylcarnitines, with the greatest elevation being C8-acylcarnitine (octanoylcarnitine). However, patients with secondary carnitine deficiency could have a relative increase, but not an absolute increase, in these acylcarnitines. Urine organic acid analysis generally shows a typical medium-chain dicarboxylic aciduria (C6-C10) in symptomatic patients, but it could be normal in asymptomatic patients. Urinary acylglycine analysis can be useful in detecting the characteristic metabolite (suberylglycine) in asymptomatic patients. Thus it is especially important that all three complementary studies be performed for asymptomatic patients.

Genetic testing is useful for confirming the diagnosis. It used to be thought that at least 90% of patients carried at least one copy of the same abnormal allele, the A985G mutation, but the frequency of this particular allele is lower in patients identified by newborn screening programs.

Patients with MCAD deficiency should avoid fasting. Infants require frequent feedings: every 3 to 4 hours. The older infant or child may be allowed to fast for progressively longer periods of time, but not for more than 8 to 12 hours. The period of nocturnal fasting should be alleviated by providing uncooked cornstarch as a source of slow-release sugar with the last bottle or meal of the day. A low-fat diet (<30%) may be beneficial, as may oral carnitine supplementation for patients with secondary carnitine deficiency. Carnitine supplementation should be monitored with periodic plasma carnitine analysis. Acute metabolic crises should be treated with intravenous glucose and carnitine. The prognosis for patients who are identified before the onset of irreversible neurologic damage is generally excellent.

PHENYLKETONURIA

Several genetic disorders produce hyperphenylalaninemia. Classic PKU and non-PKU hyperphenylalaninemia are caused by defects in phenylalanine hydroxylase, and variant PKU is caused by one of several defects in tetrahydrobiopterin (BH_4) metabolism.[39] Several nongenetic factors also produce hyperphenylalaninemia in the newborn, but this hyperphenylalaninemia disappears in the first year of life. The most common causes of transient hyperphenylalaninemia are prematurity and high protein intake. Newborn screening programs identify infants with genetic and nongenetic hyperphenylalaninemia. It is imperative that patients identified by the screening program receive a rapid, accurate, and definitive diagnosis because the clinical implications and therapies for the various forms of hyperphenylalaninemia are different.

All genetic forms of hyperphenylalaninemia are caused by defects that directly or indirectly affect the activity of the enzyme phenylalanine hydroxylase. This enzyme catalyzes the conversion of phenylalanine to tyrosine and requires BH_4 as a cofactor. Classic PKU and non-PKU hyperphenylalaninemia are caused by allelic defects of phenylalanine hydroxylase itself, whereas variant PKU is caused by defects of BH_4 biosynthesis or reutilization. BH_4 is also a cofactor for tyrosine hydroxylase and tryptophan hydroxylase, which are enzymes involved in neurotransmitter biosynthesis. Approximately 98% of patients with hyperphenylalanemia have a defect in phenylalanine hydroxylase, whereas 2% have a defect in BH_4 metabolism.

Patients with milder deficiencies of phenylalanine hydroxylase, i.e., patients with transient hyperphenylalaninemia or non-PKU hyperphenylalaninemia, usually do not require dietary treatment. However, patients with more severe deficiencies, that is, patients with classic PKU, require lifelong phenylalanine restriction. Treatment should start within the first month of life to avoid irreversible neurologic damage. When started early, treatment is generally effective in preventing the long-term neurologic sequelae of this disease. However, standard treatment appears unable to prevent more subtle intellectual and behavioral disabilities.[39] Dietary restriction should be lifelong. Women with PKU who fail to maintain the appropriate diet are at risk for having neurologically impaired offspring (maternal PKU syndrome; see "Maternal Diseases Affecting the Fetus").

In recent years, clinical trials have demonstrated that some patients with milder forms of classic PKU respond to oral supplementation with a BH_4 homologue. They appear to tolerate a higher dietary protein intake while maintaining acceptable serum phenylalanine concentrations. Further studies are needed to define better which patients are suitable candidates for this form of therapy.

Defects of BH_4 metabolism cause defective neurotransmitter synthesis as well as hyperphenylalaninemia, and lead to a more generalized neurologic syndrome known as *variant PKU*, characterized by convulsions, abnormal tone and posture, abnormal movements, hyperthermia, hypersalivation and swallowing difficulties, drowsiness, irritability, and developmental delay. Standard dietary management corrects the hyperphenylalaninemia that these patients have, but does not improve the neurologic problems related to their neurotransmitter deficiencies. Only a small percentage of patients with hyperphenylalaninemia have BH_4-related defects, and these patients must be identified early in order to initiate appropriate therapy. A variety of approaches are being used to treat these patients with some success.[39]

Newborn screening for hyperphenylalaninemia is based on measuring the concentration of phenylalanine in the blood while the newborn infant is receiving a phenylalanine-containing diet.[39,56] In the past, blood samples were obtained before discharge from the hospital, typically on the third or fourth day of life. Many newborn infants now go home from the hospital before 24 hours of age, thereby creating problems for screening programs. Screening before 24 hours increases the risk of a false-negative result, whereas delaying screening until after discharge increases the risk of poor compliance.

The rate of false-negative results is less a problem with MS/MS screening than the traditional approaches, partly because it is possible to measure the concentrations of phenylalanine and tyrosine (the product of the phenylalanine hydroxylase reaction) concurrently. Those who have a positive screening result require prompt attention, including plasma amino acid analysis. If the plasma phenylalanine concentration and the plasma phenylalanine-to-tyrosine ratio is increased, the patient should be placed on a low-phenylalanine diet. Breast feeding should be stopped. In all cases of confirmed hyperphenylalaninemia, the patient should be evaluated by a metabolic disorders specialist to rule out a defect in BH_4 metabolism.

THE ABNORMAL NEWBORN INFANT: CLINICAL PHENOTYPES

On the whole, newborn infants with inborn errors of metabolism have relatively few types of presentation. The most common clinical presentations are listed in Table 50-3, along with a differential diagnosis of the categories of metabolic disorders that may be associated with each presentation. A more detailed discussion of each presentation follows.

Prenatal Onset

Most inborn errors of metabolism do not affect the developing fetus and do not affect the woman who is carrying an affected fetus until after the birth of the baby. Similarly, most maternal illnesses, including inborn errors, do not affect the developing fetus. There are, however, several notable exceptions.[98]

MATERNAL DISEASES AFFECTING THE FETUS

The prototype of a maternal disease affecting the fetus is maternal PKU.[72] A pregnant woman who has PKU is at increased risk for spontaneous abortion. She also has an increased risk of having a child with major birth anomalies, including intrauterine growth restriction, microcephaly, mental retardation, and a congenital heart defect, as well as a broad range of minor anomalies. The risk of birth defects is proportional to the mother's serum phenylalanine concentration. There is no safe level below which the fetus is not at risk. Women with PKU should be placed on a strict low-phenylalanine diet before conception. This has proved difficult to do in practice, however, and maternal PKU syndrome remains a significant problem for women with PKU.

FETAL DISEASES AFFECTING THE MOTHER

As a rule, inborn errors of metabolism of the fetus do not affect the developing fetus or pregnant mother. However, reports began to appear in the 1990s describing mothers who had experienced *acute fatty liver of pregnancy* (AFLP) while carrying a fetus who subsequently manifested evidence of a fatty acid oxidation defect after birth.[100] AFLP is the most extreme end of a clinical spectrum of maternal complications of pregnancy that includes HELLP syndrome (*h*emolysis, *e*levated *l*iver enzymes, and a *l*ow *p*latelet count) and AFLP. HELLP syndrome and AFLP are potentially serious complications of pregnancy (see Chapter 15).

TABLE 50–3 Clinical Findings Helpful in the Differential Diagnosis of Suspected Metabolic Disease in Neonates

Diagnostic Finding	Considerations	Diagnostic Finding	Considerations
Prenatal Onset		Gastrointestinal abnormalities	Carbohydrate defects Intestinal transport defects Lysosomal storage disorders Organic acidemias
Maternal diseases affecting fetus	Phenylketonuria		
Fetal diseases affecting mother	Fatty acid oxidation defects	Hair or skin abnormalities	Amino acid disorders Menkes disease Organic acidemias
Fetal diseases affecting fetus	Lysosomal storage disorders	Hematologic abnormalities	Organic acidemias Respiratory chain defect
The "sick" neonate	Amino acid disorders Carbohydrate defects Fatty acid oxidation defects Organic acidemias Respiratory chain defects Urea cycle defects Other	Hepatic dysfunction (see Table 50-5)	Amino acid defects Bile acid biosynthetic defects Carbohydrate defects Congenital disorders of glycosylation Fatty acid oxidation defects Peroxisomal disorders Respiratory chain defects
Cardiomegaly and/or cardiomyopathy (see Table 50-4)	Fatty acid oxidation defects Glycogen storage diseases Lysosomal storage diseases Peroxisomal disorders Respiratory chain defects	Hepatomegaly/ splenomegaly	Carbohydrate defects Fatty acid oxidation defects Glycogen storage diseases Lysosomal storage disorders Peroxisomal disorders
Eye Anomalies		Sepsis	Galactosemia Respiratory chain defects
Cataracts	Carbohydrate defects Lysosomal storage disease Respiratory chain defects	Unusual odor (see Table 50-7)	Amino acid disorders Organic acidemias
Cornea	Lysosomal storage disorders	Dysmorphic syndromes (see Table 50-8)	Large-molecule disorders Small-molecule disorders
Retinal anomalies	Fatty acid oxidation defects Lysosomal storage disorders Peroxisomal disorders		

Clinical, biochemical, and histologic evidence of hepatic dysfunction mark both disorders. Patients with HELLP syndrome commonly develop epigastric pain, nausea, vomiting, headache, and biochemical findings of elevated serum liver enzymes, and they occasionally develop disseminated intravascular coagulation. AFLP is less common than HELLP syndrome and shows a greater degree of hepatic dysfunction. It often produces a severe coagulopathy, hypoglycemia, and fulminant hepatic failure. Microvesicular fatty deposits in the liver characterize both disorders. Both disorders can have life-threatening consequences for the fetus and mother. Women with either of these disorders improve remarkably after delivery, suggesting that the fetus is causing a toxic effect that resembles that seen in patients with inborn errors of fatty acid oxidation.

There is convincing evidence that a specific defect of fatty acid oxidation, long-chain 3-hydroxyacyl-CoA dehydrogenase (LCHAD) deficiency, is associated with the HELLP syndrome and AFLP spectrum.[6,35] LCHAD is part of a trifunctional multimeric enzyme complex that performs the three terminal steps in the fatty acid β-oxidation cycle: long-chain 2,3-enoyl-CoA hydratase, LCHAD, and long-chain 3-ketoacyl-CoA thiolase. LCHAD deficiency can be seen as an isolated deficiency or as part of trifunctional protein deficiency that affects all three enzyme activities. Both disorders are inherited as autosomal recessive traits.

Isolated LCHAD deficiency is marked by relative genetic homogeneity. More than 50% of the mutant alleles found in patients who have this disease carry the same mutation: a G1528C change in the gene that encodes for the α-subunit of LCHAD. Other mutations in the same gene that predispose a heterozygous mother to AFLP have also been identified. A relatively large number of at-risk pregnancies have now been identified and reviewed after the birth of a child with LCHAD deficiency.[6] These studies show that a woman who is heterozygous for LCHAD deficiency is at risk for developing HELLP syndrome or AFLP during a pregnancy in which she is carrying a fetus who is homozygous for the same deficiency. Thus a heterozygous mother is only at risk if her fetus inherits a second LCHAD mutation from the father. The baby, in turn, is at risk for significant postnatal problems associated with his or her enzyme deficiency. The diagnosis and care of a child with LCHAD deficiency is discussed later under Hypoglycemia.

The fraction of women who develop AFLP as a consequence of LCHAD deficiency is greater than 50%. The current recommendation is to evaluate all pregnant women who develop AFLP for LCHAD deficiency by biochemical and genetic testing. This recommendation does not extend to women who develop HELLP syndrome because it is more common than AFLP and less likely to be associated with LCHAD deficiency. Rarely, other inborn errors of fatty acid β-oxidation can also produce AFLP.

FETAL DISEASES AFFECTING THE FETUS

The fetus does not generally suffer prenatally detectable consequences of its own inborn error of metabolism until after birth because the abnormal metabolites that it produces are removed by the maternal circulation, or conversely, deficiency states caused by the inborn error are replenished by the maternal circulation. The primary exceptions to this rule are disorders of large-molecule metabolism in which macromolecules are not degraded appropriately and therefore accumulate in fetal organs (see "Dysmorphic Syndromes").

The most common of these inborn errors are the lysosomal storage disorders, which can produce congenital ascites or hydrops fetalis.[89] The lysosomal storage disorders that can lead to these problems include β-glucuronidase deficiency and Morquio syndrome (i.e., mucopolysaccharidoses); Farber disease and G_{M1}-gangliosidosis (glycolipidoses); galactosialidosis and sialidosis (oligosaccharidoses); and free sialic storage disease, a lysosomal transport defect. Several other disorders can also cause hydrops, including carbohydrate-deficient glycoprotein syndrome (known as *congenital disorder of glycosylation*), glycogen storage disease IV, Niemann-Pick disease type C (i.e., a defect of intracellular cholesterol transport), and several inborn errors of red cell glycolytic enzymes (see Chapter 22).

The Sick Newborn Infant

Newborn infants have a limited number of ways to respond to an acute illness such as an inborn error of metabolism.[11,45] These responses generally include cardiorespiratory, feeding, and neurologic difficulties. Symptoms generally do not appear on the first day of life but usually begin later in the first week. The initial symptoms are often poor feeding associated with a poor suck and irritability. Muscle tone is decreased, sometimes marked by a fluctuating pattern of decreased and increased tone. Reflexes are often abnormal, and seizures can develop. The poor feeding is sometimes accompanied by vomiting. Diarrhea is uncommon.

Disorders accompanied by a metabolic acidosis (i.e., the lactic acidemias or organic acidemias) can lead to a compensatory increase in respiratory rate. In the case of urea cycle defects, hyperammonemia increases the respiratory drive, leading to hyperpnea. The neonate shows lethargy, which can progress to coma and death. These symptoms often progress rapidly, sometimes within a matter of hours but more often during the course of a few days. It is important to suspect a metabolic disorder as early as possible in its course to interrupt the progression of symptoms, because many of these disorders are life threatening.

Many inborn errors of metabolism are associated with what appears to be a cascade of effects. A number of specific metabolites are overproduced as a result of a specific enzymatic deficiency. In excess, these normal metabolites serve as endogenous toxins that impair a relatively narrow range of metabolic or physiologic processes. When disrupted, these other processes lead to production of additional metabolites, which impair other cellular processes. Early interruption of the cascade through such relatively simple measures as fluid and caloric support might abort episodes of metabolic decompensation. Physicians who care for older children with metabolic disorders often receive a retrospective history of "sepsis" in the neonatal period that was never confirmed by culture and that resolved spontaneously; these episodes might have represented an interrupted metabolic intoxication syndrome. Early nonspecific supportive treatment can abort the pathologic cascade or delay the onset of a more fulminant course until a provisional metabolic diagnosis, upon which more specific treatment can be based, becomes available.

So-called sick newborns should be evaluated for a defect in amino acid metabolism, carbohydrate metabolism, fatty acid β-oxidation, organic acid metabolism, the mitochondrial respiratory chain, and the urea cycle (see Table 50-3). As a rule, the differential diagnosis for these patients can be narrowed by the presence of other clinical findings or by a characteristic laboratory finding, such as acidosis, hyperammonemia, hypoglycemia, ketosis, or lactic acidemia (see "The Abnormal Newborn Infant: Laboratory Phenotypes").

ERRORS OF METABOLISM NOT DETECTABLE BY STANDARD SCREENING

There is a limited but ever-growing number of inborn errors of metabolism that might not be identified by the standard laboratory approach presented later in this chapter. These disorders must, therefore, be considered and pursued independently and specifically. They include the carbohydrate-deficient glycoprotein syndromes (known as *congenital disorders of glycosylation*), folinic acid–responsive seizures, glucose transporter type 1 (GLUT-1) deficiency, Menkes disease, nonketotic hyperglycinemia, the peroxisomal disorders, pyridoxine-dependent seizures, and sulfite oxidase deficiency. The congenital disorders of glycosylation and the peroxisomal disorders are diverse groups of conditions and are discussed later under Dysmorphic Syndromes. Menkes disease is discussed under Hair and Skin Abnormalities.

Folinic Acid–Responsive Seizures
Folinic acid–responsive seizures is a poorly understood disorder or group of disorders that appear to be related to defects in neurotransmitter metabolism.[33,64] The diagnosis can be facilitated by biochemical analysis of cerebrospinal fluid (CSF). Practically, the patient can be evaluated for the possibility of folinic acid–responsive seizures by monitoring the response to a challenge of intravenous folinic acid (5 mg per day). It can take several weeks to see a response.

Glucose Transporter Type 1 Deficiency
GLUT-1 deficiency sometimes manifests in the neonatal period with seizures that are refractory to standard anticonvulsants, opsoclonus, and intermittent hemiplegic episodes.[43,57] With time, affected children develop ataxia, apraxia, and developmental delay. The disorder is caused by deficiency of the protein that facilitates glucose transport across the blood-brain barrier.

Once considered, the diagnosis can be readily established by concurrently measuring glucose, lactate, and pyruvate in the blood and CSF. The characteristic finding is a low CSF glucose concentration (less than 40 mg/dL) (hypoglycorrhachia) and a decreased CSF glucose-to-blood glucose concentration ratio (less than 0.35; normal, 0.65). The blood and CSF lactate and pyruvate concentrations are normal. The diagnosis can be confirmed by measuring erythrocyte uptake of a nonmetabolizable glucose homologue, 3-methylglucose, or by mutational analysis of the *GLUT-1* gene.

GLUT-1 deficiency can be treated successfully with a low-carbohydrate, high-fat diet (a ketogenic diet), which provides ketones as an alternative fuel source for the brain. It is important that the diagnosis be made as early as possible in order to initiate treatment before irreversible neurologic damage occurs.

Nonketotic Hyperglycinemia
Nonketotic hyperglycinemia is an autosomal recessive disorder caused by a defect in the glycine cleavage enzyme.[27,30] In the first few days of life, the infant has profound hypotonia, poor feeding, hiccupping, lethargy often leading to coma, and severe (generally myoclonic) seizures. Electroencephalographic analysis initially shows a burst-suppression pattern, which evolves with time into hypsarrhythmia. The disorder often leads to early death.

Standard laboratory analysis of plasma amino acids might not suffice to establish the diagnosis because the plasma glycine concentration might only be minimally elevated. Diagnosis of this disorder requires amino acid analysis on concurrently collected plasma and CSF samples; the biochemical hallmark of nonketotic hyperglycemia is an elevated CSF glycine-to-plasma glycine ratio. In addition, patients with nonketotic hyperglycinemia must be distinguished from those with ketotic hyperglycinemia, which accompanies many of the organic acidemias. Thus urinary organic acid analysis should be performed to determine whether the patient has characteristic organic aciduria (see "Specialized Biochemical Testing").

Treatment for nonketotic hyperglycinemia is poor, although efforts to block the action of glycine on the N-methyl-D-aspartate receptor are being evaluated.

Pyridoxine-Dependent Seizures
Another disorder that should be considered in the evaluation of a newborn infant with unexplained seizures accompanied by negative findings on a standard metabolic evaluation is pyridoxine-dependent seizures.[25,64] This disorder typically begins in the neonatal period, although in some cases, the seizures begin in utero.

The biochemical basis of this disorder was thought to be an inborn error in glutamic acid decarboxylase, which is the rate-limiting step in the synthesis of γ-aminobutyric acid (GABA). GABA is a critical neurotransmitter. Patients with this disorder have a decreased CSF GABA concentration. Pyridoxine (vitamin B_6) is a cofactor for the decarboxylase and was thought to augment the activity of the deficient enzyme. However, recent studies have shown that the mechanism of action is more complicated. It now appears that pyridoxine-dependent seizures are due to a genetic defect in the *ALDH7A1* gene, which encodes for a protein called *antiquitin*. Antiquitin is an enzyme involved in the lysine (a dibasic amino acid) degradation pathway. Antiquitin deficiency leads to accumulation of pipecolic acid and Δ^1-piperide 6-carboxylic acid, which react with and inactivate the active form of pyridoxine in brain, pyridoxal phosphate. Thus patients with pyridoxine-dependent seizures have an autosomal recessive disorder in lysine metabolism that inactivates pyridoxal phosphate, which is required for GABA synthesis. Pyridoxine supplementation compensates for the increased loss of pyridoxal phosphate.

The disorder is generally diagnosed by demonstrating clinical and electroencephalographic responses to a pharmacologic challenge dose of pyridoxine rather than by biochemical analysis of lysine metabolites in the CSF or genetic analysis of the *ALDH7A1* gene, because the clinical approach is more easily performed and provides a more rapid answer. The response to parenteral pyridoxine (50 to 100 mg) is often dramatic, with normalization of the electroencephalographic pattern within minutes. This pyridoxine challenge test must, however, be done with caution because patients can experience apnea, hypotonia, and hypotension. The test should be done in an intensive care setting with electroencephalographic monitoring (see Chapter 40, Part 5). Once the diagnosis is established, daily oral pyridoxine supplementation (5 to 10 mg/kg) is effective treatment for this disorder. The prognosis for this disorder, once recognized and treated, is favorable.

A variant of pyridoxine-dependent seizures has been recognized in which the patient does not respond (or responds partially) to parenteral or oral pyridoxine, but responds to oral pyridoxal 5′-phosphate (pyridoxal phosphate).[25,64] Pyridoxal phosphate is the "active" form of vitamin B_6; that is, it serves as the cofactor for the enzymes involved in neurotransmitter biosynthesis. The patients who respond to pyridoxal phosphate have a clinical presentation similar to that of patients with pyridoxine-dependent seizures. However, they have a number of unique biochemical findings: decreased CSF concentrations of homovanillic acid (an L-dopa metabolite) and 5-hydroxyindoleacetic acid (a serotonin metabolite), increased CSF concentrations of two other L-dopa metabolites (3-O-methyldopa and vanillactic acid), and increased CSF concentrations of two amino acids (glycine and threonine). These changes are thought to be secondary to a generalized dysfunction of three vitamin B_6-dependent enzymes, aromatic L-amino acid decarboxylase, glycine cleavage enzyme, and threonine dehydratase. The underlying genetic defect is a deficiency of pyridox(am)ine 5′-phosphate oxidase (PNPO), which is required for the conversion of dietary pyridoxine and pyridoxamine phosphate to pyridoxal 5′-phosphate.

A patient suspected of having this disorder can be evaluated biochemically for the CSF abnormalities enumerated above or, more simply, by using pyridoxal phosphate in place of pyridoxine in an oral challenge test (pyridoxal phosphate is not available in a parenteral form). The patient should receive 50 mg of pyridoxal phosphate by nasogastric tube, while in an intensive care unit with EEG monitoring because of the risk of apnea, hypotonia, and hypotension. In some cases, the EEG response was relatively rapid (within an hour), but the patient remained unresponsive for several days following administration of pyridoxal phosphate. If the challenge test is successful, the patient should continue to receive pyridoxal phosphate (10 mg/kg every 6 hours). See Chapter 40 for further details on evaluating and managing patients with this disorder.

Sulfite Oxidase Deficiency

Sulfite oxidase deficiency exists in two forms: (1) an isolated genetic deficiency of sulfite oxidase and (2) a genetic defect in the molybdenum cofactor, which is required for the function of sulfite oxidase and xanthine dehydrogenase/aldehyde oxidase. Sulfite oxidase is involved in the degradation of the sulfur-containing amino acids, methionine, homocysteine, and cysteine to sulfate, whereas xanthine dehydrogenase and aldehyde oxidase are involved in the purine degradation

pathway leading to uric acid.[3] Both disorders are characterized clinically by early onset, refractory seizures, hypotonia leading to hypertonia, and if the patients survive long enough, microcephaly, lens dislocation, and severe psychomotor delay. Many affected infants die in the first year of life. There is no proven treatment for this disorder, although a low-methionine, low-cystine diet has been tried and may have been beneficial in a few patients with mild disease.

The key biochemical findings of sulfite oxidase deficiency, either in cases of isolated deficiency or in cases of molybdenum cofactor deficiency, are increased excretion of urinary sulfite and thiosulfate, increased plasma and urinary S-sulfocysteine, and decreased plasma cystine. In addition, the plasma homocysteine concentration is very low in these patients and provides a unique biochemical marker that can be obtained rapidly. Patients with molybdenum cofactor deficiency produce the same set of metabolites as patients with the isolated deficiency, plus they excrete increased amounts of xanthine and hypoxanthine and decreased amounts of uric acid. As in the case of homocysteine, the serum uric acid is sometimes very low in patients with molybdenum cofactor deficiency and provides an easily measured marker for this form of the disease.

Cardiomegaly and Cardiomyopathy

See also Chapter 45.

Inborn errors of metabolism that are manifested by cardiomegaly, cardiomyopathy, or both in the neonatal period can be divided into five diagnostic categories: fatty acid β-oxidation defects, glycogen storage disorders, lysosomal storage disorders, mitochondrial oxidative defects, and other defects (Table 50-4). The pathogenesis for cardiac disease differs among these different diagnostic categories. The glycogen storage disorders and the lysosomal storage disorders are infiltrative processes resulting from the accumulation of partial breakdown products of glycogen and complex carbohydrates, respectively, whereas the fatty acid β-oxidation defects and the mitochondrial oxidative defects compromise energy production in the heart or lead to production of toxic metabolites.[21,24,75]

GLYCOGEN STORAGE DISORDERS

The glycogen storage disorder that most commonly causes cardiomyopathy in early infancy is Pompe disease, also known as *acid maltase deficiency* or *glycogen storage disease type II*. Acid maltase is the only enzyme involved in glycogen metabolism that is located within the lysosome. Pompe disease can also be considered a lysosomal storage disorder, and it is probably helpful to consider its pathogenesis from this perspective. Acid maltase is a key enzyme responsible for degrading glycogen; it cleaves the α-1,4-glucoside linkages of the glycogen polymer, converting glycogen to glucose.

Generalized hypotonia, failure to thrive, and cardiomyopathy characterize the neonatal form of Pompe disease. Hepatomegaly does not develop in patients with Pompe disease (except as a consequence to heart failure), as it does in patients with some other glycogen storage disorders. The diagnosis can be confirmed by specific enzyme analysis using skeletal muscle, cardiac muscle, or more conveniently, cultured skin fibroblasts, or by genetic testing. Enzyme replacement therapy for Pompe disease appears promising.

TABLE 50–4   Disorders Associated with Cardiomegaly or Cardiomyopathy

Category of Disorder	Disorder
Fatty acid oxidation	Carnitine-acylcarnitine translocase deficiency
	Carnitine palmitoyltransferase II deficiency
	Long-chain 3-hydroxyacyl-CoA dehydrogenase deficiency
	Multiple acyl-CoA dehydrogenase deficiency
	Very-long-chain acyl-CoA dehydrogenase deficiency
Glycogen storage	GSD type II (Pompe disease)
	GSD type IX (phosphorylase bkinase deficiency)
Lysosomal storage	Glycolipidoses
	Mucopolysaccharidoses
	Oligosaccharidoses
Respiratory chain	nDNA defects
	Complex I
	Complex III
	Complex IV
	Barth syndrome
	Leigh syndrome
	mtDNA defects
	Leigh syndrome
	mtDNA depletion syndromes
	$tRNA^{Ile}$, $tRNA^{Leu}$
Other	Congenital disorders of glycosylation

GSD, glycogen storage disease; mtDNA, mitochondrial DNA; nDNA, nuclear DNA; $tRNA^{Ile}$, transfer RNA for isoleucine; $tRNA^{Leu}$, transfer RNA for leucine.

Cardiomyopathy is not generally seen in the neonatal period in association with the other glycogen storage disorders, except in rare cases of cardiac-specific phosphorylase b kinase deficiency.[21,24]

LYSOSOMAL STORAGE DISORDERS

The lysosomal storage disorders produce cardiomegaly, valvular disease, or cardiomyopathy (dilated or hypertrophic).[21,24,89] Lysosomal storage disorders should be considered in the differential diagnosis of the newborn infant with cardiac disease who also has physical findings suggestive of a lysosomal storage disorder, such as craniofacial dysmorphism, corneal clouding or retinal abnormalities, hepatosplenomegaly, or skeletal anomalies (see "Dysmorphic Syndromes"). The lysosomal storage disorders that may be associated with cardiomyopathy in the newborn period include glycolipidoses (e.g., G_{M1}-gangliosidosis and G_{M2}-gangliosidosis), mucopolysaccharidoses (e.g., Hurler disease and Sandhoff disease), and oligosaccharidoses (e.g., I-cell disease and fucosidosis).

FATTY ACID β-OXIDATION AND MITOCHONDRIAL RESPIRATORY CHAIN DEFECTS

The myocardium derives a significant fraction of its energy from the mitochondrial oxidative metabolism of fatty acids, especially long-chain fatty acids.[21,44] The oxidation of these fatty acids requires a carnitine-mediated system to transport long-chain fatty acids into the mitochondrion, a β-oxidation pathway to break down the fatty acids, and the mitochondrial oxidation phosphorylation system to extract energy from the breakdown products. Cardiomyopathy would be expected to develop in the context of a defect in carnitine-mediated transport of long-chain fatty acids into the mitochondrion, defects of the fatty acid β-oxidation pathway, and defects of the respiratory chain itself. Studies have demonstrated that defects of long-chain fatty acid oxidation are a significant cause of cardiac disease, whereas defects affecting primarily medium-chain or short-chain fatty acid oxidation are less so.

Two defects of carnitine transport have been found to cause cardiomyopathy in the neonatal period: carnitine-acylcarnitine translocase deficiency and carnitine palmitoyltransferase II deficiency. A third defect of carnitine transport, deficiency of the plasma membrane carnitine transporter, does not commonly cause cardiomyopathy in the neonatal period, although it often produces cardiomyopathy in infancy and childhood.

Several defects of the β-oxidation pathway can cause cardiomyopathy: LCHAD deficiency, trifunctional protein deficiency, and very-long-chain acyl-CoA dehydrogenase deficiency.[21] These disorders can also cause life-threatening cardiac arrhythmias, presumably because of the accumulation of toxic long-chain acylcarnitines in the myocardial cells. Multiple acyl-CoA dehydrogenase deficiency (glutaric aciduria type II), a defect in the transfer of reducing equivalents from the enzymes of the β-oxidation pathway to the respiratory chain, can produce also cardiomyopathy (see "Dysmorphic Syndromes").

Several respiratory chain defects are associated with cardiomyopathy in the neonatal period.[38,75,80,90] These disorders may be classified according to whether they are the consequence of an error in a nuclear-encoded component (nDNA) or in a mitochondrial-encoded component (mtDNA) of the respiratory chain, or a nuclear-encoded gene involved in the synthesis, structural integrity or function of the mitochondrion (see "Lactic Acidemia"). These disorders can produce isolated cardiomyopathy or a highly diverse multisystem disease.

Nuclear-encoded defects that produce cardiomyopathy include defects of complex I (NADH-coenzyme Q reductase), complex III (reduced ubiquinone cytochrome c reductase), and complex IV (cytochrome c oxidase), as well as nuclear-encoded defects that affect protein required for the assembly of the oxidative phosphorylation complexes, such as SCO2, which is involved in the assembly of complex IV.[62,91] Barth syndrome is an X-linked disorder that impairs production of the lipid membrane required for normal mitochondrial function. This disorder is characterized by cardiomyopathy, cataracts, deafness, and neutropenia.[5] Leigh syndrome is characterized by a broad and variable clinical pattern that can include hypotonia, optic atrophy, nystagmus, developmental delay, myopathy, cardiomyopathy, and hepatic dysfunction. It is also a genetically heterogeneous disorder that can be caused by several different mutations, some involving nDNA and others involving mtDNA.

Lastly, several mtDNA defects can cause cardiomyopathy, including mutations affecting the mitochondrially encoded components of the oxidative phosphorylation complexes, as well as the transfer ribonucleic acids for glycine (tRNA^{Gly}), isoleucine (tRNA^{Ile}), and leucine (tRNA^{Leu}) (see "Lactic Acidemia").[9,75,80]

OTHER DISORDERS

The main consideration in the miscellaneous category of inborn errors that may be associated with cardiomyopathy is the congenital disorders of glycosylation (CDG). The CDG syndrome is a highly pleiotropic disorder that can result in pericardial effusions, cardiomyopathy, or both, in addition to a broad range of other abnormalities, including neurologic abnormalities, hepatic dysfunction and, in some cases, a characteristic pattern of malformation (see "Dysmorphic Syndromes").

Eye Anomalies

Many inborn errors of metabolism manifest with unusual ophthalmologic findings (see Table 50-3). A careful ophthalmologic examination is a crucial part of the clinical evaluation for a suspected inborn error of metabolism; conversely, patients with unusual ophthalmologic findings might require a metabolic evaluation (see Chapter 53).

Inborn errors of metabolism can affect any of the structural components of the eye.[66] Cataracts are classically associated with carbohydrate disorders (e.g., galactosemia) and lysosomal storage disorders, but they are also associated with Lowe syndrome (oculocerebrorenal syndrome), peroxisomal defects (e.g., Zellweger syndrome, neonatal adrenoleukodystrophy), and respiratory chain defects (e.g., Barth syndrome, Senger syndrome).[5,66] The cornea is often affected by lysosomal storage diseases, which can cause corneal clouding, as in G$_{M1}$-gangliosidosis, β-glucuronidase deficiency, I-cell disease, and sialidosis. Lens dislocation does not generally occur

during the neonatal period in patients with homocystinuria or sulfite oxidase deficiency.

Several inborn errors of metabolism affect retinal development.[66] The so-called cherry-red spot found in several of the lysosomal storage disorders (Farber disease, galactosialidosis, G$_{M1}$-gangliosidosis, and sialidosis) is the best known of these retinal anomalies. Abnormal deposits in the retinal pigment epithelial layer can be found in older patients who have an unusual defect of mitochondrial fatty acid oxidation (LCHAD deficiency) and in patients with CDG syndrome, peroxisomal disorders, and respiratory chain defects.

Gastrointestinal Abnormalities

Newborn infants with inborn errors of metabolism might have various gastrointestinal abnormalities. Common findings include poor feeding, jaundice, and hepatomegaly (see "Hepatomegaly and Splenomegaly"). Many of the organic acidurias and urea cycle disorders are associated with vomiting. A number of patients with an organic acidemia have undergone surgery for and been found to have pyloric stenosis. Researchers hypothesize that the organic acidemias produce toxic metabolites that affect pyloric sphincter tone. Similarly, pancreatitis is a well-documented problem in a minority of patients with several organic acidemias, fatty acid oxidation disorders, or respiratory chain defects.[37]

Diarrhea is a relatively uncommon finding, but it can occur in patients who have defects of bile acid synthesis (see "Hepatic Dysfunction"), respiratory chain defects (see "Lactic Acidemias"), CDG syndrome (see "Dysmorphic Syndromes"), deficiencies of the intestinal disaccharidases or monosaccharide transport systems, congenital chloride diarrhea, and Wolman disease, a lysosomal storage disorder (see "Hepatomegaly and Splenomegaly"). Several lysosomal storage disorders can also produce congenital ascites and hydrops fetalis (see "Prenatal Onset").

Hair and Skin Abnormalities

See also Chapter 52.

Abnormalities of the skin and hair are characteristic of several inborn errors of metabolism. Menkes disease, an X-linked disorder involving intracellular copper metabolism, leads to defects in a number of copper-dependent enzymes. Menkes disease is a highly pleiotropic disorder characterized by sparse and kinky scalp hair—hence the name kinky-hair disease. The disorder causes hypotonia, hypothermia, intractable seizures, profound developmental delay, and early death. The disorder may be associated with lactic acidosis caused by impaired activity of cytochrome c oxidase, a copper-dependent enzyme. The hair is also brittle and coarse in the childhood-onset forms of argininosuccinic aciduria, a urea cycle defect, but this is not seen in neonates with this disease (see "Hyperammonemia").

A number of disorders include abnormalities of skin pigmentation. PKU may be associated with fair hair and skin pigmentation in affected white neonates. Similarly, newborn infants with cystinosis also have fairer hair and skin than their unaffected siblings. However, cystinosis, an autosomal recessive defect affecting lysosomal transport of cystine, a sulfur-containing amino acid, does not produce symptoms until several months of age, when it results in renal Fanconi syndrome and, ultimately, renal failure caused by cystine crystal deposits in the kidney.

Rash and partial alopecia may be associated with multiple carboxylase deficiency, an organic aciduria caused by defects in biotin metabolism: holocarboxylase synthetase deficiency and biotinidase deficiency (see "Newborn Screening").[102] Both defects can produce severe ketoacidosis, feeding difficulties, apnea, lethargy, hypotonia, and coma in the newborn period. Holocarboxylase synthetase and, in some cases, biotinidase deficiency can be detected by urinary organic acid analysis. Both conditions respond to biotin therapy, biotinidase deficiency more so than holocarboxylase synthase deficiency.

Hematologic Abnormalities

Several organic acidemias, including isovaleric acidemia, propionic acidemia, and methylmalonic acidemia, are characterized by neutropenia, thrombocytopenia, anemia, or pancytopenia.[40,93] The thrombocytopenia may be severe enough to lead to clinically significant bleeding. The precise pathophysiologic basis of these findings is not well understood, but is thought to be caused by direct bone marrow suppression of the metabolic imbalance associated with these disorders.

Hematologic abnormalities may be associated with respiratory chain defects, including Barth syndrome[5] (see "Cardiomegaly and Cardiomyopathy") and Pearson syndrome.[80] In contrast to the neutropenia and cardiomyopathy found in Barth syndrome, Pearson syndrome is characterized by sideroblastic anemia, pancreatic exocrine insufficiency, and lactic acidosis. Pearson syndrome is the consequence of a heteroplasmic mutation (deletion) of the mtDNA (see "Lactic Acidemia"). Neutropenia is a characteristic feature of glycogen storage disease type Ib, and this diagnosis should be considered in the patient who presents with hypoglycemia, hepatomegaly, triglyceridemia, neutropenia, and recurrent infections (see "Hypoglycemia").[96]

Hepatic Dysfunction

A number of inborn errors of metabolism are associated with hepatic disease. Excluding disorders that are associated primarily with defects in bilirubin metabolism (see Chapter 48), several groups of disorders lead to hepatic dysfunction and some degree of hepatomegaly. One approach to categorizing these disorders is to divide them into those that impair one or more aspects of hepatic function to a more significant degree than they produce liver enlargement and those for which the reverse is true. The former group of disorders is discussed in this section; the latter group, composed primarily of lysosomal storage disorders, is discussed under Hepatomegaly and Splenomegaly.

The inborn errors of metabolism that cause hepatic dysfunction can be categorized further according to the function or functions that they impair: defects that cause hypoglycemia, defects that cause hepatocellular damage leading to liver failure and cirrhosis, and defects that cause cholestatic disease. Although this approach is useful from a physiologic

perspective, many inborn errors affect more than one of these hepatic functions, and an alternative scheme based on biochemical classification may be applied more practically. The biochemically based approach has been adopted in organizing this section. It is recommended that defects of the following biochemical categories be considered in evaluating patients with hepatic dysfunction: amino acid metabolism, bile acid metabolism, carbohydrate metabolism, fatty acid β-oxidation, peroxisomal disorders, respiratory chain defects, and a miscellaneous group of disorders (Table 50-5).[14] The clinical aspects of these disorders are presented in greater detail in Chapter 48.

AMINOACIDOPATHY

Tyrosinemia Type I

Tyrosinemia type I, also known as hepatorenal tyrosinemia, is the classic aminoacidopathy that can produce a fulminant disorder characterized by progressive hepatocellular damage leading to cirrhosis, proximal renal tubular dysfunction, and peripheral neuropathy.[83] The biochemical basis of this disorder is a defect in fumarylacetoacetate hydratase, an enzyme

TABLE 50-5   Disorders Associated with Abnormal Liver Function

Category of Disorder	Defect
Amino acid metabolism	Tyrosinemia type I Citrin deficiency Urea cycle defects
Bile acid biosynthesis	See text for specific disorders
Carbohydrate metabolism	Galactosemia Hereditary fructose intolerance
Fatty acid oxidation	Carnitine palmitoyltransferase II deficiency Long-chain 3-hydroxyacyl-CoA dehydrogenase deficiency Multiple acyl-CoA dehydrogenase deficiency Very-long-chain acyl-CoA dehydrogenase deficiency
Peroxisomal disorders	Neonatal adrenoleukodystrophy Zellweger syndrome
Respiratory chain	Complex I, III, or IV, or combined deficiencies mtDNA depletion syndromes
Other	α_1-Antitrypsin deficiency Congenital disorders of glycosylation Glycogen storage disease type IV Niemann-Pick disease type C

mtDNA, mitochondrial DNA.

acting late in the tyrosine degradative pathway. Fumarylace-toacetate accumulates secondary to this enzyme deficiency and is nonenzymatically converted to succinylacetone, which is the characteristic urinary metabolite identified in patients with this disorder. Succinylacetone can be identified by urine organic acid analysis.

Until recently, the only treatment for this disorder that appeared to be effective was liver transplantation. A new treatment based on pharmacologic inhibition of 4-hydroxyphenylpyruvate dioxygenase (an enzyme upstream of the hydratase in the tyrosine catabolic pathway) with 2-(2-nitro-4-trifluoromethylbenzoyl)-1,3-cyclohexanedione (NTBC) appears to be effective, especially when therapy is begun before the onset of acute liver failure.

Citrin Deficiency

Urea cycle defects are generally associated with mild hepatocellular dysfunction during their acute presentation, but the neurologic manifestations of these disorders are the predominant signs (see "Hyperammonemia"). The degree of hepatocellular disease can become more significant later in the course of these diseases, especially in argininosuccinic aciduria. There is, however, a urea cycle defect, citrin deficiency, that produces neonatal intrahepatic cholestasis.[60]

Citrin deficiency is a genetic disorder caused by deficiency of the mitochondrial aspartate glutamate carrier, which plays a key role in the urea cycle, gluconeogenesis, and the malate shuttle (which moves NADH between intracellular compartments). Impaired citrin function would limit the conversion of citrulline and aspartate to argininosuccinic acid, a key component of the urea cycle. Absent aspartate, citrulline accumulates and urea production is impaired. Hence, citrin deficiency is also known as citrullinemia type II. Citrullinemia type II was previously thought to be a relatively mild adult-onset form of hyperammonemia, whereas citrullinemia type I was a serious neonatal or pediatric disorder associated with argininosuccinic acid synthetase deficiency (see the discussion under "Hyperammonemia" in "Approaches to Specific Abnormal Laboratory Findings").

Subsequently, citrin deficiency was identified as a self-limited disorder that resolves by 1 year of age and can be treated successfully with a low-lactose diet and support for the hepatic dysfunction. However, more severe, progressive cases were also identified that produced neonatal intrahepatic cholestasis.[60] Patients with this form of citrin deficiency had increased serum concentrations of citrulline, methionine, and phenylalanine, as well as galactose. These patients were often ascertained by newborn screening that identified the increased amino acid concentrations and by programs that measure serum galactose as their screen for galactosemia (but not by programs that measure GALT activity) (see "Newborn Screening"). Neonatal citrin deficiency is primarily a cause of cholestatic liver disease rather than hyperammonemia. It is a treatable disease.

BILE ACID BIOSYNTHESIS DEFECTS

Heritable defects in bile acid biosynthesis can cause severe hepatobiliary disease (cholestatic jaundice and intestinal malabsorption) in the newborn infant.[14,28] These defects are probably underdiagnosed because they are not ascertained by the standard methods of metabolic screening of the sick neonate. However, once considered, they can be diagnosed with relative ease. Recognition of these disorders is especially important because effective treatment exists for many of these defects.

In simple terms, bile acid biosynthesis involves conversion of cholesterol to two bile acids, cholic acid and chenodeoxycholic acid. The first steps in this conversion involve transformation of the cholesterol nucleus, and the last few steps involve transformation of the cholesterol side chains. Several defects in conversion of the cholesterol nucleus to bile acids have been described including: 3β-hydroxy-Δ^5-C_{27}-steroid dehydrogenase deficiency and 3-oxo-Δ^4-steroid-5β-reductase deficiency.[14,28] Both of these disorders can result in severe cholestatic disease in the newborn period and can lead in later months to steatorrhea, clinically significant malabsorption of fat-soluble vitamins D and K, failure to thrive, and chronic hepatitis. The patients generally have no or relatively mild hepatomegaly, mildly elevated hepatic aminotransferase values, and nonspecific findings on liver biopsy. If untreated, many patients progress to irreversible liver disease and die in early childhood. Early recognition is crucial because it permits institution of bile acid replacement therapy using a combination of cholic and chenodeoxycholic acids, which is effective in reversing the hepatotoxic manifestations of these enzyme deficiencies.

Several of the peroxisomal disorders also impair bile acid biosynthesis because they affect enzymes required for the final steps of cholesterol side-chain oxidation.[28,99] These enzymes (i.e., the bifunctional enzyme and the thiolase) are also involved in peroxisomal oxidation of very-long-chain fatty acids, and their deficiency leads to a highly pleiotropic dysmorphic syndrome associated with severe neurologic consequences. Bile acid replacement therapy does not ameliorate the neurologic consequences of these disorders. The peroxisomal disorders, including those that produce cholestatic disease, are discussed further under "Dysmorphic Syndromes".

CARBOHYDRATE METABOLISM DISORDERS

Two disorders of carbohydrate metabolism, galactosemia (see "Newborn Screening") and hereditary fructose intolerance, are associated with hepatocellular disease. These disorders manifest only when the newborn's diet contains the monosaccharide to which the newborn is intolerant, such as galactose in the case of galactosemia and fructose in the case of hereditary fructose intolerance. Similarly, these disorders are detectable by urinary screening tests only when the affected newborn is receiving a diet containing the offending monosaccharide. Because fructose is not a component of breast milk and is a component of only the infant formulas that contain sucrose, hereditary fructose intolerance usually does not manifest in the neonatal period. Both disorders can be detected by the presence of reducing substances other than glucose in urine (see "Specialized Biochemical Testing"). The diagnosis of galactosemia[19] or hereditary fructose intolerance must be confirmed by specific biochemical analysis or genetic testing.

Treatment of these disorders consists of dietary restriction of the hepatotoxic monosaccharide. Such restriction is not easily managed because of the nearly ubiquitous presence of galactose (in the form of lactose) and fructose (in the form of sucrose) in many processed foods. Nevertheless, dietary restriction can be successful and is associated with improved long-term outcomes.

Other disorders of carbohydrate metabolism can also cause hepatic dysfunction, including the glycogen storage diseases (especially types I and III), fructose-1,6-diphosphatase deficiency, and pyruvate carboxylase deficiency. These disorders affect gluconeogenesis and, in contrast to galactosemia and hereditary fructose intolerance, result primarily in hypoglycemia rather than generalized hepatocellular dysfunction (see "Hypoglycemia").

FATTY ACID OXIDATION DEFECTS

Several defects of fatty acid oxidation are associated with fat accumulation in the liver and with hepatocellular dysfunction (see Table 50-5). A defect of fatty acid oxidation should be suspected in patients with unexplained hepatocellular disease that is accompanied by nonketotic or hypoketotic hypoglycemia.

One defect of fatty acid oxidation that is a well-established cause of hepatic dysfunction is multiple acyl-CoA dehydrogenase deficiency. This deficiency is a genetically heterogeneous disorder caused by deficiency of one of two proteins that serve as intermediates between several acyl-CoA dehydrogenases that are involved in fatty acid β-oxidation or amino acid degradation, and the mitochondrial respiratory chain. This disorder can also be classified as an organic aciduria and is also called glutaric aciduria type II because glutaric acid is often the principal metabolite observed on urinary organic acid analysis (see "Specialized Biochemical Testing"). Some forms of this disorder are associated with dysmorphic features (see "Dysmorphic Syndromes").

PEROXISOMAL DISORDERS

Several of the peroxisomal disorders cause significant hepatocellular disease in the neonatal period. These syndromes can also produce dysmorphic manifestations and are discussed later.

RESPIRATORY CHAIN DEFECTS

Several respiratory chain defects are associated with hepatocellular disease, but there is no simple rule for predicting which defects cause hepatocellular disease and which do not. The respiratory chain defects that cause hepatic dysfunction in the neonatal period can involve a nuclear-encoded component (nDNA) or a mitochondrial-encoded component (mtDNA) of the respiratory chain (see "Lactic Acidemia"). Respiratory chain defects may be manifested as isolated hepatopathies, in which generalized hepatic dysfunction is the main feature, or as highly diverse multisystem disease, in which hepatic dysfunction occurs with encephalopathy, cardiomyopathy, skeletal myopathy, renal tubular dysfunction, or hematologic abnormalities (see "Lactic Acidemia").[15,88]

A particular group of nuclear-encoded defects has received increasing attention as a cause of hepatic dysfunction—the mitochondrial DNA depletion syndromes.[53,76,80] This is a group of autosomal recessive disorders characterized by reduced mtDNA copy number. Several nuclear genes have been identified as the cause of these disorders including two genes that encode for proteins involved in the mitochondrial nucleotide salvage pathway, deoxyyguanosine kinase (DGUOK) and thymidine kinase (TK2), or mitochondrial DNA replication, polymerase γ (POLG), or encode for an inner mitochondrial membrane protein (MPV17). DGUOK, POLG, and MPV17 mutations have been identified as a cause of neonatal liver disease. In some cases, the patients also had encephalopathy. Mutations in the TK2 gene are associated with severe neonatal skeletal myopathy rather than liver dysfunction. The relative contribution of the mitochondrial depletion syndromes to neonatal liver disease, as well as other phenotypes, remains to be established.

OTHER DISORDERS

Three disorders must be considered in the miscellaneous category of inborn errors of metabolism that cause hepatic dysfunction in the newborn period: congenital disorders of glycosylation (CDG), glycogen storage disease type IV, and Niemann-Pick disease type C. The CDG syndromes are discussed under "Dysmorphic Syndromes". Another disorder, neonatal hemochromatosis, can produce severe liver dysfunction, but is not understood to be an inborn error of metabolism.

Glycogen storage disease type IV is a rare disorder that can cause isolated hepatic dysfunction. Niemann-Pick disease type C is a disorder of intracellular cholesterol trafficking that generally causes benign transient neonatal jaundice although it occasionally causes fulminant hepatic failure. The disease subsequently manifests in adolescence or adulthood as a progressive neurodegenerative disorder.

Hepatomegaly and Splenomegaly

Several inborn errors of metabolism are associated with hepatomegaly in the newborn period. In many of these disorders, liver enlargement develops as a result of primary hepatocellular disease. Another group of disorders, the lysosomal storage disorders, result in hepatomegaly because of excessive storage of incompletely metabolized macromolecules in the liver.

Lysosomes contain a large number of enzymes involved in degrading macromolecules. In the absence of one or more of these enzymes, the macromolecules are only partially degraded. Depending on the origin and nature of the macromolecules, the partially degraded products accumulate in one or more tissues or organs and produce a range of clinical phenotypes. The lysosomal storage disorders can be classified according to the types of macromolecules that accumulate in the lysosome: glycogen, glycolipids or other complex lipids, mucopolysaccharides, or oligosaccharides (Table 50-6). Another group of lysosomal storage diseases is associated with defects of lysosomal transport (e.g., cystinosis), but these disorders generally do not manifest in the neonatal period.

Several lysosomal storage disorders manifest in the neonatal period and should be considered in the differential diagnosis of patients who present with hepatomegaly, with or without other signs of storage disease (see Table 50-6).[11,89] Type II glycogen storage disease (Pompe disease) is the only glycogen storage disease caused by a defect in a lysosomal enzyme, but it generally is associated with hypotonia or cardiomyopathy rather than hepatomegaly (see "Cardiomegaly and Cardiomyopathy"). Other glycogenoses, such as glycogen storage disease types I, III, IV, and VI, may be associated with hepatomegaly and, especially in the case of type I disease (von Gierke disease), with hypoglycemia.

TABLE 50-6   Lysosomal Storage Disorders in Neonates

Category of Disorder	Substrate	Disorders
Glycogenoses	Glycogen	GSD type II (Pompe disease) GSD type IV
Lipidoses	Glycolipids or other complex lipids	Farber disease G_{M1}-gangliosidosis Gaucher disease Krabbe disease Niemann-Pick disease Wolman disease
Mucopolysaccharidoses	Mucopolysaccharides	β-Glucuronidase deficiency
Oligosaccharidoses	Glycoproteins Glycolipids	Fucosidosis I-cell disease Sialidosis

GSD, glycogen storage disease.

Several glycolipidoses or related disorders of complex lipid catabolism can manifest with hepatomegaly or splenomegaly in the newborn period.[11,89] Farber disease is an untreatable autosomal recessive defect of acid ceramidase. There are different clinical forms of this disorder, and patients can have joint swelling and pain, hoarseness, disturbance in swallowing, macular cherry-red spots, or central nervous system (CNS) dysfunction. An acute neuronopathic form of Gaucher disease results in hepatosplenomegaly during the first months of life. In these patients, the characteristic neurologic picture includes trismus, strabismus, and retroflexion of the head, followed by inexorable neurologic deterioration. This autosomal recessive disorder is caused by a deficiency of glucosylceramidase. Niemann-Pick disease (i.e., sphingomyelinase deficiency) can begin at birth with hepatosplenomegaly and progress with failure to thrive, psychomotor retardation, pulmonary infiltrates, macular cherry-red spots, and early death. One of the most striking of these disorders is Wolman disease, which is characterized by hepatomegaly, abdominal distention, vomiting, diarrhea, anemia, failure to thrive, and adrenal calcifications. This disorder, caused by lysosomal acid lipase deficiency, invariably leads to early death.

β-Glucuronidase deficiency (i.e., mucopolysaccharidosis type VII) occasionally manifests in the neonatal period, although it usually begins later. It occurs rarely with hydrops fetalis in addition to the more common signs of a mucopolysaccharidosis: hepatosplenomegaly, inguinal or umbilical hernias, skeletal dysplasia, corneal clouding, and coarse facial features.

Four oligosaccharidoses are manifested in the neonatal period. I-Cell disease is characterized by coarse facies and disproportionate craniofacial features, limitation of joint movement, hepatosplenomegaly, corneal clouding, and gingival hypertrophy. Severe forms of fucosidosis, galactosialidosis, and sialidosis may have a similar manifestation. Patients with these defects of mucopolysaccharide or oligosaccharide catabolism might also present with hydrops fetalis.

Two other lysosomal storage disorders can manifest in the neonatal period, but neither is associated with hepatomegaly

in the first month of life. Patients with the infantile form of G_{M1}-gangliosidosis (i.e., β-galactosidase deficiency) have psychomotor delay and coarse facial features but do not develop hepatomegaly until later in the first year of life. These patients might also have cherry-red spots.[66] Rarely, Krabbe disease (i.e., galactosylceramidase deficiency) begins in the neonatal period with progressive psychomotor retardation, but hepatomegaly does not develop in affected patients.

Preliminary clinical assessment of a patient with a suspected lysosomal storage disease should include a careful eye examination to detect corneal clouding, cataracts, or abnormal retinal pigment changes; a cardiac evaluation, including an electrocardiogram and echocardiogram; a peripheral blood smear to detect leukocyte inclusions; and a radiologic study of the skeleton for identification of dysostosis multiplex. Leukocyte inclusions are characteristic of the oligosaccharidoses (i.e., fucosidosis, I-cell disease, α-mannosidosis, and sialidosis), are the exception in the glycolipidoses (e.g., Niemann-Pick disease), and are not found in glycogen storage disease type II. Laboratory evaluation of lysosomal disorders is presented in "Specialized Biochemical Testing".

Other than supportive care, organ transplantation appears to offer the only possibility for definitive treatment for lysosomal storage disorders. Bone marrow transplantation, and possibly cord blood transplantation, can arrest or even reverse some of the somatic disease and neurologic degeneration associated with some of these disorders.[61,89]

Sepsis

A newborn infant with a metabolic disease may be at greater risk for sepsis than other neonates, and the presence of documented sepsis does not exclude the possibility of an underlying metabolic disorder. Several inborn errors of metabolism predispose the newborn infant to infections. The best-documented of these associations is the risk of *E. coli* infection in patients with galactosemia. Infections with other bacteria can also develop, but an *E. coli* infection is relatively specific. The diagnosis of galactosemia should be suspected in all neonates with *E. coli* sepsis, and these infants might need a galactose-free formula until the diagnosis has been excluded.

Unusual Odor

Several inborn errors of metabolism are characterized by unusual odors (Table 50-7). In many of these disorders, the odor is an inconstant finding and can be detected only during episodes of acute metabolic decompensation. In some cases, the odor is difficult to appreciate during a bedside examination and can more easily be detected by smelling a urine specimen that has been kept at room temperature for several hours or a paper sheet that has been stained with urine and air dried.

Dysmorphic Syndromes

Newborn infants with inborn errors of metabolism usually are not dysmorphic, and therefore metabolic evaluations of dysmorphic patients are not likely to be fruitful (see Chapter 29). However, many inborn errors of metabolism cause dysmorphic syndromes. Most of these disorders affect large-molecule metabolism or organelle biogenesis and function, but increasing numbers of inborn errors of small-molecule metabolism are being identified that also produce dysmorphic syndromes.

DEFECTS IN LARGE-MOLECULE METABOLISM

Two groups of inborn errors of large-molecule metabolism produce dysmorphic syndromes: defects of glycoconjugate biosynthesis and the lysosomal storage disorders (Table 50-8). The defects of glycoconjugate biosynthesis are commonly referred to as the congenital disorders of glycosylation syndromes. From a pathogenetic perspective, the CDG syndromes represent the mirror image of the lysosomal storage disorders. The CDG syndromes are the consequence of enzyme deficiencies that impair the biosynthesis of glycoconjugates, whereas the lysosomal storage disorders are primarily the consequence of enzyme deficiencies that impair the biodegradation of glycoconjugates.

Congenital Disorders of Glycosylation

The CDG are a highly pleiotropic group of disorders, which are caused by genetic deficiencies in the biosynthesis of glycoconjugates. The prototypic form of this disorder, which is now referred to as *CDG type Ia* (CDG-Ia), has a characteristic pattern of dysmorphism plus multisystem disease.[36,48] Most patients with this form of CDG present in the neonatal period or in early infancy with neurologic abnormalities, including strabismus or other eye movement abnormalities, hypotonia, ataxia, and with time, developmental delay. Other problems at presentation can include failure to thrive (usually attributed to poor feeding, vomiting, or diarrhea), cardiac problems (cardiomegaly, cardiomyopathy, or pericardial effusion), hepatomegaly (associated with mild elevations in liver enzyme values and hypoalbuminemia), proteinuria, skeletal anomalies, and recurrent infections, especially of the pulmonary tree.

The dysmorphism characteristically associated with this disorder includes an abnormal pattern of fat distribution, with an especially prominent fat pad in the buttocks, doughy skin texture, and inverted nipples. This pattern of dysmorphism can be recognized in the neonatal period.

Cranial imaging demonstrates cerebellar or olivopontocerebellar hypoplasia and a milder degree of cerebral hypoplasia. Microscopic examination of liver biopsy specimens reveals a characteristic form of fibrosis, whereas ultrastructural studies demonstrate a characteristic pattern of lysosomal inclusions and changes in the endoplasmic reticulum.

About 20% of patients with neonatal onset of the disease die in the first year of life as a result of cardiac failure, liver failure, or infection. Those who survive the first year of life manifest severe mental retardation, ataxia, peripheral neuropathy, retinal pigmentary degeneration, and skeletal dysplasia.

The characteristic biochemical marker of this disease is a generalized abnormality of glycosylation of circulating and cell membrane glycoproteins. The diagnosis of CDG-Ia is made by isoelectric focusing of transferrin, a circulating glycoprotein that contains two carbohydrate side-chains attached by N-glycosidic linkage to the peptide backbone of the protein. Patients with CDG type Ia show an immunoisoelectric focusing pattern consistent with underglycosylation. The underlying cause of this syndrome is an autosomal recessive defect in phosphomannomutase, which is one of the enzymes required for biosynthesis of mannose-containing glycoconjugates. There is no effective treatment for type Ia disease.

Approximately two dozen forms of CDG have been described since type Ia was identified and the transferrin immunoisoelectric focusing analysis was developed.[36,48] The immunoisoelectric focusing test has provided a useful method for identifying additional forms of CDG with a remarkable range of clinical phenotypes. For example, CDG-Ib is one of the most distinctive of these variants, because it manifests with hepatic and intestinal problems rather than neurologic problems. This variant produces hypoglycemia, protein-losing enteropathy, failure to thrive, vomiting, diarrhea, hepatomegaly and hepatic dysfunction associated with congenital hepatic fibrosis, and thrombosis or an increased bleeding tendency. Type Ib is caused by deficiency of another enzyme involved in mannose metabolism, phosphomannose isomerase. Unlike the situation for CDG-Ia, patients with CDG-Ib can be treated effectively with oral mannose supplementation. The clinical problems of several patients with type Ib disease have been reversed with this form of therapy. The other CDG disorders are primarily neurologic disorders associated

TABLE 50–7	Characteristic Odors of Several Neonatal Inborn Errors of Metabolism	
Disorder	**Nature of Odor**
Isovaleric acidemia	Sweaty feet
Maple syrup urine disease	Maple syrup
β-Methylcrotonyl-CoA carboxylase deficiency	Male cat urine
Multiple acyl-CoA dehydrogenase deficiency (glutaric aciduria type II)	Sweaty feet
Multiple carboxylase deficiency	Male cat urine
Phenylketonuria	Musty

TABLE 50–8   Inborn Errors of Metabolism That Cause Dysmorphic Syndromes

Category of Disorder	Syndrome
Large-Molecule Metabolism	
Disorder of glycoconjugate biosynthesis	Congenital disorders of glycosylation
Lysosomal storage diseases	Glycolipidoses Mucopolysaccharidoses Oligosaccharidoses
Small-Molecule Metabolism	
Cholesterol biosynthesis	Conradi-Hunermann syndrome Desmosterolosis Smith-Lemli-Opitz syndrome
Organic acidurias	3-Hydroxyisobutyryl-CoA deacylase deficiency Mevalonic aciduria* Multiple acyl-CoA dehydrogenase deficiency
Peroxisomal Disorders	
Biogenesis disorders	Chondrodysplasia punctata, rhizomelic type Zellweger syndrome and its variants Infantile Refsum disease Neonatal adrenoleukodystrophy
Single-enzyme defects	Acyl-CoA oxidase deficiency Bifunctional enzyme deficiency Thiolase deficiency

*Mevalonic aciduria has been classified as an organic acidemia on the basis of the method used for its diagnosis, but it can also be classified as a peroxisomal single enzyme disorder or as a defect in cholesterol biosynthesis because of its intracellular location and function, respectively.

with severe developmental delay and mental retardation, but many of them also have distinguishing features.

In addition to the forms of CDG that involve N-linked glycoconjugates, analogous defects in O-linked glycoconjugates have been identified. Patients with these defects cannot be ascertained by the transferrin isoelectric focusing test, because it only detects abnormalities of N-linked glycoconjugates. Several defects in O-linked glycoconjugation have been identified, including Walker-Warburg syndrome (a neuronal migration abnormality associated with malformations of the brain and eye, and congenital muscular dystrophy) and hereditary multiple exostosis (multiple osteochondromas). There is every reason to expect that additional disorders of N-linked and O-linked glycosylation will be identified in the future.

Lysosomal Storage Diseases

Several lysosomal storage disorders begin in the neonatal period with cardiomegaly, characteristic ocular abnormalities, or hepatomegaly (Staretz-Chacham). Many of the patients have dysmorphic features, including coarse facies, macroglossia, and skeletal dysplasia (dysostosis multiplex). At least one mucopolysaccharidosis (β-glucuronidase deficiency), four oligosaccharidoses (fucosidase deficiency, galactosialidosis, I-cell disease, and sialidase deficiency), and one glycolipidosis (G_{M1}-gangliosidosis) begin in this way. The laboratory evaluation of these disorders is presented

under "Tests for Lysosomal Storage Disorders". Definitive diagnosis requires specific enzyme analysis.

DEFECTS IN SMALL-MOLECULE METABOLISM

The inborn errors of small-molecule metabolism that produce dysmorphic syndromes are a highly heterogeneous group of disorders (see Table 50-8). As a class, this group represents disorders of endogenous teratogenesis. The pathogenesis of each disorder appears to be unique. Further study of these disorders should enhance our understanding of the mechanisms of teratogenesis and development in general.

Cholesterol Biosynthesis

Several defects of cholesterol biosynthesis manifest in infancy. The best understood defects of steroid biosynthesis are those that lead to the congenital adrenal hyperplasia syndromes. The most common of these syndromes, 21-hydroxylase deficiency, is associated with dysmorphogenesis (i.e., ambiguous genitalia) and electrolyte imbalances. This class of disorders is discussed more fully in Chapter 49.

Inborn errors of cholesterol biosynthesis include defects in the early steps of the pathway and defects in the late steps. Mevalonic aciduria is caused by a defect in an early step in cholesterol biosynthesis (i.e., mevalonate kinase deficiency) and is discussed in the next section (see "Organic Acidurias").

Smith-Lemli-Opitz (SLO) syndrome is a prominent example of a recognizable malformation disorder that is caused by a defect in a late step in cholesterol biosynthesis.[41,67,95] SLO syndrome was recognized in the 1970s as a highly variable malformation syndrome. In its mild form the disorder is characterized by prenatal and postnatal growth restriction, microcephaly, characteristic craniofacial dysmorphism (including ptosis, low-set ears, epicanthal folds, and micrognathia), strabismus, syndactyly of the second and third toes, hypospadias, and mental retardation. In its most severe form, patients also exhibit postaxial polydactyly, cleft palate, eye malformations, holoprosencephaly, cardiac defects, and, in boys, pseudohermaphroditism ranging from hypospadias to sex reversal. At autopsy, a range of severe malformations of the brain, heart, and kidneys can be identified. The mild phenotypes are designated SLO syndrome type I, and the severe phenotypes are designated SLO syndrome type II; however, the distinction between the two types was arbitrary, and the pathogenetic relationship between the two types was unknown.

In 1994, the genetic basis of SLO syndrome was shown to be a heritable defect in cholesterol biosynthesis.[41,95] Patients were found to have an abnormally low plasma cholesterol concentration and a markedly increased concentration of 7-dehydrocholesterol and, to a lesser degree, 8-dehydrocholesterol in plasma and cultured skin fibroblasts. Further work established the enzymatic basis of this syndrome as an autosomal recessive defect affecting the synthesis of 7-dehydrocholesterol reductase. SLO types I and II appear to be allelic forms of this enzyme deficiency. After recognition of the underlying defect causing the SLO syndrome and development of specific methods for diagnosis, SLO syndrome has been recognized as a relatively common inborn error of metabolism, with a frequency of approximately one case in 20,000 persons.

The diagnosis of SLO syndrome should be investigated in patients with suggestive clinical phenotypes. Because the clinical phenotype is so variable and may be difficult to recognize in female patients without obvious genital anomalies, the diagnosis should also be pursued in patients with low plasma cholesterol concentrations. The diagnosis should also be pursued in patients who have a suggestive clinical phenotype but normal plasma cholesterol concentrations, because many of the methods in standard clinical use for measuring the plasma cholesterol concentration are relatively nonspecific and could yield false-negative results for patients with SLO syndrome. SLO syndrome can be diagnosed more specifically by measuring 7-dehydrocholesterol in plasma or cultured skin fibroblasts using gas chromatography or gas chromatography with mass spectrometry.

Efforts to treat SLO patients with supplemental cholesterol were begun immediately after recognition of the biochemical basis of the disease. Cholesterol supplementation could improve some aspects of the outcome, including the behavioral aspects of the disease, especially when treatment is begun very early in infancy.[41] As expected, the outcome appears to be better for patients with milder forms of the disease than for those with the severe forms (patients with significant defects in prenatal morphogenesis). However, the long-term intellectual outcome of this form of treatment remains poor.

Other defects of cholesterol biosynthesis have been identified subsequent to the discovery of the genetic basis of SLO syndrome, including Conradi-Hunermann syndrome,

the rhizomelic form of chondrodysplasia punctata, lathosterolosis, desmosterolosis, Greenberg skeletal dysplasia, and CHILD (congenital hemidysplasia, ichthyosiform erythroderma, and limb defects) syndrome.[41,67]

Patients with Conradi-Hunermann syndrome have chondrodysplasia punctata and rhizomelic skeletal dysplasia. Chondrodysplasia punctata is a distinctive radiologic finding, which refers to the abnormal pattern of punctate calcification of epiphysial cartilage and related tissues. This finding can be seen in some of the neonatal forms of peroxisomal disease (e.g., Zellweger syndrome) as well as SLO syndrome.

Rhizomelic dysplasia is a pattern of proximal limb shortening that is found in several malformation syndromes. Using the same analytic methods required to diagnose and evaluate patients with SLO syndrome, a previously unrecognized defect in sterol biosynthesis was identified in a fraction of patients with the rhizomelic form of chondrodysplasia punctata and in patients with Conradi-Hunermann syndrome.

Desmosterolosis has an osteosclerotic form of skeletal dysplasia and malformations similar to SLO syndrome. It appears that defects of sterol biosynthesis will prove to be responsible for a family of recognizable malformation syndromes, including many characterized by unusual skeletal dysplasia.

Organic Acidurias

Three organic acidurias (or acidemias) are associated with dysmorphic syndromes: 3-hydroxyisobutyryl-CoA deacylase deficiency, mevalonate kinase deficiency (mevalonic aciduria), and multiple acyl-CoA dehydrogenase deficiency (glutaric aciduria type II).

3-HYDROXYISOBUTYRYL-CoA DEACYLASE DEFICIENCY

3-Hydroxyisobutyryl-CoA deacylase deficiency is a rare disorder that produces craniofacial dysmorphism, vertebral anomalies, tetralogy of Fallot, and agenesis of the corpus callosum.[8] The deficient enzyme plays a role in valine catabolism. In the absence of this enzyme, the precursor of 3-hydroxyisobutyryl-CoA, methacrylyl-CoA, accumulates and is conjugated with cysteine to form two unusual metabolites that are excreted in the urine. This disorder is detected by urinary amino acid analysis, which reveals the unusual cysteine conjugates.

This disorder appears to be caused by intracellular accumulation of methacrylyl-CoA or methacrylate, which is formed by nonenzymatic hydrolysis of methacrylyl-CoA. Methacrylate is a potent teratogen in various animal models. In addition to this defect, several patients with 3-hydroxyisobutyric aciduria did not have deacylase deficiency or another recognizable enzyme deficiency in the valine pathway. The clinical phenotype of these patients was similar to that of the patient with deacylase deficiency, including significant craniofacial and cerebral dysmorphism, which was accompanied in some cases by intracerebral calcifications. Although the underlying defect has not been identified in these patients, the presumption is that a defect in the metabolism of 3-hydroxyisobutyric acid led to the intracellular accumulation of methacrylate or a related teratogen.

MEVALONATE KINASE DEFICIENCY

Mevalonic aciduria is caused by a rare defect, mevalonate kinase deficiency, in an early step in cholesterol biosynthesis.[29] It is classified as an organic aciduria because it is diagnosed by urine organic acid analysis. It can also be classified as a peroxisomal single enzyme disorder because mevalonate kinase is located within the peroxisome (see "Peroxisomal Disorders").

The pathogenesis of this disorder is complex because mevalonic acid has a role in several key pathways. In addition to its role as a precursor of cholesterol, mevalonic acid is a precursor of dolichol, which is required for complex carbohydrate biosynthesis; heme, which plays a key role in oxygen transport; and ubiquinone, a component of the respiratory chain (see "Lactic Acidemia").

Mevalonate kinase deficiency is a highly pleiotropic disorder associated in the newborn period with dysmorphic features (e.g., nonspecific craniofacial anomalies, cataracts), hepatosplenomegaly, lymphadenopathy, diarrhea, hypotonia, and anemia. In severe cases, it leads to profound failure to thrive, developmental delay, and early death. Although the defect would be expected to lead to lactic acidosis because of decreased synthesis of ubiquinone and malfunctioning of the respiratory chain, lactic acidosis is not a common feature of the disorder. The hypocholesterolemia seen in these patients is generally mild. Alternatively, mevalonate kinase deficiency can produce a very different clinical phenotype, hyper IgD syndrome, which is one of the periodic fever disorders. Mevalonic aciduria and hyper IgD syndrome appear to be allelic forms of mevalonate kinase deficiency.

The characteristic diagnostic feature is mevalonic aciduria, which can be documented by urinary organic acid analysis. No effective treatment exists for this disorder, although corticosteroids might be of some benefit.

MULTIPLE ACYL-CoA DEHYDROGENASE DEFICIENCY

Multiple acyl-CoA dehydrogenase deficiency was originally known as glutaric aciduria type II because of the very large urinary excretion of glutaric acid, a product of amino acid catabolism (lysine, hydroxylysine, and tryptophan) (see "Newborn Screening"). The organic acid pattern also shows many other metabolites, and the disorder came to be called multiple acyl-CoA dehydrogenase deficiency when it was recognized that the pattern reflected deficient activity of several flavin-dependent acyl-CoA dehydrogenases. These dehydrogenases are required for amino acid catabolism and fatty acid oxidation. The biochemical defect affects one of two proteins (electron-transfer flavoprotein [ETF] or ETF dehydrogenase) involved in transferring electrons generated by flavin-dependent acyl-CoA dehydrogenases to the respiratory chain.

Multiple acyl-CoA dehydrogenase deficiency is a clinically heterogeneous disorder; the most severe form is associated with metabolic consequences (e.g., acidosis, hypoglycemia, ketosis) and dysmorphic consequences (e.g., craniofacial dysmorphism, polycystic kidneys, cerebral cortical dysplasia, intrahepatic biliary hypoplasia). A less-severe form is associated with similar metabolic consequences but no dysmorphism. The dysmorphic form of the disease is found in some patients with ETF dehydrogenase deficiency, and the nondysmorphic form is associated with ETF deficiency. It is unclear how ETF dehydrogenase deficiency leads to dysmorphism.

Peroxisomal Disorders

Many of the peroxisomal disorders produce dysmorphic syndromes. The peroxisomal disorders are a highly diverse group of disorders, reflecting the metabolic diversity of the enzymes contained within this small organelle.[99] In contrast to the lysosome, which primarily contains a large number of degradative enzymes, the peroxisome contains biosynthetic and catabolic enzymes. Many of these enzymes are involved in unusual oxidation reactions; the name of this organelle was derived from one such reaction involving hydrogen peroxide.

The peroxisomal disorders are classified into two groups: defects of peroxisome biogenesis and defects affecting a single enzyme (see Table 50-8; see "Test for Peroxisomal Disorders").[99]

BIOGENESIS DISORDERS

The first group consists of disorders associated with absent or severely reduced numbers of peroxisomes and multiple enzyme deficiencies. These disorders are caused by defects in peroxisomal biogenesis, which lead to impaired import of proteins and enzymes into the peroxisome.[54] The paradigm of this group of disorders is Zellweger syndrome, an autosomal recessive trait characterized by craniofacial dysmorphism, severe psychomotor retardation, renal cortical cysts, epiphyseal stippling, failure to thrive, and early death. Epiphyseal stippling is an unusual radiographic finding of ectopic calcification found most characteristically in the ankle, patella, vertebrae, hips, and trachea (see "Cholesterol Biosynthesis" earlier). Other peroxisomal assembly disorders include neonatal adrenoleukodystrophy, infantile Refsum disease, and rhizomelic chondrodysplasia punctata.

Genetic studies have identified approximately 20 different genetic loci associated with peroxisomal biogenesis defects. Genetic complementation studies have shown that Zellweger syndrome, neonatal adrenoleukodystrophy, and infantile Refsum disease represent allelic variants at many of these loci. Zellweger syndrome is the most severe variant, and infantile Refsum disease is the least severe variant. There is no cure or effective treatment for this group of disorders.

Rhizomelic chondrodysplasia punctata is the consequence of mutations at one of the other loci involved in peroxisomal biogenesis. Peroxisomal deficiencies have been found only in the rhizomelic form of chondrodysplasia punctata, which is an autosomal recessive disorder characterized by severe shortening of the proximal extremities (hence the term *rhizomelic*), craniofacial dysmorphism, congenital cataracts, joint contractures, and severe psychomotor retardation. The skeletal abnormalities of this form of dwarfism are evident in the neonatal period. There is no treatment for this disorder.

SINGLE-ENZYME DEFECTS

The second group of peroxisomal disorders includes defects associated with a normal number of peroxisomes and a single enzyme deficiency. The best-known disorder in this group is X-linked adrenoleukodystrophy, which does not produce dysmorphism and does not manifest in the neonatal period, and it therefore is not discussed further. However, several other peroxisomal monoenzymopathies with onset in the neonatal period have been recognized.[99] Several of these disorders have been identified in patients who appear to have the physical stigmata of Zellweger syndrome or its variants but have normal numbers of peroxisomes. The best characterized of these disorders are acyl-CoA oxidase deficiency, bifunctional enzyme deficiency, and thiolase deficiency. These three enzymes share a common biochemical role in peroxisomal (rather than mitochondrial) fatty acid oxidation and bile acid biosynthesis. The predominantly dysmorphic abnormalities and many of the laboratory abnormalities associated with Zellweger syndrome and its variants therefore can be attributed to abnormal fatty acid metabolism or abnormal bile acid metabolism. Similarly, defects affecting the enzymes that catalyze plasmalogen biosynthesis produce a clinical phenotype that resembles rhizomelic chondrodysplasia punctata.

Several other single-enzyme deficiencies have been described that do not involve the peroxisomal pathways of fatty acid oxidation or plasmalogen biosynthesis. One of these disorders, mevalonic aciduria, is a defect in cholesterol biosynthesis and is described under "Organic Acidurias."

VITAMIN K METABOLISM

Vitamin K epoxide reductase deficiency is an autosomal recessive disorder that produces a phenocopy of the fetal warfarin embryopathy syndrome.[63] The enzyme deficiency is characterized by persistent coagulopathy, stippled epiphyses, nasal hypoplasia, brachydactyly with distal digital hypoplasia, and conductive hearing loss. Vitamin K epoxide reductase is the site of warfarin's pharmacologic action. The various dysmorphic features of fetal warfarin syndrome and vitamin K epoxide reductase deficiency are consequences of impaired activity of the vitamin K-mediated carboxylation reactions, which include proteins of the bone matrix and circulating coagulation factors. Vitamin K supplementation is an effective therapy for the coagulopathy associated with this disorder but might not be effective for the other manifestations because of their prenatal onset.

THE ABNORMAL NEWBORN INFANT: LABORATORY PHENOTYPES
Biochemical Testing

The laboratory evaluation plays a key role in the differential diagnosis of the metabolic disorders of infancy. The laboratory investigation of these patients should be staged. It should begin with broadly focused screening tests, which are then followed by more specialized examinations. Laboratory findings helpful in the differential diagnosis of suspected metabolic disease are listed in Table 50-9. A complete discussion of each of these findings is provided in the next section.

SCREENING STUDIES

The precise composition of the metabolic screen varies from one institution to another. There should be, however, a core of tests available at all institutions that care for sick neonates.[2,11] A suggested list of tests is presented in Table 50-10. These laboratory tests are chosen because they provide a relatively rapid, inexpensive evaluation for a wide range of disorders. It is strongly recommended that the specific details of collection and handling of all samples be clearly understood before samples are obtained and that there be collaboration with laboratory personnel throughout the process.

Blood Studies

A number of blood studies are indicated, many of which are routinely performed during the care of sick neonates. The complete blood cell count should include examination of cell morphology and a differential cell count. Neutropenia and thrombocytopenia may be associated with a number of the organic

TABLE 50–9	Laboratory Findings Helpful in the Differential Diagnosis of Suspected Metabolic Disease in Neonates	
Finding	**Diagnostic Considerations**
Acidosis (see Figs. 50-1 and 50-2)	Fatty acid oxidation defects Gluconeogenesis defects Glycogen storage diseases Ketogenesis defects Ketolytic defects Krebs cycle defects Organic acidemias Respiratory chain defects
Alkalosis: respiratory	Urea cycle defects
Alkalosis: metabolic	Steroid biosynthetic defects
Hepatic dysfunction (see Table 50-5)	Amino acid defects Bile acid biosynthesis defects Carbohydrate defects Fatty acid oxidation defects Peroxisomal disorders Respiratory chain defects Other
Hyperammonemia (see Box 50-2 and Fig. 50-4)	Amino acid disorders Fatty acid oxidation defects Organic acidemias Urea cycle defects
Hypoglycemia (see Table 50-17 and Fig. 50-3)	Fatty acid oxidation defects Gluconeogenesis defects Glycogen storage disease Ketogenesis defects Organic acidemias
Ketosis/ketonuria	Amino acid defects Gluconeogenic defects Glycogen storage diseases Ketolytic defects Organic acidemias
Pancytopenia	Organic acidemias Respiratory chain defects
Proximal renal tubular dysfunction (see Table 50-14)	Amino acid defects Carbohydrate defects Respiratory chain defects

acidemias, including isovaleric acidemia, methylmalonic acidemia, and propionic acidemia (see "Hematologic Abnormalities").[40] Neutropenia may be found with glycogen storage disease type Ib, an uncommon variant of glucose-6-phosphatase deficiency.[96] This variant is caused by a defect of the glucose-6-phosphate translocase associated with the phosphatase rather than the phosphatase itself (see "Hypoglycemia"). Barth syndrome can also be a cause of neonatal neutropenia (see "Cardiomegaly and Cardiomyopathy").[5] Pearson syndrome, a respiratory chain defect, can cause pancytopenia (see "Lactic Acidemia"). Megaloblastosis may be found in disorders of purine biosynthesis, such as some rare forms of homocystinuria or orotic aciduria.

TABLE 50–10	Initial Laboratory Screening of Neonates with Suspected Metabolic Disease
Body Fluid	**Laboratory Studies**
Blood	Blood cell count
	Electrolytes
	Blood gases
	Lactate and pyruvate
	Glucose
	Ketones (β-hydroxybutyrate and acetoacetate)
	Ammonia
	Uric acid
Urine	Smell
	Crystalluria
	Reducing substances
	pH
	Acetone
	α-Ketoacids (diphenylhydrazone)
	Ferric chloride
Cerebrospinal fluid	Glucose
	Lactate and pyruvate

Electrolytes and blood gases are required to determine whether acidosis or alkalosis exists and, if so, whether the abnormality is associated with an increased anion gap. Lactate and pyruvate analysis should be measured to identify the nature of any excess anions (see "Lactate and Pyruvate Analysis"). Lactic acidemia may be present without frank acidosis.

Hypoglycemia is a frequent finding in sick neonates, especially premature infants, but is also a critical finding in some metabolic disorders. Hypoglycemia should be investigated further when it is severe, when accompanied by other signs of metabolic disease, or when it proves refractory to conventional therapy.

Ketones (i.e., β-hydroxybutyrate and acetoacetate) are useful in developing a differential diagnosis for newborns with hypoglycemia. In particular, nonketotic or hypoketotic hypoglycemia is the hallmark of defects of fatty acid oxidation.

The blood ammonia concentration should be determined in all neonates with evidence of unexplained lethargy and neurologic intoxication. Early recognition of the congenital hyperammonemias is crucial because they are a rapidly progressive group of disorders that can quickly lead to irreversible damage after hours rather than days. Effective treatment is available for many of these disorders, but it must be instituted early in the course of the disease.

A blood uric acid test is a convenient screen for the few inborn errors of metabolism that are associated with hypouricemia or hyperuricemia. Type I glycogen storage disease is probably the most common inherited disorder associated with hyperuricemia (see "Hypoglycemia"), whereas xanthine dehydrogenase deficiency caused by molybdenum cofactor deficiency causes hypouricemia (see "The Sick Newborn Infant").

Urine Studies

A urine sample should be sent for metabolic screening using simple colorimetric agents or strips, if such testing is still available at one's institution (Table 50-11).[2,11] However, this approach to testing has been abandoned or replaced by more specialized forms of testing in most institutions, and it is no longer possible to obtain. In this event, a urine specimen should be sent directly for the more specialized testing. In any event, an aliquot of urine should be collected, covered, and set aside by the infant's incubator when possible. After a few hours at room temperature, the specimen should be smelled for evidence of an unusual odor. Several inborn errors of metabolism, especially the organic acidurias, are associated with characteristic odors (see Table 50-7).

Urine specimens should be tested for reducing substances, which include principally the monosaccharides (i.e., simple sugar molecules). The Clinitest reaction detects excess excretion of galactose and glucose but not fructose. False-positive reactions are found with ampicillin and related penicillin derivatives and with some other drugs that are excreted as their glucuronide conjugates. A specimen that shows a positive reaction with the Clinitest reaction should be investigated further by means of the Clinistix reaction (i.e., glucose oxidase), which is specific for the monosaccharide glucose. A specimen with positive Clinitest and negative Clinistix results should be analyzed specifically for galactose.

The urine pH should be determined in order to characterize the renal response to an alteration in blood pH. In the face of a significant acidemia, the kidneys should produce an acidic urine (pH less than 5). A renal acidification disorder should be considered in the absence of an appropriate urine pH.

Spot tests may be used to detect excessive urinary excretion of ketones, α-ketoacids, or other metabolites. Ketonuria should be investigated, especially in patients with hypoglycemia. The Acetest or Ketostix reactions are used for acetone and acetoacetate, and the 2,4-dinitrophenylhydrazone (DNP) reaction is used for α-ketoacids.

TABLE 50–11	Characteristic Urinary Findings in Inborn Errors of Metabolism
Finding	**Disorder**
Reducing substance	Hereditary fructose intolerance
	Galactosemia
	Hereditary tyrosinemia
Acetonuria	Organic acidemias
DNP (α-ketoacids)	Maple syrup urine disease
	Phenylketonuria
	Tyrosinemia type I
Ferric chloride	Phenylketonuria
	Tyrosinemia type I
Nitrosonaphthol	Tyrosinemia type I
p-Nitroaniline	Methylmalonic acidemia
Sulfitest	Sulfite oxidase deficiency

DNP, 2,4-dinitrophenylhydrazone.

The ferric chloride reaction is also a useful test, although it is relatively insensitive and subject to potentially misleading false-positive reactions with several drugs. It is helpful when used in conjunction with other screening studies, such as in detecting PKU and tyrosinemia.

Several other screening studies are recommended for use in special circumstances. These studies include the nitrosonaphthol reaction, which detects certain tyrosine metabolites; the *p*-nitroaniline reaction, which is relatively specific for methylmalonic aciduria; and the Sulfitest, which detects excess sulfite excretion in patients with sulfite oxidase deficiency.

Cerebrospinal Fluid Studies

Many sick infants undergo lumbar puncture for CSF analysis as part of a sepsis evaluation. In addition to obtaining the standard samples for CSF glucose and protein analysis, additional samples for more specialized testing, such as lactate and pyruvate analysis or amino acid analysis, should also be obtained if clinically indicated. When possible, appropriate blood samples should be collected at the same time as the lumbar puncture is performed to permit comparison of blood and CSF concentrations. For example, concurrent plasma and CSF glycine measurements are required for the diagnosis of nonketotic hyperglycinemia (see "The Sick Newborn Infant").

SPECIALIZED BIOCHEMICAL TESTING

Screening studies help determine whether further metabolic testing is indicated and, if so, what testing should be done next (Table 50-12). In general, the more specialized tests require relatively sophisticated equipment and personnel to perform and interpret, take longer to perform (sometimes days to weeks), are more expensive, and are usually available in only a few centers. All physicians who might care for a sick neonate with a suspected inborn error of metabolism should develop their own referral system for patients with various metabolic abnormalities. It is a good idea to set up a referral system in advance of a specific emergency so that appropriate referral can be obtained more easily when the time comes.

Because not all patients require transfer or tolerate transfer to a tertiary care center, plans should also be on hand for collecting samples for various specialized tests. It is truly unfortunate when the often extraordinary and well-intentioned efforts of those caring for a sick newborn infant are subverted by improper collection or handling of samples. Detailed requirements for collection and handling of samples for various metabolic analysis should be available in the nursery, and they should be kept in a place where they can be found in an emergency.

The distinction between a screening study and a specialized follow-up test is not always clear. In some circumstances, the physician would proceed directly to performing a specialized study. For example, a urinary organic acid analysis should be performed as soon as a neonate is thought to have a metabolic acidosis or has an unusual odor typical of one of the neonatal organic acid disorders. Similarly, it is generally best to perform some of the specialized studies during an episode of acute metabolic decompensation, such as hypoglycemia, when they are most

TABLE 50–12	Specialized Laboratory Tests That May Be Required for the Care of Neonates with Suspected Metabolic Disease
Body Fluid or Tissue	**Laboratory Tests**
Blood	Amino acids
	Carnitine (total, free, and acylcarnitine profile)
	Lactate and pyruvate
	Tests for congenital disorders of glycosylation:
	Transferrin immunoelectrophoresis or mass spectrometry
	Tests for peroxisomal disorders:
	Very-long-chain fatty acids
	Phytanic acid
Urine	Amino acids
	Carnitine (total, free, and acylcarnitine profile)
	Organic acids
	Tests for lysosomal storage disorders:
	Glycolipids
	Mucopolysaccharides
	Oligosaccharides
Cerebrospinal fluid	Amino acids
	Lactate and pyruvate
Other	
Cultured skin fibroblasts	Enzyme studies
	Genetic studies
	Metabolite analysis
White blood cells	Enzyme studies
	Genetic studies

likely to be informative, rather than waiting until the results of the screening tests become available. As a rule, the sequence of ordering tests should be compressed in an acutely ill patient.

Amino Acid Analysis

The most commonly performed of the specialized studies is probably quantitative plasma and urinary amino acid analysis.[2,10,11] Some laboratories provide a qualitative amino acid screening study performed by paper or thin-layer chromatography as part of their screening protocol. Although this study may be useful, it does not substitute for a quantitative determination when the clinical findings suggest a disorder that is reflected in an abnormal amino acid pattern (Table 50-13). In most cases, a complete quantitative analysis is required, whereas in other situations, specific amino acids should be the focus of attention.

It is important to provide the laboratory performing the quantitative analysis with all relevant clinical and laboratory data so that it can focus on specific amino acids as needed.

TABLE 50–13	Neonatal-Onset Inborn Errors of Metabolism Characterized by Abnormal Plasma Amino Acid Patterns
Disorder	**Finding**
Amino Acid Disorders	
Maple syrup urine disease	↑Isoleucine, leucine, valine
Nonketotic hyperglycinemia*	↑Glycine
Phenylketonuria	↑Phenylalanine
Sulfite oxidase deficiency	↑S-Sulfocysteine
Hereditary tyrosinemia	↑Tyrosine, methionine
Lactic Acid Disorders	
Respiratory chain defects	↑Alanine (± proline)
PC deficiency	↑Alanine, citrulline, lysine
Organic Acidemias	
Methylmalonic acidemia	↑Glycine
Isovaleric acidemia	↑Glycine
Propionic acidemia	↑Glycine
Urea Cycle Disorders	
Urea cycle defects	↑Glutamine, ↓arginine, plus . . .
Argininosuccinic aciduria†	↑ASA, ↓citrulline
Citrullinemia	↑↑Citrulline
CPS and OTC deficiency	↓Citrulline

*Glycine concentrations are elevated in plasma and, to an even greater extent, in the cerebrospinal fluid.
†ASA is present in very large amounts in urine but is only marginally increased in plasma because of efficient renal clearance.
ASA, argininosuccinic acid (including its two anhydrides); CPS, carbamyl phosphate synthetase; OTC, ornithine transcarbamylase; PC, pyruvate carboxylase; ↑, increased; ↑↑ very increased; ↓, decreased; ±, with or without ↑.

For example, when evaluating a patient with hyperammonemia, it is important to inform the laboratory personnel so that they will look for argininosuccinic acid and its anhydrides; otherwise, these metabolites could be overlooked or misinterpreted. This recommendation to inform the laboratory of the clinical context of the investigation applies equally to the other specialized studies discussed here.

Quantitative amino acid analysis of CSF is not indicated as a rule, but it should be performed when appropriate, such as in the context of a hypotonic newborn infant who has seizures and an elevated plasma glycine level that is not accompanied by acidosis or ketosis. These findings suggest the diagnosis of nonketotic hyperglycinemia (see "The Sick Newborn Infant"). The plasma glycine level may be only minimally elevated in some patients with nonketotic hyperglycinemia. The biochemical hallmark of this disorder is an elevated ratio of CSF glycine to plasma glycine.

Carnitine Analysis

Plasma and urinary carnitine analysis is indicated for patients who show evidence of unexplained acidosis, hyperammonemia, hypoglycemia, or ketonuria when there might be a disorder accompanied by an abnormal organic aciduria, defect in fatty acid oxidation, or respiratory chain defect. In these settings, carnitine insufficiency or frank carnitine deficiency can develop.

Many of the organic acidurias or fatty acid oxidation defects are associated with overproduction of intracellular acyl-CoAs (i.e., CoA esters of an acid molecule). As they accumulate, these acyl-CoAs are transesterified with free carnitine to form acylcarnitines and free CoA. Many of these acylcarnitines then leave the cell, circulate in the bloodstream, and are ultimately excreted in the urine. If the production of a particular acyl-CoA is very large, comparably large amounts of the corresponding acylcarnitines are excreted in the urine, resulting initially in intracellular carnitine insufficiency and ultimately in carnitine deficiency (i.e., secondary carnitine deficiency). Abnormal acylcarnitines can also inhibit renal reabsorption of carnitine. Carnitine analysis should be performed whenever possible on samples of plasma and urine obtained concurrently.

Carnitine analysis should include measurement of total carnitine, free carnitine, total acylcarnitines, as well as the individual acylcarnitine profile. Measurement of total carnitine, free carnitine, and total acylcarnitines will help determine whether the patient has carnitine insufficiency or deficiency, while a quantitative acylcarnitine profile will help identify which, if any, acyl-CoA are accumulating, and hence identify the locus of the patient's metabolic defect.

Lactate and Pyruvate Analysis

Blood lactate analysis is indicated when acidosis or an increased anion gap is found, and it is used to investigate the possibility of a defect in carbohydrate metabolism, fatty acid oxidation, organic acid metabolism, or the respiratory chain (see Lactic Acidemia).[2,11] Lactate should also be measured in patients who have skeletal myopathy, cardiomyopathy, encephalopathy, retinal pigmentary deposits, neutropenia, or thrombocytopenia and in patients with hypoglycemia or ketosis even if they do not have frank acidosis. Many inborn errors of metabolism result in lactic acidemia without lactic acidosis.

When possible, the concentration of lactate and pyruvate should both be determined. These metabolites should be measured concurrently in blood and CSF, when a lumbar puncture is being performed for other reasons or the patient's presentation suggests the possibility of a CNS-specific defect. Measuring CSF lactate and pyruvate concentrations does not generally add useful information when the blood lactate and pyruvate concentrations have already been found to be elevated. Lactic acid is the reduction product of pyruvic acid. The lactate-to-pyruvate (L:P) ratio is a useful measure of the intracellular redox potential and is useful in approaching the differential diagnosis of the lactic acidemias (see Lactic Acidemia). Lactic acidemia and pyruvic acidemia are often accompanied by lactic aciduria and pyruvic aciduria, which can be detected, but poorly quantitated, by urinary organic acid analysis.

The significance of the finding of lactic acidemia can be investigated further by reviewing a quantitative plasma amino acid analysis for evidence of an increased alanine concentration, because alanine is the transamination product of pyruvate. The evaluation for lactic acidemia should include measurement of lactate, pyruvate, and alanine.

Urine Organic Acid Analysis

Urinary organic acid analysis was originally used to document defects in amino acid metabolism distal to the removal of the amino group from the amino acid. As currently performed, urinary organic acid analysis detects and quantitates a large number of metabolites that represent intermediates of carbohydrate and fatty acid oxidation, as well as those of amino acid catabolism.[2,10,11] Accordingly, urinary organic acid analysis is a highly useful study and is performed in a wide variety of clinical contexts. Urinary organic acid analysis is indicated for patients who have unexplained acidosis, lactic acidemia, hyperammonemia, hypoglycemia, or ketonuria.

A partial list of the organic acidurias with onset in the neonatal period is presented in Box 50-1. The organic acid disorders are called *-emias* or *-urias* for historical reasons. In most cases, abnormal metabolites accumulate in blood and urine in these disorders, and the terms *organic acidemia* and *organic aciduria* are used interchangeably in this chapter. Isovaleric acidemia, methylmalonic acidemia, and propionic acidemia appear to be the most common of the organic acid disorders that appear in the newborn period. The incidence of the organic acidemias that are detected by MS/MS newborn screening differs from the incidence of disorders that appear in the newborn period. Urinary organic acid analysis is generally performed by gas-liquid chromatography or, with increasing incidence, by combined gas-liquid chromatography and mass spectrometry.

Tests for Congenital Disorders of Glycosylation

The possibility of a CDG syndrome should be suspected in a newborn infant with the characteristic dysmorphism of CDG-Ia (e.g., abnormal fat pads of the buttocks and inner thighs, orange peel skin, inverted nipples) or a child with pericardial effusion or cardiomyopathy, hepatomegaly, diarrhea, an increased bleeding tendency or thrombosis, or neurologic abnormalities (e.g., strabismus, hypotonia, developmental delay). Several clinical forms of CDG syndrome have been described, each having a different genetic basis. Fortunately, most of the disorders described can be diagnosed using the transferrin immunoisoelectric focusing assay or the mass spectrometric adaption of this method to identify patients with an abnormal pattern of glycosylation.[36,48] Patients found to have a positive test result will require further testing to determine their particular disorder.

Tests for Lysosomal Storage Disorders

Patients with coarse facial features, corneal clouding, cataracts, hepatomegaly, or dysostosis multiplex should be evaluated for a possible lysosomal storage disorder. Urine screening tests are available for quantitation of total mucopolysaccharides. The test results should be interpreted with caution since many of the tests have significant false-positive and false-negative rates. If the quantitative mucopolysaccharide screening test result is positive, chromatographic separation and identification of the individual mucopolysaccharides should be performed. Alternatively, selective analysis of the enzymes involved in mucopolysaccharide metabolism whose deficiency would be consistent with the patient's clinical phenotype can be performed as the next step. The enzyme analyses can be performed using white blood cells or cultured skin fibroblasts.[2]

Patients with clinical features suggestive of an oligosaccharidosis can be evaluated using one of the available chromatographic systems for separating and quantitating various oligosaccharides. A positive result can be investigated by performing a selective battery of enzyme assays using white blood cells or cultured skin fibroblasts.

Tests for Peroxisomal Disorders

Peroxisomal disorders include defects of biogenesis (group 1) and defects of individual enzymes (group 2). Almost all of the disorders in group 1 (Zellweger syndrome and its milder variants) and many of the disorders in group 2 (defects of peroxisomal fatty acid oxidation: acyl-CoA oxidase deficiency, bifunctional enzyme deficiency, and thiolase deficiency) have impaired very-long-chain fatty acid oxidation and are characterized by increased plasma concentrations of very-long-chain fatty acids (chain length longer than 22 carbons). In most cases, measurement of individual plasma very-long-chain fatty acids is the most useful single measure of peroxisomal function and serves as a useful initial test for these disorders.[99] Very-long-chain fatty acids can also be measured in cultured fibroblasts, thereby permitting premortem or postmortem diagnosis from a skin biopsy specimen established in culture.

Other measurements are required to diagnosis some forms of peroxisomal disease, such as rhizomelic chondrodysplasia punctata, and to distinguish between the various forms of peroxisomal disease. These additional tests include plasma phytanic acid analysis, erythrocyte plasmalogen analysis, and plasma dihydroxycholestanoic and trihydroxycholestanoic acid analysis. Mevalonic aciduria is diagnosed with urinary organic acid analysis. More definitive testing, including complementation analysis or assays

---

BOX 50–1   Organic Acidurias with Onset in the Neonatal Period

3-Hydroxyisobutyric aciduria
3-Hydroxy-3-methylglutaryl-CoA lyase deficiency
Isovaleric acidemia*
3-Ketothiolase deficiency
Maple syrup urine disease
3-Methylcrotonyl-CoA carboxylase deficiency
Methylmalonic aciduria*
Mevalonic aciduria
Multiple acyl-CoA dehydrogenase deficiency (glutaric aciduria type II)
Multiple carboxylase deficiency (biotinidase deficiency; holocarboxylase synthetase deficiency)
Propionic acidemia*
Pyroglutamic acidemia
Succinyl-CoA 3-ketoacid transferase deficiency

*Most commonly seen disorders.

of peroxisomal fatty acid β-oxidation, is often required to establish a specific diagnosis.[99]

Definitive Biochemical Diagnosis

Judicious application of the various biochemical tests described above will in many cases, but not all, allow the physician to establish a diagnosis. However, it is important to remember that the diagnosis must be confirmed by definitive testing because the same metabolite pattern (i.e., biochemical phenotype) can be associated with more than one inborn error of metabolism, which might differ in their treatment, prognosis and inheritance pattern. Definitive diagnosis is generally done by specific enzyme analysis or genetic testing. Relatively few laboratories perform many of the enzyme studies that are required to confirm the diagnosis of a rare genetic disorder. As a rule, these enzyme analyses are time consuming, relatively difficult to perform, and expensive. Specific enzyme analysis can often be done using blood cells (most commonly, white blood cells), but often require cultured skin fibroblasts or other tissue specimens.

It is therefore not surprising that laboratories performing these studies prefer (or require) evidence that there is a significant likelihood that the test being performed will demonstrate an abnormality. It behooves the physician caring for a sick neonate to obtain the preliminary evidence suggesting that a specific defect is likely before proceeding to specific enzyme analysis. This is often done in consultation with local experts in metabolic disease, but when such expertise is not available, the laboratories performing such assays usually are willing to give advice that will ultimately maximize the benefit of their efforts.

Genetic Testing

The discussion in this chapter focuses almost exclusively on the classic methods of biochemical genetics, which include analysis of metabolites, structural macromolecules, and enzymes. For the most part, little consideration is given to the role that recent advances of molecular genetics are playing in facilitating the diagnosis, improving our understanding of the pathogenesis, and expanding the possibilities for treatment of inborn errors of metabolism. This has been an intentional omission, because a discussion of the tools of molecular genetics is presented in Chapter 8 and molecular diagnosis is generally performed after a clinical diagnosis has been confirmed biochemically or enzymatically. The reasons for this omission notwithstanding, there are five clinical circumstances in which molecular testing comes to the forefront, and the clinician should be aware of them.

First, diagnosis can be accomplished easily and rapidly by mutational analysis for diseases that are characterized by relative genetic homogeneity (i.e., a few mutations account for most cases of the disease). Medium-chain acyl-CoA dehydrogenase (MCAD) deficiency provides an excellent example. Approximately 90% of the disease-causing alleles found in affected patients have the same mutation (i.e., an A to G change at nucleotide 985). Second, diagnosis can be provided by mutational analysis, but not by conventional biochemical studies. This is the situation for disorders caused by mutations of the mitochondrial DNA; DNA-based mutation analysis can provide a specific diagnosis, whereas classic metabolite or enzymatic studies cannot. Third, mutation analysis can provide useful prognostic information. For example, in cases of galactosemia ascertained by newborn screening, mutation analysis can assist the clinician in determining the patient's tolerance for galactose and the need to restrict dietary galactose intake. Fourth, mutation analysis of postmortem samples can be used to diagnose the condition in patients who have died without a diagnosis. Fifth, knowledge of a patient's mutation can facilitate evaluation of other family members and prenatal testing.

Postmortem Evaluation

Although the management of a very sick newborn who is at imminent risk of dying is a familiar issue in neonatal care, certain points must be considered in the case of a newborn infant with a suspected inborn error of metabolism. Samples of blood, urine, and, if possible, CSF should be obtained before death. Serum and plasma samples should be obtained; a total of 10 mL should be collected, aliquoted, and saved for metabolite studies and for preparation and storage of DNA. As much urine as possible should be saved. All samples should be frozen at −20°C and preferably at −70°C.

A thoughtful but direct discussion should be arranged before death with the parents, during which the reasons for a postmortem examination are presented. It should be explained that an autopsy performed for the purpose of investigating a suspected metabolic disorder is different from autopsies performed for other purposes in that the autopsy examination must be performed within hours of death, preferably within less than 4 hours. This urgency is dictated by the need to obtain tissue before postmortem changes compromise the integrity of enzyme systems.

If the performance of a complete autopsy is not acceptable to the parents, the option of a limited autopsy should be discussed.[20,71] The selection of tissues or organs requested in a limited postmortem examination vary with the clinical situation but in general should include specimens of liver and skeletal muscle and a skin biopsy specimen for establishing a fibroblast cell culture. These specimens can be obtained with minimal disfigurement. Several small (1 cm³) specimens of liver and skeletal muscle should be obtained. Similar specimens of heart tissue should be obtained from patients with cardiomyopathy. If permission for a limited postmortem examination is refused, permission for premortem percutaneous liver and open skeletal muscle biopsies should be sought; these procedures can be performed at the bedside. All specimens should be stored at −70°C for future study.

Similar arrangements should also be made for neonates who die suddenly in the hospital or at home, because inborn errors have become a well-recognized cause of sudden death. Approximately 2% of sudden, unexpected deaths in the neonatal period are the consequence of a metabolic disorder.[16] It is understandably more difficult to make arrangements that comply with the recommendations for the sick infant, but experience has shown that a modified protocol can be successful.[7,71] These modifications are dictated in part by the logistics of arranging for a prompt autopsy after an unexpected death, but equally important are the requirements dictated by the differential diagnosis of inborn errors that cause sudden death of the neonate.

The diagnostic entities that have to be considered primarily include defects in energy metabolism: glycogen storage diseases, defects in fatty acid oxidation, and electron transport chain defects. The most common pathogenetic mechanism that leads to sudden death in these disorders is cardiomyopathy or cardiac arrhythmia, which is the consequence of myocardial energy deficiency or disruption of the electrical conduction system by toxic metabolites that accumulate in these disorders.

Practically, recommendations are that a full autopsy be done within 72 hours of death. The autopsy should include particular attention to examination of the heart, liver, and skeletal muscle for evidence of glycogen or lipid storage. The following specimens should be obtained and stored frozen: liver, urine from the bladder (no matter how small the sample size), and bile from the gallbladder.[7,71] A skin biopsy should be obtained for establishing a cell line of cultured fibroblasts.

The results of the metabolite studies are dictated in part by the results of the standard pathologic evaluation. For example, findings consistent with a possible fatty acid oxidation defect should include measurement of glucose, free fatty acids, and total and free acylcarnitines in the liver specimen; organic acids and an acylcarnitine profile in urine; and an acylcarnitine profile in bile. The possibility of two specific inborn errors of fatty acid oxidation, MCAD deficiency and LCHAD deficiency, can be evaluated by molecular techniques that identify the mutations most commonly associated with these disorders. The specific requirements for other diagnostic possibilities are outlined in the relevant sections of this chapter.

Approaches to Specific Abnormal Laboratory Findings

Most newborn infants with an inborn error of metabolism have one or more of only a handful of key laboratory findings: metabolic acidosis, lactic acidemia, hypoglycemia, and hyperammonemia. An approach to differential diagnosis of inborn errors with each of these findings will now be presented. As with all attempts to develop a useful approach to differential diagnosis, it is important to remember that the algorithm never quite fits all patients. Such probably will be the case for these algorithms as well because of the range of diagnostic possibilities and the considerable genetic heterogeneity that characterizes all inborn errors of metabolism. Nevertheless, the approaches presented should serve as useful first approximations.

METABOLIC ACIDOSIS

Metabolic acidosis is a common laboratory finding in sick neonates. It is most often a consequence of shock or severe organ failure of the kidney or liver. In other cases, acidosis is a discrete finding suggesting that the patient has an inborn error affecting acid production or renal acid excretion. It is important to determine the cause of the acidosis because many cellular functions rapidly deteriorate at reduced pH. The most common treatment of acidosis is to "correct" the acidosis with bicarbonate; however, the most effective treatment of acidosis is to correct the cause of the acidosis. It is often possible to correct the acidosis caused by an inborn error of metabolism by reducing endogenous overproduction of specific acids.

Differential Diagnosis

The evaluation of metabolic acidosis should begin with an investigation for systemic shock, renal failure, and generalized liver disease. In the case of shock, the patient should be reevaluated for recurrent acidosis after restoration of normal cardiopulmonary function. Shock might have been the consequence of an inborn error of metabolism. Similarly, patients with severe liver disease should be evaluated for an underlying inborn error of metabolism as the cause of their liver disease (see Table 50-5).

After assessing the patient's cardiopulmonary, renal, and hepatic status, the physician should initiate a diagnostic study for a possible inborn error of metabolism by measuring serum electrolytes, blood gases and pH, and urine pH. The anion gap should be calculated. Acidosis that is associated with a normal anion gap and an inappropriate renal response to systemic acidosis (urine pH greater than 5) implicates a renal tubular defect. The presence of a normal kidney response to the systemic acidosis (urine pH less than 5) and an increased anion gap suggests that the excess acid load is systemic in origin rather than renal (see Chapter 36, Part 2). However, an increased anion gap is not always present in disorders associated with excessive production of abnormal acidic metabolites, and additional studies should be performed before concluding that a patient with a normal anion-gap metabolic acidosis has a renal defect rather than another disorder.

Additional studies that should be performed include determinations of blood lactate and pyruvate, serum glucose, plasma amino acids, plasma and urinary ketones, blood ammonia, plasma and urinary carnitine, and urinary organic acids. The results of these studies can be used to develop the algorithm for the differential diagnosis of metabolic acidosis shown in Figure 50-1. This algorithm uses the blood lactate concentration as the discriminant at its first branch point, thereby dividing the causes of metabolic acidosis into the lactic acidemias and other acidemias. The advantage to this approach is that a discrete algorithm can then be used to evaluate patients with lactic acidemias. One disadvantage is that many categories of disease (e.g., the organic acidemias) include a subset of disorders that produce lactic acidemia and a subset that does not; another is that the same disease might produce lactic acidemia in some patients but not in others. On balance, the presence of lactic acidemia is a useful discriminant. The disorders associated with lactic acidemia are discussed later under "Lactic Acidemia".

The serum glucose concentration is then used in Figure 50-1 to differentiate among the disorders that cause metabolic acidosis without lactic acidemia. Several groups of disorders are associated with a normal or increased serum glucose concentration at onset, whereas other groups of disorders are associated with hypoglycemia. These groups of disorders can be divided further into those that exhibit ketosis and those that do not. Ketosis is a relatively uncommon finding in the neonate. The possibility of ketosis should be searched for carefully in blood and urine in the sick newborn infant. If present, ketosis should be taken as strong evidence that the neonate has a metabolic disorder.[2,11] However, if ketosis is not present, especially in the premature newborn infant, the possibility of an underlying ketotic metabolic disorder should not be dismissed, because the pathways of ketone synthesis might not have developed sufficiently.

Figure 50–1. Approach to neonatal metabolic acidosis. AC:FC, ratio of acylcarnitine to free carnitine; FAO, fatty acid oxidation; RTA, renal tubular acidosis.

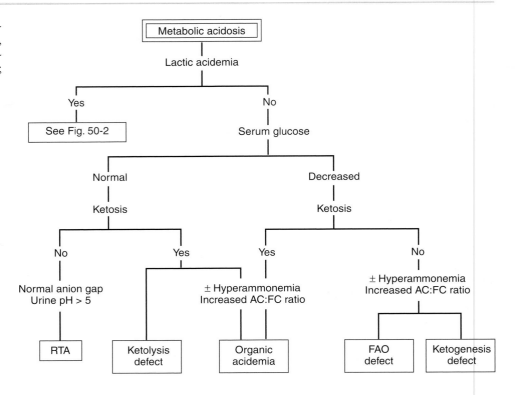

Other information from the initial screening studies should also be considered at this point. Serum electrolyte concentrations should be used to calculate the anion gap. The blood ammonia concentration should be assessed because it has diagnostic and therapeutic implications. Plasma amino acid analysis and plasma and urine carnitine analyses should be reviewed because they also might have diagnostic and therapeutic implications.

Patients who have a normal serum glucose concentration with ketosis might have an organic acidemia or a ketolytic defect. Approximately a dozen organic acidemias can have their onset in the neonatal period (see Box 50-1). Many of the organic acid disorders have a common set of features, including ketoacidosis, vomiting, convulsions, coma, and in some disorders, an unusual smell (see Table 50-7). Because the main diagnostic test for the organic acid disorders—urinary organic acid analysis—can detect essentially all of these defects, the physician need only consider this diagnostic category and order the appropriate analysis.

In general, analysis of a urine sample collected early in the course of an acute episode of metabolic decompensation has the best chance of revealing the characteristic pattern of organic aciduria. In other cases, the sample obtained during an acute episode contains too many metabolites, and the primary defect is obscured. Accordingly, it is advisable to send at least two samples to the laboratory, one obtained during and the other after an acute episode, when an organic acid disorder is suspected.

In addition to an abnormal urinary organic acid pattern, patients with many of the relatively common organic acidemias generally have an increased serum anion gap, reflecting the accumulation of abnormal organic acids, and hyperammonemia. The degree of hyperammonemia may be so great (500 to 1000 µmol/L)[85] that it generates concern and possibly

confusion about whether the patient has a primary urea cycle defect (see "Hyperammonemia"). However, the organic acidemias can generally be distinguished from the urea cycle defects. The organic acidemias are associated with a more significant metabolic acidosis than is seen in the urea cycle defects, especially early in the course of the illness; an abnormal organic acid pattern; and an increased acylcarnitine-to-free carnitine ratio, which is often accompanied by a pathognomonic acylcarnitine profile. The clinical features of individual organic acidemias are discussed later.

Defects of Ketolysis

The other causes of ketotic normoglycemic acidosis are defects in ketolysis (i.e., the degradation of ketone bodies once they are formed). Ketolytic defects constitute a subset of organic acidemias. They are identified by urinary organic acid analysis but are considered separately here because their pathogenesis is unique. In normal individuals, ketone bodies are formed in the liver and then transported to peripheral tissues, where they are used as a glucose-sparing energy source.

Ketolytic defects are primarily defects in extrahepatic ketone use rather than ketone body synthesis by the liver. These defects are characterized by normoglycemia or even hyperglycemia. Ketolytic defects are relatively rare, especially in the neonate. Two ketolytic defects with onset in the newborn period are succinyl-CoA:3-ketoacid CoA-transferase deficiency and β-ketothiolase deficiency.[85] Both result in lethargy, hypotonia, a normal or increased serum glucose concentration, and marked ketosis during the fed state and the fasted state.

The diagnosis of succinyl-CoA:3-ketoacid CoA-transferase deficiency should be considered in a patient with negative findings on organic acid analysis except for markedly increased concentrations of β-hydroxybutyrate, acetoacetate, and β-hydroxyisovalerate. Confirmation of the diagnosis requires specific enzyme studies.

β-Ketothiolase deficiency impairs ketone body use and isoleucine metabolism because the enzyme is involved in both pathways. The urinary organic acid pattern seen in patients with this disorder shows increased amounts of 2-butanone, 2-methyl-3-hydroxybutyrate, and tiglylglycine, as well as increased excretion of acetoacetate and β-hydroxybutyrate. This disorder can be confused with diabetic ketoacidosis or salicylism when it occurs in the older child.

The treatment for both disorders is a low-protein diet and possibly a low-fat diet, especially during intercurrent illnesses. Carnitine supplementation might also be helpful.

Renal Tubular Defects

The most likely diagnosis when metabolic acidosis is associated with a normal serum glucose concentration, the absence of ketosis, a normal blood ammonia concentration, a normal anion gap, and an inappropriate renal response to systemic acidosis (urine pH greater than 5) is a renal tubular defect.

Renal tubular acidosis (RTA) is not discussed here because it is more appropriately considered in Chapter 51. However, certain inborn errors of metabolism are associated with RTA. In general, there are two forms of RTA that reflect the anatomic and functional locus of the defect: proximal RTA and distal RTA. The inborn errors of metabolism that are discussed in this chapter are associated with defects causing proximal RTA but not distal RTA. Most inborn errors of metabolism that cause proximal RTA also affect other components of proximal renal tubular function, producing the renal Fanconi syndrome (i.e., generalized aminoaciduria, glucosuria, phosphaturia, and RTA). Inborn errors of metabolism that cause renal Fanconi syndrome include defects of amino acid, carbohydrate metabolism, organic acid metabolism, and the respiratory chain (Table 50-14). The diagnostic approach and general treatment of these disorders are discussed in the respective parts of this chapter.

The next category to consider is the disorders that are associated with hypoglycemia (see Fig. 50-1), for which the presence or absence of ketosis provides the most discriminating laboratory clue. Patients who have hypoglycemia without ketosis (i.e., nonketotic or hypoketotic hypoglycemia) have a defect in mitochondrial fatty acid β-oxidation or in ketogenesis unless another cause is found. Patients with defects of mitochondrial fatty acid β-oxidation are unable to generate acetyl-CoA for ketone body synthesis, whereas patients with defects in ketogenesis are unable to use acetyl-CoA for ketone body synthesis. These disorders can also be associated with hyperammonemia, an increased anion gap, and disordered carnitine homeostasis. Defects in mitochondrial fatty acid β-oxidation are discussed in more detail under "Hypoglycemia".

Defects of Ketogenesis

The most common ketogenesis defect is 3-hydroxy-3-methylglutaric aciduria, which is the result of an autosomal recessive deficiency of 3-hydroxy-3-methylglutaryl-CoA lyase.[85] This enzyme deficiency affects ketone body formation from fatty acid oxidation and leucine (a branched-chain amino acid) catabolism. This disorder, therefore, can be classified as an amino acid disorder or as a fatty acid oxidation defect. The defect interferes with the major pathways of ketone body formation and consequently is a cause of severe nonketotic acidosis and hypoglycemia in the newborn infant. Patients generally have vomiting, hypotonia, or lethargy at presentation, but others present with seizures caused by the profound hypoglycemia associated with this disorder. This disorder can be diagnosed by urinary organic acid analysis and is treated with a leucine-restricted, low-protein diet.

ORGANIC ACIDEMIAS

Patients who have hypoglycemia with ketosis should be evaluated for an organic acidemia. Methylmalonic acidemia and propionic acidemia, two of the most common organic acid disorders, are often associated with ketosis. This is also true of several other branched-chain organic acidemias. These common organic acidemias may be associated with hypoglycemia, an increased anion gap, hyperammonemia, hyperglycinemia, and an increased ratio of acylcarnitine to free carnitine with an abnormal pattern of specific acylcarnitines, but none of these findings is present invariably.[11,85] Definitive diagnosis can be accomplished by urinary organic acid analysis and plasma carnitine analysis with an acylcarnitine profile, followed by enzymatic or other specialized biochemical testing.

Defects in Branched-Chain Amino Acid Metabolism

The most common organic acidurias in the newborn period are isovaleric acidemia, methylmalonic acidemia, and propionic acidemia (see Box 50-1).[11,85] These three disorders share many of the same clinical and biochemical features. All three disorders are the consequence of defects in branched-chain amino acid metabolism, affecting the catabolism of isoleucine, leucine, or valine. The clinical phenotype fits the classic description of a newborn infant who is healthy at birth and then becomes inexplicably ill on the second or third day of life (see "The Sick Newborn Infant"). Standard supportive management might not halt the progression of the disease, and the neurologic status deteriorates until the patient becomes comatose and, in many cases, dies.

Biochemically, these disorders are characterized by a combination of many or all of the following features: severe

TABLE 50–14	Disorders That Cause Renal Fanconi Syndrome
Category of Disorder	**Disorder**
Amino acid defects	Tyrosinemia type I
Carbohydrate defects	Galactosemia Glycogen storage disorder type I Hereditary fructose intolerance
Organic acidemia	Pyroglutamic aciduria
Respiratory chain defects	Complex I, II, or IV, or combined defects mtDNA depletion syndromes

mtDNA, mitochondrial DNA.

ketoacidosis, hyperammonemia, lactic acidemia, hyperglycinemia, abnormal carnitine metabolism (i.e., relative carnitine insufficiency with an increased acylcarnitine-to-free carnitine ratio and abnormal acylcarnitine profile), hypocalcemia, and neutropenia, thrombocytopenia, or pancytopenia. Occasionally, patients with an organic acidemia do not present with acidosis. The blood sugar level may be decreased, normal, or increased.

Other relatively less common defects in branched-chain amino acid metabolism (e.g., 3-methylcrotonyl-CoA carboxylase deficiency) have similar clinical and biochemical phenotypes. MSUD also has a similar phenotype, except that hypoglycemia is not usually present (see "Newborn Screening"). Many of these patients are first ascertained by the alert nurse or parent who notices an abnormal odor emanating from the sick newborn infant's bed or diaper (see Table 50-7).

Ketone Body Metabolism Defects

The other organic acidurias with onset in the newborn period have certain clinical or biochemical features that distinguish them from the branched-chain organic acidurias. The defects in ketone body metabolism have already been discussed. The defects in ketolysis (i.e., succinyl-CoA:3-ketoacid CoA-transferase deficiency and β-ketothiolase deficiency) and the defects in ketogenesis (i.e., 3-hydroxy-3-methylglutaric aciduria) are diagnosed and subsequently treated as organic acidemias. Another organic aciduria, mevalonic aciduria, is associated with hepatosplenomegaly, diarrhea, anemia, hypocholesterolemia, and craniofacial dysmorphism. The underlying defect in this disorder is deficiency of mevalonate kinase, which is a peroxisomal enzyme that catalyzes the first committed step in the biosynthesis of cholesterol and nonsterol isoprenoids (see "Dysmorphic Syndromes").[29]

Pyroglutamic Acidemia

Pyroglutamic acidemia is caused by a defect in glutathione synthetase, an enzyme required for the biosynthesis of glutathione. Glutathione is a tripeptide involved in maintaining the redox status within the cell. This rare disorder produces acidosis but not ketosis or hypoglycemia in the newborn period. Clinically, it causes type I RTA (see Table 50-14), hemolysis, and hyperbilirubinemia in the newborn period. It leads to acidosis during intercurrent illnesses later in childhood and progressive neurologic abnormalities, including ataxia, spasticity, and mental retardation. The primary objective of treatment is to correct the acidosis and electrolyte imbalances associated with the disorder, especially during acute illnesses. In the neonatal period, it is also important to aggressively treat any anemia or hyperbilirubinemia that develops. Antioxidants, such as vitamin E and vitamin C, may be of long-term benefit.

Multiple Carboxylase Deficiency

Several organic acidurias represent compound phenotypes because the genetic defect affects the synthesis or functioning of several enzymes. The most common of these compound disorders is multiple carboxylase deficiency, which may be the consequence of either of two genetically distinct defects: biotinidase deficiency and holocarboxylase synthetase deficiency (see "Newborn Screening"). Both enzyme deficiencies lead to functional deficiencies of four enzymes, all carboxylases: acetyl-CoA carboxylase, which is involved in fatty acid synthesis; β-methylcrotonyl-CoA carboxylase deficiency, which is involved in branched-chain amino acid metabolism; propionyl-CoA carboxylase, which is also involved in branched-chain amino acid metabolism; and pyruvate carboxylase deficiency, which is involved in gluconeogenesis. Both forms of multiple carboxylase deficiency can cause lactic acidemia and a complex organic aciduria; both are also considered in the algorithm for lactic acidemia (see "Lactic Acidemia").

Both forms of multiple carboxylase deficiency can be diagnosed in the sick child by means of urinary organic acid analysis, although false-negative results may be obtained in biotinidase deficiency. Direct enzyme analysis of biotinidase deficiency is the best method of establishing this diagnosis.

Multiple Acyl-CoA Dehydrogenase Deficiency

Another disorder that represents a compound organic aciduria is multiple acyl-CoA dehydrogenase deficiency, or glutaric aciduria type II (see "Dysmorphic Syndromes").[85] This disorder is the consequence of a defect in ETF or ETF dehydrogenase, which are enzymatic components in the pathway that transfers reducing equivalents from the flavin-dependent dehydrogenases involved in mitochondrial fatty acid β-oxidation and the oxidation of several amino acids to the respiratory chain. This disorder is characterized by dysmorphogenesis of the brain, face, and kidneys, as well as the more expected clinical and biochemical phenotype of a fatty acid oxidation defect. This disorder is also associated in many cases with lactic acidosis, especially during acute phases of the illness.

MANAGEMENT

Management of a patient with an organic acidemia should include supportive care (i.e., administration of bicarbonate, mechanical ventilation, and reduced protein or fat intake with concomitantly increased glucose administration). If the patient has a severe neurologic intoxication, hemodialysis should be considered.[31,73,79,85] Centers unable to provide hemodialysis to newborn infants should consider transferring such patients because exchange transfusion, peritoneal dialysis, and hemofiltration are considerably less efficient than hemodialysis for managing many of these disorders.

Treatment should be modified as soon as a provisional diagnosis is available. For example, branched-chain amino acid–free parenteral nutrition and specially designed enteral formulas have been used to manage acutely ill patients with MSUD. Insulin can be used to augment the anabolic state, starting at 0.05 to 0.10 units/kg per hour.

Carnitine is used in many of these disorders to remove toxic metabolites during the acute phase. Carnitine can be given orally or intravenously. During an acute crisis, it is probably best to provide intravenous carnitine at 100 to 200 mg/kg per day (larger doses are sometimes given) as a continuous drip or in four divided doses. If parenteral carnitine is unavailable, carnitine should be given PO at comparable amounts in three or four divided doses. Glycine has been given for similar reasons to patients with isovaleric acidemia and related disorders.[85] Glycine should be given PO at a dosage of 250 to 500 mg/kg per day in three divided doses during the acute crisis. Intralipid can be started after carnitine supplementation has begun and once it is certain that the patient does not have a defect of fatty acid β-oxidation.

After the patient's condition is stabilized, oral feedings should be initiated. In the absence of a specific diagnosis, a high-carbohydrate formula that contains proportionately reduced amounts of protein and fat should be started. The diet should be modified after the neonate's diagnosis has been established. As a rule, it is necessary to limit only protein intake or, more correctly, the intake of certain amino acids, but restriction of protein and fat intake may be required for some disorders. A range of special formulas are commercially available for these patients, but specialized diets should always be designed with the assistance of a dietitian experienced in managing patients with inborn errors of metabolism.

Efforts to reduce the endogenous production of toxic metabolites could also include antibiotic suppression of gut flora that produce metabolites that enter the patient's bloodstream (e.g., long-term metronidazole in patients with methylmalonic and propionic acidemias).[94] Specific vitamins may be provided as cofactors for certain enzyme deficiencies, possibly including biotin (10 mg PO), hydroxycobalamin (1 mg/day IM), pyridoxine (10 mg/day PO), riboflavin (20 mg/day PO), or thiamine (10 mg/day PO). Carnitine (100 mg/kg per day) and glycine (250 mg/kg per day) are also used during the maintenance phase of treatment.

The various approaches to the acute and long-term management of organic acidemias have led to improved survival and outcome. However, the prognosis for patients with these disorders still varies widely for different disorders and for patients with the same disorder.[85] Efforts to establish correlations of genotype and phenotype for these disorders are underway and may soon provide a rational basis for providing prognostic information.

LACTIC ACIDEMIA

The lactic acidemias are a complex group of inborn errors of metabolism. The classification, diagnosis, and treatment of these disorders will almost certainly change as understanding of their pathogenesis improves. In particular, current understanding of the pathogenesis of defects of the respiratory or electron transport chain is evolving rapidly.

Lactic acidemia may be the consequence of overproduction of lactate, underuse of lactate, or both. A prerequisite for evaluating a patient with lactic acidemia is to assess the adequacy of tissue oxygenation. After it has been established that tissue oxygenation is adequate, several laboratory studies should be performed to determine the cause of the lactic acidemia, including those for blood lactate and pyruvate, blood gases and electrolytes, serum glucose, blood ammonia, plasma amino acids, plasma and urinary ketones, plasma and urinary carnitine, and urinary organic acids. If a lumbar puncture is planned to investigate the possibility of sepsis, a sample of CSF should be obtained for lactate and pyruvate analysis, along with samples for the more routine studies; a blood sample should be obtained concurrently for blood lactate and pyruvate analysis. The results of these studies can be used to generate an algorithm for establishing the diagnosis for a neonate with lactic acidemia (Fig. 50-2).

Differential Diagnosis

The differential diagnosis of the primary genetic lactic acidemias with onset in the neonatal period includes defects of gluconeogenesis, glycogenolysis, or pyruvate metabolism; defects of the Krebs (or tricarboxylic acid) cycle; and defects of the respiratory chain (Table 50-15). Many defects of fatty acid oxidation, organic acid metabolism, and the urea cycle are associated with lactic acidemia because of relationships

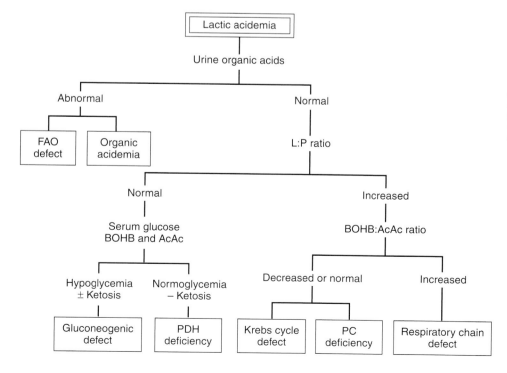

Figure 50–2. Approach to neonatal lactic acidemia. AcAc, acetoacetate; BOHB, β-hydroxybutyrate; BOHB:AcAc, β-hydroxybutyrate-to-acetoacetate ratio; FAO, fatty acid oxidation; L:P, lactate-to-pyruvate ratio; PC, pyruvate carboxylase; PDH, pyruvate dehydrogenase complex.

TABLE 50–15   Disorders Associated with Lactic Acidemia in Neonates

Category of Disorder	Disorder
Defects in gluconeogenesis, glycogenolysis, or pyruvate metabolism	Fructose-1,6-diphosphatase deficiency GSD type I (glucose-6-phosphatase deficiency) GSD type III (debrancher deficiency) Phosphoenolpyruvate carboxykinase deficiency Pyruvate carboxylase deficiency Pyruvate dehydrogenase complex deficiency
Krebs cycle defects	Dihydrolipoamide dehydrogenase deficiency Fumarase deficiency α-Ketoglutarate dehydrogenase deficiency
Organic acidemias	See Box 50-1
Respiratory chain (RC) defects	
mtDNA mutations	
Point mutations	
mRNA	Maternally inherited Leigh syndrome (ATPase 6)
rRNA	Aminoglycoside-induced nonsyndromic deafness
tRNA	Isolated cardiomypathy (tRNA^{Leu}, tRNA^{Ile})
Large deletions/duplications	Pearson syndrome
nDNA mutations	
Mutations that directly affect subunits of the RC complexes	Complex I, II, III, IV and V, or combined deficiencies
Mutations that affect nuclear genes required for transport, assembly or stabilization of the RC complexes	Complex III (BCS1L) Complex IV (SURF, SCO1, SCO2, COX10, COX15)
Mutations that affect nuclear genes required for replication or maintenance of the mitochondrial genome	Mitochondrial DNA depletion syndromes Mitochondrial polymerase γ deficiency Deoxyguanosine kinase deficiency Thymidine kinase 2 deficiency
Mutations that affect genes involved in other mitochondrial processes required for normal RC function	Barth syndrome (tafazzin)

ATPase 6, subunit 6 of ATP synthase; COX, cytochrome oxidase; GSD, glycogen storage disorder; nDNA, nuclear DNA; mtDNA, mitochondrial DNA; RC, respiratory chain; tRNA^{Leu}, transfer RNA for leucine (UUR); tRNA^{Ile}, transfer RNA for isoleucine.

among the various pathways of intermediary metabolism. These disorders are more properly considered secondary lactic acidemias and are discussed elsewhere in this chapter. Multiple carboxylase deficiency is an exception to this rule because the underlying defect impairs biotin metabolism, which may produce pyruvate carboxylase deficiency and lactic acidemia.

The urinary organic acid pattern, along with the blood ammonia concentration and plasma and urine carnitine analyses, provides a practical means for discriminating between the primary and secondary lactic acidemias. The urinary organic acid pattern is by definition abnormal in patients with an organic acidemia and is abnormal in many of the disorders of fatty acid β-oxidation. Patients with fatty acid oxidation defects often excrete increased amounts of dicarboxylic acids, 3-hydroxydicarboxylic acids, or both. In contrast, the primary lactic acidemias are associated with a normal organic acid pattern or a nonspecific pattern of increased excretion of lactate and pyruvate, various Krebs cycle intermediates, dicarboxylic and 3-hydroxydicarboxylic acids, or 3-methylglutaconic acid.

The dicarboxylic and 3-hydroxydicarboxylic acids are the consequence of secondarily impaired mitochondrial fatty acid β-oxidation.

Despite the potential overlap between the patterns of urinary organic acids produced by these disorders, urinary organic acid analysis generally provides a useful means of discriminating between the primary and secondary lactic acidemias because qualitative and quantitative differences exist between the patterns seen in the two groups of disorders. The concentrations of urinary metabolites excreted in the primary lactic acidemias are generally less than that produced by the organic acidurias and fatty acid oxidation defects.

The plasma ammonia concentration and the plasma and urine carnitine analyses also provide useful information for distinguishing between the primary and secondary lactic acidemias. Patients with an organic aciduria or a fatty acid β-oxidation defect often have hyperammonemia and relative carnitine insufficiency, with an increased acylcarnitine-to-free carnitine ratio and specific acylcarnitine abnormalities.[59,70]

In contrast, patients with one of the primary lactic acidemias generally have a normal plasma ammonia concentration and relatively mild and nonspecific changes in their plasma and urinary carnitine values.

The exception to this rule is the severe neonatal form of pyruvate carboxylase deficiency, because these patients can have hyperammonemia. Similarly, patients with a primary urea cycle defect could have lactic acidosis, but the degree of acidosis is relatively mild, especially early in the course of the disease, when respiratory alkalosis rather than metabolic acidosis is generally present (see "Hyperammonemia").

Primary Lactic Acidemias

In practical terms, the first step in discriminating among the primary lactic acidemias is to examine the results of the lactate (L) and pyruvate (P) analyses in terms of the absolute and relative values of this pair of metabolites. The L:P ratio is a reflection of the redox state of the cytoplasm. The L:P ratio is normally between 10:1 and 20:1. Defects of gluconeogenesis or the pyruvate dehydrogenase complex are generally associated with a normal L:P ratio, whereas defects of the Krebs cycle, pyruvate carboxylase, or the respiratory chain are often associated with an increased L:P ratio.[55]

Pyruvate carboxylase (PC) is an exceptional case because it is a gluconeogenic enzyme, but its metabolic deficiency has different consequences than other gluconeogenic enzymes. The pathophysiology of PC deficiency is reviewed in the next section. The second exception to this rule is that many respiratory chain defects are associated with normal blood lactate and pyruvate concentrations and a normal L:P ratio. The reasons for this are not well understood, although the normal L:P ratio is considered to be the consequence of partial deficiencies or tissue-specific defects that exist in many patients. The possibility of a respiratory chain defect should not be ignored in patients with a normal blood lactate concentration or a normal L:P ratio when the patient's clinical picture otherwise suggests a respiratory chain disorder.

Further differentiation of the primary lactic acidemias can be made with the results of the plasma β-hydroxybutyrate (BOHB) and acetoacetate (AcAc) analysis and the serum glucose analysis. As discussed in regard to the results of the blood lactate and pyruvate analyses, the results of plasma BOHB and AcAc analyses should be evaluated in terms of the absolute and relative values of this pair of metabolites. Whereas the L:P ratio is a reflection of the redox state of the cytoplasm, the BOHB:AcAc ratio is a reflection of the redox state within the mitochondrion. Both ratios must be examined to appreciate the redox state within the cell.

The presence of different redox states in these two cellular compartments is the consequence of impaired production of reducing equivalents (i.e., in Krebs cycle defects), impaired shuttling of reducing equivalents between the cytosolic and the mitochondrial compartments (i.e., in PC deficiency and the Krebs cycle defects), or impaired oxidation of reducing equivalents within the mitochondrion (i.e., in respiratory chain defects). Normally, shuttling of reducing equivalents between the cytosolic and mitochondrial compartments is mediated by an oxaloacetate-dependent pathway. Shuttling of reducing equivalents is impaired in PC deficiency and Krebs cycle defects because these disorders lead to oxaloacetate deficiency. In the case of PC deficiency, the role of this enzyme is to form oxaloacetate from pyruvate and carbon dioxide; in the case of the Krebs cycle defects, oxaloacetate is the last step in each turn of the tricarboxylic acid cycle, and oxaloacetate deficiency develops when enzymes earlier in the cycle do not function normally.

The primary lactic acidemias associated with a normal L:P ratio include defects of gluconeogenesis and defects of the pyruvate dehydrogenase complex (see Fig. 50-2). These two groups of disorders can be distinguished from each other by the presence or absence of hypoglycemia and ketosis. Defects of gluconeogenesis are generally associated with hypoglycemia and ketosis, whereas patients with pyruvate dehydrogenase complex deficiency are generally normoglycemic and do not have ketosis (see "Hypoglycemia").

PYRUVATE DEHYDROGENASE DEFICIENCY

Patients with pyruvate dehydrogenase complex deficiency can present in the neonatal period with severe lactic acidosis and rapidly progressive deterioration. Less severe deficiencies are compatible with survival but lead to psychomotor retardation. Most patients with pyruvate dehydrogenase complex deficiency have an X-linked form of the disease, in which male patients are more severely affected than female patients. In many cases, patients with pyruvate dehydrogenase complex deficiency are born with structural CNS malformations, including agenesis of the corpus callosum and cystic lesions of cerebral cortex; in other patients, lesions of the basal ganglia and brainstem that are consistent with Leigh disease are present or develop later in infancy. However, the Leigh disease phenotype is not pathognomonic for pyruvate dehydrogenase deficiency because Leigh disease is genetically heterogeneous; it can also be the consequence of PC deficiency or defects of nuclear- or mitochondrial-encoded subunits of the respiratory chain.[17,80]

Efforts to treat patients with pyruvate dehydrogenase complex deficiency have included a high-fat, low-carbohydrate diet with thiamine and lipoic acid supplementation. The rationale for this therapy is that glucose is catabolized through the glycolytic pathway to pyruvate and then requires the action of the pyruvate dehydrogenase complex before it can enter the Krebs cycle, whereas fatty acids enter the Krebs cycle without passing through the pyruvate dehydrogenase complex. Thiamine and lipoic acid are cofactors for the first and second components of the pyruvate dehydrogenase complex, respectively. Some patients have been treated with dichloroacetate, a drug that maintains the pyruvate dehydrogenase complex in its activated state. These treatment efforts have met with mixed success.

As shown in Figure 50-2, the primary lactic acidemias associated with an increased L:P ratio can be distinguished by considering the absolute and relative concentrations of BOHB and AcAc. Patients with PC deficiency, a Krebs cycle defect, or a respiratory chain defect all exhibit postprandial ketosis. However, for the reasons explained previously, severe PC deficiency and Krebs cycle defects are accompanied by a decreased or a normal BOHB:AcAc ratio, whereas respiratory chain defects are accompanied by an increased BOHB:AcAc ratio.

KREBS CYCLE DEFECTS

Krebs cycle defects are rare. Four defects affecting the Krebs cycle have been described: α-ketoglutarate dehydrogenase complex deficiency, fumarase deficiency, succinate dehydrogenase deficiency, and dihydrolipoamide dehydrogenase deficiency. The clinical presentations of α-ketoglutarate dehydrogenase deficiency and fumarase deficiency are variable but always affect neurologic function. They can cause hypotonia, ataxia, and, in some cases, CNS malformations. Succinate dehydrogenase deficiency behaves clinically and biochemically as a respiratory chain defect, which is not surprising because succinate dehydrogenase forms part of complex II of the respiratory chain.

Dihydrolipoamide dehydrogenase deficiency affects a protein that is a component of three different α-ketoacid dehydrogenase complexes: the α-ketoglutarate dehydrogenase complex (i.e., Krebs cycle component), the pyruvate dehydrogenase complex (i.e., the enzyme that converts pyruvate to acetyl-CoA and thereby permits its entry into the Krebs cycle), and the branched-chain α-ketoacid dehydrogenase complex (i.e., the enzyme that is deficient in MSUD). Dihydrolipoamide dehydrogenase deficiency is therefore a compound deficiency of these three α-ketoacid dehydrogenase complexes and is associated with severe ketoacidosis and a pathognomonic organic aciduria. The Krebs cycle defects can be detected by urinary organic acid analysis.

Effective treatment does not exist for these Krebs cycle disorders.

The severe neonatal form of PC deficiency is associated with acidosis, hyperammonemia, hypercitrullinemia (citrulline is an amino acid component of the urea cycle), and hyperlysinemia (lysine is a dibasic amino acid). This disorder is characterized by postprandial ketosis, a normal or decreased BOHB:AcAc ratio, and an increased L:P ratio. It has a fulminant course of progressive neurologic deterioration. Less severe forms of PC deficiency are not associated with hyperammonemia, hypercitrullinemia, or hyperlysinemia, and the L:P ratio and BOHB:AcAc ratios are normal. PC deficiency is discussed further under "Hypoglycemia."

DEFECTS OF THE RESPIRATORY CHAIN

Defects of the respiratory chain are a complex group of disorders reflecting the large number of genes involved in this metabolic system.[13,17,55,80] The respiratory chain is composed of five multimeric protein units: complex I, II, III, IV and V. The number of protein subunits in these complexes ranges from 4 to 43 proteins. An additional level of complexity is that some subunits are encoded by nuclear DNA (nDNA) and others are encoded by mitochondrial DNA (mtDNA). The nDNA encodes for approximately 85% of the subunits, while mtDNA encodes for approximately 15%. Complexes I, III, IV, and V contain subunits encoded by both genomes, while complex II contains only nuclear-encoded subunits. The common names, composition, and genetic origin of the subunits of the five respiratory chain complexes are listed in Table 50-16.

The mitochondrial genome differs in several key ways from the nuclear genome.[17,55,80] There are both structural and biologic differences between the two genomes. The structural differences include the following:

- mtDNA is much smaller than nDNA. It is a circular, double-stranded genome that contains about 16,500 basepairs (16.5 kb), which encode for 37 genes (compared with the 30,000 genes that are encoded by the nuclear genome). The mtDNA encodes for 13 mRNAs, two rRNAs, and 22 tRNAs. The mRNAs encode for the polypeptide subunits of the respiratory chain complexes. The two rRNAs and 22 tRNAs are necessary for translation of mtDNA.
- The genetic codes of the mtDNA and nDNA differ in several key codons, such that the two genomes require their own translational apparatus.
- Almost all regions of mtDNA are part of coding sequence, that is, the mtDNA has few introns. This is very different from the situation for nDNA, which contains a high proportion of noncoding regions.
- The mutation rate for mtDNA is approximately 10-fold greater than that of nDNA, in part because it does not have histones and in part because it has a poor mutation repair apparatus.

Combining the high mtDNA mutation rate with the high proportion of coding sequence in mtDNA, mtDNA mutations are thought to account for a disproportionate percentage (based on their relative size) of human disease compared with the nuclear genome. Conversely, the number of nuclear genes involved in mitochondrial structure and function is far greater than the number of mitochondrial encoded genes, supporting the clinical observation that nuclear mutations are also a significant cause of mitochondrial disease, especially in children.

TABLE 50–16   The Respiratory Chain Complexes

| Complex | Name | COMPOSITION AND GENETIC ORIGIN | | |
		nDNA	mtDNA	Total
I	NADH-CoQ reductase	37	7	43
II	Succinate-CoQ reductase	4	0	4
III	CoQH$_2$-cytochrome c reductase	10	1	11
IV	Cytochrome c oxidase	10	3	13
V	ATP synthase	12	2	14

CoQ, coenzyme Q (ubiquinone); CoQH$_2$, reduced coenzyme Q (ubiquinol); nDNA, nuclear DNA-encoded subunits; mtDNA, mitochondrial DNA-encoded subunits; NADH, reduced nicotinamide adenine dinucleotide.

In addition to these structural differences, there are also several key biologic differences between the mitochondrial and nuclear genomes:

- mtDNA is inherited exclusively from the mother, leading to maternal or matrilineal inheritance of mitochondrial encoded disorders.
- Each mitochondrion contains multiple copies of mtDNA, varying between two and 10 copies per organelle. Each cell, in turn, contains a variable number of mitochondria, leading to hundreds to thousands of copies of mtDNA per cell. In contrast, each cell (except mature germ cells) contains two copies of nDNA.
- Each cell may contain only one form of mtDNA ("normal" or "abnormal") or more than one form of mtDNA ("normal" or "abnormal"). The presence of only one form of mtDNA is called *homoplasmy*; the presence of more than one form is called *heteroplasmy*. The cell can contain any proportion of abnormal mtDNA. The clinical consequences of abnormal mtDNA are proportional to the degree of heteroplasmy of that mutation. The phenomenon of mtDNA heteroplasmy differs sharply from that for nDNA, wherein an individual is either homozygous or heterozygous for a normal or abnormal allele.
- The proportion of normal and abnormal mtDNA in a cell can change over time because mtDNA replication is not synchronous with nuclear division. A shift in the degree of heteroplasmy can occur prenatally or postnatally, can lead to improvement or worsening of the clinical phenotype, or can produce a change in the pattern of tissue and organ involvement.
- The clinical consequences of a mtDNA defect (homoplasmic or heteroplasmic) vary in different tissues and organs, depending on the mitochondrial (aerobic) energy requirements of each tissue or organ. This phenomenon has been termed the *threshold effect*.

The unique biologic properties of mtDNA provide a rationale for the unusual mode of inheritance, pattern of clinical involvement, and sometimes evolving clinical picture of some respiratory chain disorders.

An extraordinarily broad range of clinical phenotypes has been described among patients with respiratory chain defects.[13,17,80] This is not surprising given the almost universal requirement that different cells, tissues, and organs have for mitochondrial energy production. The clinical abnormalities primarily observed in newborns with respiratory chain disorders involve the CNS (lethargy, apnea, hypotonia, near miss episodes, coma), skeletal muscle (decreased spontaneous movements, atrophy, hypertonia or hypotonia, recurrent myoglobinuria), heart (hypertrophic cardiomyopathy), liver (hepatomegaly, hepatic failure), kidney (proximal tubular dysfunction), exocrine pancreas, and hematopoietic system (sideroblastic anemia, neutropenia, thrombocytopenia). In some cases, other clinical abnormalities can be identified (e.g., ocular abnormalities), which often provide a clue that facilitates further diagnostic evaluation. Thus, all patients suspected of having a respiratory chain disorder should undergo a comprehensive clinical evaluation to delineate the full pattern of organ involvement.

Similarly, all patients suspected of having a respiratory chain disorder should undergo a metabolic evaluation for lactic acidemia and related biochemical abnormalities, as discussed in the beginning of this section (see "Lactic Acidemia"). These studies should be done in both the fasting and fed state (1 hour postprandial). The metabolic evaluation should include measurement of blood lactate and pyruvate, plasma and urine ketones (β-hydroxybutyrate and acetoacetate), plasma amino acids (focusing on alanine, the transamination product of pyruvate), plasma carnitine analysis (including total carnitine, free carnitine and the acylcarnitine profile), plasma coenzyme Q10 (which is required for normal functioning of the respiratory chain), and urine organic acid analysis. In addition to measuring the blood lactate and pyruvate concentrations, these metabolites should also be measured in the CSF (especially in patients with CNS symptoms) if they are normal in blood. Magnetic resonance spectroscopy (MRS) of the brain may also be helpful in identifying increased lactate. It is important to remember that the absence of lactic acidemia, or any of the other aforementioned biochemical findings, does not exclude the diagnosis of a respiratory chain disorder.

More specialized diagnostic evaluation for a suspected respiratory chain disorder entails a combination of enzyme and morphologic analysis of tissues, polarographic analysis of intact mitochondria, and genetic analysis of mtDNA or nDNA encoded genes.[17,26] Polarographic analysis measures oxygen consumption by intact mitochondria using a variety of substrates. It requires freshly isolated mitochondria and is available in only a few centers. Interpretation of the results of these diagnostic studies is complicated by the fact that many defects are tissue specific. In particular, many defects are not expressed biochemically in blood cells or cultured skin fibroblasts, which mandates the need for invasive studies to obtain a skeletal muscle, cardiac, or liver biopsy. Enzyme and polarographic analysis can implicate deficiency of one or more of the respiratory chain complexes, but they do not permit the clinician to determine whether the patient has a defect in a nuclear- or mitochondrial-encoded subunit. Genetic analysis of the mitochondrial genome is available, but many mtDNA defects are not detectable in all tissues because of heteroplasmy. In recent years, considerable progress has been made in identifying the nuclear genes that encode for the respiratory chain subunits and related mitochondrial processes, and genetic analysis is becoming increasingly available for many nuclear-encoded defects. Genetic analysis of nuclear defects is not limited by the tissue-specificity issue that plays a role in the genetic evaluation of mtDNA-encoded defects.

A general consensus seems to have developed about the diagnostic evaluation of patients with a suspected respiratory chain disorder.[13,17,26] As noted earlier, the first step is to perform a comprehensive clinical evaluation and a noninvasive metabolic evaluation to establish whether the patient is likely to have a respiratory chain disorder. If the patient appears likely to have a respiratory chain disorder and the clinical phenotype is characteristic of a specific, well-defined mitochondrial disorder that can be confirmed by genetic testing of a blood sample, then proceeding with such genetic testing is generally indicated. If, on the other hand, it appears that the patient has a mitochondrial respiratory chain disorder that does not have a recognizable clinical pattern, then performing additional, more specialized, invasive biochemical testing to define the underlying metabolic defect before initiating genetic testing is the preferred route to pursue. The choice of diagnostic pathway is also influenced by the patient's clinical status, including transfusion history, ability to tolerate anesthesia or an invasive procedure such as an open skeletal muscle biopsy, and expected survival.

The key to learning the well-characterized clinical phenotypes that can be diagnosed by focused genetic testing using blood samples is to acquire an understanding of the current classification scheme for respiratory chain disorders. The traditional approach to classifying mitochondrial disorders was based on clinical phenotypes, pathologic findings and biochemical findings. This approach is still useful. However, a clinically based classification system is limited by two well-established characteristics of mitochondrial respiratory chain disorders: a particular clinical phenotype can be caused by more than one genetic defect, and conversely, the same genetic defect can produce more than one clinical phenotype. Recognition of these limitations led to efforts to classify mitochondrial disorders according to their genetic bases. This approach to classification is also imperfect, but it is improving as current understanding of the genetic bases of these disorders becomes greater.

The genetic classification divides the mitochondrial disorders into two broad categories, mtDNA defects and nDNA defects (see Table 50-15). The mitochondrial encoded disorders can be classified into those caused by point mutations and those caused by large deletions or duplications that affect multiple genes of the mitochondrial genome. Mitochondrial point mutations can be suclassified into those that affect mRNA, rRNA or tRNA. The nuclear-encoded disorders can be divided further into mutations that directly affect the genes that encode for subunits of the respiratory chain complexes; genes required for transport, assembly, or stabilization of the respiratory chain complexes; genes required for replication or maintenance of the mitochondrial genome; and genes involved in other mitochondrial processes required for normal respiratory chain function.

The differential diagnosis of several respiratory chain disorders that produce recognizable clinical syndromes in the newborn period are listed in Table 50-15. Most patients whose respiratory chain disorder manifests in the newborn period have a nDNA defect; when the disorder manifests later in childhood or adulthood, mtDNA defects predominate. Many of the most common and best characterized respiratory chain disorders that manifest in late childhood or adulthood do not appear in early infancy or manifest as much more severe, markedly different clinical phenotypes. The list of disorders is not comprehensive; rather it includes disorders that are relatively well-characterized and illustrate the basic approaches to diagnosis of these disorders.

Maternally inherited Leigh syndrome (MILS) is an example of a point mutation that affects a mtDNA structural gene (an mRNA) that encodes for a subunit of a respiratory chain complex (see Table 50-15). MILS is associated with a point mutation (generallyT8993C, T8993G, or T9176C) in the gene that encodes for subunit 6 of complex V (ATPase 6). Leigh syndrome was originally defined as a subacute necrotizing encephalopathy that involves the thalamus, brainstem, and posterior columns of the spinal cord. Typically, it has a mean age of onset of 2 years of age and is characterized by psychomotor regression, tremor, dystonia, optic atrophy, ophthalmoplegia, and respiratory difficulty with apnea. Death usually occurs by 4 years of age. Some patients have a Leigh syndrome–like disorder that is associated with hypertrophic cardiomyopathy, skeletal myopathy, or renal proximal tubular dysfunction. The defects that produce Leigh syndrome or a Leigh syndrome–like disorder include (but are not limited to) nuclear-encoded subunits of complex I, II, or IV, nuclear-encoded assembly genes for complex I or complex IV, nuclear-encoded subunits of the pyruvate dehydrogenase complex, or mtDNA encoded tRNAs.[13,17,91] MILS is an early onset, severe form of Leigh syndrome that is caused by mutations in the mitochondrially encoded subunit 6 of complex V. Patients without the ATPase 6 mutations listed should be evaluated for the other causes of Leigh syndrome. Detailed biochemical studies might refine the diagnosis to a specific complex or protein and direct further genetic studies.

Aminoglycoside-induced nonsyndromic deafness is caused by the A1555G mutation in the mitochondrial rRNA gene that encodes for the 12S ribosomal complex component. The aminoglycoside-induced nonsyndromic deafness disorder is a pharmacogenetic disorder that physicians should be aware of when obtaining a family history of maternally inherited hearing loss thought to be attributable to aminoglycoside use. The use of aminoglycosides in neonates with this mutation may produce irreversible deafness. This mutation is not the cause of aminoglycoside associated renal toxicity, but it can cause cardiomyopathy.

Isolated hypertrophic cardiomyopathy has been found in association with several tRNA mutations, principally involving the tRNA for leucine (tRNA^{Leu}) and the tRNA for isoleucine (tRNA^{Ile}). The tRNA^{Leu} defects include the A3243G mutation and the C3305T mutation. The A3243G mutation is probably the most commonly identified mtDNA mutation, and is the most common cause of MELAS (mitochondrial encephalomyopathy, lactic acidosis, and strokelike episodes), which manifests rarely in the newborn period as a severe encephalopathy syndrome. The C3305T mutation generally produces an infantile-onset hypertrophic cardiomyopathy with or without skeletal myopathy. Three tRNA^{Ile} mutations, A4269G, A4295G, and A4300, can produce isolated cardiomyopathy and should be considered in the evaluation of patients with this finding (also see multiple mtDNA depletion syndromes in Table 50-15).

Pearson syndrome is an example of a mitochondrial encoded disorder associated with large deletions or duplications of mtDNA. Pearson syndrome is characterized clinically by refractory sideroblastic anemia, neutropenia, thrombocytopenia, exocrine pancreatic dysfunction, and lactic acidosis. Patients with Pearson syndrome who survive the neonatal period can subsequently have gradual regression of the symptoms and signs of Pearson syndrome, and then develop Kearns-Sayre syndrome, which is an encephalomyopathy associated with progressive external ophthalmoplegia, hearing loss, cardiac arrhythmias, diabetes mellitus, and renal dysfunction.[17] The Kearns-Sayre syndrome is an alternate expression of the same mtDNA mutation, and is an example of how the phenotypes of mtDNA-encoded disorders can evolve dramatically with time.

Nuclear-encoded defects that produce recognizable clinical phenotypes in the newborn period are also listed in

Table 50-15. The first group of such disorders involves genes that encode for a specific subunit of the respiratory chain complexes. These disorders are often characterized by severe ketoacidosis that is associated with seizures, apnea, severe hypotonia, hepatomegaly, and renal proximal tubular dysfunction. Detailed enzymatic and polarographic studies are required to identify the deficient respiratory chain complexes. The specific deficiency can then be investigated by genetic analysis. For example, genetic testing is now available clinically for 7 of the 37 nuclear-encoded subunits of complex I.

The second group of nuclear disorders involves genes that encode for proteins that are required for transport, assembly, or stabilization of the respiratory chain complexes. For example, defects of several genes involved in assembly of complex IV (cytochrome oxidase, COX) have been identified. These defects appear to produce distinctive clinical phenotypes. SURF1 mutations produce Leigh syndrome. As noted earlier, Leigh syndrome does not manifest until later in infancy, but Leigh syndrome–like disorders can manifest in the newborn period.[13,17,91] SCO1 mutations can lead to encephalomyopathy and hepatic failure. COX10 mutations also lead to a Leigh syndrome–like phenotype (or encephalopathy), which is sometimes accompanied by hypertrophic cardiomyopathy, renal proximal tubular dysfunction, or anemia. SCO2 mutations and COX 15 mutations lead to encephalopathy or hypertrophic cardiomyopathy. Mutations of the assembly factors required for the other respiratory chain complexes have also been described. GRACILE syndrome, an eponymic association of growth *r*estriction, *a*mino aciduria, *c*holestasis, *i*ron overload, *l*actic acidosis, and *e*arly death, is the best described of these disorders; it is caused by mutations of the BCS1L gene, which is required for assembly of complex III.[13]

The third group of nuclear-encoded disorders involves genes that are required for replication or maintenance of the mitochondrial genome. These disorders are characterized by a reduction in mtDNA copy number, a condition known as mitochondrial DNA depletion syndrome. This syndrome can result from a deficiency of the mitochondrial DNA polymerase γ (POLG), an enzyme responsible for mitochondrial replication. It can also be the consequence of deoxyguanosine kinase (dGK) deficiency or thymidine kinase 2 (TK2) deficiency; dGK and TK2 are enzymes required for synthesis or recycling of the deoxyribonucleotides necessary for DNA replication. In brief, mitochondrial DNA is wholly dependent on the nucleus for production of the enzymes and deoxyribonucleotides it requires for its own replication. Absent these materials, the mitochondrion cannot replicate and its numbers decline. POLG deficiency leads to isolated encephalopathy or seizures, or to liver failure, hepatoencephalopathy, or Alpers syndrome (hepatopathic poliodystrophy). dGK deficiency presents with encephalopathy and liver failure, whereas TK2 presents with encephalopathy and severe skeletal myopathy.[13,76]

The fourth group of nuclear-encoded disorders are caused by mutations in genes required for other mitochondrial processes that are necessary for normal respiratory chain function. Barth syndrome is an example of such a disorder.[5] The clinical features of Barth syndrome include hypertrophic cardiomyopathy, cyclic neutropenia, and cataracts. It is an

X-linked recessive disorder caused by a mutation in the *tafazzin* gene, which encodes for a protein required for synthesis of the lipid milieu of the mitochondrial membranes. Mutations in the *tafazzin* gene can also produce an unusual form of cardiomyopathy known as left ventricle noncompaction.

Treatment of patients with a respiratory chain defect is largely supportive.[13,17,80] Therapy includes symptomatic management, such as treating acute or chronic acidosis with bicarbonate or citrate, and treating cardiac, renal, and other systemic disease with standard methods. It also includes avoiding certain drugs, such as valproate and barbiturates, which may be mitochondrial toxins. There is no dietary therapy of proven benefit for patients with respiratory chain disease, although vitamins or other nutritional supplements are generally tried using the rationale that they might stabilize or augment residual enzyme activity of the respiratory chain complexes, or serve as artificial electron acceptors or antioxidants. Coenzyme Q10 is administered because it is a structural homologue of ubiquinone, which accepts electrons from complex I and complex II and passes them on to complex III. Riboflavin is used based on the rationale that complexes I and II contain flavin. Vitamins C and K are used in combination based on the rationale that they could provide an electron transfer shuttle to bypass a complex III deficiency. Thiamine is a cofactor in the pyruvate dehydrogenase complex, which serves as the point of entry for glucose into the Krebs cycle. The daily dietary supplements in use for a neonate include coenzyme Q10 (20 mg), vitamin B_1 (thiamine, 20 mg), vitamin B_2 (riboflavin, 25 mg), vitamin C (250 mg), and vitamin K_3 (menadione, 5 mg). Carnitine may also be used, especially in patients with secondary carnitine deficiency (50 to 100 mg/kg per day). The doses cited are at the lower end of the range of doses recommended by various physicians; some investigators have recommended doses up to 10 times greater than these. However, none of these recommendations are based on controlled studies.

Dichloroacetate has been tried in patients with respiratory chain defects, and several groups are investigating its clinical use. The rationale for using dichloroacetate (50 mg per day) is that it maintains the pyruvate dehydrogenase complex in its activated state, thereby permitting entry of pyruvate, the final product of anaerobic oxidation of glucose, into the Krebs cycle and fueling the respiratory chain. It is unclear whether dichloroacetate is of any clinical benefit to patients with respiratory chain defects, and it can produce peripheral neuropathy in some patients.

Finally, all patients must receive a thorough clinical evaluation to determine whether they may have an organ-specific defect that would be amenable to organ transplantation. For example, heart transplantation was reportedly successful in a patient with cardiomyopathy caused by a tissue-specific mtDNA depletion syndrome.[74]

HYPOGLYCEMIA

See also Chapter 49, Part 1.
Recognizing hypoglycemia in the newborn may be difficult because the symptoms of hypoglycemia (i.e., lethargy, poor feeding, hypothermia, and seizures) are nonspecific. Frequent blood sugar determinations are often required to confirm the suspicion of hypoglycemia. Because inborn errors of metabolism are a relatively infrequent cause of

neonatal hypoglycemia, other diagnostic possibilities should be investigated concurrently.[77]

The first possibility to consider is neonatal stress secondary to perinatal asphyxia, hypothermia, or intrauterine malnutrition (e.g., placental abnormalities, prematurity, multiple gestations). The second consideration is the possibility of a hormonal abnormality affecting insulin and cortisol production or regulation. Third, the possibility of a malformation syndrome, such as Beckwith-Wiedemann syndrome, should be considered. The endocrine disorders and malformation syndromes associated with hypoglycemia are discussed more fully in Chapter 49, Part 1, as is the treatment of hypoglycemia. The fourth possibility is that the patient has a severe hepatocellular or cirrhotic liver disease that leads nonspecifically to fasting hypoglycemia.

The inborn errors that can produce this degree of liver damage include hereditary tyrosinemia, galactosemia (if the patient is receiving a diet containing galactose), hereditary fructose intolerance (if the patient is receiving a diet containing fructose), glycogen storage disease type IV, and respiratory chain defects (see Table 50-5). If liver disease is present, evaluation for these disorders should be performed (see "Hepatic Dysfunction").

Differential Diagnosis

Hypoglycemia may be associated with five categories of inborn errors of metabolism: fatty acid oxidation defects, gluconeogenesis defects, glycogen storage diseases, ketogenesis defects, and organic acidemias (Table 50-17). The diagnostic approach to hypoglycemia therefore must give consideration to entities belonging to each of these categories. Usually, Krebs cycle defects and respiratory chain defects do not produce hypoglycemia, but these defects should be considered when other evidence points in their direction. The diagnostic approach must quickly narrow the field of possible diagnoses so that specific treatment can be instituted.

The classic approaches to the differential diagnosis of hypoglycemic disorders in children are the fasting study and special challenge tests. These studies are, however, not feasible in newborn infants because of the significant risks and technical difficulties associated with performing such studies and because of the lack of control data derived from normal neonates. Alternatively, efforts to determine the cause of hypoglycemia in the newborn infant should include hormonal and biochemical studies before and after feeding and especially during an acute episode of hypoglycemia. Definitive diagnosis might have to be postponed several months until the child is old enough to tolerate a formal fasting study or specialized in vitro cell studies.

An algorithm (Fig. 50-3) for diagnosing the disorders that cause neonatal hypoglycemia can be generated from the results of the following studies: blood electrolytes and pH, plasma and urinary ketones, plasma free fatty acids, blood lactate and pyruvate, blood ammonia, liver function tests, plasma and urinary carnitine and acylcarnitine analysis, and urinary organic acids. A specific diagnosis might not be made by these studies, but they are necessary for providing a provisional diagnosis that can be confirmed by specific enzyme analysis.

The first laboratory finding that is used to discriminate between the disorders that cause hypoglycemia is the presence or absence of ketosis (see Fig. 50-3), because the physiologic response to fasting or hypoglycemia should be increased lipolysis, fatty acid oxidation, and ketone body formation. Defects of gluconeogenesis, glycogenolysis, and organic acid metabolism (especially the common branched-chain disorders) are generally accompanied by ketosis, whereas defects in fatty acid β-oxidation and ketogenesis are accompanied by increased plasma free fatty acids without a

---

TABLE 50–17   Metabolic Defects Associated with Neonatal Hypoglycemia

Category of Disorders	Disorder
Fatty acid oxidation	Carnitine-acylcarnitine translocase deficiency Carnitine palmitoyltransferase II deficiency Long-chain 3-hydroxyacyl-CoA dehydrogenase deficiency Short-chain acyl-CoA dehydrogenase deficiency Very-long-chain acyl-CoA dehydrogenase deficiency
Gluconeogenesis	Fructose-1,6-diphosphatase deficiency Hereditary fructose intolerance Phosphoenolpyruvate carboxykinase deficiency Pyruvate carboxylase deficiency
Glycogen storage disease (GSD)	GSD type I (glucose-6-phosphatase deficiency) GSD type III (debrancher deficiency)
Ketogenesis	3-Hydroxy-3-methylglutaryl-CoA lyase deficiency
Organic acidemias	Isovaleric acidemia Maple syrup urine disease Methylmalonic acidemia Multiple acyl-CoA dehydrogenase deficiency Multiple carboxylase deficiency Propionic acidemia

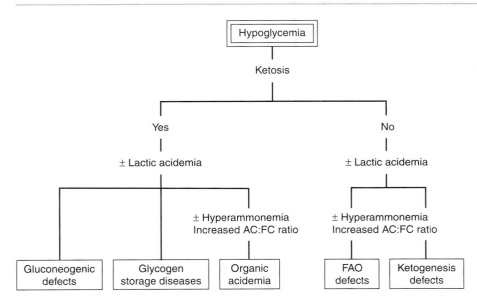

Figure 50–3. Approach to neonatal hypoglycemia. AC:FC, ratio of acyl-carnitine to free carnitine; FAO, fatty acid oxidation.

concomitant increase in plasma β-hydroxybutyrate and acetoacetate concentrations.

The second laboratory finding used to distinguish among the neonatal hypoglycemias is lactic acidemia (see Fig. 50-3). Although the simple presence or absence of lactic acidemia is not useful for discriminating among these disorders because they all can exhibit some degree of lactic acidemia depending on the physiologic circumstances, the relative degree of lactic acidemia and its relationship to feeding are important discriminating factors. For example, the magnitude of the lactic acidemia seen in the organic acidemias is generally less than that seen in the gluconeogenesis defects and glycogen storage diseases. The lactate concentration decreases in the fed state for patients with glycogen storage disease type I, whereas it increases for patients with glycogen storage disease type III. Similarly, lactic acidemia becomes more pronounced with fasting in patients with fatty acid oxidation defects and organic acidemias but is greater in the fed state than in the fasted state for those with the glycogen storage disorders associated with hypoglycemia. Hyperammonemia often accompanies hypoglycemia in patients with fatty acid oxidation defects, ketogenesis defects, and organic acidemias, but it is not seen in defects of gluconeogenesis (except severe PC deficiency) or the glycogen storage diseases.

Glycogen Storage Disorders

Glycogen storage disease type I is the most common defect of gluconeogenesis or glycogenolysis.[12] This diagnosis should be considered if, in addition to increased plasma free fatty acid and ketone body concentrations, clinical examination demonstrates hepatomegaly and additional laboratory studies reveal lactic acidosis, hypertriglyceridemia, and hyperuricemia.

The most common form of glycogen storage disease type I is von Gierke disease, which is caused by deficiency of glucose-6-phosphatase. Von Gierke disease may be more accurately called *glycogen storage disease type Ia*, because there are several subtypes of this disorder. For example, the disorder caused by deficiency of glucose-6-phosphate

translocase is type Ib. In addition to the clinical features of type Ia disease, glycogen storage disease type Ib is also characterized by neutropenia and neutrophil dysfunction, which lead to a propensity for serious bacterial infections. The long-term complications of both forms of type I glycogen storage disease include intellectual delay as a result of unrecognized or untreated hypoglycemia, short stature, gout, renal disease, and hepatic adenoma.

Type III glycogen storage disease may also occur in the neonatal period. Type III disease may be as severe as type I disease.

Definitive diagnosis of glycogen storage disease type I requires detailed enzymatic analysis of a liver biopsy specimen; the liver specimen must be fresh if studies for subtype Ib are to be done. Type III disease can be diagnosed by enzyme analysis of cultured skin fibroblasts. Alternatively, the diagnosis of glycogen storage disease Ia, Ib, and III can be established by genetic testing.

The mainstay of treatment for these forms of glycogen storage disease is to avoid prolonged fasting. Older affected patients should be provided with continuous nasogastric infusion or uncooked cornstarch at night. These treatments appear to be successful in controlling the hypoglycemia and other metabolic consequences associated with these disorders, but they might not eliminate the long-term sequelae (e.g., development of hepatic adenoma in glycogen storage disease type Ia).[12]

Gluconeogenesis Defects

Gluconeogenesis is the pathway by which glucose is synthesized from noncarbohydrate metabolites. The principal gluconeogenic precursors are pyruvate and lactate, certain gluconeogenic amino acids, and glycerol, which is derived mainly from fat metabolism. Several inborn errors of gluconeogenesis cause hypoglycemia (see Table 50-17).

Fructose-1,6-diphosphatase deficiency is an autosomal recessive disorder characterized by hyperventilation associated with severe ketoacidosis, hypoglycemia, seizures, and lethargy sometimes leading to coma. Hepatomegaly and the degree of liver dysfunction are generally mild. The defect in gluconeogenesis leads to lactic acidosis. Diagnosis requires a liver, intestine, or kidney biopsy for specific enzyme analysis. Acute episodes are treated with glucose administration, which is generally successful in correcting the hypoglycemia and ketoacidosis. Long-term treatment requires avoidance of fasting and removal of most fructose from the diet. As discussed for the glycogen storage diseases, patients with fructose-1,6-diphosphatase deficiency benefit from continuous nighttime feedings or the use of uncooked starch.

Pyruvate carboxylase (PC) deficiency can manifest in the neonatal period with hepatomegaly, lactic acidosis, citrullinemia, and hyperlysinemia, and structural CNS malformations. Patients who present in the newborn period might not survive beyond the first few months of life. Patients with less severe forms of PC deficiency may do well when they avoid fasting, have nighttime feedings, and receive supplementation with citrate, which yields oxaloacetate, the missing product of the PC enzyme reaction.

Phosphoenolpyruvate carboxykinase (PEPCK) deficiency is a rare disorder with an incompletely described phenotype.

Organic Acidemias

Several organic acidurias or acidemias cause neonatal hypoglycemia (see Table 50-17; see also "Metabolic Acidosis"). These disorders should be suspected when there is a metabolic acidosis, an anion gap, ketosis, abnormal results on urine spot tests for α-ketoacids, or an abnormal smell. Urinary organic acid analysis is the key diagnostic study. Many patients with an organic acid disorder have significant hyperammonemia. Plasma and urinary carnitine measurements are useful in diagnosing and possibly managing these disorders. Many of the organic acidurias are characterized by an increased acylcarnitine-to-free carnitine ratio in plasma and urine and overproduction of a particular acylcarnitine.

Fatty Acid Oxidation Disorders

Two groups of disorders cause neonatal hypoglycemia without ketosis: defects of fatty acid oxidation and defects of ketogenesis. It should be pointed out that inborn errors of metabolism that cause severe hepatocellular or cirrhotic liver disease also produce nonketotic or hypoketotic hypoglycemia associated with lactic acidosis. The disorders of fatty acid oxidation are discussed further in this section, whereas the defects of ketogenesis (e.g., 3-hydroxy-3-methylglutaryl-CoA lyase deficiency) are discussed in the preceding section on metabolic acidosis.

The primary pathway of fatty acid oxidation takes place within the mitochondrion.[44,70] Most forms of dietary fat contain primarily long-chain fatty acids (chain length of 14 to 20 carbons). For these long-chain fatty acids to be oxidized, they must be transported across the mitochondrial membranes into the mitochondrial matrix. The system for transporting these fatty acids across the mitochondrial membranes includes three components: carnitine palmitoyltransferase I (CPT I), carnitine-acylcarnitine translocase, and carnitine palmitoyltransferase II (CPT II). Medium-chain and short-chain fatty acids do not require this special system for transport across the mitochondrial membranes. Another transporter facilitates the uptake of free carnitine across the plasma membrane into the cytoplasm.

Inside the mitochondrion, fatty acids exist as their acyl-CoA derivatives. These fatty acid acyl-CoAs are degraded by the mitochondrial fatty acid β-oxidation system to form acetyl-CoA. The acyl-CoAs are degraded sequentially by a series of four enzymes: acyl-CoA dehydrogenase, enoyl-CoA hydratase, 3-hydroxyacyl-CoA dehydrogenase, and 3-ketothiolase. Different forms of these enzymes exist for fatty acid acyl-CoAs of different chain-lengths. These enzymes sequentially degrade the acyl-CoAs two carbon groups per turn of the β-oxidation cycle, from long-chain acyl-CoAs, to medium-chain acyl-CoAs, and finally to short-chain acyl-CoAs. An intact mitochondrial respiratory chain is required for normal functioning of the fatty acid β-oxidation pathway because it replenishes the oxidized forms of flavin adenine dinucleotide and nicotinamide adenine dinucleotide needed by the acyl-CoA dehydrogenases and the 3-hydroxyacyl-CoA dehydrogenases, respectively. Disorders caused by deficiency of almost all these enzymes have been described.[44,70,78]

As a rule, defects of long-chain fatty acid oxidation are more likely to manifest in the neonatal period and to cause serious problems than are defects of medium- or short-chain fatty acids.[70,78] Defects in long-chain fatty acid oxidation that manifest in the neonatal period include CPT II deficiency (but not CPT I deficiency), carnitine-acylcarnitine translocase deficiency, very-long-chain acyl-CoA dehydrogenase deficiency, long-chain 3-hydroxyacyl-CoA dehydrogenase (LCHAD) deficiency and the related disorder, mitochondrial trifunctional protein deficiency. Plasma membrane carnitine transporter deficiency (the cause of primary carnitine deficiency) does not generally manifest in the neonatal period.[6,35]

These disorders are a recognized cause of hypoglycemia, liver disease, cardiomyopathy, cardiac arrhythmias, and sudden death. The association of these defects with cardiomyopathy is consistent with the role of long-chain fatty acids as the chief energy source for the myocardium. The cause of the arrhythmias is less certain but may be a toxic effect of the long-chain acylcarnitines that accumulate in these disorders. Hyperammonemia may be seen in patients with the most severe forms of these deficiencies, for example, carnitine-acylcarnitine translocase deficiency and LCHAD deficiency. Neonatal CPT II deficiency is also associated with renal microcysts and CNS malformations. One of these defects, long-chain 3-hydroxyacyl-CoA dehydrogenase deficiency, is gaining attention as a cause of acute fatty liver of pregnancy in pregnant women who are carrying a fetus that is homozygous for this deficiency (see "Prenatal Onset").[6,35]

Defects of medium-chain or short-chain fatty acid β-oxidation include medium-chain acyl-CoA dehydrogenase (MCAD) deficiency, short-chain acyl-CoA dehydrogenase (SCAD) deficiency, and short-chain 3-hydroxyacyl-CoA dehydrogenase (SCHAD) deficiency.[70,78] MCAD deficiency is the most common of the fatty acid oxidation defects when all age groups are considered, but it does not generally appear in the neonatal period (see "Newborn Screening"). Similarly, SCHAD deficiency does not generally appear in newborns. SCAD deficiency, however, can manifest in the neonatal period with metabolic acidosis. Neonates with MCAD deficiency or SCAD deficiency do not develop cardiomyopathy.

Acute management of the newborn with a suspected fatty acid oxidation defect should begin with prompt infusion of high concentrations of glucose to correct the hypoglycemia and the underlying energy deficit. The patient should receive glucose at a rate of 10 mg/kg per minute or greater to maintain the serum glucose concentration above 100 mg/dL. The patient should not be given any formula that contains fat or parenteral intralipids until it is determined whether the patient has a defect of fatty acid oxidation.

A related consideration is the use of carnitine in patients with a suspected or proven fatty acid oxidation disorder. Carnitine has been used in patients with these disorders because they are often carnitine depleted. However, there is also concern that carnitine supplementation could increase the production of long-chain acylcarnitines, which can be arrhythmogenic.[44] The relative merits of using carnitine in the acute or chronic care of these patients with long-chain fatty acid β-oxidation defects are uncertain, but judicious use of a moderate carnitine dose (50 mg/kg per day) is often used until a diagnosis is established, and then adjusted depending on the diagnosis, the patient's clinical status, and the patient's plasma carnitine analysis.

Once the initial hypoglycemic episodes are controlled, the patient should be started on a high-carbohydrate, low-fat diet, while making certain to avoid fasting. Formulas enriched with medium-chain triglycerides should not be started before the infant's diagnosis has been established, because they can be dangerous to patients with defects in medium-chain fatty acid oxidation. Ultimately, a decision will have to be made regarding the infant's tolerance for fat. Riboflavin supplementation (50 mg/day) should be tried and its benefit evaluated. Long-term carnitine supplementation may be of benefit in some patients.

HYPERAMMONEMIA

The neonate with a hyperammonemia syndrome generally does well for the first few hours or days of life and then develops poor feeding, lethargy, vomiting, and tachypnea. If unrecognized and untreated, the illness generally progresses rapidly to coma, seizures, autonomic instability, and death. When hyperammonemia is suspected, the possibility should be investigated immediately because these illnesses are life threatening, and they can produce irreversible neurologic sequelae.

Differential Diagnosis

More than a dozen disorders can cause significant hyperammonemia in the newborn infant, and an attempt must be made to quickly reach a provisional diagnosis (Box 50-2). By convention, the primary hyperammonemias include deficiencies of the enzymes that make up the urea cycle itself plus N-acetylglutamine synthetase, which is required for activation of the first step in the urea cycle, carbamyl phosphate synthetase. The secondary hyperammonemias include enzyme or protein deficiencies that interfere with the normal functioning of the urea cycle: amino acid transport defects, fatty acid oxidation disorders, lactic acidemias, and organic acidurias.

A systematic approach to the differential diagnosis of these disorders is presented in Figure 50-4. It is imperative that the possibility of a primary hyperammonemia syndrome (a urea cycle defect) be distinguished from a secondary hyperammonemia syndrome (e.g., an organic aciduria), because

---

> **BOX 50–2** Genetic Disorders Associated with Hyperammonemia in Neonates
>
> **AMINO ACID TRANSPORT DEFECTS**
> Hyperornithinemia-hyperammonemia-homocitrullinemia (HHH syndrome)
> Lysinuric protein intolerance
>
> **FATTY ACID OXIDATION DEFECTS**
> Carnitine-acylcarnitine translocase deficiency
> Carnitine palmitoyltransferase II deficiency
> Long-chain acyl-CoA dehydrogenase deficiency
> Long-chain 3-hydroxyacyl-CoA dehydrogenase deficiency
>
> **LACTIC ACIDEMIA**
> Pyruvate carboxylase deficiency
>
> **ORGANIC ACIDURIAS**
> 3-Hydroxy-3-methylglutaryl-CoA lyase deficiency
> Isovaleric acidemia
> 3-Ketothiolase deficiency
> Methylmalonic acidemia
> Multiple acyl-CoA dehydrogenase deficiency
> Propionic acidemia
>
> **UREA CYCLE DEFECTS**
> Argininosuccinic acid lyase deficiency
> Argininosuccinic acid synthetase deficiency
> Carbamyl phosphate synthetase deficiency
> Ornithine transcarbamylase deficiency
> N-Acetylglutamate synthetase deficiency

---

the best way of treating the hyperammonemia in the latter would be to treat the underlying disorder.

The first step in evaluating a suspected hyperammonemia is to obtain an accurate plasma ammonia concentration. The plasma sample for ammonia determination must be collected and stored on ice and then rapidly analyzed. The plasma ammonia concentration may be as high as 150 μmol/L in a sick newborn. A plasma ammonia concentration greater than 150 μmol/L is the consequence of an inborn error of metabolism until proved otherwise.

Most primary disorders of the urea cycle do not begin in the first 24 hours of life. Hyperammonemia that develops within the first 24 hours of life is generally associated with prematurity or a secondary hyperammonemia, usually a disorder of organic acid metabolism or fatty acid oxidation.[11,45,92] The severe hyperammonemia associated with prematurity has been designated transient hyperammonemia of the newborn. It is a mistake to believe that transient means that this disorder is benign. The degree of hyperammonemia found in this disorder can be as great as that found in many of the primary hyperammonemia syndromes, sometimes exceeding 1000 μmol/L. This disorder therefore requires the same rapid and vigorous therapy as the other defects of the urea cycle.

The key to distinguishing between a primary and a secondary hyperammonemia syndrome is the presence or absence of acidosis, ketosis, or hypoglycemia. The urea cycle defects generally are associated with respiratory alkalosis in response to the increased ventilatory rate induced by the hyperammonemia itself. A urea cycle disorder such as argininosuccinic aciduria, which accumulates an acidic metabolite,

Figure 50-4. Approach to neonatal hyperammonemia. AL, argininosuccinic acid lyase; AS, argininosuccinic acid synthetase; ASA, argininosuccinic acid; CPS, carbamyl phosphate synthetase; NAGS, N-acetylglutamate synthetase; OTC, ornithine transcarbamylase. (*Adapted from Brusilow SW, Horwich AL: Urea cycle enzymes. In Scriver CR, et al, editors: The metabolic and molecular bases of inherited disease, 8th ed. New York, 2001, McGraw-Hill, p 1909, reproduced with permission of The McGraw-Hill Companies.*)

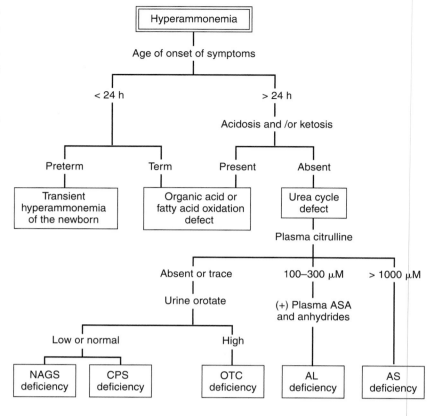

can be associated with a mild acidosis, but the acidosis is rarely the predominant feature of presentation. Similarly, a component of metabolic acidosis can be superimposed on the respiratory alkalosis as the patient deteriorates. In contrast, the organic acidemias are generally associated with a metabolic acidosis of greater magnitude and an increased anion gap from their onset (see "Metabolic Acidosis"). Several fatty acid oxidation defects and the severe neonatal form of PC deficiency are also associated with a metabolic acidosis.

The second feature that distinguishes the organic acidemias from the urea cycle defects is the presence of ketosis in the organic acidemias. Ketosis can be detected rapidly by the screening studies outlined previously (see Tables 50-11 and 50-12). Definitive diagnosis of an organic acidemia requires quantitative urinary organic acid analysis. The distinguishing features of a fatty acid oxidation disorder are nonketotic or hypoketotic hypoglycemia. The presence of ketotic hypoglycemia and lactic acidosis, as well as the plasma amino acid pattern, distinguish PC deficiency from a urea cycle defect.

Urea Cycle Defects

In the absence of severe acidosis, ketosis, or hypoglycemia, a provisional diagnosis of a urea cycle defect should be made. The first step in the urea cycle is the formation of carbamyl phosphate from ammonia by carbamyl phosphate synthetase I (CPSI, but hereafter referred to simply as CPS). The next enzyme in the cycle, ornithine transcarbamylase (OTC), converts carbamyl phosphate and ornithine to citrulline. Citrulline is converted to argininosuccinate by argininosuccinate synthetase (ASS). Argininosuccinate is then cleaved by argininosuccinate

lyase (ASL) to produce arginine. Finally, arginine is cleaved by arginase to form urea and ornithine. The urea is excreted in the urine, and the ornithine is available to restart the cycle. A fifth enzyme, N-acetylglutamate synthetase (NAGS), must be available to form N-acetylglutamine, which is required for the activation of CPS. Ornithine, citrulline, argininosuccinate, and arginine are all amino acids.

Urea cycle disorders can be differentiated from each other by performing amino acid analysis and urine orotic acid analysis (see also Specialized Biochemical Testing).[92] Typically, the amino acids proximal to the enzyme deficiency are increased, while the amino acids distal to the enzyme deficiency block are decreased. Except in the case of arginase deficiency, all of the urea cycle disorders are characterized by an increased plasma concentration of glutamine (a storage form for ammonia) and a decreased plasma arginine concentration.

The plasma citrulline and argininosuccinate concentrations provide the keys to distinguishing among the urea cycle defects that manifest with hyperammonemia in the neonatal period (see Fig. 50-4). The plasma citrulline concentration is generally low in NAGS deficiency, CPS deficiency, and OTC deficiency because citrulline synthesis requires the sequential action of these enzymes. Measurement of urinary orotic acid, which is formed from excessive amounts of carbamyl phosphate that leave the mitochondrion and enter the cytosolic pyrimidine biosynthetic pathway, can be used to distinguish among NAGS deficiency, CPS deficiency, and OTC deficiency. The urinary orotic acid concentration is low or normal in NAGS deficiency and CPS deficiency, but elevated in OTC deficiency.

Once formed, citrulline is converted to argininosuccinate by ASS. In the absence of ASS, citrulline produced by the earlier steps of the urea cycle accumulates in high concentration. For this reason, ASS deficiency is commonly called citrullinemia. ASL deficiency leads to increased excretion of argininosuccinate (and its anhydrides) and moderate elevation of plasma citrulline. Deficiency of the last step in the urea cycle, arginase, is not a cause of hyperammonemia in the neonatal period but is a cause of neurologic disease in later childhood. NAGS deficiency resembles CPS deficiency, and it requires enzyme analysis of a liver biopsy or genetic testing to distinguish between the two disorders.[92]

Treatment for the acute phase of the urea cycle defects includes stopping dietary protein intake, suppressing endogenous protein catabolism through parenteral administration of glucose, providing drugs that serve as alternate pathways for ammonia detoxification and excretion, and, in severe cases, hemodialysis.[46] Physicians who are unable to offer these forms of therapy should consider transferring their patients to centers that have such capability.

The protocols for detoxifying ammonia employ drugs that form excretable compounds with amino acids that accumulate during hyperammonemic crisis. The first drug to be developed was benzoate, which conjugates with glycine to form benzoylglycine (hippurate); formation and excretion of one molecule of hippurate eliminates one molecule of ammonia. The second drug to be developed was sodium phenylacetate, which conjugates with glutamine to form phenylacetylglutamine; formation and excretion of one molecule of phenylacetylglutamine eliminates two molecules of ammonia. Sodium phenylacetate is still available for intravenous use, but it has been replaced by sodium phenylbutyrate for oral use because sodium phenylbutyrate has a less offensive odor than sodium phenylacetate.

In addition to these drugs, arginine is provided to prime the urea cycle (i.e., regenerate ornithine), which is the precursor for the next turn of the cycle. N-carbamylglutamate is an analogue of N-acetylglutamate that can be taken orally and appears to be an effective treatment for N-acetylglutamate synthetase deficiency. Long-term management of these disorders after the acute illness entails modification of this basic plan.[92]

The prognosis for neonates who present with a urea cycle defect in the newborn period is guarded.[4,47] Without treatment, the mortality rate is high. With treatment, the mortality is reduced, but survivors are often left with significant neurologic impairments and a lifelong illness that predisposes them to recurrent life-threatening metabolic crises. The prognosis is particularly guarded for patients with defects affecting the early part of the cycle, namely NAGS deficiency, CPS deficiency, and OTC deficiency. The prognosis for patients with more distal defects in the urea cycle, ASS deficiency, and ASL deficiency, is better, although these patients also experience recurrent hyperammonemic crises. The guarded prognosis for all these patients has led many groups to perform early liver transplantation for these patients. The results of these efforts appear promising.[51]

Other Causes of Hyperammonemia

Four groups of disorders are associated with secondary hyperammonemia in neonates (see Box 50-2). We have already discussed fatty acid β-oxidation disorders, PC

deficiency, and organic acidemias. The remaining group consists of two amino acid transport defects, the hyperornithinemia-hyperammonemia-homocitrullinuria (HHH) syndrome and lysinuric protein intolerance. The mechanism of the hyperammonemia in these disorders is impaired intracellular transport of one or more of the amino acids that make up the urea cycle. Treatment of these disorders is aimed at overcoming the defects in transport.[92,103]

TREATMENT

It is not possible in an overview of inborn errors of metabolism to discuss treatment of all the individual diseases that might be encountered. Treatments for some inborn errors of metabolism were discussed in the relevant sections of this chapter. General principles that are relevant to many of these diseases are discussed in the following section.

With few exceptions, the inborn errors of metabolism expressed in the newborn period are inherited as recessive traits. Disorders inherited in this manner generally have a common mechanism of pathogenesis, which is depicted in Figure 50-5. In simple terms, patients with these metabolic diseases are lacking a specific enzyme that converts substance B to substance C. In some cases, the enzyme requires one or more cofactors for its activity. Deficient enzyme activity may be caused by an error in apoenzyme function or cofactor availability.

The absence of enzyme activity can produce disease in a number of different ways. First, there is accumulation of substance B proximal to the enzyme block, leading to increased concentrations of substance B that might be toxic. The congenital hyperammonemias are a good example of this mechanism. Without one of the urea cycle enzymes, ammonia accumulates and causes significant neurotoxic effects. Second, there is overproduction of substance B, which is converted by alternate pathways to toxic metabolites E and F. It is thought that tyrosinemia type I, for example, produces its hepatotoxic and neurotoxic effects through overproduction of toxic secondary metabolites. Third, the disease state may be caused by deficiency of substance C or D, which is distal to the enzyme block. Defects of gluconeogenesis, such as pyruvate carboxylase deficiency, presumably work through this mechanism. Hypoglycemia results from impaired production of gluconeogenic precursors.

The disease state may be produced by a combination of these mechanisms. It is thought that many of the organic acidemias produce their toxic effects through a combination of mechanisms. In many of these disorders, acyl-CoA molecules accumulate proximal to the enzyme block and interfere

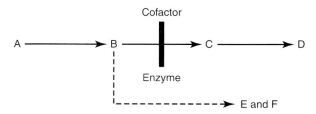

Figure 50-5. Schematic depiction of the pathogenesis of many inborn errors of metabolism. See text for details.

with a number of other metabolic pathways (e.g., the urea cycle), and there is underproduction of metabolites distal to the enzyme deficiency that are essential for other cellular processes.

Treatment at the Metabolite Level

Traditional approaches to treating inborn errors of metabolism have focused on this model of pathogenesis. The two general approaches in use are manipulation at the metabolite level and manipulation at the protein (or enzyme) level (Table 50-18).

The most common form of metabolite manipulation is dietary restriction, which decreases the amount of precursor A that the impaired enzyme must handle. The dietary management of PKU is an example of successful application of this approach. Dietary restriction is often combined with other treatment approaches, such as metabolite diversion.

The therapy for the urea cycle defects is perhaps the best studied of the metabolite diversion strategies. Two drugs, sodium phenylacetate and sodium benzoate, are provided to these patients to serve as ammonia traps (see also "Hyperammonemia"). Phenylacetate conjugates with glutamine to form phenylacetylglutamine, eliminating two ammonia molecules as the nitrogen component of glutamine; benzoate conjugates with glycine to form benzoylglycine (hippurate), eliminating one ammonia molecule as the nitrogen component of glycine. Arginine is also provided to prime the urea cycle because it is the last amino acid in the urea cycle and is split to release urea and ornithine, the precursor for the next turn of the cycle.

Other forms of diversion therapy include carnitine and glycine supplementation for the organic acidurias. Carnitine and glycine are transesterified with acyl-CoAs to form acylcarnitines and acylglycines, respectively. These transesterifications release free CoA, making it available for essential intracellular processes, while the potentially toxic acyl groups are excreted in the urine as acylcarnitines and acylglycines.

The deficiency of substances distal to the enzyme block (e.g., C or D) can be overcome by supplementing with exogenous C or D. An example of this approach is the feeding of uncooked cornstarch to patients with the hepatic forms of glycogen storage disease who cannot generate glucose from endogenous glycogen and are predisposed to fasting hypoglycemia.[12] The uncooked cornstarch is metabolized slowly to

TABLE 50–18	Approaches to Treatment of Inborn Errors of Metabolism
Approach	**Examples**
Metabolite manipulation	Dietary restriction Diversion Supplementation
Protein manipulation	Inhibition Replacement Stimulation of residual activity Transplantation
Gene manipulation	Somatic cell gene therapy

provide a steady source of glucose while these patients are sleeping.

Treatment at the Protein Level

There are several approaches to treating at the protein level. Historically, the first example of this approach was to stimulate residual enzyme activity by providing pharmacologic amounts of cofactor required by the deficient enzyme. This approach has been used successfully to reduce the clinical severity of several vitamin-dependent enzymopathies, including vitamin B_6 and homocystinuria, vitamin B_{12} and methylmalonic acidemia, and thiamine and MSUD. It is important to understand that only a fraction of patients with any of these disorders respond to vitamin supplementation, for reasons that are still not completely understood.

The converse of the first approach is to inhibit enzyme activity and block production of toxic metabolites. The use of NTBC to treat tyrosinemia type I is an example of this approach. Tyrosinemia type I is a defect in the distal portion of the catabolic pathway for tyrosine. The enzyme deficiency that causes tyrosinemia type I leads to overproduction of toxic metabolites that produce the hepatic and neurologic complications of the disease. NTBC is a drug that inhibits an enzyme, p-hydroxyphenylpyruvate dioxygenase, which is proximal in the catabolic pathway to the enzyme deficiency that causes tyrosinemia type I. NTBC successfully suppresses overproduction of the toxic metabolites that produce the hepatic and neurologic complications of tyrosinemia type I.

A more direct approach to treating an enzyme deficiency is to replace the dysfunctional enzyme. This approach has been the focus of biochemical genetics for some time and has been tried from two directions: providing direct enzyme replacement and providing enzyme through organ transplantation. It has been very difficult to provide enzyme in a bottle for a number of reasons, including the need to produce large amounts of pure enzyme; the need to direct the enzyme to the organ, cell, or organelle where it is needed; the tendency of the body to reject foreign proteins; and the great expense of such efforts. The greatest success of this approach has been for some of the hematologic clotting disorders, such as factor VIII deficiency (see Chapter 46).

Direct enzyme replacement therapy has been available for several years for two inborn errors of metabolism, Gaucher disease and α_1-antitrypsin deficiency. In the case of Gaucher disease, enzyme replacement therapy has been successful in treating the hematologic and visceral manifestations and somewhat less successful in treating the skeletal manifestations of children and adults with the non-neuronopathic form of this disease. In the case of α_1-antitrypsin deficiency, enzyme replacement therapy is effective for the adult-onset pulmonary manifestations of the disease but not for the hepatic problems expressed in the neonatal period. The lessons learned in treating these diseases are being applied to other inborn errors of metabolism, especially the lysosomal storage disorders.

The second approach to enzyme replacement therapy is organ transplantation. This approach is being pursued vigorously for a number of inborn errors of metabolism (Table 50-19). Perhaps the best studied approach is liver transplantation, which has been performed successfully

TABLE 50–19 Experience with Organ Transplantation for Treating Inborn Errors of Metabolism

Organ	Disorder
Bone marrow	Lysosomal storage disorders
	Severe combined immunodeficiency
Heart	Dilated cardiomyopathy
	Familial hypercholesterolemia
Heart and lung	Cystic fibrosis
Kidney	Cystinosis
	Fabry disease
Liver	α_1-Antitrypsin deficiency
	Glycogen storage disorders
	Tyrosinemia type I
	Ornithine transcarbamylase deficiency

for about two dozen different inborn errors of metabolism.[51,86] This approach has been particularly successful for disorders in which the liver is the sole source of the enzyme and the only organ affected by the disease.

Many inborn errors of metabolism cannot be treated with liver transplantation or even multiple organ transplantation because the abnormal genotype produces a multisystem disease. This appears to be the case for many patients with a respiratory chain disorder, but not all.[74,87] Bone marrow transplantation is sometimes used to treat multiorgan disease because pluripotent bone marrow cells provide precursors for many related cell types in different organs. The benefit of bone marrow transplantation or stem cell transplantation for the lysosomal storage diseases appears promising and is an area of intense interest.[61,68]

Treatment at the Genetic Level

Treatment of inborn errors of metabolism has focused on modification of the phenotype rather than the genotype, but vigorous efforts are underway to develop methods for manipulating the genotype of somatic cells (i.e., cells other than germ cells). Efforts have focused on somatic cell gene therapy rather than altering germ cells for numerous ethical reasons. Additionally, there is the very practical reason that most children born with inborn errors of metabolism are not known to be at risk before they manifest symptoms of disease.

Somatic cell gene therapy requires insertion of a functional gene into a patient's somatic cells in such a way that they are introduced into the appropriate target organs, are functionally active, and are appropriately regulated. Somatic cell gene therapy has the goal of treating the affected patient's disease; it cannot correct the affected patient's germline. Successful somatic cell gene therapy has not been demonstrated conclusively for any inborn error of metabolism. The approaches to somatic cell gene therapy employ viral vectors or physicochemically modified DNA as a means of delivering a suitably tailored normal gene to its appropriate target. In vivo and ex vivo approaches also are being used to introduce the corrective gene. One source of concern with this approach

has been that gene insertion into the patient's genome would be random and could lead to harmful mutagenesis. Homologous recombination is being explored as a means of circumventing this risk. In homologous recombination, a new gene (or DNA fragment) is inserted in exchange for the defective gene (or DNA fragment) rather than inserted randomly into the patient's genome. Homologous recombination could therefore provide a means of selectively excising the deleterious gene in exchange for the normal gene without the risk of producing harmful random insertional mutagenesis.

A novel pharmacogenetic approach for treating X-linked adrenoleukodystrophy was explored based on studies that showed genetic redundancy for many genes and many pathways.[42] In particular, the mammalian genome contains a gene that encodes for a protein that is functionally related to the protein that is abnormal in X-linked adrenoleukodystrophy. This protein is called adrenoleukodystrophy-related protein (ALDRP). Using sodium phenylbutyrate, which is known to activate a subgroup of latent genes, the investigators were able to activate the gene that encodes for the ALDRP protein in cultured cells from patients with X-linked adrenoleukodystrophy and in X-linked adrenoleukodystrophy knockout mice, and correct the biochemical lesion. Human trials with sodium phenylbutyrate or similar drugs are anticipated for the future. It is also anticipated that further studies will identify and capitalize on other instances of genetic redundancy for treating other inborn errors of metabolism.

Along with these efforts to develop somatic gene therapy, considerable effort is being expended to address the larger clinical, ethical, and societal issues of this form of treatment. These issues will undoubtedly prove to be as formidable a challenge as the technical issues, and they deserve the same attention.

CONCLUSION

Inborn errors of metabolism are an important cause of morbidity and mortality in newborn infants. These disorders are probably underdiagnosed because of their rarity, the nonspecific way many of them are expressed, and the difficulty clinicians have with their diagnosis. This chapter reduces this difficulty by providing a practical approach to the diagnosis of these disorders based on sets of common clinical and laboratory findings.

REFERENCES

1. AAP Newborn Screening Task Force: Newborn screening: a blueprint for the future, *Pediatrics* 106(suppl):389, 2000.
2. Applegarth DA, et al: Laboratory detection of metabolic disease, *Pediatr Clin North Am* 36:49, 1989.
3. Arnold GL, et al: Molybdenum cofactor deficiency, *J Pediatr* 123:595, 1993.
4. Bachmann C: Outcome and survival of 88 patients with urea cycle disorders: a retrospective evaluation, *Eur J Pediatr* 162:410, 2003.
5. Barth PG, et al: X-linked cardioskeletal myopathy and neutropenia (Barth syndrome): an update, *Am J Med Genet* 126A:349, 2004.
6. Bellig LL: Maternal acute fatty liver of pregnancy and the associated risk for long-chain 3-hydroxyacyl-coenzyme a dehydrogenase (LCHAD) deficiency in infants, *Adv Neonatal Care* 4:26, 2004.

7. Boles RG, et al: Retrospective biochemical screening of fatty acid oxidation disorders in postmortem livers of 418 cases of sudden death in the first year of life, *J Pediatr* 132:924, 1998.

8. Brown GK, et al: β-Hydroxyisobutyryl CoA deacylase deficiency: a defect in valine metabolism associated with physical malformations, *Pediatrics* 70:532, 1982.

9. Bruno C, et al: The mitochondrial DNA C3303T mutation can cause cardiomyopathy and/or skeletal myopathy, *J Pediatr* 135:197, 1999.

10. Burlina AB, et al: Clinical and biochemical approach to the neonate with a suspected inborn error of amino acid and organic acid metabolism, *Semin Perinatol* 23:162, 1999.

11. Burton BK: Inborn errors of metabolism in infancy: a guide to diagnosis, *Pediatrics* 102:E69, 1998.

12. Chen Y-T, et al: Type 1 glycogen storage disease: nine years of management with corn starch, *Eur J Pediatr* 152:S56, 1993.

13. Chinnery PF: *Mitochondrial disorders overview* (website). www.genetests.org. Accessed February 21, 2010.

14. Clayton PT: Diagnosis of inherited disorders of liver metabolism, *J Inherit Metab Dis* 26:135, 2003.

15. Cormier-Daire V, et al: Neonatal and delayed-onset liver involvement in disorders of oxidative phosphorylation, *J Pediatr* 130:817, 1997.

16. Cote A, et al: Sudden unexpected deaths in infancy: what are the causes? *J Pediatr* 135:437, 1999.

17. DiMauro S, Schon EA: Mitochondrial respiratory-chain diseases, *N Engl J Med* 348:2656, 2003.

18. Ellaway CJ, et al: Clinical approach to inborn errors of metabolism presenting in the newborn period, *J Paediatr Child Health* 38:511, 2002.

19. Elsas LJ II: *Galactosemia* (website). www.genetests.org. Accessed September 27, 2007.

20. Ernst LM, et al: The value of the metabolic autopsy in the pediatric hospital setting, *J Pediatr* 148:779, 2006.

21. Exil VJ, et al: Metabolic basis of pediatric heart disease, *Prog Pediatr Cardiol* 20:143, 2005.

22. Fernandes J, et al, editors: *Inborn metabolic diseases: diagnosis and treatment*, 4th ed. Heidelberg, 2006, Springer-Verlag.

23. GeneReviews: *Genetic Disease Online Reviews at GeneTests-GeneClinics* (website). http:/www.genetests.org. Accessed July 15, 2010.

24. Gilbert-Barness E: Review: Metabolic cardiomyopathy and conduction system defects in children, *Ann Clin Lab Sci* 34:15, 2004.

25. Gospe SM Jr: *Pyridoxine-dependent seizures* (website). www.genetests.org. Accessed July 24, 2007.

26. Haas RH, et al: The in-depth evaluation of suspected mitochondrial disease, *Molec Genet Metab* 94:16, 2008.

27. Hamosh A: *Glycine encephalopathy* (website). www.genetests.org. Accessed July 26, 2010.

28. Heubi JE, et al: Inborn errors of bile acid metabolism, *Semin Liver Dis* 27:282, 2007.

29. Hoffmann GF, et al: Clinical and biochemical phenotypes in 11 patients with mevalonic aciduria, *Pediatrics* 91:915, 1993.

30. Hoover-Fong JE, et al: Natural history of glycine encephalopathy in 65 patients, *J Inher Metab Dis* 26:64, 2003.

31. Horster F, Hoffmann GF: Pathophysiology, diagnosis, and treatment of methylmalonic aciduria—recent advances and new challenges, *Pediatr Nephrol* 19:1071, 2004.

32. Hughes J, et al: Outcomes of siblings with classical galactosemia, *J Pediatr* 154:721, 2009.

33. Hyland K, Arnold LA: Value of lumbar puncture in the diagnosis of infantile epilepsy and folinic acid-responsive seizures, *J Child Neurol* 17(suppl 3):S48, 2002.

34. Iafolla A, et al: Medium-chain acyl-coenzyme A dehydrogenase deficiency: clinical course in 120 affected children, *J Pediatr* 124:409, 1994.

35. Ibdah JA, et al: A fetal fatty-acid oxidation disorder as a cause of liver disease in pregnant women, *N Engl J Med* 340:1723, 1999.

36. Jaeken J: Congenital disorders of glycosylation (CDG): It's all in it! *J Inherit Metab Dis* 26:99, 2003.

37. Kahler SG, et al: Pancreatitis in patients with organic acidemias, *J Pediatr* 124:239, 1994.

38. Kane JM, et al: Metabolic cardiomyopathy and mitochondrial disorders in the pediatric intensive care unit, *J Pediatr* 151:538, 2007.

39. Kaye CI and the Committee on Genetics: Newborn Screening Fact Sheets, *Pediatrics* 118:e934, 2006.

40. Kelleher JF, et al: The pancytopenia of isovaleric acidemia, *Pediatrics* 65:1023, 1980.

41. Kelley RI: Inborn errors of cholesterol biosynthesis, *Adv Pediatr* 47:1, 2000.

42. Kemp S, et al: Gene redundancy and pharmacologic gene therapy: implications for X-linked adrenoleukodystrophy, *Nat Med* 4:1261, 1998.

43. Klepper J, Voit T: Facilitated glucose transporter protein type 1 (GLUT1) deficiency syndrome: impaired glucose transport into the brain, *Eur J Pediatr* 161:295, 2002.

44. Kompare M, et al: Mitochondrial fatty-acid oxidation disorders, *Semin Pediatr Neurol* 15:140, 2008.

45. Leonard JV, Morris AAM: Inborn errors of metabolism around time of birth, *Lancet* 356:583, 2000.

46. Leonard JV: The nutritional management of urea cycle disorders, *J Pediatr* 138(suppl 1):S40, 2001.

47. Maestri NE, et al: Neonatal onset ornithine transcarbamylase deficiency: a retrospective analysis, *J Pediatr* 134:268, 1999.

48. Marquardt T, et al: Congenital disorders of glycosylation: review of their molecular bases, clinical presentations and specific therapies, *Eur J Pediatr* 162:359, 2003.

49. Marsden D, et al: Newborn screening for metabolic disorders, *J Pediatr* 148:577, 2006.

50. Matern D, Rinaldo P: *Medium-chain acyl-coenzyme A dehydrogenase deficiency* (website). www.genetests.org. Accessed August 2, 2010.

51. McBride KL, et al: Developmental outcomes with early orthotopic liver transplantation for infants with neonatal-onset urea cycle defects and a female patient with late-onset ornithine transcarbamylase deficiency, *Pediatrics* 114:e523, 2004.

52. McCandless SE: A primer on expanded newborn screening by tandem mass spectrometry, *Prim Care* 1:583, 2004.

53. Morris AAM, et al: Liver failure associated with mitochondrial DNA depletion, *J Hepatol* 28:556, 1998.

54. Moser H, et al: Phenotype of patients with peroxisomal disorders divided into sixteen complementation groups, *J Pediatr* 127:13, 1995.

55. Munnich A: Defects of the respiratory chain. In Fernandes J, et al, editors: *Inborn metabolic diseases: diagnosis and treatment*, 3rd ed. Berlin, 2000, Springer-Verlag, p 157.

56. NIH Consensus Development Conference Statement: Phenylketonuria: screening and management, *Pediatrics* 108:972, 2000.

57. Nordli DR Jr, De Vivo DC: Classification of infantile seizures: Implications for identification and treatment of inborn errors of metabolism, *J Child Neurol* 17(suppl 3):S3, 2002.

58. Nyhan WL, et al: Treatment of the acute crisis in maple syrup urine disease, *Arch Pediatr Adolesc Med* 152:593, 1998.

59. Ogier de Baulny H, et al: Neonatal hyperammonemia caused by a defect of carnitine-acylcarnitine translocase, *J Pediatr* 127:723, 1995.

60. Ohura T, et al: A novel inborn error of metabolism detected by elevated methionine and/or galactose in newborn screening: Neonatal intrahepatic cholestasis caused by citrin deficiency, *Eur J Pediatr* 162:317, 2003.

61. Orchard P, et al: Hematopoietic cell therapy for metabolic disease, *J Pediatr* 151:340, 2007.

62. Papadopoulou LC, et al: Fatal infantile cardioencephalomyopathy with COX deficiency and mutations in SCO2, a COX assembly gene, *Nat Genet* 23:333, 1999.

63. Pauli RM, et al: Association of congenital deficiency of multiple vitamin K dependent coagulation factors and the phenotype of the warfarin embryopathy, *Am J Hum Genet* 41:566, 1987.

64. Pearl PL, et al: The pediatric neurotransmitter disorders, *J Pediatr Neurol* 22:606, 2007.

65. Picker JD, Levy HL: *Homocystinuria caused by cystathionine beta-synthase deficiency* (website). www.genetests.org. Accessed August 2, 2010.

66. Poll-The BT, et al: The eye as a window to inborn errors of metabolism, *J Inherit Metab Dis* 26:229, 2003.

67. Porter FD: Malformation syndromes due to inborn errors of cholesterol synthesis, *J Clin Invest* 110:715, 2002.

68. Prasad VK, et al: Emerging trends in transplantation of inherited metabolic diseases, *Bone Marrow Transplant* 41: 99, 2008.

69. Rashed MS, et al: Diagnosis of inborn errors of metabolism from blood spots by acylcarnitines and amino acids profiling using automated electrospray tandem mass spectrometry, *Pediatr Res* 38:324, 1995.

70. Rinaldo P, et al: Clinical and biochemical features of fatty acid oxidation disorders, *Curr Opin Pediatr* 10:615, 1998.

71. Rinaldo P, et al: Sudden and unexpected neonatal death: A protocol for the postmortem diagnosis of fatty acid oxidation disorders, *Semin Perinatol* 23:204, 1999.

72. Rouse B, et al: Maternal PKU syndrome: congenital heart defects, microcephaly, and developmental outcomes, *J Pediatr* 136:57, 2000.

73. Rutledge SL, et al: Neonatal hemodialysis: effective therapy for the encephalopathy of inborn errors of metabolism, *J Pediatr* 116:125, 1990.

74. Santorelli FM, et al: Hypertrophic cardiomyopathy and mtDNA depletion. Successful treatment with heart transplantation, *Neuromusc Dis* 12:56, 2002.

75. Santorelli FM, et al: The emerging concept of mitochondrial cardiomyopathies, *Am Heart J* 141:e1, 2001.

76. Sarzi E, et al: Mitochondrial DNA depletion is a prevalent cause of multiple respiratory chain deficiency in childhood, *J Pediatr* 105:531, 2007.

77. Saudubray JM, et al: Genetic hypoglycemia in infancy and childhood: pathophysiology and diagnosis, *J Inherit Metab Dis* 23:197, 2000.

78. Saudubray JM, et al: Recognition and management of fatty acid oxidation defects: a series of 107 patients, *J Inherit Metab Dis* 22:488, 1999.

79. Schaefer F, et al: Dialysis in neonates with inborn errors of metabolism, *Nephrol Dial Transplant* 14:910, 1999.

80. Schapira AHV: Mitochondrial disease, *Lancet* 368:70, 2006.

81. Schulze A, et al: Expanded newborn screening for inborn errors of metabolism by electrospray ionization-tandem mass spectrometry: results, outcome, and implications, *Pediatrics* 111: 1399, 2003.

82. Schweitzer S, et al: Long-term outcome in 134 patients with galactosemia, *Eur J Pediatr* 152:36, 1993.

83. Scott CR: The genetic tyrosinemias, *Am J Med Genet Part C* 142C:121, 2006.

84. Scriver CR, et al, editors: *The metabolic and molecular bases of inherited disease,* 8th ed. New York, 2001, McGraw-Hill.

85. Seashore MR: *The organic acidemias: An overview.* www.genetests.org. Accessed August 2, 2010.

86. Sokal EM: Liver transplantation for inborn errors of metabolism, *J Inherit Metab Dis* 29:426, 2006.

87. Sokal EM, et al: Liver transplantation in mitochondrial respiratory chain disorders, *Eur J Pediatr* 158(Suppl 2):S81, 1999.

88. Sokol RJ, Treem WR: Mitochondria and childhood liver disease, *J Pediatr Gastroenterol Nutr* 28:4, 1999.

89. Staretz-Chacham O, et al: Lysosomal storage disorders in the newborn, *Pediatrics* 123:1191, 2009.

90. Sue CM, et al: Neonatal presentations of mitochondrial metabolic disorders, *Semin Perinatol* 23:113, 1999.

91. Sue CM, et al: Differential features of patients with mutations in two COX assembly genes, Surf-1 and SCO2, *Ann Neurol* 47:589, 2000.

92. Summar ML: *Urea cycle disorders overview* (website). www.genetests.org. Accessed August 2, 2010.

92a. Talele SS, Xu K, Pariser AR, et al: Therapies for inborn errors of metabolism: what has the orphan drug act delivered? *Pediatrics* 126(1):101, 2010. Epub 2010 Jun 21.

93. Tavil B, et al: Haematologic findings in children with inborn errors of metabolism, *J Inherit Metab Dis* 29:607, 2006.

94. Thompson GN, et al: The use of metronidazole in management of methylmalonic and propionic acidemias, *Eur J Pediatr* 169:408, 1991.

95. Tint GS, et al: Defective cholesterol biosynthesis associated with the Smith-Lemli-Opitz syndrome, *N Engl J Med* 330:107, 1994.

96. Visser G, et al: Neutropenia, neutrophil dysfunction, and inflammatory bowel disease in glycogen storage disease type Ib: results of the European Study on Glycogen Storage Disease Type I, *J Pediatr* 137:187, 2000.

97. Waisbren SE, et al: Effect of expanded newborn screening for biochemical genetic disorders on child outcomes and parental stress, *JAMA* 290:2564, 2003.

98. Walter JH: Inborn errors of metabolism and pregnancy, *J Inherit Metab Dis* 23:229, 2000.

99. Wanders RJA, et al: Metabolic and molecular basis of peroxisomal disorders: A review, *Am J Med Genet* 126A:355, 2004.

100. Wilcken B, et al: Pregnancy and fetal long-chain 3-hydroxyacyl-CoA dehydrogenase deficiency, *Lancet* 341:407, 1993.

101. Wilcken B, et al: Screening newborns for inborn errors of metabolism by tandem mass spectrometry, *N Engl J Med* 348:2304, 2003.

102. Wolf B: *Biotinidase deficiency* (website). http://www.genetests.org. Accessed September 25, 2008.

103. Zammarchi E, et al: Neonatal onset of hyperornithinemia-hyperammonemia-homocitrullinuria syndrome with favourable outcome, *J Pediatr* 131:440, 1997.

CHAPTER 51

The Kidney and Urinary Tract

Beth A. Vogt and Katherine MacRae Dell

In the past two decades, the field of clinical neonatal nephrology has broadened significantly, due to a variety of factors. For instance, the widespread use of invasive vascular catheters has resulted in a new set of complications, including acute kidney injury and renovascular hypertension related to thromboembolic disease. The improved survival of infants with extremely low birthweight and bronchopulmonary dysplasia has led to the relatively new complication of neonatal nephrocalcinosis. The advent of prenatal ultrasonography created new paradigms for the prenatal management of urinary tract anomalies (see Chapter 11).

The goals of this chapter are to review the anatomic and functional development of the kidney, outline the recommended approach to the evaluation of the neonate with suspected renal disease, and provide an overview of the common nephrologic and urologic problems seen in preterm and term neonates.

KIDNEY AND URINARY TRACT DEVELOPMENT

Kidney and urinary tract development is a complex process involving interactions between genes involved in the formation and maturation of the renal blood vessels, glomeruli, tubules, extracellular matrix, and uroepithelium. This carefully coordinated process involves the regulated activation and inactivation of hundreds of genes that encode transcription factors, growth factors and receptors, structural proteins, adhesion molecules, and other regulatory proteins.[39] Since the mid-1990s, the rapidly expanding fields of molecular genetics and proteomics have provided important new insights into the mechanisms involved in renal and urinary tract development. This section highlights some of the important pathways involved in these processes and provides examples of human diseases resulting from abnormalities in normal development.

Development of the Kidney

Three different kidney systems, the pronephros, mesonephros, and metanephros, form in succession during intrauterine development and are illustrated in Figure 51-1. The pronephros, a vestigial structure of 7 to 10 solid or tubular cell groups called *nephrotomes*, develops in the cervical region and disappears by the end of the fourth week of gestation. As the pronephros regresses, the mesonephros appears and is characterized by excretory tubules that form an S-shaped loop, with a glomerulus and Bowman capsule at the proximal end. At the distal portion, the tubule enters the collecting duct (also referred to as the *mesonephric*, or *wolffian*, duct), which does not drain into the coelomic cavity. During the second month of gestation, the urogenital ridge, which is the forerunner of the gonads, develops. By the end of the second month of gestation, most portions of the mesonephros disappear. However, a few caudal tubules remain in close proximity to the testes and ovaries, developing into the vas deferens in males and remaining as remnant tissue in females.

The formation of the metanephric, or definitive, kidney begins at 5 weeks of gestation, when the ureteric bud, an outgrowth of the dorsomedial wall of the mesonephric duct, invades a cord of mesenchymal cells called the *metanephric blastema*. The ureteric bud grows into the metanephric blastema and undergoes a series of divisions to form the major and minor caliceal system of the renal pelvis and collecting ducts of the kidney. At the tip of the branches, the mesenchymal cells of the metanephric blastema are induced by the advancing ureteric bud to differentiate into the epithelial cells that eventually become the glomeruli and renal tubules. Foci of the metanephric blastema become condensed adjacent to the branching ureteric bud to form "comma"-shaped bodies that then elongate to form S-shaped bodies (Fig. 51-2). The lower portion of the S-shaped body becomes associated with a tuft of capillaries to form the glomerulus, while the upper portion forms the tubular elements of the nephron.

Figure 51–1. A, Schematic diagram showing the relation of the intermediate mesoderm of the pronephric, mesonephric, and metanephric systems. In the cervical and upper thoracic regions, the intermediate mesoderm is segmented; in the lower thoracic, lumbar, and sacral regions, it forms a solid, unsegmented mass of tissue known as the nephrogenic cord. Note the longitudinal collecting duct, initially formed by the pronephros but later taken over by the mesonephros. **B,** Schematic representation of the excretory tubules of the pronephric and mesonephric systems in a 5-week-old embryo. The ureteric bud penetrates the metanephric tissue. Note the remnant of the pronephric excretory tubules and longitudinal collecting duct. (*From Langman J, editor:* Medical embryology, *3rd ed, Baltimore, 1975, Williams & Wilkins, p 162.*)

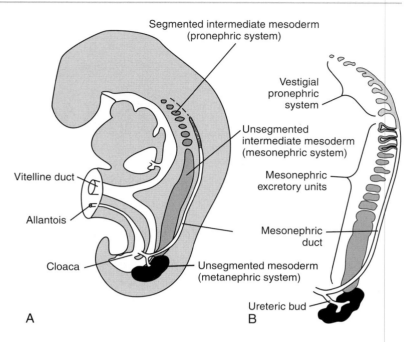

The metanephric kidney ascends from the pelvic to the thoracolumbar region. This process is thought to occur as the result of a decrease in body curvature and body growth of the lumbar and sacral regions. In the pelvis, the metanephric kidney receives its blood supply from a pelvic branch of the aorta. During ascent, the metanephric kidney receives its blood supply from arterial branches at higher levels of the aorta. Although the pelvic vessels usually degenerate, the persistence of these early embryonic vessels leads to supernumerary renal arteries. The metanephric kidney becomes functional during the second half of pregnancy. Nephrogenesis, which is the formation of new nephron units, is complete at 34 weeks of gestation, when each kidney contains its definitive complement of approximately 800,000 to 1,200,000 nephrons.[2]

Studies of transgenic mice that carry mutations in certain developmentally expressed genes have provided important insights into the key proteins involved in renal development (Table 51-1). For example, mice lacking the transcription factor Wilms tumor (WT)-1 fail to develop kidneys or gonads due to the impaired development of the metanephric mesenchyme. Those lacking the glial derived neurotrophic growth factor (GDNF) develop renal agenesis due to the failure of ureteric bud formation. Those lacking α8-integrin, a cell-cell adhesion molecule, have impaired collecting tubule branching morphogenesis. Mice with mutations in the type 2 angiotensin II receptor gene develop a variety of structural abnormalities of the urinary tract, possibly due to abnormal vascular tone.

Specific mutations have now been identified in several congenital and inherited monogenic kidney diseases, which have provided important clues to the pathogenesis of disease (Table 51-2). For example, patients with congenital nephrotic syndrome of the Finnish type have mutations in the gene encoding nephrin, an important component of the glomerular basement membrane. Renal coloboma

syndrome results from mutations in the transcription regulator PAX-2. Bartter syndrome, a disorder that may present in the newborn period with hypokalemia, metabolic alkalosis, and severe dehydration, is caused by mutations in the ion transport proteins responsible for sodium and potassium handling in the loop of Henle.

For some of these disorders, the pathogenesis may be evident from the nature of the abnormal protein product, such as impaired renal water handling in patients with nephrogenic diabetes insipidus who harbor mutations in genes encoding aquaporin 2 and the antidiuretic hormone receptor, the key proteins in regulating water handling in the collecting tubule.[45] However, there are several disorders, such as polycystic kidney disease, for which the causative genes have been identified but the precise mechanisms by which the mutated gene and its aberrant protein product actually cause disease have not been fully delineated.

Development of the Bladder and Urethra

The bladder and urethra are formed during the second and third months of gestation, which is summarized in Figure 51-3. During the fourth to seventh week of development, the cloaca, which is located at the proximal end of the allantois and is the precursor to the urinary bladder and urethra, is divided by the urorectal septum into the primitive urogenital sinus (anterior portion) and the anorectal canal (posterior portion). The primitive urogenital sinus develops into the bladder (upper portion), prostatic and membranous urethra (pelvic portion) in males, and the penile urethra (males) or urethra and vestibule (females). As the cloaca develops, the caudal portion of the mesonephric ducts is absorbed into the bladder wall. Similarly, the caudal portions of the ureters, which originate from the mesonephric ducts, enter the bladder. During these processes, the ureteral orifices move cranially and the

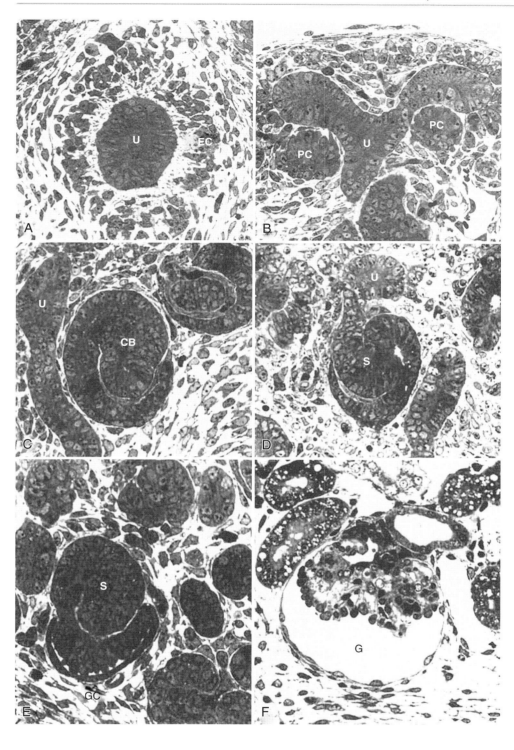

Figure 51–2. Micrographs of semithin sections made from 11- to 14-day-old mouse kidneys. **A,** Ureter (U) and early condensation (EC) of mesenchymal cells from metanephric blastema. **B,** Ureter and pretubular condensation (PC) of metanephric blastema mesenchyme. **C,** Ureter and "comma"-shaped body (CB). **D,** Ureter and S-shaped body (S). **E,** S-shaped body and glomerular capillary (GC). **F,** Glomerulus (G). *(From Saxen L: Organogenesis of the kidney. In Barlow PW, Green PB, editors: Developmental and cell biology series. Cambridge, UK, 1987, Cambridge University Press, p 26.)*

mesonephric ducts move closer together to enter the prostatic urethra, forming the trigone of the bladder. At the end of the third month of gestation, the epithelial proliferation of the prostatic urethra forms outbuddings that constitute the prostate gland in males. In females, the cranial portion of the urethra forms buds that develop into the urethral and paraurethral glands.

Physiology of the Developing Kidney

During intrauterine life, the kidneys play only a minor role in regulating fetal salt and water balance because this function is maintained primarily by the placenta. The most important functions of the prenatal kidneys are the formation and excretion of urine to maintain an adequate amount of amniotic fluid. After birth, there is a progressive maturation in renal

TABLE 51-1   Examples of Mouse Models of Developmental Kidney Diseases

Mutant Gene/Protein	Mutant Mouse Phenotype	Abnormal Kidney/Urinary Tract/Process
AGTR2/angiotensin type II receptor	Varied urinary tract abnormalities	Altered vascular tone/renal bloodflow
GDNF/glial-derived growth factor	Renal agenesis	Ureteric bud absent
HNF1B/hepatocyte nuclear factor 1β	Polycystic kidneys	Collecting tubule hyperplasia
Inv/inversin	Cystic kidneys	Altered left-right polarity
ITGA8/integrin, α8	Renal dysplasia	Abnormal ureteric bud induction and impaired collecting tubule branching
LMX1B/Lim homeobox transcription	Massive proteinuria/glomerular	Altered glomerular basement membrane architecture
PDGFB/platelet-derived growth factor-β	Hemorrhage and capillary leak	Abnormal glomeruli; impaired angiogenesis
PKHD1/fibrocystin	Polycystic kidneys	Collecting tubule hyperplasia
WT1/Wilms tumor suppressor gene protein	Renal agenesis; glomerulosclerosis	Absence/loss of metanephric mesenchyme

From the Kidney Development Database at http:golgi.ana.ed.ac.uk/kidhome.html and the OMIM Database at http:www.ncbi.nlm.nih.gov/entrez/query.fcgi?db=OMIM.

function, which appears to parallel the needs of the neonate for growth and development (Table 51-3).

RENAL BLOOD FLOW

Absolute renal blood flow (RBF) and the percentage of cardiac output directed to the kidneys increase steadily with advancing gestational age. The kidneys of a human fetus weighing more than 150 g receive approximately 4% of the cardiac output, compared with approximately 6% in the term infant. The relatively low RBF of the fetus is related to high renovascular resistance caused by the increased activity of the renin-angiotensin-aldosterone and sympathetic nervous systems. The renal blood flow dramatically increases postnatally, reaching 8% to 10% of the cardiac output at 1 week of life, and achieves adult values of 20% to 25% of the cardiac output at 2 years of age. This rise in renal blood flow is caused primarily by decreasing renovascular resistance and increasing cardiac output and perfusion pressure.

GLOMERULAR FILTRATION

The glomerular filtration rate (GFR) in the fetal kidney increases steadily with advancing gestational age (Fig. 51-4). By 32 to 34 weeks after conception, a GFR of 14 mL/min per 1.73 m² is achieved, which further increases to 21 mL/min per 1.73 m² at term (see Table 51-3). The GFR continues to increase postnatally, achieving adult values of 118 mL/min per 1.73 m² by the age of 2 years. The achievement of adult GFR may be delayed in preterm infants, especially those with very low birthweights and those with nephrocalcinosis.[52] The progressive increase in GFR during the initial weeks of postnatal life primarily results from an increase in glomerular perfusion pressure. Subsequent increases in GFR during the first 2 years of life are caused primarily by increases in renal blood flow and the maturation of superficial cortical nephrons, which lead to an increase in the glomerular capillary surface area.

CONCENTRATION AND DILUTION OF URINE

Newborn infants have a limited capacity to concentrate their urine, with maximal urinary osmolality of 800 mOsm/kg in a term infant; compared to that of a 2 year old, which approximates adult values of 1400 mOsm/kg (see Table 51-3). In contrast, the term newborn infant has full ability to maximally dilute urine in response to a water load, achieving adult values of 50 mOsm/kg. Preterm infants are unable to fully dilute their urine, but can achieve urine osmolalities of 70 mOsm/kg. However, the response of premature infants to an acute water load may be limited because of their low GFR and the decreased activity of sodium transporters in the diluting segment of the nephron. The excessive administration of water may place the newborn infant at a high risk for dilutional hyponatremia and hypervolemia. Urinary diluting and concentrating capacity in term and preterm infants is discussed in more detail in Chapter 36.

EVALUATION OF THE NEONATE WITH RENAL DISEASE

History

The results of prenatal ultrasonography should be carefully reviewed, with particular attention devoted to kidney size, echogenicity, structural malformations, amniotic fluid volume, and bladder size and shape (Box 51-1). Although the bladder may be identified and its volume discerned at 15 weeks of gestation, the kidneys are not visualized until after the 16th to 17th week of gestation in most fetuses. The presence of small or enlarged kidneys, renal cysts, hydronephrosis, bladder enlargement, or oligohydramnios suggests significant renal or urologic pathology.

The antenatal history should be reviewed thoroughly, with particular attention devoted to medications, toxins, and unusual environmental exposures during the pregnancy.

TABLE 51–2	Examples of Inherited Renal Disorders with a Known Genetic Basis That Present in Infancy		
Disease	**Mutated Gene/Protein**	**Kidney Disease Phenotype**	**Protein Function**
Autosomal recessive polycystic kidney disease	PKHD1/fibrocystin	Polycystic kidneys	Receptor-like properties; function unknown
Bartter syndrome, neonatal/infantile	CCKb/kidney chloride channel B ROMK/inwardly rectifying potassium channel	Hypokalemic metabolic alkalosis, recurrent dehydration	Sodium, potassium and/or chloride transport in the loop of Henle
Branchio-oto-renal syndrome	EYA1/eyes absent, Drosophila, homologue of, 1	Renal dysplasia	Regulator of gene transcription factors
Congenital nephrotic syndrome, Finnish type	NPHS1/nephrin	Nephrotic syndrome	Glomerular filtration barrier component
Denys-Drash/Beckwith-Wiedemann/aniridia/hemihypertrophy	WT1/Wilms tumor suppressor gene	Progressive renal failure/hypertension/Wilms tumor	Transcription factor
Distal renal tubular acidosis with sensorineural deafness	ATP6N1B/H$^+$-ATPase	Metabolic acidosis	Hydrogen ion transport
Fanconi-Bickel syndrome	GLUT2/solute carrier family 2 protein	Fanconi syndrome (global proximal tubular dysfunction)	Facilitative glucose transporter
Infantile nephronophthisis	INV/nephrocystin 2	Polyuria, small kidneys	Determination of left-right asymmetry
Infantile nephropathic cystinosis	CTNS/cystinosin	Cystinosis, renal failure	Cystine transporter
Nail-patella syndrome	LMX1B/Lim homeodomain protein	Glomerulonephritis, nephrotic syndrome	Regulator of type IV collagen production
Nephrogenic diabetes insipidus, X-linked	AVPR2/ADH receptor	Diabetes insipidus	ADH receptor
Renal coloboma syndrome	PAX2/PAX2 protein	Hypoplastic kidneys, renal failure	Induction/regulation of WT1
Simpson-Golabi-Behmal overgrowth syndrome	GPC3/glypican 3	Nephromegaly/renal dysplasia	Control of cell division and growth

ADH, antidiuretic hormone.
From the OMIM Database at http:www.ncbi.nlm.nih.gov/entrez/query.fcgi?db=OMIM.

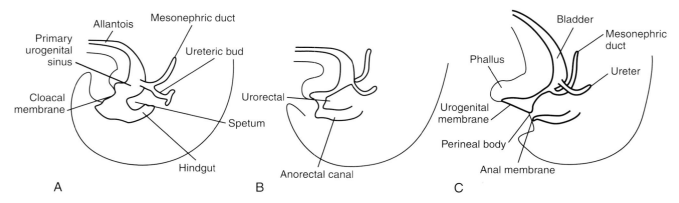

Figure 51–3. Diagrams showing the division of the cloaca into the urogenital sinus and anorectal canal. Note that the mesonephric duct is gradually absorbed into the wall of the urogenital sinus and that the ureters enter separately. **A,** At the end of 5 weeks. **B,** At the end of 7 weeks. **C,** At the end of 8 weeks. (*From Langman J, editor: Medical embryology, 3rd ed, Baltimore, 1975, Williams & Wilkins, p 168.*)

TABLE 51–3   Normal Values for Renal Function

Age	Glomerular Filtration Rate (mL/min/1.73 m²)	Renal Bloodflow (mL/min/1.73 m²)	Maximum Urine Osmolality (mOsm/kg)	Serum Creatinine (mg/dL)	Fractional Excretion of Sodium (%)
Newborn					
32-34 weeks' gestation	14 ± 3	40 ± 6	480	1.3	2–5
Term	21 ± 4	88 ± 4	800	1.1	<1
1-2 weeks	50 ± 10	220 ± 40	900	0.4	<1
6 months-1 year	77 ± 14	352 ± 73	1200	0.2	<1
1-3 years	96 ± 22	540 ± 118	1400	0.4	<1
Adult	118 ± 18	620 ± 92	1400	0.8–1.5	<1

IUGR, intrauterine growth restriction.
Adapted from Avner ED, et al: Normal neonates and maturational development of homeostatic mechanism. In Ichikawa I, editor: *Pediatric textbook of fluids and electrolytes*. Baltimore, 1990, Williams & Wilkins, p 109.

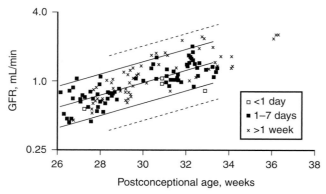

Figure 51–4. Scatterplot showing an increase in the glomerular filtration rate (GFR) as a function of postconceptional age. It was measured by using the single-injection method to determine the clearance of polyfructosan-S. (*From Wilkins BH: Renal function in sick, very low birth weight infants. I. Glomerular filtration rate,* Arch Dis Child 67:1140, 1992, *with permission.*)

Structural and functional alterations of the newborn kidney have been described in infants with antenatal exposure to angiotensin-converting enzyme (ACE) inhibitors, angiotensin receptor blockers (ARBs), nonselective nonsteroidal anti-inflammatory drugs, and selective COX-2 inhibitors.[12] Classic ACE fetopathy (renal failure, limb deformities, hypotension, pulmonary hypoplasia, and hypocalvaria) is seen following second and third trimester exposure to ACE inhibitors, while first-trimester exposure to ACE inhibitors has been associated with increased risk of cardiovascular and central nervous system malformations.[19] Maternal exposure to immunosuppressive agents including tacrolimus and aminoglycosides including gentamicin have been associated with neonatal renal dysfunction.[12]

A review of the medical history of the family is important, including any prior fetal or neonatal deaths. Although there is no established genetic basis for many congenital renal anomalies, certain disorders such as renal hypoplasia/dysplasia, multicystic dysplastic kidney, and vesicoureteral reflux may have familial clustering. There is a clear genetic basis for certain diseases, including polycystic kidney disease and congenital nephrotic syndrome.

Physical Examination

The evaluation of blood pressure and volume status is critical in the newborn with suspected renal disease. Hypertension may be present in infants with polycystic kidney disease, acute kidney injury, renovascular or aortic thrombosis, or obstructive uropathy. Hypotension usually results from volume depletion, hemorrhage, or sepsis, any of which may lead to acute kidney injury. Edema may occur in infants with acute kidney injury, hydrops fetalis, or congenital nephrotic syndrome. Ascites may be present in infants with urinary tract obstruction congenital nephrotic syndrome, or volume overload. Special attention should be paid to the abdominal examination. In the neonate, the lower pole of each kidney is easily palpable because of the neonate's reduced abdominal muscle tone. The presence of an abdominal mass in a newborn should be assumed to involve the urinary tract until proven otherwise because two thirds of neonatal abdominal masses are genitourinary in origin.[16] The most common renal cause of an abdominal mass is hydronephrosis, followed by a multicystic dysplastic kidney. Less common causes of an abdominal mass include polycystic kidney disease, renal vein thrombosis, ectopic or fused kidneys, and renal tumors. The abdomen should be examined for the absence of or laxity in the abdominal muscles, which may suggest Eagle-Barrett ("prune-belly") syndrome. Distention of the newborn bladder may suggest lower urinary tract obstruction or an occult spinal cord lesion.

A number of anomalies should alert the physician to the possibility of underlying renal defects, including abnormal external ears, aniridia, microcephaly, meningomyelocele, pectus excavatum, hemihypertrophy, a persistent urachus, bladder or cloacal exstrophy, an abnormality of the external genitalia, cryptorchidism, imperforate anus, and limb

KIDNEYS
Dilated renal pelvis
   Physiologic
   Hydronephrosis: vesicoureteral reflux, urinary tract
      obstruction
Multicystic dysplastic kidney (prenatal differentiation from
   hydronephrosis may be difficult)
Hyperechoic kidney (renal dysplasia, autosomal recessive
   polycystic kidney disease)
Renal duplication, malposition
Lack of visualization: renal agenesis, hypoplasia, malposition
Renal tumors

URETER
Hydroureter
Ureterocele

BLADDER
Dilation
   With thickened wall: urethral valves
   Without thickened wall: megacystis-megaureter
      syndrome, neurogenic bladder
Bladder exstrophy, cloacal exstrophy
Lack of visualization despite prolonged observation and
   maternal furosemide administration

COMPROMISED FETUS:
severe intrauterine growth restriction, fetal stress, bilateral
   renal agenesis, cystic disease, ureteral obstruction

ASCITES
Urinary ascites probable if bladder wall thickened or
   kidneys abnormal

HYDROPS FETALIS
Most often due to nonrenal causes; occasionally caused by
   bilateral renal cystic disease, urinary tract obstruction,
   nephrotic syndrome

OLIGOHYDRAMNIOS
Bilateral renal malformations, urinary tract obstruction
Rupture of membranes, postmaturity, subacute fetal distress

POLYHYDRAMNIOS
Renal tubular disorder with urinary concentrating defect
Multiple pregnancy, upper gastrointestinal tract obstruction,
   neurologic disorders, maternal diabetes, fetal hydrops
Pearlman syndrome

PLACENTAL EDEMA
Congenital nephrotic syndrome of the Finnish type

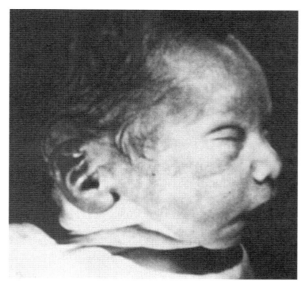

Figure 51–5. Potter facies. Characteristic findings include epicanthal folds, hypertelorism, low-set ears, a crease below lower lip, and a receding chin.

characteristic facial features include wide-set eyes, depressed nasal bridge, beaked nose, receding chin, and posteriorly rotated, low-set ears. Other associated anomalies include a small, compressed chest wall, with resulting pulmonary hypoplasia, and arthrogryposis (see Chapter 44). The condition is uniformly fatal. "Potter-like" features may be seen in infants with significant renal impairment and oligohydramnios related to severe antenatal urinary tract obstruction or disorders such as autosomal recessive polycystic kidney disease. Such patients often have pulmonary hypoplasia and spontaneous pneumothorax or pneumomediastinum resulting from their requirement for high ventilator pressures.

Laboratory Evaluation

URINALYSIS

The examination of a freshly voided specimen of urine provides immediate, valuable information about the condition of the kidneys. The collection of an adequate, uncontaminated specimen from the neonate can be very difficult. A specimen collected by cleaning the perineum and applying a sterile adhesive plastic bag may be useful in screening, but it may result in a false-positive urine culture because of fecal contamination. Bladder catheterization is more reliable but may be technically difficult in preterm infants. Suprapubic bladder aspiration is an alternative urinary collection method in preterm infants without intra-abdominal pathology or bleeding disorders.

Analysis of the urine should include inspection, measurement of specific gravity, urinary dipstick assessment, and microscopic analysis. The newborn urine is usually clear and nearly colorless. Cloudiness may represent a urinary tract infection or the presence of crystals. A yellow-brown to deep olive-green color may represent large amounts of conjugated bilirubin. Porphyrins, certain drugs such as phenytoin, bacteria, and urate crystals may stain the diaper pink and be confused with

deformities. A single umbilical artery raises the suspicion of renal disease. In one study, 7% of otherwise normal infants with a single umbilical artery were found to have significant renal anomalies.[13] The utility of screening all infants with a single umbilical artery, however, remains controversial.

A constellation of physical findings, designated the *oligohydramnios (Potter) sequence*, may be seen in infants with bilateral renal agenesis (Fig. 51-5). The complete absence of fetal kidney function results in anhydramnios, which causes fetal deformation from compression by the uterine wall. The bleeding. Brown urine suggests bleeding from the upper urinary tract, hemoglobinuria, or myoglobinuria.

Urinary specific gravity may be measured by using a clinical refractometer or a urinary dipstick method. The specific gravity of neonatal urine is usually very low (less than 1.004) but may be factitiously elevated by high-molecular-weight solutes such as contrast agents, glucose or other reducing substances, or large amounts of protein. Urinary osmolality may be a more reliable measurement of the concentrating and diluting capacity of the kidney.

Urinary dipstick evaluation can also detect the presence of heme-containing compounds (i.e., red blood cells, myoglobin, and hemoglobin), protein, and glucose. White blood cell products such as leukocyte esterase and nitrite may also be detected on urinary dipstick evaluation and should raise the suspicion of urinary tract infection, mandating collection of a urine culture. The microscopic examination of urinary sediment may detect the presence of red blood cells, casts, white blood cells, bacteria, or crystals.

ASSESSMENT OF RENAL FUNCTION

Although 98% of term infants void during the first 30 hours of life,[17] a delay in urination for up to 48 hours should not be a cause for immediate concern in the absence of a palpable bladder, abdominal mass, or other signs or symptoms of renal disease. A failure to void for longer than 48 hours may suggest impairment of renal function and should prompt further investigation.

The serum creatinine level is the simplest and most commonly used indicator of neonatal kidney function. The serum creatinine concentration immediately after birth reflects the maternal creatinine concentration, neonatal muscle mass, and GFR at the time of delivery. In term infants, the serum creatinine level gradually decreases from 1.1 mg/dL to a mean value of 0.4 mg/dL within the first 2 weeks of life. However, in preterm infants, the plasma creatinine level does not fall steadily from birth but instead rises in the first 48 hours before beginning to fall to equilibrium levels.[38]

Failure of the serum creatinine level to fall or a persistent increase in serum creatinine suggests impairment of renal function. In general, each doubling of the serum creatinine level represents an approximately 50% reduction in GFR; for example, a rise in serum creatinine from 0.4 to 0. 8 mg/dL represents a 50% reduction in GFR. A reasonably accurate estimate of GFR can be made from the serum creatinine concentration by using an empirically derived formula that has been applied to normal preterm and term infants.[11]

Estimated GFR (mL/min per 1.73 m²):
Preterm infants:

$$0.33 \times length\ (cm)/serum\ creatinine\ (mg/dL)$$

Term infants:

$$0.45 \times length\ (cm)/serum\ creatinine\ (mg/dL)$$

Radiologic Evaluation

Ultrasonography has become the most common method of imaging the neonatal urinary tract. It offers a noninvasive evaluation without exposure to contrast agents or radiation.

Ultrasonography is indicated in infants with a history of any renal abnormality noted on antenatal ultrasound, as well as abdominal mass, acute kidney injury, hypertension, hematuria, oliguria, congenital malformations, or specific findings on physical examination that suggest anomalies of the urinary tract. Ultrasonography can identify hydronephrosis, cystic kidney disease, and abnormalities of kidney size and position. It also may be used as a screening tool for nephrocalcinosis and nephrolithiasis in preterm infants who have been receiving long-term loop diuretic therapy. A Doppler flow study of the renal arteries and aorta may be helpful in the evaluation of thrombosis in infants with suspected renovascular hypertension or acute kidney injury.

A diagnostic voiding cystourethrogram (VCUG) should be considered an important part of the radiologic examination in infants with significant hydronephrosis, renal dysplasia or anomaly, or documented urinary tract infection. This study is the procedure of choice to evaluate the urethra and bladder and to ascertain the presence or absence of vesicoureteral reflux. Voiding cystourethrography involves the instillation of a radiopaque contrast agent into the bladder by urinary catheterization. Films of the urethra during voiding and of the bladder and ureters toward the end of voiding are essential.

Other radiologic tests may occasionally be used for diagnostic purposes in the neonate (see Chapter 37). Radioisotopic renal scanning is of value in locating anomalous kidneys, determining kidney size, and identifying obstruction or renal scarring. Radioisotopic scans may also provide information about the relative blood flow to each kidney and the contribution of each kidney to overall renal function. Abdominal computed tomography is useful in the diagnosis of renal tumors, renal abscesses, and nephrolithiasis.

CLINICAL PROBLEMS

Hematuria

Hematuria is defined as five or more red blood cells per high-powered field on microscopic evaluation of a centrifuged urine sample. Blood can enter the urine from any location in the urinary tract, from the kidney to the urethra. The most frequent cause of hematuria in the neonate is acute tubular necrosis (ATN), which is caused by perinatal asphyxia, the administration of nephrotoxic drugs, or sepsis. Another important cause of hematuria is renal venous thrombosis, which must be considered in the infants of diabetic mothers, those with cyanotic congenital heart disease, those who are dehydrated, and those with indwelling umbilical venous catheters. Other causes of neonatal hematuria include urinary tract infection, trauma from catheterization or suprapubic aspiration, neoplasia, obstructive uropathy, coagulopathy, and thrombocytopenia. Extraurinary (e.g., vaginal, rectal, perineal, preputial) sources may also lead to apparent hematuria.

Several conditions can simulate hematuria, including myoglobinuria, hemoglobinuria, and pigmenturia. In infants with myoglobinuria and hemoglobinuria, the urine may look red or brown and test dipstick-positive for blood, but red blood cells are not present on microscopic examination of the urine. Myoglobinuria may be seen in infants with inherited metabolic myopathy, infectious myositis, or rhabdomyolysis. Hemoglobinuria may be present in infants with erythroblastosis fetalis or other forms of hemolytic disease. Urine discolored by bile pigments, porphyrins, or urate crystals may also raise the suspicion of hematuria, but in these conditions the urinary dipstick tests negative for blood and the microscopic examination reveals no red blood cells.

Proteinuria

Proteinuria is defined as a urinary dipstick value of at least 1+ (30 mg/dL), with a specific gravity of 1.015 or less, or a urinary dipstick value of at least 2+ (100 mg/dL), with a specific gravity of more than 1.015. Nearly any form of injury, whether glomerular or tubular, can result in an increase in urinary protein excretion. Common causes of neonatal proteinuria include ATN, fever, dehydration, cardiac failure, high doses of penicillin, and the administration of a contrast agent. Persistent massive proteinuria and edema in a neonate should prompt the consideration of congenital nephrotic syndrome, an autosomal recessive disorder characterized by proteinuria, failure to thrive, a large placenta, and chronic renal dysfunction. False-positive dipstick values for protein may be the result of highly concentrated urine, alkaline urine, infection, and detergents.

Glycosuria

The diagnosis of glycosuria is established by the presence of glucose on a urinary dipstick. Glycosuria frequently occurs when the serum glucose concentration exceeds the renal threshold, such as that in neonates with hyperglycemia related to sepsis or to the administration of total parenteral nutrition. It is important to measure the serum glucose concentration in neonates in whom glucose has been detected by urinary dipstick evaluation. The correction of hyperglycemia normalizes the urinary dipstick findings.

Isolated glycosuria with a normal serum glucose concentration is defined as renal glycosuria, a benign condition caused by an abnormality in the transport of proximal tubular glucose. Two forms of inherited renal glycosuria have been described. In type A, the defect involves a depression in the threshold and the maximum capacity of the renal tubule to reabsorb glucose (TmG). Type B renal glycosuria is characterized by a low threshold and a normal TmG. The inheritance pattern of renal glycosuria is autosomal recessive in most patients, although an autosomal dominant mode of transmission has been described. No therapy is necessary other than the recognition of the condition, avoidance of confusion with diabetes mellitus, and provision of a normal intake of carbohydrates.

If glycosuria is accompanied by other evidence of renal tubular dysfunction, such as an excessive urinary loss of potassium, phosphorus, and amino acids, a generalized proximal tubulopathy (i.e., Fanconi syndrome) should be considered. Glycosuria may also be seen in infants with congenital renal diseases such as renal dysplasia, in which there is significant tubular dysfunction. Glycosuria in an infant with severe, watery diarrhea should raise the suspicion of congenital intestinal glucose-galactose malabsorption syndrome.

Acute Kidney Injury

Acute kidney injury is an increasingly common condition in the neonatal intensive care unit, ranging from mild dysfunction to complete anuric kidney failure. Acute kidney injury is characterized by a deterioration in kidney function over hours to days, leading to an inability of the kidneys to excrete nitrogenous waste products and maintain fluid and electrolyte homeostasis. Although the criteria for neonatal acute kidney injury have varied among studies, a frequently used definition is a serum creatinine level of more than 1.5 mg/dL.[7] Oliguric acute kidney injury is characterized by a urine flow rate of less than 1 mL/kg per hour, whereas in nonoliguric acute kidney injury the urine flow rate is maintained above this level. Data on the incidence of acute kidney injury in the hospitalized neonatal population are variable, mainly because of the different criteria used to define the condition, ranging from 8% to 24%.[6,29] Risk factors for development of neonatal acute kidney injury include very low birthweight (less than 1500 g), low 5-minute APGAR score, maternal drug administration [(nonsteroidal anti-inflammatory drugs and antibiotics)], intubation at birth, respiratory distress syndrome, patent ductus arteriosus, phototherapy, and neonatal medication administration (nonsteroidal anti-inflammatory drugs, antibiotics, diuretics).[14]

The signs of acute kidney injury may include oliguria, systemic hypertension, cardiac arrhythmia, evidence of fluid overload or dehydration, decreased activity, seizure, vomiting, and anorexia. Laboratory evidence may include elevated serum creatinine and blood urea nitrogen, hyperkalemia, metabolic acidosis, hypocalcemia, hyperphosphatemia, and a prolonged half-life for medications excreted by the kidney (e.g., aminoglycosides, vancomycin). The causes of neonatal acute kidney injury are multiple and can be divided into prerenal, renal, and postrenal categories (Box 51-2).

PRERENAL AZOTEMIA

Prerenal azotemia is the most common type of acute kidney injury in the neonate and may account for up to 85% of all cases. Prerenal azotemia is characterized by inadequate renal perfusion, which, if promptly treated, is followed by improvements in renal function and urine output. The most common causes of prerenal azotemia are dehydration, hemorrhage, septic shock, necrotizing enterocolitis, patent ductus arteriosus, and congestive heart failure. The postnatal administration of medications that reduce renal blood flow, such as indomethacin or ibuprofen, angiotensin-converting enzyme inhibitors, and phenylephrine eyedrops can result in prerenal azotemia. In utero exposure to nonselective nonsteroidal anti-inflammatory drugs, COX2 inhibitors, angiotensin-converting enzyme inhibitors, and angiotensin receptor antagonists can also induce neonatal acute kidney injury.[12]

INTRINSIC (RENAL) ACUTE KIDNEY INJURY

ATN is the most common cause of intrinsic acute kidney injury in neonates. The causes of ATN include perinatal asphyxia, sepsis, cardiac surgery, a prolonged prerenal state, and nephrotoxic drug administration. The pathophysiology of ATN is complex and appears to involve renal tubular cellular injury, alterations in adhesion molecules, and changes in renal

PRERENAL
Dehydration
Hemorrhage
Sepsis
Necrotizing enterocolitis
Congestive heart failure
Drugs: angiotensin-converting enzyme inhibitors, indomethacin, ibuprofen, amphotericin, tolazoline

RENAL
Acute tubular necrosis
Renal dysplasia
Polycystic kidney disease
Renal venous thrombosis
Uric acid nephropathy
Transient acute renal insufficiency of the newborn

POSTRENAL
Posterior urethral valves
Bilateral ureteropelvic junction obstruction
Bilateral ureterovesical junction obstruction
Neurogenic bladder
Obstructive nephrolithiasis

hemodynamics. Other causes of intrinsic acute kidney injury in the newborn include renal dysplasia, autosomal recessive polycystic kidney disease, and renal arterial or venous thrombosis. Transient acute kidney injury of the newborn is a poorly understood, rapidly reversible syndrome characterized by oliguric acute kidney injury and hyperechogenic renal medullary pyramids on ultrasound.[37] This syndrome has been reported in otherwise healthy term infants with sluggish feeding and is thought to be related to the deposition of Tamm-Horsfall protein or uric acid in the renal tubular collecting system.

OBSTRUCTIVE (POSTRENAL) ACUTE KIDNEY INJURY

Obstructive acute kidney injury is caused by bilateral urinary tract obstruction and can usually be reversed by relief of the obstruction. Obstructive acute kidney injury in the neonate may be related to a variety of congenital urinary tract conditions, including posterior urethral valves, bilateral ureteropelvic or ureterovesical junction obstruction, obstructive urolithiasis, and a neurogenic bladder. Extrinsic compression of the ureters or bladder by a congenital tumor such as a sacrococcygeal teratoma or intrinsic obstruction by renal calculi or fungus balls is a rare cause of obstructive acute kidney injury.

EVALUATION

A careful history should focus on prenatal ultrasound abnormalities, perinatal asphyxia, the prenatal or postnatal administration of potentially nephrotoxic drugs, and a family history of renal disease. The physical examination should focus on signs of volume depletion or volume overload, the abdomen, genitalia, and a search for other congenital anomalies or signs of the oligohydramnios (Potter) sequence. Levels of electrolytes, blood urea nitrogen, creatinine (Cr), calcium,

phosphorus, albumin, and uric acid should be monitored frequently if significant metabolic abnormalities are present. Urine should be sent for urinalysis, urine culture, and urine sodium and creatinine determination. The fractional excretion of sodium (FE_{Na}), as well as other diagnostic indexes, may be useful in differentiating prerenal from intrinsic acute kidney injury (Table 51-4):

$$FE_{Na} \, (\%) = (UNa \times PCr)/(PNa \times UCr) \times 100\%$$

Neonates with an FE_{Na} value of more than 3.0% generally have intrinsic acute kidney injury, whereas those with an FE_{Na} value of less than 2.5% have prerenal acute kidney injury. Renal ultrasound is helpful in the identification of congenital renal disease and urinary tract obstruction.

MEDICAL MANAGEMENT

The prevention of acute kidney injury in newborn infants requires maintenance of an adequate circulatory volume, careful fluid and electrolyte management, prompt diagnosis and treatment of hemodynamic or respiratory abnormalities, and close monitoring of potentially nephrotoxic medications. In the case of established oliguric acute kidney injury, a urinary catheter should be placed to exclude lower urinary tract obstruction. If there is no improvement in urine output after bladder drainage is established, a fluid challenge of 10 to 20 mL/kg should be administered over 1 to 2 hours to exclude prerenal acute kidney injury.

A lack of improvement in urine output and serum creatinine suggests intrinsic acute kidney injury. The goal of medical management of intrinsic acute kidney injury is to provide supportive care until there is spontaneous improvement in renal function. Fluids should be restricted to insensible losses (500 mL/m² per day, or 30 mL/kg per day) plus urine output and other measured losses (see Chapter 36). Daily weights and careful intake and output measurements are essential to follow volume status. Nephrotoxic drugs

TABLE 51–4 Diagnostic Indexes in Acute Kidney Injury

Test	Prerenal AKI	Intrinsic AKI
BUN/Cr ratio (mg/mg)	>30	<20
FE_{Na} (%)	≤2.5	≥3.0
Urinary Na (mEq/L)	≤20	≥50
Urinary Osm (mOsm/kg)	≥350	≤300
Urinary specific gravity	>1.012	<1.014
Ultrasonography	Normal	May be abnormal
Response to volume challenge	UO >2 mL/kg/h	No increase in UO

AKI, acute kidney injury; BUN, blood urea nitrogen; Cr, creatinine; FE_{Na}, fractional excretion of sodium (Na); Osm, osmolality; UO, urinary output.

should be discontinued to reduce the risk of additional renal injury. Medications should be adjusted by dose, interval, or both according to the degree of renal dysfunction. Potassium and phosphorus should be restricted in those neonates with hyperkalemia or hyperphosphatemia. Metabolic acidosis may require treatment with intravenous or oral sodium bicarbonate. Loop and thiazide diuretics may prove helpful in augmenting the urinary flow rate. The role of low-dose dopamine in therapy for neonatal acute kidney injury has not been determined.

RENAL REPLACEMENT THERAPY

Renal replacement therapy should be considered if maximum medical management fails to maintain acceptable fluid and electrolyte levels. The two purposes of renal replacement therapy are ultrafiltration (removal of water) and dialysis (removal of solutes). The indications for the initiation of renal replacement therapy include hyperkalemia, hyponatremia with symptomatic volume overload, acidosis, hypocalcemia, hyperphosphatemia, uremic symptoms, and an inability to provide adequate nutrition due to the need for fluid restriction in the face of oliguria (Box 51-3).

Peritoneal dialysis is the most commonly used renal replacement modality in the neonatal population because it is technically less difficult and does not require vascular access or anticoagulation. For this procedure, hyperosmolar dialysate is repeatedly infused into and drained out of the peritoneal cavity through a surgically placed catheter, accomplishing ultrafiltration and dialysis. Cycle length, dwell volume, and the osmolar concentration of the dialysate can be varied to accomplish the goals of therapy. The relative contraindications to peritoneal dialysis include recent abdominal surgery, necrotizing enterocolitis, pleuroperitoneal leakage, and ventriculoperitoneal shunting.

Continuous renal replacement therapy (CRRT) is becoming a more frequently used therapeutic modality in the neonate whose condition is unstable.[51] For this procedure, the patient's blood is continuously circulated through a pump-driven extracorporeal circuit containing a highly permeable hemofilter. In continuous venovenous hemofiltration (CVVH), an ultrafiltrate of plasma is removed, a portion of which is returned to the patient in the form of a physiologic replacement fluid. In continuous venovenous hemodialysis (CVVH-D), countercurrent dialysate is used rather than replacement fluid to achieve solute removal. CRRT can be employed in conjunction with extracorporeal membrane oxygenation (ECMO) by putting the CRRT circuit in line with the ECMO circuit. The chief advantage of CRRT is the ability to carefully control fluid

removal, which makes this modality especially useful in the neonate with hemodynamic instability. The main disadvantages are the need to achieve and maintain central vascular access and the need for continuous anticoagulation.

Intermittent hemodialysis is a less commonly used but technically feasible mode of renal replacement therapy in the neonatal population. Hemodialysis involves intermittent 3- to 4-hour treatment periods in which fluids and solutes are rapidly removed from the infant by using an extracorporeal dialyzer, with clearance achieved by the use of countercurrent dialysate. The chief advantage of hemodialysis is the ability to rapidly remove solutes and fluids, a characteristic that makes this modality the therapy of choice in neonatal hyperammonemia.[41] The main disadvantages are the requirement for central vascular access and the hemodynamic instability and osmolar shifts that may occur with rapid solute and fluid shifts.

The ability to provide renal replacement therapy may be limited by ability to place and maintain intravascular or peritoneal dialysis access in the very small premature neonate. If dialysis access cannot be established, care of the infant with acute kidney injury is limited to maximal supportive medical management with meticulous attention to fluid and electrolyte balance.

PROGNOSIS

The prognosis for neonates with acute kidney injury is variable, and largely related to the infant's underlying medical condition, with mortality rates ranging from 14% to 73%.[6] In general, those infants with prerenal acute kidney injury who receive prompt treatment for renal hypoperfusion have an excellent prognosis. Infants with postrenal acute kidney injury related to congenital urinary tract obstruction have a variable outcome, which depends on the degree of associated renal dysplasia.

Infants with intrinsic acute kidney injury have significant risks of morbidity and mortality. A study of 23 infants who received peritoneal dialysis during the first month of life showed that at 1 year 30% were on dialysis, 9% had chronic renal failure, 26% had made a full renal recovery, and 35% had died in the neonatal period.[9] There was a substantial difference in outcome according to the underlying cause of acute kidney injury; neonates with renal structural anomalies had a 17% mortality rate, and those with ATN had a 55% mortality rate.[9] A long-term study of infants with extremely low birthweight with neonatal acute kidney injury showed that 45% developed progressive renal disease, highlighting the need for long-term nephrology follow-up care.[1] Prominent risk factors for progressive kidney disease included proteinuria (urine protein/Cr ratio greater than 0.6 at 1 year of age), serum Cr greater than 0.6 mg/dL at 1 year of age, and body mass index greater than the 85th percentile. Other long-term sequelae seen in survivors of neonatal acute kidney injury include hypertension, an impaired capacity for urinary concentration, renal tubular acidosis, and impaired renal growth.

Hypertension

DEFINITION AND INCIDENCE

The incidence of hypertension in term or preterm neonates is estimated to be approximately 2%.[25] However, the determination of the true incidence of neonatal hypertension is

---

BOX 51–3   **Indications for Dialysis**

Hyperkalemia
Hyponatremia
Acidosis
Hypocalcemia
Hyperphosphatemia
Volume overload
Uremic symptoms
Inability to provide adequate nutrition

problematic because of inconsistencies in the definition of hypertension, variations in blood pressure measurement techniques, and normal changes in blood pressure with gestational age and weight. Many other factors affect blood pressure readings, including the level of wakefulness, abdominal palpation, crying, and pain (see Chapter 43).

Useful data on normal infant blood pressures were published by Zubrow and colleagues, who prospectively measured blood pressure in nearly 700 infants.[54] From these data, the investigators were able to define mean blood pressure and 95% confidence limits for infants according to birthweight, gestational age, and postconceptional age (Figs. 51-6 to 51-8). Infants with blood pressure readings that consistently exceed the 95th percentile are defined as having significant hypertension (see Appendix B).

CAUSES

The causes of neonatal hypertension are varied and are outlined in Box 51-4. A number of risk factors for neonatal hypertension have been identified, including antenatal steroid administration, maternal hypertension, umbilical artery catheterization, acute kidney injury, patent ductus arteriosus, indomethacin treatment, and chronic lung disease.[47]

Renovascular hypertension is the most frequent cause of neonatal hypertension and accounts for up to 80% to 90% of all cases. The most common cause of renovascular hypertension is renal arterial thromboembolism related to umbilical artery catheterization. Risk factors for complications from umbilical artery catheters include maternal diabetes, sepsis, dehydration, birth trauma, perinatal asphyxia, patent ductus arteriosus, and cocaine exposure. Hypertension occurs in approximately 25% of patients with renal arterial thrombosis and may be associated with hematuria, oliguria, renal failure, congestive heart failure, and ischemia of the lower extremities.

Other causes of neonatal hypertension include hypervolemia related to oliguric acute kidney injury, structural renal disease, including autosomal recessive polycystic kidney disease, aortic coarctation, and obstructive uropathy. Medications such as corticosteroids, endocrine disorders, abdominal wall closure, and treatment with ECMO have been associated with elevation of blood pressure in the neonate. Neurologic causes of hypertension include intracranial hypertension and drug withdrawal. Twelve percent of infants with bronchopulmonary dysplasia develop hypertension, which is probably multifactorial in origin but may involve effects of umbilical

Figure 51–6. Linear regression of mean systolic and diastolic blood pressures (BP) by birthweight on the first day of life. CL, confidence limits. (*From Zubrow AB, et al: Determinants of blood pressure in infants admitted to neonatal intensive care units: a prospective multicenter study, Philadelphia Neonatal Blood Pressure Study Group, J Perinatol 115:470, 1995, with permission.*)

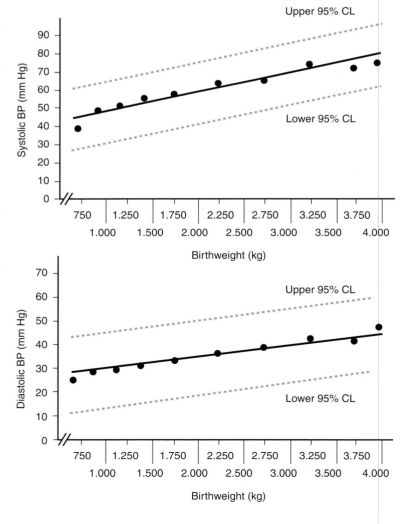

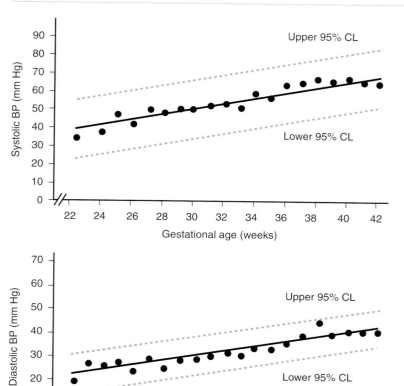

Figure 51–7. Linear regression of mean systolic and diastolic blood pressures (BP) by gestational age on the first day of life. CL, confidence limits. (*From Zubrow AB, et al: Determinants of blood pressure in infants admitted to neonatal intensive care units: a prospective multicenter study, Philadelphia Neonatal Blood Pressure Study Group,* J Perinatol *15:470, 1995, with permission*).

artery catheterization and the administration of corticosteroids and bronchodilators.[5]

CLINICAL PRESENTATION

The clinical presentation of hypertension in the neonate is variable. Although some babies may be asymptomatic, nonspecific symptoms such as poor feeding, irritability, and lethargy are common. Significant cardiopulmonary symptoms may include tachypnea, cyanosis, impaired perfusion, vasomotor instability, congestive heart failure, and hepatosplenomegaly. Neurologic symptoms such as tremors, hypertonicity, hypotonicity, opisthotonos, asymmetric reflexes, hemiparesis, seizures, apnea, or coma may also occur. The renal effects of hypertension may include acute kidney injury and sodium wasting related to pressure natriuresis.

EVALUATION

The first step is to determine whether the hypertension persists when the infant is quiet and relaxed. A complete physical examination is imperative, including four blood pressure measurements of the extremities to diagnose or rule out aortic coarctation. The infant should be examined carefully for signs of volume overload, including peripheral edema, cardiac gallop, or rales. Ambiguous genitalia in a hypertensive infant should raise the suspicion of congenital adrenal hyperplasia. Initial laboratory studies should include a urinalysis

and determinations of serum electrolytes, blood urea nitrogen, serum creatinine, and serum calcium. Although the measurement of plasma renin activity is advocated by some investigators, the findings are often variable and difficult to interpret in neonates.

Ultrasonography of the kidneys with a Doppler flow study of the aorta and renal arteries should be performed to exclude a renal arterial or aortic thrombus or structural anomalies of the urinary tract. Magnetic resonance angiography may be considered, although its use may be limited in the very small infant. Angiography may be necessary for a sick infant with vascular insufficiency of the lower extremities, congestive heart failure, or acute kidney injury. Echocardiography should be performed to exclude aortic coarctation and evaluate the left ventricular mass. Thyroid function studies and urinary studies for catecholamines, 17-hydroxysteroids, and 17-ketosteroids should be reserved for those rare instances when the results of the previously mentioned studies are normal.

TREATMENT

The clinician has a wide variety of intravenous and oral antihypertensives that may be used in the management of neonatal hypertension (Tables 51-5 and 51-6). In general, treatment should be individualized according to the suspected underlying cause of the hypertension. Neonates with signs

Figure 51–8. Linear regression of mean systolic and diastolic blood pressures (BP) by postconceptional age. CL, confidence limits. *(From Zubrow AB, et al: Determinants of blood pressure in infants admitted to neonatal intensive care units: a prospective multicenter study, Philadelphia Neonatal Blood Pressure Study Group, J Perinatol 15:470, 1995, with permission).*

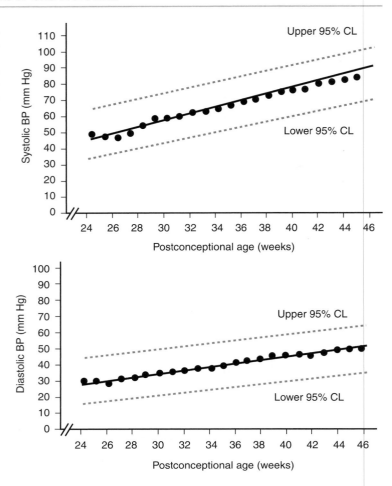

BOX 51–4	**Causes of Neonatal Hypertension**

RENOVASCULAR DISEASE
Renal arterial thrombosis
Renal arterial stenosis
Renal venous thrombosis

CONGENITAL RENAL MALFORMATIONS

OBSTRUCTIVE UROPATHY
Hydronephrosis

RENAL PARENCHYMAL DISEASE
Acute tubular necrosis
Polycystic kidney disease

COARCTATION OF THE AORTA

NEUROLOGIC DISORDERS
Seizures
Intracranial hypertension
Drug withdrawal

MISCELLANEOUS CAUSES
Bronchopulmonary dysplasia
Drug exposure (e.g., corticosteroids, catecholamines)
Abdominal wall closure
Extracorporeal membrane oxygenation

---

and symptoms of a hypertensive emergency such as cardiopulmonary failure, acute neurologic dysfunction, and renal insufficiency are best treated with a continuous intravenous infusion of an antihypertensive agent such as nitroprusside, nicardipine, esmolol, or labetalol. The chief advantage of a continuous infusion is the ability to quickly increase or decrease the rate of infusion to achieve the desired blood pressure. The goal of therapy is a gradual decrease in blood pressure to minimize injury to the brain, heart, and kidneys. Blood pressure should not be lowered below the 95th percentile for at least 24 to 48 hours to avoid the possibility of cerebral and optic disc ischemia.

Oral antihypertensive agents are best used in infants with less severe hypertension or in those whose acute hypertension has been controlled with intravenous infusions and who are ready to switch to chronic oral therapy. Captopril is widely used in the treatment of hypertensive infants and is quite effective, given the high incidence of renovascular hypertension. Careful attention to urine output and the levels of serum creatinine and potassium is recommended when initiating treatment with angiotensin-converting enzyme inhibitors because neonates may be extremely sensitive to the reduction in renal blood flow associated with the administration of these agents. Other useful oral agents include diuretics, beta blockers, calcium channel blockers, and vasodilators (see Table 51-6).

TABLE 51–5   Intravenous Antihypertensive Medications

Drug	Dose	Interval	Action
Diazoxide	2 to 5 mg/kg/dose	q 5 min prn; then q 4 to 24 h	Vasodilator
Esmolol	100 to 300 μg/kg/min	IV infusion	Beta blocker
Hydralazine	0.1 to 0.4 mg/kg/dose	q4 to 6 h	Vasodilator
Labetalol	0.25 to 3.0 mg/kg/hr	IV infusion or bolus	Alpha and beta blocker
Nicardipine	1 to 3 μg/kg/min	IV in fusion	Calcium channel blocker
Sodium nitroprusside	0.5 to 8.0 μg/kg/min	IV infusion	Vasodilator

IV, intravenous; prn, as required.

TABLE 51–6   Oral Antihypertensive Medications

Drug	Dose	Interval	Class
Amlodipine	0.1 to 0.3 mg/kg/dose	q 12	Calcium channel blocker
Captopril	0.01 to 0.5 mg/kg/dose	q 6 to 12 h	Angiotensin-converting enzyme inhibitor
Chlorothiazide	5 to 15 mg/kg/dose	q 12 h	Distal tubule diuretic
Furosemide	1 to 6 mg/kg/dose	q 8 to 24 hr	Loop diuretic
Labetalol	1 to 3 mg/kg/dose	q 8 to 12 hr	Alpha and beta blocker
Propranolol	0.25 to 1.0 mg/kg/dose	q 6 to 8 hr	Beta blocker

In infants with suspected renovascular hypertension, the umbilical artery catheter should be removed as soon as possible. Systemic heparinization may be considered to prevent the extension of the clot. If the hypertension cannot be controlled medically or massive aortic thrombosis results in major complications, thrombolysis with urokinase, streptokinase, or tissue plasminogen activator may be considered. If severe hypertension persists, surgical thrombectomy or nephrectomy may be contemplated.

PROGNOSIS

Hypertension related to umbilical artery catheters usually resolves with time and infants do not typically require antihypertensive medications beyond 12 months of age. Infants may require increases in their antihypertensive medications following discharge from the hospital due to rapid growth, but over time antihypertensive agents may be weaned by maintaining a stable medication dose as the infant grows in size. Despite blood pressure normalization, long-term consequences of neonatal renovascular hypertension have been described. In a report of 12 children studied at a mean follow-up of almost 6 years, Adelman found that 5 of 11 patients displayed unilateral renal atrophy on ultrasound or intravenous pyelography despite having normal rates of creatinine clearance.[3] Follow-up radionuclide scans remained abnormal for all patients studied, even for those without renal atrophy identified on ultrasound. Although the long-term significance of these findings is unknown, long-term nephrology follow-up is indicated to survey for chronic hypertension and kidney disease.

Nephrocalcinosis

Renal medullary calcifications were first described in the premature infant in 1982 by Hufnagle and coworkers.[31] Since then, nephrocalcinosis has become a well-known complication in the neonatal population, occurring in 27% to 65% of hospitalized premature infants weighing less than 1500g.[32,49] Infants with nephrocalcinosis may present with microscopic or gross hematuria, granular material in the diaper, acute kidney injury related to ureteral obstruction, or urinary tract infection. Nephrocalcinosis may also be discovered incidentally on abdominal imaging studies.

Nephrocalcinosis, defined as calcium deposition in the renal interstitium, develops as the consequence of an imbalance between stone-promoting and stone-inhibiting factors. The primary risk factor in neonates is hypercalciuria (excessive urinary calcium excretion), which is commonly caused by chronic treatment with loop diuretics. Other risk factors include low gestational age, low birthweight, severe respiratory disease, low urine volume, the hypercalciuric effect of corticosteroids or xanthine derivatives, hypocitraturia, hyperuricosuria, long duration of parenteral hyperalimentation, metabolic acidosis, and a familial history of nephrolithiasis.[28]

Routine ultrasonographic screening should be considered for all infants who receive diuretics for chronic lung or heart disease. In those with documented nephrocalcinosis or nephrolithiasis, the use of agents that increase urinary calcium excretion, such as loop diuretics and corticosteroids, should be minimized or discontinued if possible. A high urinary flow rate should be maintained to reduce the probability of urinary crystallization. Oral calcium supplements should be discontinued, and metabolic acidosis, if present, should be treated with potassium citrate because chronic acidosis enhances urinary calcium excretion. Thiazide diuretics such as chlorothiazide may be effective in reducing urinary calcium excretion, although serum calcium should be monitored closely to avoid hypercalcemia. The goal of therapy should be the maintenance of the spot urinary calcium to creatinine ratio less than 0.86 for infants younger than 7 months of age.[44]

The usual outcome for infants with neonatal nephrocalcinosis is spontaneous resolution over time. In one study, nephrocalcinosis persisted in 34% of preterm infants at 15 months of age, and in only 15% at 30 months of age.[46] However, there is evidence that neonatal nephrocalcinosis is associated with impairment in kidney function (GFR less than 85 mL/min/1.73 m^2) and tubular function (phosphaturia and renal tubular acidosis),[34] highlighting the importance of long-term nephrology follow-up care.

Renal Venous Thrombosis

Renal venous thrombosis, once a common occurrence, is now infrequent, possibly because of the better obstetric management of mothers with diabetes, prevention of polycythemia, and prevention and treatment of dehydration. Risk factors for renal venous thrombosis include poorly controlled maternal diabetes mellitus, dehydration, perinatal asphyxia, inherited prothrombotic states, and the presence of an umbilical venous catheter. Thrombosis begins in the small renal veins and propagates toward the main renal vein, ultimately reaching the inferior vena cava. Thrombosis is usually unilateral but may be bilateral and is associated with adrenal infarction in a minority of patients.

The classic clinical triad of symptoms in renal venous thrombosis includes a flank mass, gross hematuria, and thrombocytopenia, although all elements of the triad may not be present in each patient. Additional signs may include oliguric acute kidney injury, hypertension, vomiting, lethargy, anorexia, fever, and shock. Ultrasonography reveals a typical image, characterized by nephromegaly, the loss of corticomedullary differentiation, and increased renal echogenicity. A Doppler study may reveal renal venous or vena caval thrombosis. Uptake may be absent or severely diminished on a radionuclide scan.

There are no evidence-based guidelines for management of neonatal renal venous thrombosis. Supportive medical treatment consists of the correction of fluid and electrolyte imbalances as well as the treatment of acute kidney injury, possibly including dialysis support. Anticoagulation (unfractionated heparin, low molecular weight heparin) and fibrinolytic therapies (streptokinase, urokinase, and recombinant tissue plasminogen activator) have been used with anecdotal success.[35] Surgical thrombectomy is considered in patients with thrombosis of the inferior vena cava, and nephrectomy may be necessary in infants with severe refractory hypertension. The perinatal mortality rate in infants with renal venous thrombosis has decreased progressively during the past few decades. However, the prognosis for the affected kidney is poor, with progressive atrophy in up to 70% of kidneys.[35] The long-term consequences in infants with renal venous thrombosis include chronic kidney disease, renal tubular dysfunction, and systemic hypertension.

CONGENITAL AND INHERITED DISORDERS OF THE KIDNEY AND URINARY TRACT

Many of the disorders of the kidney and urinary tract that present in infancy are the result of congenital malformations or inherited disorders (Box 51-5). Most of the congenital disorders occur sporadically, and the pathogenesis of many of these disorders is not well defined. Alternatively, some patients may have clinical findings consistent with well-defined genetic diseases that display classic mendelian inheritance patterns, such as autosomal dominant, autosomal recessive, or X-linked inheritance. In many cases, the mutated genes in these diseases have been identified. The following commentaries review some of the more common of these disorders.

BOX 51–5 Overview of Congenital and Inherited Disorders of the Kidney and Urinary Tract That Present in Infancy

UROLOGIC ANOMALIES
Ureteropelvic junction or ureterovesical junction obstruction
Posterior urethral valves
Eagle-Barrett syndrome
Vesicoureteral reflux

CYSTIC AND DYSPLASTIC DISORDERS
Dysplasia/hypoplasia
  Hypoplasia
  Dysplasia
  Multicystic dysplastic kidney
  Unilateral or bilateral renal agenesis
Polycystic kidney disease
  Autosomal recessive polycystic kidney disease
  Autosomal dominant polycystic kidney disease
  Glomerulocystic kidney disease
Other cystic disorders
  Infantile nephronophthisis
  Cystic dysplasia associated with congenital abnormalities

TUBULAR TRANSPORT DISORDERS
Renal tubular acidosis
Fanconi syndrome
Bartter syndrome
Nephrogenic diabetes insipidus
Tubular disorders associated with syndromes such as oculocerebrorenal syndrome of Lowe, cystinosis, and galactosemia
Pseudohypoaldosteronism

MISCELLANEOUS DISORDERS
Congenital nephrotic syndrome
Teratogen fetopathies (e.g., angiotensin-converting enzyme inhibitors)
Tumors (e.g., Wilms tumor, neuroblastoma, congenital mesoblastic nephroma)

Congenital Urinary Tract Malformations

RENAL AGENESIS

Unilateral renal agenesis, or the congenital absence of the kidney, occurs in 1 in 500 to 3200 live births and bilateral renal agenesis occurs in 1 in 4000 to 10,000.[42] Renal agenesis occurs when the ureteric bud fails to induce proper differentiation of the metanephric blastema, an event that may be related to both genetic and environmental factors. Renal agenesis may be seen in infants with the VACTERL association (i.e., *v*ertebral abnormalities, *a*nal atresia, *c*ardiac abnormalities, *t*racheoesophageal fistula or *e*sophageal atresia, *r*enal agenesis and dysplasia, and *l*imb defects), caudal regression syndrome, branchio-oto-renal syndrome, and multiple chromosomal defects, but it may also occur in otherwise healthy infants.[42] Because contralateral urinary tract abnormalities, including vesicoureteral reflux, ureteropelvic junction obstruction, renal dysplasia, and ureterocele, occur in up to 90% of individuals with unilateral renal agenesis,[8] a thorough evaluation of the urinary tract, including a voiding cystourethrogram, should be considered in all patients.

RENAL DYSPLASIA

Renal dysplasia is characterized by abnormal renal development in the fetus, leading to replacement of the renal parenchyma by cartilage and disorganized epithelial structures. The pathogenesis of renal dysplasia may involve mutations in developmental genes, altered interaction of the ureteric bud with the extracellular matrix, abnormalities of renal growth factors, and urinary tract obstruction. Renal dysplasia frequently occurs in infants with obstructive uropathy and a variety of congenital disorders, including Eagle-Barrett syndrome; the VACTERL association; branchio-oto-renal syndrome; CHARGE syndrome (i.e., *c*oloboma, *h*eart disease, choanal *a*tresia, *r*estricted growth and developmental delay with or without anomalies of the central nervous system, *g*enital hypoplasia, and *e*ar anomalies or deafness); Jeune syndrome; and trisomies 13, 18, and 21. The function of dysplastic kidneys is variable, and infants with bilateral dysplasia may exhibit signs of renal insufficiency as early as the first few days of life. Concentration and acidification defects may also be present, but hematuria, proteinuria, and hypertension are unusual findings. Children with bilateral renal dysplasia generally develop progressive renal insufficiency during childhood and adolescence.

MULTICYSTIC DYSPLASTIC KIDNEY

The multicystic dysplastic kidney (MCDK) is a nonfunctional kidney, devoid of normal renal architecture, composed of multiple large cysts that resemble a cluster of grapes (Fig. 51-9).[43] Its incidence is estimated at 1 in every 4300 live births and occurs twice as often on the left side as the right side. The pathogenesis is poorly understood but may involve failure of the ureteric bud to integrate and branch appropriately into the metanephros. Although, in the past, infants with MCDK were primarily identified after detection of an abdominal mass in the neonatal period, the widespread use of prenatal ultrasonography has led to identification of many cases of MCDK in utero. Historically, a full evaluation of the urinary tract, including a VCUG, was advised for all infants with MCDK to rule out abnormalities of the contralateral urinary tract including

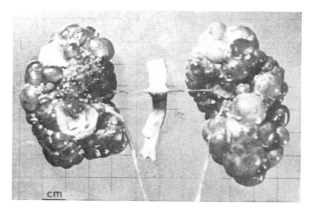

Figure 51–9. Bilateral multicystic dysplastic kidneys in a newborn infant. Kidneys are enlarged and irregularly cystic; the usual reniform configuration is barely apparent. Both ureters are atretic, and the renal arteries are extremely small. This condition is one cause of the total absence of renal function.

vesicoureteral reflux. However, many clinicians now reserve this study for infants with "complex MCDK," defined as MCDK with contralateral renal dysplasia, hydronephrosis, bladder abnormality, ureterocele, or cryptorchidism.[24]

The majority of MCDKs undergo partial or complete spontaneous involution over time. The contralateral kidney, if unaffected by other urologic malformations, generally grows larger than expected because of compensatory hypertrophy, allowing the child to maintain normal renal function. It is common practice to use serial ultrasonography to follow up patients with MCDKs to ensure involution over time and appropriate compensatory growth of the contralateral kidney. Infants with complex MCDK have a higher incidence of urinary tract infection and progression to kidney failure and should be followed up closely after discharge from the hospital. Although an MCDK poses a theoretical risk of hypertension and malignancy, surgical removal is reserved for children in whom the MCDK fails to involute or grows larger over time.

HYDRONEPHROSIS

Hydronephrosis, defined as significant dilation of the upper urinary tract (Fig. 51-10), is the most common congenital condition detected by prenatal ultrasonography, and with the advent of improved ultrasonography technology, it is being detected at a higher rate.[4] Mild dilation of the renal pelvis is frequently reported in late gestation (see Chapter 9). The most common causes of hydronephrosis are physiologic hydronephrosis, ureteropelvic or ureterovesical junction obstruction, posterior urethral valves, Eagle-Barrett syndrome, and vesicoureteral reflux.

Prenatal Management

A finding of prenatal hydronephrosis raises many questions, including those about the underlying cause of the abnormality and potential treatment options. The ability of prenatal ultrasonography to predict the specific urinary tract anatomy and the long-term renal prognosis remains limited. Certain

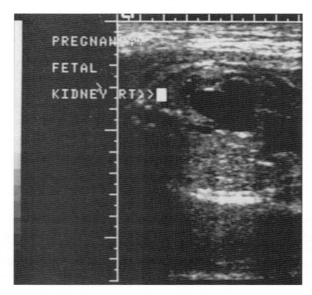

Figure 51–10. Sonogram of the right kidney in a 32-week-old fetus. Notice the large dilation of the collecting system.

findings on prenatal ultrasonography, such as increased renal echogenicity, bilateral disease, and oligohydramnios raise concern for long-term renal dysfunction. Early identification of a urinary tract abnormality allows consideration of prenatal consultation with nephrology or urology, enables coordination of prompt postnatal care, and affords the parents an opportunity to adjust to the possibility of a congenital anomaly. Prenatal intervention including percutaneous vesicoamniotic shunt placement, bladder aspiration, and drainage of a severely distended kidney remains an unproved therapy that involves significant risks, including preterm labor and chorioamnionitis.

Postnatal Management
After delivery, many clinicians advise the administration of prophylactic antibiotics to newborns with hydronephrosis to prevent urinary tract infection. Common choices of antibiotics are ampicillin and amoxicillin (20 mg/kg per day in two divided doses) administered until a VCUG is performed to determine the presence or absence of vesicoureteral reflux.[4,23] Ultrasonography of the kidneys and urinary tract should be performed within the first few days of life for all infants with moderate to severe hydronephrosis on prenatal ultrasound. Because the degree of hydronephrosis may be significantly underestimated because of the low GFR during the first 3 days of life, repeat ultrasonography is mandatory within several weeks. Infants with only mild hydronephrosis on prenatal ultrasonography should have their initial postnatal ultrasound scans performed at 2 weeks of age. A pediatric nephrologist or urologist should coordinate further evaluation, possibly to include a VCUG and/or radionuclide renal scan to determine the precise cause of the hydronephrosis.

Physiologic Hydronephrosis
Up to 15% of all prenatally detected hydronephrosis ultimately resolves spontaneously and is not associated with an anatomic abnormality of the urinary tract. Physiologic hydronephrosis

may be caused by a delay in the maturation of the ureter, which leads to transient urinary flow obstruction. The hydronephrosis in these patients generally resolves within the first 2 years of life.

Ureteropelvic Junction Obstruction
Ureteropelvic junction obstruction is the most common cause of moderate to severe congenital hydronephrosis and may be the result of incomplete recanalization of the proximal ureter, abnormal development of the ureteral musculature, abnormal peristalsis, or polyps. Ureteropelvic junction obstruction is more common in boys and may be associated with other congenital anomalies, syndromes, or other genitourinary malformations. The diagnosis is confirmed by an obstructive pattern observed on a diuretic-enhanced radionuclide scan. Many clinicians advocate antibiotic prophylaxis to prevent urinary tract infection, although this practice remains somewhat controversial in cases of ureteropelvic junction obstruction without reflux. Definitive treatment involves surgical repair.

Ureterovesical Junction Obstruction
Ureterovesical junction obstruction is the second most common cause of congenital hydronephrosis and is characterized by hydronephrosis with associated ureteral dilation. This disorder may be related to the deficient development of the distal ureter or the presence of a ureterocele. The diagnosis is confirmed by a radionuclide scan and voiding cystourethrogram. Ureterovesical junction obstruction is usually not associated with other congenital malformations. Antibiotic prophylaxis to prevent urinary tract infection remains somewhat controversial in cases of ureterovesical junction obstruction without associated reflux. Definitive treatment involves surgical repair.

Posterior Urethral Valves
Posterior urethral valves represent the most common cause of lower urinary tract obstruction, with an incidence of 1 in 5000 to 8000 live male births. A posterior urethral valve is composed of a congenital membrane that obstructs or partially obstructs the posterior urethra. The prenatal ultrasound scan may show hydronephrosis; dilated ureters; a thickened, trabeculated bladder; a dilated proximal urethra; and oligohydramnios. The antenatal presentation may include a palpable, distended bladder; a palpable prostate on rectal examination; a poor urinary stream; and signs and symptoms of renal and pulmonary insufficiency. The voiding cystourethrogram is diagnostic for posterior urethral valves and reveals associated vesicoureteral reflux in 30% of patients.

Treatment is centered on securing adequate drainage of the urinary tract, initially by placement of a urinary catheter and later by primary ablation of the valves; vesicostomy; or upper urinary tract diversion. The long-term outcome for infants with posterior urethral valves depends on the degree of associated renal dysplasia and correction of the obstruction postnatally does not necessarily result in subsequent normal kidney growth. As many as 30% of the boys with posterior urethral valves who present in infancy are at risk for progressive renal insufficiency in childhood or adolescence.

Eagle-Barrett Syndrome

Eagle-Barrett syndrome is characterized by a dilated, unobstructed urinary tract; deficiency of abdominal wall musculature; and bilateral cryptorchidism (Fig. 51-11). The estimated incidence is 1 in 35,000 to 50,000 live births, with more than 95% of the cases occurring in boys. Two theories of pathogenesis are in utero urinary tract obstruction and a specific mesodermal injury between the 4th and 10th weeks of gestation.[50] The most common urinary tract abnormalities in infants with Eagle-Barrett syndrome are renal dysplasia or agenesis, vesicoureteral reflux, and a large-capacity, poorly contractile bladder. Cardiac, pulmonary, gastrointestinal, and orthopedic anomalies are present in a large percentage of patients with Eagle-Barrett syndrome. Treatment in the neonatal period involves the optimization of urinary tract drainage, the management of renal insufficiency, and antibiotic prophylaxis. Management later in childhood may include the surgical repair of reflux, orchiopexy, reconstruction of the abdominal wall, and renal transplantation.

Vesicoureteral Reflux

Vesicoureteral reflux is defined as the retrograde propulsion of urine into the upper urinary tract during bladder contraction. The underlying cause of vesicoureteral reflux is believed to be ectopic insertion of the ureter into the bladder wall, resulting in a shorter intravesicular ureter, which acts as an incompetent valve during urination. Vesicoureteral reflux is graded from I to V, with grade I indicating the lowest and grade V the highest. In infants and children evaluated for their first urinary tract infection, at least one third have vesicoureteral reflux identified on a voiding cystourethrogram.

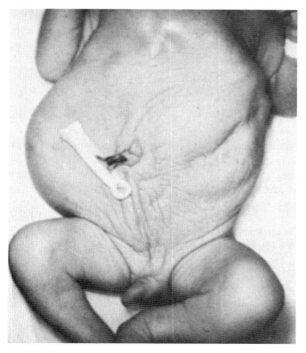

Figure 51–11. Eagle-Barrett syndrome (i.e., "prune-belly" syndrome). Notice the distinct, flabby abdomen that is indicative of absent or deficient abdominal musculature.

Although the exact genetic basis of this condition has not been determined, there appears to be a genetic component because the incidence of vesicoureteral reflux is at least 30% in first-degree relatives.[40]

Primary vesicoureteral reflux tends to resolve over time as the intravesical segment of the ureter elongates with growth. The rate of spontaneous resolution is dependent on the grade of vesicoureteral reflux, the child's age at presentation, and whether the reflux is unilateral or bilateral. Daily oral antibiotic prophylaxis is thought to be important for the prevention of urinary tract infection, although this is somewhat controversial in patients with low-grade vesicoureteral reflux. Surgical repair is considered in children with high-grade vesicoureteral reflux or breakthrough urinary tract infections despite antibiotic prophylaxis. Long-term complications of vesicoureteral reflux include hypertension, renal scarring, and chronic kidney disease ("reflux nephropathy").

EXSTROPHY-EPISPADIAS COMPLEX

The exstrophy-epispadias complex (EEC) includes a spectrum of malformations that ranges from the mildest form, epispadias, through classic bladder exstrophy, to the most severe form, exstrophy of the cloaca, which may encompass omphalocele, bladder exstrophy, imperforate anus, and spinal defects.[22]

The incidence of EEC is estimated at 1 in 10,000 births with a male predisposition of 1.5:1.[10,15,36] Epispadias occurs at a rate of 2.4 per 100,000; classic bladder exstrophy varies from 2.1 to 4.0 per 100,000 live births (the highest rate of 8.1 per 100,000 is found in Native American Indians);[15] exstrophy of the cloaca ranges from 0.5 to 1 per 200,000 live births.[22]

Enlargement or mechanical disruption of the cloacal membrane (bladder portion of the cloaca and the overlying ectoderm) prevents the invasion of mesodermal cells along the infraumbilical midline, resulting in exstrophy. Deformities of the cloacal membrane may result in hypospadias, epispadias, vesical and cloacal exstrophy, double urethra, and cloacal membrane agenesis. If rupture of the membranes occurs before the fourth week of gestation, exstrophy of the cloaca ensues. If the rupture occurs after 6 weeks of gestation, epispadias or classic bladder exstrophy occurs. This is a multifactorial disorder with a strong genetic predisposition that is still under investigation.[10,36,53] This disorder has a small risk of recurrence within families, and maternal smoking appears to enforce the severity.[26]

The clinical presentation of classic bladder exstrophy is characterized by an evaginated bladder plate with urine dripping from the ureteric orifices on the bladder surface. Bilateral inguinal hernias are usually present as well. Pubic bones can be felt on both sides of the bladder. The penis appears shorter and the epispadic urethra covers the dorsum of the penis. Testes are usually descended. In females, the clitoris is completely split next to the open urethra.[22]

Epispadias is categorized by three degrees of severity, with severe forms involving the entire urethra and bladder.[22] Cloacal exstrophy is the more severe form and can easily involve different organs that require immediate surgical attention.[22]

A renal sonogram is mandatory for every infant with exstrophy-epispadias complex to obtain a baseline examination of both kidneys before repair. Spine ultrasound and radiographs are required to define individual abnormalities. Hip radiographs and possibly magnetic resonance imaging of the pelvis help estimate the symphysis gap and hip localization.[22]

Treatment is surgical and patients require long-term follow-up and a multidisciplinary team that includes a pediatric urologist, pediatric orthopedic surgeon, and appropriate support team.[22]

Inherited Renal Disorders

Inherited renal disorders include a spectrum of abnormalities involving the glomeruli or renal tubules. Monogenic diseases (those with single gene defects) that may present in the newborn period include congenital nephrotic syndrome, polycystic kidney diseases, and tubular transport abnormalities.

CONGENITAL NEPHROTIC SYNDROME

Congenital nephrotic syndrome is a rare condition that is defined as the development of nephrotic syndrome within the first 3 months of life.[33] As in other forms of nephrotic syndrome, the clinical characteristics include massive proteinuria, hypoalbuminemia, hyperlipidemia, and edema. Most of the reported cases of primary congenital nephrotic syndrome occur in infants with Finnish ancestry (CNS-F); in Finland, the estimated incidence of CNS-F is 1 in 8200 live births. CNS-F is a well characterized autosomal recessive disorder and is the primary focus of this section. However, congenital nephrotic syndrome has also been described in infants of non-Finnish ancestry, in infants with other forms of kidney disease including diffuse mesangial sclerosis, and in infants with congenital infections.

A prenatal diagnosis of congenital nephrotic syndrome should be suspected in mothers with a high serum or amniotic fluid α-fetoprotein concentration because the amniotic fluid contains large amounts of protein resulting from urinary protein losses. The ultrasonographic detection of placental edema, ascites, or fetal hydrops should also raise the suspicion of this disorder (see Chapters 8 and 9).

Infants with CNS-F, in whom the disease process begins during intrauterine life, typically have full-blown nephrotic syndrome at birth, with massive proteinuria, profound hypoalbuminemia, hyperlipidemia, and edema. Forty-two percent of the infants with CNS-F are delivered prematurely; the mean gestational age is 36.6 weeks. Many infants, particularly those born after 37 weeks, are small for their gestational age. The placenta is always large, weighing greater than 25% of the infant's birthweight.

CNS-F is caused by mutations in *NPHS1*, the gene encoding nephrin, which is located on the long arm of chromosome 19. Nephrin is a key component of the slit diaphragm, an epithelial cell structure that plays a major role in the glomerular filtration barrier. Alterations in nephrin cause disruption of the filtration barrier, leading to massive urinary protein loss and the clinical characteristics of nephrotic syndrome. The renal histopathology of CNS-F includes mesangial hypercellularity, tubular microcysts, and variably sized glomeruli, many of them very small and having a characteristic fetal appearance, with prominent, cuboidal epithelial cells (Fig. 51-12). Although CNS-F with *NPHS1* mutations accounts for the majority of patients with CNS, other genetic forms of CNS

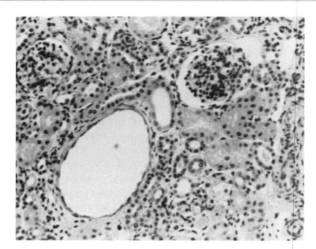

Figure 51–12. Congenital nephrotic syndrome of the Finnish type. Notice the glomerular mesangial hypercellularity and tubular microcysts.

have been identified, including disorders associated with mutations in *NPHS2* (podocin), *WT-1* (Wilms tumor suppressor gene), and *LAMB2* (laminin beta-2 gene).

The treatment of congenital nephrotic syndrome is complex. The clinician should first exclude congenital infections such as syphilis, human immunodeficiency virus, cytomegalic inclusion disease, hepatitis, rubella, and toxoplasmosis, all of which have been associated with treatable forms of nephrotic syndrome in neonates. Unlike other forms of nephrotic syndrome occurring later in life, CNS-F is resistant to therapy with corticosteroids and immunosuppressive agents. Current treatment includes intravenous albumin supplementation, aggressive nutritional support, correction of associated hypothyroidism, prompt treatment of infectious and thromboembolic complications, bilateral nephrectomy for the management of protein loss, peritoneal dialysis support, and early renal transplantation.

AUTOSOMAL RECESSIVE POLYCYSTIC KIDNEY DISEASE

Autosomal recessive polycystic kidney disease (ARPKD) is an inherited disorder characterized by polycystic kidneys and congenital hepatic fibrosis; it occurs in approximately 1 in 40,000 live births.[20] ARPKD is distinct from renal dysplasia (including cystic dysplasia), a disorder usually seen in patients with chromosomal or syndromic conditions. The majority of patients with ARPKD present in the newborn period, although rare presentations in later childhood are described. Prenatal ultrasonography shows enlarged, echogenic kidneys. Although the amniotic fluid volume is initially normal, oligohydramnios is often noted in the late middle trimester. The newborn infant with ARPKD may present with palpable abdominal masses, severe hypertension, and renal insufficiency. Respiratory failure related to pulmonary hypoplasia and marked abdominal distention from the massively enlarged kidneys are common in neonates with ARPKD.

ARPKD is caused by mutations in *PKHD1*, located on chromosome 6p21. *PKHD1* encodes encodes fibrocystin, a very large, novel protein with receptor-like properties for which the exact function is unknown. Renal histopathology reveals that after a transient phase of proximal tubular cyst formation, the principal site of subsequent cyst formation is the collecting duct (Fig. 51-13). Progressive interstitial fibrosis is an additional histopathologic feature of ARPKD. In addition, virtually all infants with ARPKD have some degree of congenital hepatic fibrosis with biliary dysgenesis, although clinical evidence of hepatic involvement is present in only 40% of patients.

The management of the neonate with ARPKD is largely supportive. Ventilatory support is critical in neonates with pulmonary hypoplasia or respiratory embarrassment (see Chapter 44). Hypertension is often a primary concern and may require the administration of continuous intravenous infusions of several antihypertensive agents. Patients may require correction of electrolyte imbalances, notably hyponatremia. Most patients with ARPKD ultimately require dialysis or kidney transplantation. The long-term consequences of hepatic fibrosis may include portal hypertension, bleeding varices and ascending cholangitis. Hepatic synthetic function typically remains intact even in patients with significant liver disease.

AUTOSOMAL DOMINANT POLYCYSTIC KIDNEY DISEASE

Autosomal dominant polycystic kidney disease (ADPKD) is the most common inherited renal disorder, occurring at an incidence of 1 in 1000 live births; however, neonatal presentation is relatively rare.[18] ADPKD is characterized by progressive bilateral renal cyst formation, although the dyssynchronous development of cysts may account for unilateral or asymmetric involvement in the neonate. The clinical spectrum of neonatal ADPKD ranges from severe neonatal manifestations that are indistinguishable from those of ARPKD to variable degrees of renal insufficiency and hypertension to asymptomatic cysts seen on renal ultrasonography. Because the clinical presentation of neonatal ARPKD and ADPKD can be very similar, an examination of the patient's parents for the presence of renal cysts is important in establishing the correct diagnosis. However, approximately 10% of patients with ADPKD will have a new mutation. Therefore, the absence of cysts in either parent does not completely exclude the diagnosis of ADPKD.

ADPKD results from mutations in two genes, *PKD1* and *PKD2*.[27] Mutations in the *PKD1* gene, located on chromosome 16, account for approximately 85% of the cases of ADPKD. The *PKD1* gene encodes polycystin 1, a large protein of unknown function that may play a role in cell-cell or cell-matrix interactions. Mutations in the *PKD2* gene, located on the long arm of chromosome 4, account for only 15% of the cases of ADPKD. The *PKD2* gene product polycystin 2 is a voltage-gated ion channel.

The prognosis for an infant with ADPKD presenting in the neonatal period or antenatally was initially thought to be poor. However, a recent study suggests that over 90% of these patients maintain intact renal function during childhood.[48] Although ADPKD is a systemic disease that can affect the liver, gastrointestinal tract, aorta and cerebral vessels, extrarenal manifestations in children are rare. Approximately 50% of all patients with ADPKD ultimately develop end-stage renal disease requiring dialysis or kidney transplantation.

NEONATAL BARTTER SYNDROME

Neonatal Bartter syndrome (previously known as *hyperprostaglandin E syndrome*) is one of the inherited hypokalemic tubulopathies that also includes classic Bartter syndrome and Gitelman syndrome.[21] Bartter syndrome is inherited as an autosomal recessive trait; the incidence of neonatal Bartter syndrome is 1 in 50,000 to 100,000 live births. Newborn infants with neonatal Bartter syndrome typically present with profound salt wasting, polyuria, hypokalemia, and hypercalciuria. Bartter syndrome is discussed in detail in Chapter 36.

RENAL TUBULAR ACIDOSIS

Renal tubular acidosis is caused by a defect in the reabsorption of bicarbonate or in the secretion of hydrogen ions that is not related to a decrease in GFR. Renal tubular acidosis should be suspected in infants with persistent hyperchloremic (i.e., nonanion gap) metabolic acidosis. There are three forms of renal tubular acidosis: proximal (type II), distal (type I), and hyperkalemic (type IV). Type II renal tubular acidosis is caused by impaired proximal tubular bicarbonate reabsorption, with a relatively normal distal tubular ability to acidify the urine. Type I renal tubular acidosis is characterized by an inability to acidify the urine (excrete H^+ ions) despite the presence of metabolic acidosis. Type IV renal tubular acidosis manifests a defect in ammoniagenesis, which is due to hyperkalemia from mineralocorticoid deficiency or tubular resistance to aldosterone. There are primary and secondary forms of renal tubular acidosis; they may be sporadic or inherited as classic mendelian traits. Renal tubular acidosis is discussed in detail in Chapter 36.

TUMORS OF THE KIDNEY

Renal tumors in the newborn infant are uncommon and include congenital mesoblastic nephroma, multilocular cystic nephroma, and Wilms tumor (i.e., nephroblastoma). Other renal neoplasms, including renal cell carcinoma, rhabdoid tumor, lymphoma, and teratoma, are rare in the newborn

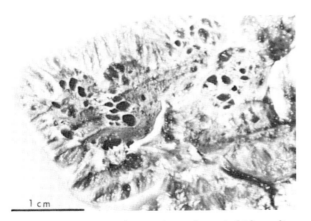

Figure 51–13. Autosomal recessive polycystic kidney disease in a newborn infant showing preservation of lobar structure and corticomedullary differentiation. The cortex is thick and spongy, and the medullary pyramids contain grossly apparent cysts; the latter are sometimes visible radiographically. (*From Elkin M, et al: Cystic diseases of the kidney—radiological and pathological considerations, Clin Radiol 20:65, 1969, with permission.*)

infant. The clinical presentation of a renal tumor in the neonatal period is usually that of abdominal swelling or a palpable mass. There may be hypertension, hematuria, fever, and feeding intolerance.

Congenital mesoblastic nephroma is the most common renal neoplasm in the first year of life. Approximately 60% of all congenital mesoblastic nephromas are diagnosed before 6 months of age; the clinical presentation is an abdominal mass. Congestive heart failure and hypertension are less common manifestations. Nephrectomy is curative, with the exception of infrequent local recurrences and rare pulmonary metastases.

Multilocular cystic nephroma is a benign renal tumor that consists of large cysts separated by fibrous septa. This tumor arises from metanephric blastema and has features of immature blastema, tubules, and skeletal muscle on histopathologic examination. The prognosis is excellent with surgical removal alone for these patients.

Wilms tumor is a malignancy that accounts for 90% of all renal tumors diagnosed in the pediatric population. However, 80% of all Wilms tumors are diagnosed in patients between the ages of 1 and 5 years, making its appearance uncommon in the first year of life and rare in the first month of life.[30] Most of these tumors occur sporadically, but 15% are associated with congenital anomalies or syndromes, including congenital aniridia, hemihypertrophy, WAGR syndrome (i.e., Wilms tumor, aniridia, genitourinary anomalies, and mental retardation), Denys-Drash syndrome (i.e., Wilms tumor, male pseudohermaphroditism, and nephrotic syndrome caused by diffuse mesangial sclerosis), and Beckwith-Wiedemann syndrome (i.e., omphalocele, macroglossia, and visceromegaly). Two candidate genes for Wilms tumor have been localized: WT-1, which is located on chromosome 11p13, and another gene on chromosome 11p15.

Definitive therapy for a localized renal mass begins with surgical exploration, and in most cases the primary treatment is nephrectomy. Infants with multilocular cystic nephromas or congenital mesoblastic nephromas require no postoperative therapy. Infants with malignant tumors such as Wilms tumor are treated according to well established oncologic protocols. The prognosis for most infants with neonatal renal tumors is good, although an infant with an aggressive Wilms tumor, an atypical congenital mesoblastic nephroma, or a renal sarcoma may have a poor prognosis.

REFERENCES

1. Abitbol CL, et al: Long-term follow-up of extremely low birth weight infants with neonatal renal failure, *Pediatr Nephrol* 18:887, 2003.
2. Abrahamson D: Glomerulogenesis in the developing kidney, *Semin Nephrol* 11:375, 1991.
3. Adelman RD: Long-term follow-up of neonatal renovascular hypertension, *Pediatr Nephrol* 1:35, 1987.
4. Aksu N, et al: Postnatal management of infants with antenatally detected hydronephrosis, *Pediatr Nephrol* 20:1253, 2005.
5. Alagappan A, Malloy M: Systemic hypertension in very low-birth weight infants with bronchopulmonary dysplasia: incidence and risk factors, *Am J Perinatol* 15:3, 1998.
6. Andreoli SP: Acute renal failure in the newborn, *Semin Perinatol* 28:112, 2004.
7. Ashkenazi D: Acute kidney injury in critically ill newborns: what do we know? What do we need to learn? *Pediatr Nephrol* 24:265, 2009.
8. Atiyeh B, et al: Contralateral renal abnormalities in patients with renal agenesis and noncystic renal dysplasia, *Pediatrics* 91:812, 1993.
9. Blowey DL, et al: Peritoneal dialysis in the neonatal period: outcome data, *J Perinatol* 13:59, 1993.
10. Boyadjiev SA, Dodson JL, Radford CL, et al: Clinical and molecular characterization of the bladder exstrophy-epispadias complex: analysis of 232 families, *BJU Int* 94:1337, 2004.
11. Brion LP, et al: A simple estimate of glomerular filtration rate in low birth weight infants during the first year of life: noninvasive assessment of body composition and growth, *J Pediatr* 109:698, 1986.
12. Boubred F, et al: Effects of maternally administered drugs on the fetal and neonatal kidney, *Drug Saf* 29:397, 2006.
13. Bourke WG, et al: Isolated single umbilical artery—the case for routine renal screening, *Arch Dis Child* 68:600, 1993.
14. Cataldi L, et al: Potential risk factors for the development of acute renal failure in preterm newborn infants: a case-control study, *Arch Dis Child Fetal Neonatal Ed* 90:F514, 2005.
15. Caton AR, Bloom A, Druschel CM, Kirby RS: Epidemiology of bladder and cloacal exstrophies in New York State, 1983-1999, *Birth Defects Res A Clin Mol Teratol* 79(11):781, 2007.
16. Chandler JC, Gauderer MW: The neonate with an abdominal mass, *Pediatr Clin North Am* 51:979, 2004.
17. Clark DA: Times of first void and first stool in 500 newborns, *Pediatrics* 60:457, 1977.
18. Cole B, et al: Polycystic kidney disease in the first year of life, *J Pediatr* 111:693, 1987.
19. Cooper WO, et al: Major congenital malformations after first-trimester exposure to ACE inhibitors, *N Engl J Med* 354:2443, 2006.
20. Dell KM, Avner ED: *Autosomal recessive polycystic kidney disease*. Gene Clinics: Clinical Genetic Information Resource [database online]. Copyright, University of Washington, Seattle (website). http://www.geneclinics.org. Initial posting July 2001, updated March 2006, 2001.
21. Dell KM, Guay-Woodford LM: Inherited tubular transport disorders, *Semin Nephrol* 19:364, 1999.
22. Ebert AK, Reutter H, Ludwig M, Rösch WH: The exstrophy-epispadias complex, *Orphanet J Rare Dis* 4:23, 2009.
23. Estrada CR, Jr.: Prenatal hydronephrosis: early evaluation, *Curr Opin Urol* 18:401, 2008.
24. Feldenberg L, Siegel N: Clinical course and outcome for children with multicystic dysplastic kidneys, *Pediatr Nephrol* 14:1098, 2000.
25. Flynn JT: Neonatal hypertension: diagnosis and management, *Pediatr Nephrol* 14:332, 2000.
26. Gambhir L, et al: Epidemiological survey of 214 families with bladder exstrophy-epispadias complex, *J Urol* 179(4):1539, 2008.
27. Grantham JJ: Clinical practice. Autosomal dominant polycystic kidney disease, *N Engl J Med* 359:1477, 2008.
28. Hein G, et al: Development of nephrocalcinosis in very low birth weight infants, *Pediatr Nephrol* 19:616, 2004.
29. Hentschel R, et al: Renal insufficiency in the neonatal period, *Clin Nephrol* 46:54, 1996.
30. Hrabovsky EE, et al: Wilms' tumor in the neonate: a report from the National Wilms' Tumor Study, *J Pediatr Surg* 21:385, 1986.

31. Hufnagle KG, et al: Renal calcifications: a complication of long-term furosemide therapy in preterm infants, *Pediatrics* 70:360, 1982.
32. Jacinto JS, et al: Renal calcification incidence in very low birth weight infants, *Pediatrics* 81:31, 1988.
33. Jalanko H: Congenital nephrotic syndrome, *Pediatr Nephrol* epub ahead of print, 2007.
34. Kist-van Holthe JE, et al: Is nephrocalcinosis in preterm neonates harmful for long-term blood pressure and renal function? *Pediatrics* 119:468, 2007.
35. Lau KK, et al: Neonatal renal vein thrombosis: review of the English-language literature between 1992 and 2006, *Pediatrics* 120:e1278, 2007.
36. Ludwig M, Ching B, Reutter H, Boyadjiev SA: Bladder exstrophy-epispadias complex, *Birth Defects Res A Clin Mol Teratol* 85:509, 2009.
37. Makhoul IR, et al: Neonatal transient renal failure with renal medullary hyperechogenicity: clinical and laboratory features, *Pediatr Nephrol* 20:904, 2005.
38. Miall LS, et al: Plasma creatinine rises dramatically in the first 48 hours of life in preterm infants, *Pediatrics* 104:e76, 1999.
39. Moritz KM, Wintour EM: Functional development of the meso- and metanephros, *Pediatr Nephrol* 13:171, 1999.
40. Murer L, et al: Embryology and genetics of primary vesico-ureteric reflux and associated renal dysplasia, *Pediatr Nephrol* 22:788, 2007.
41. Picca S, et al: Medical management and dialysis therapy for the infant with an inborn error of metabolism, *Semin Nephrol* 28:477, 2008.
42. Robson WL, et al: Unilateral renal agenesis, *Adv Pediatr* 42:575, 1995.
43. Robson WL, et al: Multicystic dysplasia of the kidney, *Clin Pediatr (Phila)* 34:32, 1995.
44. Sargent JD, et al: Normal values for random urinary calcium to creatinine ratios in infancy, *J Pediatr* 123:393, 1993.
45. Scheinman SJ, et al: Genetic disorders of renal electrolyte transport, *N Engl J Med* 340:1177, 1999.
46. Schell-Feith EA, et al: Preterm neonates with nephrocalcinosis: natural course and renal function, *Pediatr Nephrol* 18:1102, 2003.
47. Seliem WA, et al: Antenatal and postnatal risk factors for neonatal hypertension and infant follow-up, *Pediatr Nephrol* 22:2081, 2007.
48. Shamshirsaz AA, et al: Autosomal-dominant polycystic kidney disease in infancy and childhood: progression and outcome, *Kidney Int* 68:2218, 2005.
49. Short A, Cooke RW: The incidence of renal calcification in preterm infants, *Arch Dis Child* 66:412, 1991.
50. Sutherland RS, et al: The prune-belly syndrome: current insights, *Pediatr Nephrol* 9:770, 1995.
51. Symons J, et al: Continuous renal replacement therapy in children up to 10 kilograms, *Am J Kidney Dis* 41:984, 2003.
52. Vanpee M, et al: Renal function in very low birth weight infants: normal maturity reached during early childhood, *J Pediatr* 121:784, 1992.
53. Wood HM, Babineau D, Gearhart JP: In vitro fertilization and the cloacal/bladder exstrophy-epispadias complex: a continuing association, *J Pediatr Urol* 3:305, 2007.
54. Zubrow AB, et al: Determinants of blood pressure in infants admitted to neonatal intensive care units: a prospective multicenter study, Philadelphia Neonatal Blood Pressure Study Group, *J Perinatol* 15:470, 1995.

CHAPTER 52

The Skin

Steven B. Hoath and Vivek Narendran

The skin, as the perceived surface of the body, comes into being at the moment of birth. The intersection between genetics and environment is amply demonstrated by the phenotype of newborn skin. The initial evaluation of a newly born infant includes drying the baby to prevent heat loss and an informed assessment of skin color, perfusion, and integrity. Pathologic processes visible on the skin surface range from general signs of internal organ dysfunction (cyanosis, pallor, jaundice) to clinical evidence of specific diseases (vesicles, petechiae) to cutaneous determinants of gestational age (breast buds, plantar creases, desquamation). Maternal-infant bonding is, in large part, a complex dynamic interaction between skin surfaces.[42]

At birth, the skin of the term infant must perform multiple physiologic functions critical for survival in an extrauterine environment (Box 52-1).[22] Many of these functions depend on structural development of the skin during the last trimester of pregnancy. The development of a competent epidermal barrier, for example, is essential for temperature regulation, maintenance of fluid homeostasis, infection control, and prevention of penetration of environmental toxins and drugs.

The epidermal permeability barrier primarily resides in the outermost layer of the epidermis, the stratum corneum. This layer, approximately one fourth the thickness of this sheet of paper, develops in utero during the third trimester of pregnancy in conjunction with a protective mantle of vernix caseosa. Preterm infants with extremely low birthweight (less than 1000 grams birthweight) lack a well-developed stratum corneum and pose special problems for newborn caregivers. The stratum corneum is necessary for the adherence of thermistors, cardiorespiratory monitors, and endotracheal tubes and forms the primary environmental interface with caregivers and parents. Box 52-2 gives a summary of general principles of skin care drawn from the literature.[8,38]

In addition to prematurity, a host of diseases and disorders of the fetus and newborn present with cutaneous manifestations. The advantage of the accessibility of the skin to physical examination is counterbalanced by the extreme structural and functional diversity of this organ. The caregiver must distinguish benign and transient lesions of newborn skin, such as erythema toxicum, from potential life-threatening diseases such as herpes simplex neonatorum. A basic understanding of the structural development of the skin, as well as the multiple functions subserved by the skin during transition to extrauterine life, is of basic importance to all newborn caregivers.[20,22]

This chapter provides an overview of the principles of newborn skin care followed by a summary of the many diseases of the newborn presenting with primary or secondary cutaneous manifestations. It is important to recognize that many common cutaneous findings in the newborn, such as sebaceous gland hyperplasia and neonatal pustular melanosis, point clearly to an intrauterine etiology. Thus far, however, an understanding of the biology of the fetus and its amniotic fluid environment is not sufficiently advanced to offer definitive explanatory mechanisms.

THE STRUCTURAL BIOLOGY OF FETAL AND NEONATAL SKIN

Development of the Epidermis

Human skin has two distinct but interdependent components—the epidermis and the dermis (Fig. 52-1). The epidermis has marked regional variations in thickness, color, permeability, and surface chemical components. It consists of a highly ordered, compact layering of keratinocytes and melanocytes. Traditionally, the epidermis is segmented into distinct structural and functional compartments called the stratum germinativum (basale), stratum spinosum, stratum granulosum, and stratum corneum (see Fig. 52-1). Intermixed is a third distinct cell type, the Langerhans cell, which is derived from bone marrow precursors and migrates into the primitive epidermis.

The process of cutaneous morphogenesis can be divided into embryonic and fetal periods (Fig. 52-2).[23,37] This transition, which occurs at approximately 2 months or 60 days, is an important time in skin development because many critical morphogenetic events occur during this transitional period. Between 30 and 40 days of development, the embryonic skin consists of a two-layered epidermis: the basal layer associated with the basal lamina and the periderm, which serves as a cover and a presumptive nutritional interface

---

BOX 52–1 | Multiple Physiologic Roles of the Skin at Birth

Barrier to water loss
Thermoregulation
Infection control
Immunosurveillance
Acid mantle formation
Antioxidant function
Ultraviolet light photoprotection
Barrier to chemicals
Tactile discrimination
Attraction to caregiver

BOX 52–2 | Principles of Newborn Skin Care

DELIVERY ROOM
Provide immediate drying and tactile stimulation.
Remove blood and meconium.
Leave vernix intact and spread to allow absorption.

BATHING
Limit frequency.
Use neutral pH cleansers.
Use only water for infants weighing less than 1000 g.
Avoid antibacterial soaps.

EMOLLIENTS
Avoid petrolatum-based ointments in infants with very
  low birthweight during the first week of life.
Use emollients as needed for dryness in older infants.

DISINFECTANTS
Use chlorhexidine, and remove excess after procedure.
Use of isopropyl alcohol and alcohol-based disinfectants is
  discouraged in infants with very low birthweight until
  the stratum corneum has formed.

ADHESIVES
Minimize use of adhesives.
Use hydrogel electrodes.
Avoid solvents and bonding agents.
Counsel patience during tape removal.

TRANSEPIDERMAL WATER LOSS
For infants younger than 30 weeks' gestation, select high incubator humidity (>60%) and transparent, semipermeable
  dressings to reduce evaporative water and heat loss.
Use incubators and supplemental conductive heat to
  avoid drying effects of radiant warmers.
Measure humidity routinely.

CORD CARE
Allow natural drying.
Avoid the routine use of isopropyl alcohol.

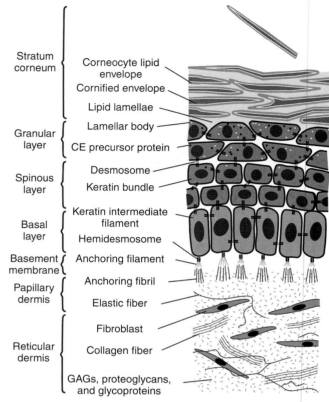

Figure 52–1. Structure of the skin. The normal term infant's skin is composed of three separate layers: dermis, basement membrane, and epidermis. The epidermis can be subdivided into four further strata (basal, spinous, granular, corneum), each representing a specific stage in terminal differentiation. CE, cornified envelope; GAG, glycosaminoglycan (GAG). *(From Hardman MJ, Byrne C: Skin structural development. In Hoath SB et al, editors: Neonatal skin: structure and function, 2nd ed, New York, 2003, Marcel Dekker.)*

---

with the amniotic fluid. The basal layer includes cells that give rise to the future definitive epidermis, whereas the periderm is a transient layer that covers the embryo and fetus until the epidermis keratinizes at the end of the second trimester. Basal cells join with each other and peridermal cells by a relatively few desmosomes but do not yet form hemidesmosomes with the basement membrane. Small numbers of keratin intermediate filaments are associated with these junctions. Matrix adhesion of the embryonic epidermis is likely mediated by actin-associated $\alpha6\beta4$ integrin.[37]

Langerhans cells and melanocytes migrate into the embryonic epidermis and are identifiable at 40 and 50 days of gestation, respectively. At this stage, the Langerhans cells do not express CD1 antigen on their cell surfaces, nor are Langerhans cell granules identifiable. Likewise, at this time, the melanocyte lacks the characteristic cytoplasmic organelle, the melanosome. A third immigrant cell, the Merkel cell, does not appear to be present in embryonic epidermis and may differentiate at a later stage from keratinocytes in situ.

At the time of embryonic-fetal transition (60 days' gestation), the epidermis begins to stratify, forming an intermediate layer of cells. These young keratinocytes still contain a high volume of glycogen in their cytoplasm and produce large amounts of intermediate filaments in association with the desmosomes. At this time, new keratins are identifiable as markers of differentiation as well as the pemphigus antigen, which is detectable on the cell surface. These cells, unlike

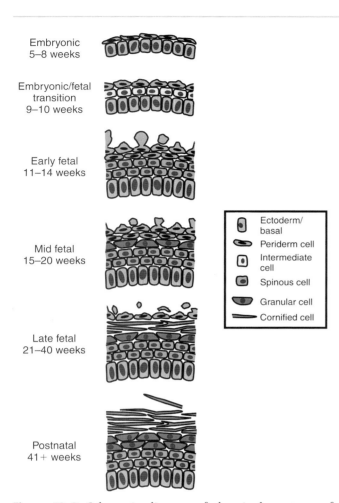

Embryonic
5–8 weeks

Embryonic/fetal
transition
9–10 weeks

Early fetal
11–14 weeks

Mid fetal
15–20 weeks

Late fetal
21–40 weeks

Postnatal
41+ weeks

	Ectoderm/basal
	Periderm cell
	Intermediate cell
	Spinous cell
	Granular cell
	Cornified cell

Figure 52–2. Schematic diagram of the six key stages of epidermal differentiation and development. The epidermis develops from a single layer of undifferentiated ectoderm (5-8 weeks) to a multilayered stratified differentiated epithelium with a competent epidermal barrier (40 weeks). The periderm undergoes intense proliferation (11-14 weeks) and forms characteristic blebs and microvilli thought to be functionally important. Regression and disaggregation of the periderm occurs concomitant with formation of the vernix caseosa (not shown). *(From Hardman MJ, Byrne C: Skin structural development. In Hoath SB et al, editors:* Neonatal skin: structure and function, *2nd ed, New York, 2003, Marcel Dekker pp 1-19.)*

adult spinous cells, remain proliferative and continue to express epidermal growth factor receptors on their surfaces. Two to three additional layers of intermediate cells are added during the second trimester. These cells show a progressive increase in the number of keratin filaments but do not further differentiate until the onset of keratinization in the interappendageal epidermis around 22 to 24 weeks' gestation.

The Langerhans cells in the embryonic epidermis begin to express CD1 antigen and contain Langerhans granules after the embryonic-fetal transition. The numbers of Langerhans cells increase significantly during the third trimester; however, the function of these cells in fetal skin remains unknown.

Between 80 and 90 days' gestation, melanocytes also increase in density at a time when keratinocytes in the epidermis are forming appendages, and melanin synthesis begins at the end of the first trimester. Transfer of melanosomes to keratinocytes occurs in the fifth month of gestation.

Melanin production is low in the newborn, who is not as pigmented as the older child and is more sensitive to sunlight, but there is no significant difference in the number of melanocytes in light, medium, or deeply pigmented skin or in infant or adult skin. Difference in color is the result of the shape, size, chemical structure, and distribution of melanosomes and the activity of individual melanocytes. Color variations in human skin have a presumptive sun protective function and may serve as camouflage.

DEVELOPMENT OF THE APPENDAGES

The appendages derive from embryonic invaginations of epidermal germinative buds into the dermis.[24] They include hair, sebaceous glands, apocrine glands, eccrine glands, and nails. The arrector pili muscle is attached to the hair follicle. Lanugo (i.e., fine, soft, immature hair) frequently covers the scalp and brow of the premature infant. The scalp line may be poorly demarcated, and lanugo also may cover the face. Scalp hair is usually somewhat coarser and matures earlier in dark-haired infants.

The growth phases of the hair follicle are usually synchronous at birth. Eighty percent of the follicles are in the resting state. During the first few months of life, the synchrony between hair loss and regrowth is altered so that 20% of scalp hairs are growing in the same phase at the same time. Hair may become coarse and thick, acquiring an adult distribution, or there may be temporary alopecia.

There are sex differences in hair growth; boys' hair grows faster than girls' hair. In both sexes, scalp hair growth is slower at the crown. The normal pattern of hair growth is disturbed in many chromosomal disorders. Evidence supports a genetic link between the formation of clockwise posterior parietal hair whorls and specific (right) handedness of the individual.[30] This finding supports an unexpected association between gene-based hair patterning and human brain development. Evidence has shown the human hair follicle can synthesize cortisol de novo and is a functional equivalent of the hypothalamic-pituitary-adrenal axis.[27] The significance of this skin-brain connection remains to be elucidated.

The eccrine sweat glands are coiled structures that form during the first trimester as a downgrowth from epidermal cellular clones.[50] No new glands are formed after birth. They are distributed over the entire body surface and are innervated by sympathetic cholinergic nerves. During the first 24 hours of life, term infants usually do not sweat; on approximately the third day, sweating begins on the face. Palmar sweating begins later. Thermal sweating as a function of body or environmental temperature should be distinguished from emotional sweating associated with crying or pain. The latter is best assessed on the palms and soles.[50]

The sebaceous glands differentiate primarily from the epithelial portion of the hair follicle at approximately 13 to 15 weeks of life and almost immediately produce sebum in all hairy areas.[58] The glands develop as solid outpouchings from the upper third of the hair follicle. These solid buds become filled with liquid centrally where the cells disintegrate; acini and ducts develop, opening most frequently into the canals between the hair follicle wall and hair shaft. Ectopic glands occur occasionally on the lips, buccal mucosa, esophagus, and vagina.

Surprisingly little is know about the regulation of the rapid growth and activity of sebaceous glands up to and immediately after birth. Hypothetically, secretion by the fetal adrenal gland of weak androgens such as dehydroepiandrosterone (DHEA) is followed by intrasebocyte conversion to testosterone and production of products of the pilosebaceous unit such as vernix caseosa.[58] This hypothesis remains to be fully tested, but it has the singular advantage of functionally integrating two disparate and unexplained facts: the mutual hyperplasia of the sebaceous gland and the adrenal cortex during the latter half of gestation in the human fetus. Androgens are the only hormones that unequivocally have a stimulating effect on the sebaceous glands; estrogens depress their growth. Between 2 months and 2 years, the sebaceous glands of the normal infant begin a period of quiescence that lasts until puberty.

The apocrine glands are relatively large organs that originate from and empty into a hair follicle. Embryologically, they develop somewhat later than the eccrine glands. Apocrine development is advanced by 7 or 8 fetal months, when the glands begin to produce a milky-white fluid containing water, lipids, protein, reducing sugars, ferric iron, and ammonia. In the newborn, the acini are well formed. The biologic function of the gland is unknown in infants, but it is related to pheromone production in other animal species.

VERNIX BIOLOGY

Vernix caseosa, a unique material that coats the fetal skin surface during the last trimester of pregnancy, contains lipids of sebaceous origin as well as numerous water-laden fetal corneocytes. A growing body of evidence supports the hypothesis that vernix caseosa participates in regionally "waterproofing" the skin surface, thereby allowing cornification to occur, initially around the hair follicles and then over the interfollicular skin.[21] A better understanding of vernix caseosa and fetal sebaceous gland physiology is biologically relevant and may be applicable to care of the infant with very low birthweight and to clinical situations in which the epidermal surface is inadequately developed, burned, or traumatized.

Physiologically, vernix is a hydrophobic material containing wax esters, cholesterol, ceramides, and squalene in addition to other minor lipid components. Vernix has high water content ($\sim 80\%$), with the water primarily distributed within flat, polygonal, cornified squames. As term approaches, vernix detaches from the fetal skin surface under the influence of pulmonary surfactant and is swallowed by the fetus. In close analogy to breast milk, vernix contains multiple molecules associated with the innate immune system, including lysozyme, lactoferrin, and defensins, as well as antioxidants such as alpha-tocopherol.[21,57] Vernix possesses both emollient (moisturizing) as well as cleansing functions. Thus, at birth the human infant is covered with a complex material possessing endogenous anti-infective, antioxidative, moisturizing, and cleansing capabilities. Extreme prematurity, as well as postmaturity, are associated with diminished vernix on the skin surface at birth.

Development of the Dermis

The fetal dermis acquires some of the characteristics of adult dermis around 20 weeks' gestation. However, it is only in the more mature fetus that the true structural and biochemical qualities of the newborn dermis are detectable. The dermis contains three identifiable zones: the region adjacent to the basement membrane, the papillary, and the reticular dermis (see Fig. 52-1). The superficial dermis has finer collagen fibers and is biochemically more active than the deeper zone. The papillary dermis also is more susceptible to light injury and elastic tissue degeneration than the reticular dermis. The dermis has a symbiotic relationship with and may exert a controlling influence on the epidermis. It is a metabolically active tissue that contains fibrous elements, amorphous ground substance, free cells, nerves, blood vessels, and lymphatics.

The fibrous elements are collagen and elastic tissue. Collagen types I, III, V, and VI comprise the dermal collagens, whereas type IV is present in the basement membrane of the dermal-epidermal junction and dermal vessels, and type VII occurs in anchoring fibrils and basal keratinocytes. With increasing age, collagen becomes progressively less soluble, and thicker bundles predominate. The morphologic characteristics and chemical properties of cutaneous elastic fibers differ from those of collagen. Elastic fibers are first detectable in the skin by histochemical means and electron microscopy at around 20 weeks' gestation.

The fibroblasts are the most numerous cells in the dermis. They produce collagen and the glycosaminoglycans of the ground substance. Mast cells (which produce heparin and histamine), histiocytes, macrophages, lymphocytes, neutrophils, and an occasional plasma cell and eosinophil are also present in the dermis. The major glycosaminoglycans in the ground substance of skin are hyaluronic acid and dermatan sulfate (i.e., chondroitin sulfate B). An increase in age brings a shift from hyaluronic acid toward dermatan sulfate and a decrease in water content of the dermis.

BLOOD AND LYMPHATIC VESSEL DEVELOPMENT

The vascular network supplying the skin develops in early embryonic life from the mesoderm.[51] In 60- to 70-day-old fetuses, there are two vascular networks: a superficial one that appears to correspond to the subpapillary plexus of adult skin and a deeper network that represents the deep reticular vascular network of adult skin. New capillary beds organize to supply the developing epidermal appendages from the fifth month of gestation. These two networks persist into the newborn period; however, the arrangement of vessels remains unstable for the first year of life, and further organization of the vascular network occurs postnatally.

Vasomotor tone is controlled by a delicate and complex series of neural and pharmacologic mechanisms that involve the sympathetic nervous system, norepinephrine, acetylcholine, and histamine and may involve serotonin, vasoactive polypeptides, corticosteroids, and prostaglandins. The physiologic requirements of skin vary considerably; skin blood flow ranges from 0.1 to 150 mL/mm³ of tissue per minute.⁵¹

DEVELOPMENT OF CUTANEOUS INVERVATION

The nerve networks in the dermis develop at a very early embryologic age and appear to be distributed in a random fashion. The most superficial nerves have the smallest diameter and are the least myelinated. In addition to the dermal nerve network, which may show considerable regional variation, nerve fibers may serve particular regions or structures such as hair follicles, eccrine glands, arrector pili muscles, and the subepidermal zone. Superficial nerves conduct mechanosensory stimuli from the specialized Merkel cells within the epidermis. The sebaceous glands are not innervated.

Special neurologic structures include a dense perifollicular nerve network with exquisite tactile sensory properties and mucocutaneous end organs highly concentrated in erogenous zones. Meissner tactile organs are found in newborn skin as undeveloped structures that mature after birth. Merkel corpuscles probably govern two-point tactile discrimination on palms and fingertips; they are disk-shaped terminals that are seen during the 28th week of fetal life. After birth, these receptors undergo little alteration. Vater-Pacini corpuscles are found around the digits, palms, and genitals; they are fully formed and numerous at birth.²²

The arrector pili muscles are innervated by sympathetic nerves, and norepinephrine acts as the neurotransmitter. The eccrine glands are innervated by sympathetic fibers, but acetylcholine acts as the neurotransmitter. Parasympathetic fibers may accompany the sensory nerves in the vessel walls and cause vasodilation. The axon reflex is poorly developed in the newborn; in the neonate of low birthweight, axon-reflex sweating may be difficult to elicit.⁵⁰

DISORDERS AND DISEASES OF FETAL AND NEONATAL SKIN

This section provides a cursory synopsis of normal and abnormal aspects of newborn skin. An accurate description of primary and secondary skin lesions underlies the proper identification of skin condition and whether appropriate treatment is needed. Tables 52-1 and 52-2 describe the basic lesional morphology of infant skin with specific examples. More definitive treatises on normal skin structure, function, development, and specific disease states are available.¹²,²⁰ The remainder of this chapter delineates specific conditions of newborn skin ranging from transient lesions to definitive cutaneous diseases and diagnostic categories.

Transient Cutaneous Lesion

A number of benign and transient lesions of the skin are commonly observed in a normal nursery population. It is important for the infant caregiver to distinguish such ephemeral lesions from significant life-threatening diseases with cutaneous manifestations.

TABLE 52–1   Primary Cutaneous Lesions*

Type	Description	Clinical Examples
Macule	A circumscribed, flat lesion with color change, up to 1 cm in size; by definition, they are not palpable	Ash leaf macules, café-au-lait spots, capillary ectasias
Patch	Same as macule but greater than 1 cm in size	Nevus depigmentosus, nevus simplex, mongolian spots
Papule	A circumscribed, elevated, solid lesion, up to 1 cm in size; elevation may be accentuated with oblique lighting	Verrucae, milia, juvenile xanthogranuloma
Plaque	A circumscribed, elevated, plateau-like, solid lesion, greater than 1 cm in size	Mastocytoma, nevus sebaceous
Nodule	A circumscribed, elevated, solid lesion with depth, up to 2 cm in size	Dermoid cysts, neuroblastoma
Tumor	Same as a nodule but greater than 2 cm in size	Hemangioma, lipoma, rhabdomyosarcoma
Vesicle	A circumscribed, elevated, fluid-filled lesion up to 1 cm in size	Herpes simplex, varicella, miliaria crystallina
Bulla	Same as a vesicle but greater than 1 cm in size	Sucking blisters, epidermolysis bullosa, bullous impetigo
Wheal	A circumscribed, elevated, edematous, often evanescent lesion, due to accumulation of fluid within the dermis	Urticaria, bite reactions, drug eruptions
Pustule	A circumscribed, elevated lesion filled within purulent fluid, less than 1 cm in size	Neonatal pustular melanosis, erythema toxicum neonatorum, infantile acropustulosis
Abscess	Same as a pustule but greater than 1 cm in size	Pyodermas

*These lesions arise de novo and are therefore most characteristic of the disease process.
Modified from Yan AC et al, editors Lesional morphology and assessment. In Eichenfeld LF et al, editors: *Textbook of neonatal dermatology*. Philadelphia, 2008, Saunders, p 33.

TABLE 52–2   Secondary Cutaneous Lesions*

Type	Description	Clinical Examples
Crust	Results from dried exudates overlying an impaired epidermis. Can be composed of serum, blood, or pus.	Epidermolysis bullosa, impetigo
Scale	Results from increased shedding or accumulation of stratum corneum as a result of abnormal keratinization and exfoliation. Can be subdivided further in pityriasiform (branny, delicate), psoriasiform (thick, white, and adherent), and ichthyosiform (fish scale–like).	Ichthyoses, postmaturity desquamation, seborrheic dermatitis
Erosion	Intraepithelial loss of epidermis. Heals without scarring.	Herpes simplex, certain types of epidermolysis bullosa
Ulcer	Full thickness loss of the epidermis with damage into the dermis. Will heal with scarring.	Ulcerated hemangiomas, aplasia cutis congenita
Fissure	Linear, often painful break within the skin surface, as a result of excessive xerosis.	Inherited keratodermas, hand and foot eczema
Lichenification	Thickening of the epidermis with exaggeration of normal skin markings caused by chronic scratching or rubbing.	Sucking callus, atopic dermatitis
Atrophy	Localized diminution of skin. *Epidermal atrophy* results in a translucent epidermis with increased wrinkling, whereas *dermal atrophy* results in depression of the skin with retained skin markings. Use of topical steroids can result in epidermal atrophy, whereas intralesional steroids may result in dermal atrophy.	Aplasia cutis congenita intrauterine scarring, and focal dermal hypoplasia
Scar	Permanent fibrotic skin changes that develop as a consequence of tissue injury. In utero scarring can occur as a result of certain infections or amniocentesis or postnatally from a variety of external factors.	Congenital varicella, aplasia cutis congenita

*These lesions arise as characteristic modifications of primary lesions through environmental interaction (e.g., drying) or subject interaction (e.g., scratching).
Modified from Yan AC et al: Lesional morphology and assessment. In Eichenfeld LF et al, editors: *Textbook of neonatal dermatology*, Philadelphia, 2008, Saunders, 2008, p 33.

SEBACEOUS GLAND HYPERPLASIA AND MILIA

Approximately 40% of infants have multiple, white, 1-mm cysts (i.e., milia) scattered over the cheeks, forehead, nose, and nasolabial folds. These milia may be few or numerous, but they frequently occur in clusters. Milia are often confused with the smaller, flatter, more yellow dots of sebaceous gland hyperplasia seen on the midface as well (Fig. 52-3). Histologically, milia are keratogenous cysts similar to Epstein pearls, which are distributed along the midpalatal raphe. Bohn nodules are cysts that occur on the palate and the buccal and lingual aspects of the dental ridges and represent remnants of mucous gland tissue. Intraoral lesions are found in 75% to 80% of newborns. Because all these cysts exfoliate or involute spontaneously within the first few weeks of life, no treatment is required.

PIGMENTARY LESIONS[53]

The most frequently encountered pigmented lesion is the mongolian spot (cutaneous melanosis), which occurs frequently in African-American, Asian, and Native American infants and, infrequently, in white infants. Although most of these lesions are found in the lumbosacral area, occurrence at other sites is not uncommon. The pigmentation is macular and gray-blue, lacks a sharp border, and may cover an area 10 cm or larger in diameter. Pigmentary lesions result from delayed disappearance of dermal melanocytes.

Most of these lesions gradually disappear during the first few years of life, but aberrant lesions in unusual sites are

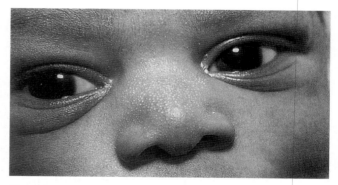

Figure 52–3. Sebaceous gland hyperplasia is manifested by tiny yellow-white follicular papules without inflammation over the nose and surrounding area. (*From Lucky AW: Transient benign cutaneous lesions in the newborn. In Eichenfield LF et al, editors:* Neonatal dermatology, *Philadelphia, 2008, Saunders.*)

more likely to persist. Because of their distinctive color and morphology, mongolian spots are not easily confused with congenital pigmented melanocytic nevi or café-au-lait spots, which have their onset later in infancy or in early childhood, although occasionally they may be present at birth.

Abnormal hyperpigmentation of the areolas and genitals may be evidence of the existence of an in utero glucocorticoid insufficiency associated with defects in the biosynthesis of hydrocortisone.

TRANSIENT MACULAR STAINS OR SALMON PATCHES[41]

Salmon patches or transient macular stains are present in up to 70% of normal newborns (Fig. 52-4A-B). They are usually found on the nape, the eyelids, and the glabella. In a prospective study of affected infants, most of the facial lesions had faded by 1 year of age, but those on the neck were more persistent. Surveys of adult populations confirm the persistence of the nuchal lesions in approximately one fourth of the population.

HARLEQUIN COLOR CHANGE

Harlequin color change is a phenomenon observed in the immediate neonatal period and is more common in the infant with low birthweight. The dependent side of the body becomes intensely red, and the upper side pales, with a sharp midline demarcation. The peak frequency of attacks in one series occurred on the second, third, and fourth days, but episodes were observed during the first 3 weeks of life. These episodes are of no pathologic significance. They have been attributed to a temporary imbalance in the autonomic regulatory mechanism of the cutaneous vessels; there are no accompanying changes in the respiratory rate, muscle tone, or response to external stimuli.

ERYTHEMA TOXICUM

Erythema toxicum is a benign and self-limited eruption that usually develops between 24 and 72 hours of age, but new lesions may appear until 2 to 3 weeks of age.[45] The disorder is more common in term infants than in premature infants, which suggests that it may represent an inflammatory reaction requiring mature skin. These lesions may vary considerably in character and number; they may be firm, 1- to 3-mm, pale yellow-to-white papules or pustules on an erythematous base resembling flea bites or erythematous macules as large as 3 cm

in diameter. Individual lesions are evanescent, often lasting only a matter of hours. They may be found on any area of the body but occur only rarely on the palms and soles. They are asymptomatic with no related systemic involvement, and their cause is unknown, although a variety of specific cytokines have been implicated in the pathogenesis.[39] A microscopic examination of a Wright-stained or Giemsa-stained smear of the pustule contents demonstrates numerous eosinophils; Gram stains are negative for bacteria, and cultures are sterile. No treatment is necessary, because spontaneous resolution occurs in 6 days to 2 weeks.

TRANSIENT NEONATAL PUSTULAR MELANOSIS

Transient neonatal pustular melanosis is a distinctive eruption that consists of three types of lesions. First-stage lesions are small, superficial vesiculopustules with little or no surrounding erythema.[45] These rapidly progress to the second stage, which consists of collarettes of scale or scale crust surrounding a hyperpigmented macule (third stage) (Fig. 52-5A-C). All three types of lesions may be present at birth, but the macules are observed more frequently. The lesions may be profuse or sparse and occur on any body surface, including the palms, soles, and scalp. Sites of predilection are the forehead, submental area and anterior neck, and lower back. When intact pustules rupture, a pigmented macule often is discernible central to the collarette of scale, which represents the margin of the unroofed pustule. Presumably, the macules result from postinflammatory hyperpigmentation, and those present at birth may be the sequelae of in utero pustular lesions.

Pustular melanosis may be confused with erythema toxicum, congenital cutaneous candidiasis, or staphylococcal pyoderma.[45,53] Cultures and Gram stains of smears prepared from intact pustules are devoid of organisms; Wright stains of intralesional contents demonstrate cellular debris, polymorphonuclear leukocytes, and a few or no eosinophils, in contrast to those of erythema toxicum. Although the pustules disappear in 48 hours, the hyperpigmented macules may

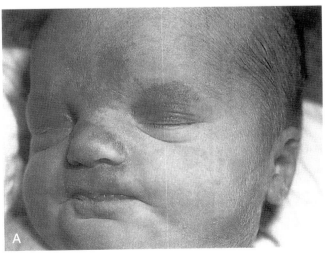
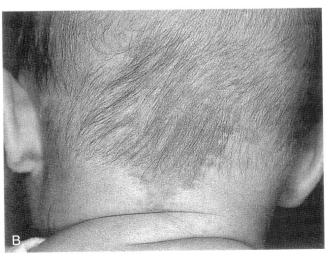

Figure 52–4. Capillary ectasias or transient macular stains (salmon patches). Also called a nevus simplex, these lesions appear on the glabella, eyelids, nose, and upper lip (**A**). The most common location for a nevus simplex is the nape of the neck (**B**). (*From Lucky AW: Transient benign cutaneous lesions in the newborn. In Eichenfield LF et al, editors:* Neonatal dermatology, *Philadelphia, 2008, Saunders.*)

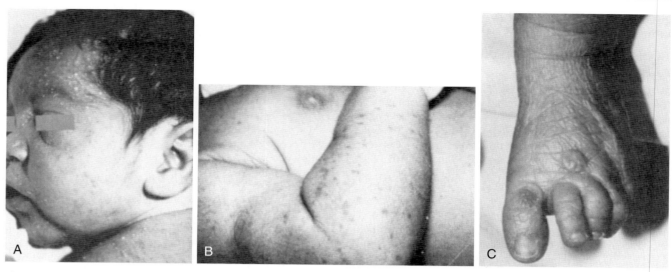

Figure 52–5. Transient neonatal pustular melanosis. **A,** Superficial pustules on the face and shoulders of a 1-day-old infant. Some have ruptured, leaving a collarette of scale. **B,** Pigmented macules on the arm and chest of a newborn. **C,** Large pustule on the dorsum of the foot and hyperpigmented macule on the toe of a neonate.

persist for as long as 3 months. Neither type of lesion requires therapy, and although the cause is unknown, parents may be reassured that the disorder is benign and transient.

MILIARIA

Miliaria is an eruption resulting from eccrine sweat duct obstruction leading to sweat retention.[45] The three types of lesions are superficial thin-walled vesicles without inflammation (i.e., miliaria crystallina); small, erythematous grouped papules (i.e., miliaria rubra); and nonerythematous pustules (i.e., miliaria pustulosis or profunda).

The eruption most frequently develops in the intertriginous areas and over the face and scalp. It is exacerbated by exposure to a warm and humid environment. Miliaria sometimes can be confused with erythema toxicum; rapid resolution of the lesions when the infant is placed in a cooler environment differentiates them from pyoderma. A Wright-stained smear of vesicular lesions demonstrates only sparse squamous cells or lymphocytes, permitting exclusion of infectious vesicular eruptions. No topical therapy is indicated.

NEONATAL ACNE AND INFANTILE ACNE

Neonatal acne (i.e., neonatal cephalic pustulosis) is a relatively common condition that affects both sexes. It consists of small red papules and pustules on the face during the first weeks of life (Fig. 52-6). Comedones and cysts are usually absent. The lesions are asymptomatic and resolve spontaneously over several weeks. It has been suggested that occurrence of these lesions is coincident with colonization by the yeast *Pityrosporon ovale.*

In contrast, infantile acne is an uncommon but distressing facial eruption (usually in male infants) that has its onset somewhat later, during the first few months of life.[19,45] This condition resembles acne in the adolescent patient and is characterized by comedones, papules, pustules, and, rarely, nodules. The duration may vary, but the disorder usually clears spontaneously during the latter portion of the first year

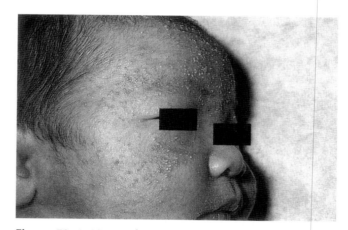

Figure 52–6. Neonatal acne (cephalic pustulosis). Commonly seen on the cheeks and scalp during the first 2 to 4 weeks after birth; usually manifested by small red papules and pustules without comedones. *(From Lucky AW: Transient benign cutaneous lesions in the newborn. In Eichenfield LF et al, editors: Neonatal dermatology, Philadelphia, 2008, Saunders.)*

of life. This condition probably represents a heightened response of the sebaceous glands to neonatal androgens.[19] No treatment or treatment with mild topical acne preparations to produce drying and peeling should suffice. Occasionally, the infant may be left with pitted scarring, and some may experience severe acne as adolescents.

INFANTILE ACROPUSTULOSIS

Infantile acropustulosis consists of pruritic papules and vesiculopustules with onset from birth to 10 months of age. The lesions appear in crops every 2 to 3 weeks and last 7 to 10 days. They involve the hands and feet primarily but occasionally may affect the limbs as well. Because of the distribution, it is often confused with scabies. It is more common in African-American and in male infants. The condition resolves spontaneously. A subcorneal pustule filled with neutrophils is seen on skin biopsy. Therapy consists of topical steroids and antihistamines.

Disorders of Cornification: The Scaly Baby

The most common causes of excessive scaling in the neonate are physiologic desquamation and dysmaturity, neither of which is of long-term significance. Less common causes include the congenital ichthyoses and the ectodermal dysplasias (particularly hypohidrotic ectodermal dysplasia), all of which are chronic, heritable disorders.[32] Disorders of cornification that may manifest during the first weeks of life are given in Table 52-3.

PHYSIOLOGIC DESQUAMATION AND DYSMATURITY

The gestational age of a newborn with accentuated physiologic desquamation usually is 40 to 42 weeks (see Chapter 27); peak shedding occurs near the eighth day of life. These infants are otherwise normal in physical appearance and behavior. In contrast, the dysmature infant (see Chapter 14) has distinctive characteristics. The body is lean, with thin extremities and decreased subcutaneous fat. The ponderal index is low and indicates diminished body weight in relation to length. The skin is often scaly with parchment-like desquamation, especially of the distal extremities. There is often meconium staining of the skin as well as the nails and umbilical cord. The hair is abundant, and the nails are abnormally long. In the normal infant with accentuated physiologic scaling and the dysmature infant, desquamation is a transient phenomenon, and the integument continues to serve its intended protective function. In contrast, the infant with congenital ichthyosis may have serious difficulties early in life because of impaired barrier function and subsequent risks of secondary infection.

ICHTHYOSES

The term *ichthyosis* derives from the similarity of the skin condition to the scales of a fish. It refers to a complex and often confusing plethora of conditions characterized by disorders of cornification with or without systemic symptoms. Ichthyosis in the newborn period may manifest as scaling only, scaling and erythroderma, a collodion membrane, or the thickened plates of harlequin ichthyosis. Two descriptive terms have been used for ichthyotic conditions that occur only in the newborn: *harlequin ichthyosis* and *collodion baby*. Attempts to classify this complex set of disorders based on phenotypic and genotypic criteria recognize three main groups: (1) bullous ichthyosis and related disorders due to keratin mutations, (2) nonbullous ichthyosiform erythroderma and lamellar ichthyosis mainly due to transglutaminase 1 mutations, and (3) syndromic ichthyosis, namely, systemic (multiorgan) diseases with many different causes.[55] Selected conditions with particular relevance to the newborn are highlighted below, followed by a general overview of treatment strategies.

Harlequin Ichthyosis

Harlequin ichthyosis (i.e., harlequin fetus) is a rare, very severe disorder of keratinization inherited as an autosomal recessive trait in most families, although a dominant form may exist, and sporadic cases occur frequently. This clinical phenotype represents a heterogeneous group of disorders characterized by perturbations of epidermal intercellular lipid, altered lamellar granules, and variation in expression or processing of structural proteins involved in normal epidermal keratinization. Although the histologic, ultrastructural, and biochemical findings of the various subtypes differ, their clinical features are indistinguishable. The skin of affected infants is markedly thickened, hard (armor-like), and hyperkeratotic, with deep crevices running transversely and vertically. The fissures are most prominent over areas of flexion. Rigidity of the skin around the eyes results in marked ectropion, although the globe is usually normal. The ears and nose are underdeveloped, flattened, and distorted, and the lips are everted and gaping, producing a "fish-mouth" deformity. The nails and hair may be hypoplastic or absent. Extreme inelasticity of the skin is associated with flexion deformity of all joints. The hands and feet are ischemic, hard, and waxy in appearance, with poorly developed distal digits.

Most harlequin fetuses are born prematurely, usually between 32 and 36 weeks' gestation, adding to their morbidity and mortality. Complications include sepsis, distal gangrene, and difficulties with feeding and respiration. Most infants die in the neonatal period; however, therapeutic trials of oral retinoids combined with intensive nursing care have resulted in survival of several of these infants. All surviving infants have had chronic, severe ichthyosis.

Collodion Baby

The collodion baby is less severely affected than the infant with harlequin ichthyosis and may represent a phenotypic expression of several genotypes. This condition eventuates in lamellar ichthyosis or congenital ichthyosiform erythroderma in approximately 60% of patients. Sjögren-Larsson syndrome, Conradi-Hünermann syndrome, trichothiodystrophy, dominant lamellar ichthyosis, and neonatal Gaucher disease account for the remainder of the infants born with a collodion membrane. Rarely, shedding of the collodion membrane results in a normal underlying integument (i.e., lamellar exfoliation of the newborn). Collodion babies often are born prematurely. The infant is covered with a cellophane-like membrane, which by its tautness may distort the facial features and the digits (Fig. 52-7). Less commonly, only part of the integument is involved. The membrane is shiny and brownish-yellow, resembling an envelope of collodion or oiled parchment, and may be perforated by hair. The presence of ectropion, eclabium, and crumpled ears causes these infants to resemble one another for the first few days of life. Fissuring and peeling begin shortly after birth, and large sheets may desquamate, revealing erythema of variable intensity. After the membrane has fissured, no respiratory difficulties are encountered. Complete shedding of the collodion membrane may take several weeks. Pedigree information and histopathologic examination of a skin biopsy are additional aids in the delineation of the specific type of ichthyosis.

Despite the apparent thickened skin, these infants have an abnormal epidermal barrier, which may lead to complications such as dehydration, electrolyte imbalance, temperature instability, and cutaneous and systemic infection. Pneumonia from aspiration of squamous cells found in the amniotic fluid is another potential complication.

TABLE 52–3 Disorders of Cornification That Usually Manifest during the First Weeks

Disorder (Inheritance)	Clinical Features	Mutation	Protein/function
CHILD syndrome (XD)	Unilateral ichthyosiform erythroderma, chondrodysplasia punctata, cataracts, limb reduction defects, aymmetric organ hypoplasia	3β-Hydroxysteroid delta isomerase	Enzyme involved in cholesterol synthesis
CHIME syndrome (Zunich-Kaye syndrome) (AR)	Ichthyotic erythematous plaques, cardiac defects; typical facies, retinal colobomas, mental retardation, hearing loss, anomalous dentition	Unknown	Unknown
Congenital ichthyosiform erythroderma (AR)	Fine white scales, background erythema	Ichthynin, member of DUF803 protein family	Uncertain, likely membrane receptor
Conradi-Hünermann: X-linked chondrodysplasia punctata (XD)	Striated ichthyosiform hyperkeratosis, alopecia, cataracts, frontal bossing, short proximal limbs, stippled calcifications of the epiphyseal regions	Emopamil binding protein	Enzyme involved in cholesterol synthesis
Epidermolytic hyperkeratosis (AD)	Scaling and blistering	Keratins 1, 10	Cytoskeleton structural protein
Familial peeling skin (AR)	Superficial acral skin peeling	Keratinocye transglutaminase 5	Stratum corneum cross-linking enzyme
Gaucher disease (AR)	Collodion membrane with later mild scaling, hepatoslenomegaly, neurologic abnormalities	β-Glucocerebrosidase	Enzyme
Harlequin ichthyosis (AR)	Thick armored scale with fissuring, ectropion, eclabion	ATP-binding cassette	ABC transporter
Ichthyosis follicularis (usually X-linked recessive)	Follicular hyperkeratosis, nail dystrophy, alopecia, photophobia, short stature, psychomotor delay	Unknown	Unknown
Ichthyosis hystrix (AD)	Plaques of hyperkeratosis Superficial peeling	Keratin 1	Cytoskeleton structural protein
KID syndrome (may be AD, AR)	Verrucous plaques, stippled pattern of keratoderma, vascularizing keratitis, deafness	Connexin 26	Gap junction protein
Lamellar ichthyosis (usually AR)	Collodion membrane with large adherent plates	Transglutaminase 1 or ATP-binding cassette	Stratum corneum cross-linking enzyme or ABC transporter
Netherton syndrome (AR)	Erythroderma in infancy, scant hair (bamboo hair), often failure to thrive, atopic diathesis, food allergies	SPINK5	Serine protease inhibitor
Neutral lipid storage disease (AR)	Collodion membrane or ichthyosiform erythroderma, liver abnormalities, mental retardation, muscle atrophy	CGI-58	Enzyme in esterase/lipase family
Recessive X-linked ichthyosis	Collodion membrane, large dark scales, corneal opacities, cryptorchidism	Steroid sulfatase	Metabolic enzyme
Sjögren-Larsson (AR)	Fine lamellar scale, spastic diplegia, seizures, retinal "glistening white dots"	Fatty aldehyde dehydrogenase gene	Metabolic enzyme
Trichothiodystrophy (AR)	Collodion membrane, broken hair, photosensitivity, short stature, decreased fertility, susceptibility to infection	Xeropigmentosum protein	DNA repair enzymes, regulation of transcription

ABC, ATP-binding cassette; AD, autosomal dominant; AR, autosomal recessive; CHILD, congenital hemidysplasia, ichthyosiform erythroderma, limb defects; KID, keratitis, ichyosis, deafness; XD, X-linked dominant.

Adapted from Irvine AD, Paller AS: Disorders of cornification (ichthyosis). In Eichenfield LF et al, editors: *Textbook of neonatal dermatology*, Philadelphia, 2008, Saunders, p.285.

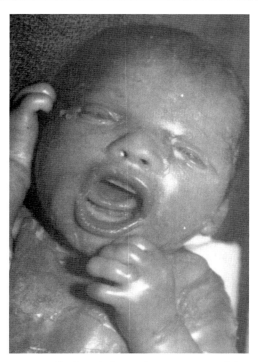

Figure 52–7. Collodion baby with ectropion, eclabium, and deformed digits.

X-Linked Ichthyosis

X-linked ichthyosis is the most common form of ichthyosis in the newborn period affecting approximately 1/2500 males.[55] In contrast, ichthyosis vulgaris occurs with a frequency of 1/300 but appears first in early childhood and will not be discussed. Steroid sulfatase (arylsulfatase) deficiency is the cause of the clinical manifestations of X-linked ichthyosis, which may include alterations in the skin, eye, and testes of affected infants. Most patients have cutaneous findings at birth, and 80% to 90% show scaling by 3 months of age. Rarely, a collodion membrane may be present. The hyperkeratosis is variable, but the scales typically are large, thick, and dark and are prominent over the scalp, neck, anterior trunk, and extensor extremities. Sparing of palms and soles and partial sparing of the flexures are helpful diagnostic features. Systemic manifestations are generally absent, and complications are rare. Skin biopsy is helpful (although the histologic pattern resembles that of lamellar ichthyosis), showing hyperkeratosis, a well-developed granular layer, hypertrophic epidermis, and a perivascular lymphocytic infiltrate. This form of ichthyosis is clinically apparent in affected homozygous males and not in heterozygous females. Because of the steroid sulfatase enzyme deficiency in the somatic tissues of affected males, increased levels of cholesterol sulfate can be documented by serum lipoprotein electrophoresis, and assays of steroid sulfatase activity show depressed levels of enzyme in cultured leukocytes, fibroblasts, amniocytes, and scales, confirming the diagnosis. Cryptorchidism is seen in approximately 25% of affected males; these patients may be at increased risk for testicular cancer. Deep stromal corneal opacities have also been found in about 50% of male

infants with the disorder and in a smaller percentage of female carriers, but they do not affect vision. Female carriers of the gene for X-linked ichthyosis, when pregnant with an affected male fetus, have a deficiency of placental steroid sulfatase reflected by low maternal urinary estriol excretion and a difficult or prolonged labor that often requires intervention.

Babies affected with the rare condition of multiple sulfatase deficiency may have similar cutaneous findings but also have systemic features of a storage disease (i.e., metachromatic leukodystrophy), because they have a deficiency of several other sulfatases. Approximately 10% of patients have a contiguous gene deletion syndrome; this condition results from a larger deletion of the terminal short arm of the X chromosome. Deletion of the genes that are contiguous with the steroid sulfatase gene may result in mental retardation, Kallmann syndrome, and a bone dysplasia (i.e., X-linked recessive chondrodysplasia punctata).

Management of Ichthyosis

Management of ichthyotic patients in the newborn period runs the gamut from amelioration of mild cosmetic problems with excessive dryness and scaling to treatment of potentially life-threatening illness due to deficits in the epidermal barrier and subsequent infection. Table 52-4 lists the primary signs, symptoms, and pathogenetic mechanisms that form the primary targets of therapy for ichthyosis. Severely affected infants require aggressive topical care, liberal use of bland emollients, and careful monitoring of electrolyte needs. The infant should be placed in an environment with increased humidity, and prompt attention should be paid to signs of infection. Often the long-term goal of ichthyotic therapy is to eliminate scaling due to excessive cornification and to reduce dryness (xerosis) of the skin without inducing irritation. Keratolytic agents should be used with caution in the neonatal period and during the first 6 months of life, however. Although the stratum corneum is often thick and scaly, the barrier is compromised, and the risks of systemic absorption of potentially toxic substances, such as lactic acid and salicylic acid, are significant (see Table 52-8). Liberal use of

TABLE 52–4   Primary Targets for Ichthyosis Therapy

Signs and Symptoms	Pathogenetic Mechanisms
Dryness	Abnormal quality or quantity of scales
Scaling	Abnormal thickness of stratum corneum
Fissures and erosions	Skin inflammation
Keratoderma	Barrier failure
Erythema	Secondary infections
Pruritus	Obstruction of adnexal ducts
Anhidrosis	Stiffness of the skin
Ectropion	

Adapted from Vahlquist A et al: Congenital ichthyosis: an overview of current and emerging therapies. *Acta Derm Venereol* 88:4, 2008.

bland emollients generally suffice for lubrication during the neonatal period.

Future Prospects

At present there is no definitive cure for ichthyosis, and current therapies are generally palliative. Over the past decade, however, the molecular bases of many of these predominately monogenetic disorders have been elucidated (see Table 52-3). Identification of the affected genes opens the door for prenatal diagnosis and genetic counseling for these potentially lethal conditions. Unusual associations between skin and brain have been described, including a link between steroid sulfatase deficiency in X-linked ichthyosis and attention-deficit/hyperactivity disorder. Rapid progress in this field is anticipated, including the possibility of cutaneous gene therapy.[55] Parents are referred to an extensive online support group for families of infants with cornification disorders, the Foundation for Ichthyosis and Related Skin Types, FIRST (www.scalyskin.org).

Vesicobullous Eruptions

Blistering eruptions in the neonatal period may be caused by infections, congenital diseases, or infiltrative processes or may be of unknown origin.[25] The proper management of infants with such eruptions depends on knowledge of the cause of the disease or, when this is not possible, on an understanding of the pathogenesis of the type of blister encountered. Establishing the pathogenesis often depends on determining at which level within the skin the blister has occurred.

Blister sites may be intraepidermal or subepidermal. In the epidermis, the blister can be very high (subcorneal), midepidermal, or basal. The midepidermal blister may be formed by primary separation of intercellular contacts (e.g., acantholysis), by secondary edematous disruption of intercellular contacts (e.g., spongiosis), or by intracellular injury as seen in patients with viral infections. The diagnosis of a blistering disease usually requires a family history, an immediate past history of the infant and mother, laboratory studies to exclude infectious agents, evaluation of the infant's general state of health, consideration of the morphologic characteristics of the eruption, and often a biopsy of the affected skin. The biopsy should be obtained from a fresh, typical, small lesion and should include some surrounding skin.

BACTERIAL AND YEAST INFECTIONS

Colonization of the newborn's skin begins at birth. The organisms acquired at birth are similar to those found on adult skin.[8] *Staphylococcus epidermidis* (coagulase negative) predominates, but diphtheroids, streptococci, and coliform bacteria also are found. The newborn skin affords an excellent culture medium for *Staphylococcus aureus;* the groin and other skin sites may become colonized before the umbilicus. *Candida albicans* usually is not found on normal skin but may be present in the oral mucosa or in the diaper area as a result of fecal contamination (see Chapter 39).

SEPSIS

Bacterial sepsis in the neonate can manifest with vesicles, pustules, or bullae. The most common cause of sepsis manifesting with pustules is *S. aureus*. Group B *Streptococcus*

agalactiae is a leading cause of neonatal sepsis, pneumonia, and meningitis, but it rarely manifests in the neonate at birth with vesicles, pustules, or bullae.[31] In an attempt to decrease the frequency of Group B *Streptococcus agalactiae* infection, maternal prophylaxis is recommended before delivery under certain conditions. Other occasional causes of pustules and sepsis in neonates include *Listeria monocytogenes, Haemophilus influenzae, Pseudomonas aeruginosa,* and *Klebsiella pneumoniae.*

STAPHYLOCOCCAL INFECTION AND IMPETIGO

Superficial skin infections due to *S. aureus* range from localized bullous impetigo to generalized cutaneous involvement with systemic illness. In contrast to congenital blistering diseases, which are often present at birth, skin infections with *S. aureus* usually develop after the first few days of life.[26,52] They may be bullous, crusted, or pustular. Typical lesions are small vesicles or pustules or large, fragile bullae filled with clear, turbid, or purulent fluid. They rupture easily, leaving red, moist, denuded areas, often with a superficial varnish-like crust. Although they may develop anywhere on the body, the blisters and pustules commonly occur in the diaper area and on axillae and periumbilical skin. When the epidermis is shed in large sheets, staphylococcal scalded skin syndrome should be suspected. The diagnosis is made by Gram stain and culture of the blister fluid, which can distinguish this eruption from streptococcal impetigo and other bullous disorders of the neonatal period. Blood cultures should be obtained from affected infants before initiating systemic antibiotic therapy, even if the infants are usually otherwise well. Contacts and nursery personnel should be investigated for a source of the infectious organism. The infant should be placed in isolation and observed carefully for early signs of sepsis. A high index of suspicion during examination of other infants in the nursery is the most effective means of preventing epidemic spread of this infection (see Chapter 39).

Compresses of physiologic saline solution and systemic antibiotics to cover the principal etiologic possibilities are indicated until culture results are available. Fluid and electrolyte replacement therapy may be required if the disease is extensive. Recovery is usually complete in several days, and there is no residual scarring.

STAPHYLOCOCCAL SCALDED SKIN SYNDROME

The staphylococcal scalded skin syndrome is a severe bullous eruption heralded by a bright erythema that resembles a scald. The erythema begins on the face and gradually spreads downward to involve the remainder of the skin, with accentuation in the flexural areas. The level of cleavage is superficial, occurring in the granular layer of the epidermis; the bullae, therefore, are flaccid and easily ruptured and rapidly progress into areas of denudation. The infant is febrile, irritable, and has marked cutaneous tenderness. The face, neck, and flexural areas are the first to be eroded (Fig. 52-8A). The entire upper epidermis may be shed from the limb like a glove (see Fig. 52-8B). Crusting around the mouth and eyes results in a typical facies. Conjunctivitis is common, as is hyperemia of the mucous membranes, but oral ulcerations do not occur. Infants with a milder form of the disease display a scarlatiniform eruption, with perioral and flexural desquamation but without bullae or denudation. Like staphylococcal bullae are sterile, cultures should be obtained from the nasopharynx, conjunctival sac, umbilicus, abnormal skin, blood, urine, and any other suspected focus of infection that might have provided a portal of entry for the organism.

Treatment consists of prompt systemic administration of penicillinase-resistant semisynthetic penicillin and fluid and electrolyte replacement if necessary. Flaky desquamation occurs during the healing phase. Scarring never occurs because the blister cleavage plane is intraepidermal.

STREPTOCOCCAL INFECTION

Infection with group B β-hemolytic streptococci rarely produces skin lesions, but vesicles, bullae, and erosions have been reported. Epidemics of group A streptococcal infection may occur primarily as omphalitis or, rarely, as isolated pustules. Infants with these infections should be treated aggressively with parenteral antibiotics because sepsis, cellulitis, meningitis, and pneumonia have been documented.

MISCELLANEOUS BACTERIAL INFECTIONS

Listeria, Haemophilus, and congenital syphilis may also be the cause of cutaneous vesicles or pustules in the newborn. *P. aeruginosa* may cause large hemorrhagic bullae in the neonatal period. This is usually a nosocomial infection seen primarily in infants with low birthweights. The skin lesions result from septicemia and hematogenous spread to the skin. In older children, the pustules and bullae are in the perineal region, but in the newborn, they may occur anywhere. The lesions rapidly ulcerate, leaving "punched-out" erosions. Diagnosis can be made by performing a Gram stain or culture of the bullae or the base of the ulcer. Parenteral antibiotics should be administered immediately; the prognosis is usually poor.

VIRAL LESIONS

One of the most important causes of blistering in the neonatal period is herpes simplex infection.[25] Frequently, an inconspicuous cutaneous lesion heralds severe systemic infection. The infection may be acquired in utero or perinatally. Intrauterine herpes simplex infection typically manifests with vesicles at birth or within 24 hours. The vesicular eruption may be widespread or even bullous, resembling epidermolysis bullosa. Rarely, congenital scars may be present. Additional findings include low birthweight, microcephaly, chorioretinitis, and neurologic changes. Neonatal herpes simplex may be limited to the skin, eyes, and mouth or may be disseminated with multiple organ involvement. The cutaneous lesions usually develop at 6 to 13 days of life, concurrent with or after nonspecific systemic signs and symptoms. Typically, the lesions are 1- to 3-mm vesicles usually occurring on the scalp or face. Vesicles may be present on the torso or buttocks, especially in a breech delivery. Rarely, pustules, erosions, or oral ulcerations may be the only cutaneous findings. In infants with cutaneous lesions suggestive of herpes simplex infection, antiviral therapy should be administered immediately, and the diagnosis can be confirmed by scraping the base of a fresh vesicle and staining with Giemsa or Wright stain (i.e., Tzanck test), immunofluorescence, or viral culture. Current recommendations for prevention of herpes simplex infections include caesarean section for women

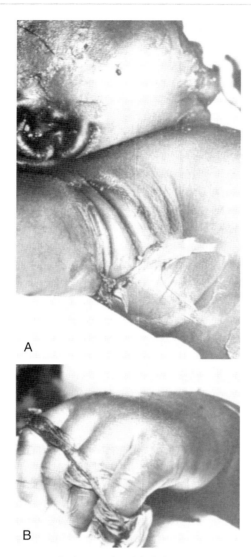

Figure 52–8. Staphylococcal scalded skin syndrome. **A,** Extensive denudation in the axilla. **B,** Glovelike shedding of the superficial portion of the epidermis.

pyoderma, staphylococcal scalded skin syndrome is rarely seen at birth, with most neonatal cases presenting between 3 and 7 days of life.

The infecting organism in scalded skin syndrome is *S. aureus,* usually a group 2 phage type, although other phage types occasionally have been incriminated. These organisms produce an exotoxin (i.e., exfoliatin) that has proteolytic activity on desmoglein-1, a molecule found within the desmosomes of keratinocytes, that is responsible for the cutaneous manifestations.[34,52] Two major serotypes of the toxin, A and B, cause bullous impetigo and scalded skin syndrome. In cases of the former, the toxin produces exfoliation and blisters locally, whereas in the latter, the toxin circulates systemically with widespread epidermal necrolysis. Histologic examination of the skin demonstrates separation at the level of the granular layer with cell death and acantholysis; there is a striking absence of inflammatory infiltrate. Because intact with active lesions or prodromal symptoms consistent with herpes. Vaccines against herpes simplex virus 2 have been of low efficacy. High-dose, prolonged acyclovir therapy remains the treatment of choice for neonatal herpes simplex infections.

Primary varicella may occur in the newborn if the mother has a primary varicella infection in the last 3 weeks of the pregnancy. The onset of this diffuse vesicular disease is 5 to 10 days of age, and the lesions may be numerous and monomorphic, given the infant's impaired ability to mount an immune response. Varicella zoster has also been reported in the neonatal period in infants of mothers who have had primary varicella during pregnancy. These vesicles are unilateral and occur in a dermatomal distribution. The vesicles of varicella, herpes zoster, and herpes simplex have a similar histologic pattern (see Chapter 39, Part 4), with cleavage in the midepidermis. Acantholysis and marked destruction of individual cells result in the ballooning type of degeneration characteristic of viral vesicles.

Table 52-5 lists common viral infections of the neonate that may appear with cutaneous manifestations. Diagnostic workup and characteristic histology and laboratory findings are given.

CANDIDIASIS

(See also Chapter 39, Part 3)

Candida species are commensal organisms commonly found in the gastrointestinal and female genital tracts. Roughly one third of health care workers in neonatal intensive care units test positive for *Candida* on routine surveillance cultures, and up to 40% of women are culture positive for *Candida* at the time of delivery. Candidiasis in the first 4 weeks of life is usually benign and is localized most often to the oral cavity (thrush) or the diaper area. If maternal vaginal organisms are acquired during the birth process, the infant may manifest symptomatic mouth lesions or become an intestinal carrier. Fecal contamination is the usual source of the organism in candidal dermatitis. Paronychial lesions also may occur, particularly in thumb-sucking infants. The lesions of thrush are detectable as creamy white patches of friable material on the buccal mucosa, gums, palate, and tongue. Early cutaneous lesions consist of erythematous papules and vesicopustules that become confluent, forming a moist, erosive, scaly dermatitis surrounded by satellite pustules. Candidiasis in the preterm infant may manifest as a different erythema.

Rarely, cutaneous candidiasis may be congenital as a result of ascending infection from a vaginal or cervical focus. Risk factors for this type of candidiasis include a foreign body in the uterus or cervix, premature birth, and a history of vaginal candidiasis. Affected infants usually have a widespread eruption with pustules on the palms and soles and, occasionally, nail dystrophy (Fig. 52-9). Distinctive yellow-white papules on the umbilical cord and placenta represent *Candida* granulomas. *C. albicans* may be demonstrable on histologic examination of these tissues and may be cultured from the amniotic fluid.

Although candidal infection is usually localized to skin, infants who weigh less than 1500 g are also at risk for systemic infections. In addition to birthweight less than 1500 g, risk factors for disseminated candidiasis include central line placement, respiratory therapy, antibiotic use, and parenteral nutrition. Marked differences in the rate of systemic candidiasis among centers has been described. Use of cefotaxime appears to increase the incidence.[2a]

In the chronic mucocutaneous or granulomatous forms of candidiasis (rare in the neonatal period), the scalp, lips, hands, and nails may be sites of chronically scaling, heaped-up lesions. These two forms of infection often are associated with a defect in the immune response, multiple endocrinopathies, or both.

The diagnosis is aided by identification of budding yeast spores on Gram stain or of spores and pseudohyphae on a potassium hydroxide preparation. Growth of the organism is rapid on Sabouraud dextrose or Mycosel agar.

Treatment depends on the extent of involvement. Topical antifungal agents from the imidazole group are the most effective for disease limited to the skin. Systemic administration of amphotericin B, 5-fluorocytosine, or an imidazole should be reserved for patients with evidence of disseminated disease. Fluconazole or itraconazole for disseminated candidiasis in the neonate with low birthweight may provide an alternative to systemic amphotericin B and 5-fluorocytosine.

HEREDITARY BLISTERING DISEASES

Epidermolysis Bullosa

Epidermolysis bullosa (EB) refers to a group of heterogeneous diseases that are characterized by simplex (intraepidermal), junctional (lucidolytic), or dystrophic (subepidermal) subtypes with blisters produced by minor degrees of trauma and heat.[5] These disorders are the result of a variety of inherited defects of the proteins that maintain skin integrity. The clinical phenotypes vary according to the region within the skin that the defective protein is expressed and at what depth the resultant blister occurs. Traditionally, EB has been classified by clinical phenotype, histologic and ultrastructural features (i.e., depth of blister), and inheritance pattern. Advances have made molecular analysis of the defect available as well.[15] At present, 10 distinct genes are linked etiologically to EB subtypes. First trimester prenatal diagnosis is available, and preimplantation genetic testing is possible in select centers.[15]

The clinical features may be quite variable in the newborn period, making it difficult to identify the specific subtype of EB and the expected prognosis. The subtypes of EB that may manifest in the neonatal period are listed in Table 52-6. Some subtypes of EB are severe, life-threatening diseases, and others are mild and do not manifest until adolescence. Friction-induced blistering of the skin is the classic feature of EB. If there is friction in utero, the baby may be born with large areas of denuded skin. In the past, this was referred to as Bart syndrome, but further delineation of the molecular defects has shown that several subtypes of EB can result in this clinical picture (see Table 52-6). More frequently, the birth process or minor perinatal trauma causes blistering of the skin. The more severe, dystrophic, recessive form of EB is associated with low birthweight.

Junctional EB of the Herlitz type deserves special mention because it is almost always present at birth and is a very severe form of EB. The epidermis loosens after minimal trauma, and bullae of various sizes are formed anywhere on

TABLE 52–5 Diagnosis of Selected Neonatal Viral Infection with Cutaneous Manifestations

Virus	Culture	Histology of Skin Lesion	PCR	Serology
CMV	Widely available; reliable, culture urine, saliva; shell vial technique yields results in 48-72 hours	Skin lesions are due to extramedullary hematopoiesis, not due to viral replication in skin	Highly sensitive; well studied in plasma as a marker of disseminated CMV infection in immune compromised hosts	Rising antibody titer to CMV IgG is a sensitive and specific test; CMV IgM is not a sensitive test in the newborn
Enterovirus	Available in reference laboratories; culture vesicular lesions, pharynx (during the acute phase of illness), and stool (up to 6 weeks following the illness)	Nonspecific	Highly sensitive; not widely available	Not usually helpful, as no class specific antibody response can be measured and type-specific serologies are not widely available
HIV	Available; not highly sensitive in newborn, repeat culture at 1 month of age	Nonspecific	Sensitive means of diagnosis, can be repeated at 1-2 months, 4-6 months, and at 18 months of age	Nonspecific passive maternal antibody present at birth persists
HSV	Widely available; reliable; culture skin lesions	Tzanck stain of epithelial cells from the bottom of a vesicle: specific for herpesviruses HSV and VZV; direct fluorescent antibody stains for HSV 1 or 2	Highly sensitive; best studied on CSF (sensitivity of skin lesions not well studied)	Rising antibody titer to HSV IgG is a sensitive and specific test; HSV IgM is not a sensitive test in the newborn
Rubella	Not usually available; culture pharynx	Skin lesions are due to extramedullary hematopoiesis, not due to viral replication in skin	Not well studied	Rising antibody titer to rubella IgG is a sensitive and specific test; rubella IgM is not a sensitive test in the newborn. Compare mother's prenatal serology test results with those at the time of birth
VZV	Available in many reference laboratories; culture skin lesions	Tzanck stain (see above): specific Stains available for VZV	Highly sensitive, but not well studied on skin lesions; not widely available	Rising antibody titer to VZV IgG is a sensitive and specific test; VZV IgM is not a sensitive test in the newborn

CMV, cytomegalovirus; CSF, cerebrospinal fluid; HIV, human immunodeficiency virus; HSV, herpes simplex virus; IgG, IgM, immunoglobulin G, M; PCR, polymerase chain reaction; prn, as required; VZV, varicella-zoster virus.
Adapted from SF Friedlander, JS Bradley: Viral Infections. In Eichenfield LF et al, editors: *Textbook of neonatal dermatology*, Philadelphia, 2008, Saunders, p 193.

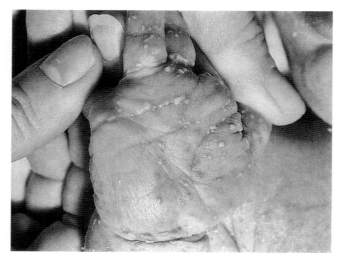

Figure 52–9. Congenital candidiasis with typical circumscribed lesions on the palm.

the body (Fig. 52-10). The nails are frequently involved. Oral and anal lesions also occur. Many lesions heal spontaneously, but large bullae may fail to heal and result in moist, chronic vegetative lesions consisting of exuberant granulation tissue. There may be significant loss of electrolytes and protein through these erosions.

Blisters and erosions may also be severe and widespread in the Dowling-Meara subtype of EB simplex. This subtype may be distinguished clinically by the characteristic grouping of the blisters and the formation of milia. In all forms of EB, blisters may be elicited readily by gentle rubbing (Nikolsky sign). Mild trauma can result in a blister within a few minutes to hours, and the resulting fresh lesions may be used for histopathologic examination. Treatment is aimed at protecting the skin from trauma and secondary infection.

Scarring or dystrophic EB has recessive and dominant forms. In contrast to the simplex and junctional groups (except the Dowling-Meara type), milia may mark the site of healed blisters. In the severe form of recessive dystrophic EB, hemorrhagic erosions and blisters may be present at birth, especially on the feet. The toe and finger lesions may heal with fusion of digits and loss of nails, resulting in a characteristic mitten-like envelope of the hands. As the fingers fuse (this usually takes several years), the hands and arms become fixed in a flexed position, and contractures develop. Repeated episodes of blistering, infection, and scar formation lead to severe deformities, loss of hair, mucosal scarring, dysphagia, anemia, and retarded physical and sexual development. Visceral amyloidosis, hyperglobulinemic purpura, clotting abnormalities, and squamous cell carcinoma are associated with this severe, life-limiting disease.

The dominant forms of scarring EB usually are less severe than the major recessive type. Lesions may be generalized or localized at birth, or they may appear later and may be limited to the elbows, knees, hands, feet, and sacrum (see Fig. 52-10B). Oral involvement is common but is usually not severe. Nails may be lost, but deforming scars and contractures occur infrequently. Red plaques rather than blisters may result from injury. The lesions heal with soft, wrinkled scars. Pigmentary change and milia may be formed at old blister sites. The general health is usually unimpaired.

The initial diagnosis of EB is a clinical one, and other disorders that cause blistering, particularly infections, should be excluded. Clinical differentiation of EB subtypes is difficult or impossible; for this reason, all infants with the diagnosis should undergo skin biopsy to obtain a more precise diagnosis. Light microscopy may be helpful in determining the level of cleavage, but results can often be difficult to interpret. Immunofluorescence mapping of biopsied EB skin specimens is the currently recommended primary laboratory method of diagnosing EB subtypes.[15] If available, electron microscopy, immunofluorescence mapping, and DNA mutational analysis are used simultaneously to confirm the diagnosis.

Unfortunately, there is no effective cure for infants with EB. Treatment is aimed at protecting the skin from trauma and secondary infection. Management strategies for treating neonatal EB are given in Box 52-3. Recent progress using gene-based and cell-based molecular therapies holds hope for future approaches that may cure or ameliorate specific EB subtypes.[54]

Incontinentia Pigmenti

Incontinentia pigmenti (IP) is a rare, X-linked, dominant genodermatosis that affects the skin, skeletal system, eyes, and central nervous system (CNS).[11] IP results from mutations in the *NEMO* gene that inhibit expression of NF-kappa B essential modulator. Molecular analysis of the *NEMO* gene is now possible, as is analysis of skewed X-chromosome inactivation, although the diagnosis of IP is typically based on characteristic clinical findings.[11] Almost all patients are female, but affected male patients have been reported and are thought to represent genetic mosaicism or Klinefelter syndrome.

The cutaneous lesions usually are present at birth and have three morphologic stages. Initially, there are inflammatory, clear-to-yellow vesicles, which are arranged linearly and appear in crops during the first few weeks of life. The vesicular lesions occur on the trunk and limbs and vary in density from few to many. They sometimes appear distinctly pustular or crusted. Gray-to-brown, warty excrescences develop next, usually on the distal limbs. The third stage consists of patterned, macular hyperpigmentation in streaks and whorls on the trunk and extremities. Occasionally, pigmentation may accompany some of the early lesions. A fourth stage consisting of atrophic, hypopigmented streaks has been described in some individuals. Nail hypoplasia, areas of alopecia, and ocular and skeletal abnormalities also may be detected. There is often peripheral eosinophilia during the vesicular phase of the disease. The diagnosis should be considered when inflammatory vesicles arranged in lines are seen in a newborn female infant. Delayed dentition, partial anodontia, and abnormalities of the CNS can occur but may not be apparent during the neonatal period. Biopsy of a small blister demonstrates a subcorneal vesicle filled with eosinophils. The differential diagnosis includes herpes simplex infection and other blistering diseases. The clinical evolution of the cutaneous process, the demonstration of a large number of eosinophils in the skin lesions and peripheral blood, and the presence of pigment-laden macrophages in the upper dermis of end-stage lesions establish the diagnosis. No specific therapy is required for the skin lesions; if inflammation becomes excessive during the vesicular phase, treatment with compresses and topical

TABLE 52–6   **Clinical Presentation and Diagnosis of Selected Epidermolysis Bullosa Subtypes in the Neonatal Period**

EB Subtype (Usual Inheritance)	CLINICAL FEATURES		Protein System	Prognosis
	Cutaneous	Extracutaneous		
Dystrophic EB, dominant (AD)	Mild to moderate blistering (may be more severe in newborn period), milia, scarring, CLAS, nail dystrophy	Mild mucosal blistering	Type VII collagen	Good, improvement with age
Dystrophic EB, recessive (Hallopeau-Siemens) (AR)	Severe blistering, milia, scarring, CLAS	Severe mucosal blistering GI involvement common Urological involvement	Type VII collagen	Disability, reduced life expectancy
EB simplex, Dowling-Meara (AD)	Moderate to severe blistering, starts generalized, then grouped (herpetiform), milia, nail dystrophy, shedding, CLAS	Mild mucosal blistering	Keratin 5 or 14	Good, improvement with age
EB simplex, Koebner (AD)	Mild to moderate blistering, often generalized, rare scarring, milia, CLAS	Occasional mucosal blistering	Keratin 5 or 14	Good, some patients improve after puberty
EB simplex, Weber-Cockayne (AD)	Mild blistering, often localized, sometimes in first 24 mo, but often not until later infancy or childhood, rare scarring, milia	Rare mucosal involvement	Keratin 5 or 14	Good
Junctional, Herlitz type (AR)	Severe generalized blistering which heals poorly, granulation tissue, scarring, nail dystrophy, CLAS	Severe mucosal blistering GI involvement common Laryngeal involvement with airway obstruction Urologic involvement	Laminin 5 (α3/β3/γ2 chain)	Death mostly within first 2 years of life
Junctional EB, non-Herlitz type (AR)	Moderate blistering, atrophic scars, nail dystrophy	Mild mucosal blistering Enamel hypoplasia	Laminin 5 or type XVII collagen	Good
Pyloric atresia-junctional EB (AR)	Severe blistering, CLAS	Pyloric atresia, urologic involvement: ureterovesicular obstruction, hydronephrosis	α6/β4 Integrin	Often early death, in some patients good prognosis

AD, autosomal dominant; AR, autosomal recessive; CLAS, congenital localized absence of skin; EB, epidermolysis bullosa; GI, gastrointestinal.
Adapted from Bruckner AL: Epidermolysis bullosa. In Eichenfield LF et al, editors: *Textbook of neonatal dermatology*, Philadelphia, 2008, Saunders, p 159.

steroids may be helpful. An ophthalmologic examination is indicated for all infants with this disorder.

Zinc Deficiency

Zinc deficiency occurs in the genetic disorder acrodermatitis enteropathica and as an acquired condition attributable to inadequate zinc intake.[40] Acrodermatitis enteropathica, a rare disorder, is inherited as an autosomal recessive trait. The gene for this disorder has been localized to chromosomal region 8q24.3 and encodes for a member of the ZIP family of metal transporters.[40] It is characterized by acute vesicobullous, eczematous, and psoriasiform eruptions around the eyes, mouth, and genitals and on the peripheral extremities (Fig. 52-11). Secondary infection with *C. albicans* is a common complication. The onset may be as early as the third week of life, but more frequently it occurs later in infancy. Failure to thrive, hair loss, ocular changes, marked irritability, and paronychial lesions are additional features of the disease. Chronic, severe, and intractable diarrhea is the most serious manifestation and may be life threatening. The disease is caused by a defect in zinc absorption or transport, and extremely low plasma zinc levels have been documented in untreated patients. The exact nature of the defect is unknown. Oral zinc sulfate is the treatment of choice and has induced dramatic remissions of the disease.

A similar eruption has been observed in premature infants maintained on total parenteral nutrition inadequately supplemented with zinc. These infants suffer from relative zinc

Figure 52–10. A, Denudation as a result of blistering in an infant with junctional epidermolysis bullosa. B, Large intact bulla and ruptured bulla on the leg of an infant with dominant dystrophic epidermolysis bullosa.

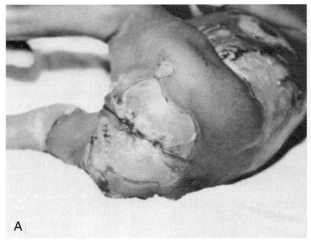
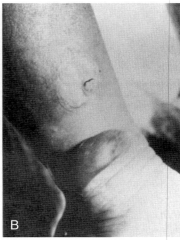

deficiency caused by high metabolic demands. Premature and term infants receiving breast milk with low levels of zinc and infants with malabsorption syndrome or cystic fibrosis also have developed symptomatic zinc deficiency. Maternal zinc deficiency in pregnancy may result in fetal malformation, growth restriction, prematurity, postmaturity, and perinatal death.

Pigmentary Abnormalities

The melanocyte system of the newborn skin usually is not at maximum functional maturity. As a result, all babies regardless of racial pigmentation may look pink or tan at birth. Within the first few weeks, pigmentation becomes more evident because melanin production has been stimulated by exposure to light.

DIFFUSE HYPERPIGMENTATION

The intensity of pigmentation must be considered in light of the infant's genetic and racial background. Diffuse hyperpigmentation in the newborn is unusual. It may be caused by a gene whose main effect is on the melanocyte, by a hereditary disease that has secondary pigmentary consequences, by endocrinopathy, by a nutritional disorder, or by hepatic disease.[53] Although in such cases hyperpigmentation may be described as diffuse, it may be accentuated in certain areas such as the face, over bony prominences, or in the flexural creases.

LOCALIZED HYPERPIGMENTATION

Café-au-Lait Macules

Café-au-lait spots are pigmented macules that may be present in the newborn infant, and they are light brown in whites and dark brown in African Americans. Whereas lesions are seen in 24% to 36% of older children, most commonly on the trunk, they are present in 0.3% to 18% of newborns, usually over the buttocks.[16] Lesions vary with ethnicity and race. Lesions that are larger than 0.5 cm in diameter and more than six in number, especially when accompanied by "freckling" in the flexures, strongly suggest neurofibromatosis. The axillary freckles really represent tiny café-au-lait macules. Café-au-lait spots are usually the first cutaneous

lesions to appear in a patient with neurofibromatosis, but additional genetic and clinical investigations may be required to establish a diagnosis. For example, small, pigmented spots (i.e., Lisch nodules) may be detected on the iris by slit-lamp examination in most patients older than the age of 6 years with classic neurofibromatosis. Patients with tuberous sclerosis also may have café-au-lait spots that are identical in appearance to those of neurofibromatosis, but they are usually accompanied by white macules, which are discussed later.

McCune-Albright Syndrome

In a patient with McCune-Albright syndrome (i.e., polyostotic bone dysplasia, café-au-lait spots, and multiple endocrine disorders), the pigmented patches may be solitary or multiple, unilateral, elongated, and large (>10 cm) and often have a ragged, irregular border. It is caused by a mutation of the *GNAS1* gene leading to increased stimulation of the adenylate cyclase system.[16]

Congenital Melanocytic Nevi

Congenital nevi represent nested proliferations of melanocytes that are present at birth or appear in the first months of life. Small nevi (<1.5 cm) are seen in 1% to 2% of newborns, intermediate nevi (1.5 to 20 cm) in 0.6%, and large nevi (see below) in less than 0.02%.[16] Small lesions (as opposed to giant pigmented nevi) are flat and light to dark brown, often with variegated color or speckling and an accentuated epidermal surface ridge pattern. These lesions vary in site, size, and number but are most often solitary. Histologically, they are characterized by the presence of nevus cells in the dermis, and most have nevus cells extending into the deeper dermis, fat, and perivascular, periappendageal, and perineural sites. There is no clearcut evidence that the small congenital nevus is a premalignant lesion, and conservative management consisting of serial observation with photographic documentation may be appropriate.[16] Decisions about surgical excision are based on location, size of lesion and expected surgical result. Laser treatment may lighten small nevi but does not completely remove the melanocytes, and its use for this indication is controversial.

BOX 52–3   Management of Epidermolysis Bullosa in the Neonatal Period

MINIMIZE TRAUMA TO SKIN AND PROMOTE COMFORT

Use gentle handling and reduce friction.

When possible, use wrapping or suturing instead of taping when applying instruments or monitors; if taping is necessary, leave probes in place.

Use oral sucrose with dressing changes.

Administer acetaminophen or opiate agonist for extreme discomfort.

PROVIDE IDEAL (MOIST) WOUND-HEALING ENVIRONMENT

Open and drain tense vesicles with sterile needle.

Perform gentle daily débridement of crust in bathtub.

Apply emollients and nonstick primary dressing.

Protect wound and secure primary dressing with secondary dressing such as gauze wrap and stockinette or Coban tape.

Tape dressing to itself and not to skin.

PREVENT SEPSIS AND BACTERIAL SUPERINFECTION OF WOUNDS

Observe wounds for purulence and foul smell.

Monitor colonization with weekly surveillance cultures.

Apply topical antibiotics combined with emollient on open erosions to control colonization.

Cover gram-positive organisms with intravenous antibiotics if there are signs or symptoms of sepsis.

MAXIMIZE NUTRITION WITH MINIMAL TRAUMA FOR OPTIMAL WOUND HEALING AND GROWTH

Breast feed if there is mild oral involvement and the infant can feed through pain.

If not, have mother pump breast milk, and bottle feed with high-flow nipple or drip feeds.

Add breast milk fortifier to maximize caloric intake.

For formula-fed baby, use high-calorie formulas.

Obtain dietary consultation and follow up to ascertain energy needs and how to meet them.

MONITOR FOR EXTRACUTANEOUS COMPLICATIONS

Eye: Request ophthalmology consultation for redness or photophobia.

Gastrointestinal: If oral involvement, watch for feeding intolerance.

Genitourinary: Look for gross hematuria, meatal narrowing in boys; consider urinary source if infant is febrile.

Polyhydramnios: Look for pyloric atresia.

Respiratory: Monitor airway for hoarse cry or stridor as a sign of laryngeal involvement.

PROVIDE PSYCHOSOCIAL SUPPORT

Provide counseling regarding prognosis once diagnosis is known. Emphasize unpredictability of course even when subtype is known.

Discuss usual short-term complications in general terms.

Provide access to peer counseling through Internet sites and local chapters of national patient advocacy groups.

Expanded from AL Bruckner: Epidermolysis bullosa. In Eichenfield LF et al, editors: *Textbook of neonatal dermatology*, Philadelphia, 2008, Saunders, p 159.

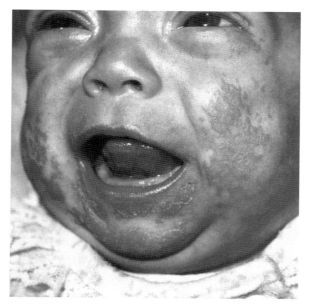

Figure 52–11. Recalcitrant perioral eruption in a premature, breast-fed infant with zinc deficiency. The eruption cleared rapidly with oral zinc replacement.

Congenital Giant Melanocytic Nevi

The giant (>20 cm) nevus (Fig. 52-12) is the most important of the congenital melanocytic (pigmented) nevi.[16] The lifetime risk of malignant transformation and melanoma is estimated to be 6% to 8%.[16] The onset of melanoma in utero has been reported. These nevi may occupy 15% to 35% of the body surface, most commonly involving the trunk. The pigmentation often is variegated from light brown to black. The

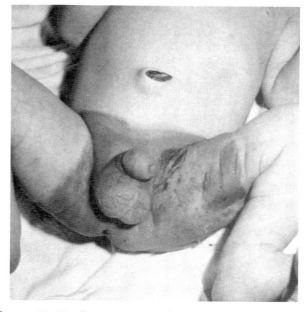

Figure 52–12. Giant pigmented nevus on the bathing trunk area.

affected skin may be smooth, nodular, or leathery in consistency. Prominent hypertrichosis is often present. Almost invariably, numerous satellite nevi coexist elsewhere on the body. Leptomeningeal melanocytosis has been documented in some of these patients, and this complication may manifest as seizures.

Because of the significant incidence of malignant degeneration, the hideous deformity, and the intense pruritus that may accompany them, it is desirable, when feasible, to excise these lesions surgically as soon as possible. Lasers, dermabrasion, and tissue expansion techniques have been used in conjunction with surgical excision for removal and cosmesis of large lesions.[17]

Peutz-Jeghers Syndrome

The cutaneous lesions of the Peutz-Jeghers syndrome may be present at birth or develop soon thereafter. They consist of brown to blue-black macules, somewhat darker than freckles, that develop around the nose and mouth. The lips and oral mucosa often are involved, as are the hands, fingertips, and toes. Macular hyperpigmentation is the only visible sign of this autosomal dominant disorder until adolescence, when the patient begins to suffer from attacks of intussusception, bleeding, and subsequent anemia secondary to coexisting small bowel polyposis.

Xeroderma Pigmentosum

Xeroderma pigmentosum is transmitted by an autosomal recessive gene and results in marked hypersensitivity to ultraviolet light. The skin is normal at birth, but changes develop soon thereafter depending upon the degree of exposure to ultraviolet light. The infant develops erythema, speckled hyperpigmentation, atrophy, actinic keratoses, and all known types of cutaneous premalignant and malignant lesions. The outcome is often fatal by the second decade of life as a result of metastatic disease. The underlying abnormality in most cases is a deficiency in an endonuclease that is responsible for the repair of DNA damaged by ultraviolet light. Approximately 20% of patients have neurologic problems. Protection from ultraviolet light exposure is mandatory to prevent skin damage and tumor development. Prenatal diagnosis of xeroderma pigmentosum is possible using autoradiography to measure DNA repair of amniotic fluid cells or chorionic villi fibroblasts.

Postinflammatory Hyperpigmentation

Hyperpigmentation may result secondarily from any inflammatory process in the skin and may have many causes, including primary irritant dermatitis, infectious processes, panniculitis, and hereditary diseases such as EB. The hyperpigmentation may result from enhanced melanosome production, larger melanin deposits in basal cells, greater numbers of keratinocytes, an increase in the thickness of the stratum corneum, or deposits of melanin in dermal melanophages. Hyperpigmentation usually fades gradually over weeks to months without treatment although a low-potency topical steroid may decrease residual inflammation.

Blue Nevus

Occasionally, a blue nevus (so called because of its Prussian blue color), or dermal melanocytoma, may be present at birth. It usually is a 1- to 3-cm, oval, dome-shaped, black-blue tumor found on the upper half of the body. It grows very slowly and has little tendency to become malignant but may be difficult to differentiate clinically from vascular tumors. Excisional biopsy is diagnostic and curative.

HYPOPIGMENTATION

Diffuse or localized reduction or absence of cutaneous pigment in the neonate may be caused by a heritable or developmental disorder or may result from a nutritional disease or postinflammatory change.[6] Decrease in cutaneous melanin may be caused by an absence or destruction of melanocytes or by a defect in one of four biologic processes: formation of melanosomes, formation of melanin, transfer of melanosomes to keratinocytes, and transport of melanosomes by keratinocytes.

Albinism

Albinism (e.g., complete albinism, oculocutaneous albinism), which occurs in all races, has an incidence of 1 case per 17,000 persons in the United States. The phenotypic picture is caused by an autosomal recessive gene. Several forms of this disorder have been delineated.[46] The affected infant usually has markedly reduced skin pigment, yellow or white hair, pink pupils, gray irides, photophobia, and cutaneous photosensitivity. Melanocytic nevi can be present in patients with albinism, and the nevi may or may not be pigmented. In African Americans, the skin may be tan, the hair may have a yellow or orange color, and freckles can appear on exposure to light. The usual eye findings are photophobia, nystagmus, and a central scotoma with reduced visual acuity. Other associated abnormalities reported in certain types of albinism are small stature and coagulation disorders.

The biochemical defect responsible for oculocutaneous albinism type 1 is a deficiency of tyrosinase, the enzyme responsible for converting tyrosine to dopa, an early step in the formulation of melanin. The range of tyrosinase deficiency correlates well with the spectrum of color seen in affected individuals. Structurally, the melanosomes appear to be normal. In oculocutaneous albinism type 2, however, mutations in the P gene affect function of a melanosomal protein. Molecular analyses of the tyrosinase and P genes are necessary for precise diagnosis. Treatment in all cases is aimed at protection from ultraviolet light because early actinic keratoses and squamous cell carcinoma are common occurrences in these patients.

Partial Albinism

Partial albinism (i.e., piebaldism) is an inherited disease caused by mutations of the autosomal dominant KIT gene coding for the tyrosine kinase transmembrane cellular receptor for mast/stem cell growth factor, a critical factor for melanoblast migration and function. This leads to defective cell proliferation and melanocyte migration during embryogenesis.[6] This condition is present at birth but may not be evident in fair-skinned infants because of a lack of contrast in skin color. In piebaldism, the hair and skin are affected. The amelanotic areas usually involve the midline frontal scalp (i.e., widow's peak), resulting in the characteristic white forelock, forehead to the base of the nose, chin, thorax, trunk, back midarm, and midleg. There are normal islands of pigment within the amelanotic areas, and the distribution pattern is fairly constant. Examination of an affected area by electron microscopy shows an absence of melanocytes or melanocytes with markedly deformed melanosomes. Repigmentation does not take place. The differential diagnosis may include vitiligo, achromic nevus, nevus anemicus, and the hypomelanotic macules of tuberous sclerosis.

Phenylketonuria

Phenylketonuria, caused by an absence of phenylalanine hydroxylase, results in a variety of neurologic and cutaneous abnormalities, which include mental retardation, seizures, diffuse hypopigmentation, eczema, and photosensitivity (see Chapter 50).

Chédiak-Higashi Syndrome

The Chédiak-Higashi syndrome is a rare, fatal disorder resulting from mutations in the autosomal recessive lysosomal trafficking regulator (*LYST*) gene.[28] The clinical features include diffuse to moderate reduction in cutaneous and ocular pigment, photophobia, hepatosplenomegaly, and recalcitrant, recurrent infections. Seizures and progressive neurologic deficits have occurred in some patients in early childhood. The leukocytes and other cells contain large granules, and this finding has its parallel in the melanocyte, which produces giant melanosomes. These abnormal granules are unable to discharge their lysosomal and peroxidative enzymes into phagocytic vacuoles. The diagnosis can be made by the characteristic family history, physical findings, laboratory demonstration of abnormal leukocytes and melanosomes, and the usual course, which leads to death in childhood. Death results from a lymphoma-like process (i.e., accelerated phase) or infection. Treatment is palliative, but bone marrow transplantation has been used successfully to reverse the immunologic defects.

Waardenburg Syndrome

Waardenburg syndrome is an auditory-pigmentary syndrome inherited as an autosomal-dominant condition secondary to mutations in the *PAX3* gene controlling neural crest differentiation.[6] The most constant features are lateral displacement of the inner canthi, a prominently broad nasal root, confluent eyebrows, variegation of pigment in the iris (i.e., heterochromia iridis) and fundus, congenital deafness, a white forelock, and cutaneous hypochromia. The clinical picture is quite striking, and the diagnosis usually is not difficult. Although usually limited to small areas, the hypopigmentation may be severe and extensive enough to resemble that of piebaldism.

Nevus Anemicus

Nevus anemicus is a congenital vascular anomaly that appears as a permanently pale, mottled lesion that occurs most often on the trunk. The lesions appear hypopigmented but contain normal amounts of pigment. The nevus is best characterized as a pharmacologic abnormality rather than an anatomic one. Pallor results from increased local reactivity to catecholamines, which results in vasoconstriction and subsequent pallor. When rubbed, the lesion does not redden like the surrounding skin. There is no effective treatment.

Nevus Achromicus

Present at birth but often not visible until 1 to 2 years of age, nevus achromicus is usually a unilateral, hypopigmented, irregularly shaped lesion. The hypopigmented area is quite uniform in color, and, in contrast to nevus anemicus, the vessels within it react normally to rubbing. The melanocytes in the affected epidermis seem to function poorly or not at all.

White Macules in Tuberous Sclerosis

Tuberous sclerosis is a condition with multisystem involvement characterized by hamartomas, often in association with mental retardation and seizures. Between 50% and 90% of infants with tuberous sclerosis have white macules that become apparent at birth or soon thereafter.[33,49] In fair-skinned infants, the hypopigmented areas may be demonstrated more easily by examining the skin with a Wood lamp. These lesions are often leaflet shaped, are variable in number, and occur more frequently on the trunk and buttocks. The melanocytes within areas of macular hypopigmentation contain poorly pigmented melanosomes. A single, hypopigmented macule in an infant without other features of tuberous sclerosis does not warrant extensive investigation.

Hemangiomas and Vascular Malformations

Vascular lesions are a common problem in the neonate.[2,13,29] They can be divided into two major categories: hemangiomas and vascular malformations (Table 52-7). Hemangiomas are benign tumors of the vascular endothelium characterized by a proliferative and an involutional phase. Malformations are developmental defects derived from the capillary, venous, arterial, or lymphatic vessels. These lesions remain relatively static, and growth is commensurate with growth of the child.

HEMANGIOMAS

Hemangiomas are the most common soft tissue tumors of infancy, occurring in approximately 1% to 3% of newborns and up to 12% by the end of the first year, although reported incidences vary.[2,29] True hemangiomas are characterized by a growth phase and marked by endothelial proliferation and hypercellularity and by an involutional phase. Hemangiomas are clinically heterogeneous, with their appearance dictated by the depth, location, and stage of evolution. In the newborn, hemangiomas may originate as a pale macule with threadlike telangiectases (Fig. 52-13A). As the tumor proliferates, it assumes its most recognizable form—a bright red, slightly elevated, noncompressible plaque (see Fig. 52-13B). Hemangiomas that lie deeper in the skin are soft, warm masses with a slightly bluish discoloration (see Fig. 52-13C). Frequently, hemangiomas have superficial and deep components. They range from a few millimeters to several centimeters in diameter and usually are solitary, but up to 20% of infants have multiple lesions. A female predominance (3:1) and an increased incidence among premature infants have been documented. Approximately 55% of these tumors are present at birth, and the remainder develop in the first weeks of life. Rarely, they may appear as fully grown tumors at birth, and these "congenital hemangiomas" resolve rapidly, often leaving pronounced atrophic skin changes in their wake. Generally, superficial hemangiomas have reached their maximum size by 6 to 8 months, but deep hemangiomas may proliferate for 12 to 14 months or, rarely, up to 2 years.

Despite the benign nature of most cutaneous hemangiomas, a significant number cause functional compromise or

TABLE 52–7   Major Differences between Hemangiomas and Vascular Malformations

	Hemangiomas	Vascular Malformations*
Clinical	Variably visible at birth Subsequent rapid growth Slow, spontaneous involution	Usually visible at birth (AVMs may be quiescent) Growth proportionate to the skin's growth (or slow progression); present lifelong
Sex ratio (F:M)	3:1 to 5:1 and 7:1 in severe cases	1:1
Pathology	Proliferating stage: hyperplasia of endothelial cells and SMC-actin+ cells Multilaminated basement membrane Higher mast cell content in involution	Flat endothelium Thin basement membrane Often irregularly attenuated walls (VM, LM)
Radiology	Fast-flow lesion on Doppler sonography Tumoral mass with flow voids on MR Lobular tumor on arteriogram	Slow flow (CM, LM, VM) or fast flow (AVM) on Doppler ultrasonography MR: Hypersignal on T2 when slow flow (LM, VM); flow voids on T1 and T2 when fast flow (AVM) Arteriography of AVM demonstrates AV shunting
Bone changes	Rarely mass effect with distortion but no invasion	*Slow-flow* VM: distortion of bones, thinning, underdevelopment *Slow-flow* CM: hypertrophy *Slow-flow* LM: distortion, hypertrophy, and invasion of bones *High-flow* AVM: destruction, rarely extensive lytic lesions *Combined malformations* (e.g., slow-flow [CVLM = Klippel-Trenaunay syndrome] or fast-flow [CAVM = Parkes-Weber syndrome]): overgrowth of limb bones, gigantism
Immunohisto-chemistry on tissue samples	*Proliferating hemangioma*: high expression of PCNA, type IV collagenase, VEGF, urokinase, and bFGF *Involuting hemangioma*: high TIMP-1, high bFGF	Lack expression of PCNA, type IV collagenase, urokinase, VEGF, and bFGF One familial (rare) form of VM linked to a mutated gene on 9p (*VMCM1*)
Hematology	No coagulopathy (Kasabach-Merritt syndrome is a complication of other vascular tumors of infancy, e.g., kaposiform hemangioendothelioma and tufted angioma, with a LM component)	Slow-flow VM or LM or LVM may have an associated LIC with risk of bleeding (DIC).

*Capillary (C), venous (V), lymphatic (L), arterial (A), and arteriovenous (AV), pure or complex-combined malformation (M).
bFGF, basic fibroblast growth factor; DIC, disseminated intravascular coagulation; LIC, localized intravascular coagulopathy; MR, magnetic resonance; PCNA, proliferating cell nuclear antigen; SMC, smooth muscle cell; VEGF, vascular endothelial growth factor.

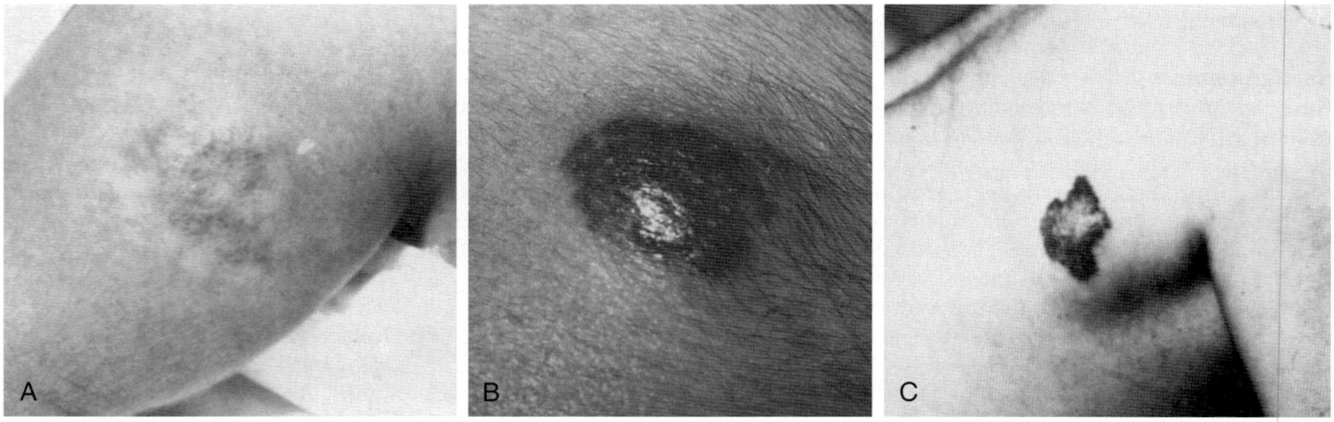

Figure 52–13. A, Hemangioma on the thigh of a preterm infant. Areas of pallor, often an initial sign, are still present. B, Superficial, bright red hemangioma. C, Mixed superficial and deep hemangioma on the back.

permanent disfigurement. Approximately 20% to 40% of patients have residual skin changes; nasal tip, lip, and parotid hemangiomas are notorious for slow involution, and very large superficial facial hemangiomas often leave disfiguring scarring. Ulceration, the most frequent complication, can be excruciatingly painful and carries the risk of infection, hemorrhage, and scarring. Occasionally, hemangiomas manifest as congenital ulcerations with only a very small rim of typical hemangioma, making the diagnosis difficult.

The Kasabach-Merritt phenomenon, a complication of a rapidly enlarging vascular lesion, is characterized by hemolytic anemia, thrombocytopenia, and coagulopathy. The differences between the vascular lesions that induce this phenomenon and classic infantile hemangiomas have been emphasized. These massive tumors are usually a deep redblue color, are firm, grow rapidly, have no sex predilection, tend to proliferate for a longer period (2 to 5 years), and have a different histologic pattern. Most patients with Kasabach-Merritt phenomenon do not have typical hemangiomas but rather have other proliferative vascular tumors, usually kaposiform hemangioendotheliomas or tufted angiomas.[13] The Kasabach-Merritt phenomenon requires aggressive, often multimodal treatment, such as transcutaneous arterial embolization, and carries a significant mortality rate (see also Chapter 46).

Periorbital hemangiomas pose considerable risk to vision and should be carefully monitored. Hemangiomas involving the ear may decrease auditory conduction, which ultimately may cause speech delay. Multiple cutaneous (i.e., diffuse hemangiomatosis) and large facial hemangiomas may be associated with visceral hemangiomas. Subglottic hemangiomas manifest with hoarseness and stridor, and progression to respiratory failure may be rapid. Approximately 50% of infants with subglottic hemangiomas have associated cutaneous hemangiomas, and "noisy breathing" by an infant with a cutaneous hemangioma involving the chin, lips, mandibular region, and neck warrants direct visualization of the airway. Sixty percent of young infants with extensive facial hemangiomas in the "beard" distribution develop symptomatic airway hemangiomas.

Extensive cervicofacial hemangiomas may be associated with multiple anomalies, including vascular malformations, known as PHACES syndrome (*p*osterior fossa malformation, *h*emangiomas, *a*rterial anomalies, *c*ardiac anomalies, *e*ye abnormalities, *s*ternal anomalies). This syndrome has a marked female predominance (9:1) and is thought to represent a developmental field defect that occurs during the 8th to 10th weeks of gestation. Lumbosacral hemangiomas may be markers for occult spinal dysraphism and anorectal and urogenital anomalies. Imaging of the spine is indicated in all patients with midline hemangiomas in this region.

Most hemangiomas require "active nonintervention" coupled with a careful discussion of the natural history of the lesions and photographic documentation of involution.[13] Ulceration is the most common complication and should be treated promptly. Oral systemic corticosteroids are the mainstay of therapy. Recombinant interferon-α, an inhibitor of angiogenesis, has been used successfully in treating lifethreatening hemangiomas, but response is slow, and a particularly worrisome side effect, spastic diplegia, has been reported in as many as 20% of infants. Pulsed dye laser

treatment has been approved by the U.S. Food and Drug Administration, but its use is limited by concerns of efficacy and potential scarring.[10]

BLUE-RUBBER BLEB NEVUS SYNDROME

The blue-rubber bleb nevus syndrome is a rare disorder consisting of multiple venous malformations of the skin and bowel.[13] Cutaneous lesions sometimes are present at birth, and their appearance is characteristic as the descriptive name of this syndrome suggests. The lesions are blue to purple, rubbery, compressible protuberances that vary from a few millimeters to 3 to 4 cm in diameter. They are diffusely distributed over the body's surface and may be sparse or may number in the hundreds. Gastrointestinal lesions are common in the small bowel but also may involve the colon. Occasionally, lesions in the liver, spleen, and CNS have been observed. Severe anemia may result from recurrent episodes of gastrointestinal bleeding. Neither the skin nor the bowel lesions regress spontaneously. Surgery is sometimes palliative, but it is frequently impossible to resect all of the affected bowel.

Vascular malformations also have been reported as a congenital feature of Bannayan-Riley-Ruvalcaba syndrome. Maffucci syndrome (i.e., vascular malformations and dyschondroplasia) and Gorham disease (i.e., vascular malformations and disappearing bones) usually are not apparent in the neonatal period.

PORT-WINE STAIN

Port-wine stains (i.e., nevus flammeus), which represent capillary malformations, are almost always present at birth and should be considered permanent developmental defects.[13] These lesions may be only a few millimeters in diameter or may cover extensive areas, occasionally affecting up to half the body's surface. They do not proliferate after birth; any apparent increase in size is caused by growth of the child. A port-wine stain may be localized to any body surface, but facial lesions are the most common. Port-wine stains usually are sharply demarcated and flat in infancy but with time develop a pebbly or slightly thickened surface. Color ranges from pale pink to purple.

The most successful treatment modality in use is the pulsed dye laser, which is effective in fading these lesions, although only 15% to 20% clear completely.[13] Some studies report treatment is more effective if undertaken in infancy, whereas others have found no difference.

Most port-wine stains occur as isolated defects and do not indicate involvement of other organs, but they occasionally may be a clue to the presence of defects in the eye or certain vascular syndromes. Children with facial port-wine stains involving skin innervated by the V1 or V2 branches of the trigeminal nerve should have a thorough ophthalmologic examination in infancy.

STURGE-WEBER SYNDROME

Sturge-Weber syndrome (i.e., encephalofacial angiomatosis) consists of a facial port-wine stain, usually in the cutaneous distribution of the first branch of the trigeminal nerve, a leptomeningeal venous malformation, mental retardation, seizures, hemiparesis contralateral to the facial lesions, and ipsilateral intracortical calcification.[13] Ocular manifestations are frequent and include buphthalmos, glaucoma, angioma of the choroid, hemianoptic defects, and optic atrophy (see Chapter 53). Roentgenograms of the skull of the older child show pathognomonic "tramline," double-contoured calcifications in the cerebral cortex on the same side as the port-wine stain. Magnetic resonance imaging with gadolinium enhancement is the diagnostic modality of choice. Electroencephalography may demonstrate unilateral depression of cortical activity, with or without spike discharges.

The prognosis depends on the extent of cerebral involvement, rapidity of progression, and response to treatment. Anticonvulsant therapy and neurosurgical procedures have been of value in treating some patients.

KLIPPEL-TRÉNAUNAY-WEBER SYNDROME

Klippel-Trénaunay-Weber syndrome is characterized by a cutaneous vascular malformation (usually a port-wine stain), venous varicosities, and overgrowth of the bony structures and soft tissues of the affected part.[13] The vascular lesions are apparent at birth. Some patients with this syndrome also have venous malformations, lymphatic anomalies, and arteriovenous shunts. Complications include severe edema, phlebitis, thrombosis, ulceration of the affected area, and vascular malformations involving the viscera. The prognosis depends on the extent of involvement, which can be assessed by peripheral vascular studies and scans. Management includes careful orthopedic assessment of limb growth. Surgery may be effective in treating severe limb hypertrophy in some patients. Compressive clothing (Jobst garments) may be helpful, but proper fitting is difficult in infants with rapid growth.

Port-wine stains also occur with moderate frequency in Beckwith-Wiedemann syndrome (i.e., macroglossia, omphalocele, macrosomia, and cytomegaly of the fetal adrenal gland) (see Chapter 49, Part 1), Robert syndrome, and Cobb syndrome (i.e., cutaneomeningospinal angiomatosis).

CONGENITAL LYMPHATIC MALFORMATIONS

Lymphangiomas are hamartomatous malformations composed of dilated lymph channels that are lined by normal lymphatic endothelium.[4,13] They may be superficial or deep and often are associated with anomalies of the regional lymphatic vessels. In addition to surgery, recent trials using intralesional injection of sclerosing agents have proven effective.

Milroy's primary congenital lymphedema is present at birth and often affects the dorsal aspects of the feet. The condition arises from a congenital dysgenesis of the lymphatic microvessels possibly secondary to mutation in the *VEGFR3* gene. This condition is rarely associated with significant complications.

Lymphangioma circumscriptum is probably the most common type of lymphangioma and may be present at birth or may appear in early childhood. Areas of predilection are the oral mucosa, the proximal limbs, and the flexures (Fig. 52-14). This malformation consists of clustered, small, thick-walled vesicles resembling frog spawn; it is often skin colored but may have a red or purple cast because of the presence of blood mixed with lymph in the vesicles. Treatment is excision, with attention to removal of the deep component of the lesion. Large lesions may require full-thickness skin grafting. Recurrence has been observed even with full-thickness grafts.

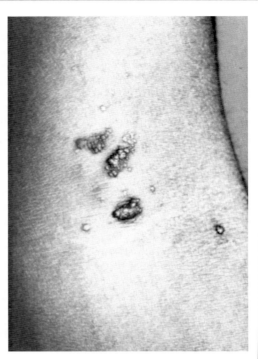

Figure 52–14. Lymphangioma circumscriptum on the upper arm.

Simple lymphangioma appears in infancy as a solitary, skin-colored, dermal or subcutaneous nodule. After trauma, it may exude serous fluid. Occasionally, it has been associated with more extensive lymphatic involvement. Uncomplicated lesions can be removed by simple excision.

Deep lymphangiomas are more diffuse and consist of large, cystic dilations of lymphatics in the dermis, subcutaneous tissue, and intermuscular septa. Surgery is impractical in most cases.

CYSTIC HYGROMA

Cystic hygroma is a benign, multilocular tumor usually found in the neck region. The tumors tend to increase in size and should be treated by surgical excision.

Epidermal Nevi

Epidermal nevi are a group of lesions that are found commonly in the neonatal period. Most of them consist of an overgrowth of keratinocytes and often have an identifiable differentiation toward one of the appendages normally found in skin.[47] They vary considerably in their size, clinical appearance, histologic characteristics, and evolution, depending on their topographic location. Lesions occurring in sites normally rich in sebaceous glands (e.g., the scalp) may look like sebaceous nevi, whereas others, found in areas where the epidermis is thick (e.g., the elbow), look primarily warty.

The most common type of epidermal nevus in the newborn infant is the sebaceus nevus, a hairless, papillomatous, yellow or pink, slightly elevated plaque on the scalp, forehead, or face.[47] These lesions have a characteristic oval or lancet shape. Because a significant incidence of basal cell epitheliomas occurs in these lesions after puberty, they should be removed surgically.

The treatment of large, verrucous epidermal nevi is generally unsatisfactory. The only effective treatment is removal of the lesion together with its underlying dermis. This is only possible in localized lesions, and treatment should be delayed beyond the neonatal period because these lesions may extend over a period of years.

Patients with epidermal nevi may have associated abnormalities, but there are three well-defined entities: Proteus syndrome, CHILD syndrome (i.e., *congenital hemidysplasia with ichthyosiform nevus and limb defects*), and nevus sebaceous syndrome.[47]

Inflammatory Diseases of the Skin

Several inflammatory skin conditions may occur in the neonate. Irritant contact dermatitis, seborrheic dermatitis, and atopic dermatitis are the most frequently encountered.[3] and may be difficult to distinguish because their clinical features have a significant degree of overlap. There are four phases of cutaneous inflammation, any one of which may persist as the dominant feature, depending on the age of the patient, the local physiologic characteristics of the skin involved, and the persistence of the underlying cause. The initial stage is erythema, which proceeds to microvesicle formation, weeping, or oozing. The epidermal response to the injurious process then causes a burst of rapid epidermal mitotic activity that leads to scaling. Lichenification (i.e., thickening of the skin) and pigmentary disturbances supervene. In the young infant, the first three stages predominate; lichenification, which results from scratching or rubbing, is not seen.

IRRITANT CONTACT DERMATITIS

Primary irritant contact dermatitis (as opposed to allergic contact dermatitis) is probably the most common exogenous cause of dermatitis in the newborn. The distribution of the eruption varies somewhat, depending on the precipitating agent. Saliva may be irritating to the face and fecal excretions to the buttocks. Detergent bubble bath, antiseptic proprietary agents, and soap zealously used to clean the perianal area may cause acute eczematous diaper dermatitis, which may become generalized.[56] Obtaining precise information about what has been applied to the skin and how it has been applied is imperative in making an accurate diagnosis. Diaper dermatitis is usually initiated from an irritant but can have a variety of causes. Its proper management should include obtaining a culture for bacteria and yeast, the discontinuance of all ointments containing irritants, and conservative treatment for 1 or 2 weeks. If no improvement follows, a skin biopsy may be indicated.

SEBORRHEIC DERMATITIS

Seborrheic dermatitis is characterized by greasy scaling associated with patchy redness, fissuring, and occasional weeping, usually involving the scalp, ears, axillary, and perineal folds (Fig. 52-15). There is controversy about whether seborrheic dermatitis is a distinct entity or presages the advent of atopic dermatitis. Some infants never progress beyond the seborrheic phase of the dermatitis, which in its

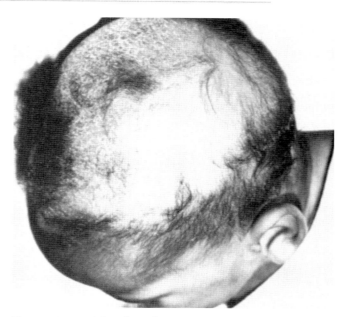

Figure 52–15. Seborrheic dermatitis on the scalp of an infant that resulted in partial alopecia.

classic form rarely is seen in the first month. Cradle cap is probably a minor variant of seborrheic dermatitis. Treatment of seborrheic dermatitis consists of a mild shampoo containing selenium zinc with gentle brushing to remove scales. A low-potency topical corticosteroid or antifungal shampoo such as ketoconazole may be efficacious. The usual course of seborrheic dermatitis is one of rapid regression after 1 or 2 weeks of therapy. Occasionally, a seborrheic-like process may affect the entire body, resulting in full-blown exfoliative dermatitis, which has been called *Leiner disease* when associated with failure to thrive and chronic diarrhea.

ATOPIC DERMATITIS

Atopic dermatitis generally does not appear in the immediate newborn period. Onset during the first year of life occurs in 60% of affected individuals, but most commonly it occurs between 3 and 6 months.[3] Atopic dermatitis is characterized by red, scaling patches and plaques on the face, particularly the cheeks, and on the extensor surfaces of the extremities. Like seborrheic dermatitis, the eruption may be generalized. Infants with atopic dermatitis are often agitated because of the severe pruritus. Clear diagnostic criteria have been established for the diagnosis of atopic dermatitis and include pruritus, chronicity, typical family history, and distribution. Skin barrier dysfunction is prominent in atopic dermatitis, along with an abnormal stratum corneum, increased turnover time, and elevated transepidermal water loss with overproduction of specific cytokines, notably interleukin (IL)-4 and IL-13. Elevated levels of IL-13 in cord blood are associated with increased atopic symptoms during early childhood.[35] Several studies have demonstrated that certain dietary and environmental interventions in the first months of life may decrease the incidence of atopic dermatitis in babies at risk for the disease. These include exclusive breast feeding for 3 months, delayed weaning beyond 6 months, and elimination of house dust mites and passive smoking.

Dermatitis resembling atopic dermatitis may be a feature of a number of systemic conditions, including ataxia-telangiectasia, X-linked agammaglobulinemia, phenylketonuria, gluten-sensitive enteropathy, and long-arm 18 deletion syndrome.[3] Many patients with hypohidrotic ectodermal dysplasia have an eczematous eruption identical to that of atopic dermatitis. Purpura is a frequent additional component of eczema, particularly in Langerhans cell histiocytosis (LCH) and Wiskott-Aldrich syndrome.

Atopic children have a much higher prevalence of staphylococcal colonization than nonatopic children.[3] When bacterial or fungal infection exists, appropriate antibacterial or antifungal therapy is indicated based on the results of culture and sensitivity studies. Weeping lesions should be treated with compresses or bathing in tepid water; protective ointments such as simple zinc oxide paste should be applied after each diaper change; soiled ointments and pastes should be removed with mineral oil. A more extensive eruption may be treated for short periods with a 1% to 2.5% hydrocortisone ointment. A scaly eruption in the scalp may be treated by frequent washing with a shampoo that contains zinc pyrithione or salicylic acid. Bathing should be done in tepid water containing water-dispersible oil. Infants with diffuse dermatitis lose heat readily and are intolerant of even mild changes in environmental temperature or humidity. Humidification of the bedroom in winter and air conditioning in summer is desirable. The efficacy of dietary management of atopic eczema remains controversial.

Subcutaneous and Infiltrative Dermatoses

JUVENILE XANTHOGRANULOMA

Juvenile xanthogranuloma is a benign, non-LCH characterized by solitary or multiple yellow-red cutaneous papules that may enlarge to become nodules.[47] One fifth of infants with juvenile xanthogranuloma are affected at birth, and two thirds have onset of lesions before 6 months of age. There is no predilection for race or sex, and no familial predisposition has been observed for this self-limited disorder, which usually remains confined to the skin. The skin lesions often are restricted to the head, neck, and upper trunk. Involution occasionally leaves a flat atrophic pigmented scar. Serum lipid levels are normal, but histologically, the lesions result from an infiltrate of fat-laden histiocytes, giant cells, and mixed inflammatory cells. Ocular lesions are the most frequent complication (although involvement of other organs may occur rarely) and may result in tumors, unilateral glaucoma, hyphema, uveitis, heterochromia iridis, and proptosis. Ophthalmologic consultation is required for management of the ocular lesions, but the best treatment for the skin lesions is expectant observation.

Several unusual variants may occur, such as giant juvenile xanthogranuloma or bony involvement. There is an increased incidence of juvenile xanthogranulomas among patients with neurofibromatosis type 1, and they may be markers for acute granulocytic leukemia in these patients.

MASTOCYTOSIS

Mast cell disease, or mastocytosis, refers to a spectrum of conditions characterized by mast cell infiltration of the skin or other organs.[48] It may be present at birth and result in a solitary mast cell tumor, a disseminated maculopapular or nodular eruption, a bullous eruption, or a diffuse infiltration of the skin.[25] The disseminated form may be complicated by mast cell infiltrates in internal organs. The diagnosis can be made by demonstration of excessive numbers of mast cells on skin biopsy. Measurement of urinary histamine metabolites or the major urinary metabolite or prostaglandin D_2 can help quantify the total body mast cell load, particularly during systemic symptoms, and may have prognostic significance.

The most common form seen at birth is the firm, solitary mast cell tumor. These tumors usually are ovoid, are pink or tan, and rarely exceed 6 cm in diameter. The lesions are conspicuous by their tendency to form wheals when rubbed (Darier sign) and, in the newborn, to develop overlying blisters. Solitary lesions involute spontaneously within months to years. Urticaria pigmentosa manifests as numerous pink-brown 1- to 2-cm, oval macules and papules. The lesions are usually located centrally and often develop later in infancy. Systemic manifestations of histamine release, such as flushing attacks or generalized pruritus, are caused by mechanical or chemical factors or overheating. Treatment is usually unnecessary, but in symptomatic patients, distressing cutaneous symptoms such as dermatographism and pruritus may be helped with oral antihistamines. Hot water bathing and vigorous toweling must be avoided, as must histamine releasers such as codeine, morphine and its derivatives, aspirin, alcohol-containing elixirs, and certain anesthetics. The prognosis for most infants with mastocytosis, even in its disseminated cutaneous form, is good. The genetics of this condition are unclear. A few pedigrees have been reported with multiple affected family members.

LANGERHANS CELL HISTIOCYTOSIS

LCH is a rare proliferative disorder with skin involvement in 50% of affected children. In 10%, skin is the only affected site, and it is often the first site of involvement. LCH can manifest at anytime from birth to adulthood. Commonly affected areas include the scalp, followed by the skin flexures, including the perineum, but any part of the skin can be affected, including the palms, soles, and nails. The appearance of skin LCH is very diverse with scaly papules, vesicles, nodules, eroded nodules, tumors, and purple plaques.[48] The majority of infants with LCH show multisystem involvement. Single or multifocal bone lesions with lymph node involvement are common, and intracranial disease may manifest with exophthalmos or diabetes insipidus. Definitive diagnosis is made on skin biopsy. CD1a-positive Langerhans cells are seen infiltrating the skin. Langerhans granules (Birbeck granules) within the cells on electron microscopy are also a common finding. LCH with multisystem organ involvement is most often a rapidly fatal disease. Various chemotherapeutic regimens have been used for treatment.

Hashimoto and colleagues described a pure cutaneous form of LCH that occurs only in the neonate or infant.[18] The characteristic features of this congenital, self-healing reticulosis are skin lesions in an otherwise well infant, a histopathology demonstrating Langerhans cell infiltrate, and spontaneous involution of the skin lesions. The pathology is said to be typical with histiocytic infiltration limited to the dermis, sparing of the epidermis, and so-called myelin-dense bodies seen on electron microscopy.

More recently, this entity is considered a mild form of LCH, as progression to severe LCH has now been reported in children who initially met the above criteria. The diagnosis of purely cutaneous LCH should only be made after several years of follow-up.

SUBCUTANEOUS FAT NECROSIS AND SCLEREMA NEONATORUM

Subcutaneous fat necrosis and sclerema neonatorum occur within the first 3 months of life. They may be variants of the same basic disorder of fat metabolism.[7] Sclerema neonatorum usually affects the preterm or debilitated newborn. It manifests by diffuse hardening of the subcutaneous tissue, resulting in a tight, smooth skin that feels bound to the underlying structures. The skin is cold and stony hard. The joints become immobile and the face masklike. The affected infant also may have multiple congenital anomalies or may develop sepsis, pneumonia, or severe gastroenteritis. CNS abnormalities, autonomic dysfunction, and respiratory distress frequently complicate the course of the disease. The mortality rate is high, but the cutaneous changes rarely last longer than 2 weeks if the infant survives. For infants who are severely ill, exchange transfusion and systemic administration of steroids have been used, but their efficacy has not been confirmed.

The lesions of subcutaneous fat necrosis are localized and sharply circumscribed (see Chapters 28 and 49, Part 2). They appear 1 to 4 weeks after delivery as small nodules or large plaques and are found on the cheeks, buttocks, back, arms, and thighs. The affected fat is firm, and the overlying skin may appear reddish or violaceous and occasionally has the texture of orange peel. Histologically, there is a granulomatous reaction in the fat, with formation of needle-shaped crystals, foreign body giant cells, fibroblasts, lymphocytes, and histiocytes. Resolution of the lesion results in fibrosis. Possible precipitating causes of fat necrosis include cold exposure, trauma, asphyxia, and peripheral circulatory collapse. The lesions usually resolve in several weeks or months without complications. Serum calcium levels should be monitored since subcutaneous fat necrosis has been associated with hypercalcemia and its complications.

COLD PANNICULITIS

Cold-induced fat necrosis of the cheeks may occur in the small infant. Warm, red, indurated plaques appear a few hours to a few days after the episode of cold exposure.[7] The lesions resolve in 2 to 3 weeks. An ice cube applied to normal skin of these patients for 2 minutes results in formation of a nodule in 3 to 72 hours at the site of application. The induced nodule parallels the course of the spontaneous lesion. The histologic picture is one of perivascular inflammation and aggregation of lipids from the rupture of fat cells. Postinflammatory hyperpigmentation may mark the site of a healed nodule.

Miscellaneous Congenital Diseases Affecting the Skin

A multitude of hereditary diseases affect the skin. Some of the congenital diseases with prominent cutaneous findings are reviewed here.

APLASIA CUTIS CONGENITA

Aplasia cutis congenita is a rare group of disorders of varying etiology characterized by the focal absence of skin at birth.[32] Most frequently, the lesions are on the scalp in the midline, but other areas of the body may be affected, including the trunk and extremities. Several theories have been proposed to explain the pathogenesis of this disorder, but a single unifying mechanism seems unlikely. Possible etiologies include incomplete closure of the neural tube, localized vascular insufficiency, amniotic membrane adhesions, teratogenic agents, and intrauterine infections. Large scalp defects are associated with trisomy 13. The diagnosis is usually based on clinical findings. Increased levels of acetylcholinesterase and α-fetoprotein have been reported in the amniotic fluid of mothers with children with aplasia cutis. Prognosis and management should be individualized based on the size, location, and presence or absence of ulceration or underlying bony defect. Management strategies include simple observation, prevention of infection in the case of ulceration, and surgical excision or skin grafting in the case of large defects.

CUTIS LAXA

Cutis laxa (i.e., generalized elastolysis) is a heterogeneous group of congenital and acquired disorders and is a feature of several malformation syndromes.[32] There are three major forms of congenital cutis laxa: one inherited as an autosomal dominant trait and two inherited in an autosomal recessive fashion. In all forms of the disease, affected infants have diminished resilience of the skin, which hangs in folds, resulting in a bloodhound appearance. The joints are not hypermobile, and there is no tendency to increased bruising as in Ehlers-Danlos syndrome (EDS). Elastic tissue may be greatly diminished in the dermis and is of poor quality. The collagen has normal tensile properties. In the autosomal dominant form, there are few complications, and the life span is usually normal. In the generalized recessive type of cutis laxa, elastic fibers elsewhere in the body are defective, resulting in inguinal, diaphragmatic, and ventral hernias; rectal prolapse; diverticula of the gastrointestinal and genitourinary tracts; pulmonary emphysema; and aortic aneurysms. Cardiorespiratory complications may cause death during childhood. The other recessive form, cutis laxa with retarded growth and skeletal dysplasia, is typified by intrauterine growth restriction, congenital dislocation of the hips, and a peculiar facies with frontal bossing, antimongoloid slanting of the palpebral fissures, and widening of the fontanelles. Unlike other loose skin syndromes, persons with cutis laxa have almost normal wound healing. These children are good candidates for cosmetic plastic surgery and its attendant psychological benefits.[32]

EHLERS-DANLOS SYNDROME

EDS is a group of inherited connective tissue disorders with the common features of hyperextensible skin, joint laxity, and soft tissue fragility (Fig. 52-16).[43] Bleeding episodes and cardiovascular complications are characteristic of some forms of the disorder. The skin of patients with EDS is hyperextensible when stretched but snaps back with

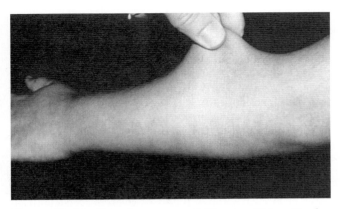

Figure 52–16. Skin hyperextensibility in Ehlers-Danlos syndrome.

normal resiliency, in contrast to the skin of patients with cutis laxa, which hangs in redundant folds. Cutis laxa is not associated with hypermobile joints or easy bruisability. In some forms, the skin also is excessively fragile. Associated findings may include short stature, scoliosis, soft tissue contractures, multiple dislocations, periodontosis, and eye defects. Involvement of the gastrointestinal tract may lead to episodes of acute blood loss or megacolon. Aortic aneurysms also may develop. All forms of the disease are inherited; some are autosomal dominant traits, others are autosomal recessive, and two forms are X-linked. Identified gene mutations include various collagens, collagen-processing genes and tenascin-X, a connective tissue protein. Forty percent of newborns with EDS are delivered prematurely.[43]

ECTODERMAL DYSPLASIA

The term *ectodermal dysplasia* describes a group of more than 100 rare congenital disorders with abnormal development of ectodermally derived tissues, of which the hypohidrotic type is the most common.[43] Diminution or absence of sweating, hypotrichosis, and defective dentition are the most striking features of hypohidrotic ectodermal dysplasia, which usually is inherited in an X-linked recessive fashion. The facies are distinctive because of frontal bossing and depression of the bridge of the nose. Eyebrows and lashes are absent or sparse. The skin around the eyes is wrinkled and frequently hyperpigmented. The skin elsewhere is thin, dry, and hypopigmented, and the cutaneous vasculature is more visible. The scalp and body hair is sparse and the ears and chin prominent. The lips are thick and everted and may show pseudorhagades. Dental anomalies range from total anodontia to hypodontia with peg-shaped teeth.

The most striking physiologic abnormality is the diminution or absence of sweating. Sweat pores usually are decreased to absent on the fingertips. Absence or hypoplasia of eccrine glands can be confirmed by skin biopsy. Other glandular structures also may be absent or hypoplastic. Less constant ancillary findings include conductive hearing loss, gonadal abnormalities, stenotic lacrimal

puncta, corneal dysplasia, and cataracts. Mental development is normal. Marked heat intolerance is caused by an inability to regulate the body temperature adequately by sweating. Fever occurs with increases in ambient temperature and exercise and should respond quickly to environmental cooling and rest. Some febrile reactions, however, may be caused by recurrent upper respiratory tract infections. Because the respiratory mucosa also may be deficient in mucus-secreting glands, viral respiratory tract infections in these patients tend to linger and become complicated by secondary bacterial infections in the bronchial tree. It is imperative to diagnose children with ectodermal dysplasia in infancy.

Every effort should be made to moderate extreme environmental temperatures by using air conditioning. Deficient lacrimation can be palliated by the regular use of artificial tears. The nasal mucosa also must be protected by intermittent saline solution irrigations and application of petrolatum. It is imperative that children with this disorder have a thorough dental evaluation during the first years of life, and dental prostheses should be provided even for toddlers so that adequate nutrition is maintained. Reconstructive procedures can be performed later in life to improve the facial configuration. A wig may be required for patients with scant scalp hair.

The incidence of atopic diseases—asthma, allergic rhinitis, and atopic dermatitis—is increased significantly among patients with anhidrotic ectodermal dysplasia. Atopic manifestations should be managed as they would be in otherwise healthy infants and children. Accurate carrier detection and early neonatal and prenatal diagnoses are feasible for many families at risk for this condition.

Numerous other types of ectodermal dysplasia have been defined, including hidrotic ectodermal dysplasia, the ectrodactyly ectodermal dysplasia cleft palate syndrome, the ankyloblepharon ectodermal dysplasia cleft palate syndrome, the ectodermal dysplasia cleft palate midfacial hypoplasia (Rapp-Hodgkin) syndrome, and chondroectodermal dysplasia (Ellis–van Creveld syndrome). Some of these conditions may manifest with scalp erosions or impetiginous lesions in the neonate. Isolated lack of sweat glands occurs in congenital familial anhidrosis.

PORPHYRIAS

The inherited porphyrias are a diverse group of inborn errors of heme biosynthesis, resulting from the deficient activity of a specific enzyme in the pathway. They are classified as hepatic or erythropoietic according to the organ site in which the underlying heme synthetic defect is predominantly expressed. The erythropoietic porphyrias include congenital erythropoietic porphyria and erythropoietic protoporphyria. The erythropoietic porphyrias are present at birth, infancy, or early childhood, whereas the hepatic porphyrias manifest after puberty or in adulthood.[44]

Erythropoietic protoporphyria is the most common childhood porphyria, caused by a deficient activity of ferrochelatase; it usually manifests by age 2 years. Erythropoietic protoporphyria is inherited as an autosomal dominant condition with incomplete penetrance. Clinical diagnosis is made with a history of crying or skin pain following sun exposure. Some patients are photosensitive to fluorescent lighting. Hemolytic anemia is absent. The diagnosis is made by the elevated levels of protoporphyrin in erythrocytes, plasma, and feces. The treatment includes sun avoidance; oral administration of β-carotene, cysteine, and antihistamines to increase tolerance to sunlight; and liver transplantation.

Congenital erythropoietic porphyria, also called Gunther disease, is a rare autosomal recessive disorder caused by deficient activity of uroporphyrinogen III synthase. The gene for congenital erythropoietic porphyria has been mapped to chromosome 10, allowing prenatal diagnosis to be made with chorionic villus sampling. Diagnosis is also suspected when a reddish-brown amniotic fluid is noticed at amniocentesis. Clinical presentation includes severe photosensitivity from birth or early infancy with formation of vesicles and bullae on areas exposed to sun, phototherapy, or fluorescent lighting. There is also marked skin fragility. Diagnosis is made by elevated levels of uroporphyrin I in urine and erythrocytes and increased levels of coproporphyrin I in feces. Treatment modalities include oral super-activated charcoal, hypertransfusion, splenectomy, and bone marrow transplantation.

Transient porphyrinemias have been described in newborns with hemolytic disease with unclear etiology. These infants present with erythema, violaceous discoloration, purpura, erosions, and blisters on areas exposed to phototherapy. The elevated levels of porphyrins normalize spontaneously after the first few months.

NEONATAL LUPUS ERYTHEMATOSUS

Neonatal lupus erythematosus (NLE) is a disease caused by transplacental passage of maternal autoantibodies. Pregnant women whose sera contain anti-Ro/SSA or anti-La/SSB are at risk of having a child with NLE. Permanent congenital heart block and transient skin lesions are the hallmark of this condition. Mean age at the onset of skin rash is 6 weeks, but it may be present at birth.[36]

Clinically, the skin lesions are primarily annular and papulosquamous. They are widespread but most commonly seen on the face and scalp, predominantly affecting the periorbital and malar areas and often causing a "raccoon eyes" appearance. Sun exposure precipitates or aggravates these lesions. Telangiectasia may be a presenting sign and a more permanent sequela. Between 30% and 50% of mothers of infants with NLE have a connective tissue disease, most commonly systemic lupus erythematosus or Sjögren syndrome.

Many questions regarding the pathogenesis of NLE remain unanswered. Serologic studies for autoantibodies are confirmatory for diagnosis. It is unclear why less than 5% of mothers with anti-Ro and anti-La antibodies give birth to affected children and why mothers of affected infants are often asymptomatic despite having the same antibodies. Diagnosis of NLE in the infant, therefore, may lead to diagnosis of lupus in the mother. Treatment of skin lesions is primarily aimed at sun protection along with topical steroids. Development of rheumatic disease later in childhood can occur and warrants long-term follow up. The risk of a subsequent child having any manifestation of NLE is roughly 25%.

PRINCIPLES OF NEWBORN SKIN CARE

It is reported that nearly 80% of normal newborns develop a skin problem, for example, a "rash" during the first month of life. Despite the desire of parents and caregivers to promote good skin care and the ubiquity of skin problems, particularly in the preterm infant, there is a surprising lack of evidence on which to base infant skin care recommendations. Studies, for example, have provided evidence that natural drying of the umbilical cord in term and preterm infants is a safe and effective means of postnatal cord care and results in earlier detachment of the cord compared with the result with alcohol use.[14] Basic principles of skin care were cited earlier in Box 52-2.

The gross appearance of the skin at birth is related in part to the maturity of the infant. The premature infant's skin may be readily distinguished from the term infant's skin. At birth, it is more transparent and gelatinous and tends to be free of wrinkles. The premature infant may be covered with fine lanugo hair. Sexual hormonal effects are less conspicuous in the premature infant; the scrotum is less rugose and pigmented, and the labia majora are less prominent and not approximated, nipples and areolas are less pigmented, and breast tissue is less palpable.

The extremely premature infant (<750 g) is at particular risk secondary to a poorly developed epidermal permeability barrier. The stratum corneum becomes multilayered during the third trimester. However, it represents a less effective barrier than adult stratum corneum. Transepidermal water losses may be 10- to 15-fold higher in preterm infants with extremely low birthweight compared with those in term infants. Each milliliter of water lost via evaporation expends 0.58 kilocalories. Epidermal permeability is highest in the premature infant immediately after birth. Heat and water loss can be a significant source of morbidity in the preterm infant and should be prevented beginning in the delivery room. The difference between cutaneous permeability in premature infants and term infants decreases with each postnatal day. At 2 weeks after birth, however, the epidermal barrier of the infant with very low birthweight still has markedly increased transepidermal water loss compared with that in infants born at the same corrected gestational age.[1]

An immature permeability barrier can lead to increased absorption of environmental toxins (Table 52-8). The normal acid mantle of the skin develops more slowly in preterm infants, and the expression of cationic antimicrobial peptides, such as those associated with the protective coating of vernix caseosa at birth, may be diminished.

Strategies for improving epidermal barrier function in preterm infants with very low birthweight are listed in Box 52-4. Studies have shown that postnatal massage of moderately preterm infants with traditional oils reduces infection and mortality.[9] An overview of the complicated interplay between genotype and environment in affecting skin condition is shown in Figure 52-17. This interaction is illustrated in the etiology of common skin disorders such as diaper dermatitis.[56] It is anticipated that increasing understanding of the molecular basis of the skin disorders and diseases covered in this chapter will shed new light on the mechanisms of more common and less serious skin problems in the newborn.

TABLE 52–8   Potential Untoward Effects from Application of Topical Products in Neonates

Compound	Function	Toxicity
Adhesive remover solvents	Skin preparations to aid in adhesive removal	Epidermal injury, hemorrhage, and necrosis
Alcohols	Skin antiseptic	Cutaneous hemorrhagic necrosis, elevated blood alcohol levels
Ammonium lactate	Keratolytic emollient	Possible lactic acidosis
Aniline	Dye used as a laundry marker	Methemoglobinemia
Benzethonium chloride	Skin cleansers	Poisoning by ingestion, carcinogenesis
Benzocaine	Mucosal anesthetic (teething products)	Methemoglobinemia
Boric acid	Baby powder, diaper paste	Vomiting, diarrhea, erythroderma, seizures, death
Calcipotriol	Topical vitamin D_3 analogue	Hypercalcemia, hypercalcemic crisis
Chlorhexidine	Topical antiseptic	Systemic absorption but no toxic effects
Coal tar	Shampoos, anti-inflammatory ointment	Excessive use of polycyclic aromatic hydrocarbons are associated with an increased risk of cancer
Corticosteroids	Topical anti-inflammatory	Skin atrophy, striae, adrenal suppression
Diphenhydramine	Topical antipruritic	Central anticholinergic syndrome
Glycerin	Emollients, cleansing agents (Aquanil)	Hyperosmolality, seizures
Lidocaine	Topical anesthetic	Petechiae, seizures
Lindane	Scabicide (Kwell)	Neurotoxicity
Mercuric chloride	Diaper rinses, teething powders	Acrodynia, hypotonia
Methylene blue	Amniotic fluid leak diagnosis	Methemoglobinemia
Neomycin	Topical antibiotic (Neosporin)	Neural deafness
Phenolic compounds (pentachlorophenol, hexachlorophene, resorcinol)	Laundry disinfectant, topical antiseptic (PHisoHex)	Neurotoxicity, tachycardia, metabolic acidosis, methemoglobinemia, death
Phenylephrine	Ophthalmic drops	Vasoconstriction, periorbital pallor
Povidone-iodine	Topical antiseptic (Betadine)	Hypothyroidism
Prilocaine	Topical anesthetic (EMLA)	Methemoglobinemia
Propylene glycol	Topical vehicles, emollients, cleansing agents (Cetaphil)	Hyperosmolality, neurotoxicity, seizures
Salicylic acid	Keratolytic emollient	Metabolic acidosis, salicylism
Silver sulfadiazine	Topical antibiotic (Silvadene)	Kernicterus (sulfa component), agranulocytosis, argyria (silver component)
Triclosan	Deodorant and antibacterial soaps	Toxicities seen with other phenolic products
Triple dye (brilliant green, gentian violet, proflavine hemisulfate)	Topical antiseptic for umbilical cord	Ulceration of mucous membranes, skin necrosis, vomiting, diarrhea
Urea	Keratolytic emollient	Uremia

Compiled from Gilliam AE, Williams ML: Skin of the premature infant, p 45, and Bree AF, Siegfried EC: Neonatal skin care and toxicology, p 59. Both in Eichenfield LF et al, editors: *Textbook of neonatal dermatology*. Philadelphia, 2008, Saunders.

BOX 52–4	Strategies to Improve Epidermal Barrier Function in Preterm Infants

Topical application of one or more nonphysiologic lipids (e.g., petrolatum)

Topical application of natural oils (e.g., sunflower oil) or mixtures of physiologic lipids (ceramides, cholesterol, free fatty acids)

Topical dressings
- Vapor-permeable: allow metabolic (repair) processes to continue in the underlying epidermis
- Vapor-impermeable (occlusive): delay metabolic responses in the underlying epidermis

Xeric stress: postnatal transition to low-humidity (~60%) environment accelerates barrier development

Adapted from Hoath SB: Physiologic development of the skin. In Polin RA et al, editors: *Fetal and neonatal physiology*, 3rd ed, Philadelphia, 2004, Saunders, p 597.

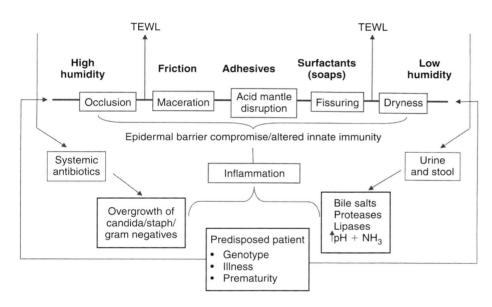

Figure 52–17. Range of factors affecting infant skin condition. The phenotype of infant skin results from the complex interplay of genotype and multiple environmental factors (humidity, friction, adhesive trauma, soap exposure). Conditions such as prematurity, illness (e.g., diarrhea), or the use of systemic antibiotics may affect regional skin health and lead to altered epidermal barrier function. TEWL, transepidermal water loss.

REFERENCES

1. Agren J, et al: Transepidermal water loss in infants born at 24 and 25 weeks of gestation, *Acta Paediatr Scand* 87:1185, 1998.
2. Atherton DJ: Infantile haemangiomas, *Early Hum Dev* 82:789, 2006.
2a. Benjamin DK Jr, Stoll BJ, Fanaroff AA, et al; National Institute of Child Health and Human Development Neonatal Research Network: Neonatal candidiasis among extremely low birth weight infants: risk factors, mortality rates, and neurodevelopmental outcomes at 18 to 22 months, *Pediatrics* 117(1):84, 2006.
3. Bernard LA, et al: Eczematous and papulosquamous disorders. In Eichenfield LF, et al, editors: *Textbook of neonatal dermatology*, Philadelphia, 2008, Saunders.
4. Blei F: Congenital lymphatic malformations, *Ann N Y Acad Sci* 1131:185, 2008.
5. Bruckner AL: Epidermolysis bullosa. In Eichenfield LF, et al, editors: *Textbook of neonatal dermatology*, Philadelphia, 2008, Saunders.
6. Chan Y-C, et al: Hypopigmentation disorders. In Eichenfield LF, et al, editors: *Textbook of neonatal dermatology*, Philadelphia, 2008, Saunders.
7. Cohen BA: Disorders of the subcutaneous tissue. In Eichenfield LF, et al, editors: *Textbook of neonatal dermatology*, Philadelphia, 2008, Saunders.
8. Darmstadt GL, et al: Neonatal skin care, *Pediatr Clin North Am* 47:757, 2000.
9. Darmstadt GL, et al: Effect of skin barrier therapy on neonatal mortality rates in preterm infants in Bangladesh: a randomized, controlled, clinical trial, *Pediatrics* 121:522, 2008.
10. Drolet BA, et al: Infantile hemangiomas: an emerging health issue linked to an increased rate of low birth weight infants, *J Pediatr* 153:712, 2008.
11. Ehrenreich M, et al: Incontinentia pigmenti (Bloch-Sulzberger syndrome): a systemic disorder, *Cutis* 79:355, 2007.
12. Eichenfield LF, et al, editors: *Textbook of neonatal dermatology*, Philadelphia, 2001, Saunders.
13. Enjolras O, et al: Vascular Stains, Malformations, and Tumors. In Eichenfield LF, et al, editors: *Textbook of neonatal dermatology*, Philadelphia, 2008, W.B. Saunders Co.

14. Evens K, et al: Does umbilical cord care in preterm infants influence cord bacterial colonization or detachment? *J Perinatol* 24:100, 2004.

15. Fine JD, et al: The classification of inherited epidermolysis bullosa (EB): Report of the Third International Consensus Meeting on Diagnosis and Classification of EB, *J Am Acad Dermatol* 58:931, 2008.

16. Gibbs NF, et al: Disorders of hyperpigmentation and melanocytes. In Eichenfield LF, et al, editors: *Textbook of neonatal dermatology*, Philadelphia, 2008, Saunders.

17. Gosain AK, et al: Giant congenital nevi: a 20-year experience and an algorithm for their management, *Plast Reconstr Surg* 108:622, 2001.

18. Hashimoto K, et al: Self-healing reticulohistiocytosis: a clinical, histologic, and ultrastructural study of the fourth case in the literature, *Cancer* 49:331, 1982.

19. Herane MI, et al: Acne in infancy and acne genetics, *Dermatology* 206:24, 2003.

20. Hoath SB, et al, editors: *Neonatal skin: structure and function*, 2nd ed, New York, 2003, Marcel Dekker.

21. Hoath SB, et al: *The biology of vernix. Neonatal skin: structure and function*, 2nd ed, New York, 2003, Marcel Dekker.

22. Hoath SB: Physiologic development of the skin. In Polin RA, et al, editors: *Fetal and neonatal physiology*, 3rd ed, Philadelphia, 2004, Saunders.

23. Holbrook K: Structure and function of the developing human skin. In Goldsmith LA, editor: *Physiology, biochemistry, and molecular biology of the skin*. Oxford: Oxford University Press, 1991.

24. Holbrook KA: Structural and biochemical organogenesis of skin and cutaneous appendages in the fetus and newborn. In Polin RA, et al, editors: *Fetal and neonatal physiology*, Philadelphia, 1998, Saunders.

25. Howard R, et al: Vesicles, pustules, bullae, erosions, and ulcerations. In Eichenfield LF, et al, editors: *Textbook of neonatal dermatology*, Philadelphia, 2008, Saunders.

26. Howell ER, et al: Cutaneous manifestations of *Staphylococcus aureus* disease, *Skinmed* 6:274, 2007.

27. Ito N, et al: Human hair follicles display a functional equivalent of the hypothalamic-pituitary-adrenal axis and synthesize cortisol, *FASEB J* 19:1332, 2005.

28. Kaplan J, et al: Chediak-Higashi syndrome, *Curr Opin Hematol* 15:22, 2008.

29. Kilcline C, et al: Infantile hemangiomas: how common are they? A systematic review of the medical literature, *Pediatr Dermatol* 25:168, 2008.

30. Klar AJ: Human handedness and scalp hair-whorl direction develop from a common genetic mechanism, *Genetics* 165:269, 2003.

31. Kline A, et al: Group B streptococcus as a cause of neonatal bullous skin lesions, *Pediatr Infect Dis J* 12:165, 1993.

32. Kos L, et al: Developmental abnormalities. In Eichenfield LF, et al, editors: *Textbook of neonatal dermatology*, Philadelphia, 2008, Saunders.

33. Kwiatkowski DJ, et al: Tuberous sclerosis, *Arch Dermatol* 130:348, 1994.

34. Ladhani S: Understanding the mechanism of action of the exfoliative toxins of *Staphylococcus aureus*, *FEMS Immunol Med Microbiol* 39:181, 2003.

35. Lange J, et al: High interleukin-13 production by phytohaemagglutinin- and Der p 1-stimulated cord blood mononuclear cells is associated with the subsequent development of atopic dermatitis at the age of 3 years, *Clin Exp Allergy* 33:1537, 2003.

36. Lee LA: The clinical spectrum of neonatal lupus, *Arch Dermatol Res*, 2008.

37. Loomis AC, et al: Fetal skin development. In Eichenfield LF, et al, editors: *Textbook of neonatal dermatology*, Philadelphia, 2008, Saunders.

38. Lund CH, et al: Neonatal skin care: evaluation of the AWHONN/NANN research-based practice project on knowledge and skin care practices, *J Obstet Gynecol Neonatal Nurs* 30:30, 2001.

39. Marchini G, et al: AQP1 and AQP3, psoriasin, and nitric oxide synthases 1-3 are inflammatory mediators in erythema toxicum neonatorum, *Pediatr Dermatol* 20:377, 2003.

40. Maverakis E, et al: Acrodermatitis enteropathica and an overview of zinc metabolism, *J Am Acad Dermatol* 56:116, 2007.

41. McLaughlin MR, et al: Newborn skin: Part II. Birthmarks, *Am Fam Physician* 77:56, 2008.

42. Moore ER, et al: Early skin-to-skin contact for mothers and their healthy newborn infants, *Cochrane Database Syst Rev*:CD003519, 2007.

43. Morrell DS, et al: Selected hereditary diseases. In Eichenfield LF, et al, editors: *Textbook of neonatal dermatology*, Philadelphia, 2008, Saunders.

44. Murphy GM: Diagnosis and management of the erythropoietic porphyrias, *Dermatol Ther* 16:57, 2003.

45. O'Connor NR, et al: Newborn skin: Part I. Common rashes, *Am Fam Physician* 77:47, 2008.

46. Okulicz JF, et al: Oculocutaneous albinism, *J Eur Acad Dermatol Venereol* 17:251, 2003.

47. Prendiville JS: Lumps, bumps, and hamartomas. In Eichenfield LF, et al, editors: *Textbook of neonatal dermatology*, Philadelphia, 2008, Saunders.

48. Prose NS, et al: Neoplastic and infiltrative diseases. In Eichenfield LF, et al, editors: *Textbook of neonatal dermatology*, Philadelphia, 2008, Saunders.

49. Roach ES: Neurocutaneous syndromes, *Pediatr Clin North Am* 39:591, 1992.

50. Rutter N: Eccrine sweating in the newborn. In Hoath SB, et al, editors: *Neonatal skin: structure and function*, 2nd ed, New York, 2003, Marcel Dekker.

51. Ryan T: The cutaneous vasculature in normal and wounded neonatal skin. In Hoath SB, et al, editors: *Neonatal skin: structure and function*, 2nd ed, New York, 2003, Marcel Dekker.

52. Stanley JR, et al: Pemphigus, bullous impetigo, and the staphylococcal scalded-skin syndrome, *N Engl J Med* 355:1800, 2006.

53. Taieb A, et al: Hypermelanoses of the newborn and of the infant, *Dermatol Clin* 25:327, 2007.

54. Uitto J: Epidermolysis bullosa: prospects for cell-based therapies, *J Invest Dermatol* 128:2140, 2008.

55. Vahlquist A, et al: Congenital ichthyosis: an overview of current and emerging therapies, *Acta Derm Venereol* 88:4, 2008.

56. Visscher MO, et al: Diaper dermatitis. In Lean Chen AI, Maibach HI, editors: *Handbook of irritant dermatitis*. New York, 2003, Springer-Verlag.

57. Yoshio H, et al: Antimicrobial polypeptides of human vernix caseosa and amniotic fluid: implications for newborn innate defense, *Pediatr Res* 53:211, 2003.

58. Zouboulis C, et al: Sebaceous glands. In Hoath SB, et al, editors: *Neonatal skin: structure and function*, 2nd ed, New York, 2003, Marcel Dekker.

CHAPTER 53

The Eye

PART 1

Examination and Common Problems

Lawrence M. Kaufman, Marilyn T. Miller, and Balaji K. Gupta

Clinicians should develop the ability to recognize the signs and symptoms of serious eye diseases or complications of diseases early in their course to prevent visual loss and, in some cases, preserve life. For example, early detection and treatment of congenital cataracts and congenital glaucoma are critical for visual rehabilitation. Malignant orbital tumors and intraocular tumors such as retinoblastoma are life threatening. Ocular findings can also assist in the diagnosis of a systemic illness such as type 1 neurofibromatosis (NF1) and CHARGE syndrome (coloboma, heart anomaly, choanal atresia, retardation, genital anomaly, ear anomaly).[68]

The visual system is not completely developed at birth but progressively matures during the neonatal period.[16] The neonatologist must recognize normal ocular findings during different stages of the infant's growth to understand what is abnormal. Some ocular and visual milestones are shown in Table 53-1.

A screening eye examination should be performed during the newborn physical examination and during routine well-baby checkups.[2] The screening examination should include the assessments listed in Box 53-1.[13] Fortunately, the screening examination identifies most problems such as glaucoma, cataract, infection, or tumor. However, if abnormalities are suspected because of the history, presence of systemic anomalies, or abnormal result of the screening examination, a more detailed ocular evaluation is mandatory, preferably by a pediatric ophthalmologist.[23]

NEONATAL EYE EXAMINATION

A screening ocular examination begins with a careful history, especially of ocular diseases in the family.[13] For example, a family history of retinoblastoma necessitates a comprehensive ocular examination of the fundus shortly after birth. Information about maternal diseases (e.g., rubella), injuries, medications, or use of drugs or alcohol during the prenatal period should be obtained. It is also important to document the duration and abnormalities of pregnancy, labor, and delivery. Premature birth suggests potential retinopathy of prematurity (ROP), and difficult delivery with obstetric forceps can result in direct ocular trauma.

The examination should be done under comfortable circumstances and with the proper equipment (Fig. 53-1). Much can be learned if the examiner takes a few moments initially to observe the infant for facial anomalies, the external ocular appearance, and ocular motility while taking the history. The examination is most easily performed with the baby in a parent's arms; the more difficult parts of an examination often can be accomplished while a baby is nursing or sucking on a bottle or pacifier.

The screening eye examination should include an evaluation of visual function, preferably, one eye at a time. For infants less than 4 to 6 weeks of age, visual function is assessed by withdrawal or blinking to light, or pupil constriction to light.[13]

Maintenance of the eyes on an object is called *fixation*. The infant's ability to fixate and follow a target can be an approximate guide to the amount of visual function present. Beyond 4 to 6 weeks of age, visual function is assessed in terms of the quality of the fixation and following. By experience, the clinician must develop an age-appropriate scale that assesses this quality of fixation and following, paying attention to the intensiveness, steadiness, and maintenance of the fixation and the smoothness and duration of the following.

Visual acuity refers to the subjective response from the patient of the ability to discern images of set sizes, such as the tumbling "E" or Snellen letters. Most normally developing children can participate in some form of visual acuity testing by the age of 30 months.

If additional information regarding visual function is desired, some ancillary visual tests are available and used in indicated situations. 1) *Optokinetic nystagmus* describes a reflex ocular response to a moving target. As a target moves across the visual field, a pursuit motion occurs, followed by a rapid return motion in the opposite direction to regain fixation. We experience this response when telephone poles or fence posts are watched from a fast-moving vehicle. With an optokinetic drum, which consists of black and white stripes on a spinning cylinder, if the examiner can elicit optokinetic nystagmus in the infant, this establishes that the child has enough visual function to discern the stripes. The stripe

TABLE 53–1 Visual System Milestones

Description	Age
Pupillary light reaction present	30-wk gestation
Pupillary light reaction well developed	1 mo
Lid closure in response to bright light	30-wk gestation
Blink response to visual threat	2-5 mo
Visual fixation present	Birth
Fixation well developed	2 mo
Visual following well developed	3 mo
Accommodation well developed	4 mo
Visual evoked potential acuity at adult level	6 mo
Grating acuity preferential looking at adult level	2 yr
Snellen letter acuity at adult level	2 yr
Color vision present	2 mo
Color vision at adult level	6 mo
Stereopsis developed	6 mo
Stereoacuity at adult level	7 yr
End of critical period for monocular visual deprivation	10 yr
Conjugate horizontal gaze well developed	Birth
Conjugate vertical gaze well developed	2 mo
Vestibular (doll's eye) rotations well developed	34-wk gestation
Optokinetic nystagmus well developed	Birth
Ocular alignment stable	4 mo
Fusional convergence well developed	6 mo
Eyeball 70% of adult diameter	Birth
Eyeball 95% of adult diameter	3 yr
Cornea 80% of adult diameter	Birth
Cornea 95% of adult diameter	1 yr
Differentiation of fovea completed	4 mo
Myelination of optic nerve completed	7 mo-2 yr
Iris stromal pigmentation well developed	6 mo

From Edward DP, Kaufman LM: Anatomy, development, and physiology of the visual system, *Pediatr Clin N Am* 50:1, 2003.

BOX 53–1 Screening Assessments

Reaction to light or visual stimuli to estimate visual function
Craniofacial dysmorphism
Orbits
Eyelids
Lashes
Ocular motility
Globes
Conjunctiva
Sclera
Cornea
Iris
Pupils
Red reflex test

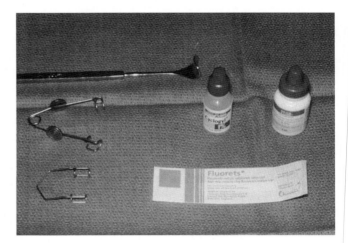

Figure 53–1. Basic equipment for ocular examination: eye speculum or Desmarres retractors, fluorescein strips, 2.5% phenylephrine (ophthalmic), 0.5% cyclopentolate (ophthalmic), and direct ophthalmoscope (not shown).

and white stripes instead of a uniformly gray target. For the test, infants are quickly shown a card that has stripes on one end and a gray target on the opposite end. The examiner watches the infant's eyes to see whether the baby looks right or left to find the stripes. If the infant's visual function is high enough to distinguish the stripes from the gray target, the infant will look consistently toward the stripes. If the infant's visual function is less than the ability to distinguish the stripes from the gray target, the infant will look randomly right or left. By varying the size of the stripes, the examiner can grade the visual acuity equivalent. The disadvantages of this procedure include the number of people necessary to administer the test, the time involved, and the need for the cooperation of an alert infant. 3) Unfortunately, most estimations of an acuity equivalent in the infant rely heavily on adequate motor responses as part of the visual evaluation. Immature or underdeveloped motor systems can reduce or interfere with eye or head movements and decrease the estimation of the visual acuity equivalent. Visual evoked potentials, which measure the electrical cortical responses to

widths can be calibrated, so as to yield a *visual acuity equivalent*. Optokinetic nystagmus can be evident in term newborns.[55] 2) Another quantitative technique to measure a visual acuity equivalent in the infant older than 3 months is *forced preferential looking*.[84] An infant prefers to look at black a visual stimulus, eliminate the need for patient cooperation or motor control.[24] Electrodes are placed over the occipital cortex to monitor activity in the brain as the eyes are visually stimulated with graded stripes or checkerboard patterns, and a computer-averaged tracing is made.

Continuing with the screening eye examination, the general facial configuration and the structure of the orbits are inspected next. Note any facial dysmorphism that could affect ocular health, or be part of an ocular syndrome, such as clefts or abnormal head shape. The orbits should be proportional and symmetric compared with the overall craniofacial configuration. Palpation is performed to examine the orbital margin, the contents of the upper and lower lids, and the round contour of the globes. The orbital rims should be sharply outlined. In the newborn infant, the rims are initially round, and increase in vertical diameter with normal growth. The area of the lacrimal sac is palpated for abnormal masses or increased size by pressing the sac against the bones of the nose and medial orbital wall. Mucopurulent material expressed from the lacrimal puncta is a symptom of obstruction of the nasolacrimal system.

The eyelids are examined grossly and are compared for symmetry of horizontal and vertical placement. Spontaneous opening and closing of the lids should be observed. The lid margins should be inspected for regularity of contour, apposition to the globe, and the presence of lacrimal puncta. The punctum, the proximal opening into the nasolacrimal drainage system, is a minute hole in each lid margin a short distance from the inner corner of the eye. A rapid up-and-down movement of the lid during nursing indicates a jaw-winking phenomenon.[44]

The examiner should view the lashes, which normally are directed outward in an orderly row. Abnormalities include distichiasis, an additional row of lashes posterior to the gray line, and trichiasis, an inward turning of the lashes. Epiblepharon is a common condition of the lower lid in which a horizontal fold of skin rotates the lashes of the lid in toward the eye. Lashes that contact the cornea can cause continued irritation and predispose the eye to infection and abrasion of cornea.

The ocular motor system is evaluated with a motility examination. This includes ocular alignment, conjugate ocular movements, and range of movement. Infants younger than 4 months may show small physiologic misalignments of the eyes. Misaligned eyes beyond the age of 4 months should be considered pathologic.[23]

Alignment is tested with the corneal reflex test (Hirschberg test). The examiner shines a well-focused light at the patient's eyes and notes the spot on the cornea where the light is reflected back. If the patient is properly fixating, the light reflex should appear in the same location on each cornea, slightly nasal to the anatomic center of the cornea. If the light reflex is centered in one eye and deviated laterally in the fellow eye, esotropia is present. If the light reflex is centered in one eye and deviated nasally in the fellow eye, exotropia is present. A positive cover-uncover test will support the impression of strabismus.

If the patient does not appear to move the eyes well enough into the periphery, either spontaneously or by following an object, these movements can be driven by the doll's head maneuver (vestibulo-ocular reflex [VOR]). The reflex is tested by turning the infant's head to one shoulder, producing an opposite movement of the eyes (Fig. 53-2). The eyes appear stationary as the head turns. This reflex may be reduced in severely brain damaged infants but normal in blind infants.[9]

Another rotational reflex is elicited by holding the infant vertically and rotating the infant in an arc around the examiner (Fig. 53-3). The infant's eyes will then tonically rotate in the direction of the spin, with short quick movements (saccades) in the direction opposite the spin. This ocular reflex may be a form of optokinetic nystagmus and is reduced in infants with major defects of the vestibular system, lower motor pathways to the extraocular muscles, visual system, or central nervous system.[9]

Examination of the globes may be difficult owing to inability of the examiner to open the neonates' eyelids sufficiently. Various pediatric eye speculums, such as an Alfonso speculum (Bausch and Lomb, STORZ, San Dimas, CA), can be used to maintain the lids open and allow for adequate inspection of the ocular surface, anterior segment, or posterior segment. Before placing the eye speculum, topical ocular anaesthesia can be achieved with a drop of tetracaine 0.5% eye drops. Oral sucrose can also relieve some of the discomfort of an ocular speculum.[25]

The conjunctiva is inspected after the lids are separated with the use of a pediatric ocular speculum or fingers. The bulbar and palpebral conjunctivae are normally moist and

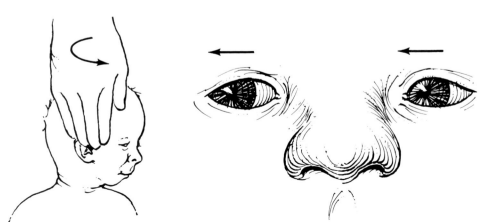

Figure 53–2. Doll's head rotation. As the head is turned toward the shoulder, a tonic neck muscle reflex produces corresponding ocular rotation in the opposite direction as though the eyes were remaining in their original position as the head moves.

Figure 53–3. Rotational nystagmus. The infant's head is inclined slightly forward with eyes open. With rotation, the eyes move in the opposite direction as in doll's eye rotation. When rotation stops, the recovery movement occurs in the reverse direction.

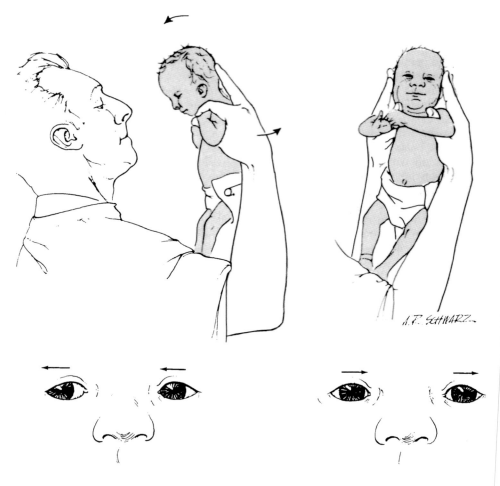

pinkish. Redness or exudate is abnormal and can indicate infection. The conjunctivae of the lids overlying the tarsal plates should be examined after the lids are everted. Eversion is usually simple to perform with the examiner's fingers, particularly if the infant is attempting to squeeze the lids shut.

The normally white sclera is evaluated for changes of color. A bluish coloration, however, is present in premature infants and in other small babies because of their very thin sclera.

The cornea is inspected with a penlight, paying attention to corneal size, shape, clarity, and luster. Magnification with loupes or an ophthalmoscope with the +10-diopter lens in place may be used. During the first few days of life, premature and term infants might demonstrate a slightly hazy cornea, which is thought to be the result of corneal edema. Thereafter, the surface of the cornea should have good luster and be absolutely transparent even to the extreme periphery. Any opacity or translucency is abnormal after the first few days of life, and referral to an ophthalmologist is indicated. Changes in transparency or opacification in the peripheral cornea may be associated with a local mesenchymal abnormality or glaucoma.

The irides are usually similar in appearance. Although normally incomplete for the first 6 months of life, pigmentation of both irides develops simultaneously. In a normal infant, the iris is often blue or blue-gray for the first few weeks or months of life. However, darkly pigmented babies can show pigmentation at birth or within the first week. Heterochromia (dissimilarity in pigmentation between the two eyes or within one eye) can indicate a normal hereditary pattern, congenital Horner syndrome, or one of several syndromes (e.g., Waardenburg) discussed later in this chapter. These syndromes might not become apparent until the end of the neonatal period or even later in life when the iris is fully pigmented.

The pupils should be central, round, and equal in diameter. The pupillary space should be uniformly black. Any amount of a white reflection is abnormal and could indicate an abnormality within the lens, vitreous, or retina. The neonate's pupils are typically miotic in ambient light, perhaps related to prolonged sleep.[38] A penlight or a transilluminator is used to shine a light at each pupil. Beyond a corrected gestational age of 30 weeks, pupils should constrict to both direct and contralateral stimulation.[38] First, the reaction of the illuminated pupil is observed. It should constrict briskly (although the response in the neonate may be slower than in an older child) and should remain constricted as long as the illumination is maintained. If a poor response is observed, the contralateral pupil's reaction is studied. If the contralateral pupil constricts, the directly illuminated eye must have intact photoreceptors and optic nerve pathways. Failure of constriction in the directly illuminated eye in this instance could result from abnormalities in the iris. If neither pupil constricts on direct illumination to one eye, the first eye may be severely deficient in vision.[51]

The swinging flashlight test is used to check for a relative afferent pupillary defect. Normally, if the light is quickly shifted from one eye to the other, the newly illuminated eye's pupil should show an initial small constriction movement. If illumination is maintained on the eye, small rhythmic constriction and dilation movements may follow—called *hippus*, a normal phenomenon. If, however, the shift of light is followed by dilation of the newly stimulated eye, a Marcus Gunn (or relative afferent pupillary defect) is present. This result indicates decreased vision in the eye that inappropriately dilated. Pupillary reflexes should be completely normal in patients with central (cortical) visual impairment.

The red reflex test is an essential part of the infant screening eye examination.[3,87] Examination starts with a +0 diopter setting in the direct ophthalmoscope, and the child is examined at arm's length, with both pupils illuminated (Fig. 53-4). The red reflex of each eye should be clearly distinct, with no shadows or alterations. Look for any asymmetry of the intensity of the red reflex within each pupil and between the two pupils. If a red reflex cannot be seen, the pupils can be dilated with Cyclomydril eye drops[72] (Alcon Laboratories), and if a clear and equal red reflex is still not seen, the baby should be referred to an ophthalmologist.[23]

Precise viewing of the anterior chamber and crystalline lens requires a slit-lamp examination, instrumentation that is usually not available to the neonatologist or primary care physician. An indirect assessment of the clarity of the cornea, anterior chamber, lens, and vitreous is performed during the red reflex test, which measures the ability of light to enter the eye and reflect back out of the eye off the retina. Similarly, the red reflex test indirectly assesses the intactness of the retina. The adventurous neonatologist or primary care physician can attempt direct viewing of the infant's retina with a direct ophthalmoscope. Viewing the retina of the undilated infant's eye with a direct ophthalmoscope is a challenge, even to the pediatric ophthalmologist. If a view of the retina is required, such as for retinopathy of prematurity screening, the consulting ophthalmologist would dilate the infant's eyes and use more sophisticated examination instrumentation such as the indirect ophthalmoscope.

Certainly, the use of the direct ophthalmoscope to directly view the retina is not considered part of the screening eye examination in the infant.[64] However, if a direct ophthalmoscope examination is attempted, attention should be directed to the clarity of the vitreous cavity and the appearance of the optic disc, major retinal vessels, the macula, and the surrounding retina.

NORMAL OCULAR FINDINGS

The eye of the newborn infant differs from the adult eye primarily in function, although structural differences also exist.[16] The growth of the eye, which parallels that of the brain, continues at a rapid rate for the first 3 years of life, especially during the first year. The anteroposterior dimension of the eye at birth is about 16.5 mm and grows to about 24 mm in adulthood. Normal values in the neonate fall within a very wide range. Suspected abnormalities in size often are substantiated only by comparison with measured values in the fellow eye or by ultrasound, computed tomography (CT), or magnetic resonance imaging (MRI). The horizontal and vertical diameters of the cornea of the newborn are about 9 to 10 mm. Enlarged corneas suggest the diagnosis of congenital glaucoma.

The lid fissures of the term infant are usually narrow and often widely separated horizontally by prominent epicanthal folds. Normal horizontal measurement of the lid fissures in the newborn can range from 17 to 27 mm (Table 53-2). These measurements should be symmetric. The term *telecanthus* indicates a disproportionate increase in the distance between the medial canthal angles. It is particularly noticeable in fetal alcohol syndrome and Waardenburg syndrome. Measurements between the two medial canthi in the term newborn vary from 18 to 22 mm. *Hypertelorism* is defined as an increase in distance between the orbits, observed clinically as a large interpupillary distance, which is often seen in many craniofacial syndromes. A secondary telecanthus is observed in patients with hypertelorism.

Reflex tearing to irritants is evident shortly after birth. However, emotional tearing begins at about 3 weeks of age and is developed at 2 to 3 months. The newborn infant possesses a strong blink reflex in response to light and to stimulation of the lids, lashes, or cornea. The reflex response to a threatening gesture does not appear until 7 or 8 weeks of age in the term infant. Repetitive eye opening is evident at birth.[33]

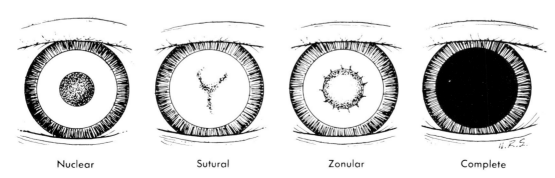

| Nuclear | Sutural | Zonular | Complete |

Figure 53–4. Appearance of the red reflex with various types of cataracts. The normal eye has a clear, round red reflex. Lens opacities (cataracts) interrupt the red reflex, producing the black shadows.

TABLE 53–2 Normal Ocular Measurements		
	TERM NEONATE	PREMATURE*
Measurement	*(mm)*	*(mm)*
Intermediate canthal distance	18-22	12-16
Medial canthus to lateral canthus	17-27	12-16
Anteroposterior diameter of eye at birth	16	10-16
Horizontal diameter of cornea	10 (average), 9 (lower limits)	7.5-8 (lower limits)

*Neonates weighing 1000 to 1300 g.

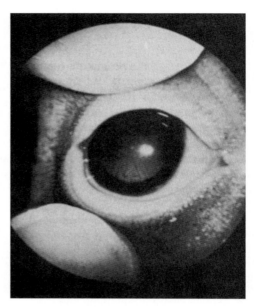

Figure 53–5. Persistent pupillary membrane in a premature infant. Notice the remnants of vascular loops of the anterior hyaloid system anterior to the lens. They will continue to atrophy during the first months of extrauterine life.

After birth, the eyes should appear straight for the most part, although erratic, purposeless, and independent movements can be observed during the first few months of life. Any constant strabismus beyond the age of 4 months requires further evaluation.[4] Conjugate horizontal gaze should be evident in the newborn; vertical conjugate gaze develops by 2 months of age. Convergence spasms are a normal transient phenomenon of infancy.

The ability to maintain a steady gaze or to fixate and follow an object is only weakly initiated at 4 to 6 weeks of age. At first, the eyes pursue a moving visual stimulus with short saccades. By 3 months of age, the infant can fixate and follow in both vertical and horizontal directions. At about 4 months of age, central fixation is associated with the motor activity of grasping. Binocular vision is present at about 6 months of age.

Prematurity

The ocular findings of the premature infant differ from those of the term neonate. At 28 weeks of gestation, the globe is only 10 to 14 mm in diameter. The anterior and posterior hyaloid vascular systems are usually present to some degree, although their involution continues for the next several months (Fig. 53-5). Remnants of this system may be seen in the form of persistent blood vessels or fibrous strands anterior and posterior to the lens. The main hyaloid artery coursing from the optic disc to the posterior lens surface may be patent or appears as a white strand in the vitreous. A moderate amount of vitreous haze is often present at this time, interfering with visualization of the fundus.

Vascularization of the retina begins with the ophthalmic artery entering the eye through the posterior edge of the eye's embryonic fissure at 4 months of gestation. Retinal vessels then grow anteriorly to vascularize the peripheral retina, a process that is not complete until near term. Thus, premature infants have incomplete retinal vascularization, creating the basis for retinopathy of prematurity.

Pupil constriction to light is not seen until 30 weeks of gestational age.[38] Lack of pupil response to light should not be considered abnormal until at least 32 weeks after conception.

Premature infants have a higher incidence of myopia, amblyopia, and strabismus in childhood. Careful follow-up of all children born prematurely is advisable to ensure early detection of these ocular conditions.

REQUESTING OPHTHALMOLOGIC CONSULTATION

Routine ophthalmologic consultation for all infants in the nursery is not warranted.[23] Pathologic ocular findings in normal neonates are sufficiently unusual that evaluation should be requested only after a screening ocular examination indicates the presence of an abnormality or for patients who for some reason are at increased risk for ocular problems. Indications for ophthalmologic consultation include a family history of congenital cataracts, retinoblastoma, congenital glaucoma, or other serious ocular diseases. Intrauterine infectious disease such as rubella, toxoplasmosis, or cytomegalovirus necessitates a thorough eye evaluation. For preterm infants, ophthalmologic consultation is necessary to exclude retinopathy of prematurity.

ORBITAL ABNORMALITIES

The contents of the orbit are confined to a conical shape by its bony walls. At the posterior apex of the orbit, the extraocular muscles originate, and the vascular and nerve structures enter the orbit. The bone structures of the lateral wall do not protect the orbital contents as far anteriorly as do the remaining sides of the orbit, which leaves the eye more susceptible to trauma on its lateral side. In the neonate, the orbital rims form a circular outline at the anterior base of the cone. Box 53-2 lists systemic syndromes with orbital abnormalities.

BOX 53–2	Syndromes Associated with Abnormal Orbits

HYPOTELORISM
Cebocephaly
Oculodentodigital dysplasia
Trisomy 13
Scaphocephaly
HYPERTELORISM
Cerebral gigantism
Cerebrohepatorenal syndrome
Chromosome deletions
Craniosynostosis
Frontonasal dysplasia and median cleft face syndrome
Infantile hypercalcemia
Smith-Lemli-Opitz syndrome
Isolated finding

The terms *proptosis, exophthalmos,* and *exorbitism* are often used interchangeably to describe forwardly displaced eyes. In the strictest sense, proptosis results from an increase in orbital contents within a normal bony orbit, exophthalmos from Graves disease, and exorbitism from shallow bony orbits.

Proptosis

The diagnosis of proptosis can be confirmed if the examiner observes the infant's eyes and lids from above, over the prominence of the eyebrows. A more anterior protrusion of the orbital contents is observed in comparison with the opposite side. In proptosis, the eye frequently also has a widened palpebral fissure.

Masses within the orbital cavity can expand most easily anteriorly, producing proptosis. Those located within the cone of extraocular muscles produce a symmetric anterior displacement, whereas tumors located outside the cone of extraocular muscles displace the eye outward and away from the area of origin of the tumor. A tumor in the inferior portion of the orbit displaces the eye upward and forward, whereas one located medially displaces the eye laterally and forward. A diffuse, extensive tumor can produce sufficient changes to affect the eye's movement, whereas a localized tumor often does not interfere with rotation of the eye. If a tumor is located anterior to the equator of the globe, it can extend anteriorly into the lids without producing proptosis.

An orbital encephalocele or meningocele producing proptosis may be evident at birth or may be delayed until later years. This abnormality results from a defect in the wall between the cranial cavity and the orbit, usually located at the suture lines. Pressure within the cranium causes herniation of brain tissue, meninges, or both into the orbit, most often at the inner angle of the orbit at the root of the nose. Diagnosis is made by identifying the bone defect in association with the area of the orbital cyst. Clinically, an encephalocele is suggested by the presence of a pulsating, fluctuant cyst that can be reduced somewhat with digital pressure or that increases with coughing or crying. Excessive manipulation of the encephalocele can cause pulse and respirations to

slow or can cause convulsions. Neurosurgical consultation and intervention are necessary.

Proptosis also can occur from venous engorgement of the orbital cavity such as that produced by a carotid-cavernous fistula. A cephalic bruit is often heard in the infant but is not pathognomonic of a carotid-cavernous sinus fistula.

A false diagnosis of proptosis might be made when there is a slight ptosis of one eye, which gives the opposite, normal eye an appearance of a wide palpebral fissure. Marked enlargement of the eye, as in congenital glaucoma or high myopia, makes the eye appear proptotic because of the increased size of the globe. Facial abnormalities that produce shallow orbits, as in Crouzon disease, simulate proptosis because the normal amount of orbital structure appears to protrude in an abnormally shallow orbit

Hyperthyroid Exophthalmos

Hyperthyroid exophthalmos, a rare neonatal sequela of hyperthyroidism, can occur as the result of maternal Graves disease during the last trimester of pregnancy. The infant is born with classic hyperthyroidism, including exophthalmos, upper lid retraction, and extraocular muscle involvement. Symptoms usually subside during the first 2 months of life.[28]

Enophthalmos

Enophthalmos refers to eyes that look sunken into the orbit. Causes in infants include orbital asymmetry, microphthalmos, trauma resulting in an orbital blow-out fracture, congenital fibrosis of the extraocular muscles, and congenital Horner syndrome.[12] Numerous syndromes, and many infants with unclassifiable facial dysmorphisms, feature deep set eyes, such as Lowe syndrome, Cockayne syndrome and Cornelia de Lange syndrome.

Ocular Hypotelorism or Hypertelorism

Abnormal spatial relationships between the two orbits create excessively wide or excessively narrow intraorbital distances.[54] These abnormalities are caused by a variety of related cranial abnormalities involving the disproportionate growth or lack of development of the body and lesser wing of the sphenoid and ethmoid sinuses and of the maxillary processes. Hypotelorism (narrowing of the intraorbital distance) may be associated with central nervous system malformation.

Ocular hypertelorism is a term indicating increased separation between the bony orbits, usually greater than 2 standard deviations above the mean. It is an anatomic description rather than a diagnostic entity, and is noted with varying severity in many syndromes such as the craniosynostosis syndromes. One condition with marked hypertelorism is frontonasal dysplasia (median facial cleft syndrome), which may be the result of morphokinetic arrest during embryogenesis. Characteristic findings of frontonasal dysplasia are medial cleft nose, lip, and palate, widow's peak, and cranium bifidum occultum. Common other ocular abnormalities include exotropia, dacryostenosis, epibulbar dermoids, palpebral fissure changes, and optic atrophy.[77]A phenotypically similar but probably distinct clinical entity within the fronto-nasal dysplasia spectrum has been reported with the features of facial midline defects, basal encephalocele, callosal agenesis, endocrine dwarfism, and morning glory disc anomaly.[75]

EYELID ABNORMALITIES
Colobomas

Colobomas of the lids are partial-thickness or complete defects that can range from a small notching of the lid borders to involvement of the entire length of the lid. Most lid colobomas occur in the medial aspect of the upper lid (Fig. 53-6). When the lower lid is involved, the defect is more often in its lateral aspects. The cause of lid colobomas is often unknown unless associated with a craniofacial syndrome. It has been suggested that these isolated colobomas arise from the localized failure of adhesion of the lid folds that results in a lag of growth, or from mechanical effects of amniotic bands. Syndromes with associated lower lid colobomas are mandibulofacial dysostosis (Treacher Collins syndrome), Goldenhar syndrome (more often upper lid), amniotic band syndrome, and Burn-McKeown syndrome.[99]

The treatment of lid colobomas is important when the lid defect prevents adequate lid closure and allows exposure of the cornea. Subsequent thickening, opacification, infection, ulceration, or perforation of the unprotected cornea can occur. Vision can be degraded by the amblyopia that develops. Early surgical correction is often required when the coloboma is greater than one third of the eyelid margin.[81]

Congenital Blepharophimosis

The term *blepharophimosis* describes eyelids that are too narrow horizontally and vertically (Fig. 53-7). There is usually an associated ptosis, and strabismus is frequently present. Lid fissure measurements commonly are reduced to about two thirds of normal, whereas the space between the medial canthi is considerably widened. Surgical repair to widen the medial and lateral canthal angles, elevate the upper lid, and correct the strabismus is available.

Blepharophimosis can occur in isolation, as a feature of BPES (blepharophimosis, ptosis, and epicanthus inversus syndrome), or in multiple systemic syndromes such as fetal alcohol syndrome, Saethre-Chotzen syndrome, and van den Ende-Gupta syndrome. BPES has been mapped to the *FOXL2* gene encoding a fork head transcription factor. BPES is divided into type 1 and type 2, with and without premature ovarian failure, respectively.[5]

Epicanthus

Epicanthus is the most commonly encountered lid abnormality. A skin fold originating in the upper lid extends over the medial end of the upper lid, the medial canthus and the caruncle, and ends in the skin of the lower lid. It gradually disappears with the growth of the bridge of the nose as the child loses its baby face. Epicanthal folds can give a false appearance of crossed eyes (pseudostrabismus). Epicanthus inversus is similar except that the predominance of the skin fold arises in the lower lid and runs diagonally upward toward the root of the nose to overlie the medial canthus. These folds are benign and generally do not require treatment.

Congenital Ectropion, Entropion, and Epiblepharon

Congenital ectropion is an eversion of the lid margin, most commonly of the lower lid. It may be associated with other eye abnormalities or syndromes such as Duane syndrome. If the ectropion is mild, no treatment is necessary. A more severely everted lid might require surgical correction. The integrity of the cornea requires monitoring and will determine the treatment.

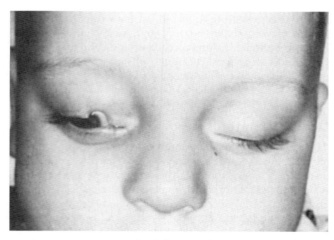

Figure 53–6. Atypical coloboma of the right upper lid.

Figure 53–7. Congenital blepharophimosis, ptosis, and epicanthus inversus (bilateral).

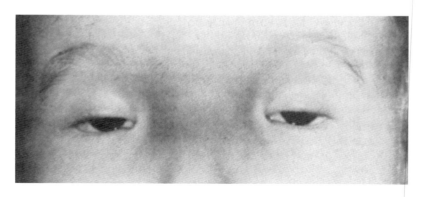

Often associated with other lid or ocular abnormalities, congenital entropion is an in-turning of the lid margin, most often of the lower lid. If the lashes on the lid margin rub the cornea and cause corneal abrasions, surgery is necessary.

Epiblepharon is an extra fold of skin along the lower lid that can cause lashes to turn inward. This condition usually requires no treatment and is most often seen in infants of Asian ancestry. This condition usually improves spontaneously during the first 4 years of life, but if it persists, consideration should be given to surgical correction.[12a]

Blepharoptosis

Blepharoptosis, often shortened to *ptosis*, is defined as an upper lid that cannot or does not rise to a normal level (Fig. 53-8). When looking straight ahead, the normal lid should elevate to a point at least midway between the pupil and the upper margin of the cornea. Neonates may have a transient self-limited droopy or closed lid as a result of facial edema or lid trauma during normal vaginal delivery. A temporary, simulated ptosis (protective ptosis or guarding) can result from irritation or infection of the cornea or conjunctiva.

Congenital ptosis most often results from the dysfunction of the levator palpebrae muscle, mostly seen as an idiopathic or familial disorder. Although occlusion of the pupil is rare, the ptotic lid can induce a corneal astigmatism and refractive amblyopia. Occlusive patching and glasses may be needed.

Mild, unilateral ptosis should prompt a comparison of pupil size to evaluate for Horner syndrome. Congenital Horner syndrome is often a result of trauma at birth, although it may be associated with mediastinal disease or neuroblastoma. The involved iris may be hypopigmented.

Ptosis also may be associated with a jaw-winking phenomenon. This syndrome is caused by anomalous motor innervation of the levator palpebrae muscle from nerve twigs to the pterygoid, masseter, or lingual muscles. The affected patient has an up-and-down rhythmic movement of the upper lid during nursing activity. The jaw-winking portion of the syndrome is thought to decrease or disappear in early adulthood, but the ptosis remains. Many surgical procedures have been designed to mitigate the ptosis.

Two forms of myasthenia gravis can produce ptosis in the neonatal period. In about 15% of neonates born to mothers with myasthenia gravis, a transient form of myasthenia occurs shortly after birth. Affected children have a weak cry and poor suck and can develop weakness in all muscle groups. Ocular symptoms are rare and most commonly involve ptosis.[31] A variety of congenital myasthenia syndromes linked to genetic disorders of the neuromuscular junction or acetylcholine production can display ptosis and ophthalmoparesis, which are often variable and related to the level of fatigue.

Pseudoptosis, or false ptosis, may be apparent when the globes are of different sizes or if enophthalmos or proptosis is present. Microphthalmia is a common congenital defect that can be mildly expressed. In such situations, the lid will look drooped even if it is functioning properly. A unilateral large globe due to monocular myopia can produce a relative ptosis in the contralateral normal eye.

EYELASH ABNORMALITIES

Excessive eyelash growth can result, as a side effect, from multiple medications, including topical prostaglandin analogues and epidermal growth factor receptor inhibitors.[18] The term *distichiasis* describes an additional row of lashes posterior to the center of the lid margin. This condition usually results in contact of the lashes with the cornea, producing corneal irritation and abrasions. Trichiasis is a lash that grows from a normal location but is misdirected toward the ocular surface.

Hypertrichosis

Excessive hair on the lids and forehead can occur as a dominant characteristic in male infants and, on occasion, may be extreme. Hypertrichosis involving the eyebrows, forehead, and upper lid appears in the Cornelia de Lange syndrome, a pathologic dwarfism associated with multiple congenital anomalies. Hypertrichosis lanuginosa is transmitted as an autosomal dominant condition. The fetal lanugo persists into adult life, creating an abundant covering of hair on the eyebrows, forehead, eyelids, and other areas of the body.

LACRIMAL ABNORMALITIES
Watery Eye

Epiphora (excess tearing) usually does not occur until after the first 3 weeks of life, when the major portion of the lacrimal gland has become functional. Although the usual cause of epiphora is a blockage of the nasolacrimal ducts (dacryostenosis), the possibility of congenital glaucoma is the most important consideration in the differential diagnosis. Less commonly, tearing can result from an obstruction of the common canaliculus, from congenital absence of the lid puncta, or from dacryocystitis. Congenital absence of the entire lacrimal drainage apparatus is extremely rare. Reflex tearing may be produced by any stimulation of the fifth cranial nerve. Epiphora can occur as the result of corneal abrasion, corneal foreign body, or nasal and facial lesions that irritate the fifth cranial nerve. Chronic nasal congestion also may produce epiphora by mechanically blocking the nasolacrimal duct.

Dacryostenosis may be present in up to 7% of neonates and creates a stagnant pooling of tears in the lacrimal sac that contributes to chronic or recurrent dacryocystitis. The inflammation is marked by a purulent exudate in the medial

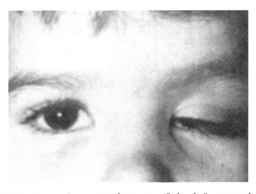

Figure 53–8. Congenital ptosis of the left upper lid.

canthal area of the conjunctiva. Severe dacryocystitis can produce swelling and induration of the lacrimal sac medial and inferior to the medial canthus.

Treatment of mild nasolacrimal infection consists of topical antibiotic drops or ointment. If surrounding cellulitis is suspected, systemic administration of medication and locally applied heat may be required. Repeated massage of the lacrimal sac at the medial canthal area serves to flush out the stagnant tears, decrease the risk for infection, and "pop" open the nasolacrimal obstruction. If the epiphora continues, a lacrimal probe passed through the nasolacrimal duct to the nose usually creates an adequate opening. Probing before 6 months of age is sometimes performed in an office setting under topical anesthesia with the baby swaddled in a sheet. In children with extensive purulent discharge and frequent infections, office probing can be considered as early as 2 months of age.

In more than 90% of children with congenital dacryostenosis, the obstructions spontaneously correct during the first year of life. If persistent, treatment is then offered, but requires general anesthesia because these children are too large to swaddle for an office probing. Surgical options include simple probing, silicone tube intubation, or balloon dilation of the lacrimal system.[53]

Dacryocystocele

A congenital dacryocystocele presents within the first week of life as a bluish mass adjacent to the medial canthus. The distended lacrimal sac is filled with clear fluid, feels firm or fluctuant to palpation, and does not pulsate like a frontal encephalocele. Initiating oral antibiotics is recommended as soon as a dacryocystocele is identified to prevent infection of the dacryocystocele, which can occur in up to two thirds of these patients.[101] If the patient presents with signs of a dacryocele infection, admission to a pediatric intensive care unit for intravenous antibiotics is required. Surgical treatment with a nasolacrimal probing should be considered within the next 2 to 4 days.

Dry Eye

The normal newborn will have moist eyes from basal secretion of tears. Reflex tearing from ocular irritation or psychogenic (emotional) tearing may not develop for weeks to months after birth. Infants do not usually have symptoms from dry eyes unless in rare conditions such as alacrima from a congenital lack of tear glands or Riley-Day syndrome. Recognition of alacrima in the infant is important in preventing corneal abrasions, infections, and perforations, the inevitable sequelae of dry eye. During the first month of life, an infant with alacrima from any cause might not appear different from the normal infant because tear production is minimal during this period. The usual time of discovery is at 6 to 12 months of age after the lack of tears has produced changes such as scarring or ulceration of the cornea.

At 1 to 2 months of age, early symptoms of dry eye are conjunctival hyperemia and photophobia. Instead of the ample tears expected with conjunctival irritation, a sticky mucoid secretion is produced, and the cornea shows punctate

staining with fluorescein solution application. Treatment includes frequent use of artificial tears (as often as every 15 to 30 minutes), punctal occlusion, or tarsorrhaphy.

Isolated congenital lack of tears, usually bilateral, is a rare anomaly. The cause is unknown, but it has been suggested to result from hypoplasia of the lacrimal gland or from an absence of innervation of the lacrimal gland structures.

The ocular findings in familial dysautonomia (Riley-Day syndrome) are characteristic and can produce the initial criteria for diagnosis. They include alacrima and corneal anesthesia. These ocular changes and constriction of the pupil by instillation of 0.125% pilocarpine should establish the diagnosis. The onset of major systemic symptoms occurs when the child is about 2 years old. An abnormal swallowing mechanism, inappropriate blood pressure and respiratory control, decreased sensitivity to pain, deficient taste perception, and abnormal ocular findings in this syndrome are the result of sympathetic, parasympathetic, and sensory neuronal abnormalities. Additional ocular findings are myopia, anisometropia (different refractive error in the two eyes), exotropia, tortuosity of the retinal vessels, and occasionally ptosis. Familial dysautonomia results from a mutation in the *IKBKAP* gene encoding elongation protein 1, resulting in defective splicing.[66]

GLOBE ABNORMALITIES
Anophthalmia

Anophthalmia is a rare sporadic phenomenon in which there is total absence or a minute rudiment of the globe, and it can present either unilaterally or bilaterally. It occurs as a developmental failure of the optic vesicle. It is often accompanied by other congenital anomalies, such as central nervous system defects and mental retardation, and has been observed in isolation, in genetic defects (e.g., *SOX2, STRA6, PAX6* genes), and in chromosomal syndromes (e.g., trisomy 13).[96] Because lid formation does not depend on ocular formation, the lids are fully formed. However, the lids remain closed and can be partially fused, and they are smaller and sunken without the support of the eye.

Treatment involves reconstruction of the orbit to improve the appearance of the face. Plastic molds of the conjunctival sac of gradually enlarging sizes are used to stretch the lids and sac sufficiently to hold an ocular prosthesis. In unilateral situations, orbital reconstruction using tissue expanders can dramatically improve the overall facial appearance.

Cryptophthalmia

In cryptophthalmia, the eyelids fail to cleave, and uninterrupted skin runs from the forehead to the malar area. The eyelids and eyelashes usually are absent; however, the eye can be palpated beneath the skin and might even be observed to move with the stimulation of a strong light.

The anterior segment of the eye is invariably disorganized into fibrovascular tissue adherent to the subcuticular tissue of the lids. Because the conjunctival sac is absent or small, attempts to separate the lids from the ocular structures are usually unsuccessful, and surgical correction is not advisable

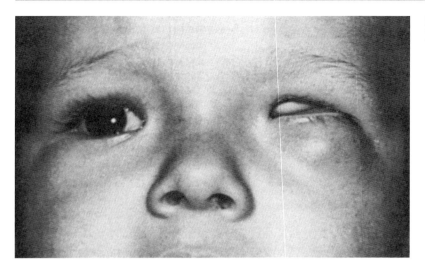

Figure 53–9. Congenital microphthalmia with a large cyst of the left eye.

in most circumstances. Although a globe is present, only rarely is vision obtainable.

Cryptophthalmia is frequently associated with systemic abnormalities such as urogenital malformations (Fraser syndrome) linked to defects of the *FRAS1* and *FREM2* genes, and a thorough genetic evaluation is indicated.[37,95]

Microphthalmia

Microphthalmia describes a variety of conditions in which the axial length of the neonatal eye is less than two thirds of the normal 16 mm. Causes include familial, syndromic, and chromosomal abnormalities and environmental influences during gestation. Simple microphthalmia is a condition in which there is an abnormally small eye but with intact internal organization. It may be associated with other ocular features of importance: a high degree of hypermetropia, retinal folds, a tendency for choroidal effusions, and the late occurrence of glaucoma.[98]

Complex microphthalmia describes small eyes with internal disorganization, such as anterior segment dysgenesis, cataract, coloboma, or persistent fetal vasculature.[97] Colobomatous microphthalmia occurs when the embryonic cleft of the optic vesicle fails to close. Typically, this form is associated with other ocular anomalies such as colobomas of the iris, ciliary body, fundus, or optic nerve, or colobomatous orbital cysts.

Microphthalmia can also be associated with other ocular and systemic syndromes, including intrauterine infections such as rubella and cytomegalovirus, craniofacial anomalies, anterior segment dysgenesis syndromes, or chromosomal abnormalities. Because of the heterogenicity of associated findings, infants with microphthalmia should be evaluated by both an ophthalmologist and geneticist.

Large Eye

An abnormally enlarged eye in the neonatal period is rare but is extremely important to recognize. An apparently enlarged eye may be caused by colobomatous microphthalmia with an associated large cyst (Fig. 53-9), congenital megalocornea (see later), or congenital glaucoma (see later). Colobomatous microphthalmia results when the embryonic optic vesicle fails to close. Tissue that originally should have become intraocular is encased in a cystic structure outside the eye in the orbit. If the cyst becomes sufficiently large that proptosis occurs, the microphthalmic eye simulates an enlarged eye.

SCLERA ABNORMALITIES

The normal term neonate has a glistening white sclera. The overlying conjunctiva and the conjunctival vessels superimpose a filmy, vascular pattern. A generalized bluish discoloration of the underdeveloped sclera is normal in premature infants. Rarely, a congenital weakness in a small area of the sclera produces a bluish bulge called a *staphyloma*. The light-blue color is caused by thinness of the sclera that transmits the darker color of the underlying uveal tissue. Osteogenesis imperfecta may be associated with a similar bluish discoloration of the sclera in the term neonate because of inadequately developed scleral collagen. Blue sclera may also be seen in other systemic diseases such as Marfan syndrome, Ehlers-Danlos syndrome, and Crouzon syndrome.

Pigmentation of the conjunctiva and sclera is common in darkly pigmented people. Intrascleral nerve loops appear as darkly pigmented dots about 3 to 4 mm from the limbus. Congenital ocular melanosis and oculodermal melanosis (nevus of Ota) occur as a unilateral slate-blue pigmentation in infancy.

CORNEA ABNORMALITIES
Cloudy Cornea

The normal premature infant might have a slightly hazy cornea for the first few weeks of life, caused by temporary excess hydration of the cornea. In the normal term infant, a similar appearance may be seen for the first 48 hours after delivery.

A persistently hazy or cloudy cornea suggests congenital glaucoma or birth injury. Anterior segment dysgenesis syndromes, corneal dystrophies, infection, or systemic disease should also be considered.

Enlarged Cornea

Most newborn infants have a corneal diameter of about 9 to 10 mm. If this measurement exceeds 12 mm, congenital glaucoma must be considered, especially if corneal haze, tearing, and photophobia are present.

Megalocornea is an enlarged cornea exceeding 13 mm in diameter. The cornea is usually clear, with distinct margins and thin iris stroma. There are no other features of congenital glaucoma, such as elevated intraocular pressure, tearing, photophobia, or conjunctival injection. Megalocornea as an isolated finding is usually inherited in an autosomal dominant manner. Megalophthalmia, which is commonly inherited as an X-linked recessive trait, is characterized by deep anterior chambers, subluxation of the lens, hypoplastic iris, and cataract formation in early adult life.

A corneal diameter of less than 10 mm may be an isolated finding or may be associated with other ocular anomalies. Cases of autosomal dominant and recessive inheritance of microcornea have been described.

Anterior Segment Dysgenesis Syndromes

A wide spectrum of clinical findings is observed in the anterior segment dysgenesis syndromes, including abnormalities of the cornea, anterior chamber, iris, and lens. Corneal opacities, adhesions of the iris, and glaucoma can occur. Although a continuous spectrum of findings can be evident in a family pedigree, or between the two eyes of one patient, eyes are often assigned into the distinct subgroups of posterior embryotoxon, Axenfeld anomaly, Rieger anomaly, or Peters anomaly.

Corneal Dystrophies

Most corneal dystrophies become apparent in adolescence or early adult life. However, congenital hereditary endothelial dystrophy may be present at birth. This condition is characterized by bilateral cloudy corneas, normal corneal diameter, and normal intraocular pressure. Early cornea transplantation may be helpful, but the prognosis is guarded.

Corneal Manifestations of Systemic Disease

Corneal opacities and haze can occur because of inborn errors of metabolism. Most are not associated with corneal opacities in the neonatal period. Systemic diseases that cause corneal opacities include the mucopolysaccharidoses, mucolipidoses, Fabry disease, hypophosphatasia, cystinosis, and Wilson disease.

CONGENITAL GLAUCOMA

Although congenital glaucoma is uncommon, the devastating effects of uncontrolled ocular pressure are sufficiently important to keep this disease uppermost in the mind of the examining physician. The classic symptoms of congenital glaucoma include epiphora, photophobia, and blepharospasm. As the disease progresses, the increased intraocular pressure produces stretching of the eye, creating an increased corneal diameter greater than 12 mm (buphthalmos, Fig. 53-10), cloudy cornea, progressive myopia, and loss of vision. Symptoms can be apparent at birth or weeks to months later.

Congenital glaucoma can occur as a primary disease or secondary to numerous other ocular conditions or systemic syndromes. A list of diseases associated with congenital glaucoma is shown in Box 53-3.

In addition to visual impairment from glaucomatous damage, amblyopia from visual deprivation or anisometropia can prevent a successful visual outcome. The prognosis depends on the age of onset, time to diagnosis, and associated ocular and systemic conditions.

IRIS ABNORMALITIES
Aniridia

Aniridia (absence of the iris) is a rare congenital anomaly, usually bilateral, that is almost invariably associated with poor vision and nystagmus. A small rudimentary cuff of peripheral iris can be observed grossly or microscopically. Associated ocular findings include glaucoma, corneal pannus, cataract, abnormal optic discs, and foveal hypoplasia. Because the fovea subserves our best vision, its maldevelopment causes the nystagmus and poor visual acuity.

Aniridia is caused by a defect in the *PAX6* gene on chromosome 11 at 11p13.[33] *WAGR* syndrome, a contiguous gene syndrome, results from a larger deletion in the area that involves the Wilms tumor gene (*WT1*), and includes Wilms

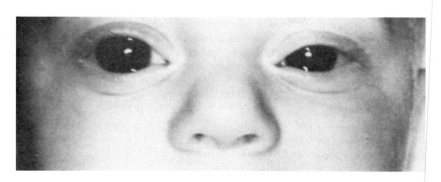

Figure 53–10. Bilateral congenital glaucoma with buphthalmos, with the right eye larger than the left.

SEEN IN ISOLATED (CONGENITAL) CONDITIONS
Aniridia
Rubella syndrome
Hallermann-Streiff syndrome
Lowe syndrome
Axenfeld or Rieger syndrome
Sturge-Weber syndrome

UNCOMMONLY SEEN IN THESE CONDITIONS
Chromosome abnormalities
Down syndrome
Homocystinuria
Marfan syndrome
Neurofibromatosis
Ocular-dental-digital syndrome
Persistent hyperplastic primary vitreous
Rubinstein-Taybi syndrome
Weill-Marchesani syndrome

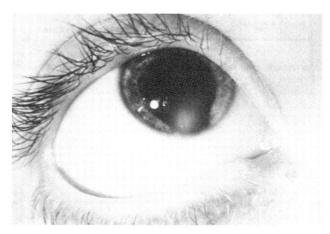

Figure 53–11. Typical iris coloboma with an inferonasal iris defect.

tumor, aniridia, genitourinary abnormalities, and mental retardation.[22]

All infants with nonfamilial aniridia should undergo chromosomal analysis to detect small deletions; if a deletion exists, the infant should be carefully monitored for early detection of Wilms tumor.[49]

Coloboma

Iris coloboma is one of the most common congenital abnormalities of the eye. It can occur as a single ocular finding, have a mendelian mode of inheritance, be associated with a chromosomal abnormality, or be associated with other malformation syndromes (Box 53-4). Typical colobomas occur in the inferonasal quadrant, where the embryonic fissure closes (Fig. 53-11). Because typical iris colobomas result from an abnormal closure of the embryonic fissure, they also may be associated with a coloboma of the ciliary body, fundus, or optic nerve. Associated microphthalmia is common. When the optic nerve or macula is involved in the coloboma, visual difficulty occurs. It is always wise to evaluate the fundus for a pathologic condition when an iris coloboma is detected.

Atypical iris colobomas occur away from the inferonasal quadrant. Atypical colobomas, which vary from a small notch in the pupil to the absence of an entire segment of the iris, are not usually associated with visual difficulties.

Coloboma of the iris, uvea, or retina, with or without microphthalmia, is a feature of CHARGE association.

Persistent Pupillary Membrane

Persistent pupillary membranes are common in the neonate, particularly in the premature infant. The membranes are remnants of the anterior fetal vascular supply of the lens that failed to atrophy in the seventh month of gestation. If these persistent vessels adhere to the lens, a localized cataract can form.

Iris Heterochromia

Heterochromia indicates a difference in pigmentation in the irides. For example, one eye may have a blue iris, and the other iris may be brown; or one iris may have a wedge of lighter or darker pigmentation. The heterochromia itself does not affect ocular health or vision but may secondarily result from other pathologic ocular conditions, such as trauma or inflammations.

Heterochromia can occur as an isolated autosomal dominant trait. It also is associated with several syndromes such as Waardenburg syndrome. Congenital Horner syndrome produces heterochromia, usually after the neonatal period, resulting from the failure of normal pigmentation to develop in the iris on the sympathetically denervated side. Aganglionic megacolon (Hirschsprung disease) can also be associated with iris heterochromia.

Congenital colobomatous microphthalmia
CHARGE association
Trisomy 13
Trisomy 18
Rieger syndrome
Iris coloboma and anal atresia syndrome
Lowe syndrome (infrequent)
Rubinstein-Taybi syndrome (uncommon)
Multiple chromosome anomalies

CHARGE, *coloboma, heart anomaly, choanal atresia, retardation, genital
anomaly, ear anomaly.*

ABNORMAL RED REFLEX

This is one of the most important abnormalities that requires immediate evaluation. The term *leukocoria* is used to describe a white pupil seen by the naked eye or during the red reflex test. Leukocoria is not a diagnosis but rather a description of an observation. Because the infant sleeps much of the time and because the pupils are small, a white pupil often is not noticed until the infant becomes more alert and active. False-positive red reflex test results are commonly due to small pupils, shifting gaze, limited patient cooperation, poor illumination from the ophthalmoscope, and examiner inexperience. Regardless, these patients should be over-referred to the ophthalmologist to ascertain the true-positive results.

Causes of leukocoria in infants include opacities of the cornea, lens, and vitreous, as well as retinal diseases such as retinoblastoma, chorioretinal coloboma, persistent hyperplastic primary vitreous, endophthalmitis, Coats disease, congenital retinal fold, retinoschisis, or scarring from ROP.

Abnormal red reflexes can also result from misaligned eye or from high or asymmetric refractive errors.

LENS ABNORMALITIES

Cataract

The size and shape of a cataract depends on the area of the lens that is being formed at the time the damage or developmental defects occur. The lens grows continuously during life, laying down new lens fibers on its external surface much as an onion does. Damage that occurs in the early embryonic period produces opacifications in the center of the lens. Such nuclear cataracts have clear layers in the periphery of the lens. Later periods of damage produce ringlike opacifications surrounded by central and peripheral clear areas (zonular cataracts). Recent damage produces peripheral opacifications near the surface of the lens (cortical cataracts). Dense opacities near the central axis cause greater visual disturbance, especially if they are located in the central visual axis.

Cataracts may be grouped according to cause: idiopathic, genetic, viral, inborn errors of metabolism, trauma, association with other eye malformations, and generalized syndromes. However, most congenital cataracts are genetic or isolated and idiopathic. A list of causes of juvenile cataracts is shown in Table 53-3.

Genetically determined cataracts often are isolated abnormalities and bilateral. Many genetic loci have been mapped.[80] The lens opacities are often present at birth but occasionally become evident later in childhood. The primary mode of transmission is autosomal dominant. Recessive transmission and X-linked transmission have been recorded. Because there is variable expressivity, parents should be examined for mild cataracts.

The rubella embryopathy syndrome is rare in the era of rubella vaccination but is still seen in developing countries. The syndrome comprises multiple congenital anomalies that result from maternal viremia during the first trimester of pregnancy. Cataracts are present in about 20% of children with the congenital rubella syndrome (Fig. 53-12). The rubella virus may remain dormant in lens material in the offspring for as long as several years. Microphthalmia, pupil abnormalities, congenital glaucoma, and anterior uveitis also may result. A cloudy, edematous, or white cornea may be found with normal intraocular pressure as part of the rubella embryopathy. Rubella retinopathy is a pigmentary disturbance of the retina without demonstrable effect on visual function. A TORCH (*t*oxoplasmosis, *o*ther agents, *r*ubella,

TABLE 53–3 Neonatal Cataracts	
Type	**Incidence**
Genetic	
Dominant	N/A
Recessive	N/A
X-linked recessive	N/A
Viral	
Rubella	Frequent
Cytomegalic inclusion disease	Infrequent
Inborn Errors of Metabolism	
Galactosemia	Frequent
Galactokinase deficiency	Frequent
Lowe syndrome	Frequent
Trauma	
Birth trauma	Infrequent
Blunt trauma	Frequent
Perforating injuries	Frequent
Battered child syndrome	Infrequent
Endocrine	
Congenital hypoparathyroidism	Frequent
Albright hereditary osteodystrophy	Infrequent
Neurologic	
Marinesco-Sjögren syndrome	Infrequent
Smith-Lemli-Opitz syndrome	Rare
Miscellaneous	
Aniridia (sporadic or associated with Wilms tumor)	Infrequent
Treacher Collins syndrome	Infrequent
Pierre Robin syndrome	Infrequent
Rubinstein-Taybi syndrome	Infrequent
Hallermann-Streiff syndrome	Frequent
Chromosome Anomalies	
Trisomy 13	Infrequent
Trisomy 18	Infrequent
Trisomy 21	Infrequent
Turner syndrome	Infrequent
Associated with Other Eye Malformations	
Microphthalmia	Frequent
Rieger anomaly	Infrequent

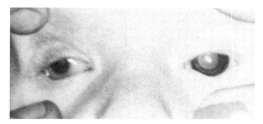

Figure 53–12. Congenital rubella syndrome with a cataract of the left eye, microphthalmia of the right eye, and exotropia.

cytomegalovirus, *h*erpes simplex) titer should be obtained from all infants with nongenetic congenital cataracts.

Galactosemia is a hereditary inborn error of metabolism with deficiency of the enzymes responsible for galactose metabolism: galactose-1-phosphate uridyltransferase, galactokinase, or uridine diphosphategalactose-4-epimerase. The affected neonate may appear normal at birth. Cataracts usually develop during the first 2 months of life. The cataracts may be zonular or may appear as vacuoles (classically described as "drop of oil") in the center of the lens owing to an accumulation of galactose and galactitol. Early diagnosis and a regimen of a galactose-free diet can prevent development or further progression of cataracts.

All congenital forms of infantile cataracts require a prompt evaluation by an ophthalmologist. Dense cataracts are treated surgically to prevent irreversible amblyopia and strabismus. Removal of the lens, followed by optical correction and amblyopia therapy, provides the best hope of restoring vision. The prognosis for vision is poorer in the involved eye when the cataract is monocular. Intraocular lens implantation, especially in older infants, is often used to restore the focusing ability of the eye.[83] Long-term follow-up is necessary to monitor vision development, treat strabismus and amblyopia, and detect glaucoma.

Subluxed Lens

The discovery of a subluxed lens (ectopia lentis) in an eye helps in identifying systemic disease processes associated with this abnormality. Although lens dislocation may be present during the neonatal period, it typically develops in the first or second decade of life. Marfan syndrome is the most common cause, but homocystinuria, sulfite oxidase deficiency, hyperlysinemia, Ehlers-Danlos syndrome, Weill-Marchesani syndrome, and trauma can also produce this finding. There is also an isolated genetic form. The dislocation results from a laxity, absence, or defect of the zonular attachments that suspend the lens from the ciliary body. A subluxed lens usually is not treated during the neonatal period unless there is the complication of cataract formation or glaucoma.

By dilating the pupil, the examiner can visualize the edge of a dislocated lens in the pupillary space (Fig. 53-13). Ectopia lentis may also be suggested by iridodonesis (shaking of the iris), which occurs when the posterior surface of the iris lacks the normal support of the lens.

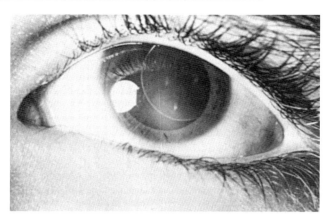

Figure 53–13. Ectopia lentis (dislocated lens) of the left eye.

RETINAL AND VITREOUS DISEASES

During the neonatal period, nonvascular structures of the fundus are nearly transparent because uveal pigmentation is not fully developed. The neonatal retina does have a sheen to its inner surface, but the macular region appears flattened. Retinal transparency is disturbed when abnormalities are present. The retina resembles a pale, ghostlike sheet when it is detached. Retinal edema gives a slightly raised, opalescent appearance. Infection obscures the underlying structures with a fuzzy, white thickening of the retinal tissue. In pathologic processes characterized by a lack or an excess of pigment, retinal abnormalities may become evident only after the first few months of life. The choroid is the deepest layer normally visible with the ophthalmoscope. Pathologic processes that prevent its development or that destroy areas of choroid expose areas of bare sclera, which appear glistening white.

Persistent Hyperplastic Primary Vitreous

Persistent hyperplastic primary vitreous (PHPV), also known as *persistent fetal vasculature*, is a congenital anomaly that produces a white pupil usually evident at birth. It results from the failure of the embryonic vitreous to regress. The embryonic vitreous system develops as a complex network of vessels that grows anteriorly from the disc to surround the developing lens, and normally involutes during the third trimester.

At birth, PHPV may appear as a strand or plaque of white tissue immediately behind a clear lens. Vessels are frequently seen to radiate from the plaque's center, and the retrolental mass may therefore be pinkish white. When the pupil is dilated, the ciliary processes are often drawn centrally along the posterior surface of the lens toward the central mass.

Almost always unilateral, PHPV occurs in term infants without a history of oxygen therapy. The involved eye is commonly microphthalmic. The anterior chamber is shallow owing to fibrous contraction of the primary vitreous, which pulls the ciliary body centrally, forcing the lens forward. With continued organization and contraction of the primary vitreous, the lens capsule may be involved, and a cataract may form. At this stage in the development of the disease, glaucoma, posterior chamber hemorrhages, or hemorrhages into the lens may occur. Retinal detachment occurs in the final stages, with continued vitreous traction. Persistent hyperplastic primary vitreous should be suspected in the neonate with a rapidly progressive unilateral cataract.

Differentiation of PHPV from ROP is usually possible because of the unilateral involvement and occurrence of PHPV in a term infant. Differentiation from retinoblastoma is important. The absence of calcification within the eye, as occurs in retinoblastoma, is a critical finding. A persistent embryonic iris vessel or one that notches the pupil suggests the presence of PHPV, even when an opaque lens obscures its presence. CT, MRI, and ultrasound can help in the diagnosis of difficult cases. Surgical removal of the lens and vitreous with optical correction and amblyopia treatment must be attempted very early to achieve any degree of success in recovering vision.

Retinal Dysplasia

Retinal dysplasia is a usually bilateral, congenital anomaly of term infants showing congenital retinal folds and retinal detachments. Histopathologically, the retina shows disorganization and dysplasia. The retinal detachments may clinically resemble a mass and should be considered in the differential diagnosis of retinoblastoma. Rather than a distinct clinical entity, retinal dysplasia may represent a common final pathway of many different developmental disorders of retinal differentiation and organization. Retinal dysplasia can occur as part of a group of congenital anomalies—including defects of the central nervous system, cardiovascular system, and skeletal system—that are sufficiently severe to produce early death of the infant. Specific conditions that result in retinal dysplasia include trisomy 13, Norrie disease, and Walker-Warburg syndrome.

Norrie Disease

A rare genetic disorder transmitted as an X-linked recessive trait, Norrie disease is characterized by the presence of bilateral total retinal detachments that result in a white pupil. Organization of the retinal detachment can disrupt the lens, producing cataract, or can affect the anterior chamber angle, producing congenital glaucoma. The usual result is atrophy of the globe. Norrie disease maps to the *NDP* gene on chromosome Xp11.4, most commonly due to mutations of the cysteine-knot motif.[102] Patients with Norrie disease may also develop progressive mental disorders often with psychotic features, and about one third of patients develop sensorineural deafness.

Mutations of the *NDP* gene away from the cysteine-knot motif often result, not in Norrie disease, but in a clinically distinct entity termed *familial exudative vitreoretinopathy* (FEVR). FEVR is characterized by avascularity of the peripheral retina, abnormal retinal neovascularization, retinal traction, and detachment. FEVR is actually a genetically diverse disorder, having been also mapped to the *FZD4* and *LRP5* genes, both of which encode for receptors for the *NDP* gene product.[7]

Retinoschisis

Retinoschisis is a hereditary abnormality in which the superficial layers of the retina are split from the deeper layers and are elevated into the vitreous. This splitting creates a veil-like appearance in front of the retina. Visual function is absent in the affected tissue. Juvenile X-linked retinoschisis is a progressive, degenerative disorder that has an X-linked recessive transmission. Macular changes and vitreous hemorrhages can occur as associated findings. Both lead to loss of vision. Early diagnosis offers a better chance in improving prognosis.

Leber Congenital Amaurosis

Leber congenital amaurosis often produces symptoms of blindness shortly after birth. Children with this disorder sometimes rub or poke their eyes excessively, called *blindism* behavior. Nystagmus usually appears after a few months. The fundus often has a normal appearance in the neonatal period. Electroretinography is a diagnostic test that measures the electrical responses of the photoreceptors to light stimulation and can confirm the severely deficient retinal function in this disorder. Leber congenital amaurosis is most commonly transmitted as an autosomal recessive disease and represents a similar phenotype in response to many different known genetic defects.[30]

Albinism

The diagnosis of albinism in the neonatal period is difficult to substantiate because the uveal pigment is underdeveloped during this period. The diagnosis may be suggested when pigmentation of the skin, hair, and irises fails to progress during the first several months in comparison with that of parents and siblings. Lack of pigmentation is more apparent earlier in darker races. The fundus remains blonde, and choroidal vessels are prominent. Photophobia, nystagmus, and abnormal transillumination of the irides are characteristic features of albinism. Moderately to severely reduced vision is characteristic as a result of foveal hypoplasia.

Chorioretinal Coloboma

A coloboma of the fundus is visible as a defect in the retinal and choroidal layers through which the underlying sclera is visible. Leukocoria may result. Typical coloboma occur inferonasally, which is the site of the closure of the embryonic fissure. The fissure usually begins to close at the globe's equator and then extends posteriorly toward the optic disc and anteriorly toward the periphery. Any part or all of this region may be involved in the colobomatous defect. The visual prognosis depends on how much of the macula or optic disc is involved.

Abnormal Macula

Several of the lysosomal storage diseases alter the appearance of the macula, a fact that may be useful in detecting these disorders (Table 53-4). The stored material accumulates in

TABLE 53–4   Neonatal Macular Changes

Condition	Defect
Tay-Sachs disease	Cherry-red spot
Niemann-Pick disease	Cherry-red spot
GM1 gangliosidosis	Cherry-red spot
Neuraminidase deficiency	Cherry-red spot and corneal clouding
Farber disease	Gray macula
Best vitelliform degeneration	Cystic macula (rare)
Toxoplasmosis	Chorioretinal scar
Coloboma	Absence of retina and choroid

Myelinated Nerve Fibers

Normal myelinization of the optic nerve fibers occurs in fetal development in reverse direction to the growth of the axons themselves. Development of myelin sheaths progresses from the geniculate bodies through the optic tracts, optic chiasm, and optic nerves to end just posterior to the optic disc. This process is usually complete at birth or within the first month of life.

Myelination of the nerve fibers occasionally proceeds aberrantly through the disc and into the retina, seen as a glistening white, opaque area involving the peripapillary retina. The edges of the myelinated areas are feathered, and the involved areas are sometimes arcuate. This process is stable after the first several months of life, and vision is unimpaired except for an enlarged blind spot or scotoma of the involved retinal area. Small areas may sometimes be confused for the cotton-wool spots seen in retinal vascular diseases. A large area of myelinated nerve fibers may result in leukocoria.

OPTIC DISC ABNORMALITIES

The optic disc should appear flat and pink, even in the newborn. Mild degrees of pallor or hypoplasia can be difficult to establish in the neonate because of a lack of patient cooperation with the examination. Disc margins should, however, be clear and distinct. The sharp margins of the optic disc are created by the abrupt ending of the choroid and retinal pigment epithelium at the disc borders. Occasionally, as a variation of normal, these structures fail to extend to the immediate edge of the disc, creating a peripapillary crescent of visible underlying sclera. This crescent is sometimes bordered by a darkly pigmented line.

Coloboma of the Optic Disc

Coloboma of the optic disc is another manifestation of failure of the globe's embryonic fissure to close adequately, in this case at its posterior limit. The optic disc might appear enlarged and elongated, usually inferiorly. The coloboma may include adjacent retina and choroid. The blood vessels may be distributed normally, or they may be displaced to the periphery of the optic disc and appear disorganized. Colobomas of the optic disc often are associated with defective vision, but the appearance of the optic disc does not correlate with potential acuity. Coloboma of the optic nerve should be differentiated from optic nerve cupping due to glaucoma, requiring a more extensive evaluation by an ophthalmologist and consideration of associated genetic syndromes.

Morning Glory Disc Anomaly

Morning glory disc describes a congenital anomaly of the optic disc showing a colobomatous-like excavation of the optic disc but with the additional findings of central glial hyperplasia, peripapillary depigmentation, and anomalous retinal vasculature. It can be distinguished from other congenital optic disc lesions, such as optic nerve coloboma, by pattern recognition. Morning glory discs can be associated with intracranial and systemic disorders such as basal encephalocele, agenesis of the corpus callosum, and moyamoya disease.[48]

the ganglion cells of the retina, which decreases the transparency of the retina except at the very center of the macula, where no ganglion cells exist. The center of the macula retains its normal cherry-red appearance, in sharp contrast to the surrounding grayish involved fundus.

Sphingolipidoses that may produce a cherry-red spot are Tay-Sachs disease, in which a cherry-red spot may be present shortly after birth or may develop during the first year, and Niemann-Pick disease (infantile), in which about 50% of patients have a cherry-red spot in the macula during the neonatal period. Of the lipidoses, Farber disease shows a grayish discoloration of the macula at 6 to 8 weeks of age, and GM1-gangliosidosis demonstrates a cherry-red spot in the macula in about 30% of patients before 2 months of age. The mucopolysaccharidoses are characterized by the abnormal deposition of mucopolysaccharides in the cornea, but the macula appears normal.

Persistence of Hyaloid Artery

Persistence of the central hyaloid artery is a common but clinically insignificant developmental abnormality. Its presence in the premature infant is sufficiently common to be considered normal. It is most often seen as a fine thread of nearly transparent tissue extending from the optic disc toward the posterior surface of the lens; it rarely may be patent and contain blood. The artery commonly continues to atrophy during the neonatal period, with rare persistence into adulthood.

Bergmeister Papilla

The persistence of the mesodermal supporting elements of the hyaloid vascular system at the disc might leave a small protuberance of gray-white tissue extending from the disc forward into the vitreous—a so-called Bergmeister papilla. A small retinal artery might course into this area and return to the disc before supplying the retina, or the papilla may be associated with one or several small, round, pearl-gray cysts of glial tissue. Vision and optic nerve function are unaffected.

Optic Pit

The surface of the optic disc occasionally shows a sharply defined hole or pit. This pit usually is situated near the lower temporal quadrant of the optic disc at its border and can vary in size, shape, and depth. It is thought to be a minimal expression of an optic disc coloboma. Visual defects may be present with this finding.

Oblique Discs

The optic nerve commonly enters the posterior aspect of the eye from a slightly nasal angle. If this angle is accentuated, the nerve head or disc may be tilted obliquely, with its temporal margin considerably more posterior than its nasal margin. This gives the optic disc an ovoid appearance.

Optic Nerve Hypoplasia

Hypoplasia of the optic nerve is a congenital anomaly in which there are a reduced number of axons within an optic nerve. The optic disc is smaller than normal and may be pale, but the retinal vessels usually are normal. A hypopigmented ring around the hypoplastic nerve creates the double-ring sign. Optic nerve hypoplasia can occur unilaterally or bilaterally. Visual impairment can range from mild to severe. In bilaterally severely affected patients, the nystagmus that develops makes the retinal and optic nerve examination difficult.

Optic nerve hypoplasia can occur as an isolated finding or in association with other ocular or systemic abnormalities. CT or MRI of the brain can reveal midline abnormalities, a disorder referred to as *septo-optic dysplasia* (de Morsier syndrome) if there is absence of the septum pellucidum. Endocrine abnormalities can occur in patients with this syndrome because of coexisting defects of the infundibulum or pituitary gland.[39] Neonatal hypoglycemia has been reported in these patients resulting from growth hormone deficiency.[73]

Most cases of optic nerve hypoplasia occur sporadically and idiopathically. Minor associations include young maternal age, nulliparity, maternal diabetes, fetal alcohol syndrome, or other maternal ingestions.[93]

Optic Nerve Atrophy

Optic nerve atrophy is a condition in which the nerve fibers have formed and subsequently atrophied in response to some insult. The optic disc shows regional or diffuse pallor, but has a normal size and configuration. Significant visual impairment is common and may be associated with nystagmus if the atrophy occurs before 6 months of age. The most common cause in the infant is perinatal hypoxia. Many other causes have been described (Box 53-5).

PUPIL ABNORMALITIES

Abnormalities of the pupil can result from structural disease of the iris or from neurologic abnormalities. Neurologic abnormalities may be described in terms of pupil size (i.e., miosis or mydriasis) or abnormal function.

Miosis can result from paralysis of the sympathetic pathways, as in Horner syndrome, or from irritation of the

---

BOX 53–5   Causes of Childhood Optic Atrophy

Compressive intracranial lesions
Compressive bony disorders
   Craniosynostosis
   Fibrous dysplasia
Hydrocephalus
Post–papilledema optic atrophy
Infectious
Hereditary
   Leber hereditary optic neuropathy
   Dominant optic atrophy (Kjer)
   Recessive optic atrophy
   Behr optic atrophy
   DIDMOAD (diabetes insipidis, diabetes mellitus, optic
      atrophy, deafness) (Wolfram) optic atrophy
Toxic or nutritional optic neuropathy
Hypoxia
Trauma
Postoptic neuritis
Radiation optic neuropathy
Paraneoplastic syndromes
Neurodegenerative disorders with optic atrophy
   Krabbe disease
   Canavan disease
   Leigh disease
   Mitochondrial encephalomyopathy, lactic acidosis, and
      stroke-like (MELAS) episodes
   Neonatal adrenoleukodystrophy
   Metachromic leukodystrophy
   Riley-Day syndrome
   Lactic acidosis
   Spinocerebellar degeneration
   Mucopolysaccharidosis
Ocular disorders
   Glaucoma
   Retinal disease
   Vascular disease
   Uveitis
   Optic nerve hypoplasia

---

parasympathetic pathways, as in central nervous system inflammation.

Mydriasis most often is caused by a paralysis of the parasympathetic pathways, which can occur in third-nerve palsy or with increased intracranial pressure. Local trauma, such as that caused by a difficult forceps delivery, can also damage the iris sphincter and result in mydriasis.

Anisocoria describes a difference in the size of the two pupils. When this condition is seen, the physician should examine the patient in bright and dim illumination to determine the abnormal pupil. If more anisometropia is evident in dim light, the pathologic pupil is the more miotic pupil because this pupil has failed to fully dilate. If more anisometropia is evident in bright light, the pathologic pupil is the more mydriatic pupil because this pupil has failed to fully constrict. Many infants have a small degree of "physiologic" anisocoria.[76]

A relative afferent pupillary defect, as detected by the swinging flashlight test, occurs when an optic nerve defect is present anterior to the lateral geniculate body.

NEUROMUSCULAR ABNORMALITIES

Strabismus

Strabismus refers to any type of ocular misalignment or inability to move the eye fully. Various classification schemes have been proposed to help organize the different forms to aid diagnosis and treatment. We favor a system that considers etiology in the first order of the classification scheme. These etiologic groups include the following:

Comitant strabismus—sometimes referred to as *benign childhood strabismus*. This is the most common type of strabismus, with onset typically from 4 months to 6 years of age. The globes, extraocular muscles, and cranial nerves to the eye are normal. The cause is idiopathic, but the fault lies in purported central nervous system ocular alignment centers.

Sensory strabismus—the oculomotor system requires a certain level of vision in both eyes to maintain ocular alignment. If vision is lost in one or both eyes, an ocular misalignment may follow.

Paralytic strabismus—resulting from lower motor neuron lesions of the third, fourth, or sixth cranial nerve.

Restrictive strabismus—resulting from lesions within the orbit that limit free movement of the extraocular muscles; for example, orbital blow-out fractures and orbital tumors

Syndromic strabismus—this group includes a variety of entities, each with distinct and stereotypical patterns, with causes that may overlap the aforementioned four groups, such as for Duane syndrome and Brown syndrome.

Central nervous system strabismus—due to lesions of the oculomotor pathways above the level of the lower motor neuron[9]

Small horizontal ocular misalignments, but with full right and left gaze movements, are a common transient feature of infancy. Persistent abnormalities in alignment beyond 3 to 4 months of age should be referred for a complete ophthalmic assessment.[4] A more prominent strabismus and a lack of full movement of an eye are suggestive of a congenital palsy of the extraocular muscles, typically a lower motor neuron lesion of the sixth or third cranial nerve.

Pseudostrabismus is present in infants who appear cross-eyed because the bridge of the nose is wide and the epicanthal folds cover some of the medial sclera. True strabismus is excluded when the corneal light reflex is found to be symmetrically placed in both pupils and alternate cover testing reveals no deviation. It is important to remember that epicanthal folds may exist with true esotropia, and if there is an intermittent esotropia, the eye may be straight on one examination. Infants with severe ROP causing a dragging of the macula may appear to have strabismus when the dystopic maculae are aligned.

Treatment of strabismus begins with a complete ocular examination and a careful cycloplegic refraction. Treatment includes prevention of amblyopia, reconstruction of the normal ocular alignment and movement, and development of binocular vision. The chances of diagnosing and successfully treating amblyopia and strabismus are better the earlier therapy is begun. Treatment should be undertaken well before the child is of school age to eliminate a visual or cosmetic disability.

Nystagmus

Nystagmus refers to an oscillation of one or both eyes. It may be horizontal, vertical, or torsional (rotary). Nystagmus is described by its waveform, direction, rate, amplitude, laterality, and intensity in different positions of gaze.[8] The most common types of nystagmus are pendular and jerk nystagmus. Pendular nystagmus is a to-and-fro movement of the eyes of equal amplitude and velocity in both directions. Jerk nystagmus is characterized by a slow component in one direction and a fast component in the opposite direction. Patients may maintain an abnormal head posture as an adaptation to the nystagmus.[1]

Physiologic nystagmus, usually a jerk nystagmus, may be seen in several situations. The optokinetic phenomenon of a target moving past the eyes causes a slow-moving component as the eyes fixate on an object, followed by a rapid refixation movement in the opposite direction. Vestibular nystagmus occurs with rotation of the body or with irrigation of the ear, causing a movement of the fluid within the semicircular canals. Positional or end-gaze nystagmus is seen in extreme gaze, usually in a horizontal direction.

Pathologic forms of nystagmus can result from ocular, neurologic, or vestibular defects. If onset is before 6 months of age, it is classified as congenital nystagmus; later onset is classified as acquired. Nystagmus due to ocular pathology (termed *sensory nystagmus*) results from a primary, profound bilateral loss of vision in an infant younger than 6 months. It can be caused by a lesion in the eyes or in the pathways leading back to the lateral geniculate. Common ocular defects causing sensory nystagmus include optic nerve hypoplasia or atrophy, macular scars, retinal disorders, cataracts, aniridia, and albinism.[50] Infants born blind typically start to show sensory nystagmus at 1 to 2 months of age.

Nonsensory congenital nystagmus (commonly called *motor nystagmus*) requires a workup that includes central nervous system imaging and a neurologic evaluation to exclude an identifiable etiologic lesion. Most cases of congenital motor nystagmus are either idiopathic in otherwise neurologically intact infants or familial.

An interesting form of benign acquired nystagmus, called *spasmus nutans*, usually develops within the first 2 years of life and disappears within months to several years after its onset. The nystagmus of spasmus nutans is often very fine and rapid and may be asymmetric or even monocular. The classic triad of spasmus nutans includes nystagmus, head nodding, and torticollis, although the diagnosis is often made when one or two of the features are absent. Optic pathways gliomas can have similar characteristics.[27] Careful follow-up is essential, and further diagnostic studies may be advisable.

AMBLYOPIA

Amblyopia is a decrease in vision in one or both eyes that is not caused by organic disease. This is a central process, an expression of brain plasticity, in response to any ocular condition that prevents a clear image from reaching the retina. The main causes are strabismus, refraction, occlusion, and deprivation. Amblyopia can develop at any time during the "sensitive period" of visual development, usually during the first 7 years in humans, and can be treated if discovered within this same time frame of plasticity.

Strabismic amblyopia occurs in children who first develop strabismus and then favor one eye. The constantly deviated eye will then develop amblyopia; hence, strabismic amblyopia is always unilateral. Refractive amblyopia results from large refractive errors that create significant blurry vision. This can be a bilateral or unilateral process. Occlusion amblyopia is caused by opacities in the visual axes, such as cataracts or corneal scars. Deprivation amblyopia is a special form of occlusion amblyopia in infants younger than 3 months. If the visual obstruction is not cleared by 3 or 4 months of age, the amblyopia becomes very dense and unresponsive to treatment—hence the urgency to identify and treat congenital cataracts.

Treatment of amblyopia is accomplished by patching or optically penalizing the better-seeing eye and prescribing the appropriate optical correction. The patching regimen is tapered as visual improvement is noted. If bilateral amblyopia is present because of high refractive error, glasses are prescribed.

EYE FINDINGS IN CHROMOSOMAL SYNDROMES

Any alteration of gene dosage often results in multiple systemic anomalies. Many ocular abnormalities have been reported in patients with chromosomal aberrations; often they are not diagnostic of a specific chromosomal syndrome. The following are examples of common chromosomal syndromes or defects associated with ocular findings of particular importance.

Trisomy 13

Ocular findings are very common in trisomy 13, with iris coloboma and underlying sectoral cataracts very suggestive of the syndrome. Other eye findings include hypotelorism, microphthalmia or anophthalmia, synophthalmia, colobomas of the iris or choroid, corneal opacities, persistent hyperplastic primary vitreous, retinal dysplasia, cataracts, and many low-incidence anomalies.[52]

Trisomy 18

Trisomy 18 is characterized by micrognathia, flexed fingers with the index finger overlapping the third finger, generalized hypertonicity of skeletal muscles, mental retardation, ventricular septal defect, umbilical hernia, rocker-bottom feet, and malrotation of the gut. Ankyloblepharon filiforme adnatum (strands joining the upper and lower lids together) are very suggestive of trisomy 18.[11] Other ocular abnormalities include retinal folds, cornea and lens opacities, ptosis, strabismus, epicanthal folds, abnormal orbital ridges, hypertelorism, microphthalmia, glaucoma, myopia, and congenital optic atrophy.

Trisomy 21

Down syndrome is a well-recognized entity comprising typical facies, mental retardation, small but obese habitus, large tongue, and cardiac, genitourinary, and gastrointestinal abnormalities. The ocular findings associated with this entity are extensive. They include epicanthus, hypertelorism, and upward slant of the palpebral fissures. Brushfield spots might be found on the unusually thin, lightly colored irises. Because strabismus, nystagmus, cataracts, glaucoma, high refractive errors, keratoconus, and blepharitis are also seen, children with Down syndrome should be examined by an ophthalmologist during infancy. Systemic or topical therapy with atropine may result in unusual and sometimes dangerous systemic responses in infants with Down syndrome.[61]

Turner Syndrome

Strabismus, ptosis, congenital cataracts, and occasionally corneal nebulae and blue sclerae in the neonatal period have been described associated with Turner syndrome.

11p Abnormalities

Infants with a deletion of the short arm of chromosome 11 involving the *PAX6* gene and the adjacent *WT1* gene on the 11p13 band have the WAGR syndrome of aniridia, genitourinary abnormalities, and mental retardation.[22] Wilms tumor has been diagnosed in a significant percentage of children with this chromosomal deletion and must be evaluated with periodic ultrasounds of the abdomen for a number of years.

13q Abnormalities

Patients with a deletion of 13q often have a characteristic facial anomaly with microcephaly, micrognathia, large malformed ears, a wide nasal bridge with hypertelorism, and protruding upper incisors. Other findings include urogenital, thumb, and congenital cardiac defects. Ocular abnormalities are almost always present and severe, including microphthalmia, iris and choroidal colobomas, ptosis, cataracts, and down-slanting palpebral apertures and epicanthus. However, the most important possible finding that requires a comprehensive retinal examination is retinoblastoma.

EYE FINDINGS IN CRANIOFACIAL SYNDROMES

Eye abnormalities associated with congenital anomalies of the face, skull, or head can occur as an isolated finding or in conjunction with well-recognized syndromes.

Craniosynostosis Syndromes

Premature closure of the cranial sutures can occur in the embryonic period or early childhood. The involved suture determines the shape of the skull because growth is inhibited perpendicular to the closed suture. Compensatory growth occurs at the open sutures and in weakened areas of the cranial vault. Premature craniosynostosis can exist as a primary isolated anomaly or may be associated with systemic or metabolic malformations. If more than one suture is involved, there is a greater chance for increased intracranial pressure resulting in papilledema or optic nerve atrophy.

Crouzon syndrome is an autosomal dominant craniosynostosis syndrome characterized by maxillary hypoplasia, shallow orbits, parrot-beak nose, moderate hypertelorism, highly arched palate, and a variety of abnormal skull conformations depending on the pattern of suture involvement. Ocular complications are stereotypic, mostly resulting from the abnormalities of the bony orbit or skull: shallow orbits, compression of the optic nerves, and papilledema from elevated intracranial pressure.[60] Visual acuity may be reduced because of amblyopia, optic nerve atrophy, or exposure keratitis.[92] Strabismus is common, as a mechanical limitation of ocular rotations within the abnormal orbit, or from anomalous or missing extraocular muscles. Shallow orbits produce exorbitism, leading to exposure keratopathy and globe subluxation. Eyelids may be ptotic or retracted. Midface abnormalities often result in symptomatic dacryostenosis. Infrequent anomalies include iris and corneal malformations, cataracts, and retinal pigmentary changes.

Because of similar cranial and orbital anomalies, eye findings can be similar in the other craniosynostosis syndromes such as Apert syndrome, Saethre-Chotzen syndrome, and Pfeiffer syndrome.[41,45]

Cornelia de Lange Syndrome

The typical facial appearance in infants with Cornelia de Lange syndrome is a low hairline, eyebrows that are joined in the middle (synophrys), long eyelashes, and a small upturned nose. Skeletal deformities ranging from syndactyly to phocomelia may be present. Eye disorders, which are less frequently encountered, include hypertelorism and downslanting palpebral fissures, dacryostenosis, strabismus, nystagmus, ptosis, severe myopia, and pupillary abnormalities.[65] Some patients with this diagnosis resemble children with fetal alcohol syndrome.

Hemifacial Microsomia

Hemifacial microsomia describes a group of patients with microtia, macrostomia, and mandibular anomalies. Most patients show unilateral involvement. Ocular manifestations can range from clinical anophthalmia to minor fissure asymmetry. Goldenhar syndrome is probably a variant of this group, with characteristic dermoids of the limbus (interface between the sclera and the cornea) or lipodermoids of the lateral canthal angle.[88] Limbal dermoids are reported more frequently than lipodermoids and are occasionally bilateral. Another common finding is an upper eyelid coloboma almost always on the more affected side. Less frequent findings are Duane syndrome and microphthalmia. Children with Goldenhar variant should have a comprehensive eye examination.

Hallermann-Streiff Syndrome

Oculomandibulofacial dyscephalia (Hallermann-Streiff syndrome) is characterized by hypoplasia of the mandible, a thin, prominent nose (parrot-beak nose), and congenital cataracts. Other common eye findings include spontaneous resorption of the crystalline lens, microphthalmia, and glaucoma.[6]

Terminal Transverse Defects with Orofacial Malformations and Oromandibular-Limb Hypogenesis

These are a heterogeneous collection of syndromes with a wide variety of facial and limb anomalies probably resulting from a variety of etiologies.[39] They include the aglossia-adactylia syndrome, Hanhart syndrome, ectrodactyly with orofacial malformations, ankyloglossia syndrome, Möbius syndrome, and a few others. The pattern of craniofacial anomalies noted in this complex includes oral and facial clefts, micrognathia, microglossia, pectoral muscle malformations with ipsilateral hand malformations (Poland syndrome), dental and oral anomalies, and hypoplastic limb anomalies. The minimal findings of Möbius syndrome are abduction weakness (sixth cranial nerve palsy) and facial nerve palsy, with frequent limb and tongue anomalies. Möbius syndrome has been reported frequently in South America following unsuccessful abortion attempts using misoprostol (Cytotec).[14]

Pierre Robin Sequence

The Pierre Robin sequence is characterized by micrognathia, glossoptosis, and cleft palate. Pierre Robin sequence can occur in isolation or in a variety of multiple-defect syndromes. About 10% of patients with Pierre Robin sequence have Stickler syndrome as well, with the additional features of high myopia, propensity for retinal detachment, cataracts, deafness, and arthritis.[20] Stickler syndrome is further subdivided into types 1 and 2, linked to defects of the genes COL2A1 and COL11A1, respectively.[17]

Waardenburg Syndrome

Waardenburg syndrome is transmitted as an autosomal dominant trait and has been divided into four types based on clinical attributes. The most common is Waardenburg syndrome type 1. It is associated with lateral displacement of the medial canthi (i.e., telecanthus), abnormal position of the lacrimal puncta, coalescing of eyebrows, white forelock, heterochromia irides, retinal pigmentary changes, and sensorineural deafness.

EYE FINDINGS IN NEUROCUTANEOUS DISODERS
Sturge-Weber Syndrome

Port-wine stains (capillary angiomas or nevus flammeus) can occur in isolation or as a feature of Sturge-Weber syndrome, with the additional finding of leptomeningeal angiomas, hemiparesis, epilepsy, mental retardation, and other ocular problems.[71] Patients with port-wine stains of the upper or lower lids have a very high likelihood of having Sturge-Weber syndrome.[90] Ocular complications of Sturge-Weber syndrome include glaucoma and chorioretinal angioma. The associated choroidal angioma is usually indistinct and difficult to visualize without indirect ophthalmoscopy. If present, it may lead to macular edema and decreased visual acuity. There is no apparent hereditary pattern. Congenital glaucoma frequently occurs and can lead to blindness.

Neurofibromatosis Type 1

NF1 (von Recklinghausen disease) is a congenital, autosomal dominant disease that is characterized by hamartomatous growths of neural crest origin. It is rarely diagnosed in the neonate. Lid abnormalities in NF1 can include neurofibromas, plexiform neurofibromas (sometimes presenting early in life), or café-au-lait spots. A plexiform neurofibroma of the upper lid greatly increases the chances of developing glaucoma. Other ocular findings in NF1 include Lisch nodules of the iris, retinal astrocytic hamartomas, sphenoid wing dysplasia resulting in pulsatile exophthalmos, and thickened corneal nerves. About 20% of NF1 patients develop optic glioma. The characteristic Lisch nodules are rarely present at birth but develop in more than 90% of affected individuals by puberty.[68] NF1 results from a germline mutation of the tumor suppressor *NF1* gene on chromosome 17q11.2.[94]

OCULAR TRAUMA

Birth trauma to the eyes is associated with the duration of labor and difficulty of delivery.[74] Lid petechiae and hemorrhages, observed more often with face presentations than with vertex presentations, usually resolve rapidly without treatment. Subconjunctival hemorrhages are also common and require no treatment. Such findings, however, should increase the suspicion of associated intraocular injuries. Retinal hemorrhages are common after delivery, occurring in 78% of newborns after vacuum delivery, 30% after normal vaginal delivery or with forceps assists, and only 8% after cesarean delivery.[35] These retinal hemorrhages are usually small, multiple, and scattered throughout the retina, but they may persist for months and must be considered in the differential diagnosis of later suspected intentional injury or shaken baby syndrome.[35] More profound retinal and vitreous hemorrhages requiring treatment with vitrectomy can also occur from birth trauma.[82]

Bleeding into the orbital contents (retrobulbar hemorrhage) can result from birth trauma. This bleeding produces a unilateral proptosis that tends to increase gradually in size during the first 3 or 4 hours after birth. Ecchymoses of the lids can be associated findings at birth or can occur 1 or 2 days later. The differential diagnosis includes dermoid cysts, teratomas, and other congenital tumors of the orbit. The hematoma usually absorbs spontaneously over 1 to 2 weeks. It is important during this time to ensure that the cornea is not abraded and that the retinal circulation is not compromised. A detailed examination of ocular findings is indicated, and if it shows compression of the arterial or venous supply at the optic disc, immediate surgical decompression of the orbit is required.

Rarely, the eye may be completely dislocated during birth, resulting when the orbit is shallow in conditions such as the craniosynostosis syndrome. This condition constitutes an emergency because the cornea is exposed.

Forceps deliveries, particularly when associated with improper application, can produce bruises and lacerations of the lid or globe.[34] A forceps mark or lid laceration requires a careful and complete examination of the orbit and globe for associated injuries.[56] Forceps application can produce a rupture in the cornea's endothelial basement membrane

(Descemet membrane). Seen with magnification, these ruptures appear as diagonal lines in the posterior portion of the cornea. They are rapidly followed by excess hydration of the cornea, with a subsequent cloudy appearance that must be differentiated from congenital glaucoma, infections of the cornea, or diseases associated with cloudy cornea such as the mucopolysaccharidoses. Children with Descemet membrane ruptures can rapidly develop astigmatism and dense amblyopia. Traumatic forceps delivery has been known to cause a variety of other ocular injuries, including Purtscher retinopathy, choroid ruptures, and traumatic optic neuropathy.[40]

Ocular injury in the newborn has also been reported as a result of fetal monitors,[46] surgical instruments,[62,86] phototherapy lights,[70] prenatal maternal injury, and amniocentesis.[67]

Blunt trauma from any cause to the ocular area of the infant can produce blood in the anterior chamber (hyphema), rupture of the globe, dislocation of the lens, vitreous hemorrhage, contusion cataract, traumatic retinal detachment, retinal hemorrhage or edema, rupture of the choroid, and arterial or venous occlusion in the retina. A history of minimal trauma with extensive multilayer retinal hemorrhages may be an indication of shaken baby syndrome.

Shaken baby syndrome can result in devastating and blinding ocular injuries. The examiner might see vitreous, preretinal, intraretinal, or subretinal hemorrhages. Peripheral, dome-shaped hemorrhagic lesions with white retinal borders could represent peripheral retinoschisis. The retina can even be folded in a circumferential manner around the macula. Retinal hemorrhages may resolve without sequelae, but involvement of the optic nerve, macula, or occipital cortex can produce profound lifelong visual loss.[43] The extent and type of retinal hemorrhages that occur in shaken baby syndrome can be pathognomonic of the syndrome and may support the legal prosecution of the offender.[91] Accidental head trauma and cardiopulmonary resuscitation in infants do not result in the type and extent of retinal hemorrhage seen in shaken baby syndrome.[69,89] Thermal and chemical burns around the eyes must be treated with extreme care. Treatment by an ophthalmologist is required after the usual first-aid measures of cooling and providing protective covering. Of immediate priority in the first-aid management of a chemical burn of the eye is copious irrigation with tap water or normal saline solution.

Abrasions of the cornea are suggested by tearing, redness, or protective forced closure of the eyes. Diagnosis is made by observing an irregularity in the smooth corneal surface or by staining the cornea with a fluorescein-impregnated strip. This is done by moistening a sterile fluorescein strip with a drop of sterile saline solution and touching it to the lower conjunctival fornix. The area of corneal abrasion turns light green in ordinary illumination but is best seen with a cobalt-blue filter. Treatment can include antibiotic ointment, cycloplegic eye drops, and oral analgesics. Prolonged patching of an injured eye should be avoided to prevent the development of amblyopia.

Lacerations can involve the conjunctiva, the cornea, or the sclera. All conjunctival lacerations should be assumed associated with a laceration of the globe until proved otherwise. Treatment of ocular lacerations requires a full and careful evaluation of the extent of damage, particularly of the globe. Treatment usually requires microscopic evaluation and repair, with the infant under general anaesthesia. Lid lacerations should be repaired properly to minimize permanent deformity. Involvement of the lacrimal canaliculi, the lid margin, and the lacrimal gland requires special attention. Avulsion of or tissue loss from the lids necessitates urgent treatment to prevent exposure injuries to the cornea.

Orbital or ocular foreign bodies require specialized and precise localization to determine the proper therapeutic approach. Fortunately, they occur rarely in the neonate.

NEONATAL OCULAR INFECTIONS
Conjunctivitis

Neonatal conjunctivitis may be caused by a variety of agents, including chemical, bacterial, chlamydial, and viral. If the condition is undiagnosed and untreated, permanent scarring and loss of vision may occur. If chlamydia or *Neisseria gonorrhoeae* is in the differential diagnosis, it is essential to culture the conjunctiva and to perform whatever chlamydia test is available at your facility.

One cause of a red eye in the neonate can occur after the instillation of silver nitrate, or other antibiotic, for gonorrhea prophylaxis into the eyes at birth. In this chemical conjunctivitis, the conjunctiva is congested and edematous, but purulence is not present, and the redness clears spontaneously in 3 or 4 days. Alternative treatments for neonatal prophylaxis other than silver nitrate include erythromycin and tetracycline ointments.

A bacterial infection is suspected if the conjunctivitis persists or progresses, or if discharge develops. Cultures with sensitivity tests identify the organism and suggest appropriate treatment. Conjunctivitis caused by *N. gonorrhoeae* is an acute, severe, purulent conjunctivitis with an incubation period of 2 to 5 days. If *N. gonorrhoeae* is the cause of the conjunctivitis, immediate treatment with systemic and topical antibiotics is necessary. In cases of infection with organisms resistant to penicillin, a third-generation cephalosporin is indicated.[79]

Ophthalmia neonatorum also can result from other common pathogens such as staphylococci, pneumococci, streptococci, or gram-negative bacteria. These bacterial infections usually appear several days after birth. Most respond well to topical antibiotics or ointment.

Chlamydial conjunctivitis is now a common infection in the neonatal period. The infection is typically acquired from the mother as the child passes through the birth canal. The usual cultures and Gram staining are unhelpful in the diagnosis of chlamydia. Diagnosis can be made by Giemsa staining of a conjunctival scraping or by a variety of commercially available antibody tests.

Chlamydial conjunctivitis is treated with erythromycin or sulfacetamide ointment three times a day for 2 to 3 weeks. Systemic antibiotics are necessary because chlamydia can cause pneumonia, otitis, and persistent nasolacrimal duct obstruction.[78] The mother may also require treatment.

Older infants with chronic or recurrent conjunctivitis usually have a blocked nasolacrimal duct as the underlying cause. The duct frequently opens spontaneously during the first year of life. Treatment with topical antibiotics and massage of the lacrimal sac can help resolve the problem.

Intrauterine Ocular Infections

Intrauterine ocular infections result from maternal infections that cross the placental barrier. Neonates with a TORCH infection should have a complete eye examination to identify ocular involvement. One of the most common is congenital toxoplasmosis, which can result in chorioretinal scars in the retina in response to an in utero chorioretinitis. These scars appear as white areas of exposed sclera, with prominent, darkly pigmented borders. When seen in the neonatal fundus, scars are usually a sign of inactive disease. A significant number of these patients have bilateral blinding macular lesions.[57]

Congenital syphilis may involve the eye with chorioretinitis, interstitial keratitis, uveitis, and optic atrophy. Typically, the corneal changes of interstitial keratitis are not apparent until after the age of 5 years. Neonatal herpes infection is most often acquired during passage through the birth canal and can cause typical herpetic eye disease such as blepharoconjunctivitis, keratitis, iritis, or chorioretinitis. Ocular involvement with either congenital cytomegalovirus disease or varicella is unusual but can result in chorioretinitis, keratitis, or cataract. Ocular involvement in congenital rubella was discussed previously.

Transmission of the human immunodeficiency virus (HIV), causing acquired immunodeficiency syndrome (AIDS), may occur prenatally or postnatally. Chorioretinitis may occur in an HIV-infected child as a result of secondary infection with herpes zoster or simplex. Other causes of retinitis in HIV/AIDS patients, such as toxoplasma, *Mycobacterium avium–intracellulare*, cryptococcus, histoplasma, nocardia, and *Treponema pallidum* and cytomegalovirus are uncommonly seen in children.[15]

Orbital Cellulitis

Cellulitis of the orbital tissue is rare in the neonate but is a common cause of proptosis in children. In children, the infection most often originates in the paranasal sinuses and produces swelling of the orbital contents. Infections caused by penetrating orbital wounds or endogenous spread from remote locations are much less common in children.

The disease is characterized by the rapid onset of progressive proptosis, often with erythema of the lids, chemosis of the conjunctiva, limited motility, and systemic signs of toxicity and hyperpyrexia. Rapid loss of vision caused by compression of the orbital structures can occur.

Diagnosis is made by clinical appearance and radiologic evaluation of the orbits and sinuses. Treatment includes admission to a hospital, CT scan of the orbits, intravenous administration of antibiotics, application of warm compresses, and surgical drainage of persistent orbital abscesses if necessary.[21]

In preseptal cellulitis, the infection is limited to the lids and does not extend past the orbital septum to involve the orbital contents. It is usually caused by streptococcal and staphylococcal bacteria and can be treated on an outpatient basis with oral antibiotics. Widespread vaccination has dramatically decreased *Haemophilus*-associated orbital and preseptal cellulitis.

OCULAR TUMORS IN INFANTS

Ocular tumors of the lids and conjunctivae are often easily diagnosed based on clinical history and pattern recognition. Diagnosing intraocular tumors requires a more detailed examination, often under anesthesia, and ancillary testing such as fluorescein angiogram and MRI. Biopsy is only rarely considered in these circumstances. Diagnosing orbital tumors can be more challenging.

Orbital tumors may be benign or malignant and can develop from ectodermal, mesodermal, and neural crest tissues or by metastasis from distant sites. They also can originate from the intracranial cavity or paranasal sinuses and enter the orbit by growing through natural or acquired bone defects in the orbital walls. Ultrasound, MRI, and CT are particularly valuable in the diagnosis of orbital disease.

Hemangioma

Infantile hemangioma is the most common primary orbital tumor that produces proptosis. In infants, the hemangioma usually is not well encapsulated and often involves the lids as well as the orbit. Although observation of lid involvement assists in making the diagnosis, a biopsy might be required to exclude other orbital tumors if the hemangioma lacks a superficial component. Crying or straining by the infant often causes the mass to increase in size and assume a bluish coloration.

Treatment initially should be confined to expectant observation because spontaneous resolution is the rule. However, some tumors require therapy because of growth that produces a refractive error (astigmatism) or obstruction of the pupillary axis, resulting in amblyopia. Glasses and patching might be necessary to prevent or treat amblyopia. Promising new therapy with oral propranolol has recently been described.[47] In the past, treatment involved systemic, injectable, or topical corticosteroids, or other drugs.[19] Occasionally, surgery is indicated.[85]

Another type of hemangioma is the port-wine stain of the face (nevus flammeus) associated with Sturge-Weber syndrome.

Lymphangioma

Lymphangiomas are slowly progressive, diffuse, soft tumors that may be present at birth or gradually develop during the first several years of life. They tend to enlarge slowly and cease growing by early adulthood. An upper respiratory tract infection may be associated with an increase in the size of the lesion. Spontaneous hemorrhage into an orbital lymphangioma can cause sudden proptosis. Lymphangiomas are composed of thin-walled vascular channels that can involve the orbit and lids as well as other tissues in the body. The tumors can cause proptosis, ptosis, strabismus, or anisometropia. Amblyopia is common and must be aggressively treated. The lesion itself is difficult to treat because it does not regress spontaneously or respond to radiation or corticosteroid therapy. Although surgery is the treatment of choice, results are not always satisfactory.

MRI can be exceedingly helpful in diagnosing a lymphangioma. Surgical removal of the tumor might be necessary for cosmetic or functional reasons, but recurrence is common. Picibanil (OK-432), a sclerosing agent, can be injected directly into lymphangiomas.[103]

Dermoid Cysts

Dermoid cysts are thought to arise from a congenital rest of primitive ectoderm at the site of closure of a fetal cleft. They usually contain connective tissue, sebaceous glands, and hair follicles. Cysts are often located near the orbital rim, where they are attached to bone at suture sites. The most frequent location is in the lateral third of the brow or upper lid. The skin overlying the soft cyst is freely movable, although the cyst remains attached to the periosteum at the site of the embryonic cleft. The cysts can connect with the cranial cavity, paranasal sinuses, or orbit, and can produce local bone changes. Cysts located within the orbit produce proptosis and vertical or horizontal displacement of the globe. Radiographic examination might document bone erosion where the cyst is attached. Local trauma can produce a hemorrhage into a dermoid cyst or cyst rupture, leading to a clinical picture resembling cellulitis. Surgical excision is recommended and is usually curative, especially for the dermoids external to the orbit.

Teratoma

Teratoma is a primary orbital tumor composed of the three embryonic cell layers. It can differentiate into a variety of tissues containing cartilage, connective tissue, skin, hair, and sebaceous glands or into endodermal epithelium. Bone is a common component and can be identified by orbital roentgenograms. Orbital teratomas that are present at birth produce a striking massive proptosis. Treatment is early excision of the teratoma. Malignant transformation can occur but is rare in the orbit.

Rhabdomyosarcoma

Rhabdomyosarcoma is the most common malignant tumor of the orbit in children (Fig. 53-14). Although it may be found in the neonatal period, the average age of occurrence is 6 to 10 years. Rhabdomyosarcoma develops in the orbit more often than elsewhere in the body. Orbital involvement produces proptosis that develops over a few weeks. Diagnosis is made by biopsy. Treatment in the past involved orbital

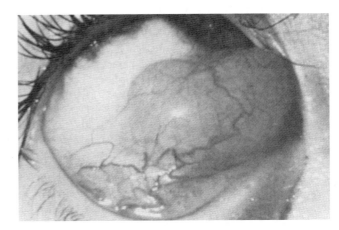

Figure 53–14. Rhabdomyosarcoma of the right orbit.

exenteration, but this is now replaced by chemotherapy and radiation therapy.

Histiocytoses

Children with histiocytoses (eosinophilic granuloma, Hand-Schüller-Christian disease, and Letterer-Siwe disease) may have proptosis or ptosis. Involvement is usually painful, with features of inflammation.

Retinoblastoma

Retinoblastoma is the most frequent malignant intraocular tumor affecting the neonatal eye. In the United States, about 50% of retinoblastoma cases are diagnosed by leukocoria detected by primary care physicians or a parent (Fig. 53-15).

Retinoblastoma occurs in about 1 in 20,000 births, with no predilection for race or sex. The tumor arises sporadically or may be familial.

The genetic basis for retinoblastoma has been widely studied. The gene, located on the q14 band of chromosome 13, is a tumor suppressor gene. Mutation or inactivation of both alleles in a vulnerable retina cell results in transformation of the cell into retinoblastoma.[100]

The tumor originates in the retina and grows anteriorly into the vitreous or posteriorly into the choroid. If the tumor disrupts vision, a sensory strabismus may result. Hence, all infants with strabismus require a fundus examination with dilated pupils to exclude retinoblastoma. With further enlargement, the tumor produces secondary glaucoma, which may be associated with pain and photophobia or symptoms identical to those of congenital glaucoma. With extension into the anterior chamber, an opaque layer of leukocytes (pseudo-hypopyon) or spontaneous bleeding (hyphema) can occur.

The diagnosis of retinoblastoma is supported by the detection of one or more solid white masses in the fundus of the eye. Small, whitish opacities in the vitreous, representing an anterior seeding of the tumor, may be present. Calcification identified within the eye on CT scan, ultrasound, and MRI findings help to confirm the diagnosis. The differential diagnosis may be exceedingly difficult if the tumor is advanced or atypical, and enucleation may be required for histologic

study and positive identification. Other lesions that rarely can simulate retinoblastoma are coloboma of the fundus, congenital retinal fold, retinal dysplasia, persistent hyperplastic primary vitreous, retinoschisis, organizing vitreous hemorrhage, or scarring from ROP.

The treatment of retinoblastoma is determined by its size and location. Examination should be performed with the infant under anesthesia, and accurate documentation of all lesions should be done with drawings or photography.

The treatment of retinoblastoma involves a team approach between pediatric oncologists, radiologists, and ophthalmologists. A variety of chemotherapeutic regimens are now used with increasing success.[10,42] Other local treatment modalities for unilateral and bilateral retinoblastoma include external-beam irradiation, plaque radiotherapy, thermotherapy, photocoagulation, and cryotherapy.

The most significant factor in the prognosis is the stage of disease when treatment is instituted. When retinoblastoma is limited to the eye, 98% of patients can expect a 5-year disease-free survival.[10] With extension beyond the globe, the cure rate is reduced. Because radiation therapy has many side effects, adjuvant chemotherapy is increasingly being used to avoid enucleation and to prevent metastatic disease.

Patients with the familial form of retinoblastoma also are at risk for developing secondary malignancies.[63] The most common secondary malignancy is osteogenic sarcoma, usually occurring in the teen years. Pinealoblastoma forms the third part of what is called *trilateral retinoblastoma*. This malignancy usually occurs during the first 4 years of life.

OCULAR CHANGES FROM MATERNAL SUBSTANCE ABUSE

An increasing number of infants are born bearing the physical, mental, and social consequences of maternal drug and alcohol abuse. Miller and colleagues described many of the ocular findings of fetal alcohol syndrome, including refractive errors, strabismus, anterior segment abnormalities, cataract, ptosis, long eyelashes, telecanthus, and optic nerve hypoplasia.[58] Maternal ingestion of cocaine can result in optic nerve abnormalities, delayed visual maturation, and prolonged eyelid edema.[26] Maternal cigarette smoking has been identified as a risk factor for strabismus.[29] As more information is gathered, additional evidence of the teratogenicity of various illicit drugs may be obtained.

REFERENCES

1. Abadi RV, Whittle J: The nature of head postures in congenital nystagmus, *Arch Ophthalmol* 109:216, 1991.
2. American Academy of Pediatrics Committee on Practice and Ambulatory Medicine, Section on Ophthalmology: Eye examination and vision screening in infants, children, and young adults, *Pediatrics* 98:153, 1996.
3. American Academy of Pediatrics, Section on Ophthalmology; American Association for Pediatric Ophthalmology and Strabismus; American Academy of Ophthalmology; American Association of Certified Orthoptists. Red reflex examination in neonates, infants, and children. Pediatrics 122:1401, 2008, *Erratum in: Pediatrics* 123:1254, 2009.

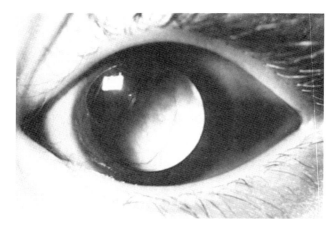

Figure 53–15. Leukokoria in a patient with advanced retinoblastoma.

4. Archer SM, et al: Strabismus in infancy, *Ophthalmology* 96:133, 1989.

5. Beysen D, et al: FOXL2 mutations and genomic rearrangements in BPES, *Hum Mutat* 30:158, 2009.

6. Bitoun P, et al: A new look at the management of the oculo-mandibulo-facial syndrome, *Ophthalmol Paediatr Genet* 13:19, 1992.

7. Boonstra FN, et al: Clinical and molecular evaluation of probands and family members with familial exudative vitreoretinopathy, *Invest Ophthalmol Vis Sci* 50:4379, 2009.

8. Buckley EG: The clinical approach to the pediatric patient with nystagmus, *Int Pediatr* 5:225, 1990.

9. Cassidy L, et al: Abnormal supranuclear eye movements in the child: a practical guide to examination and interpretation, *Surv Ophthalmol* 44:479, 2000.

10. Chantada G, et al: Results of a prospective study for the treatment of retinoblastoma, *Cancer* 100:834, 2004.

11. Clark DI, Patterson A: Ankyloblepharon filiforme adnatum in trisomy 18 (Edwards's syndrome), *Br J Ophthalmol* 69:471, 1985.

12. Cline RA, Rootman J: Enophthalmos: a clinical review, *Ophthalmology* 91:229, 1984.

12a. Crawford JS: Congenital eyelid anomalies in children, *J Pediatr Ophthalmol Strabismus* 21:140, 1984.

13. Curnyn KM, Kaufman LM: The eye examination in the pediatrician's office, *Pediatr Clin North Am* 50:25, 2003.

14. da Silva Dal Pizzol T, et al: Prenatal exposure to misoprostol and congenital anomalies: systematic review and meta-analysis, *Reprod Toxicol* 22:666, 2006.

15. Du LT, et al: Incidence of presumed cytomegalovirus retinitis in HIV-infected pediatric patients, *J AAPOS* 3:245, 1999.

16. Edward DP, Kaufman LM: Anatomy, development, and physiology of the visual system, *Pediatr Clin North Am* 50:1, 2003.

17. Edwards AO: Clinical features of the congenital vitreoretinopathies, *Eye* 22:1233, 2008.

18. Elgin U, et al: The comparison of eyelash lengthening effect of latanoprost therapy in adults and children, *Eur J Ophthalmol* 16:247, 2006.

19. Elsas FJ, Lewis AR: Topical treatment of periocular capillary hemangioma, *J Pediatr Ophthalmol Strabismus* 31:153, 1994.

20. Evans AK, et al: Robin sequence: a retrospective review of 115 patients, *Int J Pediatr Otorhinolaryngol* 70:973, 2006.

21. Ferguson MP, McNab AA: Current treatment and outcome in orbital cellulitis, *Aust N Z J Ophthalmol* 27:375, 1999.

22. Fischbach BV, et al: WAGR syndrome: a clinical review of 54 cases, *Pediatrics* 116:984, 2005.

23. Friedman LS, Kaufman LM: Guidelines for pediatrician referrals to the ophthalmologist, *Pediatr Clin North Am* 50:41, 2003.

24. Fulton AB, et al: Development of rod function in term born and former preterm subjects, *Optom Vis Sci* 86:E653, 2009.

25. Gal P, et al: Efficacy of sucrose to reduce pain in premature infants during eye examinations for retinopathy of prematurity, *Ann Pharmacother* 39:1029, 2005.

26. Good WV, et al: Abnormalities of the visual system in infants exposed to cocaine, *Ophthalmology* 99:341, 1992.

27. Gottlob I, et al: Signs distinguishing spasmus nutans (with and without central nervous systems lesions) from infantile nystagmus, *Ophthalmology* 97:1166, 1990.

28. Grüters A: Ocular manifestations in children and adolescents with thyrotoxicosis, *Exp Clin Endocrinol Diabetes* 107:S172, 1999.

29. Hakim RB, Tielsch JM: Maternal cigarette smoking during pregnancy: A risk factor for childhood strabismus, *Arch Ophthalmol* 110:1459, 1992.

30. Hanein S, et al: Leber congenital amaurosis: comprehensive survey of the genetic heterogeneity, refinement of the clinical definition, and genotype-phenotype correlations as a strategy for molecular diagnosis, *Hum Mutat* 23:306, 2004.

31. Hantaï D, et al: Congenital myasthenic syndromes, *Curr Opin Neurol* 17:539, 2004.

32. Hentschel J, et al: Neonatal facial movements in the first minutes of life-eye opening and tongue thrust: an observational study, *Am J Perinatol* 24:611, 2007.

33. Hingorani M, et al: Detailed ophthalmologic evaluation of 43 individuals with PAX6 mutations, *Invest Ophthalmol Vis Sci* 50:2581, 2009.

34. Holden R, et al: External ocular trauma in instrumental and normal deliveries, *Br J Obstet Gynaecol* 99:132, 1992.

35. Hughes LA, et al: Incidence, distribution, and duration of birth-related retinal hemorrhages: a prospective study, *J AAPOS* 10:102, 2006.

37. Ide CH, Wollschlaeger PB: Multiple congenital abnormalities associated with cryptophthalmia, *Arch Ophthalmol* 81:638, 1969.

38. Isenberg SJ, et al: The pupils of term and preterm infants, *Am J Ophthalmol* 15:75, 1989.

39. Kaufman LM, et al: Magnetic resonance imaging of pituitary stalk hypoplasia. A discrete midline anomaly associated with endocrine abnormalities in septo-optic dysplasia, *Arch Ophthalmol* 107:1485, 1989.

40. Khalil SK, et al: Traumatic optic nerve injury occurring after forceps delivery of a term newborn, *J AAPOS* 7:146, 2003.

41. Khong JJ, et al: Ophthalmic findings in Apert syndrome prior to craniofacial surgery, *Am J Ophthalmol* 142:328, 2006.

42. Kim H, et al: Clinical results of chemotherapy based treatment in retinoblastoma patients: a single center experience, *Cancer Res Treat* 40:164, 2008.

43. Kivlin JD: Manifestations of the shaken baby syndrome, *Curr Opin Ophthalmol* 12:158, 2001.

44. Koelsch E, Harrington JW: Marcus Gunn jaw-winking synkinesis in a neonate, *Mov Disord* 30:871, 2007.

45. Kreiborg S, Cohen MM Jr: Is craniofacial morphology in Apert and Crouzon syndromes the same? *Acta Odontol Scand* 56:339, 1998.

46. Lauer AK, Rimmer SO: Eyelid laceration in a neonate by fetal monitoring spiral electrode, *Am J Ophthalmol* 125:715, 1998.

47. Léauté-Labrèze C, et al: Propranolol for severe hemangiomas of infancy, *N Engl J Med* 358:2649, 2008.

48. Lee BJ, Traboulsi EI: Update on the morning glory disc anomaly, *Ophthalmic Genet* 29:47, 2008.

49. Lee H, et al: Aniridia: current pathology and management, *Acta Ophthalmol* 86:708, 2008.

50. Lorenz B, Gampe E: Analysis of 180 patients with sensory defect nystagmus (SDN) and congenital idiopathic nystagmus (CIN), *Klin Monatsbl Augenheilkd* 218:3, 2001.

51. Lowenfeld IE: *The Pupil*, 1st ed, Detroit, 1993, Iowa State University Press.

52. Lueder GT: Clinical ocular abnormalities in infants with trisomy 13, *Am J Ophthalmol* 141:1057, 2006.

53. Lueder GT: Balloon catheter dilation for treatment of older children with nasolacrimal duct obstruction, *Arch Ophthalmol* 120:1685, 2002.

54. MacLachlan C, Howland HC: Normal values and standard deviations for pupil diameter and interpupillary distance in subjects aged 1 month to 19 years, *Ophthalmic Physiol Opt* 22:175, 2002.

55. Marmur R, et al: Optokinetic nystagmus as related to neonatal position, *J Child Neurol* 22:1108, 2007.

56. McDonald MB, Burgess SK: Contralateral occipital depression related to obstetric forceps injury to the eye, *Am J Ophthalmol* 114:318, 1992.

57. Mets MB, et al: Eye manifestations of congenital toxoplasmosis, *Am J Ophthalmol* 123:1, 1997.

58. Miller MT, et al: Anterior segment anomalies associated with fetal alcohol syndrome, *J Pediatr Ophthalmol Strabismus* 21:8, 1984.

59. Miller MT, et al: Möbius and Möbius-like syndromes (TTV-OFM, OMLH), *J Pediatr Ophthalmol Strabismus* 26:176, 1989.

60. Miller MT: Craniofacial syndromes and malformations. In Wright K, editor: *Pediatric ophthalmology and strabismus,* St Louis, 1995, Mosby-Year Book.

61. Mir GH, Cumming GR: Response to atropine in Down's syndrome, *Arch Dis Child* 46:61, 1971.

62. Miyashiro MJ, Mintz-Hittner HA: Penetrating ocular injury with a fetal scalp monitoring spiral electrode, *Am J Ophthalmol* 128:526, 1999.

63. Mohney BG, et al: Second nonocular tumors in survivors of heritable retinoblastoma and prior radiation therapy, *Am J Ophthalmol* 126:269, 1998.

64. Morad Y, et al: Fundus anomalies: what the pediatrician's eye can't see, *Int J Qual Health Care* 16:363, 2004.

65. Nallasamy S, et al: Ophthalmologic findings in Cornelia de Lange syndrome: a genotype-phenotype correlation study, *Arch Ophthalmol* 124:552, 2006.

66. Naumanen T, et al: Loss-of-function of IKAP/ELP1: could neuronal migration defect underlie familial dysautonomia? *Cell Adh Migr* 2:236, 2008.

67. Naylor G, et al: Ophthalmic complications of amniocentesis, *Eye* 4:845, 1990.

68. Nichols JC, et al: Characteristics of Lisch nodules in patients with neurofibromatosis type 1, *J Pediatr Ophthalmol Strabismus* 40:293, 2003.

69. Odom A, et al: Prevalence of retinal hemorrhages in pediatric patients after in-hospital cardiopulmonary resuscitation: a prospective study, *Pediatrics* 99:E3, 1997.

70. Ostrowski G, et al: Do phototherapy hoods really protect the neonate? *Acta Paediatr* 89:874, 2000.

71. Pascual-Castroviejo I, et al: Sturge-Weber syndrome: study of 55 patients, *Can J Neurol Sci* 35:301, 2008.

72. Patel AJ, et al: Cycloplegic and mydriatic agents for routine ophthalmologic examination: a survey of pediatric ophthalmologists, *J AAPOS* 8:274, 2004.

73. Pinto G, et al: Idiopathic growth hormone deficiency: presentation, diagnostic and treatment during childhood, *Ann Endocrinol (Paris)* 60:224, 1999.

74. Regis A, et al: Ocular injuries and childbirth, *J Fr Ophtalmol* 27:987, 2004.

75. Richieri-Costa A, Guion-Almeida ML: The syndrome of frontonasal dysplasia, callosal agenesis, basal encephalocele, and eye anomalies-phenotypic and aetiological considerations, *Int J Med Sci* 1:34, 2004.

76. Roarty JD, Keltner JL: Normal pupil size and anisocoria in newborn infant, *Arch Ophthalmol* 108:94, 1990.

77. Roarty JD, et al: Ocular manifestations of frontonasal dysplasia, *Plast Reconstr Surg* 93:25, 1994.

78. Salpietro CD, et al: Chlamydia trachomatis conjunctivitis in the newborn, *Arch Pediatr* 6:317, 1999.

79. Sandstrom I: Treatment of neonatal conjunctivitis, *Arch Ophthalmol* 105:925, 1987.

80. Santana A, et al: Mutation analysis of CRYAA, CRYGC, and CRYGD associated with autosomal dominant congenital cataract in Brazilian families, *Mol Vis* 15:793, 2009.

81. Seah LL, et al: Congenital upper lid colobomas: management and visual outcome, *Ophthal Plast Reconstr Surg* 18:190, 2002.

82. Simon J, et al: Vitrectomy for dense vitreous hemorrhage in infancy, *J Pediatr Ophthalmol Strabismus* 42:18, 2005.

83. Simons BD, et al: Surgical technique, visual outcome, and complications of pediatric intraocular lens implantation, *J Pediatr Ophthalmol Strabismus* 36:118, 1999.

84. Sireteanu R, et al: The development of peripheral visual acuity in human infants. A preliminary study, *Hum Neurobiol* 3:81, 1984.

85. Slaughter K, et al: Early surgical intervention as definitive treatment for ocular adnexal capillary haemangioma, *Clin Experiment Ophthalmol* 31:418, 2003.

86. Slobodian TV: A case of penetrating injury of the eye in a fetus during Caesarean section, *Oftalmol Zh* 1:60, 1988.

87. Sotomi O, et al: Have we stopped looking for a red reflex in newborn screening? *Ir Med J* 100:398, 2007.

88. Strömland K, et al: Oculo-auriculo-vertebral spectrum: associated anomalies, functional deficits and possible developmental risk factors, *Am J Med Genet A* 15:1317, 2007.

89. Sturm V, et al: Rare retinal haemorrhages in translational accidental head trauma in children, *Eye* 23:1535, 2009.

90. Tallman B, et al: Location of port-wine stains and the likelihood of ophthalmic and/or central nervous system complications, *Pediatrics* 87:323, 1991.

91. Tang J, et al: Shaken baby syndrome: a review and update on ophthalmologic manifestations, *Int Ophthalmol Clin* 48:237, 2008.

92. Tay T, et al: Prevalence and causes of visual impairment in craniosynostotic syndromes, *Clin Exp Ophthalmol* 34:434, 2006.

93. Tornqvist K, et al: Optic nerve hypoplasia: risk factors and epidemiology, *Acta Ophthalmol Scand* 80:300, 2002.

94. Trovó-Marqui AB, Tajara EH: Neurofibromin: a general outlook, *Clin Genet* 70:1, 2006.

95. van Haelst MM, et al: Molecular study of 33 families with Fraser syndrome: new data and mutation review, *Am J Med Genet A* 146A:2252, 2008.

96. Verma AS, Fitzpatrick DR: Anophthalmia and microphthalmia, *Orphanet J Rare Dis* 26:47, 2007.

97. Weiss AH, et al: Complex microphthalmos, *Arch Ophthalmol* 107:1619, 1989.

98. Weiss AH, et al: Simple microphthalmos, *Arch Ophthalmol* 107:1625, 1989.

99. Wieczorek D, et al: Two brothers with Burn-McKeown syndrome, *Clin Dysmorphol* 12:171, 2003.

100. Wiggs JL, Dryja TP: Predicting the risk of hereditary retinoblastoma, *Am J Ophthalmol* 106:346, 1988.

101. Wong RK, VanderVeen DK: Presentation and management of congenital dacryocystocele, *Pediatrics* 122:e1108, 2008.

102. Wu WC, et al: Retinal phenotype-genotype correlation of pediatric patients expressing mutations in the Norrie disease gene, *Arch Ophthalmol* 125:225, 2007.

103. Yoo JC, et al: OK-432 sclerotherapy in head and neck lymphangiomas: long-term follow-up result, *Otolaryngol Head Neck Surg* 140:120, 2009.

PART 2

Retinopathy of Prematurity

Dale L. Phelps

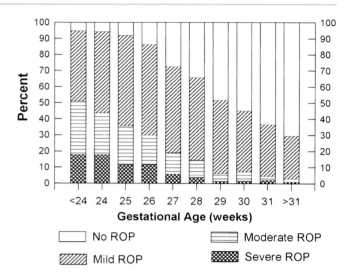

Retinopathy of prematurity (ROP) is a postnatal disorder of the retinal vessels that develops only in the incompletely vascularized retinas of premature infants. It leads to a wide range of outcomes from normal vision to blindness. First described in the early 1940s, *retrolental fibroplasia*, as it was first named, almost disappeared between 1954 and 1970, when oxygen use for preterms was severely restricted,[41] but it returned in a second epidemic in the 1970s to plague neonatal intensive care units (NICUs) as one of the major causes of disability in surviving infants with extremely low gestation.[12,26] Effective interventions have reduced its toll of vision loss in developed countries, but worldwide, ROP now appears as a third epidemic in developing countries as they begin to provide neonatal intensive care.[13]

INCIDENCE

ROP is common among extremely low gestation infants (especially those <29 weeks), but severe ROP causing vision loss is fortunately the minority of cases. The Cryotherapy for Retinopathy of Prematurity Natural History Study of 4099 infants born in the late 1980s and weighing less than 1251 g at birth prospectively followed these infants in the NICU and importantly after discharge until the final outcome of their ROP was known. The overall incidence of ROP of any severity was 66%; moderately severe ROP, 18%; and severe ROP, 6%.[26] The rates by gestational age are shown in Figure 53-16.[8,28] Among studies with similarly complete follow-up, little changed in the 1990s[36] or early 2000s.[15]

Lower gestational age and birthweight have always been the strongest predictors of ROP. After controlling for these parameters in regression analyses, the strongest additional risk factors for severe stages of ROP are prolonged administration of oxygen, duration of mechanical ventilation, and other indicators of a complicated hospital course, such as hypotension (e.g., hypovolemic shock, pneumothorax, severe intraventricular hemorrhage, septic shock), number of transfusions, multiple birth, out-born status, nonblack race for the more severe stages of ROP, and small for gestational age status at birth.[3,4,16,23,24,26,34]

PATHOGENESIS

Only infants whose retinal vessels have not yet completed their centrifugal growth from the optic disc to the ora serrata may develop ROP. Retinal vessel growth begins from the optic disc at 14 to 18 weeks' gestation, proceeding outward as the retina differentiates. Primitive future endothelial cells form cords that canalize into a network of evenly spaced primitive capillaries, which further remodel into primitive and then mature arterioles and venules. Each of these steps can be seen simultaneously at any moment in time because

Figure 53–16. Incidence of mild (less than prethreshold), moderately severe (prethreshold), and severe (threshold) retinopathy of prematurity (ROP). (*Data from Phelps DL: Retinopathy of prematurity: history, classification, and pathophysiology,* Neoreviews 2:e153, 2001; *and the ROP definitions from Cryotherapy for Retinopathy of Prematurity Cooperative Group: Multicenter Trial of Cryotherapy for Retinopathy of Prematurity: 32-year outcome-structure and function,* Arch Ophthalmol 111:339, 1993.)

they are sequentially proceeding from the disc outward toward the ora serrata in the immature retina (Fig. 53-17A).

When any injury occurs to these developing vessels, the natural progress is arrested. Prolonged hyperoxia, shock, asphyxia, hypothermia, acidosis, and vitamin E deficiency are among the factors that have been implicated as possible reasons for the initial injury. Inhibition of vascularization in this early phase 1 of ROP has been attributed to suppression of vascular endothelial growth factor (VEGF), and possibly erythropoietin, by hyperoxia. Lack of insulin-like growth factor-1 (IGF-1) in this phase of ROP and associated poor postnatal growth may also prevent normal retinal vascular growth.[17,18] After initial injury, vessel growth can resume in a near-normal fashion (i.e., no ROP), or for poorly understood reasons, the progress of primitive vessels can remain arrested, piling up within the retina, growing without forward progress, and forming a ridge of tissue that can become quite thick (see Fig. 53-17B). This tissue might subsequently regress or resolve, and the vessels again progress toward the periphery, or the ROP can worsen through the growth of fibrovascular tissue into the vitreous cavity, leading in some cases to retinal detachment.

In phase 2 of ROP, pathologic vascular proliferation appears to be associated with hypoxia-induced rising levels of VEGF, erythropoietin, and IGF-1.[17] This is consistent with the recent clinical observation that a higher incidence of intermittent hypoxemic episodes is associated with severe retinopathy of prematurity.[8a] In some infants, the regrowing vessels become inflamed, with vitreous haze, exudate along the retinal vessels, and engorgement and tortuosity of the

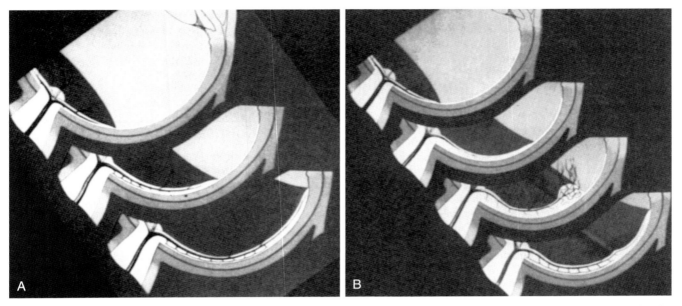

Figure 53–17. A, Cross sections of normally developing retina and retinal vasculature. From the *top left* to the *bottom right*, the area of the normally vascularizing retina increases with age from 24 weeks' gestation to term as the retina centrifugally differentiates. Retinal thickness and vessels have been exaggerated for illustration. B, Cross sections of the retina across time as the retinal vessels ablate after preterm delivery, revascularize to an excessive degree with intravitreal extension (retinopathy of prematurity), and finally regress, leaving a residual visible ridge of tissue (mild cicatrix) where the retinopathy had been. (*From Phelps DL: Retinopathy of prematurity. In* Mead Johnson Symposium on Perinatal and Developmental Medicine: the tiny baby, *held at Marco Island, Florida, Nov. 16-20, 1988; No. 33. Printed in 1990.*)

posterior pole vessels as well as the remnants of the tunica vasculosa lentis on the lens and in the iris. This condition is called *plus disease*, and recent data suggest it is linked to high levels of VEGF and associated growth factors in the retina and vitreous cavity.[1,2,5] As infants mature, rising levels of IGF-1 may allow VEGF-stimulated neovascularization to occur. When extraretinal neovascularization and plus disease occur, this "threshold" ROP can still heal spontaneously in nearly 50% of infants[7]; however, in the others, the tissue forms a scar (cicatrix) that contracts and distorts the retina, leading to a displaced macula, retinal folds, or retinal detachments. This sequence occurs as early as 8 to 10 weeks after birth but most often 3 to 5 months after birth. (An animated illustration of this sequence can be viewed at http://www.nei.nih.gov/photo.)

Oxygen was inexorably linked to ROP with the publication of the randomized, cooperative trial of oxygen restriction published in 1956. It showed that the then-common practice of administering more than 50% inspired oxygen for longer than 4 weeks resulted in an incidence of severe retinopathy of 23% in survivors, compared with just 7% in infants given oxygen just sufficient to relieve cyanosis.[22] That study randomized subjects weighing less than 1500 g at 48 hours after birth and occurred at a time when ventilators, continuous positive airway pressure, and even intravenous fluids had not yet entered the nursery. In the era that followed this study, oxygen use was severely restricted without the benefit of blood gas determinations, resulting in an increased preterm mortality rate; however, ROP was nearly eliminated for a time.[41] The resurgence of ROP in the second epidemic was attributed to the increased survival rate of

infants with retinas so immature at birth that the controlled use of oxygen did not appear to contribute to disease, and other complications of the perinatal period, in addition to the extreme immaturity, were believed to be primarily responsible.[12]

The oxygen story, however, continues to haunt us. Case series restricting oxygen at the turn of the century suggested that further restriction or control of oxygen in the modern intensive care unit could further reduce the incidence of ROP.[6,44] Although some quietly questioned whether these reports had merely demonstrated that giving oxygen carefully with attention to controlled saturation at all times around the clock would reduce ROP (i.e., were we finally just doing what our policies said we should do), others were pointing out that we did not know whether lowering pulse oximetry goals below 95% or 90%, or even 85%, was safe. Today, solid evidence is still lacking on the safe upper and lower limits of oxygenation in the preterm infant who has left in utero conditions of 60% to 70% saturation for ex utero conditions of 80% to 100% saturation.[45] Ongoing research aimed at answering those questions is being conducted cooperatively around the world.

In developing countries, however, the third epidemic of ROP is appearing as, for the first time, extremely preterm infants begin to survive. The beginning intensive care units do not initially have technology or sufficient staffing to carefully monitor oxygen administration.[13,47] The effect on vision loss is further complicated by lack of organized ophthalmic examination and treatment programs for a disorder previously unrecognized because such immature infants had not survived.

CLASSIFICATION

In 1984 and 1987, the International Classification of Retinopathy of Prematurity (ICROP) was developed to facilitate communication about ROP among physicians and investigators. It was published in two parts after years of work by ophthalmologists studying this disorder throughout the world[19,20] and was revisited in 2005.[21]

The classification has three novel new features. First, it locates the disease (anterior to posterior) by defining three zones that have strong prognostic significance (Fig. 53-18). ROP located in the most immature zone I has a much worse prognosis. Second, the extent of the disease is described by the number of clock hours (maximum of 12) involved within the zone. Third, the change in posterior pole venous dilation and arterial tortuosity that occurs in aggressive disease is identified by the designation of plus disease (or "preplus disease" if it is not normal, but does not meet criteria for plus disease).

As in previous classifications, the degree of vasculopathy at the vascular-avascular transition is divided into stages 1 through 5. Stages 1 through 3 are increasing degrees of abnormal blood vessel growth (neovascularization) at this transition, with vessels actually leaving the retina and growing in the vitreous in stage 3. Stage 4 is partial retinal detachment, and stage 5 is complete retinal detachment, both of which carry a grim prognosis for normal vision.

The international classification captures these degrees of disease and permits some early prognostication. For instance,

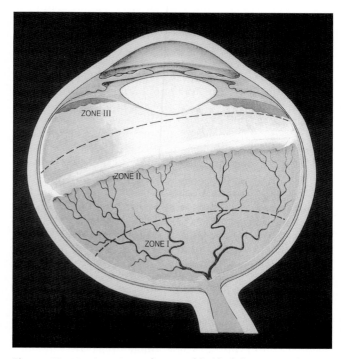

Figure 53–18. Artist's rendering of half of the eye with zone II, stage 3, retinopathy of prematurity with plus disease. The view is from the top of the head, with the temporal side of the retina to the reader's left, and the nasal side to the right. Zones I, II, and III are drawn onto the retina to assist in visualizing their positions within the eye.

ROP occurring in zone I (the most immature or posterior zone) has a greater chance of progressing to retinal detachment than does zone II disease, and rarely does zone III disease ever result in any permanent damage.[26,37] For investigators, the classification has been critical for improving communications and standardizing entry criteria for multicenter studies.

CLINICAL COURSE

When infants with ROP are examined regularly from 31 to 33 weeks' postmenstrual age (PMA), they demonstrate the sequential development of the stages of ROP until they reach a turning point when the ROP regresses (heals) or goes on to advanced disease. This turning point can occur after just stage 1, 2, or 3, and most often has turned by 36 to 42 weeks' PMA.[35]

Rates of progression are variable, and the worst prognosis is associated with onset in zone I (most immature) followed by rapid progression in time through stages 1, 2, and 3 to plus disease and retinal detachment. When this progression proceeds over a few weeks, the Japanese named it *rush disease*. Onset in zone II, or a slower evolution of the disorder, leads more often to complete resolution or to just a partial cicatrix (retinal scar). This slower resolution can take as long as a year to stabilize, but most often results in full recovery. ROP with an onset in zone III has a good prognosis for full recovery.[37]

Infants who develop only mild ROP (i.e., stage 1 or 2 without plus component) and heal without a residual cicatrix have a slightly increased incidence of myopia, strabismus, and amblyopia compared with term infants.[38] However, for those infants who develop threshold ROP and receive cryotherapy or laser ablation, severe myopia, glaucoma, and associated sequelae are common.[32] The infants who have a residual cicatrix without retinal detachment are also more likely to have any of these problems and are at risk for very slowly progressive retinal degeneration that can lead to retinal detachment and acuity loss in later decades.[27,42,43]

Infants who develop total retinal detachment are at risk for secondary glaucoma, entropion, and infections caused by eye rubbing. Even if they have no vision, they may benefit from referral for cosmetic treatment if phthisis (shrunken eye) begins to develop. Physicians must refer infants to early intervention programs and support their families.

THERAPY

The only completely effective prophylaxis for ROP is the prevention of premature deliveries. Meticulous oxygen monitoring is necessary to reduce the incidence of ROP to a minimum, but it cannot eliminate ROP,[11] nor has early administration of vitamin E[33] or restricting light exposure prevented ROP.[30,36] Lower oxygen saturation goals might prove useful in the future in reducing severe ROP.[6,44,45] These approaches are being investigated in controlled trials. The SUPPORT trial showed that management with oxygen targets of 89-91% vs 92-95% reduced ROP, but resulted in a statistically significant increase in mortality.[41a] Two additional trials are in progress and will further clarify optimal targets.

Fortunately, established ROP of a moderately severe degree (see new definition in Box 53-6) can be arrested effectively in

BOX 53–6   **Criteria for Peripheral Ablative Therapy for Retinopathy of Prematurity**

Zone II: Plus disease with stage 2 or 3 ROP
Zone I: Plus disease with stage 1 or 2 ROP
Zone I: Stage 3 ROP

ROP, retinopathy of prematurity.
Adapted from Early Treatment for Retinopathy of Prematurity Cooperative Group: Revised indications for the treatment of retinopathy of prematurity: results of the Early Treatment for Retinopathy of Prematurity Randomized Trial, *Arch Ophthalmol* 121:1684, 2003.

many cases by applying laser therapy or cryotherapy to ablate the entire peripheral avascular retina, which we believe is overproducing the angiogenic factors driving the vessels to grow abnormally. One of these factors has been identified as VEGF,[1,9] which is almost certainly representative of a group or cascade of factors involved in the control of retinal vascularization.[17] Although this treatment does not always succeed in preventing retinal detachment, it reduces the incidence of poor retinal outcomes at 2 years from 15.4% to 9.1%,[14] a further improvement from the poor outcome rate of 26% in the treated eyes in the CRYO-ROP study.[8] At 15 years' follow-up, the benefit of cryotherapy persists, although the effect on the appearance of the fundus is again greater than the benefit for visual function.[27] The criteria for laser treatment established by the ETROP multicenter trial first published in 2003 are shown in Box 53-6.

Use of supplemental oxygen to reduce the hypoxic stimulus for neovascularization has been studied in a multicenter trial. Although there was no harm to eyes that already had moderately severe ROP, there was no clear ophthalmic benefit, and there was increased pulmonary morbidity from maintaining oxygen saturations at 96% to 99% compared with 89% to 94%.[29]

With the development of effective humanized mouse antibody fragments that block VEGF in colorectal cancer and wet macular degeneration[48] (intravitreal injection), this approach has been tried in small case series of ROP patients with promising short-term results.[25] Controlled trials to study the effectiveness, and most importantly the short- and long-term safety, of an antiproliferative drug in the rapidly growing infant are needed.

When total or subtotal retinal detachment occurs, the usual prognosis is that there will be no useful vision, even when heroic vitrectomy is performed to reattach the retina.[31,46] With these discouraging results, some retinal surgeons perform scleral buckle procedures, early lens-sparing vitrectomy, or both, in an attempt to stabilize a partial detachment. However, there are no controlled trials of such interventions, and long-term follow-up outcomes are not yet available.

RECOMMENDATIONS FOR EXAMINATION SCHEDULE

Examinations to identify infants who have ROP must be done by a clinician skilled with indirect ophthalmoscopy of premature infants and must begin early enough to permit the application of laser therapy (or cryotherapy) to prevent progression of the disease if it meets treatment criteria.[10,39,40] The ophthalmic and pediatric societies periodically publish joint recommendations for the screening guidelines (Box 53-7).

Each infant at risk (i.e., those weighing less than 1500 g or born at 30 weeks' gestation or less, and those more mature preterm infants with birthweight of 1500 to 2000 g who had an unstable medical course) should be examined initially by the later of 31 weeks' PMA, or 4 weeks' chronologic age. If the retinal vasculature is complete to the ora serrata, repeated examinations are not needed. If the vessels are in zone III, ROP could develop or might be present but likely will be only mild, and repeated examinations are done at 2- to 4-week intervals to ensure complete vascularization. Infants with retinal vessels that have grown only into zone II should be followed at least every 2 weeks to observe for the development of ROP, which may require therapy. Infants with vessels only as far as zone I are at greatest risk for severe ROP and should be followed closely on the basis of the presence, severity, and rate of progression of any ROP.

Neonatologists and ophthalmologists must work closely together to ensure an efficient tracking system for timely examination of these infants and to be certain that follow-up examinations occur at the best times both in the hospital and after discharge or transfer. The examinations are technically challenging to perform, and vitreal cloudiness or poor dilation of the pupil can result in an imprecise judgment of the zone where vessels end. Moreover, the diagnosis of "no ROP" must be regarded as incomplete and vigorously followed with the question, "In what zone, or mature?" An infant can have zone I vessels and no ROP but be blind 6 weeks later because of ROP. Generally, because ROP develops in more than 90% of infants born at less than 26 weeks' gestation, the index of suspicion must be high, and follow-up examinations must be particularly adhered to in these babies. At 26 to 28 weeks' gestation, 70% develop ROP, and at 29 to 30 weeks' gestation, the incidence is lower (45%). The goal is to ensure that infants who reach criteria for surgery are offered this opportunity to minimize vision loss.

BOX 53–7   **Schedule for First Indirect Ophthalmoscopy in Premature Infants**

WHO
All infants 30 weeks' gestation or less, or weighing less than 1500 g at birth
Infants born at 1500 to 2000 g who have a medically unstable course

WHEN
By the later of 31 weeks' postmenstrual age* or 4 weeks after birth
Recommend first examination before discharge from the hospital

*Postmenstrual age in weeks is equal to the gestational age at birth plus the chronologic age in weeks after birth.
Adapted from American Academy of Pediatrics, American Association for Pediatric Ophthalmology and Strabismus, and American Academy of Ophthalmology: Screening examination of premature infants for retinopathy of prematurity, *Pediatrics* 117:152, 2006 and 118:1324, 2006.

After the acute process has resolved, continued follow-up is dictated by the worst degree of ROP that occurred in the acute course. For infants who have had laser or cryotherapy for ROP, close observation of the retina is usually provided by the retinal surgeon who has treated the infant. Pediatric ophthalmic care for corrective eyeglasses and possible strabismus or amblyopia therapy is also extremely important, and such treatment is often needed in the first year for infants with moderate ROP who did not need laser treatment, and frequently for those who needed such treatment.[32] Patients who have significant residual retinal scars (cicatrix) require regular ophthalmologic follow-up care for life because of the incidence of late retinal detachments that can sometimes be effectively treated.[42]

Neonatologists and ophthalmologists can offer hope of preserving vision in most premature infants with severe acute ROP. However, this requires an organized system of tracking each preterm birth and arranging examinations in a timely fashion both in the intensive care unit and its associated referral units to which infants return after initial care, and when infants are discharged home without full resolution of their ROP. Research must continue in order to learn about the basic mechanisms involved in the control of retinal vascular development and neovascularization. When understood and applied in appropriate clinical settings, such knowledge may permit the ultimate complete control of ROP.

REFERENCES

1. Aiello LP, et al: Vascular endothelial growth factor in ocular fluid of patients with diabetic retinopathy and other retinal disorders, *N Engl J Med* 331:1480, 1994.
2. Aiello LP, et al: Suppression of retinal neovascularization in vivo by inhibition of vascular endothelial growth factor (VEGF) using soluble VEGF-receptor chimeric proteins, *Proc Natl Acad Sci U S A* 92:10457, 1995.
3. Allegaert K, et al: Threshold retinopathy at threshold of viability: the EpiBel study, *Br J Ophthalmol* 88:239, 2004.
4. Allegaert K, et al: Perinatal growth characteristics and associated risk of developing threshold retinopathy of prematurity, *J AAPOS* 7:34, 2003.
5. Chen J, Smith LEH: Retinopathy of prematurity, *Angiogenesis* 10:133, 2007.
6. Chow LC, et al: Can changes in clinical practice decrease the incidence of severe retinopathy of prematurity in very low birth weight infants? *Pediatrics* 111:339, 2003.
7. Cryotherapy for Retinopathy of Prematurity Cooperative Group: Multicenter trial of cryotherapy for retinopathy of prematurity: preliminary results, *Pediatrics* 81:697, 1988.
8. Cryotherapy for Retinopathy of Prematurity Cooperative Group: Multicenter trial of cryotherapy for retinopathy of prematurity: 3 1/2-year outcome—structure and function, *Arch Ophthalmol* 111:339, 1993.
8a. Di Fiore JM, Bloom JN, Orge F, et al: A higher incidence of intermittent hypoxemic episodes is associated with severe retinopathy of prematurity, *J Pediatr* 157:69, 2010.
9. Donahue ML, et al: Retinal vascular endothelial growth factor (VEGF) mRNA expression is altered in relation to neovascularization in oxygen induced retinopathy, *Curr Eye Res* 15:175, 1996.
10. ETROP Cooperative Group: Revised indications for the treatment of retinopathy of prematurity: results of the early treatment for retinopathy of prematurity randomized trial, *Arch Ophthalmol* 121:1684, 2003.
11. Flynn JT, et al: Retinopathy of prematurity. A randomized, prospective trial of transcutaneous oxygen monitoring, *Ophthalmology* 94:630, 1987.
12. Gibson DL, et al: Retinopathy of prematurity-induced blindness: birth weight-specific survival and the new epidemic, *Pediatrics* 86:405, 1990.
13. Gilbert C: Retinopathy of prematurity: a global perspective of the epidemics, population of babies at risk and implications for control, *Early Hum Dev* 84:77, 2008.
14. Good WV, et al: The Early Treatment for Retinopathy of Prematurity Study: structural findings at age 2 years, *Br J Ophthalmol* 90:1378, 2006.
15. Good WV, et al: The incidence and course of retinopathy of prematurity: findings from the early treatment for retinopathy of prematurity study, *Pediatrics* 116:15, 2005.
16. Gunn TR, et al: Risk factors in retrolental fibroplasia, *Pediatrics* 65:1096, 1980.
17. Hellstrom A, et al: IGF-I is critical for normal vascularization of the human retina, *J Clin Endocrinol Metab* 87:3413, 2002.
18. Hellstrom A, Hard AL, Engstrom E, et al: Early weight gain predicts retinopathy in preterm infants: new, simple, efficient approach to screening, *Pediatrics* 123:e638, 2009.
19. International Committee for Classification of ROP: An international classification of retinopathy of prematurity, *Pediatrics* 74:127, 1984.
20. International Committee for Classification of ROP: An international classification of retinopathy of prematurity. II. The classification of retinal detachment. [published erratum appears in *Arch Ophthalmol* 105:1498, 1987.] *Arch Ophthalmol* 105:906, 1987.
21. International Committee for Classification of ROP: The International Classification of Retinopathy of Prematurity revisited. [commentary, errata, *Arch Ophthalmol* 124:1669, 2006], *Arch Ophthalmol* 123:991, 2005.
22. Kinsey VE, et al: Retrolental fibroplasia: cooperative study of retrolental fibroplasia and the use of oxygen, *Arch Ophthalmol* 56:481, 1956.
23. Lin HJ, et al: Risk factors for retinopathy of prematurity in very low birth-weight infants, *JCMA* 66:662, 2003.
24. Liu PM, et al: Risk factors of retinopathy of prematurity in premature infants weighing less than 1600 g, *Am J Perinatol* 22:115, 2005.
25. Mintz-Hittner HA, et al: Intravitreal injection of bevacizumab (Avastin) for treatment of stage 3 retinopathy of prematurity in zone I or posterior zone II, *Retina* 28:831, 2008.
26. Palmer EA, et al: Incidence and early course of retinopathy of prematurity. Cryotherapy for Retinopathy of Prematurity Cooperative Group, *Ophthalmology* 98:1628, 1991.
27. Palmer EA, et al: 15-year outcomes following threshold retinopathy of prematurity: final results from the multicenter trial of cryotherapy for retinopathy of prematurity, *Arch Ophthalmol* 123:311, 2005.
28. Phelps DL: Retinopathy of prematurity: history, classification, and pathophysiology, *Neoreviews* 2:e153, 2001.
29. Phelps DL, et al: Supplemental therapeutic oxygen for prethreshold retinopathy of prematurity (STOP-ROP), a randomized, controlled trial. I: Primary outcomes, *Pediatrics* 105:295, 2000.

30. Phelps DL, et al: Early light reduction for preventing retinopathy of prematurity in very low birth weight infants, *Cochrane Database Syst Rev* 1:CD000122, 2001.

31. Quinn GE, et al: Visual acuity of eyes after vitrectomy for retinopathy of prematurity: Follow-up at 5½ years, *Ophthalmology* 103:595, 1996.

32. Quinn GE, et al: Prevalence of myopia between 3 months and 5½ years in preterm infants with and without retinopathy of prematurity, *Ophthalmology* 105:1292, 1998.

33. Raju TNK, et al: Vitamin E prophylaxis to reduce retinopathy of prematurity—a reappraisal of published trials, *J Pediatr* 131:844, 1997.

34. Regev RH, et al: Excess mortality and morbidity among small-for-gestational-age premature infants: a population-based study, *J Pediatr* 143:186, 2003.

35. Reynolds JD, et al: Evidence-based screening criteria for retinopathy of prematurity: natural history data from the CRYO-ROP and LIGHT-ROP studies, *Arch Ophthalmol* 120:1470, 2002.

36. Reynolds JD, et al: Lack of efficacy of light reduction in preventing retinopathy of prematurity. Light Reduction in Retinopathy of Prematurity (LIGHT-ROP) Cooperative Group, *N Engl J Med* 338:1572, 1998.

37. Schaffer DB, et al: Prognostic factors in the natural course of retinopathy of prematurity. Cryotherapy for Retinopathy of Prematurity Cooperative Group, *Ophthalmology* 100:230, 1993.

38. Schaffer DB, et al: Sequelae of arrested mild retinopathy of prematurity, *Arch Ophthalmol* 102:373, 1984.

39. Section on Ophthalmology American Academy of Pediatrics, American Academy of Ophthalmology, and American Association for Pediatrics Ophthalmology and Strabismus: Correction of errata, *Pediatrics* 118:1324, 2006.

40. Section on Ophthalmology American Academy of Pediatrics, American Academy of Ophthalmology, and American Association of Pediatric Ophthalmology and Strabismus: Screening examination of premature infants for retinopathy of prematurity, *Pediatrics* 117:572, 2006.

41. Silverman WA: *Retrolental fibroplasia: a modern parable,* New York, 1980, Grune & Stratton.

41a. SUPPORT Study Group of the Eunice Kennedy Shriver NICHD Neonatal Research Network, Carlo WA, Finer NN, Walsh MC, et al: Target ranges of oxygen saturation in extremely preterm infants, *N Engl J Med* 362(21):1959, 2010. Epub 2010 May 16.

42. Tasman W: Late complications of retrolental fibroplasia, *Ophthalmology* 86:1724, 1979.

43. Tasman W, et al: Retinopathy of prematurity: the life of a lifetime disease, *Am J Ophthalmol* 141:167, 2006.

44. Tin W, et al: Pulse oximetry, severe retinopathy, and outcome at one year in babies of less than 28 weeks gestation, *Arch Dis Child Fetal Neonatal Ed* 84:F106, 2001.

45. Tin W, et al: Giving small babies oxygen: 50 years of uncertainty, *Semin Neonatol* 7:361, 2002.

46. Trese MT: Visual results and prognostic factors for vision following surgery for stage V retinopathy of prematurity, *Ophthalmology* 93:574, 1986.

47. Wheatley CM, et al: Retinopathy of prematurity: recent advances in our understanding, *Arch Dis Child Fetal Neonatal Ed* 87:F78, 2002.

48. Yoganathan P, et al: Visual improvement following intravitreal bevacizumab (Avastin) in exudative age-related macular degeneration, *Retina* 26:994, 2006.

CHAPTER **54**

Neonatal Orthopedics

Musculoskeletal abnormalities of the extremities, spine, and pelvis are common in the neonate. Some are pathologic and others physiologic in origin from normal in utero positioning. The congenital absence of all or part of a limb, deformities of the feet or hands, and abnormalities of the spine are rarely diagnostic problems, whereas others, such as developmental dysplasia of the hip (DDH), may escape diagnosis even after repeated screenings by experienced examiners. Bone and joint infections in the neonatal period produce few of the diagnostic signs and symptoms present in the older child and require a high index of suspicion and careful diagnostic evaluation. When an infection is diagnosed early and prompt treatment rendered, the growth potential of the neonate yields an excellent prognosis for normal development and function.

PART 1

Musculoskeletal Disorders
Daniel R. Cooperman and George H. Thompson

NORMAL EMBRYOLOGY

Because many neonatal musculoskeletal disorders are congenital in origin, it is important to understand the basic aspects of musculoskeletal embryology. Prenatal development is divided into two major stages: the embryonic period, consisting of the first trimester, and the fetal period, consisting of the middle and last trimesters of pregnancy. The components of the musculoskeletal system differentiate during the first trimester; the second and third trimesters are periods of further growth and development.[28,37,50,74] Abnormalities during the embryonic period produce congenital malformations, whereas the fetal period produces deformations and alterations in the configuration of essentially normal parts.

Embryonic Development

The early embryonic development of the musculoskeletal system is oriented around the notochord, a tubular column of cells running cranially and caudally along the long axis of the embryo. During the third week of gestation, the neural crests develop dorsally and on either side of the notochord. These crests fold over and are joined dorsally to produce the neural tube, from which the spinal cord and associated spinal nerves develop. At the same time, paraxial collections of mesodermal tissue develop on either side of the notochord and segment cranially and caudally into 44 distinct condensations called *somites*. From the primitive mesodermal tissue comprising the somites, the skeletal tissues, muscle, and dermal elements of the body develop.

EXTREMITIES

The upper and lower extremities develop from the limb buds. They become recognizable during the fourth week of gestation. These buds grow and differentiate rapidly in a proximal to distal sequence during the next 4 weeks. The cells differentiate into three segments: the dermatomes, which become skin; the myotomes, which become muscle; and the sclerotomes, which become cartilage and bone. By the fifth week, the hand plate forms, and mesenchymal condensations occur in the limbs. By the sixth week, the digits become evident, and chondrification of the mesenchymal condensations occurs. Notches appear between the digit rays during the seventh week. The failure of the rays to separate at this time results in syndactyly. Also during the seventh week, the upper and lower limbs rotate in opposite directions. The lower limbs rotate internally to bring the toes to the midline, whereas the upper limbs rotate 90 degrees externally to the position of the thumb on the lateral side of the limb.

SPINE

The differentiation of the spinal column begins during the fourth week of the embryonic period. The somites first appear in the occipital region of the embryo; further development occurs simultaneously in a cranial-to-caudal direction. Dorsal and anterolateral migrations of the mesodermal tissue derived from the somites give rise to the connective tissue elements of the trunk and limbs. Anteromedial extensions of the somatic mesoderm migrate to surround the notochord, separating it from the neural tube and forming the primitive anlage of the vertebral bodies. The differentiation of the neural and vascular elements of the spinal column occurs simultaneously to somite development.

Definitive formation of the spinal column occurs from the fourth through the sixth week of gestation. The somatic

1771

mesodermal tissue surrounding the notochord differentiates into a less cellular and dense upper portion and a more dense and cellular lower portion. The somites cleave together, the lower portion of the superior somite joining with the upper portion of the inferior somite. The intervertebral disc develops at the site of the cleavage. The notochord, which is contained within the newly joined primitive vertebral bodies, degenerates, and those portions at the site of cleavage become the nucleus pulposus of the intervertebral disc. The neural arches and ribs develop from the dense portions of the somite, and the vertebral body develops from the less dense portions.

Chondrification begins in the primitive mesodermal vertebrae during the sixth week of pregnancy. It progresses rapidly to form cartilaginous models of the vertebral body by the end of the first trimester. Ossification of the cartilaginous models begins during the second trimester. The ossification of each side of the neural arch and of the body at each level proceeds separately. In the neonate, the ossified vertebral body and neural arches at each level are clearly visible radiographically, separated as they are by the nonossified synchondritic junctions. The ossification centers of the neural arches and body coalesce during the first 3 years of postnatal development.

The first and second cervical segments are embryologically and anatomically distinct from the remainder of the spinal column. The first cervical vertebra—the atlas—lacks the physical form characteristic of other vertebrae, having instead only a narrow anterior arch. This arch is not ossified at birth or during the neonatal period but is most often visible by 1 year of age.

The most striking feature of the second cervical vertebra—the axis—is the prominent odontoid process, derived from the caudal portion of the first cervical somite. The odontoid process joins with the remainder of the C2 body through synchondritic links with each neural arch and the vertebral body. The synchondrosis with the centrum lies below the level of the neural arches and may be radiographically confused with a fracture line; it closes by 3 years of age. The vertical synchondroses separating the centrum from the neural arches of C2 close by 7 years of age.

The radiographic evaluation of the neonatal spine requires experience. In the lateral view, the vertebral bodies are often notched at their waists and are trapezoidal rather than rectangular. In the anteroposterior view, the synchondritic links between the neural arches and vertebral bodies are not ossified and may give the false impression of a fracture. In the cervical region, the odontoid process may be confusing to those not familiar with the normal developmental anatomy of the region. Fortunately, fractures of the cervical spine are uncommon in the neonatal period and, when present, are usually associated with a suggestive history and other signs on physical examination.

Fetal Development

The appendicular and axial skeletons are preformed in cartilage. By the end of the first trimester, primary ossification centers are present in the long bones of the extremities. Further increases in length occur through endochondral growth at the ends of the long bones. This growth continues in the postnatal period until the end of adolescence, when growth plates close and the epiphyseal regions fuse with the remainder of the long bone.

CONGENITAL ABNORMALITIES

Teratogenic influences and genetic abnormalities occurring during the embryonic period can adversely affect the normal differentiation of the musculoskeletal system, resulting in malformations of the extremities or spine. Other organ systems differentiating at the same time are often concomitantly affected, such as the association of cardiac and genitourinary abnormalities with congenital spinal deformities (see also Chapter 29).

Teratogenic Abnormalities

It has been estimated that 5% of all malformations are the result of the action of known teratogens on the developing embryo. Irradiation, industrial chemicals, therapeutic drugs, and certain maternal infections produce primary musculoskeletal malformations or secondarily affect the growth and development of the musculoskeletal system. Thalidomide is the best known cause of musculoskeletal malformation. Rubella, cytomegalic inclusion disease, and congenital herpes produce lesions of the central nervous system that may secondarily affect the musculoskeletal system.

Genetic Disorders

Genetic disorders that affect the musculoskeletal system may be divided into three categories: mendelian, chromosomal, and multifactorial.

MENDELIAN DISORDERS

Mendelian disorders are characterized by an abnormality in a single gene obeying the rules of mendelian inheritance. Skeletal dysplasias, such as achondroplasia and diastrophic dwarfism, Marfan syndrome, hemophilia, and rickets resistant to vitamin D, are examples of mendelian disorders. Skeletal dysplasias are usually diagnosed in the neonate, whereas other entities do not become clinically recognizable until later in childhood.

CHROMOSOMAL ABNORMALITIES

Chromosomal abnormalities are characterized by morphologic changes detectable on ultrastructural analysis. Trisomies are common examples. Although they are striking, the musculoskeletal manifestations of these conditions are frequently the least serious of the child's problems.

MULTIFACTORIAL CONDITIONS

These conditions are determined by a combination of genetic predisposition and intrauterine environmental influences. Such conditions typically occur in families with a frequency that is greater than expected but do not follow the obvious rules of mendelian inheritance. Talipes equinovarus (clubfoot) is such a disorder. The overall incidence of clubfoot is 1 case per 1000 live births, but the incidence of deformity among first-degree relatives is 20 to 30 times higher than that in the general population. Three percent of dizygous twins and 40% of monozygous twins share the deformity.

An increased incidence of clubfoot occurs among breech and twin births.

Congenital Limb Malformations

Congenital limb malformations are relatively common among neonates. Some are grossly obvious, such as a congenital amputation, whereas others are subtle and perhaps unrecognizable for years, such as a congenital proximal radioulnar synostosis (fusion). Congenital limb malformations are classified according to the parts that have been primarily affected by embryologic failure. Swanson and colleagues[102] developed a seven-group classification system.

1. Failure of formation of parts (i.e., arrested development)
2. Failure of differentiation (i.e., separation) of parts
3. Duplication
4. Overgrowth (i.e., hyperplasia, gigantism)
5. Undergrowth (i.e., hypoplasia)
6. Congenital constriction band syndrome
7. Generalized skeletal abnormalities

These various malformations are caused by alterations in the organization of the limb mesenchyme; the time of the insult, the sequential development of the part, and the location of the destructive process determine the type of ensuing deformity. The presentation, diagnosis, and treatment of the more common congenital limb malformations are discussed in later sections.

FAILURE OF FORMATION OF PARTS

This group of failures of part formation is subdivided into transverse and longitudinal deficiencies. A transverse deficiency is manifested as an amputation type of stump that is classified by naming the level at which the remaining limb terminates. All elements distal to the level are absent. Longitudinal deficiencies represent all other skeletal limb deformities. In identifying longitudinal deficiencies, all completely or partially absent bones are named. Bones not named are considered to be present. These deficiencies are separated into preaxial and postaxial divisions of the limb and include longitudinal failure of the formation of an entire limb segment, such as phocomelia, or of the preaxial (i.e., radius, tibia), central, or postaxial (i.e., ulna, fibula) components of the limb. The more common deformities include phocomelia, an absent radius (i.e., radial clubhand), and an absent fibula (i.e., fibular hemimelia).[13,36,41]

FAILURE OF DIFFERENTIATION OF PARTS

In failure of the differentiation of parts, the basic units of the extremity developed, but the final form was not completed. The common disorders of this group include an undescended scapula (i.e., Sprengel deformity), proximal radioulnar synostosis, and syndactyly of the fingers and toes.

DUPLICATION

Duplication occurs as the result of a particular insult to the limb bud at an early stage such that the splitting of the original embryonic part occurs. Polydactyly of the thumb, fingers, great toe, and lesser toes represents duplications of this most common of the neonatal musculoskeletal disorders.

OVERGROWTH

Overgrowth can result from an excess of skeletal growth or soft tissues. The overgrowth frequently increases in size because of the asymmetric growth of the involved part.

UNDERGROWTH

Undergrowth usually represents the defective or incomplete development of parts. It can involve an entire extremity or only a portion of it. Overgrowth disorders, such as congenital hemihypertrophy, are more common than undergrowth disorders.

CONGENITAL CONSTRICTION BAND SYNDROME

Congenital constriction band syndrome may represent focal necrosis of the limb after the embryonic period or an acquired deformity due to amniotic bands. Deformity resulting from amniotic bands is thought to be the most common cause.

GENERALIZED SKELETAL ABNORMALITIES

Generalized skeletal abnormalities manifest generalized disorders, some of which may be inherited. Examples include skeletal dysplasia and syndromes such as Marfan syndrome and neurofibromatosis.

Spinal Defects

Errors in the embryologic derivation of the spine cause a number of congenital defects of the spine and spinal cord. These errors range in severity from isolated hemivertebrae to the complex errors of vertebral formation and segmentation associated with massive defects of the neural tube or spinal cord. When such errors result in asymmetric vertebral formation or produce asymmetric vertebral growth potential, structural spinal curves such as congenital scoliosis or kyphosis develop. Partial or complete failure of the formation of a vertebra (i.e., hemivertebra) or errors in the normal pattern of vertebral segmentation and recombination (i.e., unsegmented bars and trapezoidal, butterfly, and block vertebrae) may occur as single anomalies or be associated with other malformations of the osseous, neural, and organ systems. When vertebral defects are unbalanced and have growth potential, striking spinal deformities may occur. The nature of the deformity depends on the growth potential of the abnormal segments and their positions in the spinal column. For example, lateral abnormalities produce congenital scoliosis, and anterior or posterior midline defects result in congenital kyphotic or lordotic deformities.

Malformations of the head and neck, especially the internal and external auditory apparatuses, maxillae, and mandibles, occur frequently in patients with high thoracic and cervical curves. The association of a short neck, low posterior hairline, and restriction in neck motion caused by the congenital fusion of cervical vertebrae represents Klippel-Feil syndrome. Renal anomalies, the congenital elevation of the scapulae (i.e., Sprengel deformity), impaired hearing, and congenital heart disease are common associated anomalies in affected patients. The VATER syndrome (vertebral defects, imperforate anus, tracheoesophageal fistula, and radial and renal dysplasia), in association with limb defects, underscores the complex nature of the relationships between the rapidly evolving organ systems and the musculoskeletal system during the first trimester of pregnancy.

The association of vertebral anomalies with neural tube or spinal cord defects is to be expected, given the intimate relationships of their embryonic development. Spina bifida occulta is the most common and least serious and myelomeningocele the most severe of such anomalies. Not all anomalies are easily identified on physical or radiographic examination. McMaster[69] reported a 20% incidence of occult intraspinal abnormality in patients with congenital scoliosis. Possible anomalies included intradural and extradural lipoma, cysts, teratoma, spinal cord tethers, diplomyelia, and meningocele. In some instances, the spinal cord may be split by a bony, fibrous, or cartilaginous bar extending from the posterior aspect of the vertebral body to the vertebral arches. This condition, known as diastematomyelia, commonly occurs in association with defects at the thoracolumbar junction. Unless the spurs are ossified, they are not easily visualized by conventional radiographic techniques. The physical signs of underlying spinal dysraphism include hairy patches, midline dimpling, nevi, inequality in the length of the lower extremities or circumferential asymmetry, and asymmetry in foot size.

IN UTERO POSITIONING

The imprint of in utero positioning is frequently seen in the neonate. It can produce joint and muscle contractures and torsional and angular variations in the long bones, especially those of the lower extremities. It can also produce craniofacial distortion and positional contracture of the neck. The upper extremities are usually less affected.

The expression of in utero positioning depends on fetal position and the amount of compressive force applied. Intrinsic and extrinsic factors contribute to these variables. The intrinsic factors include oligohydramnios, multiple fetuses, a large fetus, and uterine deformities (i.e., bicornuate). The extrinsic factors may include a small maternal pelvis, abnormal fetal positioning (i.e., breech and transverse), and abnormal fetal muscle tone. These factors can lead to increased uterine compression and secondary changes in the neonate. Some of the more common problems related to in utero positioning include DDH, metatarsus adductus, the calcaneovalgus foot, tibial bowing, internal and external tibial torsion, and hyperextended knees. Craniofacial abnormalities, which are much less common, may include plagiocephaly, mandibular asymmetry, flattened facies, and crumpled ears. Therefore, most of these abnormalities are physiologic rather than pathologic in origin and resolve with normal growth and development. Others, such as DDH, may not resolve and may cause significant disability unless they are recognized and appropriately managed. The speed of resolution depends on the severity of the deformity and the rate of growth of the involved area.

It is a common misconception that the bowed appearance of the neonate's lower extremities is an abnormality. All term neonates have 20- to 30-degree hip and knee flexion contractures that decrease to the neutral position by 4 to 6 months of age. The newborn hip is externally rotated in extension to 80 to 90 degrees and has a limitation of internal rotation

of 0 to 10 degrees. Metatarsus adductus results from the tucked-under position, in which each foot is wrapped around the posterolateral aspect of the opposite thigh. The same position also produces lateral tibial bowing and inward (internal) rotation of the tibia. Tibial bowing and internal tibial torsion contribute to the bowed appearance of the lower extremity during the first year of life as well as a mild pigeon-toed or in-toed gait during the second year. However, this condition must be recognized as a normal variation resulting from the in utero position; it resolves with normal growth and development.

TRAUMA

See also Chapter 28.
Neonatal musculoskeletal injuries are frequently the result of a difficult or traumatic delivery. An abnormal intrauterine presentation and forcible extraction are associated with clavicular fractures, brachial plexus injuries, and occasionally long-bone fractures or epiphyseal separations (i.e., proximal humeral epiphysis) in otherwise healthy term infants. Prematurity, low birthweight, and underlying systemic disease may also predispose an infant to birth trauma and neonatal injury. Sometimes the minimal force involved in the daily care of a significantly premature infant is sufficient to produce a long-bone fracture. Infants receiving total parenteral alimentation may develop disorders of ossification that lead to pathologic fractures. These fractures are not usually associated with neurologic injury, and the prognosis for healing and subsequently normal function is excellent. Those fractures associated with neurologic injuries are more complex and have a more guarded prognosis.

Neonatal fractures resulting from abuse are uncommon but do unfortunately, occur. Long-bone fractures in association with vague histories or suspicious causes must be investigated.

Spine

Neonatal spinal trauma may be classified as an injury directly to the spine (i.e., vertebrae, intervertebral discs, and supporting ligamentous structures) or indirectly to the surrounding structures. The latter includes injuries to the brachial plexus and the sternocleidomastoid muscle (i.e., muscular torticollis) of the neck.

SPINAL INJURY

Difficult delivery is the most frequent cause of neonatal spinal injury. Breech presentation, especially when associated with intrauterine neck hyperextension, excessive traction during delivery, and forceps traction, puts the spine and enclosed neural elements at risk for injury. Injuries of the cervical spine are more common in neonates than those of the thoracic or lumbar spine; upper cervical injuries are more common than lower ones.

Spinal cord injury may occur with or without vertebral fracture. Excessive ligamentous laxity and the relative weakness of supporting musculature predispose the neonate to stretch injuries of the spinal cord without obvious skeletal damage. This stretch can produce spinal cord ischemia due to vertebral artery or segmental vessel injuries and result in neurologic abnormality in some neonates. Extensive areas of vascular damage in the spinal cord have been reported in neonates who died as the result of obstetric trauma.

Fractures, dislocations, and subluxations of the occipitoatlantal, atlantoaxial, and second and third cervical articulations have been reported. The neonatal spine is incompletely ossified, and skeletal injury may be difficult to detect on routine radiography. Radioisotope scanning or magnetic resonance imaging maybe useful for documenting injury in questionable cases.

Injuries of the brainstem and spinal cord may be fatal if the respiratory centers are compromised. For infants who survive, the goal of treatment is to improve function. When fracture or dislocation is documented, reduction and immobilization may be necessary to achieve segmental stability. Unfortunately, reduction rarely improves neurologic function.

BRACHIAL PLEXUS INJURY

See also Chapter 28.
Injuries of the brachial plexus have long been recognized as a consequence of difficult labor and delivery.[90] In this kind of paralysis, the arm falls motionless alongside the body and is rotated inward; the forearm remains extended, but the movements of the hand are preserved.

In 1877, Wilhelm Heinrich Erb described isolated upper plexus palsy and localized the site of damage to the junction of the C5 and C6 nerve roots, known thereafter as the *Erb point*. Erb's description remains an accurate assessment of the most common variety of plexus injury, with traction damage to spinal nerves C5, C6, and C7.

Other patterns of brachial plexus injury are less common but well documented. Isolated injuries to the lower portion of the brachial plexus described by Klumpke are uncommon in infants. Wickstrom[114] reported 11 such cases in his series of 87 patients. Hoffer and associates[47] observed four cases of posterior plexus damage in their series of 39 patients. Total or mixed plexus involvement is reported to be the most common pattern of injury after isolated upper plexus palsy.

The incidence of brachial plexus injury at birth is 0.1% to 0.3% of live births. Risk factors include elevated birthweight, prolonged labor, shoulder dystocia, and breech presentation, as well as high maternal body mass index and fetal asphyxia. Additionally, a humerus fracture is a risk factor for brachial plexus injury, whereas a clavicle fracture is not. Cesarean delivery does not fully protect children from birth palsy[2]; 10% of the affected patients have a history of cesarean delivery.

Upper brachial plexus injury is the most common pattern of damage. Combined upper and lower plexus injuries occur in a small percentage of patients. Isolated lower plexus injuries and posterior plexus injuries occur much less commonly.

Traction damage of the plexus may occur at any level from the origins of the cervical nerve roots at the spinal cord to the terminal branches of the plexus and may range in severity from stretch with intact neural tissues to avulsion of nerve roots. The physical findings at birth reflect the degree of involvement. The affected limb shows little or no spontaneous motion and is held in a position of elbow extension, internal rotation, and adduction. With lesions of the upper plexus,

active wrist flexion and finger flexion may be present. In complete injuries, these motions are absent. The injury must be differentiated from other causes of decreased active motion in the neonatal period, such as fracture of the clavicle or upper humerus and septic arthritis or osteomyelitis. The diagnosis can usually be established from a history of difficult delivery, physical examination, and radiographic evaluation of the upper limb and trunk.

The prognosis varies with the extent of damage to neural tissues. Up to 90% of patients with incomplete lesions involving the upper plexus can expect full recovery with no treatment. In general, these children recover biceps function within 1 month of life and quickly become normal. Patients with complete injuries or injuries of the lower plexus do not fare as well. Most recovery occurs within the first 3 months of life, but continued slow improvement for up to 5 years after birth has been reported by Tada and colleagues[103] for patients with complete injury. Partial recovery occurs in most cases. Surgical repair of the brachial plexus has been recommended by Waters[112] for children who have no return of biceps function by 6 months of age. Compared with the natural history of the lesion, improved but not normal function is possible. Shoulder contracture and osseous deformity (nonspherical humeral heads and abnormal glenoids) are common in patients with birth palsies. They commonly occur in children who have incomplete recovery and are also seen in those who have eventually complete neurologic recovery if that recovery does not start within the first 3 weeks of life.[46]

Infants with nerve root avulsion have the worst prognosis; no motor recovery can be expected in such cases, although some sensory recovery may occur. Fortunately, such injuries are uncommon. Surgical repair of nerve root avulsion has been recommended by some investigators, including Solonen and coworkers,[97] who reported good results in three infants with complete avulsion of the cervical nerve roots who underwent surgery within the first 3 months of life. Such an approach is theoretically justified when there is convincing evidence of complete avulsion on examination and no recovery has been seen on repeated examination, although such cases are uncommon.

In most cases of neonatal brachial plexus palsy, no treatment is necessary. Abduction splinting of the limb in the first few months of life is unnecessary and may further complicate lower plexus injury. Gentle range-of-motion exercises may be used to prevent adduction and internal rotation contracture. Infants with incomplete recovery may require later reconstructive surgery to minimize deformity and functional disability. In young children without fixed contractures and secondary bony deformities, tendon transfers may be used to balance asymmetric forces.[47,110] In older children, humeral osteotomy is occasionally necessary to correct internal rotational deformity.[58]

MUSCULAR TORTICOLLIS

Torticollis, or wryneck, in the neonatal period is most commonly associated with abnormalities of the sternocleidomastoid muscle. Shortening of the sternocleidomastoid muscle results in tilting of the head toward the affected muscle and rotation of the chin toward the opposite side. Birth trauma, intrauterine malposition, muscle fibrosis, and venous abnormality within the muscle have all been implicated, but no single cause has been identified. Davids and associates[23] demonstrated that the sternocleidomastoid muscle is contained within a separate fascial compartment. They thought that a stretch or tear of the sternocleidomastoid muscle that caused bleeding could result in a compartment syndrome, leading to significant muscle damage and contracture. A palpable mass is sometimes present within the affected muscle during the first few weeks of life. Flattening of the head and slight facial asymmetry or plagiocephaly are usually present. If the deformity is not corrected, contractures of the soft tissues on the side of the affected muscle occur, and pronounced plagiocephaly may develop. The disorder, occasionally associated with a case of developmental dysplasia of the hip (DDH) severe enough to require treatment, varies between 3.7% and 10% of patients, depending on the study.[73,107,111] It is also seen in association with metatarsus adductus.[49] Both these conditions are often the consequence of in utero positioning.

Torticollis may also be the result of congenital cervicovertebral anomalies (Fig. 54-1). Ballock and colleagues[5] reported that Klippel-Feil syndrome and congenital scoliosis were diagnosed in 5% of all torticollis patients referred to a large tertiary children's hospital. The severity of the curvature and associated head deformity depend on the nature of the vertebral defect. Cervical hemivertebrae are sometimes less deforming than unsegmented, unilateral cervical bars. As in all cases of congenital spinal curvature, a careful search for other systemic anomalies, such as those involving the cardiac and genitourinary systems, must be made.

The cause of torticollis should be established before treatment is initiated. Careful radiographic examination of the cervical spine is recommended. Anteroposterior and lateral views of the neck should be obtained initially; computed tomography may be necessary in some cases. Particular attention should be given to the upper cervical spine, especially the occipitoatlantal (occiput-C1) and the atlantoaxial (C1-C2) regions. If no underlying skeletal abnormalities are identified,

a program of stretching exercises is indicated to lengthen the contracted sternocleidomastoid muscle. The head is first tilted toward the opposite shoulder, and the chin is then rotated toward the affected side. Exercises should be performed gently, and the corrected position should be maintained for 5 to 10 seconds on each repetition. A program of 10 to 15 repetitions performed four times daily is sufficient in most cases. Stretching should begin early. This procedure seldom fails if begun during the first 3 months of life, but seldom succeeds if begun after 18 months of age.[24] Positioning the infant's crib with the normal side of the neck toward the wall sometimes stimulates an infant who lies prone to turn his head and stretch the sternocleidomastoid muscle. However, it is not a reliable method of treatment.

The surgical release of sternocleidomastoid contracture is indicated if there is significant deformity after 6 months of vigorous therapy or for older children with untreated torticollis.[16] Early surgery provides the best outcome, although children can benefit from surgery up to 10 years of age.[17] Delay results in significant plagiocephaly that will not be completely corrected after the release of contracture. Recurring contracture is a problem in older children.

The treatment of torticollis resulting from congenital cervical scoliosis is difficult because the primary cause of torticollis in these patients is skeletal, and soft tissue stretching cannot provide lasting correction. Surgical fusion of the affected area may be necessary to halt progression. It may be impossible to reverse the facial asymmetry that has developed because of head tilting.

Fractures

See also Chapter 28.

Neonatal fractures usually involve the upper extremity, particularly the shoulder region, and are the result of a difficult delivery. Fractures of the lower extremity are less common

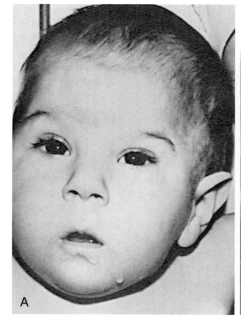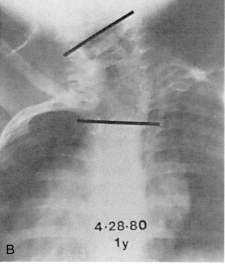

Figure 54–1. Congenital scoliosis may be manifested as torticollis. **A,** Clinical photograph of a 1-year-old child with congenital cervical scoliosis. The chin is tilted toward the right and the occiput toward the left. **B,** Radiographic views of the cervical spine in this patient show multiple hemivertebrae formation and an unsegmented congenital bar on the left side of the lower cervical spine. By convention, scoliosis films are viewed as if the examiner is facing the patient's back.

and may be indicative of an underlying neuromuscular disorder, especially those that limit joint mobility, such as arthrogryposis multiplex congenita. Fractures may also result from a bone disorder, such as osteogenesis imperfecta.

CLAVICLE

Fractures of the clavicle are the most common type of fracture in neonates. The incidence of clavicular fractures ranges from 2 to 7 cases per 1000 live births. McBride and coworkers[68] reported 9106 newborns prospectively screened for clavicular fracture. In this study, the risk factors included high birthweight, shoulder dystocia, and mechanically assisted delivery. Breech positioning was a factor in previous decades but not in this study. The liberal use of cesarean delivery appears protective. Of the 9106 babies reviewed, 1789 were delivered by cesarean section for various indications, including breech positioning. There were no clavicular fractures in these patients, although other authors have reported clavicular fractures after cesarean delivery.[48]

Fractures may be complete or incomplete (i.e., greenstick fracture). Complete fractures are more likely to be accompanied by classic symptoms and signs. Irritability and pseudoparalysis (i.e., decreased motion due to pain) of the involved limb are common. Discoloration, tenderness, and crepitation at the fracture site are common physical findings. Brachial plexus palsy, neonatal sepsis, traumatic separation of the proximal humeral epiphysis, humeral shaft fracture, and shoulder dislocation must be considered in the differential diagnosis.

The treatment of clavicular fracture is simple; asymptomatic patients with incomplete fractures need no immobilization. Symptomatic infants, usually those with complete fractures, should be treated. The treatment can include applying a figure-of-8 harness of gauze and tape or securing the affected arm to the chest with a bandage for 7 to 10 days. Pinning the sleeve of the infant's shirt to the front is often sufficient. An elastic bandage loosely applied around the chest and involved extremity after a cotton pad has been placed in the axilla can be considered for larger infants.

LONG-BONE FRACTURES

Fractures of other long bones are occasionally seen after a difficult delivery. Fractures or separations of the proximal humeral epiphysis may occur with the same force that produces clavicular fracture and brachial plexus injury. Symptoms and signs may be similar; pseudoparalysis, swelling, pain on passive motion, and crepitation with shoulder joint motion are usually present. The diagnosis of clavicular fracture can be made radiographically; however, because the proximal humeral epiphysis is not ossified at birth, routine radiography cannot demonstrate fracture or epiphyseal separation (Fig. 54-2). Ultrasonography can be used to establish the diagnosis in some cases, but most often the diagnosis is not confirmed until callus formation is seen radiographically 7 to 14 days later. Arthrography and magnetic resonance imaging can also be used to establish the diagnosis. When the diagnosis is confirmed soon after injury, the affected limb should be immobilized in a Velpeau bandage. Treatment is unnecessary if the diagnosis is delayed until callus formation has occurred. Scaglietti[90] pointed out that late contractures of the shoulder in patients with fractures or

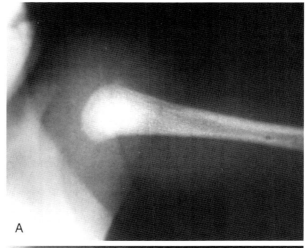

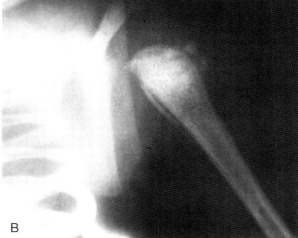

Figure 54–2. A, Normal-appearing radiograph of the humerus in a female newborn who had pseudoparalysis and appeared to have pain with passive motion of the left shoulder. B, Repeated radiograph 1 week later demonstrates subperiosteal new bone formation, indicating that there had been a traumatic separation of the proximal humeral epiphysis at delivery. The arm is now asymptomatic, and voluntary shoulder motion has returned.

separations resulting from a severely displaced proximal humerus may be difficult to distinguish from contractures caused by brachial plexus injury.

Fractures of the humeral and femoral shafts occasionally occur during delivery or with the routine management of a premature infant or an infant with a severe metabolic or neurologic disorder. Such injuries are the result of an underlying weakness of the bone rather than traumatic handling, and accompanying soft tissue injury is rarely severe. Such fractures can usually be treated successfully with the application of a simple plaster splint until radiographic callus formation occurs. A spica cast may be necessary for fractures of the proximal femur. A Pavlik harness is occasionally used for treating quite proximal femoral fractures.[99] The remodeling potential of the neonatal skeletal system is extraordinary, and long-term sequelae from long-bone fractures are not common.

PART 2

Bone and Joint Infections

Daniel R. Cooperman and George H. Thompson

Bacterial infections of the neonatal skeletal system are potentially disabling because of damage to the articular cartilage and epiphysis. Prompt diagnosis and treatment are imperative to prevent sequelae.[9,80] Unfortunately, neonates with skeletal infections do not usually have the classic symptoms or laboratory findings of sepsis because of their immature immune systems. Diagnosis requires a high index of suspicion and appropriate evaluation. When infections involve the bone, the disease process is called *osteomyelitis*. When the synovium (the membrane lining of the joint) is the primary site of infection, the process is called *septic arthritis* (see also Chapter 39).[39]

OSTEOMYELITIS

Pathology and Etiology

Bone infection, or osteomyelitis, occurs by three mechanisms: bacteremia or hematogenous; direct inoculation from a puncture wound, such as a heel or femoral vein stick; and a contiguous spread from an adjacent focus of infection. In neonates, as in infants and children, most bone infections are hematogenous in origin. The most common site of osteomyelitis is the metaphysis, the region of the bone immediately beneath the physis, or growth plate. The anatomic arrangement of metaphyseal vessels and the dynamics of blood flow in this region permit bacteria to lodge and proliferate. The nutrient artery ascends to the metaphysis from a central location within the bone. When the arterioles reach the physis, they make 180-degree turns and empty into the venous sinusoids. This process creates an area of sluggish blood flow and an opportunity for bacteria to become trapped and proliferate. A separate set of vessels nourishes the epiphysis.

In childhood, there is no connection between the epiphyseal and metaphyseal blood supply. The physis creates a barrier that is seldom penetrated by the spread of infection from the metaphysis to the epiphysis or from the epiphysis to the metaphysis. However, during the first 12 to 18 months of life, this barrier to the spread of infection does not exist because there are vessels passing through the physis that connect the epiphyseal and metaphyseal circulations.[9,12,77] These vessels allow infections to cross the physis, which may account for the increased incidence of physeal damage seen in neonatal osteomyelitis when compared with childhood osteomyelitis.[9,39,80] Peters and associates[80] observed the late onset of growth disturbance after neonatal osteomyelitis and recommended that the affected neonates be followed to skeletal maturity to monitor for growth disturbances.

When bacteria lodge in the metaphyseal vessels and begin to proliferate, inflammation followed by abscess formation occurs. The pressure from the purulent material causes extrusion of the pus through the haversian canals to the cortex and subsequently into the subperiosteal space. The continued subperiosteal accumulation of purulent material strips the periosteum from the bone. Because the periosteum supplies blood to the cortex, this stripping process interrupts cortical blood flow. As a result, large areas of cortical bone may become devascularized. This dead bone, or sequestrum, can serve as a site for chronic infection, which is isolated from limited neonatal defense mechanisms and antibiotics.[77] The elevated periosteum produces new bone in an attempt to repair the injured bone. This process in turn produces the involucrum, which surrounds the sequestrum.

Draining cutaneous sinuses may arise when pus ruptures through the periosteum, adjacent soft tissues, and skin. Infection may occasionally spread into an adjacent joint space, causing secondary septic arthritis. The destruction of the epiphysis may occur through the direct spread of infection into it. This process can result in subsequent shortening, angular deformity, or both, of the involved extremity.[80] In neonates, complete physeal closure can occur, resulting in shortening.[9] Damage to the articular surface of the joint may result in the loss of motion and ultimately degenerative osteoarthritis.

The etiologic organisms responsible for neonatal osteomyelitis are variable. *Staphylococcus aureus* has traditionally been the most common causative organism.[9] Recently, methicillin-resistant *S. aureus* (MRSA) has been reported in neonates, which is especially destructive.[62] Streptococci and enteric aerobic bacilli account for much of the remaining responsible organisms. *Candida albicans* can also cause osteomyelitis in those neonates at high risk for infection.

Diagnosis

The clinical manifestations of osteomyelitis in children vary with age. In previously healthy neonates, it usually occurs during the first 2 weeks of life. Limitation of spontaneous movement with pseudoparalysis of the involved extremity is the most common sign. Localized tenderness, erythema, increased warmth, and swelling may occur. Associated septic arthritis with accompanying joint effusion and increased warmth occurs in many cases. Term neonates usually appear less ill than would be expected because of the persistence of maternal antibodies. They have less fever, leukocytosis, and elevation of the erythrocyte sedimentation rate[9] than older children with similar infections. Less commonly, neonatal osteomyelitis presents as septicemia. The presentation and course of osteomyelitis are strongly correlated with the health of the infant before presentation. Infants with multiple sites of infection are usually ill before its onset and have an increased incidence of placement of umbilical catheters or other lines. They are also more ill than those neonates presenting with only one site of infection.[9]

Some neonates are at increased risk for osteomyelitis; they also have a more severe course of the disease. Bergdahl and colleagues[9] identified the following risk factors in a study of 40 neonates with osteomyelitis: a birthweight of less than 2500 g or gestational age of less than 37 weeks, emergency cesarean delivery, a congenital malformation requiring neonatal surgery, respiratory distress syndrome, hyperbilirubinemia, large vessel (usually umbilical) catheterization, perinatal asphyxia, scalp laceration after vacuum extraction, and renal vein thrombosis. Twenty-one neonates were found to have risk factors, but 19 did not. Of the 21, most had multiple sites of infection; 13 of the 21 (62%) neonates with risk factors had serious skeletal sequelae. In the remaining 19 neonates, multiple sites of infection were uncommon, and serious skeletal sequelae occurred in less than 20%.

The early diagnosis of osteomyelitis is based on obtaining purulent material, blood, or both for cultures and antibiotic sensitivities. Early in the course of the disease, radiographs and bone scans may be normal.[4,12,25] Bone aspiration is usually positive. The cultures of subperiosteal metaphyseal pus yield a pathogen in about 70% of cases. The point of maximal swelling, bone tenderness, and fluctuation on physical examination is the most appropriate location for needle aspiration. The skin overlying the affected region should be prepared with an antiseptic solution and draped with sterile towels. After infiltration of the area with local anesthetic, an 18-gauge spinal needle, with the stylet in place, is passed through the skin to the bone. The subperiosteal space is aspirated first. If the tap is dry, the needle with the stylet should be gently twisted through the bone cortex into the metaphysis, which is then aspirated. The aspirated fluid or blood should be immediately Gram stained and cultured. The organism may also be recovered from other sources. Blood cultures are positive in 60% of the children with osteomyelitis. When osteomyelitis complicates meningitis, the organism may be recovered from cultures of the cerebrospinal fluid.

Imaging

See also Chapter 37.

A diagnosis cannot be easily made by bone aspiration during the inflammatory phase before abscess formation. At this point, imaging can be helpful. Plain radiographs of the suspected bone are often a valuable procedure. Within a few days of the onset of infection, deep edema, joint effusion, and sometimes bone destruction can be detected.[9] The edema is visible sooner in neonates than in children because the neonate has very porous bones and a loosely attached periosteum (Fig. 54-3), which permits the earlier collection of subperiosteal abscesses in neonates than in children. This fact also accounts for the relatively favorable results of diagnostic aspiration in neonates.

If radiographs are unproductive, ultrasound can be useful in localizing the areas of deep edema and joint effusion, as can magnetic resonance imaging. Technetium bone scanning is also recommended.[44] There is some controversy over the merits of bone scanning in neonates because of their decreased inflammatory response and the large amount of isotope uptake from the very active adjacent epiphysis. In 1980, Ash and Gilday[4] concluded that it was very unreliable. However, Bressler and coworkers[12] and others[25] have suggested that technetium bone scans can be helpful. Bressler's group scanned 33 infants suspected of having osteomyelitis. Each of the 25 sites of proven osteomyelitis in 15 infants was demonstrated on bone scanning. Another 10 sites that were radiographically negative were also demonstrated to be positive on bone scanning. The bone scan, if negative, does not exclude osteomyelitis.

The results of indium and gallium scans for acute osteomyelitis in neonates have not been reported. A concern about

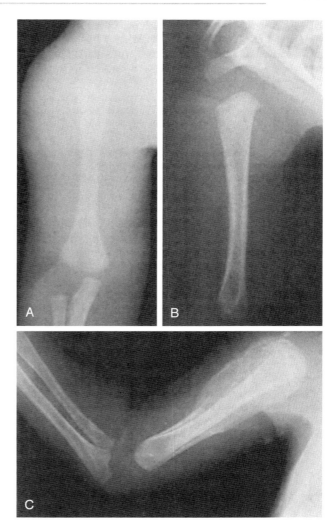

Figure 54–3. Radiologic changes in neonatal osteomyelitis. **A,** Early proximal humeral osteomyelitis. Soft tissue has become swollen around the affected bone. **B,** Periosteal elevation is manifested by subperiosteal bone formation. **C,** Massive subperiosteal new bone formation. The humeral shaft has become surrounded by new bone.

gallium scans is related to the pathology of osteomyelitis. If there is extensive septic embolization of metaphyseal vessels, labeled blood cannot penetrate the metaphysis. If the periosteum is stripped off the cortex, devascularizing the cortical bone, there can be no blood flow in the cortex. Under these circumstances, the uptake by bone may be difficult to predict. However, Demopulos and associates[25] recommended an indium scan if the technetium bone scan in the neonate is not highly suggestive of osteomyelitis.

Another concern in the assessment of osteomyelitis is the determination of whether metaphyseal aspiration can produce a positive bone scan. Canale and colleagues[14] assessed the effects of bone and joint aspiration on the bone scan results in healthy dogs. They used multiple aspiration techniques on the bones and joints of 15 dogs and scanned them between 5 hours and 10 days of aspiration. In no case did joint aspiration lead to a positive bone scan. Metaphyseal drilling and periosteal scraping with needles occasionally led to positive bone scans after a 2-day delay. Thus, bone aspiration does not initially affect a technetium bone scan.

Treatment

Treatment must not be delayed for neonates with suspected osteomyelitis. Antimicrobial therapy should be initiated, usually with a combination of agents, as soon as a presumptive diagnosis is made and appropriate material for cultures has been obtained. Treatment can later be appropriately altered according to culture results and antibiotic sensitivities. For neonates, optimal coverage is provided by a penicillinase-resistant penicillin coupled with an aminoglycoside. The new third-generation cephalosporins have been successfully used in the treatment of a form of osteomyelitis caused by enteric bacilli. However, these agents should not be used alone as the initial treatment because their activity against group B streptococci is inadequate. When these drugs are used as part of the initial therapeutic regimen, a penicillinase-resistant penicillin should be used concomitant with them. After an organism is isolated, focused antibiotic treatment is possible. The duration of treatment should be at least 3 weeks and probably not more than 6 weeks for acute hematogenous osteomyelitis. Nelson[75] suggests a clinical approach to antibiotic management. After local inflammation subsides and measures of inflammation such as erythrocyte sedimentation rate return to normal, he recommends 14 more days of antibiotics for group A streptococci and encapsulated bacteria such as pneumococci and 21 more days for staphylococcal infection.

Primary surgical treatment depends on the results of bone aspiration. If grossly purulent material is recovered from the subperiosteal space or the metaphysis, an abscess has formed. In these cases, surgical drainage is necessary to decompress the abscess. This procedure facilitates blood flow and the subsequent delivery of antibiotics. Surgical drainage also allows the removal of the bone sequestrum. When pus is not recovered at the time of initial aspiration, the patient's infection is in the cellulitic or inflammatory phase. The aspirated blood is used to obtain blood cultures, and antibiotic therapy is initiated. It is assumed that the bone blood flow is still adequate in the cellulitic phase to deliver antibiotics to the site of infection because there is no pus under pressure. The affected limb should be immobilized with splints. Neonates must be carefully followed during the early phases of treatment. Surgical intervention may become necessary if an adequate clinical response is not obtained within 48 hours of initial antimicrobial therapy.[64] An inadequate response implies that an abscess is forming. Reassessment, including repeated aspiration, is indicated. If an abscess is identified, surgical drainage will be necessary.

La Mont and coworkers[64] reviewed 69 children (15 neonates) retrospectively and 44 children (4 neonates) prospectively, all with acute hematogenous osteomyelitis. They concluded that surgery was seldom necessary because most of the prospective group improved clinically after 48 hours of appropriate intravenous antibiotics, and few of them had abscesses aspirated. In their study, surgery was infrequently used, and the results were excellent. It was their impression that the aspiration of pus from the bone was an indication for surgery but was seldom encountered. Drainage was also recommended for an extraosseous abscess.

It is believed that the surgical decompression of long bones such as the femur, tibia, humerus, radius, and ulna is necessary if pus is aspirated from bone or the subperiosteal space.[9] Decompression consists of drilling a hole in the metaphysis or removing a small cortical window. The wound is then left open to drain. It is closed later or allowed to close spontaneously, and dressings are changed two or three times a day. Surgical decompression is also necessary if there is not a good clinical response to antibiotics within 48 to 72 hours, even if no pus is aspirated from the bone.

If osteomyelitis is localized to flat bones, such as the pelvis or vertebrae, the administration of antibiotics without surgical decompression is usually sufficient treatment. However, caution is necessary because Bergdahl and associates[9] reported one death and one case of tetraparesis resulting from neonatal vertebral osteomyelitis.

SEPTIC ARTHRITIS
Pathology and Etiology

The mechanisms responsible for joint or synovial infections in neonates and children parallel those for osteomyelitis: septicemia, contiguous spread from an adjacent focus of infection, and traumatic penetration of the joint space. The risk factors include prematurity, umbilical catheterization, perinatal asphyxia, and a difficult birth.[51] Regardless of the source, the ensuing inflammatory response results in synovial hypertrophy and altered capillary permeability. Purulent material accumulates within the joint, and fibrinous clots may coat the joint surfaces. The diffusion of nutrients across the articular cartilage of the joint is interrupted, and the normal lubrication processes are altered. Lysosomal enzymes, which are released in neutrophil degeneration, attack the mucopolysaccharide components of articular cartilage. Hypertrophic granulation tissue forms a pannus that can erode articular cartilage and may allow the extension of infection to subchondral bone. Fibrous ankylosis of the joint may develop, with a permanent loss of motion.[86] Increased intra-articular pressure may occlude the vessels that supply the epiphyses and the physis, resulting in epiphyseal death or avascular necrosis. This process is especially applicable to the hip. The rupture of pus through the synovial membrane and into the surrounding tissues produces soft tissue abscesses that may later develop into draining sinuses.

Neonatal septic arthritis often results from osseous infection, and the bacterial agents responsible for the joint infections are similar to those previously described for neonatal osteomyelitis: S. aureus, streptococci, and enteric bacilli. Septic arthritis occurs less frequently as a primary entity; the Enterobacteriaceae family, the species of Pseudomonas, and Neisseria gonorrhoeae may be isolated in these cases. Fink and Nelson[33] reported septic arthritis from Haemophilus influenzae in neonates as young as 3 days of age. About 25% of the neonates with H. influenzae septic arthritis also have meningitis.

Diagnosis

The clinical presentation of neonatal septic arthritis is similar to that described for neonatal osteomyelitis. Joint effusion, increased warmth, and limited motion are often observed on physical examination.

The definitive diagnosis of septic arthritis requires aspiration of the affected joint. The causative agent can be recovered in about 60% of cases. The procedure should be performed under sterile conditions by an experienced physician because repeated attempts to penetrate the joint may further damage the joint surface and the underlying bone. After culture and Gram staining of the fluid, determinations of the cellular count as well as glucose and protein concentrations should be obtained. Infected synovial fluid typically contains more than 50,000 white blood cells per cubic millimeter (primarily polymorphonuclear leukocytes); a glucose concentration of less than 40 mg/dL, or less than 30% of the serum concentration; and an elevated protein concentration. Blood cultures should also be obtained.

Imaging

Neonatal septic arthritis has the same recommendations as those for osteomyelitis (Fig. 54-4). Of special interest are the findings of Canale and colleagues[14] that joint aspiration in dogs is never associated with a positive technetium bone scan. Consequently, the aspiration of joints should never be discouraged on the basis of a belief that it may affect a later bone scan.

Treatment

Neonatal septic arthritis, like osteomyelitis, requires prompt treatment. Irreversible joint damage may occur unless intra-articular pus is evacuated and effective antimicrobial therapy initiated.[76,100] Neonates should be managed jointly by pediatricians and orthopedic surgeons.

Combinations of antibiotics are selected to cover the most likely pathogens. A penicillinase-resistant penicillin and an aminoglycoside or cephalosporin usually provide adequate coverage pending the results of the cultures and antibiotic sensitivities (see Chapter 39).

Joint decompression is an essential component of successful therapy for pyogenic arthritis. However, opinions vary on the most effective method, specifically surgical drainage compared with repeated aspiration. Primary decompression is usually accomplished at the time of initial joint aspiration and may be sufficient in peripheral joints such as the knee, ankle, and elbow, which are easily aspirated and in which blood flow to intra-articular epiphyses is not at risk. Needle aspiration is not sufficient for decompression of the hip because increased intra-articular pressure may occlude blood flow to the femoral head, resulting in avascular necrosis. Immediate surgical drainage is mandatory for septic arthritis of the hip.

The repeated aspiration of joints other than that of the hip may be appropriate. The morbidity for careful aspirations is less than that for arthrotomy, but persistent infection after repeated aspiration is probably more harmful than the risk for primary arthrotomy. Poorly executed needle aspiration may damage the articular surfaces and inoculate underlying bone with purulent fluid.

Like the therapy for osteomyelitis, effective antimicrobial therapy for pyogenic arthritis is a function of the agent, route, and duration of drug administration. After the

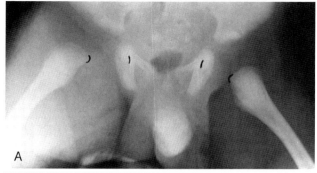
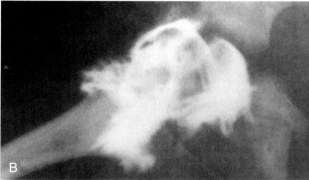

Figure 54–4. A, Anteroposterior pelvic radiograph of a 2-week-old boy who had been irritable during diaper changes for 1 week. There were no systemic symptoms, such as fever, although the child had been quite irritable and not feeding normally. The femoral heads are not visible because they do not begin to ossify until 4 to 6 months of age. Observe the widening between the acetabulum and the ossified medial corner of the proximal femoral metaphysis, which indicates lateral displacement or subluxation of the femoral head. B, Arthrocentesis revealed only a small amount of purulent material. An attempted arthrogram revealed gross distortion of the hip joint due to inspissated purulent material. At the time of hip arthrotomy, clotted, purulent material was removed. This child subsequently developed avascular necrosis as a consequence of septic arthritis with subluxation. Fortunately, he made a satisfactory recovery and regained essentially normal hip function.

pathogen has been isolated and antibiotic sensitivities are known, a single agent may be used. Intra-articular antibiotic instillation is unnecessary because adequate drug concentrations are achieved in synovial fluid by the intravenous and parenteral routes.

Joint infections caused by *H. influenzae* require 2 to 3 weeks of therapy, whereas infections caused by other agents or those complicated by osteomyelitis may require up to 6 weeks of therapy. The treatment of neonatal gonococcal arthritis differs significantly from that of arthritis caused by other pathogens. Penicillin G, ampicillin, amoxicillin, tetracycline, and erythromycin have all been used successfully in therapy for gonococcal arthritis in 7- to 10-day courses. Other than diagnostic arthrocentesis, no surgical intervention is necessary for this disease.

PART 3

Congenital Abnormalities of the Upper and Lower Extremities and Spine

Daniel R. Cooperman and George H. Thompson

UPPER EXTREMITIES

Congenital anomalies of the upper extremities are those that occur during the embryonic period. Developmental deformities are those that occur primarily in the fetal or neonatal period. Because a developmental deformity may have a prenatal association, such as in utero positioning, it could be misinterpreted as a congenital deformity. Congenital and developmental disorders of the upper extremities are less common than those affecting the lower extremities.

Shoulder

The failure of the scapula and the upper extremities to descend to their normal locations is called *Sprengel deformity*, which can vary from mild to severe. The scapula is typically located abnormally elevated with respect to the child's neck and thorax, producing webbing of the skin at the base of the neck and a low posterior hairline. In the severe form, an accessory bone, the omovertebral bone, may connect the scapula to the spinous processes of the cervical spine and allow virtually no scapulothoracic motion. The severe forms are more likely than the mild forms to be diagnosed in the neonate. Associated muscle contractures that further limit the strength and stability of the shoulder girdle may also be present. In the mild form, the scapula is slightly elevated with less than normal motion. There may be an association with congenital cervicovertebral anomalies, particularly Klippel-Feil syndrome, and this association suggests the possibility of other congenital abnormalities, such as those in the cardiovascular and genitourinary systems. When Sprengel deformity is diagnosed, abnormalities in these other systems must be assessed.

Treatment is usually delayed until middle childhood and depends on the function of the child's shoulder and extremity. For a severe form, surgical repositioning and occasionally partial resection of the scapula may be necessary.

Elbow

Congenital radioulnar synostosis is an uncommon disorder that represents a failure of separation or congenital fusion between the proximal radius and ulna. It occurs from the fifth to the eighth week of gestation, when there is separation of the humerus, radius, and ulna from a common block of cartilage in the limb bud. This disorder is bilateral in about 50% of all patients and limits forearm pronation and supination. It is rarely recognized during the neonatal period because there is no obvious deformity, only a loss of forearm rotation. In most cases, the forearm is in a physiologic position of 45 to 60 degrees of pronation. Only if there is extreme supination may the disorder be recognized. The diagnosis of this disorder, which is confirmed radiographically, should be suspected in any neonate with restricted forearm pronation or supination.

Treatment is rarely indicated unless there is an abnormal position of the forearm that interferes with the function of the hand. The method of treatment, a rotational osteotomy through the synostosis, is usually delayed until middle childhood so that an adequate assessment of function can be determined. Attempts at restoring forearm pronation and supination by excising the synostosis have been unsuccessful.

Forearm and Wrist

RADIAL HYPOPLASIA AND CLUBHAND

Hypoplasia of the radius is a commonly discussed and infrequently encountered entity, occurring in 1 of 100,000 live births. It is bilateral in 50% of cases. The deformity can vary from mild shortening of the radius to its complete absence (i.e., radial clubhand). As the radius shortens, the deformity becomes more apparent. In complete absence of the radius, the hand is radially angulated 90 degrees to the long axis of the forearm. The ulna is markedly bowed, and the ulna and humerus can be half the length of the opposite normal side by maturity. As the deformity becomes profound, so does thumb involvement (i.e., an absent first ray, thumb hypoplasia) (Fig. 54-5).

The entire extremity may be involved, including the scapula and clavicle. The radially based muscles of the forearm are also hypoplastic or absent. There is hypoplasia or the absence of the radial artery, leaving the ulnar artery as the main blood

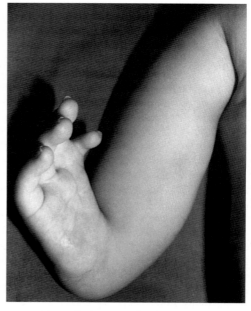

Figure 54–5. Clinical photograph of a 1-year-old boy with a right radial clubhand and hypoplastic index finger.

supply to the hand. There is no radial nerve innervation to the skin distal to the elbow, leaving the median and ulnar nerve to anastomose to provide dorsal sensation. Radial clubhand is not simply a bony defect.

The most frequently associated anomalies are blood dyscrasia and heart defects. Fanconi syndrome is a pancytopenia seen in some children with radial clubhand (see also Chapter 50). TAR syndrome (i.e., thrombocytopenia with an absent radius) is also seen. Holt-Oram syndrome, in which the primary manifestation is an absent thumb with atrioseptal defects, has a well recognized association with radial clubhand.

Radial hypoplasia alone is inherited sporadically. There is no definitely identifiable inheritance pattern; the careful scrutiny of relatives seldom yields another affected individual. Radial hypoplasia as part of a syndrome frequently has a defined inheritance pattern. Holt-Oram syndrome is inherited in a dominant fashion, and Fanconi pancytopenia is inherited as a recessive pattern.

Treatment comprises both operative and nonoperative options and is recommended for cosmetic and functional reasons. The treatment begins with stretching. During the first 6 months of life, casts and splints are used to stretch the radially deviated hand to conform to a more neutral alignment. If the deformity is corrected, the patient wears a splint all the time for the first 6 years of life and then after that only at night. If the deformity is not corrected, the hand is centralized onto the ulna. At surgery, the carpus is impaled onto the ulna after an osteotomy to straighten the ulna. If the patient has a useless thumb, the index finger occasionally undergoes pollicization—in essence it is turned into a thumb. The surgery is frequently performed when the patient is between 6 months and 1 year of age. After surgery, bracing is maintained 24 hours each day for the first 6 years of life. In bilateral cases, the hands are staged, with one operated on at 6 months and the other at about 3 years of age.

The contraindications to surgery are serious blood dyscrasia, heart problems, and profound muscle imbalance. If the elbow flexors are overpowered by the elbow extensors such that a child cannot touch the hand to the face even after physical therapy, surgery is not likely to provide a useful hand in a functional sense.

CONSTRICTION BANDS

Congenital constriction band syndrome, also known as *Streeter dysplasia* or *annular bands*, features defects of the skin resulting in ringlike strictures around the limbs and occasionally the trunk (Fig. 54-6).[35] It is seen in 1 of 15,000 live births, and multiple extremities are usually involved. The upper extremities, especially the hands, are involved more frequently than the lower extremities. The cause appears to be early amniotic rupture followed by temporary oligohydramnios with resulting intrauterine compression and the subsequent constriction of the fetal appendages by cords or bands of torn amnion (see also Chapter 22).[108]

Patterson[79] developed diagnostic criteria for congenital constriction ring syndrome. These criteria include simple ring constrictions, ring constrictions accompanied by deformity of the distal part with or without lymphedema, ring constrictions accompanied by fusions of distal parts ranging from fenestrated or terminal syndactyly (i.e., acrosyndactyly) to exogenous syndactyly, and intrauterine amputations. Other congenital anomalies frequently occur, such as clubfoot (30%), pseudarthrosis, peripheral hand palsy, and lower extremity length discrepancies.[35]

Rigid clubfoot distal to deep constriction bands may be difficult to correct.[1] Treatment involves the surgical release of the bands if the distal aspect is swollen and has lymphedema. The surgery is usually performed in two stages, although Greene[40] demonstrated that a complete one-stage release can be performed safely.

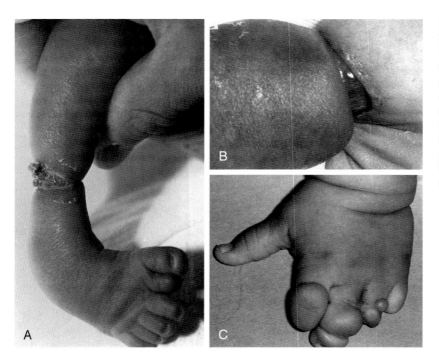

Figure 54–6. Clinical photographs of a newborn girl with multiple annular bands. **A,** The right lower extremity demonstrates a band with complete transection of the skin and subcutaneous tissue. The associated talipes equinovarus (clubfoot) deformity has a duplication of the great toe. **B,** A similar lesion is present in the right upper extremity, with a significant amount of distal edema from lymphatic and venous obstruction. **C,** The left hand shows multiple bands with segmented edema and partial amputations.

Fingers and Thumb of the Hand

CONGENITAL AMPUTATIONS

Congenital amputation is the best example of a failure of formation. In general, the greater the loss of length, the rarer the lesion. For instance, a child with a congenital amputation at the forearm level is encountered in 1 of 20,000 live births, and one with a missing arm is encountered in 1 of 270,000 live births.

When treating patients with congenital amputations of the upper extremities, it is necessary to define a goal for the patient. The arm serves as a positioning device for the hand. Consequently, treatment revolves around providing the patient with some sort of terminal device at the end of the usable arm. In the early stages, as the child achieves sitting balance, a soft terminal device is fitted. This device allows "two-handed" activities and is used to help pin objects against the normal hand. As the child reaches 2 to 3 years of age, prehension by means of a terminal device becomes possible. Early training allows children to become quite comfortable with these devices.

SYNDACTYLY

Syndactyly is the most common form of congenital anomaly in the upper extremities and represents a failure of separation of two fingers (Fig. 54-7). This failure of separation occurs sometime between weeks 5 and 8 of gestational life and is seen in 1 of 2250 live births. The anomaly appears to be sporadic in 80% of cases; the other 20% are the result of genetic transmission. Because all forms of genetic transmission have been linked to syndactyly, genetic counseling is quite difficult. The classification of syndactyly is defined by the degree of interconnection between the fingers. In complete syndactyly, the webbing extends from the tip of the fingers to the hand; in incomplete syndactyly, it does not. Simple syndactyly involves only the skin, whereas complex syndactyly includes bony fusion. Abnormalities of the blood vessels, nerves, and tendons are also seen in this anomaly.

Treatment is aimed at separating the digits to improve function. The affected digits are usually separated early, when they are of unequal length. If the thumb and index finger are syndactylized, the longer digit becomes tethered and deformed by the shorter digit.[119] Surgery within the first year of life is suggested. When the digits are of nearly equal length, such as the long finger and the index finger, the surgery can wait until 2 or 3 years of age without difficulty.

POLYDACTYLY

See also Chapter 29.

Polydactyly is a common duplication deformity of the hand (Fig. 54-8). This deformity is seen in 1 of 300 African-American and 1 of 3000 white live births in the United States. The incidence of thumb polydactyly is identical in African Americans and whites (0.8 of 1000 live births). Little-finger polydactyly is common in African Americans, with 1 of 300 affected. It is usually seen without associated abnormalities. In white infants, little-finger polydactyly is infrequent and often associated with other skeletal abnormalities, including syndactyly, coalescence of carpal bones, radioulnar synostosis, hypoplasia and aplasia of the tibia and fibula, hemivertebrae, and dwarfism. Other disorders also

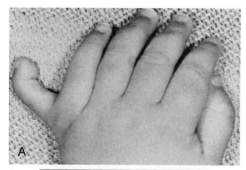
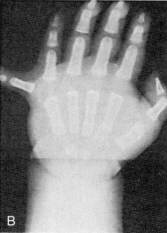

Figure 54–8. Clinical photograph (A) and radiograph (B) show congenital polydactyly, the most common digit duplication, with complete bones, tendons, and nerves. The recommended treatment is early ablation by amputation.

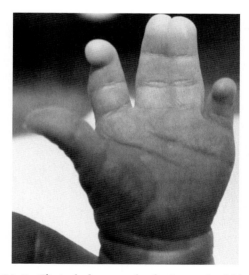

Figure 54–7. Clinical photograph of a 3-month-old boy with complete syndactyly between the third and fourth fingers. There is hypoplasia of the distal phalanges of the index and small fingers.

seen are hydrocephalus, cleft lip, hypogonadism, kidney abnormalities, and imperforate anus.

The surgical approach to polydactyly is based on the vascular and bony anatomy of the digits, and it is individualized. The surgery is usually performed sometime after 6 months but before 18 months of age to minimize the anesthetic risks.

MACRODACTYLY

Macrodactyly of the hand, also known as *idiopathic local gigantism*,[109] may involve one or more fingers and is bilateral in 5% of cases. All structures in the affected finger are enlarged, including the bone, blood vessels, nerves, and other soft tissues. True macrodactyly must be differentiated from other processes that create gigantism because the treatment is different. Local enlargement of the hand occurs in neurofibromatosis, lymphedema, hemangioma, lymphangioma, arterial vascular fistulas, fibrous dysplasia, aneurysmal bone cysts, and lipomas. The treatment for these disorders is individualized to the process. In typical macrodactyly, the child is followed carefully until the affected digit is about adult size, which usually happens between 7 and 8 years of age. At this point, growth arrests of all the bones in the affected digit are performed, and soft tissues are debulked. Occasionally, the growth is uncontrollable, and cosmesis is so poor that the parents and child prefer amputation. In contrast, ray resection with soft tissue reduction is the method of choice for managing macrodactyly of the foot, especially when it affects only the lesser toes.[15]

SPINE

Spinal disorders diagnosed during the neonatal period are uncommon.[78] Most are congenital in origin. Some, such as myelodysplasia and sacral agenesis, are obvious at birth, but others, such as congenital scoliosis and kyphosis, may not be recognized for months or years. Idiopathic spinal deformities can also occur but are rare.

Infantile Idiopathic Scoliosis

Scoliosis without a known causation is called *idiopathic*. Idiopathic spinal deformities are classified as infantile, with the onset between birth and 3 years of age; juvenile, with the onset between 4 and 10 years of age; and adolescent, with the onset at 11 years of age or older. The adolescent type is the most common form of scoliosis, and the infantile type is the least common. The infantile type is more common in the United Kingdom than in North America, the reason for which is unknown.

When a neonate or infant is found to have a spinal deformity, a very careful physical examination and radiographic assessment are necessary to determine an underlying reason. Physical examination includes evaluation of the spine for mobility and areas of tenderness. The skin should be inspected for cutaneous lesions that may indicate underlying spinal dysraphism. The lower extremities need to be carefully evaluated for symmetry and neurologic function.

Plain radiographs usually determine whether there is a spinal deformity. However, additional studies, such as magnetic resonance imaging (MRI), may be necessary to evaluate the spinal canal and spinal cord for possible lesions.

The treatment of infantile scoliosis is variable. Some curves may be observed and even improve with growth. However, others are progressive and require cast or orthotic management and possibly surgical intervention. It is important that all neonatal spinal abnormalities be referred to an orthopedic surgeon experienced in the management of pediatric spinal deformities.

CONGENITAL SPINAL DEFORMITIES

Abnormalities of vertebral formation can result in structural deformities of the spine that may be evident in the neonate or become more obvious during the first year of life. Deformities in the coronal plane produce congenital scoliosis, whereas those in the sagittal plane produce congenital kyphosis. The failure of formation, total or partial, of the sacrum is called *sacral agenesis*. If the lower lumbar spine is also absent, it is called *lumbosacral agenesis*.

CONGENITAL SCOLIOSIS

Congenital scoliosis is classified as a failure of formation (i.e., hemivertebrae), failure of segmentation (i.e., unsegmented bars), or mixed (Fig. 54-9). A failure of formation and segmentation can be partial or complete and may occur as a single abnormality or in combination with other bone, soft tissue, or neurologic abnormalities of the axial or appendicular skeleton.[28] Congenital genitourinary malformations occur in 20% of children with congenital scoliosis. Unilateral renal agenesis is the most common abnormality. Most genitourinary abnormalities do not require treatment, but about 6% of the affected patients have a silent obstructive uropathy.[37] Renal ultrasound should be performed on all neonates with congenital scoliosis to search for possible urinary tract abnormalities. Congenital heart disease (10% to 15%) and spinal dysraphism (20%) occur in neonates with congenital scoliosis. These abnormalities include a tethered spinal cord, an intradural lipoma, syringomyelia, and diastematomyelia (Fig. 54-10).[8,11,67,69,117] They are frequently associated with cutaneous lesions of the back, such as hairy patches, skin dimples, and hemangiomas, and with abnormalities of the feet and lower extremities, such as cavus feet, calf atrophy, asymmetric foot size, and neurologic changes. An ultrasound examination and MRI can be useful in the evaluation of spinal dysraphism in a neonate with congenital scoliosis. Congenital scoliosis may also occur in association with syndromes such as Klippel-Feil and VATER (vertebrae, anus, trachea, esophagus, and renal abnormalities) and with spinal dysraphic disorders such as myelodysplasia.[118]

The risk for the progression of congenital scoliosis depends on the growth potential of the malformed vertebrae.[116] Defects such as block vertebrae have little growth potential, whereas unilateral unsegmented bars invariably produce progressive deformities.[70] About 75% of children with congenital scoliosis demonstrate some progression that typically continues until skeletal growth stops. About 50% require treatment.[71] Rapid progression can be expected during periods of rapid growth, such as those between birth and 2 years of age and after 10 years of age. Orthotic management is usually contraindicated because the disorder is a growth abnormality. When progression occurs, surgery is necessary. It usually consists of a combined anterior and posterior convex hemi-epiphysiodesis

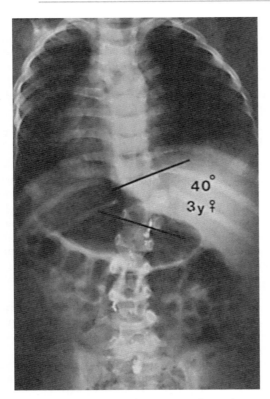

Figure 54–9. Radiograph of congenital scoliosis in a 3-year-old girl. A hemivertebra at T12 produces a 40-degree curve over a short segment of the spine. The mixed formation and segmentation defects in the upper thoracic spine are balanced and have not produced a significant curve.

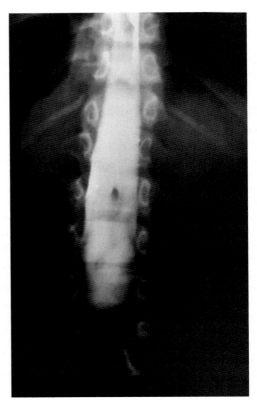

Figure 54–10. Metrizamide myelogram demonstrates cartilaginous diastematomyelia at L2 in a 3-year-old boy. Observe the midline filling defect and the increased widening or interpedicular distance in the middle lumbar region.[42,88]

to halt progression and allow for some correction from growth on the concavity of the curvature.

CONGENITAL KYPHOSIS

Congenital kyphosis includes congenital failure of the formation of all or part of the vertebral body but preservation of the posterior elements and failure of the anterior segmentation of the spine (i.e., anterior unsegmented bar). The more severe deformities are usually recognized in the neonate, and they rapidly progress. The less obvious deformities may not appear until several years later. After progression begins, it does not cease until the end of growth. The most important factor regarding congenital kyphosis is the possibility that a progressive deformity in the thoracic spine can result in paraplegia.[72] This potential outcome is usually associated with failure of the formation of the vertebral body. When necessary, the treatment of congenital kyphosis is operative.[57]

SACRAL AGENESIS

Sacral agenesis comprises a group of disorders with partial or complete absence of the sacrum. If the lower lumbar spine is also involved, it is called *lumbosacral agenesis*.[3,6,81] Motor function is typically lacking below the level of the remaining spine; however, sensation tends to present at a much more caudal level. The disorder can be classified by the amount of

sacrum remaining and the articulation between the spine and pelvis. It is a rare disorder, occurring in about 1 of 25,000 live births, and the exact cause is unknown. The incidence is increased among the children of diabetic mothers (see also Chapter 16 and Chapter 49, Part 1).[42,88]

The presentations of neonates with sacral agenesis can vary considerably. In the severe forms, there is a small pelvis, with pterygia anteriorly at the hip and posteriorly at the knees, and bilateral foot deformities, typically clubfoot. There may be spinopelvic instability. The neurologic examination tends to show no motor function below the last existing vertebra or sacral segment. However, sensation can be more variable. Children with sacral agenesis also have other visceral anomalies similar to those seen in congenital scoliosis.

The treatment of sacral agenesis is variable. Patients with only partial agenesis and a stable spinopelvic articulation can be observed. Those who are unstable may require a spinopelvic fusion in childhood for stabilization. This operation can enhance sitting balance and improve the function of the upper extremities. The problems associated with the lower extremities also require orthopedic intervention. If a child has the potential for ambulation, these problems need to be corrected to allow the child to assume an upright posture. Orthotics is usually necessary to support the extremities after they have been corrected.

LOWER EXTREMITIES

Most common neonatal congenital and developmental abnormalities of the lower extremities include torsional and angular deformities; developmental dysplasia of the hip (DDH); proximal femoral focal deficiency (PFFD); congenital hyperextension, subluxation, and dislocation of the knee; clubfoot; metatarsus adductus; vertical talus; the calcaneovalgus foot; and less serious toe deformities, such as syndactyly and polydactyly of the toes.

Torsional and Angular Deformities

PHYSIOLOGIC BOWLEG

The lower extremities of neonates commonly have mild to moderate bowing (i.e., genu varum) and internal rotation of the lower leg because of in utero positioning. The bowed appearance is actually a torsional combination of the external rotation of the hip (i.e., tight posterior capsule) and internal tibial torsion from in utero positioning. With the onset of standing and independent walking, the bowing and torsion are spontaneously corrected over a 6- to 12-month period. Significant improvement does not occur during the neonatal period or the first year of life. The typical neonate has 15 degrees of genu varum, which decreases to about 10 degrees by 1 year of age. By 2 years of age, most children have straight or neutrally aligned lower extremities. Treatment is indicated for children older than 2 to 3 years of age who have had no documented improvement with growth.

TIBIAL TORSION

Torsional changes of the tibia may be internal or external, depending on in utero positioning. The degree of tibial torsion may be measured by the thigh-foot angle. With the child in the prone position, the knee is flexed to 90 degrees to neutralize the normal tibiofemoral rotation. The foot is placed in a neutral or simulated weight-bearing position. The long axis of the foot is compared with the long axis of the thigh. An inwardly rotated foot is assigned a negative value and represents internal tibial torsion. An outwardly rotated foot represents external tibial torsion and is given a positive value. It is important that the measurements be recorded on each visit to document the improvement. Radiographic evaluation is of no value in the assessment of tibial torsion.

Internal Tibial Torsion

Internal tibial torsion is the most common cause of pigeon-toed children from birth to 2 years of age. It is the major component of physiologic bowleg, or genu varum. Because this condition is physiologic, spontaneous resolution can be anticipated with normal growth and development. The persistence of internal tibial torsion in the older child or adolescent is uncommon.

External Tibial Torsion

External tibial torsion is a common deformity and is always associated with a calcaneovalgus foot. It is caused by a variation in the normal in utero position. The sole of the foot lies pressed against the wall of the uterus, forcing the limb into a hyperdorsiflexed, everted position. This physiologic configuration produces the calcaneovalgus foot and secondarily the external tibial torsion. When these two conditions are combined with a normally externally rotated hip from a tight posterior hip capsule, they produce a very externally rotated or out-toed position. Because they are also physiologic in origin, both undergo spontaneous resolution and follow a clinical course similar to that of internal tibial torsion.

CONGENITAL ANGULAR DEFORMITIES OF THE TIBIA AND FIBULA

Congenital angular deformities of the tibia and fibula are uncommon neonatal problems. They are classified according to the direction of angulation—posteromedial or anterolateral. Posteromedial angulation is the least common but is characterized by spontaneous resolution with growth and development. Anterolateral angulation is more common and is typically associated with other underlying congenital abnormalities, such as the congenital absence of the fibula (i.e., fibular hemimelia), the congenital absence of the tibia (i.e., tibial hemimelia), and congenital pseudarthrosis of the tibia (i.e., neurofibromatosis).

Posteromedial Angulation

Posteromedial angulation has three associated clinical problems: angular deformity, the calcaneovalgus foot, and length discrepancy of the lower extremities. The angular deformity occurs at the junction of the middle and distal thirds of the shafts. The deformity is usually unilateral (Fig. 54-11). The neonates are normal and healthy, and there is no increased incidence of other congenital anomalies. The degree of angulation varies between 25 and 65 degrees and is equal in both directions. The foot is hyperdorsiflexed and has a marked calcaneovalgus posture. Radiographs are necessary to confirm the diagnosis. The cause of congenital posteromedial angulation in the tibia and fibula is unknown.

Posteromedial angulation resolves with growth, especially during the first 3 years of life. The posterior bowing tends to resolve more quickly than the medial bowing, which may not resolve until 5 years of age. However, the associated shortening of the tibia and fibula persists and progresses during growth. The fibula tends to be slightly shorter than the tibia. The appearance of the foot also improves, although a pes planovalgus appearance may persist.

Nonoperative treatment is indicated in the neonatal period.[104] If the bowing does not resolve by 3 or 4 years of age, a tibial or fibular osteotomy may be necessary. The most common sequela of posteromedial angulation is a discrepancy in leg length. Most of these children have enough discrepancy to require equalization. An appropriately planned epiphysiodesis (physeal closure) is the most common procedure. Lengthening may sometimes need to be considered.

Anterolateral Angulation

When anterolateral bowing is encountered, it is usually associated with a significant underlying pathologic disorder, such as congenital pseudarthrosis of the tibia or congenital longitudinal deficiencies of the tibia or fibula. Careful clinical and radiographic evaluation is necessary to establish the correct

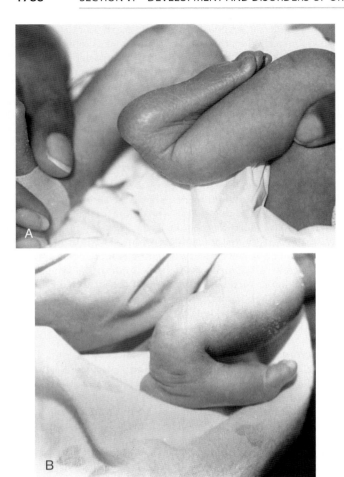

Figure 54–11. A, One-month-old boy with posteromedial angulation of the left tibia. This condition resembles a calcaneovalgus foot because the dorsum of the foot comes in contact with the lower leg. However, there is posterior angulation of the tibia in this case. B, The medial angulation is visible when viewed from the front.

diagnosis. Congenital pseudarthrosis of the tibia is typically associated with neurofibromatosis.

Hip

The most common neonatal hip disorders include DDH and septic arthritis and osteomyelitis. Septic arthritis and osteomyelitis were discussed in Part 2, "Bone and Joint Infections". Another congenital abnormality, although uncommon, is proximal femoral focal deficiency (PFFD).

DEVELOPMENTAL DYSPLASIA OF THE HIP

DDH is the most common neonatal hip disorder.[91,113] It was initially thought to be congenital in origin but is now recognized as developmental, hence the change in terminology to DDH. At birth, an involved hip is rarely dislocated; instead, it is dislocatable. Whether the hip stabilizes, subluxates, or ultimately dislocates depends on postnatal factors. Most developmental dislocations are postnatal in origin; however, the exact time of their occurrence is controversial.

Neonatal hip dislocations are classified into two major groups: the typical, which is found in a neurologically normal infant, and the teratologic, which is found in an infant with an underlying neuromuscular disorder, such as myelodysplasia, arthrogryposis multiplex congenita, or a complex of syndromes. Teratologic dislocations occur in utero and are therefore truly congenital in origin. This section concentrates on typical DDH because it is the most common form.

Pathology and Etiology

The pathogenesis and causes of typical DDH are multifactorial; genetic, physiologic, and mechanical factors are involved. The genetic factors include a positive family history (20%) and generalized ligamentous laxity, an inherited trait. The physiologic factors include female predominance (9:1) and maternal estrogen and other hormones associated with pelvic relaxation during labor and delivery. The mechanical factors include primigravida, breech presentation, and postnatal positioning. Positioning has a significant effect in determining which hip stabilizes and which may progress to dislocation.

The genetic and physiologic aspects are related etiologic factors. Most neonates with DDH have generalized ligamentous laxity, which can be a predisposition to hip instability. The maternal estrogen and other hormones associated with pelvic relaxation at delivery cross the placenta and result in further, albeit temporary, relaxation of the newborn hip joint.

About 60% of children with typical DDH are first born, and 30% to 50% develop it as a result of the breech position. In this position, there is extreme hip flexion and a limitation of hip motion that results in the stretching of an already lax hip capsule and ligamentum teres and in the posterior uncovering of the femoral head. Decreased hip motion results in the lack of normal stimulation for the growth and development of the cartilaginous acetabulum.

Congenital muscular torticollis and metatarsus adductus are associated with DDH. The presence of either of these two conditions necessitates a careful examination of the hips.

Postnatal factors are important determinants in ultimate hip stability. Positioning an unstable hip in adduction and extension may lead to dislocation. These positions put the unstable hip under abnormal pressure as a result of the normal hip flexion and abduction contracture. Consequently, an unstable femoral head can be displaced from the acetabulum over several days or weeks.

Because the hips are not dislocated at birth, the components of the hip joints, excluding the hip capsule and ligamentum teres, are usually relatively normal. There may be some variation in the shape of the cartilaginous acetabulum. If a subluxation or dislocation is not recognized, it will lead to progressive acetabular dysplasia and maldirection, excessive femoral anteversion (i.e., torsion), and hip muscle contracture. It is critical that an early diagnosis be made and appropriate treatment instituted. The longer a dislocation continues, the more complex the treatment becomes.

Diagnosis

The physical findings in neonates with DDH include a positive Barlow test (i.e., dislocatable hip), a positive Ortolani test (i.e., dislocated hip), asymmetric thigh skin folds, uneven knee levels (i.e., Allis or Galeazzi sign), and the absence of normal knee flexion contractures.

The Barlow and Ortolani tests are the most sensitive for neonatal hip instability (Fig. 54-12). The Barlow[7] test is a provocative means of diagnosing an unstable hip and is the most important maneuver in examining the neonatal hip. With the infant supine, this test is performed by stabilizing the pelvis with one hand, flexing and adducting each hip separately, and applying a posterior force with the other hand (Fig. 54-13). If a hip is dislocatable, it is usually felt as a

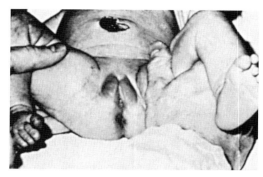

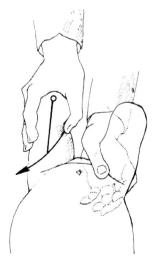

Figure 54–12. Positioning of the hip in the newborn to perform two diagnostic tests. The Ortolani sign, or click of reduction, is elicited when abducting the hip in this manner. The reverse Ortolani, or Barlow, maneuver is performed by bringing the femur into adduction with flexion, causing a click of exit or dislocation.

"clunk." After release of the posterior pressure, the hip usually spontaneously relocates. It has been estimated that about 1 in 100 newborns has a clinically unstable hip (i.e., subluxatable or dislocatable) and that 1 in 800 to 1000 infants eventually develops a true dislocation.

The Ortolani test is a procedure to reduce a recently dislocated hip (Fig. 54-14). It is most likely to be positive in infants who are 1 to 2 months of age because adequate time must have passed for true dislocation to occur. This test is performed concomitant with the Barlow test. With the hip flexed, the thigh is abducted and the femoral head lifted anteriorly into the acetabulum. If a reduction occurs, it is felt as a clunk. Clunks should not be confused with hip "clicks," which are common in neonates. A variety of normal factors produce a clicking sensation during examination of the hip, including the breaking of surface tension across the hip joint, the snapping of gluteal tendons, patellofemoral motion, and femorotibial (knee) rotation. These normal characteristics are commonly misinterpreted as a sign of instability. After 2 months of age, the Ortolani test usually becomes negative. It is no longer possible to relocate a dislocated hip because of the development of soft tissue contractures.

When the hip is dislocated, its abduction is limited by soft tissue contractures (Fig. 54-15). There is also an increased number of thigh skinfolds on the involved side because of redundant soft tissues, the appearance of a shortened extremity, and a positive Allis or Galeazzi sign. The latter sign is demonstrated by placing the feet of the supine neonate together on the examining table and assessing the relative heights of the knees. An apparent shortening is observed on

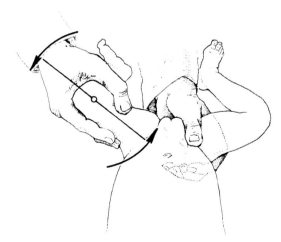

Figure 54–13. The Barlow test permits the early diagnosis of hip instability. It is a provocation test for dislocatability. The pelvis is steadied with one hand while the leg to be tested is grasped with the other. The thumb of the examiner's hand should lie over the lesser trochanter and the tip of the middle finger over the greater trochanter. With the hip and knee in flexion, gentle pressure is exerted with the thumb over the lesser trochanter. Dislocatability is manifested by a sudden shift of the proximal femur. Dislocation may be reduced with the Ortolani test.

Figure 54–14. In the Ortolani test, the pelvis is held steady with one hand while the limb to be examined is grasped with the other. The hip and knee are flexed. While gently pulling the femur forward, the examiner abducts the limb under examination, using the greater trochanter as a fulcrum. Reduction of dislocation is manifested by a sudden shift in the position of the proximal femur, often accompanied by a palpable or audible click. There must be sufficient ligamentous laxity to permit relocation of the proximal femur into the acetabulum; therefore, the test is useful primarily in the neonatal period.

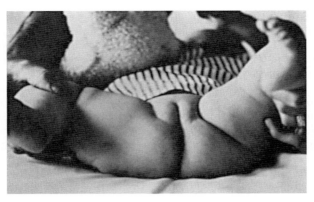

Figure 54–15. Clinical photograph showing the limitation of abduction of the thighs when the hips are flexed at 90 degrees.

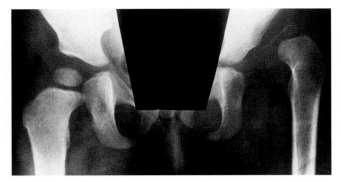

Figure 54–16. Anteroposterior pelvic radiograph of a 9-month-old girl with a complete dislocation of the left hip. Observe the hypoplasia of the proximal femur and ossific nucleus of the femoral head. The right hip is normal.

the involved side. With a proximal displacement of the femoral head, the quadriceps and hamstrings become relaxed. This effect can be demonstrated best by the so-called "hamstring" test. Both hips are flexed and abducted with the knees flexed. Attempts to extend the knee are resisted on the normal side because of increased tightness in the hamstrings. If a dislocated hip is present, the knee can come into full extension because of the lack of proximal stability, which produces a fixed fulcrum for the hamstring muscles.

Imaging

The imaging of neonatal DDH is best accomplished with ultrasonography and plain radiographs. Ultrasonography[43] is becoming an increasingly popular method for the evaluation and assessment of the neonatal hip because the femoral head does not ossify until 4 to 7 months of age. Hip stability and acetabular and femoral head development can be accurately assessed by an experienced ultrasonographer. Ultrasonography allows avoidance of the effects of ionizing radiation but is very user dependent and expensive. It is so sensitive that false-positive results are common. In large screening programs in which all births are screened, it is common to identify 7.5% of neonates with abnormal results.[18] This percentage decreases to a more appropriate level of 0.4% by 6 weeks, but the expense, anxiety, and administrative stress of retesting can be considerable. At present, there is no agreement about the efficacy of routine screening for all infants. Some large centers suggest it,[66] whereas others claim that selective ultrasonography is as effective as universal screening when it is accompanied by a good clinical screening program.[29] Additionally, a stable, normal ultrasound does not ensure normal hips after 6 months of age. Jones has reported on seven developmental dislocations in five babies (age 6 to 22 months) in whom ultrasound demonstrated stable and reduced hips. The Pediatric Orthopedic Society of North America warns that late-onset dislocation can be expected in 1 in 5000 infants who are clinically stable in the newborn period.[91] Anteroposterior and frog lateral radiographs of the pelvis may also be obtained. The limitation of plain radiographs is due to the lack of ossification of the femoral head, which may be further delayed in DDH (Fig. 54-16). Line measurements are drawn to determine the development of

the acetabulum and the relationship between the femoral head and acetabulum (see also Chapter 27 and Chapter 37).

Treatment

The treatment of neonatal DDH is simple and effective. The most important factor in the treatment of this disorder is an accurate and early diagnosis. When an unstable or dislocatable hip is recognized at birth, maintenance of the hip in the position of flexion and abduction, or the "human position," for 1 to 2 months is usually sufficient. This position maintains a reduction of the femoral head in the acetabulum and allows the progressive tightening of the ligamentous structures as the child grows. It also stimulates the normal growth and development of the acetabulum. The methods that can be used to maintain the hip in this position include double or triple diapers, the Pavlik harness, the Frejka pillow splint, and a variety of abduction orthoses. Double or triple diapers, although controversial, are commonly used in early infancy because the harness, pillow splint, and abduction orthoses usually do not fit satisfactorily. Treatment is continued until there is clinical stability of the hip and the ultrasonographic or radiographic results are normal, both of which usually take place within 3 to 4 months. There may be a true dislocation during the neonatal period. As a consequence, treatment is directed toward the reduction of the femoral head in the true acetabulum.[30,38,45]

The Pavlik harness is the major mode of treatment in this age group (Fig. 54-17). The harness places the hips in the human position by flexing them more than 90 degrees (preferably 100 to 110 degrees) and maintaining relatively full but gentle abduction (50 to 70 degrees). This position redirects the femoral head toward the acetabulum. A spontaneous relocation usually occurs within 3 to 4 weeks. The Pavlik harness is about 95% successful for dysplastic or subluxated hips and 80% successful for true dislocations. If true dislocations are initially irreducible, treatment with the Pavlik harness may not be effective. Lerman and coworkers[65] reported on 93 DDH patients treated with a Pavlik harness. There were 82% who were successfully treated. Six patients had initially irreducible hips and less than 20% ultrasound coverage; all six failed treatment with the Pavlik harness. If the reduction of a dislocated hip is achieved, treatment is continued until

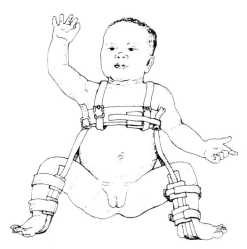

Figure 54–17. The Pavlik harness is a safe, reliable means of treating hip instability and dislocation in the neonate.

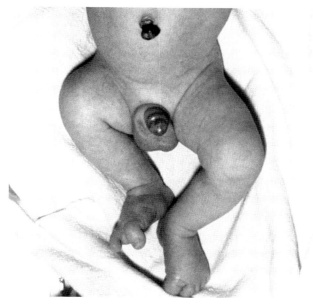

Figure 54–18. Clinical photograph of a newborn boy with significant shortening of the right thigh caused by proximal femoral focal deficiency.

ultrasonography or the radiographic parameters have returned to normal. If a spontaneous reduction does not occur, closed reduction by surgery will be necessary. This approach consists of preliminary skin traction for 1 to 3 weeks to stretch the existing soft tissue contractures followed by an examination under anesthesia, percutaneous adductor tenotomy, closed reduction, an arthrogram to assess the concentricity of the reduction, and the application of a hip spica cast in the human position. Treatment is continued until the radiographic parameters are within normal limits. The indications for an open reduction in the neonate and up to the first 6 months of life are limited.[45] Follow-up for at least 1 year is necessary because dysplastic hips that improve with treatment can deteriorate after it is withdrawn.[30] If this deterioration occurs, more treatment is indicated.

The complications attending the treatment of neonatal DDH include reduction failure and redislocation.[38] Avascular necrosis of the capital femoral epiphysis, which is the most devastating complication of this disorder, develops in about 5% of infants no matter how careful the initial management has been.

PROXIMAL FEMORAL FOCAL DEFICIENCY

PFFD is a congenital abnormality affecting the development of the proximal end of the femur and possibly the acetabulum. There is considerable variation, ranging from a mildly shortened femur to severe shortening with an absence of the femoral head and acetabulum. It may be bilateral or unilateral; bilateral cases tend to have more severe involvement. The cause of PFFD is unknown, but it results from an embryologically abnormal formation of the hip that occurs during limb bud formation.

The clinical examination is usually diagnostic. The thigh is shortened and the hip held in flexion, abduction, and external rotation (Fig. 54-18). There are usually hip- and knee-flexion contractures. Because of the proximity of the lower leg to the trunk, the entire extremity appears similar to a funnel. There may also be abnormalities of the lower leg. About 50% to 70% of affected neonates also have fibular

hemimelia with or without the absence of the lateral portion of the foot.

Radiographs are necessary in the assessment of children with PFFD. However, the components may not be fully visualized owing to the lack of ossification. If an acetabulum is present, there will usually be a femoral head. MRI scans can be helpful in difficult cases to determine the shape of the proximal femur and acetabulum.

The most important therapeutic component of the treatment of neonatal PFFD is observation. It is important that a careful evaluation be performed to search for other associated congenital abnormalities. The ultimate treatment depends on the length of the extremity, the stability of the hip, the presence or absence of a functional foot, and a determination of whether the disorder is unilateral or bilateral. Possible treatment options include prosthetic fitting; knee fusion, Syme amputation, and prosthesis; surgical reconstruction; and lengthening of the femur. The lengthening of the femur is considered only if the hip and knee are relatively normal and the degree of predicted shortening is less than 15 to 20 cm at skeletal maturity.

Knee

HYPEREXTENSION, SUBLUXATION, AND DISLOCATION OF THE KNEE

The congenital disorder comprising hyperextension, subluxation, and dislocation of the knee is uncommon. The tibia is displaced anterior to the femur, and the knee is hyperextended. The cause is multifactorial, with mechanical and genetic elements. Most cases are sporadic, with no particular predisposition; however, patients with inherited Larsen disease frequently demonstrate congenital subluxation and dislocation of the knee. Breech positioning is more frequently seen in children with congenital subluxation and dislocation of the knee, suggesting that mechanical factors are also important.

The pathologic picture is complex, and associated anomalies are common. Curtis and Fisher[22] reported on 11 patients, and in every case they noted congenital hip deformities. Seven patients had clubfoot, and seven were thought to have arthrogryposis multiplex congenita. Fibrosis of the quadriceps muscle was found in all surgical cases. The quadriceps muscle in effect runs from the anteroinferior iliac spine to the tibial tubercle. Progressive fibrosis would provide pressure for anterior subluxation of the tibia and for hip deformity as well as a tendency to hyperextend the knee.

The diagnosis is made on physical examination. Recurvatum at the knee sometimes approaches 90 degrees (Fig. 54-19). A lateral radiograph can demonstrate that the tibia is anterior to the femur. A line is drawn down the long axis of the tibia and the long axis of the femur; it does not meet at the normal axis of the knee joint.

In benign hyperextension of the knee, recurvatum of 15 to 30 degrees is common. Flexion is frequently limited to a few degrees. In this "packing deformity," the radiographs demonstrate that the tibia is not anterior to the femur and that the center of rotation of the knee joint is normal, unlike congenital dislocation and subluxation of the knee. It is important to obtain the radiographs of knees that hyperextend considerably to determine whether an epiphyseal fracture is responsible for hyperextension of the knee. The results of treatment are very different when benign hyperextension of the knee is compared with congenital dislocation of the knee. In benign hyperextension of the knee and, to a certain extent, congenital subluxation of the knee, manipulation and serial casting provide an adequate result. Early manipulation and casting are often successful in uncomplicated congenital knee dislocation if treatment is begun during the first few weeks of life. The prognosis is much worse when the knee dislocation is associated with Larsen disease or arthrogryposis multiplex congenita.[60] Children with congenital dislocation of the knee who fail casting may benefit

from traction delivered through skeletal pins in the tibia and femur. The goal of treatment is to achieve at least 100 to 110 degrees of knee flexion and full, stable knee extension before the child reaches walking age. If these objectives cannot be attained with casting, splinting, or traction, surgery before the child reaches walking age is recommended.

Foot and Toes

The most common foot and toe disorders include metatarsus adductus, the calcaneovalgus foot, talipes equinovarus (clubfoot), congenital vertical talus, and syndactyly and polydactyly of the toes.

METATARSUS ADDUCTUS

Metatarsus adductus, or forefoot adduction, is probably the most common neonatal foot problem. It results from in utero positioning, occurring equally in boys and girls,[31] and is bilateral in about 50% of neonates. The disorder has hereditary tendencies and is more common in the first-born than subsequent children because of an increased molding effect from the primigravid uterus and abdominal wall. It is also associated with hip dysplasia. About 10% of children with metatarsus adductus have DDH, and careful examination of the hips is necessary in any neonate with metatarsus adductus.[63]

Diagnosis

Clinically, the forefoot is adducted and occasionally supinated. The hindfoot and midfoot are normal. The lateral border of the foot is convex, and the base of the fifth metatarsal appears to be prominent (Fig. 54-20). The medial border of the foot is concave. There is usually an increased interval between the first and second toes, with the great toe being held in a greater varus position. Ankle dorsiflexion and plantar flexion are normal. These characteristics distinguish metatarsus adductus from a congenital clubfoot. Forefoot flexibility is variable. This flexibility can be passively assessed by stabilizing the hindfoot in a neutral position with one hand and applying pressure over the first metatarsal head with the other. Active flexibility is

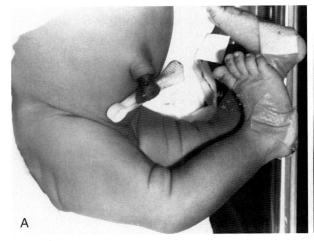
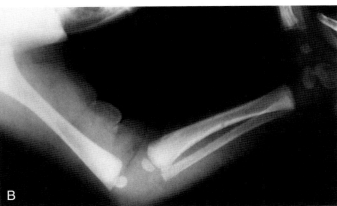

Figure 54–19. **A,** Clinical photograph of a newborn boy with bilateral congenital or developmental subluxation of the knees. The knees are hyperextended and have limited flexion. **B,** Lateral radiograph demonstrating the hyperextension or subluxation of the right knee.

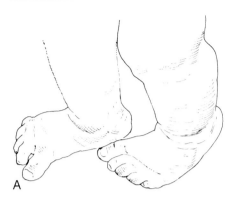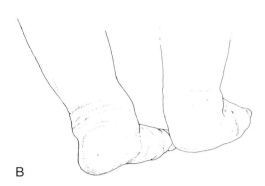

Figure 54-20. Bilateral metatarsus adductus. **A,** Dorsomedial and dorsolateral views. The medial border of the foot is concave; the lateral border is convex. The medial arch may be accentuated. **B,** Posterior view. A slightly valgus hindfoot may be present in the standing position.

assessed by gently stroking the lateral border of the involved foot. This approach induces reflex activity in the peroneal muscles along the lateral aspect of the calf. The forefoot is typically classified as flexible, moderately flexible, or rigid.[21] In flexible metatarsus adductus, the forefoot achieves the overcorrected position actively and passively. In moderately flexible metatarsus adductus, the forefoot can be brought to the neutral position; in the rigid deformity, the forefoot cannot be corrected to achieve the neutral position.

Imaging

Routine radiographs are unnecessary in the evaluation of metatarsus adductus. Radiographs do not demonstrate forefoot mobility; however, anteroposterior and lateral simulated weight-bearing radiographs of the foot are necessary to assist in the diagnosis of rigid deformities and those in which a diagnosis by other means is uncertain.

Treatment

About 85% of the neonatal metatarsus adductus deformities resolve spontaneously by 3 years of age,[31,83,87] and 95% resolve by 16 years of age.[115] Treatment is seldom recommended for metatarsus adductus because most patients develop normal foot position and mobility without treatment, and even those with some residual deformity generally have normal function.[31]

CALCANEOVALGUS FOOT

The calcaneovalgus foot is a common physiologic variant.[103] It results from in utero positioning. This condition is manifested by a hyperdorsiflexed foot, with an abducted forefoot and increasingly valgus hindfoot. It is usually associated with external tibial torsion and typically occurs unilaterally but occasionally bilaterally. In utero, the plantar surface of the foot was against the wall of the uterus, forcing it into a hyperdorsiflexed, abducted, and externally rotated position (Fig. 54-21). This position produces the calcaneovalgus foot and external tibial torsion. When these two conditions are combined with the normal, increased external rotation of the hip (i.e., tight posterior capsule) in the neonate, the result is a lower extremity that appears excessively externally rotated.

Diagnosis

The neonate typically presents with external rotation of the involved extremity and a calcaneovalgus foot. The forefoot is abducted, and the heel is everted or in the valgus position.

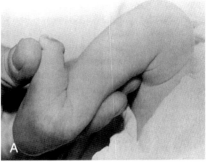

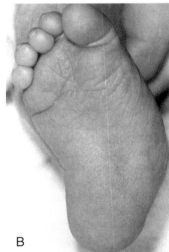

Figure 54-21. A, A 3-month-old boy with a calcaneovalgus foot. The foot can be dorsiflexed to allow the dorsum to come in contact with the anterior aspect of the lower leg. **B,** There is abduction of the forefoot and increased valgus alignment of the hindfoot. This condition is always associated with external tibial torsion.

The foot can be hyperdorsiflexed to bring its dorsal surface in contact with the anterior aspect of the lower leg. This condition should not be confused with the neonatal maturity classification of Dubowitz. External tibial torsion of 20 to 50 degrees is common. Ankle motion usually shows normal to nearly normal plantar flexion.

Three conditions must be distinguished from the benign calcaneovalgus foot: congenital vertical talus; posteromedial bowing of the tibia; and neuromuscular abnormalities, with paralysis of the gastrocnemius muscles.[103] This differentiation can usually be established by clinical examination.

Imaging

Routine imaging of a benign calcaneovalgus foot is unnecessary; it is predominantly a clinical diagnosis. However, in severe deformities or in those with limited mobility, anteroposterior and lateral simulated weight-bearing radiographs of the foot and possibly the lower leg are necessary. These radiographs allow the recognition of a congenital vertical talus or posteromedial bowing of the tibia.

Treatment

The benign calcaneovalgus foot does not require treatment. This deformity usually resolves during the first 6 months of life. However, external tibial torsion follows the same natural history as that of internal tibial torsion. Spontaneous improvement does not take place until the child begins to pull to stand and walk independently. It takes 6 to 12 months thereafter to achieve complete correction. Most neonates presenting with a benign calcaneovalgus foot and external tibial torsion have a normally aligned foot and lower extremity by 2 years of age.

TALIPES EQUINOVARUS (CLUBFOOT)

A congenital clubfoot is one of the most common pathologic deformities affecting the neonatal foot. It is a deformity of the foot and the entire lower leg. It is classified as congenital, teratologic, or positional. The congenital clubfoot is usually an isolated abnormality, whereas the teratologic form is associated with an underlying neuromuscular disorder, such as myelodysplasia or arthrogryposis multiplex congenita. Positional clubfoot refers to a normal foot that has been held in the equinovarus position in utero.

The cause of congenital clubfoot is unknown. There are hereditary factors, and they are considered multifactorial, with a major influence from a single autosomal dominant gene. It develops more commonly in boys (2:1) and is bilateral in 50% of cases. The probability of the deformity occurring randomly is 1 in 1000 live births, but within affected families, the probability is about 3% for subsequent siblings and 20% to 30% for the offspring of affected parents. Muscle biopsies of the extrinsic muscles, electromyographic studies of these muscles, and histologic analysis of the associated connective tissue have indicated a probable neuromuscular etiology.[32,50] There are disproportionate fiber types and increased neuromuscular junctions within these muscles. These findings contrast with previous etiologic theories in which the deformity of the talus was thought to be the primary abnormality. These findings also suggest why clubfoot is ubiquitous in syndromes and neuromuscular disorders, and any child with a clubfoot deformity requires a careful musculoskeletal and neurologic evaluation to search for other abnormalities.

Diagnosis

A congenital clubfoot is characterized by equinovarus deformity of the foot and ankle; variable rigidity of the deformity; mild calf atrophy; and mild hypoplasia of the tibia, fibula, and bones of the foot (Fig. 54-22).[84,101,106]

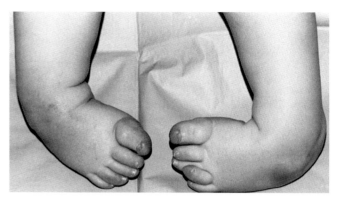

Figure 54-22. Clinical photograph of a 9-month-old boy with bilateral talipes equinovarus (clubfoot) deformity.

Imaging

Anteroposterior and lateral standing or simulated weight-bearing radiographs are used in the assessment of clubfoot.[106] Multiple different radiographic measurements can be made. The navicular bone, which is the primary site of the deformity, does not ossify until 3 years of age in girls and 4 years of age in boys. Line measurements are required to determine the position of the unossified navicular bone and the overall alignment of the foot.

Treatment

Both nonoperative and operative methods are used in the treatment of clubfoot deformities.[84] Nonoperative methods include taping, malleable splints, and serial plaster casts. Taping and malleable splints are particularly useful in premature infants until they attain an appropriate size for casting. Serial plaster casting is the major nonoperative method of treatment. For each cast change, the foot is gently manipulated toward the corrected position. Casts are changed at 1- to 2-week intervals to allow for progressive correction. Complete clinical and radiographic correction should be achieved by 3 months of age. If this expectation is realized, holding casts are used for an additional 3 to 6 months and followed by orthoses or corrective shoes until the child is walking well. The failure to achieve clinical and radiographic correction by 3 months of age is an indication for surgical treatment. Further attempts at casting may result in articular damage or a midfoot breech (i.e., rocker-bottom deformity). The rate of success for the nonoperative treatment of a congenital clubfoot is low. Previously, most children required a complete soft tissue release, which was usually performed between 6 and 12 months of age. Satisfactory long-term results were anticipated for 80% to 90% of cases.[106] However, the Ponseti method of casting[84] (augmented with percutaneous tendo Achilles tenotomy when necessary) has become widely accepted. The Ponseti casting technique and tendo Achillis tenotomy are followed by a prolonged period of bracing, which lasts from 2 to 4 years. Strict adherence to the bracing protocol is mandatory for a positive outcome.[26]

CONGENITAL VERTICAL TALUS

Congenital vertical talus is an uncommon neonatal foot deformity, but its etiology is similar to that of clubfoot.[19,27] It must be distinguished from the benign calcaneovalgus foot, which is a much more common deformity. Congenital vertical talus typically presents as a rigid rocker-bottom deformity. Most of these deformities are associated with an underlying disorder such as teratologic malformation, myelodysplasia, or arthrogryposis multiplex congenita or a syndrome such as trisomy 18.

Diagnosis

The clinical characteristic of congenital vertical talus is a rocker-bottom foot (Fig. 54-23). There is an equinus hindfoot, a valgus hindfoot, a convex plantar surface, forefoot abduction and dorsiflexion, and rigidity. A careful musculoskeletal and neurologic examination must be performed on all neonates to search for associated disorders or syndromes.

Imaging

The radiographic evaluation of congenital vertical talus is similar to that of clubfoot. Anteroposterior and lateral simulated weight-bearing radiographs of the feet are obtained (Fig. 54-24) and typically reveal a vertically oriented talus, dorsal displacement of the midfoot on the hindfoot, and a valgus hindfoot.

Treatment

As in clubfoot, nonoperative treatment is the initial method of management. Serial casting begins at birth. The forefoot is manipulated in the equinus position in an attempt to reduce

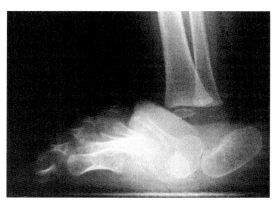

Figure 54–24. Radiograph of a 9-month-old infant showing the vertical alignment of the talus, equinus hindfoot, and dorsal angulation of the midfoot and forefoot.

the dorsally dislocated navicular bone onto the head of the talus. The rate of success for nonoperative treatment is low; most infants require an extensive soft tissue release.

The goals for the treatment of congenital vertical talus are modest and include the achievement of a plantigrade, painless foot on which a shoe can be worn. Orthotic management is frequently necessary postoperatively to maintain alignment and minimize the risk for recurrent deformity.

SYNDACTYLY AND POLYDACTYLY OF THE TOES

Syndactyly and polydactyly are common disorders of the toes.[34,105] Syndactyly of the toes is almost always asymptomatic and rarely requires treatment but may be associated with a positive family history. Syndactyly may be classified as *zygodactyly*, a complete or incomplete webbing usually involving the second and third toes, and *polysyndactyly*, with polydactyly of the fifth toe and syndactyly between the duplicated toes.[105] Zygodactyly does not interfere with wearing shoes or normal function and does not require treatment; polysyndactyly usually requires treatment.

Polydactyly of the toes can be preaxial (i.e., great toe), central, or postaxial (i.e., fifth toe).[105] It occurs in about 2 of 1000 live births and is more common among African Americans than whites. Postaxial deformities are the most common (80%) and can be subdivided into type A (articulated) and type B (rudimentary). About 30% of the neonates with polydactyly have a positive family history. It is usually an isolated disorder with autosomal dominant inheritance. Polydactyly of the hands and associated metatarsal deformities are common.

The goal of treatment is to restore a relatively normal contour to the forefoot to allow the appropriate fitting of shoes. The rudimentary digits are ligated at birth, whereas the articulated ones are removed at 9 to 12 months of age.[105] The most central of the involved digits are usually preserved and the more peripheral ones amputated.

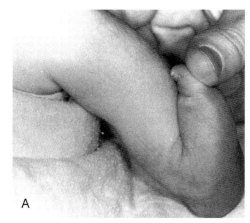

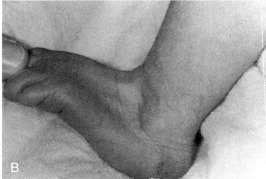

Figure 54–23. A, Newborn girl with congenital vertical talus. The dorsum of the foot also comes in contact with the anterior aspect of the lower leg. The foot has a rocker-bottom appearance. B, Attempted plantar flexion shows the tightness of the anterior musculature and a persistent rocker-bottom appearance of the midfoot and hindfoot.

SYNDROMES

See also Chapter 29.

Skeletal Dysplasias

Skeletal dysplasias constitute a group of disorders that produce short stature. Diagnoses are typically made antenatally. Many of these disorders are recognizable at birth, whereas others are manifested during growth and development. The defects can occur in the epiphyses of the physeal or growth plates or as abnormalities of bone remodeling that may affect the metaphysis or diaphysis.

The most common skeletal dysplasia is achondroplasia, which produces short-limb dwarfism that is caused by a defect in a gene that encodes one of the fibroblast growth factor receptors. Diagnostic and prenatal testing is available. It is inherited as an autosomal dominant trait, but about 80% of cases are new mutations. It is caused by abnormal endochondral ossification in the physes. Achondroplasia produces a rhizomelic pattern of shortening, with the proximal segments (i.e., humerus and femur) more involved than the lower segments (i.e., radius and ulna or tibia and fibula). Periosteal and intramembranous ossification is normal.

The diagnosis of achondroplasia is confirmed by characteristic features of the head, face, and short extremities. The head is typically enlarged; there are disproportionately short limbs and a normal trunk. Facial features include frontal bossing, flattening of the nasal bridge, midfacial hypoplasia, and prominence of the mandible. The trunk appears relatively normal, but the abdomen is usually protuberant. The hands characteristically have a space between the long and ring fingers, producing a trident hand. The thoracolumbar spine may show a gibbous or kyphotic deformity before the onset of walking. The lower extremities are usually bowed, and the musculature appears enlarged. It is important to make an early diagnosis so that genetic counseling can be performed.

Treatment is usually not indicated in the neonatal period or during the first year. The one possible exception is the presence of a gibbous deformity of the thoracolumbar spine, which may benefit from orthotic management.

Osteogenesis Imperfecta

Osteogenesis imperfecta is an inherited disorder of connective tissues. It is caused by mutations in the *COL1A1* and *COL1A2* genes, which code for type I procollagen.[61] More than 150 separate mutations have been identified. Because type I collagen is the primary matrix protein for bone, dentin, sclerae, and ligaments, there is a heterogeneous mix of phenotypes. All children with osteogenesis imperfecta have increased bone fragility and susceptibility to fracture. Some children also present with blue sclerae, defective dentinogenesis, growth restriction, presenile hearing loss, scoliosis and kyphosis, and multiple angular deformities of bone (Fig. 54-25). Osteogenesis imperfecta is uncommon, occurring in fewer than 1 of 20,000 children. In its mildest form, children have a few fractures, normal teeth, sclerae with a slightly blue tinge, minimal hearing loss, and somewhat short stature. In its most severe form, perinatal death is the rule. These children have blue sclerae, and their bones crumble in utero.

Silence and Danks[95] and Silence[94] suggested a comprehensive classification scheme based on genetic inheritance and clinical manifestation. In osteogenesis imperfecta type I, patients have increased bone fragility, distinct blue sclerae,

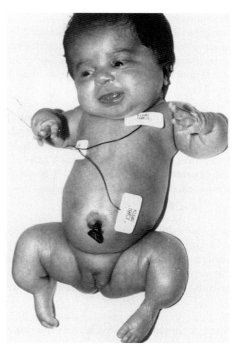

Figure 54–25. Clinical photograph of a newborn girl with severe congenital osteogenesis imperfecta. The child had multiple fractures at birth. Observe the severe shortening of the extremities. Darkened (blue) sclera were present.

and presenile hearing loss. Some of these patients have defective dentinogenesis, whereas others do not. The inheritance pattern is autosomal dominant. In type II, the children are severely affected. Most die perinatally, and their bones crumble in utero. The inheritance pattern is autosomal recessive. At present, efforts to establish a relationship between genotype and phenotype are ongoing, but complex. Recently, Bodian and associates analyzed 63 subjects with type II osteogenesis imperfecta.[10] They found 61 distinct heterozygous mutations in type I collagen, of which 43 had not been previously seen. To say that osteogenesis imperfecta is heterogeneous would be an understatement.[10] In type III, the bone fragility is quite marked but compatible with survival. The children are born with multiple fractures and have progressive bowing of bones throughout life. Early on, their sclerae are quite blue but become less blue as they mature, and by adolescence, the sclerae are essentially normal in appearance. The inheritance pattern is autosomal recessive. In type IV, the bone fragility is modest. These patients usually have white sclerae; some have defective dentinogenesis, whereas others do not. They have modest bowing of bones. Some of these children may be difficult to differentiate from the normal population early in life.

The goal of orthopedic treatment in osteogenesis imperfecta is to maximize comfort and function. In modestly affected children, this approach frequently focuses on the closed treatment of fractures. The management of fractures in modestly affected children is not dissimilar from that in the average population. Children with increased bone fragility frequently benefit from orthotics, which is used to protect their bones as they are mobilized. Intravenous pamidronate has shown promise for increasing bone density in children with moderate to severe osteogenesis imperfecta. Investigators also report reduced bone pain, a decreased incidence of fracture, and improved ambulation.[82,85,120] Children occasionally develop severe angular deformities from the poorly developed union of fractures or the insidious collapse of bones. As the deformities increase in magnitude, stress is concentrated at the angular deformities, and children become increasing susceptible to fracture. Osteotomies to straighten bones and intramedullary rods to maintain alignment may be helpful in assisting these children with their mobility. The rod provides internal support for the bone, and the elimination of angular deformities decreases stress within the bones.

Children with osteogenesis imperfecta may be quite bright. Every effort should be made to maximize their ability to attend school and interact with their peers.

Neurofibromatosis

Neurofibromatosis is a relatively common disorder that may or may not be diagnosable in the neonatal period. The presence of multiple café au lait spots or anterolateral bowing of the tibia suggests neurofibromatosis (Fig. 54-26). The café au lait spots frequently do not appear until the child is at least 2 years of age. The criteria for diagnosis have been outlined by Crawford[20] and include at least two of the following: multiple café au lait spots; a positive family history; a definitive biopsy; and characteristic bony lesions such as pseudarthrosis of the tibia, hemihypertrophy, or short and angulated spinal curvature. The café au lait spots are typically smooth;

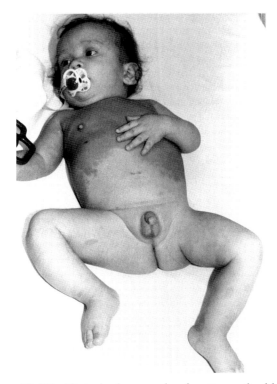

Figure 54–26. Clinical photograph of a 6-month-old boy with multiple café-au-lait spots due to neurofibromatosis.

the presence of at least five spots larger than 0.5 cm in diameter is considered diagnostic.

Arthrogryposis Multiplex Congenita

Arthrogryposis multiplex congenita refers to a symptom complex (syndrome) characterized by multiple joint contractures that are present at birth. The involved muscles are replaced partially or completely by fat and fibrous tissue. However, it is not a single disease because there are about 150 different syndromes that are associated with multiple congenital contractures. The major form of arthrogryposis multiplex congenita is known as *amyoplasia*,[89,92] which refers to the classic syndrome in which the upper and lower extremities are involved. It accounts for about 40% of all children with multiple congenital contractures. Its cause is unknown. Children with this disorder have a decreased number of anterior horn cells in their spinal cords, suggesting a neuropathic origin. The distribution of joint contractures is variable; the classic presentation is involvement of the upper and lower extremities. The clinical features include adduction, internal rotation, and contractures of the shoulders; fixed flexion and extension contractures of the elbow; rigid volar flexion and ulnar deviation or dorsiflexion and radial deviation contractures of the wrist; thumb and palm deformities; rigid interphalangeal joints of the thumb and fingers; flexion, abduction, external rotation, and hip contractures, with dislocation of one or both hips; fixed extension or flexion contractures of the knees; and severe, rigid, bilateral clubfoot (Fig. 54-27). Radiographs of all involved joints are obtained to assess their development; specialized studies are ordered as necessary.

Treatment modalities during the neonatal period consist of physical therapy and serial casting. Occasionally, orthotics and surgical intervention may be necessary; however, surgery is usually delayed until early childhood.[96]

FIBRODYSPLASIA OSSIFICANS PROGRESSIVA

With acknowledgement to Joseph A. Kitterman and Frederick S. Kaplan

Fibrodysplasia ossificans progressiva (FOP) is a rare genetic disease (incidence about 1 in 1.6 million) characterized by skeletal malformations and episodic heterotopic bone formation leading to progressive loss of mobility. Although FOP was first described in the 17th century, most individuals with FOP are initially misdiagnosed, and many suffer permanent disability from inappropriate diagnostic or therapeutic interventions. Two likely causes for these harmful diagnostic errors are the lack of teaching exposure to FOP in most medical schools and the lack of coverage of FOP in most medical textbooks.

The mode of inheritance of FOP is autosomal dominant with complete penetrance, but almost all cases result from a spontaneous activating mutation in the gene encoding activin receptor IA/activin like kinase-2 (ACVR1/ALK2), a bone morphogenetic protein type I receptor. Only seven small multigenerational families are known worldwide.[52-56,59,93]

Figure 54–27. A, A 1-month-old girl with arthrogryposis multiplex congenita involving the upper and lower extremities. The elbows are stiff in extension, whereas the wrist, fingers, and thumb are flexed. The hips are flexed and externally rotated. There are knee flexion contractures and bilateral talipes equinovarus club-foot deformities. B, Serial casting is initiated at birth to improve the alignment of the lower extremities. Occupational therapy and splinting are used at a later time on the upper extremities.

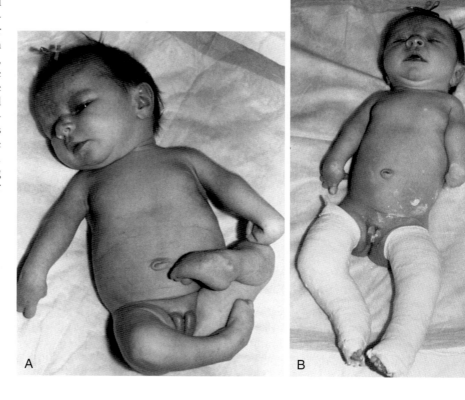

The two classic findings in FOP are distinctive malformations of the great toes and episodic "flare-ups" characterized by soft tissue tumor-like swellings that often result in heterotopic ossification at the lesional site. The invariant malformations of the great toes are due to hypoplasia or agenesis of the proximal phalanges that result in short great toes with a valgus deformity (Fig. 54-28A). The toe malformations are present at birth and may be the only congenital sign of FOP. Flare-ups, especially in the occipital region, may commence in the neonatal period, and are often mistaken for cephalohematomas. However, flare-ups are usually recognized later in the first decade and typically appear on the head, neck, back, or shoulders (see Fig. 54-28B). The onset of a tender soft tissue swelling often appears overnight, triggered by soft tissue trauma or viral illnesses or may occur spontaneously. The soft tissue swellings may resolve completely but most often result in heterotopic bone formation.

Microscopically, perivascular lymphocytic, mast cell, and macrophage infiltration occurs in striated muscle, followed by widespread death of muscle cells. Subsequently, an angiogenic fibroproliferative lesion forms, evolving through a cartilage stage and finally into mature heterotopic bone through a characteristic endochondral mechanism. This process involves striated muscles, ligaments, tendons, and aponeuroses, but spares the diaphragm, tongue, extraocular muscles, and cardiac and smooth muscle.

Figure 54–28. A, See color insert. Photograph of the feet of an infant with fibrodysplasia ossificans progressiva (FOP) showing the characteristic findings of short great toes and hallux valgus. B, Photograph of the back of a very young child with a tumor-like swelling on his back that represents an early FOP flare-up. Note the surgical scar from an unnecessary biopsy that exacerbated the disease process.

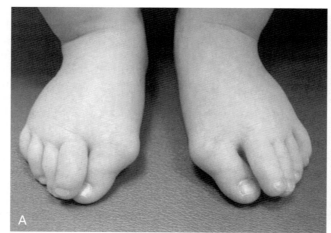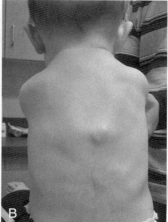

Additional common findings may include short thumbs, short broad femoral necks, proximal medial tibial osteochondromas, tall narrow cervical vertebra, and ankylosis of facet joints of the cervical spine. Findings later in life include hearing loss and a typical facies, which usually develops in the second decade of life and is due to mandibular hypoplasia.[53]

FOP can be diagnosed clinically and with great accuracy when the clinician recognizes the pathognomonic combination of great toe malformations with the presence of rapidly appearing soft tissue tumors in characteristic anatomic locations (see Fig. 54-28C). In most cases, the swellings are misdiagnosed, most commonly as cancer or aggressive fibromatosis, often because the physician is unfamiliar with FOP. In newborns, FOP should be suspected when the typical malformations of the great toes are present. For suspected cases, diagnostic genetic testing is readily available from a simple blood test.[55]

There is no effective treatment for FOP. The process of heterotopic ossification is often accelerated by trauma, including traumatic medical interventions. These include biopsies, intramuscular injections (including neonatal vitamin K), immunizations, and surgical procedures, all of which should be avoided. For flare-ups involving major joints or the airway, a brief (3 to 4 days) course of high-dose corticosteroids will reduce soft tissue swelling and may prevent ossification.

OUTCOME

Episodic heterotopic bone formation in FOP leads to progressive immobilization of the joints and restrictive disease of the chest wall.[56] Malnutrition is common if there is ossification of the jaw muscles leading to restricted mouth opening and swallowing. Average life expectancy is 40 years (range, 3 to 77 years). Identification of the responsible gene provides hope for future effective treatment of FOP.

SUGGESTED READINGS

Herring JA (ed): *Tachdjian's pediatric orthopaedics*, 3rd ed, Philadelphia, 2002, WB Saunders.

Morrissy RT, Weinstein SL (eds): *Lovell and Winter's pediatric orthopaedics*, 6th ed, Philadelphia, 2006, Lippincott Williams & Wilkins.

REFERENCES

1. Allington NJ, et al: Clubfeet associated with congenital constriction bands of the ipsilateral lower extremity, *J Pediatr Orthop* 15:599, 1995.
2. Al-Qattan MM: Obstetric brachial plexus palsy associated with breech delivery, *Ann Plast Surg* 51:257, 2003.
3. Andrish J, et al: Sacral agenesis: a clinical evaluation of its management, heredity, and associated anomalies, *Clin Orthop* 139:52, 1979.
4. Ash JM, Gilday DL: The futility of bone scanning in neonatal osteomyelitis: concise communication, *J Nucl Med* 21:417, 1980.
5. Ballock RT, et al: The prevalence of nonmuscular causes of torticollis in children, *J Pediatr Orthop* 16:500, 1996.
6. Banta JV, et al: Sacral agenesis, *J Bone Joint Surg Am* 51:693, 1969.
7. Barlow TG: Early diagnosis and treatment of congenital dislocation of the hip, *J Bone Joint Surg Br* 44:292, 1962.
8. Basu PS, et al: Congenital spinal deformity: a comprehensive assessment at presentation, *Spine* 15:2255, 2002.
9. Bergdahl S, et al: Neonatal hematogenous osteomyelitis: risk factors for long-term sequelae, *J Pediatr Orthop* 5:564, 1985.
10. Bodian DL, et al: Mutation and polymorphism spectrum in osteogenesis imperfecta type II: implications for genotype-phenotype relationships, *Hum Mol Genet* 18:463, 2009.
11. Bradford DS, et al: Intraspinal abnormalities and congenital spinal deformities: a radiographic and MRI study, *J Pediatr Orthop* 11:36, 1991.
12. Bressler EL, et al: Neonatal osteomyelitis examined by bone scintigraphy, *Radiology* 152:685, 1984.
13. Burtsh RL: Nomenclature of congenital skeletal limb deficiencies: a revision of the Frantz and O'Rahilly classification, *Artif Limbs* 10:24, 1966.
14. Canale ST, et al: Does aspiration of bones and joints affect results of later bone scanning? *J Pediatr Orthop* 5:23, 1985.
15. Chang CH, et al: Macrodactyly of the foot, *J Bone Joint Surg Am* 84:1189, 2002.
16. Cheng JC, et al: Outcome of surgical treatment of congenital muscular torticollis, *Clin Orthop* 362:190, 1999.
17. Cheng JC, et al: Clinical determinants of the outcome of manual stretching in the treatment of congenital muscular torticollis in infants: a prospective study of eight hundred and twenty-one cases, *J Bone Joint Surg Am* 83:679, 2001.
18. Clegg J, et al: Financial justification for routine ultrasound screening of the neonatal hip, *J Bone Joint Surg Br* 81:852, 1999.
19. Coleman SS, et al: Pathomechanics and treatment of congenital vertical talus, *Clin Orthop* 70:62, 1970.
20. Crawford AH: Neurofibromatosis in childhood, *Instr Course Lect* 30:56, 1981.
21. Crawford AH, et al: Foot and ankle problems, *Orthop Clin North Am* 18:649, 1987.
22. Curtis BH, Fisher RL: Congenital hyperextension with anterior subluxation of the knee: surgical treatment and long-term observations, *J Bone Joint Surg Am* 51:255, 1969.
23. Davids JR, et al: Congenital muscular torticollis: sequela of intrauterine or perinatal compartment syndrome, *J Pediatr Orthop* 13:141, 1993.
24. Demirbilek S, et al: Congenital muscular torticollis and sternomastoid tumor: result of nonoperative treatment, *J Pediatr Surg* 34:549, 1999.
25. Demopulos GA, et al: Role of radionuclide imaging in the diagnosis of acute osteomyelitis, *J Pediatr Orthop* 8:558, 1988.
26. Dobbs MB, et al: Factors predictive of outcome after use of the Ponseti method for the treatment of idiopathic clubfeet, *J Bone Joint Surg Am* 86:22, 2004.
27. Drennan JC: Congenital vertical talus. In Drennan JC, editor: *The child's foot and ankle*, New York, 1992, Raven Press.
28. Dubousset J: Congenital kyphosis and lordosis. In Weinstein SL, editor: *The pediatric spine*, New York, 1994, Raven Press.
29. Eastwood DM: Neonatal hip screening, *Lancet* 361:595, 2003.
30. Falliner A, et al: Sonographic hip screening and early management of developmental dysplasia of the hip, *J Pediatr Orthop* 8B:112, 1999.
31. Farsetti P, et al: The long term functional and radiographic outcomes of untreated and nonoperatively treated metatarsus adductus, *J Bone Joint Surg Am* 76:257, 1994.

32. Feldbrin Z, et al: Muscle imbalance in the etiology of idiopathic clubfoot, *J Bone Joint Surg Br* 77:596, 1995.

33. Fink CW, Nelson JD: Septic arthritis and osteomyelitis in children, *Clin Rheum Dis* 12:423, 1986.

34. Flatt AE: Practical factors in the treatment of syndactyly. In Littler JW, et al, editors: *Symposium on reconstructive hand surgery,* St Louis, 1977, Mosby-Year Book.

35. Foulkes GD, et al: Congenital constriction band syndrome: a seventy-year experience, *J Pediatr Orthop* 14:242, 1994.

36. Frantz CH, et al: Congenital skeletal limb deficiencies, *J Bone Joint Surg Am* 43:1202, 1961.

37. Fuller DJ, et al: The timed appearance of some congenital malformations in orthopaedic abnormalities, *Instr Course Lect* 23:53, 1974.

38. Gabuzda GM, et al: Current concept review: reduction of congenital dislocation of the hip, *J Bone Joint Surg Am* 74:624, 1992.

39. Green NE, et al: Bone and joint infections in children, *Orthop Clin North Am* 18:555, 1987.

40. Greene WB: One-stage release of congenital circumferential constriction bands, *J Bone Joint Surg Am* 75:650, 1993.

41. Grogan DP, et al: Congenital malformation of the lower extremities, *Orthop Clin North Am* 18:537, 1987.

42. Guille JT, et al: Lumbosacral agenesis: a new classification correlating spinal deformity and ambulatory potential, *J Bone Joint Surg Am* 84:32, 2002.

43. Harcke HT, et al: Current concepts review: the role of ultrasound in the diagnosis and management of congenital dislocation and dysplasia of the hip, *J Bone Joint Surg Am* 73:622, 1991.

44. Harcke HT: Role of imaging in musculoskeletal infections in children, *J Pediatr Orthop* 15:141, 1995.

45. Hensinger RN: Congenital dislocation of the hip: treatment in infancy to walking age, *Orthop Clin North Am* 18:597, 1987.

46. Hoeksma AF, et al: Shoulder contracture and osseous deformity in obstetrical brachial plexus injuries, *J Bone Joint Surg Am* 85:316, 2003.

47. Hoffer MM, et al: Brachial plexus birth palsies: results of tendon transfers to the rotator cuff, *J Bone Joint Surg Am* 60:691, 1978.

48. Hsu TY, et al: Neonatal clavicular fracture: clinical analysis of incidence, predisposing factors, diagnosis, and outcome, *Am J Perinatol* 19:17, 2002.

49. Hummer CD, et al: The coexistence of torticollis and congenital dislocation of the hip, *J Bone Joint Surg Am* 54:1255, 1972.

50. Ippolito E, et al: Congenital clubfoot in the human fetus: a histological study, *J Bone Joint Surg Am* 62:8, 1980.

51. Kabak S, et al: Septic arthritis in patients followed up in neonatal intensive care unit, *Pediatr Int* 44:652, 2002.

52. Kaplan FS, et al: The phenotype of fibrodysplasia ossificans progressiva, *Clin Rev Bone Min Metab* 3:209, 2005.

53. Kaplan FS, et al: The craniofacial phenotype in fibrodysplasia ossificans progressiva, *Clin Rev Bone Min Metab* 3:183, 2005.

54. Kaplan FS, et al: Fibrodysplasia ossificans progressiva, *Best Pract Res Clin Rheumatol* 22:191, 2008.

55. Kaplan FS, et al: Early diagnosis of fibrodysplasia ossificans progressiva, *Pediatrics* 121:e1295, 2008.

56. Kaplan FS, et al: Early mortality from cardiorespiratory failure in patients with fibrodysplasia ossificans progressiva, *J Bone Joint Surg* 2010;92:686-691.

57. Kim YJ, et al: Surgical treatment of congenital kyphosis, *Spine* 26:2251, 2001.

58. Kirkos JM, et al: Late treatment of brachial plexus palsy secondary to birth injuries: rotational osteotomy of the proximal part of the humerus, *J Bone Joint Surg Am* 80:1477, 1998.

59. Kitterman JA, et al: Iatrogenic harm caused by diagnostic errors in fibrodysplasia ossificans progressiva, *Pediatrics* 116:e654, 2005.

60. Ko JY, et al: Congenital dislocation of the knee, *J Pediatr Orthop* 19:252, 1999.

61. Kocher MS, et al: Osteogenesis imperfecta, *J Am Acad Orthop Surg* 6:225, 1998.

62. Korakaki E, et al: Methicillin-resistant Staphylococcus aureus osteomyelitis and septic arthritis in neonates: diagnosis and management, *Jpn J infect Dis* 60:129, 2007.

63. Kumar SJ, et al: The incidence of hip dysplasia with metatarsus adductus, *Clin Orthop* 164:234, 1982.

64. La Mont RL, et al: Acute hematogenous osteomyelitis in children, *J Pediatr Orthop* 7:579, 1987.

65. Lerman JA, et al: Early failure of Pavlik harness treatment for developmental hip dysplasia: clinical and ultrasound predictors, *J Pediatr Orthop* 21:348, 2001.

66. Lewis K, et al: Ultrasound and neonatal hip screening: the five-year results of a prospective study in high-risk babies, *J Pediatr Orthop* 19:760, 1999.

67. MacEwen GD, et al: Evaluation of kidney anomalies in congenital scoliosis, *J Bone Joint Surg Am* 54:1451, 1972.

68. McBride MT, et al: Newborn clavicle fractures, *Orthopedics* 17:317, 1998.

69. McMaster MJ: Occult intraspinal anomalies and congenital scoliosis, *J Bone Joint Surg Am* 66:558, 1984.

70. McMaster MJ: Congenital scoliosis. In Weinstein SL, editor: *The pediatric spine,* New York, 1994, Raven Press.

71. McMaster MJ, et al: The natural history of congenital scoliosis: a study of 251 patients, *J Bone Joint Surg Am* 64:1128, 1982.

72. McMaster MJ, et al: Natural history of congenital kyphosis and kyphoscoliosis, *J Bone Joint Surg Am* 81:1367, 1999.

73. Minihane KP, et al: Developmental dysplasia of the hip in infants with congenital muscular torticollis, *Am J Orthop* 37:E155, 2008.

74. Moore KL: *The developing human: clinically oriented embryology,* 4th ed, Philadelphia, 1988, WB Saunders.

75. Nelson JD: Bugs, drugs, and bones: a pediatric infectious disease specialist reflects on management of musculoskeletal infections, *J Pediatr Orthop* 19:141, 1999.

76. Netrawichien P: Radial clubhand-like deformity resulting from osteomyelitis of the distal radius, *J Pediatr Orthop* 15:157, 1995.

77. Ogden JA, et al: The pathology of neonatal osteomyelitis, *Pediatrics* 55:474, 1975.

78. Parke WW: Development of the spine. In Rothman RH, et al, editors: *The spine,* Philadelphia, 1975, WB Saunders.

79. Patterson TJS: Congenital constriction rings, *Br J Plast Surg* 14:1, 1961.

80. Peters W, et al: Long-term effects of neonatal bone and joint infection on adjacent growth plates, *J Pediatr Orthop* 12:806, 1992.

81. Phillips WA: Sacral agenesis. In Weinstein SL, editor: *Pediatric spine,* New York, 1994, Raven Press.

82. Plotkin H, et al: Pamidronate treatment of severe osteogenesis imperfecta in children under 3 years of age, *J Clin Endocrinol Metab* 85:1846, 2000.

83. Ponseti IV, et al: Congenital metatarsus adductus: the results of treatment, *J Bone Joint Surg Am* 48:702, 1966.

84. Ponseti IV: Current concepts review: treatment of congenital clubfoot, *J Bone Joint Surg Am* 74:448, 1992.

85. Rauch F, et al: Bone mass, size, and density in children and adolescents with osteogenesis imperfecta: effect of intravenous pamidronate therapy, *J Bone Miner Res* 18:610, 2003.

86. Regev E, et al: Ankylosis of the temperomandibular joint as a sequela of septic arthritis and neonatal sepsis, *Pediatr Infect Dis J* 22:99, 2003.

87. Rushforth GF: The natural history of hooked forefoot, *J Bone Joint Surg Br* 60:520, 1978.

88. Rusnak SL, et al: Congenital spinal anomalies in infants of diabetic mothers, *Pediatrics* 35:99, 1965.

89. Sarwark JF, et al: Current concepts review. Amyoplasia: a common form of arthrogryposis, *J Bone Joint Surg Am* 72:465, 1990.

90. Scaglietti O: The obstetrical shoulder trauma, *Surg Gynecol Obstet* 66:868, 1938.

91. Schwend RM, et al: Pediatric Orthopaedic Society of North America. Screening the newborn for developmental dysplasia of the hip: now what do we do? *J Pediatr Orthop* 27:607, 2007.

92. Shapiro F, et al: Current concepts review. The diagnosis and orthopaedic treatment of childhood spinal muscular atrophy: Peripheral neuropathy, Friedreich ataxia, and arthrogryposis, *J Bone Joint Surg Am* 75:1699, 1993.

93. Shore EM, et al: A recurrent mutation in the BMP type I receptor ACVR1 causes inherited and sporadic fibrodysplasia ossificans progressiva, *Nat Genet* 38:525, 2006.

94. Sillence DO: Osteogenesis imperfecta: an expanding panorama of variants, *Clin Orthop* 159:11, 1981.

95. Sillence DO, Danks DM: The differentiation of genetically distinct varieties of osteogenesis imperfecta in the newborn period, *Clin Res* 26:178, 1978.

96. Smith DW, et al: Arthrogryposis wrist deformities: results of infantile serial casting, *J Pediatr Orthop* 22:44, 2002.

97. Solonen KA, et al: Early reconstruction of birth injuries of the brachial plexus, *J Pediatr Orthop* 1:367, 1981.

98. Staheli LT, et al: Congenital hip dysplasia, *Instr Course Lect* 33:350, 1984.

99. Stannard JP, et al: Femur fractures in infants: a new therapeutic approach, *J Pediatr Orthop* 15:461, 1995.

100. Strong M, et al: Septic arthritis of the wrist in infancy, *J Pediatr Orthop* 15:152, 1995.

101. Sullivan JA: The child's foot. In Morrissey RT, Weinstein SL, editors: *Lovel and Winter's pediatric orthopaedics*, 4th ed, Philadelphia, 1996, JB Lippincott, p 1077.

102. Swanson AB, et al: Classification of limb malformations on the basis of embryological failures, *Surg Clin North Am* 48:1169, 1968.

103. Tada K, et al: Birth palsy: Natural recovery course and combined root avulsion, *J Pediatr Orthop* 4:279, 1984.

104. Thompson GH: Angular deformities of the lower extremities. In Chapman MW, editor: *Operative orthopaedics*, 2nd ed, Philadelphia, 1993, JB Lippincott.

105. Thompson GH: Instructional course lecture: bunions and toe deformities in adolescents and children, *J Bone Joint Surg Am* 77:12, 1995.

106. Thompson GH, et al: Congenital talipes equinovarus (clubfeet) and metatarsus adductus. In Drennan JC, editor: *The child's foot and ankle*, New York, 1992, Raven Press.

107. Tien YC, et al: Ultrasonographic study of the coexistence of muscular torticollis and dysplasia of the hip, *J Pediatr Orthop* 21:343, 2001.

108. Torpin R: *Fetal malformations caused by amniotic rupture during gestation*, Springfield, 1968, IL, Charles C Thomas.

109. Tsuge K: Treatment of macrodactyly, *J Hand Surg Am* 10:968, 1985.

110. Van Egmond C, et al: Steindler flexorplasty of the elbow in obstetrical brachial plexus injuries, *J Pediatr Orthop* 21:169, 2001.

111. Von Heideken J, et al: The relationship between developmental dysplasia of the hip and congenital muscular torticollis, *J Pediatr Orthop* 26:805, 2006.

112. Waters PM: Comparison of the natural history, the outcome of microsurgical repair, and the outcome of operative reconstruction in brachial plexus birth palsy, *J Bone Joint Surg Am* 81:649, 1999.

113. Weinstein S: Natural history of congenital hip dislocation and hip dysplasia, *Clin Orthop* 225:62, 1987.

114. Wickstrom JL: Birth injuries of the brachial plexus: treatment of defects in the shoulder, *Clin Orthop* 23:187, 1962.

115. Widhe T: Foot deformities at birth: a longitudinal prospective study over a 16-year period, *J Pediatr Orthop* 17:20, 1997.

116. Winter RB, et al: Congenital scoliosis: a study of 234 patients treated and untreated, *J Bone Joint Surg Am* 50:15, 1968.

117. Winter RB, et al: Diastematomyelia and congenital spine deformities, *J Bone Joint Surg Am* 56:27, 1974.

118. Winter RB, et al: The incidence of Klippel-Feil syndrome in patients with congenital scoliosis and kyphosis, *Spine* 9:363, 1984.

119. Wood VE: Congenital thumb deformities, *Clin Orthop* 195:7, 1985.

120. Zeitlin L, et al: Modern approach to children with osteogenesis imperfecta, *J Pediatr Orthop* 12B:77, 2003.

Therapeutic Agents

Thomas E. Young

Agent	Dosage	Comments
Anti-infective Agents		
Antibacterials		
For drugs marked by *, exact dose and dosing interval are dependent on postmenstrual and postnatal age.		
Amikacin*	15-18 mg/kg/dose every 24-48 hr	Monitor serum concentrations if treating >48 hr
Ampicillin*	Meningitis: 100 mg/kg/dose IV, IM every 6-12 hr Non-CNS infections: 25-50 mg/kg/dose IV, IM every 6-12 hr	
Azithromycin	Pertussis infections: 10 mg/kg/dose PO every 24 hr	IV administration has not been evaluated in pediatric patients
Aztreonam*	30 mg/kg/dose IV, IM every 6-12 hr	Adequate glucose must be provided to prevent hypoglycemia
Cefazolin*	25 mg/kg/dose IV, IM every 6-12 hr	First-generation cephalosporin; use is limited to perioperative prophylaxis and treatment of urinary tract and soft tissue infections
Cefepime	30-50 mg/kg/dose IV, IM every 12 hr	Fourth-generation cephalosporin; reserved for treatment of infections caused by multidrug-resistant organisms
Cefotaxime*	50 mg/kg/dose IV, IM every 6-12 hr Gonococcal ophthalmia: 100 mg/kg IV, IM single dose	Broad spectrum third-generation cephalosporin; may use to treat gram-negative meningitis
Cefoxitin*	25-33 mg/kg/dose IV every 6-12 hr	Do not use to treat meningitis
Ceftazidime*	30 mg/kg/dose IV, IM every 8-12 hr	Only cephalosporin effective against *Pseudomonas* species
Ceftriaxone*	50-100 mg/kg/dose IV, IM every 24 hr Gonococcal ophthalmia: 50 mg/kg (maximum 125 mg) IV, IM single dose	Not recommended for infants with hyperbilirubinemia; do not administer concurrently with calcium-containing solutions
Chloramphenicol	Loading dose: 20 mg/kg IV over 30 min Maintenance dose (begin 12 hr after loading dose) Premature <1 month old: 2.5 mg/kg IV every 6 hr Full term <1 week old, premature >1 month old: 5 mg/kg IV every 6 hr Full term >1 week old: 12.5 mg/kg IV every 6 hr	Monitor serum concentrations; concentrations >50 µg/mL associated with gray baby syndrome; can cause bone marrow suppression, aplastic anemia

Continued

Agent	Dosage	Comments
Clindamycin*	5-7.5 mg/kg/dose IV, PO every 6-12 hr	Do not use to treat meningitis; may cause pseudomembranous colitis
Erythromycin	10-12.5 mg/kg/dose PO every 6 hr	Higher dose used to treat pertussis and chlamydial pneumonitis and conjunctivitis
Gentamicin*	4-5 mg/kg/dose every 24-48 hr IV	Monitor serum concentrations if treating >48 hr
Imipenem	20 to 25 mg/dose IV every 12 hr	Seizures may occur if treating meningitis
Linezolid	10 mg/kg/dose IV every 8 hr (premature infants <7 days of age: dose every 12 hr)	Do not use to treat meningitis; do not use for empirical therapy if suspecting gram-negative infection
Meropenem*	Sepsis: 20 mg/kg/dose IV every 8-12 hr Meningitis and pseudomonal infections: 40 mg/kg/dose every 8 hr	Reserve for infections caused by multidrug-resistant organisms
Metronidazole*	Loading dose: 15 mg/kg IV, PO Maintenance dose: 7.5 mg/kg/dose IV, PO every 8-48 hr	Measure CSF concentrations when treating meningitis
Nafcillin*	25-50 mg/kg/dose IV every 6-12 hr	Greatest CSF penetration of antistaphylococcal penicillins; predominantly biliary excretion; irritating to veins
Oxacillin*	25-50 mg/kg/dose IV every 6-12 hr	
Penicillin G*	25,000-100,000 IU/kg/dose IV, IM every 6-12 hr	Higher doses are suggested for severe group B streptococcal infections
Piperacillin/ tazobactam*	50-100 mg/kg/dose IV every 8-12 hr	For non-CNS infections caused by susceptible β-lactamase–producing bacteria
Quinopristin, dalfopristin	7.5 mg/kg/dose IV every 12 hr	Reserve for multidrug-resistant gram-positive infections
Rifampin	PO: 10-20 mg/kg every 24 hr IV: 5-10 mg/kg/dose every 12 hr Prophylaxis against meningococcal disease: 5 mg/kg/dose PO every 12 hr for 2 days Prophylaxis against *Haemophilus influenzae* type B disease: 10 mg/kg/dose PO every 24 hr for 4 days	Used in combination with vancomycin or aminoglycosides for treatment of persistent staphylococcal infections
Ticarcillin, clavulanate*	75-100 mg/kg/dose IV every 6-12 hr	For non-CNS infections caused by susceptible β-lactamase–producing bacteria
Tobramycin*	4-5 mg/kg/dose every 24-48 hr	Serum concentrations should be monitored and doses adjusted to achieve peak concentrations of 8-10 μg/mL and trough concentrations of <2 μg/mL
Vancomycin*	10-15 mg/kg/dose IV every 6-18 hr	Trough concentrations 5-10 μg/mL for most infections, 15-20 μg/mL when treating endocarditis, pneumonia, bone and joint infections; may not be effective against organisms with MIC >2 μg/mL
Antifungals		
Amphotericin B	1-1.5 mg/kg/day IV infusion over 2-6 hr	Serum potassium and creatinine clearance values should be monitored closely; alternate-day therapy may permit better control of electrolyte status
Amphotericin B liposome (AmBisome)	5-7 mg/kg/dose every 24 hr	Less nephrotoxic than amphotericin B, but also not indicated for treating renal candidiasis

Agent	Dosage	Comments
Amphotericin B lipid complex (ABELCET)	5 mg/kg/dose every 24 hr	Less nephrotoxic than amphotericin B, but also not indicated for treating renal candidiasis
Caspofungin	25 mg/m²/dose (about 2 mg/kg/dose) IV every 24 hr	Limited data in neonates—reserve for treatment of refractory candidemia or patients intolerant of amphotericin
Fluconazole*	Loading dose: 12-25 mg/kg Systemic infections: 6 to 12 mg/kg IV or PO every 24-72 hr Prophylaxis: 3 mg/kg/dose IV twice weekly Thrush: 6 mg/kg PO on day 1, then 3 mg/kg/dose PO every 24 hr	Reversible elevations of transaminases have occurred in 12% of children. Interferes with metabolism of barbiturates and phenytoin; may also interfere with metabolism of aminophylline, caffeine, theophylline, and midazolam
Flucytosine	12.5-37.5 mg/kg/dose PO every 6 hr	Use only in conjunction with amphotericin B to treat fungal CNS infections
Micafungin	7-10 mg/kg IV every 24 hr	Limited data in neonates—reserve for treatment of refractory candidemia or patients intolerant of amphotericin
Nystatin	Topical: apply to affected area every 6 hr, continue treatment for 3 days after symptoms subside Thrush: 1 mL (premature) to 2 mL (full term) of 100,000 units/mL suspension, swab inside mouth every 6 hr	

Antivirals

Agent	Dosage	Comments
Acyclovir	20 mg/kg/dose IV every 8 hr for 14-21 days Chronic suppression: 75 mg/kg/dose PO every 12 hr	Neutropenia, phlebitis may occur; use slow infusion rates to avoid transient renal dysfunction
Ganciclovir	6 mg/kg/dose IV every 12 hr Chronic suppression: 30-40 mg/kg/dose PO every 8 hr	Significant neutropenia occurs in most patients
Lamivudine	2 mg/kg/dose PO every 12 hr	Refer to the Perinatal Guidelines at http://www.aidsinfo.nih.gov/ for the latest treatment information
Nevirapine	2 mg/kg PO single dose	Refer to the Perinatal Guidelines at http://www.aidsinfo.nih.gov/ for the latest treatment information
Valganciclovir	16 mg/kg/dose PO every 12 hr	Neutropenia occurs frequently
Zidovudine*	IV: 1.5 mg/kg/dose every 6-12 hr PO: 2 mg/kg/dose every 6-12 hr	Initiate treatment within 12 hr of birth; anemia and neutropenia may occur

Cardiovascular Drugs

Antiarrhythmics

Agent	Dosage	Comments
Adenosine	Give 50 μg/kg as a rapid IV bolus followed by a flush; if there is no response in 1-2 min, double the dose and continue to double it every 1-2 min until a response is obtained (usual maximum dose of 250 μg/kg)	Resolution of SVT is usually short lived, so it must be followed by the use of a more long-acting agent such as digoxin
Amiodarone	Loading dose: 5 mg/kg IV over 30-60 min IV infusion: Start at 7 μg/kg/min, may increase to 15 μg/kg/min PO: 5-10 mg/kg/dose every 12 hr	For treatment of refractory supraventricular arrhythmia; long elimination half-life; may cause hypothyroidism and corneal microdeposits; may increase plasma concentrations of digoxin and phenytoin

Continued

Agent	Dosage	Comments
Digoxin	Preterm, loading dose: IV: 15-20 μg/kg divided into 3 doses over 24 hr PO: 20-25 μg/kg divided into 3 doses over 24 h Maintenance dose: IV: 4-5 μg/kg daily PO: 5-6 μg/kg daily	Be aware of drug interactions; obtain periodic ECGs to assess for both desired effects and signs of toxicity
	Full term, loading dose: IV: 30-40 μg/kg divided into 3 doses over 24 hr; PO: 40-50 μg/kg divided into 3 doses over 24 hr Maintenance dose: IV: 4-5 μg/kg every 12 hr PO: 5-6 μg/kg every 12 hr	
Digoxin immune Fab (Digibind)	Dose (# of vials) = [(serum digoxin concentration) × (weight in kg)]/100	Each vial contains 38 mg and will bind 0.5 mg digoxin; once administered, digoxin serum concentrations can no longer be determined accurately
Flecainide	Begin at 2 mg/kg/dose PO every 12 hr; adjust dose based on response and serum concentrations to a maximum of 4 mg/kg/dose PO every 12 hr	Used for treatment of SVT not responsive to conventional therapies; can cause new or worsened arrhythmias
Lidocaine	0.5-1 mg/kg/dose by slow IV push; may be repeated every 10 min as needed; maintenance IV infusion: 10-50 μg/kg/min	Contraindicated in infants with cardiac failure and heart block; adverse effects include hypotension, seizures, respiratory arrest, and asystole
Procainamide	Initial IV loading dose: 7-10 mg/kg/dose Maintenance IV infusion: 20-80 μg/kg/min	Treatment of SVT refractory to vagal maneuvers and adenosine

Propranolol	Starting oral dose: 0.25 mg/kg/dose PO every 6 hr
	  Maximum: 3.5 mg/kg/dose PO every 6 hr
	Starting IV dose: 0.01 mg/kg/dose IV every 6 hr
	  Maximum: 0.15 mg/kg/dose IV every 6 hr
		Preferred therapy for SVT if associated with Wolff-Parkinson-White syndrome; adverse effects related to β-receptor blockade

Sotalol	1 mg/kg PO every 12 hr, may increase to 4 mg/kg every 12 hr	For tetralogy spells; indicated for ventricular arrhythmias; has properties that prolong both β-blockade and action potentials
Vasodilators/Vasoconstrictors		
Alprostadil	Initial dose: 0.05-0.1 mcg/kg/min IV Maintenance doses may be as low as 0.01 mcg/kg/min	Apnea is most common adverse effect and occurs more frequently in premature infants
Captopril	0.01-0.05 mg/kg/dose PO every 8 hr	Angiotensin-converting enzyme inhibitor; may be effective in high renin hypertension and severe CHF; must monitor renal function; contraindicated in infants with bilateral renovascular disease
Dobutamine	2-20 μg/kg/min IV	Titrate dose to target effect; in young infants, increased heart rate may occur; tolerance may develop with prolonged use (>3 days)
Dopamine	2-20 μg/kg/min IV	Doses in the lowest part of the range cause an increase in glomerular filtration rate, renal blood flow, and Na^+ excretion; as dose is increased, cardiotonic effects predominate at first, followed by increased systemic vascular resistance; effects vary depending on gestational and postnatal age and disease process

Agent	Dosage	Comments
Epinephrine	Resuscitation: 0.1-0.3 mL/kg/dose of 1:10,000 concentration IV push, or IC (equal to 0.01-0.03 mg/kg [10-30 μg/kg]) Continuous infusion: 0.1-1 μg/kg/min IV	Higher doses, up to 0.1 mg/kg (100 μg/kg), may be given intratracheally immediately followed by 1 mL NS Monitor for hyperglycemia, tachycardia, and lactic acidemia
Hydralazine	IV: begin with 0.1-0.5 mg/kg/dose every 6 to 8 hr Gradually increase as needed to a maximum of 2 mg/kg/dose every 6 hr PO: 0.25-1 mg/kg/dose	Use with a β-blocker to enhance antihypertensive effect and decrease the magnitude of reflex tachycardia Administer with food to enhance absorption
Ibuprofen	First dose: 10 mg/kg IV Second and third doses: 5 mg/kg IV Administer at 24-hr intervals	Less renal effects than indomethacin
Indomethacin	Initial dose: 0.2 mg/kg IV Subsequent doses: If <2 days, 0.1 mg/kg/dose every 12-24 hr for 2 doses If 2-7 days, 0.2 mg/kg/dose every 12-24 hr for 2 doses If >7 days, 0.25 mg/kg/dose every 12-24 hr for 2 doses	Prostaglandin synthase inhibitor used for PDA closure; monitor renal function; avoid concomitant steroid therapy to decrease risk for GI perforation
Isoproterenol	0.05-2 μg/kg/min IV	Continuous ECG and blood pressure monitoring essential to prevent hypotension and tachycardia
Milrinone	Loading dose: 50-75 μg/kg IV over 60 min Begin infusion at 0.5 μg/kg/min May titrate to 0.75 μg/kg/min	Has both inotropic and vasodilatory properties; hypotension more likely with bolus doses
Nitric oxide	Begin at 20 ppm, wean over several days	Monitor for methemoglobinemia; use in premature infants for indications other than pulmonary hypertension is controversial
Phentolamine	Inject a 0.5-mg/mL solution SC into the periphery of the affected area	Prevention of dermal necrosis caused by extravasation of vasoconstrictive agents
Sodium nitroprusside	Start at 0.25-0.5 μg/kg/min continuous IV infusion, increase dose every 20 min as needed Maintenance dose is usually <2 μg/kg/min For hypertensive crisis, can use doses as high as 10 μg/kg/min for ≤10 min	Must have continuous intra-arterial blood pressure monitoring; may produce profound hypotension, metabolic acidosis, thrombocytopenia, and/or CNS symptoms; cyanide toxicity can occur

Central Nervous System Drugs

Analgesics and Narcotics

Agent	Dosage	Comments
Acetaminophen*	PO: 20-25 mg/kg loading dose, then 12-15 mg/kg every 6-12 hr Rectal: 30 mg/kg loading dose, then 12-18 mg/kg every 6-12 hr	Dosing intervals dependent on postmenstrual age
Fentanyl	1-4 μg/kg IV, may be repeated as needed Continuous IV infusion: 1-5 μg/kg/hr	Synthetic opioid; may cause chest wall rigidity at the higher doses or with rapid infusion Continuous infusions are associated with development of tolerance
Methadone	0.05-0.2 mg/kg/dose every 12-24 hr PO	Reduce dose based on signs and symptoms of withdrawal

Continued

Agent	Dosage	Comments
Morphine	IV: 0.05-0.2 mg/kg/dose every 3-4 hr Neonatal narcotic abstinence: begin at 0.03 to 0.1 mg/kg/dose PO repeated every 3-4 hr as needed Adjust dose based on abstinence scoring	May exacerbate hypotension; repetitive or continuous infusion dosing associated with ileus and urinary retention Paregoric not recommended because it contains alcohol and benzoic acid
Anticonvulsants		
Fosphenytoin	Loading dose: 15-20 PE/kg IV, IM Maintenance dose: 4-8 PE/kg IV, IM every 24 hr	Fosphenytoin 1 mg PE = phenytoin 1 mg; monitor trough serum phenytoin concentrations; term infants >1 week of age may require more frequent dosing; use with caution in neonates with hyperbilirubinemia
Levetiracetam	10 mg/kg/dose IV, PO every 24 hr Increase dosage every 1-2 wk as needed to attain seizure control, to a maximum of 30 mg/kg/dose every 12 hr	Very limited data in neonates
Lidocaine	Loading dose: 2 mg/kg IV over 10 minutes, followed immediately by a Maintenance infusion: 6 mg/kg/hr for 6 hr, then 4 mg/kg/hr for 12 hr, then 2 mg/kg/hr for 12 hr	Preterm newborns and term newborns undergoing hypothermia treatment are at risk for drug accumulation due to slower drug clearance; precise dosing in these infants is uncertain
Phenobarbital	Loading dose: 20 mg/kg slow IV push, additional 5 mg/kg doses may be given up to a total of 40 mg/kg Maintenance dose: 3-4 mg/kg IV, IM, or PO as a single daily dose	Serum concentrations should be monitored and doses adjusted to maintain concentrations at 15-40 μg/mL; the long half-life of the drug suggests that single daily doses will be sufficient; little information is available on oral absorption in the first month of life
Phenytoin	Loading dose: 15-20 mg/kg IV over 30 min Maintenance dose: 4-8 mg/kg daily IV slow push or PO	Unstable in solution and may precipitate in central lines
Neuromuscular Blockers		
These agents must be used in conjunction with an effective sedative/hypnotic agent. They do not provide any analgesia or amnesia.		
Pancuronium	0.04-0.15 mg/kg/dose IV, repeat as needed	Prolonged use may be associated with delayed recovery of muscle tone; may cause an increase in heart rate
Rocuronium	0.3-0.6 mg/kg/dose IV, repeat as needed	Shortest duration of action in this group
Vecuronium	0.03-0.15 mg/kg IV, repeat as needed	Minimum cardiovascular side effects; prolonged use may result in delayed recovery of muscle strength
Sedatives/Tranquilizers		
Chloral hydrate	25-75 mg/kg/dose PO, PR	No analgesic properties; for short-term use only
Lorazepam	0.05-0.1 mg/kg/dose IV	May cause respiratory depression; may be used acutely to stop seizures
Midazolam	0.05-0.15 mg/kg/dose IV, IM: every 2-4 hr Continuous IV infusion: 0.01-0.06 mg/kg/hr	Dosage requirements are decreased by concurrent use of narcotics; monitor for respiratory depression and hypotension; may cause myoclonic seizure-like activity
Pentobarbital	2-6 mg/kg IV	Short-acting barbiturate for short-term use

Agent	Dosage	Comments
Diuretics		
Bumetanide	0.005-0.1 mg/kg per dose IV, IM, or PO every 24 hr in preterm infants <34 weeks' gestation in the first 2 mo of life and more mature infants in the first month, then every 12 hr thereafter	Water and electrolyte imbalances occur frequently, especially hyponatremia, hypokalemia, and hypochloremic alkalosis; potentially ototoxic, but less so than furosemide; may displace bilirubin from albumin binding sites when given in high doses or for prolonged periods; may be used at the same dose PO and IV because of excellent bioavailability
Chlorothiazide	10-20 mg/kg/dose PO every 12 hr	May cause hypokalemia, alkalosis, and hyperglycemia; effective in the treatment of nephrocalcinosis secondary to loop diuretics
Furosemide	IV: 1-2 mg/kg/dose PO: 2-6 mg/kg/dose Premature infants: every 24 hr Term infants in the first month of life: every 12 hr Afterward: every 6-8 hr	Potentially ototoxic; may cause hypokalemia, alkalosis, and dehydration; consider alternate-day therapy for long-term use
Spironolactone	1-3 mg/kg/dose PO every 24 hr	May require several days of therapy before effect is seen; monitor serum potassium
Endocrine Agents		
Dexamethasone	0.075 mg/kg/dose IV or PO, every 12 hr for 3 days, then wean over 7 days (DART [Dexamethasone: a randomized trial] protocol)	Treat only those infants at highest risk for chronic lung disease; adverse effects include growth failure and increased risk for cerebral palsy; do not use concurrently with indomethacin due to risk for GI perforation
Hydrocortisone	Physiologic dose: 6-10 mg/m^2/day divided into 2 or 3 doses Stress dose: 20-50 mg/m^2/day (3 mg/kg/day) divided into 2 or 3 doses	Doses for physiologic replacement and stress remain controversial; adverse effects include hyperglycemia, hypertension, water and salt retention; there is an increased risk for GI perforations when treating concurrently with indomethacin
Insulin	0.01-0.1 U/kg/hr continuous IV infusion	For hyperglycemia; titrate rate of infusion to achieve desired serum glucose concentration; may be used to treat hyperkalemia
Levothyroxine	Start with 10-14 μg/kg/dose PO or 5-8 μg/kg/dose IV daily, adjust dose to desired TSH level	Oral doses changed in 12.5-μg increments; assess thyroid function 2 weeks after a dosing change
Octreotide	Treatment of hyperinsulinemic hypoglycemia: starting dose: 1 μg/kg/dose IV or SC every 6 hr; titrate to desired effect, maximum dose is 10 μg/kg Treatment of chylothorax: 1-7 μg/kg/hr continuous infusion	Decreases chyle production
Gastrointestinal Agents		
Cimetidine	2.5-5 mg/kg/dose PO, IV every 6-12 hr	May increase risk for NEC
Erythromycin	10-12 mg/kg/dose PO every 6 hr	Treatment of feeding intolerance due to GI dysmotility; may also lessen parenteral nutrition-associated cholestasis

Continued

Agent	Dosage	Comments
Famotidine	IV: 0.25-0.5 mg/kg/dose every 24hr PO: 0.5-1 mg/kg/dose every 24 hr	May increase risk for NEC due to alterations in GI flora; continuous infusion of the daily dose in adults provides better gastric acid suppression than intermittent dosing
Lansoprazole	0.73 to 1.66 mg/kg/dose PO every 24 hr	
Metoclopramide	0.1-0.3 mg/kg/day IV, PO divided every 8 hr	May reduce gastric aspirates and reflux; may improve feeding tolerance; observe for dystonic reactions
Nizatidine	2 to 5 mg/kg/dose PO every 12 hr	
Omeprazole	0.5 to 1.5 mg/kg/dose PO every 24 hr	
Ranitidine	PO: 2 mg/kg/dose every 8 hr IV preterm: 0.5 mg/kg/dose every 12 hr IV full term: 1.5 mg/kg/dose every 8 hr IV infusion: 0.0625 mg/kg/hr	May increase risk for NEC due to alterations in GI flora; continuous infusion of the daily dose in adults provides better gastric acid suppression than intermittent dosing
Ursodiol	10-15 mg/kg/dose PO every 12 hr	
Hematologic Agents		
Alteplase (t-PA)	Dissolution of intravascular thrombi: 200 μg/kg/hr for 6 to 48 hr Restoration of patency for central venous catheter: instill a 1-mg/mL solution into the catheter	Dose is an average of that used in case reports—range 20 to 500 μg/kg/hr
Enoxaparin	Term: 1.7 mg/kg/dose SC every 12 hr Preterm: 2 mg/kg/dose SC every 12 hr	Adjust dosage to maintain anti–factor Xa level between 0.5 and 1 U/mL
Epoetin alfa	300 units/kg/dose SC daily for 10 days	May also be given IV over at least 4 hr in a protein-containing solution; patient should be on supplemental iron therapy
Heparin	0.5-1 U/mL of IV fluid	
IVIG	500 to 750 mg/kg/dose IV over 2-6 hr	Usually given as a single dose; if subsequent doses are used, administer at 24-hr intervals
Minerals/Vitamins		
Calcium gluconate 10%	Acute treatment: 1-2 mL/kg/dose IV (100-200 mg/kg CaCl salt, 10-20 mg/kg elemental calcium) Maintenance treatment: 2-8 mL/kg/day by continuous IV infusion (200-800 mg/kg CaCl salt, 20-80 mg/kg elemental calcium)	May also be given orally at the same daily dosage
Ferrous sulfate (15 mg/mL Fe)	2-6 mg/kg/day elemental iron divided into 2-3 doses PO	Higher dose for infants on epoetin therapy
Iron dextran	0.4-1 mg/kg/day continuous IV infusion in hyperalimentation solution	For infants unable to tolerate oral iron therapy
Potassium chloride	Acute treatment of symptomatic hypokalemia: begin with 0.5-1 mEq/kg IV over 1 hr, then reassess Initial oral replacement: 0.5-1 mEq/kg/day PO divided and administered with feedings	Maximum concentrations: 40 mEq/L for peripheral, 80 mEq/L for central venous infusions Small, more frequent aliquots preferred; adjust dosage based on serum potassium concentrations
Pyridoxine (vitamin B_6)	Initial diagnostic dose: 50-100 mg IV push, or IM Maintenance dose: 50-100 mg PO every 24 hr	Risk for profound sedation; ventilator support may be necessary

Agent	Dosage	Comments
Sodium bicarbonate	1-2 mEq/kg/dose IV over at least 30 min Maximum concentration used is 0.5 mEq/mL	Treatment of normal anion gap metabolic acidosis caused by renal or GI losses; sodium bicarbonate is not a recommended therapy in neonatal resuscitation; administration during brief CPR may be detrimental
THAM acetate	1-2 mmol/kg (3.3-6.6 mL/kg) per dose IV in a large vein over at least 30 min	Do not use in patients who are anuric or uremic
Vitamin A	5000 IU IM 3 times/wk for 4 weeks	Administer using 29-g needle and insulin syringe. DO NOT ADMINISTER IV.
Vitamin D	Supplementation: 400 U/day PO Treatment of deficiency: 1000 U/day PO	Vitamin D_3 (cholecalciferol; fish derived) has been shown to be more effective in raising 25(OH)-D levels when compared with vitamin D_2 (ergocalciferol; plant derived)
Vitamin E	5 to 25 U/day PO	Dilute with feedings; impairs iron absorption if administered simultaneously
Vitamin K_1	Prophylaxis: term and late preterm: 0.5-1 mg IM at birth Preterm <32 weeks' gestational age: >1000 g birthweight: 0.5 mg IM <1000 g birthweight: 0.3 mg/kg IM Treatment of HDN: 1-10 mg IV slow push	

Ophthalmic Agents

Agent	Dosage	Comments
Cyclopentolate	1-2 drops in the eye 10-30 min before funduscopy	Use solutions with concentrations of 0.5% or less in neonates; anticholinergic effects if absorbed systemically; apply pressure to lacrimal sac during and for 2 min after instillation
Phenylephrine	1 drop in the eye 10-30 min before funduscopy	Use only the 2.5% solution in neonates
Tropicamide	1 drop in the eye 10-30 min before funduscopy	Use only the 0.5% solution in neonates; anticholinergic effects if absorbed systemically; apply pressure to lacrimal sac during and for 2 min after instillation

Pulmonary Agents

Agent	Dosage	Comments
Beractant (Survanta)	4 mL/kg/dose intratracheally in 2 aliquots; may administer 3 subsequent doses at 6-hr intervals	
Calfactant (Infasurf)	3 mL/kg/dose intratracheally in 2 aliquots; may administer 3 subsequent doses at 12-hr intervals	
Poractant alfa (Curosurf)	2.5 mL/kg intratracheally in 2 aliquots; may administer 2 subsequent doses of 1.25 mL/kg/dose at 12-hr intervals	
Albuterol	0.1-0.5 mg/kg/dose every 2-6 hr through nebulization	Selective β_2-agonist; may be used every 2 hr for treatment of hyperkalemia
Aminophylline (IV)	Loading dose: 20-25 mg/kg IV or PO (10-12.5 mg/kg caffeine base)	If changing from IV to PO aminophylline—increase dose by 20%
Theophylline (PO)	Maintenance dose: 1.5-3 mg/kg/dose every 8-12 hr IV or PO	If changing from IV aminophylline to PO theophylline—no change in dose

Continued

Agent	Dosage	Comments
Caffeine citrate	Loading dose: 20-25 mg/kg IV or PO (10-12.5 mg/kg caffeine base) Maintenance dose: 5-10 mg/kg/dose every 24 h IV or PO (2.5-5 mg/kg/dose caffeine base)	Therapeutic serum caffeine levels are in the range of 5-20 μg/mL
Dornase alpha	1.25 mL-2.5 mL via nebulizer, or 0.2 mL/kg instilled directly into the endotracheal tube Administer once or twice per day	Desaturation and/or airway obstruction may occur due to rapid mobilization of secretions
Ipratropium bromide	2 puffs (34 μg)-4 puffs (68 μg) via MDI with spacer device placed in the inspiratory limb of the ventilator circuit	Precise dosing is uncertain, although therapeutic margin is wide

CHF, congestive heart failure; CNS, central nervous system; CPR, cardiopulmonary resuscitation; CSF, cerebrospinal fluid; ECG, electrocardiogram; GI, gastrointestinal; HDN, hemolytic disease of the newborn; IC, intracardiac; IV, intravenous; IVIG, intravenous immunoglobulin; IM, intramuscular; MDI, metered-dose inhaler; MIC, minimum inhibitory concentration; NEC, necrotizing enterocolitis; NS, normal saline; PDA, patent ductus arteriosus; PE, phenytoin equivalent; PO, per oral route; SC, subcutaneous; SVT, supraventricular tachycardia; TSH, thyroid-stimulating hormone.

Tables of Normal Values

Mary L. Nock

PHYSIOLOGIC PARAMETERS
Blood Pressure

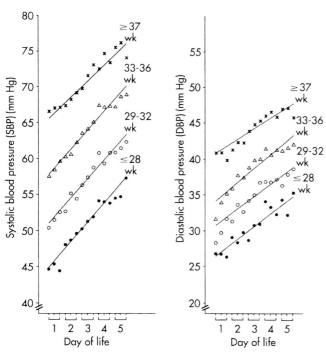

Figure B–1. Systolic and diastolic blood pressures plotted for the first 5 days of life, with each day subdivided into 8-hour periods. Infants are categorized by gestational age into 4 groups: ≤28 weeks (*n* = 33), 29 to 32 weeks (*n* = 73), 33 to 36 weeks (*n* = 100), and ≥37 weeks (*n* = 110). (*From Zubrow AB et al: Determinants of blood pressure in infants admitted to neonatal intensive care units: a prospective multicenter study. Philadelphia Neonatal Blood Pressure Study Group,* J Perinatol *15:470, 1995.*)

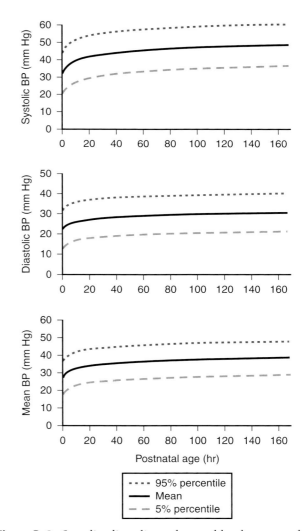

95% percentile
Mean
5% percentile

Figure B–2. Systolic, diastolic, and mean blood pressure during the first postnatal week in 86 infants of gestational ages 23 to <26 weeks who did not receive blood pressure support. (*From Batton B et al: Blood pressure during the first 7 days in premature infants born at postmenstrual age 23 to 25 weeks,* Am J Perinatol *24:109, 2007.*)

Time of First Void and Stool

TABLE B–1	Time of First Void in 500 Infants					
	395 TERM INFANTS		**80 PRETERM INFANTS**		**25 POST-TERM INFANTS**	
Hours	No. of Infants	Cumulative %	No. of Infants	Cumulative %	No. of Infants	Cumulative %
In delivery room	51	12.9	17	21.2	3	12
1-8	151	51.1	50	83.7	4	38
9-16	158	91.1	12	98.7	14	84
17-24	35	100	1	100	4	100
>24	0	—	0	—	0	—

From Clark DA: Times of first void and first stool in 500 newborns, *Pediatrics* 60:457, 1977.

TABLE B–2	Time of First Stool in 500 Infants					
	395 TERM INFANTS		**80 PRETERM INFANTS**		**25 POST-TERM INFANTS**	
Hours	No. of Infants	Cumulative %	No. of Infants	Cumulative %	No. of Infants	Cumulative %
In delivery room	66	16.7	4	5	8	32
1-8	169	59.5	22	32.5	9	68
9-16	125	91.1	25	63.8	5	88
17-24	29	98.5	10	76.3	3	100
24-48	6*	100	18[†]	98.8	0	—
>48	0	—	1[‡]	100	0	—

*At 25, 26, 27, 28, 33, and 37 hours.
[†]Five infants produced a stool more than 36 hours after birth: at 38, 39, 40, 42, and 47 hours.
[‡]At 59 hours.
From Clark DA: Times of first void and first stool in 500 newborns, *Pediatrics* 60:457, 1977.

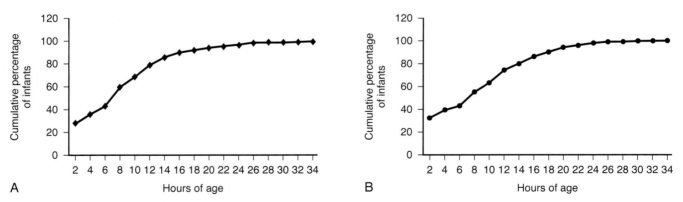

Figure B–3. Graphs depicting the cumulative percentage of infants ≥34 weeks' gestational age who had their first stool (**A**) or first urine (**B**) by a certain hour of age (*n* = 979). (*From Metaj M et al: Comparison of breast- and formula-fed normal newborns in time to first stool and urine, J Perinatol 23:627, 2003.*)

GROWTH CHARTS

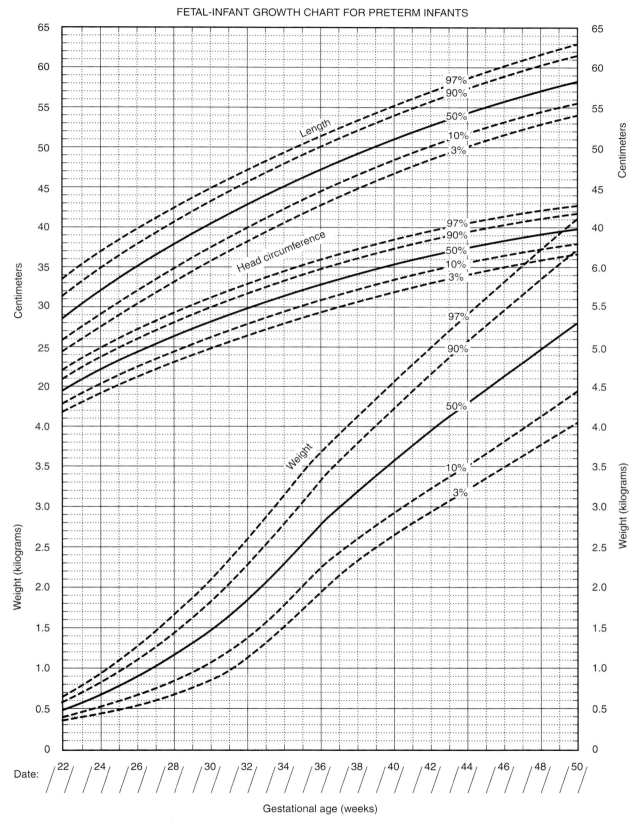

FETAL-INFANT GROWTH CHART FOR PRETERM INFANTS

Gestational age (weeks)

Figure B–4. Fetal-infant growth chart developed through a meta-analysis of published reference studies. (*From Fenton TR: A new growth chart for preterm babies: Babson and Benda's chart updated with recent data and a new format,* BMC Pediatr 3:13, 2003.)

CHEMISTRY VALUES
Blood

TABLE B–3	Serum Electrolytes and Other Measured Variables in Term Neonates			
	CORD BLOOD		2- TO 4-HOUR BLOOD	
	Mean ± SD	Range of Values	Mean ± SD	Range of Values
pH	7.35 ± 0.05	7.19-7.42	7.36 ± 0.04	7.27-7.45
P_{CO_2}	40 ± 6	24.5-56.7	43 ± 7	30-65
Hct (%)	48 ± 5	37-60	57 ± 5	42-67
Hb (g/L)	1.65 ± 0.16	1.29-2.06	1.90 ± 0.22	0.88-2.3
Na^+ (mmol/L)	138 ± 3	129-144	137 ± 3	130-142
K^+ (mmol/L)	5.3 ± 1.3	3.4-9.9	5.2 ± 0.5	4.4-6.4
Cl^- (mmol/L)	107 ± 4	100-121	111 ± 5	105-125
iCa (mmol/L)	1.15 ± 0.35	0.21-1.5	1.13 ± 0.08	0.9-1.3
iMg (mmol/L)	0.28 ± 0.06	0.09-0.39	0.30 ± 0.05	0.23-0.46
Glucose (mmol/L)	4.16 ± 1.05	0.16-6.66	3.50 ± 0.67	5.11-16.10
Glucose (mg/dL)	75 ± 19	2.9-120	63 ± 12	29-92
Lactate (mmol/L)	4.6 ± 1.9	1.1-9.6	3.9 ± 1.5	1.6-9.8
BUN (mmol/L)	2.14 ± 0.61	1.07-3.57	2.53 ± 0.71	1.43-4.28
BUN (mg/dL)	6.0 ± 1.7	3.0-10.0	7.1 ± 2.0	4-12

BUN, blood urea nitrogen; Hb, hemoglobin; Hct, hematocrit, iCa, ionized calcium, iMg, ionized magnesium.
From Dollberg S et al: A reappraisal of neonatal blood chemistry reference ranges using the Nova M electrodes, *Am J Perinatol* 18:433, 2001.

TABLE B–4	Serum Electrolyte Values in Preterm Infants											
	AGE 1 WK			AGE 3 WK			AGE 5 WK			AGE 7 WK		
Constituent	Mean	SD	Range	Mean	SD	Range	Mean	SD	Range	Mean	SD	Range
Na (mEq/L)	139.6	±3.2	133-146	136.3	±2.9	129-142	136.8	±2.5	133-148	137.2	±1.8	133-142
K (mEq/L)	5.6	±0.5	4.6-6.7	5.8	±0.6	4.5-7.1	5.5	±0.6	4.5-6.6	5.7	±0.5	4.6-7.1
Cl (mEq/L)	108.2	±3.7	100-117	108.3	±3.9	102-116	107.0	±3.5	100-115	107.0	±3.3	101-115
CO_2 (mmol/L)	20.3	±2.8	13.8-27.1	18.4	±3.5	12.4-26.2	20.4	±3.4	12.5-26.1	20.6	±3.1	13.7-26.9
Ca (mg/dL)	9.2	±1.1	6.1-11.6	9.6	±0.5	8.1-11.0	9.4	±0.5	8.6-10.5	9.5	±0.7	8.6-10.8
P (mg/dL)	7.6	±1.1	5.4-10.9	7.5	±0.7	6.2-8.7	7.0	±0.6	5.6-7.9	6.8	±0.8	4.2-8.2
BUN (mg/dL)	9.3	±5.2	3.1-25.5	13.3	±7.8	2.1-31.4	13.3	±7.1	2.0-26.5	13.4	±6.7	2.5-30.5

BUN, blood urea nitrogen.
From Thomas JL et al: Premature infants: analysis of serum during the first seven weeks. *Clin Chem* 14:272, 1968.

TABLE B–5   Whole Blood Ionized Calcium

	TERM NEONATES			PREMATURE NEONATES	
Age (hr)	Ca^{2+}, mEq/L*	Ca^{2+}, mmol/L*	Age (hr)	Ca^{2+}, mEq/L*	Ca^{2+}, mmol/L*
1-12	2.48 ± 0.22	1.24 ± 0.11	5-12	2.42 ± 0.32	1.21 ± 0.16
13-24	2.38 ± 0.24	1.19 ± 0.12	13-19	2.34 ± 0.24	1.17 ± 0.12
25-48	2.42 ± 0.26	1.21 ± 0.13	25-48	2.41 ± 0.32	1.21 ± 0.16
49-72	2.44 ± 0.28	1.22 ± 0.14	51-72	2.56 ± 0.36	1.28 ± 0.18
73-99	2.58 ± 0.34	1.29 ± 0.17	77-99	2.68 ± 0.28	1.34 ± 0.14
99-120	2.70 ± 0.24	1.35 ± 0.12	108-140	2.76 ± 0.26	1.38 ± 0.13
121-144	2.74 ± 0.24	1.37 ± 0.12	150-185	2.80 ± 0.32	1.40 ± 0.16
146-168	2.76 ± 0.32	1.38 ± 0.16			
178-264	2.80 ± 0.20	1.40 ± 0.10			

* Values given as mean ± SD.
Data from Wandrup J et al: Age-related reference values for ionized calcium in the first week of life in premature and full-term neonates, *Scand J Clin Lab Invest* 48:255, 1988; Wandrup J: Critical analytical and clinical aspects of ionized calcium in neonates, *Clin Chem* 35:2027, 1989.

TABLE B–6   Serum Calcium (mg/100 dL) and Phosphate (mg/dL) Levels in Infants with Very Low Birthweight Receiving Parenteral and Enteral Nutrition*

	Calcium Levels		Phosphate Levels	
Age (days)	500-1000 g	1001-1500 g	500-1000 g	1001-1500 g
1	8.39 ± 1.21	8.48 ± 0.65	6.16 ± 1.33	5.73 ± 0.90
2	8.50 ± 0.91	8.68 ± 1.07	5.96 ± 1.55	6.14 ± 1.13
3	9.36 ± 0.96	9.28 ± 0.98	5.21 ± 1.53	6.15 ± 1.22
4	9.28 ± 1.59	9.56 ± 0.56	4.84 ± 1.60	5.86 ± 1.07
5	9.50 ± 1.42	10.06 ± 0.74	4.41 ± 1.69	5.66 ± 1.39
12	9.52 ± 1.77	10.05 ± 0.55	5.13 ± 1.23	6.79 ± 1.16
19	9.70 ± 0.58	10.05 ± 0.86	5.97 ± 1.17	7.35 ± 0.91
26	9.46 ± 2.03	10.07 ± .055	5.98 ± 1.12	6.79 ± 0.71
33	9.71 ± 0.47	9.96 ± 0.69	5.37 ± 1.21	6.58 ± 0.60

* Included are 24 neonates of birthweight 500-1000 g, 28 neonates of birthweight 1001-1500 g. All* values are mean ± standard deviation.
Modified from El Hassan et al: Premature infants: analysis of serum phosphate during the first 4 weeks of life, *Am J Perinatol* 24:327, 2007.

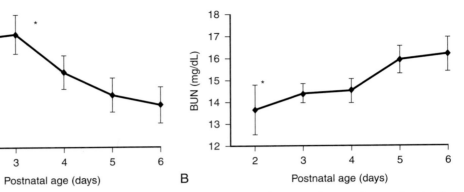

Figure B–5. Serum creatinine (A) and serum blood urea nitrogen (B) values in infants with very low birthweight (≤1500 g) during their first days of life. Data are presented as mean ± standard error of the mean, n = 138. Asterisk (*) indicates a statistically significant difference with day 6 of life. BUN, blood urea nitrogen. (*From Auron A et al: Serum creatinine in very low birth weight infants during their first days of life, J Perinatol 26:756, 2006.*)

TABLE B–7	Plasma Creatinine (mg/dL) in Premature Babies <28 Weeks' Gestational Age During the First 8 Weeks of Life*		
Age	22-24 wk (*n* = 33)	25-26 wk (*n* = 55)	27-28 wk (*n* = 73)
Birth	0.9 (0.67, 1.15)	0.87 (0.68, 1.18)	0.87 (0.69, 1.1)
12 hr	1.08 (0.8, 1.3)	1.03 (0.8, 1.27)	1 (0.77, 1.29)
24 hr	1.2 (1.02, 1.4)	1.18 (0.94, 1.41)	1.12 (0.9, 1.36)
36 hr	1.3 (1.11, 1.58)	1.25 (0.96, 1.41)	1.15 (0.9, 1.43)
48 hr	1.34 (1.12, 1.58)	1.27 (0.94, 1.6)	1.13 (0.93, 1.38)
3 days	1.32 (1.1, 1.64)	1.28 (0.89, 1.58)	1.12 (0.9, 1.43)
4 days	1.33 (1.09, 1.63)	1.26 (0.95, 1.64)	1.08 (0.84, 1.39)
7 days	1.28 (0.95, 1.71)	1.16 (0.71, 1.5)	1 (0.78, 1.22)
2 week	1.24 (0.78, 1.96)	0.95 (0.59, 1.3)	0.84 (0.64, 1.06)
3 week	1.04 (0.69, 1.49)	0.84 (0.55, 1.07)	0.71 (0.57, 0.87)
4 week	0.8 (0.6, 1.02)	0.76 (0.51, 0.94)	0.63 (0.5, 0.79)
5 week	0.79 (0.54, 1.1)	0.64 (0.46, 0.81)	0.59 (0.49, 0.67)
6 week	0.62 (0.5, 0.79)	0.59 (0.41, 0.7)	0.54 (0.44, 0.64)
7 week	0.6 (0.46, 0.78)	0.54 (0.41, 0.68)	0.51 (0.43, 0.6)
8 week	0.58 (0.44, 0.81)	0.52 (0.35, 0.62)	0.5 (0.41, 0.59)
Peak creatinine	1.5 (1.2, 1.83)	1.43 (1.01, 1.71)	1.24 (0.98, 1.52)

*Values are mean (10th, 90th percentile).
Modified from Thayyil S et al: A gestation- and postnatal age-based reference chart for assessing renal function in extremely premature infants, *J Perinatol* 28:227, 2008.

TABLE B–8   Capillary Blood Gas Reference Values in Healthy Term Neonates

Variable	No. of Patients	Mean ± SD	2.5 Percentile	97.5 Percentile
pH	119	7.395 ± 0.037	7.312	7.473
Pco_2 (mm Hg)	119	38.7 ± 5.1	28.5	48.7
Po_2 (mm Hg)	119	45.3 ± 7.5	32.8	61.2
Lactate (mmol/L)	114	2.6 ± 0.7	1.4	4.1
Hemoglobin (g/dL)	122	20.4 ± 11.6	14.5	23.9
Glucose (mg/dL)	122	69 ± 14	38	96
iCa (mmol/L)	118	1.21 ± 0.07	1.06	1.34

Samples collected at 48 ± 12 hours of life.
Modified from Cousineau J et al: Neonate capillary blood gas reference values, *Clin Biochem* 38:906, 2005.

TABLE B–9   Reference Serum Amino Acid Concentrations That Have Been Proposed as Standards for Neonates

Amino Acids	Term Infant Fed Human Milk (mmol/L)	Cord Blood (mmol/L)
Isoleucine	26-93	21-76
Leucine	53-169	47-120
Lysine	80-231	181-456
Methionine	22-50	8-42
Phenylalanine	22-71	24-87
Threonine	34-168	108-327
Tryptophan	18-101	19-98
Valine	88-222	98-276
Alanine	125-647	186-494
Arginine	42-148	28-162
Aspartic acid	5-51	18 ± 17
Glutamic acid	24-243	92 ± 57
Glycine	77-376	123-312
Histidine	34-119	42-136
Proline	82-319	72-278
Serine	0-326	57-174
Taurine	1-167	41-461
Tyrosine	38-119	34-83
Cysteine	35-132	4-37

Modified from Hanning RM et al: Amino acid and protein needs of the neonate: effects of excess and deficiency, *Semin Perinatol* 13:131, 1989.

TABLE B–10   Plasma Ammonia Levels in Preterm Infants ≤32 Weeks' Gestational Age

Age (days)	AMMONIA LEVEL* μmol/L	μg/dL
Birth	71 ± 26	121 ± 45[†]
1	69 ± 22	117 ± 37
3	60 ± 19	103 ± 33
7	42 ± 14	72 ± 24
14	42 ± 18	72 ± 30
21	43 ± 16	73 ± 28
28	42 ± 15	72 ± 25
Term infants at birth	45 ± 9	77 ± 16

*Values represent mean ± SD.
[†]Significant decline in plasma ammonia level from birth to 7 days of age (P < .01).

Modified from Usmani SS et al: Plasma ammonia levels in very low birth weight preterm infants, *J Pediatr* 123:798, 1993.

TABLE B–11 **Tests of Liver Function**

Test	Unit of Measurement	Age	Value
Albumin	g/L	0-5 days (<2.5 kg)	20-36
		0-5 days (>2.5 kg)	26-36
		1-30 days	26-43
		31-182 days	28-46
		183-365 days	28-48
PT	sec	1 days (30-36 wk of gestation)	10.6-16.2
		5 days (30-36 wk of gestation)	10.0-15.3
		30 days (30-36 wk of gestation)	10.0-13.6
		90 days (30-36 wk of gestation)	10.0-14.6
		180 days (30-36 wk of gestation)	10.0-15.0
	sec	1 day	11.6-14.4
		5 day	10.9-13.9
		30 day	10.6-13.1
		90 day	10.8-13.1
		180 day	11.5-13.1
PTT	sec	1 days (30-36 wk of gestation)	27.5-79.4
		5 days (30-36 wk of gestation)	26.9-74.1
		30 days (30-36 wk of gestation)	26.9-62.5
		90 days (30-36 wk of gestation)	28.3-50.7
		180 days (30-36 wk of gestation)	21.7-53.3
	sec	1 day	37.1-48.7
		5 day	34.0-51.2
		30 day	33.0-47.8
		90 day	30.6-43.6
		180 days	31.8-39.2
Ammonia	μmol/L	1-90 days	42-144
		3-11 mo	34-133
AST	U/L	0-5 days	35-140
		1-3 yr	20-60
ALT	U/L	0-5 days	6-50
		1-30 days	1-25
		31-365 days	3-35
ALP	U/L	0-5 days	110-300
		1-30 days	48-406
		31-365 days	82-383
γGT	U/L	0-5 days	34-263
		1-182 days	12-132
		183-365 days	1-39

For full-term infants unless otherwise noted.
ALP, alkaline phosphatase; ALT, alanine aminotransferase; AST, aspartate aminotransferase;
γ GT, γ-glutamyltransferase; PT, prothrombin time; PTT, partial thromboplastin time.
Adapted from Rosenthal P: Assessing liver function and hyperbilirubinemia in the newborn, National Academy of Clinical Biochemistry, *Clin Chem* 43:228, 1997.

TABLE B–12 Plasma Albumin and Total Protein in Preterm Infants from Birth to 8 Weeks

Gestation (wk)	26	27	28	29	30	31	32	33	34	35	36	37	38	39	40	41	42
Albumin (g/dL)																	
Reference range (95% confidence limits)	—	1.18–3.06	1.09–2.87	1.20–2.74	1.21–2.75	1.63–2.75	1.08–3.20	1.38–3.14	1.44–3.34	0.53–3.87	1.15–3.87	1.96–3.44	1.50–4.10	1.89–4.15	2.07–4.05	2.04–3.90	2.08–3.90
Corrected Age																	
26-28 wk		2.13	2.10	2.58	2.29	2.39				2.73							
29-31 wk					2.02	2.14	2.44	2.44	2.54								
32-34 wk								2.35	2.42	2.46	2.38	2.44	2.82			3.35	
Total Protein (g/dL)																	
Reference range (95% confidence limits)	—	1.28–7.94	3.03–5.03	2.18–5.84	2.64–5.80	3.26–5.66	3.63–5.81	3.57–5.87	3.57–6.59	1.52–8.62	3.85–6.91	4.69–6.95	3.32–9.16	4.17–8.25	4.26–8.08	3.73–8.47	3.24–8.76
Corrected Age																	
26-28 wk		4.07	4.45	4.84	4.49	4.45	4.70			4.41							
29-31 wk					3.93	4.42		4.82	4.51								
32-34 wk								4.54	4.93	4.78	4.86	4.81	4.55			4.96	

Modified from Reading RF et al: Plasma albumin and total protein in preterm babies from birth to eight weeks, *Early Human Dev* 22:81, 1990.

TABLE B–13	Cardiac Troponin T (cTnT) and Cardiac Troponin I (cTnI) Levels in 869 Healthy Term Newborns with Respect to Gender*			
	cTnT (μg/L)		cTnI (μg/L)	
	Male	*Female*	*Male*	*Female*
Mean	0.017	0.012	0.011	0.007
Median	0.01	0	0	0
Minimum	0	0	0	0
Maximum	1.26	0.58	0.71	0.98
99th percentile[†]	0.093	0.101	0.206	0.094

*Cardiac troponin T measured with Roche Elecsys® 2010 3rd generation assay; cardiac troponin I measured on a DadeBehering Dimension RxL assay.
[†]Diagnostic cutoff value for adults with possible myocardial damage is at 99th percentile of apparently healthy reference population; the same cutoff has been proposed for neonates.
Modified from Baum H et al: Reference values for cardiac troponins T and I in healthy neonates, *Clin Biochem* 37:1080, 2004.

Hormone Levels

TABLE B–14	Serum Growth Hormone (GH) Levels in Control Infants and Infants with Intrauterine Growth Restriction (IUGR)		
	GH (ng/mL) (Mean ± SD)		
	Cord Blood	*3 days*	*1 month*
Term	19 ± 9	29 ± 17	10 ± 8
Preterm	28 ± 16		
Term IUGR	46 ± 44	39 ± 31	12 ± 8
Preterm IUGR	55 ± 49	53 ± 34	20 ± 14

From Leger J et al: Growth factors and intrauterine growth retardation. II. Serum growth hormone, insulin-like growth factor, (IGF) I, and IGF-binding protein 3 levels in children with intrauterine growth retardation compared with normal control subjects: prospective study from birth to two years of age. Study Group of IUGR, *Pediatr Res* 40:101, 1996.

TABLE B–15	Range of Serum Testosterone Levels in Newborn Male and Female Infants		
	SERUM TESTOSTERONE (ng/mL)		
	Cord Blood	*0-48 hr*	*48 hr to 1 wk*
Male	0.25-0.6	1-5	<1
Female	0.2-0.5	0.05-0.8	<0.25

From Forest MG et al: Pattern of plasma testosterone and delta 4-androstenedione in normal newborns: evidence for testicular activity at birth, *J Clin Endocrinol Metab* 41:977, 1975.

TABLE B–16 Pooled Luteinizing Hormone (LH) and Follicle-Stimulating Hormone (FSH) Values from Male and Female Newborns*

Age (days)	No. of Patients	LH	FSH
Male			
1-5	30	0.39 ± 0.48, median 0.20	0.96 ± 0.60, median 0.85
6-10	15	2.31 ± 2.29, median 1.50	2.91 ± 4.38, median 1.40
11-15	17	3.55 ± 2.84, median 2.90	3.71 ± 2.69, median 3.00
16-20	14	4.13 ± 2.76, median 3.65	2.63 ± 1.45, median 2.15
21-25	7	2.86 ± 1.51, median 2.70	2.50 ± 1.51, median 2.10
26-28	8	2.22 ± 2.37, median 1.40	2.25 ± 0.81, median 2.40
Female			
1-5	31	0.48 ± 0.66, median 0.20	2.00 ± 1.37, median 1.80
6-10	17	0.45 ± 0.33, median 0.30	2.44 ± 2.52, median 1.40
11-15	8	1.58 ± 1.28, median 1.60	8.16 ± 4.27, median 8.95
16-20	6	1.03 ± 1.39, median 0.35	1.62 ± 1.05, median 1.90
21-25	3	0.46 ± 0.25, median 0.50	7.07 ± 5.92, median 3.90
26-28	8	2.75 ± 2.39, median 2.80	9.74 ± 9.89, median 6.15

*All values are mIU/mL, mean ± standard deviation unless otherwise indicated.
From Schmidt H, Schwarz HP: Serum concentration of LH and FSH in the healthy newborn, *Eur J Endocrinol* 143:214, 2000.

TABLE B–17 Reference Ranges of Sex Steroids in Infants*

Steroid	Age†	FEMALE			MALE		
		2.5th	50th	97.5th	2.5th	50th	97.5th
Estradiol (pmol/L)	1-7 days	25	81	116	<20	55	229
	8-15 days	42	88	134	31	66	126
	16 days-3 yr	21	48	113	<20	37	65
Prolactin (mIU/L)	1-7 days	475	4102	8003	1028	3445	8658
	8-15 days	919	3074	7018	854	2650	5889
	16 days-3 yr	126	319	1343	208	477	1559
Progesterone (nmol/L)	1-7 days	0.8	2.2	9.6	1	3.2	12.5
	8-15 days	1	2.8	4.7	1	2.8	8.2
	16 days-3 yr	0.3	0.9	3.2	0.3	1.2	3.6
SHBG (nmol/L)	1-7 days	7.4	22.8	34.8	8.8	24.1	50.7
	8-15 days	10.1	22.8	51.2	13.7	27.4	68.7
	16 days-3 yr	12.9	34.9	96.6	19.8	55.4	114.4
DHEAS (μmol/L)	1-7 days	1.87	4.29	12.8	2.32	4.42	11.47
	8-15 days	0.91	3.11	9.49	0.82	2.15	4.77
	16 days-3 yr	<0.2	0.47	3.33	<0.2	3.3	2.69

*Reference range is between 2.5th and 97.5th percentiles.
†For infants 1-7 days, 28 were male, and 17 were female; for infants 8-15 days, 20 were male, 20 were female; for infants 16 days-3 year, 42 were male, 44 were female.
DHEAS, dehydroepiandrosterone sulfate; SHBG, sex hormone–binding globulin.
Adapted from Elmlinger MW et al: Reference ranges for serum concentrations of lutropin (LH), follitropin (FSH), estradiol (E2), prolactin, progesterone, sex-hormone binding globulin (SHBG), dehydroepiandrosterone sulfate (DHEAS), cortisol and ferritin in neonates, children and young adults, *Clin Chem Lab Med* 40:1154, 2002.

TABLE B–18 Reference Ranges for Serum Cortisol in Well Preterm Infants*

Gestational Age (wk)	Cortisol (nmol/L†)
24	110-744
25	100-671
26	90-605
27	81-545
28	73-491
29	66-443

*n = 37, 31 were exposed in prenatal steroids.
†See Table B-31 for conversion to μg/dL.
From Heckmann M et al: Reference range for serum cortisol in well preterm infants, *Arch Dis Child Fetal Neonatal Ed* 81:F172, 1999.

TABLE B–19 Cortisol Concentration Quartiles in Infants with Extremely Low Birthweight (<1000 g)

Age	n	CORTISOL CONCENTRATION (μg/dL)		
		Lower Quartile	Median	Upper Quartile
12-48 hr	332	8.9	16	31
5-7 days	153	8.7	13.1	18.1

Adapted from Aucott SW et al: Do cortisol concentrations predict short-term outcomes in extremely low birth weight infants? *Pediatrics* 122:777, 2008.

TABLE B–20 Plasma 17-Hydroxyprogesterone (17-OHP) in Healthy and Ill Term and Preterm Infants*

	Healthy Term	Ill Term	Healthy Preterm	Ill Preterm
Plasma 17-OHP (nmol/L)	4.4 ± 2.6	10.6 ± 7.5	13.6 ± 11.4	24.39 ± 27.5

*All values are mean ± standard deviation.
From Murphy JF et al: Plasma 17-hydroxyprogesterone concentrations in ill newborn infants, *Arch Dis Child* 58:533, 1983.

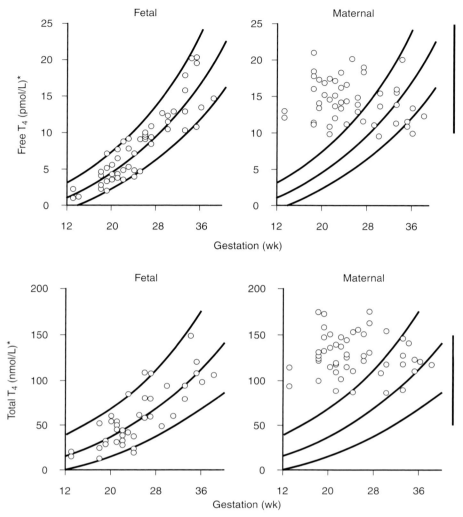

Figure B–6. Scatterplots showing individual fetal and maternal serum free and total thyroxine (T_4) concentrations during gestation. *Curved lines* represent the mean and the 5th and 95th percentile values. *Vertical lines* on the right indicate normal ranges in nonpregnant adults*. See Table B-31 for conversion from pmol/L to ng/dL and from nmol/L to μg/dL. (*From Thorpe-Beeston JG et al: Maturation of the secretion of thyroid hormone and thyroid-stimulating hormone in the fetus,* N Engl J Med *324:534, 1991.*)

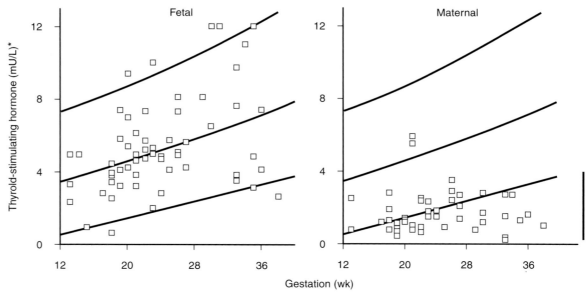

Figure B–7. Scatterplots showing individual fetal and maternal serum thyroid-stimulating hormone concentrations during gestation. *Sloping lines* are the mean and 5th and 95th percentile values. *Vertical line* on the right is the normal range in nonpregnant adults*. See Table B-31 for conversion of mU/L to μU/mL. (*From Thorpe-Beeston JG et al: Maturation of the secretion of thyroid hormone and thyroid-stimulating hormone in the fetus, N Engl J Med 324:533, 1991.*)

TABLE B–21	Reference Intervals for Thyroid Hormones*			
	Age†	2.5th	50th	97.5th
T4 (nmol/L)	1-7 days	114.5	207.9	399
	8-15 days	178.5	319.2	534.1
	1 mo-3 yr	75.4	126.8	155.5
Free T4 (nmol/L)	1-7 days	29.6	62.4	79.2
	8-15 days	18	42.3	63.6
	1 mo-3 yr	11.1	19.7	27.3
T3 (nmol/L)	1-7 days	2.7	6	8
	8-15 days	2.4	4.7	5.1
	1 mo-3 yr	1.9	3	3.4
Free T3 (nmol/L)	1-7 days	2.76	6.91	11.67
	8-15 days	2.84	5.53	11.86
	1 mo-3 yr	3.28	6.08	11.06
TSH (μIU/mL)	1-7 days	1.79	4.63	9.69
	8-15 days	1.8	3.71	7.97
	1 mo-3 yr	0.63	2.04	4.12
TBG (nmol/L)	1-7 days	116.6	196.1	399.6
	8-15 days	220	320.8	442.9
	1 mo-3 yr	235.1	450.5	571.7

*Reference range is range between the 2.5th and 97.5th percentiles.
†Sample included 45 infants aged 1-7 days, 40 aged 8 to 15 days, and 86 aged 1 month to 3 years.
TBG, thyroxine-binding globulin; TSH, thyroid-stimulating hormone.
Adapted from Elmlinger MW et al: Reference intervals from birth to adulthood for serum thyroxine (T4), triiodothyronine (T3), free T3, free T4 thyroxine binding globulin (TBG), and thyrotropin (TSH), *Clin Chem Lab Med* 39:976, 2001.

Cerebrospinal Fluid

TABLE B–22   Cerebrospinal Fluid Values in Infants with Birthweight of ≤1000 Grams

| | POSTNATAL AGE (DAYS) | | | | | |
| | 0-7 | | 8-28 | | 29-84 | |
	Mean ± SD	Range	Mean ± SD	Range	Mean ± SD	Range
Birthweight (g)	822 ± 116	630-980	752 ± 112	550-970	750 ± 120	550-907
Gestational age at birth (wk)	26 ± 1.2	24-27	26 ± 1.5	24-28	26 ± 1.0	24-27
Leukocytes/mm³	3 ± 3	1-8	4 ± 4	0-14	4 ± 3	0-11
Erythrocytes/mm³	335 ± 709	0-1780	1465 ± 4062	0-19050	808 ± 1843	0-6850
PMN (%)	11 ± 20	0-50	8 ± 17	0-66	2 ± 9	0-36
Glucose (mg/dL)	70 ± 17	41-89	68 ± 48	33-217	49 ± 22	29-90
Protein (mg/dL)	162 ± 37	115-222	159 ± 77	95-370	137 ± 61	76-260

PMN, polymorphonuclear cells.
Modified from Rodriguez AF et al: Cerebrospinal fluid values in the very low birth weight infant, *J Pediatr* 116:971, 1990.

TABLE B–23   Cerebrospinal Fluid Values in Infants with Birthweight of 1001 to 1500 Grams

| | POSTNATAL AGE (DAYS) | | | | | |
| | 0-7 | | 8-28 | | 29-84 | |
	Mean ± SD	Range	Mean ± SD	Range	Mean ± SD	Range
Birthweight (g)	1428 ± 107	1180-1500	1245 ± 162	1020-1480	1211 ± 86	1080-1300
Gestational age at birth (wk)	31 ± 1.5	28-33	29 ± 1.2	27-31	29 ± 0.7	27-29
Leukocytes/mm³	4 ± 4	1-10	7 ± 11	0-44	8 ± 8	0-23
Erythrocytes/mm³	407 ± 853	0-2450	1101 ± 2643	0-9750	661 ± 1198	0-3800
PMN (%)	4 ± 10	0-28	10 ± 19	0-60	11 ± 19	0-48
Glucose (mg/dL)	74 ± 19	50-96	59 ± 23	39-109	47 ± 13	31-76
Protein (mg/dL)	136 ± 35	85-176	137 ± 46	54-227	122 ± 47	45-187

PMN, polymorphonuclear cells.
Modified from Rodriguez AF et al: Cerebrospinal fluid values in the very low birth weight infant, *J Pediatr* 116:971, 1990.

TABLE B–24   Cerebrospinal Fluid Values in Term Neonates*

| | | | WBC/mm³ | | | | | | |
Wk	Age (days)	No. of Patients	Mean ± SD	95% CI per Mean	Median	Range	90th Percentile	Protein mg/dL	Glucose mg/dL
1	0-7	17	15.3 ± 30.3	12.5-18.1	6	1-130	18	80.8 ± 30.8	45.9 ± 7.5
2	8-14	33	5.4 ± 4.4	4.6-6.1	6	0-18	10	69 ± 22.6	54.3 ± 17
3	15-21	25	7.7 ± 12.1	6.3-9.1	4	0-62	12.5	59.8 ± 23.4	46.8 ± 8.8
4	22-30	33	4.8 ± 3.4	4.1-5.4	4	0-18	8	54.1 ± 16.2	54.1 ± 16.2
All		108	7.3 ± 13.9	6.6-8	4	0-130	11	64.2 ± 24.2	51.2 ± 12.9

*All neonates represented were suspected of having an infection, and no central nervous system infection was found.
Modified from Ahmed A et al: Cerebrospinal fluid values in the term neonate, *Pediatr Infect Dis J* 15:301, 1996.

Immunoglobulin Values

TABLE B–25	Plasma Immunoglobulin (Ig) Concentrations in Premature Infants at 25 to 28 Weeks' Gestation			
Age (mo)	No. of Patients	IgG* (mg/dL)	IgM* (mg/dL)	IgA* (mg/dL)
0.25	18	251 (114-552)†	7.6 (1.3-43.3)	1.2 (0.07-20.8)
0.5	14	202 (91-446)	14.1 (3.5-56.1)	3.1 (0.09-10.7)
1.0	10	158 (57-437)	12.7 (3.0-53.3)	4.5 (0.65-30.9)
1.5	14	134 (59-307)	16.2 (4.4-59.2)	4.3 (0.9-20.9)
2.0	12	89 (58-136)	16 (5.3-48.9)	4.1 (1.5-11.1)
3	13	60 (23-156)	13.8 (5.3-36.1)	3 (0.6-15.6)
4	10	82 (32-210)	22.2 (11.2-43.9)	6.8 (1-47.8)
6	11	159 (56-455)	41.3 (8.3-205)	9.7 (3-31.2)
8-10	6	273 (94-794)	41.8 (31.1-56.1)	9.5 (0.9-98.6)

*Geometric mean.
†The normal ranges in parentheses were determined by taking the antilog of the mean logarithm ± 2 standard deviations of the logarithms.
From Ballow M et al: Development of the immune system in very low birth weight (less than 1500 g) premature infants: concentrations of plasma immunoglobulins and patterns of infections, *Pediatr Res* 20:899, 1986.

TABLE B–26	Plasma Immunoglobulin (Ig) Concentrations in Premature Infants 29 to 32 Weeks' Gestation		
Age (mo)	IgG* (mg/dL)	IgM* (mg/dL)	IgA* (mg/dL)
0.25	368 (186-728)†	9.1 (2.1-39.4)	0.6 (0.04-1)
0.5	275 (119-637)	13.9 (4.7-41)	0.9 (0.01-7.5)
1	209 (97-452)	14.4 (6.3-33)	1.9 (0.3-12)
1.5	156 (69-352)	15.4 (5.5-43.2)	2.2 (0.7-6.5)
2	123 (64-237)	15.2 (4.9-46.7)	3 (1.1-8.3)
3	104 (41-268)	16.3 (7.1-37.2)	3.6 (0.8-15.4)
4	128 (39-425)	26.5 (7.7-91.2)	9.8 (2.5-39.3)
6	179 (51-634)	29.3 (10.5-81.5)	12.3 (2.7-57.1)
8-10	280 (140-561)	34.7 (17-70.8)	20.9 (8.3-53)

*Geometric mean.
†The normal ranges in parentheses were determined by taking the antilog of the mean logarithm ± 2 standard deviations of the logarithms.
From Ballow M et al: Development of the immune system in very low birth weight (less than 1500 g) premature infants: concentrations of plasma immunoglobulins and patterns of infections, *Pediatr Res* 20:899, 1986.

HEMATOLOGIC VALUES

TABLE B–27   Red Blood Cell Parameters of Infants with Very Low Birthweight During the First 6 Weeks of Life Derived from Arterial or Venous but Not Capillary Blood Samples

			PERCENTILES								
	Day of Life	No. of Patients	3	5	10	25	Median	75	90	95	97
Hemoglobin (g/dL)	3*	559	11.0	11.6	12.5	14.0	15.6	17.1	18.5	19.3	19.8
	12-14	203	10.1	10.8	11.1	12.5	14.4	15.7	17.4	18.4	18.9
	24-26	192	8.5	8.9	9.7	10.9	12.4	14.2	15.6	16.5	16.8
	40-42	150	7.8	7.9	8.4	9.3	10.6	12.4	13.8	14.9	15.4
Hematocrit (%)	3	561	35	36	39	43	47	52	56	59	60
	12-14	205	30	32	34	39	44	48	53	55	56
	24-26	196	25	27	29	32	39	44	48	50	52
	40-42	152	24	24	26	28	33	38	44	47	48
Red blood cells (10^{12}/L)	3	364	3.2	3.3	3.5	3.8	4.2	4.6	4.9	5.1	5.3
	12-14	196	2.9	3.0	3.2	3.5	4.1	4.6	5.2	5.5	5.6
	24-26	188	2.6	2.6	2.8	3.2	3.8	4.4	4.8	5.2	5.3
	40-42	148	2.5	2.5	2.6	3.0	3.4	4.1	4.6	4.8	4.9
Corrected reticulocytes (%)	3	283	0.6	0.7	1.9	4.2	7.1	12.0	20.0	24.1	27.8
	12-14	139	0.3	0.3	0.5	0.8	1.7	2.7	5.7	7.3	9.6
	24-26	140	0.2	0.3	0.5	0.8	1.5	2.6	4.7	6.4	8.6
	40-42	114	0.3	0.4	0.6	1.0	1.8	3.4	5.6	8.3	9.5

*On day 3, all infants are included regardless of antenatal steroids and transfusions up to that time. Thereafter, infants who did not receive erythropoietin were studied regardless of the use of antibiotics and steroids.
From Obladen M et al: Venous and arterial hematologic profiles of very low birth weight infants. European Multicenter rhEPO Study Group, *Pediatrics* 106:709, 2000.

TABLE B–28   Iron Parameters of Infants with Very Low Birthweight Infants During the First 6 Weeks of Life

			PERCENTILES								
	Day of Life	No. of Patients	3	5	10	25	Median	75	90	95	97
Ferritin (ng/mL)	3*	431	27	35	48	80	140	204	279	360	504
	12-14	130	43	65	89	128	168	243	329	410	421
	24-26	128	27	44	57	93	153	234	300	355	383
	40-42	93	17	20	35	62	110	191	290	420	457
Serum iron (μmol/L)	3	181	0.8	1.0	1.6	3.5	7.5	13.8	18.6	22.4	26.7
Transferrin saturation (%)	3	179	2.6	2.7	4.2	9.6	22.7	39.4	54.9	62.1	79.8

*On day 3, all infants are included regardless of antenatal steroids and transfusions up to that time. Thereafter, infants who did not receive erythropoietin were studied regardless of the use of antibiotics and steroids.
From Obladen M et al: Venous and arterial hematologic profiles of very low birth weight infants. European Multicenter rhEPO Study Group, *Pediatrics* 106:710, 2000.

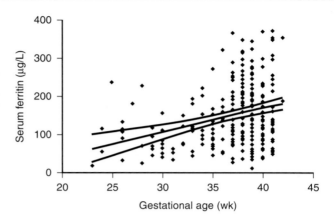

Figure B–8. Ferritin concentrations as a function of gestational age. Regression line and its 5th and 95th percentile confidence limits for the mean regression are shown. (*From Siddappa AM et al: The assessment of newborn iron stores at birth: a review of the literature and standards for ferritin concentrations,* Neonatology 92:77, 2007.)

TABLE B–29	Reference Values For Nucleated Red Blood Cell (NRBC) Count from Umbilical Vein Sampling at Birth in 695 Newborns Divided into Four Groups According to Gestational Age			
	No. of Patients	Birthweight (g) Mean ± SD 25th-75th Percentiles	Gestational Age (wk) Mean ± SD 25th-75th Percentiles	NRBC* Mean ± SD Median 25th-75th Percentiles
Group 1	120	954 ± 234 780-1105	26.7 ± 1 26-28	5643 ± 7228 2601 1147-7790
Group 2	128	1413 ± 398 1100-1720	30.4 ± 1 29-31	3328 ± 3577 1901 492-5970
Group 3	215	2189 ± 473 1940-2520	34.7 ± 1 34-36	1099 ± 1275 696 0-1672
Group 4	232	3201 ± 669 2905-3590	38.6 ± 1 38-40	442 ± 807 0 0-638

*Absolute count (NRBC/mm^3).
Adapted from Perrone S et al: Nucleated red blood cell count in term and preterm newborns: reference values at birth, *Arch Dis Child* 90:F174, 2005.

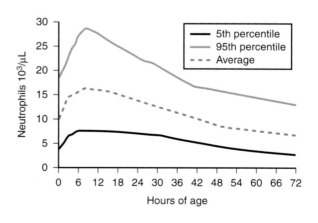

Figure B–9. Neutrophils per microliter of blood during the first 72 hours after the birth of term and near-term (>36 weeks' gestation) neonates. A total of 12,149 values were obtained for the analysis. The 5th percentile, the mean, and the 95th percentile values are shown. (*From Schmutz N et al: Expected ranges for blood neutrophil concentrations of neonates: the Manroe and Mouzinho charts revisited,* J Perinatol 28:275, 2008.)

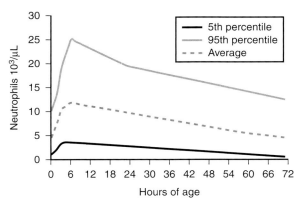

Figure B–10. Neutrophils per microliter of blood during the first 72 hours after the birth of 28- to 36-week gestation pre-term neonates. A total of 8896 values were obtained for the analysis. The 5th percentile, the mean, and the 95th percentile values are shown. (*From Schmutz N et al: Expected ranges for blood neutrophil concentrations of neonates: the Manroe and Mouzinho charts revisited,* J Perinatol 28:275, 2008.)

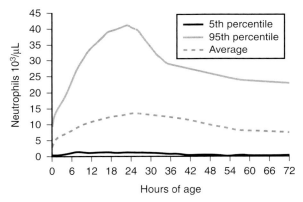

Figure B–11. Neutrophils per microliter of blood during the first 72 hours after the birth of <28-week gestation preterm neonates. A total of 852 values were obtained for the analysis. The 5th percentile, the mean, and the 95th percentile values are shown. (*From Schmutz N et al: Expected ranges for blood neutrophil concentrations of neonates: the Manroe and Mouzinho charts revisited,* J Perinatol 28:275, 2008.)

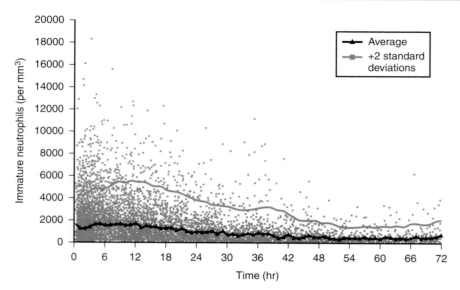

Figure B-12. Immature neutrophils (band neutrophils plus metamyelocytes) per microliter of blood during the first 72 hours after the birth of term and near-term (>36 weeks' gestation) neonates. A total of 12,857 values were obtained for the analysis. The average and 2 standard deviations above the mean value are shown. (*From Schmutz N et al: Expected ranges for blood neutrophil concentrations of neonates: the Manroe and Mouzinho charts revisited, J Perinatol 28:275, 2008.*)

TABLE B-30	**Neutrophil Values in Healthy Term Neonates at 4 Hours of Age**		
	Mean	**±SD**	**Range, 10%-90%**
I/T ratio	0.16	0.10	0.05-0.27
I/M ratio	0.21	0.25	0.06-0.35
ANC (/mm³)	15,622	4685	9500-21,500
Immature	2484	1777	700-4300
Total leukocytes	24,060	6110	16,200-31,500

ANC, absolute neutrophil count; I/T, immature to total neutrophils; I/M, immature to mature neutrophils.
Modified from Schelonka RL et al: Peripheral leukocyte count and leukocyte indexes in healthy newborn term infants, *J Pediatr* 125:604, 1994.

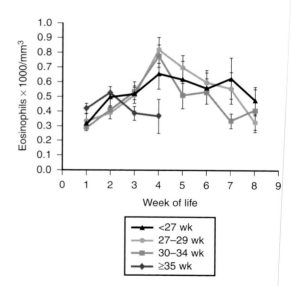

Figure B-13. Mean eosinophil counts (± standard error of the mean) plotted against postnatal age (weeks) for infants born at different gestational ages. (*From Juul SE et al: Evaluation of eosinophilia in hospitalized preterm infants, J Perinatol 25:185, 2005.*)

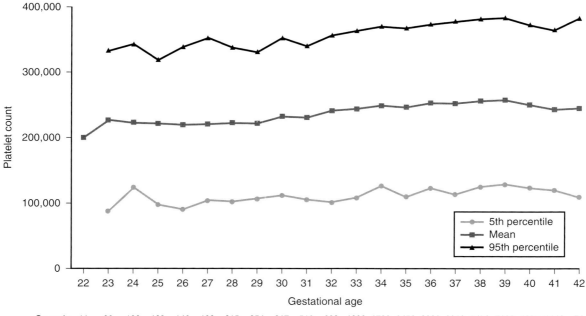

A

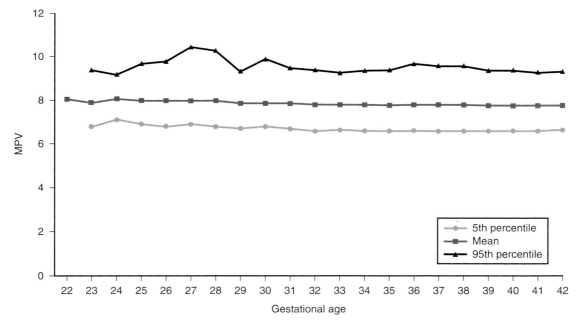

B

Figure B–14. First platelet counts (A) and concurrent mean platelet volume determinations (B) for neonates of 22 to 42 weeks' gestation. Samples obtained in the first 3 days after birth. *(From Wiedemeier SE et al: Platelet reference ranges for neonates, Platelet reference ranges for neonates, defined using data from over 47,000 patients in a multihospital healthcare system, J Perinatol 29:132, 2009.)*

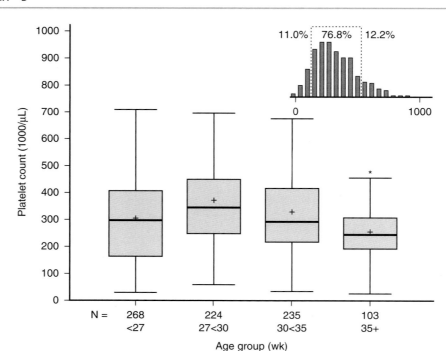

Figure B–15. Box and whisker plot showing distribution of platelet counts from 237 noninfected, non–pregnancy-induced hypertension-exposed infants in a neonatal intensive care unit separated by gestational age at birth. Box plots show mean (± standard error of the mean), median (center line), 25th and 75th percentile quartiles (box ends), and range of values (whiskers). *Inset* shows frequency distribution histogram of 830 platelet counts in increments of 50. *Dotted box* shows 76.8% were normal (>150,000 and <500,000). (*From McPherson RJ, Juul SE: Patterns of thrombocytosis and thrombocytopenia in hospitalized neonates, J Perinatol 25:167, 2005.*)

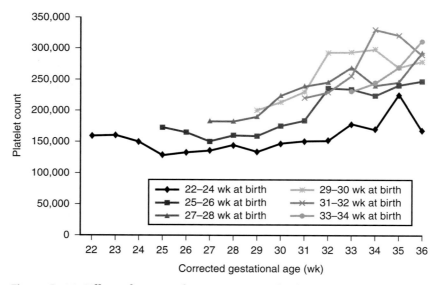

Figure B–16. Effect of postnatal age on mean platelet counts of premature infants. Mean platelet counts are plotted according to gestational age at birth. (*From Wiedmeier SE, Henry E, Sola-Visner MC, Christensen RD: Platelet reference ranges for neonates, defined using data from over 47,000 patients in a multihospital healthcare system, J Perinatol 29(2):130, 2009). Epub 2008 Sep 25.*)

CONVERSION TABLES
Standard International Units

TABLE B–31	Conversion Table to Standard International Units				
Component	Present Unit of Measurement	×	Conversion Factor	=	SI Unit
Clinical Hematology					
Erythrocytes	/mm³		1		10^6/L
Hematocrit	%		0.01		(1)vol RBC/vol whole blood
Leukocytes	/mm³		1		10^6/L
Mean corpuscular volume	μm^3		1		fL
Platelet count	10^3/mm³		1		10^9/L
Reticulocyte count	%		10		10^{-3}
Clinical Chemistry					
Acetone	mg/dL		0.1722		mmol/L
Aldosterone	ng/dL		27.74		pmol/L
Ammonia	μg/dL		0.7139		μmol/L
Bicarbonate	mEq/L		1		mmol/L
Bilirubin	mg/dL		17.10		μmol/L
Calcium	mg/dL		0.2495		mmol/L
Calcium ion	mEq/L		0.50		mmol/L
Carotenes	μg/dL		0.01836		μmol/L
Chloride	mEq/L		1		mmol/L
Cholesterol	mg/dL		0.02586		mmol/L
Copper	μg/dL		0.1574		μmol/L
Cortisol	μg/dL		27.59		nmol/L
Creatine	mg/dL		76.25		μmol/L
Creatinine	mg/dL		88.40		μmol/L
Digoxin	ng/mL		1.281		nmol/L
Epinephrine	pg/mL		5.458		pmol/L
Folate	ng/mL		2.266		nmol/L
Fructose	mg/dL		0.05551		mmol/L
Galactose	mg/dL		0.05551		mmol/L
Gases					
Po_2	mm Hg (=Torr)		0.1333		kPa
Pco_2	mm Hg (=Torr)		0.1333		kPa
Glucose	mg/dL		0.05551		mmol/L
Glycerol	mg/dL		0.1086		mmol/L
Insulin	μg/L		172.2		pmol/L
	mU/L		7.175		pmol/L
Iron	μg/dL		0.1791		μmol/L
Iron-binding capacity	μg/dL		0.1791		μmol/L
Lactate	mEq/L		1		mmol/L
Lead	μg/dL		0.04826		μmol/L

Continued

TABLE B–31   Conversion Table to Standard International Units—cont'd

Component	Present Unit of Measurement	×	Conversion Factor	=	SI Unit
Lipoproteins	mg/dL		0.02586		mmol/L
Magnesium	mg/dL		0.4114		mmol/L
	mEq/L		0.50		mmol/L
Osmolality	mOsm/kg H_2O		1		mmol/kg H_2O
Phenobarbital	mg/dL		43.06		μmol/L
Phenytoin	mg/L		3.964		μmol/L
Phosphate	mg/dL		0.3229		mmol/L
Potassium	mEq/L		1		mmol/L
	mg/dL		0.2558		mmol/L
Pyruvate	mg/dL		113.6		μmol/L
Sodium	mEq/L		1		mmol/L
Steroids					
17-hydroxycorticosteroids	mg/24 h		2.759		μmol/d
17-ketosteroids	mg/24 h		3.467		μmol/d
Dehydroepiandrosterone sulfate	μg/dL		0.02714		μmol/L
Estradiol	pg/ml		3.671		pmol/L
Progesterone	ng/mL		3.18		nmol/L
Prolactin	ng/mL		21.2		mIU/L
Testosterone	ng/mL		3.467		nmol/L
Theophylline	mg/L		5.550		μmol/L
Thyroid tests	ng/mL		21.2		mIU/L
Thyroid-stimulating hormone	μU/mL		1		mU/L
Thyroxine	μg/dL		12.87		nmol/L
Free thyroxine	ng/dL		12.87		pmol/L
Triiodothyronine	ng/dL		0.01536		nmol/L
Triglycerides	mg/dL		0.01129		mmol/L
Blood urea nitrogen	mg/dL		0.3570		mmol/L
Uric acid (urate)	mg/dL		59.48		μmol/L
Vitamin A (retinol)	μg/dL		0.03491		μmol/L
Vitamin B_{12}	pg/mL		0.7378		pmol/L
Vitamin C (ascorbic acid)	mg/dL		56.78		μmol/L
Vitamin D					
Cholecalciferol	μg/mL		2.599		nmol/L
25-OH-cholecalciferol	ng/mL		2.496		nmol/L
Vitamin E (α-tocopherol)	mg/dL		23.22		μmol/L
D-Xylose	mg/dL		0.06661		mmol/L
Zinc	μg/dL		0.1530		μmol/L
Energy					
Kilocalorie	kcal		4.1868		kJ
Blood Pressure					
	mm Hg (=Torr)		1.333		mbar

OH, hydroxylase; RBC, red blood cell(s); SI, Standard International.
Modified from Young DS: Implementation of SI units for clinical laboratory data: style specifications and conversion tables, *Ann Intern Med* 106:114, 1987 (erratum: published in *Ann Intern Med* 114:172, 1991).

Metric Units

Atomic Weight and Valence

TABLE B–32 Conversion Tables for Metric Units

A. Metric System Weights

1 kilogram (kg)	=	1000 grams (g)
1 milligram (mg)	=	0.001 gram (g)
1 microgram (μg)	=	10^{-6} g or μ
1 nanogram (ng)	=	10^{-9} g or mμ
1 picogram (pg)	=	10^{-12} g or $\mu\mu$
1 femtogram (fg)	=	10^{-15} g or m$\mu\mu$

B. Metric and Avoirdupois Systems of Volume (Fluid)

1 liter (L)	=	1000 milliliters (mL)
1 milliliter (mL)	=	1000 microliters (μL)
1 deciliter (dL)	=	100 mL

C. Standard Prefixes

	Less than 1			More than 1	
atto	10^{-18}	a	deka	10^1	da
femto	10^{-15}	f	hector	10^2	h
pico	10^{-12}	p	kilo	10^3	k
nano	10^{-9}	n	mega	10^6	M
micro	10^{-6}	μ	giga	10^9	G
milli	10^{-3}	m			
centi	10^{-2}	c			
deci	10^{-1}	d			

D. Conversion Factors

1 kg	=	2.2046 pounds (usually rounded to 2.2)
1 pound	=	0.4536 kilogram
1 ounce	=	28.35 g (usually rounded to 30)
1 L	=	1.06 quarts
1 fluid ounce	=	29.57 mL (usually rounded to 30)
1 inch	=	2.54 cm
1 cm	=	0.394 inch
Degrees Celsius	=	($^\circ$F − 32) $\times$ $^5/_9$
Degrees Fahrenheit	=	($^\circ$C $\times$ $^9/_5$) + 32

Parts per million (ppm) to percent:

1 ppm	=	0.0001%
10 ppm	=	0.001%
100 ppm	=	0.01%
1000 ppm	=	0.1%

TABLE B–33 Atomic Weight and Valence for Common Elements

Element	Atomic Weight	Valence
Calcium	40	2
Sodium	23	1
Potassium	39	1
Chlorine	35.5	1
Magnesium	24.3	2
Phosphorus	31	*

Conversion of Common Elements from Milligrams (mg) to Milliequivalents (mEq)

To convert mg to mEq:

$$\frac{mg \times valence}{atomic\ weight} = mEq$$

To convert mEq to mg:

$$\frac{mEq \times atomic\ weight}{valence} = mg$$

*The valence of phosphorus varies. For nutritional purposes, it is convenient to express quantities in moles.

Schedule for Immunization of Preterm Infants

Jill E. Baley

ALL PRETERM INFANTS

- Vaccine doses should not be reduced for preterm infants.
- Use thimerosal-free vaccines.
- Intramuscular injections to preterm infants might require a shorter needle than the standard $^5/_8$- to 1-inch needle.
- Immunizations may be given during corticosteroid administration.
- Palivizumab (Synagis) should be given according to the respiratory syncytial virus (RSV) policy.
- Preterm infants should receive a full dose of diphtheria and tetanus toxoids and acellular pertussis (DTaP), *Haemophilus influenzae* type B (Hib) conjugate, inactivated poliovirus (IPV), and pneumococcal conjugate (PC7) at 60 days' chronologic age, regardless of birthweight and gestational age, as long as they are medically stable and consistently gaining weight.
- The 13-valent pneumococcal conjugate vaccine (PCV 13) should be substituted for PCV 7 when it becomes available.
- Immunizations for preterm infants may be given over 2 or 3 days to minimize the number of injections at a single time.
- Hospitalized infants with birthweight lower than 1000 g should be observed for apnea for 72 hours after the primary series of immunizations.
- Breast feeding by a mother who is positive for hepatitis B surface antigen (HBsAg) poses no additional risk for acquisition of hepatitis B virus (HBV) infection by the infant.
- Infants with chronic respiratory tract disease should receive the influenza immunization annually, before or during the influenza season, once they are 6 months postnatal age or older:
  - The infant should receive two doses of vaccine, 1 month apart.
  - Family and other caregivers should also receive influenza vaccine annually in the fall to protect the infant from exposure.

- The American Academy of Pediatrics recommends routine immunization of infants in the United States with rotavirus vaccine. There is no preference for either the live oral human-bovine reassortant vaccine (RV5) or the liver oral, human attenuated rotavirus vaccine (RVI).
  - Preterm infants who are clinically stable should be immunized on the same schedule and with the same precautions as term infants. The infant's postnatal age must be between 6 weeks and 14 weeks, 6 days postnatal age.
  - Preterm infants who are in the NICU or nursery may be immunized at the time of discharge if they are clinically stable and age-eligible for the vaccine. The AAP believes that the risk of shedding vaccine virus in the stool, and theoretically transmitting vaccine virus to another acutely ill or non–age-eligible infant outweighs the benefit of immunizing eligible infants who remain in the NICU or nursery.
  - Any rotavirus vaccine-immunized infant who requires readmission to the NICU or nursery within 2 weeks of vaccination should remain under contact precautions for 2 to 3 weeks after vaccine administration.

PRETERM INFANTS WITH BIRTHWEIGHT OF 2000 GRAMS OR MORE

- If mother is HBsAg positive:
  - Administer hepatitis B vaccine and hepatitis B immune globulin (HBIG) within 12 hours of birth.
  - Immunize with three doses at 0, 1, and 6 months' chronologic age.
  - Check antibody to hepatitis B surface antigen (anti-HBs) and HBsAg at 9 to 15 months of age.
  - If infant is anti-HBs and HBsAg negative, reimmunize with three doses at 2-month intervals and retest.
- If mother is HBsAg unknown:
  - Administer HBV by 12 hours of age.

- If the mother tests positive, give HBIG within 7 days of birth and proceed as for HBsAg-positive mother.
- If mother is HBsAg negative:
  - Administering HBV vaccine at birth is preferable to waiting for the first pediatric visit.
  - Immunize with three doses at 0 to 2, 1 to 4, and 6 to 18 months of chronologic age.
  - Follow-up anti-HBs and HBsAg titers are not needed.

PRETERM INFANTS WITH BIRTHWEIGHTS LESS THAN 2000 GRAMS

- If mother is HBsAg positive:
  - Administer HBV and HBIG within 12 hours of age.
  - Immunize with four vaccine doses at 0, 1, 2 to 3, and 6 to 7 months' chronologic age.
  - Check anti-HBs and HBsAg at 9 to 15 months of age.
  - If anti-HBs and HBsAg are negative, reimmunize with three doses of vaccine at 2-month intervals and retest titers.
- If mother is HBsAg unknown:
  - Administer both HBV and HBIG by 12 hours of age because HBV is less reliable as a single agent under these conditions.
  - Test the mother immediately.

- If mother is HBsAg negative:
  - Administer the first dose of HBV at 30 days' chronologic age regardless of gestational age, or at discharge if the infant is discharged before 30 days of age. The infant must be medically stable and consistently gaining weight before receiving the vaccine.
  - Immunize with three doses at 1 to 2, 2 to 4, and 6 to 18 months' chronologic age.
  - HBV-containing combination vaccine may be given after 6 to 8 weeks' chronologic age.
  - Follow-up titers are not needed.

Adapted from
1. American Academy of Pediatrics, Hepatitis B. In: Pickering LK, Baker CJ, Kimberlin DW, Long SS, eds. Red Book: 2009 Report of the Committee on Infectious Diseases. 28th ed, Elk Grove Village, IL: *American Academy of Pediatrics,* 337-356, 2009.
2. Committee on Infectious Diseases, American Academy of Pediatrics. Prevention of rotavirus disease: updated guidelines for use of rotavirus vaccine, *Pediatrics* 123:1-9, 2009.
3. Committee on Infectious Diseases, American Academy of Pediatrics. Recommendations for the prevention of *Streptococcus pneumoniae* infections in infants and children: use of 13-valent pneumococcal conjugate vaccine (PCV 13) and pneumococcal polysaccharide vaccine (PPSV 23), *Pediatrics* 126:186-189, 2010.

Index

A

A cells, 1377
ABCA3 deficiency, 1108
Abdomen
  circumference of, in gestational age assessment, 153-155, 154f
  congenital anomalies of, 543-544
  examination of, 487
  mass in, renal causes of, 1686
Abdominal radiography. *See* Radiography, abdominal.
Abdominal situs abnormalities, 1266-1267
Abdominal wall defects, 1408-1412. *See also* Gastroschisis; Omphalocele.
  anterior, 165, 166f, 167f
Abducens nerve palsy, birth-related, 510
Abetalipoproteinemia, 1390
Ablative therapy
  for retinopathy of prematurity, 1766-1767, 1767b
  transcatheter, for tachycardia, 1286-1287b
ABO blood group
  incompatibility of, RhD isoimmunization and, 358
  pretransfusion testing of, 1367-1368
ABO hemolytic disease, 1314, 1456
ABO heterospecificity, unconjugated hyperbilirubinemia in, 1455-1456
Abortion
  previous, preterm delivery and, 308
  spontaneous
    after amniocentesis, 142
    amniotic fluid volume abnormalities and, 382-383
    in antiphospholipid antibody syndrome, 340
    after chorionic villus sampling, 142
    congenital anomalies and, 535, 535t
    after cordocentesis, 142
Abrasions
  birth-related, 501
    of ear, 511
  of cornea, 1758
Abruptio placentae, 155-156
  labor anesthesia and, 446
Abscess, 1709t
  brain
    macrocephaly in, 1025
    in meningitis, 806
  breast, 818-819
  soft tissue, 817
Absence anomalies, 545
Abuse, substance. *See* Substance abuse.
Acarbose, in pregnancy, 298t
Accelerations, in fetal heart rate monitoring, 182, 184
Accessory pathway reentrant tachycardia, 1278t, 1279-1280, 1280f
  treatment of, 1287-1288
Acebutolol, in breast milk, 731
Acetaminophen
  in breast milk, 730
  fetal effects of, 719-721t
  fetal protection against, 223
Acetate
  in fetal oxygen consumption, 249, 249t, 250f
  in parenteral nutrition, 650
Acetazolamide, for posthemorrhagic hydrocephalus, 1021-1022
Acetoacetate, in lactic acidemia, 1665
Acetylation, 726-727

Acetylcholine receptors, autoantibodies against, in myasthenia gravis, 340
Acetylcholinesterase, amniotic fluid, in neural tube defect screening, 139
N-Acetylglutamate synthetase deficiency, 1674-1675
Acheiria, 545
Acheiropodia, 545
Achondroplasia, 1796
  evaluation of, 544, 544f
  heterozygous, 170
  macrencephaly in, 1017
Acid elution technique, in fetal-maternal hemorrhage, 1312
Acid maltase deficiency, 1007
Acid-base balance, 677-683
  buffer systems in, 677
  developmental aspects of, 678-679
  long-term maintenance of, 677-678, 678f
  during mechanical ventilation, 1130-1131
  in neonate, 600, 677
  with neuraxial blocks, 442
Acid-base disorders. *See also* Acidosis; Alkalosis.
  diagnosis of, 679-680, 679f, 679t
  expected compensation in, 679-680, 679f, 679t
  treatment of, 680-681
Acid-base therapy, in respiratory distress syndrome, 1114
Acidemia, organic. *See* Organic acidemia/aciduria.
Acidification, distal urinary, 678, 678f, 682
Acidosis
  differential diagnosis of, 1653t
  hyperammonemia and, 1673-1674
  metabolic. *See* Metabolic acidosis.
  in neonatal asphyxia, 453-454
  renal tubular. *See* Renal tubular acidosis.
  respiratory, 681
    expected compensation in, 679-680, 679f, 679t
    in respiratory distress syndrome, 1114
  seizures and, 986
  ventilatory response to, 1151-1153
Aciduria, organic. *See* Organic acidemia/aciduria.
Acinus, appearance of, during lung development, 1076, 1078f
Acne
  infantile, 1712
  neonatal, 1712, 1712f
Acquired immunodeficiency syndrome (AIDS). *See* HIV infection.
Acrocephalosyndactyly
  type 1 (Apert syndrome), 604-606t, 1030-1031, 1030f
  type 3 (Saethre-Chotzen syndrome), 1031
  type 5 (Pfeiffer syndrome), 1031, 1031f
Acrocephaly, 1026t
Acrodermatitis enteropathica, 1395, 1721, 1723f
Acromelia, 169, 545
Acropustulosis, infantile, 1712-1713
Action potential, cardiac, 577-578, 578f
Activated partial thromboplastin time (aPTT), reference values for, 1338t, 1339t
Acupuncture, for back pain during labor, 435
Acute-phase response, in sepsis, 798
Acyclovir
  for herpes simplex virus infection, 407, 844-845
  for pneumonia, 810

Acyclovir (*Continued*)
  prophylactic
    for herpes simplex virus infection, 844-845
    for varicella-zoster virus infection, 851
  for varicella-zoster virus infection, 405, 852
Acylcarnitines
  disorders of, laboratory findings in, 1624-1626, 1625-1626t
  in inborn errors of metabolism, 1656
Acyl-CoA dehydrogenase deficiency. *See also* 3-Hydroxyacyl-CoA dehydrogenase deficiency.
  multiple, 1647, 1652, 1662
Acyl-CoAs, degradation of, 1672
Adenoma, in nesidioblastosis-adenoma spectrum, 1510-1511, 1511f
Adenomatoid malformation, cystic. *See* Cystic adenomatoid malformation.
Adenosine
  in respiratory control, 1144
  for tachycardia, 1284t, 1286-1287b
Adenovirus infection, 879-880
Adhesion
  of neutrophils, 763-765, 764f
  of phagocytes, 767
    disorders of, 1331-1332, 1332f
Adrenal crisis, in 21-hydroxylase deficiency, 1610, 1612
Adrenal glands
  congenital hyperplasia of, 675, 1607-1615
    endocrine imbalances in, 1607-1608, 1609f
    from 11β-hydroxylase deficiency, 1612-1613
    from 17α-hydroxylase deficiency, 1614
    from 21-hydroxylase deficiency, 1609-1612, 1609f, 1610f
    from 3β-hydroxysteroid dehydrogenase deficiency, 1613-1614
    hypertensive, 1612-1613
    hypoglycemia in, 1513
    lipoid, 1614
    from P-450 oxidoreductase deficiency, 1614-1615, 1615f
  insufficiency of
    in bronchopulmonary dysplasia, 1184
    hypoglycemia in, 1513
Adrenal hemorrhage
  birth-related, 521-522, 522f
  diagnostic imaging in, 702
Adrenocorticotropic hormone
  in 21-hydroxylase deficiency, 1610
  normalization of, for congenital adrenal hyperplasia, 1611-1612
  unresponsiveness to, 1513
Adrenogenital syndrome, anesthetic implications of, 604-606t
Adrenoleukodystrophy, X-linked, 1652-1653, 1677
Adult-onset disease, developmental origins of, 229-242. *See also* Fetal origins of adult disease.
Advanced practice neonatal nurses, supervision of, liability of physicians for, 52
Aeromonas hydrophila infection, ecthyma gangrenosum from, 817
Aerophore pulmonaire, 10-11
Aerosolized drugs, maternal absorption of, 709-710
African Americans
  congenital malformation rate for, 536, 537t
  infant mortality in, 21, 21f

Page numbers followed by b, f, and t indicate boxes, figures, and tables, respectively.

Volume One pp 1-758 • Volume Two pp 759-1840

i

Breast milk (Continued)
  cytomegalovirus transmission via, 846
  drug distribution into, milk-to-plasma ratio of, 714, 730
  endocrine system drugs in, 731-732
  in enteral nutrition, 658-660, 659t, 663-664
  environmental pollutants in, 732-733
  ethanol in, 732
  exogenous compounds in
    delivery and disposition of, 730
    passage of, 729-730
    types of, 730-733
  fat in, 653-654, 659t
  fatty acids in, 653-654
  fortifiers for, 658-660, 659t
    calcium in, 1525-1526, 1526t
    magnesium in, 1526t
    phosphorus in, 1525-1526, 1526t
  hepatitis B transmission via, 868
  histamine H_2 receptor antagonists in, 732
  HIV transmission via, 860-861
  immunologic properties of, 788-790, 789t
  industrial byproducts in, 733
  iron in, 1322
  jaundice from, 1461
  lactose in, 653
  lead in, 732
  magnesium in, 1526t
  mercury in, 732-733
  narcotics in, 732
  necrotizing enterocolitis and, 1434, 1435t
  nicotine in, 732
  nutrient composition of, 658-660, 659t
  pesticides in, 733
  phosphorus in, 1525-1526, 1526t
  protein in, 651-652, 659t
  proton pump inhibitors in, 732
  radiopharmaceuticals in, 732
  theophylline in, 732
Breast-feeding failure jaundice, 1460-1461
Breath sounds, in respiratory distress syndrome, 1109
Breathing. See also Respiration.
  examination of, 487
  initiation of, 1097-1098
  pattern of
    fetal, 1141-1142
    neonatal, 1142
  periodic, 599
  postnatal development of, 1142-1144, 1143f
  regulation of
    astrocytes in, 1144
    central, under anesthesia, 598
    laryngeal and pulmonary afferent reflexes in, 1143
    neurotransmitters and neuromodulators in, 1143-1144
  spontaneous
    delayed, hypoxic-ischemic encephalopathy outcome and, 970
    first breath in, 451, 451f, 459, 459f, 460f
  techniques of, for labor pain, 434
  temporary cessation of. See Apnea.
  work of
    under anesthesia, 598-599
    imposed, in mechanical ventilation, 1138
    in pulmonary function testing, 1093, 1093f, 1099f, 1102
Breech delivery
  developmental dysplasia of hip and, 1788
  germinal matrix hemorrhage–intraventricular hemorrhage risk and, 939
  phrenic nerve paralysis after, 516-517, 516f
  spine and spinal cord injuries from, 518-520
Broad ligament, 1586
Brock operation, 1293t
Bronchiolitis
  in human metapneumovirus infection, 859
  in respiratory syncytial virus infection, 856
Bronchodilators
  for bronchopulmonary dysplasia, 1187
  fetal effects of, 719-721t
  for respiratory syncytial virus infection, 857
Bronchogenic cyst, 1156

Bronchopulmonary dysplasia, 1179-1190
  adrenal insufficiency in, 1184
  airway obstruction in, 1184
  atypical (new), 1179-1180, 1181f
  chest radiography in, 689, 689f, 1179, 1180f, 1181f
  clinical presentation in, 1179-1181, 1180f, 1181f
  definition of, 1179, 1180t
  extracorporeal membrane oxygenation and, 1195
  genetic factors in, 1184
  gestational age and, 305t
  incidence of, 1179, 1180f
  infection and inflammation in, 1183-1184
  inhaled nitric oxide and, 1202-1203
  management of, 1186-1189
    bronchodilator therapy in, 1187
    corticosteroids in, 1188
    fluid therapy in, 1186-1187
    infant stimulation in, 1188-1189
    infection control in, 1187-1188
    nutritional therapy in, 1187
    parental support in, 1189
    respiratory support in, 1186
    vasodilators in, 1188
  after mechanical ventilation, 1137, 1137f, 1182
  neonatal anesthesia and, 603
  outcome of, 1189
  oxygen toxicity in, 1183, 1183f
  patent ductus arteriosus in, 1184
  pathogenesis of, 1182-1185, 1185f
  pathology of, 1181-1182, 1181f, 1182f
  prediction of, 1185
  premature lung development and, 1182
  prevention of, 1189-1190
  α_1-proteinase inhibitor in, 1184
  pulmonary edema in, 1184
  pulmonary function in, 1185-1186, 1189
  risk factors for, 1184f
  surfactant therapy and, 1110-1111
  vascular abnormalities in, 1220-1221
  vitamin A deficiency in, 1184
Bronchopulmonary sequestration, 1154t, 1155-1156
Bronchoscopy
  fiberoptic, in neonatal anesthesia, 608
  in tracheoesophageal fistula, 1402-1403, 1403f
Bronze baby syndrome, in phototherapy, 1474-1475
Buffer systems, 677
Buffy coat examination, in sepsis, 797
Bulla, 1709t
Bullous lesions, 817
Bumetanide
  for seizures, 993
Buprenorphine, as substitute in opioid abuse, 745
Burden of proof, in malpractice, 56
Butorphanol
  during labor, 439
  umbilical vein to maternal vein ratio of, 436t
Butyrate, for congenital chloride diarrhea, 1391

C

Cadmium, maternal exposure to, pregnancy outcome in, 220t
Café-au-lait spots, 1722
  in neurofibromatosis, 1797, 1797f
Caffeine
  for apnea of prematurity, 1148, 1148f
  in breast milk, 732
  fetal effects of, 718
  pharmacokinetics of, 726
Calcaneovalgus deformities
  of ankle, 547
  of foot, 1793-1794, 1793f
Calcidiol, 1532-1533
Calcification
  in adrenal hemorrhage, 521, 522f
  in cephalhematoma, 504-505, 505f
  in hypoxic-ischemic encephalopathy, 955
Calcitonin
  action of, 1558
  effects of, 1535
  fetal, 1535
  for hypercalcemia, 1548
  neonatal, 1535

Calcitonin (Continued)
  secretion of, regulation of, 1535
  synthesis and metabolism of, 1535
Calcitonin gene-related peptide (CGRP), 1535
Calcitriol, 1532-1533
Calcium
  absorption of, 1525-1526, 1526t
  atomic weight and valence of, 1837t
  in breast milk and breast milk fortifiers, 659t
    absorption and retention of, 1525-1526, 1526t
  deposition of, nephrocalcinosis and, 1548
  disturbances of, 1539-1548. See also
    Hypercalcemia; Hypocalcemia.
  in enteral nutrition, 656-657, 657t
  excessive administration of, hypercalcemia from, 1544-1545
  excretion of, 1527, 1528f
  in fetal body composition, 247, 248t
  in infant formula, 661-662t
  intake of, 1527
  ionized
    for hypocalcemia, 1544
    whole blood, 1817t
  metabolism of, 1528f
  in parenteral nutrition, 650
  physiology of, 1523-1527
  placental transport of, 1524-1525
  in preterm formulas, absorption and retention of, 1525-1526, 1526t
  regulation of, 1523, 1524f
  serum, 1523-1524, 1524f, 1524t
    in very low birthweight infants, 1817t
  in synaptogenesis, 899
  thyroid hormone effects on, 1558
Calcium channel blockers
  for preterm labor, 323-324
  for tachycardia, 1286-1287b
Calcium gluconate
  complications of, 1543
  for hypocalcemia, 1543-1544
  for seizures, 992
Calcium-sensing receptor (CaSR)
  mutations of, 1532
  in parathyroid hormone regulation, 1531-1532
California Perinatal Quality Care Collaborative, 83
  quality improvement methods of, 84
Caloric intake, maternal, fetal growth and, 255, 255f
Camptodactyly, 547
Camptomelic dysplasia, 1602-1603
Campylobacter spp. infection, diarrhea from, 813-814
Canadian Transport Risk Index of Physiologic Stability (TRIPS), 74
Canaliculus, bile, 1481-1482, 1481f, 1482f
Canavan disease, 1017
  screening for, 140, 141t
Cancer
  adult, fetal origins of, 233-234
  fetal radiation exposure and, 221, 222f
  infant, 1356-1358, 1356f
  paternal occupation and, 216
Candida albicans, 794t, 830-831
Candida parapsilosis, 794t, 830-831
Candidiasis, 830-833
  catheter-associated, 831, 831b
  clinical manifestations of, 831-832
  cutaneous, 817, 1718
    congenital, 831, 1718, 1720f
  diagnosis of, 832
  incidence of, 830
  invasive, risk factors for, 831, 831b
  microbiology of, 830-831
  osteomyelitis in, 814
  pathology and pathogenesis of, 831
  prevention of, 833
  pseudomembranous, 831
  septic, 794t
  systemic, 831-832, 831b
  treatment of, 832-833, 833t
  urinary tract infection in, 816
Cannabis sativa, 744
Capillary hemangioma, 489
Capnography, 584-585
  during neonatal anesthesia, 607
  in respiratory distress syndrome, 1113

Congenital anomalies (*Continued*)
  of musculoskeletal system. *See* Musculoskeletal
    system, congenital abnormalities of.
  oligohydramnios and, 383, 385, 385f
  parental reactions to, 625-626, 625f
  paternal age and, 217
  paternal occupation and, 217
  phenotypic variants as, 536, 536t
  polyhydramnios and, 383, 388-389, 389f
  preterm labor and, 311-312
  radiation exposure and, 137, 137t
  screening for, 138-140
    in neonatal resuscitation, 482-483
  sequences as, 531-532
  serious, prevalence of, 489t
  skeletal radiography in, 705
  of spine, 162, 162f, 163f
  support organizations for, 550-551
  syndromic, anesthetic implications of, 602-603,
    604-606t
  teratogens and, 135-138, 136f, 137t
  terminology related to, 531-532
  ultrasonography in, 138, 159-164
  of upper extremities, 1782-1785
Congenital diaphragmatic hernia. *See* Diaphragmatic
  hernia, congenital.
Congenital heart disease
  acyanotic, with no or mild respiratory distress,
    1243b, 1244, 1259-1263
  approach to, 1237-1244
  blood pressure measurement in, 1238
  cardiac catheterization in, 1243
  CHARGE association and, 1225
  chest radiography in, 691-692, 1239-1240, 1239b,
    1240f
  chromosomal abnormalities in, 1222-1223, 1223t
  classification of, 1243-1244, 1243b
  computed tomography in, 1241-1243
  in congenital rubella syndrome, 876
  cyanotic
    chest radiography in, 692
    classification of, 1243-1244, 1243b
    complete mixing in, 1243b, 1244, 1250-1253
    physical examination in, 1237-1238, 1238b
    poor mixing in, 1243b, 1244, 1245-1247
    restricted pulmonary blood flow in, 1243b,
      1244, 1247-1250
    systemic hypoperfusion and congestive heart
      failure in, 1243b, 1244, 1254-1259
    variable physiology in, 1253-1254
  diagnostic groups in, 1243-1244, 1243b
  diagnostic techniques in, 1237-1241
  in duodenal atresia, 1417
  echocardiography in, 1240-1241
    antibiotic prophylaxis and, 1293
    of cardiac function, 1241-1243, 1242b, 1242t
    of cardiac structures, 1241, 1241b
    Doppler, 1241
    of pulmonary hypertension, 1242t
  electrocardiography in, 1240, 1240b
  environmental toxins in, 1224
  fetal interventional catheterization for, 1299
  fetal surgery for, 195
  gender and, 1224
  genetic influences in, 1224
  genetic testing in, 549t
  hyperoxic test in, 1239
  hypoglycemia and, 1510
  magnetic resonance imaging in, 1241-1243
  management of, 1289-1299
    afterload in, 1291-1292
    bacterial endocarditis prophylaxis in, 1292-1293
    blood transfusion in, 1290
    contractility in, 1292
    for cyanotic spells, 1292, 1292b
    heart rate maintenance in, 1291
    heart transplantation in, 1294-1295
    interventional catheterization in, 1295-1299
    oxygen and ventilation in, 1290
    preload in, 1291
    principles of, 1289-1295
    prostaglandin E₁ in, 1290-1291
    surgery in, 1293-1294, 1293t
  maternal diseases and, 1224

Congenital heart disease (*Continued*)
  neonatal anesthesia and, 603
  neonatal physical examination for, 492
  nonimmune hydrops fetalis in, 393
  physical examination in, 1237-1238, 1238b
  presentation of, 1237
  in preterm infant, 1275
  prevalence of, 489t
  prevention of, 1215
  pulse oximetry in, 1239
  race and, 1224
  risk factors for, 1228, 1228b
  single gene defects in, 1223, 1223t
  VACTERL association and, 1224-1225
Congenital high airway obstruction syndrome
  (CHAOS), 1177
Congestive heart failure. *See* Heart failure, congestive.
Conjunctiva
  examination of, 1739-1740
  laceration of, 1758-1759
Conjunctivitis, 811-813, 1759
  chemical, 811
  chlamydial, 417, 811-813
  clinical manifestations of, 812
  diagnosis of, 812
  etiology of, 811
  gonococcal, 412
    clinical manifestations of, 812
    prevention of, 813
    treatment of, 812
  incidence of, 811
  pathogenesis of, 811-812
  prevention of, 813
  treatment of, 812-813
Conradi-Hunermann syndrome, 1651
Consanguinity, microcephaly and, 1011
Consciousness, level of, in neurologic assessment, 494
Consent, 37
  for neonatal research, 45
Constriction band syndrome, 1773, 1783, 1783f
Contact dermatitis, irritant, 1729
Continuous distending pressure, 1117
Continuous positive airway pressure (CPAP), 1117-1119
  for apnea of prematurity, 1148
  bubble, 1118
  complications of, 1117
    after extubation, 1118
  flow-driven, 1117
  high-flow nasal cannula, 1118
  indications for, 1118, 1118b
  methods of generating, 1117-1119, 1118b
  nasal, 1117
    bilevel, 1118-1119
      indications for, 1119
    for bronchopulmonary dysplasia, 1186
    in developing countries, 123
    problems with, 1118
    trauma from, 1171
  for neonatal resuscitation, 462-465, 1118
  physiology of, 1117
  for respiratory distress syndrome, 123, 1118
  ventilator-derived, 1118
Continuous renal replacement therapy, 1691
Contraction stress test, 176-177, 353t
  in intrauterine growth restriction, 265
Controlled clinical trial (RCT), history of, 14
Convection, heat exchange through, 556
Conversion tables
  atomic weight and valence, 1837t
  for metric units, 1837t
  for standard international units, 1835-1836t
Coombs test, in unconjugated hyperbilirubinemia, 1467
Copper
  in breast milk and breast milk fortifiers, 659t
  in enteral nutrition, 657t
  in infant formula, 661-662t
  in parenteral nutrition, 650
Cor pulmonale, 1267-1268
  diagnosis of, 1267-1268
  prognosis in, 1268
  treatment of, 1268
Cordocentesis, 142
  in alloimmune thrombocytopenia, 338
  in intrauterine growth restriction, 263

Cordocentesis (*Continued*)
  in nonimmune hydrops fetalis, 395
  pregnancy loss after, 142
Cornea
  abnormalities of, 1747-1748
  abrasions of, 1758
  birth injuries to, 510
  clouding of, 1747-1748
    in inborn errors of metabolism, 1644
  dystrophy of, 1748
  enlarged, 1748
  examination of, 1740
  leukoma of, birth-related, 510
  systemic disease manifestations in, 1748
Corneal reflex test, 1739
Cornelia de Lange syndrome, 532
  anesthetic implications of, 604-606t
  eye findings in, 1757
Cornification disorders, 1713-1716, 1714t
Coronal synostosis
  bilateral, 1028, 1029f
  unilateral, 1027-1028, 1028f
Corpus callosum, agenesis of, 159-160, 160f, 907-908,
  908f, 977, 1012-1013
  septo-optic dysplasia with, 908f
Cortical development. *See* Brain, development of.
Cortical dysplasia, in migrational anomalies,
  1012-1013, 1013f
Cortical folding, 898-899, 898f
Cortical lamination, 890-895
Corticosteroids. *See also* Glucocorticoids;
  Mineralocorticoids.
  antenatal
    for germinal matrix hemorrhage–intraventricular
      hemorrhage prophylaxis, 939, 944
    for respiratory distress syndrome, 103, 103f
    sodium balance and, 670
  for bronchopulmonary dysplasia, 1188
  for Diamond-Blackfan anemia, 1323
  effects of, on lung maturation, 1090
  fetal effects of, 719-721t
  in fetal growth, 252
  for hypoxic-ischemic encephalopathy, 968
  for meconium aspiration syndrome, 1160
  plus thyrotropin-releasing hormone, for respiratory
    distress syndrome, 1090, 1107
  postnatal systemic, neuronal apoptosis and, 901
  for preeclampsia/eclampsia, 284
  for preterm labor prevention, 327-328
  for respiratory distress syndrome, 1107
  for tuberculosis, 827
Corticotropin-releasing hormone, in preterm labor
  prediction, 313
Cortisol
  concentration quartiles of, in extremely low
    birthweight infants, 1824t
  deficiency of
    in 21-hydroxylase deficiency, 1610
    hypoglycemia in, 1513
  replacement of
    for congenital adrenal hyperplasia, 1611
    for 11β-hydroxylase deficiency, 1613
    for 17α-hydroxylase deficiency, 1614
    for P-450 oxidoreductase (POR) deficiency, 1615
  serum, reference ranges for, 1824t
  synthesis of, 1608
Cough medicines, fetal effects of, 719-721t
"Couney babies," 9, 11f
Couveuse, 8
Court system, 50, 51f
Coxsackievirus infection. *See* Enterovirus infections.
Crack cocaine, 748-749. *See also* Cocaine abuse.
Cradle cap, 1729
Cranial meningocele, versus cephalhematoma, 504
Cranial nerves, examination of, 496-497, 496t
Craniofacial anomalies. *See under* Face.
Craniofacial dysostosis, 1029-1030, 1030f
Craniofacial syndromes, eye findings in, 1756-1757
Craniorachischisis totalis, 905
Craniosynostosis, 490, 1025-1031, 1026b, 1026t
  classification of, 1025-1026
  coronal
    bilateral, 1028, 1029f
    unilateral, 1027-1028, 1028f

Extracorporeal membrane oxygenation *(Continued)*
  follow-up for, 1198-1199
  future considerations in, 1200
  hypercalcemia after, 1544-1545
  for meconium aspiration syndrome, 1160
  patient selection for, 1194-1198, 1194b
    absence of complex congenital heart disease in, 1194-1195
    cranial ultrasonography in, 1194
    failure of medical therapy in, 1197-1198
    gestational age in, 1194
    mechanical ventilation duration in, 1195
    reversible lung disease in, 1195-1197
  for persistent pulmonary hypertension of the newborn, 1192, 1197
  personnel needs in, 1194
  referral for, 1198, 1198b
  simulation-based learning for, 94
  transfusion during, 1371
  venoarterial, 1192-1193
  venovenous, 1193-1194
Extremely low birthweight. *See under* Low birthweight.
Extremity(ies). *See also specific parts, e.g.,* Foot (feet).
  birth injuries to, 523-526
  congenital anomalies of, 1773
    classification of, 1773
    from constriction band syndrome, 1773, 1783, 1783f
    from duplication, 1773
    examination of, 544-547
    from failure of part differentiation, 1773
    from failure of part formation, 1773
    generalized, 1773
    lower, 1787-1795
    from overgrowth, 1773
    from undergrowth, 1773
    upper, 1782-1785
  disorders of, in utero positioning and, 1774
  embryology of, 1771
  examination of, 488
  hypertrophy of, 545
  joint deformities of, 547
  long bones of, shortening of, 545, 545f
  lower
    congenital anomalies of, 1787-1795
    torsional and angular deformities of, 1787-1788
  thanatophoric dysplasia of, 543, 544f, 545
  upper
    amputations of, congenital, 1784
    congenital anomalies of, 1782-1785
Extubation, 1128-1129
Eye(s)
  abnormalities of, 490, 492
    in chromosomal syndromes, 1756
    in congenital rubella syndrome, 876
    in craniofacial syndromes, 1756-1757
    from maternal substance abuse, 1761
    in neurocutaneous disorders, 1757-1758
    ophthalmologic consultation for, 1742
    in small for gestational age, 268
  alignment of, 1739
  birth trauma to, 1758-1759
  congenital anomalies of
    examination of, 539, 540f, 541f
    in inborn errors of metabolism, 1639t, 1644
    minor, 536t
  corneal abnormalities of, 1747-1748
  dislocation of, 1758
  dry, 1746
  examination of, 486-487, 1737-1741, 1738b, 1738f, 1739f, 1740f, 1741f
  fixation of, 1737
  globe abnormalities of, 1746-1747, 1747f
  growth of, 1741
  herpes simplex virus infection of, 843
  infections of, 1759
  iris abnormalities of, 1748-1749, 1749b
  lacrimal abnormalities of, 1745-1746
  large, 1747, 1747f
  lens abnormalities of, 1750-1751, 1751f
  measurements of, 1741, 1742t
  movements of, assessment of, 496, 1739
  neuromuscular abnormalities of, 1755
  normal findings for, 1741-1742, 1742t
    in preterm infant, 1742, 1742f

Eye(s) *(Continued)*
  optic disc abnormalities of, 1753-1754
  orbital abnormalities of, 1742-1744, 1743b
  pupillary abnormalities of, 1754
  red, 1759
  retinal and vitreous diseases of, 1751-1753. *See also* Retina; Retinopathy.
  scleral abnormalities of, 1747
  sticky, 488
  trauma to, 1758-1759
  tumors of, 1759-1761, 1760f
  visual milestones for, 1738t
  watery, 1745-1746
Eyebrows, fusion of, 539
Eyelashes
  abnormalities of, 1745
  examination of. 1739
  hypertrichosis of, 1745
Eyelids
  abnormalities of, 1744-1745, 1744f, 1745f
  birth injuries to, 509
  coloboma of, 1744, 1744f
  epicanthus of, 1744
  examination of, 1739
  laceration of, 1758-1759
  ptosis of, 1745, 1745f
  swollen, 488-489

F

Face
  appearance of
    in congenital hypothyroidism, 1574, 1574f
    in fetal alcohol syndrome, 736, 737f
    in neonatal physical examination, 486
  asymmetry of, in unilateral coronal synostosis, 1027-1028, 1028f
  birth injuries to, 507-509
  congenital anomalies of
    examination of, 539
    hearing loss in, 1052
    minor, 536t
    phenotypic variants of, 536t
  fetal, ultrasonography of, 149f, 162, 163f
Facemasks, in neonatal resuscitation, 463-464, 464f
Facial bones, fractures and dislocations of, birth-related, 508-509, 508f
Facial diplegia, in neuromuscular disease, 998
Facial nerve
  examination of, 496t, 497
  palsy of, birth-related, 507-509
Facioscapulohumeral muscular dystrophy, 1005
Factor I. *See* Fibrinogen.
Factor II, deficiency of, 1343
Factor V Leiden
  and factor VIII, combined deficiency of, 1343
  thrombosis and, 1347, 1347t
Factor VII, deficiency of, 1343-1344
Factor VIIa, in revised hypothesis of coagulation, 1336, 1336f
Factor VIII
  deficiency of, 1342-1343. *See also* Hemophilia A.
  elevation of, 1347-1348
  and factor V, combined deficiency of, 1343
Factor IX, deficiency of, 1342-1343. *See also* Hemophilia B.
Factor XI, deficiency of, 1343
Factor XIII, deficiency of, 1343
Famciclovir, for herpes simplex virus infection, 407
Familial dysautonomia. *See* Riley-Day syndrome.
Family-centered neonatal intensive care, 37-38, 624-625
Fanconi anemia, 1324, 1324t
  group C, screening for, 140, 141t
  thrombocytopenia in, 1355
Fanconi syndrome, 682
  radial clubhand in, 1783
  renal, 1661, 1661t
Fanconi-Bickel syndrome, 1685t
Farber disease, 1648
Fasciitis, necrotizing, in omphalitis, 818
Fat
  body, drug distribution and
    in neonate, 724
    in pregnancy, 711, 711t
  dietary. *See* Lipid(s).

Fat *(Continued)*
  subcutaneous, necrosis of, 1731
    at birth, 502-503, 503f
Father. *See* Paternal *entries.*
Fatty acids
  in breast milk, 653-654
  free, in fetal oxygen consumption, 249, 249t, 250f
  in infant formula, 654
  oxidation of
    disorders of
      cardiomegaly/cardiomyopathy in, 1643-1644
      hypoglycemia and, 1672-1673
      liver disease in, 1647
      summary of, 1627-1634t
      in small for gestational age, 269, 270f
  placental transfer of, 1497
Febrile nonhemolytic transfusion reactions, 1364-1365
Fecal retention, in spinal cord injury, 520
Feces. *See* Stool.
Federal court system, 50, 51f
Federal law, 50
Feeding
  difficulties with, in late preterm infant, 638
  gavage, history of, 8
Feeding cup (paladai), for preterm infant in developing countries, 117-118, 118f
Femoral nerve, palsy of, birth-related, 526
Femoral pulses, evaluation of, 487
Femur
  fracture of, birth-related, 523-524, 524f, 1777
  length of, in gestational age assessment, 351
  proximal, focal deficiency of, 1791, 1791f
Fentanyl
  during EXIT procedure, 207
  intravenous patient-controlled, 438
  during labor, 438
  in neonatal anesthesia, 610
  pharmacokinetics of, 436
  umbilical vein to maternal vein ratio of, 436t
Ferric chloride test, in inborn errors of metabolism, 1655
Ferritin
  serum, by gestational age, 1830f
  in very low birthweight infants, 1829t
Fetal activity log, in intrauterine growth restriction, 265
Fetal alcohol spectrum disorder, 738, 739f
Fetal alcohol syndrome. *See also* Alcohol, fetal exposure to.
  clinical features of, 736, 737f
  congenital anomalies in, 534, 534f
  diagnosis of, 738, 739f
  eye findings in, 1761
  growth restriction in, 257
  neuronal migration disorders in, 913, 914f
  prevalence of, 736-738, 737f
  prevention of, 740-741
  risk factors for, 737-738
Fetal circulation, 449-450, 450f
  persistent. *See* Pulmonary hypertension, persistent.
  physiology of, 1226
  transition of, to extrauterine circulation, 1227
Fetal death
  incidence of, 175
  as indicator of perinatal care effectiveness, 30
  in multiple gestations, 346
  placental pathology associated with, 428-429, 428b
  in post-term pregnancy, 351-352
  in small for gestational age, 267t, 268, 271-272
Fetal distress
  on Doppler velocimetry, 264
  labor anesthesia and, 445-446
Fetal DNA, from maternal serum, for prenatal diagnosis, 143
Fetal growth
  aberrant patterns of, 261-262, 262f, 263f
    maternal contributions to, 253-257
  alcohol exposure and, 738
  body composition and, 246-247, 247f, 247t, 248t, 249f, 644, 644f
  chronic disease affecting, 255-256, 256f
  corticosteroids in, 252
  in diabetic pregnancy, 292-293
  fetal determinants of, 259-261, 260b
  fluid space distribution in, 247, 247f, 248t

Heart surgery (*Continued*)
  open
    extracorporeal membrane oxygenation after,
      1200
    types of, 1293t
Heart-hand syndrome. *See* Holt-Oram syndrome.
Heat exchange
  in heated beds, 557
  in incubators, 557
  between infant's body surface and environment,
    555-556
    calculation of, 556
  between infant's respiratory tract and environment,
    556, 563-565, 564f, 564t
    calculation of, 557
    through convection, 557
    through evaporation, 557
  between infant's skin and environment, 557-563
    during care on heated beds, 561
    during care under radiant heaters, 560
    at different ambient humidities, 559-560, 560f,
      561f
    during first day after birth, 559, 559f
    during first hours after birth, 557-558, 558f
    during first weeks after birth, 559-560, 561f
    during phototherapy, 560-561
    during skin-to-skin care, 561-563
    during mechanical ventilation, 564-565
    under radiant heaters, 557
  routes of, 555
  through conduction, 556
  through convection, 556
  through evaporation, 556
    ambient humidity and, 559, 560f
  through radiation, 556
Heat exposure, teratogenicity of, 221-222
Heat loss. *See also* Hypothermia.
  prevention of, 566-567
    in delivery room, 566
    in nursery, 566-567
    in very preterm infant, 563
Heated beds, heat exchange in, 557, 561
Heinz bodies, 1321
Helium dilution technique, 1097
Hellin-Zellany rule, in multiple gestations, 343
HELLP syndrome, inborn errors of metabolism and,
  1639-1640
Helmets, skull-molding, for deformational
  plagiocephaly, 1033
Hemangioma, 1725-1727, 1726f, 1726t
  capillary, 489
  cervicofacial, 1727
  hyperbilirubinemia in, 1459
  lumbosacral, 1727
  myocardial, 1273-1274
  periorbital, 1727, 1760
  subglottic, 1176-1177, 1176f, 1727
Hematocrit
  normalization of, partial exchange transfusion for,
    1371
  postnatal changes in, 1309t
  in very low birthweight infants, 1829t
Hematologic abnormalities, in inborn errors of
  metabolism, 1645
Hematologic values, 1829
Hematoma, of external ear, birth-related, 511
Hematopoiesis
  anatomic and functional shifts in, 1303-1304
  development of, 1303-1304, 1304f
  fetal, 762
  overview of, 761-762
Hematopoietic growth factors, 762, 766, 1304, 1305t
Hematopoietic stem cells, 761-762, 1303-1304, 1304f
  transplantation of, for dyskeratosis congenita, 1330
Hematuria, 1688-1689
Heme
  biosynthesis of, inborn errors of, 1732-1733
  catabolism of, to bilirubin, 1443-1445, 1444f
Heme oxygenase inhibitors, for unconjugated
  hyperbilirubinemia
    metalloporphyrin, 1477
    nonmetalloporphyrin, 1477
Heme oxygenase-1, in heme conversion to biliverdin,
  1443, 1444f

Hemifacial microsomia, 541, 542f
  eye findings in, 1757
Hemimegalencephaly, 910
Hemiplegia
  after arterial ischemic stroke, 948
  after germinal matrix hemorrhage–intraventricular
    hemorrhage, 942-943, 943f
Hemivertebra, 162, 162f
Hemodialysis, intermittent, 1691
Hemoglobin, 1304-1307
  at birth, 1309t
  developmental expression of, 1304-1306, 1306t
  embryonic, 1306, 1306t
  fetal, 1304-1306, 1306t
    neonatal anesthesia and, 600
  globin chain composition of, 1304-1306, 1306t
    switching of, 1306, 1307f
  in infants, 1307-1308, 1308f, 1309t
  light absorption by, 586, 586f
  oxygen dissociation curve of, 1094, 1094f, 1304-
    1306, 1306f
  unstable, 1321
  in very low birthweight infants, 1829t
Hemoglobin A, 1304-1306, 1306t
Hemoglobin A₂, 1306, 1306t
Hemoglobin E, 1321
Hemoglobin F, 1304-1306, 1306t
Hemoglobin M, in methemoglobinemia, 1325
Hemoglobin S, and sickle cell anemia, 1320
Hemoglobin variants, 1319-1321, 1320b, 1321f
Hemoglobinopathies, screening for, 139-140
Hemoglobinuria, 1688-1689
Hemolysis, 1308
Hemolytic anemia, 1313
  alloimmune, 1313-1315, 1314t
  autoimmune, 1315
  erythrocyte structural defects in, 1315-1316, 1316f,
    1317f
  glucose-6-phosphate dehydrogenase deficiency and,
    1317-1318
  hemoglobin E and, 1321
  hemoglobin S and, 1320
  hemoglobin variants and, 1319-1321, 1320b, 1321f
  hereditary elliptocytosis and, 1316, 1316f, 1317f
  hereditary pyropoikilocytosis and, 1316, 1316f,
    1317f
  hereditary spherocytosis and, 1316, 1316f
  infectious causes of, 1313t
  inherited enzymatic defects in, 1317-1318, 1318b
  membrane lipid defects in, 1316-1317
  nonimmune, 1315-1318
  thalassemias and, 1318-1319
  unstable hemoglobins and, 1321
  vitamin E deficiency and, 1318
Hemolytic disease
  of newborn
    ABO, 1314, 1456
    alloimmune, 1313-1315
    minor blood group, 1314-1315
    natural history of, 1315
    Rh, 1314, 1314t
    thrombocytopenia in, 1353-1354
  in utero. *See* Erythroblastosis fetalis.
Hemolytic transfusion reactions, 1365
Hemophagocytic lymphohistiocytosis syndrome, 1358
Hemophilia A, 1342-1343
Hemophilia B, 1342-1343
Hemophilia C, 1343
Hemorrhage
  adrenal
    birth-related, 521-522, 522f
    diagnostic imaging in, 702
  cerebellar, 938, 943
  cerebral, in immune thrombocytopenic purpura,
    335-336
  fetal-maternal, anemia and, 1312-1318
  germinal matrix–intraventricular. *See* Germinal matrix
    hemorrhage–intraventricular hemorrhage.
  intracranial
    antenatal, in alloimmune thrombocytopenia,
      337-338
    in immune thrombocytopenic purpura, 335-336
    seizures and, 987
    traumatic, macrocephaly in, 1025, 1025f

Hemorrhage (*Continued*)
  neonatal, causes of, 1313
  orbital, 1758
  pulmonary, 1163-1164
    chest radiography in, 688-689
    in small for gestational age, 267t
    after surfactant therapy, 1111
    treatment of, 1163-1164
  retinal, 1758
    birth-related, 510
    after delivery, 1758
    in shaken baby syndrome, 1758
  retrobulbar, 1758
  subarachnoid, 944
    seizures and, 987-988
  subconjunctival, 489
    at birth, 509-510
  subdural, 944, 945f
    macrocephaly in, 1025, 1025f
    seizures and, 987-988
  subependymal, 702-703, 703f
  subgaleal, 505-506, 505f
  vitreous, birth-related, 510
Hemorrhagic disease of the newborn, 1344
Hemostasis, 1334-1355
  anticoagulant strategies and proteins in, 1336-1337
  blood vessels in, 1334-1335
  coagulation and fibrinolysis in, physiologic
    alterations of, 1337-1338, 1338t, 1339t, 1340t
  coagulation factors in, 1335-1336, 1336f
  components of, 1334-1338
  defects in, 1338-1345
    acquired, 1344-1345
    congenital, 1342-1344, 1342t
  endothelium in, 1334-1335, 1335f
  fibrinolytic system in, 1337, 1337f
  laboratory testing of, 1340-1341, 1341f, 1342t
  platelets in, 1334-1335, 1335f
  thrombotic disorders and, 1346-1351
  von Willebrand factor in, 1335, 1335f
Henderson-Hasselbach equation, 677
Heparin
  for antiphospholipid antibody syndrome, 340
  in breast milk, 730
  intravenous lipid emulsions and, 648
  for thrombosis
    low-molecular-weight, 1348-1349, 1349b
    unfractionated, 1348, 1349b
Heparin cofactor, reference values for, 1340t
Heparin sulfate deficiency, protein-losing enteropathy
  in, 1389
Hepatitis, 409-411, 867-871
  conjugated hyperbilirubinemia in, 1486-1489
  in enterovirus infections, 866
  idiopathic neonatal, 1486-1488
    causes of, 1484
    clinical manifestations of, 1485
    definition of, 1483
    liver biopsy in, 1486, 1486f
    prognosis in, 1484
    treatment of, 1486-1487
Hepatitis A, 409, 867
  transfusion-transmitted, 1363
Hepatitis B, 409, 867-869
  blood tests for, 868
  clinical manifestations of, 409f, 410, 868
  diagnosis of, 409, 409f
  epidemiology of, 409
  immunization for, 410, 869
  maternal-fetal transmission of, 409-410, 410t
  perinatal transmission of, 868
  screening for, 410
  transfusion-transmitted, 1363-1364
Hepatitis B core antigen, antibody against, 868
Hepatitis B immune globulin, 410, 869
Hepatitis B surface antigen, 868
  maternal transmission of, 1488
Hepatitis B vaccine, 869
Hepatitis C, 410-411
  HIV coinfection with, 870
  maternal transmission of, 1488-1489
  perinatal, 869-870
  in pregnancy, 411
  transfusion-transmitted, 1364

Hydrocephalus (*Continued*)
classification of, 1018
clinical presentation of, 1018-1019
communicating, 1018
Dandy-Walker malformation and, 1019-1020, 1020f
external, 1022, 1022f
in germinal matrix hemorrhage–intraventricular hemorrhage, 937, 937f
intracranial cysts and, 1023-1024, 1024f
in meningitis, 806
noncommunicating, 1018
posthemorrhagic, 1021-1022, 1021f, 1022f
postinfectious, 1022
prenatal imaging of, 1019, 1019f
X-linked, 1019
Hydrochloric acid, secretion of, 1377-1378
Hydrocodone
abuse of, 745
in breast milk, 732
Hydrocortisone
for congenital adrenal hyperplasia, 1611
for preterm labor prevention, 328
Hydrogel, 579
Hydrogen electrodes, 578-579
Hydronephrosis, 1697-1699
Eagle-Barrett syndrome and, 1699
fetal surgery for, 189-191
physiologic, 1698
of pregnancy, 399
posterior urethral valves and, 1698
postnatal management of, 1698
prenatal diagnosis of, 1697, 1698f
prenatal management of, 1697-1698
ultrasonography in, 138
ureteropelvic junction obstruction and, 1698
ureterovesical junction obstruction and, 1698
vesicoureteral reflux and, 1699
Hydrops fetalis, 1315, 1319
in fetal anemia, 359-361, 360f
in fetal parvovirus infection, 412, 873
immune. *See* Erythroblastosis fetalis.
lysosomal storage disorders and, 1640
neonatal resuscitation and, 482
nonimmune, 390-397
delivery indications for, 397
diagnosis of, 391, 391f, 391t, 393-396, 395b
etiology of, 391-393, 392b, 394t
fetal echocardiography in, 393
fetal surgery for, 396-397
incidence of, 390
invasive fetal testing in, 395
maternal laboratory testing in, 393-395
pathophysiology of, 391
postnatal evaluation of, 395-396, 396b
prognosis of, 397
related to cardiovascular function, 1230-1231, 1231b
treatment of, 396-397, 396b
conservative, 396
experimental, 396-397
ultrasonography in, 391, 391f, 391t, 393, 395f
parvovirus-induced, 1323
polyhydramnios in, 389
Hydrothorax, fetal, thoracoamniotic shunting for, 191-193, 191f, 191t, 192f, 193f
3-Hydroxy-3-methylglutaric aciduria, 1627-1634t, 1661
3-Hydroxyacyl-CoA dehydrogenase deficiency
long-chain, 1627-1634t
maternal disease associated with, 1640
medium-chain, 1627-1634t, 1637-1638
short-chain, 1627-1634t
very-long-chain, 1627-1634t
β-Hydroxybutyrate
in lactic acidemia, 1665
placental transfer of, 1497-1498
3-Hydroxyisobutyryl-CoA deaclyase deficiency, 1651
11β-Hydroxylase deficiency, 1612-1613
17α-Hydroxylase deficiency, 1614
21-Hydroxylase deficiency, 1609-1612, 1609f, 1610f
diagnosis of, 1610-1611
gender assignment in, 1612
genetics of, 1612
hormonal abnormalities in, 1610

21-Hydroxylase deficiency (*Continued*)
newborn screening for, 1611
pathology of, 1610
prenatal diagnosis and treatment of, 1612, 1613f
salt-wasting form of, 1610, 1610f
simple virilizing form of, 1609
treatment of, 1611-1612
ultrasonography in, 1611
17α-hydroxyprogesterone (17-OHP)
in 21-Hydroxylase deficiency, 1610
measurement of, 1611
normal values for, 1824t
serum, in sex development disorders, 1596
3β-Hydroxysteroid dehydrogenase deficiency, 1613-1614
17β-Hydroxysteroid dehydrogenase deficiency, 1604
Hydroxyzine, during labor, 437
Hygroma, cystic, 162-163, 163f, 1728
Hyperammonemia, 1673-1675
differential diagnosis of, 1653t, 1673-1674, 1673b, 1674f
secondary, 1675
urea cycle defects and, 1674-1675
Hyperbilirubinemia
conjugated, 1481-1490, 1481f, 1482f
causes of, 1483-1490
infectious, 1488-1489
miscellaneous, 1490
definition of, 1450
diseases manifested as, 1483, 1483b
hepatic metabolic disease and, 1489
hepatitis and
idiopathic, 1486-1488. *See also* Hepatitis, idiopathic neonatal.
infectious, 1488-1489
laboratory tests for, 1485, 1485b
liver biopsy in, 1485-1486
maternal, 1451
mechanical obstruction and, 1489-1490
sepsis and, 1489
total parenteral nutrition–induced hepatic injury and, 1489
in hemolytic disease of newborn, 1315
in late preterm infant, 638
neonatal, 1451-1453, 1451f, 1452f
transient familial neonatal, 1460
unconjugated
causes of, 1454-1461
conjugation disorders as, 1459-1460
enterohepatic circulation disorders as, 1460-1461
excretion disorders as, 1460
hepatic uptake disorders as, 1459
production disorders as, 1454-1459, 1454b
Crigler-Najjar syndrome and
kernicterus in, 1464
type I, 1449f, 1459-1460
type II, 1460
definition of, 1450
diagnosis of, 1465-1468, 1465t
bilirubin-to-albumin molar ratio in, 1468, 1469t
end-tidal carbon monoxide measurements in, 1468
total bilirubin measurements in, 1450f, 1465-1468, 1466f
transcutaneous bilirubinometry in, 1468
encephalopathy in, transient, 1462, 1462f
exchange transfusion for, 1478-1480, 1479f, 1480b
genetic, ethnic, and cultural differences in, 1453
glucose-6-phosphate dehydrogenase deficiency and, 1456-1458
hypothyroidism and, 1460
infection and, 1458
intravenous immunoglobulin for, 1469b, 1478
isoimmunization and, 1455-1456
kernicterus in, 1462-1464, 1463f
in late preterm neonate, 1453
Lucey-Driscoll syndrome and, 1460
metalloporphyrins for, 1477
nonpathologic, 1450-1453, 1450f
pathologic, 1453-1481
zones of risk for, 1450, 1450f

Hyperbilirubinemia (*Continued*)
pharmacologic therapy for, 1476-1478
phenobarbital for, 1476-1477
phototherapy for, 1470-1476. *See also* Phototherapy.
polycythemia and, 1459
postdischarge follow-up for, 1480-1481, 1481b
in post-term neonate, 1453
in preterm neonate, 1452-1453
pyloric stenosis and, 1460
red blood cell enzymatic defects and, 1456
red blood cell structural defects and, 1458
sequelae of, 1461-1464
sequestration and, 1458-1459
severe, risk factors for, 1467, 1467b
in term neonate, 1451-1452, 1451f
treatment of, 1468-1480, 1469b
guidelines for, 1466f, 1475f, 1479f, 1480, 1481t
Hypercalcemia, 1544-1548
blue diaper syndrome and, 1547
carbohydrate malabsorption and, 1546-1547
causes of, 1545b
clinical manifestations of, 1544, 1547
definition of, 1544
diagnosis of, 1545b, 1547
familial hypocalciuric, 1546
hyperparathyroidism and, 1545-1547
primary, 1545-1546
secondary, 1545
hypophosphatasia and, 1547
hypophosphatemic, 1544-1545
hypothyroidism and, 1547
iatrogenic, 1544-1545
idiopathic infantile, 1546
Jansen metaphyseal chondrodysplasia and, 1547
maternal, fetal hypoparathyroidism from, 1542
renal tubular acidosis and, 1547
from subcutaneous fat necrosis, 1546
treatment of, 1547-1548
tumor-related, 1547
in Williams syndrome, 1546
Hypercapnia
in bronchopulmonary dysplasia, 1186
fetal, 1142
permissive
for congenital diaphragmatic hernia, 1197
as lung protective strategy, 1137
ventilatory response to, 1151-1153
in apnea of prematurity, 1146, 1146f
Hypercarbia, germinal matrix hemorrhage–intraventricular hemorrhage risk and, 939
Hypercholesterolemia, maternal, atherosclerosis and, 236
Hyperekplexia, 980-982
Hyperglycemia, 1518-1519
definition of, 1518
in extremely low birthweight, 648
in low birthweight, 1518-1519
in neonate, 600
parenteral nutrition and, 648
in small for gestational age, 267t
Hyperglycinemia, nonketotic, 1627-1634t, 1641
Hyperimmune globulin, cytomegalovirus, 850
Hyperinsulinemia
hypoglycemia with, 1510-1512, 1511f
in infant of diabetic mother, 292-293
Hyperkalemia
in perinatal asphyxia, 676
renal tubular acidosis with, 681b, 682
from transfusion, 1361
Hypermagnesemia
clinical manifestations of, 1550
etiology of, 1549b, 1550
neuromuscular disorders in, 1001
treatment of, 1550
Hypernatremia, 675-676
seizures in, 987
Hyperoxemia
detection of, 601
iatrogenic, 600-601
Hyperoxia test, 1096
in congenital heart disease, 1239

Marijuana use, 744
    fetal and neonate effects of, 744
    neurobehavioral and developmental effects of, 744
    pharmacology of, 744
    prevalence of, 744
Masks
    face, in neonatal resuscitation, 463-464, 464f
    laryngeal
        in neonatal anesthesia, 608
        in neonatal resuscitation, 465
Mass spectrometry, screening for inborn errors of
    metabolism based on, 1624, 1627-1634t
Mast cell tumor, 1730
Mastitis, 818-819
Mastocytosis, 1730
Materials safety data sheets, 225
Maternal. *See also* Parent(s); Pregnancy.
Maternal age
    advanced, late preterm birth and, 633
    genetic disorders and, 129-130, 131f
    preterm delivery and, 307
Maternal artery(ies)
    occlusion of, 426
    rupture of, 426
    stenosis of, 426
Maternal genes, fetal growth and, 253
Maternal morbidity, in preeclampsia/eclampsia, 285
Maternal mortality
    cultural beliefs and, 110
    global burden of, 107
    global interventions for reducing, 107-108, 109t
    as indicator of perinatal care effectiveness, 30-31
    in preeclampsia/eclampsia, 285
Maternal-fetal hemorrhage, anemia and, 1312-1318
Maternal-fetal substrate hormone relationship,
    1497-1498, 1498f
Maternal-fetal-placental unit
    drug disposition in, 709-712, 710f, 711t, 712t
    pharmacology of, 709-716, 710f
    substrate hormone relationship in, 1497-1498,
        1498f
Maternally inherited Leigh syndrome (MILS), 1668
Matrix metalloproteinases, in preterm labor
    prediction, 314
Maxillary hypoplasia
    in Apert syndrome, 1030, 1030f
    in Crouzon syndrome, 1029-1030, 1030f
    in Pfeiffer syndrome, 1031, 1031f
Maximal expiratory flow volume relationship,
    1100-1102, 1102f
Maximum vertical pocket
    measurement of, 379, 379t
    perinatal mortality related to, 382-383, 383f
    in twin gestation, 381-382, 382f
Mayer-Rokitansky-Küster-Hauser (MRKH) syndrome,
    1616
May-Hegglin anomaly, platelet abnormalities in, 1355
McArdle disease, 1008, 1647
McCune-Albright syndrome, 1722
MDMA (methylenedioxymethamphetamine; Ecstasy),
    753
Mead Whittenberger technique, in pulmonary
    function testing, 1100, 1101f
Mean airway pressure, determinants of, 1119-1120,
    1119b, 1120f
Mean corpuscular hemoglobin, postnatal changes in,
    1309t
Mean corpuscular volume, postnatal changes in,
    1309t
Measles, 854-855
    German. *See* Rubella virus infection.
MEB (muscle-eye-brain) syndrome, 912-913
Mechanical stimulation program, for osteopenia of
    prematurity, 1553
Mechanical ventilation, 1116-1138
    air leaks in, 1135-1136
    alveolarization and, 1078-1079, 1079f, 1080f
    assist/control, 1122
    base deficit during, 1131
    brain injuries from, 1138
    bronchopulmonary dysplasia after, 1137, 1137f,
        1182
    chest radiography in, 1131
    clinical evaluation during, 1130

Mechanical ventilation (*Continued*)
    complications of, 1079b, 1134-1137
        airway, 1134
        lung, 1134-1137, 1137f
        neurologic, 1138
    control variables in, 1121
    duration of, extracorporeal membrane oxygenation
        and, 1195
    endotracheal intubation for. *See* Endotracheal
        intubation.
    endotracheal tube leak in, 1134f
    end-tidal carbon dioxide monitoring during, 1131
    extubation in, 1128-1129
    gas exchange assessment during, 1130-1131
    guidelines for, 1126-1127, 1127t
    heat exchange during, 564-565
    high-frequency. *See* High-frequency ventilation.
    history of, 10-12, 12f, 13-14t
    imposed work of breathing in, 1138
    indications for, 1119, 1119b
    intermittent mandatory, 1122, 1122f
    monitoring during, 1130-1131
    during neonatal anesthesia, 607-608
    noninvasive. *See* Continuous positive airway pressure
        (CPAP); Nasal intermittent positive-pressure
        ventilation.
    oxygenation determinants in, 1119-1120, 1119b,
        1120f
    patent ductus arteriosus after, 1138
    phase variables in, 1121-1122
    positive-pressure. *See* Positive pressure ventilation.
    postextubation care in, 1128-1129
    pressure augmentation, 1126
    pressure control, 1123
    pressure support, 1122-1124, 1123f
        volume assured, 1126
    pressure-limited, 1123
    principles of, 1119-1126
    prolonged, after neonatal resuscitation, 480
    pulmonary function monitoring during, 583-584,
        1103
    pulmonary graphic monitoring during, 1131-1134,
        1131f, 1132f, 1133f, 1134f
    pulmonary time constant in, 1121
    in respiratory distress syndrome, 1110
    retinopathy of prematurity after, 1138
    strategies for
        for bronchopulmonary dysplasia, 1186, 1189
        for congenital diaphragmatic hernia, 1152
        for meconium aspiration syndrome, 1160
        pneumothorax associated with, 1164
        for pulmonary hemorrhage, 1163-1164
    synchronized intermittent mandatory, 1122,
        1122f
    during transport, 603
    ultrasonography during, 1131
    ventilation determinants in, 1120-1121, 1120b
    ventilatory modalities in, 1121
        hybrid volume-targeted, 1125-1126
        pressure-targeted, 1123-1124, 1124t
        volume-targeted, 1124-1125, 1125f
    ventilatory modes in, 1121-1123, 1128
    volume control, 1124-1125, 1125f, 1127, 1127t
        as lung protective strategy, 1137
        pressure-regulated, 1126
    volume guarantee, 1125-1126, 1127
    volume support, 1126
    weaning from, 1127-1128, 1127b
        strategies for, 1128
        ventilatory modes and, 1128
Meconium, infant, substance abuse and, 736
Meconium ascites, 1422
Meconium aspiration
    neonatal resuscitation and, 481
    versus pneumonia, 810
Meconium aspiration pneumonia, in small for
    gestational age, 267t
Meconium aspiration syndrome, 1157-1160
    amniotic fluid volume assessment in, 381
    chest radiography in, 688, 688f, 1158, 1159f
    clinical features of, 1158-1159, 1159f
    definition of, 1157
    in dysmaturity syndrome, 352
    incidence of, 1157

Meconium aspiration syndrome (*Continued*)
    management of, 1159-1160, 1159b
        in delivery room, 1159-1160
        in neonatal intensive care unit, 1160
    pathophysiology of, 1157-1158, 1158f
Meconium ileus
    in cystic fibrosis, 1383, 1421-1422
    diagnostic imaging in, 695, 695f
Meconium peritonitis, 165, 165f, 1422
Meconium plug syndrome, 694-695, 695f, 1422-1423
Meconium pseudocyst, 1422
Meconium staining, 1157
    amnioinfusion for, 388
    seizures and, 986
Medical errors, in neonatal intensive care unit, 68,
    86-87, 87b
Medical ethics. *See* Ethics.
Medical Injury Compensation Reform Act of 1975
    (MICRA), 58
Medical malpractice stress syndrome, 57
Medical personnel. *See* Health care personnel.
Medical Subject Headings (MeSH terms), 100
Medical uncertainty, communication of, 36
Medium-chain 3-hydroxyacyl-CoA dehydrogenase
    (MCAD) deficiency, 1627-1634t, 1637-1638
Medium-chain fatty acid oxidation disorders, 1672
Medium-chain triglycerides, for chylothorax, 1154
MEDLINE, 100, 100t
Megakaryocytic leukemia, acute, 1356-1357
Megakaryocytopoiesis, 1351
Megalencephaly. *See* Macrencephaly.
Megalocornea, 1748
Meissner tactile organs, 1709
Melanocytes, development of, 1706-1707
Melanocytic nevi
    congenital, 1722
    congenital giant, 1723-1724, 1723f
Melanocytoma, dermal, 1724
Melanosis, pustular, transient neonatal, 1711-1712,
    1712f
Membranes
    rupture of
        artificial, for labor induction, 354-355
        premature. *See* Premature rupture of membranes.
    stripping of, for labor induction, 354
    thickness of, 712-713
Mendelian disorders, 131-133, 133f, 134f
    affecting musculoskeletal system, 1772
    screening for, 139-140, 140t, 141t
Meningitis, 113, 806-809
    bacterial, hydrocephalus after, 1022
    in candidiasis, 831-832
    clinical manifestations of, 806-807
    diagnosis of, 807-808, 807t, 808t
    etiology of, 806
    hearing loss in, 1052
    incidence of, 806
    pathogenesis of, 806
    pathology of, 806
    prognosis in, 808-809
    treatment of, 808
Meningocele
    cranial, versus cephalhematoma, 504
    orbital, 1743
Meningoencephalitis, 809
    in enterovirus infections, 866
Meningomyelocele. *See* Myelomeningocele.
Menkes disease, hair abnormalities in, 1644
Mental Developmental Index, in Bayley Scales of
    Infant Development, 1043
Meperidine
    intravenous patient-controlled, 438
    during labor, 438
    umbilical vein-to-maternal vein ratio of, 436t
Meprobamate, in breast milk, 731
Mercury
    in breast milk, 732-733
    fetal exposure to, 219-221
    maternal exposure to, pregnancy outcome in, 220t
Merkel corpuscles, 1709
Merosin-deficient muscular dystrophy, 1002-1003
Mesentericoaxial volvulus, 1412
Mesocardia, 1267
Mesomelia, 169, 545

Mitral valve, abnormalities of, in multiple left heart defects, 1259
Mixed gonadal dysgenesis, 1600
Möbius syndrome
  anesthetic implications of, 604-606t
  versus facial nerve palsy, 507-509
Mole, cutaneous. See Nevus(i).
Molybdenum, in enteral nutrition, 657t
Molybdenum cofactor deficiency, seizures in, 991, 1642
Mondini dysplasia, 1052
Mongolian blue spots, 489, 1710
Monitoring. See Fetal monitoring; Neonatal monitoring.
Monoamine oxidase inhibitors, fetal effects of, 719-721t
Monoclonal antibody testing, in oligohydramnios, 387
Monocyte deactivation, 777
Monocyte monolayer assay, in erythroblastosis fetalis, 364
Mononuclear phagocytes. See Phagocytes.
Monosodium glutamate, metabolic dysfunction and, 224-225
Monosomy, 130
Monosomy X. See Turner syndrome.
Montalvo case, on neonatal resuscitation, 63
Moral dilemma, 33
Moral distress, 34
Moral uncertainty, 33
Morgagni hernia, 1406
Morning glory disc anomaly, 1753
Moro reflex, 488, 498-499, 499t
Morphine
  in breast milk, 732
  during labor, 438
  for neonatal abstinence syndrome, 746
  in neonatal anesthesia, 610
  umbilical vein-to-maternal vein ratio of, 436t
Mortality. See Fetal death; Infant mortality; Maternal mortality; Neonatal mortality; Perinatal mortality.
Mosaicism, 130t, 131
  placental, 428
Mother. See Maternal entries.
Mother-Baby Package, 108, 109t
Motility disorders, diarrhea and malabsorption in, 1395
Motor and sensory neuropathy, hereditary, 999-1000
Motor cortex, watershed injury to, 954
Motor system. See also Musculoskeletal system.
  development of, environmental influences on, 1059, 1059f
  examination of, 497-498, 497f
  in preterm infant, 1061-1063, 1061t
Mouth
  congenital anomalies of, examination of, 539f, 541-543, 541f, 543f
  examination of, 487
  herpes simplex virus infection of, 843
  lesions of, 1171-1173
Movement disorders, nonepileptic, 979-982
Mucolipidosis, screening for, 140, 141t
Mucopolysaccharidoses, 1648
  anesthetic implications of, 604-606t
Mucosal obstruction, nasal, 1171
Müllerian anomaly, 157, 157f
  preterm delivery and, 308
Müllerian ducts
  development of, 1586
  dysgenesis of, 1616-1617
  persistent, 1606-1607
Müllerian-inhibiting substance. See Antimüllerian hormone.
Multifactorial genetic disorders, 135
  screening for, 139
Multi-minicore myopathy, 1006
Multiple acyl-CoA dehydrogenase deficiency, 1647, 1652, 1662
Multiple carboxylase deficiency, 1662
Multiple gestations, 343-350. See also Twin(s).
  amniotic fluid volume in, 381-382, 382f
  biology in, 343-344
  birthweight discordance in, 347-348
  chorionicity in, 344
  chromosomal anomalies in, 345
  delivery considerations in, 348
  embryonic and fetal demise in, 346
  fetal and neonatal consequences of, 344-348
  fetal growth in, 347-348

Multiple gestations (Continued)
  growth restriction in, 253, 254f
  Hellin-Zellany rule in, 343
  late preterm birth and, 633
  malformations in, 345-346, 345t
  maternal consequences of, 344, 345b
  multifetal pregnancy reduction in, 349
  outcome of, 348-349
  placental insufficiency in, 259, 259f
  preterm delivery in, 309
  prevention of, 349
  twin-twin transfusion syndrome in, 345-347, 346b
  ultrasonography of, 150-151, 152-153, 154f
  zygosity in, 343-344
Multiple interruption technique, in pulmonary function testing, 1099-1100, 1100f, 1101f
Multiple organ dysfunction, in intrauterine growth restriction, 269
Multiple-hit hypothesis, of brain lesions, 920-921, 921f
Mumps virus, 854
Murmurs. See Heart murmurs.
Muscle biopsy
  for congenital muscular dystrophy, 1002, 1002f
  fetal, for Duchenne muscular dystrophy, 196
  for spinal muscular atrophy, 999, 999f
Muscle tone
  abnormalities of. See Hypertonia; Hypotonia.
  examination of, 488, 497
    in high-risk neonate, 1043
Muscle-eye-brain disease, 912-913, 1004
Muscular atrophy, spinal, 998-999, 999f
Muscular dystrophy
  congenital, 1002-1004, 1002b, 1002f, 1003f
  Duchenne, 1005
  facioscapulohumeral. 1005
  Fukuyama, 1004
  merosin-deficient, 1002-1003
  with rigid spine, 1003
  syndromic forms of, 1003-1004
  Ullrich, 1003
Muscular torticollis, 1775-1776, 1776f
  birth-related, 517-518, 517f
Musculoskeletal system
  bone and joint infections in, 1778-1781
  congenital abnormalities of, 1772-1774
    genetic, 1772-1773
    limb malformations as, 1773
    in lower extremities, 1787-1795
    spinal defects as, 1773-1774, 1785-1786
    syndromes associated with, 1795-1797
    teratogenic, 1772
    in upper extremities, 1782-1785
    in utero positioning and, 1774
  embryology of, 1771-1772
  trauma to, 1774-1777
  ultrasonography of, 169-171, 171f, 172f
Mustard operation, 1293t
Myasthenia gravis, 340-341
  autoimmune, 1000
  ptosis in, 1745
  transient acquired, 1000-1001
Myasthenic syndromes, congenital, 1001, 1001b
Mycobacterium tuberculosis, 826
Mydriasis, 1754
Myelination, 890f, 903-904, 903t, 1059
  absence of
    from germinal matrix hemorrhage–intraventricular hemorrhage, 942-943, 943f
    from white matter injury, 926, 928f, 929-932, 932f
  imaging characteristics of, 890f, 904
  sequence of, 903-904, 903t
Myeloblasts, 762
Myelocytes, 762
Myelogenous leukemia, acute, 1356-1357
Myelokathexis, neutropenia in, 1330
Myelomeningocele, 160, 160f, 161f, 905-906, 906f
  in Chiari II malformation, 1020-1021
  fetal surgery for, 190t
    fetoscopic, 198
    open, 201-202
  surgical closure of, 906
Myelomonocytic leukemia, juvenile, 1357
Myelopathy, from cervical spinal cord injury, 999

Myeloperoxidase deficiency, 1334
Myeloschisis, 905
Myocardial dysfunction, 1272
  diagnosis of, 1272, 1273b
  fetal echocardiography in, 1230-1231
  in hypoxic-ischemic encephalopathy, 966
  treatment of, 1272
Myocarditis, 1272
  in adenovirus infection, 880
  in enterovirus infections, 866
Myocardium
  performance of, assessment of, 1235-1237
  structure of, developmental changes in, 1235
  tumors of, 1272-1274, 1274f
Myoclonic encephalopathy, early, 991
Myoclonic epilepsy with ragged red fibers (MERRF), 134t
Myoclonic seizures, 979, 980f
Myoclonus, without electroencephalographic seizures, 980-982, 981f
Myocytes, development of, 1235
Myofibromatosis, infantile, 1358
Myoglobinuria, 1688-1689
Myoneurogastrointestinal disorder and encephalopathy (MNGIE), 134t
Myopathy. See also Cardiomyopathy.
  congenital, 1005-1007
  mitochondrial, 1007
  multi-minicore, 1006
  myotubular, 1006-1007, 1006f
  nemaline, 1005-1006, 1006f
Myotomy, in esophageal atresia/tracheoesophageal fistula, 1403
Myotonic dystrophy, congenital, 1004-1005
Myotubular myopathy, 1006-1007, 1006f
Myxedema, thyroid hormone replacement and, 1579

N

Nafcillin
  for pneumonia, 1162
  for sepsis, 802t, 803t
  for skin infections, 817
Nail-patella syndrome, 1685t
Nalbuphine
  during labor, 439
  umbilical vein-to-maternal vein ratio of, 436t
Naloxone
  during labor, 439
  in neonatal abstinence syndrome, 746-747
  in neonatal resuscitation, 477t, 479
Naphthalene, fetal exposure to, 219
Narcotics. See Opioids.
Nasal. See also Nose.
Nasal continuous positive airway pressure. See Continuous positive airway pressure (CPAP), nasal.
Nasal flaring, in pulmonary function testing, 1093
Nasal intermittent positive-pressure ventilation, 1118-1119
Nasal septum
  dislocation of, birth-related, 508, 508f
  fracture of, birth-related, 509
Nasal stenosis, anterior, 1170
Nasal tube, single, in neonatal resuscitation, 465
Nasolacrimal duct cysts, 1170, 1170f
Nasopharyngeal lesions, 1170-1171
Nasopharyngeal teratoma, 1171
National Aeronautics and Space Administration (NASA), simulation-based learning at, 93
National Institute of Child Health and Human Development (NICHD)
  Neonatal Network database of, 74
  Neonatal Research Network, 82-83
National Organization for Rare Disorders (NORD), 551
National Perinatal Information Center, 82
National Quality Forum (NQF), perinatal care standards of, 74, 75-80t, 75t
Natural childbirth, for labor pain, 434
Natural killer cells, 768-769
  function of, transcription factors in, 769
  g-c chain mutation of, 769
  in neonates, 769
  phenotypic and functional characteristics of, 768
  production and differentiation of, 769

PHACES syndrome, 1727
Phagocytes, 766-768, 1326-1334. *See also* Neutrophil(s).
  abnormalities of, 1327-1331
  adhesion of, 767
    disorders of, 1331-1332, 1332f
  in breast milk, 790
  chemotaxis of, 767
    disorders in, 1332
  function of, 767-768, 1326
    extrinsic defects of, 1327-1328
    intrinsic defects of, 1331-1334
  in inflammatory response, 775, 775f
  ingestion and degranulation disorders of, 1332-1333
  kinetics of, 1326, 1327t
  microbicidal activity of, 767-768
  in neonates, 768
  number of, 1326, 1326t
  oxidative killing disorders of, 1333-1334, 1333b, 1334t
  phagocytosis by, 767
  physiology of, 1326
  production and differentiation of, 766-767
Phagocytosis
  by neutrophils, 765, 766f
  by phagocytes, 767
Phagolysosome, 765-766
Phakomatoses, macrencephaly in, 1017
Pharmacokinetics
  fetal, 222-223, 223f, 436-437, 436t
  neonatal, 728-729, 728f
Pharmacology. *See also* Drug(s).
  developmental, 709-733
  of maternal-fetal-placental unit, 709-716, 710f
Phenobarbital
  in breast milk, 731
  in Crigler-Najjar syndrome, 1460
  fetal effects of, 719-721t
  for germinal matrix hemorrhage–intraventricular hemorrhage prophylaxis, 944
  in hypoxic-ischemic encephalopathy, 967
  during labor, 437
  for neonatal abstinence syndrome, 746
  for preterm labor, 328
  for seizures, 992-993
  therapeutic monitoring of, 729
  for unconjugated hyperbilirubinemia, 1476-1477
Phenothiazines, during labor, 437
Phenotype, definition of, 531
Phenotypic effects
  of environmental exposures, 224, 224b
  of nutritional deficiency during gestation, 229. *See also* Fetal origins of adult disease.
  of toxins, 235
  transgenerational persistence of, 235-236
Phenotypic variants, 536, 536t
Phenylacetate, for urea cycle defects, 1675
Phenylalanine, in parenteral amino acid solutions, 646t
Phenylalanine hydroxylase deficiency, 1638
Phenylbutyrate, for urea cycle defects, 1675
Phenylephrine
  fetal effects of, 719-721t
  for tachycardia, 1284t
Phenylketonuria, 1627-1634t, 1638, 1725
  congenital heart disease and, 1224
  maternal, 1639
    teratogenicity of, 534
  variant, 1638
Phenylpropanolamine, fetal effects of, 719-721t
Phenytoin
  in breast milk, 731
  fetal effects of, 719-721t
  in hypoxic-ischemic encephalopathy, 967
  pharmacokinetics of, 726
  for seizures, 992-993
Phosphate. *See* Phosphorus.
Phosphate-sodium cotransporter, 1528-1530
Phosphatidylcholine
  endotoxin exposure and, 1090, 1091f
  in surfactant, 1081, 1081t
Phosphatidylglycerol, in surfactant, 1081, 1081t
Phosphatidylinositol, in surfactant, 1081, 1081t
Phosphatonin peptides, in phosphorus regulation, 1528-1530

Phosphoenolpyruvate carboxykinase deficiency, 1672
Phosphofructokinase, deficiency of, 1008
Phosphorus
  absorption of, 1526t, 1528
  atomic weight and valence of, 1837t
  in breast milk and breast milk fortifiers, 659t
    absorption and retention of, 1525-1526, 1526t
  deficiency of, hypercalcemia from, 1544-1545
  in enteral nutrition, 656-657, 657t
  excess of, hypocalcemia and, 1541
  excretion of, 1528-1530, 1529f, 1530f
  in fetal body composition, 247, 248t
  in infant formula, 661-662t
  intake of, 1530
  metabolism of, 1528f
  in parenteral nutrition, 650
  physiology of, 1527-1530
  placental transport of, 1528
  in preterm formulas, absorption and retention of, 1526t
  regulation of, 1523, 1524f
  serum, 1527
    in osteopenia of prematurity, 1552
    in very low birthweight infants, 1817t
Phosphorylase, muscle, deficiency of, 1008
Phototherapy
  body surface area for, 1473
  complications of, 1474-1476
  for Crigler-Najjar syndrome, 1459
  guidelines for, 1473-1474, 1475f, 1476t
  heat exchange during, 560-561
  home-centered, 1474
  intermittent versus continuous, 1474
  irradiance in, 1472, 1473f
  for kernicterus in erythroblastosis fetalis, 371-372
  lamp variables in, 1472-1473, 1473f
  LED technology in, 1474
  light emission spectra in, 1471-1472, 1472f, 1473f
  management of newborn readmitted for, 1469b
  mechanism of action of, 1470, 1470f, 1471f
  respiratory water and heat exchange during, 564-565
  technique of, 1471-1474, 1472f, 1473f
  for unconjugated hyperbilirubinemia, 1470-1476
PHOX activity, in chronic granulomatous disease, 1333-1334, 1334t
Phrenic nerve paralysis, 1167-1168
  birth-related, 516-517, 516f
  chest radiography in, 1167-1168, 1168f
Physical activity. *See also* Exercise(s).
  preterm delivery and, 307-308
Physical examination, neonatal, 485-500
  general observations in, 486, 487f
  gestational age assessment in, 494, 495f
  health promotion during, 493-494
  introduction of examiner to mother in, 485
  limitations of, 492-493
  measurements in, 486
  neurologic assessment in, 494-499, 496b, 496t, 497f, 499t
  order of examination in, 485
  preparation for, 485, 486b
  repeat, 494
  routine, 485-488, 486b, 487f
  significant abnormalities detected in, 489-492, 489t, 491b
  spontaneously resolving conditions detected in, 488-489
Physician
  ethical responsibilities of, 45-46, 45b
  liability of, for supervision of others, 51-52
Physician assistants, supervision of, liability of physicians for, 52
Physician-patient relationship, optimal, 37
Physicians' offices, in perinatal care services, 27
Physiologic dead space, 1098
Phytosterols, in intravenous lipid emulsions, 649t
Piebaldism, 1724-1725
Pierre Robin syndrome, 531-532
  anesthetic implications of, 604-606t
  congenital anomalies in, 543, 543f
  eye findings in, 1757
  genetic testing in, 549t

Pigmentation abnormalities, 1722-1725
  in congenital anomalies, 538
  in inborn errors of metabolism, 1644-1645
  transient, 1710-1711
Pinna
  congenital anomalies of, 540, 541f, 542f
  normal, 540, 541f, 542f
Pinocytosis, 767
  calcium transport by, 1525
Pioglitazone, in pregnancy, 298t
Pituitary gland
  congenital hypothyroidism related to, 1573
  development of, 1564
  insufficiency of, hypoglycemia in, 1512-1513
  thyrotropin synthesis and storage in, 1560
Pityriasis versicolor, 836
Placenta. *See also* Maternal-fetal-placental unit.
  chromosomal abnormalities of, 428
  circumvallate, 427
  development of, 712-713
  as environmental exposure pathway, 221
  examination of, 423, 424f, 424b
  in fetal growth, 257-259, 257f, 258f, 259f
  human
    versus animal placenta, 713
    metabolic capability of, 714-715
  infection and inflammation of, 426-427
  insufficiency of
    low birthweight in, 258
    multiple gestations producing, 259, 259f
    osteopenia of prematurity and, 1551
    in post-term pregnancy, 351-352
  lesions of
    developmental and structural, 427-428
    seizures and, 986-987
  location of, ultrasonography of, 155-156, 155f, 156f
  membranes of. *See* Membranes.
  pathology of, 423-430
    clinical correlations in, 428-429, 428b
    examination for, 423, 424f, 424b
    overview of, 423-428, 424f, 425f
  perfusion of, 423-424
  structure and function of, 423-428, 424f
  thickening of, in erythroblastosis fetalis, 365-366, 366f, 367t
  transport across
    of anesthetic drugs, 436, 436t
    of calcium, 1524-1525
    of drugs, 713-714, 713b
    of immunoglobulin, 788
    of magnesium, 1530
    of maternal antibodies, 335
    of nutrients, 1497-1498, 1498f
    of phosphorus, 1528
    physiochemical factors influencing, 714, 714b
  tumors of, 428
  urea clearance in, 257-258, 258f
  vascular injury to
    fetal, 426
    maternal, 426
  vascular obstruction of, 424, 425f
  villitis of unknown etiology of, 425, 427
  villous surface area of, 257-258, 257f, 712-713
  weight of, gestational age and, 257-258, 258f
Placenta accreta, 155, 155f, 427
Placenta percreta, 427
Placenta previa, 155, 155f
  labor anesthesia and, 446
Placental abruption, 155-156
  labor anesthesia and, 446
Placental aromatase deficiency, 1615
Placental capillaries, pathology of, 426
Placentitis, chronic, 427
Plagiocephaly, 1026t
  deformational, 1032-1033, 1032f
  in unilateral coronal synostosis, 1027-1028, 1028f
Plantar grasp reflex, 498-499
Plaque, 1709t
Plasma, fresh frozen, transfusion of, 1369
Plasma disappearance curve, for drugs, 728, 728f
Plasma volume, in pregnancy, drug distribution and, 711, 711t
Plasmapheresis, for myasthenia gravis, 340

Preeclampsia/eclampsia (Continued)
definition of, 277
delivery in, 283-284
differential diagnosis of, 282-283
fetal growth and, 255-256, 256f
germinal matrix hemorrhage–intraventricular
hemorrhage risk and, 939
hepatic vascular changes in, 280t, 281
intrapartum treatment of, 283-284, 284t
labor anesthesia and, 445
management of, 283-284, 284t
maternal morbidity and mortality in, 285
in multiple gestations, 344
outcome in, 285
pathophysiology of, 278-281, 279f
perinatal morbidity and mortality in, 285
predisposing factors in, 282
prevention of, 284
progression of, variability in, 283, 283f
remote prognosis in, 285
renal vasculature in, 280t, 281
renin-angiotensin system in, 278-279, 279f
seizure prophylaxis in, 284
severity of, 283
superimposed, 277, 282, 288
uterine blood flow in, 278
uterine vasculature in, 278, 280-281, 280t
uteroplacental circulation in, 278-279, 280-281
Pregnancy. See also Maternal entries.
acute fatty liver of
inborn errors of metabolism and, 1639-1640
preeclampsia/eclampsia with, 281
acute pyelonephritis in, 400
adverse outcome of, agents associated with, 220t
air travel in, 138
bacterial vaginosis in, 402-403
body composition in, drug distribution and,
711, 711t
body weight in
drug distribution and, 711, 711t
fetal growth and, 253-254, 254f
target gain of, 254
chlamydial infection in, 416-417, 416t
cystitis in, 400
cytomegalovirus infection in, 407-409, 408f
diabetes mellitus in. See Diabetes mellitus, maternal.
drug absorption in, 709-710
drug disposition in, 709-712, 710f, 711t, 712t
drug distribution in, 711, 711t
drug excretion in, 712
drug metabolism in, 711-712, 712t
drug safety in, 135-138, 136f, 137t
enterovirus infections in, 866
environmental exposures concurrent with, 219-221.
See also Environmental exposures.
evaluation of, ultrasonography in, 153-157
fetal death in. See Fetal death.
first-trimester screening in, 138-139, 139t, 150f,
152, 153f
gonorrhea in, 412
group B streptococcal infection in, 412-414
hepatitis in, 409-411. See also Hepatitis.
herpes gestationis in, 341
herpes simplex virus infection in, 406-407
high-risk. See also High-risk neonate.
factors associated with, 20b
transport services in, 29
HIV infection in, 403-404. See also HIV infection.
hypertension in, 277-290. See also Hypertension, in
pregnancy; Preeclampsia/eclampsia.
immune thrombocytopenic purpura in, 335-336,
336t
infections during, 399-422
bacterial, 412-418
viral, 403-412
intra-amniotic infection in, 401-402, 401b
iodine during, 1573
listeriosis in, 415-416
loss of. See Abortion, spontaneous.
maternal acceptance of, 616
maternal-infant attachment in, 616-617. See also
Parent-infant attachment.
multifetal. See Multiple gestations.

Pregnancy (Continued)
nutrition in, fetal growth and, 253-255, 254f, 255f,
256b
parvovirus infection in, 411-412
physiologic hydronephrosis of, 399
post-term, 351-356. See also Post-term pregnancy.
protein binding in, drug distribution and, 711
radiation exposure in, 137, 137t
reduction of, in multiple gestations, 345-346, 349
refusal of treatment during, 38-39
rejection of, 616
rubella in, 406
second-trimester screening in, 139
substance abuse during. See Substance abuse.
syphilis in, 414-415
tobacco effects on, 742. See also Tobacco use.
toxoplasmosis in, 417-418
trauma during, birth injuries related to, 527, 527f
urinary tract infection in, 399-400
varicella-zoster virus infection in, 404-405, 405t
vitamin D during, 1533-1534
Preimplantation diagnosis, in erythroblastosis fetalis,
362
Prekallikrein, reference values for, 1338t, 1339t
Preload, in congenital heart disease, 1291
Premature beats
atrial, 1283
causes of, 1283
supraventricular, 1283
treatment of, 1289
ventricular, 1283, 1289
Premature rupture of membranes, 425
infections associated with, 400
oligohydramnios versus, 385
placental α-microglobulin-1 in, 387
preterm, 400-401
antibiotics for, 326-327, 400-401
in group B streptococcal infection, 413
pulmonary hypoplasia in, 1150-1151
Prematurity. See also Preterm infant.
anemia of, 1322-1323
necrotizing enterocolitis and, 1434
obstetric management of, 303-334. See also
Preterm delivery; Preterm labor.
osteopenia of. See Osteopenia of prematurity.
thrombocytopenia and, 1352
Prenatal care. See Antenatal care.
Prenatal diagnosis
of congenital diaphragmatic hernia, 1195-1196
of congenital hypothyroidism, 1579-1580
of cytomegalovirus infection, 849
of gastroschisis, 1410
of genetic disorders, 140-143. See also Genetic
disorders, prenatal diagnosis of.
of HIV infection, 863
of hydronephrosis, 1697, 1698f
of 21-hydroxylase deficiency, 1612, 1613f
of intrauterine growth restriction, 262-264, 264f
of nonimmune hydrops fetalis, 393-396, 395b
of omphalocele, 1410
of rubella infection, 877
Prenatal screening
for erythroblastosis fetalis, 362-364, 363f
for genetic disorders, 138-140
for hepatitis B, 410
for HIV infection, 403
for RhD status, 362-364, 363f
Prerenal azotemia, 1689
Pressure, in cardiovascular hemodynamics, 1233-1234
Pressure delivering devices, in neonatal resuscitation,
462-463, 463f
Pressure measurements, in pulmonary function testing,
1098
Pressure palsies, hereditary neuropathy with liability to,
999-1000
Pressure sensor/transducer, 581-582, 583
Pressure support ventilation, 1122-1123, 1123f
synchronized intermittent mandatory ventilation
with, 1122-1123, 1123f, 1128
Pressure waveforms, during mechanical ventilation,
1132
Pressure-volume curves, in surfactant therapy for
preterm lung, 1086-1088, 1088f

Pressure-volume loops, during mechanical ventilation,
1131-1132, 1131f, 1133f
Preterm delivery. See also Preterm labor.
behavioral factors in, 307
cervical and uterine factors in, 307-308
cocaine exposure and, 750
definition of, 303
demographic factors in, 307-308
frequency of, 303
incidence of, 1057
infection and, 309-311
in multiple gestations, 309, 344
recurrence risk of, 308, 308t
risk factors for, 303, 307-312, 308b
risk scoring system for, 312, 313t
vaginal bleeding and, 309
Preterm infant. See also High-risk neonate;
Prematurity.
anemia in, 1322-1323
Apgar score of, 1067
apnea in, 1144-1150. See also Apnea, of
prematurity.
postoperative, 599, 611-612
autonomic nervous system of, 1061-1063, 1061t
behavioral assessment of
comprehensive, 1069-1071
direct, 1067-1068
time sampling sheet for, 1061-1063, 1062f
behavioral language of, 1061-1064, 1061t, 1062f,
1064f
cerebral palsy in, 305
childhood test profiles associated with, 1071, 1071f
chronic adult diseases in, 230
classification of, 629-630, 630f
congenital heart disease in, 1275
developmental care model for, 1063-1067, 1064f,
1065f. See also Newborn Individualized
Developmental Care and Assessment Program
(NIDCAP).
early, 304
definition of, 629-630, 630f
epidemiology of, 630-631, 630f
extremely, 629
formula for
nutrient composition of, 660, 661-662t, 1526t
postdischarge, 660, 661-662t
specialized, 660
frontal lobe vulnerability in, 1070-1072
hypoglycemia in, 1518
immunization of, 1839
with birthweights of 2000 grams or more, 1839
with birthweights of less than 2000 grams,
1839-1840
incubators for. See Incubators.
inhaled nitric oxide in, 1202-1203, 1202b
late, 304
admission criteria for, 640, 640b
brain of, 634, 634f
clinical outcomes in, 631, 633t, 636-638, 636f
definition of, 629-630, 630f
discharge criteria for, 640b, 641
economic impact of, 639
epidemiology of, 630-631, 630f, 631f
etiology of, 631-633, 632b
advanced maternal age in, 633
assisted reproduction in, 633
gestational age assessment in, 632
medical interventions in, 631-632, 633f, 633t
multiple gestations in, 633
obstetric practice guidelines in, 632
gastrointestinal tract of, 634, 638
hospitalizations and rehospitalizations after
discharge of, 638-640
hyperbilirubinemia in, 638
hypoglycemia in, 634, 636f, 638
immunity and infection in, 638
long-term outcomes in, 639-640
management of, 640-641, 640b
mortality in, 636, 637t
pathophysiology of, 633-636
fetal lung fluid clearance in, 634-636, 635f
immaturity in, 633-634, 634f
respiratory distress in, 634, 636-637, 636f

Respiratory syncytial virus infection, 855-859
  clinical manifestations of, 856
  prevention and treatment of, 857-859, 858t
  respiratory sequelae of, 856
  risk factors for, 856
  transmission of, 855
Respiratory tract, 1075-1206. *See also* Lung *entries;*
    Pulmonary *entries.*
  in acid-base balance, 677
  time constant of, 1100-1102, 1101f, 1102f
  water/heat exchange between environment and,
    556, 563-565, 564f, 564t
    calculation of, 557
    through convection, 557
    through evaporation, 557
Respondeal superior doctrine of liability, 51
Resuscitation, neonatal, 443-444, 449-484
  airway clearance in, 457
  alpha-methylnorepinephrine in, 478
  anticipation of, 454-455
  Apgar score and, 7, 7f, 455, 455t
  birth transition and, 450-452, 451f, 451t, 452f
  chest compressions in, 475-476, 475f
  congenital anomaly screening in, 482-483
  congenital diaphragmatic hernia and, 482
  continuous positive airway pressure in, 462-465,
    1118
  in developing countries, 116-117, 117f
    equipment for, 123
  dopamine in, 477t, 479
  drug-depressed infant in, 479
  elements of, 455-457, 456b
  endotracheal intubation in, 465-467, 465b,
    466t
  epinephrine in, 476-478, 477t
  equipment for, 455, 462-465, 828
  erythroblastosis fetalis and, 482
  extremely low gestational age and, 472, 480
  facemasks in, 463-464, 464f
  fetal circulation and, 449-450, 450f
  history of, 6-7, 13-14t
  hydrops and, 482
  hypoxic-ischemic encephalopathy and, 965,
    965b
  initial steps in, 456-457
  laryngeal mask in, 465
  legal issues in, 62-64, 64b
    Messenger case and, 63
    Miller case and, 62-63
    Montalvo case and, 63
  at limits of viability, ethics of, 39-40
  meconium aspiration and, 481
  medications in, 476-479, 477t
  naloxone in, 477t, 479
  overview of, 455-456, 456f
  oxygen therapy in, 468-474
    free-flow, 457
    optimal strategy for, 472-473
    oxidative stress and, 468-470, 469f, 470f
  personnel for, 455
  pneumothorax and, 481
  positive end-expiratory pressure in, 461-467
  positive pressure ventilation in, 458-468
    first breath lessons for, 459, 459f, 460f
    initiation of, 459-460
    peak inflation pressures and tidal volumes during,
      460-461
    prevention of lung injury from, 460
    prolonged initial inflation during, 461, 461f
  preparation for, 454-455
  pressure delivering devices in, 462-463, 463f
  simulation-based learning for, 94
  single nasal tube in, 465
  sodium bicarbonate in, 477t, 478-479
  stabilized infant in, 479-480
    feeding of, 480
    fluid restriction for, 480
    glucose infusion for, 480
    prolonged assisted ventilation for, 480
  tactile stimulation in, 457
  thermal management in, 456-457
  very low birthweight and, 480
  volume expanders in, 477t, 478, 478b
Reticular dysgenesis, neutropenia in, 1330-1331

Reticulocytes
  in autoimmune hemolytic anemia, 1315
  corrected, in very low birthweight infants, 1829t
  count of, in anemia, 1310, 1312f
  postnatal changes in, 1309t
Reticulocytopenia, in Diamond-Blackfan anemia,
    1323
Reticulogranular pattern, in respiratory distress
    syndrome, 1109, 1109f
Retina
  anomalies of, in inborn errors of metabolism, 1644
  degeneration of, after phototherapy, 1474
  detachment of
    in familial exudative vitreoretinopathy, 1752
    in Norrie disease, 1752
  dysplasia of, 1752
  vascularization of, 1742
Retinoblastoma, 1761, 1761f
Retinoid signaling defect, in congenital diaphragmatic
    hernia, 1196
Retinoids, in heart development, 1211
Retinopathy
  in diabetic pregnancy, 294
  in familial exudative vitreoretinopathy, 1752
  of prematurity, 1764-1768
    classification of, 1766, 1766f
    clinical course of, 1766
    examination schedule for, 1755, 1767b
    incidence of, 1764, 1764f
    incubators and, 10
    legal issues related to, 54
    after mechanical ventilation, 1138
    neonatal anesthesia and, 601
    observed minus expected number of cases (O-E)
      values for, 72-73, 72f
    pathogenesis of, 1764-1765, 1765f
    plus disease in, 1764-1765
    treatment of, 1766-1767, 1767b
  rubella, 1750-1751
Retinoschisis, 1752
Retractions
  in pulmonary function testing, 1093
  in respiratory distress syndrome, 1109
Retrobulbar hemorrhage, 1758
Retrognathia, fetal, 163f
Reviews
  Cochrane, 101
  in evidence-based medicine, 100-101
Rewarming, for hypothermia, 567-568
Rh blood group system
  CDE nomenclature in, 1455
  genetics of, 358
Rh disease, 1314, 1314t
  unconjugated hyperbilirubinemia in, 1455
Rh immunoglobulin prophylaxis
  for erythroblastosis fetalis, 361-362
  pretransfusion, 1368
Rhabdomyoma, 1272-1273
Rhabdomyosarcoma, 1358
  of orbit, 1760-1761, 1760f
RhD genotyping, fetal, 362-364
RhD isoimmunization
  hydrops fetalis in, 359-361, 360f
  pathophysiology of, 358-361, 359t
  sensitization in, 358-359, 359t
  ultrasonography of, 365-369, 366f, 367t
RhD status
  preimplantation diagnosis of, 362
  prenatal screening for, 362-364, 363f
  pretransfusion testing of, 1367
Rheotrauma, ventilator-induced, 1136
Rhinovirus, 877-878, 878f
Rhizomelia, 169, 545
Rhizomelic chondrodysplasia, 1652
Rhizomelic dysplasia, 1651
Rh-negative antigens, prevalence of, 1314, 1314t
Rhor's equation, 1098
Rib cage abnormalities, 1167, 1167f
Rib fracture, birth-related, 512-513, 513f
Ribavirin, for respiratory syncytial virus infection, 857
Riboflavin
  in breast milk and breast milk fortifiers, 659t
  in enteral nutrition, 658t
  in infant formula, 661-662t

Rickets
  in bronchopulmonary dysplasia, 1187
  of prematurity. *See* Osteopenia of prematurity.
  radiography in, 705
Rifampin
  fetal effects of, 719-721t
  for tuberculosis, 826-827, 827t
Right aortic arch, 1239b
Riley-Day syndrome, 1000
  familial, 1000
  ocular findings in, 1746
  screening for, 140, 141t
Risk, relative, 102, 102t
Risk adjusters, in neonatal databases, 71-74, 72f, 73f
Ritodrine
  antenatal, for germinal matrix hemorrhage–
    intraventricular hemorrhage prophylaxis, 944
  fetal complications of, 320
  metabolic effects of, 320
  placental transport of, transient neonatal
    hypoglycemia from, 1502
  for preterm labor, 319-320
  side effects of, 319-320
Ritter disease, 817
Robertsonian translocation, 131, 132f
Rocker-bottom foot, 545, 547f, 1795, 1795f
Rocket catheter, for fetal shunting procedures, 193,
    193f
Rocuronium
  in neonatal anesthesia, 610
Rombam-Hasharon syndrome, 1332
Rooting reflex, 498-499, 499t
Rosiglitazone, in pregnancy, 298t
Rotational reflex, ocular, 1739, 1740f
Rotavirus, 871-872
  clinical manifestations of, 872
  epidemiology and transmission of, 871
Rubella syndrome, congenital, 876-877
  cataracts in, 1750-1751, 1751f
  retinopathy in, 1750-1751
Rubella virus infection, 406, 875-877
  clinical manifestations of, 406
  cutaneous, 1719t
  diagnosis of, 877
  epidemiology of, 406, 876
  in fetus, 406
  intrauterine growth restriction and, 261
  maternal-fetal transmission of, 406
  prevention of, 406, 877
  transmission of, 876
  treatment of, 877
  vaccine for, 406
Rubeola (measles), 854-855

S

Sacral agenesis/dysgenesis, 1786
  in infant of diabetic mother, 291-292, 1504, 1506f
Sacrococcygeal pits, 491
Sacrococcygeal teratoma, 162, 163f, 1357
  fetal surgery for, 190t
    fetoscopic, 197-198
    open, 201, 204f
Saethre-Chotzen syndrome, 1031
Safe Motherhood Initiative, 107-108, 109t
Safflower oil
  in infant formula, 661-662t
  in intravenous lipid emulsions, 649t
Sagittal synostosis, 1026-1027, 1027f
Salicylates
  fetal effects of, 719-721t
  placental transport of, transient neonatal
    hypoglycemia from, 1502
Saline
  infusion of
    for congenital adrenal hyperplasia, 675
    for neonatal resuscitation, 478
  injection of, for back pain during labor, 435
Salmon patches, 1711, 1711f
Salmonella enterica infection, diarrhea from, 813-814
Saltatory syndrome, in germinal matrix hemorrhage–
    intraventricular hemorrhage, 940
Sandhoff disease, 1018
Sano operation, 1258, 1293t